CLINICAL NURSING SKILLS & TECHNIQUES

ANNE GRIFFIN PERRY RN, MSN, EdD
Professor
Saint Louis University School of Nursing
Coordinator, Adult Nursing Specialty
Saint Louis University Health Sciences Center
St. Louis, Missouri

PATRICIA A. POTTER RN, MSN
Doctoral Student
Saint Louis University School of Nursing
(formerly) Director of Nursing Practice
Barnes-Jewish Hospital
St. Louis, Missouri

FOURTH EDITION
with 990 illustrations

Mosby
A Harcourt Health Sciences Company
St. Louis London Philadelphia Sydney Toronto

Mosby
A Harcourt Health Sciences Company
Dedicated to Publishing Excellence

Vice President and Publisher: Nancy L. Coon
Senior Editor: Susan R. Epstein
Senior Developmental Editor: Beverly J. Copland
Project Manager: John Rogers
Project Specialist: Kathleen L. Teal
Designer: Jeanne Wolfgeher, Liz Fett
Cover Designer: E. Rohne Rudder
Manufacturing Manager: Linda Ierardi
Photographer: Michael Clement, MD

A NOTE TO THE READER
The practice of nursing is a field that is continually advancing and, as a result, our knowledge base continues to expand. Therefore we highly recommend that the reader *always* consult current literature and/or institutional policy, especially regarding delegation to unlicensed assistive personnel, infection control guidelines, or other dynamic areas of practice.

FOURTH EDITION

Printed in the United States of America

Mosby, Inc.
11830 Westline Industrial Drive
St. Louis, Missouri 63146

ISBN 0-8151-4305-2

00 01 / 9 8 7 6 5 4 3

CONTRIBUTORS

Elizabeth A. Ayello, RN, BSN, MS, PhD, CS, CETN

Clinical Assistant, Professor of Nursing
New York University School of Education, Nursing
New York, New York

Peggy Breckinridge, RN, BSN, MSN, FNP

Associate Professor of Nursing
College of Health Sciences
Roanoke, Virginia

Victoria M. Brown, RN, BSN, MSN, PhD

Associate Professor, School of Nursing
Georgia College and State University
Milledgeville, Georgia

Gina Bufe, RN, BSN, MSN(R), PhD, CS

Psychiatric Clinical Nurse Specialist
Private Practice
Hyannis, Massachusetts

Sheila A. Cunningham, RN, BSN, MSN

Assistant Professor of Nursing
Neumann College
Aston, Pennsylvania

Rick Daniels, RN, BSN, MSN, PhD

Associate Professor of Nursing
Oregon Health Sciences University at Southern
Ashland, Oregon

Patricia A. Dettenmeier, RN, BSN, MSN(R), CCRN

Assistant Clinical Professor, School of Nursing
Instructor in Medicine, School of Medicine
Saint Louis University
St. Louis, Missouri

Carolyn Ruppel d'Avis, RN, BSN, MSN

Director, Baccalaureate Program/Adjunct Assistant Professor
The Catholic University of America
Washington, DC

Wanda Cleveland Dubuisson, RN, BSN, MN

Assistant Professor of Nursing
University of Southern Mississippi
Hattiesburg, Mississippi

Deborah Oldenburg Erickson, RN, BSN, MSN

Instructor, School of Nursing
Methodist Medical Center of Illinois
Peoria, Illinois

Linda Fasciani, RN, BSN, MSN

Assistant Professor of Nursing
County College of Morris
Randolph, New Jersey

Susan Jane Fetzer, RN, BA, BSN, MSN, MBA, PhD(c), CCRN

Assistant Professor of Nursing
University of New Hampshire
Durham, New Hampshire

Carl Kirton, RN, BSN, MA, CCRN, ACRN, ANP

Clinical Assistant, Professor of Nursing
New York University
New York, New York

Marilee Kuhrik, RN, BSN, MSN, PhD

Associate Professor of Nursing
Jewish Hospital College of Nursing & Allied Health
St. Louis, Missouri

Nancy S. Kuhrik, RN, BSN, MSN, PhD

Associate Professor of Nursing
Jewish Hospital College of Nursing & Allied Health
St. Louis, Missouri

Diane M. Kyle, RN, BSN, MS, PhD(c)

Supervisor of Clinical Services/Clinical Nurse Specialist
East Hartford Visiting Nurse Association, Inc.
East Hartford, Connecticut

Louise K. Leitao, RN-C, BSN, MA

Director of Clinical Services
East Hartford Visiting Nurses Association, Inc.
East Hartford, Connecticut

Ruth E. Ludwick, BSN, MSN, PhD, RNC

Associate Professor of Nursing
Kent State University
Kent, Ohio

Mary Kay Knight Macheca, RN, BSN, MSN(R), CS, CDE

Adult Nurse Practitioner
The Health Care Group of St. Louis, P.C.
St. Louis, Missouri

Jill Malen, RN, BSN, MS

Pulmonary Clinical Nurse Specialist
Barnes-Jewish Hospital at Washington University Medical Center
St. Louis, Missouri

Mary Dee Miller, RN, BSN, MS, CIC

Nurse Epidemiologist
Mercy Hamilton/Fairfield Hospitals
Hamilton, Ohio

Kathleen Mulryan, RN, BSN, MSN

Professor of Nursing
LaGuardia Community College
Long Island City, New York

Elaine K. Neel, RN, BSN, MSN

Instructor, School of Nursing
Methodist Medical Center of Illinois
Peoria, Illinois

Marsha Evans Orr, RN, BS, MS, CS

Zone Clinical Manager
Apria Healthcare
Phoenix, Arizona

Sharon Phelps, RN, BSN, MS

Nursing Practice Consultant
Barnes-Jewish Hospital
St. Louis, Missouri

Jacqueline A. Raybuck, RN, BSN, MSN(R), PhD, CS

Assistant Professor of Nursing
Jewish Hospital College of Nursing and Allied Health
St. Louis, Missouri

Linette M. Sarti, RN, BSN, CNOR

OR Charge Nurse
Bayfront Medical Center
St. Petersburg, Florida

April Sieh, RN, BSN, MSN

Assistant Professor
Delta College
University Center, Michigan

Sharon Souter, RN, BSN, MSN

Director of Nursing Programs
New Mexico State University at Carlsbad
Carlsbad, New Mexico

Sandra Ann Szekely, RN, BSN

Director, Clinical & Infusion Services
Comfort Care of Michigan
Troy, Michigan

Anne Falsone Vaughan, RN, BSN, MSN, CCRN

Nursing Practice Consultant
Barnes-Jewish Hospital
St. Louis, Missouri

Pamela Becker Weilitz, RN, MSN(R), CS

Director, Nursing Practice
Barnes-Jewish Hospital
St. Louis, Missouri

REVIEWERS

Marianne Adam, RN, BSN, MSN

Faculty, School of Nursing
St. Luke's Hospital
Bethlehem, Pennsylvania

Phyllis C. Adams, RN, BSN, MSN, EdD, CNS

Assistant Professor, School of Nursing
University of Texas at Arlington
Arlington, Texas

Pamela Adamshick, RN, BSN, MSN

Instructor of Nursing
St. Luke's Hospital School of Nursing
Bethlehem, Pennsylvania

Maria Ahrens, RN, BS, MSN

Clinical Faculty, School of Nursing
University of Tulsa
Tulsa, Oklahoma

Marguerite Ambrose, RN, BSN, MSN, CCRN

Assistant Professor of Nursing
La Salle University
Philadelphia, Pennsylvania

Janice L. Arbour, RN, BN

Instructor, Faculty of Nursing
University of Calgary
Calgary, Alberta, Canada

Michele August-Brady, RN, BSN, MSN, CCRN

Assistant Dean for Academics, School of Nursing
St. Luke's Hospital
Bethlehem, Pennsylvania

Tracy C. Babcock, RN, BSN, MSN

Adjunct Assistant Professor, College of Nursing
Montana State University
Bozeman, Montana

Doris Bartlett, RN, BSN, MS

Assistant Professor Nursing
Bethel College
Mishawaka, Indiana

Margaret W. Bellak, RN, BSN, MN

Associate Professor of Nursing
Indiana University of Pennsylvania
Indiana, Pennsylvania

Julie Beshore Bliss, RN, BSN, MA, MEd, EdD

Assistant Professor of Nursing
William Paterson College
Wayne, New Jersey

Teri Boese, RN, BSN, MSN

Learning Resource Services Coordinator, College of Nursing
University of Iowa
Iowa City, Iowa

Sheila Bollinger, RN, BSN, MSN, EdD, CNS

Faculty of Nursing
Houston Community College
Houston, Texas

Jean Brannon, RN, BSN, MA

Associate Professor of Nursing
San Antonio College
San Antonio, Texas

Sister Mary Rosita Brennan, CSSF, BSN, MSN, DNSc

Chair, Department of Associate Nursing
Felician College
Lodi, New Jersey

Margie E. Brown, RNC, BSN, MS, ANP

Professor of Nursing, School of Health/Science
Long Beach City College
Long Beach, California

Jeanie Burt, RN, BSN, MA

Assistant Professor of Nursing
Harding University
Searcy, Arkansas

Gale Carli, RN, MEd, MSN(c)

Instructor of Nursing
Ohlone College
Fremont, California

Amy Deutschendorf, RN, BSN, MN, OCN

Clinical Nurse Specialist, Franklin Square Hospital
Faculty Associate, University of Maryland School of Nursing
Baltimore, Maryland

Ingeborg Haug DiGiacomo, RN, BS, MA, EdD

Associate Professor of Nursing
County College of Morris
Randolph, New Jersey

Martha A. Donagrandi, BSN, MSN, RNC

Instructor of Nursing
Madonna University
Livonia, Michigan

Heyward Michael Dreher, RN, BSN, MN

Assistant Professor of Nursing
LaSalle University
Philadelphia, Pennsylvania

Patricia A. Eagan, BSN, MSN, RNC

Doctoral Student
University of Arkansas
Little Rock, Arkansas

Linda Kay Evans, RN, BSN, MSN

Instructor of Clinical Nursing
University of Missouri
Columbia, Missouri

Rosemary Fliszar, RN, BSN, MSN

Instructor of Nursing
St. Luke's Hospital School of Nursing
Bethlehem, Pennsylvania

Cynthia S. Goodwin, RN, BSN, MSN

Instructor of Nursing
University of Southern Indiana
Evansville, Indiana

Thelma L. Halberstadt, RN, BSN, MSN, EdD

Professor of Nursing
Northern Essex Community College
Lawrence, Massachusetts

John Harper, RN, BSN, MSN

Instructor of Nursing
Neumann College
Aston, Pennsylvania

Gladys Jackson, RN, BSN, MSN, MEd

Professor of Nursing
Florida Community College
Jacksonville, Florida

Karen Jensen, RN, BSN, MN

Lecturer, Faculty of Nursing
University of Manitoba
Winnipeg, Manitoba, Canada

Susan N. Junaid, RN, BA, MSN

Assistant Professor of Nursing
Allen College
Waterloo, Iowa

Catherine C. Kaiser, RN, BSN, MS

Consultant
Allentown, Pennsylvania

Barbara S. Kiernan, RN, BSN, MSN, PhD, CS, PNP

Assistant Professor of Nursing
Medical College of Georgia
Augusta, Georgia

Erica Lambert, RN, BNA, MRCNA

Assistant Director of Nursing–Staff Development
Toowoomba Hospital
Queensland, Australia

Joan Leach, RN, BSN, MSN, CAGS

Professor of Nursing
Capital Community Technical College
Hartford, Connecticut

Marian MacKinnon, RN, BSN, MSN

Assistant Professor
University of Prince Edward Island
Charlottetown, Prince Edward Island, Canada

Rhonda Martin, RN, BS, MS

Clinical Instructor of Nursing
University of Tulsa
Tulsa, Oklahoma

Rita G. Mertig, RN, BSN, MS, CCE

Associate Professor of Nursing
John Tyler Community College
Chester, Virginia

Claudia Louth Mitchell, RN, BSN, MSN

Professor/Director, ADN Program
Santa Barbara City College
Santa Barbara, California

Kimberly A. Nickischer, RN, MSN, CCRN

Faculty, School of Nursing
St. Luke's Hospital
Bethlehem, Pennsylvania

Martina Obenski, RN, BSN, MSN

Assistant Professor of Nursing
Cedar Crest College
Allentown, Pennsylvania

Elizabeth Phillip, RN, BSN, MSN

Faculty, School of Nursing
St. Luke's Hospital
Bethlehem, Pennsylvania

Melissa Powell, RN, BSN, MSN

Assistant Professor of Nursing
Eastern Kentucky University
Richmond, Kentucky

Cheryl M. Prandoni, RN, BSN, MSN

Director of Learning Resources, School of Nursing
The Catholic University of America
Washington, DC

Lee W. Richard, RN, BSN, MS, PhD, CNAA

Assistant Professor of Nursing
University of Texas Health Sciences Center at San Antonio
San Antonio, Texas

Vanice W. Roberts, RN, BSN, MSN, DSN

Professor of Nursing
Kennesaw State University
Kennesaw, Georgia

Catherine A. Robinson, RN, BA

Clinical Nursing Manager
Barnes-Jewish Hospital
St. Louis, Missouri

Paula D. Saliba, RN, BSN, MSN

Nursing Instructor
Wallace Community College
Selma, Alabama

Ellen Shannon, RNS, BSN, MSN

Instructor of Nursing
St. Luke's Hospital School of Nursing
Bethlehem, Pennsylvania

Ruth A. Shearer, RN, BSN, MS, MSN

Assistant Professor of Nursing
Bethel College
Mishawaka, Indiana

Janet A. Sipple, RN, BSN, MSN, EdD

Dean, School of Nursing
St. Luke's Hospital
Bethlehem, Pennsylvania

Elizabeth Speakman, RN, BSN, MEd

Assistant Professor of Nursing
Community College of Philadelphia
Philadelphia, Pennsylvania

Susan Speraw, RN, BSN, MN, PhD

Associate Professor of Pediatrics
Director, Division of Psychology
University of Tennessee College of Medicine—Chattanooga Unit
Chattanooga, Tennessee

Dorothy Thomas, RN, BSN, MSN

Associate Professor of Nursing
St. Louis Community College at Florissant Valley
St. Louis, Missouri

Paige Thompson, RN, BSN, MSN

Instructor, School of Nursing
St. Luke's Hospital
Bethlehem, Pennsylvania

Jane Threatt, RN, BSN, MSN, RN, CS

Assistant Professor of Nursing
North Georgia College & State University
Dahlonega, Georgia

Bridget Whitmore, RNC, BSN, MSN, WHCNP

Clinical Instructor of Nursing
Indiana University at Kokomo
Kokomo, Indiana

Annie M. Wilson, RN, BS, MS, DrPH, FNP

Associate Professor of Nursing
Prairie View A & M University
Houston, Texas

Leah Wichmann Wilson, RN, BSN, MS, CIC

Infection Control Practitioner
Infection Control Consultants
Phoenix, Arizona

Rosemary H. Wittstadt, RN, BS, MS, EdD

Assistant Professor of Nursing
Towson State University
Towson, Maryland

Leanne J. Wyrostok, RN, BN, MN

Psychomotor Skills Clinician, Faculty of Nursing
University of Calgary
Calgary, Alberta, Canada

To my children, Rebecca Lacey Perry and Chip Perry, who have taught me how to enjoy life to its fullest.

To the invaluable friends who are my family.

PREFACE

The fourth edition of *Clinical Nursing Skills and Techniques* has been developed to continue the commitment to excellence of the first three editions. This market-leading skills text has been the favorite of nursing faculty and practitioners for its

- Current, comprehensive coverage of skills using the nursing process framework
- Readable, easy-to-follow 2-column format with rationales
- Hundreds of illustrations that show accurately and visually "how-to"

This edition includes over 220 procedures that cover basic, intermediate, and advanced skills. It has been designed to be used throughout the nursing program, including the medical-surgical courses and clinicals. It is also a valuable resource for today's nurses working in acute, community-based settings, and home care agencies who may encounter clients with needs that encompass many of these procedures.

ORGANIZATION

The 45 chapters have been logically grouped into 15 units. Each chapter begins with objectives and key terms along with a list of the skills to be covered. A brief introduction of pertinent information and **Guidelines** for implementing the skills provide a foundation for the skills in the chapter.

A new feature, **Delegation Considerations,** provides guidelines for the nurse's responsibilities when assigning the skill to unlicensed assistive personnel. Professional nurses are becoming more involved with client assessment and delivery of complex therapies requiring problem solving and individualization of approaches. For this reason, the appropriate delegation of nursing tasks to unlicensed assistive personnel is crucially important. Delegation is not based on which client requires care but rather on what tasks can safely be delivered by unlicensed personnel. In developing the **delegation considerations** for this textbook, it is assumed that registered nurses work collaboratively with personnel and that unlicensed staff have received appropriate training. Several principles were followed in selecting tasks suitable for delegation:

Right task—Includes those tasks that are repetitively performed, involve little or no invasive procedures, and require minimal supervision. This includes monitoring *not* assessment activities.

Right supervision—The RN is available for monitoring, evaluation, and intervention.

Right direction—The RN is responsible for providing a clear description of any task, including its purpose, limits, and expectations. Client variations must be communicated to personnel.

Delegation requires decision making. The recommendations for delegation are guidelines only and should not be applied if, in the RN's judgment, a client requires professional nursing intervention.

The presentation of each skill is attractive and easy to follow, using the 5-step nursing process as the organizational framework. Each skill begins with a brief description of the purpose and the equipment needed. The steps of the skill are then presented in a clear, easy to understand 2-column format with rationales for every step. Hundreds of large, clear drawings and photographs help students visualize key techniques. The Planning section focuses on **Expected Outcomes,** with possible **Unexpected Outcomes** noted under the Evaluation section. **Critical Decision Points** appear throughout the skills to alert the nurse to key information to consider while performing the skill to ensure safe and effective outcomes. Each skill ends with **Recording and Reporting** that provides a sample of what and how to record. **Follow-up Activities** provide further learning and aid critical thinking development. Individual client considerations are presented at the conclusion of each skill that cover **Special, Teaching, Pediatric, Gerontologic and Home Care Considerations.** This expanded section provides comprehensive coverage of care of specific client needs. Each chapter concludes with **Critical Thinking Activities,** based on realistic clinical situations, that promote development of decision-making abilities and integrate the knowledge covered within the chapter. References and Additional Readings for each chapter provide the sources of content and suggested resources for further study.

FEATURES

The comprehensive, current, and accurate coverage of skills needed by students and practitioners has made *Clinical Nursing Skills and Techniques* a favorite of bo faculty and health-care agencies. Current resea well as input from practitioners and educa vided direction for this new edition. Ke clude:

- Comprehensive, current coverage of more than 220 skills
- A 5-step **nursing process** format that provides a consistent, clear presentation to help students learn to apply the process while learning each skill
- Easy-to-follow two-column format that features a spacious two-color design and clear, bold print
- Clearly written scientifically based **rationales** for every step to promote learning and understanding
- **Expected outcomes** that reflect the results of effective nursing interventions
- **Unexpected outcomes** that alert students to potential problems
- Nearly **1000 drawings and photographs** that add visual understanding of the performance of specific steps
- **Critical Thinking Exercises** at the end of each chapter integrate the knowledge covered within the chapter with real-life situations and promote the development of clinical decision-making abilities

NEW TO THIS EDITION

- **Delegation Considerations** discuss the nurse's responsibilities when assigning skills to unlicensed assistive personnel
- **Critical Decision Points** focus on key information to consider while performing skills to ensure safe and effective outcomes
- **Unit on Home Care** focuses on the teaching and safety aspects of skills often performed in the home. Home Care Considerations are also integrated in all skills.
- **Chapter on Communication** provides helpful guidelines for this vital aspect of nursing care
- **New skills** cover:
  - Skill 2-1 Establishing Therapeutic Communication
  - Skill 2-2 Establishing Communication Throughout the Phases of the Nurse-Client Relationship
  - Skill 2-3 Communication with the Anxious Client
  - Skill 2-4 Verbally Deescalating the Potentially Violent Client
  - Skill 4-1 Fall Prevention
  - Skill 4-2 Designing a Restraint-Free Environment
  - Skill 4-4 Seizure Precautions
  - Skill 20-8 Discontinuing Peripheral Intravenous Access
  - Skill 22-3 Aspiration Precautions
  - Skill 30-5 Assisting with Ambulation
  - Skill 35-1 Preparing the Client for Surgery
  - Skill 42-5 Enteral Nutrition in the Home

TEACHING-LEARNING PACKAGE

The complete teaching-learning package includes:

Instructor's Resource Manual that provides an outline of the key content in each chapter with page reference, answers to the critical thinking questions, educational strategies to assist in teaching the skills, and independent learning activities for students

Skills Performance Checklists, which students may purchase separately or at a special price when packaged with the text.

Mosby's Nursing Skills Video Series that parallels the content of the text. Adopters of the text receive a special discount on the series.

Mosby-FITNE Applying Critical Thinking to Nursing Skills: An Interactive Videodisc Series teaches students to learn to *think* about the procedure they are performing and to be prepared for the unexpected. Simulations take place in hospital, extended care, and home settings. The four titles are: Activity and Mobility, Promoting Oxygenation, Nutrition and Elimination, and Shift Assessment. For information or to order, contact FITNE, Inc. at 1-800-337-4107.

ACKNOWLEDGMENTS

To the nursing editorial staff. We wish to acknowledge our editor, Suzi Epstein, for her attention to the trends that are influencing nursing today and recognizing the need to create innovative and well-designed textbooks. She offers the guidance and support necessary to craft a text that we can be proud to publish.

To Bev Copland, Senior Developmental Editor, who provides wise counsel in the review and critique of manuscript and who recognizes the elements of a quality text. Her focus, direction, and patience ensures that we attend to the details necessary to develop an excellent product.

To our contributors, excellent educators and clinicians, who share their invaluable experiences and knowledge in the chapters they create. It is they who help us to achieve a "state-of-the-art" skills text.

To the professional nursing staffs and faculty at Barnes-Jewish Hospital, Jewish College of Nursing and Allied Health, and Saint Louis University. They continue to provide us with many ideas for the text as a result of their commitment to nursing. Their assistance has helped us achieve high quality for the textbook's photographic design.

To Mike Clement, M.D., for his excellent photography. Mike is a colleague who is easy to work with and who understands the richness of detail we try to show visually within the text.

To the Angelica Uniform Co. for their very kind donation of uniforms for select photographic sessions.

To our reviewers whose expertise and astute recommendations helped develop a text of high standards that reflects the current practice of nursing today.

To you, our readers, who continue to challenge us to make the very best textbook. We appreciate your insight, your ideas, and your continued desire to have the best information available for the care of your clients.

To our continued relationship as friends and coauthors. The experience of writing texts for over 15 years has taught us a great deal about one another. We look forward to continuing to collaborate so as to remain innovative and creative. The challenge is easier with the rewarding friendship that we have.

Anne G. Perry
Patricia A. Potter

CONTENTS

UNIT I

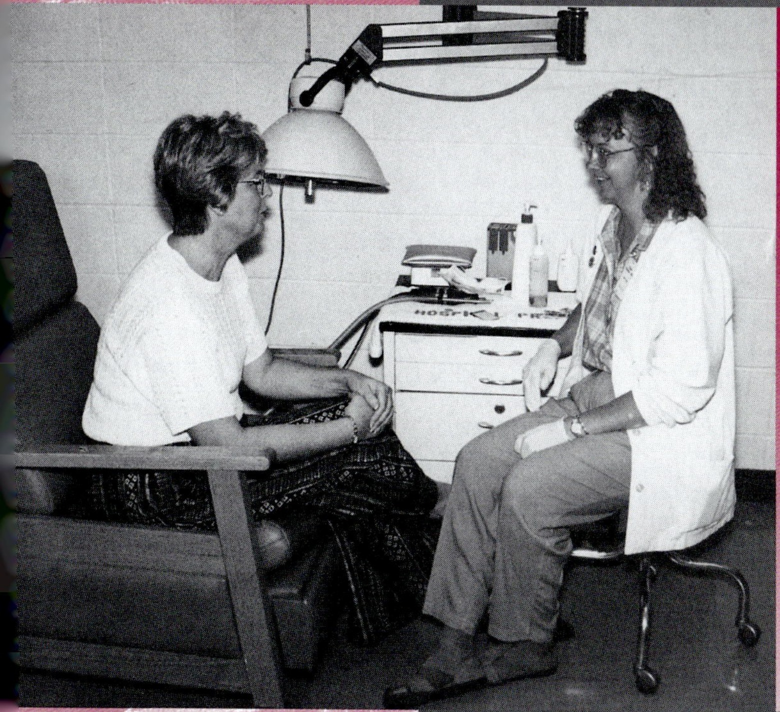

Supporting the Client Through the Health Care System

CHAPTER 1

Admitting, Transfer, and Discharge

OBJECTIVES

Mastery of content in this chapter will enable the nurse to:

- Define key terms.
- Describe the nurse's role in maintaining continuity of a client's care through admission, transfer, and discharge from an acute care facility.
- Explain the purpose and importance of advance directives.
- Identify clients in need of comprehensive discharge planning.
- Explain the importance of including the client's family in the admission, transfer, or discharge process.
- Describe the role of the nurse in discharge planning.
- Perform the following skills: admit a client to an agency, admit a client to a nursing division, transfer a client to a different agency, discharge a client.

KEY TERMS

Advance directives
American Hospital Association (AHA)
Diagnosis-related groups (DRGs)
Discharge planning
Extended care facility/skilled nursing facility
Joint Commission on Accreditation of Healthcare Organizations (JCAHO)
Nursing home (long-term care facility)
Patient's Bill of Rights
Patient Self-Determination Act

SKILLS

A client's needs and their complexity influence the efficiency of movement through the health care system. In the acute care setting a variety of services are provided by multiple care givers, and the nurse plays a key role in coordinating the client's care from admission to discharge. The nurse spends more time with clients than do other care givers. Therefore the nurse has the best perspective of the holistic approach needed in a client's care. The nurse coordinates the many resources required to ensure a smooth transition from the hospital to the home. To separate the processes of admission and discharge is a critical error; the two are simultaneous and continuous. The nurse identifies clients' health care needs: anticipates physical, psychological, and social deficits that have implications for resuming normal activities; involves family members in a plan of care; provides for health education; and assists in making health care resources available both in the hospital and at home. Ultimately the client and family should be prepared to understand the implications of any health problems and the responsibilities for continued care in the home setting.

Discharge planning is a process that facilitates a client's transition from a health care agency to the most independent level of care, whether that is home or another agency.

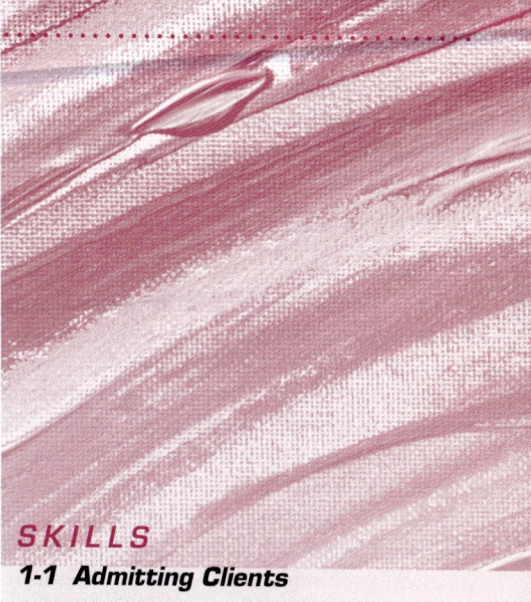

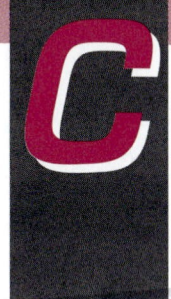

The overall goal of discharge planning is to provide the best quality of care throughout all stages of the client's illness. Research has demonstrated, however, that nurses may be confused about discharge planning policies in their hospitals (Lowenstein and Hoff, 1994). The discharge planning process must be clearly stated so that all nurses are aware of its standards of practice and of their professional responsibility.

Federal requirements mandate all hospitals to have a discharge planning process (see box below). Although the federal requirements were originally established for Medicare clients, they are generally applied to all clients within hospitals. The discharge planning process should be multidisciplinary and comprehensive.

Discharge from an agency can be stressful if a client and family members feel unprepared to resume normal activities or unable to adapt the hospital's therapeutic regimens to living at home. Before a client is discharged, the client and family members must know how to manage care in the home and what to expect in regard to any continuing physical problems. Without the necessary equipment and professional resources to care for continuing health problems, the client risks loss of any rehabilitation gains made before discharge. Failure to understand restrictions or implications of health problems may cause a client to develop complications after leaving the health care setting. For example, to control blood glucose levels, an adolescent newly diagnosed with diabetes mellitus must receive education on diabetes self-management, supplies (such as insulin, syringes, and a blood glucose monitor), and information regarding community resources. Without any one of these components, the adolescent is at risk for developing hyperglycemia, hypoglycemia, or long term vascular complications associated with the disease. Poor discharge planning ignores the client's needs within the home and increases the chance of the client needing to reenter the health care system prematurely. An emphasis in current health care is to anticipate the client's discharge needs before the client enters the health care system.

FEDERAL REQUIREMENTS FOR DISCHARGE PLANNING PROCESS

- Hospitals must identify at an early stage of hospitalization clients who are likely to suffer adverse health consequences upon discharge if there is no planning.
- The hospital must provide a discharge planning evaluation.
- A registered nurse, social worker, or other qualified person must develop or supervise development of the evaluation.
- Discharge planning must include an evaluation of the likelihood of needing posthospital services and of the availability of the services.
- Discharge planning must include an evaluation of the likelihood of a client's capacity for self-care.
- Upon request of the client's physician, the hospital must arrange for development and implementation of the client's discharge plan.
- The evaluation must be completed on a timely basis so that appropriate arrangements for posthospital care are made before discharge.
- The discharge planning evaluation must be in the client's medical record, and the results must be discussed with the client and/or significant others.

Modified from *Federal Register*, 59:238, December 13, 1994.

GUIDELINES

1. Identify as early as possible those clients who require discharge planning to foster continuity of care throughout their stay in the health care setting.
2. Include the client, family, and relevant health professionals in early planning for all moves through the health care system.
3. Consider the client's past experiences in health care settings.
4. Consider the client's cultural, socioeconomic, and educational background when discharge planning.
5. Document and communicate a plan of care to all health care personnel assuming responsibility for the client's care.
6. Assist other health care personnel in assessing appropriate resources needed as clients move through the health care system.

DELEGATION CONSIDERATIONS

The skills of admitting, transferring, and discharging clients require problem solving and knowledge application unique to a registered nurse (RN). However, the following aspects of each skill may be delegated by an RN to a licensed practical nurse (LPN) or unlicensed assistive personnel: preparation of the client's room prior to admission, transfer, or discharge; gathering and securing the client's personal care items; assisting with escorting the client on admission, transfer, or discharge; and measuring vital signs and height and weight.

SKILL 1-1 Admitting Clients

A client can access the health care system in a variety of ways (e.g., hospital, emergent care center, clinic, or physician's office), and commonalities exist for all settings (see box below). However, each institution follows a different set of policies and procedures for admitting a client, and a client's condition determines the extent of the admitting procedure. For example, a client entering through the emergency department may not be in a condition to undergo the same interview process that takes place in a hospital admitting office. In this case, family members provide pertinent information for the hospital's records while the client is transported directly to a nursing division. In contrast, an older adult client who can no longer attend to daily chores but who is still independent enough to perform some self-care undergoes extensive screening before being accepted as a **nursing home** resident.

Admitting officers, secretaries, and technicians are the personnel primarily involved with the preliminary admission procedures, such as interviewing clients and reviewing information about insurance, demographic data, and general agency procedures. Technicians and nurses can collect routine specimens and perform screening procedures such as electrocardiograms (ECGs). Some hospitals have a small satellite admitting office within the emergency department.

Clients experience considerable anxiety about the admission process, so all personnel should treat them courteously and professionally. If a client is shown an uncaring attitude, all personnel may be assumed to be unprofessional. By making clients and families feel welcome, nurses and other staff members begin to establish a therapeutic relationship with the client.

COMMON PROCEDURES FOR ADMISSION TO A HEALTH CARE AGENCY

- Placement of client in appropriate receiving area
- Assessment of client's health care problems and needs
- Determination of client's payment source for health care
- Explanation of client's rights
- Orientation to the health care agency's policies and procedures
- Preliminary testing and screening (specific for each agency)
- Development of an individualized plan of care

ROLE OF THE ADMITTING CLERK OR SECRETARY

The role of the admitting clerk or secretary includes specific activities such as initiating and maintaining a professional relationship with the client, providing for the client's safety, and providing for the client's legal rights. Each of these activities is an essential and important part of the admission process.

A courteous welcome by an admission clerk helps relieve the client's anxiety of a first encounter with agency personnel. Privacy can be maintained by escorting the client and family to an admitting interview area where important identifying information is collected (Fig. 1-1). This information includes the client's full legal name, age, birthdate, address, next of kin, physician, religious preference, occupation, and type of insurance. At this time, an identification band legibly stating the client's full legal name, hospital or agency number, physician, and birthdate should be applied securely to the client's wrist to identify the client when therapies or procedures are performed. If a client is unconscious, identification may not be made until family members arrive. Also, a client who has been a victim of crime may be safer by retaining an anonymous name under an agency's blackout procedure.

The admitting clerk or secretary should provide for the client's legal rights and instruct the client or legal guardian to read the general consent form for treatment, assess whether the form is understood, and request that the client or family member sign the form if there is agreement to be admitted for treatment. For the consent form to be valid, the client or guardian must be mentally and physically competent, be a legal adult, give voluntary consent, understand the risks and benefits of hospitalization, and

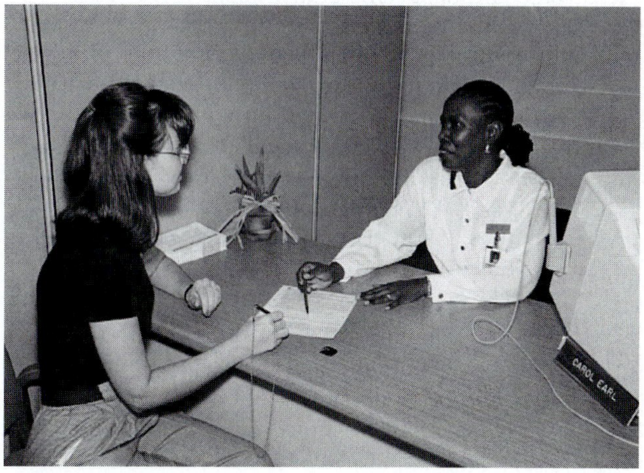

Fig. 1-1 The admitting clerk gathers important identifying information from client.

A PATIENT'S BILL OF RIGHTS

Introduction

Effective health care requires collaboration between patients and physicians and other health care professionals. Open and honest communication, respect for personal and professional values, and sensitivity to differences are integral to optimal patient care. As the setting for the provision of health services, hospitals must provide a foundation for understanding and respecting the rights and responsibilities of patients, their families, physicians, and other caregivers. Hospitals must ensure a health care ethic that respects the role of patients in decision making about treatment choices and other aspects of their care. Hospitals must be sensitive to cultural, racial, linguistic, religious, age, gender, and other differences, as well as the needs of persons with disabilities.

The American Hospital Association presents *A Patient's Bill of Rights* with the expectation that it will contribute to more effective patient care and be supported by the hospital on behalf of the institution, its medical staff, employees, and patients. The American Hospital Association encourages health care institutions to tailor this bill of rights to their patient community by translating and/or simplifying the language of this bill of rights as may be necessary to ensure that patients and their families understand their rights and responsibilities.

Bill of Rights*

1. The patient has the right to considerate and respectful care.
2. The patient has the right to and is encouraged to obtain from physicians and other direct caregivers relevant, current, and understandable information concerning diagnosis, treatment, and prognosis.

   Except in emergencies when the patient lacks decision-making capacity and the need for treatment is urgent, the patient is entitled to the opportunity to discuss and request information related to the specific procedures and/or treatments, the risks involved, the possible length of recuperation, and the medically reasonable alternatives and their accompanying risks and benefits.

   Patients have the right to know the identity of physicians, nurses, and others involved in their care, as well as when those involved are students, residents, or other trainees. The patient also has the right to know the immediate and long-term financial implications of treatment choices, insofar as they are known.
3. The patient has the right to make decisions about the plan of care prior to and during the course of treatment and to refuse a recommended treatment or plan of care to the extent permitted by law and hospital policy and to be informed of the medical consequences of this action. In case of such refusal, the patient is entitled to other appropriate care and services that the hospital provides or transfer to another hospital. The hospital should notify patients of any policy that might affect patient choice within the institution.
4. The patient has the right to have an advance directive (such as a living will, health care proxy, or durable power of attorney for health care) concerning treatment or designating a surrogate decision maker with the expectation that the hospital will honor the intent of that directive to the extent permitted by law and hospital policy.

   Health care institutions must advise patients of their rights under state law and hospital policy to make informed medical choices, ask if the patient has an advance directive, and include that information in patient records. The patient has the right to timely information about hospital policy that may limit the hospital's ability to implement fully a legally valid advance directive.
5. The patient has the right to every consideration of privacy. Case discussion, consultation, examination, and treatment should be conducted so as to protect each patient's privacy.
6. The patient has the right to expect that all communications and records pertaining to care will be treated as confidential by the hospital, except in cases such as suspected abuse and public health hazards when reporting is permitted or required by law. The patient has the right to expect that the hospital will emphasize the confidentiality of this information when it releases it to any other parties entitled to review information in these records.
7. The patient has the right to review the records pertaining to medical care and to have the information explained or interpreted as necessary, except when restricted by law.
8. The patient has the right to expect that, within its capacity and policies, a hospital will make reasonable response to the request of a patient for appropriate and medically indicated care and services. The hospital must provide evaluation, service, and/or referral as indicated by the urgency of the case. When medically appropriate and le-

These rights can be exercised on the patient's behalf by a designated surrogate or proxy decision maker if the patient lacks decision-making capacity, is legally incompetent, or is a minor.

A Patient's Bill of Rights was first adopted by the American Hospital Association in 1973. This revision was approved by the AHA Board of Trustees on October 21, 1992.

A PATIENT'S BILL OF RIGHTS—cont'd

gally permissible, or when a patient has so requested, a patient may be transferred to another facility. The institution to which the patient is to be transferred must first have accepted the patient for transfer. The patient must also have the benefit of complete information and explanation concerning the need for, risks, benefits, and alternatives to such a transfer.

9. The patient has the right to ask and be informed of the existence of business relationships among the hospital, educational institutions, other health care providers, or payors that may influence the patient's treatment and care.
10. The patient has the right to consent to or decline to participate in proposed research studies or human experimentation affecting care and treatment or requiring direct patient involvement, and to have those studies fully explained prior to consent. A patient who declines to participate in research or experimentation is entitled to the most effective care that the hospital can otherwise provide.
11. The patient has the right to expect reasonable continuity of care when appropriate and to be informed by physicians and other caregivers of available and realistic patient care options when hospital care is no longer appropriate.
12. The patient has the right to be informed of hospital policies and practices that relate to patient care, treatment, and responsibilities. The patient has the right to be informed of available resources for resolving disputes, grievances, and conflicts, such as ethics committees, patient representatives, or other mechanisms available in the institution. The patient has the right to be informed of the hospital's charges for services and available payment methods.

The collaborative nature of health care requires that patients, or their families/surrogates, participate in their care. The effectiveness of care and patient satisfaction with the course of treatment depend, in part, on the patient fulfilling certain responsibilities. Patients are responsible for providing information about past illnesses, hospitalizations, medications, and other matters related to health status. To participate effectively in decision making, patients must be encouraged to take responsibility for requesting additional information or clarification about their health status or treatment when they do not fully understand information and instructions. Patients are also responsible for ensuring that the health care institution has a copy of their written advance directive if they have one. Patients are responsible for informing their physicians and other caregivers if they anticipate problems in following prescribed treatment.

Patients should also be aware of the hospital's obligation to be reasonably efficient and equitable in providing care to other patients and the community. The hospital's rules and regulations are designed to help the hospital meet this obligation. Patients and their families are responsible for making reasonable accommodations to the needs of the hospital, other patients, medical staff, and hospital employees. Patients are responsible for providing necessary information for insurance claims and for working with the hospital to make payment arrangements, when necessary.

A person's health depends on much more than health care services. Patients are responsible for recognizing the impact of their life-style on their personal health.

Conclusion

Hospitals have many functions to perform, including the enhancement of health status, health promotion, and the prevention and treatment of injury and disease; the immediate and ongoing care and rehabilitation of patients; the education of health professionals, patients, and the community; and research. All these activities must be conducted with an overriding concern for the values and dignity of patients.

have the opportunity to ask questions. Signature on the consent form will then give the agency the right to perform routine procedures and therapies, select room placement, and provide required nursing care.

Brochures pertinent to the admission should be provided to the client at this stage of the admission process. For instance, the **American Hospital Association's (AHA) "Patient's Bill of Rights"** (see box on pp. 6-7) cites the client's right to have access to information describing the purpose of the health care agency, organization, and policies and rules that affect the person's conduct as a client. In addition, the **Patient Self-Determination Act,** effective December 1, 1991, requires all Medicare- and Medicaid-recipient hospitals to provide clients with information about their right to accept or reject medical treatment, to form **advance directives;** document the existence of advance directives; and provide community and staff education on the law, hospital policy, and advance directives (see box on p. 8). This information is also available in a brochure. Clients may want to discuss advance directives or need help in completing an advance directive document (Burke, 1993).

ADVANCE DIRECTIVES

- Advance directives convey the client's choice in continuing medical care when the client is unable to speak or make decisions.
- Advance directives include a living will, power of attorney for health care, or a notarized handwritten document.
- Document should be available in the client's medical record.
- Attending physician is notified of the client's advance directive.
- Witnesses for an advance directive document should not be medical personnel, nor should they be related to the client or heirs to the client's estate.

ROLE OF THE NURSE

Nurses should be directly involved in assigning clients to rooms, ensuring that the necessary diagnostic testing is completed, and providing for continuity of care when the client is admitted through the emergency department. Admitting personnel should confer with nursing staff to ensure that a client's room is assigned based on the client's condition, health care needs, and personal preferences. Consideration of these factors during room selection minimizes the client's anxiety and prevents conflict with other clients.

When a client is admitted through the emergency department, the nurse should notify the nursing division in a report of the client's admission information, including the client's name, assigned room and bed, admitting physician, diagnosis, and pertinent information related to the client's condition (e.g., level of consciousness, intravenous fluid infusing, need for oxygen). A full report ensures adequate preparation for the client's arrival and prompt treatment. The client and family members should be transported to the nursing division with a nursing escort and introduced to the nurse assuming the client's care. Any pertinent observations about the client's behavior (e.g., anxiety or fear, or level of knowledge regarding need for health care) can be shared with the nursing staff at this time to foster continuity of care and assist the client and family in coping with a new environment and procedures.

Clients admitted the morning of a surgical procedure or treatment are called "same day" admissions. The nurse should provide them with basic instructions regarding the purpose of the surgery or treatment, preparatory procedures, and postsurgical or posttreatment care. Admission forms, consent forms, diagnostic tests, and instruction may be completed before the actual day of surgery. Often, family members are offered informational booklets pertaining to the client's surgery or treatment.

The nurse plays an active role in coordinating the client's movement through the admission process and on to a nursing division. As is the case with the initial admission process, a client's condition influences the extent and type of admission activities. When a critically ill client reaches a hospital's nursing division, the client must undergo extensive examination and treatment procedures almost immediately. Little time is available for the nurse to orient the client and family to the division or learn of their fears or concerns. This may be a situation where the nurse delegates orientation of the family to another staff member. When a client enters a hospital for elective treatment, the nurse has time to prepare the client psychologically for hospitalization. The client often undergoes diagnostic studies, but the process is less urgent than that for an emergency admission.

The nurse must always be conscious of the client's level of fatigue and comfort. The admission process can be exhausting, especially when being delayed in the admitting office for a room assignment. When the client is experiencing physical or psychological symptoms, the nurse determines whether any portion of the admission process can be completed later.

EQUIPMENT

Prepare assigned room with necessary equipment and personal care items:

- **Bedpan and urinal**
- **Washbasin**
- **Bath towel and washcloth**
- **Toiletry items (e.g., soap, toothpaste, hand lotion; optional in some hospitals)**
- **Tissue paper**
- **Water pitcher and drinking glass**
- **Kidney or emesis basin**
- **Thermometer**
- **Sphygmomanometer**
- **Stethoscope**

STEPS	RATIONALE
ROOM PREPARATION	
1. Wash hands and prepare room equipment and furniture. Prepare bed by adjusting it to lowest horizontal position. Turn down top sheet and spread. Arrange room furniture for easy access to bed.	Promotes client's comfort by preventing delays during care. Proper position of bed lessens likelihood of client falls and of back injuries to staff assisting the client into the bed.

STEPS	RATIONALE
2. Assemble any special equipment such as suction, oxygen supplies, or intravenous (IV) pole. Be sure equipment is in working order.	Prevents delays in case immediate treatment is needed.
ASSESSMENT	
3. Greet client and family cordially. Introduce yourself by name and job title; explain your responsibilities in the client's care. (Primary nurse may be assigned at this time.)	Reduces anxiety about admission and expedites client requests.
4. Escort client and family to assigned room. Introduce them to roommate if semiprivate room is assigned.	Orientation begins with introduction to roommate.
5. Assess client's general appearance, noting signs or symptoms of physical distress.	Provides baseline assessment.
CRITICAL DECISION POINT **If client is experiencing acute physical problems, postpone routine admission procedures until client's immediate needs are met.**	
6. Assess client's and family's psychological status by noting nonverbal behaviors and verbal responses to greetings and explanations.	Anxiety influences how well a client adapts to a health care environment and retains instruction.
7. Check physician's orders for treatment measures that should be initiated immediately.	Delay can cause deterioration of condition.
8. Orient client to nursing division.	
a. Introduce staff members who enter room. Always introduce client by last name.	Promotes ability to recognize caregivers.
b. Tell client and family the name of head nurse or charge nurse of division and explain that person's role in solving problems.	Provides means for client to communicate problems.
c. Explain visiting hours and their purpose.	Willingness to observe visiting hours policy ensures client will receive adequate rest.
d. Discuss smoking policy and identify smoking areas for client and family.	The Joint Commission for Accreditation of Healthcare Organizations (JCAHO) has a standard requiring dissemination and enforcement of a hospital-wide smoking policy that prohibits the use of smoking materials throughout the hospital. Exceptions are authorized for a client by a physician prescription (JCAHO, 1996).
e. Demonstrate equipment use (e.g., bed, overbed table, lighting).	Client's safety depends on understanding correct use of equipment.
f. Show client how to use nurse call light and position it in a convenient place. Have client demonstrate use of light.	Ensures client knows how to call for assistance.
g. Escort client to bathroom (if able to ambulate).	Client's safety depends in part on understanding how to use toilet facilities.
CRITICAL DECISION POINT **Ensure that client knows how to call for assistance while in bathroom.**	
h. Explain hours for mealtime and nourishments.	
i. Describe services available (e.g., chaplain, beauty shop, activity therapy).	Offers client options for making decisions.
9. Assess vital signs (see Chapter 10) and height and weight (see Chapter 11).	Provides baseline measurement to compare future findings. Determines alterations from normal range.

STEPS	RATIONALE
10. Have family or friends leave room unless they choose to assist client with undressing. Close door and curtains. Help client undress and assist client into comfortable position.	Provides for privacy and prepares client for examination.
11. Obtain nursing history organized by standards of nursing care adopted by hospital, (e.g., functional health patterns). Data will include:	
a. Client's perception of illness	
b. Past medical history	
c. Presenting signs and symptoms	
d. Review of health status based on standards such as elimination, nutrition and metabolism, activity and exercise, self-concept, values and beliefs, cultural factors, social support, and cognitive function.	A comprehensive health history provides a holistic view of the client's health problems and response to those problems.
e. Risk factors for illness	
f. History of allergies	
CRITICAL DECISION POINT **Provide client with allergy armband listing allergies to foods, drugs, or other substances; label front of chart.**	
g. Medication history	
h. Client's knowledge of health problems and expectations of care	
12. Conduct physical assessment of appropriate body systems (see Chapter 11). If not obtained in admitting, instruct client to provide a urine specimen. Inform client as to blood specimens to be collected or tests to be performed.	Provides objective data for identifying health problems. Preparation of client can relieve anxiety that is created when unannounced procedures are performed.

NURSING DIAGNOSIS

Clustering of defining characteristics from the assessment data may reveal the following nursing diagnoses for clients requiring this skill:

- Anxiety
- Knowledge deficit regarding hospital procedures and planned therapies
- Fear
- Ineffective individual coping
- Powerlessness

Related factors are individualized based on client's condition or needs.

PLANNING

1. Expected outcomes following completion of procedure:	
➤ Client is able to explain purpose and schedule of planned treatments and procedures.	Understanding provides client with a better sense of control and reduces anxiety about the unknown.
➤ Client will demonstrate how to call for nurse when assistance is needed.	Falls commonly occur when clients attempt to reach toilet facilities or a chair without assistance.
➤ Client will be able to ambulate (if condition permits) in room free of obstacles and safely and efficiently use equipment in the room such as the bedside table, lights, and bed adjustment controls.	Equipment used in care of client can pose hazards.
➤ Client is able to verbalize understanding of smoking policy, visiting hours, mealtimes, and services available.	Knowledge of hospital policies assists client in adapting to the health care environment.

IMPLEMENTATION

1. Inform client about procedures or treatments scheduled for the next shift or day (e.g., visits by physician or dietitian). These vary based on nature of client's condition.	Client has right to be informed of any scheduled procedures or treatments. Being able to anticipate planned therapies minimizes anxiety.

STEPS	RATIONALE
2. Give client chance to ask questions about procedures or therapies.	Provides opportunity to clarify expectations and misconceptions.
3. Collect valuables client chooses to keep at facility. Complete listing sheet (see agency policy) and have client or family member sign it. Place valuables in safe.	Accounts for placement of valuables and prevents loss.
4. Ensure client and family have time together alone, if desired.	Admission can be stressful and fatiguing. Allows time for decision making.
5. Be sure call light is within easy reach, bed is in low position, and side rails are raised.	Provides for client's safety.
6. Wash hands.	Reduces spread of microorganisms.

EVALUATION

1. Confirm client's understanding of hospital policies, tests, and procedures through discussion and questions.	Learning and understanding are demonstrated through client feedback.
2. Observe client for nonverbal signs (e.g., restlessness, poor eye contact, facial tension).	Such signs may indicate anxiety.
3. Monitor client's ability to ambulate independently.	Provides data to judge client's ability to ambulate without injury.
4. Check client's room setup regularly.	Determines if care area is free of obstacles.
5. **Unexpected outcomes** that may occur include:	
➤ Client denies understanding hospital policies or knowing purpose or schedule for tests and procedures.	Reinstruction or clarification needed.
➤ Client becomes restless, expresses concerns, displays tension in body movements.	
➤ Client falls or is injured.	Safety measures unsuccessful. Nurse must attend to client's immediate physical needs, inform physician of the injury or fall, reassess the client's environment, ensure that the environment is free of safety hazards, and complete incident report.

RECORDING AND REPORTING

1. Record history and assessment findings on appropriate forms.	Prompt and thorough documentation prevents omission of data (Fig. 1-2).
2. Notify physician of client's arrival; report any unusual findings. Secure admission orders.	Client's condition may require immediate attention.
3. Begin to develop nursing plan of care. Confer with client and family as needed.	Provides for continuity of care.

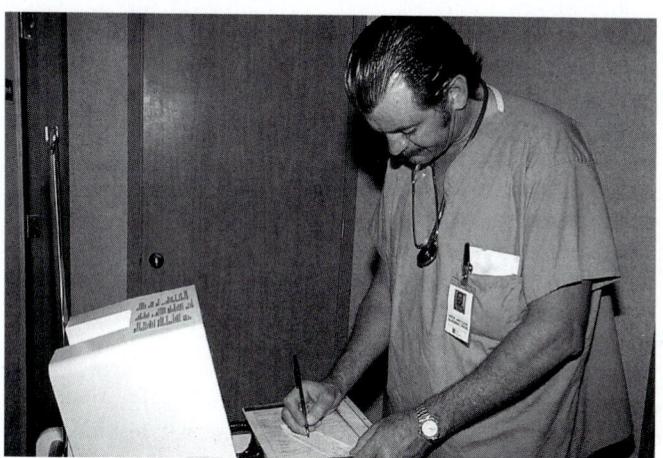

Fig. 1-2 Nurse gathering assessment.

Follow-up Activities

1. Review physician's orders and initiate all ordered interventions, (e.g., diet, medication administration, preparation for diagnostic tests).

• • • • •

Special Considerations

- Clients admitted to hospital room after surgery or from emergency department may require special equipment. Unit aides or nursing assistants often prepare the following room equipment:
  Intravenous (IV) pole
  Suction equipment
  Oxygen wall regulator and tubing
  Overhead frame with trapeze bar
- Client should be informed that a different nurse provides care on each shift. (Explain time frame for day, evening, and night shifts.) When primary nursing is method of care delivery, primary nurse coordinates nursing activities throughout the hospital stay.
- **The Joint Commission on Accreditation of Healthcare Organizations (JCAHO)** requires each client to have an admission assessment prepared by a registered nurse (JCAHO, 1996). The nurse is required to prioritize the client's needs. Each institution must set a time frame for completion of the admission assessment.
- Each client's condition is confidential. Do not tell one client another client's diagnosis or discuss the client's condition in nonpatient care areas such as elevators or cafeterias. Similarly, do not share client information with the client's family or friends unless the client's permission is obtained. When the client is unable to give permission, an immediate family member (e.g., spouse, parent) is kept informed.
- Examples of conditions that dictate temporary postponement of admitting procedure are respiratory distress, acute pain, vital sign alterations, loss of consciousness, hemorrhaging.
- Clients unable to use bedside equipment or call light will require more frequent monitoring by nurse.
- Clients admitted to a psychiatric facility are required to sign a voluntary admission form and should receive explanation of an additional set of rights pertaining to psychiatric admissions.

Teaching Considerations

- Teaching can occur throughout the admission process. A nurse can provide information regarding physical assessment findings, planned diagnostic procedures, or hospital routines. A formal teaching plan should not begin until assessment is completed and a care plan is developed.
- Teaching begins early in a client's hospitalization. The nurse introduces instruction when the client is able to be attentive and learn from the information. This can be difficult in an acute care setting. Information should be specific, focusing on topics such as the nature of the client's illness, medications needed for treatment, and use of equipment in self-care (e.g., dressings, ambulatory devices).
- In an emergency situation instruct family members on the rationale for any procedures and routines to be used in the client's care.

Pediatric Considerations

- Hospitalization is a major crisis for children with stress resulting from separation, loss of control, bodily injury, and pain. Separation anxiety is most evident during the ages of 6 to 30 months. The child experiences protest, despair, and detachment. Preschoolers are better able to tolerate brief periods of separation, but their protest behaviors are more subtle than in younger children. School-aged children are able to cope with separation but have an increased need for parental security and guidance (Wong, 1995).
- The nurse can play an important role in making the hospital experience a chance for children to develop new socialization skills and to broaden their interpersonal relationships. The nurse fosters parent-child relationships, offers educational opportunities, and provides for socialization with other children (Wong, 1995).

Gerontologic Considerations

- The stress of hospitalization can be serious for older adults because of a reduction in adaptive capacity. Helplessness, lack of control, and dependency often emerge, although some degree of personal control can be restored (Ebersole and Hess, 1994).
- Vision changes that occur with aging, along with certain medications and unfamiliarity with the surroundings can lead to falls in the hospitalized older adult client (Ebersole and Hess, 1994).

SKILL 1-2 Transferring Clients

Clients transfer to new agencies to receive different forms of therapy, to have care continued closer to home, and to continue care elsewhere when financial resources prohibit receiving care in the current facility. When clients transfer, many aspects of nursing care should continue as before. However, changes in care occur if the medical plan of treatment is revised or if the agency's policies and procedures differ from those of the previous institution. The client and family expect care to continue as smoothly as possible without interruptions in therapy that may hinder progress toward recovery.

Because nurses from the two agencies have minimal opportunity to communicate, the client's plan of care must be documented thoroughly in the medical record and on the transfer form. It is particularly important for members of the receiving staff to have a clear understanding of the client's progress and current status. Telephone reports are often given between referring physicians. In the case of nursing, it may be difficult to know which nurse will be responsible for the client's care following transfer. Primary nurses should take an active role in assuring that the client's plan of care is clearly communicated either orally or in written form.

EQUIPMENT

Gather special equipment needed in support of client during transport, such as:

- **Wheelchair or stretcher**
- **Emesis basin**
- **Bedpan and/or urinal**
- **Oxygen tank and tubing**
- **IV pole**
- **Cardiac monitor**

STEPS	RATIONALE
ASSESSMENT	
1. In collaboration with physician, assess reason for client's transfer (e.g., change in condition, resources available at agency, client or family preferences regarding client's location).	Client should have access to agency with best resources to meet health care needs.
2. Assess client's physical condition and determine vehicle for transport (consult agency policy).	Determines if client is stable for transfer.
CRITICAL DECISION POINT **Determine if client's status and safety require a vehicle equipped with life-support equipment.**	
3. Determine client's level of understanding regarding purpose of transfer and feelings about the change in care setting.	Transfers are sometimes planned quickly. Client requires adequate psychological preparation.
4. Assess method of transport to transferring vehicle (e.g., wheelchair or stretcher).	Ensures client's safety.
5. Assess if client requires pain relief or antiemetics prior to transfer.	Ensures client's comfort.
6. Assess whether client's family or significant others have been notified of transfer.	Provides adequate communication with family or significant others to assist with client's emotional and psychological adjustment to the transfer.

NURSING DIAGNOSIS

Clustering of defining characteristics from the assessment data may reveal the following nursing diagnoses for clients requiring this skill:

- Anxiety
- Fear
- Knowledge deficit regarding transfer procedure
- Pain
- Powerlessness
- Relocation stress syndrome

Related factors are individualized based on a client's condition or needs.

STEPS	RATIONALE
PLANNING	
1. **Expected outcomes** following completion of procedure:	
➤ Client's vital signs and physiological status are unchanged following transfer.	Treatments planned so as not to interrupt physical support of client during transfer.
➤ Client incurs no injury during transport procedures.	Safety measures used in transferring client from wheelchair or stretcher to transport vehicle.
➤ Client is able to explain purpose of transfer and procedure for transport.	Understanding provides client with sense of control.
➤ Receiving nursing staff acquires and confirms written plan of care.	
2. Arrange for client's transport to agency by chosen vehicle (may require support from social worker).	Transfer should occur without delays so that client has access to all needed resources at all times.
3. Obtain transfer order from sending physician. Order should include name of receiving agency and physician, and statement of client's stability for transfer.	Physician is legally responsible for releasing client from medical care and arranging for receiving physician. Client has legal right to refuse transfer against medical advice.
IMPLEMENTATION	
1. Explain to client and family reason for transfer, when it is to occur, and what procedures are planned. Encourage questions.	Explanation of transfer procedures minimizes client's and family's anxiety.
2. Make sure documentation in client's record is complete and accurate.	Accurate information is necessary for receiving agency to assume client's care.
3. Obtain from client a signature on a release form giving permission to have a copy of the medical record made for the receiving agency.	Medical personnel from receiving agency rely on client's medical record as primary resource in resuming client's care plan.
➤ ***CRITICAL DECISION POINT*** **Be sure client has signed the release form. Information in the client's record is confidential, and its use requires client's signed release.**	
4. Complete the nursing care transfer form according to agency policy.	Form provides summary of client's pertinent nursing care needs to ensure continuity of care.
5. Gather client's personal care items, clothing, and valuables. Secure in suitcase or container.	Articles can be easily lost in transfer.
6. Anticipate problems client may develop just before or during transfer. Perform necessary nursing therapies such as suctioning or changing a dressing.	Ensures client's comfort and safety in transport.
7. Assist in transferring client to stretcher or wheelchair using proper body mechanics.	Client transported to outside agency is more easily moved by stretcher into transport vehicle.
8. Perform final assessment of client's physical stability.	Minimizes risk of client developing complications during transfer.
➤ ***CRITICAL DECISION POINT*** **Be sure to check vital signs, check for clear airway, inspect patency of intravenous lines, and note client's level of consciousness.**	
9. Accompany client to transport vehicle.	Ensures medically qualified personnel are in attendance until client leaves agency.
10. Call receiving agency and notify of impending transfer and client's status (optional; check agency policy).	

STEPS	RATIONALE
EVALUATION	
1. During the final assessment compare data with previous findings.	Determines if client's condition is changing.
2. Inspect client's alignment and positioning in transport vehicle.	Proper alignment and positioning reduces risk of an injury occurring during transport.
3. Confirm client's understanding of transfer and procedures through discussion and questions.	Learning is demonstrated through client feedback.
4. Call receiving agency to inquire if they have questions about client's care.	Chart information can be misinterpreted.
5. **Unexpected outcomes** that may occur include:	
➤ Client's physical status deteriorates during preparation.	May lead to postponement of transfer.
➤ Client sustains injury during transfer to wheelchair or stretcher.	
➤ Client confused or uncertain about transfer.	Requires clarification or additional explanation.
➤ Receiving staff misinterprets directions for client's care.	Often results in duplication of diagnostic or treatment measures.

Recording and Reporting

1. Receiving nurse documents client's arrival at agency by recording date and time of arrival, reason for transfer, method of transport, client's condition, and care provided at time of arrival.	Nurse is legally responsible for documenting admission of client.

Follow-up Activities

1. Notify housekeeping of need to clean client's room.

• • • • •

Special Considerations

- Multidisciplinary conference can be useful in selecting best agency for a transfer.
- Clients who are relatively stable may be transported in van or car. Clients requiring more physical monitoring should transfer in well-equipped ambulance. Emergency transfers over long distances may occur by helicopter.
- Some institutions may require an order for certain members of the staff to accompany client during transfer.
- Agency policies dictate what portion of a client's medical record is copied, because record is property of agency.
- Recording routine nursing care measures on transfer form is not as important as recording individualized therapies. Nurse may ask client to assist in providing information.
- Measures nurse may implement just before transfer include suctioning of airway, changing soiled dressing, administering prescribed medications, bathing incontinent client, and emptying drainage collection devices.
- In many states, a nurse or therapist from the receiving agency visits client before transfer to conduct a personal assessment of client. This facilitates treatment and reduces client anxiety.

Pediatric Considerations

- Information sharing is critical whenever a child is transferred either within a hospital or between facilities. Children need their parents' comfort and security, thus the parents need to be well informed. Older children need to be involved in any discussion regarding transfers.

Gerontologic Considerations

- When an older adult client is transferred to a new facility, relocation is stressful. The nurse should ensure that significant support persons are still accessible, and that the client is thoroughly oriented to new surroundings, is allowed to take important memorabilia, and has opportunity to make decisions about care.

SKILL 1-3 Discharging Clients

Successful discharge planning is a centralized, coordinated, multidisciplinary process that ensures that the client has a plan for continuing care after leaving the hospital (American Hospital Association, 1983). Discharge planning facilitates the transition of the client from one environment to another. The following levels of outcomes must be ensured for a client's successful discharge plan (AHA, 1985).

1. Client and family understand the diagnosis, anticipated level of functioning, discharge medications, anticipated medical follow-up, use of new equipment, diet and exercise regimens, and available support systems.
2. Specialized instruction or training is provided to the client and family to ensure proper care after discharge.
3. Community support systems are coordinated to enable the client to return home.
4. Relocation of the client and coordination of support systems or transfer to another health care facility are performed.

All care givers who care for a client with a specific health problem must participate in discharge planning. Development of a plan with outcomes mutually accepted by the client and care givers, and ongoing communication about its progress are essential. For example, a client admitted to the hospital for a major surgical procedure involving the lung probably requires the collaboration of the physician, nurses, respiratory therapists, physical therapists, social workers, and home health care staff. The client needs pain control, early physical ambulation, aggressive pulmonary therapy, and training for improved exercise tolerance. The client's smooth transition from hospital to home may not be accomplished if, for example, the nurse's pain control measures are not used before physical therapy, the physician chooses to prescribe bed rest an extra day, or the social worker is not informed of the lack of family support. All care givers must work together for a discharge plan to be successful.

CLIENT RISK FACTORS FOR DISCHARGE PLANNING

- Lack of knowledge of treatment plan
- Newly diagnosed chronic disease
- Major surgery
- Radical surgery
- Prolonged recuperation from major surgery or illness
- Social isolation
- Emotional or mental instability
- Complex home care regimen
- Lack of financial resources
- Lack of available or approximate referral sources
- Terminal illness
- Lack of in home care provider

Modified from Burgess W, Ragland EC: *Community health nursing: Philosophy, process, practice,* Norwalk, Conn, 1983, Appleton-Century-Crofts.

Reimbursement pressures have resulted in shorter hospital stays for clients. It is common for health team members to direct more attention to the discharge needs of the severely debilitated client who requires continued health care in the home or an **extended care facility.** However, even a client who is hospitalized only a few days and who is without complications is often unprepared to resume a normal lifestyle immediately upon discharge.

Every hospitalized client requires discharge planning, although conditions exist that place a client at greater risk for being unable to meet continuing health care needs after discharge (see box above). When a client has one of these conditions, it is especially important to coordinate referrals to appropriate outside agencies such as a home health care agency or a rehabilitation center.

EQUIPMENT

- **Wheelchair or stretcher**

STEPS	RATIONALE
ASSESSMENT	
1. From time of admission, assess client's health care needs for discharge using nursing history, care plan, and ongoing assessments of physical abilities and cognitive function.	Plan for discharge begins at admission and continues throughout client's stay in agency.
2. Assess client's and family's need for health teaching related to home therapies, restrictions resulting from health alterations, and possible complications.	Improves understanding of health care needs and ability to achieve self-care at home. Inclusion of family member in teaching sessions provides client with available resource.

STEPS	RATIONALE
3. Assess with client and family any environmental factors within the home that might interfere with self-care (e.g., size of rooms, doorway clearances, steps, bathroom facilities). (A home health care nurse may be available on referral to assist with assessment.)	May pose risks to safety as a result of limitation created by illness or need for certain therapies.
4. Collaborate with physician and staff in other disciplines (e.g., physical therapy) in assessing need for referral for skilled home health care services or an extended care facility.	Clients eligible for home health care are confined to home as result of illness, are under physician's care, and require skilled nursing care on intermittent basis. A multidisciplinary assessment ensures a comprehensive discharge plan.
5. Assess client's and family's perceptions of continued health care needs outside the hospital.	Clients and family members may disagree on the healthcare needs required by the client after discharge. Identifying these discrepancies early may help in more accurately developing the discharge plan (Bull, 1994).

CRITICAL DECISION POINT **It may be necessary to talk with client and family separately to learn any true concerns or doubts.**

STEPS	RATIONALE
6. Assess acceptance of health problems and related restrictions.	Acceptance of health status can affect willingness to adhere to therapies and restrictions after discharge.
7. Consult other health team members about needs after discharge (e.g., dietitian, social worker, clinical nurse specialist, home health care nurse). Make appropriate referrals (see *Skill 1-2*).	Members of all health care disciplines should collaborate to determine client's needs and functional abilities.

NURSING DIAGNOSIS

Clustering of defining characteristics from the assessment data may reveal the following nursing diagnoses for clients requiring this skill:

- Anxiety
- Care giver role strain
- Fear
- Knowledge deficit regarding home care restrictions
- Relocation stress syndrome
- Self-care deficit
- Impaired home-maintenance management

Related factors are individualized based on client's condition or needs.

PLANNING

STEPS	RATIONALE
1. **Expected outcomes** following completion of procedure:	
➤ Client is able to explain how health care is to continue in home (or other facility), what treatments or medications are needed, and when to seek medical attention for problems.	Increases likelihood of care not being interrupted in home (or other facility).
➤ Client is able to demonstrate self-care activities (or family member is able to administer care measures).	Feedback ensures learning.
➤ Obstacles to client's mobility and ambulation are removed in home setting. Items that are hazards because of client's health restrictions are removed.	Client may be physically weakened or have physical changes resulting from illness that predispose client to injury.

IMPLEMENTATION

PREPARATION BEFORE DAY OF DISCHARGE

STEPS	RATIONALE
1. Suggest ways to change physical arrangement of home to meet client's needs.	Client's level of independence and ability to retain function can be maintained within safe environment.
2. Provide client and family with information about community health care resources.	Community resources may offer services client or family cannot provide.

STEPS	RATIONALE
3. Conduct teaching sessions with client and family as soon as possible during hospitalization (e.g., signs and symptoms of complications, information regarding medications, use of medical equipment, follow-up care, diet, exercise, restrictions imposed by illness or surgery). Pamphlets or books may be given to client (Fig. 1-3).	Gives client opportunities to practice new skills, ask questions, and obtain necessary feedback to ensure learning.
CRITICAL DECISION POINT Be sure printed information is written at client's reading level.	
4. Communicate client's response to teaching and the proposed discharge plan to other health team members involved in the client's care.	Facilitates the development of an individualized discharge plan.
DAY OF DISCHARGE	
CRITICAL DECISION POINT If any of the following activities can be completed before the day of discharge (eg., physician's orders for prescriptions), planning will be more effective.	
5. Let client and family ask questions or discuss issues related to home health care. A final opportunity to demonstrate learned skills may also be helpful.	Allows for final clarification of information previously discussed. Helps relieve anxiety.
CRITICAL DECISION POINT Be sure to consider any variations in the home setting (eg., resources available, room set-up in the home, etc.) to be sure skills can be performed correctly.	
6. Check physician's discharge orders for prescriptions, change in treatments, or need for special appliances. (Orders should be written as early as possible.)	Discharge is authorized only by physician. Early check of orders permits nurse to attend to any last-minute treatments or procedures well before discharge.
7. Determine whether client or family has arranged for transportation home.	Client's condition at discharge determines method of transport.
8. Offer assistance as client dresses and packs all personal belongings. Provide privacy as needed.	
9. Check all closets and drawers for belongings. Obtain copy of valuables list signed by client and have security or appropriate administrator deliver valuables to client.	Prevents loss of personal items. Client's signature verifies receipt of items. Relieves nursing department of liability for losses.
CRITICAL DECISION POINT Be sure to account for all of client's valuables.	
10. Provide client with prescriptions or medications ordered by physician.	Review of drug information provides feedback to determine client's success in learning about medications.
CRITICAL DECISION POINT Review previous instruction of medication administration with client and family.	
11. Contact agency's business office to determine whether client needs to finalize arrangements for payment of bill. Arrange for client or family to visit office.	Source of concern for many clients is whether agency has accepted insurance or other payment forms.

STEPS	RATIONALE
12. Acquire utility cart to move client's belongings. Obtain wheelchair for clients unable to ambulate. Clients leaving by ambulance are transported on ambulance stretchers.	Provides for safe transport.
13. Assist client to wheelchair or stretcher using proper body mechanics and transfer techniques. Escort client to entrance of agency where source of transportation is waiting (see agency policy) (Fig. 1-4). Lock wheelchair wheels. Assist client in transferring into automobile or transport vehicle. Help family place personal belongings in vehicle.	Prevents injury to nurse and client. Agency policy requires escort to ensure client's safe exit. Agency's liability ends once client is safely in vehicle.
14. Return to division and notify admitting or appropriate department of time of discharge.	Allows agency to prepare for admission of next client.
EVALUATION	
1. Ask client to describe nature of illness, treatment regimens, and the physical signs or symptoms to be reported to a physician.	Measures client's learning.
2. Have client (or family member) perform any treatments to be continued in the home.	Return demonstrations allow nurse to evaluate level of learning.
3. Home health nurse inspects home, identifies obstacles that pose risks for client, and recommends revisions.	Continuity of care achieved.
4. **Unexpected outcomes** that may occur include:	
➤ Client unable to explain self-care measures.	Requires clarification or reinstruction.
➤ Client demonstrates treatment incorrectly.	Requires additional practice or explanation.
➤ Risks continue to be present in the home.	Family or client may discount risk or may not have resources to make needed changes.
➤ Client or family resists discharge plans and refuses assimilation of new roles needed for home care.	Additional resources (e.g., social work, home health care, pastoral care) should be made available to client and family to assist with home care needs.

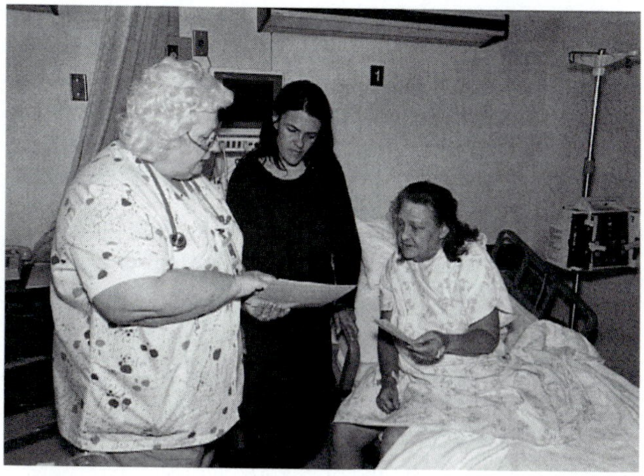

Fig. 1-3 Nurse and client participating in discharge teaching.

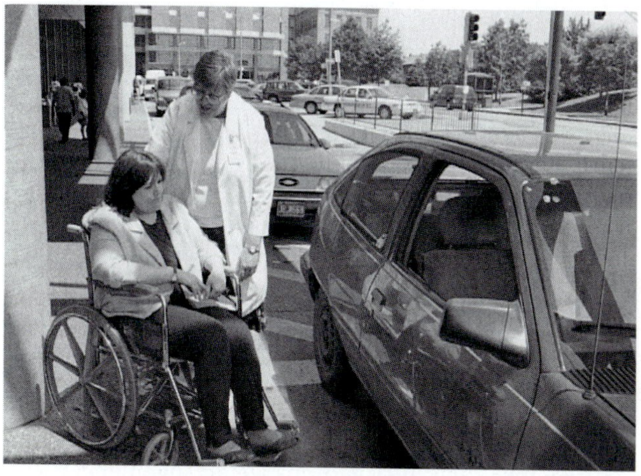

Fig. 1-4 Nurse escorts client to transport vehicle at time of discharge.

Recording and Reporting

1. Complete documentation of client's discharge on discharge summary form (Fig. 1-5). In many institutions client receives signed copy of form.

   Discharge summary is essential for documenting client's status at time client leaves health care agency. Signed copy demonstrates plan was communicated to and agreed to by client.

2. Complete documentation in nurses' notes of status of client's health problems at time of discharge.

   Allows final evaluation of client's plan of care.

Follow-up Activities

1. Notify housekeeping of need to clean client's room.

• • • • •

Special Considerations

- Potential areas to assess in planning for home care include diet management; proper, safe administration of medications; correct use of equipment; exercise limitations; wound care; risks associated with health alterations; signs and symptoms of common complications.
- Examples of environmental barriers include lack of running water, stairs, throw rugs, furniture placement, lighting, bathroom and kitchen facilities. Clients most at risk for problems in home environment include those with sensory alterations, mobility restrictions, energy limitations, or financial restrictions.
- Clients being discharged to nursing home are often fearful of new environment and potential loss of independence.
- Client must require skilled nursing care or occupational or physical therapy in the home to be eligible for third-party payment for home care. Examples of skilled care include administration of injections, changing dressings, colostomy care, tracheostomy care, administration of IVs, rehabilitative care, indwelling catheter care, teaching of injections, delivering nasogastric diet, inhalation therapy, diabetic care, care of bedridden client.
- Examples of community resources for discharge planning include medical equipment companies and rental agencies, Meals-on-Wheels program (delivery of hot meals to home), day-care centers for older adults, emergency call-for-help telephone services, community clinics, support groups.
- Some hospitals provide limited supplies of dressings, syringes, or appliances such as crutches and canes at time of discharge.
- Family members should accept valuables if client is confused, seriously weakened, or comatose.
- In some agencies, certain nurses have primary responsibility for evaluating client's adjustment after discharge. This may involve direct contact with client and family.

Teaching Considerations

- Assessment of discharge teaching needs should begin on admission and be carefully and thoroughly documented.
- Fatigue and pain levels of the client should be assessed before undertaking any teaching activity.
- Consider the client's cultural, social, and educational background when developing a discharge teaching plan.
- Clients who have short stays in health care agency may not receive teaching until day of discharge.
- Some prescriptions cannot be anticipated. Day of discharge may be only opportunity to teach client about medications. Some agencies have brochures or cards that provide specific information about individual drugs.

Pediatric Considerations

- Once family has learned how to perform any necessary care provider skills, have them assume care before the child returns home. Many hospitals incorporate a trial period requiring family to manage care before the child's discharge home (Wong, 1995).

Gerontologic Considerations

- Research has demonstrated that older adults are vulnerable to poor outcomes during the first few weeks after discharge. This reinforces the importance of either telephone or home health care follow-up for the older adults after discharge to address needs associated with functional decline and, in doing so, prevent costly readmissions (Naylor et al., 1994).
- Older adults and their families may overestimate their ability to manage care after discharge. They may also disagree about what postdischarge care includes.

BARNES

NURSING SERVICE
PATIENT DISCHARGE SUMMARY

C - 16

Date 5/00 Time ____________

Addressograph Plate

MEANS: ☑ Ambulatory ☐ Wheelchair ☐ Stretcher

DISCHARGE INSTRUCTIONS

SPECIAL INSTRUCTIONS:

Activity: ☐ Normal Limitations/Restrictions: AVOID LIFTING OBJECTS HEAVIER THAN 10 POUNDS

Modified Diet: ☑ None Directions: ____________

Medications: ☐ None Required ☑ PTA Meds Returned ☐ Scripts Given
☐ Calendar Card ☑ Pharmacy Teaching Sheets

Directions: TYLENOL #3 ÷ TAB EVERY 4 HOURS FOR PAIN

Wound Care: ☑ None Required ☐ Sent home with: ____________

Instructions: ____________

Call your doctor if you notice the following signs and symptoms of illness:

☐ Fever, drainage from incision/wound, redness or opening of wound,

☑ increased pain, ☑ other NUMBNESS OR TINGLING IN LEGS

FOLLOW-UP CARE

___ No appointment, return only if problems develop

✓ To return to doctor ASTON on 5/20 @ 10 AM

___ Other health referral made to ____________ phone ____________

Other: ____________

My discharge instructions have been explained and a copy has been given to me.

Patient/Significant Other Samuel Lee Relation ____________

Nurse Rita Wilson, RN

Original - Chart Yellow - Patient

Fig. 1-5 Discharge summary form. (Courtesy Barnes-Jewish Hospital, St Louis.)

Home Care Considerations

- The American Hospital Association (AHA, 1983) has recommended consideration of the following factors in planning for care at home:
  - Desire of client.
  - Desire and capability of family to assume responsibility and to understand and follow treatment plan.
  - Capabilities of resources in community for home health care services.
  - Physical environment of home.
  - Financial resources to provide adequate food and pay health care expenses.
- Home health care nurses require detailed information about the home environment, such as support systems and social and economic considerations that may modify and shape care, to develop complete and accurate care plans for the client. Without such information, the home health care nurse may need to assess the situation too quickly to develop a clear plan of care.
- Assess availability and skill of the primary care giver (e.g., spouse or neighbor); assess time availability, ability and willingness to give care, emotional and physical stamina, and knowledge of care giving.
- Assess attitude of immediate family members: ability to adjust to demands of client care, impact of care demands on their lives (e.g., reducing noise levels in home and preparing special diets); and potential ongoing nature of the client's needs. Family members who are not properly prepared for their role as care givers may be overwhelmed by the client's needs, which can lead to neglect or unnecessary hospital readmissions.
- Assess additional resources, including friends or neighbors who are available to help.
- Evaluate emergency preparations: a call bell or phone within client's reach, and appropriate written protocol.
- The hospital discharge planner has an obligation to warn insurance payors when they appear to be making payment decisions that adversely affect treatment needs of the client. Discharge planners must offer clients the option of paying privately for care when payors stop payment. Providers must supply in writing reasonable notice of the option to pay privately when payors stop payment.
- Assess referral for appropriateness of client admission to the home health care agency based on the following admission criteria:
  - Client is confined to place of residence (homebound).
  - Client is under care of a physician.
  - Client needs part-time or intermittent skilled nursing services.
  - Reasonable expectation exists that client's medical, nursing, and social needs can be adequately met by the home health care agency in client's place of residence.
  - Home health care services are necessary and reasonable for treatment of client's illness or injury.
- Obtain as much information as possible about the client before the nurse visits the client in the home setting; a visit to the client and family during hospitalization, if possible, permits the development of a more comprehensive plan of care.
- Document client intake information on the referral form for home health care admission to service. Ensure that information is complete. Discrepancies have been noted between the information home health care nurses deem as essential and the information that they actually receive from the agency discharging the client (Anderson and Helms, 1995).
- Review information in conjunction with established home health care agency admission criteria.
- Inform client or family member and client's physician as to the decision to accept or not accept the client for admission to the home health care agency.

CRITICAL THINKING EXERCISES

1. Why is it important to determine if a client has an advance directive at the time of admission to a hospital?
2. Mr. Williams had a total hip replacement 4 days ago and will be discharged to a skilled nursing facility in the morning. What type of information would be useful for staff at the skilled facility?
3. Describe ways the family can participate in the client's care during the admission process.
4. Identify risk factors for discharge planning that may be assessed during a client's admission and hospitalization.

REFERENCES

American Hospital Association: *Discharge planning standards–society for hospital social work directors,* Chicago, 1985, American Hospital Publishing.

American Hospital Association: *Introduction to discharge planning for hospitals,* Chicago, 1983, American Hospital Publishing.

Anderson M, Helms L: Communication between continuing care organizations, *Res Nurs and Health* 18(1):49-57, 1995.

Bull M: Elders' and family members' perspectives in planning for hospital discharge, *Appl Nurs Res* 7(4):190, 1994.

Burke M: Implementing the patient self-determination act, *Nurs Manage* 24(11):80B-C, 80F, 80H, 1993.

Discharge planning: conditions of participation, *Federal Register* 59(238), December 13, 1994. Health Care Financing Administration, DHHS.

Ebersole P, Hess P: *Toward healthy aging: human needs and nursing response,* ed 3, St Louis, 1994, Mosby.

Joint Commission on Accreditation of Healthcare Organizations: *Comprehensive accreditation manual for hospitals,* 1996, Chicago, The Commission.

Lowenstein A, Hoff P: Discharge planning: A study of nursing staff involvement, *J Nurs Adm* 24(4):45, 1994.

Naylor M, Brooten D, et al.: Comprehensive discharge planning for the hospitalized elderly: A randomized clinical trial, *Ann Intern Med* 120(12):999, 1994.

Wong DL: *Whaley and Wong's nursing care of infants and children,* ed 5, St Louis, 1995, Mosby.

ADDITIONAL READING

Barnett C, Pierson D: Advance directives: Implementing a program that works, *Nurs Manage* 25(10):58, 1994.

Brown D: Hospital discharge preparation for homeward bound elderly, *Clin Nurs Res* 4(2):181, 1995.

Calfee B: Documenting advance directives, *Nursing 1994* 24(6):17, 1994.

Congdon J: Managing the incongruities: The hospital discharge experience for elderly patients, their families, and nurses, *Appl Nurs Res* 7(3):125, 1994.

Haddock K: Collaborative discharge planning: Nursing and social services, *Clin Nurse Specialist* 8(5):248, 1994.

Jackson M: Discharge planning: issues and challenges for gerontological nursing. A critique of the literature, *J Adv Nurs* 19(3):492, 1994.

Krebs K: Discharge planning to home care: Earlier identification through automatic assessment, *J Home Care Prac* 7(2):5, 1995.

Mezey M, Latimer B: The patient self-determination act–an early look at implementation, *Hastings Center Report* 23(1):16, 1993.

Potter P, Perry A: *Fundamentals of nursing,* ed 4, St Louis, 1997, Mosby.

Wetle T: Individual preferences and advance directives, *Hastings Center Report* 24(6):55, 1994.

CHAPTER 2

Communication

OBJECTIVES

Mastery of content in this chapter will enable the nurse to:

- Define key terms.
- Identify guidelines to use in therapeutic communication.
- Explain the communication process.
- Identify the purpose of therapeutic communication, communication in various phases of the nurse-client relationship, and special issues related to communication.
- Develop skills for therapeutic communication, communication in various phases of the nurse-client relationship, and special issues related to communication.

KEY TERMS

Active listening
Cadence
Clarifying
Deescalation
Empathy
Orientation phase
Paraphrasing
Reflecting
Restating
Summarizing
Termination phase
Therapeutic silence
Working phase

SKILLS

2-1 Establishing Therapeutic Communication

2-2 Communicating Throughout the Phases of the Nurse-Client Relationship

2-3 Communicating with the Anxious Client

2-4 Verbally Deescalating the Potentially Violent Client

In nursing, effective communication extends beyond the client to include family members/significant others and members of the health care team. Therefore, nurses must possess effective communication skills as a part of their fundamental nursing knowledge base. This chapter does not intend to give a complete introduction to the complicated process of communication. The purpose of this chapter is to provide a framework by which nurses can develop a repertoire of therapeutic skills that are essential to the communication process.

Communication is an interaction between two or more persons that involves the exchange of information between a sender and a receiver (Fig. 2-1). It is an essential component of the human experience, involving the expression of emotions, ideas, and thoughts through verbal (words or written language) and nonverbal (behaviors) exchanges. Therapeutic communication is an application of the process of communication to promote the well-being of the client.

Verbal communication includes both spoken word and written word. The sender of verbal communication through the spoken word must be aware of the tone, volume, and **cadence** (pace or rate) of voice in order to send an accurate message. The sender of verbal communication through both the spoken and written word also must be aware of cultural differences between sender and receiver, such as the use of jargon or slang. Other issues the sender must consider with written communication include barriers such as cognitive and visual impairments of the receiver.

Nonverbal communication describes all behaviors that convey messages without the use of verbal language. This type of communication includes body movement, physical appearance, personal space, and touch. The sender of nonverbal communication must be aware of body language, which includes the sender's posture, body position, gestures, eye contact, facial expression, and movement (Fig. 2-2). For clarity, nonverbal communication should be consistent with the spoken word. When assessing the needs of the client, one should assess the nonverbal messages received from the client and validate them; for example, if the client is observed to be wringing his/her hands and sighing often, the nurse may ask, "You seem anxious today. Is there anything on your mind?" Problems

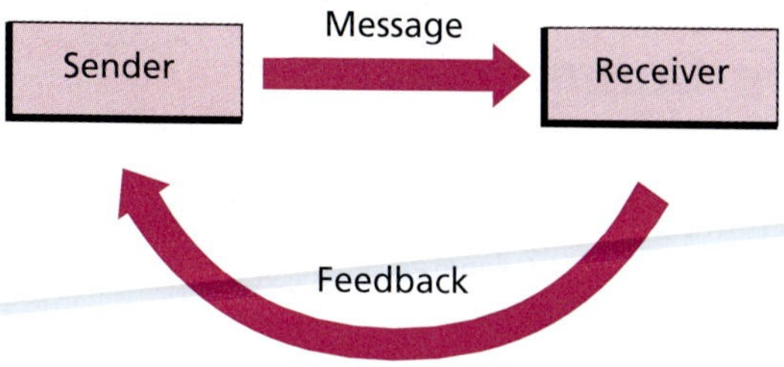

Fig. 2-1 Communication is a two-way process.

in language behavior can be avoided through the consistent use of clear, mutually understood verbal terminology and nonverbal gestures. A nurse must be aware of any cultural norms or values (e.g., eye contact) to which the client may adhere to avoid misinterpretation of nonverbal cues.

Communication is essential to nursing. Nurses use communication skills in caring for clients by providing information, promoting understanding, clarifying misinformation, assisting in developing plans of care, and facilitating wellness through client teaching. Through the relationship the nurse has with the client, a connection is made that is an essential component to the healing process. There are several key components to effective communication. One such component is self-awareness. Both the nurse and the client must be aware of the feelings they have about themselves and others as well as the feelings about the content of the messages sent and received. Other components that may affect therapeutic nurse-client communication include nonverbal cues, culture, and previous experience.

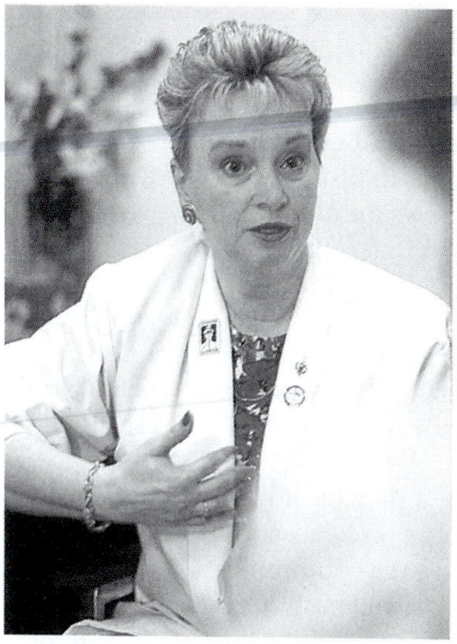

Fig. 2-2 An open, relaxed posture conveys interest.

GUIDELINES

1. Listen to what and how the client communicates, that is, content and verbal and nonverbal messages. Some clients express themselves clearly without difficulty. Often, however, indirect and nonverbal cues communicate a client's needs.
2. Nonverbal communication involves transmission of messages without the use of words. Personal appearance, tone of voice, facial expression, posture, gait, gestures, and touch are ways to convey nonverbal messages.
3. Know your own attitudes toward the client or situation. Being unaware of personal feelings can lead to negative consequences of communication. To control what and how one communicates, a person must be aware of personal feelings.
4. Control external factors in both the environmental setting and the psychological setting that influence or hinder communication. If the nurse is talking with the client about the client's personal concerns, privacy is important. If teaching, the nurse may want to have a family member/significant other present with whom to reinforce the content of the instruction. If the client is experiencing subjective distress in the form of pain or anxiety, measures should be taken to minimize these subjective experiences. Controlling noise level and interruptions may also be important.
5. Establish and understand the purpose of interaction. This is an essential quality of effective communication. Without this quality, communication is casual and superficial.
6. Guide the interaction depending on the client's condition and response. Client needs remain the focus of the interaction. For example, a nurse establishes that the purpose of the interaction is client teaching; however, the client just heard of the death of a loved one and expresses the need to talk about the death. The nurse assists the client with grieving and thus remains flexible and creative in the interaction.

SKILL 2-1 Establishing Therapeutic Communication

The primary goal of effective therapeutic communication for the nurse is to promote wellness and growth in clients. Therapeutic communication empowers clients to make decisions but differs from social communication in that it is client centered and goal directed with limited disclosure from the professional. Social communication involves equal opportunity for personal disclosure, and both participants seek to have personal needs met (Keltner et al., 1991). Nurses do not share intimate details of their personal lives with clients. Personal self-disclosure by the nurse should occur only if it may be of help to the client, such as helping the client focus on key issues. Several skills that are essential to therapeutic communication include active listening, **clarifying,** genuineness, paraphrasing, **reflecting,** restating, **summarizing,** use of **therapeutic silence,** and use of open-ended statements/questions. Some of these skills are defined with case illustrations (see box on pp. 26-27). In addition to the skills presented in the box on pp. 26-27 **paraphrasing** involves restating the client's original message by transforming the message into the nurse's own words without losing the meaning. Empathy in communication is achieved through the use of the aforementioned skills. **Empathy** is objective, nonjudgmental, and consists of insightful awareness of the feelings, emotions, and behavior of another person. It differs from sympathy in that sympathy is nonobjective and noncritical. Barriers to therapeutic communication include giving an opinion, offering false reassurance, being defensive, showing approval or disapproval, stereotyping, and asking "why?"

DELEGATION CONSIDERATIONS

Therapeutic communication is a goal of all client interactions, delegated or not. Establishing therapeutic communication is a skill that can be delegated to unlicensed assistive personnel following appropriate instruction. However, prior to delegation of this skill, the nurse should adhere to the following guidelines:

- Inform assistive care provider of proper way to interact verbally and nonverbally with the client.
- Inform assistive care provider of environmental considerations, such as privacy and confidentiality.
- Review skills with assistive care provider for communicating with the cognitively or sensorially impaired client, the older client, the pediatric client, the anxious client, and the potentially violent client if warranted according to the nursing assessment.

THERAPEUTIC COMMUNICATION TECHNIQUES

Listening

Active process of receiving information and examining one's reaction to messages received.

Example: Maintaining eye contact and receptive nonverbal communication.

Therapeutic value: Nonverbally communicates nurse's interest and acceptance to client.

Nontherapeutic threat: Failure to listen.

Broad Openings

Encouraging client to select topics for discussion

Example: "What are you thinking about?"

Therapeutic value: Indicates acceptance by nurse and value of client's initiative.

Nontherapeutic threat: Domination of interaction by nurse; rejecting responses.

Restating

Repeating main thought client has expressed.

Example: "You say that your mother left you when you were 5 years old."

Therapeutic value: Indicates nurse is listening and validates, reinforces, or calls attention to something important that has been said.

Nontherapeutic threat: Lack of validation of nurse's interpretation of message; being judgmental; defending.

Clarifying

Attempting to put into words vague ideas or unclear thoughts of client to enhance nurse's understanding or asking client to explain.

Example: "I'm not sure what you mean. Could you tell me again?"

Therapeutic value: Helps to clarify client's feelings, ideas, and perceptions and to provide an explicit correlation between them and client's actions.

Nontherapeutic threat: Failure to probe; assumed understanding.

THERAPEUTIC COMMUNICATION TECHNIQUES—cont'd

Reflecting

Directing back to client ideas, feelings, questions, and content.

Example: "You're feeling tense and anxious, and it's related to a conversation you had with your sister last night?"

Therapeutic value: Validates nurse's understanding of what client is saying and signifies empathy, interest, and respect for client.

Nontherapeutic threat: Stereotyping client's responses, inappropriate timing of reflections; inappropriate depth of feeling of reflections; inappropriate to client's cultural experience and education.

Focusing

Questions or statements that help client expand on a topic of importance.*Example:* "I think that we should talk more about your relationship with your father."

Therapeutic value: Allows client to discuss central issues related to problem and keeps communication process goal directed.

Nontherapeutic threat: Allowing abstractions and generalizations; changing topics.

Sharing Perceptions

Asking client to verify nurse's understanding of what client is thinking or feeling.

Example: "You're smiling, but I sense that you are really very angry with me."

Therapeutic value: Conveys nurse's understanding to client and has potential for clarifying confusing communication.

Nontherapeutic threat: Challenging client; accepting literal responses; testing.

Identifying Themes

Underlying issues or problems experienced by client that emerge repeatedly during nurse-client relationship.

Example: "I've noticed that in all the relationships that you have described, you've been hurt or rejected by the man. Do you think this is an underlying issue?"

Therapeutic value: Allows nurse to best promote client's exploration and understanding of important problems.

Nontherapeutic threat: Giving advice; disapproving; reassuring.

Silence

Lack of verbal communication for a therapeutic reason.

Example: Sitting with client and nonverbally communicating interest and involvement.

Therapeutic value: Allows client time to think and gain insights, slows the pace of the interaction, and encourages client to initiate conversation, while conveying nurse's support, understanding, and acceptance.

Nontherapeutic threat: Questioning client: asking for "why" responses; failure to break a nontherapeutic silence.

Humor

Discharge of energy through comic enjoyment of the imperfect.

Example: "That gives a whole new meaning to the word nervous," said with shared kidding between nurse and client.

Therapeutic value: Can promote insight by making repressed material conscious, temper aggression, reveal new options, and is socially acceptable.

Nontherapeutic threat: Indiscriminate use; belittling client; screen to avoid therapeutic intimacy.

Informing

Skill of information giving.

Example: "I think you need to know more about how your medication works."

Therapeutic value: Helpful in health teaching about relevant aspects of client's well-being and self-care.

Nontherapeutic threat: Giving advice.

Suggesting

Presentation of alternative ideas for client's consideration relative to problem solving.*Example:* "Have you thought about responding to your boss in a different way when he raises that issue with you? For example, you could ask him if a specific problem has occurred."

Therapeutic value: Increases client's perceived options or choices.

Nontherapeutic threat: Giving advice, inappropriate timing; being judgmental.

Modified from Stuart GW, Sundeen SJ: *Principles and practice of psychiatric nursing*, ed 4, St Louis, 1991, Mosby.

STEPS	RATIONALE
ASSESSMENT	
1. Determine client's need to communicate (e.g., client who constantly uses call light; client who is crying; client who does not understand an illness; client who has just been admitted to the hospital or nursing home).	Clients in need of support, comfort, knowledge, or encouragement can benefit from meaningful communication.
2. Assess reason client needs health care.	Nature of illness can affect client's coping ability and effectiveness in communicating needs and concerns.
3. Assess factors about self and client that normally influence communication: perceptions, values and beliefs, emotions, sociocultural background, severity of illness, knowledge, age level, verbal ability, roles and relationships, environmental setting, physical comfort, or discomfort (Fig. 2-3).	Communication is a dynamic process influenced by interpersonal and intrapersonal processes. By assessing factors that influence communication the nurse can more accurately assess the experiences of the client.

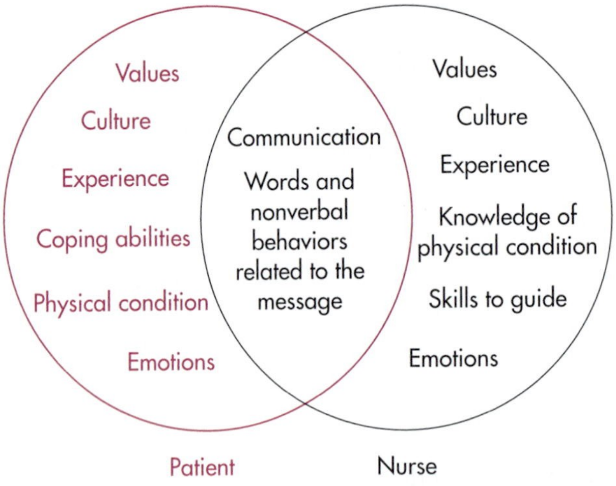

Fig. 2-3 Essential and influencing variables of the therapeutic communication environment. (From Keltner NL et al: *Psychiatric nursing,* ed 21, St Louis, 1995. Mosby.)

STEPS	RATIONALE
4. Assess client's language and ability to speak. Does the client have difficulty finding words or associating ideas with accurate word symbols? Does the client have difficulty with expression of language and/or reception of messages? What is the client's primary language?	Determines the need for special communication techniques (e.g., picture boards; aids, such as an interpreter).
5. Observe client's pattern of communication and verbal or nonverbal behavior (e.g., gestures, tone of voice, eye contact).	Client's patterns of communication may determine the type of and manner of communication used by the nurse.
6. Assess resources available in selecting communication methods:	Relying totally on information from client can restrict quality of interaction. Additional resources provide insight into best methods to communicate.
a. Review information available through chart, care plan, past experience, nursing assessment.	The greater amount or quality of information nurse has, the greater the ability to understand and communicate with client.
b. Consult with physician and other health team members concerning client's condition, problems, impression.	Collaboration with other health team members facilitates nurse's response to client based on integration of knowledge.

STEPS | **RATIONALE**

NURSING DIAGNOSIS

Clustering of defining characteristics from the assessment data may reveal the following nursing diagnoses for clients requiring this skill:

- Anxiety
- Impaired verbal communication
- Ineffective individual coping (specify)
- Decisional conflict (specify)
- Fear
- Knowledge deficit (specify)
- Noncompliance (specify)
- Impaired social interaction

Related factors are individualized based on a client's condition or needs.

PLANNING

1. **Expected outcomes** following use of these techniques:
   - Client is able to express ideas, fears, and concerns clearly and openly with relief of anxiety.
   - Client understands information communicated by nurse.
2. Prepare for communication by formulating individualized client goals, considering time allocation, formulating initial questions, and mentally preparing to keep one's mind clear of other concerns or distractions

   Rationale: Preparation is part of planned process that facilitates communication and interaction.
   Without understanding purpose of interaction, allowing adequate time, or preparing for communication, a greater risk exists of casual nongoal-oriented communication that may fail to assist client in reaching a greater potential toward physical, psychological, social, and spiritual health.
3. Prepare client and environment physically by providing a quiet environment conducive to interaction, maintaining privacy, reducing distractions or interruptions, and taking care of client's physical needs before beginning discussion.

   Rationale: Certain environments are more conducive to therapeutic interactions than others. Privacy is less threatening to client and promotes freer expression of feelings. Distractions and interruptions hinder adequate reception of the message. Taking care of basic needs decreases client distractions.

IMPLEMENTATION

1. Create a climate of warmth and acceptance. Maintain a supportive environment, considering both the environmental factors (temperature of room, noise level) and the emotional and physical state of the client (presence of pain or anxiety). Be aware of nonverbal cues that are both sent and received.

   Rationale: Facilitates open exchange without fear or anxiety.
2. Provide an introduction by addressing the client by name and introducing self and role on health care team ("Hello, my name is Sally and I am the registered nurse assigned to take care of you today. . .").

   Rationale: Conveys respect and establishes rapport.
3. Use appropriate nonverbal behaviors (e.g., good eye contact, open relaxed position, sitting eye level with client [see Fig. 2-2]).

   Rationale: This facilitates communication by providing a nonverbal message that conveys the nurse is interested in what the client has to say.
4. Observe client's nonverbal behaviors. Actively listen to the client. If the client's verbal behaviors do not match the nonverbal behaviors, the nurse should seek clarification.

   Rationale: Congruence between the client's verbal and nonverbal behaviors ensures the correct message is received by the nurse.
5. Explain purpose of interaction when information is to be shared.

   Rationale: Information and explanation can decrease anxiety about the unknown.
6. Encourage the client to ask for clarification at any time during the communication.

   Rationale: Gives client a sense of control and keeps channels of communication open.
7. Use therapeutic communication techniques when interacting with the client (see box on pp. 26-27).

   Rationale: Techniques serve to establish a greater understanding of messages sent and received.

STEPS	RATIONALE
CRITICAL DECISION POINT **Use questions carefully and appropriately. Ask one question at a time and allow sufficient time to answer. Use direct questions. Avoid asking questions about information that may not have yet been disclosed to the client (e.g., HIV status). Avoid asking "why" questions; this may cause increased defensiveness in the client and may hinder communication.**	
8. Avoid communication barriers as discussed earlier in this chapter.	Communication breakdown occurs when a message is not received, is distorted, or is not understood. Communication may be hindered by nontherapeutic responses.
9. Summarize with the client what was discussed during the interaction.	Summary signals close of the interaction, allows nurse and client to depart with the same idea, and provides a sense of closure at completion of discussion.

EVALUATION

1. Observe client's verbal and nonverbal responses toward your communication.	Both verbal and nonverbal feedback reveals the client's interest and willingness to communicate.
2. Ask client for feedback regarding message communicated. Evaluate if information obtained from client is accurate regarding client's ideas, fears, and concerns.	Determines if client clearly received message from nurse. Determines if nurse clearly received message from client.
3. **Unexpected outcomes** that may occur include:	
➤ Client continues to verbally and nonverbally express feelings of anxiety, fear, anger, confusion, distrust, and helplessness.	Communication between nurse and client has not served to allay these emotions. Client may be responding to internal and external factors and cues.
➤ Feedback between nurse and client reveals a lack of understanding.	Barriers to communication obviously exist.
➤ Nurse is unable to acquire information about client's ideas, fears, and concerns.	Techniques used by the nurse fail to promote client's willingness to communicate openly.

RECORDING AND REPORTING

1. Report any pertinent information obtained through the client's verbal and nonverbal behaviors to members of the health care team. Record in nurses' notes communication pertinent to client's health, responses to illness or therapies, and responses that demonstrate understanding or lack of understanding (include verbal and nonverbal cues).	Provides information valuable for assessment of client's needs and problems.

FOLLOW-UP ACTIVITIES

1. If there is a lack of understanding between client and nurse:
   a. Review client and nurse's communication.
   b. Identify factors that hindered communication.

• • • • •

Special Considerations

- Communication should be clear and concise for client experiencing altered levels of consciousness and cognition; repeat information, orient to surroundings, and offer reassurance.
- Clients experiencing emotionally charged situations may not comprehend the message. Focus on understanding the client, providing feedback and assisting in problem solving, and providing an atmosphere of warmth and acceptance.
- Adjust the amount and quality of time for communicating depending on clients' needs. Flexibility and adaptation of techniques may be necessary based on clients' needs.
- Be aware of cultural and gender differences when interacting with clients. Plan for identified communication difficulties associated with culture, language, age, and gender. Be alert to literacy status.

Teaching Considerations

- Client teaching should be individually tailored to meet the needs of the client. Teaching should always be conducted toward meeting the client's learning needs with a consideration for the client's preferred methods for learning. This may include, but is not limited to, communicating through return demonstrations, written information, audiovisual media, and checklists.

SKILL 2-3 Communicating with the Anxious Client

Clients in the health care setting may experience anxiety for a variety of reasons; a newly diagnosed illness, separation from loved ones, threat associated with diagnostic tests or surgical procedures, and expectations of life changes are just a few factors that can cause anxiety. How successfully a client copes with anxiety depends in part on previous experiences, the presence of other stressors, the significance of the event causing anxiety, and the availability of supportive resources. The nurse can be a support to the client. The nurse can help to decrease anxiety through effective communication. Communication methods reviewed in this skill assist the nurse in helping the anxious client clarify factors causing anxiety and cope more effectively.

DELEGATION CONSIDERATIONS

Communication with an anxious client is best managed by a professional nurse. However, therapeutic communication is important in all client interactions. Communicating effectively with the anxious client is a skill that unlicensed assistive personnel must be able to perform. However, prior to delegation of this skill, the nurse should adhere to the following guidelines:

- Inform assistive care provider in proper way to interact verbally and nonverbally with the client. Be sure staff member understands why client is anxious.
- Review skills with assistive care provider for communicating with the anxious client.

STEPS	RATIONALE
ASSESSMENT	
1. Assess for physical, behavioral, and verbal cues that indicate the client is anxious, such as dry mouth, sweaty palms, tone of voice, frequent use of call light, difficulty concentrating, wringing of hands, and statements such as "I am scared."	Anxiety can interfere with usual manner of communication and thus interfere with client's care and treatment. Extreme anxiety can interfere with comprehension, attention, and problem-solving abilities.
2. Assess for possible factors causing client anxiety (e.g., hospitalization, unknown diagnosis, or fatigue).	Client's feeling of anxiety may be unknown to the nurse. Understanding the source of anxiety can assist the nurse in client support and communication.

CRITICAL DECISION POINT Nurse may need to confer with family members about possible causes of anxiety.

STEPS	RATIONALE
3. Assess factors influencing communication with the client (e.g., environment, timing, presence of others, values, experiences, need for personal space because of heightened anxiety).	Understanding factors that influence communication helps a nurse identify effective communication strategies.
4. Assess own level of anxiety and make a conscious effort to remain calm.	Anxiety is highly contagious, and one's own anxiety can exacerbate the client's anxiety.

NURSING DIAGNOSIS

Clustering of defining characteristics from the assessment data may reveal the following nursing diagnoses for clients requiring this skill:

- Anxiety
- Impaired verbal communication
- Ineffective individual coping (specify)
- Decisional conflict (specify)
- Fear
- Knowledge deficit (specify)
- Impaired social interaction

Related factors are individualized based on a client's condition or needs.

PLANNING

1. **Expected outcomes** following use of these skills:
   - Client's anxiety is reduced through the use of effective communication techniques.
2. Prepare for communication by considering the following: client goals, time allocation, and resources.
   - *Rationale:* Effective communication allows the client to establish rapport, achieve a sense of calm, and begin to analyze the source of anxiety.
3. Recognize and control your own anxiety (breathe slowly and deeply). Be aware of nonverbal cues that indicate own anxiety (e.g., body language, posture, and tone/pace of speech).
   - *Rationale:* Anxiety of the nurse can increase the client's anxiety.
4. Prepare the environment physically by providing a quiet, calm area, allowing ample personal space.
   - *Rationale:* Decreasing stimuli can have a calming effect. Invasion of personal space is known to increase anxiety.

CRITICAL DECISION POINT First acknowledge and take care of the anxious client's physical and emotional discomfort but avoid dwelling on physical complaints. Relieving physical discomfort is important, but if treated exclusively the underlying cause of anxiety may not be discovered and anxiety continues.

IMPLEMENTATION

STEPS	RATIONALE
1. Provide brief, simple introduction; introduce yourself and explain purpose of interaction.	Anxiety may limit amount of information client can understand.
2. Use appropriate nonverbal behaviors and active listening skills, such as staying with the client at the bedside.	Nonverbal messages to client convey nurse's interest and help to alleviate anxiety.
3. Use appropriate verbal techniques that are clear and concise to respond to the anxious client. Use brief statements that both acknowledge current feeling state and provide direction to client.	Provides reassurance and prevents further escalation of anxiety.
4. Help client acquire alternate coping strategies, such as progressive relaxation, slow deep-breathing exercises, and visual imagery (see Chapter 5).	Coping mechanisms provide the foundation for effective communication so that the client can explore causes of anxiety and steps to alleviate anxious feelings.
5. Minimize noise in physical setting.	A less stimulating environment can create a calming, stress-free atmosphere that reduces anxiety.
6. Provide necessary comfort measures.	Pain can heighten client's anxiety.

STEPS	RATIONALE
EVALUATION	
1. Observe for continuing presence of physical signs and symptoms or behaviors reflecting anxiety.	Determines extent to which planned interaction relieved client's anxiety.
2. Have client discuss ways to cope with anxiety in the future and make decisions about own care.	Measures client's ability to assume more health-promoting behavior.
3. Evaluate client's ability to discuss factors causing anxiety.	Measures client's ability to attend or focus on an area of concern.
4. **Unexpected outcomes** that may occur include:	
➤ Physical signs and symptoms of anxiety continue.	Nurse's interaction may have increased client's anxiety, or source of anxiety not resolved.
➤ Client displays difficulty in decision making, and perception of facts may be altered.	Anxiety continues to prevent client from problem solving.
➤ Client avoids nurse's efforts at focusing discussion or is unable to discuss real concerns.	Therapeutic communication and interaction is hindered because of unresolved anxiety.
RECORDING AND REPORTING	
1. Record in nurses' notes cause of client's anxiety and any exhibited signs and symptoms of behaviors.	Documents nature of client's problem and response. Provides guidelines for other nurses to continue interaction.
2. Record and report methods used to relieve anxiety and client's response.	Ensures continuity of care between nurses.

FOLLOW-UP ACTIVITIES

1. If anxiety continues to escalate:
   a. Continue to use previous steps.
   b. Use refocusing or distraction skills such as relaxation and imagery to reduce anxiety. Research has indicated that imagery and relaxation are effective techniques in decreasing anxiety.
   c. Be very direct and clear when making requests.
   d. If client needs to deal with stimulus causing anxiety, reintroduce when client is less anxious.
   e. Touch, while therapeutic, requires individualized assessment of client's anxiety level and need for personal space. When used appropriately, reassurance through human touch may help control feelings of panic.
   f. As a last resort, the dependent nursing intervention of administering an antianxiety medication may be necessary.

• • • • •

Special Considerations

➤ Clients experiencing emotionally charged situations may not comprehend the message. Focus on understanding the client, providing feedback and assisting in problem solving, and providing an atmosphere of warmth and acceptance.

➤ Adjust the amount and quality of time for communicating depending on clients' needs. Flexibility and adaptation of techniques may be necessary based on clients' needs.

Teaching Considerations

➤ Teaching the client to identify possible sources of anxiety, such as illness, hospitalization, knowledge deficits, or other known stressors, gives client knowledge of anxiety and increases client's sense of control over anxiety.

Pediatric Considerations

➤ Children often demonstrate anxiety through physical and behavioral signs but are unable to express anxiety verbally. Children may express anxiety through restless behavior, physical complaints, or behavioral regression. It is important to note any changes in the child's behavior that occur during illness or hospitalization.

Gerontologic Considerations

➤ Anxiety is one of the most common symptoms seen in older adults, especially obsessive-compulsive disorder. Clients often become ritualistic and intent on performing activities a certain way. Anxiety can develop as a result of a specific event or a general pattern of change (e.g., decline in health) (Lueckenotte, 1996).

SKILL 2-4 Verbally Deescalating the Potentially Violent Client

Anger is the common underlying factor associated with potential for violence. A client can become angry for a variety of reasons. The anger may be directly related to a client's experience with illness or it can be associated with problems that existed before the client entered the health care setting. In the health care setting, the nurse has frequent contact with a client and thus often becomes the target of the client's anger. It is important for the nurse to understand that in many cases the client's ability to express anger is important to recovery. For example, when a client has experienced a significant loss, anger becomes a means to help cope with grief. A client may express anger toward the nurse, but the anger often hides a specific problem or concern. For example, a client diagnosed as having cancer may voice displeasure with the nurse's care instead of expressing a fear of dying.

It can be very stressful for a nurse to deal with an angry client. Anger can represent rejection or disapproval of the nurse's care. A nurse's efforts at satisfying the needs of one angry client can result in a failure to meet the priorities of other clients.

The nurse must allow the client to express anger openly, and the nurse must not feel threatened by the client's words. However, the client's anger should not be allowed to compromise care. Skills for communicating with an angry client or a potentially violent client allow a nurse to assist the client in dealing with anger constructively and in refocusing emotional energy toward effective problem solving. **Deescalation** skills are useful techniques that can be used to manage the potentially violent client; these skills range from using nonthreatening verbal and nonverbal messages to safely disengaging and controlling the aggressor physically (Fortinash and Holoday-Worret, 1996).

DELEGATION CONSIDERATIONS

Deescalation is a skill best performed by an R.N. However, unlicensed assistive personnel must be able to communicate effectively with the potentially violent client, provided that communication with this type of client is not beyond the skill level of the assistive personnel. Prior to delegation of this skill, the nurse should adhere to the following guidelines:

- Inform assistive care provider in proper way to interact verbally and nonverbally with the client.
- Review skills with assistive care provider for communicating with the potentially violent client and methods of deescalation.
- Review approaches that have previously been successful and unsuccessful.

STEPS	RATIONALE
ASSESSMENT	
1. Observe for behaviors that indicate the client is angry (e.g., pacing, clenched fist, loud voice, throwing objects) and/or expressions that indicate anger (e.g., repeat questioning of the nurse, nonadherence to requests, belligerent outbursts, and threats).	Anger is a normal expression of frustration or a response to feeling threatened. However, its expression can interfere or block communication and interactions.
2. Assess factors that influence communication of the angry client, such as refusal to comply with treatment goals, use of sarcasm or hostile behavior, having a low-frustration level, or being emotionally immature.	Allows nurse to accurately assess situation or experiences of client that can hinder or facilitate communication.
3. Consider resources available to assist in communicating with the potentially violent client, such as members of the health care team or family members.	May assist in clarifying cause and intervention required to deal with client's anger.

CRITICAL DECISION POINT **With some violent behaviors (e.g., physical aggression) the nurse may be able to deescalate the situation. When this potential exists the nurse must know who to call for assistance (e.g., trained techs, security staff, etc.).**

STEPS	RATIONALE

NURSING DIAGNOSIS

Clustering of defining characteristics from the assessment data may reveal the following nursing diagnoses for clients requiring this skill:

- Anxiety
- Impaired verbal communication
- Ineffective coping (specify)
- Decisional conflict (specify)
- Fear
- Risk for violence: self-directed or directed at others
- Impaired social interaction

Related factors are individualized based on a client's condition or needs.

PLANNING

STEPS	RATIONALE
1. **Expected outcomes** following use of these techniques: ➤ Client no longer exhibits verbal and nonverbal expressions of anger.	
2. Prepare for interaction with the angry client:	
a. Pause to collect own thoughts, feelings, and reactions.	Awareness of nurse's own reactions to anger removes threat to or rejection of the client expressing anger.
b. Determine what the client is saying.	Effective communication helps the nurse understand what has angered the client. Awareness and control of the nurse's reaction and responses can facilitate more constructive interaction.
c. Attempt a calm, firm, assertive approach. Attempt to talk in comfortable, reassuring voice.	
3. Prepare environment to deescalate the potentially violent client.	
a. Encourage other people, particularly those who provoke anger, to leave room or area.	Encourages the clients' expression of anger rather than provokes it.
b. Maintain adequate distance.	Avoids pressuring client; the nurse maintains safe distance if anger becomes out of control.
c. Maintain open exit. Position self closest to the door to facilitate escape from a potentially violent situation. Do not block exit so client feels escape is unattainable; this may potentiate a violent outburst.	Prevents feeling of being trapped for both nurse and client.
d. Make sure gestures are slow and deliberate rather than sudden and abrupt.	Less chance of misinterpretation of message and less threatening.
e. When anger begins to disturb others, close door. This is particularly important if the client is becoming agitated.	Agitation and anxiety can spread to others.
f. Reduce disturbing factors in room (e.g., noise, drafts, inadequate lighting).	Reduces irritating factors.
g. Take care of client's physical and emotional needs and discomforts (e.g., offer analgesic for pain).	Physical and emotional needs may be factors in client's anger; sometimes the client is not aware of these needs.

IMPLEMENTATION

STEPS	RATIONALE
1. Create climate of acceptance for client. Maintain nonthreatening verbal and nonverbal communication skills when interacting with the angry or potentially violent client.	A relaxed atmosphere may prevent further escalation.
2. Respond to the potentially violent client.	
a. Use therapeutic silence and allow client to ventilate feelings.	Often deescalates anger because anger expends emotional and physical energy; client runs out of momentum and energy to maintain anger at high level.
b. Answer questions as appropriate; if client presents with a power-struggle type of question, redirect and set limits by giving clear, concise expectations. Inform client of potential consequences and follow through with consequences if behaviors are not altered.	By setting limits on power-struggle questions, structure is provided, and anger is diffused.

STEPS	RATIONALE
c. If the client is making verbal threats to harm others, remain calm yet professional and continue to set limits with inappropriate behavior. If the strong likelihood of imminent harm to others is present upon discharge, the nurse should notify the proper authorities (e.g., nurse manager).	The angry client loses the ability to process information rationally and therefore may impulsively express anger through intimidation.
d. Maintain personal space and safety with the client who is making verbal threats of violence directed at others. Maintain nonthreatening nonverbal behaviors, including body language.	

➤ ***CRITICAL DECISION POINT*** **The potentially violent client can be impulsive and explosive, and therefore the nurse must keep personal safety skills in mind. In this case, touch should be avoided.**

e. If the client appears to be calm and anger is diffused, explore alternatives to the situation or feelings of anger.	Processing with the client may prevent future explosive outbursts and teach the client effective ways of dealing with anger.

EVALUATION

1. Observe for continuing behaviors of verbal expressions of anger.	Indicates success of communication efforts.
2. Note client's ability to answer questions and problem solve.	Determines whether anger has lessened so that client can focus on alternative coping skills.
3. Unexpected outcomes that may occur include: ➤ Client continues to demonstrate behaviors or verbal expression of anger or violence. Nurse is unable to assist the client in relieving source of anger or in expressing anger openly without violent acts.	

RECORDING AND REPORTING

1. Record in nurse's notes observations related to anger; quote client exactly. Report verbal threats of violence to the appropriate hospital personnel.	Aids in assessment and intervention of the potentially violent client while maintaining client safety.
2. Record and report nursing interventions used and client's responses.	Documents nurse's actions and promotes continuity of care.

FOLLOW-UP ACTIVITIES

1. If anger continues to escalate:
   a. Reassess factors contributing to anger.
   b. Remove or alter factors contributing to anger.

• • • • •

Special Considerations

➤ Clients experiencing emotionally charged situations may not comprehend the message. Focus on understanding the client, providing feedback and assisting in problem solving, and providing an atmosphere of warmth and acceptance.

➤ Adjust the amount and quality of time for communicating depending on clients' needs. Flexibility and adaptation of techniques may be necessary based on clients' needs.

Teaching Considerations

➤ Teaching the client to identify possible factors that contribute to angry outbursts, such as inadequate coping skills, low frustration levels, illness, hospitalization, knowledge deficits, or other known stressors, may give client a sense of control over situation. As well, one should teach the client new adaptive methods of coping with anger.

Pediatric Considerations

➤ Limit-setting for inappropriate behaviors exhibited by the child that are applied immediately are effective, especially since children tend to have less internal control over their own behaviors.

Gerontologic Considerations

➤ Clients who have cognitive impairments may exhibit tantrum-like behaviors in response to real or perceived frustration. The nurse can use distraction techniques to remove the cognitively impaired older adult client from the disturbing stimuli, or the nurse can use redirection to an activity that is pleasurable to the client.

Home Care Considerations

➤ Personal safety for the nurse against the potentially violent client extends to all health care settings, including the client's home. The nurse may be in a potentially dangerous situation while giving care to a client at home; the nurse may give care to the client without support from other staff members. The nurse must be cognizant of the verbal and nonverbal cues of the client that are indicative of escalating anger. Be aware of physical surroundings, including possible exits. Maintain a nonthreatening position, including body language, position, and tone/pace of voice, when interacting with the angry or potentially violent client. The nurse should attempt to deescalate the client. If deescalation does not occur and the nurse feels safety may be threatened, the nurse should call for assistance or remove self from situation.

CRITICAL THINKING EXERCISES

1. Identify the phase of the nurse-client relationship in the following brief scenario and state the communication technique used.
   Nurse: Mr. Jones, how can we help you to follow a low-cholesterol diet?
   Client: I don't know which foods are low in cholesterol, but I know that this diet is important to my health.
   Nurse: You don't know which foods are low in cholesterol, but know that this diet is important to your health?
2. You are attempting to do client teaching with a 70-year-old Caucasian female who is wringing her hands and continually states, "I don't know what to do first, I'm so nervous." How would you do client teaching with this person?
3. You come into Mr. Smith's room and notice him talking in a loud voice, telling you that you are incompetent, and that he is going to report you to the head nurse. How would you communicate effectively with this client?

REFERENCES

Fortinash K, Holoday-Worret P: *Psychiatric mental health nursing,* St Louis, 1996, Mosby.

Keltner N, Schwecke L, Bostrom C: *Psychiatric nursing,* ed 2, St Louis, 1991, Mosby.

Lueckenotte A, *Gerontologic nursing,* Mosby, St Louis, 1996.

Stuart GW, Sundeen SJ: *Principles and practice of psychiatric nursing,* ed. 4, St. Louis, 1991, Mosby.

ADDITIONAL READING

Clark JM, Hopper L, Jesson A: Communication skills: progression to counselling, *Nurs Times* 20(87):41-43, 1991.

Fortinash K, Holoday-Worret J: *Psychiatric mental health nursing,* St Louis, 1996, Mosby.

Fine J, Rouse-Bane S: Using validation techniques to improve communication with cognitively impaired older adults, *J Gerontol Nurs* 21:39-45, June, 1995.

Oliver S, Redfern S: Interpersonal communication between nurses and elderly patients: refinement of an observation schedule, *J Advan Nurs,* 16:30-38, 1991.

Stuart G, Sundeen S: *Principles and practice of psychiatric nursing,* ed 5, St Louis, 1995, Mosby.

Taylor C: *Essentials of psychiatric nursing,* ed 14, St Louis, 1994, Mosby.

Wilkinson S: Factors which influence how nurses communicate with cancer patients, *J Advan Nurs* 16:677-688, 1991.

CHAPTER 3

Recording and Reporting

OBJECTIVES

Mastery of content in this chapter will enable the nurse to:

- Define key terms.
- Describe guidelines for effective documentation and reporting.
- Describe a change-of-shift report given to a nursing team.
- Complete an incident report accurately.
- Write a nurse's progress note using SOAP, SOAPE, PIE, and Focus charting formats.
- Complete a nursing Kardex.
- Complete a nursing flow sheet.
- Explain guidelines used in documentation of home health care and long-term care.
- Describe the role of critical pathways in multidisciplinary documentation.
- Discuss the role of computerization in documentation.

SKILLS

3-1 Giving a Change-of-Shift Report

3-2 Documenting Nurses' Progress Notes

3-3 Incident Reporting

KEY TERMS

Acuity charting
Case management
Charting by exception
Consultation
Critical pathways
Diagnosis-related group (DRG)
Flow sheet
Focus charting
Incident report
Kardex
Objective data
PIE
POMR
Prospective reimbursement
Resident
Sign
SOAP
Subjective data
Standardized care plan
Third-party payor
Variance

Nursing documentation continues to evolve as an essential component within the burgeoning health care system. Documentation has become a vital link between the provision and evaluation of care (Iyer and Camp, 1995). One of the most challenging nursing issues is how to document quality client care within the constraints imposed by regulations, resources, and finances.

Nursing documentation has become increasingly important because of its fiscal connection in determining the cost of client care. Accreditation agencies such as the Joint Commission on Accreditation of Healthcare Organizations (JCAHO) establish standards for nurses (and other health care providers) in the monitoring and evaluation of the quality and appropriateness of client care. For example, under the prospective reimbursement system, hospitals are reimbursed a set dollar amount by Medicare and most **third-party payors** for each **diagnosis-related group (DRG).** Everything that is done by the nurse for the client must be documented to ensure recovery of cost.

In addition, the members of the health care team must be able to communicate effectively with one another in the form of documentation. Furthermore, technology has increased the variety and methods of documentation, which potentially heightens the productivity and scope of nursing practice (Mathews and Zadak, 1993). Finally, nurses are accountable for their actions, and, as a result, written information must be clear and logical, exactly describing all care delivered.

MULTIDISCIPLINARY COMMUNICATION WITHIN THE HEALTH CARE TEAM

An optimum level of client care requires proficient communication among the members of the health care team (Fig. 3-1). Records and reports communicate specific information about a client's health care so that all interventions are directed toward the client's goals.

Reports are oral or written exchanges of information shared between care givers in a number of ways. After completing a work shift, nurses give a verbal or taped report to nurses on the next shift. A physician may call a nursing unit to receive a verbal report on a client's progress for the day. The laboratory submits written reports summarizing diagnostic test results for inclusion in the medical record.

A medical record is a permanent, legal, written document that communicates information relevant to a client's health care management. An example is a clinic record or chart. After each clinic visit, information about the client's health care is recorded. With each successive visit the record is available to the physician and other members of the health care team. It is a continuing account of the client's health status and needs.

Another way that information is communicated is through discussions among team members. They allow a review of information so that problems are identified and solutions are recommended. An example is a discharge planning conference, in which members of several disciplines (e.g., nursing, social work, and physical therapy) meet to discuss the client's progress toward discharge goals. **Consultations** are another form of discussion whereby one professional care giver provides formal advice about the care of a client. For example, a dietitian may consult with the nurse on the best foods to meet a client's preferences and dietary restrictions. Consultations and conferences should be documented in a client's record so that all care givers benefit from the information and plan the client's care accordingly.

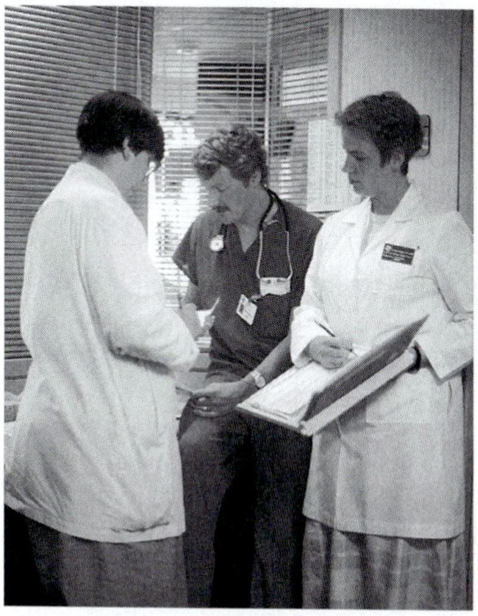

Fig. 3-1 Communication in the health care team.

Guidelines for Quality Documentation and Reporting

Quality documentation and reporting enhance efficient, individualized client care and can be achieved through use of standard guidelines.

Factuality. A factual record or report contains descriptive, objective information about what a nurse sees, hears, feels, and smells. The nurse discriminates between **objective** and **subjective data.** An objective description (e.g., "Pulse 78 per min., regular") is the result of direct observation and measurement. Factual information is less likely to be misleading or cause misinterpretation. Vague words such as *fair, good, appears,* or *seems* and phrases such as *within normal limits* are not acceptable because they lead to inferences or conclusions that cannot be supported by objective information. If a nurse makes inferences or conclusions without factual information, errors in care can occur.

Records and reports can also include subjective information (data verbalized by the client). If a client gives information to the nurse, it should be recorded as a subjective entry in the client's own words. For example, "Client states, 'I feel helpless being unable to do anything for myself.' " The nurse can then add objective findings that more clearly describe the client's emotional problem, such as crying or loss of appetite. The description "the client seems depressed" does not communicate helpful information. The description does not tell another care giver whether the client is withdrawing from conversation or threatening self-injury. A record or report should clearly explain the nurse's observations of the client's behaviors and not be an interpretation of those observations.

Accuracy. A client's record must be accurate so that precise documentation is sustained. The use of exact measurements such as "intake, 220 ml of water" rather than "client drank an adequate amount of fluid" is essential. Measurements are used to determine whether a client's condition improves or deteriorates. Use of an institution's accepted abbreviations, symbols, and system of measures (e.g., metric) ensures that all staff members use the same language in reports and records.

Correct spelling is also important for accurate documentation and reporting. Terms can easily be confused or misinterpreted (e.g., *dysphagia* versus *dysphasia*). Simple spelling mistakes can cause serious treatment errors. It is particularly important to spell medication names correctly on administration records because of the potential of a medication administration error.

An accurate entry in a record must reflect what nurses do during the time frame of the entry. Nurses never chart for anyone else or let anyone chart for them. (The exception is when nurses call their units to report on medication or therapy they had not charted while on duty.) It is acceptable for nurses to later call and ask colleagues to chart information. However, the entry must clearly show what was done and by whom (e.g., "At 8 PM Jane Parmenter, RN, called and reported that morphine sulfate 10 mg IM at 2 PM was administered for abdominal pain.").

Late entries can be made in special situations. A common example is when the medical record is not available when the nurse needs it. A client may be relocated for a diagnostic test. A medication must be entered for the time it was actually given. Late progress notes are recorded by the actual time and date of entry, but information within the note refers to actual time of occurrence or when the entry should have been made. Often the nurse may determine that important information should be added after a progress note has been completed. The nurse simply enters a follow-up progress note. Finally, a late entry may also involve a situation of the nurse omitting a progress note and later realizing the need to add information. It is important to follow agency policy when writing a late entry.

Another way to ensure accuracy is to correctly sign and countersign entries. Any descriptive entry in a record ends with the care giver's full name and title (e.g., Romero Hernandez, RN). In many institutions the first initial is accepted. Nicknames are not used. A nursing student enters the full name, and school, such as "S. Caldwell, OHSU nursing student." RNs or nurse educators may countersign a note entered into the record by a nursing student. When a nurse countersigns, it means that the entry was reviewed and the care given was approved. When a nurse countersigns an entry, it is important that the person administering care is clearly identified. If the record is inaccurate, both nurses can share liability for any client injury. Different agencies may have specific countersigning policies.

Completeness. The information within a recorded entry should be complete, containing concise and thorough information about a client. Lengthy notes are difficult to read. Sketchy or abbreviated notes may leave an impression that nursing care was hurried or incomplete. A long report wastes time and is often boring. A brief, well-written note avoids unnecessary words and irrelevant detail. Criteria are standardized for complete communication of certain health problems or nursing activities.

Whenever it becomes necessary for a nurse to notify the nurse in charge, a supervisor, or a physician of information about a client, it is important that the information be completely documented in the record. The nurse documents the time of the call, the person notified, and the information reported (e.g., "1900 Dr. Abernathy notified of BP 90/60, pulse 116, general urticaria in reaction to IV morphine sulfate, S. Jackson, RN"). To further illustrate, a negative example using this same scenario is "1900 Dr. notified of an allergic reaction to morphine sulfate." The obvious lack of completeness demonstrates its importance in documentation.

Currentness. Timely entries are essential in the client's concurrent care (JCAHO, 1996). Delays in recording or reporting can result in serious omissions and untimely delays for needed care. Legally, a late entry in a chart may be interpreted as negligence. Ongoing decisions about client care must be based on currently reported information. Activities that must be communicated *at the time they occur* include administration of medications or treatments; vital signs; clinical or physical assessment; preparation for diagnostic tests or surgery; change in a client's status and resulting treatment, if any; and admission, transfer, discharge, or death of a client. Routine activities such as bathing or giving oral hygiene do not need to be charted immediately. This information is often entered on flow sheets. The institution's accepted time system, military or civilian, (Table 3-1) should be used for reporting or documenting information. Note that military time begins at one minute after midnight and is recorded as 0001. Each minute is incrementally added until 1:00 A.M., is recorded as 0100, and so on.

Organization. The nurse communicates information in a chronological and logical format. A health team member will better understand information given in the order in which it occurred. If an institution uses a format for written notes (e.g., SOAP or PIE), follow the format according to institution standards.

Confidentiality. A confidential communication is information given by one person to another with trust and confidence that such information will not be inappropriately disclosed. The law protects information about clients that is gathered by examination, observation, conversation, or treatment. Nurses are legally and ethically obligated to keep information about clients' illnesses and treatments confidential. Only staff members who are directly involved in a client's care have legitimate access to the client's records.

Table 3-1 Comparison of Military and Civilian Times

Military	Civilian	Military	Civilian
0100	1:00 AM	1420	2:20 PM
0200	2:00 AM	1800	6:00 PM
0215	2:15 AM	2400	Midnight
1200	Noon	0001	12:01 AM

Legibility. Recorded notes that are illegible can cause treatment errors. The nurse should use the best penmanship to be sure notes are clear and easy to read. If a nurse's script is not legible, entries should be printed. Most institutions require use of black or blue ink.

Common Record-Keeping Forms

Nurses practice in a variety of settings. Consequently, different facilities use a variety of documentation forms. Many forms eliminate the need to duplicate repeated data in the nursing notes. The forms present special types of information in a format more accessible than the compilation of all progress notes. Most of the forms are self-explanatory as to the type of information required from the nurse.

Nursing History and Assessment Forms. A nursing history and assessment form is a special form completed at the time a client is admitted for nursing care. The form usually contains basic biographical data (e.g., age, method of admission, and physician), the admitting medical diagnosis or chief complaint, a brief medical-surgical history (e.g., previous surgeries or illnesses, allergies, and medication history), the client's perceptions about illness or hospitalization, and a physical assessment of all body systems (Fig. 3-2). The form allows the admitting nurse to make a thorough assessment to identify relevant nursing diagnoses or client problems. Information on history forms provides baseline data that can be compared with changes in the client's condition. The JCAHO (1996) requires that a nursing assessment be completed for each client at the time of admission to a health care agency.

Graphic Sheets and Flow Sheets. **Flow sheets** and graphic sheets are forms that allow nurses to assess the client and document the findings on a repeated basis. Common entries on flow sheets are vital signs, physical assessments, intake and output, laboratory data, integument assessment, and neurologic assessments. The checklist facilitates a thorough assessment by providing a framework instead of using open-ended narrative charting (O'Brien and Landstrom, 1994). It is unnecessary to chart a narrative progress note each time that vital signs are checked, a bath is given, or a drug is administered. The flow sheet is a quicker and more efficient way to record information. Figs. 3-3 and 3-4 give examples of nursing flow sheets.

Today flow sheets are not only available as printed forms but are also included within computer software programs. Nurses are able to enter data, which later can be printed out as a flow sheet. The computer provides continuous storage of flow sheet data, eliminating the need to review multiple pages of forms.

When completing a flow sheet, the nurse should review previous entries. This can be useful as a self-check to be sure data being entered are accurate and thorough. In the case of assessment flow sheets, a review allows the nurse to determine if the client's condition has changed. When care givers review flow sheets, the expectation follows that ongoing data are meaningful and relevant to the client's care.

Nursing Kardex. Nursing information needed for the daily care of clients is readily accessible in the nursing Kardex. The **Kardex** is a flip-over card usually kept in a portable index file or notebook at the nurses' station (Fig. 3-5). Most Kardex forms have two parts: an activity and treatment section, and a nursing care plan section. Nurses refer to a Kardex throughout the day. It organizes information in a useful manner as nurses give change-of-shift reports or make walking rounds. The Kardex contains pertinent information about clients and their ongoing care plans. An updated Kardex eliminates the need for continual referral to the chart for routine information. Information that is commonly found in the Kardex includes basic demographic data, primary diagnosis, current physician's orders, a standardized nursing care plan, progress on critical paths, nursing orders or therapies, scheduled tests or procedures, and factors related to activities of daily living. Some institutions use computerized formats that are updated daily and may be termed a patient care profile (PCP).

Charting by Exception. **Charting by exception** is an innovative approach to streamline documentation by reducing repetition and time spent in charting (Iyer, 1995). It is a shorthand method for documenting normal findings and routine care based on clearly defined standards of practice and predetermined criteria for nursing assessments and interventions. Clearly defined standards of practice that define nurses' responsibilities to clients provide the framework for routine care of all clients. With standards integrated into documentation forms, such as predefined normal assessment findings or predetermined interventions, a nurse needs only to document significant findings or exceptions to the predefined norms. In other words, the nurse writes a longhand note only when the standardized statement on the form is not met. Assessments are standardized on forms so that all care givers evaluate and document findings consistently.

Because the standard assessments are located in the chart, client data are already present on the permanent record, so nurses do not have to keep temporary notes for later transcription and care givers have easy access to current data. The assumption with charting by exception is that all standards are met with a normal or expected response unless otherwise documented. When nurses see entries in the chart, they know that something out of the ordinary has been observed or has occurred. For that reason, it is easy to track when changes in a client's condition have developed.

Twenty-Four Hour Client Care Records and Acuity Charting. A 24-hour record keeping system is often used to eliminate excess charting forms. Assessment information and documentation of activities of daily liv-

Text continued on p. 51.

Ashland Community Hospital

ADMIT FORM

Part I: Admission Routine

Date Time | Temp. Pulse Resp.

Mode ☐ amb. ☐ gurney ☐ wc ☐ other | B/P

Via ☐ admitting ☐ ER ☐ other | Height Actual Weight

Admitting Physician: | **Family Physician:**

Admitting Diagnosis:

Most Recent Adm. (hosp./date/reason)

Patient's Statement (of present complaint)

IMMUNIZATION STATUS
☐ CURRENT ☐ NOT CURRENT PHYSICIAN NOTIFIED

Allergies:

Type of Reaction

Medications Patient's significant other understands purpose ☐ yes ☐ no

Medication and strength	freq.	time last dose	Medication and strength	freq.	time last dose	**Disposition of meds:**
1.			6.			☐ did not bring
2.			7.			☐ patient has
3.			8.			☐ family has
4.			9.			☐ pharmacy
5.			10.			

Valuables List: (jewelry, clothing, etc.)

☐ glasses ☐ contact lenses ☐ dentures— ☐ bridge/partial ☐ other

Oriented to ☐ room ☐ bed ☐ phone ☐ call light/TV ☐ visiting hours ☐ safety/smoking policy
☐ doctor's orders ☐ armband

Part II: Patient/Family History

Patient History (major illnesses/operations/major injuries) include endocrine history/problems—past pregnancies

1 4 7
2 5 8
3 6 9

Use of tobacco ☐ no ☐ yes Type Daily amount

Use of alcohol ☐ no ☐ yes Type Daily amount

Organ donor ☐ no ☐ yes Living will ☐ no ☐ yes If yes, copy at ACH ☐ no ☐ yes

Other pertinent information:

Family History ☐ heart disease ☐ stroke ☐ hypertension ☐ asthma ☐ TB ☐ diabetes ☐ cancer
☐ kidney disease ☐ allergy ☐ epilepsy ☐ blood disorder ☐ mental disorder ☐ other

Socio/Economic Religion: Marital status: ☐ single ☐ married ☐ divorced ☐ widowed

Family ☐ lives with ☐ lives alone ☐ no family **Lives in** ☐ house ☐ apt. ☐ other

Occupation ☐ full time ☐ part time ☐ retired ☐ other

ADL ☐ independent ☐ needs assist with (specify what kind of help is needed and who provides it)

Anticipated Discharge Needs: ☐ self care ☐ community agency ☐ discharge planner ☐ other

Comments/plan:

Notify in emergency: relation phone

Nearest relative: relation phone

Info obtained from ☐ patient ☐ family ☐ other **Admitting Nurse:**

ACH 144

Fig. 3-2 Nurse admission note (Courtesy Ashland Community Hospital, Ashland, Ore).

Part III: System Assessment

Place an "X" in area of abnormality. If unable to assess, indicate reason.

EENT

Assess eyes, ears, nose, throat for abnormality. ☐ No problem

							(other)
impaired vision	blind	pain	reddened	drainage	gums		
hard of hearing	deaf	burning	edema	lesion	teeth		

Explain:

RESP

Assess chest configuration, resp. rate, rhythm, depth, pattern, breath sounds, comfort. ☐ No problem

							(other)
asymmetric	tachypnea	apnea	rales	cough	absent		
barrel-chest	bradypnea	shallow	rhonchi	sputum	diminished		
dyspnea	orthopnea	labored	wheezing	pain	cyanotic		

Explain:

CV

Assess heart sounds, rate rhythm, pulse, blood pressure, circulation, fluid retention, comfort. ☐ No problem

							(other)
arrhythmia	tachycardia	rub	numbness	dimin. pulses	edema		
irregular	bradycardia	murmur	tingling	absent pulses			
pain	S_3 or S_4	fatigue					

Explain:

GI

Assess weight, abdomen, bowel habits, swallowing, bowel sounds, comfort. ☐ No problem

Home diet/food habits/caffeine amount—

							stool color (other)
weight loss	N or V	anorexia	diarrhea	distention	hypoactive BS	mass	
obese	thirst	dysphagic	constipation	rigidity	hyperactive BS	pain	

Explain:

GU and GYN

Assess urine freq., control, color, consistency, odor, comfort/Gyn—bleeding, discharge, pregnancy. ☐ No problem

Birth control method last menses last Pap smear

							(other)
pain	hesitancy	oliguria	dysuria	urine color	vaginal bleeding		
frequency	incontinent	nocturia	hematuria	discharge	pregnancy		

Explain:

NEURO

Assess motor function, sensation, LOC, strength, grip, gait, coordination, orientation, speech, vision. ☐ No problem

							(other)
weakness	numbness	headache	paralysis	stuporous	pupils		
unsteady	tingling	seizures	lethargic	comatose	speech		
vertigo	pain	tremors	confused	vision	grip		

Explain:

MS and SKIN

Assess mobility, motion, gait, alignment, joint function/Skin color, texture, turgor, integrity. ☐ No problem

appliance	stiffness	itching	petechiae	hot	drainage
prosthesis	swelling	lesion	poor turgor	cool	
deformity	wound	rash	skin color	flushed	
atrophy	pain	eochymosis	diaphoretic	moist	

Explain:

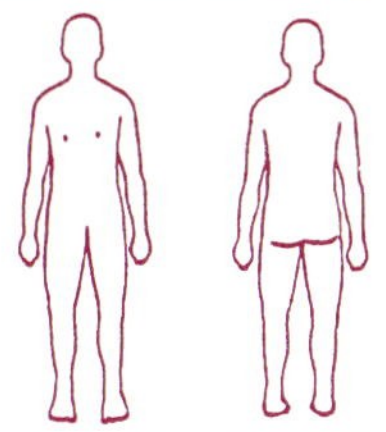

Date:__________ Time:__________ R.N. Signature____________________

Fig. 3-2, cont'd Nurse admission note.

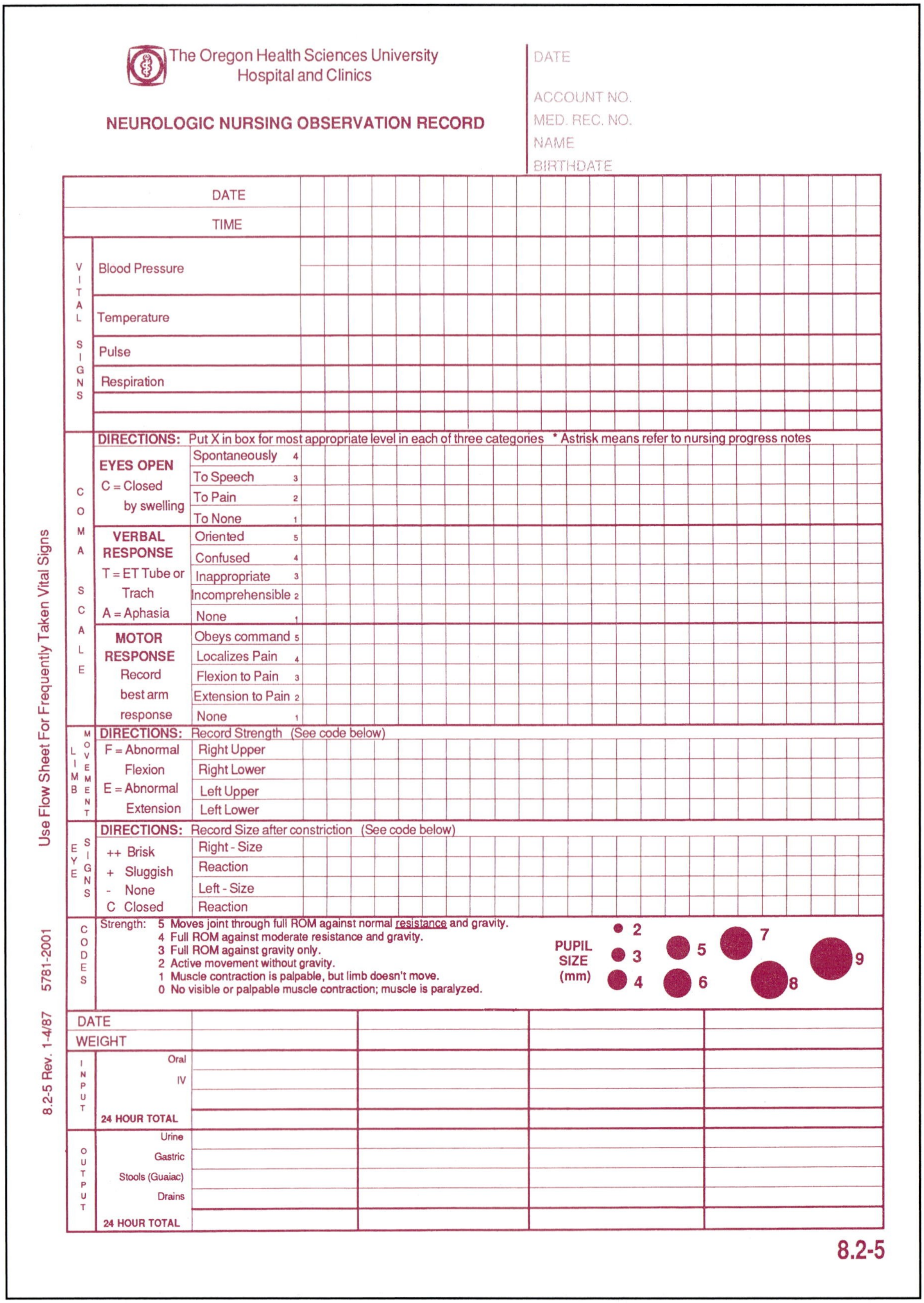

The Oregon Health Sciences University
Hospital and Clinics

NEUROLOGIC NURSING OBSERVATION RECORD

DATE

ACCOUNT NO.
MED. REC. NO.
NAME
BIRTHDATE

	DATE
	TIME
VITAL SIGNS	Blood Pressure
	Temperature
	Pulse
	Respiration

DIRECTIONS: Put X in box for most appropriate level in each of three categories * Astrisk means refer to nursing progress notes

COMA SCALE			
	EYES OPEN C = Closed by swelling	Spontaneously	4
		To Speech	3
		To Pain	2
		To None	1
	VERBAL RESPONSE T = ET Tube or Trach A = Aphasia	Oriented	5
		Confused	4
		Inappropriate	3
		Incomprehensible	2
		None	1
	MOTOR RESPONSE Record best arm response	Obeys command	5
		Localizes Pain	4
		Flexion to Pain	3
		Extension to Pain	2
		None	1

DIRECTIONS: Record Strength (See code below)

LIMB MOVEMENT		
	F = Abnormal Flexion	Right Upper
		Right Lower
	E = Abnormal Extension	Left Upper
		Left Lower

DIRECTIONS: Record Size after constriction (See code below)

EYE SIGNS		
	++ Brisk	Right - Size
	+ Sluggish	Reaction
	- None	Left - Size
	C Closed	Reaction

CODES

Strength:
5 Moves joint through full ROM against normal resistance and gravity.
4 Full ROM against moderate resistance and gravity.
3 Full ROM against gravity only.
2 Active movement without gravity.
1 Muscle contraction is palpable, but limb doesn't move.
0 No visible or palpable muscle contraction; muscle is paralyzed.

PUPIL SIZE (mm): 2, 3, 4, 5, 6, 7, 8, 9

DATE					
WEIGHT					
INPUT	Oral				
	IV				
	24 HOUR TOTAL				
OUTPUT	Urine				
	Gastric				
	Stools (Guaiac)				
	Drains				
	24 HOUR TOTAL				

Use Flow Sheet For Frequently Taken Vital Signs

8.2-5 Rev. 1-4/87 5781-2001

8.2-5

Fig. 3-3 Nursing assessment flow sheet (Courtesy Oregon Health Sciences University Hospital, Portland, Ore).

ASHLAND COMMUNITY HOSPITAL

GRAPHIC/INTAKE-OUTPUT RECORD
DAILY CARE/ACTIVITY RECORD

	DATE					
	Hosp Day / Post OP Day	/	/	/	/	/
	Bath:	PB BB Sh Tub	PB BB Sh Tub	PB BB Sh Tub	PB BB Sh Tub	PB BB Sh Tub
	Daily Care:	AM PM HS	AM PM HS	AM PM HS	AM PM HS	AM PM HS
	Hygiene Oral/Skin					
	Foley Care/PeriCare					
	Stool/GUIAC + −					
	Turn (L.B.R.) Position					
		24 04 08 12 16 20	24 04 08 12 16 20	24 04 08 12 16 20	24 04 08 12 16 20	24 04 08 12 16 20
	Temperature:					
	Pulse:					
	Respiration:					
	Blood Pressure					
	Daily Weight/Time					
	Diet/%					
	Snack/%					
		11-7 7-3 3-11 24 hr	11-7 7-3 3-11 24 hr	11-7 7-3 3-11 24 hr	11-7 7-3 3-11 24 hr	11-7 7-3 3-11 24 hr
INTAKE	ORAL					
	IV					
	TPN					
	PC = 250cc					
	8 Hr. Total					
OUTPUT	URINE-Vd					
	URINE-Cath					
	NG					
	Emesis					
	8 Hr Total					
EQUIPMENT						
	Diagnostic Studies					

ACH FORM 118

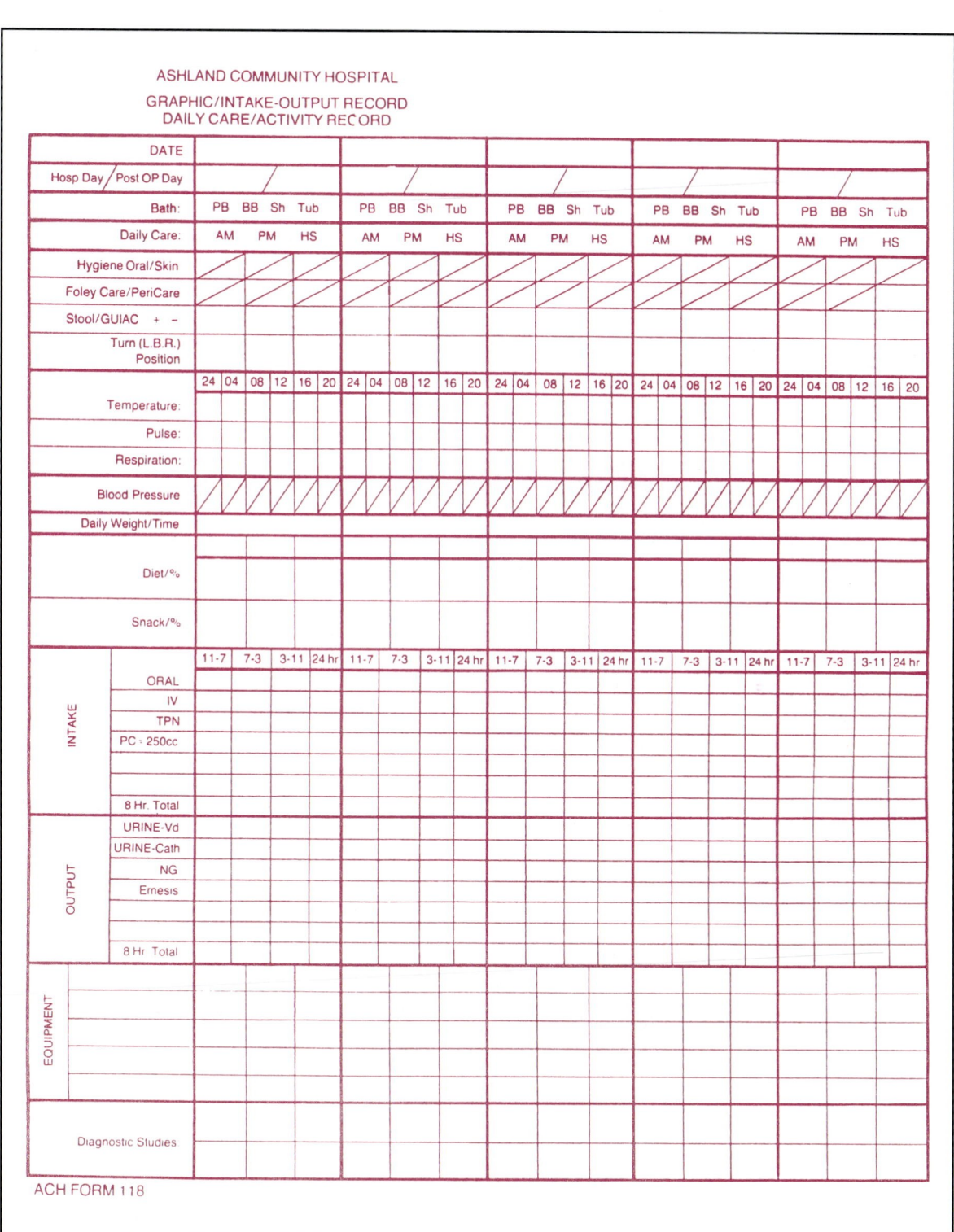

Fig. 3-4 Graphic intake-output record (Courtesy Ashland Community Hospital, Ashland, Ore).

Oregon Health Sciences University
Hospital and Clinics

ACCOUNT NO.
MED. REC. NO.
NAME
BIRTHDATE

ADMIT DATE ____________ AGE ______
DIAGNOSIS ____________
____________ CONDITION ______
ALLERGIES ____________
WEIGHT ______ HT ______ B/P ______ SERVICE ____________
ISOLATION ______ MODE OF TRANSPORTATION ______ DOCTOR# ______
DIET ____________
TF ____________
FLUID RESTRICTION ______ PER TRAY ______

IN EMERGENCY CALL

CALL HO ______

INTAKE ______	PO ______	IV ______
OUTPUT ______	7-3 ______	7-3 ______
R.C. ______	3-11 ______	3-11 ______
	11-7 ______	11-7 ______

TREATMENTS

DATE		DATE	
	VITAL SIGNS ______		
			AUTOLET
	ACTIVITY ______		

ASSISTANCE c̄ ADL'S/TURNS TOTAL ______ PARTIAL ______ SELF ______

	WT		
	GUIAC		

IV FLUIDS

	DT
	PT
	SPEECH THERAPY

DNR ______ UPDATE DUE ______

HSU-17259 (1/92)

Fig. 3-5 Nursing Kardex (Courtesy Oregon Health Sciences University Hospital, Portland, Ore).

ing are concisely maintained in 24-hour notations as opposed to shift-by-shift charting.

In addition, 24-hour formats are foundational to acuity charting systems. **Acuity charting** or documentation requires staff to document their interventions and thereby obtain an overall level of acuity for each client. Staffing patterns can then be determined by examining the acuity levels of the clients on a particular nursing unit. The client-to-staff ratio is calculated from the composite data of nursing care from the 24-hour record.

Standardized Care Plans. Nurses develop care plans on each client, and **standardized care plans** may be used to provide for continuity of care. These plans are based on an institution's standards of nursing practice, are preprinted, and specify the care for clients who have similar health problems.

Most standardized care plans also allow the nurse to individualize the written plan. Specific goals or modifications in implementations as well as desired outcomes of care may be documented. The nurse remains responsible to individualize the approach to client care.

Case Management and Critical Pathways. The **case management** model of delivering care may use its own documentation format. This model uses a multidisciplinary plan of care that is often summarized into **critical pathways.** These are usually one- to two-page formats that include key interventions and expected outcomes that allow the health care team to follow integrated care plans for client problems specific to a medical condition or surgical procedure (Fig. 3-6). The documentation is minimal as the nurse charts on a standardized form, specific to the pathway of an individual client.

The critical paths are used on each shift of care to direct and monitor the flow of client care. Due to the nature of human responses, there are variances in outcomes as the client deviates from the critical path plan. These variances refer to either the positive or negative changes in a client's progression towards expected outcomes (Acord-Szczesny, 1994). A **variance** analysis is necessary to review the data for trends and developing and implementing an action plan to respond to the identified client problems. Critical pathways will potentially lead to more accuracy of predicted outcomes, and the variations in client progress will be more easily determined.

Discharge Summary Forms. Upon discharge from inpatient care, a clinical resume is prepared by the nurse, the social worker, and other members of the health care team. The reason for hospitalization, significant findings, client's status, and any specific teaching plan is included on the discharge summary forms (JCAHO, 1996). Often a copy of the discharge form is given to the client's family member or home health care nurse. This ensures better continuity of care as the client transfers to the previous geographic location (e.g., another inpatient facility, home, respite care, or long-term care).

Home Health Care Documentation. In the home setting, documentation is the crucial element for continuity of nursing care; it represents the evidence of achieving nursing standards and provides the basis for reimbursement for home health care services. Medicare has specific guidelines for establishing eligibility for home care reimbursement. In the fulfillment of medicare guidelines, documentation by home health care nurses has become the largest problem area, with 50% of the nursing time spent in documentation (Braunstein, 1993). Meeting the challenge of controlling this very necessary documentation will continue to be imperative as charting remains foundational to home health care.

Documentation in the home has different implications than in other areas of nursing. The primary difference is the narrower scope of persons directly providing care in the home setting. In addition, both quality of care and justification for financial reimbursement depend heavily on documentation.

Home care documentation also has unique needs regarding accessing the client record. Some parts of the record are needed in the home, while other chart forms are needed in the care giver's office. Technology continues to address these access needs via computerization. Modems, laptop computers, and "electronic home visits" are just a few of the methods allowing for records availability in multiple locations (Miller, 1995).

In home care the nurses' notes should clearly identify the necessity of the nursing visit. The nurses' notes must be able to justify to the reader, usually a reimbursement reviewer, that the care provided is commensurate with the care plan of the overall health care team, the client requires the care in the home, and a necessary service is provided.

Long-Term Care Documentation. The challenges of caring for aged persons in long-term care continue to increase as geriatric clients develop more disabilities associated with their age. Correspondingly, nursing documentation is significantly different from the acute care settings (Iyer, 1995). For example, acute care charting includes frequent physical assessment findings (e.g., vital signs, breath sounds, heart sounds, neurologic checks), often specifying information on an hour-by-hour documentation format. Long-term documentation requires a multidisciplinary approach in the assessment and planning process for the clients and is not as detailed in regard to time increments (often entries may only be made on a weekly basis). Financial reimbursement for **residents** is based on the documentation of nursing care.

In addition, outside agencies determine the standards and policies for long-term care documentation. For example, the department of health in each state governs the frequency of written nursing records on the residents in long-term care facilities.

1

BARNES

CARE PATH®
501
LUNG TRANSPLANT EVALUATION

SERVICE	PHYSICIAN	
PRIMARY NURSE	PRIMARY NURSE	
DC DATE	ADM DATE	DATE OF SURGERY

A-8

Problem Number	PATIENT PROBLEMS / NURSING DIAGNOSES
#1	LACK OF KNOWLEDGE R/T LUNG TRANSPLANT EVALUATION EXPERIENCE
#2	DECREASE IN EXERCISE CAPACITY R/T IMPAIRED OXYGENATION/VENTILATION/DECONDITIONING
#3	POTENTIAL FOR ALTERATION IN COPING R/T SITUATIONAL CRISIS/TRANSITION
#4	POTENTIAL FOR ALTERATION IN FAMILY PROCESSES R/T SITUATIONAL CRISIS/TRANSITION
#5	POTENTIAL FOR ALTERATION IN NUTRITION R/T INAPPROPRIATE INTAKE/DYSPNEA
#6	IMPAIRED GAS EXCHANGE R/T ALVEOLAR-CAPILLARY MEMBRANE CHANGE/ALTERED BLOOD FLOW

*IF APPROPRIATE

#	1 - 12 ASSESSMENT / MONITORING	1 - 12 CONSULTS	1 - 2, 6 - 8, 12 PROCEDURES / TEST	2, 10, 12 TREATMENT	1 ACTIVITY
PRE ADMIT		Transplant office to preschedule following as needed for pt.: 2-D Echo, Quant. V-Q, Resting RVG, PFTs, MRI, Cardiac Cath, Chest CT, Transesophageal echocardiogram			
DAY 1	Braden scale Respiratory status Fall prevention Assess/individualize pt. problem list	Notify consults as per orders. Check with transplant P.A. for additional tests which may be needed. SMA 6 and 12, CBC, CMV, HSV, EBV, Vz titers, HbsAq, HbsAb, HIV, Hep. A, Hep. C titers, T & S, PT, PTT HLA (A,B,C,DR) Typing, incl. cytotoxic screen, u/a - routine & micro, CXR-AP & lat EKG	Apply skin tests 07, 08 } Nursing, Pulm. Rehab., & H.O. 09, 10, 11, 12 } 12 } Psychologist 13, 14 } CDL } PFTs } Chaplain 15, 16, 17, 18, 19, 20 } Cardiology Consult	Appropriate bed surface for Braden scale O_2 • At rest ______ • Activity ______ CPT x1 x2 x3 x4 by Nursing, Physical Therapy, family Aerosols x1 x2 x3 x4 (Self)	Continue activity as done at home

SIGNATURE	INIT.	SIGNATURE	INIT.	SIGNATURE	INIT.

3100-45 (REV. 10/93)

501

Fig. 3-6 Critical pathway (Courtesy Barnes-Jewish Hospital, St Louis, Mo).

2

BARNES

CARE PATH®
501
LUNG TRANSPLANT EVALUATION

CNS	DIETARY	RT
HOME HEALTH	OT	OTHER
PT	SW	OTHER

A-8

Problem Number	PATIENT PROBLEMS / NURSING DIAGNOSES
#7	POTENTIAL FOR INEFFECTIVE AIRWAY CLEARANCE R/T EXCESSIVE SECRETIONS/FATIGUE
#8	INEFFECTIVE BREATHING PATTERN R/T INCREASED WORK OF BREATHING
#9	POTENTIAL FOR INFECTION R/T ALTERED NUTRITION/CHRONIC DISEASE
#10	POTENTIAL FOR INJURY R/T PHYSICAL DECONDITIONING
#11	SPIRITUAL DISTRESS R/T CHALLENGED BELIEF AND VALUE SYSTEM
#12	POTENTIAL FOR ALTERED SKIN INTEGRITY R/T POOR NUTRITION/DECREASED MOBILITY

1	1, 5, 9, 12	1 - 12	1 - 12	1, 2, 4, 11	
MEDS / IVS	NUTRITION	PATIENT / FAMILY EDUCATION	DISCHARGE PLANNING	PSYCHOSOCIAL/ EMOTIONAL/ SPIRITUAL NEEDS	INITIALS (SEE KEY AT BOTTOM)
		Give LTE manual, 6200 pt. letter.			
Pt. to do self meds.; Initiate IV access within 2 hrs. of admission	Continue home diet	Lung transplant evaluation Review tests for day 1 & 2 Personalize instruction to pts. individual learning needs. **Pt./family able to verbalize purpose and any special preparation for follow-up care for tests.**	Plan of care has been mutually set with pt./ family. Educational and DC planning needs will be assessed. **Pt./family verbalizes understanding of care path.**	Allow pt./ family to verbalize concerns and questions and relate problems back to appropriate discipline.	

SIGNATURE	INIT.	SIGNATURE	INIT.	SIGNATURE	INIT.

Fig. 3-6, cont'd Critical pathway.

Computerized Records. Computers are used in health care facilities in a variety of ways, including computerized documentation systems (Fig. 3-7). There are many benefits to computerized documentation, such as reduction of transcription errors, standardization of nursing care, increasing nursing productivity and efficiency, and easier monitoring of quality improvement. Computerization of data results in complete legibility and offers a structure through software design that reinforces standards of nursing care.

Computerized documentation continues to change drastically with the increased use of new technological interfaces (Chu, 1993). Notebook-sized computers with pen-based reading functions, handwriting recognition capabilities, and automated speech-recognition systems are examples of technology that is influencing nursing documentation. In addition, a complete computer-based patient record (CPR) is a futuristic trend in client records (Town, 1993). The CPR will be a comprehensive system that makes use of a broad scope of computerization capabilities. The breadth of the effect of computerization on nursing documentation presents a unique challenge to nursing and overall will ultimately improve the quality of client care.

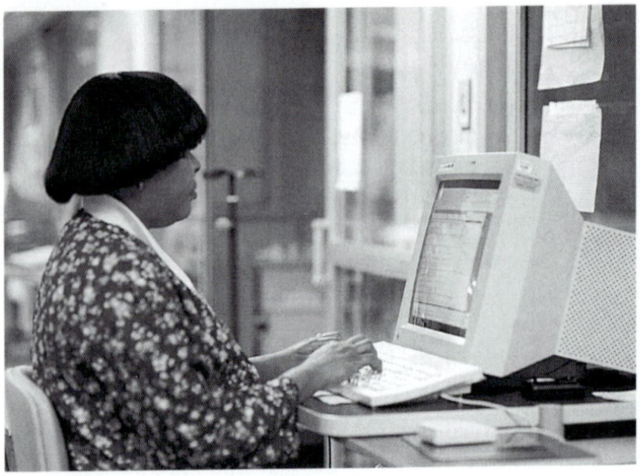

Fig. 3-7 Computerized documentation provides many benefits.

SKILL 3-1 Giving a Change-of-Shift Report

In addition to written documentation, it is a nursing responsibility to verbally convey relevant information about each client to other members of the health care team. One example is the change-of-shift report, whereby at the end of each shift, nurses report information about their assigned clients to the nurses working on the next shift. The change-of-shift report occurs two or three times a day on every type of nursing unit in all types of health care settings. The purpose of the report is to provide better quality and continuity of care among nurses caring for a client.

A change-of-shift report may be given orally in person, by audiotape recording, or during rounds at the client's bedside. Oral reports are given in conference rooms with staff from both shifts participating. If an audiotape is used, it is prepared by the nurse who has completed care for the client and left for the nurse on the next shift to review. Taped reports can improve efficiency by allowing staff to report when time is available. A disadvantage of a taped report is that it does not allow staff members to ask questions or clarify explanations. To avoid this problem, nurses from the previous shift will often wait and be available for questions from the nurse's taped report. Reports given in person or during rounds permit nurses to obtain immediate feedback when questions are raised about the client's care.

EQUIPMENT

- **Worksheets, nursing Kardex (or patient care profile), nursing care plan or multidisciplinary treatment plan or critical pathway**
- **Tape recorder**

DELEGATION CONSIDERATIONS

The skill of change-of-shift report requires problem solving and knowledge application unique to a professional nurse. For this skill, delegation is inappropriate. However, unlicensed assistive personnel (UAP) should know what to report to a nurse, (e.g., apparent change in client's level of pain, reduction in level of consciousness, change in vital signs) so that the nurse may include any pertinent information (after validation) in the report.

STEPS	RATIONALE
ASSESSMENT	
1. Gather information from worksheets, UAP report, or other relevant documents.	Nurse will not read forms during report that the next nurse can easily read independently. However, data used in reports must be current and reflect an overview of the client's progress during the shift.
PLANNING	
1. Prioritize information based on client's needs and problems.	Ensures quality of care and continuity from shift to shift.
CRITICAL DECISION POINT It is essential to decide which information is relevant to communicate to the next shift.	
IMPLEMENTATION	
1. Provide a detailed description of the client's progress during the shift, using a systematic, logical approach (such as the nursing process or functional health patterns). The following is a suggested plan:	
CRITICAL DECISION POINT Develop an organized format for delivering report that allows for thorough presentation of content related to client care.	
a. *Background information*—Include client's name, sex, age, current primary reason for hospitalization, and brief history. Also include any known allergies, code status (i.e., do not resuscitate), and special needs as related to any physical challenges (e.g., blind, hearing deficit, amputee).	Organizes data based on priorities and individualized by the reporting nurse.
b. *Assessment data*—Provide objective observations and measurements made by the nurse during the shift. Describe client's condition and emphasize any recent changes. Include any *relevant* information reported by client, family, or health care team members, such as laboratory data, diagnostic test results, etc.	Oncoming nurse will use data as a baseline for comparison during next shift.
c. *Nursing diagnoses*—Explain clearly the nursing diagnoses appropriate for client.	Clarifies client's current responses to health problems.
d. *Interventions and evaluation*—(steps can be combined in a report).	Staff learn the effect interventions are having on client's recovery and progress.
(1) Describe therapies or treatments administered during shift and expected outcomes (e.g., medication changes, lab results, consultation visits). Specify how interventions are uniquely given for this client. Explain client's response and whether outcomes are met. The format of evaluation could take the format of a critical pathway and the utilization of variance documentation. Do not explain basic steps of procedure.	
(2) Describe instructions given in teaching plan and client's ability to demonstrate learning.	Ensures continuity of teaching, minimizing repetition, but communicating any needs for reinforcement.
e. *Family information*—Report on family visitation or involvement, specifically as it influenced client. Explain if family members were included in care procedures or instruction.	Informs staff as to level of involvement family members have assumed in client's care.

STEPS	RATIONALE
f. *Discharge plan*—The client's progress in reaching discharge is reviewed on an ongoing basis during each change-of-shift report. The discharge plan identifies the interventions and outcomes needed to allow the client to have a smooth transition from hospital or health care facility to home. This plan also identifies the roles and responsibilities of the multidisciplinary team and their follow-up visits.	All team members collaborate to follow the plan of care that promotes discharge.
g. *Current priorities*—Explain clearly the priorities to which oncoming nurse must attend.	
2. *Clarify*—Ask staff from the oncoming shift if they have any questions regarding information reported.	Allows for clarification of misinterpretation and discussion of additional areas of interest.

CRITICAL DECISION POINT **Always attempt to find the specific nurses from the next shift who will be directly providing care of the clients for whom report was given.**

• • • • •

Special Considerations

- Report on the immediate treatment planned for a newly admitted client.
- Explain the status of specific preparatory activities for clients who are going for diagnostic or treatment procedures.
- Describe current physical status of clients returning from diagnostic or operative procedures.
- Discuss status of educational progress, communication with referral agencies, and preparation of family members for clients who are being discharged.
- A more in-depth report may be needed if a nurse new to a unit or an inexperienced nurse will be working the next shift.

SKILL 3-2 Documenting Nurses' Progress Notes

Documentation is anything written or printed that is relied on as a record of proof for authorized persons. A medical record is a comprehensive description of a client's health status and needs, as well as the services provided for a client's care. Accurate documentation reflects the quality of care and provides evidence of each health care team member's accountability in giving care. The purpose of the client's record is to provide information for communication, education, assessment, research, financial billing, auditing, and legal documentation (Table 3-2).

Whenever an entry is made into a record, the nurse follows certain basic guidelines to ensure correctness (Table 3-3). These guidelines are essential for a legally sound document. If the nurse fails to use these guidelines, errors can be made in how data are recorded or later interpreted.

Nurses involved in the direct care of clients are responsible for recording thorough assessments of a client's condition, descriptions of changes in a client's condition, a detailed accounting of nursing therapies delivered, and an evaluation of the client's response to care. The nursing department of each health care agency selects the method used for documentation of client care. The method should reflect the philosophy of the nursing service and incorporate the standards of care and practice for the department. For example, if a nursing department's standards of practice use nursing diagnosis or a framework such as Gordon's functional health patterns (Gordon, 1994), the documentation system uses diagnoses or health patterns in care plans and other forms.

Because the nursing process shapes a nurse's approach and direction of care, good documentation reflects the nursing process. Assessment data are recorded to offer to all health care team members a data base from which to draw conclusions about the client's problems. Information describing the client's problems or diagnoses then directs care givers to choose an appropriate care plan with nursing therapies. Evaluation of care communicates the client's status, degree of progress, and success in meeting expected outcomes of care.

The problem-oriented medical record **(POMR)** is a format for documentation that places emphasis on the client's problems. Data are organized by problem or diagnosis,

Table 3-2 Purposes of Records

Purpose	Description
Communication	The record is a means for health team members to communicate *progress* in the client's *care* (e.g., individual therapies, client education, use of referrals). In addition, it provides a description of the *client's progress*. Anyone reading the record should have a clear understanding of the plan of care.
Education	The record contains a variety of information, including medical and nursing diagnoses, successful and unsuccessful therapies, diagnostic findings, and client behaviors. Students of nursing, medicine, and other health-related disciplines use records as educational resources.
Assessment	Records provide data that nurses use to identify and support nursing diagnoses and plan proper interventions for care. Information from records adds to the nurse's own observations and assessment. Information in medical progress notes allows the nurse to anticipate the status of the client and to conduct an assessment that augments, validates, or confirms physician findings.
Research	Statistical data relating to the frequency of clinical disorders, complications, use of specific medical and nursing therapies, deaths, and recovery from illness can be gathered from client records. Records are resources for describing characteristics of the client populations in a health care agency.
Financial billing	The medical record is a document that shows the extent to which hospitals should be reimbursed for services. For the facility to obtain full reimbursement, the record must show that all physicians' orders were completed adequately and correctly, and it must reflect results of those orders.
Auditing	A regular review of information in client records gives a basis for evaluation of the quality and appropriateness of care provided in an institution. The JCAHO requires health care institutions to establish quality assessment and improvement programs to conduct objective, ongoing reviews of client care. Review of records can reveal information about the processes and outcomes of care.
Legal documentation	A medical record must be accurate because it is a legal document. In the case of a lawsuit, the medical record, not the nursing care, is on trial. Nursing care may have been excellent; however, care not documented is care not done as far as a court of law is concerned.

Table 3-3 Guidelines for Correct Recording

Guideline	Correct Action
Do not erase, apply correction fluid, or scratch out errors made while recording.	Draw a single line through the error, write the word "error" above it, and sign your name or initials. Then record the note correctly.
Do not leave blank spaces in nurses' notes.	Draw a line horizontally through the space and sign your name at its end.
Record all entries legibly and permanently.	Use black or blue ink for all entries (check agency policy for type of ink preferred); never use pencil, which can be erased.
Begin each entry with the time and end with your signature and title (students may be required to sign an abbreviation of their school).	Sign using first initial, complete last name, and title (C. Robinson, RN *or* T. Wallace, SN, U of I).

and narrative notes include assessment, planning, intervention, and evaluative information specific to the client's health status. In a true POMR system, all care givers contribute to a single list of identified client problems. Most institutions use a modified POMR system whereby nursing staff contribute to a single list of nursing diagnoses or problems. Clients benefit from a POMR charting method because all health care team members can contribute to a common plan of care. A POMR has a data base, problem list, care plan, and progress notes.

The data base is a section that contains all available assessment information about the client (e.g., the physician's report of the physical examination and medical history, the nurse's admission history, the clinical or physical assessment, the dietitian's assessment). The data base remains active and current, with revisions made as new data become available.

The problem list should include each of the client's problems or diagnoses, listed in the order in which each problem was identified. The list is comprehensive, including physiological, psychosocial, cultural, spiritual, environmental, and developmental needs. Usually the problem list is in a selected location (e.g., in front of the record), so that it is easy to find and can serve as an organizer or table of contents.

Care plans or standardized care plans are developed for each problem. These plans may be diagnostic, therapeutic, or educational and often have a multidisciplinary approach. In a diagnostic plan the physician indicates diagnostic studies to be performed. A therapeutic plan may include specific medical therapies ordered by the physician or if the therapeutic plan is based on a nursing diagnosis, the nurse outlines proposed interventions. An educational plan includes the types of information or skills required by a client to assume self-care or adapt to any health-related problems. In a POMR, all team members have access to the various plans of care so that care can be better coordinated.

Progress notes are a form of recording that document a client's progress. Often these notes follow a special format so that information about each client problem is documented and communicated clearly. The various formats used for progress notes include SOAP (acronym for Subjective data, Objective data, Assessment, and Problem); SOAPE (acronym for Subjective data, Objective data, Assessment, Plan, and Evaluation); PIE (acronym for Problem, Intervention, and Evaluation); APIE (acronym for Assessment, Plan, Intervention, and Evaluation); and the format used in focus charting, DAR (Data, Action, and Response). The nurse uses the same format whenever a progress note is entered. It then becomes easy for staff to find notes referring to each problem. Any care giver should be able to read a progress note and understand what type of problem a client has, the level of care provided, and the results of interventions.

EQUIPMENT

- **Progress note forms (manual or computer)**
- **Pen**

> **DELEGATION CONSIDERATIONS**
>
> Charting progress notes requires problem solving and knowledge application unique to a professional nurse. For this skill, delegation is inappropriate.

STEPS	RATIONALE
ASSESSMENT	
1. Review all necessary assessments and nursing interventions required by client. Evaluate client's response and status of each diagnosis.	Nursing process organizes nursing care and directs care toward appropriate client problems.
CRITICAL DECISION POINT Use documentation time as a method of reviewing and evaluating the overall scope of implemented client care.	
IMPLEMENTATION	
1. Record a summary of nursing care in progress notes:	Timely, accurate summary provides clear explanation of client's status.
a. Refer to specific problems or nursing diagnoses as a means to organize the note.	
b. Follow the guidelines for charting (see p 57) to ensure quality documentation.	
c. Begin each note with the current date and time.	
d. Use the format selected by the institution to record information.	Use of single format allows all nurses to easily locate progress notes and follow continuity of care for each client problem.
(1) *PIE charting* (acronym for Problem, Intervention, and Evaluation).	**PIE** charting is based on client problem or diagnosis.
P Statement of nursing problem or nursing diagnosis (EXAMPLE: Anxiety related to knowledge deficit of postoperative procedures, inexperience with surgery).	
I Description of interventions delivered to client (EXAMPLE: Explained to client normal postoperative monitoring and procedures to expect during return from the operating	

STEPS	RATIONALE
room [OR]. Demonstrated turning, coughing, and deep breathing [TCDB] exercises. Provided booklet to client on postoperative nursing care).	
E Evaluation of client's response to therapies and progress toward goals of care (EXAMPLE: Client able to demonstrate TCDB, discussed importance of requesting pain medication. States, "I don't have any questions now." K. Ishihara, RN).	
(2) *SOAP charting* (acronym for *S*ubjective data, *O*bjective data, *A*ssessment, and *P*lan). **SOAP** charting is based on an identified client problem or diagnosis.	
S Description of subjective data gathered during care of client (EXAMPLE: "I'm worried about what it will be like after surgery").	
O Objective data is what nurse collects through assessment skills (EXAMPLE: Client asking frequent questions about surgery. Has had no previous experience. Poor eye contact during conversation, moves restlessly in bed. Spouse present, acts as a support).	
A Assessment or conclusion of what data reveals is summarized (EXAMPLE: Anxiety related to knowledge deficit of postoperative procedures and inexperience with surgery).	
P Plan of care delivered based on assessment (EXAMPLE: Explained routine postoperative monitoring and procedures to expect on return from OR. Demonstrated TCDB and provided client with teaching booklet. E. Rademaker, RN).	
(3) *Focus charting.* **Focus charting** deals with the focus or primary subject matter of the note (EXAMPLE: Anxiety related to knowledge deficit of postoperative procedures and inexperience with surgery).	It provides format to document any client situation, even one unrelated to a client problem or diagnosis.
D Data collected regarding the focused subject (EXAMPLE: Client asking questions about what to expect after surgery. Has no previous experience. Has poor eye contact, moves restlessly in bed).	
A Actions taken by nurse (EXAMPLE: Explained routine postoperative monitoring and procedures to expect following return from OR. Demonstrated TCDB exercises).	
R Client's response to care (EXAMPLE: Client able to demonstrate TCDB correctly. Discussed importance of requesting pain medication early. States has no further questions at this time. D. Markle, RN).	
2. Sign progress note with full name and status. Do not leave an open space between this note and the previously written note.	Identifies who is accountable for client's care. Anyone could use open space to write information that changes accuracy of record.

SKILL 3-3 Incident Reporting

An incident is any event not consistent with the routine operation of a health care unit or routine care of a client. The client, visitor, or employee may be at risk when anything unusual occurs in a health care area. Examples of incidents include a client fall, accidental needle-stick injury, medication administration error, a visitor experiencing symptoms of illness, or carelessness in performance of a procedure that leads to actual or potential client injury. When an incident occurs, the nurse involved or the nurse who witnessed the incident completes an **incident report.** Reporting of incidents helps in the identification of high-risk trends in nursing care or daily unit operations that warrant correction. The report is completed even if an injury does not occur or is not apparent. The information from incident reports helps nursing staff find solutions to prevent repeated incidents. The reports are an important part of a unit's quality improvement program.

EQUIPMENT

- **Incident report form, pen**

DELEGATION CONSIDERATIONS

Incident reporting often involves unlicensed assistive personnel who actually find the client situation requiring the report. Care givers need to know their responsibility in actions to take, in reporting to the nurse what they have found, and in explaining their actions to resolve the situation. Overall, writing incident reports requires problem solving and knowledge application unique to a professional nurse. Therefore, for incident report writing, delegation is inappropriate.

STEPS / **RATIONALE**

ASSESSMENT

1. Be observant when witnessing an incident: note exactly the sequence of events involved in the incident, including time and type of incident; injury to client, nurse, or other staff; and observation of factors that may have contributed to the incident (e.g., wet floor discovered in area of client fall, loose needle in client's bed linen).

   Rationale: Report must include objective, chronologic information in the event the incident leads to a lawsuit or investigation into institutional policy and procedure. The nurse who witnessed the incident or who found the client at the time of the incident files the report.

CRITICAL DECISION POINT **Prepare an incident report on any questionable event. Do not avoid incident reporting based on the notion that punitive actions are taken whenever incident reports are filed.**

2. Assess the extent of any injury to client or others.

   Rationale: Indicates type of treatment or action needed.

IMPLEMENTATION

1. If an incident involves an injury, take steps to restore the individual's safety, such as stabilizing the client's position after a fall and assessing for further injuries.

   Rationale: A priority is to stabilize any injury to prevent worsening of individual's condition.

2. When a client sustains an injury, call a physician immediately.

   Rationale: Ensures prompt medical attention.

3. When a visitor or staff member sustains an injury, refer to emergency department or appropriate treatment setting.

4. Complete an incident report form.

   Rationale: Prompt recording ensures accurate data.

CRITICAL DECISION POINT **Document on the incident report form as quickly as possible. Do not allow this to be a type of documentation that is prolonged. The closer to the event, the more accurate the recording. (NOTE: This also necessitates that the staff readily know where the incident forms are kept.)**

STEPS	RATIONALE
a. Record time of incident and describe exactly what occurred or was observed, using objective findings and observations (Table 3-4).	Prevents inferences and misinterpreation.
CRITICAL DECISION POINT It is extremely important to use words that are objective in nature and to use language that does not allow for subjective interpretation. Do not include personal opinions or feelings.	
b. Describe objectively the client's or staff member's condition when incident was discovered or observed.	Establishes baseline for comparison with any later changes.
c. Describe measures taken by any care givers at time of incident.	Provides standard in determining appropriateness of therapies.
d. Send completed report to designated department.	Data are used for facility's risk management and quality improvement programs.
5. When a client is involved, document the events of the incident in the client's chart.	
a. Do not duplicate all information from incident report.	Incident report can include factors nurse observed that may be contrary to policy and procedure. Client's chart should include only the objective description of incident.
b. Do not record that an incident report was completed.	Client's chart is legally recoverable and can be used in court. Incident reports are property of the institution but are recoverable through a subpoena.
c. Simply enter an objective description of what happened.	Medical record is for purpose of documenting client's health status and medical care.
d. Record any assessment and intervention activities initiated as a result of incident.	
6. If client was injured, implement any ordered therapies and begin routine assessment of body systems influenced by injury.	

Table 3-4 Examples of Incident Report Entries

Proper Entry	Incorrect Entry
6 PM Client found on floor at foot of bed; able to respond to name when called. 2 cm abrasion noted across left forehead. Vital signs stable. Dr. Smith notified and arrived on floor at 6:15 PM. Placed client on fall-prevention protocol.	Client found on floor at foot of bed, probably fell on way to bathroom. Small abrasion over left forehead. Dr. Smith notified. Client instructed to use call light when needing to go to bathroom.
Administered morphine sulfate 10 mg at 4 PM; 6 mg morphine sulfate ordered. Monitored vital signs q 15 minutes; called Dr. Jones; vital signs remain stable.	Administered 10 mg morphine sulfate at 4 PM without checking order before administering. 6 mg morphine sulfate ordered.
Needle stick to right index finger, caused minimal bleeding. Notified employee health department.	Needle stick to right index finger, likely due to needle left in bed linen after blood drawing. Notified employee health.

CRITICAL THINKING EXERCISES

1. Mr. Petrosian has an ultrasound test during your time of care. When he returns from the diagnostic study, you realize that you forgot to document the abdominal dressing change you did prior to his leaving. How would you chart this late entry?
2. Your initial assessment of a client reveals that the wrong intravenous solution (.45% normal saline) is being administered (.9% normal saline is the correct fluid). Write an incident report noting the important factors.
3. Ms. Freed, a client on a medical nursing unit, recently became dyspneic upon walking from her bed to the bathroom. In addition, her pulse elevated, and she was slightly confused upon ambulating back to her bed. Write your nursing documentation using both the SOAP and DAR formats for progress notes. Does either format exclude information? If so, can it be found elsewhere in a client's record?

REFERENCES

Acord-Szczesny J: Computer tracking of critical path variations, *Inside Case Management,* 1(2):1, May 1994.

Braunstein ML: The electronic patient records solution, *Caring,* 12(7):30, 1993.

Chu S: Clinical information systems. II. The nursing interface, *Nurs Mgmt* 24:11, 1993.

Gordon M: *Nursing diagnosis: process and application,* ed 3, St Louis, 1997, Mosby.

Iyer PW, Camp NH: *Nursing documentation: a nursing process approach,* ed 2, St Louis, 1995, Mosby.

Joint Commission on Accreditation of Healthcare Organizations: *Accreditation manual for hospitals,* Chicago, 1996, The Commission.

Mathews J, Zadak K: Managerial decisions for computerized patient care planning, *Nurs Mgmt* 24:7, 1993.

Miller K: Home health care update 95, *Nursing 95* 25:7, 1995.

O'Brien K, Landstrom G: Using system integration to revise documentation, *Nurs Mgmt* 25:2, 1994.

Town J: Changing to computerized documentation—PLUS!, *Nurs Mgmt* 24(7), 44, 1993.

ADDITIONAL READING

Addy-Keller J, Mcelwaney E: A new documentation tool, *Nurs Mgmt* 24(11):46, 1993.

Crummer M, Carter V: Critical pathways: the pivotal tool, *J Cardiovas Nurs* 7(4):30, 1993.

Jost K: Psychosocial care: document it, *Am J Nurs* 95:7, 1995.

Mandell M: Not documented: not done, *Nursing 94* 24(8):62, 1994.

Martin F: Documentation tips: to help you stay out of court, *Nursing 94* 24(6):63, 1994.

Nadler G: The challenge of a paperless system, *J Nurs Admin* 4:37, 1993.

Parisi S: What to do after a med. error, *Nursing 94* 24(6):59, 1994.

Sieracki C: Organizational liability prevention: automated profiles, *Nurs Mgmt* 24:7, 1993.

Trofino J: Voice-activated nursing documentation: on the cutting edge, *Nurs Mgmt* 24:7, 1993.

Twardon C, Gartner M: The nursing plan: innovative home health documentation, *Nurs Mgmt* 24:11, 1993.

Woodyard LW, Sheetz J: Critical pathway patient outcomes: the missing standard, *J Nurs Care Qual* 8(1):51, 1993.

UNIT II

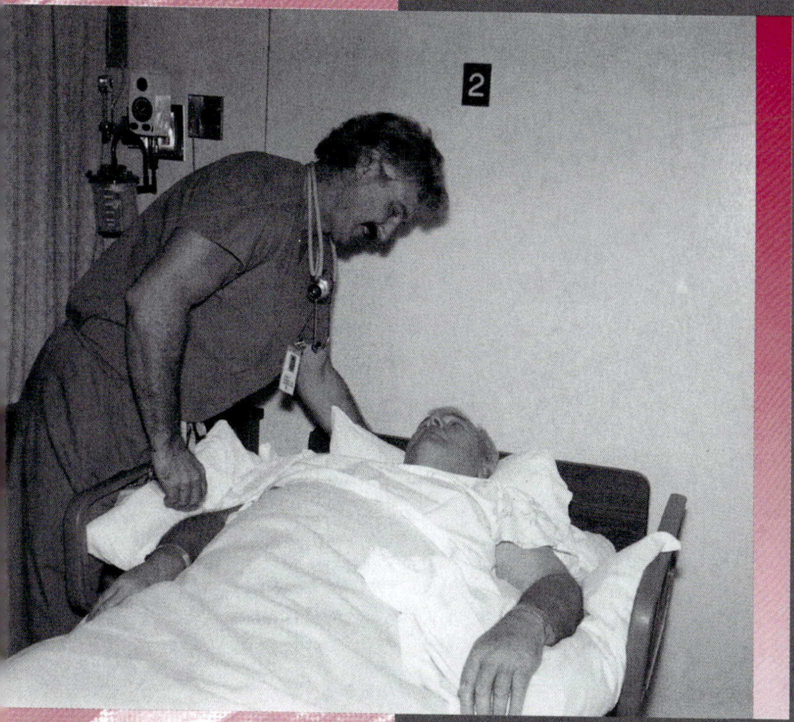

Safety and Comfort

CHAPTER 4

Safety

OBJECTIVES

Mastery of content in this chapter will enable the nurse to:

- Define key terms.
- Discuss methods to reduce physical hazards.
- State nursing diagnoses associated with a client's safety.
- Develop expected outcomes for clients whose safety is threatened.
- Discuss specific risks to safety as they pertain to the older adult client.
- Describe nursing interventions specific for reducing the risk of falls and other traumatic injuries.
- Describe steps in the design of a restraint-free environment.
- Describe nursing interventions for a client who experiences generalized seizures.
- Describe methods to evaluate interventions designed to maintain or promote a client's safety.

SKILLS

4-1 Fall Prevention
4-2 Designing a Restraint-Free Environment
4-3 Applying Restraints
4-4 Seizure Precautions

KEY TERMS

Ambularm^{Tm}
Aspiration
Belt restraints
Extremity restraints
Jacket restraints
Mitten restraints
Mummy restraints
Restraint
Seizure
Seizure precautions

Health promotion and illness prevention involve maintaining the client's safety. Maintenance of a client's safety in the home, community, and health care environment is essential.

Promoting client safety reduces the length and cost of treatment, the frequency of treatment-related accidents, the potential for lawsuits, and the number of work-related injuries to personnel. In addition, a safe environment encourages clients to assume a more active role in their health care practices.

Threats to an adult client's safety are frequently related to lifestyle habits. The client who abuses alcohol has a greater risk than other persons for motor vehicle accidents. Likewise, the long-term smoker has a greater risk of cardiovascular or pulmonary disease than do nonsmokers. In addition, the adult experiencing a high level of stress is more likely to have an accident because of the impact of stress on decision making. High levels of stress also increase the risk of illnesses such as headaches, gastrointestinal disorders, and infection.

Threats to the safety of older adults focus primarily on accidents. Beginning at about age 70, the death rate from falls increases dramatically and the rate continues to increase with age. In fact, by age 79, falls surpass motor vehicle accidents as the leading cause of accidental death (*Accident Facts,* 1994). Falls are a leading cause of injury in hospitalized older adult clients as well. Injuries to older adults can be related to psychogenic factors, physiological changes occurring because of the aging process, a pathological condition, medications, and/or environmental hazards. Ebersole and Hess (1994) identify the following areas for nurses to consider when attempting to provide a safe environment for the older adult: housing, relocation stress, institutionalization, migration patterns, transportation and mobility, community and neighborhood supports, adaptational capacity of the aged, and environmental safety and convenience.

A client's safety can be maintained by preventing client self-injury. These accidents are classified as client-inherent accidents. Examples are self-inflicted cuts, injuries, and burns; ingestion or injection of foreign substances; self-mutilation or setting fires; and pinching fingers in drawers or doors. Client-inherent accidents can occur in both oriented and disoriented clients.

Measures designed to promote client safety are the result of individualized assessment findings. Often it is the conclusion of the nurse that a client's safety is at risk, and subsequent nursing interventions are implemented. Assessment of a client's safety should occur in the home, health care facility, and community environment.

A safe environment is one in which basic needs are met, physical hazards are reduced or eliminated, transmission of organisms is reduced, and sanitary measures are carried out. Many physical hazards, especially those implicated in falls, can be minimized by adequate lighting, removal of clutter, and installation of safety features, such as grip bars and nonslip floor surfaces. In addition, in the hospital or long-term care setting, safety is enhanced by the presence of call bells or other signaling devices, side rails, and devices, such as Ambularm™, that alert staff to clients who may need assistance.

Clients at risk for injury from falling or other traumas may need restraints temporarily. Restraints are not a solution for a client problem, they are a temporary means to control behavior. Restraints do not necessarily prevent falls. In fact, it has been shown that clients may suffer fewer injuries if left unrestrained (Capezerti, Evans, Strumpf et al., 1996; Patterson, Strumpf, Evans, 1995). Many complications are associated with the use of restraints, the most severe resulting in client death. There are many alternatives to the use of restraints, and all should be employed. Ideally, nurses should collaborate to design fall-prevention programs and a restraint-free environment for clients.

When restraints are necessary for client safety, the appropriate restraint must be used and applied correctly. Measures to prevent the hazards of immobility and other complications must be instituted.

Nurses caring for clients who have a seizure disorder must be familiar with seizure precautions to provide adequate protection to the client. Nursing interventions are designed to protect a client from traumatic injury, maintain a patent airway, and maintain a positive sense of self-esteem.

GUIDELINES

1. Know the client's age, level of awareness, orientation, ability to assimilate information and make judgments, ability to communicate, sensory and motor status, usual activity patterns, and activities of daily living.
2. Know the client's medical history and present therapies. Certain illnesses, such as a stroke, and medications, such as tranquilizers, can cause physical or cognitive impairment that increases the risk of injury.
3. Be aware of environmental conditions that can affect the client's safety and increase risk of injury, for example, cluttered halls.
4. Know the proper use of safety devices, such as walkers, canes, geriatric (Geri) chairs, and restraints for a client receiving nursing care in a hospital, extended care facility, or at home.

DELEGATION CONSIDERATIONS

The skills necessary to prevent falls, establish a restraint-free environment, apply restraints, and implement routine seizure precautions can be delegated to unlicensed assistive personnel.

- Review environmental safety precautions (e.g., dry, uncluttered floors, bed locked and left in low position, call bell within reach).
- Assist in applying an ordered restraint properly.
- Review times client is to be checked and times restraints are to be released for range of motion (ROM), skin care, and repositioning.
- Stress protection from injury when a client experiences a seizure.
- Caution not to restrain or attempt to insert tongue blade or airway after client begins a tonic-clonic seizure.

SKILL 4-1 Fall Prevention

It is estimated that about 30% of the population 65 years and older living in the community falls at least once each year (Clinical News, 1995) and that falls account for up to 90% of all reported hospital incidents, with the risk for the older adult significantly greater (Brady et al., 1993). It is therefore essential for nurses to accurately assess clients and their environment for risk factors. In this way, measures may be instituted to reduce and/or eliminate hazards before client injury occurs.

In the home, older clients are more likely to fall in the bedroom, bathroom, and kitchen. These falls most often occur while transferring from beds, chairs, and toilets; get-

HOME HAZARD ASSESSMENT

Home Exterior

Are sidewalks uneven?
Are steps in good repair?
Do steps have securely fastened handrails?
Is there adequate lighting?
Is outdoor furniture sturdy?

Home Interior

Do all rooms, stairways, and halls have adequate lighting?
Are night-lights available?
Are area rugs secured?
Are wooden floors nonslippery?
Is furniture placed appropriately to permit mobility?
Is furniture sturdy enough to provide support for getting up and down?
Are temperature and humidity within normal range?
Are there any steps or thresholds that may pose a hazard?
Are step edges clearly marked with colored tape?
Are handrails available and secure?
Are extension cords used appropriately?
Are smoke, fire, and carbon monoxide detectors installed?

Kitchen

Are hand-washing facilities available?
Is the pilot light on for the gas stove?
Are the dials on the stove readable?
Are storage areas within easy reach?
Are cleaning fluids, bleach, etc., in original containers and stored properly?
Is the water temperature within normal range?
Are there clean areas for food storage and preparation?
Is refrigeration adequate?
Are appliances in good working order?
Are electrical appliances located away from water sources?
Are electrical cords in good condition?

Bathroom

Are hand-washing facilities available?
Are there skidproof strips or surfaces in the tub or shower?
Are bath mats secured?
Does the client need grip bars near the bathtub and toilet?
Does the client need an elevated toilet seat?
Is the medicine cabinet well lighted?
Are medications in their original containers?
Have outdated medications been discarded?

Bedroom

Are beds of adequate height to allow getting on and off easily?
Is day and night lighting adequate?
Are floor coverings nonskid?
Does the client have a telephone nearby?
Are emergency numbers visible near the phone?

Modified from Tideiksaar R: Home safe home: practical tips for fall-proofing, *Geriatric Nursing* 11(6):284, 1989 and Ebersole P and Hess P: *Toward healthy aging: human needs and nursing process*, ed 4, St Louis, 1994, Mosby.

ting into or out of bathtubs; tripping over carpet edges or doorway thresholds; slipping on wet surfaces; and descending stairs (Tideiksaar, 1989). Therefore it is important that the environment be carefully assessed and the client be informed of potential hazards (see box above).

In the hospital setting a tool, such as a Risk for Falls Assessment Tool, may be used to identify a client at risk for falling (see box on p. 68). The client's physical status, mental status, medications, and devices used to ambulate are assessed to determine the degree of risk.

Based on an individual client's condition and environment, nursing measures are instituted to ensure safety. The call bell/intercom system (Fig. 4-1) should be explained to the client and family, side rails used appropriately, beds and wheelchairs locked, and beds left in the low position (Fig. 4-2). Clients may be placed in Geri chairs, or wedge cushions (Fig. 4-3) may be used on chairs. Seating in lounges or dayrooms should be arranged to encourage client interaction. Various types of seating should be available, such as lounge chairs and recliners. Wheelchairs should be used only to transport clients.

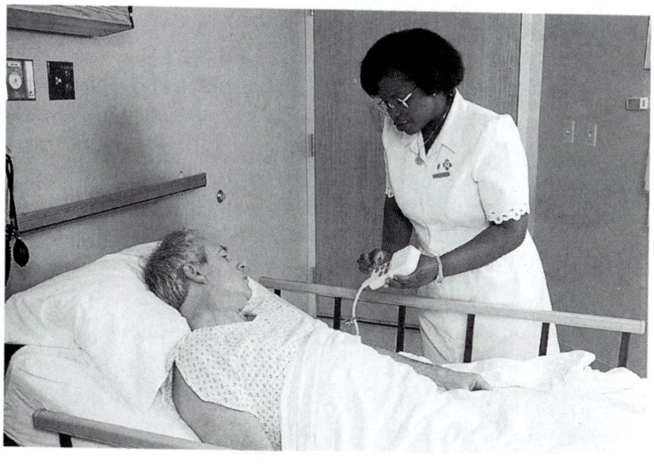

Fig. 4-1 The nurse demonstrates the use of the call bell to the client and secures it in an accessible position.

RISK FOR FALLS ASSESSMENT TOOLS

Tool 1: RISK Assessment Tool for Falls

Directions: Place a check mark in front of elements that apply to your client. The decision of whether a client is at risk for falls is based on your nursing judgment. Guideline: A client who has a check mark in front of an element with an asterisk (*) or four or more of the other elements would be identified as at risk for falls.

General Data

___ Age over 60
___ History of falls before admission*
___ Postoperative/admitted for surgery
___ Smoker

Physical Condition

___ Dizziness/imbalance
___ Unsteady gait
___ Diseases/other problems affecting weight-bearing joints
___ Weakness
___ Paresis
___ Seizure disorder
___ Impairment of vision
___ Impairment of hearing
___ Diarrhea
___ Urinary frequency

Mental Status

___ Confusion/disorientation*
___ Impaired memory or judgment
___ Inability to understand or follow directions

Medications

___ Diuretics or diuretic effects
___ Hypotensive or central nervous system suppressants (e.g., narcotic, sedative, psychotropic, hypnotic, tranquilizer, antihypertensive, antidepressant)
___ Medication that increases gastrointestinal motility (e.g., laxative, enema)

Ambulatory Devices Used

___ Cane
___ Crutches
___ Walker
___ Wheelchair
___ Geriatric (Geri) chair
___ Braces

Tool 2: Reassessment Is Safe "Kare" (RISK) Tool

Directions: Place a check in front of any element that applies to your client. A client who has a check mark in front of any of the first four elements would be identified as at risk for falls. In addition, when a high-risk client has a check mark in front of the element "Use of a wheelchair," the client is considered to be at greater risk for falls.

___ Unsteady gait/dizziness/imbalance
___ Impaired memory or judgment
___ Weakness
___ History of falls
___ Use of a wheelchair

Modified from Brians LK et al: The development of the RISK tool for fall prevention, *Rehabil Nursing* 16(2):67, 1991.

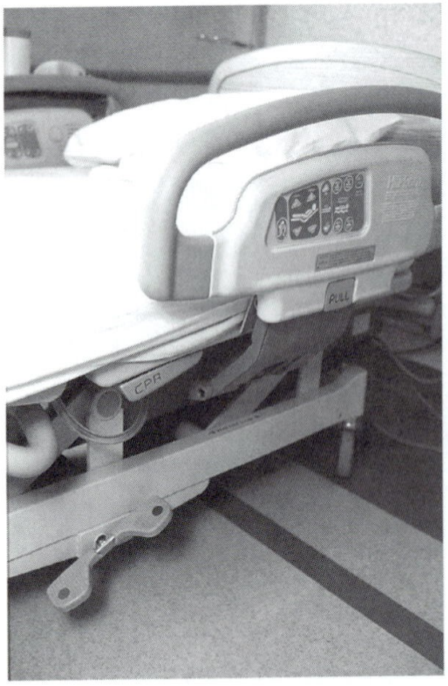

Fig. 4-2 The hospital bed should have the wheels locked, be kept in the low position, and have the side rails up.

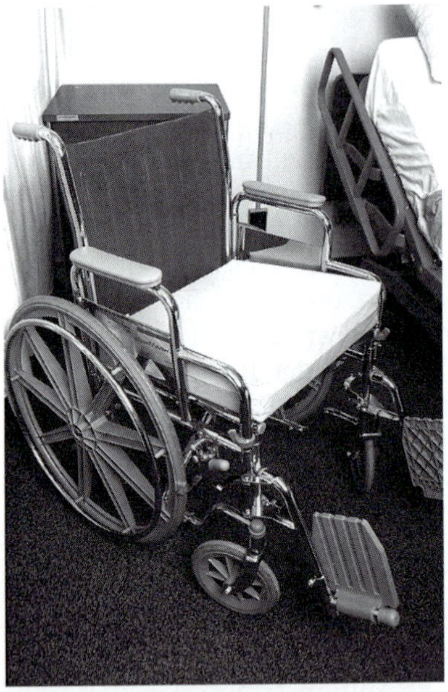

Fig. 4-3 A wedge pillow on the seat is thicker at the front, deterring the client from getting up without assistance.

For clients who continue to attempt to ambulate without the necessary assistance, a monitoring device, such as an **Ambularm**^{Tm} (see pp. 71-73), may be utilized. This electronic, battery-operated alarm is attached to a client's leg. When the client bends the leg over the edge of the bed to get out, the alarm sounds. In this way, staff can respond to the client in a timely fashion and provide assistance with ambulation and other activities of daily living.

At home or in the health care setting, it is very important that clients have adequate footwear when ambulating. Clients should have well-fitting, sturdy shoes with nonskid rubber soles. A walking shoe or sneaker is recommended. In addition, clients should wear cotton socks, which absorb moisture and prevent friction.

EQUIPMENT

- **Home Hazard Assessment**
- **Risk for Falls Assessment Tools**
- **Hospital bed with side rails**
- **Call bell**
- **Ambularm^{Tm} monitoring device**

STEPS	RATIONALE
ASSESSMENT	
1. Assess older adult directly and review medical history for physiological changes common to aging process that increase risk of falling: osteoporosis, decreased hearing, decreased night vision, cataracts or glaucoma, orthostatic hypotension, decreased balance, slowed nervous system response, osteoarthritis. A medication history is essential, as many older clients are taking antihypertensive medications and diuretics.	Physiological alterations predispose client to falls (e.g., postmenopausal woman is prone to osteoporosis and therefore at risk of breaking hip or ankle when walking: the fall results from stress fracture; fracture is not caused by fall). Antihypertensive medications and diuretics may cause hypotension and lead to falls.
2. Assess risk factors in home, health care facility, and/or community that pose a threat to older adult's safety (e.g., improperly lighted stairways or throw rugs).	Provides opportunity to decrease risk of accidents.
3. Determine client's actual or risk of injury as a result of motor, sensory, or cognitive changes.	Provides opportunity to identify factors that increase older adult's risk of injury.

NURSING DIAGNOSIS

Clustering of defining characteristics from the assessment data may reveal the following nursing diagnoses for clients requiring this skill:

- ➤ Risk for injury
- ➤ Knowledge deficit regarding use of restraints
- ➤ Risk for trauma

Related factors are individualized based on client's condition or needs.

PLANNING

1. **Expected outcomes** following completion of procedure:
   - ➤ Client's environment is free of hazards.
   - ➤ Client is able to identify safety risks.
   - ➤ Client does not suffer a fall or injury.

IMPLEMENTATION

HOME OR HEALTH CARE FACILITY

STEPS	RATIONALE
1. Provide adequate, nonglare lighting throughout.	Reduces likelihood of falling over objects or bumping into them. Glare is a major problem for older adults.
2. Remove unnecessary objects from rooms, hallways, and stairs.	Eliminates potential hazards.
3. Arrange necessary objects in a logical way, placing them consistently in easy to reach locations.	Allows the client to carry out self-care activities safely.

CRITICAL DECISION POINT Clients who follow a consistent routine feel more secure, are less confused, and can better recognize safety hazards.

STEPS	RATIONALE
4. Install secure, easily visible grip bars or handrails in hallways and bathrooms (see illustration) as well as raised toilet seats.	Provides support when stepping out of the tub, rising from the toilet, or walking down the hall.
5. Stairs:	
a. Install treads with uniform depth of 9 inches and 9-inch risers (vertical face of steps).	Eliminates need to continually adjust vision.
b. Install uniform textured or plain colored surfaces on each tread, and mark edge of tread with contrasting color (see illustration).	Provides obvious visual clue to end of step. Uniform texture or color helps to decrease vertigo.
c. Ensure proper lighting of each tread. Block sun or lightbulb glare with translucent shades or screens or use lower wattage bulbs.	Older client's vision is unable to quickly adjust to changes in lighting.
d. Ensure adequate headroom so users do not have to duck to use stairs.	Sudden changes in head position may result in dizziness.
e. Remove protruding objects from staircase walls.	Decreased peripheral vision may prevent client from seeing objects.
f. Keep outdoor walkways and stairs in good condition (free of holes, cracks, and splinters) and well lighted.	Decreased visual acuity can prevent older client from seeing structural defect.
6. Handrails:	
a. Install smooth but slip-resistant handrails at least 2 inches from wall.	Allows client to grasp handrail firmly for support.
b. Secure handrail firmly so that user's weight can be supported, especially at bottom and top of stairway.	Greatest risk of falling is at top and bottom stairs because center of gravity is being shifted and balance is unstable.
7. Floors:	
a. Secure all carpeting, mats, and tile; place nonskid backing under area rugs.	Ability to adjust to slip and to prevent fall is reduced in the elderly.
b. Dry spills on floors immediately.	Slipping occurs more readily on wet surfaces.

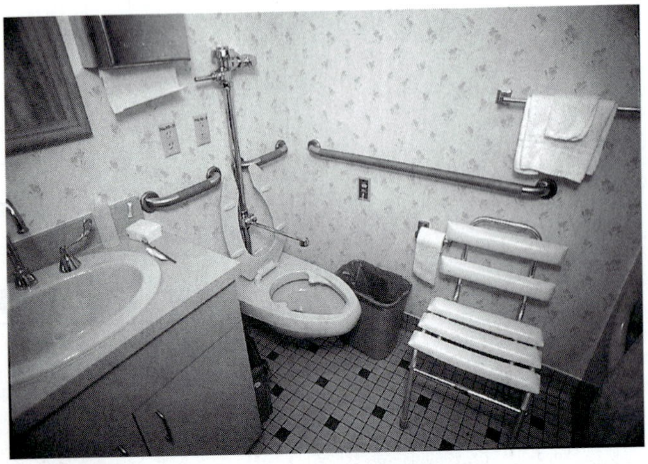

Step 4 Grip bars should be installed in bathrooms.

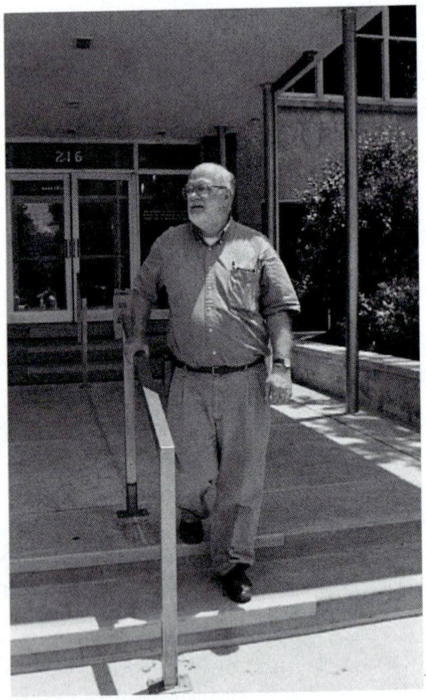

Step 5b Steps with contrasting color on edge.

STEPS	RATIONALE
HEALTH CARE FACILITY	
8. Identify client by checking armband and having client state name.	Prevents client care errors.
9. Introduce self to client, including both name and title or role, and explain what you plan to do.	Reduces client anxiety and promotes cooperation.
10. Gather equipment.	Promotes organization.
11. Wash hands.	Reduces transmission of microorganisms.
12. Provide privacy. Position and drape client as needed.	Prevents lowering of client's self-esteem.
13. Adjust bed to proper height and lower side rail on side of client contact.	Allows for proper body mechanics and prevents injury.
14. Call bell/intercom system (see Fig. 4-1, p. 67)	
a. Explain and demonstrate how to turn call bell/intercom system on and off at bedside and in bathroom.	Knowledge of location and use of call bell is essential to client safety.
➤ **CRITICAL DECISION POINT** **Observe client return demonstration to ensure learning has taken place.**	
b. Consistently secure call bell/intercom system to an accessible location.	Prevents client from searching for device, overreaching, and possibly falling out of bed.
15. Side rails (see Fig. 4-2, p. 68)	
a. Explain to client and family the two main reasons for using side rails: preventing falls and turning self in bed.	Promotes client and family cooperation.
b. Check agency policies regarding age and side rail use.	Side rails are often required on all clients 65 years and older, unless a release form is signed by the client or family.
c. Keep side rails up and bed in low position with bed wheels locked when client care is not being administered and the client is an older adult, weak, confused, sedated, or sleeping.	Prevents client from falling out of bed. With bed in low position, if client climbs over side rails and falls, trauma may be reduced.
d. Leave one side rail up and one down on the side where the oriented and ambulatory client gets out of bed.	Getting into bed is easier; client can use side rail to position self once in bed.
16. Ambularm™ monitoring device	
a. Explain the use of the Ambularm™ to the client and family (see illustration).	Promotes client cooperation.
➤ **CRITICAL DECISION POINT** **Device is not useful if client repeatedly removes it.**	

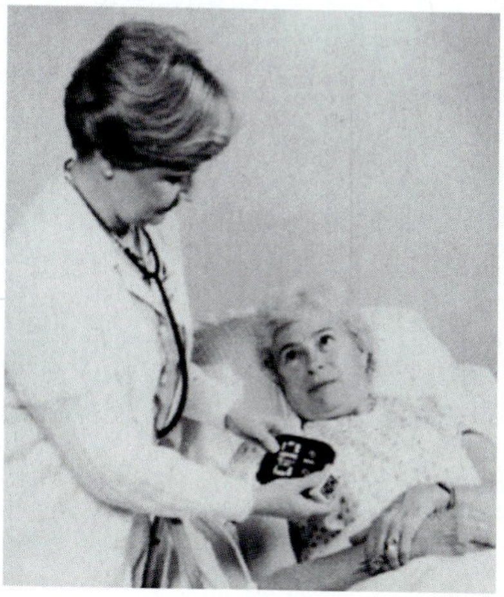

Step 16a The nurse explains the use of the Ambularm™ to the client.

STEPS	RATIONALE
b. Measure client's thigh circumference just above knee for proper size leg band.	Obtain a regular band if circumference is up to 18 inches; a large if it is 18 inches or larger.

CRITICAL DECISION POINT **A band that is too loose may slip off; a band too tight may interfere with circulation and/or cause skin irritation.**

STEPS	RATIONALE
c. Test battery and alarm by touching Ambularm^{Tm} snaps to corresponding snaps on leg band (see illustration).	Ensures proper functioning of system.
CRITICAL DECISION POINT **Use of Ambularm^{Tm} is contraindicated in clients with these conditions: Inspect client's legs for signs of impaired circulation, swelling, skin irritations, breaks in the skin, or thrombophlebitis.**	Ambularm^{Tm} band may aggravate these conditions.

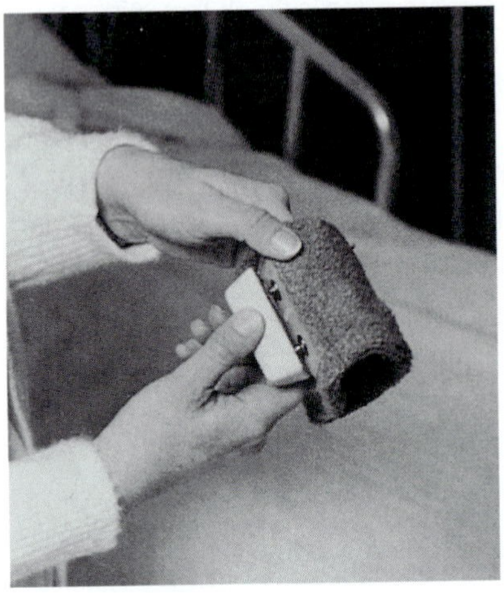

Step 16c To test the battery and sound alarm, before each use touch Ambularm^{Tm} snaps to corresponding snaps on the leg band.

STEPS	RATIONALE
d. Apply the leg band just above the knee (see illustration). Snap the Ambularm^{Tm} onto the leg band securely (see illustration). Leave client's leg in a straight horizontal position on the bed.	Ensures proper functioning of system. When the client's leg approaches a near-vertical position, a position-sensitive switch triggers an audio alarm (see illustration).

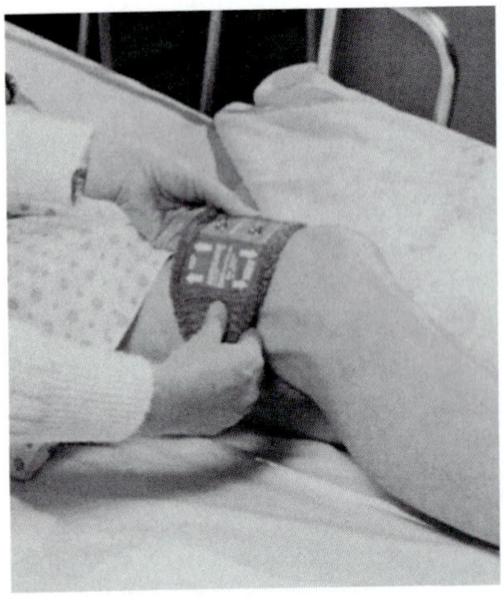

Step 16d Position leg band just above knee.

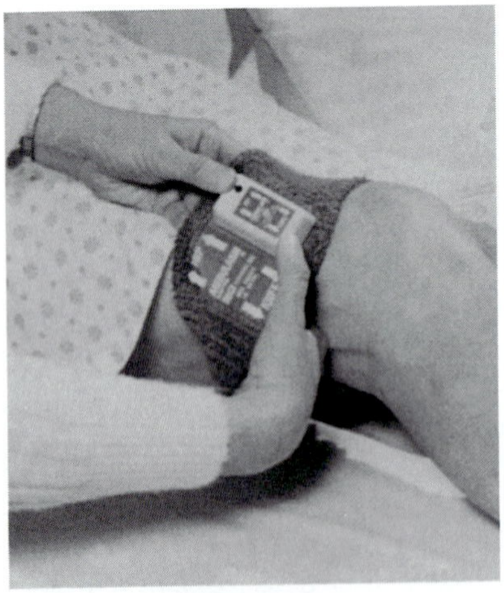

Step 16d Securely snap Ambularm^{Tm} onto leg band.

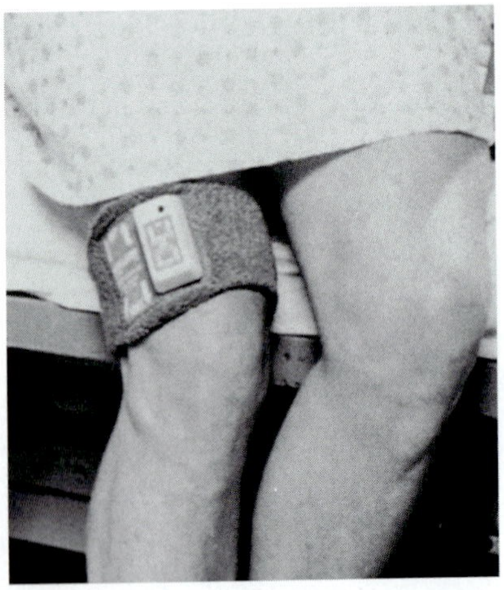

Step 16d When Ambularm^{Tm} approaches a near-vertical position, a position-sensitive switch triggers an audio alarm.

STEPS	RATIONALE
e. Deactivate the alarm by unsnapping the device from the leg band.	Alarm remains on until staff deactivate it.
f. Leave client in bed, leg in horizontal position, call bell/intercom system within reach, side rails up, and bed in lowest position.	Use of Ambularm^{Tm} is an adjunct to other safety features; it does not replace them.
g. Wash hands for at least 10 seconds.	Reduces transmission of microorganisms.

EVALUATION

STEPS	RATIONALE
1. Observe that client's living environment is modified for safety in relation to cognitive and motor needs.	Determines which modifications are needed within home or health care agency environment so that the client's safety is increased.
2. Ask client to identify safety risks.	Ensures client is able identify risks to safety.
3. Reassess motor, sensory, and cognitive status to determine client's response to modification of potential risks. Determine that no falls or injuries occur.	Determines the degree to which nursing interventions have been effective in reducing actual or potential threats to client's safety.
4. **Unexpected outcomes** that may occur include:	
➤ Client is unable to identify safety risks.	Further instruction is required.
➤ Client suffers a fall.	Not all falls can be prevented; however, the nurse must reassess client and the environment to determine if this fall could have been prevented.

RECORDING AND REPORTING

STEPS	RATIONALE
1. Record specific interventions to promote safety.	Provides a written record of specific risks to safety and what nurse did to reduce them.
2. Report to all health care personnel specific risks to client's safety and measures taken to reduce threats.	Informs all appropriate personnel that potential risks exist and what measures have been taken to minimize threats.
3. Document relevant information related to the use of Ambularm^{Tm}: client's behavior that warrants use of Ambularm^{Tm}, condition of client's leg prior to application, instructions given to client and family, time device was applied, client's response to use of device, other safety measures employed (e.g., side rails, call bell).	

FOLLOW-UP ACTIVITIES

1. Environment needs to be continually reassessed for hazards.
2. Assess client's leg frequently for presence of pulses, color, temperature, and mobility when Ambularm^{Tm} is in use. The condition of the skin under the leg band should also be assessed.
3. Nurses should disconnect the Ambularm^{Tm} prior to assisting the client out of bed

Special Considerations

- Clients taking diuretics and antihypertensive medications may have postural hypotension and dizziness.
- The Ambularm^{Tm} alarm can be heard for a distance of 100 to 200 feet, and the sound may be muted by heavy robes, closed doors, etc.
- Manufacturer's instructions for sterilization must be followed if the Ambularm^{Tm} is to be reused on another client.

Teaching Considerations

- A client should be instructed to have yearly vision and hearing examinations. Adaptive devices, such as a hearing aid or glasses, may be needed or modified.
- In a health care facility, a client and family should be thoroughly oriented to the surroundings, with special emphasis given to call lights and/or intercom devices.
- The client and family should be familiar with the purpose and use of the Ambularm^{Tm}.

Gerontologic Considerations

- In general, older clients, especially those with sensory perception and mobility problems, are prone to falls. (Lueckenotte, 1996)
- Older adults, especially postmenopausal women, are at risk for fractured hips. Fractures can cause independent clients to become more dependent or immobilized. (Lueckenotte, 1996)

Home Care Considerations

- The home environment should be assessed carefully.
- Night-lights should be used.
- Items in the home should be kept in their familiar positions.
- The client may need a hospital bed, with side rails, and a bell to signal care giver or family, especially at night.

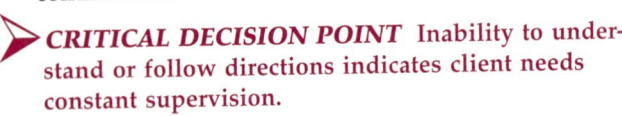

SKILL 4-2 Designing a Restraint-Free Environment

For clients who are at risk of falling or wandering, restraints should be the last resort. When necessary, clients are restrained for several reasons: to prevent falling and wandering, to protect from self-injury (pulling out tubes, removing dressings, etc.), and to prevent violence towards others.

The 1987 Omnibus Budget Reconciliation Act (OBRA) defines clients' rights and choices regarding restraints, and the reasons for the use of physical restraint are clearly stated. The use of mechanical or physical restraints must be part of the prescribed medical treatment, all less restrictive interventions must be tried first, other disciplines must be used, and supporting documentation must be provided (Health Care Financing Administration, 1990).

A restraint-free environment should be the goal for all clients, whether in a health care facility or home. Measures can be taken to ensure safety for those clients who are at risk for self-injury by interrupting therapy and those who may inflict injury on others.

STEPS	RATIONALE
ASSESSMENT	
1. Assess the client's physical and mental status, noting level of consciousness and ability to understand and communicate.	Accurate assessment ensures proper interventions.
CRITICAL DECISION POINT Inability to understand or follow directions indicates client needs constant supervision.	
2. Assess client's knowledge of condition and treatment.	Knowledge of treatment protocols and rationales may increase the client's cooperation.

NURSING DIAGNOSIS

Clustering of defining charactistics from the assessment data may reveal the following nursing diagnoses for clients requiring this skill:

- Risk for injury
- Knowledge deficit (specify area; e.g., alternatives to restraints)
- Risk for trauma

Related factors are individualized based on client's condition or needs.

PLANNING

1. **Expected outcomes** following completion of procedure:
   - Client will be injury free and/or will not inflict injury on others while in a restraint-free environment.

STEPS	RATIONALE
IMPLEMENTATION	
1. Orient client and family to surroundings, introduce to staff, and explain all treatments and procedures.	Promotes client understanding and cooperation.
2. Encourage family and friends to stay with client. Sitters or companions may be utilized.	Reduces client anxiety and increases safety when care is provided by one person and supervision is constant.
3. Place client in a room close to staff.	Allows for frequent observation.
4. Provide appropriate visual and auditory stimuli. A clock, calendar, radio, television, and family pictures may be indicated.	Orients client to day, time, and physical surroundings.
CRITICAL DECISION POINT Stimuli must be individually selected for the client to ensure appropriateness.	
5. Meet client's needs as quickly as possible.	Toileting needs, relief of pain, and other activities of daily living, provided in a timely fashion, decrease client discomfort and anxiety.
6. Approach client in a calm, nonthreatening, professional manner.	Reduces tension in the environment.
7. A limited number of care givers should interact with the client.	Reduces noise, overstimulation, and possible confusion for the client.
CRITICAL DECISION POINT A sufficient number of staff should be readily available quickly for emergency situations.	
8. Organize treatments so client has long uninterrupted periods throughout the day.	Provides for sleep and rest periods. Constant activity may irritate the client.
9. Stress reduction techniques, such as massage and imagery, may be employed.	Reduced stress allows client energy to be channeled more appropriately.
10. Various disciplines should be utilized.	Physical therapy, speech therapy, and occupational therapy may assist the client to focus on appropriate actions.
11. Review medications frequently.	Idiosyncratic reactions and drug interactions may cause changes in client behavior.
EVALUATION	
1. Observe client for any injuries.	Client should be injury free.
2. Client does not injure others.	
3. **Unexpected outcomes** that may occur include:	
➤ Client may continue to disrupt therapy or commit violent acts towards others.	Intensify supervision of client. Restraints may be indicated.

Recording and Reporting

1. Record client behaviors and all interventions to mediate these behaviors.

Follow-Up Activities

1. Check agency policies regarding restraints and obtain an order if the use of restraints is indicated (see Skill 4-3) (Fig. 4-4).

• • • • •

Special Considerations

- Overstimulation of clients is to be avoided; confusion and hostility may result. All sensory stimulation should be meaningful to the client; for example, television and radios should be on for specific programs, not all day.

Teaching Considerations

- Clients and family members should be familiar with all medications and their possible side effects.

Holy Family Hospital and Medical Center
Methuen, Massachusetts

PHYSICIAN RESTRAINT ORDER SHEET

ALLERGIES (FOOD AND/OR DRUG): ☐ NKA

HEIGHT: WEIGHT:

DIAGNOSIS(ES):

DATE	MEDICATION ORDERS	ALL OTHER ORDERS
	A physician's order is required for the use of restraint and/or seclusion. The order must be written or the telephone order countersigned by the ordering or "covering" physician within 24 hours of the order being given. "Restrain p.r.n." orders are not permitted. Orders must include a time limit not to exceed 24 hours. Physicians must review the use of restraints and reissue medical orders every 24 hours.	
		1) Restrain patient according to hospital policy.
		2) Behavior requiring restraint:
		☐ Confusion/disorientation/combative
		☐ Self harm
		☐ Harm to others/surroundings
		☐ Removing medical devices
		☐ Other
		3) Length of time (may not exceed 24 hrs):
		☐ 24 hours; ☐Other
		4) Type of restraint to be used:
		5) Additional instructions if any:
	Signature:	

✓ ORDERS CARRIED OUT (ALLERGIES, HT, WT, & DIAGNOSIS(ES) MUST BE COMPLETED ON ALL ADMISSION ORDERS AND UPDATED AS NECESSARY)

6/95 MF#682

Caritas Christi • A Catholic Health Care System • Member

A

Fig. 4-4 **A,** Restraint order form.

Holy Family Hospital and Medical Center
70 East Street, Methuen, MA 01844

BEHAVIORAL RESTRAINT FLOW SHEET

Behavior Requiring Restraint: (Check all that apply)
- ☐ Confusion/disorientation/combative
- ☐ Self Harm
- ☐ Harm to others/surroundings
- ☐ Removing medical devices
- ☐ Other: ______________________

Less Restrictive Measures Attempted: (Check all that apply)
- ☐ Pain/comfort measures
- ☐ Schedule position changes
- ☐ Schedule toileting
- ☐ Place closer to Nursing Station
- ☐ Reorient
- ☐ Encourage family/friends to visit
- ☐ Other: ______________________

Physician order obtained: ☐ Yes; ☐ No

Type of Restraint: (Check all that apply)
- ☐ Soft wrist/ankle
- ☐ Halter type vest
- ☐ Seat Belt
- ☐ Mitts
- ☐ Leather
- ☐ Other: ______________________

Patient/Family Informed: ☐ Yes; ☐ No

If no, Comment: ______________________

Date Restraint Applied: ______________ **Time:** __________

Date Restraint Ended: ______________ **Time:** __________

Date: / Time:am/pm	12	2	4	6	8	10	12	2	4	6	8	10
1. Hydration/Nutrition/Elimination												
2. Skin condition												
3. Range of motion/turn & position												
4. Communication (call light in reach)												
5. Circulation/Neurovascular Changes												
6. Assess chg. in clinical condition/behavior												
7. Assess for early release												
8. Restraint reduced/removed*												
9. Behavioral/Safety Check done q15"												
10. Vital Signs (if applicable)**												
Initials of assessor:												

Initials/Signature: Initials/Signature: Initials/Signature:

Comments:

* New order required when restraint removed or reduced. ** Temperature not required unless indicated.

KEY: ✓ = Observation / Intervention; NN = Nurses' Notes; O = Patient Off Unit; R = Restraint Removed

Note: It is not necessary to document the Behavioral/Safety Check every 15 minute but nurse must note every 2 hours in the assessment documentation #7 that the observation was performed. ***Any changes in behavior require an assessment.***

Caritas Christi · A Catholic Health Care System · Member

Written: 7/95; Revised: 16. August 1996

B

Fig. 4-4, cont'd **B,** Behavioral restraint flow sheet (Courtesy Holy Family Hospital & Medical Center, Methuen, Mass).

Gerontologic Considerations

- Older clients who become confused and attempt to disrupt therapy or become violent may be suffering from the effects of multiple drug administration, may be anoxic, or may have fluid and electrolyte imbalance. Laboratory reports, signs and symptoms of fluid and electrolyte disturbances, and the possible side effects of medications and interactions of all medications must be assessed.

Home Care Considerations

- Clients at risk for self-injury or violence to others need intensive supervision. The family and/or care giver must recognize this and be able to provide it.

SKILL 4-3 Applying Restraints

Clients at risk for injury may need to be temporarily restrained. A physical **restraint** is a device that limits a client's ability to move. The restraint must be part of the prescribed medical treatment, and all other less restrictive measures must be employed first (see Skill 4-2).

The use of restraints is associated with several serious complications. The Food and Drug Administration (FDA), which regulates restraints as medical devices and requires manufacturers to label them "prescription only," estimates that hundreds of restraint-related injuries occur each year, approximately 100 of them resulting in client death. Most client deaths have resulted from suffocation from a vest or jacket restraint (Lambert, 1992).

In addition, pressure ulcer formation, hypostatic pneumonia, constipation, incontinence, contractures, and neurovascular impairment can result from enforced immobility. Altered sensory perception and altered thought processes may also result. Humiliation, fear, anger, and a decreased sense of self-esteem may occur (Weick, 1992).

When the use of restraints is the only appropriate intervention to maintain the client's safety, both the client and the family should be informed that the restraint is temporary and protective. As with other procedures, the nurse must follow specific agency guidelines when using restraints. Most institutions require a physician's order, which should specify the type of behavior requiring restraint and the type of restraint. Orders should be renewed according to agency protocol.

EQUIPMENT

- Proper restraint
- Padding

STEPS	RATIONALE
ASSESSMENT	
1. Assess if a client needs a restraint.	Restraints are used when other measures have failed to prevent interruption of therapy such as traction, intravenous (IV) infusions, or nasogastric tube feedings; to prevent confused or combative client from self-injury by removing Foley catheters, surgical drains, or life support equipment; to reduce risk of injury to others by client; and at times to reduce the risk of a client falling out of bed or wheelchair.
2. Review agency policies regarding restraints. Check the physician's order for purpose of restraint and the type and duration of restraint.	A physician's order is necessary to apply restraints. The least restrictive type of restraint should be ordered. Because restraints limit the client's ability to move freely, the nurse must make clinical judgments appropriate to the client's condition and agency policy. If the nurse restrains a client in an emergency situation, a physician's order should be obtained as soon as possible.
3. Review the manufacturer's instructions prior to entering the client's room.	The nurse should be familiar with all devices used for client care and protection. Incorrect application of a restraining device may result in client injury or death.

STEPS	RATIONALE
4. Inspect the area where the restraint is to be placed. Assess condition of skin underlying area on which restraint is to be applied.	Restraints may compress and interfere with functioning of devices or tubes. Provide baseline assessment data regarding skin integrity. Enables nursing personnel an objective measure against subsequent skin assessments.

➤ **CRITICAL DECISION POINT** **Restraints should not interfere with IV equipment, tubes, etc. They should not be placed over access devices, such as an arteriovenous (AV) dialysis shunt.**

NURSING DIAGNOSIS

Clustering of defining characteristics from the assessment data may reveal the following nursing diagnoses for clients requiring this skill:

- Impaired physical mobility
- Risk for impaired skin integrity
- Risk for peripheral neurovascular dysfunction
- Powerlessness
- Self-care deficit
- Self-esteem disturbance
- Risk for violence: self-directed or directed at others
- Risk for injury

Related factors are individualized based on a client's condition or needs.

PLANNING

1. **Expected outcomes** following completion of procedure:
   - Client remains free from injury.
   - Client's therapy (IV tube, catheters, etc.) is uninterrupted.

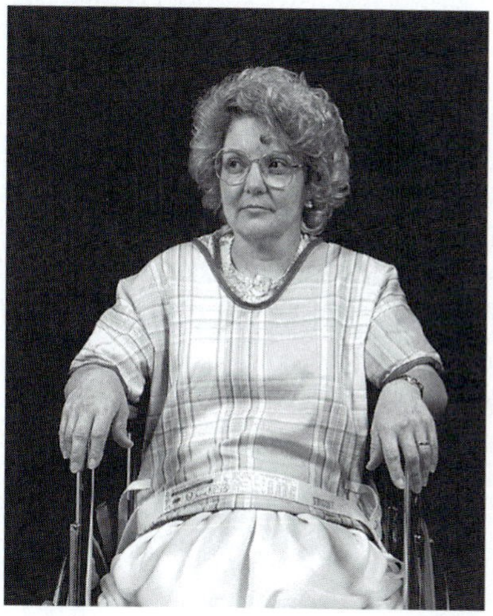

Step 9a Jacket (Vest or Posey) restraint.

IMPLEMENTATION

STEPS	RATIONALE
1. Identify client by checking the armband and having client state name, if possible.	Prevents client care errors.
2. Introduce self to client, including both name and title or role, and explain what you plan to do.	Reduces client anxiety and promotes cooperation.
3. Gather equipment.	Promotes organization.
4. Wash hands.	Reduces transmission of microorganisms.
5. Provide privacy. Position and drape client as needed.	Prevents lowering of client's self-esteem.
6. Adjust bed to proper height and lower side rail on side of client contact.	Allows nurse to utilize proper body mechanics and prevent injury.
7. Place client in correct anatomical position.	Prevents contractures and neurovascular impairment.
8. Pad skin and bony prominences that will be under the restraint.	Reduces friction and pressure from the restraint to the skin and underlying tissue.
9. Apply selected restraint:	
a. **Jacket (Vest or Posey) restraint:** vestlike garment. The front and back of the garment should be labeled as such (see illustration). Apply over clothing or hospital gown.	Restrains client while lying or reclining in bed and while sitting in chair or wheelchair. Proper application prevents suffocation or choking. Clothing or gown prevents friction against the skin.

STEPS	RATIONALE
b. **Belt restraint:** device that secures client to bed or stretcher. Avoid placing belt too tightly across client's chest or abdomen (see illustration).	Restrains center of gravity and prevents client from rolling off stretcher or sitting up while on stretcher or from falling out of bed. Tight application may interfere with ventilation.
c. **Extremity (ankle or wrist) restraint:** restraint designed to immobilize one or all extremities. Commercially available limb restraints are composed of sheepskin with foam padding (see illustration).	Maintains immobilization of extremity to protect client from injury from fall or accidental removal of therapeutic device (e.g., IV tube or Foley catheter).
d. In an emergency, if a commercial extremity restraint is not immediately available, a clove-hitch restraint can be constructed by making a figure eight with gauze and picking up loops. Place padding around extremity, then place loops of clove hitch directly over padded surface (see illustration).	

CRITICAL DECISION POINT A clove-hitch configuration should not tighten as the client moves. If tightening occurs, the device is not constructed properly.

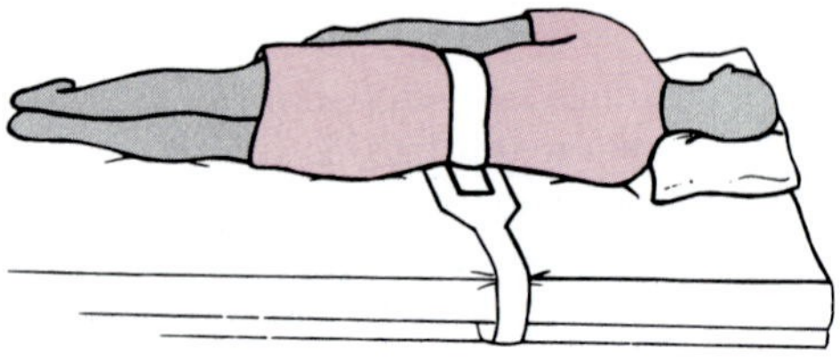

Step 9b Belt restraint tied to bed frame.

STEPS	RATIONALE
e. **Mitten restraint:** thumbless mitten device to restrain client's hands (see illustration).	Prevents clients from dislodging invasive equipment, removing dressings, or scratching, yet allows greater movement than a wrist restraint.
10. Attach restraints to bed frame, which moves when the head of the bed is raised or lowered (see illustration). **Do not attach to side rails.**	

CRITICAL DECISION POINT The client may be injured if the restraint is secured to the side rail and it is lowered.

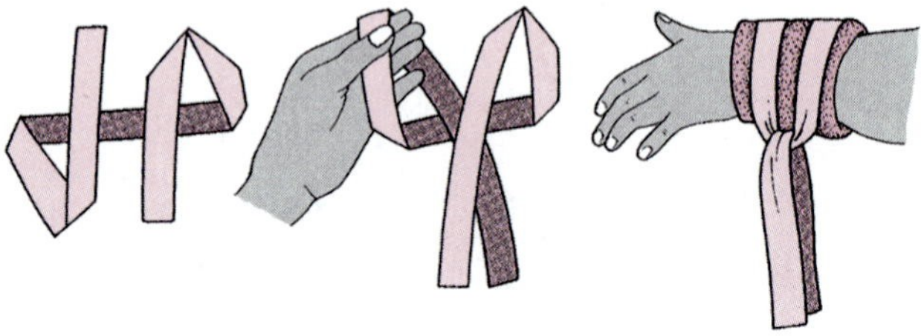

Step 9d In an emergency, a clove-hitch restraint can be constructed using gauze. Make a figure eight and pick up loops. Place loops over extremity.

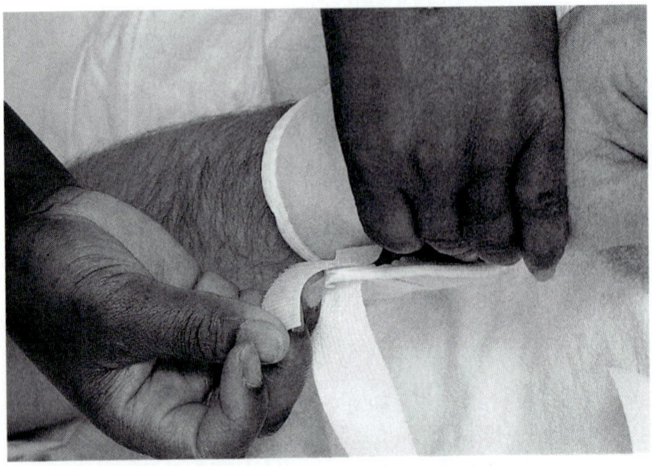

Step 9c Securing an extremity restraint.

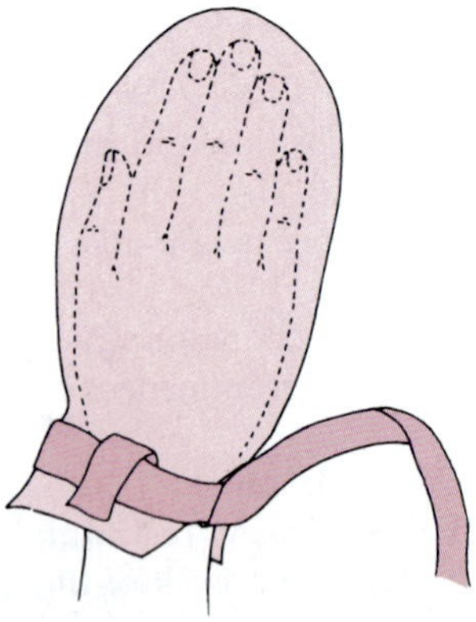

Step 9e Mitten restraint.

STEPS	RATIONALE
11. When the client is in a chair, the jacket restraint should be secured by placing the ties under the armrests and securing at the back of the chair (see illustration).	Prevents client from sliding, restraint ties up the back of the chair.
CRITICAL DECISION POINT **If the ties are not under the armrests, clients may be able to slide the ties up the back of the chair and free themselves.**	
12. Secure the restraints with a quick release tie (see illustration).	Allows for quick release in an emergency.
13. Insert two fingers under the secured restraint (see illustration).	Checking for constriction prevents neurovascular injury.
CRITICAL DECISION POINT **A tight restraint may cause contriction and impede circulation.**	

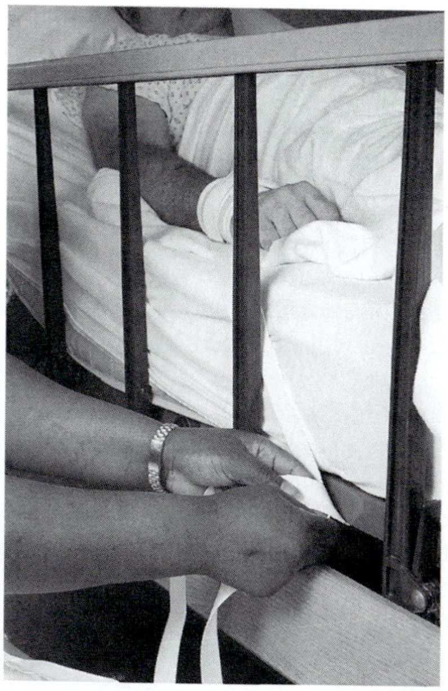

Step 10 Restraints should be tied to bed frame.

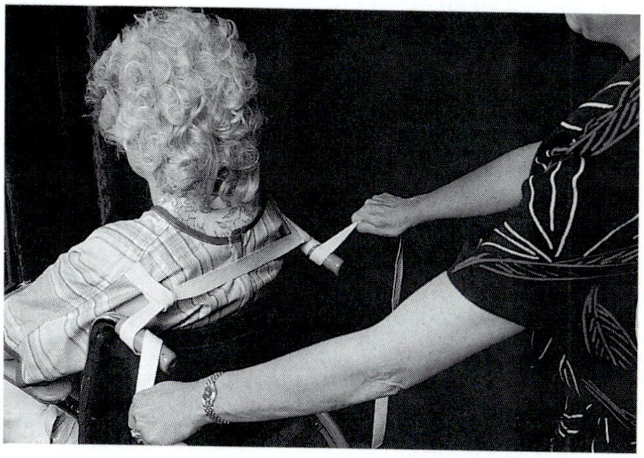

Step 11 Jacket restraint secured to back of wheelchair.

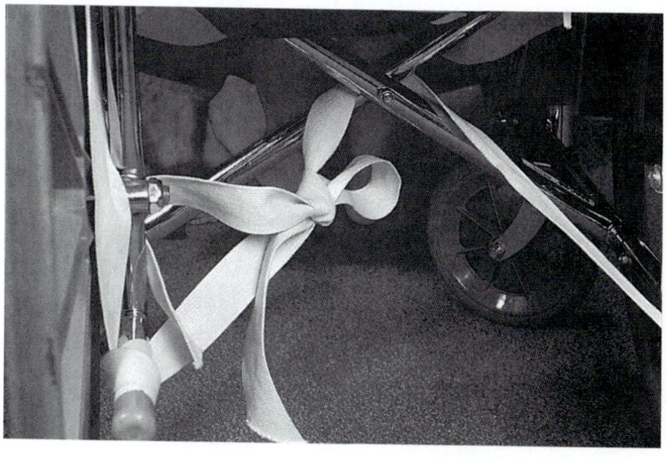

Step 12 Quick release tie.

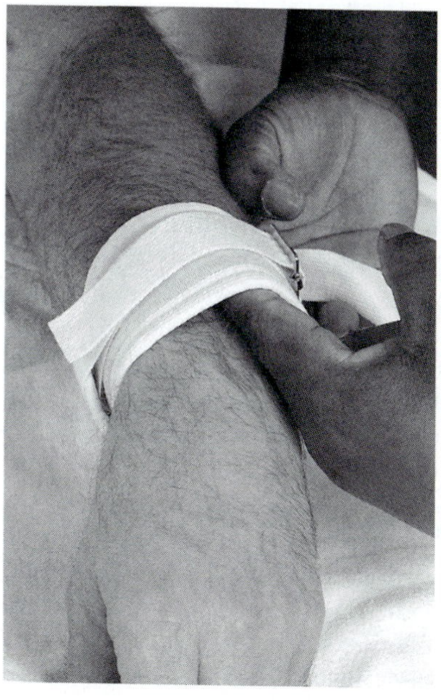

Step 13 The nurse checks restraints for constriction by inserting two fingers under the restraint.

STEPS	RATIONALE
14. Every 30 minutes, proper placement of the restraint and skin integrity, pulses, temperature, color, and sensation of the restrained body part should be assessed.	Frequent assessments prevent complications, such as suffocation, skin breakdown, and impaired circulation.
15. Restraints should be removed for 30 minutes every 2 hours. If the client is violent or noncompliant, remove one restraint at a time and/or have staff assistance while removing restraints. Client should not be left unattended at this time.	Provides opportunity to change client's position and perform full ROM.
16. Secure call bell or intercom system within reach.	Allows client, family, or care giver to obtain assistance quickly.
17. Leave bed or chair with wheels locked. Bed should be in the lowest position.	Locked wheels prevent bed or chair from moving if client attempts to get out. If client falls when bed is in the lowest position, the chances of injury are reduced.
18. Wash hands.	Reduces the transmission of microorganisms.

EVALUATION

1. Inspect client for any injury, including all hazards of immobility, while restraints are in use.	Client should be free of injury and not exhibit any signs of immobility complications.
2. Observe IV catheters and urinary catheters to determine that they are positioned correctly and that therapy remains uninterrupted.	
3. **Unexpected outcomes** that may occur include:	
➤ Impaired skin integrity related to improper or prolonged use of restraint.	Reassess proper application of restraint, ensuring adequate padding. Check skin under the restraint every 30 minutes for abrasions and remove restraint every 2 hours. Change wet or soiled restraints to prevent skin maceration.
➤ Altered neurovascular status of an extremity related to improper use of a restraint.	Tight restraints interfere with circulation. When there is any indication of neurovascular impairment, such as cyanosis, pallor, coldness of skin, and/or client's complaints of tingling sensations, pain, or numbness, the restraint should be removed immediately and the physician notified.
➤ Increased confusion and disorientation.	Use of restraints can further increase disorientation. Provide appropriate sensory stimulation and reorient as needed.
➤ The client releases the restraint and suffers a fall or other traumatic injury.	Reassess the type of restraint used for its appropriateness and its correct application.

RECORDING AND REPORTING

1. Record in nurses' notes:
   - ➤ Client's behavior before restraints were applied
   - ➤ Client's level of orientation
   - ➤ Nursing interventions employed to ensure client's safety without using restraints
   - ➤ Client's and/or family's understanding of and consent to the application of restraints
   - ➤ Type of restraint applied
   - ➤ Time the restraint was applied
   - ➤ Client's behavior after restraints were applied
   - ➤ Times client was assessed while restraints were on
   - ➤ Specific assessments related to oxygenation, skin integrity, musculoskeletal system and peripheral vascular integrity.
   - ➤ Time that the restraints were released
   - ➤ Client's response when restraints were removed

Documents that client's physical safety was at risk and that specific restraint was warranted. Documents presence or absence of any break in skin integrity and status of musculoskeletal system before and after application of restraint.

FOLLOW-UP ACTIVITIES

1. Design nursing measures to promote skin integrity and reduce risk of restricted mobility (see Chapters 8 and 31).
2. Continually attempt to utilize alternatives to restraints (see Skill 4-2) and monitor client's response.

• • • • •

Special Considerations

➤ For legal purposes, the nurse must be familiar with agency policy and procedures for the ordering and application of restraints.

➤ Clients with wrist and ankle restraints should be placed in a lateral position rather than supine. This will avoid **aspiration** should the client vomit.

➤ Client who is able to undo restraint but remains safely in bed or chair indicates to nursing personnel that restraint is no longer needed. Reassess need for use of restraints every 4 to 8 hours.

➤ Clients whose movement is restricted are unable to meet their activities of daily living without assistance. Providing fluids frequently, assisting with toileting, etc. is essential.

Teaching Considerations

➤ Teach primary care giver:
- How to correctly restrain a client
- To observe for early signs of constriction, pressure, and hazards of immobility
- How and when to change a client's position, perform ROM, and administer skin care

Pediatric Considerations

CRITICAL DECISION POINT When a child needs to be restrained for a procedure, it is best that the person applying the restraint not be the child's parent or guardian.

➤ A **mummy restraint** is a safe, efficient, short-term method to restrain a small child or infant for examination or treatment. Open a blanket and fold one corner toward the center. Place the child on the blanket with shoulders at the fold and feet toward opposite corner (Fig. 4-5, *A*).

➤ With child's right arm straight down against the body, right side of blanket is pulled firmly across

A B C D

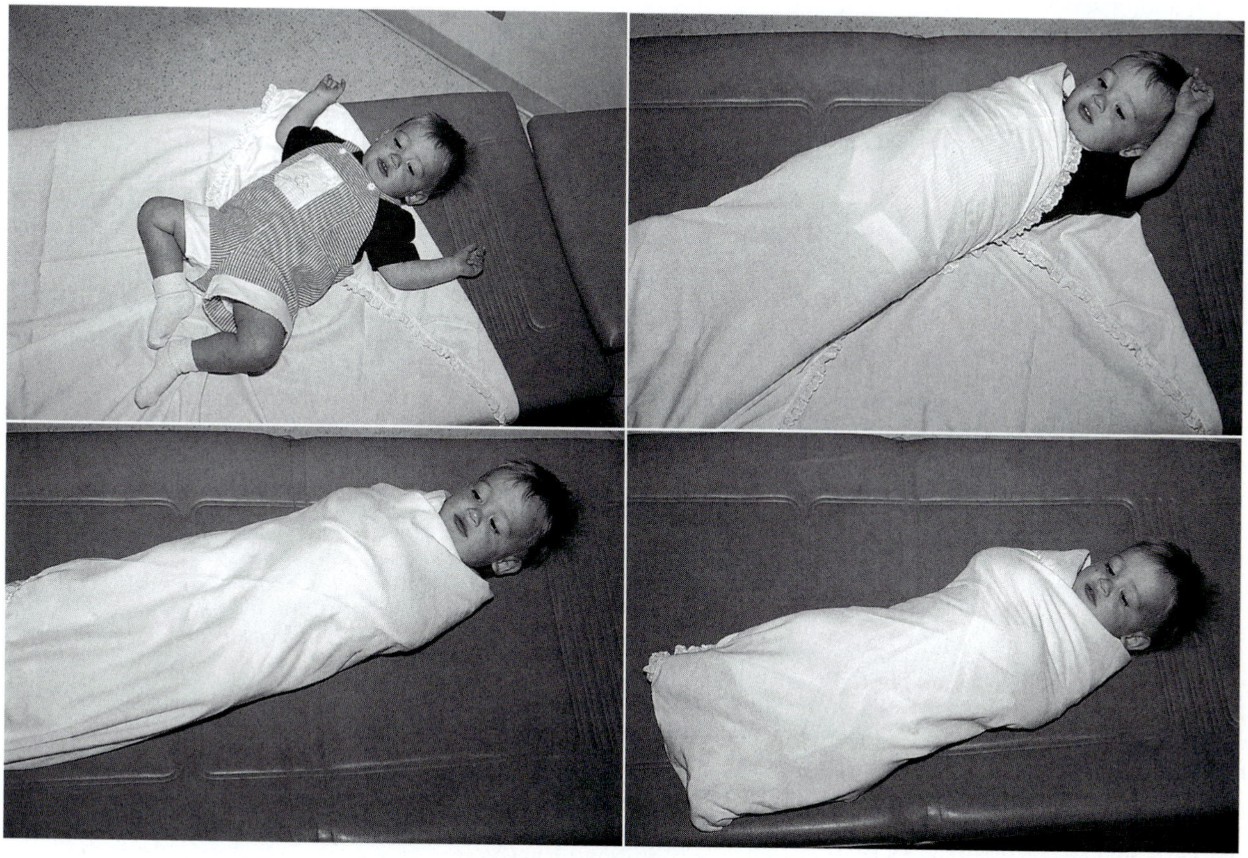

Fig. 4-5 Mummy restraint.

right shoulder and chest and secured beneath left side of body (Fig. 4-5, *B*). Left arm is placed straight against side, and left side of blanket is brought across shoulder and chest and locked beneath child's body on right side (Fig. 4-5, *C*). Lower fold is folded and brought over body and tucked or fastened securely with safety pins (Fig. 4-5, *D*) (Wong, 1995).

Gerontologic Considerations

- Advanced age is not, in itself, an indication for the use of restraints. Promoting functional restoration by performing an individual assessment of risk factors, orienting the client as needed, modifying the environment, teaching muscle strengthening exercises, and meeting the older client's needs in activities of daily living will help prevent falls and other traumatic injuries (Ebersole and Hess, 1994).

SKILL 4-4 Seizure Precautions

A **seizure** is a hyperexcitation of neurons in the brain leading to a sudden, violent, involuntary series of muscle contractions that may be paroxysmal and episodic, as in a seizure disorder, or transient and acute, as after a head injury. A generalized tonic-clonic or grand mal seizure lasts from 1 to 2 minutes (no longer than 5) and is characterized by a cry, loss of consciousness with falling, tonicity (rigidity), clonicity (jerking), and incontinence. Prior to a convulsive episode, a few clients may report an aura, which serves as a warning or sense that a seizure is about to occur. An aura may be a bright light, smell, or taste (Shantz and Spitz, 1993). Following the seizure, there is a postictal phase, during which the client may have amnesia, confusion, and may fall into a deep sleep (Seizure recognition and observation, 1992).

Status epilepticus consists of generalized tonic-clonic seizures that last longer than 5 minutes or are followed quickly by subsequent seizures. This constitutes a medical emergency and requires intensive monitoring and treatment.

Seizure precautions include all nursing interventions to protect the client from traumatic injury, positioning for adequate ventilation and drainage of secretions, providing privacy, and providing support following the seizure. It is now recommended that objects not be placed in a client's mouth to avoid injury to the oral cavity. It has been found that significant injury to the mouth is rare during a seizure, even the most violent ones (Ellis, 1993). Injury may occur from forcing an object into the mouth and from teeth biting down on a hard object. Even soft objects may come apart and be aspirated.

It is important that the nurse observe the client carefully before, during, and after the seizure so that the episode can be documented accurately.

EQUIPMENT

- Oral airway
- Padding for side rails and headboard
- Suction machine
- Oral suction equipment
- Clean disposable gloves

STEPS	RATIONALE
ASSESSMENT	
1. Assess seizure history, noting frequency of seizures, presence of aura, and sequence of events, if known.	Enables the nurse to anticipate the onset of seizure activity.
2. Assess for medical and surgical conditions that may lead to seizures or exacerbate existing seizure condition.	Neurological conditions and surgery may precipitate seizures.
3. Assess medication history.	Seizure medications must be taken as prescribed and not stopped suddenly. This may precipitate seizure activity.
4. Inspect client's environment for potential safety hazards if a seizure occurs.	An airway, suction apparatus, clean gloves, and pillows should be visible for immediate use in the hospital setting for clients with a history of seizures.

NURSING DIAGNOSIS

Clustering of defining characteristics from the assessment data may reveal the following nursing diagnoses for clients requiring this skill:

- Risk for aspiration
- Ineffective airway clearance
- Knowledge deficit regarding safety precautions during seizure activity

Related factors are individualized based on a client's condition or needs.

STEPS	RATIONALE

PLANNING

1. **Expected outcomes** following completion of procedure:
   - Client remains free of traumatic injury while experiencing a seizure.
   - Client's airway remains patent during seizure activity.
   - Client does not experience a lowered sense of self-esteem following seizure episode.

IMPLEMENTATION

STEPS	RATIONALE
1. Position client safely. If standing or sitting at the time of the seizure, guide client to floor and protect head by cradling in the nurse's lap or placing a pillow under head. Clear surrounding area of furniture. If client is in bed, raise side rails, pad, and put bed in low position.	Protects client from traumatic injury, especially head injury.
2. If possible, provide privacy. Have staff control the flow of visitors in the area.	Embarrassment is common after a seizure, especially if the seizure was witnessed by others.
3. If possible, turn the client on the side, with head flexed slightly forward.	Prevents the tongue from blocking the airway and promotes drainage of secretions, thus reducing the risk of aspiration.
4. Do not restrain client. Loosen clothing.	Prevents musculoskeletal injury.
5. Do not force any objects into the client's mouth.	Prevents injury to mouth and prevents possible aspiration.

CRITICAL DECISION POINT Injury may result from forcible insertion of a hard object. Soft objects may break or come apart and be **aspirated.**

STEPS	RATIONALE
6. Stay with the client, observing the sequence and timing of seizure activity.	Accurate, specific observations will assist in the documentation, diagnosis, and treatment of the seizure disorder.
7. After the seizure is over, explain what happened, and answer the client's questions.	Informing clients of the type of seizure activity experienced will assist them in participating knowledgeably in their care.
8. For clients experiencing status epilepticus, put on clean gloves and insert an oral airway (see illustration) when jaw is relaxed between seizure activity.	Intensive monitoring and treatment are required for this medical emergency. Frequently an oral airway must be inserted and suctioning performed (see Chapters 14 and 16). Clean gloves prevent the nurse from coming in contact with the client's saliva.

CRITICAL DECISION POINT Do not place fingers near or in the client's mouth. The client may inadvertently bite the nurse's fingers during a seizure.

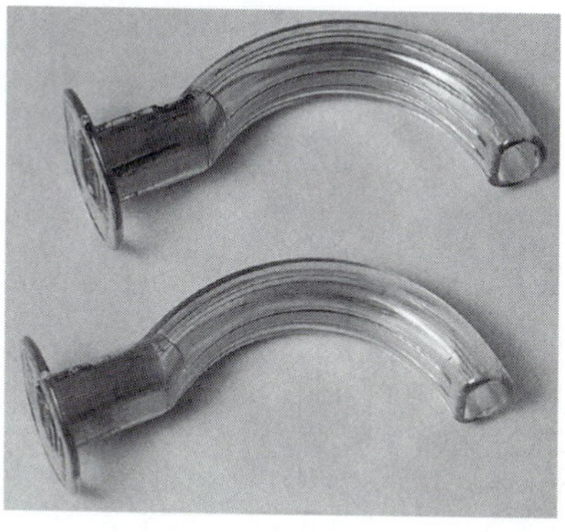

Step 8 Oral airways.

STEPS	RATIONALE
9. Pad side rails and headboard (see illustration).	Traumatic injury is avoided. Avoid use of pillows to pad side rails as suffocation could occur.
10. Following the seizure, assist client to a position of comfort in bed with padded side rails up and bed in lowest position. Place call bell or intercom system within reach.	Provides for continued client safety.
11. Wash hands.	Reduces transmission of microorganisms.

E VALUATION

1. Assess client for traumatic injury during and after seizure episode.	Injury may occur during seizure activity.
CRITICAL DECISION POINT Inspect oral cavity for breaks in the mucous membrane due to bites and broken teeth.	
2. Observe client's color and respiratory rate and pattern during and after the seizure.	The client may experience shallow irregular breathing during the seizure, but normal color and respirations should be apparent following the episode.
3. Ask client to verbalize feelings after the seizure.	Therapeutic interaction may enable client to recognize feelings associated with having a seizure disorder. Client self-esteem is maintained.
4. **Unexpected outcomes** that may occur include:	
➤ Client suffers traumatic injury.	Not all injuries can be prevented; however, the possiblity of injury will be reduced by assisting client to a supine position, guarding the head, and padding side rails.
➤ Client's airway becomes occluded, and materials are aspirated.	Insert oral airway and apply suction to maintain patent airway.
➤ Client verbalizes negative feelings following a seizure.	Confusion, anxiety, embarrassment, or disappointment may follow a seizure. The nurse needs to offer support to clients and allow them to verbalize their feelings.

RECORDING AND REPORTING

1. Record the timing of seizure activity and sequence of events. Record presence of aura (if any), level of consciousness, posture, color, movements of extremities, incontinence, and client status immediately following the seizure.	Accurate and precise recording may assist in the diagnosis and treatment of a seizure disorder.

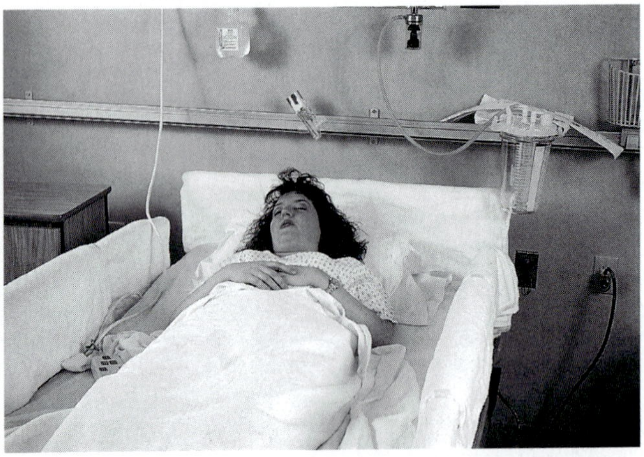

Step 9 Padded side rails and headboard.

FOLLOW-UP ACTIVITIES

1. Following the seizure, clients are often confused and sleepy and need to be protected. A quiet, nonstimulating environment should be provided.
2. Work with the client and family to identify precipitating factors.
3. Referral to a support group or the Epilepsy Foundation may be indicated.

• • • • •

Special Considerations

- Clients should never be restrained during a seizure as musculoskeletal injury may result.

Teaching Considerations

- Clients should be thoroughly familiar with prescribed medications. Medication should never be stopped suddenly as this may precipitate seizures.
- Alcohol should be avoided as it may be incompatible with anticonvulsive medications. It may intensify central nervous system depression.
- Proper oral hygiene and frequent dental care are necessary when a client takes phenytoin (Dilantin) long-term, as gingival hyperplasia is a side effect (Skidmore-Roth, 1996).
- Client should wear a Medic-Alert bracelet or an identification card noting the presence of a seizure disorder and listing the medications taken.
- Hypoglycemia, fatigue, stress, and illness have the potential to initiate seizure activity (Beare and Myers, 1994). Therefore clients should eat a balanced diet at regular intervals, get enough sleep, and consult their doctor promptly when ill.
- A seizure condition usually imposes driving limitations. It is recommended that a waiting period of 1 seizure-free year elapse before a client attempts to drive or operate dangerous equipment (Phipps et al., 1995).

Gerontologic Considerations

- Older adults may have many various symptoms that can hide the recognition of a seizure disorder. Confusion lasting several days, receptive and expressive language problems, and unusual behaviors may be the result of a seizure (Lannon, 1995).
- Older adults tend to metabolize anticonvulsants more slowly, therefore drugs may accumulate, resulting in toxicity. Many anticonvulsants have known blood levels for therapeutic ranges so blood levels should be monitored carefully (McKenry and Solerno, 1995).
- If a client has dentures, do not try to remove them during a seizure. If they loosen, tilt head slightly forward and remove after the seizure (Lannon, 1995).

Home Care Considerations

- Family members need to be familiar with the care of a client experiencing a seizure.
- The client's home should be assessed for environmental hazards in light of the seizure condition.
- Until a seizure condition is well controlled (usually for at least 1 year), the client should not take a tub bath or engage in activities such as swimming unless a knowledgeable family member is present.

CRITICAL THINKING EXERCISES

1. Mr. Lopez, 92 years old, lives with a daughter who works outside the home during the day. He has severe osteoarthritis of the spine and hips, which has begun to limit his ambulation. He is also becoming increasingly forgetful. What aspects of his environment need to be assessed? Design specific interventions to ensure his safety. What specific data would indicate that Mr. Lopez cannot stay alone in the house during the day?
2. A nurse is walking down the hospital hallway when a client walks out and says, "Help me. I see a light, and I may start to have a seizure." The client immediately cries and begins to fall to the floor. Outline, in priority order, the steps the nurse should take and give their rationale.
3. A 90-year-old, oriented, cooperative woman had surgery to repair a fractured hip yesterday. After spending one night in the intensive care unit, she returns to the floor and is very restless, confused, and attempting to remove her IV and Foley catheter. What can the nurse do to avoid restraining this client?

REFERENCES

Accident facts, Itasca, Ill., 1994, National Safety Council.

Beare P, Myers J: *Principles and practice of adult health nursing,* ed 2, St Louis, 1994, Mosby.

Brady R, Chester F, Pierce L et al: Geriatric falls: prevention strategies for the staff, *Journal of Gerontological Nursing* 19(9):26, 1993.

Brians LK et al: The development of the RISK tool for fall prevention, *Rehabil Nursing* 16(2):67, 1991.

Capezuti E, Evans I, Strumpf N et al: Physical restraint use and falls in nursing home residents, *Journal of the American Geriatrics Society* 44(6):627, 1996.

Clinical news: falls in the home—the price of prevention, *American Journal of Nursing* 95(2):10, 1995.

Ebersole P and Hess P: *Toward healthy aging: human needs and nursing process,* ed 4, St Louis, 1994, Mosby.

Ellis C: Nursing assessment and intervention for the patient experiencing seizures: a structured approach, *Clinical Nursing Practice in Epilepsy,* 1(2):4, 1993.

Health Care Financing Administration: *Federal Register* 54(21):1, 1990.

Lambert V: Patient Restraints, *FDA Consumer* 26(8):9, 1992.

Lannon S: Epilepsy in the elderly, *Clinical Nursing Practice in Epilepsy,* 2(2):5, 1995.

Lueckenotte AG: *Gerontologic nursing,* St Louis, 1996, Mosby.

McKenry L, Solerno E: *Mosby's pharmacology in nursing,* ed 19, St Louis, 1995, Mosby.

Patterson JE, Strumpf NE, Evans LK: Nursing consultation to reduce restraints in a nursing home, *Clinical Nurse Specialist* 9(4):231, 1995.

Phipps W et al: *Medical-surgical nursing: concepts and clinical practice,* ed 5, St Louis, 1995, Mosby.

Seizure recognition and observation: a guide for allied health professionals, ed 2, Landover, Md, 1992, Epilepsy Foundation of America.

Shantz D, Spitz M: What you need to know about seizures, *Nursing 93,* 23(11):34, 1993.

Skidmore-Roth L: *Mosby's drug guide for nurses,* St Louis, 1996, Mosby.

Tideiksaar R: Home safe home: practical tips for fall-proofing, *Geriatric Nursing* 11(6):280, 1989.

Weick M: Physical restraints: an FDA update, *American Journal of Nursing* 92(11):74, 1992.

Wong DL: *Whaley & Wong's nursing care of infants and children,* ed 5, St Louis, 1995, Mosby.

ADDITIONAL READING

Corr K, Corr D: Taking the gloves off, *Nursing 94* 24(9):70, 1994.

Elkin M, Perry AG, and Potter PA: *Nursing interventions and clinical skills,* St Louis, 1996, Mosby.

Leger-Krall S: When restraints become abusive, *Nursing 94* 24(3):55, 1994.

Magee R et al: Use of restraints in extended care and nursing homes, *Journal of Gerontological Nursing* 19(4):31, 1993.

Phillips C, Hawes C, Fries B: Reducing the use of physical restraints in nursing homes: will it increase costs? *American Journal of Public Health* 83(3):342, 1993.

Sandler RL: Restraining devices, *American Journal of Nursing* 95(7):34, 1995.

Stolley J: Freeing your patients from restraints, *American Journal of Nursing* 95(2):27, 1995.

Watzke J, Wister A: Staff attitudes: monitoring technology in long-term care, *Journal of Gerontological Nursing* 19(11):23, 1993.

Williams C, Burger S, Murphy K: Restraint of patients, *The Brown University Long-Term Care Quality Letter* 6(3):1, 1994.

Ziemba S: Seizures, *American Journal of Nursing* 95(2):32, 1995.

CHAPTER 5

Comfort

OBJECTIVES

Mastery of content in this chapter will enable the nurse to:

- Define key terms.
- Identify noninvasive, nonpharmacological pain relief measures.
- Identify skills appropriate for relieving a client's specific pain complaint.
- Assess a client's level of comfort.
- Plan care based on client's history and physical assessment.
- Assist client in positioning and splinting to achieve pain relief.
- Discuss mechanisms by which nonpharmacological measures relieve pain.
- Guide client through a painful procedure using anticipatory guidance.
- Assist a client through progressive relaxation.
- Perform a therapeutic massage.
- Assist client in relieving pain through the use of guided imagery and distraction.
- Deliver medication through a patient-controlled analgesia (PCA) device.
- Teach client to use a PCA device.
- Monitor and manage the client receiving epidural analgesia.
- Evaluate the effectiveness of pain management techniques.

SKILLS

KEY TERMS

Acute pain
Anticipatory guidance
Backrub
Chronic pain
Coping
Cutaneous
Distraction
Effleurage
Epidural analgesia
Friction
Guided imagery
Invasive
Massage
Noninvasive
Nonpharmacological aids
Noxious
Pain
Pain intensity
Pain threshold
Pain tolerance
Patient-controlled analgesia (PCA)
Perception
Pétrissage
Pharmacological agents
Relaxation
Sensory discrimination
Splinting
Therapeutic
Transcutaneous electrical nerve stimulation (TENS)

Pain is a complex phenomenon that cannot be defined in a purely physiological sense. The perception of pain is generally accepted to mean a sensation of unpleasantness having three components. The **sensory-discriminative** component is the recognition of a painful **(noxious)** sensation. This component involves the individual's perception of pain. The *affective-motivational* component involves the individual's behavioral and emotional responses to the pain experience. The *cognitive* component involves memory of past pain experiences, learned behaviors and responses, and the meaning of the pain to the individual. A helpful working definition of **pain** is the one proposed by the International Association for the Study of Pain in 1979: "An unpleasant sensory and emotional experience associated with actual or potential tissue damage, or described in terms of such damage" (National Institute of Nursing Research, 1994).

The nurse may use several approaches to manage pain. Because the pain an individual experiences is personal, pain management requires an individualized approach. One approach uses pharmacological agents. Timely administration is crucial to ensure that the client gains optimal relief. In some circumstances, administration of analgesic medication at regular intervals around the clock rather than on an "as-needed" basis is preferable. This pain "prevention" approach is useful in managing pain before it becomes severe (e.g., during the early postoperative period) and can facilitate an earlier recovery (Acute Pain Management Guideline Panel, 1992; Jacox et al., 1992). Although care givers often fear that frequent administration of pain medications will result in the client's psychological and physiological dependence on the medication, such dependence is rare (McCaffery and Ferrell, 1992a). Other approaches use noninvasive techniques that provide a low-risk alternative to the client with pain, an opportunity for the client to assume an active role in achieving a higher level of comfort, and, in some instances, freedom from pain. No single therapy can provide relief for all clients all the time. Therefore the Consensus Development Panel of the National Institutes of Health (Jacox et al., 1992) recommends an integrated approach that considers both pharmacological and nonpharmacological therapies in managing pain.

Promoting comfort with noninvasive, nonpharmacological techniques, as with pharmacological agents, requires careful attention to assessment and planning. Assessment of pain needs to be based on a client's age; level of cognition; personality; culture and ethnicity; coping style; emotional, physical, and spiritual needs; state of health; and past pain experiences. The effectiveness of any therapy will be minimal if clients do not receive what they perceive as helpful. It is important for clients to be active

Table 5-1 Misconceptions About Assessment of Clients Who Indicate That They Have Pain

Misconception	Correction
1. The health team is the authority about the existence and nature of the client's pain sensation.	The person with pain is the only authority about the existence and nature of that pain, since the sensation of pain can be felt only by the person who has it.
2. Our personal values and intuition about the trustworthiness of others is a valuable tool in identifying whether a person is lying about pain.	Personal values and intuition do not constitute a professional approach to the client with pain. The client's credibility is not on trial.
3. Pain is largely an emotional or psychological problem, especially in the client who is highly anxious or depressed.	Having an emotional reaction to pain does not mean that pain is caused by an emotional problem. If anxiety or depression is alleviated, the intensity of pain will not necessarily be any less.
4. Lying about the existence of pain, malingering, is common.	Very few people who say they have pain are lying about it. Outright fabrication of pain is considered rare.
5. Clients who obtain benefits or preferential treatment because of pain are receiving secondary gain and do not hurt as much as they say or may not hurt at all.	Clients who use pain to advantage are not the same as malingerers and may still hurt as much as they say they do. Also, secondary gain may be an inaccurate diagnosis.
6. All real pain has an identifiable physical cause.	All pain is real, regardless of its cause. Almost all pain has both physical and mental components. Pure psychogenic pain is rare.
7. Visible signs, either physiological or behavioral, accompany pain and can be used to verify its existence and severity.	Even with severe pain, periods of physiological and behavioral adaptation occur, leading to periods of minimal or absence of pain. Lack of pain expression does not necessarily mean lack of pain. How must the clients act for us to believe they have pain?
8. Comparable physical stimuli produce comparable pain in different people. The severity and duration of pain can be predicted accurately for everyone on the basis of the stimuli for pain.	Comparable stimuli in different people do *not* produce the same intensities of pain. Comparable stimuli in different people will produce different intensities of pain that last different periods. No direct and invariant relationship exists between any stimulus and the perception of pain.
9. People with pain should be taught to have a high tolerance for pain. The more prolonged the pain or the more experience people have with pain, the better is their tolerance for pain.	Pain tolerance is the individual's unique response, varying between clients and varying in the same client from one situation to another. People with prolonged pain tend to have an increasingly low pain tolerance. Respect for the client's pain tolerance is crucial for adequate pain control.

Modified from McCaffery M, Beebe A: *Pain: clinical manual for nursing practice.* St Louis, 1989, Mosby, p 17.

participants in any attempt to alleviate discomfort, because they are the best authority about their pain (Jacox et al., 1994; McCaffery, 1992a).

The concept of clients as authoritative participants makes pain control an ethical and legal dilemma. Pain can dehumanize, destroy autonomy, and create a sense of hopelessness and powerlessness in the client; yet the treatment of pain is regularly and systematically inadequate (Gray, 1992; McCaffery and Ferrell, 1992a; Vallerand, 1995). The goals of health care—prolonging life and alleviating suffering—often come into conflict when dealing with pain control in the clinical setting. Although pain experience is primarily subjective and qualitative, it is often treated objectively and quantitatively by health care providers who dictate dosage, frequency of administration, and length of treatment (Maxam-Moore, Wilkie, and Woods, 1994; Tittle and McMillan, 1994). Pain caused or allowed as a result of nurses' or physicians' attitudes and practices therefore becomes a matter of ethics. McCaffery and Beebe (1989) have identified common societal misconceptions about pain that health care professionals need to consider when planning client care (Table 5-1). Neglecting to provide adequate pain relief for clients under the care of health care providers is a legal issue (Copp, 1993; Cushing, 1992; Jurf and Nirschl, 1993).

Managing a client's pain can be challenging and rewarding if the nurse is knowledgeable about the nature of pain and how it might best be treated. Freedom from

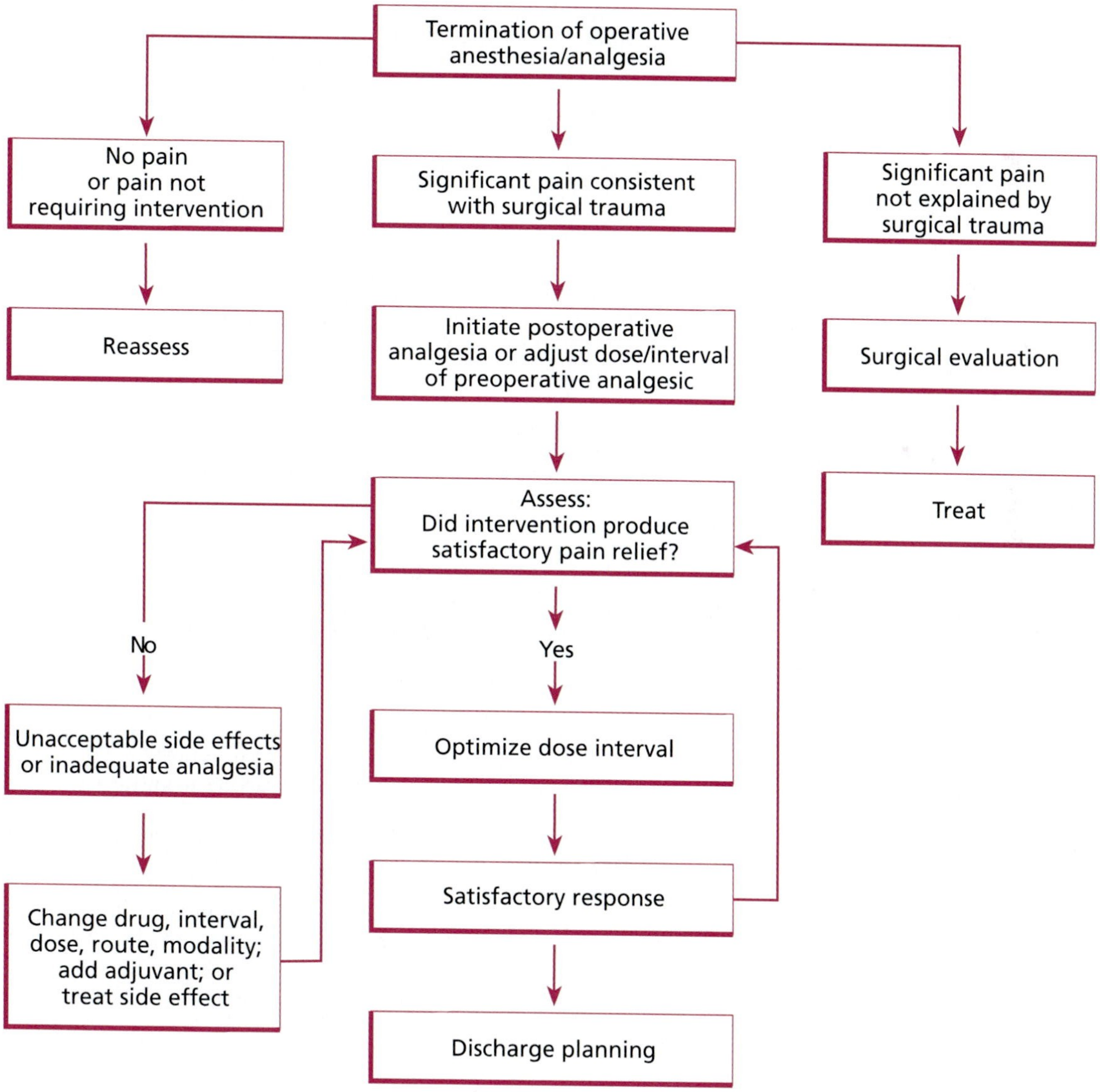

Fig. 5-1 Pain treatment flowchart: postoperative phase. (From Acute Pain Management Guideline Panel: Acute Pain Management: Operative or Medical Procedures and Trauma: Clinical Practice Guidelines, AHCPR Pub No 92-0032, Rockville, Md, 1992, Agency for Health Care Policy and Research, Public Health Service, US Department of Health and Human Services.)

Table 5-2 Pharmacological and Nonpharmacological Interventions

Interventions		Comments
Pharmacological		
Nonsteroidal anti-inflammatory drugs (NSAIDs)	Oral (alone)	Effective for mild to moderate pain. Begin preoperatively. Relatively contraindicated in clients with renal disease and risk of or actual coagulopathy. May mask fever.
	Oral (adjunct to opioid)	Potentiating effect resulting in opioid sparing. Begin preoperatively. Cautions as above for oral alone.
	Parenteral (ketorolac)	Effective for moderate to severe pain. Expensive. Useful when opioids contraindicated, especially to avoid respiratory depression and sedation.
Opioids	Oral	As effective as parenteral in appropriate doses. Use as soon as oral medication is tolerated. Route of choice.
	Intramuscular	Has been standard parenteral route, but injections are painful and absorption unreliable. Avoid this route when possible.
	Subcutaneous	Preferable to intramuscular when low-volume continuous infusion is needed and intravenous access is difficult to maintain. Injections painful and absorption unreliable. Avoid this route for long-term, repetitive dosing.
	Intravenous	Parenteral route of choice after major surgery. Suitable for titrated bolus or continuous administration (including PCA), but requires monitoring. Significant risk of respiratory depression with inappropriate dosing.
	Patient-controlled analgesia (PCA) (systemic)	Intravenous or subcutaneous routes recommended. Good steady level of analgesia. Popular with clients but requires special infusion pumps and staff education. See cautions about opioids.
	Epidural and intrathecal	When suitable, provides good analgesia. Significant risk of respiratory depression, sometimes delayed in onset. Requires careful monitoring. Use of infusion pumps requires additional equipment and staff education. Expensive if infusion pumps are employed.
Local anesthetics	Epidural and intrathecal	Limited indications. Effective regional analgesia. Opioid sparing. Addition of opioid to local anesthetic may improve analgesia. Risks of hypotension, weakness, numbness. Requires careful monitoring. Use of infusion pump requires additional equipment and staff education.
	Peripheral nerve block	Limited indications and duration of action. Effective regional analgesia. Opioid sparing.
Nonpharmacological		
Simple relaxation (begin preoperatively)	Jaw relaxation Progressive muscle relaxation Simple imagery	Effective in reducing mild to moderate pain and as adjunct to analgesic drugs for severe pain. Use when client expresses interest in relaxation. Requires 3 to 5 minutes of staff time for instruction.
	Music	Both client-preferred and "easy listening" music are effective in reducing mild to moderate pain.
Complex relaxation (begin preoperatively)	Biofeedback	Effective in reducing mild to moderate pain and operative site muscle tension. Requires skilled personnel and special equipment.
	Imagery	Effective for reduction of mild to moderate pain. Requires skilled personnel.
Education/instruction (begin preoperatively)		Effective for reduction of pain. Should include sensory and procedural information and instruction aimed at reducing activity-related pain. Requires 5 to 15 minutes of staff time.
Transcutaneous electrical nerve stimulation (TENS)		Effective in reducing pain and improving physical function. Requires skilled personnel and special equipment. May be useful as adjunct to drug therapy.

Acute Pain Management Guideline Panel. Acute Pain Management: Operative or Medical Procedures and Trauma: Clinical Practice Guidelines, AHCPR Pub No 92-0032, Rockville, MD, Agency for Health Care Policy and Research, Public Health Service, US Dept of Health and Human Services, Feb, 1992.

pain is not always a realistic goal. In these clients pain management may have to be directed toward pain control rather than complete pain relief. Although pain management has been extensively studied, research results have not been effectively implemented in clinical practice (Maxam-Moore, Wilkie, and Woods, 1994; Puntillo, 1994; Tittle and McMillan, 1994). According to McCaffery (1992b), a primary problem is that nurses have not been taught how to deal with the fact that pain is completely subjective; that is, they may not use a standardized scientific approach when assessing pain and its intensity. In 1992 the Agency for Health Care Policy and Research (AHCPR) issued a guideline for effective pain management for clients with acute pain after surgery, medical procedures, or trauma (Acute Pain Management Guideline Panel, 1992). This guideline is designed to help care givers, clients, and clients' families understand the assessment and treatment of postoperative and other acute pain in both adults and children. The guideline has four major goals:

1. Reduce the incidence and severity of clients' postoperative or posttraumatic pain.
2. Educate clients about the need to communicate unrelieved pain so that they can receive prompt evaluation and effective treatment.
3. Enhance client comfort and satisfaction.
4. Contribute to fewer postoperative complications and shorter stays after surgical procedures.

A flowchart guides care givers in making decisions about assessing and controlling client pain throughout the postoperative or postprocedure recovery period (Fig. 5-1). The AHCPR guidelines advocate a range and combination of approaches to pain management to ensure that decisions about assessment and analgesic use reflect current knowledge and provide the best possible care for the client (Table 5-2). In addition to a thorough assessment, research indicates that use of a standardized flow sheet to document assessment of pain intensity and pharmacological management may improve pain management (Voight, Pace, and Pouliot, 1995). Health care professionals still have much to learn about the unique experience pain holds for each client.

The first two skills in this chapter focus on noninvasive, nonpharmacological comfort measures. Administration of medications through patient-controlled analgesia and an epidural catheter are the focus of the last two skills. These skills may be used alone or in combination, depending on a client's needs. Many of the measures discussed can be taught to the client and family for use in the home.

GUIDELINES

1. Know the medical history and type of therapy and medications the client is receiving. Specific illnesses or procedures have predictable effects on comfort.
2. Determine the client's perception of the pain experience. A thorough assessment of factors contributing to the client's pain will enable the nurse to select appropriate therapies. In addition, assess the effects of pain on self-care abilities and sleep.
3. Demonstrate respect for the client's evaluation of the quality and quantity of pain experienced and the response to methods of pain management.
4. Control environmental factors that may influence the client's response to discomfort, such as too much stimuli or fatigue, as well as the effectiveness of comfort measures used.
5. Decide the frequency for assessing a client's comfort. It is the nurse's responsibility to determine the client's response to comfort measures and expression of discomfort. The collection of data leading to establishment of pain trends and a comparison of changes in pain patterns are useful in making therapeutic decisions.
6. Verify and communicate significant changes in comfort level. There is no firm guide for the best time to report changes in comfort. However, the nurse who knows the client well and listens to a client's response to the pain management interventions can identify when comfort measures are no longer effective or no longer necessary, as well as when the type and quality of pain have changed.

SKILL 5-1 Removing Painful Stimuli

After assessment of an individual's expression of pain, removal of the painful stimulus may be the approach chosen for management. Although this is a seemingly simple, even obvious, solution, removal of a painful stimulus is often overlooked in the search for a more complicated reason for the pain. Common sources of discomfort are damp or wet dressings, constrictive dressings, wrinkled bed linens, environmental irritants such as the noise of a television, and activity in excess of the individual's tolerance. Maintaining an uncomfortable position for a prolonged period is another common source of discomfort, particularly for dependent clients.

If a client is fatigued or anxious, even mild irritations can become significant sources of pain. The nurse should always remain observant during any contact with the client for potential sources of painful stimuli. Removal of painful stimuli, careful repositioning, and teaching splinting and breathing techniques during coughing or movement can afford clients considerable relief for extended periods of time (Guyton-Simmons and Ehrmin, 1994). The client can often suggest the most comfortable position to assume. The nurse must judge whether any position is contraindicated on the basis of the client's health status.

EQUIPMENT

- Pillows
- Dressings

DELEGATION CONSIDERATIONS

The nurse, in collaboration with the client, is responsible for the assessment, planning, initial implementation, and evaluation of needed comfort measures. The following information is necessary when delegating skills to unlicensed assistive personnel or family members:

- Assess and report changes in client's condition.
- Identify and eliminate environmental conditions that might enhance pain.
- Plan nursing care to provide maximum rest periods.
- Turning, positioning, and reducing environmental stimuli are important for comfort and pain control.

BEHAVIORAL INDICATORS OF EFFECTS OF PAIN

Vocalizations
Moaning
Crying
Screaming
Gasping

Facial Expressions
Grimace
Clenched teeth
Open, alert eyes
Biting the lips
Tightened jaw

Body Movement
Restlessness
Immobilization
Muscle tension
Rhythmic or rubbing motions
Protective movement of body parts

Social Interaction
Avoidance of conversation
Focus only on activities for pain relief
Avoidance of social contacts
Reduced attention span

STEPS	RATIONALE
ASSESSMENT	
1. Assess client's predisposition to alterations in comfort.	Certain conditions place clients at risk for alterations in comfort (e.g., postoperative clients, those with open wounds or burns, cancer clients, those undergoing invasive procedures or dental procedures, anxious clients, those suffering headache or chronic low back pain, clients in labor).
2. Assess physical and emotional signs and symptoms of acute pain of low to moderate intensity: a. Increased heart rate b. Increased respirations c. Increased blood pressure d. Pallor e. Increased blood glucose level f. Diaphoresis g. Increased muscle tension h. Dilated pupils i. Decreased GI motility j. Anxiety	Physiological responses to pain may reveal the existence and nature of pain or need for change in position or environment. Signs of sympathetic nervous system stimulation (which elicits "fight or flight" response) are often, but not universally, observed in clients experiencing acute pain of mild to moderate intensity or superficial pain (Acute Pain Management Guideline Panel, 1992; McCaffery and Ferrell, 1992b).
3. Assess physical and emotional signs and symptoms of severe or deep **acute pain:** a. Pallor b. Muscle tension c. Decreased heart rate	Signs and symptoms typically occur with pain originating from involvement of visceral organs and result from stimulation of the parasympathetic nervous system.

STEPS | **RATIONALE**

d. Decreased blood pressure
e. Rapid, irregular respirations
f. Nausea and vomiting
g. Weakness
h. Exhaustion
i. Powerlessness
j. Stoicism
k. Dilated pupils

4. Assess physical and emotional signs and symptoms of **chronic pain:**
a. Fatigue
b. Insomnia
c. Anorexia
d. Impaired mobility
e. Distorted posturing
f. Weight loss
g. Depression
h. Hopelessness
i. Anger

Clients with chronic pain often do not show overt signs and symptoms of acute pain. Signs and symptoms reflect physiological adaptation and decreased sympathetic nervous system response. Psychological distress and personality disorders are also often seen in clients with chronic pain (Basler, 1993; Jones, 1993).

CRITICAL DECISION POINT **Sustained physiological responses could cause serious harm. Most people reach a level of adaptation in which physical signs return to normal. Therefore a client will not always exhibit physical signs throughout duration of pain.**

5. Assess behavioral responses to discomfort (see box on p. 94).

Nonverbal behavior is useful in evaluating pain experienced by clients incapable of or having difficulty with communicating verbally (Duchene, 1996; Guyton-Simmons and Ehrmin, 1994). Emotional reaction to pain is variable and influences the intensity, latency, and duration of pain (Bachiocco, Morselli, and Carli, 1993; Basler, 1993; Jurf and Nirschl, 1993).

6. Assess characteristics of pain:
a. Onset and duration
b. Location

Allows nurse to identify possible causative factors from client's description of pain. Chronic pain is described in more general terms and may or may not have well-defined onset (Wilkie and Boss, 1996).

c. Intensity: ask client to rate pain on a scale of 0 to 10 (0, no pain; 10, worst pain)

Pain is a subjective experience; therefore client's evaluation should be accepted. The pain rating scale is regarded as the most reliable indicator of pain intensity (see illustration) (Cushing, 1992; McCaffery, 1992b).

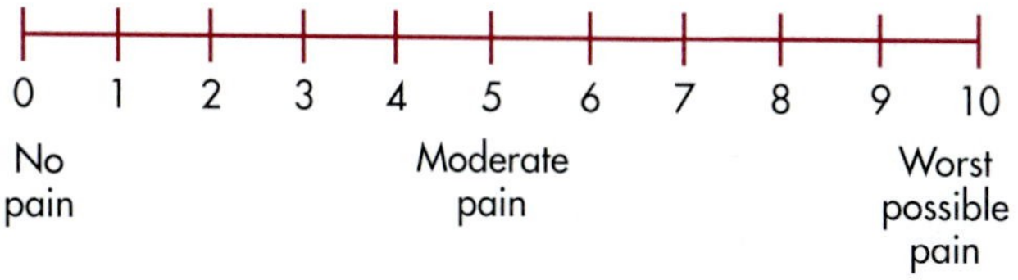

Step 6c Linear analog scale.

d. Quality (e.g., use open-ended questions such as, "Tell me what your pain feels like.")

Assessment is more accurate if client can describe sensation in own words. People describe certain types of pain consistently (e.g., myocardial infarction: vicelike or crushing; surgical incision: sharp or stabbing).

CRITICAL DECISION POINT **If the client cannot describe the pain, offer examples, such as sharp, dull, pricking, burning, stabbing, gnawing, aching, pounding.**

STEPS	RATIONALE
7. Assess environment for factors that exacerbate pain experience.	Environmental stimuli, such as loud noises, bright lights, strong odors, or temperature extremes, can alter client's response to pain.
8. Assess factors that precipitate or aggravate pain and discomfort.	Pain may be precipitated or aggravated by physical activity, diagnostic or therapeutic procedures, or change in posture or position.
9. Inspect area of pain.	Clinical observations clarify information received from client.

CRITICAL DECISION POINT May require temporary removal of dressing followed by reapplication (see Chapter 37).

10. Ask what was used for pain relief in the past or what client believes will help.	No single approach is right for every client. A combination of interventions is often the most effective approach to pain relief (Acute Pain Management Guideline Panel, 1992; Jurf and Nirschl, 1993; Woodin, 1993).
11. Check physician's orders for position restrictions.	Client's physical condition may prohibit certain positions.

NURSING DIAGNOSIS

Clustering of defining characteristics from the assessment data may reveal the following nursing diagnoses for clients requiring this skill:

- Activity intolerance
- Anxiety
- Ineffective individual coping
- Knowledge deficit regarding factors that precipitate pain
- Knowledge deficit regarding pain management techniques
- Pain

Related factors are individualized based on a client's condition or needs.

PLANNING

1. **Expected outcomes** following completion of procedure:	
➤ Client verbalizes full or partial relief from pain.	Removing painful stimulus should result in near immediate relief.
➤ Nonverbal behaviors reflect comfort is attained.	Pain may be controlled but not absent, depending on its cause.
2. Prepare environment:	
a. Temperature suited to client	Temperature extremes can alter client's response to pain.
b. Lighting	Bright or very dim lighting can aggravate pain sensation.
c. Sound	Loud or irritating sounds can aggravate pain.
d. Activity	Prevent unnecessary interruptions; allow for rest periods. Fatigue reduces tolerance for pain.
3. Close room door or curtain.	Provides privacy and reduces stimuli that may increase pain.
4. Explain to client that splinting with pillows and positioning can reduce pain.	Promotes client cooperation.
5. Explain steps to be taken to minimize pain stimuli.	Reduces anxiety.

IMPLEMENTATION

1. Wash hands. Apply gloves if exposure to body fluids or blood is likely.	Reduces spread of microorganisms.
2. Remove painful stimulus:	
a. Assist client to position that fully exposes area of discomfort.	Improves access to area and minimizes client's need to move.

STEPS	RATIONALE
b. Move bed linen aside to expose only area of discomfort.	Maintains client's privacy.
c. Remove wet dressing, if applicable.	Minimizes irritation to wound and surrounding tissues.
d. Smooth wrinkles in bed linens.	Reduces pressure and irritation to skin.
e. Loosen any constrictive bandage or device (e.g., blood pressure cuff, Ace bandages, upper band of elastic hose, IV dressings, identification bands).	Bandage or device encircling extremity may restrict circulation.
➤ ***CRITICAL DECISION POINT*** **In case of casts or pressure bandages, physician's order will be needed to loosen or adjust.**	
f. Remove underlying tubes, wires, or equipment.	Objects apply pressure directly on dependent skin surfaces.
3. Apply splinting:	Splinting immobilizes painful area.
a. Explain purpose of splinting to client.	
b. Assist client to place hands firmly over area of discomfort (see illustration).	

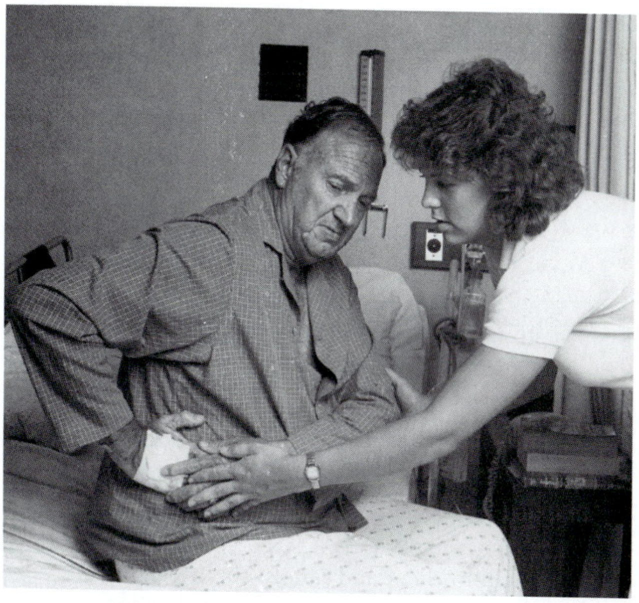

Step 3b Splinting.

STEPS	RATIONALE
c. Assist client to splint during coughing, deep breathing, and turning.	Splinting decreases movement and subsequent pain during activity.
4. Assist client to attain comfortable position within normal body alignment.	Turning and repositioning reduce stimulation of pain and pressure receptors.
a. Use pillows to support body position.	
b. Position client to prevent pressure on bony prominences.	
5. Remove and dispose of gloves. Wash hands.	Reduces transmission of microorganisms.

EVALUATION

STEPS	RATIONALE
1. Evaluate client's comfort level, using original assessment criteria.	Determines client's response to stimulus removal and positioning.
2. Unexpected outcomes that may occur include:	
➤ Client verbalizes continued discomfort or describes worsening of pain.	Pain may have changed or may have been incompletely assessed.
➤ Client continues to display nonverbal behaviors reflecting pain.	Underlying medical condition may have changed. Positioning over painful site can aggravate discomfort.

STEPS | **RATIONALE**

Recording and Reporting

1. Report change in quality or increased intensity of pain, presence of bright red blood saturating dressing, constriction of casted extremity, or change in vital signs to nurse in charge or to physician.

   If findings indicate worsening of client's condition, physician must be notified so that appropriate medical treatment can be initiated.

2. Record findings of ongoing assessment, interventions completed (including notification of physician, if done), and client's response to interventions.

   Documents client's response and provides improved continuity of care for future pain experiences (Kohr, 1995).

Follow-up Activities

1. Reassess client's pain complaint.
2. Review instructions for splinting and positioning with client and family for understanding and ability to perform.
3. Implement additional pain-relief measures if pain continues or worsens (e.g., relaxation, massage, imagery [see Skill 5-2], pharmacological support).

• • • • •

Special Considerations

- Behavioral responses to pain may not be present in cases of chronic pain.
- A verbal descriptive scale consists of a line with three- to five-word descriptions or numbers equally spaced along the line. The descriptions are ranked from "No pain" to "Most severe pain." A visual analog scale does not have labeled subdivisions. It represents a continuum of intensity along a straight line.

Teaching Considerations

- Review client's technique when using coughing and deep-breathing exercises.
- Explain relationship of emotions to pain (e.g., fear and anxiety cause vasoconstriction, which may intensify pain).
- Explain to client and family about behavioral changes that can be caused by medication.

Pediatric Considerations

- Children can rate their level of pain on the Oucher Pain Scale (Fig. 5-2) and the Wong-Baker Faces Scale (Fig. 5-3) for assessing pain in children.

Gerontologic Considerations

- Pain assessment in older adults should also include an evaluation of the effect of pain on the client's quality of life (Lueckenotte, 1996).
- Many older clients tend to have multiple sources of pain.
- Older adults require more time for repositioning.
- Pain is not a natural occurrence of aging or chronic disease. Such a belief can lead to under-reporting of pain.

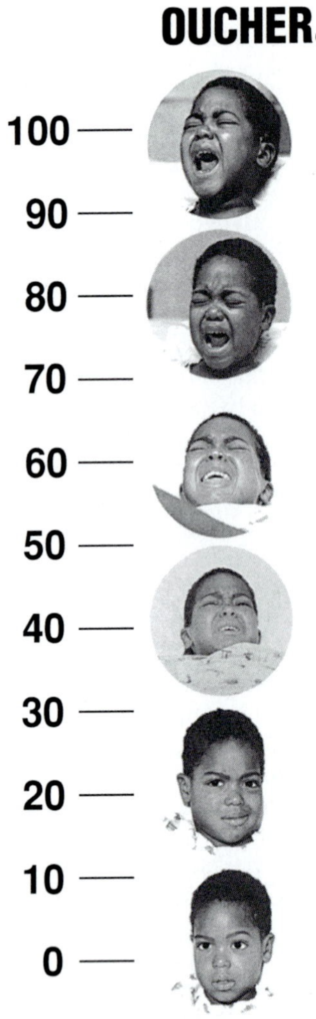

Fig. 5-2 African American version of the Oucher Pain Scale. (© Denyes, Villarruel, 1990. Used with permission.)

Home Care Considerations

- Home living conditions, such as type of bed, stairs, and environmental stimuli, should be considered. Supportive bed and quiet environment will enhance sleep and promote pain management.

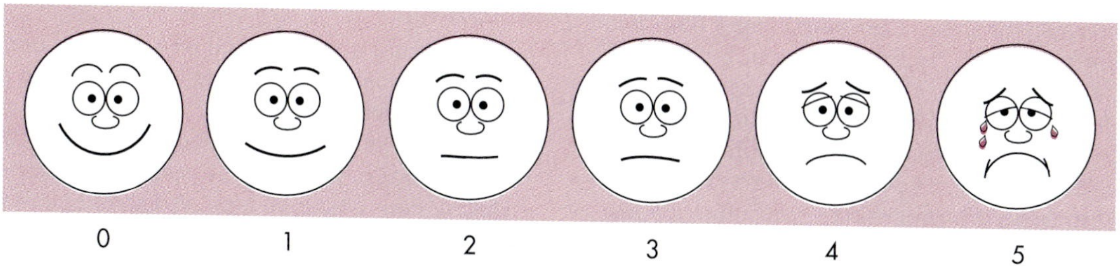

Fig. 5-3 Wong-Baker Faces Scale. (Can be duplicated for clinical practice.) (From Wong D: *Whaley and Wong's Essentials of Pediatric Nursing*, ed 5, St Louis, 1995, Mosby.)

SKILL 5-2 Nonpharmacological Aids to Promote Comfort

These cognitive or behavioral strategies are effective because they impinge on the amount of attention that can be given to painful sensory input (Stanik-Hutt, 1993; Whipple and Glynn, 1992).

ANTICIPATORY GUIDANCE

Clients often must undergo a number of painful diagnostic and therapeutic procedures. The degree of discomfort depends in large part on a client's perceptions of the experience. Because perception is greatly influenced by higher centers in the brain, the pain experience is a product of a person's past pain experiences, values, cultural expectations, and emotions. The nurse has an excellent opportunity to help clients learn to control their anxieties and fears. **Anticipatory guidance** is a cognitive strategy that involves use of descriptive sensory words and phrases the client is familiar with to talk through a painful experience or event (Stephens, 1993; Wilkie and Boss, 1996). The client gains an understanding of what to expect during a procedure. Clients should have the opportunity to ask questions about the procedure and their role during the procedure. The nurse makes the client as comfortable as possible to eliminate potential irritants. The client thus is able to direct full attention to the procedure, with the result of improved pain tolerance.

MASSAGE

Modifying the perception of pain, as well as minimizing the reaction to pain, provides a client considerable pain relief. A gentle **massage** is a form of **cutaneous** stimulation that activates large-diameter sensory nerve fibers in the skin to prevent painful stimuli from reaching the brain's conscious awareness (Jurf and Nirschl, 1993). A proper massage not only blocks perception of pain impulses but also helps relax muscle tension and spasm that otherwise might increase pain (Ferrell-Torry and Glick, 1993). Massage of a body part is often an instinctual response to pain and thus is a basic but highly effective means to control pain. The high state of relaxation often achieved with massage adds to the effects of other pain-relief measures (Ferrell-Torry and Glick, 1993; Meintz, 1995). A massage of the back, shoulders, and lower part of the neck is sometimes referred to as a **backrub.** A nurse should offer a backrub after a bath or before a client prepares for sleep to promote relaxation and comfort, relieve muscle tension, and stimulate circulation. An effective backrub takes 3 to 5 minutes and is an important intervention for decreasing pain and improving sense of well-being.

RELAXATION

Relaxation is a cognitive strategy that provides mental and physical pain relief or reduces pain to an acceptable level. By teaching clients the use of progressive relaxation techniques, the nurse offers the client a sense of self-control when pain occurs. Progressive relaxation may be used independently or with other pain-relief measures. This technique eases muscle tension and reduces anxiety associated with pain (Jurf and Nirschl, 1993). Relaxation techniques may require a physician's order if the stability of a client's condition is in question. The nurse should be available to assist the client in peforming relaxation techniques, as well as in timing procedures (such as dressing changes) so that the technique can be most beneficial. The client's full participation and cooperation are necessary for progressive relaxation to be effective. The techniques are particularly effective for chronic pain, labor pain, and relief of procedure-related pain.

GUIDED IMAGERY

Guided imagery is a creative sensory experience that can effectively reduce pain perception and minimize reaction to pain. It draws on internal experience of memories, dreams, fantasies, and visions; explores the inner world of experience; protects privacy of the client; and fosters the imagination. The goal of imagery is to have the client use one or several of the senses to create an image of the desired result. This image creates a positive psychophysiological response (Dossey, 1992; Stephens, 1993). Pain relief associated with imagery may be related to the release of endorphins (Tiernan, 1994). Thus focus of the imagination helps clients change their perceptions about their disease, treatment, and healing ability, which also helps relieve pain, tension, or stress. Choosing images that clients find pleasant requires a careful assessment by the nurse. Otherwise, the nurse may mistakenly describe images of objects or things that the client fears or dislikes. For example, a scene of rolling waves at the seashore may be restful to one client but desolate or frightening to another. Imagery may be used with progressive relaxation, massage, or as a distraction.

DISTRACTION

Distraction is a technique that diverts an individual's attention away from the pain sensation. By introducing meaningful stimuli, the nurse helps the client refocus attention. The client's pain tolerance increases as distraction lowers awareness of pain (Wilkie and Boss, 1996). Typically, distraction is most effective for mild to moderate pain, but with intense concentration even acute pain can be relieved. In most cases the pain relief lasts only as long as the distraction; when the distraction is removed, the client may have a heightened awareness of pain. Examples of distraction include music, visitors, television, breathing exercises, or active listening (Jurf and Nirschl, 1993).

EQUIPMENT

- **Anticipatory guidance: prepare supplies and equipment for specific diagnostic or therapeutic procedure to be performed**
- **Massage: lotion or oil, folded sheet, bath towel**
- **Relaxation: relaxation tape and tape player**
- **Distraction: based on type of distraction (e.g., tape player, assorted music tapes, puzzles, video games, other games)**

DELEGATION CONSIDERATIONS

The nurse, in collaboration with the client, is responsible for the assessment, planning, initial implementation, and evaluation of needed comfort measures. The following information is necessary when delegating skills to unlicensed assistive personnel or family members:

- Communicate basic principles of nonpharmacological skills such as distraction, relaxation, massage, and guided imagery.
- Encourage and reinforce the use of individualized nonpharmacological interventions for prevention and relief of pain.
- Teach family members and nursing staff how to perform appropriate interventions individualized for the client.

STEPS	RATIONALE
ASSESSMENT	
1. Have client identify level of pain or comfort.	Certain conditions place clients at risk for alterations in comfort.
2. Assess physiological and emotional responses to pain or discomfort (see Skill 5-1, Assessment step 2).	Physiological responses of individuals vary with severity and duration of pain. Responses serve as means to evaluate effectiveness of pain-relief measures. Overt signs and symptoms may not be present with chronic pain. Physical signs and symptoms may indicate change in comfort level.
3. Assess intensity and quality of pain:	
a. Intensity: ask client to rate pain on scale of 0 to 10 (0, no pain; 10, worst pain).	Pain is a subjective experience. Numerical pain rating scale allows client freedom to identify pain perception and is therefore considered the most reliable indicator of pain intensity (McCaffery, 1992b).
b. Quality: use open-ended questions, such as, "Tell me what your pain feels like." Seek clarification if description is unclear or uncertain (e.g., sharp versus dull; aching or burning versus stabbing).	Such information serves as baseline to determine change in character of pain.
4. Assess factors related to pain (e.g., environment, culture, previous pain experience, activities, knowledge of and experience with procedures to be done).	These factors can affect response to pain. Nurse can control these factors to improve effects of pain-relief therapies.

STEPS	RATIONALE
5. Assess factors that preceded or aggravated pain experience (e.g., diet, exercise, emotional stress). Ask client to describe events leading to pain. Precipitating factors to consider include timing of postoperative analgesics, fatigue, inadequate environmental stimuli, nighttime, immobilization, positioning, isolation, or end of visiting hours (absence of support persons).	Identification of factors accompanying pain response directs nurse to schedule measures to prevent pain and control factors adding to client's discomfort.
6. Examine site of client's pain or discomfort. Include inspection (discoloration, swelling, drainage), palpation (change in temperature, area of altered sensation, painful area, areas that trigger pain, areas that reduce pain), and range of motion of involved joints (if applicable).	Clinical observations clarify information from client. Site of discomfort may direct nurse to specific types of pain-relief measures.
➤ ***CRITICAL DECISION POINT*** **May require temporary removal of dressing.**	
7. Identify pain management techniques client may be using or has used in past.	Use of familiar techniques will improve cooperation. Client may be unwilling to try therapy that previously failed.
8. Assess client's willingness to participate in noninvasive, nonpharmacological pain-relief measures.	Client has right to decide about own care. Participation increases effectiveness. If client is reluctant to try activity, accept this uncertainty and provide information about suggested therapy so that client can make decision.
➤ ***CRITICAL DECISION POINT*** **It may be helpful the first time to administer an analgesic so that client can gain a level of comfort needed to practice noninvasive approaches.**	
9. Assess activities client participates in at home that may serve as distraction (e.g., jigsaw puzzles, crocheting or knitting, board games, music, imagery, relaxation tapes).	Doing these activities in health care setting increases likelihood that client will participate.
10. Assess client's language level and identify descriptive terms that will be used when employing relaxation, guided imagery, anticipatory guidance.	Provides clarification of information.

NURSING DIAGNOSIS

Clustering of defining characteristics from the assessment data may reveal the following nursing diagnoses for clients requiring these skills:

- Activity intolerance
- Anxiety
- Ineffective individual coping
- Knowledge deficit regarding nonpharmacological pain-relief measures
- Pain
- Powerlessness

Related factors are individualized based on a client's condition or needs.

PLANNING

1. Expected outcomes following completion of procedure:	
➤ Client is relaxed and comfortable after technique or diagnostic procedure as evidenced by: • Slow, deep respirations • Calm facial expressions • Calm tone of voice • Relaxed muscles • Relaxed posture	Effective guidance before and during procedure assists client to relax and experience less discomfort. Physiological response to relaxation procedures and massage is deep relaxation. Distraction promotes comfort by diverting attention from one situation to another.

STEPS	RATIONALE
➤ Client verbalizes pain relief.	Although objective physiological indicators to determine pain intensity or relief exist, they are not as reliable as client's subjective expression (Acute Pain Management Guideline Panel, 1992).
➤ Client demonstrates and describes pain-relief measures.	Demonstrates understanding.
2. Explain purpose of technique and what will be expected of client during activity. If diagnostic or therapeutic procedure is to be performed, plan to explain procedure in advance.	Proper explanation of activity results in enhanced client cooperation. Client will have time to understand nurse's explanations, avoiding anxiety associated with confusion or misunderstanding.
3. Plan to perform technique before client's rest period.	Use 2-hour intervals for rest between pain-relief activities whenever possible to maximize effects.
4. Assist client to use bathroom before performing technique, if needed.	Techniques may take 20 to 30 minutes. Client comfort enhances relaxation and decreases distraction.
5. Prepare environment by:	
a. Controlling lighting in room	Anticipatory guidance for a procedure: focus bright light on specified area. Relaxation, guided imagery, distraction: use fluorescent lighting if possible. Bright or very dim lighting can aggravate pain perception.
b. Controlling distractions by visitors or staff	Distractions prevent client from attending to pain-reduction or pain-control techniques.
c. Maintaining comfortable room temperature (sheet or light blanket prevents chilling)	Temperature extremes can alter client's response to pain.
6. Close curtains around client's bed or close door.	Maintains client's privacy, helps control lighting, and reduces anxiety.
7. Assist client to comfortable position for technique chosen, such as semi-Fowler's or Sims' position.	Client comfort enhances relaxation and participation in skills.

IMPLEMENTATION

ANTICIPATORY GUIDANCE

STEPS	RATIONALE
1. Use descriptive terms to explain steps of procedure in detail to client. Respect client's listening limitations.	Knowing what to expect helps client cope with painful or uncomfortable procedures.
2. Explain to client approximate length of time procedure will take (e.g., 10 to 20 minutes). Warn client that delays may occur (e.g., in preparing treatment room, transporting client, waiting for physician).	Knowing how long procedure will take helps eliminate anxiety.
3. Prepare by describing sensations client can anticipate during steps of procedure (e.g., pressure, cold, needle prick).	Nurse cannot assure client there will be no pain. Ability to anticipate sensation minimizes actual discomfort.
4. Verbally guide client through procedure using terms identified previously (e.g., "Physician is going to clean your skin with a cool liquid." "Now you will feel a needle stick." "It will feel like someone is pinching your skin.").	Repetition of explanation of steps during procedure helps orient client to progress.
5. Assist client in returning to comfortable position.	Some procedures require uncomfortable or immobile position; when possible, reposition client for comfort.

MASSAGE

STEPS	RATIONALE
1. Wash hands.	Reduces transmission of microorganisms.
2. Adjust bed to high, comfortable position and lower side rail.	Ensures proper body mechanics and prevents strain on nurse's back muscles.
3. Place client in comfortable position such as prone or side-lying position.	Enhances relaxation and exposes area to be massaged.

STEPS	RATIONALE
CRITICAL DECISION POINT Clients with respiratory difficulties may lie on side with head of bed elevated.	
4. Drape client to expose only area to be massaged.	Maintains client's privacy and warmth.
5. Warm lotion in hands.	Warm lotion is soothing, and warmth helps to produce local muscle relaxation (Meintz, 1995).
CRITICAL DECISION POINT Do not use lotion or oils before massaging head and scalp.	
6. Choose stroke technique based on desired effect:	
a. **Effleurage** (see illustration)	Gliding stroke, used without manipulating deep muscles, smooths and extends muscles, increases nutrient absorption, improves lymphatic and venous circulation (Meintz, 1995).
b. **Pétrissage** (see illustration)	Use on tense muscle groups to "knead" muscles, promote relaxation, and stimulate local circulation.
c. **Friction**	Strong circular strokes bring blood to surface of skin, thereby increasing local circulation and loosening tight muscle groups (Meintz, 1995).

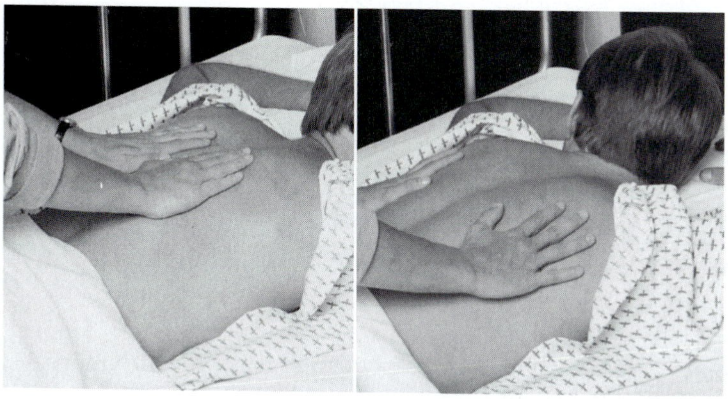

Step 6a Effleurage.

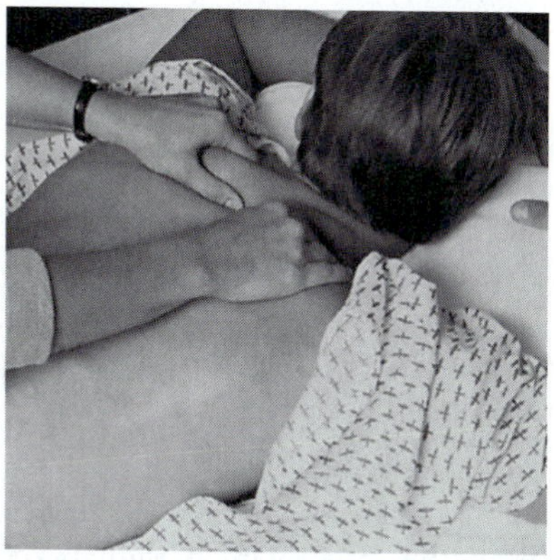

Step 6b Pétrissage.

STEPS	RATIONALE
7. Encourage client to breathe deeply and relax during massage.	
8. Massage head and scalp.	Strong circular strokes (friction) stimulate local circulation and relaxation.
9. Standing behind client, stimulate scalp and temples.	
10. Supporting client's head, rub muscles at base of head.	
11. Massage hands and arms:	Releases tension in hands and arms. Studies indicate that anxious behaviors may be significantly reduced with hand massage (Snyder and Burns, 1995).
a. Support hand and apply friction to palm using both thumbs.	Encourages relaxation; enhances circulation and venous return.
b. Support base of finger and work each finger in corkscrewlike motion.	
c. Complete hand massage using effleurage strokes from fingertips to wrist.	
d. Knead muscles of forearm and upper arm between thumb and forefinger.	

STEPS	RATIONALE
12. Massage neck:	
a. Place client in prone position unless contraindicated.	
b. Knead each neck muscle between thumb and forefinger.	Reduces tension that often localizes in neck muscles.
c. Gently stretch neck by placing one hand on top of shoulders and other at base of head and gently move hands away from each other.	Helps relax muscle body.
13. Massage back:	
a. Place client in prone or side-lying position.	Side-lying position is indicated for clients unable to lie prone.
b. Do not allow hands to leave client's skin.	Continuous contact with skin's surface is soothing and stimulates circulation to tissues. Breaking contact with skin can startle client.
c. Apply hands first to sacral area, massage in circular motion (see illustration). Stroke upward from buttocks to shoulders. Massage over scapulas with smooth, firm stroke. Continue in one smooth stroke to upper arms and laterally along sides of back down to iliac crests. Continue massage pattern for 3 minutes.	Gentle firm pressure applied to all muscle groups promotes relaxation.

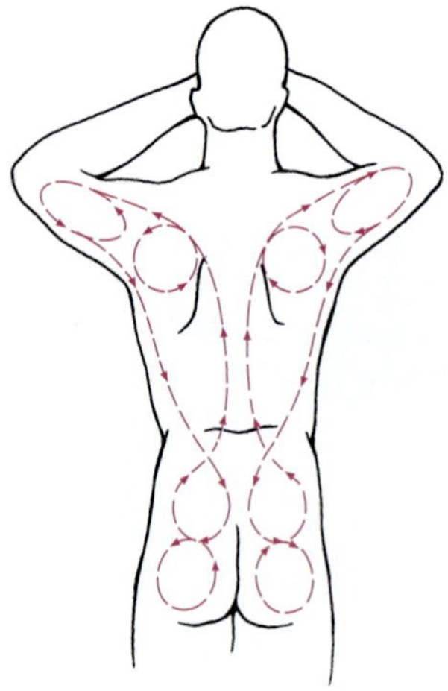

Step 13c Circular massage.

CRITICAL DECISION POINT Be certain to massage muscular region, not bruised, swollen, or inflamed areas or bones of the spine (Meintz, 1995).

d. Use long, gliding strokes along muscles of spine in upward and outward motion.	Massage follows distribution of major muscle groups.
e. Knead muscles of each shoulder toward front of client.	Area often tightens because of tension.
f. Use palms in upward and outward circular motion from lower buttocks to neck.	
g. Knead muscles of upper back and shoulder between thumb and forefinger.	These muscles are thick and can be vigorously massaged.
h. Use both hands to knead muscles up one side of back, then other.	
i. End massage with long stroking movements.	Most soothing of massage movements.
14. Massage feet:	
a. Place client in supine position.	
b. Hold foot firmly. Support ankle with one hand or support sides of foot with each hand while performing massage.	
c. Make circular motions with thumb and fingers around bones of ankle and top of foot.	
d. Trace space between tendons with firm finger pressure, moving from toe to ankle.	
e. Massage sides and top of each toe.	
f. Use top of fist to make circular motions on bottom of foot.	

STEPS	RATIONALE
g. Knead sides of foot between index finger and thumb.	
h. Conclude with firm, sweeping motions over top and bottom of foot.	Light strokes may tickle (Meintz, 1995).
15. Tell client you are ending massage.	Informs and prepares client for inhalation and exhalation (next step).
16. When procedure is complete, instruct client to inhale deeply, exhale, and then initially move about slowly after resting a few minutes.	Returns client to more awake and alert state. When deeply relaxed, client may experience dizziness on arising too rapidly.
a. Wipe excess lotion or oil from client's back with bath towel.	Excess lotion or oil can irritate skin and lead to breakdown.
17. Wash hands.	Reduces spread of microorganisms.

RELAXATION

STEPS	RATIONALE
1. Instruct client to take several slow, deep breaths.	Increased oxygen can lessen anxiety and prevent shortness of breath with relaxation. Breaths should be diaphragmatic and deep to avoid hyperventilation.
2. Have client close eyes, if desired.	Client may be less easily distracted.
3. Instruct client to follow verbal cues for relaxation; use calm, soft voice.	Relaxation is guided verbally or by tape until individual is comfortable with sequence and no longer needs verbal guidance.
a. Begin series of alternating tightening and relaxing muscle groups: (1) clench right fist, relax; (2) clench left fist, relax; (3) clench both fists, relax; (4) tighten right biceps, relax; (5) tighten left biceps, relax.	Alternating tension and relaxation in muscle groups allows client to feel difference.

CRITICAL DECISION POINT **Tension of each muscle group is maintained for 5 to 7 seconds except for the feet. Allows time to focus on the muscle group; cramps can easily occur in the feet.**

STEPS	RATIONALE
b. As each muscle group is completed, ask client to enjoy relaxed feeling and allow mind to drift and think how nice it is to be relaxed; ask client to breathe deeply.	Distracts client from perceiving pain. Enhances the relaxation response. Breathing deeply prevents Valsalva response, which can increase intrathoracic pressure and compromise cardiac function.
c. Instruct client to repeat each step two times: (1) reach with right arm, relax; (2) reach with left arm, relax; (3) reach with both arms, relax; (4) wrinkle forehead, relax; (5) squint eyes, relax; (6) tighten jaw muscles, relax; (7) press head into pillow, relax; (8) bring right shoulder to earlobe, relax; (9) bring left shoulder to earlobe, relax; (10) bring both shoulders to earlobe, relax; (11) tighten abdominal muscles, relax; (12) tighten hips and buttocks, relax; (13) press right leg into mattress, relax; (14) press left leg into mattress, relax; (15) point right toes and stretch, relax; (16) point left toes and stretch, relax; (17) stretch right leg, relax; (18) stretch left leg, relax; (19) stretch both legs, relax; (20) flex right foot, relax; (21) flex left foot, relax; (22) flex both feet, relax; (23) tense right leg, relax; (24) tense left leg, relax; (25) tense both legs, relax; (26) tense entire body, relax.	Relaxation is integrated response associated with diminished sympathetic nervous system arousal; decreased muscle tension is desired outcome. Relaxation decreases pulse and respiration rates and blood pressure and reduces anxiety.

STEPS	RATIONALE
CRITICAL DECISION POINT If muscle group tightens after relaxation has proceeded to other muscles, return to that group and repeat tension-relaxation until relaxation is achieved.	
d. Calmly explain during exercise that client may feel sensations of tingling, heaviness, floating, or warmth as relaxation occurs.	Prevents anxiety should sensation occur without warning.
e. Ask client to continue slow, deep breaths.	Allows opportunity to enjoy feelings of relaxation.
4. When exercise is complete, instruct client to inhale deeply, exhale, and then initially move about slowly after resting a few minutes.	Returns client to more awake and alert state. When deeply relaxed, client may experience dizziness on arising too rapidly.

GUIDED IMAGERY

STEPS	RATIONALE
1. Direct client through guided imagery exercise:	
a. Instruct client to imagine that inhaled air is ball of healing energy.	Development of specific images assists in removal of pain perception.
b. Imagine inhaled air travels to area of pain.	Client's ability to concentrate decreases pain perception.
2. Alternatively, nurse may direct imagery:	
a. Suggest client think about going to pleasant place such as beach or mountains.	Directs imagery after selection of restful place by nurse and client.
b. Direct client to experience all sensory aspects of restful place (e.g., for beach: warm breeze, warm sand between toes, warmth of sunshine, rhythmic sound of waves, smell of salt air, gulls gliding and swooping in air).	Helps client concentrate and relax.
c. Continue deep, slow, rhythmic breathing.	
d. Count to three, inhale, and open eyes. Move about slowly initially.	
3. Provide client time to practice exercise without interruption.	Guided imagery requires an intense level of concentration that may take time to achieve.

DISTRACTION

STEPS	RATIONALE
1. Direct client's attention away from pain with distraction techniques.	Redirection of attention alters emotional or cognitive aspects of pain, which reduces muscle tension and alters pain perception (Stanik-Hutt, 1993; Whipple and Glynn, 1992).
2. Ask client to close eyes or to focus on single object in room.	Directs attention inward and protects client from external distraction.
3. Instruct client to concentrate on slow, rhythmic breathing. Guide breathing or instruct client to control and concentrate on breathing by thinking: "in, one, two; out, one, two."	Promotes full relaxation.
4. Continue skill using chosen method.	Focusing on the skill impinges on amount of attention that can be given to painful sensory input (Stanik-Hutt, 1993; Whipple and Glynn, 1992).
a. Use music client has helped to select (Meintz, 1995).	Stimulating music blocks out all other sounds, focusing attention on stimuli other than pain. Soothing music enhances relaxation, therby increasing pain threshold (Whipple and Glynn, 1992).
(1) Emphasize listening to rhythm.	
b. Adjust volume as pain increases or decreases.	Provides auditory signal that client controls.
c. Direct client to give detailed account of an event or story.	Stress details of event to enhance distraction from pain stimulus.
d. Engage client in conversation; encourage participation of family members and visitors.	Visitors can help direct attention away from mild to moderate pain.

STEPS	RATIONALE
EVALUATION	
1. Evaluate client's physiological and behavioral response to technique. Observe character of respirations, body position, facial expression, tone of voice, mood, mannerisms, verbalization of discomfort.	Determines effectiveness of procedure, level of relaxation, degree of pain relief achieved, and which procedures were most effective.
2. Use pain rating scale to evaluate comfort level.	Objectively measures change in pain intensity.
3. Observe client perform pain control measures.	Documents learning.
4. **Unexpected outcomes** that may occur include:	
➤ Client is uncomfortable during diagnostic or therapeutic procedure, requiring procedure to be delayed or stopped.	Client movement can create risk during procedure.
➤ Client may be unable to concentrate on technique because of intense pain.	Techniques intended for use with mild to moderate pain.
➤ Client indicates continued discomfort: tense posture or muscles, increased pulse, increased or shallow respirations, splinting or holding painful body part, facial grimacing, restlessness or irritability, verbalized discomfort.	Client unable to concentrate on relaxation method, source of distraction, or image.
➤ Client is unable to describe or use pain-relief measures.	Pain may interfere with learning.
➤ Discomfort increases.	Stop technique.
RECORDING AND REPORTING	
1. Record in nurses' notes client's pain rating, procedure and technique, preparation given to client, client's response to procedure or technique, and further comfort needs related to event. Incorporate pain-relief technique into nursing care plan.	Documents therapy provided and provides guidelines to help determine client's reaction in future. Record keeping improves continuity of care.
2. Record alterations in client's condition (e.g., changes in blood pressure, pulse, respiration, condition of client's skin, complaints of dizziness).	
3. Report client's response to procedure or technique to charge nurse and to staff at change of shift.	Directs nurse to continue techniques as needed. Responses to procedure may not be limited to one shift. If further evaluation is necessary, staff members need to be aware of past experiences.
4. Report any unusual responses to techniques (e.g., uncontrolled or aggravated pain) to nurse in charge or physician.	May require continued monitoring for adverse effects or alternative therapy. Unexpected findings or occurrences during procedure should be reported, since additional assistance or time with the client may be needed.

FOLLOW-UP ACTIVITIES

1. Postprocedural restrictions should be explained to client and family.
2. Client may desire to talk with nurse about procedure or technique to help clarify events and reduce anxiety.
3. Client should be instructed to practice relaxation or guided imagery technique two or three times per day, since practice improves ability to achieve relaxation and increases comfort level more quickly.
4. Client may incorporate guided imagery into relaxation exercise.
5. Assess vital signs if dizziness results from relaxation. Encourage bed rest until dizziness subsides.
6. Do not give up a technique or strategy without adequate trial. Use a combination of techniques for more effective pain control.
7. Client may need referral to pain or behavioral therapist. Consult with physician or case manager regarding referral.

Special Considerations

- Individuals may express hearsay about techniques or diagnostic and therapeutic procedures.
- Techniques may be used as adjunct to other pain control modalities for clients suffering intense pain (Ferrell and Rhiner, 1994).
- If possible, nurse who explains procedure or technique should be with client during procedure or technique.
- Anticipatory guidance:
  - Do not attempt dialogue during procedure but use brief phrases to provide information and find out how client is tolerating procedure.
  - Procedure may not be totally pain free, but client is able to tolerate brief episodes of discomfort with appropriate explanations.
- Massage:
  - Contraindicated for individuals at risk for thromboemboli.
  - Large muscles of upper arm require more time to massage.
  - If client falls asleep, provide undisturbed time.
- Relaxation:
  - Contraindications to relaxation are not firmly established; research is not conclusive at this time. If client is at risk for thromboemboli, omit tensing component of relaxation procedure.
  - If client cannot tense specific muscle group as a result of illness or injury, omit that muscle group.
  - Periodically remind client to breathe to prevent holding breath.
  - Diaphragmatic breathing and deliberate tensing of muscles may increase pain of postoperative clients. These clients should be encouraged to control their own breathing and focus on relaxing groups of muscles with the tensing phase (Meintz, 1995).
- Guided imagery:
  - Clients may fall asleep during imagery. If this is not desired, ask client to sit in upright position or set timer or alarm.
  - Image may be vague (e.g., colored light; healthy body image; area of pain is wax, not real body part).
  - Clients may need reassurance that they are in control of their images.
- Techniques may be used in conjunction with other forms of pain management.
- Client may need referral to pain or behavioral therapist. Consult with physician or case manager regarding referral.
- Distraction:
  - Some clients experience comfort after cessation of distraction; for others comfort lasts only as long as distraction.
  - Client may require variety of distractions, depending on level of pain, availability of distraction, and experience in using distraction.
  - If client does not like music, substitute ball game or other distraction of client's choice.
  - Sensation of pain may intensify with removal of distraction, such as when visiting hours are over.

Teaching Considerations

- Clients need information about different pain therapies because participation is essential to successful outcome.
- Some diagnostic and therapeutic procedures conclude with client needing to maintain given position; explain reason before procedure and make client as comfortable as possible.
- Sometimes clients experience shortness of breath. If this occurs, ask client to take a deep breath, take shallow breaths, or breathe more slowly.
- Techniques may require more practice before results are achieved. Pharmacological intervention may be required to lessen pain so that client can achieve relaxation and augment other methods for pain control (Ferrell and Rhiner, 1994).
- Teach client to rest between periods of activity because fatigue increases pain perception.
- Discuss and practice with client possible techniques to use at home.
- Teach appropriate family member how to perform massage (if not contraindicated) as part of home care (Ferrell and Rhiner, 1994; Meintz, 1995).

Pediatric Considerations

- Since they are largely expressive tools, most pain rating scales can be reliably used by clients older than age 7 (Donovan and Miaskowski, 1992). Although validity and reliability scores of pain rating scales generally increase with age, some rating tools can be used with a child as young as 3 years if the child is verbal and can adequately understand instructions for use of the tool (Waters, 1992).
- Pain may be difficult to assess in children because they often lack the verbal or cognitive ability to express their feelings. When they are able to verbally communicate their pain, they may be reluctant to do so because they may have misconceptions about the cause of their pain or they may fear the consequences (e.g., another painful test or procedure or an injection) (Duchene, 1996; Oschenreither and Cubina, 1996; Waters, 1992).
- Infants and children experience pain but may respond to pain differently than adults do because of their different developmental levels. For example, they may cry and thrash about, have sleep disturbances, have a shortened attention span, suck or rock, refuse to eat or play, or be quiet and withdrawn. Still others become active when they are in pain; variations in activity levels are related to the child's personality, developmental level, and previous pain experiences (Duchene, 1996; Waters, 1992).

- Parents can be a helpful source of information when assessing a child's pain and when planning pain relief therapies. Most parents know how their child exhibits pain and which pain relief interventions have been successful or unsuccessful.
- A number of nonpharmacological pain management therapies can be used successfully with children. Distraction and relaxation strategies work for all ages. The technique or device used will need to be suitable to the developmental level of the child (e.g., a pacifier can be used for the infant, reading or playing a recording of a favorite story is appropriate for the preschooler, listening to music on a portable cassette or CD player with headphones may work for a teenager). Because children have an active imagination, relaxation can be a powerful adjuvant in pain control. Play therapy and art can also be effective. Parents can be very helpful in providing pain relief. They often provide comfort, for example, by their presence, by their conversation, and by holding and cuddling their child (Acute Pain Management Guideline Panel, 1992; Jacox et al., 1994; Oschenreither and Cubina, 1996).

Gerontologic Considerations

- Pain may be difficult to assess in older adults. Cognitive impairment or dementia may affect their ability to report pain severity on a visual analog scale or numerical scale. Behavioral observations (e.g., agitation, restlessness, groaning) for pain may be confused with signs of dementia (Acute Pain Management Guideline Panel, 1992).
- Visual, hearing, cognitive, and motor impairments may make it difficult for older adults to be able to effectively use procedures such as distraction, relaxation, or guided imagery (Acute Pain Management Guideline Panel, 1992).

Home Care Considerations

- Family members may need to collaborate planning time to reduce noise and other stimuli in the home to promote client's relaxation.

SKILL 5-3 Patient-Controlled Analgesia

Causes of pain are numerous, particularly in the acute care setting. The nurse's awareness of these causes is essential for choosing the best pain-control method. Parenteral administration of narcotics is the method of choice when acute or severe pain exists, when high doses of oral drugs are ineffective, or when clients have obstructive or absorptive GI alterations. One of the advances in pain-control modalities is **patient-controlled analgesia (PCA),** which allow clients to self-administer small continuous doses of IV narcotics (usually morphine) as they feel the need.

PCA is used extensively in postoperative, obstetrical, oncological, and trauma clients, as well as in those experiencing sickle cell crises (Egbert, Lampros, and Parks, 1993). The two variations of PCAs are the electronic computerized pump, which is attached to an IV pole (Fig. 5-4) or to the client's pajamas by a waist belt, and the more recent nonelectronic, non–battery operated pump, which may be attached to an IV pole or placed in a "sleeve" and attached to the client's gown or around the client's wrist (Fig. 5-5). The latter is lightweight, less costly, and more portable. However, measurement of the total, cumulative dosage is more difficult with the nonelectronic pump.

A PCA consists of three parts: an infusion pump with a chamber that houses a prefilled syringe (infuser), a timing unit linked to a switch or button that is activated by the client to deliver a preset dose of medicine (patient-control module), and tubing that delivers the medication from the infuser through the patient-control module to an indwelling IV line. Computerized PCAs can be programmed to deliver specific physician-prescribed doses of medication in a number of ways: as predetermined interval doses, as a bolus dose, as a continuous infusion (basal rate), or as a combination of the three. Overdosing is prevented by interposing a preprogrammed delay time or "lockout" (usually 5 to 10 minutes) between client-initiated doses.

The PCA has several advantages. It allows more constant serum levels of the narcotic and therefore avoids the peaks and troughs of large bolus injections (Egbert, Lampros, and Parks, 1993). Because the blood level is maintained within a narrow range of the minimum effective analgesia concentration for the individual, pain relief is enhanced and the incidence of side effects, such as sedation and respiratory depression, is decreased (Nossel, 1996). As a result, pain control and client satisfaction improve (Egbert, Lampros, and Parks, 1993). A second advantage is that fewer postoperative complications occur, probably because of diminished sedation, which can lead to cardiovascular and respiratory complications associated with immobility. Studies show improved pulmonary function tests and fewer postoperative pulmonary complications (Kaiser, 1992). Earlier and easier ambulation may also help minimize postoperative complications. Increased client control and independence are other advantages of PCA. Because the device provides medication on demand as soon as the client feels the need, the total amount of narcotic use is usually reduced. Research results demonstrate a strong

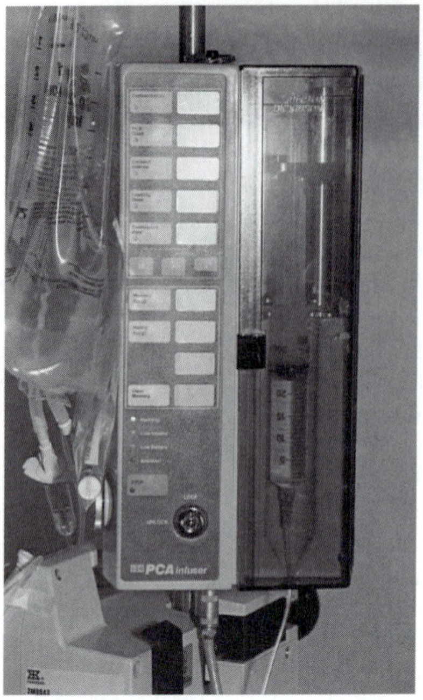

Fig. 5-4 Patient-controlled analgesia (PCA) device.

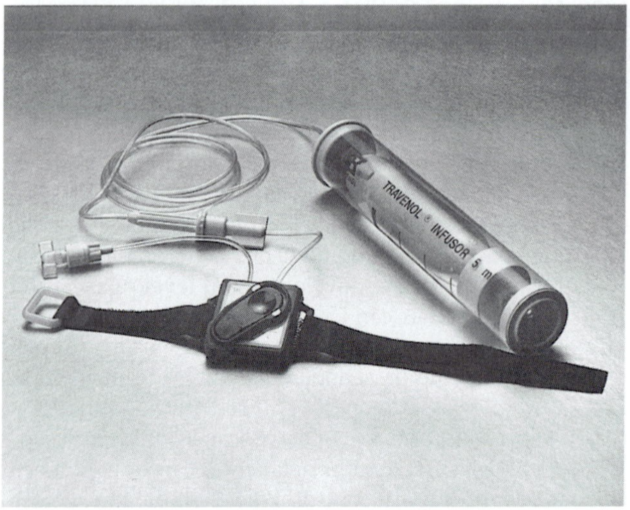

Fig. 5-5 Patient-controlled analgesia (PCA) device.

positive relationship between the client's belief in his or her ability to control pain and the pain experience. An increase in the client's self-control expectancy decreases the intensity, latency, and duration of postoperative pain (Bachiocco, Morselli, and Carli, 1993). PCA allows the client to manage pain with minimal nursing intervention and therefore also saves nursing time (Lazzara, 1993). Clients are not as dependent on the nursing staff for dosing as they are with the more conventional oral or intramuscular (IM) and subcutaneous (SQ) injectable medications. Another advantage is the superiority of patient-administered medications over IM or SQ injections. Studies show a significant statistical difference in outcomes between clients using PCA and those receiving IM pain medications from the nursing staff. Clients using PCA had a reduced incidence of severe pain, a smaller increase in sedation, a smaller drop in incentive spirometry, fewer chest film abnormalities, and a smaller total dose of medication. Clients were also better able to perform postoperative exercises; had less difficulty with adherence to pulmonary toilet, sleep, self-care, and ambulation; and were discharged home earlier (Acute Pain Management Guideline Panel, 1992; Stanik-Hutt, 1993). Less apprehension and ecchymosis were also associated with PCA. A final advantage is that PCA offers a more ethical approach to pain control: clients have some control over the frequency and timing of the administration of their pain medication and are less dependent on the attitudes and values of health care providers.

EQUIPMENT

- **PCA system (Obtain primed infuser and patient-control unit from pharmacy.)**
- **Identification label and time tape (may already be attached and completed by pharmacy)**
- **18- or 20-gauge needle**
- **Alcohol swab**
- **Adhesive tape**
- **Disposable gloves**

DELEGATION CONSIDERATIONS

The administration of PCA requires problem solving and knowledge application unique to a professional nurse. For this skill, delegation is inappropriate. However, unlicensed assistive personnel should know the signs of unrelieved pain and notify the nurse when they occur. Unlicensed personnel should *never* administer a PCA dose for the client.

STEPS	RATIONALE
ASSESSMENT	
1. Assess client's comfort level.	Certain conditions place clients at risk for alterations in comfort (e.g., trauma, postoperative states, advanced cancer, sickle cell anemia).
2. Assess client's nonverbal responses to pain (see Skill 5-1, Assessment step 3).	Nonverbal physiological responses are mediated by autonomic nervous system, vary with severity and duration of pain, and serve as means to evaluate effectiveness of medication.
3. Assess characteristics and intensity of pain through client's verbal expression and use of pain scale (see Skill 5-1, Assessment step 4).	Allows client to describe pain from experience. Pain is subjective sensation. Objective indicators are not as reliable as client's subjective expression of pain (McCaffery, 1992b).
4. Assess environment for factors that contribute to pain.	
5. If client has had surgery, inspect incision.	Tissue trauma or damage stimulates peripheral pain receptors to transmit impulses to cortex to create conscious awareness of pain (Stanik-Hutt, 1993).
6. Assess patency of existing IV infusion line (see Chapter 20).	IV line must be patent for medication to reach venous circulation.
7. Assess venipuncture site for infiltration or inflammation (see Chapter 20).	Confirmation of placement of IV needle or catheter and integrity of surrounding tissues ensures medication is administered safely.
8. Assess knowledge and effectiveness of previous pain management strategies.	Response to pain-control strategies assists in identifying learning needs and affects client's willingness to try therapy.
9. Check physician's order for name of medication dose and frequency of medication.	Narcotic medication administration is a dependent nursing function and requires physician's prescription. The most commonly prescribed medications are morphine sulfate and meperidine hydrochloride (Demerol) but fentanyl citrate (Sublimaze), hydromorphone, and buprenorphine hydrochloride (Buprenex) can be used for PCA (Lazzara, 1993).
10. Check client's history of drug allergies.	Avoids placing client at risk for allergic reaction.

NURSING DIAGNOSIS

Clustering of defining characteristics from the assessment data may reveal the following nursing diagnoses for clients requiring this skill:

- Activity intolerance
- Anxiety
- Ineffective individual coping
- Knowledge deficit regarding PCA use
- Pain
- Powerlessness
- Risk for infection

Related factors are individualized based on client's condition or needs.

PLANNING

STEPS	RATIONALE
1. **Expected outcomes** following completion of procedure:	
➤ Client verbalizes pain relief.	Drug is given safely and is effective in providing pain control.
➤ Client exhibits relaxed facial expression and body position.	
➤ Client remains alert and oriented.	
➤ Client increasingly participates in self-care activities.	
➤ Client correctly operates PCA device.	

STEPS	RATIONALE
2. Explain purpose and demonstrate function of PCA:	Effective explanations allow client participation in care and independence in pain control.
a. Designed to deliver specific type and dose of pain medication that promotes comfort yet minimizes drowsiness.	
CRITICAL DECISION POINT Be sure client is alert, attentive, and able to manipulate PCA button.	
b. Allows client to push medication demand button on timing unit instead of calling the nurse.	Gives client control of pain. Client does not have to call and wait for nurse to prepare and deliver medication.
c. Provides lockout time between doses to prevent overdosage. Client can tell when timing unit is ready to deliver another dose. If button is pressed before lockout time is complete, only partial dose will be administered.	System has built-in safeguards to help prevent accidental administration of doses or overdosing. No medication can flow between pushes.
d. Infuser will be on IV pole or attached to bed clothing or wrist.	
e. Device administers balanced amount of medication to provide comfort and minimize drowsiness.	Balanced dosing with client-controlled administration produces constant serum drug levels rather than peaks and troughs associated with PRN nurse-administered therapy (Nossel, 1996).
CRITICAL DECISION POINT Instruct client to check with nurse or physician with questions and concerns, or if medication is not controlling pain. A "rescue" dose may need to be given for breakthrough pain, or the dosage may need to be adjusted.	
3. Check infuser and patient-control module for accurate labeling or evidence of leaking.	Avoids medication error. Damage to system can occur in shipping and handling; inspect to avoid injury or harm to client, self, or others.
4. Program the computerized PCA pump to deliver the prescribed medication dose and lockout interval.	
5. Draw curtains around client's bed or close door to room.	Maintains client's privacy.
6. Position client comfortably for procedure. Maintain any postoperative position restrictions. Venipuncture site needs to be accessible.	Comfortable position enhances effectiveness of analgesia.
IMPLEMENTATION	
1. Wash hands.	Reduces transmission of microorganisms.
2. Follow the "five rights" to be sure of correct medication (see Chapter 18). Check client's identification band and call client by name.	Minimizes risk of medication error and harm to client.
3. Apply gloves.	Follow standard precautions: potential contact with blood exists when working with IV line.
4. Attach 18- or 19-gauge needle to exit tubing adapter of patient-control module or attach needleless system adaptor.	PCA medication is usually administered by IV piggyback route.
5. Wipe injection port of IV line with alcohol if closed port is being used.	Alcohol is a topical antiseptic that minimizes entry of surface microorganisms during needle insertion.
6. Insert needle into injection port nearest IV site. If using needleless system, connect exit tubing adapter to port nearest IV site.	Establishes route for medication to enter main IV line.

STEPS	RATIONALE
7. Secure connection and immobilize PCA tubing with strip of adhesive tape.	Prevents dislodging of needle from port. Facilitates ambulation.
8. Administer loading dose of analgesia as prescribed.	A one-time dose may be given manually by nurse or programmed into PCA pump. Establishes initial serum level and immediate control of pain (Lazzara, 1993).
9. Discard gloves and supplies in appropriate containers. Wash hands.	Reduces transmission of infection.
10. If client is experiencing pain, demonstrate use of PCA system; if not, have client repeat instructions given earlier (see illustrations).	Repeating instructions reinforces learning. Checking client's understanding through return demonstration helps nurse determine client's level of understanding and ability to manipulate device.

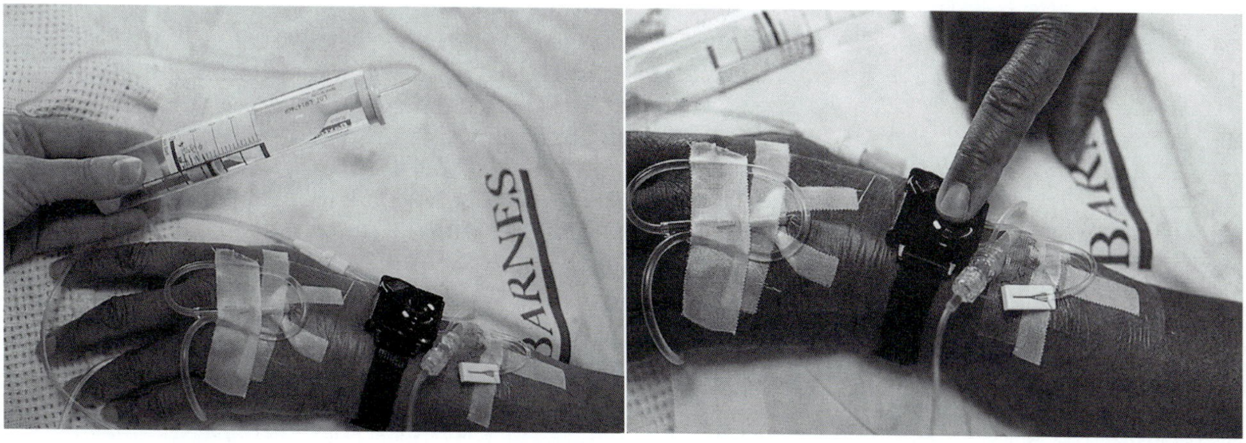

Step 10(1) and (2) Patient demonstrates PCA devices.

EVALUATION

1. Use pain rating scale to evaluate comfort level.	Determines response to PCA.
2. Observe for signs of adverse reactions.	IV medications produce rapid effects.
3. Periodically check infusion rate and condition of site (follow protocol of institution). Infusion rate may be checked by observing movement of volume indicator on infuser.	IV must remain patent for proper drug administration. Infiltration requires discontinuation of infusion.
4. Ask client to describe purpose of PCA.	Evaluates cognitive learning.
5. Have client demonstrate dose delivery.	Evaluates skill in use of PCA.
6. **Unexpected outcomes** that may occur include:	
➤ Client verbalizes discomfort is still present or is worse.	Underlying medical or postsurgical condition may have changed or client may be undermedicated.
➤ Client displays nonverbal behaviors reflective of pain.	
➤ Client is sedated and not readily arousable.	Client may be oversedated and may need to have dose regulated.
➤ Client is unable to manipulate PCA device to maintain pain control.	Alternative medication routes may be needed.

THE UNIVERSITY HOSPITAL
St. Louis University Medical Center

Patient's Dashew

PCA INFUSOR SYSTEM - DAILY MEDICATION RECORD/PCA REGIMEN

ALLERGIES: ______ PCA DAY # ______

DATE/ TIME	DRUG (SPECIFY: Concentration/ Diluent)	LOCKOUT INTERVAL	COMMENTS	NURSE'S SIGNATURE
11/1	120 mg morphine sul-	6 min	Dose = 1mg 16 min	K. Thompson, RN
1230	fate in 60 cc			
	Normal Saline			

PATIENT STATUS

DATE/ TIME	VITALS RR	HR	BP	SEDATION STATUS (a)	PAIN STATUS (b)	ACCESS STATUS (c)	AMOUNT INFUSED	AMOUNT LEFT	DRUG DOSAGE (in mg) DOSE	# HOURS	NURSES' SIGNATURE
1330	18	84	110/72	4	2	1	2cc	58cc	4 mg	1	K. Thompson, RN
1430	16	80	112/70	3	1	1	1cc	57cc	2 mg	1	K. Thompson, RN
1630	16	82	110/70	2	1	1	1cc	56cc	2mg	2	J. Harrigan RN

(a) SEDATION SCALE 1=AWAKE
2=DROWSY
3=DOZING
4=MOSTLY SLEEPING
5=SLEEPING

(b) PAIN SCALE 1=NO PAIN
2=MILD PAIN
3=MODERATE PAIN
4=SEVERE PAIN
5=UNBEARABLE

(c) ACCESS SITE 1=NORMAL
2=LOCAL TENDERNESS
3=PALPABLE CORD
4=HEAT (associated with site)
5=ERYTHEMA
6=EDEMA
7=PURULENT DRAINAGE

DRUG WASTAGE RECORD

DATE/ TIME	DRUG (SPECIFY: AMOUNT)	COMMENTS (Note: Reason for wastage; if d/c'd chart volume remaining before returning to pharm.	NURSES' SIGNATURE	
			1.	1.
			2.	2.
			3.	3.

DATE/ TIME	COMMENTS	NURSE'S SIGNATURE

DISPENSED BY: P. Smith, R.Ph RECEIVED BY: K. Thompson, RN

DATE: ______ RX.NO. ______

Fig. 5-6 PCA infuser system—daily medication record. (Courtesy St. Louis University Medical Center.)

STEPS	RATIONALE
RECORDING AND REPORTING	
1. Record drug, dose, and time begun on appropriate medication record. Specify concentration and diluent. Note lockout time (Fig. 5-6).	Timely documentation prevents errors.
2. Record regular periodic assessments of client status on PCA medication record (see Fig. 5-6) or on nurses' notes. Forms may vary from institution to institution, but information recorded is similar. Indicate: a. Vital signs b. Sedation status c. Pain rating d. Status of vascular access site e. Amount of solution infused f. Amount of solution remaining g. Amount of drug received (in milligrams) h. Time since last status check	Provides data to evaluate response of client to pain therapy.
3. When PCA syringe is empty, return copy of PCA medication record to pharmacy with used PCA system.	If PCA is discontinued before device is completely empty, record drug wastage on PCA medication record. Note date, time, amount (in milligrams) of drug wasted, and reason for wastage. Wastage must be witnessed and record signed by two registered nurses. Control and dispensation of narcotics are regulated by the Controlled Substances Act.
4. Report any adverse reactions to nurse in charge or to physician. Report client's pain status and response to PCA system during change-of-shift report.	Reaction may require therapeutic intervention or dosage regulation.

FOLLOW-UP ACTIVITIES

1. Reassess comfort level at least every 4 hours or more frequently as condition warrants.
2. When PCA is discontinued or prefilled syringe is empty, remove from infusion port, discard needle in needle box, cap exit tubing, and return entire PCA system to pharmacy.

• • • • •

Special Considerations

- The following are not candidates for PCA: clients with impaired mental status, history of chronic obstructive pulmonary disease, severe metabolic disorders (i.e., sepsis or severe fluid and electrolyte abnormalities), psychological disorders, history of narcotic abuse, allergies to morphine (or other prescribed narcotic), impaired renal or hepatic function, inability to press delivery button (e.g., clients with severe arthritis or paralysis), or poor client understanding (Lazzara, 1993).
- Because infusor syringe is filled with narcotic analgesic, syringe must be stored in narcotic box in clinical division when sent from the pharmacy if infusion will not be immediately started.
- Some nonelectronic systems must be worn next to the body to maintain correct fluid temperature. Solutions may need to be stored at room temperature before infusion. Follow manufacturer's instructions.
- Maximum dose that can be delivered in 1 hour by a PCA system depends on filling times of medication reservoirs on the patient-control module. These times are determined by the model in use. The nurse must read manufacturer's guide to obtain this information. For example, Baxter's most common PCA infuser system (model 2C1073) has a filling time of 6 minutes. When demand button is pressed, system delivers 0.5 ml of drug solution. Therefore 5 ml of solution is delivered in 1 hour:

$$60 \text{ min} \div 6 \text{ min} = 10 \text{ doses}$$

thus

$$0.5 \text{ ml} \times 10 = 5 \text{ ml/hr}$$

Suppose, for example, that a prefilled syringe contains 120 mg of morphine in a 60 ml diluent, or 2 mg/ml. Since 5 ml of fluid is delivered in 1 hour (with a filling time of 6 minutes), a maximum of 10 mg of morphine could be delivered in 1 hour:

$$2 \text{ mg/ml} \times 5 \text{ ml/hr} = 10 \text{ mg/hr}$$

Teaching Considerations

- Encourage client to push button on timing unit whenever pain is felt. Tell client not to delay interval if there is pain.
- Instructions are best given during pain-free or pain-reduced states and before initiating therapy. If preoperative client, instruct before surgery.
- Explain regimen to family so that they can support and assist client.
- Inform client of pain-management strategies that may supplement or enhance pharmacological intervention.

Pediatric Considerations

- PCA can be an effective means of pain control in children who can understand the concept. When selecting pediatric candidates for PCA use, consideration must be given to developmental level, cognitive level, and motor skills. PCA use was found to be safe and effective for clients as young as 7 years (Acute Pain Management Guideline Panel, 1992; Lazzara, 1993;). Waters (1992) reports safe use with children 5 years of age and older who have cognitive ability to understand mechanics of the PCA equipment and its use in controlling pain. From developmental perspective, use of PCA is particularly effective with adolescents, since it leads to feeling of control.
- Pharmacological pain support is safe and effective in pediatric clients when dose is calibrated according to child's weight. As with adults, doses may need adjusting after initiation of medication to obtain analgesia with minimal side effects (Acute Pain Management Guideline Panel, 1992).
- Because adolescents and young adults are more likely to be undermedicated, they tend to choose PCA pumps for pain management. Some clients report emotional discomfort with self-administration of analgesia (Vanier et al., 1993).

Gerontologic Considerations

- Older adults are more likely to be undermedicated than are middle-age adults because of ungrounded fears of respiratory depression. Older clients may not need to be medicated as frequently because of likelihood of delayed excretion of narcotic; however, their dose should still be large enough to achieve pain relief (Ferrell, Cronin, and Warfield, 1992; McCaffery and Ferrell, 1992b). Low-dose continuous infusion of PCA may be the best way to provide effective pain management in older adults, particularly those with chronic cancer pain, since they experience higher peak and longer duration of pain relief (Acute Pain Management Guideline Panel, 1992; Jacox et al., 1994).

SKILL 5-4 Epidural Analgesia

The use of epidurally administered narcotics is becoming a popular and accepted technique for management of acute postoperative and trauma pain both in intensive care units and in general medical-surgical units. The epidural route is also effective in controlling and relieving chronic pain, especially that associated with cancer (Jacox et al., 1994; Naber, Jones, and Halm, 1994). Such use requires that the nurse be familiar with the aspects of epidural therapy. Epidural narcotics are desirable for pain control because they decrease the total narcotic requirement and produce fewer side effects (Stanik-Hutt, 1993). Studies have indicated that epidurally administered narcotics provide longer lasting pain relief, increased client alertness, improved pulmonary function, decreased postoperative time on ventilators, and earlier ambulation (Naber, Jones, and Halm, 1994).

The brain and spinal cord are covered by three meninges or membranes. The dura mater is the outermost protective membrane. The epidural space lies between the dura mater and the vertebral column. When a narcotic is injected into the epidural space, it binds to opiate receptors located on the dorsal horn of the spinal cord and blocks the transmission of pain impulses to the cerebral cortex of the brain. Because the narcotic does not cross the blood-brain barrier, pain relief results from drug levels in the spinal cord rather than in the plasma, with little central or systemic distribution of the drug. Pain is relieved with smaller doses of narcotics, and side effects are less severe. As a result, postoperative clients can be mobilized earlier and the incidence of mobility-related complications can be reduced (Wild and Coyne, 1992).

For placement of the epidural catheter, the client should be placed in the lateral decubitus or sitting position with shoulders and hips squared and hips and head flexed (Naber, Jones, and Halm, 1994). The anesthesiologist or client's attending physician places a catheter into the epidural space (Fig. 5-7), generally in the lower lumbar region, to administer analgesics. Usually opiates such as morphine are used. When the epidural catheter is intended for temporary or short-term use, it may not be sutured in place and exits from the insertion site on the back (Fig. 5-8). By contrast, a catheter intended for permanent or long-term use is "tunneled" subcutaneously and exits on the side of the body or on the abdomen (Fig. 5-9). Tunneling decreases the chance of infection or dislodging of the catheter. In both cases the catheter is secured with a sterile occlusive dressing (Fig. 5-10) (Wild and Coyne, 1992). Epidural medication can be administered either intermittently by

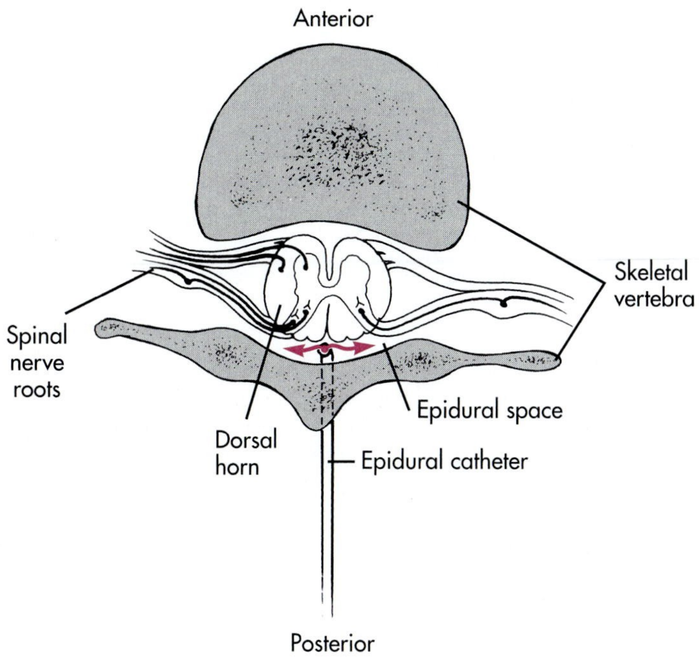

Fig. 5-7 Anatomical drawing of epidural space.

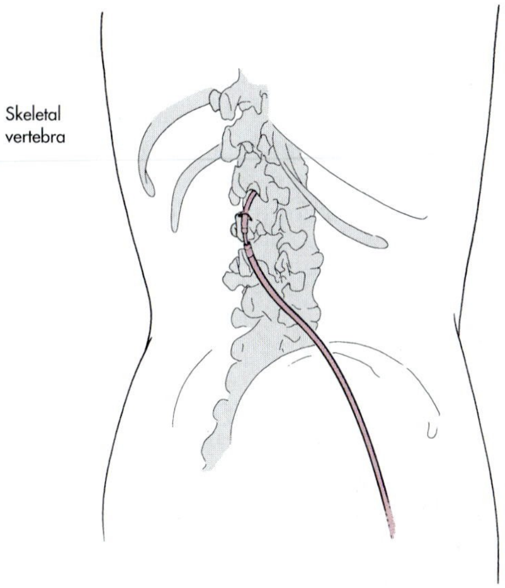

Fig. 5-8 External epidural catheter.

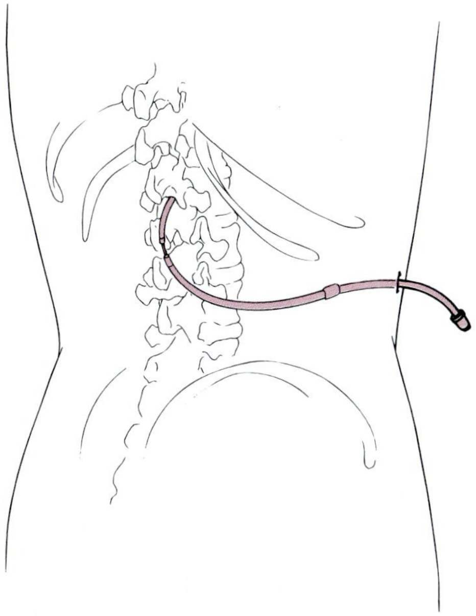

Fig. 5-9 Tunneled epidural catheter.

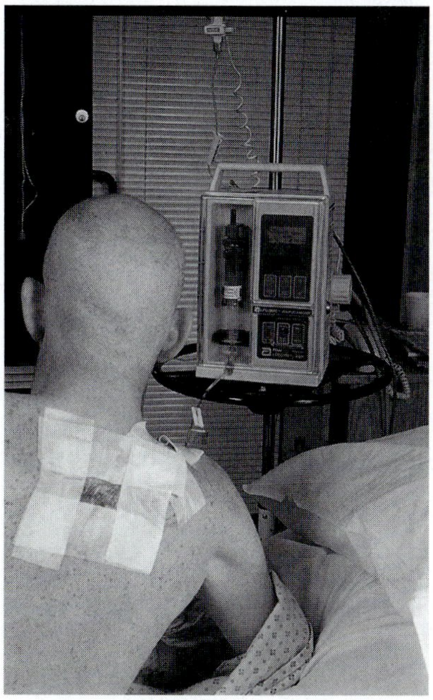

Fig. 5-10 Epidural catheter secured.

bolus injection or continuously by a controlled delivery system such as an infusion pump (see Chapter 20). Continuous infusion seems to provide more constant pain relief and fewer side effects because of the use of low dosages of medication (Jurf and Nirschl, 1993).

Although the use of epidural narcotics for pain control has many advantages for the client, it requires astute nursing observation and care. The epidural catheter poses a threat to client safety because of its anatomical location, its potential for migration through the dura, and its proximity to spinal nerves and vessels. Assisting the client in obtaining pain control or relief, evaluating the analgesic effect, and intervening appropriately in the event of a complication or occurrence of side effects are the responsibilities of the nurse caring for these clients (Jurf and Nirschl, 1993; Naber, Jones, and Halm, 1994; Wild and Coyne, 1992).

EQUIPMENT

- Disposable gloves

ADMINISTERING A BOLUS MEDICATION

- 10- to 12-ml syringe
- Filter needle
- 20-gauge, 1-inch needle
- Povidone-iodine swabs
- Prediluted preservative-free narcotic as prescribed by physician
- Label (for injection port)

ADMINISTERING MEDICATION BY CONTINUOUS INFUSION

- Prediluted preservative-free narcotic as prescribed by physician and prepared for use in IV infusion pump (usually prepared by pharmacy)
- Infusion pump
- Infusion pump and compatible IV tubing *without* Y-ports
- Tape
- Label (for tubing)

DELEGATION CONSIDERATIONS

Administration of epidural anesthesia requires problem solving and knowledge application unique to a professional nurse. Delegation to unlicensed assistive personnel is inappropriate. However, staff must be instructed on how to reposition clients so as to prevent disruption of the catheter.

STEPS	RATIONALE
ASSESSMENT	
1. Assess client's comfort level and consider presenting medical condition.	Certain conditions make epidural analgesia the method of choice for pain control: postoperative states, clients with trauma, or advanced cancer, and those predisposed to cardiopulmonary complications because of preexisting medical condition or surgery.
CRITICAL DECISION POINT **Contraindications to epidural analgesia include:** • Infection • Clotting disorders • Anticoagulant therapy • Increased intracranial pressure • Prior laminectomy with opening of the dura • Previous adverse or allergic reaction to narcotics • Spine abnormalities that may make insertion of catheter difficult • Lack of nursing personnel to monitor for side effects and complications (Naber, Jones, and Halm, 1994)	
2. Assess client's nonverbal response (see Skill 5-1, Assessment step 2).	Signs of sympathetic nervous stimulation are often, but not universally, seen in clients experiencing acute pain of mild to moderate intensity or superficial pain (McCaffery and Ferrell, 1992b). Client with chronic pain often does not show overt signs and symptoms of acute pain.

STEPS	RATIONALE
3. Assess characteristics and intensity of pain (see Skill 5-1, Assessment step 6).	Allows client to describe pain. Pain is primarily a subjective experience. Objective indicators are not as reliable as client's subjective expression of pain (McCaffery, 1992b).
4. Assess environment for factors that may be contributing to pain.	Environmental stimuli can aggravate client's response to pain.
5. Assess sedation level of client by assessing for level of orientation, motor functioning, and drowsiness.	Establishes a baseline before first dose. The first sign of altered respiratory function from opioid use is most often a change in consciousness level (Wild and Coyne, 1992).
6. Check client's history of drug allergies.	Avoids placing client at risk for allergic reaction.
7. Assess rate, pattern, and depth of respirations.	Establishes baseline. Slow, shallow, and irregular respirations are signs of respiratory depression, which may occur as late as 24 hours after epidural injection (Jurf and Nirschl, 1993).
8. Assess blood pressure.	Establishes baseline. Small drop in blood pressure may be seen in first hour after epidural injection. Hypotension after opioid use usually results, however, from a decreased circulating catecholamine level that was elevated in response to pain (Wild and Coyne, 1992).
9. Assess mobility and motor and sensory function (see Chapter 11) before assisting client into or out of bed. Check for: a. Motor weakness b. Numbness and tingling of lower extremities (paresthesias)	Prevents injury from falling that may occur from weakness, sedation, or postural hypotension. In addition, rapid onset of motor weakness is indication that epidural catheter may have migrated across dura into subarachnoid space (Wild and Coyne, 1992); if catheter puts pressure on spinal nerves, paresthesias can result (Jurf and Nirschl, 1993).
10. Check to see if epidural catheter is secured to client's skin. (If transparent dressing has been applied, note "hatch" marks on catheter.)	Aids in preventing dislodging or migration of catheter. Hatch marks indicate proper placement.
11. Assess epidural catheter insertion site for:	
a. Redness, warmth, tenderness, swelling	Local inflammation and superficial skin infection at insertion site are the most common infections resulting from epidural catheters (Wild and Coyne, 1992).
b. Drainage	Purulent drainage is sign of infection. Clear drainage may indicate puncture of dura, causing narcotic to be delivered into subarachnoid space or causing cerebrospinal fluid leakage. Bloody drainage may indicate catheter entered blood vessel.
12. Check physician's order for medication, dosage, and infusion method.	Narcotic medication administration is dependent nursing function and requires physician's prescription.
13. If continuous infusion, check infusion pump for proper calibration and operation.	Ensures client will obtain prescribed analgesic dose.
14. If continuous infusion, check patency of IV tubing.	IV tube must be patent for medication to reach epidural space.

NURSING DIAGNOSIS

Clustering of defining characteristics from the assessment data may reveal the following nursing diagnoses for clients requiring this skill:

- Pain
- Activity intolerance
- Anxiety
- Ineffective individual coping
- Knowledge deficit regarding epidural analgesia
- Powerlessness
- Risk for injury
- Risk for infection

Related factors are individualized based on a client's condition or needs.

STEPS	RATIONALE
PLANNING	
1. **Expected outcomes** following completion of procedure:	
➤ Client verbalizes pain relief.	Drug effective in relieving pain. Catheter intact. Equipment functioning properly.
➤ Catheter and injection cap or infusion pump tubing are securely taped.	Closed, intact system prevents entry of pathogens and disruption of flow of medication.
➤ Client remains normotensive.	
➤ Heart rate stays in normal range.	
➤ Client is alert and oriented.	
➤ Respirations are regular, unlabored, and equal to or greater than 8 breaths/min.	Indicates absence of respiratory depression.
➤ Client does not experience headache.	Indicates catheter in epidural space.
➤ Epidural dressing is dry and intact.	No cerebrospinal fluid leakage.
➤ Catheter and infusion tubing are free of knots and kinks.	Helps to ensure that system is patent.
➤ No redness, warmth, exudate, tenderness, or swelling are evident at catheter insertion site. Client is afebrile.	Indicates absence of inflammation or infection.
➤ Client voids without difficulty and in adequate amounts.	Indicates absence of urinary retention (a potential side effect).
➤ Client has no or minimal pruritus.	Indicates absence of potential side effect of epidurally administered narcotic.
➤ Client has no paresthesias of lower extremities.	
2. Identify client by checking arm band and asking client's name.	Ensures correct client receives ordered drug.
3. Explain purpose and function of epidural analgesia and expectations of client during procedure.	Proper explanation enhances client cooperation and effective results.
4. Attach "epidural line" label:	Labeling helps to ensure narcotic analgesic is administered into correct line and into epidural space.
a. Intermittent bolus: attach label close to injection cap on epidural catheter.	
b. Continuous infusion: attach label to IV tubing connected to epidural catheter. Use tubing *without* Y-ports.	Use of tubing without Y-ports prevents accidental injection or infusion of other medication meant for vascular space into epidural space.
5. Draw curtains around client's bed or close door to room.	Maintains client's privacy.
IMPLEMENTATION	
1. Wash hands and apply gloves.	Reduces transmission of microorganisms.
CRITICAL DECISION POINT **Follow the "five rights" in preparing the correct medication and dosage (see Chapter 18).**	
2. For bolus injection:	
a. Using large syringe, draw up prediluted preservative-free narcotic solution through filter needle.	Large volume of fluid permits narcotic to contact optimal number of receptors (Wild and Coyne, 1992). Preservative may be toxic to neural tissue and could result in nerve damage (Wild and Coyne, 1992). Filter needle removes any microscopic glass particles.
b. Change from filter needle to regular 20-gauge needle. For a needleless system, remove filter needle from syringe and place sterile cap on syringe.	Changing to regular needle is necessary to allow medication to be injected.
c. If needle system is being used, clean injection cap with povidone-iodine. (*Do not* use alcohol.)	Cleaning agent prevents introduction of microorganisms during needle insertion. Alcohol causes pain and is toxic to neural tissue.

STEPS	RATIONALE
d. Dry the injection cap with sterile 2 × 2 gauze.	Prevents formation of sticky residue and injection of disinfectant.
e. Insert needle into injection cap. For needleless system, remove cover of port and connect syringe.	
f. Aspirate, gently. Observe return.	Aspiration of clear fluid of less than 1 ml indicates correct epidural catheter placement.
➤ *CRITICAL DECISION POINT* More than 1 ml of clear fluid or bloody return means catheter may be in subarachnoid space or in a vessel (Jurf and Nirchl, 1993). Do not inject drug. Notify physician.	
g. If less than 1 ml of clear fluid returns, inject drug slowly (see Chapter 20).	Slow injection helps prevent client discomfort by lowering pressure exerted by fluid as it exits catheter (Wild and Coyne, 1992).
h. Remove needle from injection cap or disconnect needleless system from port and place sterile cap on the port.	
i. Dispose of uncapped needle and syringe in "sharps" container.	Prevents accidental needle sticks.
3. For continuous infusion:	
a. Attach container of diluted preservative-free narcotic to infusion pump tubing and prime (see Chapter 20).	Tubing should be filled with solution and free of air bubbles to avoid air embolus.
b. Attach proximal end of tubing to pump and distal end to epidural catheter. Tape all connections. Start infusion. (See Chapter 20 for use of infusion pump.)	Infusion pumps propel fluid through tubing. Taping maintains a secure, closed system to help prevent infection.
c. Check infusion pump for proper calibration and operation.	Maintains patency and ensures client is receiving proper dose and pain relief.
4. Remove and dispose of gloves. Wash hands.	Reduces transmission of microorganisms.

EVALUATION

STEPS	RATIONALE
1. Evaluate comfort level and compare with original assessment data.	Determines if response to analgesia has been effective and if catheter is securely in place.
2. Observe for signs of adverse reactions to epidurally administered narcotic.	Although pain is relieved with smaller doses and side effects are less severe with epidural narcotic analgesia, side effects can still occur (Woodin, 1993).
a. Observe respiratory rate, rhythm, and pattern; sedation level; and skin color.	Respiratory depression may result from epidural narcotic use as long as 24 hours after initiation (Jurf and Nirschl, 1993).
➤ *CRITICAL DECISION POINT* Keep an ampule of naloxone (Narcan), 0.4 mg, a strong opioid antagonist, at the bedside to use in case of emergency to counteract adverse reactions. Give naloxone in incremental doses to improve respiratory function. Reversal of analgesic effect may result in acute withdrawal and pain (Jacox et al., 1994).	
b. Monitor blood pressure and pulse.	Postural hypotension and minor heart rate changes may occur with narcotic use.
c. Monitor intake and output. Assess for bladder distention. Observe for frequency or urgency.	Urinary retention may occur as a result of effects of narcotic on spinal nerves innervating bladder.
d. Observe for pruritus, especially of face, head, neck, and torso.	Itching may be caused by histamine release or disturbances in cutaneous sensation because of binding of opiate receptors in spinal cord (Wild and Coyne, 1992).

STEPS	RATIONALE
e. Observe for nausea and vomiting.	Nausea and vomiting can begin 4 to 6 hours after a bolus because of time needed for drug to reach chemoreceptor trigger zone. Nausea from epidural analgesia is exacerbated by movement.
3. Check insertion site for clear or bloody drainage. Assess for complaints of headache.	Headache and cerebrospinal fluid leakage can occur from a dural puncture. Bloody drainage may occur if catheter has migrated into a vessel.
4. Monitor temperature. Observe insertion site for signs of inflammation.	Infection can occur from poor sterile technique or systemic bacteremia.
5. Evaluate for paresthesias.	Excessive analgesia, infusion of drugs toxic to central nervous system, or contact of catheter with neural tissue may cause sensory deficits (Acute Pain Management Guideline Panel, 1992).
6. Unexpected outcomes that may occur include:	
➤ Client states pain is still present.	Primary causes are insufficient drug dose or catheter blockage, breakage, or improper position. With continuous infusion, pump may be malfunctioning or tubing may not be patent.
➤ Client is lethargic or not easily aroused.	Client may be oversedated.
➤ Client experiences periods of apnea or respirations are less than 8 breaths/min, shallow, or irregular.	These are signs of respiratory depression from oversedation. Dosage will need adjustment (Acute Pain Management Guideline Panel, 1992).
➤ Client suddenly complains of headache. Clear drainage is present on epidural dressing or more than 1 ml of fluid can be aspirated from catheter.	Probable indication that catheter has migrated and punctured the dura. Stop infusion or injection, keep client flat, and notify physician (Naber, Jones, and Halm, 1994).
➤ Blood is present on epidural dressing or can be aspirated from catheter.	Probable indication that catheter has punctured a vessel. Stop infusion and notify physician.
➤ Redness, warmth, tenderness, swelling, or exudate is noted at catheter insertion site. Client is febrile.	These are signs of local or systemic infection. Notify physician (Woodin, 1993). Catheter will need to be removed.
➤ Client experiences minimal urinary output, urinary frequency or urgency, bladder distention, pruritus, and nausea and vomiting.	These are side effects of medication. Dosage needs to be altered or side effects managed by other treatments or medications.

Reporting and Recording

1. Record drug, dose, and time given (if injection) or time begun and ended (if infusion) on appropriate medication record. Specify concentration and diluent.	Timely documentation prevents errors.
2. Record any supplemental analgesic requirements.	Client's dosage may need to be adjusted.
3. Record medication on narcotic record.	Control and dispensation of narcotics are regulated by the Controlled Substances Act.
4. With continuous infusion, obtain and record pump "readout" hourly for first 24 hours after infusion is begun and then every 4 hours.	Frequent evaluation is necessary until nurse is certain that client has received proper dosage and is stabilized. Policy on frequency may vary from institution to institution; follow institution's guidelines.
5. Record regular periodic assessments of client's status in nurses' notes or on appropriate flow sheets (Fig. 5-11). Indicate:	Forms may vary from institution to institution, but information recorded will be the same. Follow institution's policy related to frequency of assessments.
a. Vital signs b. Intake and output c. Sedation level d. Pain status e. Neurological status f. Status of epidural site	Provides data to evaluate client's response to pain therapy by epidural route.

STEPS	RATIONALE
g. Presence or absence of adverse reactions to medication	
h. Presence or absence of complications resulting from placement and maintenance of epidural catheter	
6. Report any adverse reactions or complications to physician.	Reaction or complication may require therapeutic intervention or dosage regulation.

Follow-up Activities

1. Reassess client's comfort level and response to treatment at least every 4 hours or more frequently if condition warrants.
2. Assess sedation level and respiratory rate and depth hourly for first 24 hours after initiation and then every 4 hours, since respiratory depression from epidural analgesia can last as long as 24 hours.

MEMORIAL MEDICAL CENTER
Springfield, Illinois

EPIDURAL ANALGESIA FLOW SHEET

Analgesic Drug Used:

____ Duramorph (____mcg/ml)
✓ Fentanyl (10 mcg/ml)
____ Hydromorphone (____mcg/ml)
____ Sufentanil (____mcg/ml)

Device In Use:

____ Abbott PCA (mcg units)
____ Bard PCA (ml units)

Date	5/3	5/3													
Time	09	13													
Mode: B = Bolus, P = PCA, C = Continuous, P + C = PCA + Continuous	P+C	P+C													
Manual Bolus by MD (Drug/Dose)	3mcg	—													
Volume in Bag	100	60													
Volume Infused	—	40													
Concentration	0.0	0.0	0.0	0.0	0.0	0.0	0.0	0.0	0.0	0.0	0.0	0.0	0.0	0.0	0.0
PCA Dose (ml)	1.0	1.0													
Delay (min)	20	20													
Basal Rate	10	10													
One Hour Limit	13	13													
Sedation Level	2	3													
Analgesic Level	7	3													
Complications	—	—													
Initials	JD	JD													
RN Signature	J. Davenport, RN														

Sedation Level
1 = wide awake
2 = drowsy
3 = dozing intermittently
4 = mostly sleeping
5 = awakens only when aroused

Analgesic Level
1 2 3 4 5 6 7 8 9 10
1 = no pain; 10 = worst pain imaginable

Complications
1 = nausea
2 = vomiting
3 = pruritis
4 = unable to void
5 = headache
6 = respiratory depression
7 = ileus

Record of Waste & Spoilage

Date	Quantity	Describe in Detail	Signature #1	Signature #2

White copy to chart   Yellow copy to Pharmacy   Pink copy to Anesthesia Pain Service   Page 1 of 1

Fig. 5-11 Epidural analgesia flow sheet. (Courtesy Memorial Medical Center, Springfield, Ill.)

3. Follow institution's policy on frequency of epidural site dressing changes. (Dressings over temporary catheters are seldom changed unless complication arises, since catheter is usually left in place for only 24 to 72 hours; physician usually changes dressing in this case.)
4. With continuous infusion, monitor pump hourly for proper calibration and operation.
5. With continuous infusion, record volume of medication infused on "intake and output" record at least every 8 hours.
6. With continuous infusion, follow institution's policy on frequency of replacement of medication solution and tubing.

• • • • •

Special Considerations

- Keep patent IV or heparin lock in place until 24 hours after epidural analgesia has ended in case IV medications have to be given to counteract adverse reactions.
- A transcutaneous scopolamine patch or metoclopramide (Reglan), 10 mg IV, may be given for nausea.
- Oxygen and resuscitative equipment must be readily available in case of severe respiratory depression.
- Do not give other narcotics or other central nervous system depressants except as prescribed by the clinician responsible for epidural analgesia. Such medications may potentiate action of narcotic being administered epidurally.
- Apnea monitors and pulse oximeters may be used to detect potential respiratory depression (Naber, Jones, Halm, 1994).
- Urinary retention and bladder distention resulting from epidural analgesia may require catheterization of bladder.
- Conversion from IV morphine to epidural morphine dosing is approximately 10 to 1, although this dose varies from individual to individual. Client can experience withdrawal symptoms during conversion (Acute Pain Management Guideline Panel, 1992).

Teaching Considerations

- Describe catheter placement and use to client. Drawing or showing pictures helps.
- Teach client the purpose, action, and signs and symptoms of adverse reactions to narcotic to be administered.
- Teach client to report pain level using pain scale and to report any side effects.
- Inform client of other pain-management strategies that may supplement or enhance pharmacological intervention (e.g., imagery, distraction, relaxation).
- Explain that pain relief begins within 30 to 60 minutes of epidural injection and may last between 6 and 24 hours.
- Explain therapy to family or significant others so that they can support and assist client.
- Some clients may feel so much better after obtaining pain relief that they attempt to ambulate without assistance or to overdo their activities. Caution them to begin slowly to avoid injury.

Pediatric Considerations

- Research has demonstrated that children respond to pain in much the same way as adults. Yet pain in children is often undertreated because of unfounded concerns about narcotic dependency or potential side effects (McCaffery and Ferrell, 1992b). Undertreatment results in a deleterious postsurgical stress response in children; epidural analgesia has been shown to be safe and effective in providing postoperative analgesia in pediatric clients (Acute Pain Management Guideline Panel, 1992; Jacox et al., 1994).

Gerontologic Considerations

- Supplemental IV or IM dosages of narcotics used for breakthrough pain or inadequate analgesia must be given and titrated carefully because of possibility of additive or synergistic interactions, especially in older adults, who are sensitive to narcotics (Jacox et al., 1994).

Home Care Considerations

- Clients needing long-term or permanent therapy are discharged with a tunneled catheter. Before consideration of catheter placement in preparation for discharge and care in the home, several variables need to be assessed, including fine motor skills, cognitive ability, stage of disease and prognosis, and degree of involvement of family or significant others.
- Teach client and care giver proper dosage and administration of medication. Evaluating client's technique for catheter care and administering medication, as well as reinforcing instructions, are priorities.
- Explain pain assessment based on pain scale and available drug and dosage available for breakthrough pain. Inform client how to contact clinician for increase in dosage if highest level prescribed is ineffective.
- Teach client and care giver aseptic technique for narcotic administration and for all catheter care

procedures, including dressing changes. Instruct client to change dressing every week (policy will vary with home care agency). Teach signs and symptoms of infection and instruct client to report to nurse or physician immediately should signs and symptoms appear.

➤ Teach client and care giver about signs and symptoms of adverse reactions to narcotic being used and interventions that can be taken (Acute Pain Management Guideline Panel, 1992; Jacox et al, 1994):
- Respiratory depression: teach how to give IM naloxone.
- Urinary retention: teach how to perform straight catheterization and how to give SQ bethanechol (Urecholine) if prescribed.
- Pruritus: advise client to:
  Wear clean, lightweight cotton clothing.
  Keep room cool.
  Use cool moist compresses.
  Lubricate skin.
  Apply cornstarch.
  Use a medication if prescribed, for example, diphenhydramine (Benadryl), metoclopramide (Reglan), or prochlorperazine (Compazine).

➤ Give phone numbers of clinicians to contact in emergency.

CRITICAL THINKING EXERCISES

1. What factors that influence the pain experience make it difficult to assess accurately? What solutions can you suggest to avoid inaccuracies in assessing and evaluating a client's pain?
2. Identify the reasons nonpharmacological approaches to pain management are successful.
3. A 12-year-old client is scheduled for an appendectomy tomorrow. The child's mother tells you that the child has seldom been sick and has never had any surgery. A PCA device has been ordered after the surgery.
   a. What assessment data will be needed for determining the client's pain, methods of pain management, and teaching needs?
   b. What should be included in a teaching plan for this client?
4. A 68-year-old adult client with colon cancer has been admitted to your unit after undergoing a colon resection. An epidural catheter was inserted during surgery for postoperative pain management. The client reports having severe abdominal pain before surgery and asks if his pain is going to return.
   a. What teaching needs should be included in the nursing plan?
   b. What assessment data would you collect before giving an epidural analgesic injection?
   c. When evaluating the client receiving epidural analgesia, what signs and symptoms might indicate complications? What actions would you take?

REFERENCES

Acute Pain Management Guideline Panel: *Acute Pain Management: Operative or Medical Procedures and Trauma: clinical Practice Guideline,* AHCPR Pub No 92-0032, Rockville, Md, 1992, Agency for Health Care Policy and Research, Public Health Service, US Department of Health and Human Services.

Bachiocco V, Morselli A, Carli G: Self-control expectancy and postsurgical pain: relationships to previous pain, behavior in past pain, familial pain tolerance models, and personality, *J Pain Symptom Manage* 8(4):205, 1993.

Basler H-D: Group treatment for pain and discomfort, *Patient Educ Counsel* 20:167, 1993.

Copp L: An ethical responsibility for pain management, *J Adv Nurs* 18(1):1, 1993.

Cushing M: The legal side: pain management on trial, *Am J Nurs* 92(2):21, 1992.

Donovan MI, Miaskowski C: Striving for a standard of pain relief, *Am J Nurs* 92:106, 1992.

Dossey B: Psychophysiologic self-regulation. In Dossey B, Guzzetta C: *Cardiovascular nursing: holistic practice,* St Louis, 1992, Mosby.

Duchene P: Sensation, perception, and pain. In Hoeman S: *Rehabilitation nursing: process and application,* ed 2, St Louis, 1996, Mosby.

Egbert A, Lampros L, Parks L: Effects of patient-controlled analgesia on postoperative anxiety in elderly men, *Am J Crit Care* 2(2):118, 1993.

Ferrell B, Cronin N, Warfield C: The role of patient-controlled analgesia in the management of cancer pain, *J Pain Symptom Manage* 7(3):149, 1992.

Ferrell B, Rhiner M: Managing cancer pain: a three step approach, *Nurs 94* 24(7):57, 1994.

Ferrell-Torry A, Glick O: The use of therapeutic massage as a nursing intervention to modify anxiety and the perception of cancer pain, *Cancer Nurs* 16(2):93, 1993.

Gray B: Pain management, *Nurseweek Calif Nurs* 1:8, 1992.

Guyton-Simmons J, Ehrmin J: Problem solving in pain management by expert intensive care nurses, *Crit Care Nurse* 14(5):37, 1994.

International Association for the Study of Pain. Pain terms: a list with definitions and notes on usage, *Pain* 6:249, 1979.

Jacox A, Carr D, Payne R, et al: *Management of cancer pain: clinical practice guideline No 9,* Rockville, Md, 1994, Agency for Health Care Policy and Research, Public Health Service, US Department of Health and Human Services.

Jacox A, Ferrell B, et al: A guideline for the nation: managing acute pain, *Am J Nurs* 92:49, 1992.

Jones S: Effect of psychological processes on chronic pain, *Br J Nurs* 2(9):463, 1993.

Jurf J, Nirschl A: Acute postoperative pain management: a comprehensive review and update, *Crit Care Nurs Q* 16(1):8, 1993.

Kaiser K: Assessment and management of pain in the critically ill trauma patient, *Crit Care Nurs Q* 15(2):14, 1992.

Kohr J: Measuring your patient's pain, *RN* 58(4):39, 1995.

Lazzara D: Patient-controlled analgesia in the intensive care unit, *Crit Care Nurs Q* 16(1):26, 1993.

Lueckenotte A: *Gerontologic nursing,* St Louis, 1996, Mosby.

Maxam-Moore V, Wilkie D, Woods S: Analgesics for cardiac surgery patients in critical care: describing current practice, *Am J Crit Care* 3(1):31, 1994.

McCaffery M: Response to "Quantification of the effects of listening to music as a noninvasive method of pain control," *Scholarly Inquiry Nurs Pract* 6(1):59, 1992a.

McCaffery M: RN's assessment is critical in pain control, *Am Nurs* 24:4, 1992b.

McCaffery M, Beebe A: *Pain: clinical manual for nursing practice,* St Louis, 1989, Mosby.

McCaffery M, Ferrell BR: Opioid analgesics: nurses' knowledge of doses and psychological dependence, *J Nurs Staff Develop* 8:77, 1992a.

McCaffery M, Ferrell BR: How vital are vital signs? *Nursing* 22:43, 1992b.

Meintz S: Whatever became of the back rub? *RN* 58(4):49, 1995.

Naber L, Jones G, Halm M: Epidural analgesia for effective pain control, *Crit Care Nurse* 14(5):69, 77, 1994.

National Institute of Nursing Research: *Symptom management: acute pain,* Bethesda, Md, 1994, Public Health Service, National Institutes of Health, US Department of Health and Human Services.

Nossel M: Chronic nonmalignant pain management. In Salerno E, Willens J: *Pain management handbook: an interdisciplinary approach,* St Louis, 1996, Mosby.

Oschsenreither J, Cubina M: Pediatric pain management. In Salerno E, Willens J: *Pain management handbook: an interdisciplinary approach,* St Louis, 1996, Mosby.

Puntillo K: Dimensions of procedural pain and its analgesic management in critically ill surgical patients, *Am J Crit Care* 3(2):116, 1994.

Snyder M, Burns K: Interventions for decreasing agitation behaviors in persons with dementia, *J Gerontol Nurs* 21(7):34, 1995.

Stanik-Hutt J: Strategies for pain management in traumatic thoracic injuries, *Crit Care Nurs Clin North Am* 5(4):713, 1993.

Stephens R: Imagery: a strategic intervention to empower clients. II. A practical guide, *Clin Nurse Specialist* 7(5):235, 1993.

Tiernan P: Independent nursing interventions: relaxation and guided imagery in critical care, *Crit Care Nurse* 14(5):47, 1994.

Tittle M, McMillan S: Pain and pain related side effects in an ICU and on a surgical unit: nursing management, *Am J Crit Care* 3(1):25, 1994.

Vallerand A: Gender differences in pain, *Image: J Nurs Sch* 27(3):235, 1995.

Vanier M, Labrecque G, Lepage-Savary D, et al: Comparison of hydromorphone continuous subcutaneous infusion and basal rate subcutaneous infusion plus PCA in cancer pain: a pilot study, *Pain* 53(1):27, 1993.

Voight L, Paice J, Pouliot J: Standardized pain flowsheet: impact on patient-reported pain experiences after cardiovascular surgery, *Am J Crit Care* 4(4):308, 1995.

Waters L: Pharmacologic strategies for managing pain in children, *Orthop Nurs* 11:34, 1992.

Whipple B, Glynn N: Quantification of the effects of listening to music as a noninvasive method of pain control, *Scholarly Inquiry Nurs Pract* 6(1):43, 1992.

Wild L, Coyne C: The basics and beyond: epidural analgesia, *Am J Nurs* 92:26, 1992.

Wilkie D, Boss B: Pain: nursing assessment and role in management. In Lewis S, Collier I, Heitkemper M: *Medical-surgical nursing: assessment and management of clinical problems,* ed 4, St Louis, 1996, Mosby.

Woodin L: Cutting postop pain, *RN* 56(8):26, 1993.

ADDITIONAL READING

ANA statements focus on pain, *Am Nurs* 24:7, 1992.

Gordon S, Gaines S, Hauber, R: Self-administered versus nurse-administered epidural analgesia after cesarean section, *J Obstet Gynecol Neonatal Nurs* 23(2):99, 1994.

Greenland S: A review of the uses of epidural analgesia, *Nurs Standard* 9(32):32, 1995.

Gujol M: A survey of pain assessment and management practices among critical care nurses, *Am J Crit Care* 3(2):123, 1994.

Hekmat N, Burke M, Howell S: Preventive pain management in the postoperative hand surgery patient, *Orthop Nurs* 13(3):37, 1994.

Meehan D, McRae M, Rourke D, et al: Analgesic administration, pain intensity, and patient satisfaction in cardiac surgical patients, *Am J Crit Care* 4(6):435, 1995.

Potter P, Perry A: *Fundamentals of nursing: concepts, process, and practice,* ed 4, St Louis, 1997, Mosby.

Salerno E, Willens J: *Pain management handbook: an interdisciplinary approach,* St Louis, 1996, Mosby.

Selby T: Guidelines address pain management, *Am Nurs* 24:1, 1992.

Timmons M, Bowen F: The effect of structured preoperative teaching on patients' use of patient-controlled analgesia (PCA) and their management of pain, *Orthop Nurs* 12(1):23, 1993.

Walker J: Caring for elderly people with persistent pain in the community: a qualitative perspective on the attitudes of patients and nurses, *Health Soc Care* 2(4):221, 1993.

Unit III

Hygiene

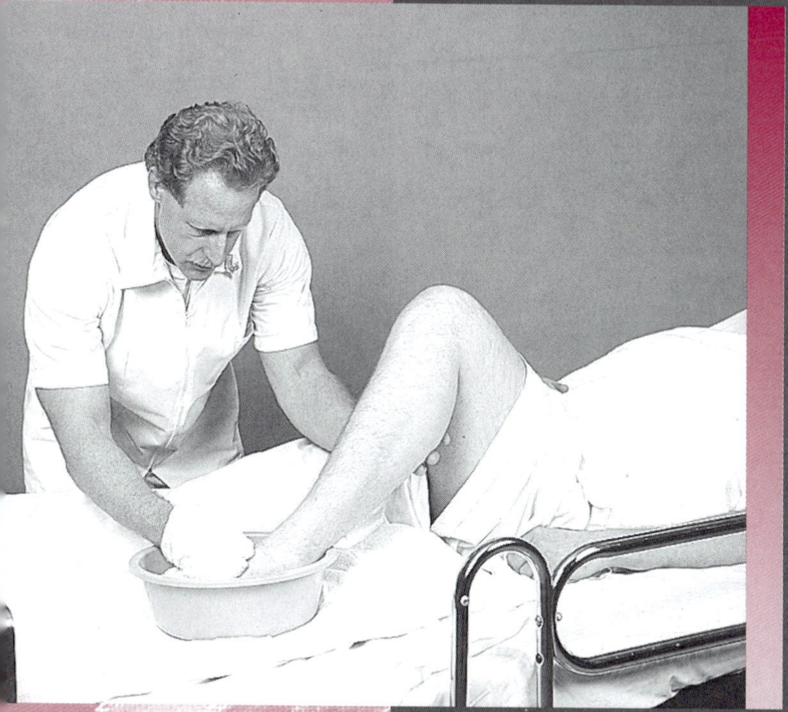

CHAPTER 6

Bathing and Skin Care

OBJECTIVES

Mastery of content in this chapter will enable the nurse to:

- Define key terms.
- Discuss guidelines used to provide hygiene care to clients.
- Identify principles of aseptic technique applied while administering a bed bath.
- Administer a complete bed bath.
- Explain precautions to take while assisting clients with a tub bath or shower.
- Record pertinent observations made while bathing clients.
- Administer perineal care to male and female clients.
- Identify guidelines to follow when administering mouth care.
- Explain differences in providing oral care to dependent versus unconscious clients.
- Administer oral hygiene correctly to a client.
- Discuss precautions used to prevent breakage of dentures.
- Identify guidelines for administering hair, nail, and foot care.
- Comb and brush a client's hair.
- Shampoo the hair of a bedridden client.
- Shave a male or female client.
- Identify risk factors for foot and nail problems.
- Safely administer nail care.

SKILLS

6-1 Bathing a Client
6-2 Providing Perineal Care
6-3 Brushing Teeth
6-4 Performing Mouth Care for the Unconscious or Debilitated Client
6-5 Cleaning Dentures
6-6 Shampooing the Hair of a Bedridden Client
6-7 Shaving a Client
6-8 Performing Nail and Foot Care

KEY TERMS

Alopecia
Aspiration
Buccal
Cerumen
Cheilosis
Conjunctivitis
Cuticle
Dandruff
Débridement
Dental caries
Dentifrice
Dermatitis
Devitalized tissue
Episiotomy
Exudate
Febrile
Flossing
Fontanel
Gag reflex
Gingivae
Gingivitis
Granulation tissue
Halitosis
Hygiene
Maceration
Mastication
Melanocyte
Microvasculature
Necrotic
NPO
Orthopedic
Pediculosis
Periodontal
Periodontitis
Plaque
Podiatrist
Pruritus
Sebaceous gland
Seborrheic dermatitis
Sebum
Stomatitis
Tartar
Tepid
Vellus

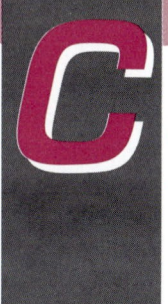

Many clients require assistance with personal hygiene or must learn hygiene techniques. **Hygiene** is the science of health. Maintenance of personal hygiene is necessary for an individual's comfort, safety, and sense of well-being.

Hygiene practices are congruent with health promotion. The nurse's role is to maintain or assist the client to maintain the integrity of skin surfaces so that skin cells receive the nutrition and hydration needed to resist injury and disease. To provide skin care, the nurse should understand the structure and function of the skin.

BATHING AND SKIN CARE

An active organ, the skin's functions include protection, secretion, excretion, temperature regulation, and sensation. Three primary layers make up the skin: the epidermis, dermis, and subcutaneous tissue. The skin covers the entire surface of the body and is continuous with mucous membranes of the mouth, eyes, ears, nose, vagina, and rectum. Thorough hygiene is essential for the integrity and function of each skin layer.

The epidermis, or outer skin layer, contains several thin layers of cells undergoing different stages of maturation. The innermost layer continually produces new cells that migrate to the outer layer, the corpus stratum, where dead cells are shed from the epidermal surface.

Bacteria reside on the skin's outer surface. These resident bacteria are normal flora that do not cause disease, but inhibit multiplication of disease-causing microorganisms. Transient bacteria that arise from objects coming in contact with the skin are also present. Bathing removes dead cells and bacteria and helps maintain skin integrity.

The dermis contains bundles of collagen and elastic fibers to support the epidermis. Nerve fibers, blood vessels, sweat glands, **sebaceous glands,** and hair follicles are found in the dermis. Sebaceous glands secrete **sebum,** an oily, odorous fluid, into the hair follicles. Sebum lubricates skin and hair. Two types of sweat glands, the eccrine and the apocrine glands, are distributed over the skin's surface. Eccrine glands secrete a watery fluid (sweat) that assists in temperature control through evaporation. The apocrine glands secrete sweat in the axillary and genital areas. Bacterial decomposition of sweat from the apocrine glands causes body odor.

The subcutaneous tissue layer contains blood vessels, nerves, lymph tissue, and loose connective tissue filled with fat cells. Fatty tissue insulates the body. Subcutaneous tissue also provides support for upper skin layers.

Because a portion of the skin is usually exposed to environmental irritants and because the skin is an active organ sensitive to physiological changes within the body, some skin problems commonly occur (Table 6-1). The nurse should look for the presence of such conditions while providing hygiene and should suggest measures to alleviate these conditions. The client is always the best resource to explain the nature and course of skin problems as they develop. Skin problems can cause changes that affect a client's appearance and body image. The nurse should be sensitive to the client's feelings while attempting to care for a skin problem.

MOUTH CARE

The oral cavity, which is lined with a normally moist, intact mucous membrane, contains the teeth and gums. The membranous lining, composed of both epithelial and connective tissue, protects underlying organs, secretes mucus to keep the oral cavity lubricated, and absorbs water, salts, and other solutes. Saliva, a clear viscous fluid secreted by the mucous and salivary glands of the mouth, moistens the oral cavity, initiates digestion of starches, provides a means for removing cellular and bacterial debris, and aids in the chewing and swallowing of food. The buffer capacity of saliva protects the gums and teeth. Normally the mucosa is light pink and moist.

The teeth are organs of chewing, or **mastication.** Dentin, a hard, ivory-like substance that surrounds the pulp cavity (Fig. 6-1), forms the major part of a tooth. A layer of enamel, visible in the oral cavity, covers the upper portion of the tooth, or crown. The **periodontal** membrane, just below the gum margins, surrounds the tooth root and holds it firmly in place. A tooth receives its blood, lymph, and nerve supply from the base of the tooth socket within the jaw. Healthy teeth are smooth, shiny, and properly aligned.

The gums, or **gingivae,** are mucous membranes with underlying supportive fibrous tissue. They encircle the necks of erupted teeth to hold them firmly in place. The gums are normally pink, moist, firm, and relatively inelastic.

Structures of the oral cavity must remain healthy for a person's comfort, sense of well-being, maintenance of nutrition, and protection from infection. Even a minor alteration of the oral cavity, such as inflammation of the gums, can create a significant health problem. Appetite is diminished, and the discomfort from inflammation can become

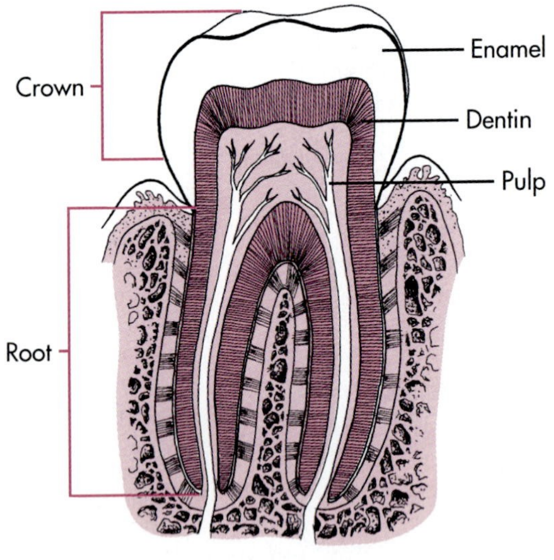

Fig. 6-1 A normal tooth.

Table 6-1 Common Skin Problems

Problem	Characteristics	Implications	Interventions
Dry skin	Flaky, rough texture on exposed areas such as hands, arms, legs, or face.	Skin may become infected if epidermal layer is allowed to crack.	Bathe less frequently. Use superfatted soap (e.g., Dove) for cleansing (Hardy, 1990). Rinse body of all soap well, because residue left can cause irritation and breakdown. Add moisture to air through use of humidifier. Increase fluid intake when skin is dry. Use moisturizing lotion to aid healing process; lotion forms protective barrier and helps maintain fluid within skin. Use creams to clean skin that is dry or irritated by soaps and detergents.
Acne	Inflammatory, papulopustular skin eruption, usually involving bacterial breakdown of sebum; appears on face, neck, shoulders, and back.	Infected material within pustule can spread if area is squeezed or picked. Permanent scarring can result.	Wash hair and skin each day with hot water and soap to remove oil. Use cosmetics sparingly because oily cosmetics or creams accumulate in pores and tend to make condition worse. Dietary restrictions may need to be implemented. Foods found to aggravate condition should be eliminated from diet. Exposure to ultraviolet rays, either from sunshine or heat lamp, may help control acne; use caution to prevent burning of skin. Use prescribed topical antibiotics for severe acne.
Hirsutism	Excessive growth of body and facial hair, especially in women.	Hirsutism may cause negative body image by giving female a male appearance.	The following may be used to remove unwanted hair: depilatories (can cause infection, rashes, or dermatitis), shaving (safest method), electrolysis (permanently removes hair by destroying hair follicles), tweezing (lasts temporarily), and bleaching (lasts temporarily).
Skin rashes	Skin eruption that may result from overexposure to sun or moisture or from allergic reaction; may be flat or raised, localized or systemic, pruritic or nonpruritic.	If skin is continually scratched, inflammation and infection may occur. Rashes can also cause discomfort.	Wash area thoroughly and apply antiseptic spray or lotion to prevent further itching and aid healing process. Warm soaks may relieve inflammation.
Contact dermatitis	Inflammation of skin characterized by abrupt onset with erythema, pruritus, pain, and appearance of scaly oozing lesions; seen on face, neck, hands, forearms, and genitalia.	Dermatitis is often difficult to eliminate because person is usually in continual contact with substance causing skin reaction. Substance may be hard to identify.	Condition usually disappears when exposure to causative agents (e.g., cleansers, soaps) is avoided.
Abrasion	Scraping or rubbing away of epidermis; may result in localized bleeding and later weeping of serous fluid.	Infection occurs easily as result of loss of protective skin layer.	Nurses should always be careful not to scratch clients with their jewelry or fingernails. Wash abrasions with mild soap and water. Dressing or bandage could increase risk of infection because of retained moisture.

an annoying irritant. Thorough oral hygiene maintains the integrity of oral cavity structures.

The nurse assists clients to maintain good oral hygiene by teaching correct techniques or by actually performing hygiene for weakened or disabled clients. Educating clients about common gum and tooth disorders and methods of prevention may motivate them to follow good oral hygiene practices. It may be necessary for the nurse to refer clients to a dentist for problems requiring special care.

HAIR CARE

Hair grows from follicles located within the dermis of the skin (Fig. 6-2). Tiny blood vessels supply each follicle with nourishment necessary for normal hair growth. Each hair

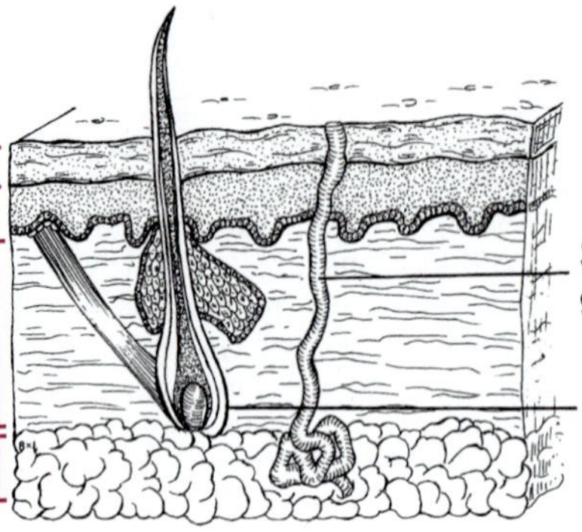

Fig. 6-2 Cross section of hair follicle and supporting structures.

has a shaft extending from the follicle. Sebaceous glands secrete sebum, an oily substance, into each follicle, which lubricates the hair and scalp. The hair shaft is normally shiny and pliant and is not excessively oily, dry, or brittle.

The primary function of hair is protection. For example, hair protects the scalp from injury and the sun's rays. Eyebrows and eyelashes protect the eyes from foreign particles.

Two types of hair cover the body. Terminal hair is the long, coarse, thick hair that is easily visible on the scalp, axillae, and pubic area. Special hair care practices focus primarily on care of terminal hair. **Vellus** is the soft, fine hair that covers the entire body except for the palms of the hands, fingertips, soles of the feet, tips of the toes, and part of the genitalia. Hair growth, distribution, and pattern can be indicators of a person's health status. Hormonal changes, emotional and physical stress, aging, gender, race, infection, and certain diseases can affect hair characteristics. The hair shaft is an inert structure; any change in its color or condition occurs as a result of hormonal activity and nutrient supply to the hair follicle. For example, a reduction in the serum protein level will result in hair becoming dry and brittle.

A person's appearance and sense of well-being often depend on the way the hair looks and feels. Illness or disability may prevent clients from maintaining daily hair care. An immobilized client's hair soon becomes tangled if not brushed or combed regularly. Dressings may leave sticky adhesive, blood, or antiseptic solutions on the hair. Diaphoresis leaves hair oily and unmanageable. Proper hair care is important to a person's body image. Brushing, combing, shampooing, and shaving are basic hygiene measures.

GUIDELINES

1. Bathe body parts as soon as they become soiled. Problems such as incontinence, wound drainage, or excessive diaphoresis may require bathing several times a day.
2. Attempt to provide baths during the time of day that the client prefers.
3. Protect clients from injury by assessing and controlling the bath water temperature.
4. Wear gloves whenever there is risk of contacting body fluids.
5. Control environmental factors that may alter skin integrity, such as moisture, heat, and external sources of pressure (wrinkled bed linen, improperly placed drainage tubing).
6. Encourage clients to participate in bathing and skin care to maintain independence with self-care.
7. If the client is unable to participate in bathing and skin care, involve the family or significant other.
8. Establish a regular routine that the client can easily follow at home. Ideal dental hygiene requires brushing after every meal and before bed and flossing at least once a day, the ideal being after each meal.
9. Use dental hygiene products of the client's choice whenever possible.
10. Remember that dental hygiene can be a means for improving the client's comfort level. Persons who are mouth breathers, are using oxygen, are unable to eat or drink, have nasogastric tubes inserted, or have had trauma or surgery of the mouth will benefit from frequent oral care.
11. Use the time spent providing mouth care to teach clients about factors that increase the incidence of dental or gum disease and the techniques that ensure good oral hygiene.
12. Consider clients' cultural preferences in regard to grooming techniques. For example, women of some cultures shave the hair on their legs, whereas others prefer to keep their legs unshaven.
13. Respect clients' preferences for grooming products. However, the nurse may have opportunities to caution against use of products that can damage or injure hair and nails.
14. Consider clients' normal grooming routines. Incorporate their schedule into the care plan.

SKILL 6-1 Bathing a Client

Nurses provide two categories of baths: cleansing and therapeutic. Cleansing baths are usually given in the morning before scheduled tests or procedures. However, some clients may prefer bathing in the evening. In addition to cleansing the skin, the bath stimulates circulation and reduces body odor by removing secretions, perspiration, and bacteria from the skin. Self-image is therefore restored. While bathing the client, the nurse can get to know the client better and interact therapeutically. Further assessments can be made, and joint range of motion (ROM) exercises can be performed.

The type of cleansing bath a nurse provides depends on the client's physical capabilities and the degree of hygiene required. The nurse is responsible for assessing what type of bath is most appropriate for the client's needs.

Bathing of skin surfaces affords a client considerable comfort. However, depending on the condition of the hair and nails, the client may not feel completely clean. When a person is unable to perform personal care during illness or disability, it becomes the nurse's responsibility to assist with cleaning and grooming hair, shaving, and soaking and trimming nails. Many of the procedures can be done during or immediately after a bath. Clients may appreciate having their hair combed or feet soaked any time during the day to maintain an attractive appearance or to promote comfort. The client should be encouraged to make decisions regarding need and frequency of hygienic care. Types of cleansing baths include:

- *Complete bed bath*—Administered to clients who are totally dependent. The nurse gives the bath with the client in bed.
- *Partial bed bath*—Consists of bathing only body parts that would cause discomfort if left unbathed, such as hands, face, axillae, and perineal area. Dependent clients in need of partial hygiene or self-sufficient bedridden clients who are unable to reach all body parts receive a partial bed bath.
- *Tub bath*—Client is immersed in a tub of water. The tub bath allows more thorough washing and rinsing than a bed bath. Client may still require the nurse's assistance. Tubs are available that facilitate lifting dependent clients into the water.
- *Shower*—Client sits or stands under a continuous stream of water. The shower provides more thorough cleansing than a bed bath.

Therapeutic baths are generally ordered by physicians for a specific effect, such as soothing the skin or promoting healing.

Types of therapeutic baths include:

- *Sitz bath*—Cleanses and reduces pain and inflammation of perineal and anal areas. Used for client who has undergone rectal or perineal surgery, childbirth, or who has local irritation from hemorrhoids or fissures. The client sits in a special tub or basin.
- *Medicated bath (oatmeal, cornstarch, sodium bicarbonate, Aveeno, Burow's solution)*—Aids in relief of skin irritation and creates an antibacterial and drying effect. Oatmeal has added effect of softening and lubricating the skin.

EQUIPMENT

- **Two washcloths**
- **Two bath towels**
- **Bath blanket**
- **Soap and soap dish**
- **Toiletry items (deodorant, powder, lotion, cologne)**
- **Warm water**
- **Clean hospital gown or client's own pajamas or gown**
- **Laundry bag**
- **Disposable gloves (when risk for contacting body fluids)**

DELEGATION CONSIDERATIONS

Skills of bathing can be delegated to unlicensed assistive personnel.

- Inform care provider about early signs of impaired skin integrity and tell provider to have nurse reassess the skin when changes are noted.
- Caution care provider to use warm water.
- Review procedure for application of moisturizing lotions.
- Do not massage reddened areas.

STEPS	RATIONALE
ASSESSMENT	
1. Assess client's tolerance for activity, discomfort level, cognitive ability, and musculoskeletal function.	Determines client's ability to perform self-care and level of assistance required from nurse. Also determines type of bath to administer (e.g., tub bath or partial bed bath).

CRITICAL DECISION POINT Clients whose levels of independence and mobility change frequently require more assistance during bathing.

STEPS	RATIONALE
2. Assess client's bathing preferences: frequency of and time of day bathing preferred, type of hygiene products used, and other factors related to cultural diversity.	Client participates in plan of care. Promotes client's comfort and willingness to cooperate.
3. Ask if client has noticed any problems related to condition of skin.	Allows nurse to direct physical assessment of skin during bathing.
4. Identify risks for skin impairment: a. Immobilization (e.g., clients who have paralysis, immobilized extremities, traction; weakened or disabled clients) b. Reduced sensation (e.g., paresthesias, circulatory insufficiency, neuropathies) c. Nutritional and hydration alterations d. Excessive moisture secretion or excretion on skin, particularly on skin surfaces that rub against each other (e.g., under breasts, in perineal area) e. Vascular insufficiency f. External devices applied to or around skin (e.g., casts, braces, restraints, dressings, catheters, tubes) g. Older adult clients h. Friction (sliding down in bed) i. Incontinence (bowel or bladder) j. Allergies	Risk factors increase the likelihood of injury to the skin because of pressure, impaired tissue synthesis, softening of or friction on tissues, and impaired circulation.
5. Assess client's knowledge of skin hygiene in terms of its importance, preventive measures to take, and common problems encountered (Table 6-1).	Determines client's learning needs.
6. Check physician's therapeutic bath order for type of solution, length of time for bath, body part to be attended.	Therapeutic baths are ordered for specific physical effect, which may include promotion of healing or soothing effect.
7. Review orders for specific precautions concerning client's movement or positioning.	Prevents accidental injury to client during bathing activities. Determines level of assistance required by client.

NURSING DIAGNOSIS

Clustering of defining characteristics from the assessment data may reveal the following nursing diagnoses for clients requiring this skill:

- Activity intolerance
- Bathing/hygiene self-care deficit
- Impaired skin integrity
- Knowledge deficit regarding skin care
- Risk for impaired skin integrity

Related factors are individualized based on a client's condition or needs.

PLANNING

STEPS	RATIONALE
1. Expected outcomes following completion of procedure:	
➤ Skin is clean, dry, elastic, well hydrated, and without areas of local inflammation.	Indicates intact integument.
➤ Previous skin lesions are cleaner, with less drainage. Sizes of lesions do not change after one bathing.	
➤ Joint ROM remains same or improves from previous measurement.	Important measure for bed rest clients prone to contractures.
➤ Client expresses sense of comfort and relaxation.	Bath relaxes client and removes sources of discomfort.
➤ Client tolerates bath without fatigue or chilling.	
➤ Client describes benefits and techniques of proper hygiene and skin care.	Demonstrates learning.

STEPS	RATIONALE
2. Explain procedure and ask client for suggestions on how to prepare supplies. If partial bath, ask how much of bath client wishes to complete.	Promotes client's cooperation and participation.
3. Adjust room temperature and ventilation, close room doors and windows, and draw room divider curtain.	Warm room that is free of drafts prevents rapid loss of body heat during bathing. Privacy ensures client's mental and physical comfort.
4. Prepare equipment and supplies.	Avoids interrupting procedure or leaving client unattended to retrieve missing equipment.

IMPLEMENTATION

COMPLETE OR PARTIAL BED BATH

STEPS	RATIONALE
1. Offer client bedpan or urinal. Provide towel and washcloth.	Client will feel more comfortable after voiding. Prevents interruption of bath.
2. Wash hands.	Reduces transmission of microorganisms.
CRITICAL DECISION POINT Apply gloves if drainage or secretions appear on client's skin.	
3. Lower side rail closest to you and assist client in assuming comfortable position, maintaining body alignment. Bring client toward side closest to nurse. Place hospital bed in high position.	Aids nurse's access to client. Maintains client's comfort throughout procedure. Nurse does not have to reach across bed, thus minimizing strain on back muscles.
4. Loosen top covers at foot of bed. Place bath blanket over top sheet. Fold and remove top sheet from under blanket. If possible, have client hold bath blanket while withdrawing sheet.	Removal of top linens prevents their becoming soiled or moist during bath. Blanket provides warmth and privacy.
5. If top sheet is to be reused, fold it for replacement later. If not, dispose in laundry bag, taking care not to allow linen to contact uniform.	Proper disposal prevents transmission of microorganisms.
6. Remove client's gown or pajamas. If an extremity is injured or has reduced mobility, begin removal from *unaffected* side. If client has IV tube, remove gown from arm *without* IV first; then lower IV container and slide gown covering affected arm over tubing and container. Rehang IV container and check flow rate (see illustrations).	Provides full exposure of body parts during bathing. Undressing unaffected side first allows easier manipulation of gown over body part with reduced ROM.

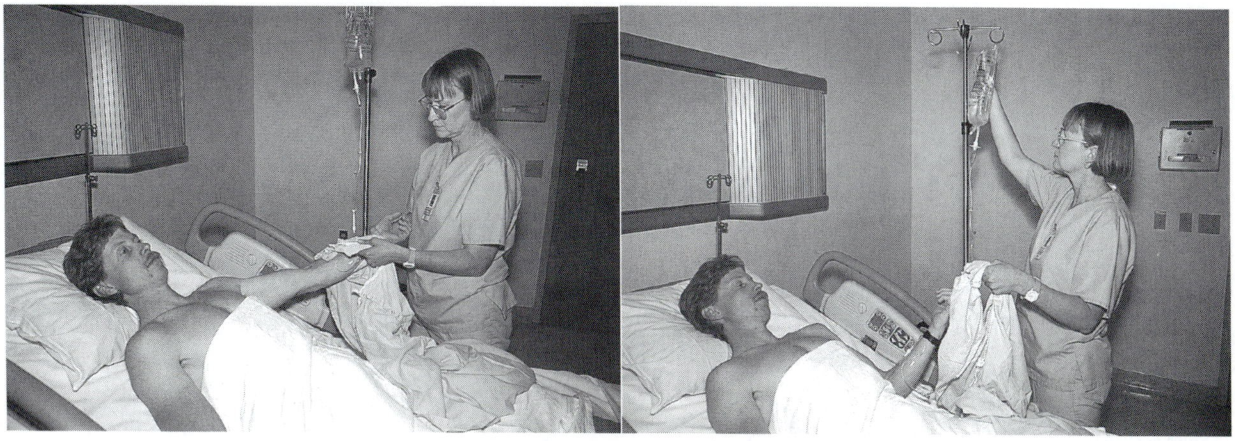

Step 6

Continued

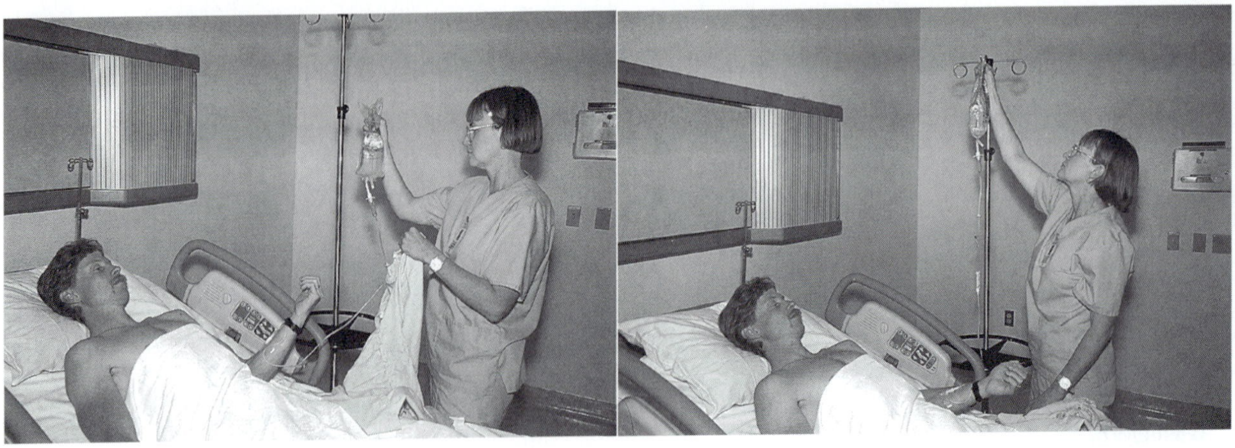

Step 6, cont'd

STEPS	RATIONALE
7. Pull side rail up. Fill washbasin two thirds full, with warm water. Have client place fingers in water to test temperature tolerance. Place plastic container of bath lotion in bath water to warm, if desired.	Raising side rail maintains client's safety as nurse leaves bedside. Warm water promotes comfort, relaxes muscles, and prevents unnecessary chilling. Testing temperature prevents accidental burns. Bath water warms lotion for application to client's skin.
8. Remove pillow if allowed and raise head of bed 30 to 45 degrees. Place bath towel under client's head. Place second bath towel over client's chest.	Removal of pillow makes it easier to wash client's ears and neck. Placement of towels prevents soiling of bed linen and bath blanket.
9. Fold washcloth around fingers of nurse's hand to form mitt (see illustration). Immerse mitt in water and wring thoroughly.	Mitt retains water and heat better than loosely held washcloth; keeps cold edges from brushing against client, and prevents splashing.
10. Wash client's eyes with plain warm water. Inquire if client is wearing contact lenses. If so, perform eye care as described in Chapter 9. Use different section of mitt for each eye. Move mitt from inner to outer canthus (see illustration). Soak any crusts on eyelid for 2 to 3 minutes with damp cloth before attempting removal. Dry eye thoroughly but gently.	Soap irritates eyes. Use of separate sections of mitt reduces infection transmission. Bathing eye from inner to outer canthus prevents secretions from entering nasolacrimal duct. Pressure can cause internal injury.

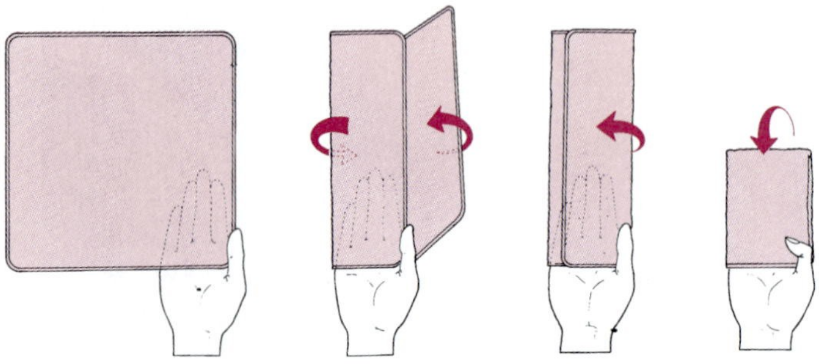

Step 9

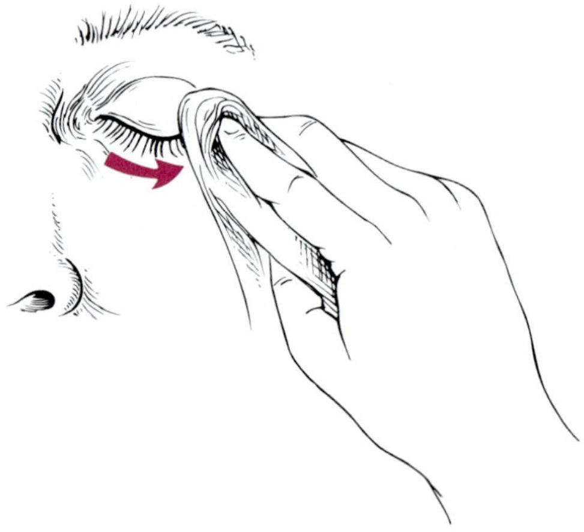

Step 10

STEPS	RATIONALE
11. Ask if client prefers to use soap on face. Wash, rinse, and dry well forehead, cheeks, nose, neck, and ears. (Men may wish to shave at this point or after bath.)	Soap tends to dry face, which is exposed to air more than other body parts.
12. Remove bath blanket from client's arm that is farthest from nurse. Place bath towel lengthwise under arm. Raise side rail and move to other side to wash arm if desired.	Bathing far side first prevents reaching over clean area.
13. Bathe arm with soap and water using long, firm strokes from distal to proximal areas (fingers to axilla). Raise and support arm above head (if possible) while thoroughly washing axilla.	Soap lowers surface tension and facilitates removal of debris and bacteria when friction is applied during washing. Long, firm strokes stimulate circulation. Movement of arm exposes axilla and exercises joint's normal ROM.
14. Rinse and dry arm and axilla thoroughly. If client uses deodorant or talcum powder, apply it.	Alkaline residue from soap discourages growth of normal skin bacteria (Barnes, 1987). Excess moisture causes skin maceration or softening. Deodorant controls body odor.
15. Fold bath towel in half and lay it on bed beside client. Place basin on towel. Immerse client's hand in water. Allow hand to soak for 3 to 5 minutes before washing hand and fingernails (see Skill 6-8). Remove basin and dry hand well.	Soaking softens cuticles and calluses of hand, loosens debris beneath nails, and enhances feeling of cleanliness. Thorough drying removes moisture from between fingers.
16. Raise side rail and move to other side of bed. Lower side rail and repeat steps 12 through 15 for other arm.	
17. Check temperature of bath water and change water if necessary.	Warm water maintains client's comfort.
CRITICAL DECISION POINT **If client is at risk for falling, be sure side rails are up before obtaining fresh water.**	
18. Cover client's chest with bath towel and fold bath blanket down to umbilicus. With one hand, lift edge of towel away from chest. With mitted hand, bathe chest using long, firm strokes. Take special care to wash skinfolds under female client's breasts. It may be necessary to lift breast upward while bathing underneath it. Keep client's chest covered between wash and rinse periods. Dry well.	Draping prevents unnecessary exposure of body parts. Towel maintains warmth and privacy. Secretions and dirt collect easily in areas of tight skinfolds. Skinfolds are susceptible to excoriation if breasts are pendulous.
19. Place bath towel lengthwise over chest and abdomen. (Two towels may be needed.) Fold blanket down to just above pubic region.	Prevents chilling and exposure of body parts.
20. With one hand, lift bath towel. With mitted hand, bathe abdomen, giving special attention to bathing umbilicus and abdominal folds. Stroke from side to side. Keep abdomen covered between washing and rinsing. Dry well.	Moisture and sediment that collect in skinfolds predispose skin to maceration and irritation.
21. Apply clean gown or pajama top.	Maintains client's warmth and comfort. Dressing affected side first allows easier manipulation of gown over body part with reduced ROM.
CRITICAL DECISION POINT **If one extremity is injured or immobilized, always dress affected side first.***	

*This step may be omitted until completion of bath; gown should not become soiled during remainder of bath.

STEPS	RATIONALE
22. Cover chest and abdomen with top of bath blanket. Expose near leg by folding blanket toward midline. Be sure perineum is draped.	Prevents unnecessary exposure.
23. Bend client's leg at knee by positioning nurse's arm under leg. While grasping client's heel, elevate leg from mattress slightly and slide bath towel lengthwise under leg. Ask client to hold foot still. Place bath basin on towel on bed and secure its position next to foot to be washed.	Towel prevents soiling of bed linen. Support of joint and extremity during lifting prevents strain on musculoskeletal structures. Sudden movement by client could spill bath water. (Omit this step if client is unable to hold leg in basin.)
24. With one hand supporting lower leg, raise it and slide basin under lifted foot. Make sure foot is firmly placed on bottom of basin. Allow foot to soak while washing leg.	Proper positioning of foot prevents pressure being applied from edge of basin against calf. Soaking softens calluses and rough skin.
CRITICAL DECISION POINT **If client is unable to hold leg, do not immerse; simply wash with washcloth (see illustration).**	
25. Unless contraindicated, use long, firm strokes in washing from ankle to knee and from knee to thigh. Dry well.	Promotes venous return.
CRITICAL DECISION POINT **Clients with history of deep vein thromboses or hypercoagulation disorders should not have their lower extremities washed with long firm strokes.**	
26. Cleanse foot, making sure to bathe between toes. Clean and clip nails as needed (see Skill 6-8). Dry well. If skin is dry, apply lotion.	Secretions and moisture may be present between toes. Lotion helps retain moisture and soften skin.
CRITICAL DECISION POINT **Do not massage any reddened area on client's skin.**	
27. Raise side rail and move to other side of the bed. Lower side rail and repeat steps 22 through 26 for other leg and foot.	
28. Cover client with bath blanket, raise side rail for client's safety, and change bath water.	Decreased bath water temperature can cause chilling. Clean water reduces microorganism transmission.
29. Lower side rail. Assist client in assuming prone or side-lying position (as applicable). Place towel lengthwise along client's side.	Exposes back and buttocks for bathing.
30. Keep client draped by sliding bath blanket over shoulders and thighs. Wash, rinse, and dry back from neck to buttocks using long, firm strokes. Pay special attention to folds of buttocks and anus. Give a backrub.	Maintains warmth and prevents unnecessary exposure. Skinfolds near buttocks and anus may contain fecal secretions that harbor microorganisms.
31. Apply disposable gloves if not done previously.	Prevents contact with microorganisms in body secretions.
32. Assist client in assuming side-lying or supine position. Cover chest and upper extremities with towel and lower extremities with bath blanket. Expose only genitalia. (If client can wash, covering entire body with bath blanket may be preferable.) Wash, rinse, and dry perineum (see Skill 6-2). Pay special attention to skinfolds. Apply water-repellant ointment to area exposed to moisture.	Maintains client's privacy. Clients capable of performing partial bath usually prefer to wash their own genitalia. Water-repellant ointments (e.g., A & D, Pericare) protect skin from moisture (Agency for Health Care Research, 1992).
33. Dispose of gloves in receptacle.	Prevents transmission of infection.
34. Apply additional body lotion or oil as desired.	Moisturizing lotion prevents dry, chapped skin.

STEPS	RATIONALE
35. Assist client in dressing. Comb client's hair. Women may want to apply makeup.	Promotes client's body image.
36. Make client's bed (see Skills 7-1 and 7-2).	Provides clean environment.
37. Remove soiled linen and place in dirty-linen bag. Clean and replace bathing equipment. Replace call light and personal possessions. Leave room as clean and comfortable as possible.	Prevents transmission of infection. Clean environment promotes client's comfort. Keeping call light and articles of care within reach promotes client's safety.
38. Wash hands.	Reduces transmission of microorganisms.
TUB BATH OR SHOWER	
1. Consider client's condition and review orders for precautions concerning client's movement or positioning.	Prevents accidental injury to client during bathing.
2. Schedule use of shower or tub.	Prevents unnecessary waiting that can cause fatigue.
3. Check tub or shower for cleanliness. Use cleaning techniques outlined in agency policy. Place rubber mat on tub or shower bottom. Place disposable bath mat or towel on floor in front of tub or shower.	Cleaning prevents transmission of microorganisms. Mats prevent slipping and falling.
4. Collect all hygienic aids, toiletry items, and linens requested by client. Place within easy reach of tub or shower.	Placing items close at hand prevents possible falls when client reaches for equipment.
5. Assist client to bathroom if necessary. Have client wear robe and slippers to bathroom.	Assistance prevents accidental falls. Wearing robe and slippers prevents chilling.
6. Demonstrate how to use call signal for assistance.	Bathrooms are equipped with signaling devices in case client feels faint or weak or needs immediate assistance. Clients prefer privacy during bath if safety is not jeopardized.
7. Place "occupied" sign on bathroom door.	Maintains client's privacy.
8. Fill bathtub halfway with warm water. Ask client to test water, and adjust temperature if water is too warm. Explain which faucet controls hot water. If client is taking shower, turn shower on and adjust water temperature before client enters shower stall. Use shower seat or tub chair and provide if needed (see illustration).	Adjusting water temperature prevents accidental burns. Older adults and clients with neurological alterations (e.g., spinal cord injury) are at high risk for burns as a result of reduced sensation. Use of assistive devices facilitates bathing and minimizes physical exertion.

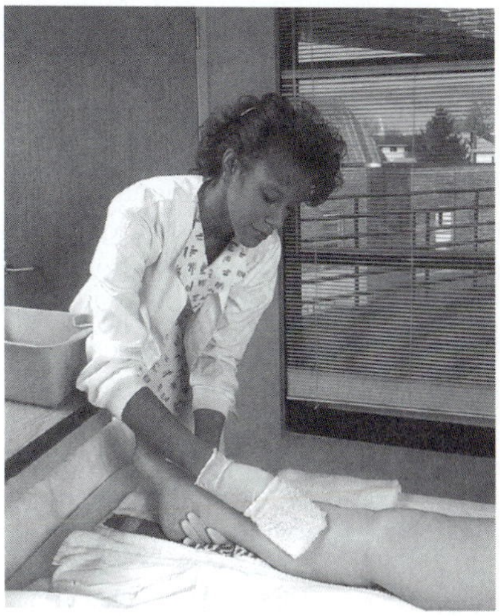

Step 24, p.138

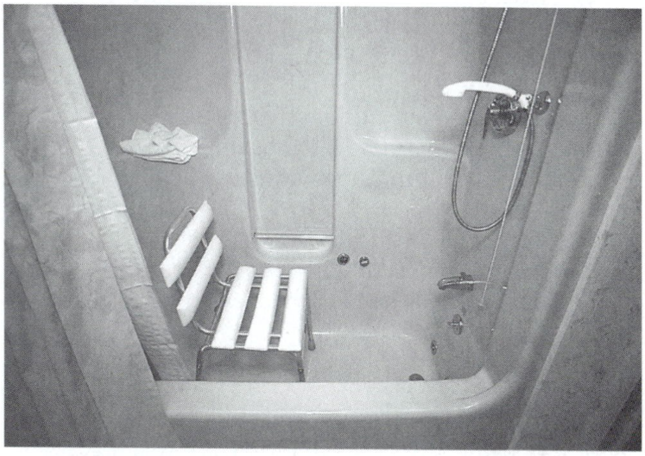

Step 8

STEPS	RATIONALE
9. Instruct client to use safety bars when getting in and out of tub or shower. Caution client against use of bath oil in tub water.	Prevents slipping and falling. Oil causes tub surfaces to become slippery.
10. Instruct client not to remain in tub longer than 20 minutes. Check on client every 5 minutes.	Prolonged exposure to warm water may cause vasodilation and pooling of blood, leading to lightheadedness or dizziness.
11. Return to bathroom when client signals, and knock before entering.	Provides privacy.
12. For client who is unsteady, drain tub of water before client attempts to get out of it. Place bath towel over client's shoulders. Assist client in getting out of tub as needed and assist with drying.	Prevents accidental falls. Client may become chilled as water drains.
CRITICAL DECISION POINT **Weak or unstable clients need extra assistance in getting out of a tub. Planning for additional personnel is essential before attempting to assist the client from the tub.**	
13. Assist client as needed in donning clean gown or pajamas, slippers, and robe. (In home setting client may don regular clothing.)	Maintains warmth to prevent chilling.
14. Assist client to room and comfortable position in bed or chair.	Maintains relaxation gained from bathing.
15. Clean tub or shower according to agency policy. Remove soiled linen and place in dirty-linen bag. Discard disposable equipment in proper receptacle. Place "unoccupied" sign on bathroom door. Return supplies to storage area.	Prevents transmission of infection through soiled linen and moisture.
16. Wash hands.	Reduces transfer of microorganisms.

EVALUATION

1. Observe skin paying particular attention to areas that were previously soiled, reddened, or showed early signs of breakdown.	Techniques used during bathing should leave skin clean and clear.
2. Observe ROM during bath.	Measures joint mobility.
3. Ask client to rate level of comfort.	
4. Ask if client feels fatigued.	Determines client's tolerance of bathing activities.
5. Ask client to explain proper hygiene techniques.	Evaluates client's knowledge level.
6. **Unexpected outcomes** that may occur include:	
➤ Areas of excessive dryness, rashes, or pressure ulcers appear on skin.	Previous bathing or skin care measures were ineffective.
➤ Joint ROM decreases.	Indicates need for more frequent ROM exercise or pain which may limit ROM.
➤ Client becomes excessively fatigued and unable to cooperate or participate in bathing.	Indicates nurse needs to offer more assistance. Client's physical tolerance to any form of exertion is minimal.
➤ Client seems unusually restless or complains of discomfort.	Assess vital signs. Factors that may alter pulse, respirations, or blood pressure include anxiety, fatigue from physical exertion, or pain.
➤ Client is unable to identify or discuss methods or advantages of proper hygiene and skin care.	Factors such as anxiety, pain, or fatigue interfere with learning. Client may not be willing or motivated to learn about hygiene care.

RECORDING AND REPORTING

1. Record bath on flow sheet. Note level of assistance required.	Quick method to document procedure.

STEPS	RATIONALE
2. Record condition of skin and any significant findings (e.g., reddened areas, bruises, nevi, or joint or muscle pain).	Timely documentation maintains accuracy of client's record. Condition of skin documents response to therapy, such as turning and positioning.
3. Report evidence of alterations in skin integrity to nurse in charge or physician.	Client may require special medical treatment.

Follow-up Activities

1. Obtain special bed surface if client is predisposed to skin breakdown or shows signs of early pressure ulcer formation.
2. Provide special skin care as needed (see Chapter 8).

• • • • •

Special Considerations

- Clients with breathing difficulties require pillow or elevated head of bed during bath.
- Avoid placing soap in washbasin; this avoids soapy rinse water.
- Diabetic clients require special attention to foot care. (See Skill 6-8).
- Conditions placing clients at risk for falls in bathtub include neurological impairment; medications, such as sedatives, antihypertensives, and narcotic analgesics; arthritis; muscular disease or weakness; amputation; and poor balance or coordination in older adult clients.
- Clients with decreased sensation need to be cautious when entering hot bath water. Whenever possible they need to use unaffected extremity to test water temperature to avoid accidental scalding.

Teaching Considerations

- Family members caring for clients in the home should be included in discussions about hygiene.
- Instruct older adults or other clients with reduced sensation on how to check temperature of bath water.
- Instruct clients on how to inspect surfaces between skinfolds for signs of irritation or breakdown.
- Teach clients that, when flossing, force should be directed toward the tooth being flossed rather than toward the gum line; otherwise, the tender gum tissue can be "sliced" (Kahn, 1986). The mouth should be rinsed after flossing to remove debris. Regular flossing helps prevent cavities and gum disease.
- Encourage clients to visit the dentist every 6 months. Even though a client may establish an effective preventive program, the dentist will screen for serious dental or periodontal problems.

Pediatric Considerations

- Adolescents may require more frequent bathing as a result of more active sebaceous glands.

Gerontologic Considerations

- Consider conditions of older adult's skin when planning hygiene routine. Because of the aging process more moisture is needed; client's skin can be rehydrated with lotions and fluids.
- Older adults with urinary incontinence need meticulous skin care to reduce skin irritation from urine and feces (see Chapters 25 and 26).
- Older adults may require less frequent baths, more frequent application of skin lotion.

Home Care Considerations

- In home setting, set up equipment according to established routines. Client is best resource for what works in terms of convenience and saving time.
- Clients at risk for falls may wish to have grab bars installed around tub and have bathroom floor carpeted. Client also may use portable shower seat.
- The three types of bath for the homebound client are the complete bed bath; the abbreviated bed bath, during which only parts of the body are washed that, if neglected, might cause illness, odor, or discomfort; and the partial bath, which may take place at the sink, in the tub, or in the shower.
- Type of bath chosen depends on assessment of the home, availability of running water, and condition of bathing facilities.
- If beds do not have side rails, positioning may be accomplished with pillows or by placing bed against wall.
- Never leave bathing client unattended. Adhesive strips on bottom of tub or shower, handrails, chairs, or stools in tub or shower will further protect client.
- Follow client's usual bathing and skin care routines.
- Determine if there is need to have home health aide or other assistance after discharge. Contact social service, or appropriate department within hospital, to obtain referral to home health agency.

SKILL 6-2 Providing Perineal Care

Perineal care involves thorough cleansing of the client's external genitalia and surrounding skin. A client routinely receives perineal care during a bath.

"Pericare" is important in promoting the client's comfort and cleanliness. Special attention is given to cleansing the skin around the genitals, since secretions can accumulate and cause skin breakdown and infection of the skin and urinary or reproductive systems. The nurse retains responsibility for doing this procedure if the client is unable to do so and determines the client's understanding of the importance of basic perineal hygiene.

Gloves must be worn during the procedure because of the risk of contacting infectious microorganisms, such as HIV or herpes virus, from perineal drainage. Certain clients require perineal care at times other than during a bath (e.g., because of fecal incontinence or as part of Foley catheter care). In addition, pericare promotes healing after perineal surgery or vaginal deliveries.

To minimize embarrassment for both the nurse and the client, it helps for the nurse to be of the same sex as the client. Embarrassment should not cause the nurse to overlook the client's hygiene needs.

EQUIPMENT

- Washbasin
- Soap dish with soap
- Two or three washcloths
- Bath towel
- Bath blanket
- Waterproof pad or bedpan
- Toilet tissue or diaper wipes
- Disposable gloves

Additional supplies are needed when pericare is given other than during a bath:

- Cotton balls or swabs
- A solution bottle or container filled with warm water or prescribed rinsing solution
- Waterproof bag

DELEGATION CONSIDERATIONS

Skills of perineal care can be delegated to unlicensed assistive personnel.

- Inform and assist care provider in proper way to position male and female clients.
- Inform care provider about proper positioning of indwelling catheter during perineal care.
- Caution care provider to use warm water.

STEPS	RATIONALE
ASSESSMENT	
1. Identify clients at risk for developing infection of genitalia, urinary tract, or reproductive tract (e.g., presence of indwelling catheter, fecal incontinence).	Secretions that accumulate on surface of skin surrounding female and male genitalia act as reservoir for infection. Tissues traumatized by surgery or by presence of foreign object provide route for introduction of infectious organisms.
2. Assess client's cognitive and musculoskeletal function.	Determines client's ability to perform self-care and determines level of assistance required from nurse.
3. Assess genitalia for signs of inflammation, skin breakdown, or infection (see Chapter 11).	Determines extent of perineal care required by client.
4. Assess client's knowledge of importance of perineal hygiene.	Clients at risk for infection in perineal area may be unaware of importance of cleanliness. Reflects client's need for education.

NURSING DIAGNOSIS

Clustering of defining characteristics from the assessment data may reveal the following nursing diagnoses for clients requiring this skill:

- Self-care deficit, bathing
- Impaired skin integrity
- Knowledge deficit regarding hygienic care
- Risk for impaired skin integrity
- Risk for infection
- Impaired physical mobility

Related factors are individualized based on a client's condition or needs.

STEPS	RATIONALE
PLANNING	
1. **Expected outcomes** following completion of procedure:	
➤ Skin and surrounding genitalia are clean, intact, and without redness or drainage.	Skin is free of irritation or infection.
➤ Client expresses sense of cleanliness and denies irritation.	Perineum is clean.
➤ Client is able to describe or perform steps of perineal hygiene.	Client acquires self-care skills.
2. Explain procedure and its purpose to client.	Helps minimize anxiety during procedure that is often embarrassing to nurse and client.
3. Prepare necessary equipment and supplies.	Used when administering a bed bath.
IMPLEMENTATION	
1. Pull curtain around client's bed or close room door. Assemble supplies at bedside.	Maintains client's privacy and ensures orderly procedure.
2. Raise bed to comfortable working position. Lower side rail and assist client in assuming side lying position, placing towel lengthwise along client's side and keeping client covered with bath blanket.	Facilitates good body mechanics. Provides easy access to genitalia.
3. Apply disposable gloves.	Eliminates transmission of microorganisms.
4. If fecal material is present, enclose in a fold of underpad or toilet tissue and remove with disposable wipes. Cleanse buttocks and anus, washing front to back (see illustration). Cleanse, rinse, and dry area thoroughly. If needed, place an absorbent pad under client's buttocks. Remove and discard underpad and replace with clean one.	Cleansing reduces transmission of microorganisms from anus to urethra or genitalia.
5. Change gloves when they are soiled.	

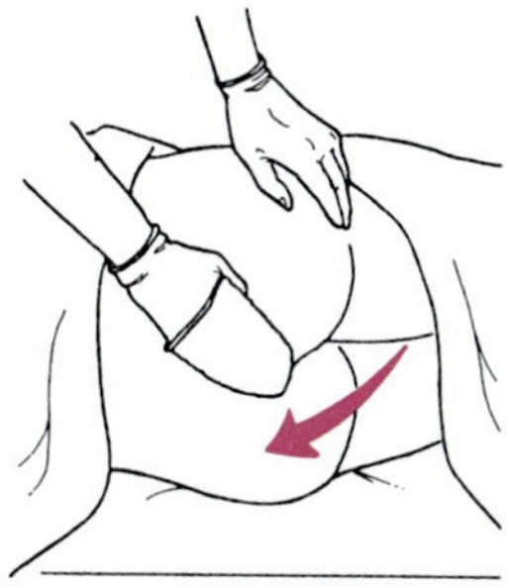

Step 4

STEPS	RATIONALE
6. Fold top bed linen down toward foot of bed and raise client's gown above genital area.	Exposes perineal area for easy accessibility.
a. "Diamond" drape client by placing bath blanket with one corner between client's legs, one corner pointing toward each side of bed, and one corner over client's chest. Tuck side corners around client's legs and under hips.	Prevents unnecessary exposure of body parts and maintains client's warmth and comfort during procedure.
b. Raise side rail. Fill washbasin with warm water.	Prevents client from falling. Proper water temperature prevents burns to perineum.
c. Place washbasin and toilet tissue on overbed table. Place washcloths in basin.	Equipment placed within nurse's reach prevents accidental spills.
7. Provide perineal care.	
a. Female perineal care:	
(1) Assist client to dorsal recumbent position.	Provides easy access to genitalia.
(2) Lower side rail and help client flex knees and spread legs. Note restrictions or limitations in client's positioning.	Provides full exposure of female genitalia. Minimize degree of abduction in female if position causes pain because of arthritis or contracture or in older adults with decreased mobility.

STEPS	RATIONALE
(3) Fold lower corner of bath blanket up between client's legs onto abdomen. Wash and dry client's upper thighs.	Minimizes transmission of microorganisms. Keeping client draped until procedure begins minimizes anxiety. Buildup of perineal secretions can soil surrounding skin surfaces.
(4) Wash labia majora. Use nondominant hand to gently retract labia from thigh; with dominant hand, wash carefully in skinfolds. Wipe in direction from perineum to rectum (front to back) (see illustration). Repeat on opposite side using separate section of washcloth. Rinse and dry area thoroughly.	Skinfolds may contain body secretions that harbor microorganisms. Wiping from perineum to rectum (front to back) reduces chance of transmitting fecal organisms to urinary meatus.
(5) Separate labia with nondominant hand to expose urethral meatus and vaginal orifice. With dominant hand, wash downward from pubic area toward rectum in one smooth stroke (see illustration). Use separate section of cloth for each stroke. Cleanse thoroughly around labia minora, clitoris, and vaginal orifice.	Cleansing method reduces transfer of microorganisms to urinary meatus. (For menstruating women or clients with indwelling urinary catheters, cleanse with cotton balls.)
(6) If client uses bedpan, pour warm water over perineal area. Dry perineal area thoroughly, using front-to-back method.	Rinsing removes soap and microorganisms more effectively than wiping. Retained moisture harbors microorganisms.
(7) Fold lower corner of bath blanket back between client's legs and over perineum. Ask client to lower legs and assume comfortable position.	
b. Male perineal care:	
(1) Lower side rails and assist client to supine position. Note restriction in mobility.	Provides full exposure of male genitalia.
(2) Fold lower corner of bath blanket up between client's legs and onto abdomen. Wash and dry client's upper thighs.	Minimizes transmission of microorganisms. Keeping client draped until procedure begins minimizes anxiety. Buildup of perineal secretions can soil surrounding skin surfaces.
(3) Gently raise penis and place bath towel underneath. Gently grasp shaft of penis. If client is uncircumcised, retract foreskin. If client has an erection, defer procedure until later.	Towel prevents moisture from collecting in inguinal area. Gentle but firm handling reduces chance of client having an erection. Secretions capable of harboring microorganisms collect underneath foreskin.
(4) Wash tip of penis at urethral meatus first. Using circular motion, cleanse from meatus outward (see illustration). Discard washcloth and repeat with clean cloth until penis is clean. Rinse and dry gently.	Direction of cleansing moves from area of least contamination to area of most contamination, preventing microorganisms from entering urethra.
(5) Return foreskin to its natural position.	Tightening of foreskin around shaft of penis can cause local edema and discomfort.

Step 7a (4)

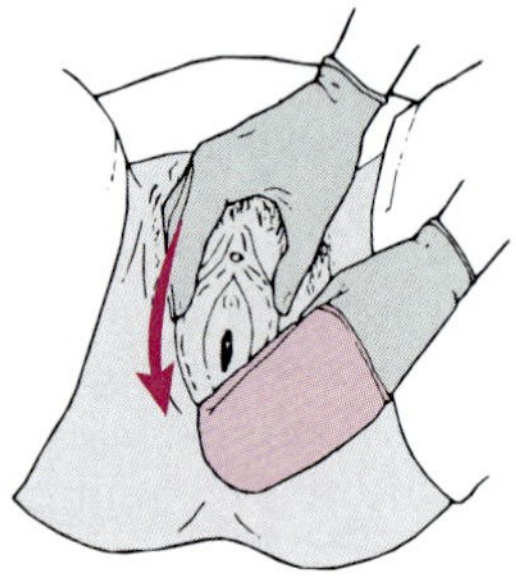

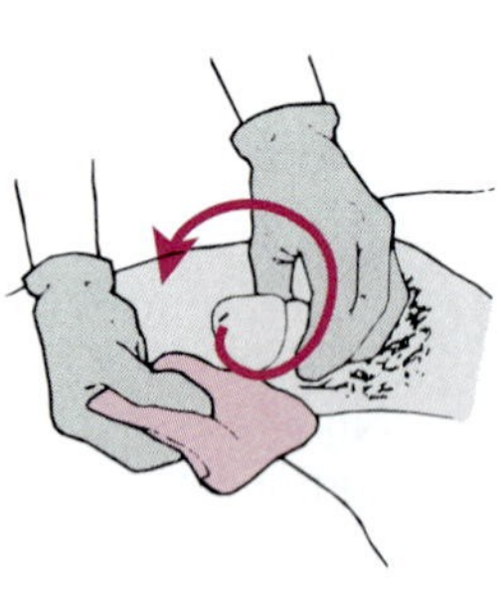

Step 7b (4)

STEPS	RATIONALE
CRITICAL DECISION POINT **After administering perineal care, the nurse needs to make sure the foreskin is in its natural position. This is extremely important in those clients with decreased sensation in their lower extremities.**	
(6) Wash shaft of penis with gentle but firm downward strokes. Pay special attention to underlying surface of penis. Rinse and dry penis thoroughly. Instruct client to spread legs apart slightly.	Vigorous massage of penis can lead to erection, which can embarrass client and nurse. Underlying surface of penis may have greater accumulation of secretions. Abduction of legs provides easier access to scrotal tissues.
(7) Gently cleanse scrotum. Lift it carefully and wash underlying skinfolds. Rinse and dry.	Pressure on scrotal tissues can be painful to client. Secretions collect between skinfolds.
(8) Fold bath blanket back over client's perineum and assist client in turning to side-lying position.	Draping promotes comfort and minimizes client's anxiety. Side-lying position provides access to anal area.
8. If client has had urinary or bowel incontinence, apply thin layer of skin barrier containing petrolatum or zinc oxide over anal and perineal skin.	Protects skin from excess moisture and toxins from urine or stool (Maklebust, 1991).
CRITICAL DECISION POINT **Clients who are incontinent or who are exposed to body secretions need more frequent skin assessment to determine risk for pressure ulcer development. Fully assess exposed skin before repositioning.**	
9. Remove disposable gloves and dispose in proper receptacle.	Moisture and body secretions on gloves can harbor microorganisms.
10. Assist client in assuming a comfortable position and cover with sheet.	Client's comfort helps to minimize stress of procedure.
11. Remove bath blanket and dispose of all soiled bed linen. Return unused equipment to storage area.	Reduces transmission of microorganisms.
EVALUATION	
1. Inspect surface of external genitalia and surrounding skin after cleansing.	Thick secretions may cover underlying skin lesions or areas of breakdown. Evaluation determines need for additional hygiene.
2. Ask if client feels sense of cleanliness.	Evaluates client's comfort level.
3. Observe for abnormal drainage or discharge from genitalia.	Evaluates presence of infection.
4. Observe client's ability to perform hygiene and ask questions about its importance.	Evaluates client's self-care ability and knowledge level.
5. **Unexpected outcomes** that may occur include:	
➤ Skin and genitalia may be inflamed, with localized tenderness, swelling, and presence of foul-smelling discharge.	Indicates infection or maceration of skin layers.
➤ Client expresses discomfort.	Perineal area is not thoroughly cleansed, or irritation is present as a result of infection.
➤ Client is unable to describe or perform perineal hygiene.	Further instruction is required at a later time.
RECORDING AND REPORTING	
1. Record procedure and presence of any abnormal findings (e.g., character and amount of discharge, condition of genitalia).	Ensures accurate and timely documentation of care (flow sheet may be used).

STEPS	RATIONALE
2. Record appearance of suture line, if present.	Documents nurse's observations of client's postoperative recovery.
3. Report any break in suture line or presence of abnormalities to nurse in charge or physician.	Additional therapy may be required as result of altered wound healing or altered skin integrity.

Follow-up Activities

1. Assist with sitz baths if client has localized inflammation of suture line or genitalia.
2. Apply antibiotic ointment to suture line if ordered.
3. Apply protective ointment and institute a more aggressive bowel or urinary control program if skin irritation from repeated incontinence continues.

• • • • •

Special Considerations

- Clients with urinary or fecal incontinence, rectal or perineal surgery, or surgery involving the lower urinary tract require special attention.
- Women who are recovering from vaginal childbirth require special attention to perineal care. It may be necessary to offer care frequently.

Teaching Considerations

- Clients most at risk for infection of perineum are taught signs and symptoms of early infection, as well as principles and techniques for cleansing perineum correctly. Clients who are physically unable to perform hygiene and who rely on family members for care must have family instructed on hygiene techniques.

Pediatric Considerations

- Young adolescent girls should learn basic perineal hygiene measures and know why they are predisposed to urinary tract infections.

Gerontologic Considerations

- Older adults with limited mobility need assistance in perineal care. Using a side-lying position increases client's comfort and provides nurse with opportunity to provide perineal care and inspect surrounding skin as well.

Home Care Considerations

- For clients who require bathing, assess perineum at every visit because of risk for infection and skin breakdown.

SKILL 6-3 Brushing Teeth

Brushing, flossing, and irrigation are necessary for proper cleansing of teeth. Brushing removes food particles, loosens plaque, and stimulates gums. **Plaque** is the cause of dental caries. **Flossing** removes **tartar** that collects at the gum line. Irrigation removes dislodged food particles and excess toothpaste. When a client becomes ill, a regular dental hygiene routine is often difficult, if not impossible, to follow. The nurse offers oral hygiene assistance as required, from preparing needed supplies to actually brushing the client's teeth.

The nurse's responsibility also includes determining the frequency with which clients require brushing. Certain conditions resulting from illness or therapy cause the oral cavity to become excessively dry or irritated. For example, clients with food or fluid restrictions often develop thick, foul-tasting secretions in the mouth because of reduced hydration. Frequent oral hygiene provides considerable relief. Frequency of care should be based on the condition of the oral cavity and the client's level of comfort. Oral hygiene may be required as often as every 1 to 2 hours.

EQUIPMENT

- Soft-bristled toothbrush (hard toothbrush damages enamel and gums)
- Nonabrasive fluoride toothpaste or dentifrice (abrasive toothpastes wear down enamel)
- Dental floss
- Water glass with cool water
- Normal saline or fluoride mouthwash (optional; follow client's preference)
- Emesis basin
- Face towel
- Paper towels
- Disposable gloves

DELEGATION CONSIDERATIONS

Skills of brushing teeth can be delegated to unlicensed assistive personnel.

- Inform and assist care provider in proper way to provide tooth brushing.
- Instruct care provider how to recognize impaired integrity of oral mucosa.

STEPS	RATIONALE
ASSESSMENT	
1. Wash hands and apply disposable gloves.	Reduces transmission of microorganisms. Gloves prevent contact with microorganisms in blood or saliva.
2. Inspect integrity of lips, teeth, buccal mucosa, gums, palate, and tongue (see Chapter 11).	Determines status of client's oral cavity and extent of need for oral hygiene.
3. Identify presence of common oral problems:	Helps determine type of hygiene client requires and information client requires for self-care.
a. **Dental caries**—chalky white discoloration of tooth or presence of brown or black discoloration	
b. **Gingivitis**—inflammation of gums	
c. **Periodontitis**—receding gum lines, inflammation, gaps between teeth	
d. **Halitosis**—bad breath	
e. **Cheilosis**—cracking of lips	
f. **Stomatitis**—inflammation of the mouth	
4. Remove gloves and wash hands.	Prevents spread of microorganisms.
5. Assess risk for oral hygiene problems:	Certain conditions increase likelihood of impaired oral cavity integrity and need for preventive care.
a. Dehydration, inability to take fluids or food by mouth **(NPO)**	Causes excess drying and fragility of mucous membranes; increases accumulation of secretions on tongue and gums.
b. Presence of nasogastric or oxygen tubes; mouth breathers	Causes drying of mucosa (Harrell and Damon, 1989).
c. Chemotherapeutic drugs	These drugs kill rapidly multiplying cells, including cancerous tumors and cells lining oral cavity and gastrointestinal tract. Drug effects can lead to stomatitis (Dudjak, 1987).
d. Radiation therapy to head and neck	Reduces salivary flow and lowers pH of saliva; can lead to stomatitis and tooth decay (Danielson, 1988).
e. Presence of artificial airway	Increases irritation to gums and mucosa. Excess secretions accumulate on teeth and tongue.
f. Blood-clotting disorders (e.g., leukemia, aplastic anemia)	Predisposes to inflammation and bleeding of gums.
g. Oral surgery, trauma to mouth	Break in mucosa increases risk of infection. Vigorous brushing can disrupt suture lines.
h. Aging	
i. Diabetes mellitus	Prone to dryness of mouth, gingivitis, periodontal disease, and loss of teeth.
6. Determine client's oral hygiene practices:	Allows nurse to identify errors in technique, deficiencies in preventive oral hygiene, and client's level of knowledge regarding dental care.
a. Frequency of tooth brushing and flossing	
b. Type of toothpaste or dentifrice used	
c. Last dental visit	
d. Frequency of dental visits	
e. Type of mouthwash or moistening preparation	Lemon-glycerine preparations can be detrimental. Glycerine is an astringent that dries and shrinks mucous membranes and gums. Lemon exhausts salivary reflex and can erode tooth enamel (Poland, 1987). Mouthwash provides pleasant aftertaste but can dry mucosa after extended use if it has an alcohol base (Blaney, 1986).
7. Assess client's ability to grasp and manipulate toothbrush. Assessment determines level of assistance required from nurse.	Older adult clients or persons with musculoskeletal or nervous system alterations may be unable to hold toothbrush with firm grip or manipulate brush.

STEPS | **RATIONALE**

NURSING DIAGNOSIS

Clustering of defining characteristics from the assessment data may reveal the following nursing diagnoses for clients requiring this skill:

- Altered oral mucous membrane
- Self-care deficit, bathing/hygiene
- Knowledge deficit regarding oral hygiene care

Related factors are individualized based on client's condition and needs.

PLANNING

STEPS	RATIONALE
1. **Expected outcomes** following completion of procedure:	
➤ Client expresses feeling of cleanliness.	
➤ Oral cavity structures have normal characteristics.	If client had degree of alteration before brushing, condition should not be worse after brushing.
• Oral mucosa is moist, intact, and of normal color.	Mucosa and gums are moist and intact.
• Gums are pink, firm, and adherent to neck of teeth.	
• Teeth are clean, smooth, and shiny.	
• Tongue is pink and without secretions or coating.	
➤ Client describes correct oral hygiene techniques and necessary frequency.	Demonstrates understanding of nurse's instructions.
➤ Client makes choices regarding hygiene procedure and assists by flossing and brushing.	Client is able to manage self-care.
2. Prepare equipment at bedside.	
3. Explain procedure to client and discuss preferences regarding use of hygienic aids.	Some clients feel uncomfortable about having the nurse care for their basic needs. Client involvement with procedure minimizes anxiety.

IMPLEMENTATION

STEPS	RATIONALE
1. Place paper towels on overbed table and arrange other equipment within easy reach.	
2. Raise bed to comfortable working position. Raise head of bed (if allowed) and lower side rail. Move client or help client move closer. Side-lying position can be used.	Raising bed and positioning client prevent nurse from straining muscles. Semi-Fowler's position helps prevent client from choking or aspirating.
3. Place towel over client's chest.	
4. Apply gloves.	Prevents contact with microorganisms or blood in saliva.
5. Apply toothpaste to brush, holding brush over emesis basin. Pour small amount of water over toothpaste.	Moisture aids in distribution of toothpaste over tooth surfaces.
6. Client may assist by brushing. Hold toothbrush bristles at 45-degree angle to gum line (see illustration). Be sure tips of bristles rest against and penetrate under gum line. Brush inner and outer surfaces of upper and lower teeth by brushing from gum to crown of each tooth. Clean biting surfaces of teeth by holding top of bristles parallel with teeth and brushing gently back and forth (see illustration on p. 149). Brush sides of teeth by moving bristles back and forth (see illustration on p. 149).	Angle allows brush to reach all tooth surfaces and to clean under gum line where plaque and tartar accumulate. Back-and-forth motion dislodges food particles caught between teeth and along chewing surfaces.
7. Have client hold brush at 45-degree angle and lightly brush over surface and sides of tongue. Avoid initiating gag reflex.	Microorganisms collect and grow on tongue's surface and contribute to bad breath. Gagging may cause aspiration of toothpaste.

STEPS	RATIONALE
8. Allow client to rinse mouth thoroughly by taking several sips of water, swishing water across all tooth surfaces, and spitting into emesis basin.	Irrigation removes food particles.
9. Allow client to gargle or rinse mouth with mouthwash as desired.	Mouthwash leaves pleasant taste in mouth.
10. Assist in wiping client's mouth.	Promotes sense of comfort.
11. Allow client to floss.	Reduces tartar on tooth surfaces.
12. Allow client to rinse mouth thoroughly with cool water and spit into emesis basin. Assist in wiping client's mouth.	Irrigation removes plaque and tartar from oral cavity.
13. Assist client to comfortable position, remove emesis basin and bedside table, raise side rail, and lower bed to original position.	Provides for client comfort and safety.
14. Wipe off overbed table, discard soiled linen and paper towels in appropriate containers, remove soiled gloves, and return equipment to proper place.	Proper disposal of soiled equipment prevents spread of infection.
15. Wash hands.	Reduces transmission of microorganisms.

EVALUATION

1. Ask client if any area of oral cavity feels uncomfortable or irritated.	Pain indicates more chronic problem.
2. Apply gloves and inspect condition of oral cavity.	Determines effectiveness of hygiene and rinsing.
3. Ask client to describe proper hygiene techniques.	Evaluates client's learning.
4. Observe client brushing.	Evaluates client's ability to use correct technique.
5. **Unexpected outcomes** that may occur include:	
➤ Mucosa is dry and inflamed.	Dry mucosa is sign of dehydration and changes resulting from local trauma, infection, or chemotherapy.
➤ Gum margins are retracted from teeth, with localized areas of inflammation. Bleeding occurs around gum margins.	Bleeding of gums or mucous membranes may result from too vigorous brushing and flossing or client's underlying bleeding tendency.
➤ Teeth show signs of dental caries.	Client's personal dental hygiene is poor.
➤ Tongue continues to have thick coating.	Several brushings are required to remove thick coating.
➤ Client is unable to describe correct oral hygiene techniques or brush properly.	Further instruction is required.

RECORDING AND REPORTING

1. Record procedure on flow sheet. Note condition of oral cavity in nurses' notes.	Documents client's response to hygiene measures and status of oral cavity.
2. Report bleeding or presence of lesions to nurse in charge or physician.	Bleeding may indicate serious systemic problems. Certain oral lesions may be cancerous.

FOLLOW-UP ACTIVITIES

1. Refer client with oral problems requiring special care to dentist.

• • • • •

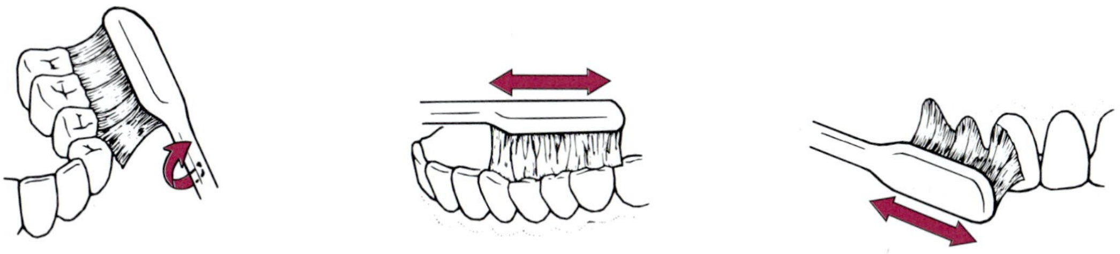

Step 6

Special Considerations

- All postoperative clients who received general anesthesia are initially given nothing by mouth after surgery and thus require frequent mouth care. Brushing may be contraindicated for these clients.
- Clients with sensitive gums or bleeding tendencies benefit from use of unflavored oral care sponges. A swab stick containing an aqueous solution of sorbitol, sodium, carboxymethylcellulose, and electrolytes may be used.
- Clients unable to grasp a toothbrush can have an enlarged handle placed on toothbrush (e.g., push handle through center of small plastic ball).
- Clients with diabetes mellitus require visits to the dentist every 3 or 4 months. They should be taught to follow rigid cleansing schedules and to handle tissues gently, since diabetes depresses the immune system and decreases circulation to mucosa (Blaney, 1986).

Teaching Considerations

- Educate clients about methods to prevent tooth decay (e.g., reduce intake of carbohydrates, especially sweet snacks between meals; brush within 30 minutes of eating sweets; rinse mouth thoroughly with water or eat acid-containing fruit such as an apple; use fluoridated water).
- Cheilosis can be prevented by applying lip ointment or lubricant and avoiding licking of lips.

Pediatric Considerations

- Early dental care is the best insurance against dental caries and disease: caring for a child's teeth begins at birth, before the first primary teeth break through the gums. Fluoride should be given to an infant from birth to help prevent cavities and to maintain gingival health. In the absence of fluoridated drinking water, a fluoride supplement with vitamins should be administered daily.
- As soon as teething begins, clean an infant's gum pads and teeth with a small piece of gauze twice a day (after breakfast and after the last meal of the day). This practice eliminates decay-producing plaque.
- Teach parents that a bottle given to a child at bedtime should contain only water. Falling asleep with a bottle of milk or juice or while breast-feeding bathes the teeth in a carbohydrate-rich fluid that can cause cavities and tooth discoloration.
- Parents and care givers need to be responsible for the child's oral hygiene for about the first 8 years, since the child does not develop the neural patterns and muscular coordination needed for performing mouth care until that age.
- Unless problems occur earlier, dental visits should begin about age 2. After the first visit, dental checkups every 6 months are encouraged (Moss, 1988).

Gerontologic Considerations

- A number of normal age-related changes occur in the oral cavity. Thinning of the oral mucosa and decreased vascularity of the gingivae predispose older adults to injury and periodontal disease. Loss of tissue elasticity and decreased mass and strength of the muscles make chewing more difficult. Resorption of the alveolar bone can loosen natural teeth. The number of taste buds declines: in an attempt to enhance the taste of food, the older adult may choose salty and sugary foods, which erode tooth enamel and expose dentin (Pettigrew, 1989).
- Even with these changes, most mouth problems are preventable with good oral hygiene practices and regular dental checkups.

Home Care Considerations

- During the initial admission visit, document the condition of the client's mouth, teeth, and gums, thus providing a baseline for assessment of the client's ability to comply with special diets and fluid intake and to carry out oral hygiene practices.
- Assess oral cavity during each visit to determine effects of medication regimen.
- Assess the state of dental health of family members and attitudes toward oral hygiene.

SKILL 6-4 Performing Mouth Care for the Unconscious or Debilitated Client

Unconscious or debilitated clients pose challenges because of their risk for having alterations of the oral cavity and because of their total dependence on the nurse for oral care. The nurse should recognize that these clients may not eat or drink orally; frequently they are mouth breathers or they have artificial airways, and they often have nasogastric or oxygen therapy. All of these factors contribute to drying of the mucosa and the formation of secretions and crusts on the tongue and mucous membranes. Some clients require mouth care as often as every 1 to 2 hours until the mucosa returns to normal. Many unconscious clients have no **gag reflex** as a result of neurological injury.

The accumulation of salivary secretions in the mouth can easily lead to **aspiration.** Because oral secretions usually contain gram-negative bacteria, aspiration may lead to pneumonia. Proper oral hygiene requires keeping the oral mucosa moist and removing secretions that can lead to infection.

EQUIPMENT

- Antiinfective solution (e.g., diluted hydrogen peroxide) that loosens crusts
- Small soft-bristled toothbrush
- Sponge toothette or tongue blade wrapped in single layer of gauze
- Padded tongue blade
- Face towel
- Paper towels
- Emesis basin
- Water glass with cool water
- Water-soluble lip lubricant
- Small-bulb syringe (optional)
- Suction machine equipment (optional)
- Disposable gloves

DELEGATION CONSIDERATIONS

Skills of brushing teeth of an unconscious or debilitated client can be delegated to unlicensed assistive personnel.

- After checking for gag reflex, inform care provider in proper way to position clients for mouth care.
- Instruct care provider on how to use the oral suction catheter for clearing oral secretions (see Skill 14-1).
- Instruct care provider on how to recognize impaired integrity of oral mucosa.

STEPS	RATIONALE
ASSESSMENT	
1. Wash hands. Apply disposable gloves.	Reduces transmission of microorganisms. Gloves prevent contact with microorganisms in blood or saliva.
2. Test for presence of gag reflex by placing blade on back half of tongue.	Reveals whether client is at risk for aspiration.
CRITICAL DECISION POINT **Clients with impaired gag reflex require oral care as well. The nurse must determine the type of suction apparatus needed at the bedside to protect the client's airway against aspiration.**	
3. Inspect condition of oral cavity (see Chapter 11).	Determines condition of oral cavity and need for hygiene.
4. Remove gloves. Wash hands.	Prevents spread of infection.
5. Assess client's risk for oral hygiene problems (see Skill 6-3).	Certain conditions increase likelihood of alterations in integrity of oral cavity structures and may require more frequent care.

NURSING DIAGNOSIS

Clustering of defining characteristics from the assessment data may reveal the following nursing diagnoses for clients requiring this skill:

- Altered oral mucous membrane
- Risk for aspiration
- Risk for injury

Related factors are individualized based on a client's condition or needs.

PLANNING

STEPS	RATIONALE
1. **Expected outcomes** following completion of procedure:	
➤ Buccal mucosa and tongue are pink, moist, and intact. Gums are moist and intact. Teeth are cleaner, smooth, and shiny. Tongue is pink and without coating. Lips are moist, smooth, and without cracks.	Degree of improvement in condition of oral cavity structures will depend on extent of secretions or changes that existed before care.
➤ Debilitated client expresses feeling of cleanliness.	Comfort achieved.
➤ Oral pharynx remains patent.	Secretions removed, thus avoiding aspiration.

STEPS	RATIONALE
2. Position client on side (Sims' position) with head turned well toward dependent side and head of bed lowered. Raise side rail.	Allows secretions to drain from mouth instead of collecting in back of pharynx. Prevents aspiration.
3. Explain procedure to client.	Allows debilitated client to anticipate procedure without anxiety. Unconscious client may retain ability to hear.

IMPLEMENTATION

STEPS	RATIONALE
1. Wash hands and apply disposable gloves.	Reduces transfer of microorganisms.
2. Place paper towels on overbed table and arrange equipment. If needed, turn on suction machine and connect tubing to suction catheter.	Prevents soiling of table top. Equipment prepared in advance ensures smooth, safe procedure.
3. Pull curtain around bed or close room door.	Provides privacy.
4. Raise bed to its highest horizontal level; lower side rail.	Use of good body mechanics with bed in high position prevents injury.
5. Position client close to side of bed; turn client's head toward mattress.	Proper positioning of head prevents aspiration.
6. Place towel under client's head and emesis basin under chin.	Prevents soiling of bed linen.
7. Carefully separate upper and lower teeth with padded tongue blade by inserting blade, quickly but gently, between back molars. Insert when client is relaxed, if possible. Do not use force (see illustration).	Prevents client from biting down on nurse's fingers and provides access to oral cavity.

➤ ***CRITICAL DECISION POINT*** **Never use fingers to separate client's teeth.**

STEPS	RATIONALE
8. Clean mouth using brush or sponge toothettes moistened with peroxide and water. Clean chewing and inner tooth surfaces first. Clean outer tooth surfaces. Swab roof of mouth, gums, and inside cheeks. Gently swab or brush tongue but avoid stimulating gag reflex (if present). Moisten clean swab or toothette with water to rinse. (Bulb syringe may also be used to rinse.) Repeat rinse several times.	Brushing action removes food particles between teeth and along chewing surfaces. Swabbing helps remove secretions and crusts from mucosa and moistens mucosa. Repeated rinsing removes peroxide that can be irritating to mucosa.
9. Suction secretions as they accumulate, if necessary.	Suction removes secretions and fluid that can collect in posterior pharynx.

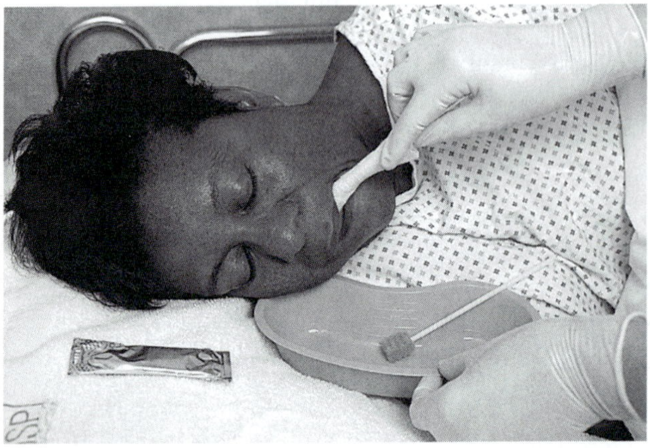

Step 7

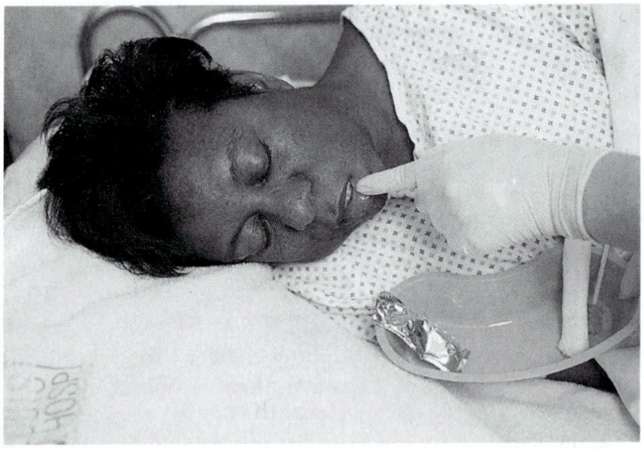

Step 10

disabilities (e.g., arthritis, neuromuscular diseases that impair motor function, diminished manual dexterity) may result in additional changes and make it more difficult for the older adult to independently carry out proper oral hygiene and denture care (Pettigrew, 1989).

Home Care Considerations

- On regular visits, assess for signs and symptoms of infection or irritation, including reddened, bleeding lesions.
- Provide special care to clients undergoing head and neck radiation, since gums may be dry and swollen and may interfere with proper denture fit.

SKILL 6-6 Shampooing the Hair of a Bedridden Client

The frequency of shampooing depends on condition of the hair and the person's daily routines. Hair condition may have gender and racial variations. Dry hair, which commonly results from aging and protein deficiency, requires less frequent shampooing than oily hair or the hair of people who exercise actively.

The nurse should remind hospitalized clients that staying in bed, excess perspiration, or treatments that leave blood or solutions in the hair may require more frequent shampoos. In a hospital setting it may be necessary to transport a client by stretcher to a special facility where a spray nozzle and sink are available for shampooing.

Clients who are allowed to sit in a chair usually can be shampooed in front of a sink. The individual should be positioned facing away from the sink, with the head and neck hyperextended over the sink's edge. A folded towel placed under the neck on the edge of the sink provides added comfort. If the client must sit at the bedside, it is possible to shampoo the hair as the client leans forward over a wash basin. Caution is needed with clients who have suffered neck injuries, since flexion and hyperextension of the neck could cause further injury.

If the client cannot sit in a chair or be transferred to a stretcher, shampooing must be done with the client in bed. The nurse may choose to do this after the bath (common in the care of infants) or later as a separate procedure.

EQUIPMENT

- Two bath towels
- Face towel or washcloth
- Shampoo
- Hair conditioner (if client requests)
- Water pitcher
- Plastic shampoo trough or board
- Washbasin
- Bath blanket
- Waterproof pad
- Clean comb and brush
- Hair dryer (optional)
- Hydrogen peroxide and saline solution (optional)
- Gloves (optional)

DELEGATION CONSIDERATIONS

The skill of shampooing can be delegated to unlicensed assistive personnel.

- Inform and assist care provider in proper way to position clients with head or neck mobility restrictions.
- Caution care provider to use warm water.
- Review procedure for use of medicated shampoo for lice; stress the steps to take to prevent transmission to other clients.

STEPS	RATIONALE
ASSESSMENT	
1. Determine if risks exist that might contraindicate shampooing. Physician's order may be needed to shampoo (consult agency policy).	Certain medical conditions such as head injury, spinal cord injury, and arthritis could place client at risk for injury during shampooing because of positioning, exposure to moisture, or manipulation of head and neck.
2. Determine if there are restrictions for positioning client.	Influences manner in which nurse prepares and positions client for procedure.
3. Review physician's orders to determine whether to use medicated shampoo.	Special shampoos may be ordered for conditions such as lice or dandruff.
4. Assess client's routine hair care practices: preferred style, type of hair care products used.	Cultural factors and gender may influence methods for grooming and hair styling.

STEPS	RATIONALE
5. Assess condition of client's hair and scalp. Note distribution of hair, degree of oiliness, and hair texture. Inspect scalp for abrasions, lacerations, lesions, areas of inflammation, and presence of infection or infestation (Table 6-2).	Determines need for further interventions (e.g., conditioners, medicated shampoo) and assesses effectiveness of previous hygiene methods.

NURSING DIAGNOSIS

Clustering of defining characteristics from the assessment data may reveal the following nursing diagnoses for clients requiring this skill:

- Self-care deficit, bathing/hygiene
- Impaired physical mobility
- Impaired skin integrity

Related factors are individualized based on a client's condition or needs.

Table 6-2 **Hair and Scalp Problems**

Problem	Characteristics	Implications	Interventions
Dandruff	Scaling of the scalp accompanied by itching; in severe cases, dandruff on eyebrows.	Dandruff causes embarrassment; if dandruff enters eyes, conjunctivitis may develop.	Shampoo regularly with medicated shampoo; in severe cases seek physician's advice.
Ticks	Small gray-brown parasites that burrow into skin and suck blood.	Ticks transmit several diseases to people; most common are Rocky Mountain spotted fever, Lyme disease, and tularemia.	Do not pull ticks from skin because sucking apparatus remains and may become infected; placing drop of oil or ether on tick or covering it with petrolatum eases removal; oil suffocates tick.
Pediculosis capitis (head lice)	Tiny grayish white parasitic insects that attach to hair strands; eggs look like oval particles, resemble dandruff; bites or pustules may be observed behind ears and at hairline.	Head lice are difficult to remove and if not treated may spread to furniture and other people.	Use medicated shampoo for eliminating lice; repeat 12 to 24 hours later; change bed linens, using isolation precautions required by agency.
Pediculosis corporis (body lice)	Tend to cling to clothing so may not be easily seen; body lice suck blood and lay eggs on clothing and furniture.	Client itches constantly; scratches on skin may become infected; hemorrhagic spots may appear on skin where lice are sucking blood.	Client should bathe or shower thoroughly; after skin is dried, apply lotion for eliminating lice; after 12 to 24 hours another bath or shower should be taken; bag infested clothing or linen until laundered.
Pediculosis pubis (crab lice)	Found in pubic hair; crab lice are grayish white with red legs.	Lice may spread through bed linen, clothing, or furniture or sexual contact.	Shave hair off affected area; cleanse as for body lice; if lice were sexually transmitted, partner must be notified.
Alopecia	Occurs in all races. Balding patches in periphery of hair line, hair becomes brittle and broken; caused by improper use of hair curlers and picks, tight braiding, hot styling tools, certain diseases.	Patches of uneven hair growth and loss alter client's appearance.	Stop hair care practices that damage hair.

STEPS	RATIONALE
P LANNING	
1. **Expected outcomes** following completion of procedure:	
➤ Client states that hair feels clean.	All soap, oil, and sediment are removed.
➤ Hair is shiny and pliant.	
➤ Scalp is clean.	
2. Explain procedure to client.	Client may be apprehensive about positioning or water entering eyes.
I MPLEMENTATION	
1. Wash hands.	Reduces transmission of microorganisms.
2. Arrange equipment in convenient place and lower side rail.	Easy access to both equipment and client prevents interruptions during procedure.
3. Place waterproof pad under client's shoulders, neck, and head (see illustration). Position client supine, with head and shoulders at top edge of bed. Place plastic trough under client's head and washbasin at end of trough. Be sure trough spout extends beyond edge of mattress.	Prevents soiling of bed linen.
4. Place rolled towel under client's neck and bath towel over client's shoulders.	Hyperextension of neck minimizes problem of water draining down back of neck.
5. Brush and comb client's hair.	Removing tangles results in more thorough cleansing.
6. Obtain warm water.	Proper water temperature prevents burns to face and scalp.
7. Ask client to hold face towel or washcloth over eyes.	Prevents shampoo or water from entering eyes.
8. Slowly pour water from water pitcher over hair until it is completely wet (see illustration). If hair contains matted blood, don gloves and apply peroxide to dissolve clots, then rinse hair with saline. Apply small amount of shampoo.	Water aids in distribution of shampoo suds over hair.

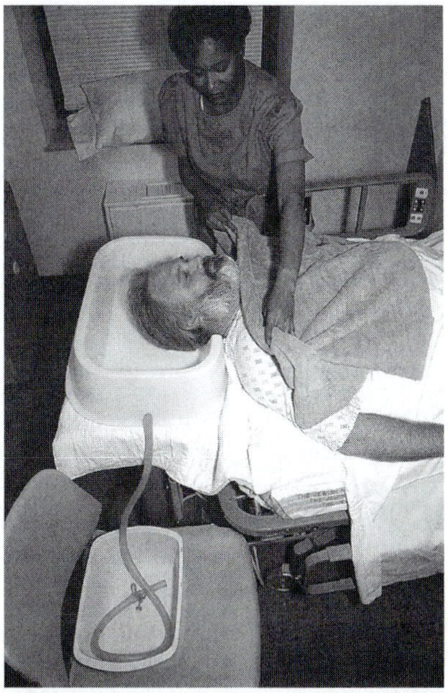

Step 3

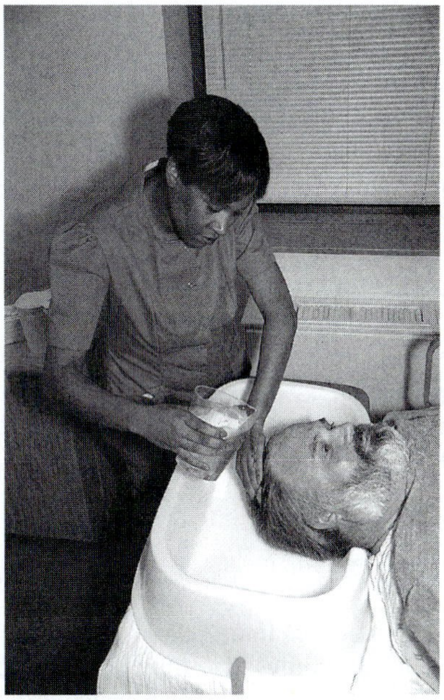

Step 8

STEPS	RATIONALE
9. Work up lather with both hands. Start at hairline and work toward back of neck. Lift head slightly with one hand to wash back of head. Shampoo sides of head. Massage scalp by applying pressure with fingertips.	Systematic progression over hair and scalp ensures thorough cleansing. Massage increases scalp circulation. Use of fingernails during massage can scratch scalp.
10. Rinse hair with water. Make sure water drains into basin. Repeat rinsing until hair is free of soap. To speed drainage from trough, press down on its spout.	Retained soap leaves dull finish on hair and may irritate scalp.
11. Repeat steps 8-10 (optional).	Ensures thorough cleansing.
12. Apply conditioner or cream rinse if requested and rinse hair thoroughly.	Conditioner prevents excess drying. Cream rinse makes combing and brushing easier.
13. Wrap client's head in bath towel. Dry client's face with cloth used to protect eyes. Dry off any moisture along neck or shoulders (see illustration).	Retained moisture may cause cooling and chills.

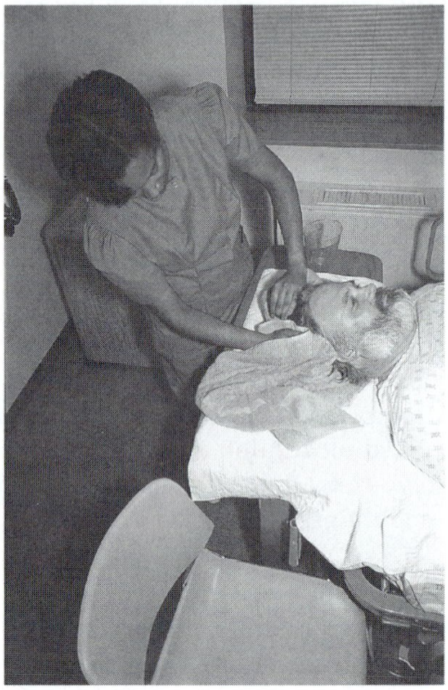

Step 13

STEPS	RATIONALE
14. Dry client's hair and scalp. Use second towel if first becomes saturated.	Drying prevents chilling.
15. Comb hair to remove tangles and dry with dryer if desired.	
16. Apply oil preparation or conditioning product to hair, if desired by client.	Oil prevents drying and breaking of hair at ends of follicles.
17. Assist client to comfortable position and complete styling of hair.	Promotes client's sense of well-being.
18. Return equipment to its proper place. Discard soiled linen in linen hamper. Wash hands.	Maintains cleanliness of environment and reduces transmission of infection.

EVALUATION

STEPS	RATIONALE
1. Ask client how hair feels.	Client will experience sense of cleanliness after shampooing.
2. Inspect condition of hair.	Shampooing should leave hair in clean condition.
3. **Unexpected outcomes** that may occur include:	
➤ Nurse may note presence of scalp lesions, dry flaky scalp, or localized areas of inflammation.	Chronic scalp conditions will not be alleviated by single shampooing.

RECORDING AND REPORTING

1. Record any pertinent findings related to condition of hair or scalp.

Documents client's response to therapy and condition of hair or scalp if further treatment is necessary.

FOLLOW-UP ACTIVITIES

1. Obtain physician's order to initiate appropriate interventions for specific hair or scalp problems.

• • • • •

Special Considerations

- Shampooing may be contraindicated for clients with increased intracranial pressure; cerebrospinal fluid leaks; open incisions of face, head, or neck; cervical neck injuries; presence of tracheostomy; severe facial edema; respiratory distress.
- Trendelenburg's position (head positioned lower than trunk and legs) is ideal for draining water away from client's face. However, many clients cannot tolerate this position.
- Hyperextension must be avoided if client has any form of neck injury.

Teaching Considerations

- Permanently disabled clients (e.g., from spinal cord injury) may require family member or friend to learn shampooing techniques.
- In clients with lice, teach measures to prevent exposure.

Pediatric Considerations

- The growth of healthy hair averages ½ inch per month; however, the rate will differ with age. The growth of scalp hair accelerates between the ages of 15 and 30 years.

Gerontologic Considerations

- Hair growth declines sharply between 50 and 60 years (Joyner, 1988).
- Hair thinning and baldness accompany aging. Although hairline recession may begin during adolescence, it more commonly begins during the forties. Coarse hair becomes finer as hair follicles decrease in size. Some hair loss is usually common in both men and women after age 60. Common baldness (not hereditary baldness) is caused by a progressive decrease in the deep dermal blood vessels of the scalp (Gallagher and Kreidler, 1987).
- Graying of the hair may begin in the thirties. Graying before this time is considered "premature" (Gallagher and Kreidler, 1987). Graying is caused by decreased melanin production in the hair follicle.

Home Care Considerations

- Assess room temperature, availability of water, and most satisfactory position for the client.
- Provide extra protection from wetness for clients with casts.
- Obtain dry shampoo preparations when a wet shampoo is contraindicated.
- Construct a trough by arranging a plastic shower curtain or tablecloth under the client's head and then tapering the cloth to form a narrow end that can drain into a bucket or basin next to the client's bed.
- In the home setting, one of the nurse's greatest challenges is to find ways the client can shampoo the hair without causing injury. For example, a client with a long leg cast may need to wash the hair at a sink until it is safe to shower or until the cast is removed and tub baths can be resumed.
- Caution clients about using chemicals and hot combs for straightening hair. Such practices can cause considerable damage to the hair. Misuse can result in scalp burns, hair loss, and allergic reactions that can cause severe skin rashes, urticaria, and conjunctivitis (Joyner, 1988).

SKILL 6-7 Shaving a Client

Shaving of facial hair can be done after a bath or shampoo. Most men prefer to do this task for themselves. However, when a client is physically unable to shave, the nurse should be able to perform the procedure as quickly and comfortably as possible. Men without beards usually shave daily. Clients with mustaches and beards require daily grooming. Keeping these areas clean is important because food particles collect easily in the hair. The beard or mustache should be trimmed, combed, or washed as needed or at the client's request. The nurse should never shave off a mustache or beard without client consent. Some religions and cultures forbid cutting or shaving any body hair (e.g., the Sikh religion) (Galanti, 1991).

Some women may wish to shave the hair under their arms or on their legs. Generally, it is not necessary for women to shave each day, but some may prefer it. The technique used to shave a woman's axillary or leg hair is the same as that for the male client's facial hair.

EQUIPMENT

Disposable razor
- Razor with new blade
- Disposable gloves (optional)
- Bath towel(s)
- Mirror
- Washcloth
- Washbasin
- Shaving cream or soap
- After-shave lotion (if client desires)

Electric razor
- Razor (with clean cutting heads)
- Bath towel
- Skin or beard conditioner
- Mirror
- After-shave lotion (if client desires)

Mustache care
- Scissors
- Brush or comb
- Bath towel
- Gooseneck lamp or overhead light
- Mirror

DELEGATION CONSIDERATIONS

The skill of shaving can be delegated to unlicensed assistive personnel.
- Inform and assist care provider in proper way to position clients with head or neck mobility restrictions.
- Caution care provider to use warm water.

STEPS	RATIONALE
ASSESSMENT	
1. Assess if client has bleeding tendency. Review medical history or laboratory values (e.g., platelet counts, prothrombin time).	Determines need to use electric razor for client's safety.
CRITICAL DECISION POINT **Clients receiving anticoagulant therapy should use an electric razor.**	
2. Assess client's ability to manipulate razor.	Determines level of assistance required.
3. Assess client's preferences for shaving products (e.g., after-shave lotion, skin conditioner, shaving cream).	Promotes client's independence through decision making.

NURSING DIAGNOSIS

Clustering of defining characteristics from the assessment data may reveal the following nursing diagnoses for clients requiring this skill:
- Grooming self-care deficit
- Impaired physical mobility
- Risk for injury

Related factors are individualized based on a client's condition or needs.

STEPS	RATIONALE
PLANNING	
1. **Expected outcomes** following completion of procedure:	
➤ Client experiences sense of comfort.	
➤ Client expresses sensation of face feeling clean and refreshed.	Hair and soap lather are removed.
➤ Skin surface is smooth, well hydrated, and free of cuts.	Client is free from injury.
➤ Client assists with procedure.	Participation provides sense of control.
2. While performing actual procedure, ask client to explain steps he or she uses to shave. Ask client to indicate if shave becomes uncomfortable.	Client can become apprehensive about being accidentally cut.

STEPS	RATIONALE

IMPLEMENTATION
DISPOSABLE RAZOR

1. Arrange supplies at bedside table and adjust lighting. Easy access to supplies prevents interruption of procedure.	Lighting provides clear view of client's face.
2. Assist client to sitting or supine position with head of bed elevated.	Provides easy access to all sides of client's face.
3. Place bath towel over client's chest and shoulders.	Prevents shaving cream or water from soiling gown.
4. Run warm water in wash basin.	Warm water will soften beard. Proper temperature prevents accidental burns.
5. Place washcloth in basin and wring out thoroughly. Apply cloth over client's entire face for several seconds.	Warm cloth helps soften skin and beard. Sensation of warmth can be relaxing.
6. Apply shaving cream or soap to client's face. Smooth cream evenly over sides of face, chin, and under nose.	Cream creates additional softening effect and lubricates skin for application of razor.

CRITICAL DECISION POINT **If client has sores, open lesions, or a tendency to bleed, the nurse should don disposable gloves.**

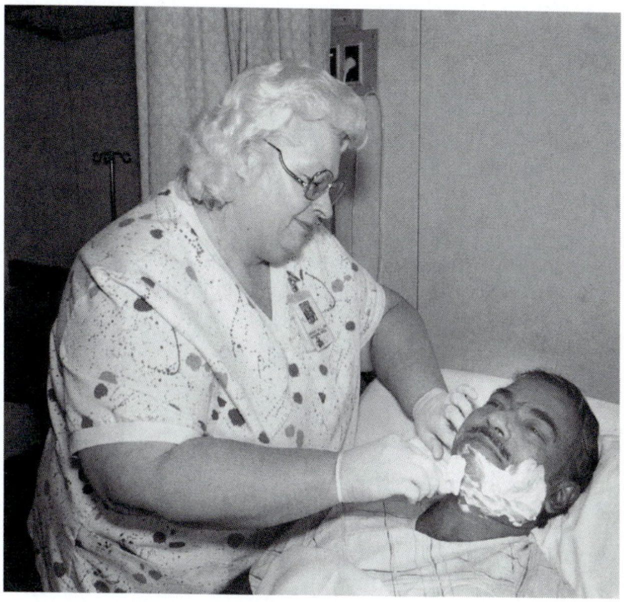

Step 7

7. Hold razor in dominant hand at 45-degree angle to the client's skin. Begin by shaving across one side of client's face. Use nondominant hand to gently pull skin taut while shaving.	Use short, firm strokes in direction hair grows (see illustration). Short downward strokes work best over upper lip. Holding skin taut prevents razor cuts and discomfort during shaving.
8. Dip razor blade in water as shaving cream accumulates on blade's edge.	Keeps cutting surface of razor blade clean.
9. After all facial hair is shaved, rinse face thoroughly with moistened washcloth.	Prevents accumulation of shaving cream, which can cause drying of skin.
10. Dry face thoroughly and apply after-shave lotion if desired.	Retained moisture may cause chapping of skin.
11. Assist client to comfortable position.	
12. Return equipment to proper place. Discard soiled linen in hamper. Wash hands.	Maintains cleanliness of client's environment and reduces transmission of infection.

STEPS	RATIONALE
ELECTRIC RAZOR	
1. Perform steps 1 through 3 for disposable razor.	
2. Apply skin conditioner or preshave preparation.	Softens skin and beard to reduce friction from razor head.
3. Turn razor on and begin by shaving across side of face. Gently hold skin taut while shaving over skin's surface. Use gentle downward stroke of razor in direction of hair growth.	Prevents pulling of beard and skin.
4. After completing shave, apply after-shave lotion as desired.	Stimulates and lubricates skin.
5. Perform steps 11 and 12 for disposable razor.	
MUSTACHE AND BEARD CARE	
1. Perform steps 1 through 3 for disposable razor.	
2. If necessary, gently comb mustache or beard.	Straightens hair that requires trimming.
3. Allow client to use mirror and direct areas to trim with scissors.	Allows client to make decisions about care; maintains sense of independence.
EVALUATION	
1. Inspect condition of shaved area and skin underneath beard or moustache.	Nurse looks for areas of localized bleeding from cuts and for areas of dryness.
2. Ask client if face feels clean and comfortable.	Evaluates level of client's comfort.
3. Ask if client is satisfied with degree of participation.	Client maintains sense of control.
4. **Unexpected outcomes** that may occur include:	
➤ Small isolated nicks or cuts may appear on skin.	Result of dull blade or improper shaving technique.
➤ Skin surface may appear dry.	Result of soap residue.
➤ Client reports burning or stinging sensation.	Result of cuts or rubbing of skin surface.
➤ Client requests permission to shave self.	Nurse plans next shave to involve client.

RECORDING AND REPORTING

1. It is not necessary to record shaving procedure unless it is included on the agency's checklist.

FOLLOW-UP ACTIVITIES

1. If client's face remains dry, apply lotion as desired to lubricate skin.

• • • • •

Special Considerations

- ➤ Conditions that place clients at risk for excessive bleeding if cut include use of anticoagulants, use of high doses of aspirin, and bleeding disorders (e.g., leukemia, hemophilia, disseminated intravascular coagulation, decreased platelets). These clients are usually restricted to using an electric razor.
- ➤ Some institutions have special policies restricting use of client's own electrical equipment. Check electrical cord for any safety hazards.
- ➤ If bleeding from nicks or cuts occurs, apply disposable gloves before rinsing, drying, and applying after-shave lotion.

Teaching Considerations

- ➤ Shaving is a simple procedure that can be taught to a family member. Instruct primary care giver in safety precautions for shaving, especially if client is receiving anticoagulant therapy.
- ➤ Instruct family member in technique to follow in the event the client is accidently nicked.

Pediatric and Gerontologic Considerations

- ➤ Usually the facial hair of adolescents and older clients does not grow quickly and thus a shave might not be necessary each day.

Home Care Considerations

- ➤ Provide adequate towels around client's neck to avoid spilling shaving cream or water on chest or bed.
- ➤ Provide adequate lighting for procedure.
- ➤ Perform procedure in comfortable setting, such as bathroom or bedroom.

SKILL 6-8 Performing Nail and Foot Care

Feet and nails often require special care to prevent infection, odors, and injury to soft tissues. Often people are unaware of foot or nail problems until discomfort or pain occurs. Common foot and nail problems are listed in Table 6-3. Problems often result from abuse or poor care of the feet and hands, such as biting nails or trimming them improperly, exposure to harsh chemicals, or wearing ill-fitting shoes. Changes in the shape, color, and texture of nails may result from various nutritional, infectious, and circulatory disorders.

The feet are important to a person's physical and emotional health. Foot pain may cause a person to change gait, resulting in strain on different muscle groups. If job performance requires a person to walk or stand comfortably, a foot disorder can become a serious problem.

Nails are epithelial tissues that grow from the root of the nail bed located in the skin at the nail groove. A normal healthy nail is transparent, smooth, and convex. Color includes variations of pink with translucent white tips. Pigment deposits or bands are common in nail beds of clients with dark skin. The nail bed angle should measure 160 degrees. The nail is surrounded by a cuticle, which slowly grows over the nail and must be regularly pushed back. The skin around the nail beds and cuticles should be smooth and without inflammation.

Nail and foot care should be included in a client's daily hygiene; the best time is during the client's bath.

EQUIPMENT

- Washbasin
- Emesis basin
- Washcloth
- Bath or face towel
- Nail clippers
- Orange stick
- Emery board or nail file
- Body lotion
- Disposable bath mat
- Paper towels
- Disposable gloves

DELEGATION CONSIDERATIONS

The skill of nail and foot care of the nondiabetic client can be delegated to unlicensed assistive personnel.

- Inform and assist care provider in proper way to use nail clippers.
- Caution care provider to use warm water.

STEPS	RATIONALE
ASSESSMENT	
1. Inspect all surfaces of fingers, toes, feet, and nails. Pay particular attention to areas of dryness, inflammation, or cracking. Also inspect areas between toes, heels, and soles of feet.	Integrity of feet and nails determines frequency and level of hygiene required. Heels, soles, and sides of feet are prone to irritation from ill-fitting shoes.
2. Assess color and temperature of toes, feet, and fingers. Assess capillary refill of nails. Palpate radial and ulnar pulse of each hand and dorsalis pedis pulse of foot; note character of pulses.	Assesses adequacy of blood flow to extremities. Circulatory alterations may change integrity of nails and increase client's chance of localized infection when break in skin integrity occurs.
3. Observe client's walking gait. Have client walk down hall or walk straight line (if able).	Painful disorders of feet can cause limping or unnatural gait.
4. Ask female clients about whether they use nail polish and polish remover frequently.	Chemicals in these products can cause excessive dryness.
5. Assess type of footwear worn by clients: Are socks worn? Are shoes tight or ill fitting? Are garters or knee-high nylons worn? Is footwear clean?	Types of shoes and footwear may predispose client to foot and nail problems (e.g., infection, areas of friction, ulcerations).
6. Identify client's risk for foot or nail problems:	Certain conditions increase likelihood of foot or nail problems.

CRITICAL DECISION POINT Clients with peripheral vascular diseases, diabetes mellitus, older adults, and clients whose immune system is suppressed may require nail care from a specialist. Professional foot care reduces their risks for infection related to improper nail care procedures.

Table 6-3 Common Foot and Nail Problems

Condition	Characteristics	Implications	Interventions
Callus	Thickened portion of epidermis, consisting of mass of horny, keratotic cells; usually flat, painless, and found on undersurface of foot or on palm of hand; caused by local friction or pressure.	Foot calluses may cause discomfort when wearing tight-fitting shoes.	Advise client to wear gloves when using tools or objects that may create friction on palms. Encourage client to wear comfortable shoes. Soak callus in warm water and Epsom salts to soften cell layers. Use pumice stone to remove callus after it softens. Applications of creams or lotions can reduce re-formation. Use of orthotic devices (e.g., foam insoles, metatarsal pads, various cushioning devices) redistributes weight and pressure away from callus area.
Corns	Keratosis caused by friction and pressure from shoes; mainly on toes, over bony prominence; usually cone shaped, round, and raised. Calluses with painful core.	Conical shape compresses underlying dermis, making it thin and tender. Pain is aggravated by tight-fitting shoes. Tissue can become attached to bone if allowed to grow. Client may suffer alteration in gait because of pain.	Surgical removal may be necessary, depending on severity of pain and size of corn. Use oval corn pads carefully, since they increase pressure on toes and reduce circulation.
Plantar warts	Fungating lesion that appears on sole of foot; caused by Papillomavirus.	Warts may be contagious, are painful, and make walking difficult.	Treatment ordered by physician may include topical applications of acids, electrodesiccation (burning with electric spark), cryotherapy (freezing) with carbon dioxide or liquid nitrogen, or laser therapy (Osterman and Stuck, 1990).
Athlete's foot (tinea pedis)	Fungal infection of foot; scaliness and cracking of skin between toes and on soles of feet; small blisters containing fluid may appear, apparently induced by constricting footwear (e.g., sneakers).	Athlete's foot can spread to other body parts, especially hands. It is contagious and frequently recurs.	Feet should be well ventilated. Drying feet well after bathing and applying powder help prevent infection. Wearing clean socks or stockings reduces incidence. Physician may order application of griseofulvin, miconazole nitrate, or tolnaftate.
Ingrown nails	Toenail or fingernail growing inward into soft tissue around nail; results from improper nail trimming, poor shoe fit, or heredity.	Ingrown nails can cause localized pain when pressure is applied.	Treatment is frequent hot soaks in antiseptic solution and removal of portion of nail that has grown into skin. Instruct client on proper nail trimming techniques. Professional débridement of offending nail border or removal of affected nail margin may be necessary.
Ram's horn nails	Unusually long curved nails.	Attempt by nurse to cut nails may damage nail bed and/or cause infection.	Refer client to podiatrist.
Paronychia	Inflammation of tissue surrounding nail after hangnail or other injury; occurs in people who frequently have their hands in water; common in diabetic clients.	Area can become infected.	Treatment is hot compresses or soaks and local application of antibiotic ointments. Paronychia can be prevented by careful manicuring.
Foot odors	Result of excess perspiration promoting microorganism growth. Faulty foot hygiene or improper footwear may also contribute.		Frequent washing, use of foot deodorants and powders, and clean footwear will prevent or reduce this problem.

STEPS	RATIONALE
a. Elderly	Poor vision, lack of coordination, or inability to bend over contribute to difficulty among elderly in performing foot and nail care. Normal physiological changes of aging also result in nail and foot problems.
b. Diabetes	Vascular changes associated with diabetes reduce blood flow to peripheral tissues. Break in skin integrity places diabetic at high risk for skin infection.
c. Heart failure, renal disease	Both conditions can increase tissue edema, particularly in dependent areas (e.g., feet). Edema reduces blood flow to neighboring tissues.
d. Cerebrovascular accident, stroke	Presence of residual foot or leg weakness or paralysis results in altered walking patterns. Altered gait pattern causes increased friction and pressure on feet.
7. Assess type of home remedies clients use for existing foot problems:	Certain preparations or applications may cause more injury to soft tissue than initial foot problem.
a. Over-the-counter liquid preparations to remove corns	Liquid preparations can cause burns and ulcerations.
b. Cutting of corns or calluses with razor blade or scissors	Cutting of corns or calluses may result in infection caused by break in skin integrity.
c. Use of oval corn pads	Oval pads may exert pressure on toes, thereby decreasing circulation to surrounding tissues.
d. Application of adhesive tape	Skin of older adult is thin and delicate and prone to tearing when adhesive tape is removed.
8. Assess client's ability to care for nails or feet: visual alterations, fatigue, musculoskeletal weakness.	Determines client's ability to perform self-care and degree of assistance required from nurse.
9. Assess client's knowledge of foot and nail care practices.	Determines client's need for health teaching.

NURSING DIAGNOSIS

Clustering of defining characteristics from the assessment data may reveal the following nursing diagnoses for clients requiring this skill:

- Altered peripheral tissue perfusion
- Dressing/grooming self-care deficit
- Impaired physical mobility
- Impaired skin integrity
- Knowledge deficit regarding foot and nail care
- Risk for infection
- Risk for injury

Related factors are individualized based on a client's condition or needs.

PLANNING

STEPS	RATIONALE
1. Expected outcomes following completion of procedure:	
➤ Nails are smooth. Cuticles and tissues surrounding nail are clear and of normal color. Surfaces of feet are smooth.	Excess skin layers are removed. Nail integrity and cleanliness are maintained.
➤ Client walks freely, without pain or unusual gait.	Sources of pressure or irritation are removed.
➤ Client explains or demonstrates nail care correctly.	Client learns skill.
2. Explain procedure to client, including fact that proper soaking requires several minutes.	Client must be willing to place fingers and feet in basins for 10 to 20 minutes. Client may become anxious or fatigued.
3. Obtain physician's order for cutting nails if agency policy requires it.	Client's skin may be accidentally cut. Certain clients are more at risk for infection, depending on their medical condition.

IMPLEMENTATION

STEPS	RATIONALE
1. Wash hands. Arrange equipment on overbed table.	Easy access to equipment prevents delays.
2. Pull curtain around bed or close room door (if desired).	Maintaining client's privacy reduces anxiety.

STEPS	RATIONALE
3. Assist ambulatory client to sit in bedside chair. Help bedfast client to supine position with head of bed elevated. Place disposable bath mat on floor under client's feet or place towel on mattress.	Sitting in chair facilitates immersing feet in basin. Bath mat protects feet from exposure to soil or debris.
4. Fill washbasin with warm water. Test water temperature.	Warm water softens nails and thickened epidermal cells, reduces inflammation of skin, and promotes local circulation. Proper water temperature prevents burns.
5. Place basin on bath mat or towel and help client place feet in basin. Place call light within client's reach.	Clients with muscular weakness or tremors may have difficulty positioning feet. Client's safety is maintained.
6. Adjust overbed table to low position and place it over client's lap. (Client may sit in chair or lie in bed.)	Easy access prevents accidental spills.
7. Fill emesis basin with warm water and place basin on paper towels on overbed table.	Warm water softens nails and thickened epidermal cells.
8. Instruct client to place fingers in emesis basin and place arms in comfortable position.	Prolonged positioning can cause discomfort unless normal anatomical alignment is maintained.
9. Allow client's feet and fingernails to soak for 10 to 20 minutes. Rewarm water after 10 minutes.	Softening of corns, calluses, and cuticles ensures easy removal of dead cells and easy manipulation of cuticle.
CRITICAL DECISION POINT **Diabetics are discouraged from soaking hands and feet.**	
10. Clean gently under fingernails with orange stick while fingers are immersed (see illustration). Remove emesis basin and dry fingers thoroughly.	Orange stick removes debris under nails that harbors microorganisms. Thorough drying impedes fungal growth and prevents maceration of tissues.

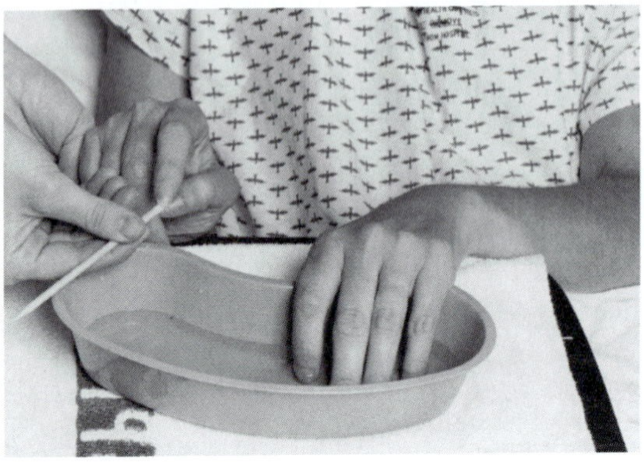

Step 10

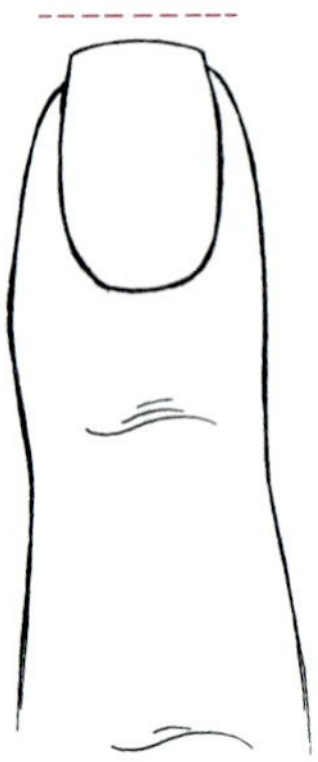

Step 11

STEPS	RATIONALE
11. With nail clippers, clip fingernails straight across and even with tops of fingers (see illustration). Shape nails with emery board or file. If client has circulatory problems, do not cut nail; file the nail only.	Cutting straight across prevents splitting of nail margins and formation of sharp nail spikes that can irritate lateral nail margins. Filing prevents cutting nail too close to nail bed.
12. Push cuticle back gently with orange stick.	Reduces incidence of inflamed cuticles.
13. Move overbed table away from client.	Provides easier access to feet.
14. Put on disposable gloves and scrub callused areas of feet with washcloth.	Gloves prevent transmission of fungal infection. Friction removes dead skin layers.
15. Clean gently under nails with orange stick. Remove feet from basin and dry thoroughly.	Removal of debris and excess moisture reduces chances of infection.
16. Clean and trim toenails using procedures in steps 11 and 12 (see illustrations on p. 169). Do not file corners of toenails.	Shaping corners of toenails may damage tissues.
17. Apply lotion to feet and hands and assist client back to bed and into comfortable position.	Lotion lubricates dry skin by helping to retain moisture.

STEPS	RATIONALE
18. Remove disposable gloves and place in receptacle. Clean and return equipment and supplies to proper place. Dispose of soiled linen in hamper. Wash hands.	Reduces transmission of infection.

EVALUATION

1. Inspect nails and surrounding skin surfaces	Evaluates condition of skin and nails. Allows nurse to note any remaining rough nail edges.
2. Ask client to explain or demonstrate nail care.	Evaluates client's level of learning techniques.
3. Observe client's walk after toenail care.	Evaluates level of comfort and mobility achieved.
4. **Unexpected outcomes** that may occur include:	
➤ Nails discolored, rough, and concave or irregular in shape.	A single hygiene measure will not improve nail condition.
➤ Cuticles and surrounding tissues may be inflamed and tender to touch. Localized areas of tenderness may occur on feet with calluses or corns at point of friction.	Repeated soakings are necessary to help relieve inflammation and remove layers of cells from calluses or corns. Change in footwear or corrective foot surgery may be needed for permanent improvement in corns or calluses.
➤ Ulcerations involving toes or feet may remain.	Foot care will not eliminate ulcers caused by vascular disease but will aid in keeping areas clean.
➤ Client unable to explain or perform foot care.	Further instruction is required.
➤ Client complains of pain while walking and has unsteady gait.	Pressure or irritation on foot remains.

RECORDING AND REPORTING

1. Record procedure and observations (e.g., breaks in skin, inflammation, ulcerations).	Documents procedure, client's response, and presence of abnormalities requiring additional therapy.
2. Report any breaks in skin or ulcerations to nurse in charge or physician.	These abnormalities can seriously increase client's risk of infection and must be carefully observed.

FOLLOW-UP ACTIVITIES

1. Clients with severe hypertrophy of nails should be referred to podiatrist for care to avoid risk of additional tissue injury.
2. Clients with chronic foot pain should be seen by physician.

• • • • •

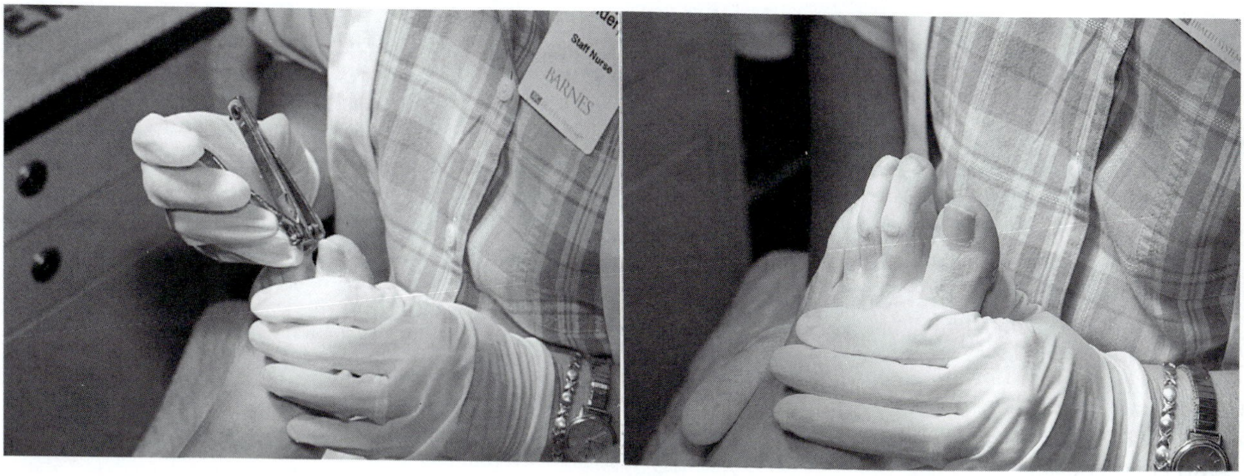

Step 16

Special Considerations

- Clients with diabetes and peripheral vascular disease may have peripheral neuropathies that reduce sensation.
- Never cut nails of clients with diabetes and other circulatory problems. File only.

Teaching Considerations

- Instruct nondiabetic client to wash and soak feet daily using lukewarm water. Thoroughly pat feet dry and dry well between toes.
- Caution client against cutting corns or calluses or using commercial removers. Consult physician or podiatrist.
- If feet tend to perspire, apply mild foot powder.
- Encouraging client to wear absorbent liners with nylon stockings will also help reduce perspiration and foot odors. Seamless white socks are preferred, since they are more absorbent (Evanski and Reinherz, 1991).
- If dryness is noted along feet or between toes, apply lanolin, baby oil, or even corn oil and rub gently into skin.
- Teach client to avoid wearing elastic stockings or constricting garters and to avoid crossing legs. Both impair circulation to lower extremities.
- Inspect feet daily: tops and soles, heels, and area between toes. Use mirror to check soles and heels.
- Encourage client to wear clean socks or stockings daily (change twice a day if feet perspire a lot).
- Check for holes or darns that might cause pressure.
- Caution client against walking barefoot. Clients with impaired foot circulation should wear protective footwear at all times and check inside of shoes daily for pebbles, foreign objects, and tears in inner liner (Osterman and Stuck, 1990).
- Encourage client to wear proper-fitting shoes. Soles of shoes should be flexible and nonslipping. Shoes should have porous uppers and be sturdy, closed in, and not restrictive to the feet.
- Minor cuts should be washed immediately and dried thoroughly. Only mild antiseptics (e.g., Neosporin ointment) should be applied to the skin. Avoid iodine or merbromin.

Gerontologic Considerations

- Changes in aging skin include thinning of epidermis and subcutaneous fat and dryness because of decreased activity of oil and sweat glands. These changes can be seen in the feet. In addition, nails become opaque, tough, scaly, brittle, and hypertrophied.
- A lifetime of limited exercise can result in laxity of foot ligaments and musculature and lead to instability and impaired mobility.
- Common foot problems of older adults include heel pain caused by tearing of plantar fascia and foot musculature, metatarsalgia (pain beneath metatarsal head), hammertoes and claw toes, corns and calluses, pathological nail conditions (e.g., ingrown toenails, fungal infections), arthritis, and neuropathies that cause diminished sensation in foot (Osterman and Stuck, 1990).
- Older persons are also more vulnerable to bunions because feet tend to spread with aging. Young people are rarely affected, although bunions sometimes occur in individuals as young as 10 to 13 years of age (Evanski and Reinherz, 1991).

Home Care Considerations

- Alternative therapies: moleskin applied to areas of feet that are under friction is less likely to cause local pressure than corn pads; spot adhesive bandages can guard corns against friction, but do not have padding to protect against pressure; wrapping small pieces of lamb's wool around toes reduces irritation of soft corns between toes.
- Assess use of bathroom sink for soaking client's hands and tub for soaking feet.

CRITICAL THINKING EXERCISES

1. You are helping a family care for an older adult relative in the home. What type of hygiene products are available in local drugstores for the special care needs of bathing the older adult?
2. Describe how you might instruct a daughter to perform perineal care for her mother who has arthritis of the hips.
3. What assessment data would you collect when caring for the foot of a 67-year-old diabetic client whose foot was cut while walking barefoot in the backyard?

REFERENCES

Agency for Health Care Policy and Research: *Pressure ulcers in adults: prediction and prevention,* Pub Nos 92-0047, 92-0050, Rockville, Md, 1992, Public Health Service, US Department of Health and Human Services.

Barnes SH: Patient and family education for the patient with a pressure necrosis, *Nurs Clin North Am* 22:463, 1987.

Blaney GM: Mouth care—basic and essential, *Geriatr Nurs* 7:242, 1986.

Danielson KH: Oral care and older adults, *J Gerontol Nurs* 14:6, 1988.

Dudjak LA: Mouth care for mucositis due to radiation therapy, *Cancer Nurs* 10:131, 1987.

Evanski PM, Reinherz RP: Easing the pain of common foot problems, *Patient Care* 25:38, 1991.

Galanti G: *Caring for patients from different cultures,* Philadelphia, 1991, University of Pennsylvania Press.

Gallagher LP, Kreidler MC: *Nursing and health: maximizing human potential throughout the life cycle,* Norwalk, Conn, 1987, Appleton & Lange.

Greifzu S, Radjeski D, Winnick B: Oral care is part of cancer care, *RN* 53:43, 1990.

Hardy M: A pilot study of the diagnosis and treatment of impaired skin integrity: dry skin in older persons, *Nurs Diagn* 90:60, 1990.

Harrell JS, Damon JF: Prediction of patients' need for mouth care, *West J Nurs Res* 11:748, 1989.

Joyner M: Hair care in the black patient, *J Pediatr Health Care* 2:281, 1988.

Kahn R: Renewing the commitment to oral hygiene, *Geriatr Nurs* 7:244, 1986.

Maklebust J: Pressure ulcer update, *RN* 41(12):56, 1991.

Meckstroth RL: Improving quality and efficiency in oral hygiene, *J Gerontol Nurs* 15:38, 1989.

Moss SJ: Preventive techniques in infant dental care, *Nurse Pract* 13:37, 1988.

Osterman HM, Stuck RM: The aging foot, *Orthop Nurs* 9:43, 1990.

Pettigrew D: Investing in mouth care, *Geriatr Nurs* 10:22, 1989.

Poland JM: Comparing Moi-Stir to lemon glycerin swabs, *Am J Nurs* 87:422, 1987.

ADDITIONAL READING

Badger F, Cameron E, Evers H: The nursing auxiliary service and the care of elderly patients, *J Adv Nurs* 14:471, 1989.

Donahue AM: Tepid sponging, *J Emerg Nurs* 9:78, 1983.

Ebersole P, Hess P: *Toward healthy aging: human needs and nursing response,* ed 4, St Louis, 1994, Mosby.

Friedman A, Barton L: Efficacy of sponging vs acetaminophen for reduction of fever, *Pediatr Emerg Care* 6(1):6, 1990.

Golden S: *Nursing a loved one at home,* Philadelphia, 1988, Running Press Book Publishers.

Kpnea NT, Scher RK: Nail abnormalities: easily observed signs of systemic disease, *Consultant* 27:47, 1987.

Patient information from your doctor: preventing common foot problems, *Patient Care* 25:54, 1991.

Wong DL: *Whaley and Wong's nursing care of infants and children,* ed 5, St Louis, 1995, Mosby.

CHAPTER 7

Care of the Client's Environment

OBJECTIVES

Mastery of content in this chapter will enable the nurse to:

- Define key terms.
- Describe equipment found in a hospitalized client's room.
- Explain bed safety features.
- Describe common bed positions.
- Make an occupied bed.
- Make an unoccupied bed.

KEY TERMS

Drawsheet
Fowler's position
Mitered corner
Reverse Trendelenburg position
Semi-Fowler position
Trendelenburg position

SKILLS

7-1 Making an Unoccupied Bed
7-2 Making an Occupied Bed

When caring for clients who need to remain in or near their bed for an extended period, it is important to try to make that environment as comfortable as possible. A calm, comfortable restorative environment can be maintained in a hospital, in an extended care facility, or in the client's home.

Rooms should be comfortable, safe, and large enough to allow clients, visitors, and care providers to move about freely. The care provider should be able to control temperature, ventilation, noise, and odors easily.

A room in a typical hospital, extended care, or long-term care facility contains the following basic pieces of furniture: overbed table, bedside stand, storage space, chairs, lights, and bed with call light. These furnishings provide a setting for the client to rest as well as safe and convenient access to all client care supplies. Behind each bed is a wall unit that may contain various power outlets, as well as receptacles for connecting oxygen and suction equipment. In most hospitals a mercury sphygmomanometer with cuff is attached to the wall. Special intensive care units often have poles extending from the ceiling on which to hang intravenous (IV) fluid bags. The room is generally designed so that all necessary supplies and equipment are easily accessible for the nurse's and physician's use.

When care is provided in the client's home, special equipment and adaptations to the client's home may be necessary. If a client is to receive home oxygen, then oxygen tanks are needed, and with some oxygen equipment, the client may need additional electrical wiring in the home. Clients and their families may need to order a hospital bed and overbed table so that physical care can be given easily. In addition, the client's bathroom is adapted with safety equipment for ease in toileting and getting into and out of the tub and shower.

ROOM EQUIPMENT

Chairs

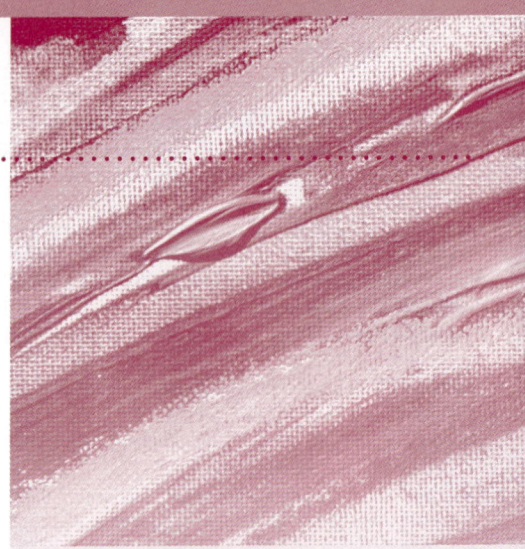

Most hospital rooms contain an armless, straight-back chair and an upholstered lounge chair with arms. When clients are recovering from surgery or illnesses resulting in abdominal pain, they often prefer the straight-back chair because less effort is needed to get into or out of it. Straight-back chairs are convenient when temporarily transferring the client from the bed, for example, during bed making. The straight-back chair is also easier to maneuver than the heavy lounge chair. However, the straight-back chair may be more uncomfortable and less safe for certain clients than the deeper lounge chair. The lounge chair often has a deeper seat and may require more effort on the part of the client to sit comfortably.

Lights

Each room has an overbed light that focuses on the client's bed. The light controls are usually on the call light apparatus. Each room also has a floor or table lamp. Special examination lights may extend over the bed from the wall or ceiling. These lights are useful during procedures such as a dressing change. They are often movable and should be positioned for easy reach but moved aside when not in use. Portable lamps provide extra illumination for bedside procedures. These are especially useful to focus light on hard-to-reach areas, for example, during urinary catheter insertion.

A call light is at each client's bedside. When a client presses a button located on the side rail of the bed or at the end of an extension cord, a light goes on at the nurses' station or outside the client's room. The call light signal indicates that a client needs assistance and is "calling" the nurse. In addition to call lights, most hospitals have intercom systems that allow clients to talk to a staff person at the nurses' station (Fig. 7-1). Many hospital units also have emergency signal lights, particularly in the client's bathroom, which nurses use to call for assistance when clients are in trouble. Clients may also be instructed to use the emergency signal lights if an emergency situation arises when they are in the bathroom alone.

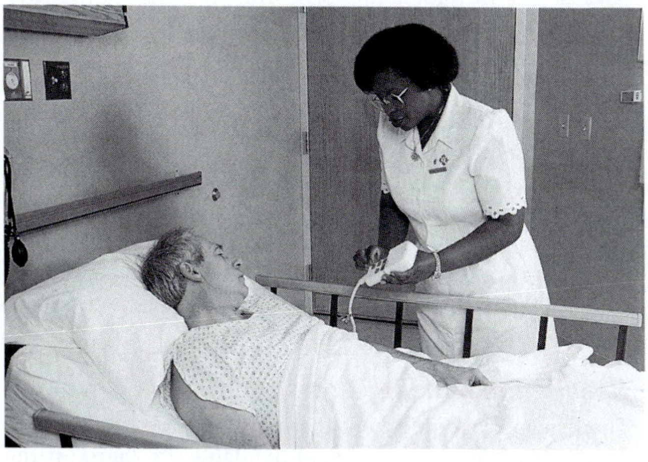

Fig. 7-1 Nurse teaching client how to use intercom to nurses' station.

Overbed Tables

The overbed table is a long, narrow table with wheels. It can be adjusted to various heights over the client's bed or chair. It usually contains two storage drawers. The table provides ideal working space for the nurse and serves as a surface on which to place meal trays, toiletry items, and objects frequently used by the client.

Bedside Stand

The bedside stand or table is a small table or cabinet located next to the bed. It is used to store the client's personal articles and hygiene equipment such as the bath basin, towels, or an emesis basin. Each table usually contains a drawer above and a cupboard below. The telephone, water pitcher, facial tissues, and drinking cup are commonly placed on the bedside table.

Beds

Because the bed is the piece of equipment used most by the client, it should be designed for comfort and safety, and it should be adaptable to various positions.

The typical hospital bed consists of a firm mattress on a metal frame that can be raised and lowered horizontally. The frame is divided into three sections so that the operator can raise and lower the head and foot of the bed separately, in addition to inclining the entire bed with the head up or down. Table 7-1 lists common bed positions. Most beds are powered by electric motors, but some beds operate manually or by hydraulic power.

Hospital beds come in two different lengths. Standard length is approximately 6 feet (a longer bed is available for taller clients). Each bed sits on four rollers, or casters, that allow the nurse to move the bed easily. Often clients who are critically ill or who are immobilized in traction are transported to different locations, such as the radiology department, in bed.

The position of a bed is usually changed by electric controls built into the side of the bed, at the foot of the bed, or on a bedside cable. Clients can thus raise or lower sections of the bed without expending much energy. It is important for nurses to instruct clients on the proper use of the controls and to caution them against positions that might cause harm. A hospital bed is usually 65 to 70 cm (26 to 28 inches) above the floor at its lowest level. In the home most beds are 50 to 55 cm (20 to 22 inches) high. The greater height of a hospital bed prevents undue musculoskeletal strain on the nurse and the client. It is unnecessary for the nurse to reach across or bend down while caring for clients, and clients can move from the bed to a chair with minimal stress on hips and knees.

Beds contain a number of safety features. Locks located on the wheels, casters, or at the center of the bed frame (Fig. 7-2) should be used whenever the bed is stationary to prevent accidental movement during performance of a procedure (e.g., transferring the client from bed to a stretcher). Side rails, located on both sides of a bed, protect clients from accidental falls, help clients position themselves, and provide upper extremity support as a client

Table 7-1 Common Bed Positions

Position	Description	Uses
Fowler's 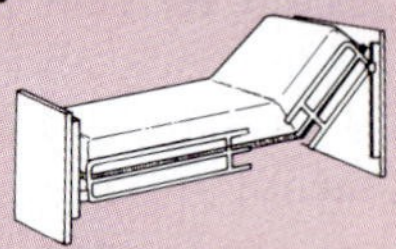	Head of bed raised to angle of 45 to 90 degrees or more; semisitting position (knees raise on most beds approximately 15 degrees).	Preferred while client eats; used during nasogastric tube insertion and nasotracheal suction; promotes lung expansion.
Semi-Fowler's 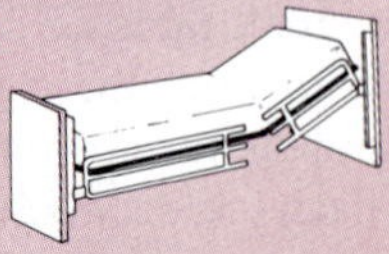	Head of bed raised approximately 30 to 45 degrees; incline is less than Fowler's position (knees raise on most beds approximately 15 degrees).	Promotes lung expansion; relieves strain on abdominal muscles.
Trendelenburg 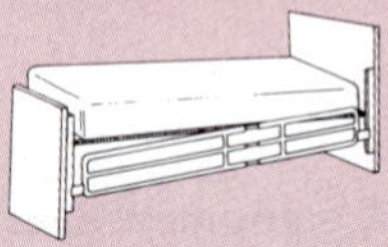	Entire bed frame tilted, with head of bed down.	For postural drainage; facilitates venous return in clients with poor peripheral perfusion.
Reverse Trendelenburg 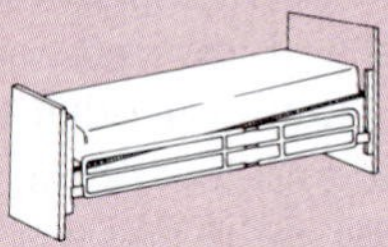	Entire bed frame tilted, with foot of bed down.	Used infrequently; promotes gastric emptying and prevents esophageal reflux.
Flat 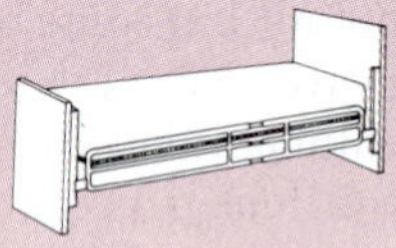	Entire bed frame parallel with floor.	For clients with vertebral injuries and in cervical traction. Position used for clients who are hypotensive, and generally preferred by clients for sleeping.

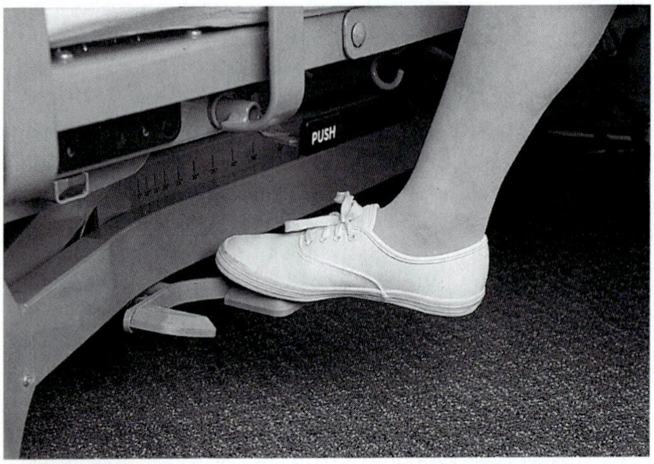

Fig. 7-2 Lock on bed wheels.

gets out of bed. Side rails are adjustable metal frames that can be raised and lowered by pushing or pulling a knob. The nurse never leaves the bedside when a side rail is lowered with the client still in bed. Each bed also has a special headboard that is removable. This feature is important in emergency situations when the medical team must have easy access to the client's head during cardiopulmonary resuscitation (see Chapter 16).

Mattresses. Most beds have firm, water-repellent mattresses. A mattress should have an even surface for the client's comfort. Most mattresses have handles on the sides to be used when the mattresses are removed or turned over. A rubber or plastic surface permits easy cleaning. Special mattresses provide extra comfort and support for clients and relieve pressure on bony prominences. Chapter 32 reviews a variety of special mattresses and indications for their use.

Special Equipment

There is special equipment that may be added to a bed or room. Examples of equipment available are listed in the box on p. 175. The nurse is responsible for knowing how to use all equipment safely.

SPECIAL ROOM EQUIPMENT

Foot Boots

Boots made of a smooth substance such as foam or sheepskin to support the foot in dorsiflexion (Fig. 7-3) may be preferred over foot boards because dorsiflexion is maintained while positioning the client in nonsupine positions. The boot stays secured with Velcro strips. Daily removal and inspection of the foot are required.

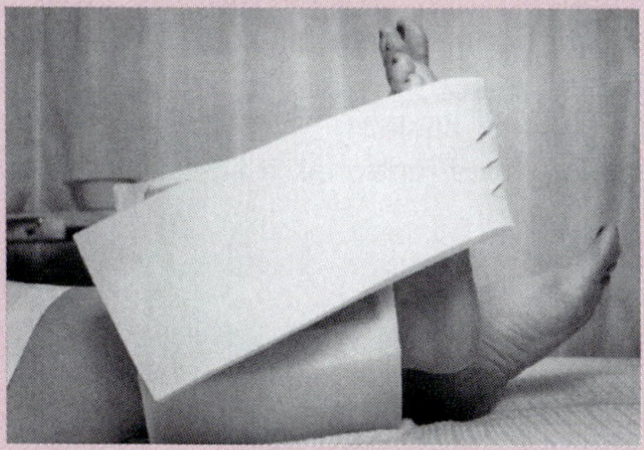

Fig. 7-3

Bed Board

A long wooden or plexiglass board, the length of a regular bed mattress, that is placed under a mattress to provide added support. Clients with back pain frequently use bed boards. The boards are hinged so that the foot or end of the bed can be elevated.

Intravenous (IV) Pole

A metal pole or stand that supports an IV fluid container while fluid is administered to a client. The rod may fit into the metal frame of a client's bed, stand on the floor, or attach to an overhead track (Fig. 7-4).

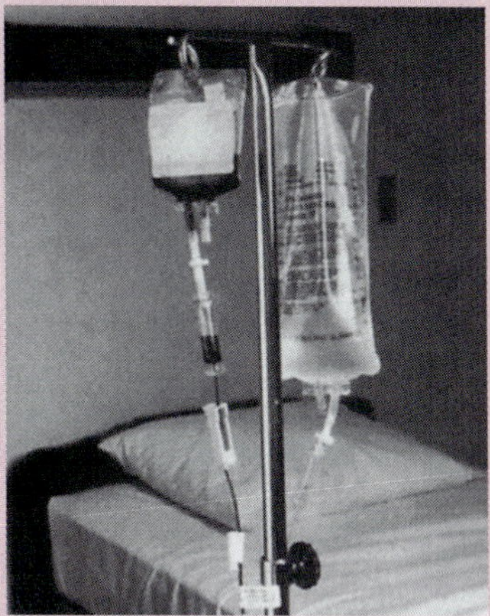

Fig. 7-4

GUIDELINES

1. Keep the environment as comfortable as possible by controlling ventilation and temperature. Depending on a client's age and physical condition, room temperature should be maintained between 20° C and 23° C (68° F and 74° F). Infants, older adults, and the acutely ill may need a warmer temperature. However, certain critically ill clients require cooler room temperatures to lower the body's metabolic demands. Controlling drafts and eliminating lingering odors from draining wounds, vomitus, bedpans, or urinals will also improve a client's comfort. Most hospitals now prohibit smoking in clients' rooms.
2. Control extraneous noises in a client's room. Ill clients are sensitive to noises in a hospital environment. A nurse should try to control noise levels by handling equipment properly; making sure equipment is in proper working order; controlling voice volume; and, unless contraindicated, closing the client's room door.
3. Make the environment as safe as possible. Keep all personal care items within the client's reach. When the head of the bed is raised, the bedside stand is usually not within easy reach and must be moved forward. If the client must leave the bed to go to the bathroom, be sure there are no objects obstructing the way.
4. Make the environment personal for the client. A picture of family members, some get well cards, or a small radio may help the client to relax. However, do not clutter the client's room with unnecessary equipment and supplies. Whenever possible remove equipment and supplies after treatments are complete.
5. Be sure the client is easily accessible to the health care team. Often a client will have numerous IV lines and drainage tubes connected to portable poles and suction machines. At times of emergency, the health care team must reach the client easily and quickly. Keep intravenous poles and portable equipment in positions that do not obstruct access to the client.

DELEGATION CONSIDERATIONS

The skills of bed making and making an occupied bed can be delegated to unlicensed assistive personnel.

- Instruct care provider how to transfer client from bed to chair. Review any precautions or activity restrictions for client.
- Inform care provider how to properly position clients during occupied bed-making procedure.
- Tell care provider what to do if wound drainage, dressing material, drainage tubes, or intravenous (IV) tubing becomes dislodged or is found in the linens.
- Instruct care provider what to do if client becomes fatigued.
- Stress safety procedures, for example, use of side rails in making an occupied bed, location of call system for easy access in the event that staff assistance is needed.

SKILL 7-1 Making an Unoccupied Bed

Clients spend much of their time in bed, eating, bathing, using bedpans or urinals, and undergoing numerous therapeutic procedures. It is essential that the nurse keep the bed as clean and comfortable as possible. Frequent inspections are necessary to be sure that the linen is clean, dry, and wrinkle free. Bed linen that becomes wet or soiled should be changed immediately.

Whenever possible the nurse should make the bed while it is unoccupied. Having the client get out of bed is an ideal way to promote ambulation. The nurse usually makes a bed in the morning after the client's bed bath or while the client is up bathing and showering. Another convenient time for bed making is when the client is out of the room for tests or procedures.

By making an unoccupied bed the nurse can ensure that the linen is smooth and free of wrinkles. It is also easier to insert any extra waterproof pads or special foam rubber mattresses (see Chapter 32) when a bed is unoccupied.

EQUIPMENT

- **Linen bag(s)**
- **Mattress pad (needs to be changed only when soiled)**
- **Bottom sheet (flat or fitted)**
- **Drawsheet (optional)**
- **Top sheet**
- **Blanket**
- **Bedspread**
- **Waterproof pads or bath blankets (optional)**
- **Pillowcases**
- **Bedside chair or table**
- **Disposable gloves (optional, if linens are soiled)**

STEPS	RATIONALE
ASSESSMENT	
1. Verify client's activity orders and assess client's ability to get out of bed (e.g., level of fatigue or discomfort, status of vital signs, coordination, strength, nausea, or dizziness).	Physician's assessment of client's medical condition determines level of activity allowed, including whether the client should be out of bed. Nursing assessment documents whether it is safe for the client to get out of bed and whether additional assistance is needed.
2. Assess potential for client incontinence or for having excess drainage on bed linen (e.g., postoperative clients with wounds or drainage tubes, clients receiving soak applications, diaphoretic clients).	Determines need for protective waterproof pads or bath blankets on bed.
3. Determine need for any special position precautions once client is out of bed (e.g., elevation of leg or arm).	Position must be maintained while client is sitting to prevent any physical complications.

NURSING DIAGNOSIS

Clustering of defining characteristics from the assessment data may reveal the following diagnoses for clients requiring this skill:

- ➤ Activity intolerance
- ➤ Impaired physical mobility

Related factors are individualized based on a client's condition or needs.

PLANNING

STEPS	RATIONALE
1. **Expected outcomes** following completion of procedure: ➤ Bed linen is taut, with a clean dry surface. ➤ Client's vital signs remain stable, and client denies fatigue or dizziness while transferring to or sitting in chair. ➤ Client's skin remains free from breakdown.	
2. Determine with the client when the best time would be to change the bed linens. Explain to the client that the bed should be changed while the client is sitting in a chair.	The client should not feel inconvenienced by the procedure. The client may feel anxious or uncomfortable if fatigued.

STEPS	RATIONALE

IMPLEMENTATION

1. Wash hands and apply gloves, if linen is soiled.
   - Reduces transmission of microorganisms.
2. Assemble and arrange equipment on bedside chair or table. Remove all unnecessary equipment, such as overbed table.
   - Assembling all equipment provides smooth flow of procedure and assists in increasing client's comfort. Placing linen on clean surface minimizes spread of infection.
3. Lower side rail on near side of bed and remove call light. Adjust bed height to comfortable working position.
   - Provides easy access to bed. Minimizes strain on back muscles.
4. On near side, loosen linen, starting at head of bed. Move along sides and then down toward the foot. Move to other side of bed, lower side rail, and loosen all linen.
   - Makes linen easier to remove.
5. Remove bedspread and blanket separately by folding each into a bundle or square. If spread and blanket are soiled, place them in linen bag. Keep soiled linen away from uniform (see illustration). Avoid fanning or shaking linen.
   - Reduces transmission of microorganisms.

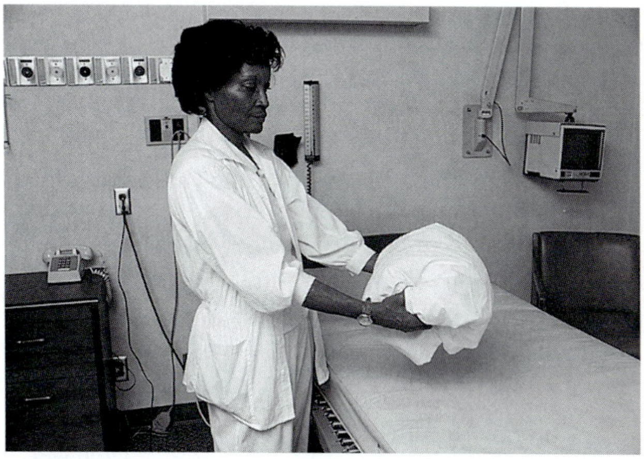

Step 5

6. If spread or blanket is to be reused, fold each by grasping top edge with both hands, one hand at the center, and other hand at the end. Fold top edge down, even with the bottom edge. Pick up spread at center and fold so that farthest side comes even with nearest side. Bring top and bottom edges together again. Place folded spread or blanket over back of chair.
   - Facilitates replacement and prevents wrinkling.
7. Remove soiled pillowcases by grasping closed end with one hand and slipping pillow out with other. Discard pillowcases in linen bag and place pillows on table.
   - Pillows slide out easily, minimizing chance of contact with soiled linen.
8. Fold each piece of remaining bed linen into bundle or folded square and discard into linen bag. Do not put linen on floor.

CRITICAL DECISION POINT **Attempting to fold all soiled linen at once creates a bulky bundle that is difficult to discard and may come in contact easily with uniform.**

9. Slide mattress toward head of bed. Wipe off any moisture on the mattress with a washcloth moistened in antiseptic solution; dry thoroughly.
   - If mattress slides toward foot of bed when head of bed is raised, it is difficult to tuck in linen. Antiseptic reduces transmission of microorganisms.

STEPS	RATIONALE
10. Stand at side of bed where clean linen is placed. Spread mattress pad over mattress. Smooth out all wrinkles in pad.	Time is saved by making half of bed first and then moving to the opposite side. Wrinkles or folds of linen are source of chronic irritation against client's skin.
11. If using flat sheet as bottom sheet, unfold lengthwise and place vertical center crease of sheet lengthwise along center of bed. Fold over sheet's top layer toward opposite side of bed. Smooth bottom layer of sheet across mattress on near side; bring edge over side of mattress. Allow it to hang about 25 cm (10 in) over mattress edge. Hem of bottom edge of sheet should lie seam down, even with bottom edge of mattress (see illustration). Pull remaining top portion of sheet over top edge of mattress.	Method of unfolding linen saves time and energy. Making one side of bed at a time avoids excess movement. Proper placement of linen ensures that adequate length will be available to cover opposite side of bed. Keeping seam edge down eliminates source of irritation to client's skin. If bottom edge of sheet is not tucked in, it can be changed later without removing top linen.

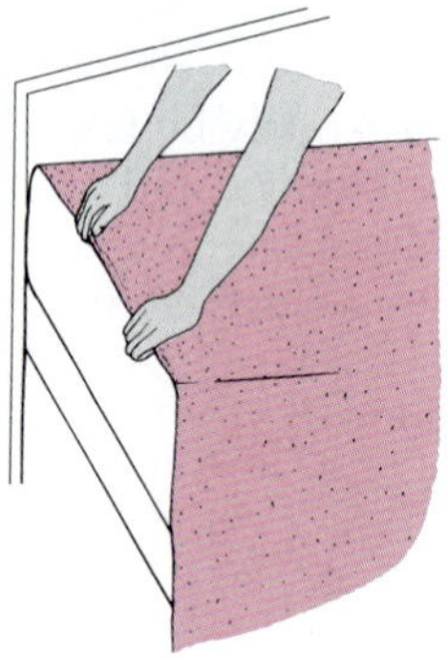

Step 11

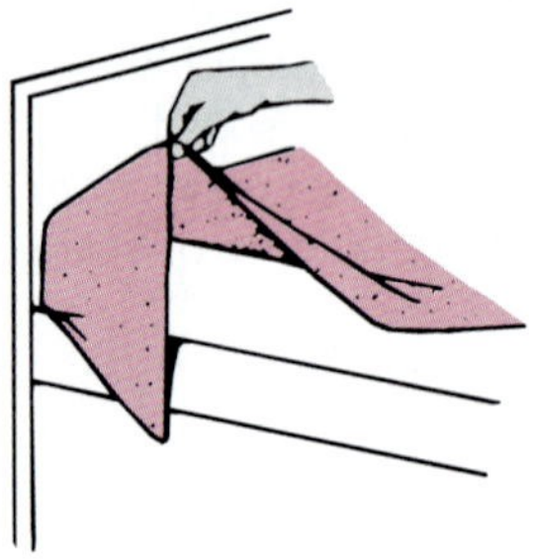

Step 12c

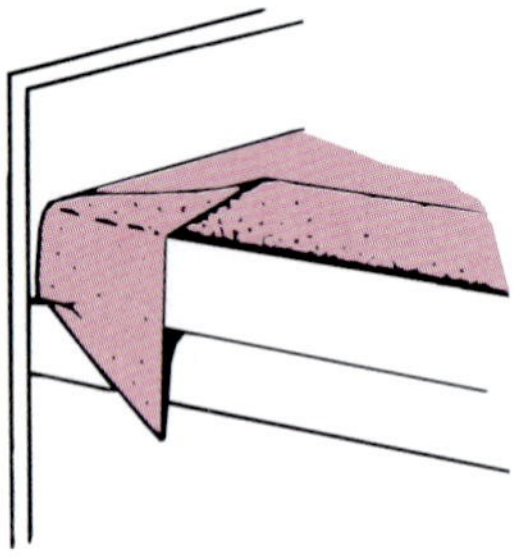

Step 12d

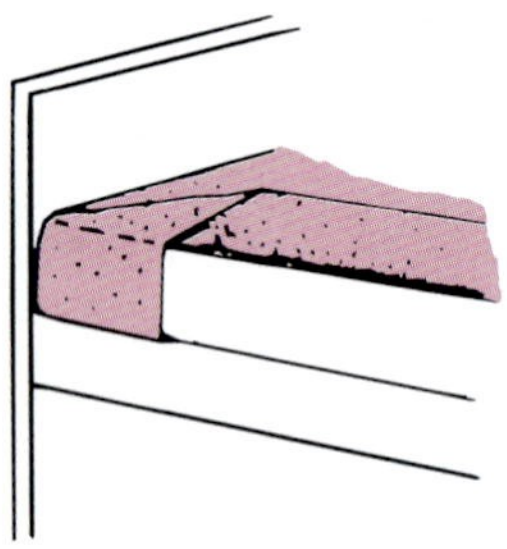

Step 12e

STEPS	RATIONALE
12. While standing at the head of the bed, **miter** top **corner** of bottom sheet:	
a. Face head of bed diagonally. Place hand that is away from head of bed under top corner of mattress near mattress edge and lift.	
b. With other hand, tuck top edge of bottom sheet smoothly under mattress so that side edges of sheet above and below mattress would meet if brought together.	
c. Face side of bed and lift edge of top sheet approximately 45 cm (18 in) down from top of mattress (see illustration).	
d. Lay sheet on top of mattress to form a triangular fold, with lower base of triangle even with mattress side edge (see illustration).	
e. Tuck lower edge of the sheet, hanging free below mattress, under mattress.	Tucking with palms down keeps the nurse from hitting knuckles on the bed frame or bedsprings. Do this without pulling the triangular fold (see illustration).
f. Hold portion of sheet covering side edge of mattress in place with one hand (see illustration). With the other hand, pick up top of triangular linen fold and bring it down over side of mattress. Tuck this portion of the sheet under mattress (see illustration).	Mitered corner is not loosened easily.

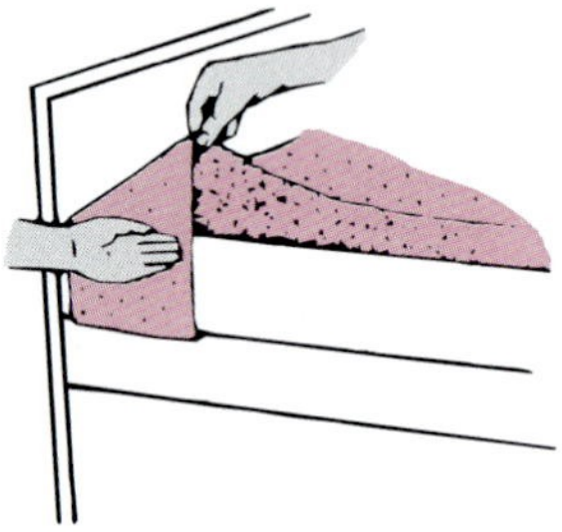

Step 12f (1)

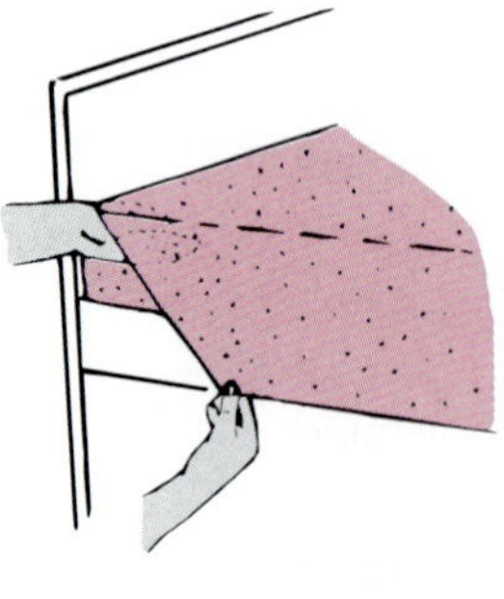

Step 12f (2)

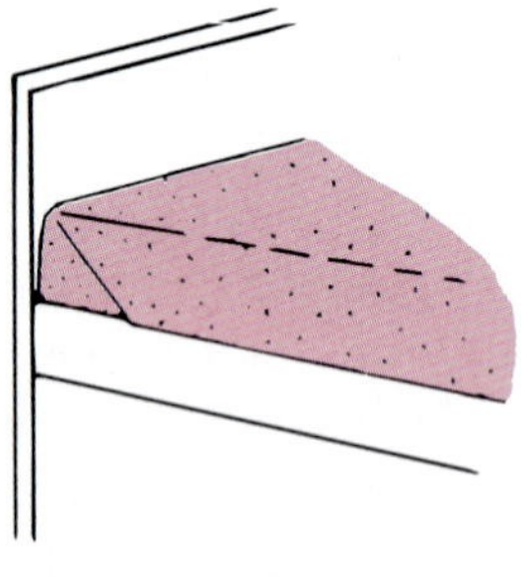

Step 13

STEPS	RATIONALE
13. Tuck remaining portion of sheet under mattress. Keep linen smooth (see illustration on p. 178). (Optional) Open drawsheet so that it unfolds in half, with seams toward mattress. Lay center fold lengthwise along the middle of the bed. Fanfold top layer at center of bed. Smooth bottom layer of drawsheet out over mattress. Tuck excess edge under mattress, keeping palms down.	Folds of linen can irritate client's skin and contribute to the development of pressure ulcers. The **drawsheet** is used to lift and reposition client. Placement under client's torso distributes most of the body weight over sheet. Tucking excess under mattress anchors the sheet in place to prevent sliding and wrinkling.
14. Move to opposite side of bed.	One side of bed is completed before moving to other side.
15. Spread fanfolded bottom sheet smoothly over edge of mattress from head to foot of bed.	Wrinkles can cause irritation.
16. Miter top corner of bottom sheet (see Step 12). When tucking corner, be sure sheet is taut.	Taut sheet eliminates wrinkles and folds that can rub client's skin.
17. Facing side of bed, grasp remaining edge of bottom sheet, lean back, keeping back straight, and while using a broad base of support, pull while tucking excess linen tightly under mattress. Proceed from head to foot of bed (see illustration). Avoid lifting mattress during tucking to ensure tight fit.	Proper use of body mechanics while tucking linen prevents back injury.

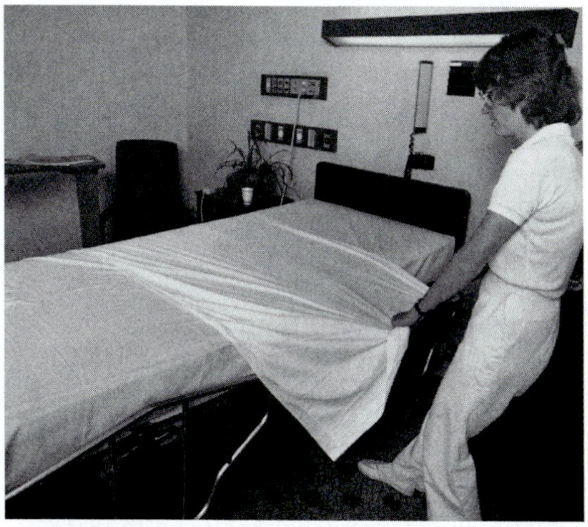

Step 17

18. Smooth folded drawsheet over bottom sheet. Grasp edge of drawsheet with palms down; lean back; and tuck sheet under mattress. Tuck first at the middle, then at the top, and then at the bottom.	Tucking first at the top or bottom may pull sheet sideways, causing poor fit. Loose bed sheets reduce friction and help prevent pressure ulcers (Hanson, et al., 1993; AHCPR, 1992).

CRITICAL DECISION POINT **Frequently observe client to determine tolerance to sitting in chair. Client should not be dizzy, fatigued, or uncomfortable.**

19. In the presence of excessive drainage, apply waterproof pad or bath blanket over drawsheet. Apply with absorbent side up.	Pad collects body secretions and drainage, protecting linen from becoming soiled.

CRITICAL DECISION POINT **Pads can cause irritation to the skin; use only what is needed to collect drainage.**

STEPS	RATIONALE
20. Move to side of bed where linen is located. Place top sheet over bed with vertical center fold lengthwise down middle of bed. Open sheet out from head to foot, being sure the seam on top edge of sheet is up and even with top edge of mattress. Spread excess sheet over bottom edge of mattress. Do not fan top sheet over bed.	Placement ensures equal distribution of sheet over bed. Positioning sheet with seam up prevents irritation of client's skin. Fanning creates air currents, which can spread microorganisms throughout the room.
21. (Optional) Make horizontal toe pleat by standing at foot of bed and fanfold sheet 5 to 10 cm (2 to 4 in) across the bed. Pull sheet up from bottom to make fold. Fold should be approximately 15 cm (6 inches) from bottom edge of mattress (see illustration).	Allows for free movement of client's feet and prevents friction against surface of toes.
22. Tuck in remaining portion of sheet under mattress.	Anchors top sheet so that client can move freely.
23. Place blanket on bed, unfolding it so that crease runs lengthwise along middle of bed. Top edge should be parallel with edge of top sheet and 15 to 20 cm (6 to 8 in) down from mattress top edge. Bottom edge should hang over mattress. Spread blanket evenly over bed.	Blanket provides adequate warmth. Cuff will be formed with sheet folded over top edge of blanket and spread.
24. Place spread over bed according to Step 23. Be sure that top edge of spread extends about 2.5 cm (1 in) above blanket's edge. Then tuck top edge of spread over and under top edge of blanket.	Spread gives bed neat appearance and provides extra warmth.
25. Make cuff by folding upper edge of top sheet down over top edge of blanket and spread.	Smooth cuff avoids irritation to client's face.
26. Standing on one side at foot of bed, lift mattress corner slightly with one hand, and with other hand, tuck top sheet, blanket, and spread under mattress. Be sure not to pull out toe pleat of sheet.	Pressure ulcers can develop on client's toes and heels if feet rub between tight-fitting bed sheets. Lifting mattress too high can loosen bottom linen.
27. Make modified mitered corner with top sheet, blanket, and spread by picking up side edge of top sheet, blanket, and spread approximately 45 cm (18 in) up from foot of mattress. Lift linens to form triangular fold and lay on bed. Tuck loose edge under side of mattress. Pick up triangular fold, and bring it down over the mattress, holding linen in place along side of mattress. Do not tuck tip of triangle (see illustration).	Modified mitered corner secures top linen but keeps even edge of top sheet, blanket, and spread draped over mattress.

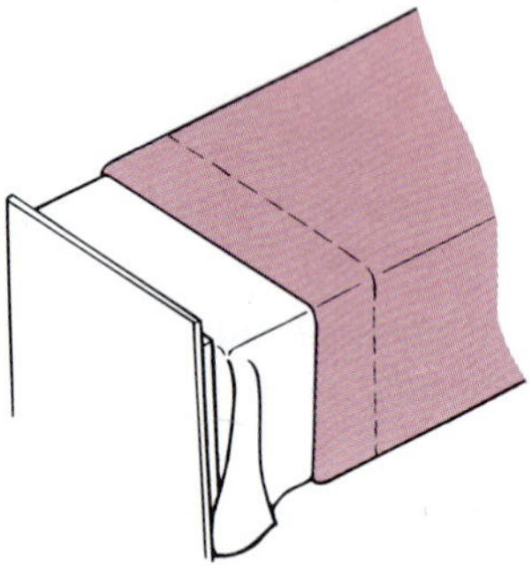

Step 21

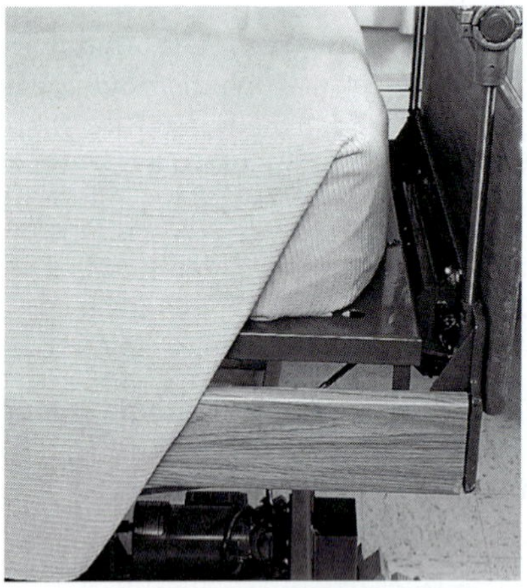

Step 27

STEPS	RATIONALE
28. Go to the other side and spread sheet, blanket, and bedspread evenly. Fold top edge of spread over blanket and make cuff with top sheet (see Step 25). Make modified mitered corner at foot of bed (see Step 27).	Completing one side of bed at a time saves time and energy.
29. Put on clean pillowcase. With one hand, grasp pillowcase at center of closed end. Gather case, turning it inside out overhand while holding it. With the same hand, pick up the middle of one end of pillow. Pull pillowcase down over pillow with the other hand. Be sure corners of case fit evenly over pillow (see illustration).	Eases sliding of case smoothly over pillow.

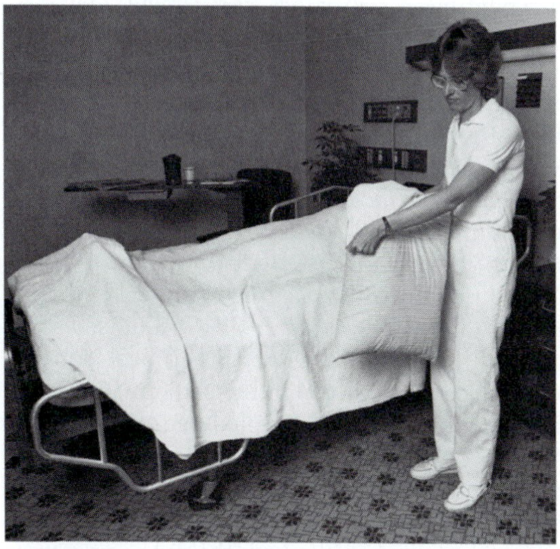

Step 29

30. Position pillows at center of head of bed, and place call light within client's reach. Return bed to comfortable height for client.	Maintains neat appearance. Provides for client safety.
31. Fold back top covers to one side, or fanfold them to bottom third of bed.	Eases client's return to bed.
32. Rearrange furniture, and place personal items within easy reach.	Promotes sense of well-being.
33. Discard dirty linen in hamper or chute. Wash hands.	Prevents transmission of microorganisms.

EVALUATION

1. Assess client's tolerance for sitting up in chair by comparing heart rate to previous resting rate; ask if client feels weak, dizzy, or fatigued; assess blood pressure if client complains of dizziness or weakness.	Client's inability to tolerate exertion or low-level exercise may be reflected in changes in vital signs or subjective report of symptoms.
2. Assess client's level of comfort and condition of skin after returning to bed.	Frequent skin assessment results in timely interventions to maintain skin integrity for those clients at risk for pressure ulcer development (see Chapter 8).
3. **Unexpected outcomes** that may occur include:	
➤ Client's blood pressure falls below baseline and heart rate is elevated.	Sitting in upright position may cause orthostatic hypotension; exertion may increase heart rate.
➤ Client complains of weakness or dizziness.	Symptoms of poor activity tolerance and orthostatic changes.

RECORDING AND REPORTING

1. Bed making need not be documented. Record client's vital signs and symptoms only if there are changes.	Document client's response to activity and position change.

STEPS **RATIONALE**

FOLLOW-UP ACTIVITIES

1. Assist client back to bed; obtain new vital signs; and ask client about any sensations of weakness, dizziness, or anxiety. Notify physician of orthostatic changes and client's present status.
2. Obtain physician's order for special skin care.

• • • • •

Special Considerations

- If the client has a circulatory impairment, elevate affected extremity while client is out of bed. This promotes venous return.
- If client is diaphoretic, bath blankets spread across bottom sheets will collect the moisture.
- Use drawsheets and waterproof pads with caution. Accumulation of moisture creates a risk for skin maceration and breakdown.
- While the client is in surgery, the nurse may choose to prepare an unoccupied surgical bed. Top linen is arranged in a manner that facilitates easy transfer of the client from stretcher to bed. Bottom sheet is placed on the bed in the same manner as it is when making an unoccupied bed. Because client often returns from surgery with a dressing, the nurse places a plastic or cloth drawsheet and absorbent pad on the bed. After top sheet, blanket, and spread are put on the bed, the nurse prepares the linen by performing the following steps:
  - Fanfold all top linen back from head of bed toward foot of mattress. Linen fold should be just above bottom edge of mattress.
  - Leave bed in high position for easy transfer of client from stretcher to unoccupied surgical bed (Fig. 7-5).
- Optional steps:
  - Fold all top linen back from foot of bed toward center of mattress. Linen fold should be flush with bottom edge of mattress.
  - Fold all top linen that is down over sides of bed toward center of mattress. Linen folds should be flush with side edges of mattress.
  - Face one side of bed; pick up nearest bottom corner of linen; and fold back and over toward opposite side of bed, forming a triangle. Repeat for other side.
  - Grasp apex of triangle and fanfold top linen over to side of bed.

Gerontologic Considerations

- Older adults have fragile skin and require more protection. Be sure bed linens are clean, dry, and free of wrinkles.
- Encourage older adults to spend as much time out of bed as possible.

Home Care Considerations

- Assess the primary care giver's ability and willingness to maintain a clean environment for the client.
- Assess home laundry facilities to plan with the primary care giver the frequency with which linens could reasonably be laundered.
- Assess the amount of linen in the home to establish with the primary care giver the number of changes of sheets that could be reserved for the client's use.

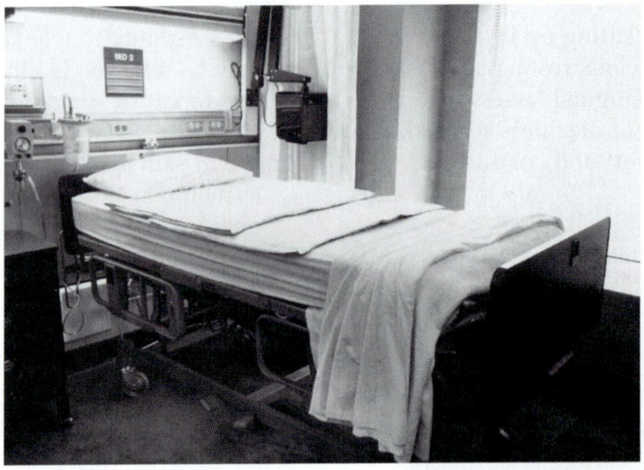

Fig. 7-5

SKILL 7-2 Making an Occupied Bed

At times it is necessary to make a bed that is occupied by a client. The client may be too weak to get out of bed; the illness may prohibit sitting up; or the client may be restricted to bed because of postprocedure precautions, traction, or heavy body or leg casts. If a client is confined to bed, bed making should be done in a way that conserves time and the client's energy. The nurse also tries to keep the client as comfortable as possible. In cases where a client experiences severe pain, an analgesic administered 30 to 60 minutes before the procedure is helpful in controlling pain and maintaining comfort.

Even though the client is unable to get out of bed, the nurse encourages self-help as much as possible. For example, the client can turn, assist in moving up in bed, or hold top sheets while linen is applied. These activities help maintain the client's strength and mobility and allow participation in hygiene care.

Making an occupied bed poses some difficulties. It is harder to prevent transfer of organisms from soiled linens to clean linens and to keep newly applied linen smooth and wrinkle-free. The procedure can be done quickly, however, if the nurse is organized.

EQUIPMENT

- Linen bag(s)
- Mattress pad (needs to be changed only when soiled)
- Bottom sheet (flat or fitted)
- Drawsheet
- Top sheet
- Blanket
- Bedspread
- Waterproof pads and/or bath blankets (optional)
- Pillowcases
- Bedside chair or table
- Disposable gloves (optional)

STEPS	RATIONALE
ASSESSMENT	
1. Assess potential for client incontinence or for excess drainage on bed linen.	Determines need for protective waterproof pads or extra bath blankets on bed.
2. Check chart for orders or specific precautions concerning movement and positioning.	Ensures client safety and use of proper body mechanics.

NURSING DIAGNOSIS

Clustering of defining characteristics from the assessment data may reveal the following diagnoses for clients requiring this skill:

- Activity intolerance
- Impaired physical mobility
- Impaired skin integrity and risk for
- Pain
- Chronic pain
- Self-care deficit, bathing/hygiene

Related factors are individualized based on client's condition or needs.

PLANNING

STEPS	RATIONALE
1. **Expected outcomes** following completion of procedure: ➤ Client's skin remains free from breakdown. ➤ Client expresses feeling of relaxation and comfort. ➤ There are no areas of redness from bed linen irritation. Bed linen is smooth and without wrinkles.	
2. Explain procedure to the client, noting that the client will be asked to turn on side and roll over linen.	Minimizes anxiety and promotes cooperation.

IMPLEMENTATION

STEPS	RATIONALE
1. Wash hands and put on gloves (gloves are worn only if linen is soiled or there is risk for contact with body secretions).	Reduces transmission of microorganisms.

STEPS	RATIONALE
2. Assemble equipment and arrange on bedside chair or table. Remove unnecessary equipment such as a dietary tray or items used for hygiene.	Assembling all equipment provides for smooth procedure and assists in increasing client's comfort. Placing linen on clean surface minimizes spread of infection.
3. Draw room curtain around bed or close door.	Maintains client's privacy.
4. Adjust bed height to comfortable working position. Lower side rail on one side of bed. Remove call light.	Minimizes strain on back. It is easier to remove and apply linen evenly to bed in flat position. Provides easy access to bed and linen.
5. Loosen top linen at foot of bed.	Makes linen easier to remove.
6. Remove bedspread and blanket separately. If spread and blanket are soiled, place them in linen bag. Keep soiled linen away from uniform.	Reduces transmission of microorganisms.
7. If blanket and spread are to be reused, fold them by bringing the top and bottom edges together. Fold farthest side over onto nearer bottom edge. Bring top and bottom edges together again. Place folded linen over back of chair.	Folding method facilitates replacement and prevents wrinkles.
8. Cover client with bath blanket in the following manner: unfold bath blanket over top sheet. Ask client to hold top edge of bath blanket. If client is unable to help, tuck top of bath blanket under shoulder. Grasp top sheet under bath blanket at client's shoulders and bring sheet down to foot of bed. Remove sheet and discard in linen bag.	Bath blanket provides warmth and keeps body parts covered during linen removal.
9. With assistance from another nurse, slide mattress toward head of bed.	If mattress slides toward foot of bed when head of bed is raised, it is difficult to tuck in linen. In addition, it is uncomfortable for the client because the client's feet may be pressed against or hang over the foot of the bed.
10. Be sure side rail in front of client is up. Position client on the far side of the bed, facing away. Adjust pillow under client's head.	Moving client to side provides space for placement of clean linen. Side rail ensures client's safety from forward falls from the bed surface and helps client in moving.
11. Loosen bottom linens, moving from head to foot.	Prepares for removal of all bottom linen simultaneously.
12. With seam side down (facing the mattress), fanfold bottom sheet and drawsheet toward client—first drawsheet, then bottom sheet. Tuck edges of linen just under buttocks, back, and shoulders. Do not fanfold mattress pad if it is to be reused (see illustration).	Provides maximum work space for placing clean linen. Later, when client turns to other side, soiled linen can be removed easily.
13. Wipe off any moisture on exposed mattress with towel and appropriate disinfectant.	Reduces transmission of microorganisms.
14. Apply clean linen to exposed half of bed:	
a. Place clean mattress pad on bed by folding it lengthwise with center crease in middle of bed. Fanfold top layer over mattress. (If pad is reused, simply smooth out any wrinkles.)	Applying linen over bed in successive layers minimizes energy and time used in bed making.
b. Unfold bottom sheet lengthwise so that center crease is situated lengthwise along center of bed. Fanfold sheet's top layer toward center of bed alongside the client. Smooth bottom layer of sheet over mattress, and bring edge over closest side of mattress. Allow edge of sheet to hang about 25 cm (10 in) over mattress edge. Lower hem of bottom sheet should lie seam down and even with bottom edge of mattress (see illustration).	Proper positioning of linen on one side ensures that adequate linen will be available to cover opposite side of bed. Keeping seam edges down eliminates irritation to client's skin.

STEPS	RATIONALE
15. Miter bottom sheet at head of bed: a. Face head of bed diagonally. Place hand away from head of bed under top corner of mattress, near mattress edge, and lift. b. With other hand, tuck top edge of bottom sheet smoothly under mattress so that side edges of sheet above and below mattress would meet if brought together. c. Face side of bed and pick up top edge of sheet at approximately 45 cm (18 in) from top of mattress. d. Lift sheet, and lay it on top of the mattress to form a neat triangular fold, with lower base of triangle even with mattress side edge. e. Tuck lower edge of sheet, which is hanging free below the mattress, under mattress. Tuck with palms down, without pulling triangular fold. f. Hold portion of sheet covering side of mattress in place with one hand. With the other hand, pick up top of triangular linen fold and bring it down over side of mattress. Tuck this portion under mattress.	Mitered corner cannot be loosened easily even if client moves frequently in bed.
16. Tuck remaining portion of sheet under mattress, moving toward foot of bed. Keep linen smooth.	Folds of linen are source of irritation.
17. (Optional) Open drawsheet so that it unfolds in half. Lay center fold along middle of bed lengthwise, and position sheet so that it will be under the client's buttocks and torso. Fanfold top layer toward client, with edge along back. Smooth bottom layer out over mattress, and tuck excess edge under mattress (keep palms down).	Drawsheet is used to lift and reposition client. Placement under client's torso distributes most of client's body weight over sheet.
18. Place waterproof pad over drawsheet, with center fold against client's side. Fanfold top layer toward client.	Protects bed linen from being soiled.

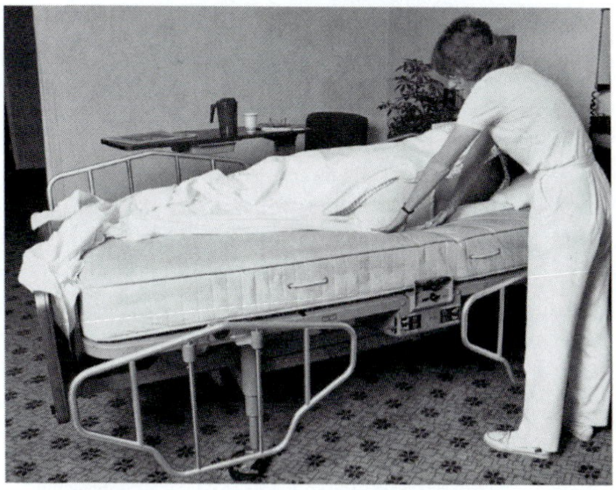

Step 12

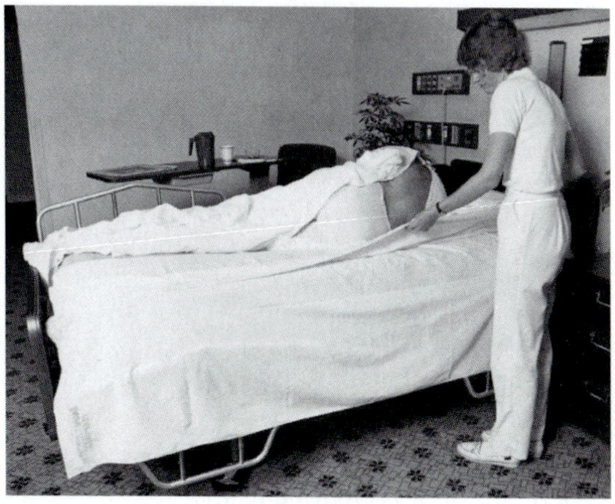

Step 14b

STEPS	RATIONALE
19. Raise side rail on working side and go to other side.	Maintains client's safety and body alignment during turning.
20. Lower side rail. Assist client to roll slowly onto other side, over folds of linen, and loosen edges of soiled linen from under mattress.	Exposes opposite side of bed for removal of soiled linen and placement of clean linen. Makes linen easier to remove.
21. Remove soiled linen by folding it into a bundle or square, with soiled side turned in. Discard in linen bag. If necessary, wipe mattress with antiseptic solution, and dry mattress surface before applying new linen.	Reduces transmission of microorganisms.
22. Pull clean, fanfolded linen smoothly over edge of mattress from head to foot of bed.	Smooth linen will not irritate client's skin.
23. Assist client in rolling back into supine position. Reposition pillow.	Maintains client's comfort.

➤ *CRITICAL DECISION POINT* Assess client's tolerance to procedure. Observe for fatigue, pain, and shortness of breath. Client may need to rest during the procedure.

24. Miter top corner of bottom sheet (see Step 15). When tucking corner, be sure that sheet is smooth and free of wrinkles.	Wrinkles and folds can cause irritation to skin.
25. Facing side of bed, grasp remaining edge of bottom sheet. Lean back; keep back straight; and pull while tucking excess linen under mattress. Proceed from head to foot of bed. (Avoid lifting mattress during tucking to ensure fit.)	Proper use of body mechanics while tucking linen prevents injury.
26. Smooth fanfolded drawsheet out over bottom sheet. Grasp edge of sheet with palms down; lean back; and tuck sheet under mattress. Tuck from middle to top and then to bottom.	Tucking first at top or bottom may pull sheet sideways, causing poor fit.
27. Place top sheet over client with center fold lengthwise down middle of bed. Open sheet from head to foot, and unfold over client.	Sheet should be equally distributed over bed by correctly positioning center fold.
28. Ask client to hold clean top sheet, or tuck sheet around client's shoulders. Remove bath blanket and discard in linen bag (see illustration).	Sheet prevents exposure of body parts. Having client hold sheet encourages client participation in care.

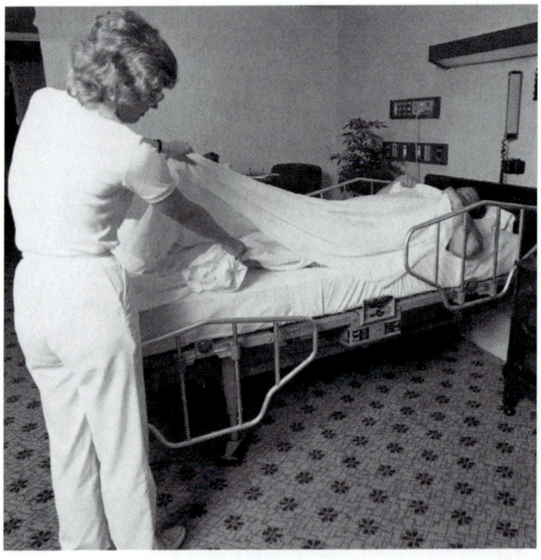

Step 28

STEPS	RATIONALE
29. Place blanket on bed, unfolding it so that crease runs lengthwise along middle of bed. Unfold blanket to cover client. Top edge should be parallel with edge of top sheet and 15 to 20 cm (6 to 8 in) from top sheet's edge.	Blanket should be placed to cover client completely and provide adequate warmth.
30. Place spread over bed according to Step 29. Be sure that top edge of spread extends about 2.5 cm (1 in) above blanket's edge. Tuck top edge of spread over and under top edge of blanket.	Gives bed neat appearance and provides extra warmth.
31. Make cuff by turning edge of top sheet down over top edge of blanket and spread.	Protects client's face from rubbing against blanket or spread.
32. Standing on one side at foot of bed, lift mattress corner slightly with one hand and tuck top linens under mattress. Top sheet and blanket are tucked under together. Be sure that linens are loose enough to allow movement of client's feet. Making a horizontal toe pleat is an option (see Skill 7-1, Step 21).	Makes neat-appearing bed. Pressure ulcers can develop on client's toes and heels from feet rubbing against tight-fitting bed sheets.
33. Make modified mitered corner with top sheet, blanket, and spread:	Secures top linen but keeps even edge of blanket and top sheet draped over mattress.
a. Pick up side edge of top sheet, blanket, and spread approximately 45 cm (18 in) from foot of mattress. Lift linen to form triangular fold, and lay it on bed.	
b. Tuck lower edge of sheet, which is hanging free below mattress, under mattress. Do not pull triangular fold.	
c. Pick up triangular fold, and bring it down over mattress while holding linen in place along side of mattress. Do not tuck tip of triangle.	
34. Raise side rail. Make other side of bed; spread sheet, blanket, and bedspread out evenly. Fold top edge of spread over blanket and make cuff with top sheet (see Step 31); make modified mitered corner at foot of bed (see Step 33).	Side rail protects client from accidental falls.
35. Change pillowcase:	
a. Have client raise head. While supporting neck with one hand, remove pillow. Allow client to lower head.	Support of neck muscles prevents injury during flexion and extension of neck.
b. Remove soiled case by grasping pillow at open end with one hand and pulling case back over pillow with the other hand. Discard case in linen bag.	Pillows slide out easily, thus minimizing contact with soiled linen.
c. Grasp clean pillowcase at center of closed end. Gather case, turning it inside out over the hand holding it. With the same hand, pick up middle of one end of the pillow. Pull pillowcase down over pillow with the other hand (see Step 29, p. 181).	Eases sliding of pillowcase over pillow.
d. Be sure pillow corners fit evenly into corners of pillowcase. Place pillow under client's head.	Poorly fitting case constricts fluffing and expansion of pillow and interferes with client comfort.
36. Place call light within client's reach and return bed to comfortable position.	Ensures client safety and comfort.
37. Open room curtains, and rearrange furniture. Place personal items within easy reach on overbed table or bedside stand. Return bed to a comfortable height.	Promotes sense of well-being.
38. Discard dirty linen in hamper or chute and wash hands.	Prevents transmission of microorganisms.

STEPS	RATIONALE

E VALUATION

1. Ask if client feels comfortable (see illustration).
2. Inspect skin for areas of irritation.
3. Observe client for signs of fatigue, dyspnea, pain, or discomfort.

   Provides the nurse with data about the client's level of activity tolerance and ability to participate in other procedures.

4. **Unexpected outcomes** that may occur include:
   - ➤ Client feels discomfort from linen fold.

     Linen is not properly smoothed.
   - ➤ Client's skin shows signs of breakdown.

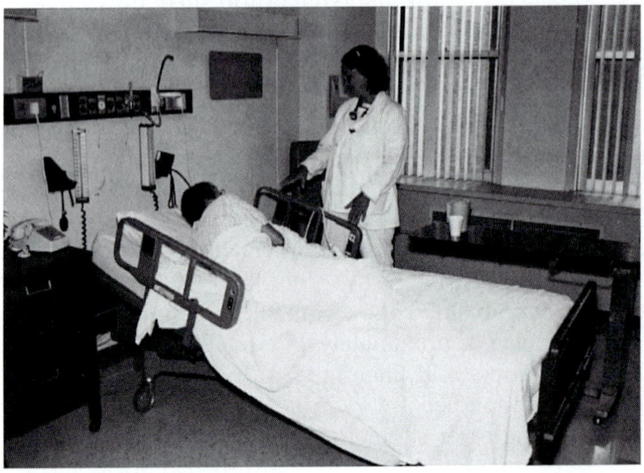

Step 1

RECORDING AND REPORTING

1. Making an occupied bed need not be recorded.

FOLLOW-UP ACTIVITIES

1. Implement skin care practices as needed.

• • • • •

Special Considerations

- ➤ Explain that the client will not fall off bed during turning procedure.
- ➤ Client with respiratory distress may be unable to tolerate lying flat during bed making.

Teaching Considerations

- ➤ Explain steps of procedure involving client's participation.

CRITICAL THINKING EXERCISES

1. Your client complains of dizziness. What assessments would you make before making the bed? What would affect your decision to make an occupied versus an unoccupied bed?
2. You have been assigned to care for a client who is incontinent. What protective measures will you implement to reduce transmission of microorganisms?
3. What are the issues that must be taken into consideration when getting an older adult with impaired mobility out of bed in order to make an occupied bed?

REFERENCES

Agency for Health Care Policy and Research (AHCPR): *Pressure ulcers in adults; prediction and prevention,* Pub Nos 92-0047, 92-0050, Rockville, Md, 1992, US Dept of Health and Human Services.

Hanson D, et al: The prevalence and incidence of pressure ulcers in home care: Are patients at risk? *J Home Health Care* 5(3):25, 1993.

ADDITIONAL READING

Ebersole P, Hess P: *Toward healthy aging: human needs and nursing response,* ed 4, St Louis, 1994, Mosby.

Rice R: *Manual of home health nursing procedures.* St Louis, 1994, Mosby.

Rousseau P: Management of pressure sores, *Postgrad Med* 83(5):51, 1988.

Rousseau P: Decubitus ulcers, *Postgrad Med* 88(2):53, 1990.

CHAPTER 8

Pressure Ulcer Care

OBJECTIVES

Mastery of content in this chapter will enable the nurse to:

- Define key terms.
- Describe guidelines to follow in preventing pressure ulcer formation.
- Identify risks for development of pressure ulcers.
- Identify outcome criteria for clients at risk for pressure ulcers or impaired skin integrity.
- Discuss the meaning of risk assessment scores for four commonly used pressure ulcer risk assessment scales.
- Describe characteristics of the entire client, as well as the pressure ulcer itself, to include in an assessment.
- Discuss implications for the use of topical agents in the treatment of pressure ulcers.
- Apply topical agents correctly to a pressure ulcer.
- Discuss teaching needs of the client and family regarding pressure ulcers.

KEY TERMS

Astringent
Capillary closing pressure
Colonized
Debridement
Erythema
Eschar
Excoriation
Exudate
Maceration
Pressure ulcer
Shearing
Slough
Tissue ischemia
Topical agents

SKILLS

Pressure ulcers (formerly called *decubitus ulcers, pressure sores,* or *bed sores*) are "localized areas of tissue necrosis that develop when soft tissue is compressed between a bony prominence and an external surface for a prolonged period of time" (National Pressure Ulcer Advisory Panel [NPUAP], 1989). Ischemia develops when pressure on the skin (32 mm Hg, or **capillary closing pressure**) is greater than the pressure inside the small, peripheral blood vessels supplying blood to the tissue. Fat and muscle tissue do not tolerate decreased blood flow and are therefore less resistant to pressure than skin (Maklebust and Sieggreen, 1996). Maklebust and Sieggreen (1996) describe the two models of **pressure ulcer** formation that have been proposed. The traditional model is that the tissue destruction first occurs in the epidermis of the skin and then later in the deeper layers of tissue. The other model suggests that the tissue nearest to the bone or muscle is injured first, before signs of tissue damage can be seen on the skin surface. Ischemia may be evident by skin discoloration such as a red spot in clients with light skin. If pressure is unrelieved or repeated, tissues will continue to break down relative to the client's general health and tolerance for pressure. This pressure, if not relieved, can cause irreversible tissue damage in as little as 90 minutes.

Pressure points over bony prominences where pressure ulcers occur are shown in Fig. 8-1. The most common sites are the sacrum, heels, elbows, lateral malleoli, greater trochanters, and ischial tuberosities (Meehan, 1994). Pressure ulcers can occur on any area of skin subjected to pressure. Non-bony locations include the nares, with pressure ulcers resulting from NG tubes or oxygen cannulas; the ears, with ulcers resulting from oxygen cannulas; or the genitalia, with ulcers resulting from Foley catheter tension. Any shearing force, the force that stretches the skin during turning or moving in bed, increases the reduction in blood flow. Circulatory impairment often is compounded by the altered body metabolism and negative nitrogen balance that commonly occur in immobilized clients.

Pressure ulcers pose serious risks to a client's health status. A break in the skin, seen in stages II to IV pressure ulcers (Table 8-1), eliminates the body's first line of defense against infection. When an ulcer is into the subcutaneous tissues, protein- and electrolyte-rich body fluids are lost through the wound. With large ulcers, serious electrolyte imbalances can occur. A pressure ulcer can prolong morbidity and interfere with the rehabilitative and supportive care the client receives.

Significant numbers of clients are at risk for or suffering from pressure ulcers; it is critical that nursing respond with an aggressive preventive approach. Care is complex because of the many variables involved in each client's risk for developing pressure ulcers. Even high-risk clients who receive thorough nursing care may develop ulcers in spite of the nurse's efforts. When a pressure ulcer develops, the nurse must explore the possible precipitating variables, vigorously attempt to minimize the effects of these variables, and propose wound care treatment utilizing current wound healing principles in the management of the ulcer (see Chapters 37 and 40).

GUIDELINES

1. Adequate nutrition is important in the prevention and treatment of pressure ulcers (AHCPR, 1994). A diet high in protein with enough calories, vitamins, and minerals can maintain normal tissue status and promote healing (AHCPR, 1994). For most clients the goal of positive nitrogen balance can be achieved by a dietary intake of 30 to 35 kcal/kg/day and 1.25 to 1.50 g of protein/kg/day (AHCPR, 1994). Clients who are suspected of having or who have actual vitamin and/or mineral deficiencies will need supplementation (AHCPR, 1994).
2. Frequently turn and position client to relieve pressure around superficial capillaries and allow tissues to compensate for temporary ischemia. Classic research (Kosiak, 1959) found that tissue ischemia begins within 1 to 2 hours after onset of pressure in paraplegic animals. Turning clients every 1 to 2 hours will help minimize formation of pressure ulcers (see Chapter 29).
3. Specialized beds and mattresses (see Chapter 32) distribute pressure on dependent body parts more evenly. Clients at high risk for pressure ulcer formation should be placed on these devices as soon as possible.

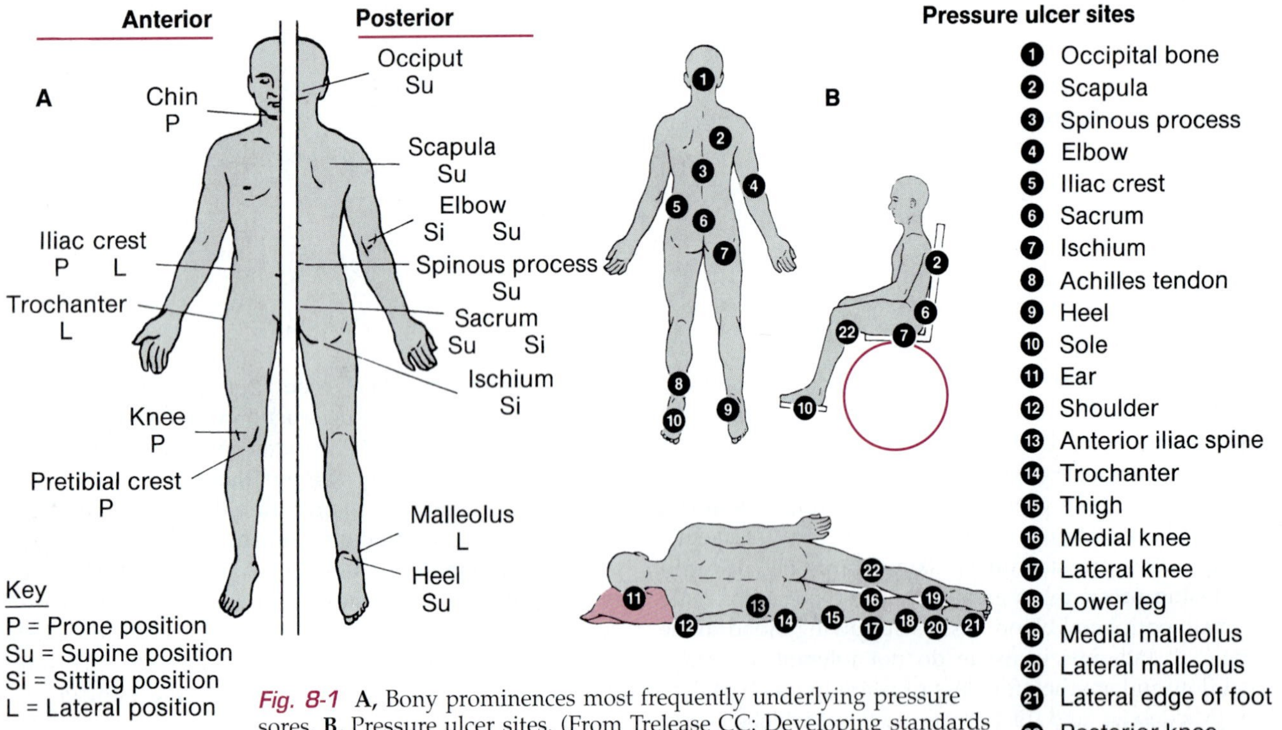

Fig. 8-1 **A,** Bony prominences most frequently underlying pressure sores. **B,** Pressure ulcer sites. (From Trelease CC: Developing standards for wound care, *Ostomy/Wound Manage* 26:50, 1988.)

Table 8-1 Staging of Pressure Ulcers

Staging Definition*

Stage I

Nonblanchable erythema of intact skin; the heralding lesion of skin ulceration. In individuals with darker skin, discoloration of the skin, warmth, edema, induration, or hardness may also be indicators.

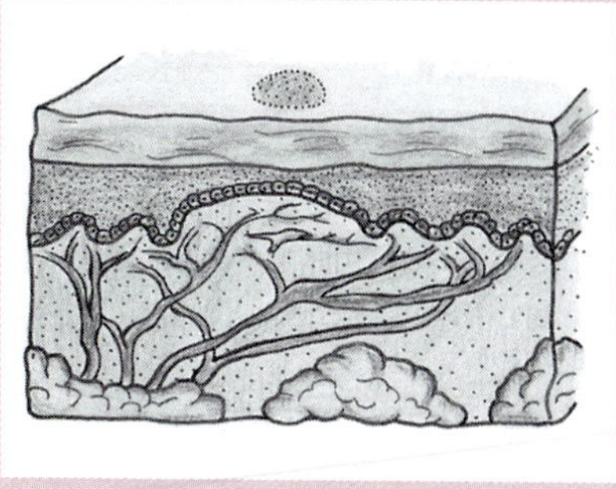

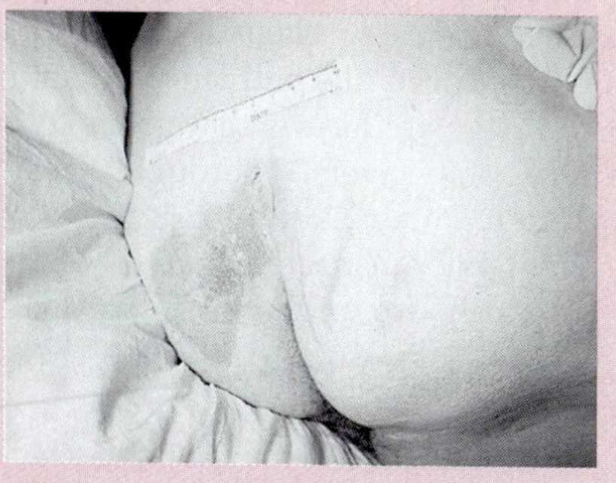

Stage II

Partial-thickness skin loss involving epidermis and/or dermis. The ulcer is superficial and presents clinically as an abrasion, blister, or shallow crater.

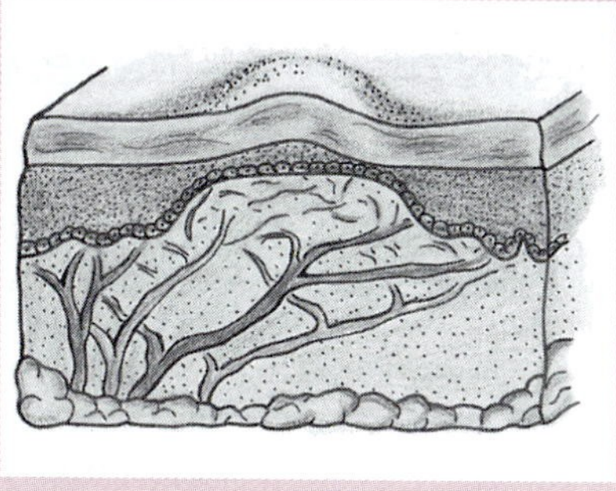

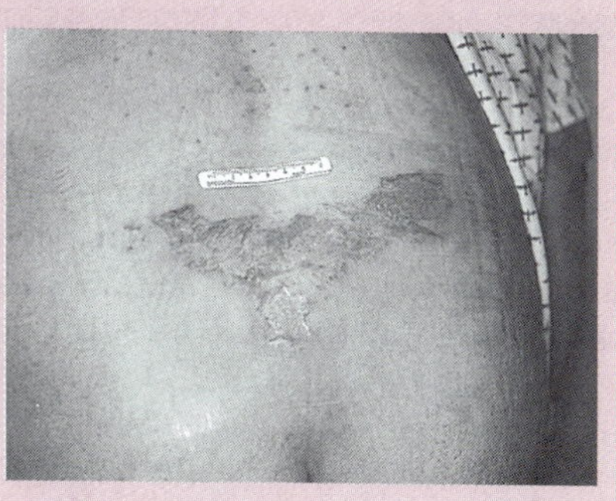

Stage III

Full-thickness skin loss involving damage or necrosis of subcutaneous tissue that may extend down to, but not through, underlying fascia. The ulcer presents clinically as a deep crater with or without undermining of adjacent tissue.

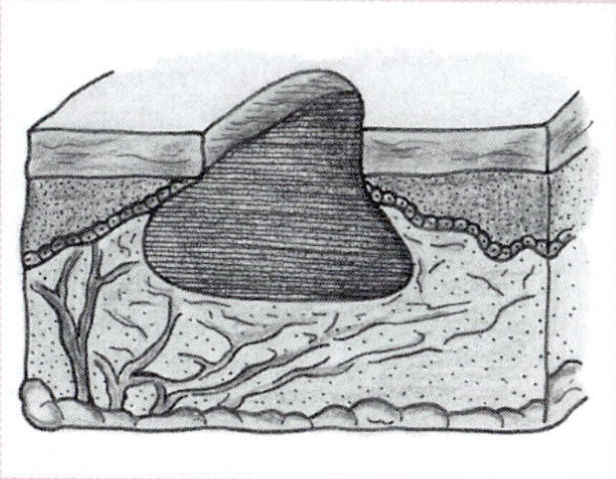

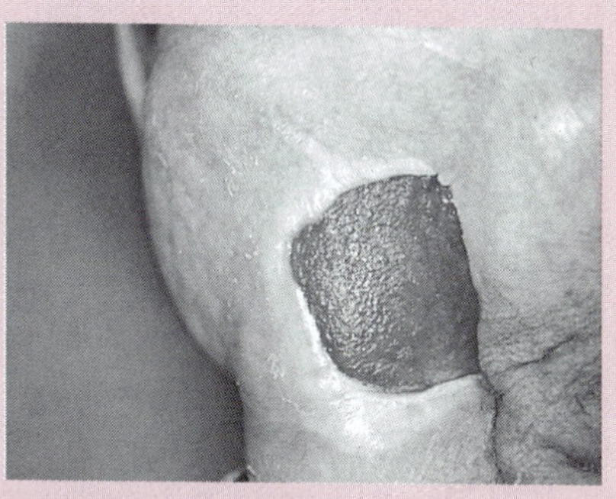

Stage IV

Full-thickness skin loss with extensive destruction, tissue necrosis, or damage to muscle, bone, or supporting structures, for example, tendon or joint capsule. (NOTE: Undermining and sinus tracts may also be associated with stage IV pressure ulcers.)

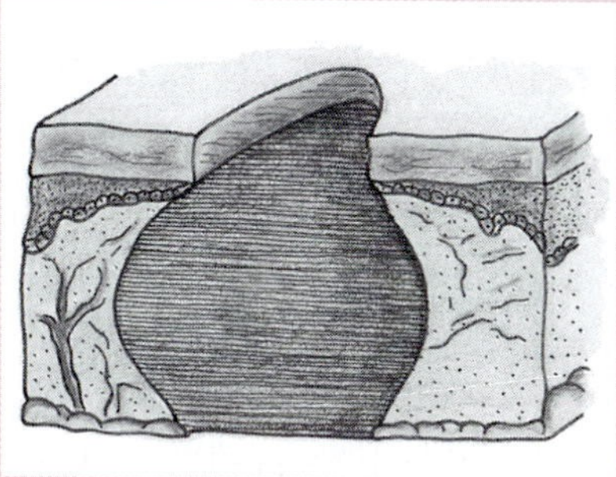

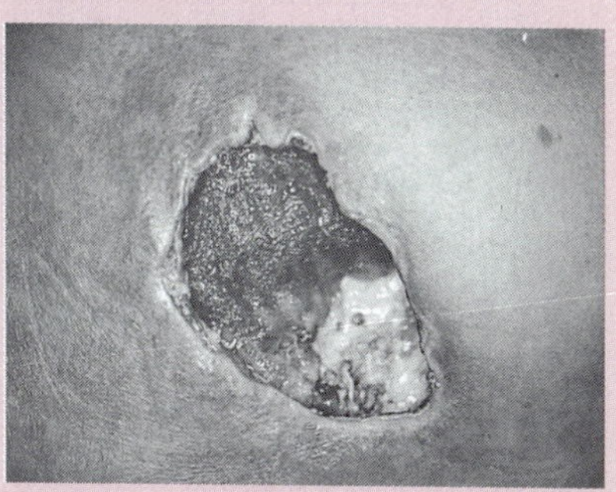

From AHCPR (1994).

*Staging definitions recognize these assessment limitations:

1. Identification of stage I pressure ulcers may be difficult in patients with darkly pigmented skin.
2. When eschar is present, accurate staging of the pressure ulcer is not possible until the eschar has sloughed or the wound has been debrided.
3. It may be difficult to assess pressure ulcers in persons with casts, other orthopedic devices, or support stockings.

4. Use chair cushions to reduce pressure when client is seated. Encourage small movement shifts every 15 to 30 minutes while client is seated.
5. Do not expose client's skin to moisture or increased temperature. Incontinence, diaphoresis, and wound drainage are factors that promote maceration of superficial skin layers. Thorough washing and drying will help maintain skin integrity.
6. Frequently inspect linen and bedclothes to be sure they are clean, dry, and wrinkle-free. Uneven underlying bed linen or bedclothes can create pressure against skin layers.
7. Eliminate anything that may increase ischemic damage, such as massage and "donuts" (air-filled or foam rings) (AHCPR, 1992, 1994).
8. Carefully monitor the pressure ulcer with regard to the process of healing. Changes in therapy are frequently indicated. Prescribed treatment for a client's pressure ulcer will vary, depending on the extent of the ulcer and the client's underlying condition.

SKILL 8-1 Risk Assessment and Prevention Strategies

The optimal treatments for pressure ulcers are the early identification of the at-risk client and the implementation of prevention strategies. The following three populations are known to be at risk for pressure ulcers: (1) clients with a neurological impairment that decreases sensation, (2) chronically ill long-term care clients, and (3) orthopedic clients. These groups can be readily identified, but *any* client exposed to the right conditions for pressure ulcer development may be at risk.

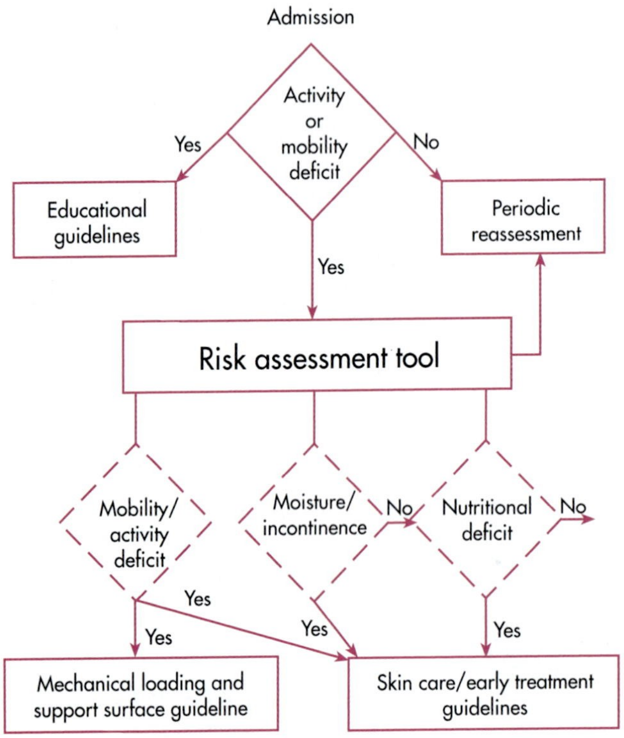

Fig. 8-2 Risk Assessment Tool. (Modified from Panel for the Prediction and Prevention of Pressure Ulcers in Adults, Agency for Health Care Policy and Research, Rockville, Md, 1992, Public Health Service, US Department of Health and Human Services.)

The AHCPR panel developed clinical guidelines for pressure ulcer prevention and treatment of stage I pressure ulcers in 1992. The guidelines recommend that clients who are bed or chair bound or who have an impaired ability to reposition should be assessed for pressure ulcer risk. The AHCPR 1994 guidelines state that additional factors that may put a client at risk for developing pressure ulcers include immobility, incontinence, nutritional factors such as inadequate dietary intake and impaired nutritional status, and altered level of consciousness. Clients with advanced age, excess body heat, and diminished sensation may also be at risk for developing pressure ulcers. Friction and shear can also contribute to pressure ulcer development.

The AHCPR 1992 panel recommended that a risk assessment tool tested for reliability and validity be used on admission and at periodic intervals after admission for all clients screened and found to have a mobility deficit (Fig. 8-2). The panel suggests the use of risk assessment tools such as the Braden scale or the Norton scale. The earliest reported scale was in 1962 with the Norton scale, which has the following five risk factors: physical condition, mental state, activity, mobility, and incontinence. The Braden scale (Table 8-2) has the following six parameters: sensory perception (recognition of pressure), friction or shear, ability to change and control body position, skin moisture, nutritional intake, and physical activity (Bergstrom, Demuth, and Braden, 1987). Although not mentioned in the AHCPR guidelines, other risk assessment tools used clinically are the Gosnell (1973) scale and the Knoll scale (which was developed by Abruzzese [1982] in 1975). It is important to understand how to interpret the meaning of the client's total score on each of these four scales.

Table 8-2 Braden Scale for Predicting Pressure Ulcer Risk*

	1 Point	2 Points	3 Points	4 Points
Sensory perception Ability to respond meaningfully to pressure-related discomfort	*Completely limited:* Unresponsive (does not moan, flinch, or grasp) to painful stimuli due to diminished level of consciousness or sedation. OR Limited ability to feel pain over most of body surface.	*Very limited:* Responds only to painful stimuli. Cannot communicate discomfort except by moaning or restlessness. OR Has a sensory impairment which limits the ability to feel pain or discomfort over half of body.	*Slightly limited:* Responds to verbal commands but cannot always communicate discomfort or need to be turned. OR Has some sensory impairment which limits ability to feel pain or discomfort in 1 or 2 extremities.	*No impairment:* Responds to verbal commands. Has no sensory deficit that would limit ability to feel or voice pain or discomfort.
Moisture Degree to which skin is exposed to moisture	*Constantly moist:* Skin is kept moist almost constantly by perspiration, urine, etc. Dampness is detected every time patient is moved or turned.	*Very moist:* Skin is often, but not always, moist. Linen must be changed at least once a shift.	*Occasionally moist:* Skin is occasionally moist, requiring an extra linen change approximately once a day.	*Rarely moist:* Skin is usually dry, linen requires changing only at routine intervals.
Activity Degree of physical activity	*Bedfast:* Confined to bed.	*Chairfast:* Ability to walk severely limited or nonexistent. Cannot bear own weight and/or must be assisted into chair or wheelchair.	*Walks occasionally:* Walks occasionally during day, but for very short distances, with or without assistance. Spends majority of each shift in bed or chair.	*Walks frequently:* Walks outside the room at least twice a day and inside room at least once every 2 hours during waking hours.
Mobility Ability to change and control body position	*Completely immobile:* Does not make even slight changes in body or extremity position without assistance.	*Very limited:* Makes occasional slight changes in body or extremity position but unable to make frequent or significant changes independently.	*Slightly limited:* Makes frequent though slight changes in body or extremity position independently.	*No limitations:* Makes major and frequent changes in position without assistance.
Nutrition Usual food intake pattern	*Very poor:* Never eats a complete meal. Rarely eats more than one third of any food offered. Eats 2 servings or less of protein (meat or dairy products) per day. Takes fluids poorly. Does not take a liquid dietary supplement. OR Is NPO and/or maintained on clear liquids or IVs for more than 5 days.	*Probably inadequate:* Rarely eats a complete meal and generally eats only about half of any food offered. Protein intake includes only 3 servings of meat or dairy products per day. Occasionally will take a dietary supplement. OR Receives less than optimal amount of liquid diet or tube feeding.	*Adequate:* Eats over half of most meals. Eats a total of 4 servings of protein (meat, dairy products) each day. Occasionally will refuse a meal, but will usually take a supplement if offered. OR Is on a tube-feeding or TPN regimen that probably meets most of nutritional needs.	*Excellent:* Eats most of every meal. Never refuses a meal. Usually eats a total of 4 or more servings of meat and dairy products. Occasionally eats between meals. Does not require supplements.

*Score client in each of the six subscales. Maximum score is 23, indicating little or no risk. A score of ≤16 indicates "at risk"; ≤9 indicates high risk.
From Barbara Braden, Ph.D., R.N., Creighton University School of Nursing, Omaha, Nebraska.

Continued

Table 8-2 Braden Scale for Predicting Pressure Ulcer Risk*—cont'd

	1 Point	2 Points	3 Points	4 Points
Friction and shear	*Problem:* Requires moderate to maximal assistance in moving. Complete lifting without sliding against sheets is impossible. Frequently slides down in bed or chair, requiring frequent repositioning with maximal assistance. Spasticity, contractions, or agitation leads to almost constant friction.	*Potential problem:* Moves feebly or requires minimal assistance. During a move skin probably slides to some extent against sheets, chair, restraints, or other devices. Maintains relatively good position in chair or bed most of the time but occasionally slides down.	*No apparent problem:* Moves in bed and in chair independently and has sufficient muscle strength to sit up completely during move. Maintains good position in bed or chair at all times.	

EQUIPMENT

- Risk assessment tool
- Documentation record
- Body chart or tracing film and/or camera
- Lanolin-based lotion
- Pressure relief mattress, bed, and/or chair cushion
- Positioning aids

DELEGATION CONSIDERATIONS

This skill requires problem solving and knowledge application unique to a professional nurse. For this skill, delegation is inappropriate.

STEPS	RATIONALE
ASSESSMENT	
1. Identify any client characteristics that might be risk factors for pressure ulcer formation.	Determines need to administer preventive care in addition to use of topical agents for existing ulcers.
a. Paralysis, paresis, or immobilization caused by restrictive devices	Client is unable to turn or reposition independently.
b. Sensory loss	Client feels no discomfort from pressure.
c. Circulatory disorders	Disorders reduce perfusion of skin's tissue layers.
d. Fever	Increases metabolic demands of tissues. Accompanying diaphoresis leaves skin moist.
e. Anemia	Decreased hemoglobin reduces oxygen-carrying capacity of blood and amount of oxygen available to tissues.
f. Malnutrition	Inadequate nutrition can lead to weight loss, muscle atrophy, and reduced tissue mass. Less tissue is available to serve as a pad between skin and underlying bone. Poor protein, vitamin, mineral, and caloric intake limit wound-healing capabilities.
g. Incontinence	Skin becomes exposed to moist environment containing bacteria. Moisture causes skin maceration.
h. Heavy sedation and anesthesia	Client is not mentally alert and does not turn or change position independently. Sedation can also alter sensory perception.
i. Age	Older skin is less elastic and drier; tissue mass is reduced.
j. Dehydration	Results in decreased skin elasticity and turgor.

STEPS	RATIONALE
k. Edema	Edematous tissues are less tolerant of pressure, friction, and shear.
l. Existing pressure ulcers	Limits surfaces available for position changes, placing available tissues at increased risk.
2. Select one of the risk assessment tools.	A valid and reliable risk assessment tool should be used to evaluate client's risk for developing a pressure ulcer (AHCPR, 1992).
3. Identify additional risks for pressure ulcer formation by assessing the particular factors that are found on the selected risk assessment tool.	To prevent pressure ulcers, individuals at risk must be identified so that risk factors can be reduced through intervention (AHCPR, 1992).
4. Obtain "risk score" (see Table 8-2).	The risk cutoff score will depend on instrument used; predicts client's need for preventive care.
5. Assess condition of client's skin over regions of pressure (see Fig. 8-1). Body weight against bony prominences places underlying skin at risk for breakdown. Look for areas of:	"Skin inspection is fundamental to any plan for preventing pressure ulcers" (AHCPR, 1992).
a. Skin discoloration (redness in light-tone skin; purplish or bluish in darkly pigmented skin) and temperature changes (warmth or coolness) (Bennett, 1995). See the box below for cultural considerations in assessing clients with darkly pigmented skin.	May indicate that tissue was under pressure; hyperemia is a normal physiological response to hypoxemia in tissues.
b. Blanching	Blanching is normal, expected response.
c. Induration	Localized edema beneath the skin surface, induration commonly occurs with abnormal hyperemia (Pires and Mueller, 1991).
d. Pallor and mottling	Persistent hypoxia in tissues that were under pressure; an abnormal physiological response.
e. Absence of superficial skin layers	Represents early pressure ulcer formation.

CULTURAL CONSIDERATIONS FOR SKIN ASSESSMENT FOR PRESSURE ULCERS: THE CLIENT WITH INTACT DARKLY PIGMENTED SKIN

Assess Localized Skin Color Changes

Any of the following may appear:

- Skin color changes
- Color darker than surrounding skin, purplish, bluish, eggplant
- Taut
- Shiny
- Induration

Assess for Edema (Nonpitting Swelling)

Importance of Lighting for Skin Assessment

- Use natural or halogen light
- Avoid fluorescent lamps, which can give the skin a bluish tone

Assess Skin Temperature

- Initially may feel warmer than surrounding skin
- Subsequently may feel cooler than surrounding skin
- Use the back of your hand and fingers and, if client condition permits, no gloves when doing this assessment

Based on Bennett MA: Report of the Task Force on the Implications for Darkly Pigmented Intact Skin in the Prediction and Prevention of Pressure Ulcers, 1995.

STEPS	RATIONALE
6. Assess client for additional areas of potential pressure.	Clients at high risk have multiple sites for pressure necrosis, in addition to bony prominences.
a. Nares: NG tube, oxygen cannula	
b. Tongue and lips: oral airway, endotracheal (ET) tube	
c. Ears: oxygen cannula, pillow	
d. Intravenous (IV) sites (especially long-term access sites)	Stress on catheter at exit site.
e. Drainage tubes	Stress against tissue at exit site.
f. Indwelling urethral (Foley) catheter	For female clients, the catheter can put pressure on the labia, especially when it is edematous. For male clients, pressure from a catheter not properly anchored can put pressure on the tip of the penis and urethra.
➤ ***CRITICAL DECISION POINT*** **Inspect skin around and beneath orthopedic devices, such as a cervical collar, braces, or a cast.**	
7. Observe client for preferred positions when in bed or chair.	Weight of body will be placed on certain bony prominences. Presence of contractures may result in pressure exerted in unexpected places. This phenomenon is best assessed through observation.
8. Observe ability of client to initiate and assist with position changes.	Potential for friction and shear increases when client is completely dependent on others for position changes.
➤ ***CRITICAL DECISION POINT*** **Assess client's and support persons' understanding of risks for pressure ulcers. This provides an opportunity to begin prevention education using the AHCPR consumer booklets on pressure ulcers.**	

NURSING DIAGNOSIS

Clustering of defining characteristics from the assessment data may reveal the following nursing diagnoses for clients requiring this skill:

- ➤ Risk for impaired skin integrity
- ➤ Impaired skin integrity
- ➤ Altered nutrition: less than body requirements
- ➤ Altered peripheral tissue perfusion
- ➤ Impaired physical mobility
- ➤ Knowledge deficit related to pressure ulcer prevention

Related factors are individualized based on a client's condition or needs.

PLANNING

STEPS	RATIONALE
1. Expected outcomes following completion of procedure:	
a. Skin is intact without discoloration (such as erythema [redness] or purplish [eggplant color]) or breakdown.	Prevention strategies are successful.
b. Client is able to change positions independently.	Turning schedule has not disrupted sleep pattern.
c. Peripheral circulation is maintained as evidenced by absence of pallor, mottling, or redness.	Adequate blood flow is maintained.
2. Explain procedure(s) and purpose to client and family.	Relieves anxiety and provides opportunity for education.
3. Wash hands and prepare equipment and supplies.	Reduces transmission of microorganisms.

IMPLEMENTATION

➤ ***CRITICAL DECISION POINT*** **Implement the NPUAP Pressure Ulcer Prevention Points (see Fig. 8-2), which are based on the AHCPR clinical guidelines. Using these may prevent the client from developing a pressure ulcer.**

STEPS	RATIONALE
1. Close room door or bedside curtain.	Maintains client privacy.
2. If client has open, draining wounds, use disposable gloves.	Prevents accidental exposure to body fluids. Using gloves is part of compliance with standard precautions.
3. Assist client to change position.	See Chapters 28 and 29 for specifics. Avoid positions that place the client directly on an area of existing ulceration. It may be helpful to use a schedule for position changes.
Use the following positions: a. Supine b. Prone c. 30-degree lateral (see illustration)	Achieved with one pillow under shoulder and one pillow under leg on the same side. Protects sacrum and trochanters.

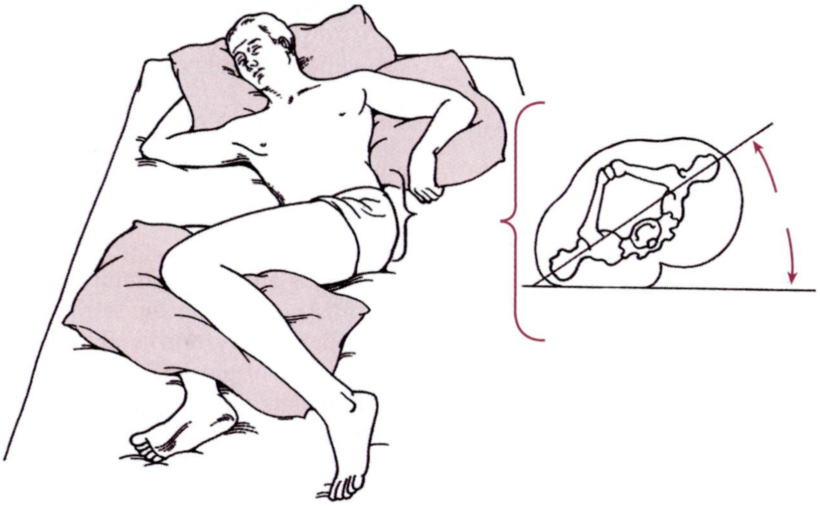

Step 3c

CRITICAL DECISION POINT **Observe for skin discoloration in area that was under pressure. In light skin clients, redness from initial flushing is expected. In darkly pigmented clients, the skin may appear purplish or bluish (Bennett, 1995). Bennett also suggests using natural or halogen light sources when assessing for discoloration on clients with darkly pigmented skin. Avoid using fluorescent lighting because it can give a bluish tint to the skin that can interfere with the accurate assessment of the skin coloring (see box on p. 195).**	Brisk capillary refill is an expected response; sluggish or absent capillary refill represents an abnormal response. Skin should be gently palpated for texture, temperature, and fluid.
4. Palpate any area of discoloration or mottling. Skin temperature changes may be an important early indicator of a stage I (see Table 8-1) pressure ulcer in clients with darkly pigmented skin (Bennett, 1995) (see box on p. 195).	Early detection of pressure indicates need for more frequent position changes.
5. Monitor length of time any area of discoloration persists.	Redness usually persists for 50% of the time hypoxia occurred.
a. Determine appropriate turning interval.	If turning interval is 2 hours, and redness lasts 15 minutes, then hypoxia was approximately 30 minutes.

STEPS	RATIONALE
b. A turning interval of less than 1½ to 2 hours may not be realistic; therefore use of a pressure relief device would be recommended (see Chapter 32).	Recommended turning interval should be the turning interval minus hypoxia time: 2 hr − 30 min = 1½ hr
6. Remove gloves, discard appropriately, and wash hands.	Reduces spread of microorganisms.

EVALUATION

1. Observe client's skin for areas at risk for change in color or texture.	Enables the nurse to evaluate success of prevention techniques.
2. Observe tolerance of client for position change.	Position changes may interfere with client's sleep and rest pattern.
3. Compare subsequent risk assessment scores.	Provides ongoing comparison of client's risk level to facilitate appropriateness of plan of care.
4. **Unexpected outcomes** that may occur include:	
➤ Skin becomes mottled, reddened, purplish, or bluish.	Early signs of pressure ulcer.
➤ Client reports sense of fatigue and inability to sleep.	Turning schedule needs to be modified to promote sleep.
➤ Areas under pressure develop persistent discoloration, induration, or temperature changes.	Impaired blood flow to an area of the skin.

RECORDING AND REPORTING

1. Record client's risk score.	Accurate and complete documentation of all risk assessments ensures continuity of care and may be used as a foundation for the skin care plan (AHCPR, 1992).
2. Record appearance of skin under pressure.	Baseline observations and subsequent inspections reveal success of prevention program.
3. Describe positions, turning intervals, pressure relieving support devices, and other prevention measures.	Documents care.
4. Report any need for additional consultations for the high-risk client.	Preventing and treating pressure ulcers requires a multidisciplinary approach. Resources include physical therapist, occupational therapist, social worker, dietitian, home health nurse, clinical nurse specialist (CNS), and enterostomal therapy nurse.

FOLLOW-UP ACTIVITIES

1. Document and communicate interval for reevaluation of risk assessment score.
2. Obtain physician's order (when needed) for identified consults such as physical therapist, dietitian, clinical nurse specialist (CNS), and enterostomal therapy nurse.

• • • • •

Special Considerations

- ➤ Body regions that receive greatest pressure in specific positions:
  - Sitting: ischial tuberosities, sacrum
  - Supine: back of skull, elbows, sacrum, ischial tuberosities, heels
  - Prone: elbows, knees, toes
  - 30-degree lateral side-lying: knees, greater trochanters
- ➤ Clients may tolerate the 30-degree lateral side-lying position for longer intervals, which would allow for minimal disturbance at night.
- ➤ Although the AHCPR (1992, 1994) recommends maintaining the head of the bed at the lowest degree of elevation consistent with medical conditions and other restrictions, clients who are receiving tube feedings will need the head of the bed elevated to prevent aspiration.
- ➤ Clients who have experienced prolonged (≥3 hours) surgical or testing procedures which require mobility restrictions should be considered to be at risk.
- ➤ If client's ability to assist with position changes is unknown or severely limited, obtain assistance be-

fore attempting position changes to minimize friction or shear to the client's skin and to reduce injury.

- Spasticity may result in pressure ulcer development in atypical locations such as between the buttocks.
- If a client requires a pressure relief surface for the bed, an appropriate pressure relief surface should also be considered for the chair.
- A client who is admitted to the hospital after having fallen and who was on the floor for an unknown period should be considered at risk.

Teaching Considerations

- Review the AHCPR 1992 and 1994 consumer booklets on pressure ulcers with the client and family (Ayello, 1993, 1995).
- Explain risks of pressure ulcer formation.
- Assist client (and family) to understand multiple factors involved in preventing and treating pressure ulcers.
- Explain and demonstrate positioning options to achieve pressure relief.
- Explain the purpose and maintenance of pressure relief devices.
- When teaching clients to change position for pressure relief, suggest using television programing and commercial intervals or a watch with an alarm as reminders.

Gerontologic Considerations

- In older adults, a risk score of 17 or 18 (rather than the usual score of 16) may be a more efficient prediction of pressure ulcer risk on the Braden scale (Braden and Bergstrom, 1994; Bryant et al., 1992).
- Sitting posture and position need to be reevaluated since body weight and muscle tone change with age.
- In the older client, the epidermal-dermal junction becomes flatter, putting the client at increased risk for epidermal peel as a result of shearing forces (Loescher, 1995).

Home Care Considerations

- The 30-degree lateral and prone positions may be useful at night to prolong the time between position changes, resulting in less sleep disruption for the client and care giver.
- Identify community resources, such as neighbors and relatives, for assistance should the client need help with position changes, including after a fall.
- Pressure relief maneuvers must be customized to the independent client. The individual may find a watch with a timer, even or odd hours, and television commercials helpful in remembering to complete pressure relief techniques.

SKILL 8-2 Treatment of Pressure Ulcers

Treatment of clients with pressure ulcers requires a holistic approach that uses the expertise of the multidisciplinary health care team (AHCPR, 1994). It involves not only assessment and local care of the pressure ulcer but also assessment and care of the entire client (AHCPR, 1994). Pressure ulcer treatment includes local care of the wound and supportive measures such as pressure relief and adequate nutrition. The basis for the development of an effective pressure ulcer treatment plan is a thorough assessment of the client and the ulcer (Fig. 8-3) (AHCPR, 1994). Local wound care principles are wound **debridement** (if ulcer is necrotic), cleaning, and dressing application (see also Chapters 37 and 40).

The best solution to use to clean most pressure ulcers is normal saline (AHCPR, 1994). **Astringents** such as alcohol and witch hazel can harm skin layers through excessive drying and vasoconstriction, which can reduce local blood flow to tissues. It is also important to avoid using topical agents such as povidone-iodine, iodophor, sodium hypochlorite solution (Dakin's solution), hydrogen peroxide, or acetic acid, which kill the cell fibroblasts that are necessary for wound healing (AHCPR, 1994).

Local treatment of pressure ulcers includes the use of a variety of dressings, which are selected on the basis of the ulcer's characteristics. Occlusive dressings are used with increasing frequency to treat pressure ulcers. Occlusive dressings (transparent dressings, hydrocolloid dressings, and hydrogels) may be used alone or in combination with topical agents (see Chapter 37). All pressure ulcers are considered **colonized;** therefore the AHCPR (1994) suggests that clean dressings and gloves, rather than sterile, be used. Swab cultures only detect surface organisms, and therefore using them routinely to detect wound infection is not recommended (AHCPR, 1994). The AHCPR Panel (1994) does recommend quantative methods of wound culture such as tissue biopsy and wound fluid aspiration.

Current research may determine additional methods useful in treating pressure ulcers. Some ongoing areas of research include topically applied growth factors, electrical stimulation (Itoh et al., 1991), and hyperbaric oxygen therapy (Surman, 1996). Growth factors occur naturally in wound fluid and may stimulate both granulation and epithelialization when applied topically. Pulsed electrical stimulation is a procedure that can be performed by physi-

Text continued on p. 204

PRESSURE SORE STATUS TOOL NAME______________________

Complete the rating sheet to assess pressure sore status. Evaluate each item by picking the response that best describes the wound and entering the score in the item score column for the appropriate date.

Location: Anatomic site. Circle, identify right (**R**) or left (**L**) and use "**X**" to mark site on body diagrams:

_____ Sacrum & coccyx _____ Lateral ankle
_____ Trochanter _____ Medial ankle
_____ Ischial tuberosity _____ Heel Other Site _____

Shape: Overall wound pattern; assess by observing perimeter and depth.

Circle and date appropriate description:

_____ Irregular _____ Linear or elongated
_____ Round/oval _____ Bowl/boat
_____ Square/rectangle _____ Butterfly Other Shape _____

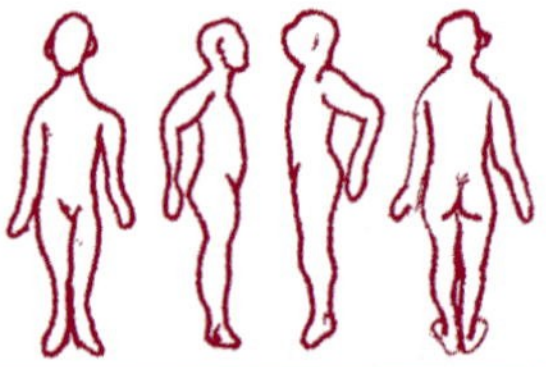

Item	**Assessment**	**Date**	**Date**	**Date**
		Score	**Score**	**Score**
1. **Size**	1 = Length x width < 4 sq cm 2 = Length x width 4 -16 sq cm 3 = Length x width 16.1 - 36 sq cm 4 = Length x width 36.1 - 80 sq cm 5 = Length x width > 80 sq cm			
2. **Depth**	1 = Non-blanchable erythema on intact skin 2 = Partial thickness skin loss involving epidermis &/or dermis 3 = Full thickness skin loss involving damage or necrosis of subcutaneous tissue; may extend down to but not through underlying fascia; &/or mixed partial & full thickness &/or tissue layers obscured by granulation tissue 4 = Obscured by necrosis 5 = Full thickness skin loss with extensive destruction, tissue necrosis or damage to muscle, bone or supporting structures			
3. **Edges**	1 = Indistinct, diffuse, none clearly visible 2 = Distinct, outline clearly visible, attached, even with wound base 3 = Well-defined, not attached to wound base 4 = Well-defined, not attached to base, rolled under, thickened 5 = Well-defined, fibrotic, scarred or hyperkeratotic			
4. **Under-mining**	1 = Undermining < 2 cm in any area 2 = Undermining 2-4 cm involving < 50% wound margins 3 = Undermining 2-4 cm involving > 50% wound margins 4 = Undermining > 4 cm in any area 5 = Tunneling &/or sinus tract formation			
5. **Necrotic Tissue Type**	1 = None visible 2 = White/grey non-viable tissue &/or non-adherent yellow slough 3 = Loosely adherent yellow slough 4 = Adherent, soft, black eschar 5 = Firmly adherent, hard, black eschar			
6. **Necrotic Tissue Amount**	1 = None visible 2 = < 25% of wound bed covered 3 = 25% to 50% of wound covered 4 = > 50% and < 75% of wound covered 5 = 75% to 100% of wound covered			

Fig. 8-3 Bates-Jensen Pressure Sore Assessment Tool. (Courtesy Barbara Bates-Jensen.)

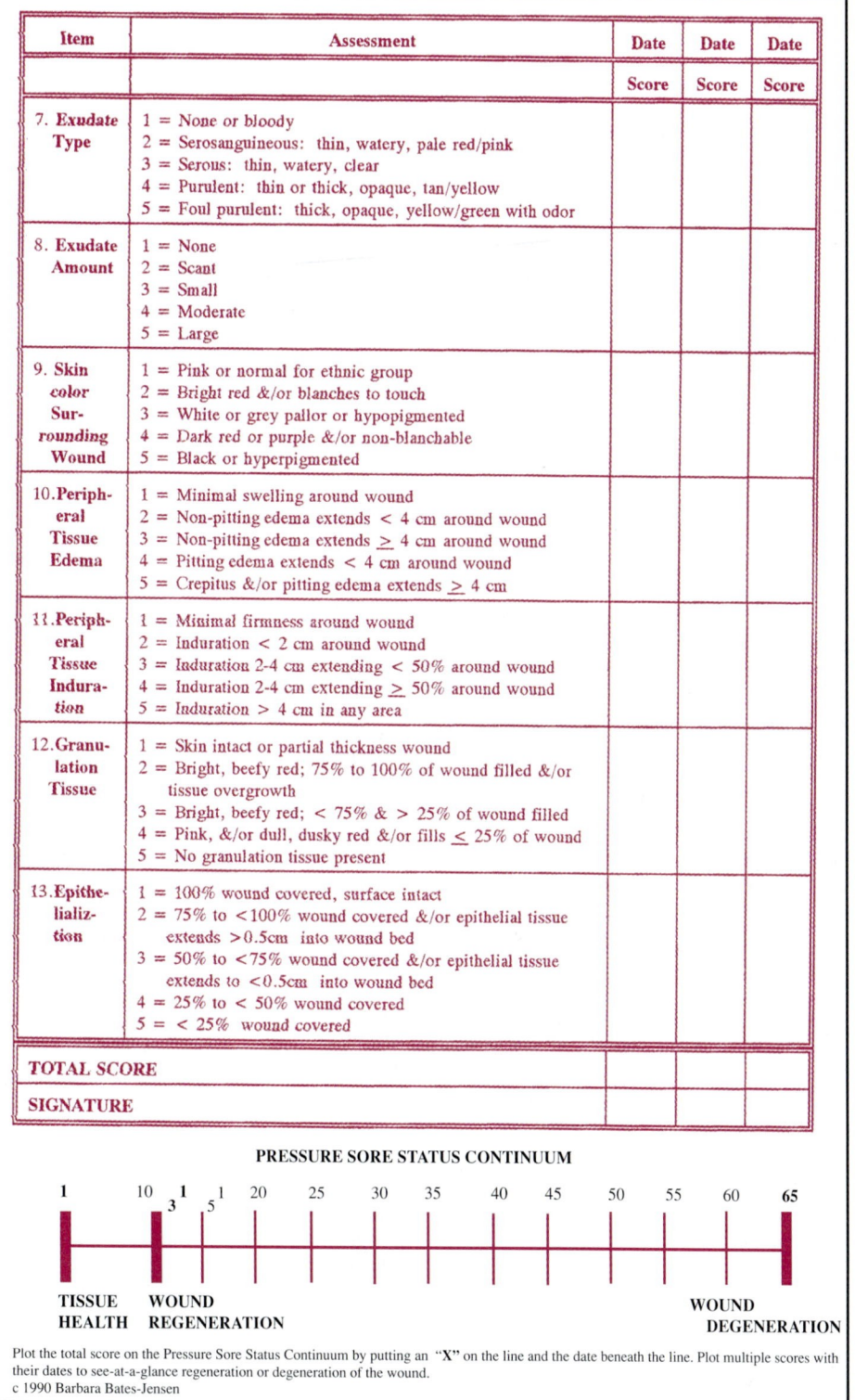

Item	Assessment	Date	Date	Date
		Score	Score	Score
7. **Exudate Type**	1 = None or bloody 2 = Serosanguineous: thin, watery, pale red/pink 3 = Serous: thin, watery, clear 4 = Purulent: thin or thick, opaque, tan/yellow 5 = Foul purulent: thick, opaque, yellow/green with odor			
8. **Exudate Amount**	1 = None 2 = Scant 3 = Small 4 = Moderate 5 = Large			
9. **Skin color Sur-rounding Wound**	1 = Pink or normal for ethnic group 2 = Bright red &/or blanches to touch 3 = White or grey pallor or hypopigmented 4 = Dark red or purple &/or non-blanchable 5 = Black or hyperpigmented			
10. **Periph-eral Tissue Edema**	1 = Minimal swelling around wound 2 = Non-pitting edema extends < 4 cm around wound 3 = Non-pitting edema extends ≥ 4 cm around wound 4 = Pitting edema extends < 4 cm around wound 5 = Crepitus &/or pitting edema extends ≥ 4 cm			
11. **Periph-eral Tissue Indura-tion**	1 = Minimal firmness around wound 2 = Induration < 2 cm around wound 3 = Induration 2-4 cm extending < 50% around wound 4 = Induration 2-4 cm extending ≥ 50% around wound 5 = Induration > 4 cm in any area			
12. **Granu-lation Tissue**	1 = Skin intact or partial thickness wound 2 = Bright, beefy red; 75% to 100% of wound filled &/or tissue overgrowth 3 = Bright, beefy red; < 75% & > 25% of wound filled 4 = Pink, &/or dull, dusky red &/or fills ≤ 25% of wound 5 = No granulation tissue present			
13. **Epithe-lializ-tion**	1 = 100% wound covered, surface intact 2 = 75% to <100% wound covered &/or epithelial tissue extends >0.5cm into wound bed 3 = 50% to <75% wound covered &/or epithelial tissue extends to <0.5cm into wound bed 4 = 25% to < 50% wound covered 5 = < 25% wound covered			
TOTAL SCORE				
SIGNATURE				

PRESSURE SORE STATUS CONTINUUM

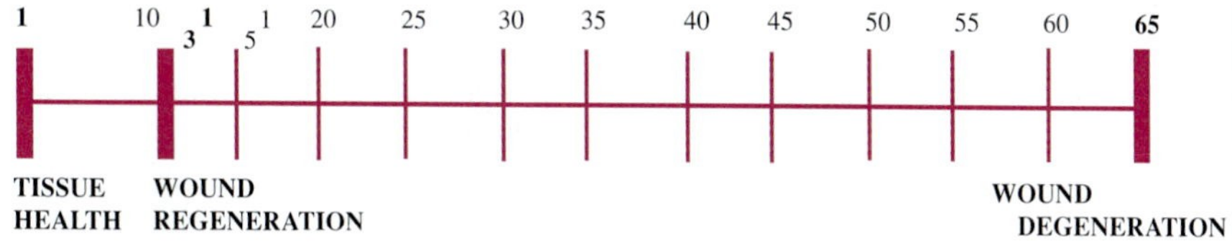

Plot the total score on the Pressure Sore Status Continuum by putting an "X" on the line and the date beneath the line. Plot multiple scores with their dates to see-at-a-glance regeneration or degeneration of the wound.

Fig. 8-3, cont'd For legend see opposite page.

Continued

PRESSURE SORE STATUS TOOL

Instructions for use

General Guidelines:

Fill out the attached rating sheet to assess a pressure sore's status after reading the definitions and methods of assessement described below. Evaluate once a week and whenever a change occurs in the wound. Rate according to each item by picking the response that best describes the wound and entering that score in the item score column for the appropriate date. When you have rated the pressure sore on all items, determine the total score by adding together the 13-item scores. The HIGHER the total score, the more severe the pressure sore status. Plot total score on the Pressure Sore Status Continuum to determine progress.

Specific Instructions:

1. **Size**: Use ruler to measure the longest and widest aspect of the wound surface in centimeters; multiply length x width.

2. **Depth**: Pick the depth, thickness, most appropriate to the wound using these additional descriptions:
   - 1 = tissues damaged but no break in skin surface.
   - 2 = superficial, abrasion, blister or shallow crater. Even with, &/or elevated above skin surface (e.g., hyperplasia).
   - 3 = deep crater with or without undermining of adjacent tissue.
   - 4 = visualization of tissue layers not possible due to necrosis.
   - 5 = supporting structures include tendon, joint capsule.

3. **Edges**: Use this guide:

Indistinct, diffuse	=	unable to clearly distinguish wound outline.
Attached	=	even or flush with wound base, no sides or walls present; flat.
Not attached	=	sides or walls are present; floor or base of wound is deeper than edge.
Rolled under, thickened	=	soft to firm and flexible to touch.
Hyperkeratosis	=	callous-like tissue formation around wound & at edges.
Fibrotic, scarred	=	hard, rigid to touch.

4. **Undermining**: Assess by inserting a cotton tipped applicator under the wound edge; advance it as far as it will go without using undue force; raise the tip of the applicator so it may be seen or felt on the surface of the skin; mark the surface with a pen; measure the distance from the mark on the skin to the edge of the wound. Continue process around the wound. Then use a transparent metric measuring guide with concentric circles divided into 4 (25%) pie-shaped quadrants to help determine percent of wound involved.

5. **Necrotic Tissue Type**: Pick the type of necrotic tissue that is predominant in the wound according to color, consistency and adherence using this guide:

White/gray non-viable tissue	=	may appear prior to wound opening; skin surface is white or gray.
Non-adherent, yellow slough	=	thin, mucinous substance; scattered throughout wound bed; easily separated from wound tissue.
Loosely adherent, yellow slough	=	thick, stringy, clumps of debris; attached to wound tissue.
Adherent, soft, black eschar	=	soggy tissue; strongly attached to tissue in center or base of wound.
Firmly adherent, hard/black eschar	=	firm, crusty tissue; strongly attached to wound base and edges (like a hard scab).

Fig. 8-3, cont'd Bates-Jensen Pressure Sore Assessment Tool. (Courtesy Barbara Bates-Jensen.)

6. **Necrotic Tissue Amount**: Use a transparent metric measuring guide with concentric circles divided into 4 (25%) pie-shaped quadrants to help determine percent of wound involved.

7. **Exudate Type**: Some dressings interact with wound drainage to produce a gel or trap liquid. Before assessing exudate type, gently cleanse wound with normal saline or water. Pick the exudate type that is predominant in the wound according to color and consistency, using this guide:

Bloody	=	thin, bright red
Serosanguineous	=	thin, watery pale red to pink
Serous	=	thin, watery, clear
Purulent	=	thin or thick, opaque tan to yellow
Foul purulent	=	thick, opaque yellow to green with offensive odor

8. **Exudate Amount**: Use a transparent metric measuring guide with concentric circles divided into 4 (25%) pie-shaped quadrants to determine percent of dressing involved with exudate. Use this guide:

None	=	wound tissues dry.
Scant	=	wound tissues moist; no measurable exudate.
Small	=	wound tissues wet; moisture evenly distributed in wound; drainage involves $\leq$ 25% dressing.
Moderate	=	wound tissues saturated; drainage may or may not be evenly distributed in wound; drainage involves > 25% to $\leq$ 75% dressing.
Large	=	wound tissues bathed in fluid; drainage freely expressed; may or may not be evenly distributed in wound; drainage involves > 75% of dressing.

9. **Skin Color Surrounding Wound**: Assess tissues within 4cm of wound edge. Dark-skinned persons show the colors "bright red" and "dark red" as a deepening of normal ethnic skin color or a purple hue. As healing occurs in dark-skinned persons, the new skin is pink and may never darken.

10. **Peripheral Tissue Edema**: Assess tissues within 4cm of wound edge. Non-pitting edema appears as skin that is shiny and taut. Identify pitting edema by firmly pressing a finger down into the tissues and waiting for 5 seconds, on release of pressure, tissues fail to resume previous position and an indentation appears. Crepitus is accumulation of air or gas in tissues. Use a transparent metric measuring guide to determine how far edema extends beyond wound.

11. **Peripheral Tissue Induration**: Assess tissues within 4cm of wound edge. Induration is abnormal firmness of tissues with margins. Assess by gently pinching the tissues. Induration results in an inability to pinch the tissues. Use a transparent metric measuring guide with concentric circles divided into 4 (25%) pie-shaped quadrants to determine percent of wound and area involved.

12. **Granulation Tissue**: Granulation tissue is the growth of small blood vessels and connective tissue to fill in full thickness wounds. Tissue is healthy when bright, beefy red, shiny and granular with a velvety appearance. Poor vascular supply appears as pale pink or blanched to dull, dusky red color.

13. **Epithelialization**: Epithelialization is the process of epidermal resurfacing and appears as pink or red skin. In partial thickness wounds it can occur throughout the wound bed as well as from the wound edges. In full thickness wounds it occurs from the edges only. Use a transparent metric measuring guide with concentric circles divided into 4 (25%) pie-shaped quadrants to help determine percent of wound involved and to measure the distance the epithelial tissue extends into the wound.

Fig. 8-3, cont'd Bates-Jensen Pressure Sore Assessment Tool. (Courtesy Barbara Bates-Jensen.)

cal therapists with the goal of increased wound healing. Although controversial, hyperbaric oxygen therapy uses increased amounts of pressurized oxygen delivered to clients in a variety of specialized methods (Surman, 1996).

EQUIPMENT

- Disposable gloves (clean)
- Goggles and cover gown
- Plastic bag for dressing disposal
- Measuring device (tape measure)
- Cotton-tipped applicators
- Camera and tracing film (optional)
- Topical agent (as ordered)
- Cleansing agent (normal saline)
- Sterile solution container
- Washbasin, washclothes, towels
- Dressing of choice
- Skin protectant
- Hypoallergenic tape (if needed)
- 35-ml syringe with 19-gauge needle
- Documentation records (e.g., graph paper)

DELEGATION CONSIDERATIONS

This skill requires problem solving and knowledge application unique to a professional nurse. For this skill, delegation is inappropriate.

STEPS	RATIONALE
ASSESSMENT	
1. Assess the client's level of comfort and need for pain medication (AHCPR, 1994; Dallam et al., 1995).	Dressing change procedure is better tolerated if pain is controlled.
2. Determine if client has allergies to **topical agents.**	Topical agents contain elements that may cause localized skin reactions.
3. Review physician's order for topical agent or dressing (in many cases physician follows nurse's recommendations for pressure ulcer care).	Ensures that proper medication and treatment are administered.
4. Wash hands, and apply clean gloves. Close room door or bedside curtains.	Reduces transmission of microorganisms and prevents accidental exposure to body fluids.
5. Position client to allow dressing removal.	Area should be accessible for dressing change. Proper disposal of old dressing promotes proper handling of contaminated waste.

AYELLO'S ASSESSMENT MNEMONIC

Anatomical location, age	A	Chronic wounds heal slower.
Size, shape, stage	S	Staging of the wound will help in selecting the appropriate healing treatments and dressing. Measuring guides can assist in determining the length and width of the ulcer. A sterile cotton-tipped application can be used to measure the depth of the ulcer.
Sinus tract	S	Gently use a sterile cotton-tipped applicator tip to locate any sinus tracts.
Exudate	E	Wound drainage must be contained to protect the surrounding skin.
Sepsis	S	Systemic infections must be treated. Routine swab culturing of pressure ulcers for local infection is not recommended (Maklebust, 1994).
Surrounding skin	S	Protect the surrounding skin from breakdown from moisture.
Margins, **maceration**	M	Identify condition of wound margins and if they are contracting. Evaluate for maceration; if present, institute measures to protect skin.
Erythema, epithelization, **eschar**	E	Evaluate for wound healing, as evidenced by these changes in the ulcer. **Erythema** in clients with dark skin tone is best assessed with good lighting. Skin may have a purplish hue (Graves, 1990).
Necrotic, nose, neovascularization	N	Necrotic tissue must be removed to stage and heal the ulcer.
Tissue bed, tenderness to touch, tension, temperature, treatments	T	Identify tissue bed and prior ulcer treatment and medicate for pain (Bergstrom et al., 1994).

Courtesy Elizabeth Ayello.

STEPS	RATIONALE
6. Assess each of the client's pressure ulcer(s) and surrounding skin to determine ulcer characteristics, including its stage (see Table 8-1).	Staging is a way of classifying a pressure ulcer. It is based on the depth of destruction of the tissue.
CRITICAL DECISION POINT **To correctly stage a pressure ulcer, the nurse must be able to see its base. Therefore, pressure ulcers that are covered with necrotic tissue cannot be staged until the eschar is debrided (AHCPR, 1994).**	Staging of the pressure ulcer is only done once on initial assessment of the wound.
7. Another way to classify pressure ulcers is by the color of the wound bed. Known as the *red-yellow-black color system,* it is quick and easy to use (Krasner 1995). Wounds that are necrotic are classified as *black wounds;* wounds that have exudate and yellow **slough** are classified as *yellow wounds;* and wounds that are in the active healing phase and are clean with pink to red granulation and epithelial tissue are classified as *red wounds* (Krasner, 1995).	The color of the wound identifies the healing phase of the wound.
8. Minimum pressure ulcer characteristics to include in assessing the wound are as follows: location, stage, size, sinus tracts, exudate, necrotic tissue (black, hard tissue is called *eschar*), granulation tissue, and epithelization. Consider using either the Bates-Jensen (1990) Pressure Sore Assessment Tool (see Fig. 8-3) or Ayello's (1992) Assessment Mnemonic (see box on p. 204). All pressure ulcers should be reassessed at least weekly (AHCPR, 1994).	
a. Note color, temperature, edema, moisture, and appearance of skin around the ulcer and of the ulcer, itself. Remember to modify the assessment technique based on the client's individual skin color (see box on p. 195).	Skin condition may indicate progressive tissue damage. Retained moisture causes maceration.
b. Measure two maximum perpendicular diameters. It is important to have the client in the same position each time pressure ulcer measurements are taken. This will provide consistency so that subsequent measurements can be compared for changes in size. Obtain the wound's length first and then its width (Surface area = Length × Width). Use either a tape or circular pressure ulcer measuring device (see illustration on p. 206).	Provides an objective measure of wound size. May influence size and type of dressing selected.
c. Measure the depth of the pressure ulcer using a sterile saline moistened, cotton-tipped applicator or other device that will allow measurement of wound depth. Place the applicator *gently* into the pressure ulcer until it touches the bottom. Mark the place on the applicator where it reaches the top of the wound, and then remove the applicator from the ulcer. Measure the distance from the tip of the applicator to the mark using a measuring tape or ruler to determine the depth of the pressure ulcer (Volume = 2[L × D] + [W × D] + [L + D]).	Depth measure is important for determining wound volume. Although surface area adequately represents tissue loss in stage I and II ulcers, volume more adequately represents tissue loss in deeper stage III and IV wounds.

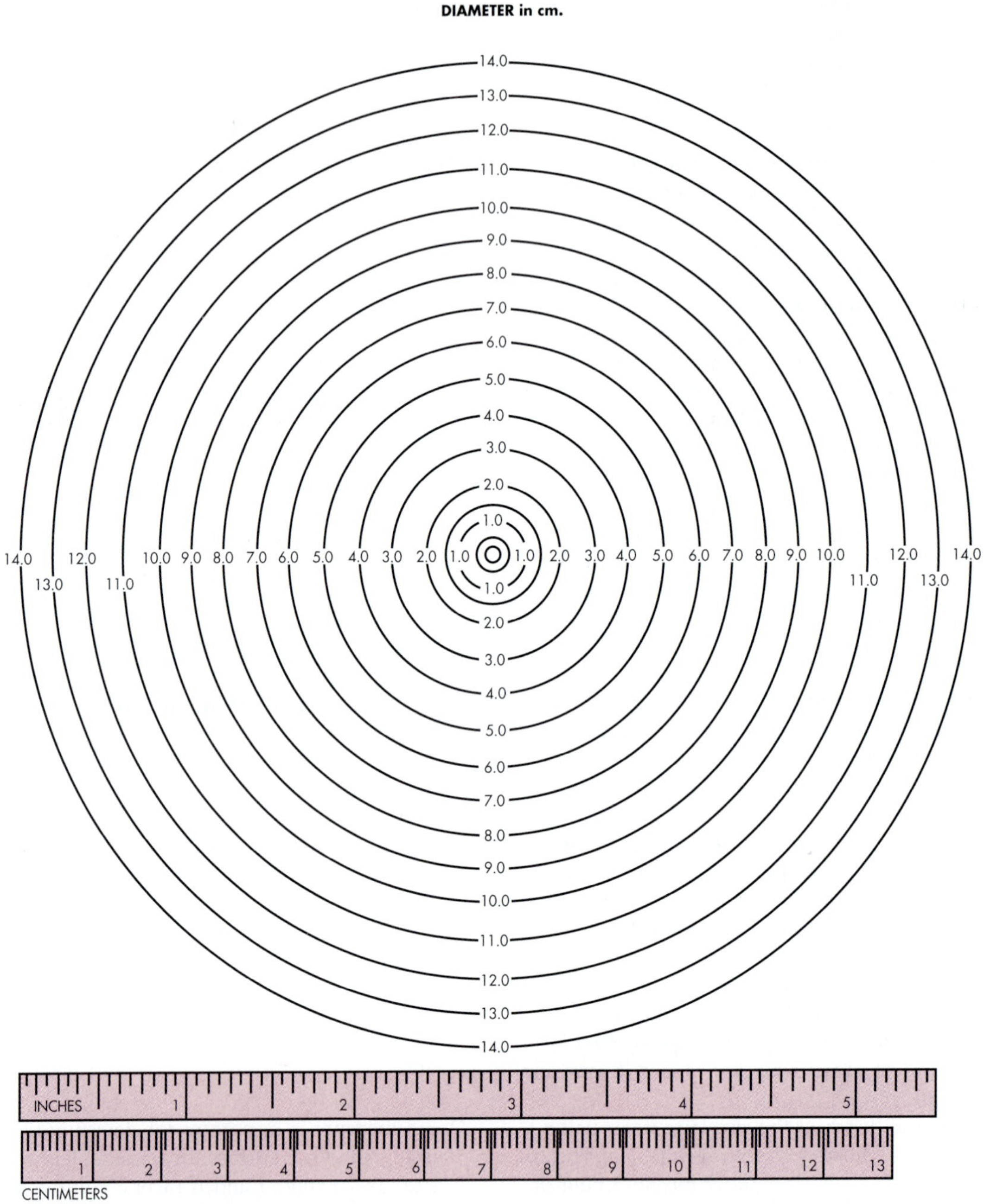

DISCARD AFTER USE

Step 8b Measuring guide. Center over wound to be measured. (Modified with permission from Maklebust J and Sieggreen M: *Pressure ulcers: guidelines for prevention and nursing management*, ed 2 Springhouse, PA, 1996, Springhouse Corporation.)

STEPS	RATIONALE
d. Measure depth (d) of undermining skin by lateral tissue necrosis. Use a cotton-tipped applicator, and gently probe under skin edges.	Undermining represents the loss of the underlying tissues (subcutaneous and muscle) to a greater extent than the skin (see illustration). Undermining may indicate progressive tissue necrosis.
9. Remove gloves; discard appropriately; and wash hands.	Reduces transmission of microorganisms.
10. Assessment of the entire client is necessary in developing a pressure ulcer treatment plan. According to the AHCPR (1994), this assessment should include (a) a complete history and physical examination, (b) the identification of complications and comorbid conditions, (c) a nutritional assessment, (d) an assessment of pain, (e) a psychosocial assessment, and (f) an evaluation of the individual's risks for additional pressure ulcers.	
11. The client's nutritional status should be assessed at least every 3 months. Clinically significant malnutrition is present if (a) serum albumin is less than 3.5 g/dl, (b) lymphocyte count is less than 1800/mm^3, or (c) body weight decrease more than 15% (AHCPR, 1994). Observe the client's mouth and skin for signs of vitamin and mineral deficiencies.	
12. Assess client's and support persons' understanding of pressure ulcer characteristics and purpose of treatment (AHCPR, 1994).	Explanations relieve anxiety and promote cooperation during procedure.

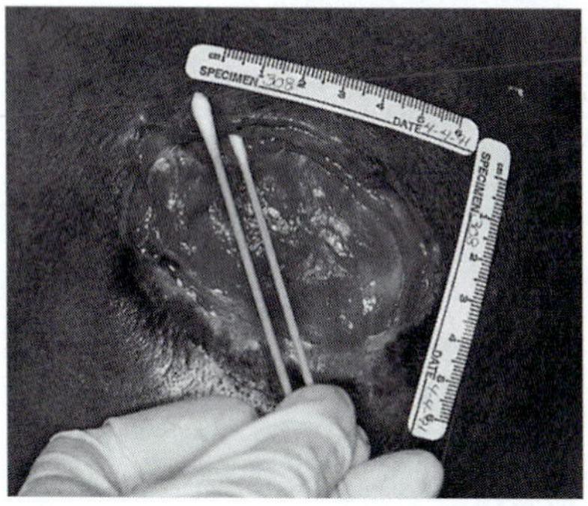

Step 8d Measuring depth of undermining of wound.

NURSING DIAGNOSIS

Clustering of defining characteristics from the assessment data may reveal the following nursing diagnosis for clients requiring this skill:

- Impaired skin integrity
- Pain
- Altered nutrition: less than body requirements
- Altered peripheral tissue perfusion
- Impaired physical mobility
- Knowledge deficit regarding pressure ulcer treatment plan

Related factors are individualized based on a client's condition or needs.

PLANNING

STEPS	RATIONALE
1. **Expected outcomes** following completion of procedure:	
➤ Ulcer drainage decreases.	Ulcer shows signs of healing.
➤ Ulcer measurements and tracings are progressively smaller.	Signs of healing. With eschar-covered wounds, size may initially increase after removal of eschar.
➤ Skin surrounding ulcer remains healthy and intact.	Surrounding tissues are not irritated.
2. Nutrition is adequate to compensate for wound fluid losses and wound repair (see illustration on p. 208).	
3. Skin surrounding the ulcer is protected from trauma.	Wound fluids and agents used in treatment may be irritating to intact skin.
4. Client's overall skin is protected from further breakdown.	Client may remain at risk for further breakdown while existing ulcer heals.

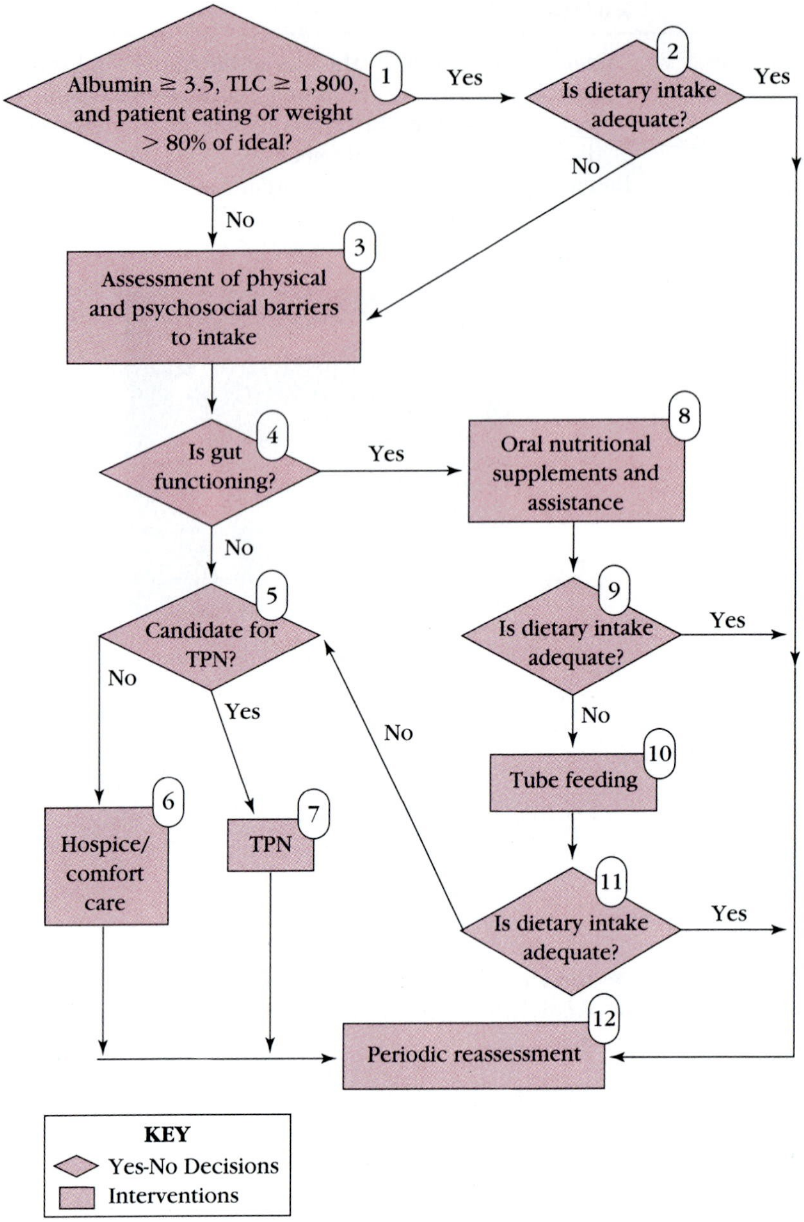

Step 2 Nutritional Assessment and Support. (From Bergstrom N et al: *Treatment of pressure ulcers*, AHCPR pub no 95-0652, Rockville, MD, 1994, DHHS, PHS, AHCPR.)

STEPS	RATIONALE
5. Explain procedure and its purpose to client and family. Use the AHCPR (1994) consumer booklet *Treating Pressure Sores* (Ayello, 1995).	Preparatory explanations relieve anxiety, correct any misconceptions about the ulcer and its treatment, and offer an opportunity for client and family education.
6. Prepare the following necessary equipment and supplies:	
a. Wash basin, warm water, soap, washcloth, and bath towel.	Used to bathe surrounding skin.
b. Normal saline or other cleansing agent in sterile solution container. Use a 19-gauge needle or angiocath with a 35-ml syringe.	Ulcer surface must be cleansed before the application of topical agents and a new dressing.
c. Prescribed topical agent:	
(1) Chemical and enzymatic agents: Santyl (collagenase), Elase (fibrinolysin and deoxyribonuclease), Panafil (papain), or Granulex (trypsin, balam Peru, and castor oil)	Proteolytic enzymes debride dead tissue to clean ulcer surface.

STEPS	RATIONALE
(2) Dextranomer beads: Debrisan (Fowler, 1987)	Cleans wounds with heavy exudate. Absorbs fluid, protein, fibrin, fibrinogen, and all products of tissue breakdown and bacterial infection.
d. Dressing (see Table 8-3 and Chapter 37):	
(1) Select an appropriate dressing based on the pressure ulcer characteristics, purpose for which the dressing is intended, and client care setting. The dressing should maintain a moist environment for the wound while keeping the surrounding skin dry (AHCPR, 1994)	
(2) Gauze type: 4 × 4 pads, fluffs	Applied over ulcers treated with enzymes, mechanical debridement with a wet to dry normal saline dressing, or dextranomer beads.
(3) Transparent membrane dressings	Applied over superficial ulcers and skin subjected to shear.
CRITICAL DECISION POINT **Transparent membrane dressings can also be used for autolytic debridement of noninfected pressure ulcers.**	
(4) Hydrocolloid	Maintains moist environment to facilitate wound healing.
CRITICAL DECISION POINT **Hydrocolloid can also be used to protect skin from friction and shear injury. Some of the brands have custom shapes available for specific anatomical parts, such as heels, elbows, and sacrum. Monitor this dressing when it is near the anus to make sure it is intact (AHCPR, 1994).**	
(5) Hydrogel	Maintains moist environment to facilitate wound healing. Very soothing to clients with painful wounds.
(6) Calcium alginate	Highly absorbent of wound **exudate** in heavily draining wounds.
(7) Exudate absorbers	Highly absorbent of wound exudate.
(8) Foam	Protective and will prevent wound dehydration; also absorbs small to moderate amounts of drainage.
e. Hypoallergenic tape or adhesive dressing sheet (Hypofix).	Used to secure nonadherent dressing. Prevents skin irritation and tearing.
IMPLEMENTATION	
1. Assemble needed supplies at bedside. Close room door or bedside curtains. Wash hands, and don gloves. Open sterile packages and topical solution containers. (Goggles and moisture-proof cover gown should be worn if potential for contamination from spray exists when cleansing the wound.)	Maintains client privacy. Supplies should be ready for easy application so that nurse can use supplies without contaminating them; reduces transmission of microorganisms.
2. Remove bed linen and client's gown to expose ulcer and surrounding skin. Keep remaining body parts draped.	Prevents unnecessary exposure of body parts.
3. Gently wash skin surrounding ulcer with warm water and soap.	Cleansing of skin surface reduces bacteria.
4. Rinse area thoroughly with water.	Soap can be irritating to skin.
5. Gently dry skin thoroughly by patting lightly with towel.	Retained moisture causes maceration of skin layers.
6. Change gloves.	Aseptic technique must be maintained during cleansing, measuring, and application of dressings. Refer to institutional policy regarding use of clean or sterile gloves.

Table 8-3 Treatment Options by Ulcer Stage

Ulcer Stage	Ulcer Status	Dressing	Comments*	Expected Change	Adjuvants
I	Intact	None	Allows visual assessment.	Resolves slowly without epidermal loss over 7 to 14 days.	Turning schedule. Support hydration. Nutritional support. Silicone-based lotion to decrease shear. Pressure relief mattress or chair cushion.
		Film, adherent	Protects from shear.		
		Hydrocolloid	May not allow visual assessment.		
II	Clean	Composite film	Viasorb, film plus telfa, Exudry. Limits shear.	Heals through reepithelialization and epithelial budding.	See previous stage. Manage incontinence.
		Hydrocolloid	Change every 7 days if occlusive seal.		
		Hydrogel sheet	Absorbent, requires secondary dressing of gauze or adherent film.		
III	Clean	Hydrocolloid	See stage II.	Heals through granulation and reepithelialization. (Note: does not become a stage II ulcer as it heals.)	See previous stages. Electrical stimulation. Evaluate pressure relief needs.
		Hydrogel foam	Apply ¼-inch thick, cover with gauze or hydrocolloid.		
		Exudate absorbers calcium alginate wound pastes	Change when strike through is noted on secondary dressing. Cover with gauze or hydrocolloid.		
		Gauze, fluffy	Use with normal saline.		
		Growth factors	Use with gauze.		
IV	Clean	Hydrogel	See stage III Clean.	Heals through granulation and reepithelialization. Because of contraction, surface may close more rapidly than base, leaving wound cavity.	Surgical consult for closure. See stages I, II, and III. Clean.
		Hydrocolloid plus hydrocolloid paste/beads	See stage III Clean; critical to treat areas of undermining.		
		Calcium alginate	See stage III Clean.		
		Gauze	Pack deeply undermined ulcers.		
		Growth factors	Use with gauze.		
	Eschar	Adherent film	Will facilitate softening of eschar.	Eschar will lift at the edges as healing progresses. Cross-hatching central area of eschar with a small blade will facilitate release from center.	See previous stages. Surgical consult for debridement. Enzymes covered with gauze dressing may be used to debride ulcer.
		Hydrocolloid	Will facilitate softening of eschar.		
		Gauze plus ordered solution	Absorb drainage and control odor if Dakins is used.		
		None	Rarely, if eschar is dry and intact, no dressing is used, allowing eschar to act as physiological cover.		

*As with *all* occlusive dressings, wounds should *not* be clinically infected.

STEPS	RATIONALE
7. Cleanse ulcer thoroughly with normal saline or prescribed wound cleansing agent. Use an adequate amount of pressure (measured in psi [pounds per square inch]) to effectively clean the wound, but do not use so much pressure that you injure the wound tissue. In a nonnecrotic wound, a psi between 4 and 15 is considered safe and effective for cleaning a pressure ulcer (AHCPR, 1994).	
a. Use a 19-gauge needle (or angiocath) with a 35-ml syringe to clean most pressure ulcers, especially deep ulcers. The psi of this type of wound cleaning system is 8, which will not harm the fragile healing tissue in the pressure ulcer (AHCPR, 1994).	
CRITICAL DECISION POINT **Be careful not to stick the client or yourself with the needle or angiocath.**	
b. Cleansing in the shower may be done with a handheld shower head.	
8. Whirlpool treatments may be used to assist with wound debridement. Keep the wound directly away from the water jets.	Removes wound debris. Previously applied enzymes may require soaking for removal.
9. Apply topical agents, if prescribed.	
a. Chemicals/enzymes:	
(1) Using a wooden tongue blade, apply a small amount of enzyme debridement ointment directly to the necrotic areas on the base of pressure ulcer. Avoid getting the enzyme on the surrounding skin. The amount of enzyme should be the same as the amount of butter you would spread on bread. A thick layer of ointment is not necessary; a thin layer absorbs and acts more effectively. Crosshatching of the eschar areas may be needed in some necrotic pressure ulcers.	
(2) Apply thin, even layer of ointment over necrotic areas of ulcer. Do not apply enzyme to surrounding skin.	Proper distribution of ointment ensures effective action. Some enzymes can cause burning, paresthesia, and dermatitis to surrounding skin.
(3) Place gauze dressing directly over ulcer, and tape it in place. Follow specific manufacturer's recommendation for type of dressing material to use to cover a pressure ulcer when using their enzyme.	Protects wound and prevents removal of ointment during turning or repositioning.
b. Dextranomer beads:	
(1) Hold the container of beads approximately 1 in (2.5 cm) above ulcer site, and lightly sprinkle a 5-mm layer over wound.	A single layer of insoluble powder is needed to absorb wound exudate.
(2) Apply gauze dressing over ulcer.	Holds beads in place and protects wound.
c. Hydrocolloid beads or paste:	
(1) Fill ulcer defect to approximately half of the total depth with hydrocolloid beads or paste.	Hydrocolloid beads or paste assist in absorbing wound drainage. Heavily draining wounds can be treated with hydrocolloid beads or granules.
(2) Cover with hydrocolloid dressing; extend dressing 1 to 1½ (2.2-4cm) inches beyond edges of wound.	Maintains wound humidity. May be left in place for up to 7 days.

STEPS	RATIONALE
d. Hydrogel agents:	
(1) Cover surface of ulcer with hydrogel using applicator or gloved hand.	Provides maintenance of wound humidity while absorbing excess drainage. May be used as carrier for topical agents.
(2) Apply dry, fluffy gauze or hydrocolloid or transparent dressing over gel to completely cover ulcer.	Holds hydrogel against wound surface; absorbent.
e. Calcium alginates:	Provides maintenance of wound humidity while absorbing excess drainage.
(1) Pack wound with alginate using applicator or gloved hand.	
(2) Apply dry gauze, foam, or hydrocolloid over alginate.	Holds alginate against wound surface.
10. Reposition client comfortably off pressure ulcer.	Avoids accidental removal of dressings.
11. Remove gloves, and dispose of soiled supplies. Wash hands.	Reduces transmission of microorganisms.

EVALUATION

CRITICAL DECISION POINT **A clean pressure ulcer should show evidence of some healing within 2 to 4 weeks.**

STEPS	RATIONALE
1. Observe skin surrounding ulcer for inflammation, edema, and tenderness.	Contact dermatitis may result from exposure to certain topical agents. Without proper preventive care, ulcer can spread to involve neighboring tissue.
2. Inspect dressings and exposed ulcers, observing for drainage, foul odor, and tissue necrosis. Monitor client for signs and symptoms of infection, including fever and elevated white blood cell count.	Ulcers can become infected.
3. Compare subsequent ulcer measurements.	Allows comparison of serial measurements to assess wound healing. It is helpful to plot surface area and volume measurements on graph paper (see illustration).
4. Do *not* use the pressure ulcer staging system to measure pressure ulcer healing (NPUAP, 1995).	Use of the staging system to measure healing rather than its intended use for depth of tissue destruction is inappropriate (NPUAP, 1995).

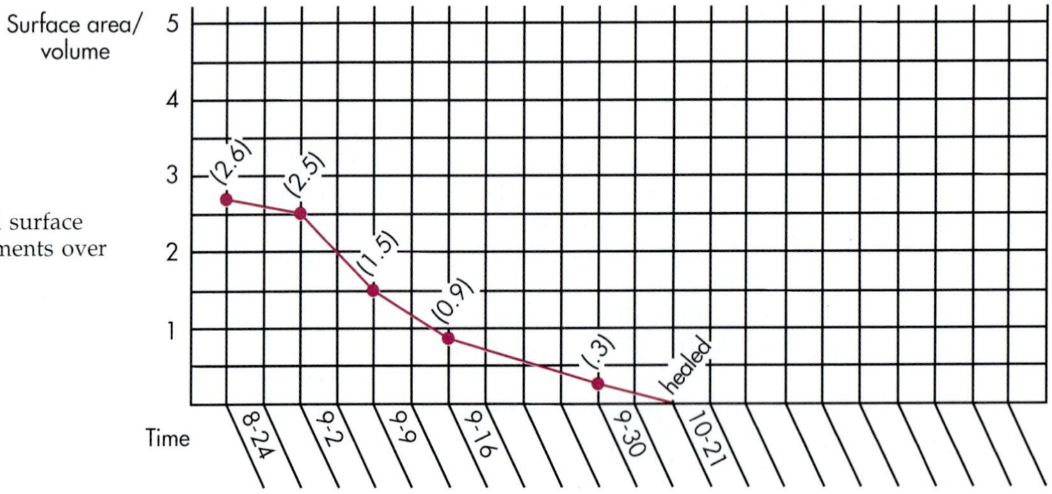

Step 3 Graph of wound surface area or volume measurements over time.

STEPS	RATIONALE
5. **Unexpected outcomes** that may occur include:	
➤ Skin surrounding ulcer becomes macerated.	Neighboring tissues become involved from exposure to topical agents and moisture.
➤ Ulcer becomes deeper with increased drainage and/or development of necrotic tissue.	With further ischemia, chances of infection increase.
➤ Pressure ulcer extends beyond original margins.	Ischemia extends to tissue layers.

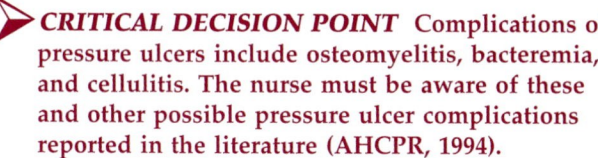

➤ ***CRITICAL DECISION POINT*** **Complications of pressure ulcers include osteomyelitis, bacteremia, and cellulitis. The nurse must be aware of these and other possible pressure ulcer complications reported in the literature (AHCPR, 1994).**

➤ ***CRITICAL DECISION POINT*** **Deterioration of the client's or the ulcer's condition indicates the need for reevaluation of the treatment plan (AHCPR, 1994).**

Recording and Reporting

1. Record appearance of ulcer in client's record.	Baseline observations and subsequent inspections reveal progress of healing.
2. Describe type of topical agent used, dressing applied, and client's response.	Documents care.
3. Report any deterioration in ulcer appearance to nurse in charge or physician.	

Follow-up Activities

1. Report need for wound debridement to physician or other appropriate staff members.
2. Obtain a physician's order (as needed) for additional consults, for example, a dietitian, physical therapist, occupational therapist, social service, or enterostomal (ET) nurse.
3. If appropriate, order supplies needed for next dressing change.
4. Monitor for systemic signs and symptoms of poor wound healing, such as abnormal laboratory results (WBC, Hgb/Hct, serum albumin, serum prealbumin total proteins), weight loss, and fluid imbalances.

• • • • •

Special Considerations

➤ All pressure ulcer staging systems are based on the depth of the tissue destroyed. The nurse must be able to see the type of tissue on the bottom of the pressure ulcer bed. Therefore, a pressure ulcer that is covered with necrotic tissue (eschar, which is black, hard necrotic tissue) or slough (yellow, stringy necrotic tissue) cannot be staged (AHCPR, 1994).

➤ The pressure ulcer staging system was designed to identify the depth of tissue destroyed. It was not created to classify wound healing. *Do not use reverse staging to describe a pressure ulcer as it heals.* It is incorrect to say that a stage IV pressure ulcer that begins to heal is now a stage III.

➤ As the pressure ulcer heals, the wound is filled with granulation tissue and not the original type of tissue that was in the ulcer. Nurses can consult the NPUAP (1995) position on reverse staging of pressure ulcers for a more in-depth explanation.

➤ A client with multiple pressure ulcers should be evaluated for appropriate pressure relief surface or bed (see Chapter 32).

➤ External devices may induce pressure areas (e.g., casts, braces, splints).

➤ An eschar-covered wound may appear or actually increase in size as the eschar is removed.

➤ Usually if necrotic tissue is present in ulcer, it should be debrided. Necrotic tissue supports the growth of pathological organisms and may interfere with the healing process (AHCPR, 1994).

➤ An exception to the debridement principal for necrotic tissue is pressure ulcers on the heel. "Heel ulcers with *dry* eschar need not be debrided if they do not have edema, erythema, fluctuance, or drainage" (AHCPR, 1994, p. 49). Fluctuance is the "wavelike motion, indicative of the presence of fluid, used to describe the appearance of wound tissue" (AHCPR, 1994, p. 110). Necrotic heel pressure ulcers should be assessed daily to monitor for these signs. If these signs of pressure ulcer complications occur, debridement would be required (AHCPR, 1994).

- Some enzymes cause a temporary redness known as the *strawberry effect* to the surrounding skin. This is a normal occurrence that does not need treatment.
- Preventing and treating pressure ulcers may require a multidisciplinary approach. Some resources for prevention and management include a physical therapist, occupational therapist, social worker, dietitian, clinical specialist, and ET nurse.
- The Kundin scale is a tool that is sometimes used for wound volume calculations (Fig. 8-4).
- Wound volume also can be calculated by covering the pressure ulcer with a transparent membrane dressing and then filling the wound with a measured amount of normal saline. After determining the amount of fluid needed to "fill" the wound, it is important to remove the saline and dressing and then proceed with the client's dressing proctocol.
- Early ulcers tend to have irregular borders. With time, borders become smooth and rounded.

Teaching Considerations

- Discuss treatment and identify individual(s) who will assist in care at home.
- Discuss process of wound healing and expected wound appearance. For example:
  - Client's and support persons' perception about appearance of the pressure ulcer. Eschar covered wounds may look like a scab that indicates wound healing to the client or support persons. After the ulcer is debrided, they may feel that nurses have caused an injury to the ulcer.
  - Client's and support persons' perceptions about size of pressure ulcer. Lay people may think that a "bedsore" is small, about the size of a wedding ring. Some of the larger wounds, especially after debridement, may be very troublesome to the client and support persons.
  - Client's and support persons' perceptions about treatment. Client and support persons may believe it is cruel for staff to keep turning and positioning the client every 2 hours. They may misunderstand some dressing change techniques such as pulling out the dried gauze dressing used for mechanical debridement.
- Identify the signs, symptoms, and four stages of ulcers to report to the health care team.
- Review prevention guidelines to halt further breakdown.
- Discuss options for maintaining good nutrition.

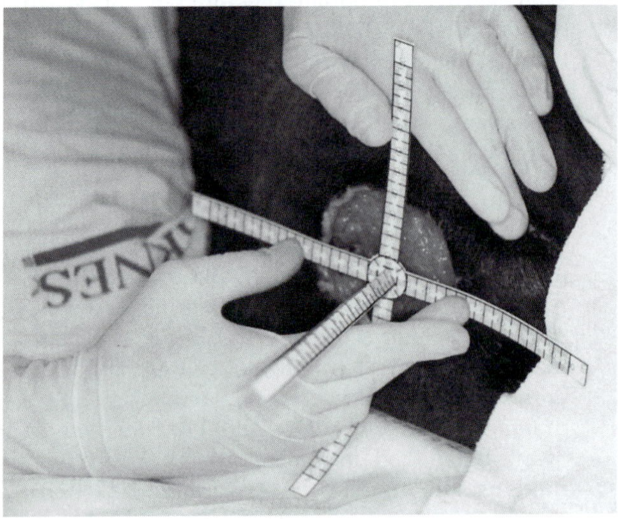

Fig. 8-4 Kundin scale.

Gerontologic Considerations

- Wound healing may be slower in the older adult.
- The normal reduction in the Langerhans' cells in the older adult's epidermis causes a decrease in T-cell function and immunity (Loescher, 1995).
- Because older skin has a slower and less intense inflammatory reaction, older clients must be monitored more closely for altered responses to skin irritants (Loescher, 1995).

Home Care Considerations

- "Consider care giver time when selecting a dressing. In the home care setting, care givers may choose more expensive dressing materials to reduce the frequency of dressing changes" (AHCPR, 1994, p. 54).
- Cost can also be a factor. Some clients have more time than financial resources. They may choose a less expensive treatment option such as dressing material, especially if there is no third-party reimbursement. Another example might be teaching the family to make normal saline rather than buying it premade.
- "Disposal of contaminated dressings in the home should be done in a manner consistent with local regulations" (AHCPR, 1994, p. 65).
- Identify clean storage area for dressing supplies.
- Determine availability of required supplies.
- Discuss need for home health nurse.
- Discuss need for home pressure relief surface or bed.
- Identify adaptive equipment needed to care for the client at home.
- Medicare regulations limit reimbursement of some types of pressure relief equipment for stage III and IV pressure ulcers.

CRITICAL THINKING EXERCISES

1. A 72-year-old African-American man is admitted to the hospital with a diagnosis of left cerebral vascular accident (CVA). He has right sided weakness and cannot turn or walk without using his walker and one person's assistance. He also has difficulty swallowing and is incontinent of urine.
   a. What risk factors, if any, for pressure ulcers does this client have?
   b. What characteristics should the nurse assess to monitor for a stage I pressure ulcer?
   c. How should this be accomplished?
   d. Can you develop a plan of care for this client?
2. On admission to the nursing home, an 86-year-old Irish woman needs a pressure ulcer risk assessment score done using the Braden scale. Using the following client assessment data, determine her pressure ulcer risk assessment score:

   Client responds to verbal commands but cannot communicate her need to be turned. She walks occasionally during the day, but only for short distances. Her mobility is slightly limited, and she can make frequent but slight changes in her extremities independently. She has sufficient strength to sit up completely and maintains a good position in the bed or chair at all times. Her skin is thin, dry, and intact, and only routine linen changes are needed. Her appetite is excellent, and she eats most of the meals offered to her.
   a. What is her risk score?
   b. One week later, her score on the Braden Scale is 16. Explain the clinical significance of each of these findings.
   c. What plan of care is indicated at this time?
3. In assessing your 66-year-old Latino client, you find he has a 3 × 2 cm wound on his sacrum that is 1 in deep. The wound is into his subcutaneous tissue but not through it. The tissue bed is pink to red, and there is scant serous exudate.
   a. What stage is this pressure ulcer?
   b. Can you classify this pressure ulcer by color? If so, what classification would you give it?
   c. What other assessments should the nurse do of this pressure ulcer?
   d. The physician order reads, "Povidone-iodine wet to dry dressings q shift to sacral pressure ulcer." What should the nurse do about this order?

REFERENCES

Abruzzese R: The effectiveness of an assessment tool in specifying nursing care to prevent decubitus ulcers. In *PRN: The Adelphi report—project for research in nursing,* 1982 Adelphi University Library.

AHCPR Panel for the Prediction and Prevention of Pressure Ulcers in Adults: *Pressure ulcers in adults: prediction and prevention. Clinical Practice Guideline* No 3, Pub No 92-0047, Rockville, Md, Public Health Service, US Department of Health and Human Services, May 1992.

AHCPR Panel for the Treatment of Pressure Ulcers in Adults: *Treatment of pressure ulcers: clinical practice guideline,* No 15, Pub No 95-0653, Rockville, Md, Public Health Service, US Department of Health and Human Services, December 1994.

Ayello, EA: Teaching the assessment of patients with pressure ulcers, *Decubitus* 5(4):53-54, 1992.

Ayello EA: A critique of the AHCPR's Preventing pressure ulcers: a patient's guide as a written instructional tool, *Decubitus* 6(3):44-50, 1993.

Ayello EA: Critique of AHCPR's Consumer Guide: Treating Pressure Sores, *Advance Wound Care* 8(5):18-32, 1995.

Bates-Jensen B: New pressure ulcer status tool, *Decubitus* 3(3):14-15, 1990.

Bennett MA: Report of the Task Force on the Implications for Darkly pigmented intact skin in the prediction and prevention of pressure ulcers, *Advanc Wound Care* 8(6):34-35, 1995.

Bergstrom N et al: Treatment of pressure ulcers: AHCPR Pub No 95-0652, Rockville, MD, Public Health Service, US Department of Health and Human Services, Agency for Health Care Policy and Research, 1994.

Bergstrom N, Braden B, Laguzza A, Holman V: The Braden Scale for predicting Pressure Sore Risk, *Nurs Research* 36(4):205, 1987.

Bergstrom N, Demuth PJ, Braden BJ: A clinical trial of the Braden Scale for predicting pressure sore risk, *Nurs Clin North Am* 22(2):417, 1987.

Braden BJ, Bergstrom N: Predictive utility of the Braden Scale for predicting pressure sore risk, *Research in Nurs and Health* 17:459, 1994.

Braden BJ, Bergstrom N: Clinical utility of the Braden scale for predicting pressure sore risk, *Decubitus,* 2(3):44, 1989.

Bryant RA, Shannon ML, Pieper B et al: Pressure ulcers. In Bryant RA, ed: *Acute and chronic wounds: nursing management,* St Louis, 1992, Mosby.

Clarke M, Kadhom HM: The nursing prevention of pressure sores in hospital and community patients, *J Adv Nurs* 13(3):365, 1988.

Dallam L, Smyth C, Jackson B et al: Pressure ulcer pain: assessment and quantification, *JWOCN,* 22(5):211-218, 1995.

Fowler EM: Equipment and products used in management and treatment of pressure ulcers, *Nurs Clin North Am* 22(7):449, 1987.

Gosnell DJ: An assessment tool to identify pressure sores, *Nurs Research* 22:55, 1973.

Gosnell DJ: Assessment and evaluation of pressure sores, *Nurs Clin North Am* 22(2):399, 1987.

Gosnell DJ: Pressure sore risk assessment: a critique Part 1: the Gosnell scale, *Decubitus* 2:3, 1989.

Gosnell DJ: Pressure sore risk assessment. Part II: analysis of risk factors, *Decubitus* 2:3, 1989.

Graves DJ: Stage I in ebony complexion. *Decubitus* 3(4):4, 1990 (letter).

Hanson D, Langemo DK, Olson B et al: The prevalence and incidence of pressure ulcers in home care: Are patients at risk? *J Home Care* 5(3):25-32, 1993.

Hentzen B, Bergstrom N, Pozehl B: Prevalence and incidence of pressure ulcers and associated risk factors in rural-based home health population. Poster presentation at 17th Annual Midwest Nursing Research Society, March 28-30, Cleveland Ohio, 1993.

Itoh M, Montemayor JS, Matsumoto E et al: Accerelerated wound healing of pressure ulcers by pulsed high peak power electromagnetic energy (Diapulse), *Decubitus* 4(1):24-34, 1991.

Jiricka MK, Ryan P, Carvalho MA, Bukvich J: Pressure ulcer risk factors in an ICU population, *Am J Crit Care* 4(5):361, 1995.

Kosiak M: Etiology and pathology of decubitus ulcers, *Arch Phys Med Rehabil 40*:62, 1959.

Krasner D: Wound care: how to use the red-yellow-black system, *Am J Nurs 5*:44, 1995.

Langemo DK, Olson B, Hunter S, et al: Incidence of pressure sore in acute care, rehabilitation, extended care, home health, and hospice in one locale, *Decubitus* 2(2):42-43, 1989.

Leshem OA, Skelskey C: Pressure ulcers: quality management, prevalence, and severity in a long term care setting, *Advanc Wound Care* 7(2):50-54, 1994.

Loescher LJ: The dynamics of aging skin, *Progressions* 7(2):3-13, 1995.

Maklebust J: Highlights AHCPR guidelines for pressure ulcer treatment, Clinical Symposium on Pressure Ulcer Wound Management, Nashville, Tenn, Oct 1994.

Maklebust J, Brunckhorst L, Cracchiolo-Caraway A et al: Pressure ulcer incidence in high-risk patients managed on a special three-layered air cushion, *Decubitus* 1(4):30, 1988.

Maklebust J, Sieggreen M: *Pressure ulcers: guidelines for prevention and nursing management,* ed 2, Springhouse, Pennsylvania, 1996, Springhouse.

Meehan M: National Pressur Ulcer Prevalence Survey, *Advanc Wound Care* 7(3):27-38, 1994.

National Pressure Ulcer Advisory Panel (NPUAP): Pressure ulcer prevalence, cost and risk assessment: consensus development conference statement, *Decubitus* 2(2):24-28, 1989.

National Pressure Ulcer Advisory Panel (NPUAP): NPUAP position on reverse staging of pressure ulcers. *Advanc Wound Care 8*(6):32-33, 1995.

Norton D: Calculating the risk: reflections on the Norton scale, *Decubitus* 2:3, 1989.

Norton D, McLaren R, Exon-Smith AN: *An investigation of geriatric nursing problems in hospital, 1962.* Reissue, 1975, Churchill Livingstone, Edinburgh.

Olson B: Effects of massage for prevention of pressure ulcers, *Decubitus* 2(4):32-37, 1989.

Pires M, Muller A: Detection and management of early tissue pressure indicators: a pictorial essay, *Progressions* 3(3):3, 1991.

Surman, MW: An introduction to hyperbaric oxygen therapy for the ET nurse, *J of WOCN* 23(2):80, 1996.

Trelease CC: Developing standards for wound care, *Ostomy/Wound Manage 26*:50, 1988.

Versluysen M: How elderly patients with femoral fracture develop pressure sores in hospital, *Br Med J 292*(6531):1311, 1986.

ADDITIONAL READING

Baharestani MM: The lived experience of wives caring for their frail, home bound, elderly husbands with pressure ulcers, *Advanc Wound Care* 7(3):40-52, 1994.

Bolton LL, van Rijswijk L, Shaffer FA: Quality wound care equals cost-effective wound care: a clinical model, *Nurs Manage* 27(7):30, 1996.

Breslow RA, Bergstrom N: Nutritional prediction of pressure ulcers, *J Amer Diet Assoc 94*(11):1301-1304, 1994.

Breslow RA, Hallfrisch J, Guy DG et al: The importance of dietary protein in healing pressure ulcers, *J Amer Geriat Soc 41*(4):357-362, 1993.

Colin D, Abraham P, Preault L et al: Comparison of 90 and 30 laterally inclined positions in the prevention of pressure ulcers using transcutaneous oxygen and carbon dioxide pressures, *Advanc Wound Care* 9(3):35, 1996.

Ebersole P, Hess P: *Toward healthy aging: human needs and nursing response,* ed 4, St Louis, 1994, Mosby.

Faller NA, Lawrence KG: Nursing to promote healing, *Ostomy/Wound Manage 32*:43, 1991.

Darkovich SL: Managing pressure ulcers: When is no treatment the right treatment? *Nursing 96* 26(7):47, 1996.

Kosiak M: Etiology of decubitus ulcers, *Arch Phys Med Rehabil 42*:19, 1961.

Seiler WO, Stahelin HB: Efficient pressure ulcer prevention using a new automatic pressure relieving mattress system, *Wounds* 4(3):108, 1992.

Stotts NA: Determination of bacterial burden in wounds. NPUAP Proceedings 1995, *Advanc Wound Care 7*(4):28-46–28-52, 1995.

Tenpas DM: Contracture and pressure necrosis, *Ostomy/Wound Manage 26*:50, 1990.

Thomas DR: Nutritional factors affecting wound healing, *Ostomy/Wound Manage,* 42(5):40, 1996.

Young ME: Malnutrition and wound healing, *Heart Lung 17*(1):60, 1988.

CHAPTER 9

Eye and Ear Care Prostheses

OBJECTIVES

Mastery of content in this chapter will enable the nurse to:

- Define key terms.
- Explain why proper care of prostheses is important to a client's self-esteem.
- Identify guidelines used in caring for lenses and prostheses.
- Explain differences in the care of soft and rigid contact lenses.
- Correctly remove, store, cleanse, and insert a contact lens.
- Explain the rationale for maintaining aseptic technique during care of an artificial eye.
- Describe techniques that determine whether a hearing aid functions properly.
- Correctly remove, cleanse, and reinsert a hearing aid.

KEY TERMS

Contact lens
Enucleation
Myopia
Ophthalmologist
Optometrist
Presbycusis
Presbyopia
Prosthesis
Refractive errors

SKILLS

9-1 Taking Care of Contact Lenses
9-2 Taking Care of an Artificial Eye
9-3 Taking Care of an In-the-Ear Hearing Aid

Many clients rely on artificially constructed devices to replace or restore lost or impaired body functions. Eyeglasses and contact lenses help to restore visual loss, and hearing aids can improve sound reception. Clients often depend on these devices to maintain an attractive appearance as well as to improve sensory function. Artificial eyes, in particular, help clients maintain a normal appearance when an eye has been lost as the result of injury or disease. Prostheses and contact lenses must fit and function properly so that clients can function normally within their environment. Clients can be extremely sensitive about lens or prosthetic care. Accidental breakage or malfunction can seriously impair sensory function and threaten self-esteem when a client becomes dependent on others for assistance.

Lenses and prostheses must be cleaned regularly to ensure proper function. Most clients have an established routine for cleaning their contact lenses or prostheses. When clients are unable to care for themselves, the nurse must understand the correct way to clean, handle, and store contact lenses and prostheses. Clients usually show great interest in the manner in which the nurse performs cleaning and maintenance procedures. Careful handling of lenses, artificial eyes, and hearing aids is vital to avoid damage to these devices or to clients' eyes or ears.

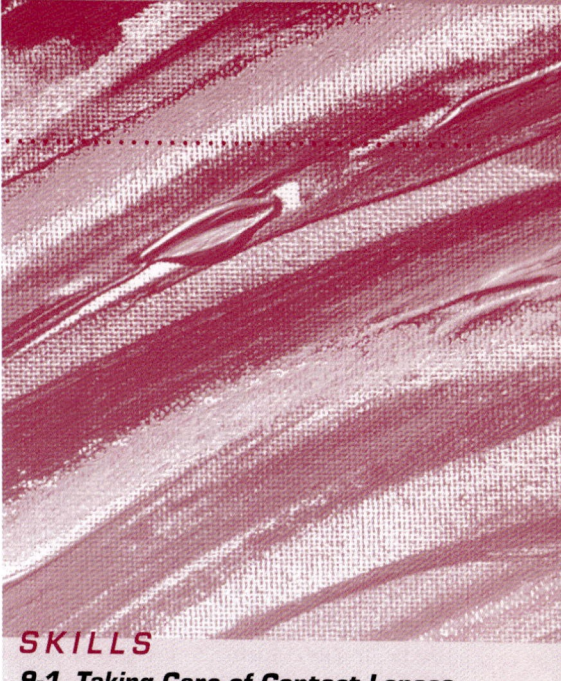

GUIDELINES

1. Let the client be a resource in the care of each device. Unless receiving lenses or a prosthesis for the first time, a client is likely to have an established routine for care and maintenance and has adapted special care techniques as well. It is the nurse's responsibility to be sure clients are not damaging the devices or injuring themselves.
2. Always protect the device from breakage. Replacement can be costly.
3. When a sensory loss exists, use techniques that facilitate interaction with the client. For example, if a client wears a hearing aid, the nurse should use communication techniques that improve the client's ability to hear and understand. If visual function is reduced, the nurse should provide visual aids to improve the client's interaction with the environment.
4. Encourage clients to express feelings about changes in body image, such as feeling unusual or different, because of reliance on an artificial device for function or appearance. For example, clients with hearing impairments are often treated as though they are mentally impaired because they do not understand what is said to them. Family members become frustrated when they cannot communicate with the client whose hearing aid malfunctions. The nurse can be supportive and demonstrate understanding when communicating with these clients and can teach families methods for interacting more effectively.

DELEGATION CONSIDERATIONS

The skills of caring for eye and ear prostheses can be delegated to unlicensed assistive personnel.

- Inform and assist care provider in proper way to care for eye and ear prostheses.
- Stress to care provider that careful handling of these devices is of utmost importance to prevent physical injury to the client and damage to the devices.
- Have care provider protect client's privacy when inserting/removing artificial assistive devices (e.g., artificial eye).
- Instruct care provider to explain steps of the procedure to client as procedure progresses.
- Encourage care provider to use appropriate communication techniques to ensure smooth completion of task at hand.
- Inform care provider of types of findings to report (e.g., eye pain, eye socket drainage).

SKILL 9-1 Taking Care of Contact Lenses

A **contact lens** is a thin, transparent, oval disk that fits directly over the cornea of the eye. Contact lenses are designed specifically to correct **refractive errors** of the eye or abnormalities in the cornea's shape. They are relatively easy to apply and remove.

There are three basic types of contact lenses: rigid (hard), soft, and rigid gas permeable (RGP), also known as oxygen permeable. They differ in size, material, and amount of oxygen flow they permit to the eye's surface. Rigid contact lenses are made of firm, durable plastic and are smaller than the cornea. These lenses ride on the tear film layer of the cornea and are held in place by surface tension. Blinking causes the tear film to move under and over the contact lens, providing oxygen to the cornea. Soft contact lenses are made of soft, flexible plastic, and because they cover the entire cornea and a small rim of the sclera, they do not ride on the corneal tear film. The cornea receives oxygen through the soft lens, which is oxygen permeable. Rigid gas-permeable lenses are similar to the rigid lens, but the plastic lens allows oxygen to pass through to the cornea. All three lenses are available as clear (untinted) or tinted.

Contact lenses are also available as daily wear, extended wear, and disposable. All lenses must be removed periodically to prevent ocular infection and corneal ulcers or abrasions. Daily-wear lenses should be removed overnight for cleaning and disinfection and should not be worn for more than 10 to 14 hours daily (Cohen and Krachmer, 1992). It is recommended that all extended-wear lenses be worn no longer than 6 consecutive nights without cleaning and disinfecting (Johnson & Johnson Vision Products, 1994). Disposable lenses are available for daily wear and extended wear and are usually replaced every 1 to 2 weeks. Pain, tearing, discomfort, and redness of the conjunctivae may be symptoms of lens overwear. Persistence of symptoms even after lens removal is abnormal, however, and may indicate serious ocular damage.

As contact lenses are worn, they accumulate secretions and foreign matter. This material deteriorates and then irritates the eye, causing distorted vision and risk for infection. Once removed, contact lenses should be cleaned and thoroughly disinfected.

Care of contact lenses includes proper cleaning, insertion and removal, and storage. Many clients wear contact lenses today. It is extremely important that nurses determine whether clients wear contact lenses, particularly when clients are admitted to hospitals or agencies in unresponsive or confused states. If a seriously ill client is wearing contact lenses and this fact goes undetected, severe corneal injury can result.

Clients usually have a preferred method for caring for their lenses. When it is necessary for the nurse to assist with lens care, the client's preferences should be considered.

EQUIPMENT

- Clean lens storage container
- Bath towel
- Suction cup (optional)
- Sterile saline solution
- Sterile lens cleaning solution
- Sterile lens rinsing solution
- Sterile lens disinfectant
- Sterile enzyme solution (depends on care regimen)
- Sterile wetting solution (depends on care regimen)
- Cotton ball or cotton-tipped applicator
- Emesis basin
- Disposable gloves

STEPS	RATIONALE
ASSESSMENT	
1. Place towel just below client's face.	Catches lens if one should accidentally fall from eye.
2. Stand at client's side. Inspect eye or ask client if contact lens is in place.	Lenses are generally comfortable to wear, and client may forget they are in place. Prolonged wear may cause injury to eye.
CRITICAL DECISION POINT Unconscious or confused clients entering the health care setting should be carefully assessed; lenses are often difficult to assess if clear (untinted).	
3. Ask if client feels any eye discomfort and assess length of time client normally wears lenses.	Scratched lens can cause corneal irritation and abrasion. Accumulation of dust or debris between lens and cornea causes irritation. Continuous wearing of certain types of lenses can irritate cornea.
4. Ask if client is able to manipulate and hold contact lens.	Determines level of assistance required in care.
CRITICAL DECISION POINT May need to assess level of assistance required later after lenses have been removed.	
5. Assess client for any unusual visual signs/symptoms (reduced visual acuity, blurred vision, halos, photophobia).	May indicate underlying visual alteration or need to change lens prescription. A reduction of visual acuity calls for referral.
6. Assess types of medications prescribed for client: sedatives, hypnotics, muscle relaxants, antihistamines, anticholinergics, and antidepressants.	Sedatives, hypnotics, and muscle relaxants reduce blink reflex and thus reduce lubrication of cornea. Antihistamines, anticholinergics, and antidepressants can reduce tear production.
7. After lenses are removed (see Implementation), inspect eye for signs of corneal irritation (e.g., redness, pain, swelling of eyelids and conjunctivae, discharge, and excess tearing).	Signs/symptoms indicate corneal irritation or abrasion.
CRITICAL DECISION POINT If pain persists or worsens after removal of lenses, an immediate referral to the ophthalmologist should be made. Severe pain may indicate corneal epithelium disruption or infection (Cohen and Krachmer, 1992).	

STEPS	RATIONALE

NURSING DIAGNOSIS

Clustering of defining characteristics from the assessment data may reveal the following nursing diagnoses for clients requiring this skill:

- Bathing/hygiene self-care deficit
- Knowledge deficit regarding contact lens care
- Pain
- Risk for infection
- Risk for injury
- Sensory perceptual alterations (visual)

Related factors are individualized based on a client's condition or needs.

PLANNING

STEPS	RATIONALE
1. **Expected outcomes** following completion of procedure:	
➤ Client verbalizes comfort after removal and reinsertion of lenses.	
➤ Client's eye shows no signs of ocular infection, such as redness, pain, swelling, discharge, blurred vision, or photophobia.	
➤ Client verbalizes improved visual perception after lens cleaning.	Lenses cleaned and positioned correctly.
➤ Client demonstrates no signs of eye injury as evidenced by irritation, foreign body sensation, redness, and tearing.	
➤ Client demonstrates the proper technique for removing, cleaning, and reinserting lenses.	Learning achieved.
2. Discuss procedure with client.	Client can assist in planning by explaining technique that may aid removal and insertion. Client may be anxious as nurse retracts eyelids and manipulates lenses.
3. Have client assume supine or sitting position in bed or chair.	Provides easy access for nurse while retracting eyelids and manipulating lenses.

➤ ***CRITICAL DECISION POINT*** **Client may assume side-lying position if movement and position are restricted for this procedure.**

STEPS	RATIONALE
4. Assemble supplies at bedside.	Provides easy access to supplies.

IMPLEMENTATION

➤ ***CRITICAL DECISION POINT*** **Standard precautions apply to tears when they contain visible blood.**

REMOVING SOFT LENSES

STEPS	RATIONALE
1. Wash hands. Apply disposable gloves if there are cuts, scratches, or dermatological lesions on nurse's hands.	Reduces transmission of microorganisms.
2. Place towel just below client's face.	Catches lens if one should accidentally fall from eye.
3. Add a few drops of sterile saline solution to client's eye.	Lubricates eye to facilitate lens removal.
4. Tell client to look straight ahead.	Eases tipping of lens during removal.
5. Using middle finger, retract lower eyelid.	Exposes lower edge of lens.
6. With pad of index finger of same hand, slide lens off cornea onto white of eye.	Positions lens for easy grasping. Use of finger pad (rather than fingernail) prevents injury to cornea and damage to lens.
7. Pull upper eyelid down gently with thumb of other hand and compress lens slightly between thumb and index finger.	Causes soft lens to double up. Air enters underneath lens to release suction.

STEPS	RATIONALE
CRITICAL DECISION POINT **Soft lenses consist primarily of water and can be easily torn.**	
8. Gently pinch lens and lift out.	Protects lens from damage. Avoid allowing lens edges to stick together.
CRITICAL DECISION POINT **If lens edges stick together, place lens in palm and soak thoroughly with sterile saline solution. Gently roll lens with index finger in back-and-forth motion. If gentle rubbing does not separate edges, soak lens in sterile saline solution, which assists in returning lens to normal shape.**	
9. Clean and rinse lens (see Cleansing and Disinfecting Contact Lenses). Place lens in proper storage case compartment: R for right lens and L for left lens (see illustration).	Ensures proper lens will be reinserted into correct eye. Proper storage prevents cracking or tearing.
10. Repeat Steps 3 through 9 for other lens. Secure cover over storage case. Label with client's name and room number.	Proper storage prevents damage to or loss of lenses.
CRITICAL DECISION POINT **Remember to assess appearance and condition of eyes after lenses are removed.**	
11. Dispose of towel, remove gloves, and wash hands.	Reduces transmission of infection.
REMOVING RIGID LENSES	
1. Wash hands and apply gloves if needed.	Reduces transmission of microorganisms.
2. Place towel just below client's face.	Catches lens if one should accidentally fall from eye.
3. Be sure lens is positioned directly over cornea.	Correct position of lens allows easy removal from eye.
CRITICAL DECISION POINT **If lens is not positioned directly over cornea, have client close eyelids, place index and middle fingers of one hand on eyelid just beside the lens and beneath, and gently but firmly massage lens back into place.**	
4. Place index finger on outer corner of client's eye and draw skin gently back toward ear (see illustration).	Tightens eyelid against lens to dislodge and pop out.
5. Tell client to blink. Do not release pressure on eyelid until blink is completed.	... clear top and bottom of lens until

Ma...

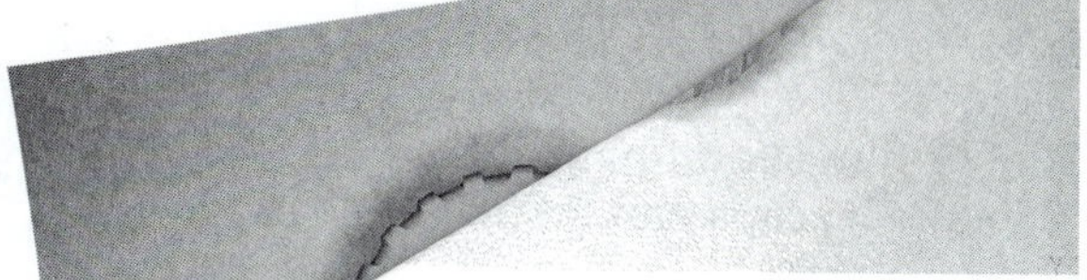

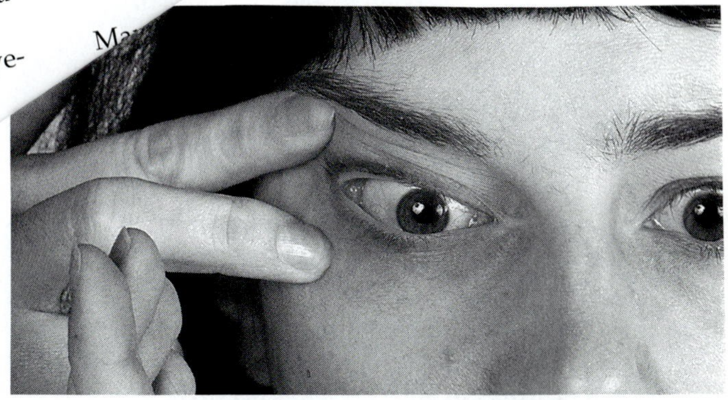

Step 4

STEPS	RATIONALE
6. If lens fails to pop out, gently retract eyelid beyond edges of lens. Press lower eyelid gently against lower edge of lens.	Pressure causes upper edge of lens to tip forward.
7. Allow both eyelids to close slightly and grasp lens as it rises from eye. Cup lens in hand.	Maneuver causes lens to slide off easily. Protects lens from breakage.
CRITICAL DECISION POINT **A lens suction cup can be used to remove lenses from the eyes of confused or unconscious clients. Gently apply suction cup to lens surface and lift out.**	
8. Clean and rinse lens (see Cleansing and Disinfecting Contact Lenses). Place lens in proper storage case compartment: R for right lens and L for left lens. Center lens in storage case, convex side down.	Both lenses may not have the same prescription. Proper storage prevents breaking, scratching, chipping, and discoloration.
9. Repeat Steps 3 through 8 for other lens. Secure cover over storage case. Label with client's name and room number.	Proper storage prevents damage to or loss of lenses.
10. Dispose of towel, remove gloves, and wash hands.	Reduces spread of infection and keeps client's environment neat.

CLEANSING AND DISINFECTING CONTACT LENSES

STEPS	RATIONALE
1. Wash hands.	Reduces transmission of microorganisms.
2. Assemble supplies at bedside. Place towel over work area.	Provides easy access to supplies. Towel helps to prevent lens breakage.
CRITICAL DECISION POINT **Check expiration dates of all solutions and discard outdated solutions to avoid adverse effects or infections.**	
3. Open lens container carefully, taking care not to flip lens caps open suddenly.	Prevents lenses from being accidentally spilled or flipped out of case.
4. After removing one lens from case, apply one or two drops of cleaning solution to lens in palm of hand (use cleanser recommended by lens manufacturer or care practitioner).	Removes tear components, including mucus, lipids, and proteins that collect on lens.
5. Ru... gently but thoroughly on both sides for 20 to 30 sec... index finger (soft lenses) or little finger or co... applicator soaked with cleaning solution (rig... clean inside lens. Be careful not to touch ... with fingernail.	It is easier to manipulate and clean lens using fingertips. Cleans microorganisms from all surfaces.
CRITICAL DECISION ... f care provider should be cut short ... ng or tearing of lens.	
6. Holding lens over emesis basin, rin... with manufacturer-recommended rinsi... (soft lenses) or cold tap water (rigid lenses).	Removes debris and cleaning solution from lens surface. ...nsing methods and solutions differ for each type of
7. Place lens in proper storage case compartme... fill with storage solution recommended by manu... turer or eye care practitioner.	
8. Repeat Steps 3 through 7 for other lens.	

INSERTING SOFT LENSES

STEPS	RATIONALE
1. Wash hands thoroughly with mild noncosmetic soap, rinse well, and dry with clean lint-free towel or paper towel. Apply gloves if needed.	Lint or ... removes residue, enhances wetability of ... odora... scratches to lens that can be caused ... eye.
2. Place towel over client's chest.	Catches lens if a... age, scratching, a...

...metic or d...

STEPS	RATIONALE
3. Remove right lens from storage case and rinse with recommended rinsing solution; inspect lens for foreign materials, tears, and other damage.	Removes disinfectant solution. Prevents irritation or damage to eye. Always begin with right lens to avoid placing wrong lens in eye.
4. Check that lens is not inverted (inside out).	Soft lens is inverted if bowl has a lip; it is in proper position if curve is even from base to rim.
5. Using middle or index finger of opposite hand, retract upper lid until iris is exposed.	Soft lenses do not adhere as easily as hard lenses. Separating lids as much as possible allows room for lens to completely contact cornea without touching lids or lashes.
6. Using middle finger of the hand holding the lens, pull down lower lid.	
7. Instruct client to look straight ahead "through" the lens and finger; then gently place lens directly on cornea and release lids slowly, starting with lower lid.	Ensures secure fit and comfort.
8. If lens is on sclera rather than cornea, tell client to slowly close eye and roll it toward the lens.	Centers soft lens over cornea.
9. Tell client to blink a few times.	Ensures lens is centered, free of trapped air, and comfortable.
10. Be sure lens is centered properly by asking client to open eyes and note if vision is blurred.	If lens slips to side of cornea or into conjunctival sac, vision will blur.
11. Repeat Steps 3 through 10 for left eye.	
12. Assist client to comfortable position.	
13. If client's vision is blurred: a. Retract eyelids. b. Locate position of lens. c. Ask client to look in direction opposite lens, and with index finger, apply pressure to lower eyelid margin and position lens over cornea. d. Have client look slowly toward lens.	Repositions lens over center of cornea as client looks toward lens.
14. Discard soiled supplies and solution from storage case, rinse case thoroughly and allow to air dry, and wash hands.	Reduces transmission of microorganisms.

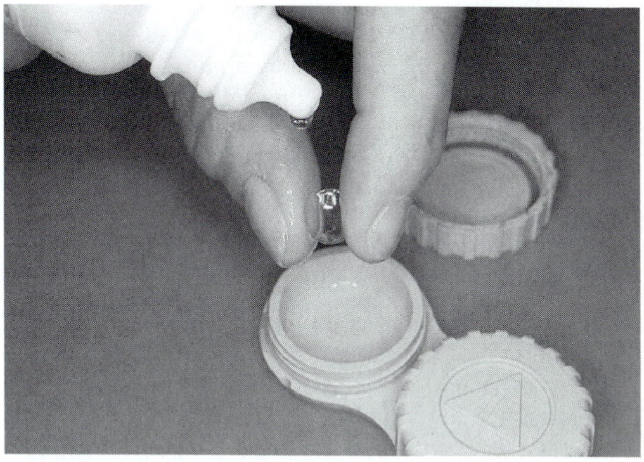

Step 3

INSERTING RIGID LENSES

STEPS	RATIONALE
1. Wash hands thoroughly with mild noncosmetic soap, rinse well, and dry with clean lint-free towel or paper towel. Apply gloves if needed.	Lint or film left on hands from towels or cosmetic or deodorant soaps can be transferred to lens and irritate eye.
2. Place towel over client's chest.	Catches lens if accidentally dropped and avoids breakage and scratching.
3. Remove right lens from storage case; attempt to lift lens straight up (see illustration).	Sliding lens out of case can cause scratches on the surface. Always begin with right lens to avoid placing wrong lens in eye.

STEPS	RATIONALE
4. Rinse with cold tap water.	Hot water causes lens to warp. Reduces transmission of microorganisms.
5. Wet lens on both sides using prescribed wetting solution.	Lubricates lens so that it slides easily and adheres to cornea.
6. Place lens concave side up on tip of index finger of dominant hand (see illustration).	Proper manipulation of lens ensures easy insertion. Inner surface of lens should face up so that it is applied against cornea.
7. Instruct client to look straight ahead while retracting lower eyelid; place lens gently over center of cornea (see illustration).	Rigid lens can be placed as client looks straight ahead. Retraction of lids promotes easy insertion between lid margins.

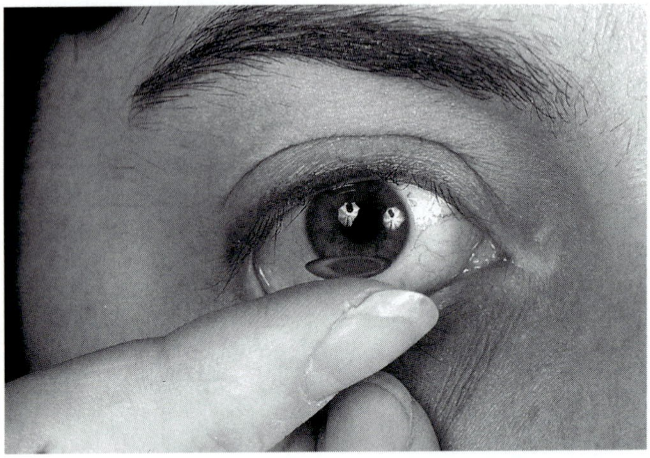

Step 6

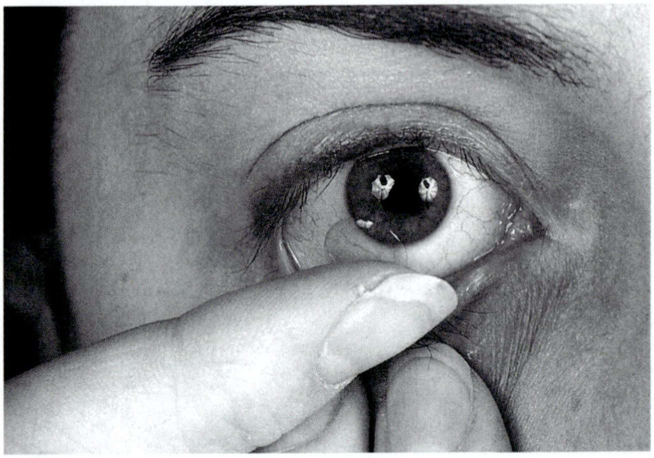

Step 7

STEPS	RATIONALE
8. Ask client to close eyes briefly and to avoid blinking.	Helps to secure position of lens.
9. Be sure lens is centered properly by asking client to open eyes and note if vision is blurred.	If lens slips to side of cornea or into conjunctival sac, vision will blur.
10. Repeat Steps 3 through 9 for left eye.	
11. Assist client to comfortable position.	
12. Discard soiled supplies and solution from storage case, rinse case thoroughly and allow to air dry, and wash hands.	Reduces transmission of microorganisms.

EVALUATION

STEPS	RATIONALE
1. Ask client if lens feels comfortable after removal and reinsertion of lenses.	Determines if any debris is caught between lens and cornea. Lens should be removed if client experiences discomfort.
2. Inspect eye (over time) for signs of ocular infection.	
3. Assess client's visual acuity (see Chapter 11).	Determines improvement in visual perception.
4. Observe client for signs of eye injury.	
5. Observe client demonstrating technique for lens care.	Evaluates client's understanding of techniques.
6. **Unexpected outcomes** that may occur include:	
➤ Client complains of burning, pain, or foreign body sensation.	Symptoms of lens overwear; lenses must be removed.
➤ Client complains of blurred vision.	Improper placement is likely cause of blurred vision.
➤ Client develops inflammation of conjunctivae, pain, discharge, excess tearing, or reduced vision.	Lens must be removed and physician notified.
➤ Client is unable to perform lens care correctly.	Further instruction is required.

Recording and Reporting

1. Record or report any signs/symptoms of visual alterations noted during procedure.

   May indicate presence of eye injury or disease.

2. Record on nursing care plan or Kardex times of lens insertion and removal if client is going to surgery or special procedure.

Follow-Up Activities

1. If client continues to feel foreign body sensation, remove, clean, rinse, and reinsert lenses.

• • • • •

Special Considerations

- Never apply direct downward pressure to eyeball because this may cause serious injury.
- Special heat-resistant cases can be placed in electric heating units for soft lens sterilization; however, units usually are not available in health care institutions.
- Soft lenses are more pliable than rigid lenses and thus less irritating. Chronic irritation should be reported to physician.
- Wearers of soft and extended-wear lenses, are at risk for ocular infections and corneal ulcers. Common infectious agents are *Pseudomonas aeruginosa* and staphylococci. Infection by *Acanthamoeba* organisms is rare but can cause a more serious infection (Cohen and Krachmer, 1992). Adherence to recommended methods of lens care should be emphasized. Advise client against using saliva, homemade saline solution, or tap water as wetting solutions because they can cause infection.
- Some women experience discomfort with contact lens wear during menstrual periods, pregnancy, menopause, or while taking oral contraceptives. Hormonal-related fluid retention may cause corneal swelling and result in ill-fitting lenses.

Teaching Considerations

- Nurse should encourage client to see a vision care specialist **(ophthalmologist** or **optometrist)** regularly: every 3 to 5 years before age 40, every 2 years after age 40, and yearly after age 65.
- Plastic lenses scratch easily. Special cleaning solutions and drying tissues are recommended.
- Never use fingernail on lens to remove dirt or debris that does not loosen during washing.
- Follow recommendations of lens manufacturer or eye care practitioner when cleaning and disinfecting lenses.
- Encourage client to remember the mnemonic RSVP: *R*edness, *S*ensitivity, *V*ision problems, and *P*ain. If one of these problems occurs, remove contact lenses immediately. If problems continue, contact vision care specialist (Lewis, Collier, and Heitkemper, 1996).
- Lenses become very slippery once cleaning solution is applied.
- If lens is dropped on a hard surface, moisten finger with cleaning or wetting solution and gently touch lens to pick it up. Then clean, rinse, and disinfect lens.
- Lens should be kept moist or wet when not worn.
- Use fresh solution daily when storing and disinfecting lenses.
- Soft lenses need to be cleaned weekly with an enzymatic cleaner to remove protein.
- Do not wipe lens with tissue or towel.
- Thoroughly wash and rinse lens storage case on a daily basis. Clean periodically with soap or liquid detergent; rinse thoroughly with warm water and air dry.
- To avoid mix-up, always start with the same lens when removing or inserting lenses.
- Disposable or planned replacement lenses should be thrown away after prescribed wearing period.

Pediatric Considerations

- Parents and/or older children can learn how to care for lenses.

Gerontologic Considerations

- When checking for visual impairment during a nursing history, consider age of the client. Some symptoms occur in people in one age group and not in another. The incidence of **myopia,** or nearsightedness, tends to increase up to the third decade of life. On the other hand, **presbyopia,** or farsightedness, resulting from loss of elasticity of the lens, occurs with advancing age; it begins to affect people around the age of 40 (Boyd-Monk and Steinmetz, 1987). Other visual changes that normally occur with aging include reduced visual fields, decreased visual acuity, delayed dark-light adaptation, impaired night vision, impaired accommodation to near objects, impaired color vision, impaired depth perception, presence of floaters, presence of opacities, and increased glare sensitivity. As a result of these changes, the older client's environment should be assessed for potential hazards (see Chapter 41) and adapted to the client's visual needs (Ebersole and Hess, 1994).

Home Care Considerations

- Rigid lenses and daily-wear soft lenses should be removed for sleeping, sunbathing, swimming, and showering.
- Clients in the home setting should be cautioned against working over sink unless towel is placed in sink or sink stopper is in place.
- Lenses must be both cleaned and disinfected. One procedure does not replace the other.
- Do not wear lenses in presence of noxious or irritating vapors or fumes because they can cause damage to contact lens surface.
- Use aerosol products (e.g., hair spray, cologne, deodorants) before lenses are inserted.
- Apply makeup after lenses are inserted and use water-based or water-soluble eyeliners only; cosmetics trapped under a lens can cause irritation.
- Do not use eye drops or medications without consulting an eye care practitioner.

SKILL 9-2 Taking Care of an Artificial Eye

As a result of tumor, infection, congenital blindness, or severe trauma to the eye, clients may have to undergo **enucleation,** a procedure involving the complete removal of the eyeball. Surgery is indicated when there is danger of an infectious or malignant process spreading to the neighboring eye or brain tissue or when trauma has caused disruption of the entire globe of the eye. All that remains after enucleation is the socket and eyelids. For obvious cosmetic purposes, clients who have undergone enucleation are often fitted with an artificial eye, or **prosthesis.** Artificial eyes are made of plastic and sometimes glass. The common plastic prosthesis is smooth and assumes the shape of the normal eyeball's anterior curvature. The prosthesis fits just behind the client's eyelids. Each prosthesis is designed to have the appearance of the client's natural iris, pupil, and sclera. Prostheses are relatively easy to remove and insert and can be worn day and night. Cleansing with soap and water can be done daily or any time up to several months based on client's preference.

EQUIPMENT

- Soft washcloth or cotton gauze square
- Washbasin with warm water or saline
- 4 × 4–inch gauze pads
- Mild soap
- Facial tissues
- Bath towel
- Suction device (e.g., rubber bulb syringe or medicine dropper bulb) (optional)
- Disposable gloves
- Covered plastic storage case

STEPS	RATIONALE
ASSESSMENT	
1. Determine which eye is artificial.	
CRITICAL DECISION POINT Care provider should avoid showing any revulsion during procedure.	
2. Inspect surrounding tissues of eyelid and eye socket for inflammation, tenderness, swelling, and drainage. (Inspect socket after removal of prosthesis.)	Infection can spread easily to neighboring eye, underlying sinuses, or brain tissue.
3. Assess client's routine for prosthetic care: frequency and methods of cleaning.	Determines compliance with and knowledge of self-care.
4. Assess client's ability to remove, clean, and reinsert prosthesis.	Determines level of assistance required during care.

NURSING DIAGNOSIS

Clustering of defining characteristics from the assessment data may reveal the following nursing diagnoses for clients requiring this skill:

- Bathing/hygiene self-care deficit
- Body image disturbance
- Risk for infection
- Risk for injury

- Knowledge deficit regarding eye prosthesis care
- Pain
- Sensory perceptual alterations (visual)

Related factors are individualized based on a client's condition or needs.

PLANNING

1. **Expected outcomes** following completion of procedure:
   - Client verbalizes feelings regarding prosthesis removal and care.
   - Client's eyelid margins are clean and of normal pink color, with lashes turned away from prosthesis. — Eyelids are cleaned and positioned correctly.
   - Client demonstrates no signs of infection, such as redness, tenderness, swelling, or discharge from socket or eyelid margins. — Eyelid margins and socket are free of infection.
   - Client verbalizes that prosthetic eye fits comfortably. — Prosthesis is inserted correctly.
   - Client demonstrates the proper technique for removing, cleaning, and reinserting prosthesis. — Learning is achieved.
2. Discuss procedure with client. — Allows client opportunity to suggest further ideas about procedure.
3. Assist client to sitting or supine position with head elevated. — Position facilitates removal of prosthesis with less chance of breakage.

IMPLEMENTATION

1. Wash hands. Apply disposable gloves. — Reduces transmission of microorganisms.
2. With thumb, gently retract lower eyelid against lower orbital ridge (see illustration). — Exposes lower edge of eye prosthesis.

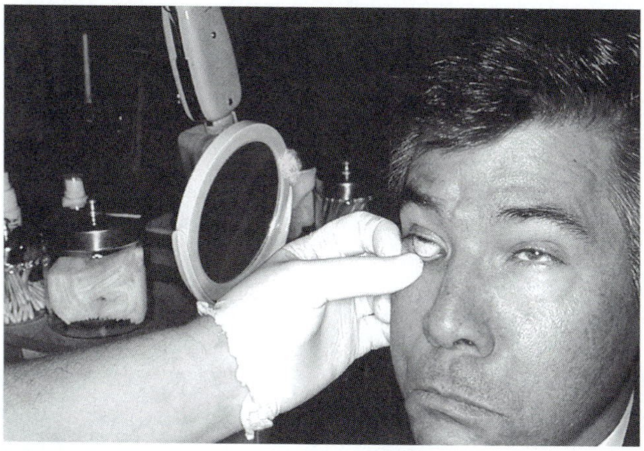

Step 2

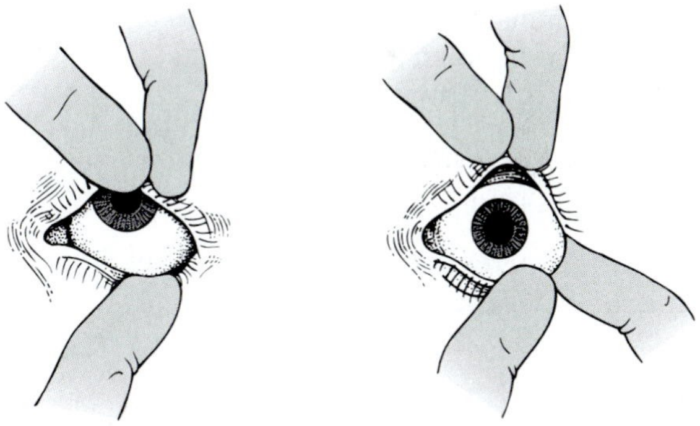

Step 3

3. Exert slight pressure below eyelid and slide prosthesis out (see illustration). If prosthesis does not slide out, use moistened rubber bulb syringe or medicine dropper bulb to apply direct suction to prosthesis. — Breaks suction, causing prosthesis to rise and slide out of socket (Bocking et al., 1990).
4. Place prosthesis in palm of hand. — Protects prosthesis from breakage.
5. Clean prosthesis:
   a. Wash with mild soap and warm water or plain saline solution by rubbing well between thumb and index finger. — Tears and secretions containing microorganisms may have collected on surface of prosthesis. Soap is less irritating than detergents.

STEPS	RATIONALE
b. Rinse well under running tap water (see illustration).	Removes soap and residue.
c. Dry and polish prosthesis with soft washcloth or facial tissue.	Maintains shiny appearance of prosthesis to resemble normal eye.

CRITICAL DECISION POINT Inspect prosthesis for rough edges, which may abrade tissue surfaces.

CRITICAL DECISION POINT Nurse should discuss importance of regular prosthesis cleaning during procedure.

STEPS	RATIONALE
6. If client is not to have prosthesis reinserted, store in sterile saline solution or water in plastic storage case. Label container and place in bedside stand.	Maintains condition of plastic prosthesis. Label prevents accidental loss of container.
7. Clean eyelid margins and socket:	
a. Retract upper and lower eyelid margins with thumb and index finger.	Exposes eye socket.
b. Wash socket with clean washcloth or gauze square moistened with warm water or saline solution.	Removes secretions that contain microorganisms.
c. Remove excess moisture with gauze pads.	Removes moisture that can harbor microorganisms.
d. Wash eyelid margins with mild soap and water. Wipe from inner to outer canthus using a clean section of cloth with each wipe.	Prevents secretions from entering tear duct in inner canthus.
e. Dry eyelids by wiping from inner to outer canthus.	
8. Moisten prosthesis in water.	Water lubricates, insertion easier.
9. Retract client's upper eyelid with index finger or thumb of nondominant hand.	Eases prosthesis insertion.
10. With dominant hand, hold prosthesis so that notched or pointed edge is positioned toward nose and iris faces outward.	Ensures proper fit (Bocking et al., 1990).
11. Slide prosthesis up under upper eyelid as far as possible and then push down lower lid to allow prosthesis to slip into place (see illustration).	Prosthesis will fit evenly into socket.

CRITICAL DECISION POINT Do not force prosthesis into socket.

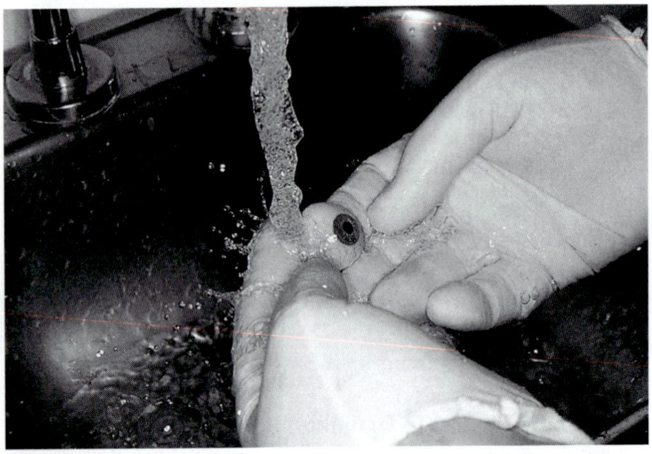

Step 5b

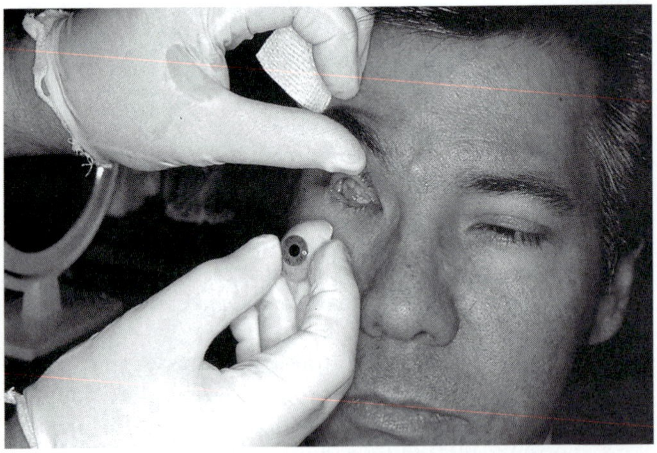

Step 11

STEPS	RATIONALE
12. Gently wipe away excess fluid if necessary.	Wipe toward nose to prevent dislodgment.
13. Help client assume comfortable position.	Maintains client's comfort.
14. Dispose of soiled supplies, remove gloves, and wash hands.	Reduces transmission of microorganisms.

EVALUATION

1. Ask client about feelings regarding prosthesis removal and care.	Evaluates client's self-concept.
2. Inspect condition of eyelids and socket.	Evaluates cleanliness and position of eyelids and presence of infection.
3. Ask client if prosthesis fits comfortably.	Determines comfort level and evaluates client's ability to perform techniques.
4. Have client explain or demonstrate prosthetic care.	Evaluates client's ability to perform procedure.
5. **Unexpected outcomes** that may occur include:	
➤ Client states prosthesis feels uncomfortable.	Prosthesis may require repositioning or may need to be inspected for any rough areas.
➤ Signs of inflammation develop in tissues of socket or lid margins.	If area of tenderness or inflammation exists in socket, it may be necessary to remove prosthesis for a few days.
➤ Excessive, purulent, or foul drainage develops.	Indicates infection.
➤ Client is unable to explain or perform prosthetic care.	Further instruction is required.

RECORDING AND REPORTING

1. Record removal of prosthesis and storage location for client going to surgery.	Prosthesis must be removed before surgery to prevent loss.
2. Record or report any alterations in integrity of tissues surrounding eye (e.g., purulent or foul drainage).	Documents condition or change in client's status.

FOLLOW-UP ACTIVITIES

1. If eyelid or socket is infected, prosthesis should remain removed. Provide client with comfortable eye patch to allow healing and to maintain client's positive body image.
2. Advise clients to consult the prosthetist annually to have the artificial eye cleaned and polished to maintain appearance and comfort.

• • • • •

Special Considerations

➤ Artificial eye will not move in socket nor will pupil respond to light reflex or accommodation.
➤ Most clients prefer to remove, clean, and insert prosthesis themselves.
➤ Soap is not used when cleaning socket because it is difficult to rinse thoroughly and may cause irritation to tissues.
➤ If crusts are difficult to remove, place moistened cloth over eyelids for several minutes during cleaning. This will loosen all crusts.

Teaching Considerations

➤ Never use alcohol, chemicals, or any solvents for cleaning; these agents can damage plastic prostheses (Bocking et al., 1990).
➤ Look for rough edges on prosthesis after removal, which may abrade tissue surfaces.
➤ Instruct primary care giver not to force artificial eye into socket.
➤ If rubbing the prosthetic eye, rub toward the nose. Wiping away from the nose may cause the eye to fall out.
➤ Wear a protective patch or goggles when swimming, diving, or water skiing or remove the prosthesis and store it.

Gerontologic Considerations

➤ Assess the manual dexterity of the older adult client. The nurse will need to assist with removal and insertion if dexterity is diminished.

Home Care Considerations

➤ Assess level of understanding of client and primary care giver regarding client's condition and need for a prosthesis.

- Assess ability and willingness of client and primary care giver to administer eye care.
- Assess physical condition for which client is being treated and determine special precautions necessary.
- Assess ability of client to cooperate with procedures.
- Client in home setting should use available equipment (e.g., clean washcloth). Procedure need not be sterile.
- Some clients may wear a prosthesis for several months before removing or cleaning. Excess tearing or crusting indicates need to clean eye and socket.

SKILL 9-3 Taking Care of an In-the-Ear Hearing Aid

Hearing is vital for normal communication and orientation to sounds in the environment. For people with hearing loss, hearing aids improve the ability to hear and understand spoken words.

Hearing aids amplify so that sound is heard at a more effective level. All aids have four basic components:

1. A microphone, which receives and converts sound into electrical signals.
2. An amplifier, which increases the strength of the electrical signal.
3. A receiver, which converts the strengthened signal back into sound.
4. A power source (batteries), which energizes the components.

In addition, programmable hearing aids are now available on the market. These aids input signals rather than just amplifying the sounds. They are programmed by an audiologist with the use of a computer specific to a client's hearing impairment. These aids are adjusted to accommodate the range of the client's residual hearing. Programmable aids independently amplify high-frequency (soft-spoken consonants) from low-frequency (loudly spoken vowels) sounds; this process occurs rapidly and continuously. Programmable hearing aids also contain a remote control that has two user-selected programs (e.g., everyday listening and "special situations"); this remote also contains the volume control (ReSound Corporation, 1994 and 1995). There are several styles of hearing aids available to clients today:

1. An in-the-canal (ITC) aid fits entirely in the ear canal (Fig. 9-1). It has cosmetic appeal, is easy to manipulate and place in the ear, does not interfere with the wearing of eyeglasses or use of the telephone, and can be worn during most physical exercise. However, obtaining a proper fit is more difficult and cerumen tends to plug this model more than others.
2. An in-the-ear (ITE or intra-aural) aid fits into the external auditory ear and allows more fine-tuning (Fig. 9-2). It is more powerful and therefore is useful for a wider range of hearing loss than the ITC aid. It is easy to position and adjust and does not interfere with eyeglass wearing. However, it is slightly more noticeable than the ITC aid and is not recommended for persons with moisture or skin problems in the ear canal. It is the most common type worn today.
3. A behind-the-ear (BTE or postaural) aid hooks around and behind the ear and is connected by a short, clear, hollow plastic tube to an ear mold inserted into the external auditory canal (Fig. 9-3). It is useful for clients with rapidly progressive hearing loss or manual dexterity difficulties and those who find partial ear occlusion intolerable. Disadvantages are that it is more visible, may interfere with eyeglasses and telephone use, and is more difficult to keep in place during physical exercise.
4. The eyeglass aid is a hearing aid that fits in the ear canal and attaches to a battery located on the arm of the eyeglass frame. The frame must be bulky to accommodate the equipment; therefore style selection is limited.

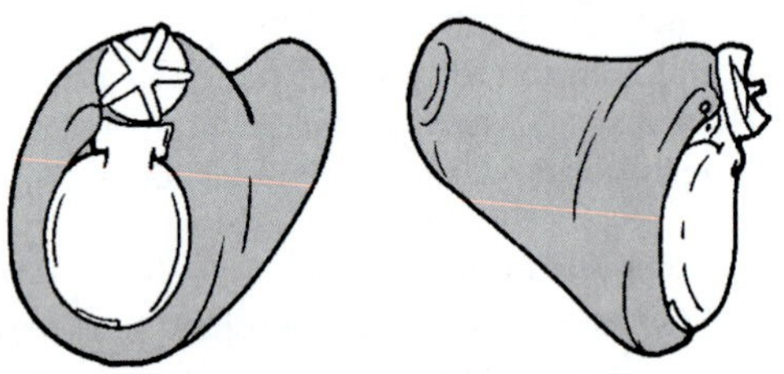

Fig. 9-1 In-the-canal (ITC) hearing aid.

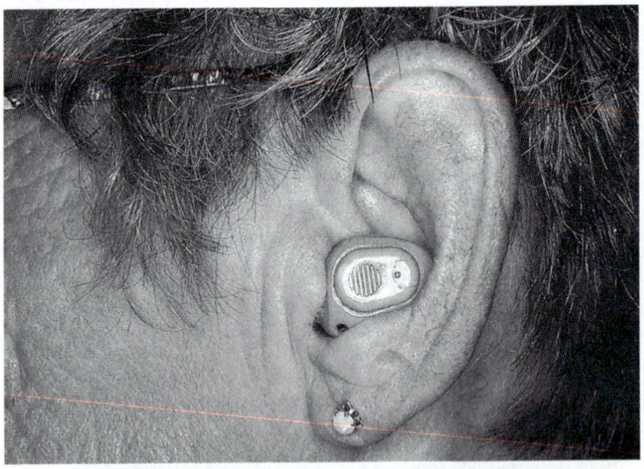

Fig. 9-2 In-the-ear (ITE or intra-aural) hearing aid.

5. The body aid is a bulky instrument used for severe hearing loss. A fitted ear mold attaches to a round receiver that connects to a transmitter the size of a cigarette case. The case may be hidden in the clothing, but the receiver and wire cannot. This type of aid is rarely used today.

Hearing aid devices can be tailored to a client's specific amplification need. Anyone caring for a hearing aid should know that the device is delicate and must be protected from moisture, heat, and breakage.

EQUIPMENT

- Soft towel and washcloth
- Brush or wax loop
- Storage case
- Disposable gloves (if drainage present)

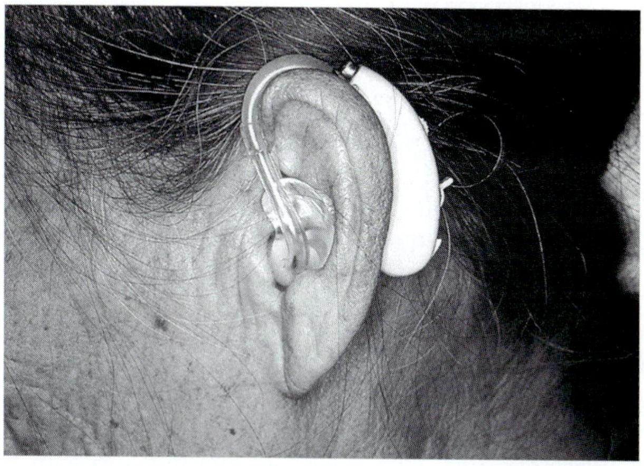

Fig. 9-3 Behind-the-ear (BTE or postaural) hearing aid.

STEPS	RATIONALE
ASSESSMENT	
1. Assess client's knowledge of and routines for cleaning and caring for hearing aid.	Determines client's understanding and need for health education. Nurse will adapt method of care to client's procedure.
2. Determine whether client can hear clearly with use of aid by talking slowly and clearly in normal tone of voice.	Inability to hear may indicate faulty function of hearing aid.
3. Assess whether hearing aid is working by removing from client's ear. Close battery case and turn volume slowly to high. Cup hand over hearing aid. If squealing or a whistling sound (feedback) is heard, it is working. If no sound is heard, replace batteries and test again.	Determines need for new battery. Feedback squeal will cause harsh whistling sound.
4. Inspect ear mold for cracked or rough edges.	Can cause irritation to external ear canal.
5. Inspect for accumulation of cerumen around aid and plugging of opening in aid.	Prevents clear sound reception and transmission.

NURSING DIAGNOSIS

Clustering of defining characteristics from the assessment data may reveal the following nursing diagnoses for clients requiring this skill:

- Impaired verbal communication
- Knowledge deficit regarding hearing aid care
- Risk for injury
- Sensory perceptual alterations (auditory)

Related factors are individualized based on a client's condition or needs.

PLANNING

STEPS	RATIONALE
1. **Expected outcomes** following completion of procedure:	
➤ Client hears conversation spoken in normal tone of voice and responds appropriately.	Batteries are operational. Aid is secure and unobstructed.
➤ Client demonstrates proper care of the hearing aid.	Demonstrates learning.
➤ Client responds appropriately to environmental sounds.	Client is able to hear warning sounds of danger.
➤ Client states that aid fits comfortably.	Aid is positioned correctly.
2. Have client suggest any additional tips for care; explain that next step is to clean and reinsert hearing aid.	Client becomes uncomfortable when unable to hear clearly. Explain all steps before removing aid to minimize confusion and anxiety.

STEPS	RATIONALE
IMPLEMENTATION	
CLEANING HEARING AID	
1. Wash hands. Apply disposable gloves only if drainage present.	Reduces transmission of microorganisms.
2. Assemble supplies at bedside table or sink area.	Procedure can be performed without delays.
3. Wipe aid with soft washcloth. Use wax loop or brush (supplied with aid) or tip of syringe needle to clean the holes in the aid.	Wax prevents clear sound reception and transmission.
CRITICAL DECISION POINT **Do not jam wax deeper into holes because this could cause damage to the aid.**	
4. Wash ear canal with washcloth moistened in soap and water. Rinse and dry.	Removes cerumen from ear canal.
5. If hearing aid is to be stored, place it in dry, safe storage case and/or a container that has a desiccant material.	Protects hearing aid against damage and breakage.
6. Open battery door and allow it to air dry.	Increases battery life and allows moisture to evaporate (Olson, 1995).
CRITICAL DECISION POINT **When hearing aid is not in use, be sure hearing aid is turned off or remove or disconnect battery.**	
7. Label case with client's name and room number.	Helps to prevent loss of client's personal belongings.
CRITICAL DECISION POINT **If client uses two aids, note right or left ear when labeling case.**	
INSERTING HEARING AID	
1. Check batteries (see Assessment) and replace batteries (if necessary) over soft surface (e.g., towel or bed).	Necessary for proper sound amplification. Protects hearing aid against damage and breakage (Olson, 1995).
2. Turn aid off and turn volume control down.	Will protect client from sudden exposure to feedback sounds.
3. Hold the aid so that the canal—the long portion with the hole(s)—is at the bottom. Guiding the aid along client's cheek, bring it to the ear.	Proper orientation is important for hearing aid insertion.
4. Insert canal portion of aid into the ear first. Use other hand to pull down and back on outer ear. Gently push the aid into ear until it is in place and fits snugly in the midline.	Opens up ear canal for easier insertion (Olson, 1995).
5. If hearing aid has volume control, gradually adjust volume to comfortable level for talking to client in regular voice at 3 to 4 feet away. Rotate volume control toward the nose to increase volume and away from the nose to decrease volume.	Gradual adjustment prevents exposing client to harsh squeal or feedback. Client should hear nurse comfortably.
CRITICAL DECISION POINT **Programmable aids have the volume control located on the remote. For most clients, hearing aids work best at lower volume settings.**	
6. Remove soiled equipment from bedside. Dispose of used supplies. Wash hands.	Maintains clean environment and reduces risk of infection.

STEPS	RATIONALE
E VALUATION	
1. Converse with client in normal tone of voice and observe response.	Determines improvement in auditory function.
2. Observe client performing hearing aid care.	Demonstrates client's understanding of techniques.
3. Observe client's response to environmental sounds.	Inability to hear environmental sounds may indicate faulty function of hearing aid.
4. Question client about comfort after insertion of hearing aid.	Determines client's comfort level.
5. **Unexpected outcomes** that may occur include:	
➤ Client is unable to hear conversations or environmental sounds clearly.	Ear canal may be obstructed. Hearing aid may be malfunctioning.
➤ Client's verbal responses are inappropriate.	Hearing is impaired.
➤ Client is unable to clean or insert hearing aid.	Further instruction is required.
➤ Client complains of ear discomfort and may complain of whistling sound.	Hearing aid not properly positioned or volume control not properly adjusted.
RECORDING AND REPORTING	
1. Document that aid is removed and stored if client is going for surgery or special procedure.	Protects nurse from liability in case of loss of hearing aid.
2. Report to nursing staff and document on plan of care the difficulties client has in communicating.	Improves continuity of care in communication techniques for client.

FOLLOW-UP ACTIVITIES

1. Regular follow-up visits with the hearing aid specialist or audiologist are needed to assess aid's effectiveness and fit, to solve problems, and to make readjustments if needed.
2. If soreness, red spots, or open sores develop in client's ear, remove the aid and refer client to the hearing aid specialist or audiologist.
3. Refer client to an audiologist or hearing aid specialist for consultation if appropriate.

• • • • •

Special Considerations

- ➤ Hearing aids offer the greatest benefit in conductive hearing loss. Common causes of conductive loss include chronic otitis media, otosclerosis, or congenital anomalies.
- ➤ Contrary to some perceptions, amplification of sound through a hearing aid may substantially help clients with sensorineural hearing loss, which may be caused by presbycusis or lesions of the cochlea or auditory nerve or may be noise induced.
- ➤ The earlier a diagnosis of hearing impairment is made and accepted, the better the prognosis for acceptance of a hearing aid.
- ➤ Hearing aid users may find that background noises are bothersome and when amplified tend to mask speech. A tone control to reduce low-frequency amplification may help.
- ➤ Two aids (binaural) may be better than one: listening with both ears increases discrimination of speech and improves sound localization.
- ➤ As the degree of hearing loss increases, the need for a good seal between the hearing aid and the ear increases to prevent feedback.

Teaching Considerations

- ➤ Nurse should discuss with client the guidelines for hearing aid use and tips for self-care.
- ➤ Never use alcohol or other chemicals as cleaning agents because they can cause cracking and drying of the mold.
- ➤ If hearing is less than "normal" after cleaning, check for the following:
  - Aid is blocked with cerumen, loose, or fitted to wrong ear.
  - Batteries are worn or dead.
- ➤ A hearing aid specialist or audiologist must clean actual hearing aid device.
- ➤ Suggest assistive listening devices for specific situations (e.g., telephone or television amplifiers).
- ➤ Teach client some methods for managing the environment through improved listening techniques (e.g., speech reading, listening in a quiet environment, close proximity to the speaker).
- ➤ Teach family better communication techniques.

Pediatric Considerations

- ➤ As children grow older, they can become self-conscious of a hearing aid (Wong, 1995). The aid can be made less conspicuous with hair styling, selection of attractive frames for glasses (over the ear aid), and placement of the on-the-body type where it is not seen.

- Child is given responsibility to care for device as soon as child is able.

Gerontologic Considerations

- Hearing aids are small in size, and that fact together with age-related neuromuscular changes (i.e., stiff fingers, enlarged joints, decreased sensory perception) often make the care and handling of the hearing aid a difficult and frustrating experience for the older adult. Clients with these conditions should contact their hearing aid specialist or audiologist for assistance.
- **Presbycusis,** hearing loss associated with aging, results in high-pitched sounds becoming inaudible, thus hearing becomes increasingly restricted to low-frequency sounds. High-frequency sounds include the consonants f, p, t, k, ch, sh, and st; these sounds are increasingly difficult for the older adult to hear. Because consonants are the letters by which spoken words are recognized, the ability of the older adult with presbycusis to understand the spoken word is greatly affected.
- Nurses need to be alert for cues of hearing loss such as inappropriate responses in conversing or responding, postural behavior, social withdrawal, volume level of radio and television, and family perception of the client's hearing ability (Taylor, 1993).

Home Care Considerations

- Assess level of understanding of client and primary care giver regarding care required for the hearing aid.
- Assess willingness and ability of client or primary care giver to perform necessary care of the hearing aid.
- Assess physical conditions for which the client is being treated and determine necessary special precautions.
- Assess ability of client to cooperate with procedures to care for the hearing aid.
- Avoid exposure of aid to extreme heat or cold. Do not leave aid in its case near stove, heater, or sunny window. Do not use with hair dryer on hot settings or with sunlamp. In humid climate, a storage case containing silica gel is ideal for absorbing moisture.
- Remove aid for bathing or when at hair stylist.
- Hair spray tends to clog the aid; therefore apply hair spray *before* fitting the aid.
- Store batteries in cool, dry place. Keep spare batteries on hand (especially on holidays). Batteries can last a few days to a few weeks depending on the type of battery, frequency of use, volume setting, and power of the aid. Dispose of used batteries properly because they are harmful if swallowed.
- Various brands of aids use different sizes of batteries, and thus batteries are not interchangeable. Insert batteries only when aid is turned off.

CRITICAL THINKING EXERCISES

1. **From a physiological point of view, what is the principle that supports the need to remove contact lenses on a regular basis?**
2. **What would you tell a client with contact lenses to do to prevent ocular infections or corneal abrasions?**
3. **You are assigned to care for a client with an artificial eye. What assessment data would you collect before implementing care of the eye?**
4. **What factors would you need to consider in evaluating the effectiveness of a client's hearing aid?**

REFERENCES

Bocking H, et al: Making sense of artificial eyes, *Nurs Times* 86(18):40, 1990.

Boyd-Monk H, Steinmetz C: *Nursing care of the eye,* Norwalk, Conn, 1987, Appleton & Lange.

Cohen E, Krachmer J: Red eyes and contact lenses, *Patient Care* 26(9):143, 1992.

Ebersole P, Hess P: *Toward healthy aging: human needs and nursing response,* ed 4, St Louis, 1994, Mosby.

Johnson & Johnson Vision Products: *Your guide to healthy contact lens wear,* New Brunswick, NJ, 1994, Johnson & Johnson.

Lewis S, Collier I, Heitkemper M: *Medical-surgical nursing: assessment and management of clinical problems,* ed 4, St Louis, 1996, Mosby.

Olson R: Now hear this! *RN* 58(8):43, 1995.

ReSound Corporation: *Hear what you've been missing,* Redwood City, Calif, 1994, ReSound Corporation.

ReSound Corporation: ReSound hearing health care, *Hearing J* 48(7):53, 1995.

Taylor K: Geriatric hearing loss: management strategies for nurses, *Geriatric Nurs* 14(2):74, 1993.

Wong DL: *Whaley and Wong's nursing care of infants and children,* ed 5, St Louis, 1995, Mosby.

Unit IV

Vital Signs and Physical Assessment

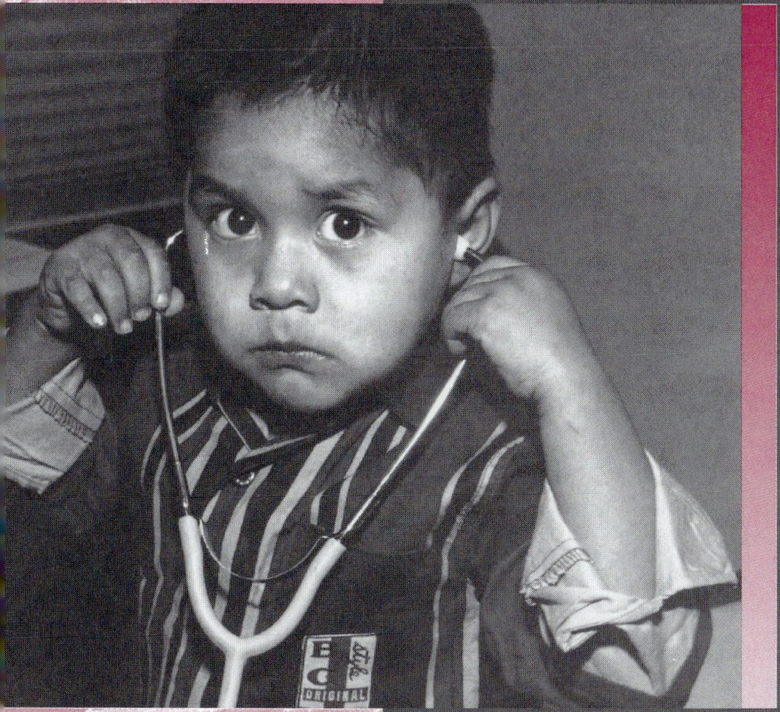

CHAPTER 10

Vital Signs

OBJECTIVES

Mastery of content in this chapter will enable the nurse to:

- Define key terms.
- Correctly record vital signs.
- Identify when it is appropriate to assess each vital sign.
- Correctly assess a client's oral, rectal, axillary, and tympanic membrane temperatures.
- Identify factors to assess in determining potential alterations in body temperature.
- Discuss factors in selecting temperature measurement sites.
- Explain nursing measures to initiate when a client's temperature is above or below normal.
- Correctly assess a client's radial and apical pulse.
- Identify factors to assess in determining potential alterations in pulse character.
- Explain implications of a pulse deficit.
- Correctly assess a client's respirations.
- Identify factors to assess in determining potential alterations in respirations.
- Correctly measure a client's blood pressure (BP) using techniques of auscultation and palpation.
- Discuss factors in selecting an extremity to measure blood pressure.
- Identify factors to assess in determining potential alterations in BP.
- Correctly assess a client's oxygenation status using pulse oximetry.
- Identify factors to assess in determining potential alterations in oxygen saturation.
- Correctly measure a client's central venous pressure using a fluid column manometer.

SKILLS

10-1 Measuring Body Temperature
10-2 Assessing Apical Pulse
10-3 Assessing Radial Pulse
10-4 Assessing Arterial Blood Pressure
10-5 Assessing Respirations
10-6 Measuring Oxygen Saturation (Pulse Oximetry)

KEY TERMS

Antipyretic
Apical pulse
Apnea
Axillary
Bradycardia
Bradypnea
Cardiac output
Centigrade
Central venous pressure (CVP)
Core temperature
Diaphoresis
Diastolic pressure
Dysrhythmia
Fahrenheit
Fever
Heat stroke
Hypertension
Hyperthermia
Hypotension
Hypothermia
Orthopnea
Orthostatic hypotension
Oximetry
Oxygen saturation
Postural hypotension
Premature ventricular contraction (PVC)
Pulse deficit
S_1
S_2
Sphygmomanometer
Stroke volume
Systolic pressure
Tachycardia
Tachypnea
Vasoconstriction
Vasodilation
Vital signs

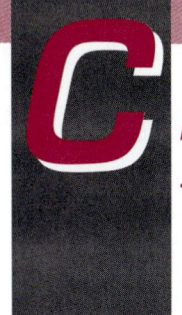

Temperature, pulse, blood pressure (BP), oxygen saturation, and respiration are the most frequent measurements obtained by health care practitioners. These measures predict the effectiveness of the circulatory, pulmonary, neural, and endocrine body functions in maintaining health. Because of their importance as indicators of the body's physiological status and response to physical, environmental, and psychological stressors they are referred to as **vital signs.** Vital signs may reveal sudden changes in a client's condition, as well as changes that occur progressively over a lengthy period of time. Any difference between a client's normal baseline measurement and present vital signs can be an indication for the nurse to initiate appropriate nursing therapies and to pursue necessary medical interventions.

Vital signs are included in a routine physical assessment (Chapter 11). The nurse's findings aid in determining whether it is necessary to assess specific body systems more thoroughly. For example, during a routine vital sign measurement the nurse notes an abnormal respiratory rate; the nurse then auscultates lung sounds. Vital sign assessment may be limited to measurement of a single vital sign for the purpose of reviewing a specific aspect of a client's condition. For example, after administering an antipyretic medication, the nurse measures the client's temperature to evaluate the drug's effects. Part of the nurse's clinical judgment involves deciding which vital signs to measure, when measurements should be made, and the frequency of assessment (see box below). The nurse should always obtain a baseline measurement of vital signs upon first contact with a client to provide a means for comparison with subsequent vital sign measurements.

WHEN TO TAKE VITAL SIGNS

1. On client's admission to a health care facility.
2. In a hospital or care facility on a routine schedule according to a physician's order or institution's standards of practice.
3. When assessing client during home health visits.
4. Before and after a surgical or invasive diagnostic procedure.
5. Before and after the administration of medications or application of therapies that affect cardiovascular, respiratory, and temperature control functions.
6. When the client's general physical condition changes (e.g., loss of consciousness or increased severity of pain).
7. Before and after nursing interventions influencing a vital sign (e.g., before and after a client previously on bed rest ambulates or before and after client performs range of motion exercises).
8. When the client reports specific symptoms of physical distress (e.g., feeling "funny" or "different").

GUIDELINES

1. The primary nurse caring for the client is responsible for vital signs. The nurse obtains baseline vital signs, interprets their significance, and makes decisions about appropriate interventions.
2. Equipment used to measure vital signs must be functional and appropriate to ensure accurate findings.
3. Knowing the normal range for all vital signs enables the nurse to detect deviations from normal.
4. A client's normal range may differ from the standard range for age or physical state. Normal values for a client serve as a baseline for comparing later findings; thus a nurse detects changes in condition over time.
5. The nurse knows the client's medical history, therapies, and prescribed medications. Some illnesses or treatments cause predictable vital sign changes. Most medications affect at least one of the vital signs.
6. The nurse controls or minimizes environmental factors that may affect vital signs. Measuring a client's BP after exercise or an emotional upset may yield values that are not clear indicators of the client's current status.
7. An organized, systematic (step-by-step) approach when taking vital signs ensures accuracy of findings.
8. Based on the client's condition the nurse collaborates with the physician to decide the minimum frequency of vital sign assessment. The nurse uses independent judgment if more frequent assessments are needed. If a client's physical condition begins to worsen, the nurse takes vital signs more often, sometimes as often as every 5 to 10 minutes. After a client returns from surgery or a major diagnostic examination, such as cardiac catheterization, frequent measurements are taken until the vital signs stabilize back to the range before the procedure. Changes or trends in vital signs are useful in making therapeutic decisions for client care.
9. The nurse analyzes results of vital sign measurements and incorporates all the clinical findings about a client in determining nursing diagnoses. Vital signs are not assessed in isolation. The nurse assesses physical signs or symptoms, as well as vital signs, to be aware of the client's ongoing health status.
10. The nurse verifies and communicates significant changes in vital signs. Baseline measurements allow a nurse to identify changes in vital signs. The nurse informs the physician when vital signs become abnormal and reports any changes to the nurse in charge.

SKILL 10-1 Measuring Body Temperature

Body temperature is the difference between the amount of heat produced by the body processes and the amount of heat lost to the external environment. The **core temperature,** or temperature of the deep body tissues, is under control of the hypothalamus and is maintained within a narrow range. Skin or body surface temperature rises and falls as the temperature of the surrounding environment changes and can fluctuate dramatically.

The body tissues and cells function best within a relatively narrow temperature range, between 36° C to 38° C (96.8° F to 100.4° F), but no single temperature is normal for all people. The temperature range for the normal adult depends on age, gender, range of physical activity, and state of health (Fig. 10-1).

Many factors affect the body temperature. Physiological and behavioral control mechanisms function to maintain a constant core temperature. For example, peripheral **vasodilation** increases blood flow to the skin, which increases the amount of heat radiated to the environment. Control mechanisms have failed when heat produced by the body is not equal to heat lost to the environment. For example, clients who lack sweat gland function are unable to tolerate warm temperatures because they cannot cool themselves adequately. At these times, the nurse may initiate measures such as controlling environmental temperatures, removing or adding external coverings, and administering ordered **antipyretics** to achieve better temperature control.

The measurement of body temperature is aimed at obtaining a representative average temperature of core body tissues. Average normal temperature varies depending on the measurement site used. Research findings from numerous studies are contradictory; however, it is generally accepted that rectal temperatures are usually 0.5° C (0.9° F) higher than oral temperatures, and **axillary** temperatures are usually 0.5° C (0.9° F) lower than oral temperatures (Pontious et al., 1994). Sites reflecting core temperature are more reliable indicators of body temperature than sites reflecting surface temperatures (see box).

To ensure accurate temperature readings each site must be measured correctly. The same site should be used when repeated measurements are necessary or temperature mea-

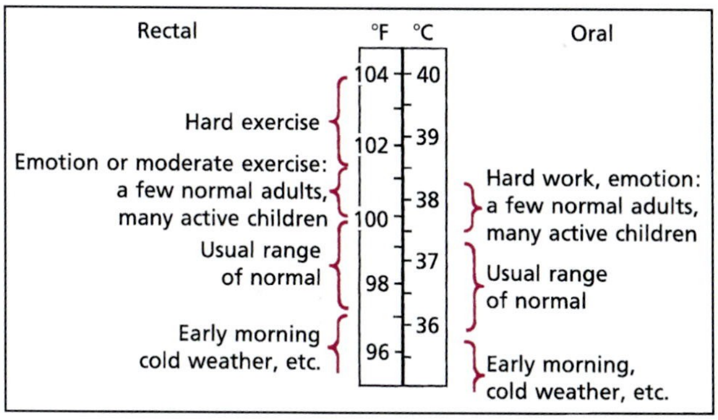

Fig. 10-1 Ranges of rectal and oral temperatures found in normal persons. (Modified from Mountcastle VB: *Medical physiology*, vol 2, ed 14, St Louis, 1980, Mosby; based on Dubois EF: *Fever and the regulation of body temperature*, Springfield, Ill, 1948, Charles C Thomas.)

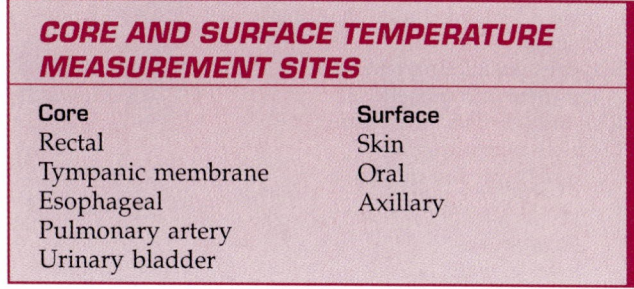

CORE AND SURFACE TEMPERATURE MEASUREMENT SITES

Core	Surface
Rectal	Skin
Tympanic membrane	Oral
Esophageal	Axillary
Pulmonary artery	
Urinary bladder	

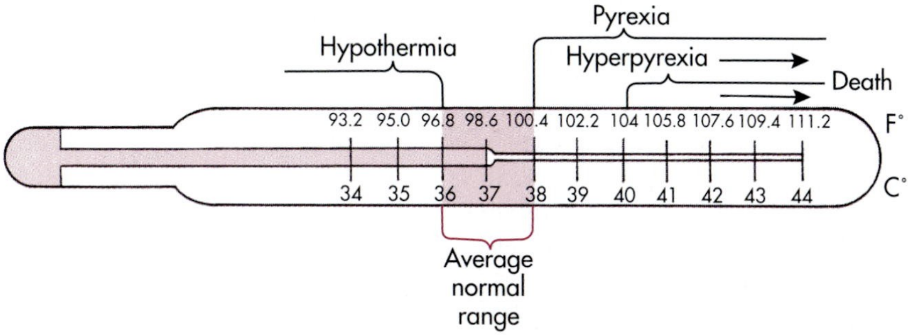

Fig. 10-2 Comparison of Fahrenheit and centigrade calibrations.

Table 10-1 Advantages and Disadvantages of Frequently Selected Temperature Measurement Sites and Methods

Tympanic membrane sensor

Advantages

Easily accessible site
Minimal client repositioning required
Provides accurate core reading
Very rapid measurement (2 to 5 seconds)
Can be obtained without disturbing or waking client
Eardrum close to hypothalamus; sensitive to core temperature changes

Disadvantages

Hearing aids must be removed before measurement
Should not be used with clients who have had surgery of the ear or tympanic membrane
Requires disposable probe cover
Expensive

Electronic thermometer

Advantages

Plastic sheath unbreakable; ideal for children
Quick readings

Disadvantages

May be less accurate by axillary route

Rectal

Advantages

Argued to be more reliable when oral temperature cannot be obtained

Disadvantages

May lag behind core temperature during rapid temperature changes
Should not be used with clients who have had rectal surgery, a rectal disorder, bleeding tendencies, and heart disease
Requires positioning and may be source of client embarrassment and anxiety
Risk of body fluid exposure
Requires lubrication
Contraindicated in newborns

Oral

Advantages

Accessible—requires no position change
Comfortable for client
Provides accurate surface temperature reading
Indicates rapid change in core temperature

Disadvantages

Affected by ingestion of fluids or foods, smoke, and oxygen delivery (Neff J, et al., 1992)
Should not be used with clients who have had oral surgery, trauma, history of epilepsy, or shaking chills
Should not be used with infants, small children, or confused, unconscious, or uncooperative clients
Risk of body fluid exposure

Axilla

Advantages

Safe and noninvasive
Can be used with newborns and uncooperative clients

Disadvantages

Long measurement time
Requires continuous positioning by nurse
Measurement lag behind core temperature during rapid temperature changes
Requires exposure of thorax

Skin

Advantages

Inexpensive
Provides continuous reading
Safe and noninvasive

Disadvantages

Lags behind other sites during temperature changes, especially during hyperthermia
Diaphoresis or sweat can impair adhesion

surements are compared over time. Each site has advantages and disadvantages (Table 10-1). The nurse chooses the safest and most accurate site for the client.

Three types of thermometers measure body temperature: mercury-in-glass, electronic, and disposable. The mercury-in-glass thermometer consists of a glass tube sealed at one end with a mercury-filled bulb at the other. Exposure of the bulb to heat causes the mercury to expand and rise in the enclosed tube. The length of the thermometer is marked with either **Fahrenheit** or **centigrade** calibrations (Fig. 10-2). Three types of glass thermometers are available: oral, or slim-tipped; stubby; and pear-shaped rectal (Fig. 10-3).

The electronic thermometer consists of a rechargeable, battery-powered display unit, a thin wire cord, and a temperature-processing probe covered by a disposable plastic sheath (Fig. 10-4). Separate probes are available for oral and rectal use. The oral probe has a blue tip, and the rectal probe has a red tip.

Another form of electronic thermometer is used exclusively for tympanic temperature. An otoscope-like speculum with an infrared sensor tip detects heat radiated from the tympanic membrane of the ear (Fig. 10-5). Within 2 to 5 seconds after placement in the auditory canal and depressing the scan button a value appears on the display and a sound signals when the peak temperature reading has been measured.

An electronic thermometer is not necessarily more accurate than a glass thermometer; factors that normally influence oral temperature measurements affect all types of thermometers. The advantages of the electronic thermometer are that their readings appear within seconds, they are easy to read, and client discomfort is minimized.

Disposable, single-use thermometers are thin strips of plastic with chemically impregnated paper (Fig. 10-6). They are used for oral or axillary temperatures, particularly with children. Chemical dots on the thermometer change color to reflect temperature reading, usually within 45 seconds. Another form of disposable temperature thermometer is a temperature sensitive patch or tape. Applied to the forehead or abdomen the patch changes colors at different temperatures. Disposable thermometers are useful for screening temperatures. However, mercury-in-glass or electronic thermometers are preferred for their accuracy.

EQUIPMENT

- **Appropriate thermometer**
- **Soft tissue**
- **Lubricant (for rectal measurements only)**
- **Pen, pencil, vital sign flowsheet or record form**
- **Disposable gloves, plastic thermometer sleeve or disposable probe cover**

DELEGATION CONSIDERATIONS

The skill of temperature measurement can be delegated to unlicensed assistive personnel.

- Inform care provider of appropriate route and device to measure temperature.
- Inform and observe care provider in proper positioning of clients for rectal temperature measurement.
- Inform care provider of factors that can falsely raise or lower temperature.

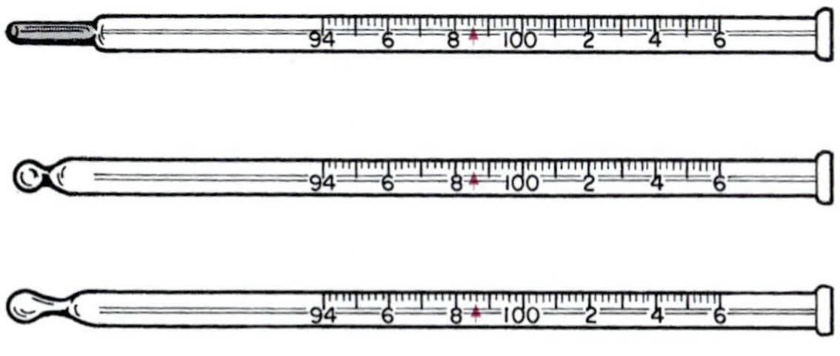

Fig. 10-3 *Top to bottom:* comparison of oral (axillary is appropriate as well); stubby (any site); and rectal thermometers.

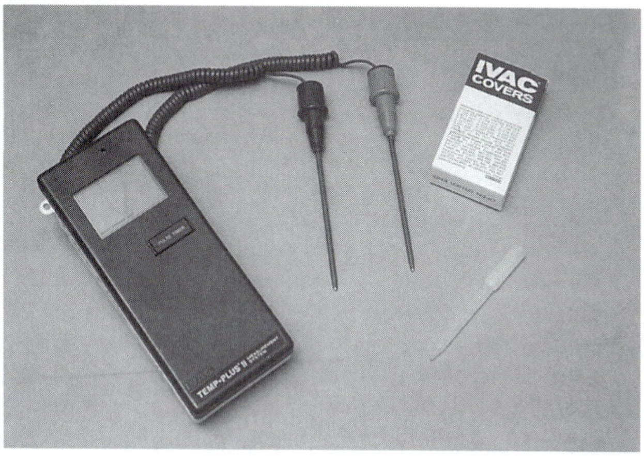

Fig. 10-4 Electronic thermometer with disposable plastic sheath.

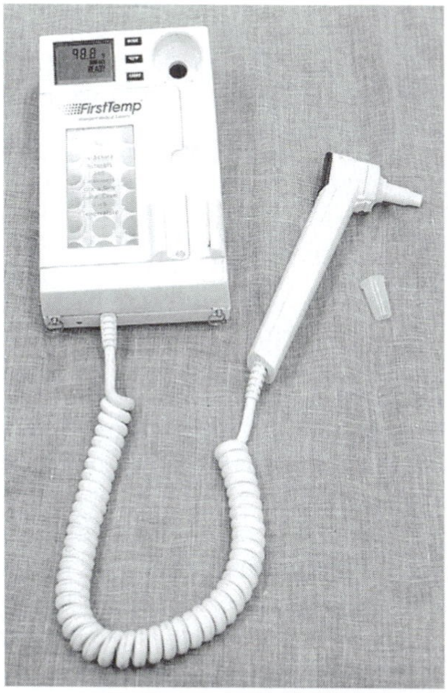

Fig. 10-5 Tympanic membrane thermometer.

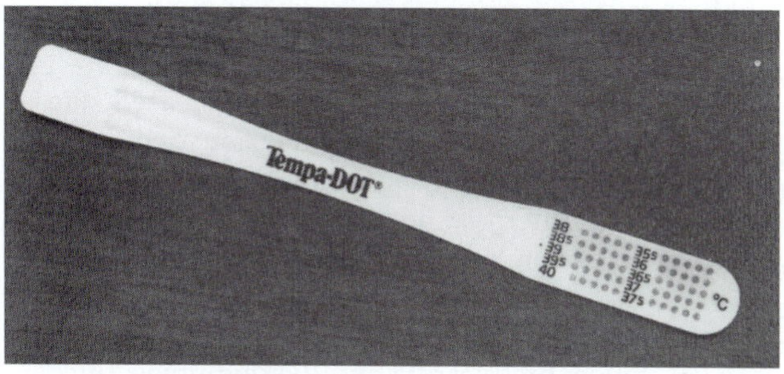

Fig. 10-6 Disposable, single-use thermometer.

STEPS	RATIONALE

ASSESSMENT

1. Determine need to measure client's body temperature:

CRITICAL DECISION POINT Oral temperature should not be assessed for at least 30 minutes after client has ingested fluids or food or has been smoking. Oral temperature should not be used if client is a mouth breather or requires continuous oxygen therapy; clients recovering from oral surgery, have a history of seizures, have uncontrollable shivering, or are confused, uncooperative, or unconscious; newborns, infants, small children, or uncooperative children; and should not be used for clients who may bite on the thermometer.

CRITICAL DECISION POINT Rectal temperature should not be used for clients who have had rectal surgery, a rectal disorder, or bleeding tendencies and are never used for newborns or infants.

CRITICAL DECISION POINT Axillary temperature requires the care provider to continually position the thermometer during assessment.

CRITICAL DECISION POINT Tympanic temperature should not be used for clients recovering from ear surgery or when ear infection or cerumen impaction is suspected.

CRITICAL DECISION POINT Diaphoresis **or sweat can impair adhesion of temperature sensitive patches to skin.**

a. Note risk factors for temperature alterations: expected or diagnosed infections, open wounds or burns, white blood cell count below 5,000 or above 12,000, immunosuppressive drug therapy, injury to hypothalamus, exposure to temperature extremes, blood product infusion, hypothermia or hyperthermia therapy, or postoperative status.

Certain conditions place clients at risk for temperature alterations and may require more frequent temperature measurement.

b. Assess for other signs and symptoms of temperature alteration:

Physical signs and symptoms may indicate alteration in body temperature. Behaviors that do not permit the use of certain temperature measurement sites may be related to temperature alterations.

(1) **Fever:** (depending on stage) pale or flushed skin; skin warm or hot to touch; skin dry or diaphoretic; dry mucous membranes; shivering with chills; piloerection or "gooseflesh" of skin; tachycardia; malaise with muscle or joint pain; nausea, vomiting, or diarrhea; feeling hot or cold; restlessness.

(2) **Heat stroke** and exhaustion: decreased skin turgor; tachycardia; hypotension; decreased venous filling; concentrated urine.

(3) **Hyperthermia:** hot, dry skin; tachycardia; hypotension; excessive thirst; muscle cramps; visual disturbances; confusion or delirium.

(4) **Hypothermia:** pale skin; skin cool or cold to touch; bradycardia and dysrhythmias; uncontrollable shivering; reduced level of consciousness; shallow respirations.

STEPS	RATIONALE
2. Assess for factors that normally influence temperature:	Allows nurse to accurately assess for presence and significance of temperature alteration.
a. Age.	Older adults have a narrower range of temperature than do younger adults.
CRITICAL DECISION POINT **No single temperature is normal for all people. A temperature within a normal range in an older adult may reflect a fever. Undeveloped temperature control mechanisms in infants and children can cause temperature to rise and fall rapidly.**	
b. Exercise.	Muscle activity raises heat production.
c. Hormones.	Women have wider temperature fluctuations than men because of menstrual cycle hormonal changes; body temperature change can vary during menopause.
d. Stress.	Stress elevates temperature.
e. Environmental temperature.	Infants and older adults are more sensitive to environmental temperature changes.
f. Medications.	Drugs may impair or promote sweating, vasoconstriction, vasodilation, or interfere with the ability of the hypothalamus to regulate temperature.
g. Daily fluctuations.	Body temperature is lowest during early morning; peaks in late afternoon; falls gradually during night.
3. Assess site most appropriate for temperature measurement (see Table 10-1): a. Oral site b. Rectal site c. Axillary site d. Tympanic membrane site	
4. Determine previous baseline temperature and measurement site (if available) from client's record.	Allows nurse to assess for change in condition. Provides comparison with future temperature measurements.

NURSING DIAGNOSIS

Clustering of defining characteristics from the assessment data may reveal the following nursing diagnoses for clients requiring this skill.

- Risk for altered body temperature
- Hyperthermia
- Hypothermia
- Ineffective thermoregulation

Related factors are individualized based on client's condition or needs.

PLANNING

STEPS	RATIONALE
1. Expected outcomes following completion of procedure:	
➤ Body temperature is within normal range for client's age group. Thermoregulation is maintained.	Nurse controls for environmental factors that could normally alter temperature.
➤ Body temperature returns to normal or baseline range following therapies for abnormal temperature.	
2. Explain to client the way temperature will be measured and importance of maintaining proper position until reading is complete.	Promotes client cooperation and increases compliance. Clients are often curious about their temperatures and should be cautioned against prematurely removing the thermometer to read results.

IMPLEMENTATION

STEPS	RATIONALE
1. Wash hands.	Reduces transmission of microorganisms.
a. Assist client to comfortable position that provides easy access to temperature measurement site.	Ensures both client's comfort and accuracy of temperature reading.

STEPS	RATIONALE
2. ORAL TEMPERATURE MEASUREMENT WITH GLASS THERMOMETER	
a. Apply disposable gloves.	Maintains standard precautions when exposed to items soiled with body fluids (e.g., saliva).
b. Hold end (if color-coded, tip will be blue) of glass thermometer with fingertips.	Reduces contamination of thermometer bulb.
c. Read mercury level while gently rotating thermometer at eye level (see illustration). If mercury is above desired level, grasp tip of thermometer securely, stand away from solid objects, and sharply flick wrist downward. Continue shaking until reading is below 35.5° C (96° F).	Mercury should be below 35.5° C (96° F). Thermometer reading must be below client's actual temperature before use. Brisk shaking lowers mercury level in glass tube.
d. Insert thermometer into plastic sleeve cover.	Protects from contact with saliva.
e. Ask client to open mouth and gently place thermometer under tongue in posterior sublingual pocket lateral to center of lower jaw (see illustration).	Heat from superficial blood vessels in sublingual pocket produces temperature reading.
f. Ask client to hold thermometer with lips closed. Caution against biting down on thermometer.	Maintains proper position of thermometer during recording. Breakage of thermometer may injure mucosa and cause mercury poisoning.
g. Leave thermometer in place for 3 minutes or according to agency policy.	Studies vary as to proper length of time for recording. Holtzclaw (1992) recommends 3 minutes.
h. Carefully remove thermometer, remove and discard plastic sleeve cover in appropriate receptacle, and read at eye level. Gently rotate until scale appears.	Prevents cross contamination. Ensures accurate reading.
i. Cleanse any additional secretions on thermometer by wiping with clean soft tissue. Wipe in rotating fashion from fingers toward bulb. Dispose of tissue in appropriate receptacle. Store thermometer in appropriate protective storage container.	Avoids contact of microorganisms with nurse's hands. Wipe from area of least contamination to area of most contamination. Glass thermometers should not be shared between clients unless terminal disinfection is performed between each measurement. Protective storage container prevents breakage and reduces risks of mercury spill.
j. Remove and dispose of gloves in appropriate receptacle. Wash hands.	Reduces transmission of microorganisms.
k. Discuss findings with client as needed.	Promotes participation in care and understanding of health status.

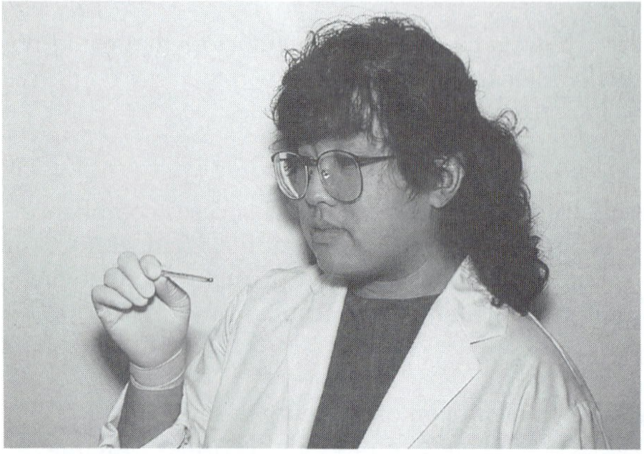

Step 2c Nurse reading mercury thermometer at eye level.

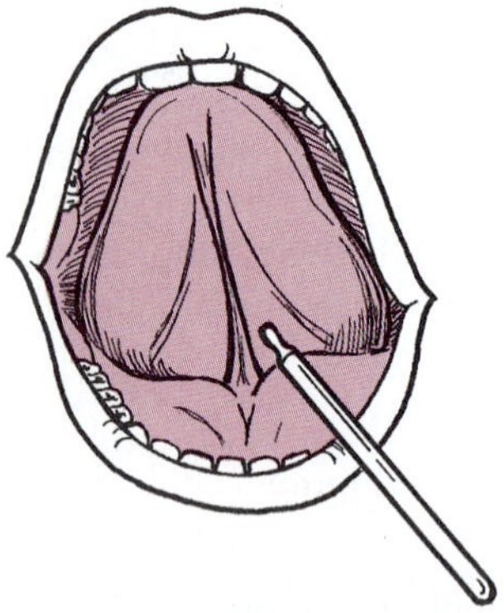

Step 2e Sublingual area of oral cavity.

STEPS	RATIONALE
3. ORAL TEMPERATURE MEASUREMENT WITH ELECTRONIC THERMOMETER	
a. Follow steps 1 and 1a.	
b. Apply disposable gloves (optional).	Use of oral probe cover, which can be removed without physical contact, minimizes need to wear gloves.
c. Remove thermometer pack from charging unit. Attach oral probe (blue tip) to thermometer unit. Grasp top of stem, being careful not to apply pressure to ejection button.	Charging provides battery power. Ejection button releases plastic cover from probe.
d. Slide disposable plastic probe cover over thermometer probe until it locks in place (see illustration).	Soft plastic cover will not break in client's mouth and prevents transmission of microorganisms between clients.

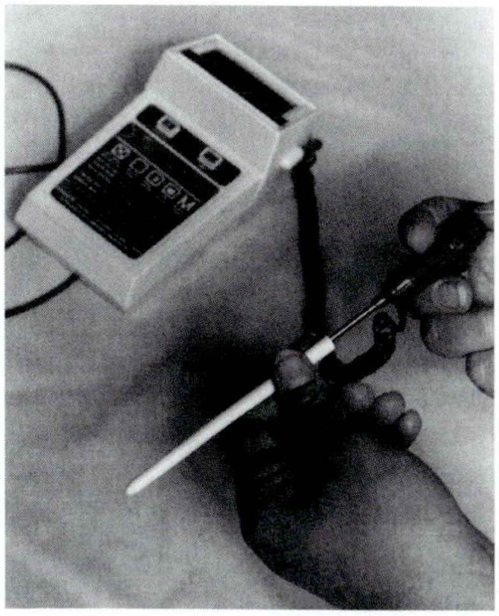

Step 3d Electronic thermometer with probe cover.

STEPS	RATIONALE
e. Ask client to open mouth; then gently place thermometer probe under tongue in posterior sublingual pocket lateral to center of lower jaw.	Heat from superficial blood vessels in sublingual pocket produces temperature reading. With electronic thermometer, temperatures in right and left posterior sublingual pocket are significantly higher than in area under front of tongue.
f. Ask client to hold thermometer probe with lips closed.	Maintains proper position of thermometer during recording.
g. Leave thermometer probe in place until audible signal occurs and client's temperature appears on digital display; remove thermometer probe from under client's tongue.	Probe must stay in place until signal occurs to ensure accurate reading.
h. Push ejection button on thermometer stem to discard plastic probe cover into appropriate receptacle.	Reduces transmission of microorganisms.
i. Return thermometer stem to storage well of recording unit.	Protects probe from damage. Automatically causes digital reading to disappear.
j. If gloves worn, remove and dispose in appropriate receptacle. Wash hands.	Reduces transmission of microorganisms.
k. Return thermometer to charger.	Maintains battery charge.
l. Discuss finding with client as needed.	Promotes participation in care and understanding of health status.

STEPS	RATIONALE
4. RECTAL TEMPERATURE MEASUREMENT WITH GLASS THERMOMETER	
a. Draw curtain around bed and/or close room door. Assist client to Sims' position with upper leg flexed. Move aside bed linen to expose only anal area. Keep client's upper body and lower extremities covered with sheet or blanket.	Maintains client's privacy, minimizes embarrassment, and promotes comfort. Exposes anal area for correct thermometer placement.
b. Apply disposable gloves.	Maintains standard precautions when exposed to items soiled with body fluids (e.g., feces).
c. Hold end (if color-coded, tip will be red) of glass thermometer with fingertips.	Reduces contamination of thermometer bulb.
d. Read mercury level while gently rotating thermometer at eye level. If mercury is above desired level, grasp tip of thermometer securely, stand away from solid objects, and sharply flick wrist downward. Continue shaking until reading is below 35.5° C (96° F).	Mercury should be below 35.5° C (96° F). Thermometer reading must be below client's actual temperature before use. Brisk shaking lowers mercury level in glass tube.
e. Insert thermometer into plastic sleeve cover.	Protects from contact with feces.
f. Squeeze liberal portion of lubricant on tissue. Dip thermometer's blunt end into lubricant, covering 2.5 to 3.5 cm (1 to 1½ inches) for adult.	Lubrication minimizes trauma to rectal mucosa during insertion. Tissue avoids contamination of remaining lubricant in container.
g. With nondominant hand, separate client's buttocks to expose anus. Ask client to breathe slowly and relax.	Fully exposes anus for thermometer insertion. Relaxes anal sphincter for easier thermometer insertion.
h. Gently insert thermometer into anus in direction of umbilicus. 3.5 cm (1½ inches) for adult. Do not force thermometer.	Ensures adequate exposure against blood vessels in rectal wall.
i. If resistance is felt during insertion, withdraw thermometer immediately. Never force thermometer.	Prevents trauma to mucosa. Glass thermometers can break.
CRITICAL DECISION POINT **If thermometer cannot be adequately inserted into rectum, remove thermometer and consider alternative method for obtaining temperature.**	
j. Hold thermometer in place for 2 minutes or according to agency policy.	Prevents injury to client. Studies vary as to proper length of time for recording. Holtzclaw (1992) recommends 2 minutes.

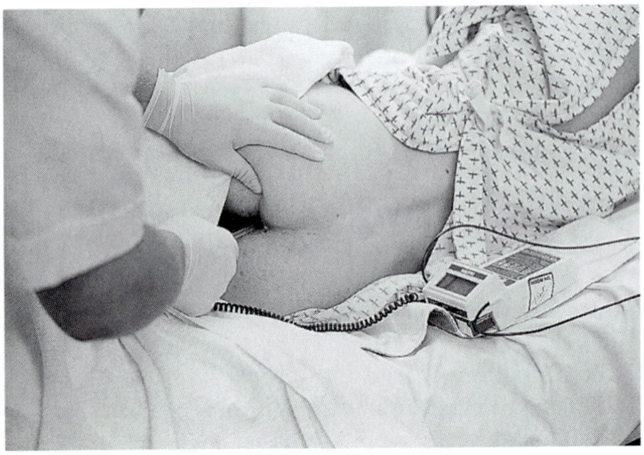

Step 5e Inserting rectal thermometer.

STEPS	RATIONALE
k. Carefully remove thermometer, remove and discard plastic sleeve cover in appropriate receptacle, and wipe off any remaining secretions with clean tissue. Wipe in rotating fashion from fingers toward bulb. Dispose of tissue in appropriate receptacle.	Prevents cross contamination. Wipe from area of least contamination to area of most contamination.
l. Read thermometer at eye level. Gently rotate until scale appears.	Ensures accurate reading.
m. Wipe client's anal area with soft tissue to remove lubricant or feces and discard tissue. Assist client in assuming a comfortable position.	Provides for comfort and hygiene.
n. Store thermometer in appropriate protective storage container.	Glass thermometers should not be shared between clients unless terminal disinfection is performed between each measurement. Protective storage container prevents breakage and reduces risks of mercury spill.
o. Remove and dispose of gloves in appropriate receptacle. Wash hands.	Reduces transmission of microorganisms.
p. Discuss findings with client as needed.	Promotes participation in care and understanding of health status.

5. RECTAL TEMPERATURE MEASUREMENT WITH ELECTRONIC THERMOMETER

STEPS	RATIONALE
a. Follow steps 4a and 4b.	
b. Remove thermometer pack from charging unit. Attach rectal probe (red tip) to thermometer unit. Grasp top of stem, being careful not to apply pressure to ejection button.	Charging provides battery power. Ejection button releases plastic cover from probe.
c. Slide disposable plastic probe cover over thermometer probe until it locks in place.	Probe cover prevents transmission of microorganisms between clients.
d. Continue as for 4 f, g, h, and i.	
e. Leave thermometer probe in place (see illustration) until audible signal occurs and client's temperature appears on digital display; remove thermometer probe from anus.	Probe must stay in place until signal occurs to ensure accurate reading.
f. Push ejection button on thermometer stem to discard plastic probe cover into appropriate receptacle.	Reduces transmission of microorganisms.
g. Return thermometer stem to storage well of recording unit.	Protects probe from damage. Automatically causes digital reading to disappear.
h. Wipe client's anal area with soft tissue to remove lubricant or feces and discard tissue. Assist client in assuming a comfortable position.	Provides for comfort and hygiene.
i. Remove and dispose of gloves in appropriate receptable. Wash hands.	Reduces transmission of microorganisms.
j. Return thermometer to charger.	Maintains battery charge.
k. Discuss findings with client as needed.	Promotes participation in care and understanding of health status.

6. AXILLARY TEMPERATURE MEASUREMENT WITH GLASS THERMOMETER

STEPS	RATIONALE
a. Draw curtain around bed and/or close room door. Assist client to supine or sitting position. Move aside bed linen or gown to expose shoulder and arm.	Maintains client's privacy, minimizes embarrassment, and promotes comfort. Exposes axilla for correct thermometer placement.

STEPS	RATIONALE
b. Prepare glass thermometer following steps 2b and c under "Oral Temperature Measurement with Glass Thermometer."	
c. Insert thermometer into center of axilla, lower arm over thermometer, and place arm across client's chest (see illustrations).	Maintains proper position of thermometer against blood vessels in axilla.
d. Hold thermometer in place for 3 minutes.	Studies vary as to proper length of time for recording. Stephen and Sexton (1987) concluded that changes after 3 minutes had little clinical significance.
e. Carefully remove thermometer, remove and discard plastic sleeve in appropriate receptacle, and wipe off any remaining secretions with clean tissue. Wipe in rotating fashion from fingers toward bulb. Dispose of tissue in appropriate receptacle.	Prevents cross contamination. Wipe from area of least contamination to area of most contamination.
f. Read thermometer at eye level. Gently rotate until scale appears.	Ensures accurate reading.
g. Store thermometer in appropriate protective storage container. Glass thermometers should not be shared between clients unless terminal disinfection is performed between each measurement.	Protective storage container prevents breakage and reduces risks of mercury spill.
h. Assist client in assuming a comfortable position replacing linen or gown.	Restores comfort and sense of well-being.
i. Wash hands.	Reduces transmission of microorganisms.
j. Discuss findings with client as needed.	Promotes participation in care and understanding of health status.

7. AXILLARY TEMPERATURE MEASUREMENT WITH ELECTRONIC THERMOMETER

STEPS	RATIONALE
a. Draw curtain around bed and/or close room door. Assist client to supine or sitting position. Move clothing or gown away from shoulder and arm.	Maintains client's privacy, minimizes embarrassment, and promotes comfort. Exposes axilla for correct thermometer placement.
b. Prepare electronic thermometer following steps 3c and d under "Oral Temperature Measurement with Electronic Thermometer."	
c. Insert thermometer into center of axilla (as shown for glass thermometer in step 6c), lower arm over thermometer, and place arm across client's chest.	Maintains proper position of thermometer against blood vessels in axilla.

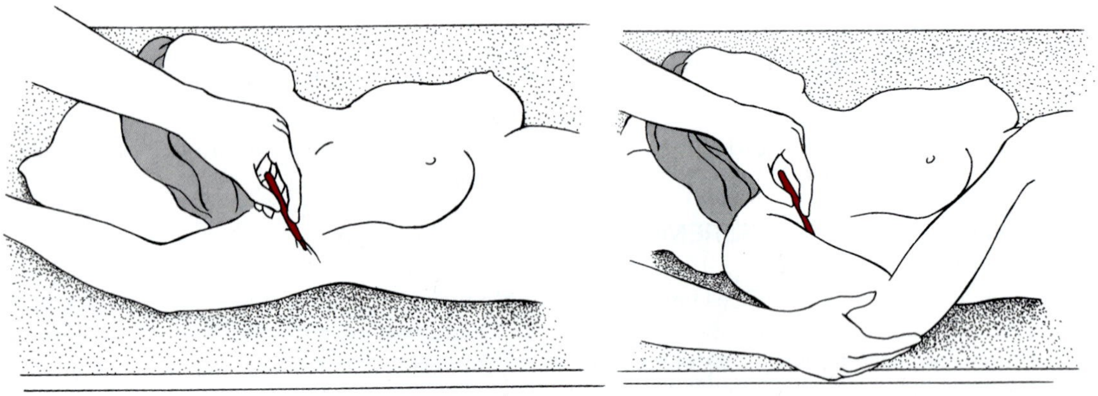

Step 6c Inserting axillary thermometer.

STEPS	RATIONALE
d. Hold thermometer in place until audible signal occurs and client's temperature appears on digital display, remove probe from axilla.	Probe must stay in place until signal occurs to ensure accurate reading.
e. Push ejection button on thermometer stem to discard plastic probe cover into appropriate receptacle.	Reduces transmission of microorganisms.
f. Return thermometer stem to storage well of recording unit.	Protects probe from damage. Automatically causes digital reading to disappear.
g. Assist client in assuming a comfortable position replacing linen or gown.	Restores comfort and sense of well-being.
h. Wash hands.	Reduces transmission of microorganisms.
i. Return thermometer to charger.	Maintains battery charge.
j. Discuss findings with client as needed.	Promotes participation in care and understanding of health status.

8. TYMPANIC MEMBRANE TEMPERATURE WITH ELECTRONIC THERMOMETER

STEPS	RATIONALE
a. Assist client in assuming comfortable position with head turned toward side, away from nurse.	Ensures comfort and exposes auditory canal for accurate temperature measurement.
b. Remove thermometer handheld unit from charging base, being careful not to apply pressure to ejection button.	Base provides battery power. Removal of handheld unit from base prepares it to measure temperature. Ejection button releases plastic cover from probe.
c. Slide disposable speculum cover over otoscope-like tip until it locks into place.	Soft plastic probe cover prevents transmission of microorganisms between clients.
d. Insert speculum into ear canal following manufacturer's instructions for tympanic probe positioning (see illustration): (1) Pull ear pinna upward and back for adult. (2) Move thermometer in a figure-eight pattern. (3) Fit probe snub in canal and do not move. (4) Point toward nose.	Correct positioning of the probe with respect to ear canal ensures accurate readings. The ear tug straightens the external auditory canal, allowing maximum exposure of the tympanic membrane. Some manufacturers recommend movement of the speculum tip in a figure-eight pattern that allows the sensor to detect maximum tympanic membrane heat radiation. Gentle pressure seals ear canal from ambient air temperature.
e. Depress scan button on handheld unit. Leave thermometer probe in place until audible signal occurs and client's temperature appears on digital display.	Depression of scan button causes infrared energy to be detected. Probe must stay in place until signal occurs to ensure accurate reading.
f. Carefully remove speculum from auditory meatus.	

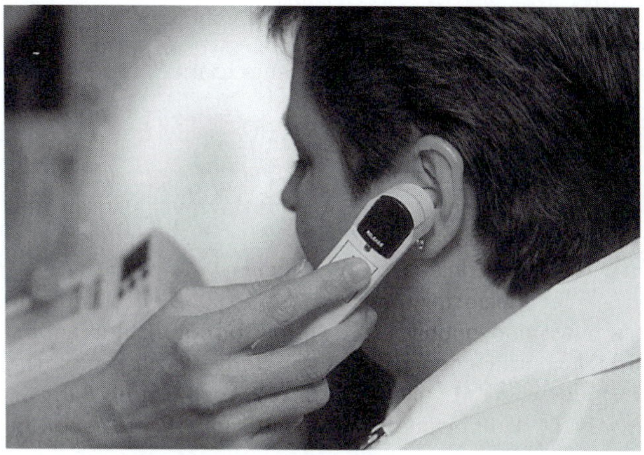

Step 8d Tympanic membrane thermometer with probe cover being placed in client's ear.

STEPS	RATIONALE
g. Push ejection button on handheld unit to discard plastic probe cover into appropriate receptacle.	Reduces transmission of microorganisms. Automatically causes digital reading to disappear.
h. Return handheld unit to charging base.	Protects probe from damage.
i. Assist client in assuming a comfortable position.	Restores comfort and sense of well-being.
j. Wash hands.	Reduces transmission of microorganisms.
k. Discuss findings with client as needed.	Promotes participation in care and understanding of health status.
EVALUATION	
1. If temperature is assessed for the first time, establish temperature as baseline if it is within normal range.	Used to compare future temperature measurements.
2. Compare temperature reading with client's previous baseline and normal temperature range for client's age group.	Normal body temperature fluctuates within narrow range; comparison reveals presence of abnormality. Improper placement or movement of thermometer can cause inaccuracies. Second measurement confirms initial findings of abnormal body temperature.
CRITICAL DECISION POINT **If temperature is abnormal, repeat measurement. If indicated select an alternative site or instrument.**	
3. **Unexpected outcomes** that may occur include:	
➤ Body temperature is above normal expected range.	Client has fever, hyperthermia, or may be experiencing heat stroke.
➤ Body temperature is below normal expected range.	Client is hypothermic.
RECORDING AND REPORTING	
1. Record temperature on vital sign flowsheet (Fig. 10-7) or nurses' notes. Also record any signs or symptoms of temperature alterations.	Vital sign measurements should be recorded promptly on flowsheets to avoid omissions from client's record.
2. Report abnormal findings to nurse in charge or physician.	Abnormalities may require immediate implementation of therapy. Measurement of body temperature after administration of specific therapies should be documented in narrative form in nurses' notes.

FOLLOW-UP ACTIVITIES

1. For temperature above normal expected range, initiate the following nursing measures:
   a. Increase fluid intake to at least 3 L daily (unless contraindicated by client's condition).
   b. Control environmental temperature at 21° to 27° C (70° to 80° F).
   c. Reduce external covering on client's body to promote heat loss. Do not induce shivering.
   d. Keep clothing and bed linen dry.
   e. Limit physical activity and sources of emotional stress.
   f. Initiate measures to stimulate appetite and provide nutrients to meet increased energy needs (Chapter 22).
   g. Encourage oral hygiene because oral mucous membranes dry easily from dehydration (Chapter 6).
   h. Implement measures to determine etiology of fever such as obtain necessary culture specimens for lab analysis (e.g., urine, blood, sputum, and wound sites) (Chapter 43).
   i. Implement measures to prevent or control spread of infection, for example, pulmonary hygiene and postural drainage (Chapter 13), wound care (Chapter 40), and adequate urinary elimination (Chapter 25).
2. If fever persists or reaches unacceptable level as defined by physician, administer antipyretics and antibiotics as ordered, and apply hypothermia blanket (Chapter 39).

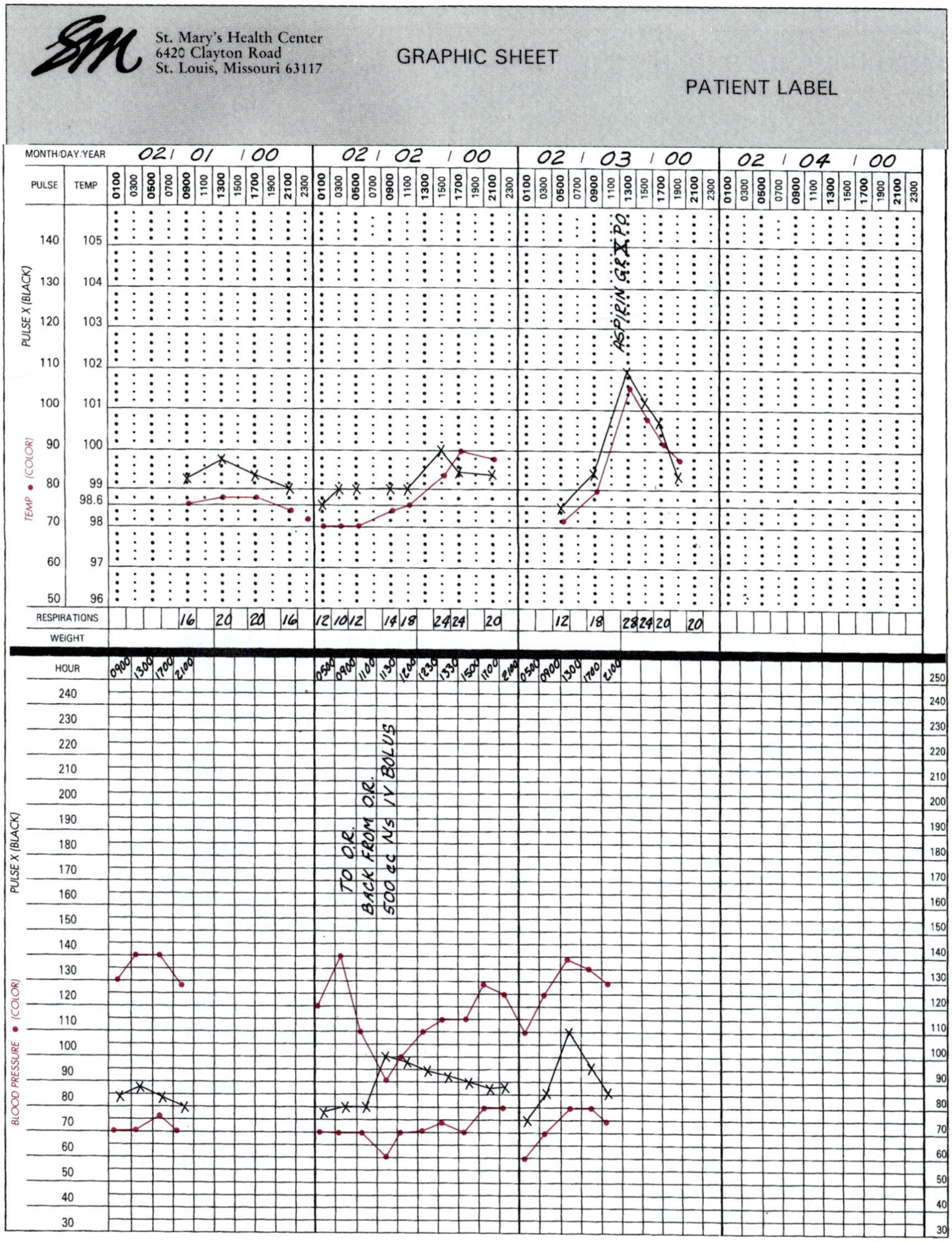

Fig. 10-7 Temperature, pulse, and respiration recording on vital signs flowsheet. (Courtesy St. Mary's Health Center, St. Louis.)

3. If heat stroke is expected initiate the following nursing measures:
   a. Remove client to cooler environment and reduce amount of clothing and bed linens.
   b. Place wet towels on skin and use an oscillating fan to increase convection heat loss.
   c. Apply hypothermia blankets as indicated (Chapter 39).
   d. Monitor for signs and symptoms of dehydration; additional intravenous fluids may be required.
4. For hypothermia, initiate the following nursing measures:
   a. Remove wet clothes and cover client with warm blankets.
   b. Close room doors or windows to eliminate drafts.
   c. Encourage warm liquids.
   d. Apply hyperthermia blankets as indicated (Chapter 39).
5. For temperature below 35° C (95° F), initiate the following additional measures:
   a. Turn client every 1 to 2 hours and take extremities through passive ROM (Chapter 30).
   b. Monitor apical pulse rate and rhythm (Skill 10-2), since hypothermia causes bradycardia, cardiac dysrhythmias, and electrolyte imbalances.

• • • • •

Special Considerations

- Compare temperatures taken during same time of day.
- Temperature should be taken approximately 30 minutes after administering antipyretics, and every 4 hours until temperature stabilizes.
- Clients with musculoskeletal alterations may be able to suggest to nurse ways for positioning to avoid discomfort during insertion of a rectal thermometer. Older adults unable to flex their legs may lie on their sides with legs straight.
- Caution clients using oral thermometer against moving mouth or repositioning thermometer.
- Do not allow client to insert rectal thermometer. Tissue trauma may easily occur if thermometer is forced.
- If client complains of rectal pain after insertion of thermometer, notify physician and observe for rectal bleeding. Localized discomfort may result from irritation of hemorrhoids.
- Instruct care provider or family to never leave client unattended when rectal thermometer is in place.

Teaching Considerations

- Identify client's ability to initiate preventative health measures and recognize alteration in body temperature. Educate clients and family members about measures to prevent body temperature alterations.
- Educate clients about risk factors for hypothermia and frostbite: fatigue; malnutrition; hypoxemia; cold, wet clothing; alcohol intoxication.
- Educate clients about risk factors for heat stroke: strenuous exercise in hot humid weather; tight-fitting clothing in hot environments; exercising in poorly ventilated areas; sudden exposures to hot climates; poor fluid intake before, during, and after exercise.
- Educate clients regarding the importance of taking and continuing antibiotics as directed until course of treatment is completed.

Pediatric Considerations

- Children may assume prone position for rectal temperature measurement.
- Axillary or tympanic temperature is safest for newborns. In an infant or young child it may be necessary to hold arm against child's side when assessing axillary temperature.
- Eoff and Joyce (1981) recommend a 5 minute axillary temperature for children.
- Temperature may be taken as the last vital sign with children who cry or become restless.
- Infants are very sensitive to slight changes in environmental temperatures.

Gerontologic Considerations

- The temperature of older adults is at the lower end of the normal temperature range 36° C (96.8° F).
- Temperatures considered within normal range may reflect a fever in an older adult.
- Older adults are very sensitive to slight changes in temperature.
- Environmental temperature plays a greater role in the older adult because their thermoregulatory systems are not as efficient.
- Older adults may need assistance in detecting cold environments and minimizing heat loss.
- Edentulous adults or older adults with poor muscle control may be unable to close their mouth tightly enough to obtain accurate oral temperature readings.
- A decrease in sweat gland reactivity in the older adult results in higher threshold for sweating at high temperatures, which can lead to hyperthermia.

- Older adults are at high risk for hypothermia because of diminished sensation to cold, abnormal vasoconstrictor responses, and impaired shivering.
- With aging, a loss of subcutaneous fat reduces the insulating capacity of the skin (Fulmer and Degutis, 1992).

Home Care Considerations

- Assess temperature and ventilation of client's environment to determine existence of any environmental condition that may influence outcome of the client's temperature.
- Assess safe storage of mercury-in-glass thermometers to protect from breakage and mercury spills.

SKILL 10-2 Assessing Apical Pulse

Each ventricular contraction ejects approximately 60 to 70 ml (stroke volume) of blood into the aorta. The heart rate is the number of ejections occurring in 1 minute. The volume of blood pumped by the heart during 1 minute is the **cardiac output** (CO). The cardiac output equals the product of the amount of blood pumped by the ventricle per stroke, or the **stroke volume** (SV), and the HR for 1 minute.

The **apical pulse** rate is the assessment of the number and quality of apical sounds in one minute. Each apical pulse is the combination of two sounds: S_1 and S_2. $\mathbf{S_1}$ is the sound of the tricuspid and mitral valves closing at the end of ventricular filling, just before systolic contraction begins. $\mathbf{S_2}$ is the sound of the pulmonic and aortic valves closing at the end of ventricular ejection. The apical pulse is the most accurate, noninvasive measurement of the frequency and rhythm of ventricular contractions of the heart.

A stethoscope is used to auscultate sound waves of the apical pulse (Fig. 10-8). It is a closed cylinder that amplifies sound waves as they reach the body's surface. The four major parts of the stethoscope are the earpieces, binaurals, tubing, and chestpiece.

The plastic or rubber earpieces should fit snugly and comfortably in the nurse's ears. Binaurals should be angled and strong enough so the earpieces stay firmly in place without causing discomfort. The earpieces follow the contour of the ear canal, pointing toward the face when the stethoscope is in place.

The polyvinyl tubing should be flexible and 30 to 40 cm (12 to 18 inches) in length; longer tubing decreases sound transmission. The tubing should be thick walled and moderately rigid to eliminate transmission of environmental noise and to prevent kinking.

The chestpiece consists of a bell and diaphragm. The diaphragm is a circular flat-surfaced portion of the chestpiece covered with a plastic disk. It transmits high-pitched sounds created by high velocity movement of air and blood. The diaphragm is positioned to make a tight seal against the client's skin. Enough pressure is exerted to complete the seal and should leave a temporary red ring on the client's skin when the diaphragm is removed.

The bell is the cone-shaped portion of the chestpiece usually surrounded by a rubber ring to avoid chilling the client. It transmits low-pitched sounds created by the low velocity movement of blood. The bell is held lightly against the skin for sound amplification. The bell and diaphragm are rotated into position on the chestpiece depending on which part the nurse chooses to use. To test, lightly tap to determine which side is functioning.

EQUIPMENT

- **Stethoscope**
- **Wristwatch with second hand or digital display**
- **Pen, pencil, vital sign flowsheet, or record form**
- **Alcohol swab**

DELEGATION CONSIDERATIONS

The skill of apical pulse measurement can be delegated to unlicensed assistive personnel.

- Inform care provider of appropriate client position when obtaining apical pulse measurement.
- Inform care provider of appropriate duration of apical pulse count.
- Any abnormalities should be reported and reconfirmed by the nurse.

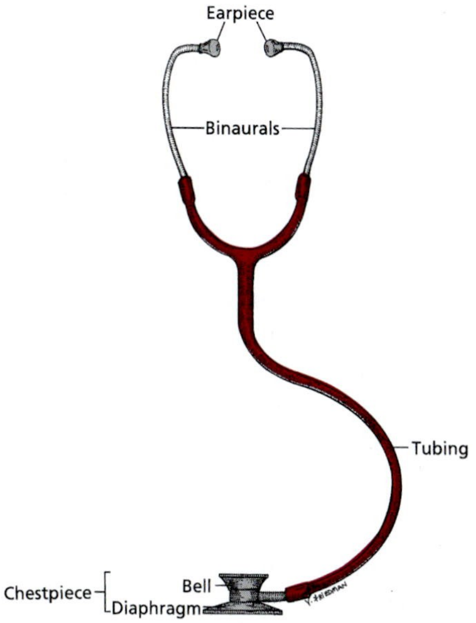

Fig. 10-8 Acoustic stethoscope.

STEPS	RATIONALE
ASSESSMENT	
1. Determine need to assess apical pulse:	
a. Note risk factors for alterations in apical pulse.	Certain conditions place clients at risk for pulse alterations. Alterations in heart rhythm can be affected by heart disease, cardiac dysrhythmias, onset of sudden chest pain or acute pain from any site, invasive cardiovascular diagnostic tests, surgery, sudden infusion of large volume of IV fluid, internal or external hemorrhage, and administration of medications that alter heart function.
b. Assess for signs and symptoms of altered SV and CO such as dyspnea, fatigue, chest pain, orthopnea, syncope, palpitations (person's unpleasant awareness of heartbeat), jugular venous distention, edema of dependent body parts, cyanosis or pallor of skin.	Physical signs and symptoms may indicate alteration in cardiac function.
2. Assess for factors that normally influence apical pulse rate and rhythm:	Allows nurse to accurately assess presence and significance of pulse alterations.
a. Age.	Infant's heart rate at birth ranges from 100 to 180 beats/min at rest; by age 2, pulse rate slows to 70 to 110 beats/min; by adolescence, rate varies between 55 to 90 beats/min and remains so throughout adulthood; no changes occur in older adults at rest and in absence of disease.
b. Exercise.	Physical activity requires an increase in CO that is met by an increased HR and SV; a well-conditioned client may have a slower than normal resting HR and returns quicker to resting rate after exercise.
c. Position changes.	Heart rate increases temporarily when changing from lying to sitting or standing position.
d. Medications.	Antidysrhythmics, sympathomimetics, and cardiotonics affect rate and rhythm of pulse; large doses of narcotic analgesics can slow HR; general anesthetics slow HR; central nervous system stimulants such as caffeine can increase HR.
e. Temperature.	Fever or exposure to warm environments increases HR; HR declines with hypothermia.
f. Sympathetic stimulation.	Emotional stress, anxiety, or fear results in stimulation of the sympathetic nervous system, which increases HR.
3. Determine previous baseline apical rate (if available) from client's record.	Allows nurse to assess for change in condition. Provides comparison with future apical pulse measurements.

NURSING DIAGNOSIS

Clustering of defining characteristics from the assessment data may reveal the following nursing diagnoses for clients requiring this skill.

- Altered cardiopulmonary tissue perfusion
- Decreased cardiac output

Related factors are individualized based on client's condition or needs.

PLANNING

STEPS	RATIONALE
1. Expected outcomes following completion of procedure:	
➤ Apical heart rate is within normal range.	Adults average 60 to 100 beats per minute.
➤ Rhythm is regular.	Cardiovascular status is stable.

STEPS	RATIONALE
2. Explain to client that apical HR is to be assessed. Encourage client to relax as much as possible. Ask client not to speak while assessing pulse. If client has been active, wait 5 to 10 minutes before assessing pulse.	Anxiety or activity can cause elevation in HR. Client's speech interferes with nurse's ability to hear sounds when apical pulse is measured. Apical pulse rate should be assessed at rest to allow for objective comparison of values.
IMPLEMENTATION	
1. Wash hands.	Reduces transmission of microorganisms.
2. Draw curtain around bed and/or close door.	Maintains privacy and minimizes embarrassment.
3. Assist client to supine or sitting position. Move aside bed linen and gown to expose sternum and left side of chest.	Exposes portion of chest wall for selection of auscultatory site.
4. Locate anatomical landmarks to identify the point of maximal impulse (PMI) also called the apical impulse. Heart is located behind and to left of sternum with base at top and apex at bottom. Find Angle of Louis just below suprasternal notch between sternal body and manubrium; can be felt as a bony prominence. Slip fingers down each side of angle to find second intercostal (ICS). Carefully move fingers down left side of sternum to fifth ICS and laterally to the left midclavicular line (MCL). A light tap felt within an area 1 to 2 cm (½ to 1 inch) of the PMI is reflected from the apex of the heart.	Use of anatomical landmarks allows correct placement of stethoscope over apex of heart. This position enhances ability to hear heart sounds clearly. If unable to palpate the PMI, reposition client on left side. In the presence of serious heart disease, the PMI may be located to the left of the MCL or at the sixth ICS.

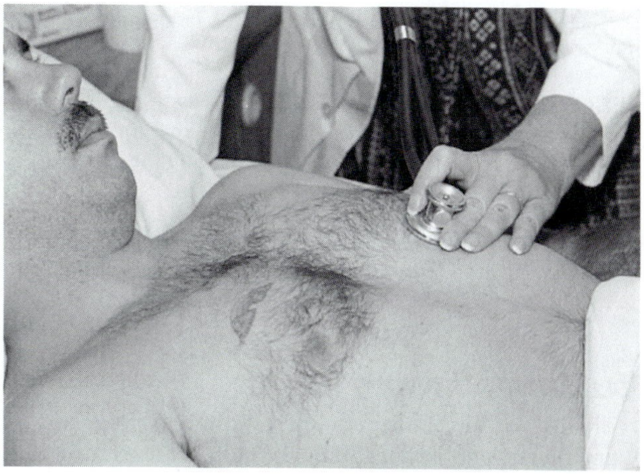

Step 6 Stethoscope over PMI.

STEPS	RATIONALE
5. Place diaphragm of stethoscope in palm of hand for 5 to 10 seconds.	Warming of metal or plastic diaphragm prevents client from being startled and promotes comfort.
6. Place diaphragm of stethoscope over PMI at the fifth ICS, a left MCL, and auscultate for normal S_1 and S_2 heart sounds (heard as "lub dub") (see illustration).	Allow stethoscope tubing to extend straight without kinks that would distort sound transmission. Normal sounds S_1 and S_2 are high pitched and best heard with the diaphragm.
7. When S_1 and S_2 are heard with regularity, use watch's second hand and begin to count rate: when sweep hand hits number on dial, start counting with zero, then one, two, and so on.	Apical rate is determined accurately only after nurse is able to auscultate sounds clearly. Timing begins with zero. Count of one is first sound auscultated after timing begins.
8. If apical rate is regular, count for 30 seconds and multiply by 2.	Regular apical rate can be assessed within 30 seconds.
9. If heart rate is irregular, or client is receiving cardiovascular medication, count for 1 minute (60 seconds).	Irregular rate is more accurately assessed when measured over longer interval.
10. Note regularity of any **dysrhythmia** (S_1 and S_2 occuring early or later after previous sequence of sounds; for example, every third or every fourth beat is skipped).	Regular occurrence of dysrhythmia within 1 minute may indicate inefficient contraction of heart and alteration in cardiac output.
11. Replace client's gown and bed linen; assist client in returning to comfortable position.	Restores comfort and promotes sense of well-being.

STEPS	RATIONALE
12. Discuss findings with client as needed.	Promotes participation in care and understanding of health status.
13. Wash hands.	Reduces transmission of microorganisms.
14. Clean earpieces and diaphragm of stethoscope with alcohol swab as needed (optional).	Controls transmission of microorganisms when nurses share stethoscope.
EVALUATION	
1. If pulse is assessed for the first time, establish apical rate as baseline if it is within normal range.	Used to compare future pulse assessments.
2. Compare apical rate and character with client's previous baseline and normal heart rate range.	Allows nurse to assess for change in client's condition and for presence of cardiac alteration.
CRITICAL DECISION POINT If apical rate is abnormal or irregular, repeat measurement or have another nurse conduct measurement.	Original measurement may result from error by assessor. Second measurement confirms initial findings of abnormal HR.
3. Unexpected outcomes that may occur include:	
➤ Apical rate under 60 **(bradycardia)** or over 100 **(tachycardia).**	Indicates potential for poor cardiac output, resulting from variety of causes: heart disease, medication side effect, blood loss, hypothermia.
➤ Rhythm is irregular.	Indicates potential for inefficient ventricular ejection, which can lead to poor CO.
RECORDING AND REPORTING	
1. Record apical rate and rhythm on vital sign flowsheet (Fig. 10-7, p. 251) or nurses' notes. Also record any signs or symptoms of alterations in CO.	Vital sign measurements should be recorded promptly on flowsheets to avoid omissions from client's record.
2. Report abnormal findings to nurse in charge or physician.	Abnormalities may require immediate implementation of therapy. Assessment of apical rate before and after administration of specific therapies should be documented in narrative form in nurses' notes.

FOLLOW-UP ACTIVITIES

1. Clients with irregular rate or rhythm may require an electrocardiogram (ECG) or Holter monitor per physician's order (Skill 45-6) to detect conduction alterations within the heart.

• • • • •

Special Considerations

- Normal pulse range for given age is best basis for comparison if client's baseline rate has been abnormal.
- Occasional **premature ventricular contractions** (PVCs) are common in most persons. However, frequency of PVCs increases with heart disease. Nurse will hear premature sequence of S_1 and S_2 and then short pause before normal S_1 and S_2 return. Numerous PVCs or PVCs that alternate with a normal heartbeat repeatedly should be reported to physician.

Teaching Considerations

- Care givers of clients taking certain prescribed cardiotonic or antiarrhythmic medications should learn to assess apical pulse rates to detect side effects of medications.

Pediatric Considerations

- Point of maximal impulse of an infant is usually located at the third to fourth ICS near the left sternal border.
- Apical pulse is best site for assessing infant's or young child's HR and rhythm.
- Breath holding in an infant or child affects apical pulse rate.

Gerontologic Considerations

- The PMI may be difficult to palpate in an older adult because the anterior-posterior diameter of the chest increases with age, and the heart becomes repositioned as a result of left ventricular enlargement.
- When assessing elderly women with sagging breasts, the breast tissue is gently lifted and the stethoscope placed at the fifth ICS or the lower edge of the breast.

➤ Heart sounds may be muffled or difficult to hear in the elderly because of an increase in air space in the lungs.

Home Care Considerations

➤ Assess home environment to determine the room that affords a quiet environment for auscultating apical rate.

SKILL 10-3 Assessing Radial Pulse

The ejection of blood from the heart, assessed by the apical pulse, distends the walls of the aorta. Because of the force of the blood exiting the heart, aortic distention creates a pulse wave that travels rapidly toward the extremities. When the pulse wave reaches a peripheral artery, it can be felt by palpating the artery lightly against underlying bone or muscle. The pulse is the palpable bounding of the blood flow. The number of pulsing sensations occurring in 1 minute is the pulse rate.

Assessing the client's peripheral pulse sites offers valuable data for determining the integrity of the cardiovascular system. Pulse rate, rhythm, and strength indirectly evaluate the heart's cardiac output (CO). An abnormally slow, rapid, or irregular pulse may indicate the heart's inability to deliver an adequate cardiac output. The strength or amplitude of a pulse reflects the volume of blood ejected against the arterial wall with each heart contraction, also called stroke volume (SV). If the heart's stroke volume falls, the pulse often becomes weak and difficult to palpate. In contrast, a full bounding pulse is an indication of increased stroke volume.

The integrity of peripheral pulses indicates the status of blood perfusion to the area distributed by the pulse (Table 10-2). For example, assessment of the right femoral pulse determines whether blood flow to the right leg is adequate. If a peripheral artery feels weak on palpation, the volume of blood reaching tissues distal to the pulse site may be inadequate.

An inefficient contraction of the heart that fails to transmit a pulse wave to the peripheral pulse site creates a pulse deficit. Pulse deficits are frequently associated with dysrhythmias and warn of potential alteration of cardiac output. To assess for a **pulse deficit,** the nurse and a colleague assess a peripheral pulse rate and the apical pulse rate (Skill 10-2) simultaneously and compare the measurements. The difference between the rates is the pulse deficit.

The radial artery pulse is the most common peripheral site for pulse rate assessment. Assessment of other peripheral pulse sites, such as the brachial or femoral artery, is unnecessary when routinely obtaining vital signs. Other peripheral pulses are assessed when a complete physical

Table 10-2 Pulse Sites

Site	Location	Assessment Criteria
Temporal	Over temporal bone of the head, above and lateral to the eye.	Easily accessible site to assess pulse in children.
Carotid	Along medial edge of sternocleidomastoid muscle in the neck.	Easily accessible site to assess character of peripheral pulse. Used during physiological shock or cardiac arrest when other sites are not palpable.
Apical	Fourth to fifth intercostal space at left midclavicular line.	Site for auscultation of heart sounds.
Brachial	Groove between biceps and triceps muscles at the antecubital fossa.	Assesses status of circulation to lower arm. Site used to auscultate blood pressure.
Radial	Radial (thumb) side of forearm at the wrist.	Common site to assess character of peripheral pulse. Assesses status of circulation to hand.
Ulnar	Ulnar side of forearm at the wrist.	Assesses status of circulation to ulnar side of hand. Used to assess an Allen test.
Femoral	Below the inguinal ligament, midway between symphysis pubis and anterior superior iliac spine.	Assesses character of pulse during physiological shock or cardiac arrest when other pulses are not palpable. Assesses status of circulation to the leg.
Popliteal	Behind the knee in popliteal fossa.	Assesses status of circulation to the lower leg.
Posterior tibial	Inner side of each ankle, below medial malleolus.	Assesses status of circulation to the foot.
Dorsalis pedis	Along top of foot between extension tendons of great and first toe.	Assesses status of circulation to the foot.

is conducted (see Chapter 11) or when the radial artery is not available for assessment because of surgery, trauma, or impaired blood flow.

EQUIPMENT

- Wristwatch with second hand or digital display
- Pen, pencil, vital sign flowsheet or record form

DELEGATION CONSIDERATIONS

The skill of radial pulse measurement can be delegated to unlicensed assistive personnel.

- Inform care provider of appropriate duration of radial pulse count.
- If client has history of or risk for irregular pulse advise care giver as to frequency of assessment.

STEPS	RATIONALE
ASSESSMENT	
1. Determine need to assess radial pulse:	
a. Note risk factors for alterations in pulse.	Certain conditions place clients at risk for pulse alterations: a history of heart disease, cardiac dysrhythmia, onset of sudden chest pain or acute pain from any site, invasive cardiovascular diagnostic tests, surgery, sudden infusion of large volume of IV fluid, internal or external hemorrhage, or administration of medications that alter cardiac function. A history of peripheral vascular disease can alter pulse rate and quality.
b. Assess for signs and symptoms of altered SV and CO such as dyspnea, fatigue, chest pain, orthopnea, syncope, palpitations (person's unpleasant awareness of heartbeat), jugular venous distention, edema of dependent body parts, cyanosis or pallor of skin.	Physical signs and symptoms may indicate alteration in cardiac function, which affects radial pulse rate and rhythm.
c. Assess for signs and symptoms of peripheral vascular disease such as pale, cool extremities; thin, shiny skin with decreased hair growth; thickened nails.	Physical signs and symptoms may indicate alteration in arterial blood flow.
2. Assess for factors that normally influence radial pulse rate and rhythm: age, exercise, position changes, medications, temperature, sympathetic stimulation.	Allows nurse to accurately assess presence and significance of pulse alterations.
3. Determine previous baseline pulse rate (if available) from client's record.	Allows nurse to assess for change in condition. Provides comparison with future pulse measurements.

NURSING DIAGNOSIS

Clustering of defining characteristics from the assessment data may reveal the following nursing diagnoses for clients requiring this skill.

- ➤ Altered cardiopulmonary tissue perfusion
- ➤ Decreased cardiac output
- ➤ Altered peripheral tissue perfusion

Related factors are individualized based on client's condition and needs.

PLANNING

STEPS	RATIONALE
1. **Expected outcomes** following completion of procedure:	
➤ Radial pulse is palpable, within normal rate range.	Adults average 60 to 100 beats per minute.
➤ Rhythm is regular.	Cardiac status is stable.
➤ Radial pulse is strong, firm, and elastic.	Radial artery is patent.

STEPS	RATIONALE
2. Explain to client that radial HR is to be assessed. Encourage client to relax as much as possible. If client has been active, wait 5 to 10 minutes before assessing pulse.	Anxiety or activity can cause elevation in HR. Radial pulse rate should be assessed at rest to allow for objective comparison of values.
IMPLEMENTATION	
1. Wash hands.	Reduces transmission of microorganisms.
2. If necessary, draw curtain around bed and/or close door.	Maintains privacy and minimizes embarrassment.
3. Assist client to assume a supine or sitting position.	Provides easy access to pulse sites.
4. If supine, place client's forearm straight alongside or across lower chest or upper abdomen with wrist extended straight (see illustration). If sitting, bend client's elbow 90 degrees and support lower arm on chair or on nurse's arm. Slightly extend wrist with palm down.	Relaxed position of lower arm and extension of wrist permits full exposure of artery to palpation.
5. Place tips of first two fingers of hand over groove along radial or thumb side of client's inner wrist (see illustration).	Fingertips are most sensitive parts of hand to palpate arterial pulsation. Nurse's thumb has pulsation that may interfere with accuracy.
6. Lightly compress against radius, obliterate pulse initially, and then relax pressure so pulse becomes easily palpable.	Pulse is more accurately assessed with moderate pressure. Too much pressure occludes pulse and impairs blood flow.
7. Determine strength of pulse. Note whether thrust of vessel against fingertips is bounding, strong, weak, or thready.	Strength reflects volume of blood ejected against arterial wall with each heart contraction.
8. After pulse can be felt regularly, look at watch's second hand and begin to count rate: when sweep hand hits number on dial, start counting with zero, then one, two, and so on.	Rate is determined accurately only after nurse is assured pulse can be palpated. Timing begins with zero. Count of one is first beat palpated after timing begins.
9. If pulse is regular, count rate for 30 seconds and multiply total by 2.	A 30-second count is accurate for rapid, slow, or regular pulse rates.

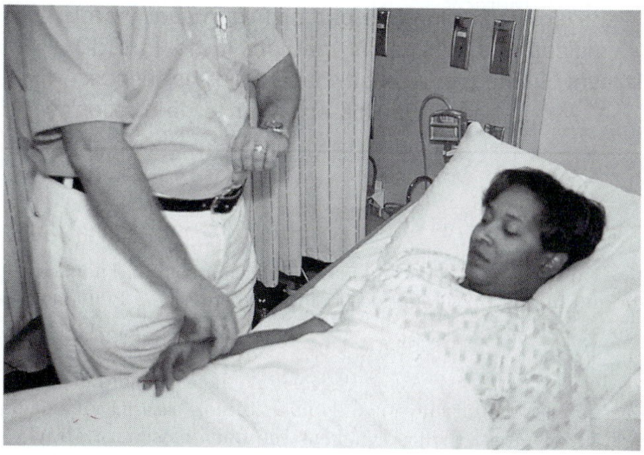

Step 4 Pulse check with client's forearm across upper abdomen with wrist extended.

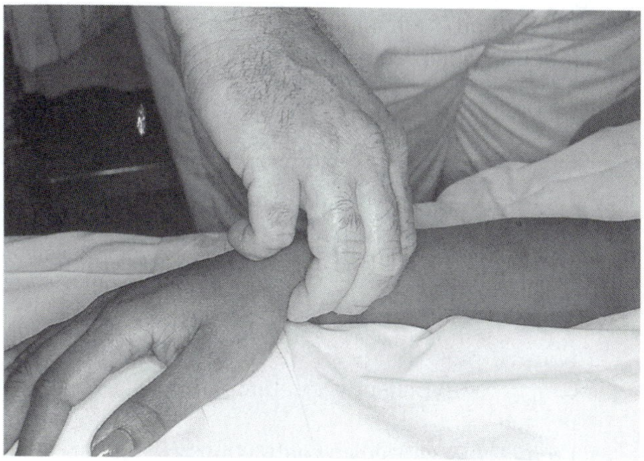

Step 5 Hand placement for pulse checks.

STEPS	RATIONALE
10. If pulse is irregular, count rate for 60 seconds. Assess frequency and pattern of irregularity.	Inefficient contraction of heart fails to transmit pulse wave, interfering with CO, resulting in irregular pulse. Longer time period ensures accurate count.
CRITICAL DECISION POINT If pulse is irregular, assess for pulse deficit. Count apical pulse (Skill 10-2) while colleague counts radial pulse. Begin apical pulse count out loud to simultaneously assess pulses.	The difference between measurements is pulse deficit and may indicate alterations in CO.
11. Assist client in returning to comfortable position.	Promotes comfort and sense of well-being.
12. Discuss findings with client as needed.	Promotes participation in care and understanding of health status.
13. Wash hands.	Reduces transmission of microorganisms.
EVALUATION	
1. If pulse is assessed for the first time, establish radial pulse as baseline if it is within normal range.	Used to compare future pulse assessments.
2. Compare pulse rate and character with client's previous baseline and normal pulse rate range.	Allows nurse to assess for change in client's condition and for presence of cardiac alteration.
3. **Unexpected outcomes** that may occur include:	
➤ Pulse rate for an adult is under 60 beats per minute **(bradycardia)** or over 100 beats per minute (tachycardia).	Indicates potential for poor CO, resulting from variety of causes: heart disease, medication side effect, blood loss, temperature alteration.
➤ Rhythm is irregular.	Indicates need to compare apical and radial pulse for pulse deficit.
➤ Radial pulse may be weak and difficult to palpate.	Reduced CO causes weak pulse. Local obstruction to blood flow (e.g., clot or edema of hand and wrist) may cause pulse to be difficult to palpate.
➤ Pulse deficit is present.	Heart contraction is not strong enough to generate a pulse wave, or overcome an occlusion in a peripheral artery. Dysrhythmia results in poor CO and diminished pulse wave.

RECORDING AND REPORTING

1. Record pulse rate and site assessed on vital sign flowsheet (see Fig. 10-7, p. 251) or nurses' notes. Also record any accompanying signs and symptoms of pulse alterations.	Vital signs should be recorded promptly on flowsheets to avoid omissions from client's record.
2. Report abnormal findings to nurse in charge or physician.	Abnormalities may necessitate immediate implementation of therapy.

FOLLOW-UP ACTIVITIES

1. Clients with irregular rate or rhythm may require an electrocardiogram (ECG) or Holter monitor per physician's order (Chapter 44) to detect conduction alterations within the heart.
2. If radial pulse absent or weak, assess radial pulse on other extremity for comparison. Perform complete assessment of all peripheral pulses (see Chapter 11).

• • • • •

Special Considerations

- ➤ Normal pulse range for given age is best basis for comparison if client's baseline rate has been abnormal.
- ➤ Premature ventricular contractions (PVCs) are common in most persons. However, frequency of PVCs increases with heart disease. Nurse will feel weak pulse followed by a pause and an exaggerated pulse. Numerous PVCs or PVCs that alternate with a normal heartbeat repeatedly should be reported to physician.
- ➤ If radial pulses are inaccessible because of dressings, bandages, casts, or IV placement, use apical pulse. Also use apical pulse when radial pulse re-

veals irregularities. Client with history of heart disease should have apical pulse assessment.

- Occasionally a nurse has difficulty palpating a pulse. A Doppler or ultrasound stethoscope is designed to amplify sounds so that low-velocity blood flow can be heard (Chapter 11). The stethoscope has a special probe applied over the pulse site. A thin layer of transmission gel covers the skin. The stethoscope transmits a "whooshing" sound that indicates arterial blood flow.

Teaching Considerations

- Clients taking certain prescribed cardiotonic or antiarrhythmic medications should learn to assess their own pulse rates to detect side effects of medications. Clients undergoing cardiac rehabilitation should learn to assess their own pulse rates to determine their response to exercise (see Chapter 42).

Pediatric Considerations

- Apical pulse is best site for assessing infant's or young child's HR and rhythm.

Gerontologic Considerations

- It is often difficult to palpate the pulse of an older adult or obese client. A Doppler device provides a more accurate reading.
- The arteries of an older adult may feel stiff and knotty because of decreased elasticity.
- Once elevated, the pulse rate of an older adult takes longer to return to normal resting rate (Wold, 1993).

SKILL 10-4 Assessing Arterial Blood Pressure

Blood pressure (BP) is the force exerted by the blood against the vessel walls. During a normal cardiac cycle, BP reaches a peak that is followed by a trough, or low point, in the cycle. The peak pressure occurs when the heart's ventricular contraction, or systole, forces blood under high pressure into the aorta. When the ventricles relax, the blood remaining in the arteries exerts a minimum or diastolic pressure. **Diastolic pressure** is the minimal pressure exerted against the arterial walls at all times.

The standard unit for measuring BP is millimeters of mercury (mm Hg). The measurement indicates the height to which the BP can sustain the column of mercury. The most common technique of measuring BP is auscultation using a stethoscope. As the BP cuff is deflated, the five different sounds heard over an artery are called Korotkoff phases. The sound in each phase has unique characteristics (Fig. 10-9). Blood pressure is recorded with the systolic reading (first Korotkoff sound) before the diastolic (beginning of the fifth Korotkoff sound). The difference between **systolic pressure** and diastolic pressure is the pulse pressure. For a BP 120/80, the pulse pressure is 40.

Blood pressure reflects various interrelated hemodynamic factors within the circulatory system: cardiac output, peripheral resistance, blood volume, blood viscosity, and vessel wall elasticity. Blood pressure has a direct relationship to cardiac output (CO) and peripheral vascular resistance (R):

$$BP = CO \times R$$

As CO increases, more blood is pumped against the arterial walls, causing systolic BP to rise. When the size of the arteries and arterioles decrease, the greater the resistance (R) to blood flow and BP rises. In contrast, as vessels dilate and vascular resistance falls, BP drops.

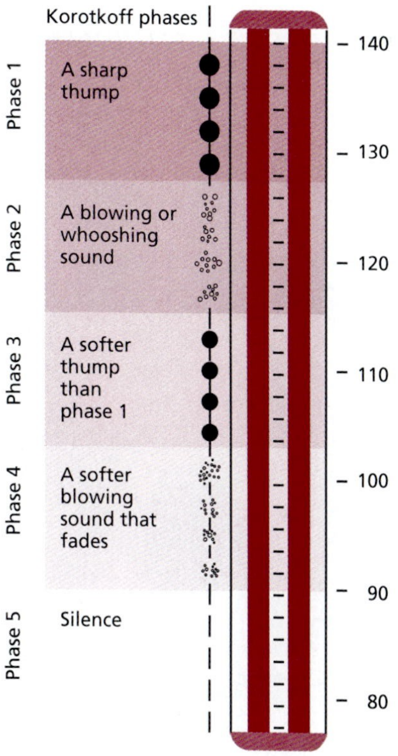

Fig. 10-9 The sounds auscultated during blood pressure measurement can be differentiated into five Korotkoff phases. In this example, the blood pressure is 140/90.

The volume of blood circulating within the vascular system affects BP. Normally blood volume remains constant: 5000 ml in an adult. However, if volume increases, such as after a rapid IV infusion, pressure exerted against arterial walls rises. When circulating blood volume falls, as in the case of hemorrhage or dehydration, BP falls. When the thickness or viscosity of the blood increases, the heart must contract more forcefully to move the blood through the circulatory system and BP rises. When vessel walls are elastic they are easily distensible and can accommodate changes in pressure. Arteriosclerotic vessels lose their elasticity, no longer yield to pressure, and the BP rises.

HYPERTENSION

Hypertension is a major factor underlying death, heart attack, and stroke in the United States and Canada. The American Medical Association's Joint National Committee on Detection, Evaluation, and Treatment of High Blood Pressure (1993) has set criteria for determining categories of hypertension (Table 10-3). The diagnosis of **hypertension** in adults is made when an average of two or more diastolic readings on at least two subsequent visits is 90 mm Hg or higher or when the average of multiple systolic BP on two or more subsequent visits is consistently higher than 140 mm Hg. One BP recording does not qualify as a diagnosis of hypertension. However, if the nurse assesses a high reading (for example, 150/90 mm Hg), the client should be encouraged to return for another checkup within 2 months (Table 10-4).

BLOOD PRESSURE EQUIPMENT

Arterial blood pressure may be measured either directly (invasively) or indirectly (noninvasively). The direct method requires electronic monitoring equipment and the insertion of a thin catheter into an artery. The risks of invasive blood pressure monitoring require care delivery in an intensive care setting.

The more common noninvasive method requires use of the sphygmomanometer and stethoscope. A **sphygmomanometer** includes a pressure manometer, an occlusive cloth cuff that encloses an inflatable rubber bladder, and a pressure bulb with a release valve that inflates the bladder (Fig. 10-10). There are two types of manometers: aneroid and mercury. The aneroid manometer has a glass-enclosed circular gauge containing a needle that registers millimeter calibrations. Metal parts in the aneroid manometer are subject to temperature expansion and contraction; thus the instrument is not as reliable as a mercury manometer. Before using the aneroid manometer, the nurse must be sure the needle points to zero and the instrument is correctly calibrated.

The mercury manometer is an upright tube containing mercury. Pressure created by inflation of the bladder moves the column of mercury upward against the force of gravity. Millimeter calibrations mark the height of the mercury column. The mercury manometer is the most ac-

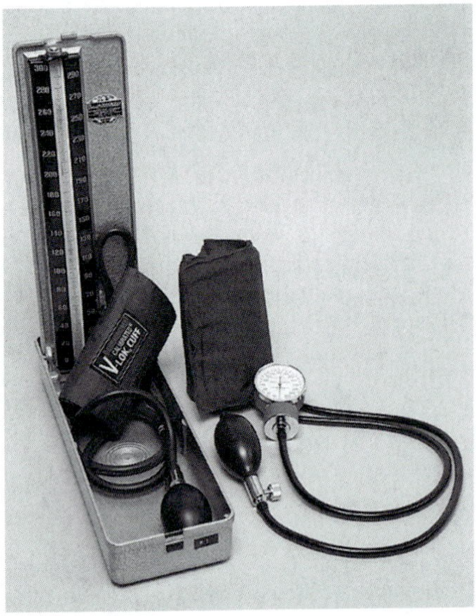

Fig. 10-10 Mercury and aneroid sphygmomanometers.

Table 10-3 Classification of Blood Pressure for Adults Age 18 Years and Older*

Category	Systolic (mm Hg)	Diastolic (mm Hg)
Normal†	<130	<85
High normal	130-139	85-89
Hypertension‡		
STAGE 1 (Mild)	140-159	90-99
STAGE 2 (Moderate)	160-179	100-109
STAGE 3 (Severe)	180-209	110-119
STAGE 4 (Very Severe)	≥210	≥120

Modified from National High Blood Pressure Education Program; National Heart, Lung and Blood Institute; National Institutes of Health: *The fifth report of the Joint National Committee on Detection, Evaluation and Treatment of High Blood Pressure.* NIH Pub No 93-1088, Bethesda, Md., NIH, January 1993.

*Not taking antihypertensive drugs and not acutely ill. When systolic and diastolic pressures fall into different categories, the higher category should be selected to classify the individual's blood pressure status. For instance, 160/92 mm Hg should be classified as Stage 2, and 180/120 mm Hg should be classified as Stage 4. Isolated systolic hypertension (ISH) is defined as SBE ≥ 140 mm Hg and DBP < 90 mm Hg and staged appropriately (e.g., 170/85 mm Hg is defined as Stage 2 ISH).

†Optimal blood pressure with respect to cardiovascular risk is SBP < 120 mm Hg and DBP < 80 mm Hg. However, unusually low readings should be evaluated for clinical significance.

‡Based on the average of two or more readings taken at each of two or more visits following an initial screening.

Note: In addition to classifying stages of hypertension based on average blood pressure levels, the clinician should specify presence or absence of target-organ disease and additional risk factors. For example, a patient with diabetes and a blood pressure of 142/94 mm Hg plus left ventricular hypertrophy should be classifed as "Stage 1 hypertension with target-organ disease (left ventricular hypertrophy) and with another major risk factor (diabetes)." The specificity is important for risk classification and management.

Table 10-4 Follow-Up Criteria for First-Occasion Measurement

Range (mm Hg)		Recommended Follow-Up
Systolic	**Diastolic**	
<130	<85	Recheck within 2 years
130-139	85 to 89	Recheck within 1 year
140-159	90 to 99	Confirm in 2 months
160-179	100 to 109	Evaluate or refer to source of care within 1 month (not to exceed 2 weeks)
180-209	110 to 119	Evaluate or refer to source of care within 1 week
≥210	≥120	Evaluate or refer to source of care immediately

Modified from National High Blood Pressure Education Program; National Heart, Lung and Blood Institute; National Institutes of Health: *The fifth report of the Joint National Committee on Detection, Evaluation, and Treatment of High Blood Pressure.* NIH Pub No 93-1088, Bethesda, Md., NIH, January 1993.

curate of the sphygmomanometers. To ensure accurate readings, the mercury column should fall freely when pressure is released and always be at zero when the cuff is deflated. Mercury manometers may be wall mounted or portable.

The release valves of both mercury and aneroid sphygmomanometers should be clean and freely movable in either direction. The valve, when closed, should hold the mercury or pressure constant. A sticky valve makes pressure cuff deflation hard to regulate. The pressure bulb and tubing should be airtight.

Cloth or disposable vinyl compression cuffs used with the sphygmomanometer come in several different sizes. The size selected is proportional to the circumference of the limb being assessed. Ideally width of the cuff should be 40% of the circumference (or 20% wider than the diameter) of the midpoint of the limb on which the cuff is to be used (American Heart Association, 1988). The bladder, enclosed by the cuff, should encircle at least two thirds of the arm of an adult and the entire arm of a child (Joint National Commission on Detection, Evaluation and Treatment of High Blood Pressure, 1993). In an adult the average bladder width is 12 to 13 cm (4.8 to 5.2 inches) and the length is 22 to 23 cm (8.5 to 9 inches). An improperly fitting cuff produces inaccurate BP readings (Table 10-5).

Electronic devices are available to determine BP without the use of a stethoscope. The device includes the appropriately sized BP cuff and either a microphone or a pressure sensor built into the automatically inflatable cuff. Automatic devices are easy to use and efficient when repeated or frequent measurements are required. However, automatic devices are more sensitive and are more susceptible to outside interference, such as movements by client, position of client.

Table 10-5 Common Mistakes in Blood Pressure Assessment

Error	Effect
Bladder or cuff too wide	False low reading
Bladder or cuff too narrow	False high reading
Cuff wrapped too loosely	False low reading
Deflating cuff too slowly	False high diastolic reading
Deflating cuff too quickly	False low systolic and false high diastolic readings
Stethoscope that fits poorly or impairment of the examiner's hearing, causing sounds to be muffled	False low systolic and false high diastolic readings
Inaccurate inflation level	False low systolic reading
Multiple examiners using different Korotkoff sounds for diastolic readings	Inaccurate interpretation of systolic and diastolic readings
Stopping during deflation then reinflating cuff to recheck systolic	False high diastolic reading
Failure to wait 30 seconds before repeating blood pressure measurement	False high diastolic reading

EQUIPMENT

- **Mercury or aneroid sphygmomanometer**
- **Cloth or disposable vinyl pressure cuff of appropriate size for client's extremity**
- **Stethoscope**
- **Alcohol swab**
- **Pen, pencil, vital sign flowsheet or record form**

DELEGATION CONSIDERATIONS

The skill of blood pressure measurement can be delegated to unlicensed assistive personnel.

- Inform care provider of appropriate client position when obtaining blood pressure measurement.
- Inform care provider if client has alterations affecting the appropriate limb for blood pressure measurement.
- Inform care provider of appropriate size blood pressure cuff for designated extremity.
- Inform care provider if client is at risk for orthostatic hypotension and how to measure.

STEPS	RATIONALE
ASSESSMENT	
1. Determine need to assess client's BP:	
a. Note risk factors for alteration in BP.	Certain conditions place clients at risk for BP alteration: history of cardiovascular disease, renal disease, diabetes, circulatory shock (hypovolemic, septic, cardiogenic, or neurogenic), acute or chronic pain, rapid IV infusion of fluids or blood products, increased intracranial pressure, postoperative, toxemia of pregnancy.
b. Observe for signs and symptoms of BP alterations: (1) High BP (hypertension) is often asymptomatic until pressure is very high. Assess for headache (usually occipital), flushing of face, nosebleed, and fatigue in older adults. (2) Low BP (hypotension) is associated with dizziness; mental confusion; restlessness; pale, dusky, or cyanotic skin and mucous membranes; cool, mottled skin over extremities.	Physical signs and symptoms may indicate alterations in BP.
2. Assess for factors that normally influence BP:	
a. Age.	Normal average BP varies throughout life (see *Pediatric* and *Gerontologic Considerations*).
b. Gender.	During and after menopause women can have higher blood pressures than men of same age.
c. Daily (diurnal) variation.	Blood pressure varies throughout day; pressure is lowest in early morning, rises during morning and afternoon, and peaks in late afternoon or evening.
d. Position.	Blood pressure can fall as person moves from lying to sitting or standing position; normally, postural variations are minimal.
e. Exercise.	Increases in oxygen demand by the body for activity increases BP.
f. Sympathetic stimulation.	Pain, anxiety, or fear stimulates the sympathetic nervous system to increase HR, CO, and vascular resistance causing BP to rise.
g. Medications.	Antihypertensives, diuretics, beta-adrenergic blockers, vasodilators, calcium channel blockers, angiotensin-coverting enzyme (ACE) inhibitors, and antiarrhythmics lower BP; narcotic analgesics and general anesthetics can also cause hypotension.
h. Smoking.	Smoking results in **vasoconstriction,** a narrowing of blood vessels, causing BP to rise.
3. Determine best site for BP assessment. Avoid applying cuff to extremity when: intravenous fluids infusing; an arteriovenous shunt or fistula is present; when breast or axillary surgery has been performed on that side; if extremity has been traumatized, diseased, or requires a cast or bulky bandage. The lower extremities may be used when the brachial arteries are inaccessible.	Inappropriate site selection may result in poor amplification of sounds, causing inaccurate readings. Application of pressure from inflated bladder temporarily impairs blood flow and can further compromise circulation in extremity that already has impaired blood flow.
4. Determine previous baseline BP (if available) from client's record.	Allows nurse to assess for change in condition. Provides comparison with future BP measurements.

NURSING DIAGNOSIS

Clustering of defining characteristics from the assessment data may reveal the following nursing diagnoses for clients requiring this skill.

- Altered cardiopulmonary tissue perfusion
- Decreased cardiac output
- Altered peripheral tissue perfusion
- Knowledge deficit regarding BP control
- Fluid volume deficit
- Fluid volume excess

Related factors are individualized based on client's condition or needs.

STEPS	RATIONALE
PLANNING	
1. **Expected outcomes** following completion of procedure:	
➤ Blood pressure is within normal expected range for client's age.	Cardiovascular status is stable.
2. Encourage client to avoid exercise and smoking for 30 minutes before assessment of BP.	Exercise and smoking can cause false elevations in BP.
3. Have client assume sitting or lying position. Be sure room is warm, quiet, and relaxing.	Maintains client's comfort during measurement. The client's perceptions that the physical or interpersonal environment is stressful affect the BP measurement (Thomas et al., 1993).
4. Explain to client that BP is to be assessed and have client rest at least 5 minutes before measurement. Ask client not to speak when BP is being measured.	Reduces anxiety that can falsely elevate readings. Blood pressure readings taken at different times can be objectively compared when assessed with client at rest. Talking to a client when the BP is being assessed increases readings 10% to 40% (Thomas et al., 1993).

IMPLEMENTATION

ASSESSING BLOOD PRESSURE BY AUSCULTATION—UPPER EXTREMITIES

STEPS	RATIONALE
1. Wash hands.	Reduces transmission of microorganisms.
2. With client sitting or lying, position client's forearm, supported if needed, with palm turned up (see illustration).	If arm is unsupported, client may perform isometric exercise that can increase diastolic pressure 10%. Placement of arm above the level of the heart causes false low reading.
3. Expose upper arm fully by removing constricting clothing.	Ensures proper cuff application.
4. Palpate brachial artery (see illustration). Position cuff 2.5 cm (1 inch) above site of brachial pulsation (antecubital space). Center bladder of cuff above artery (see illustration). With cuff fully deflated, wrap cuff evenly and snugly around upper arm (see illustration).	Inflating bladder directly over brachial artery ensures proper pressure is applied during inflation. Loose-fitting cuff causes false high readings.

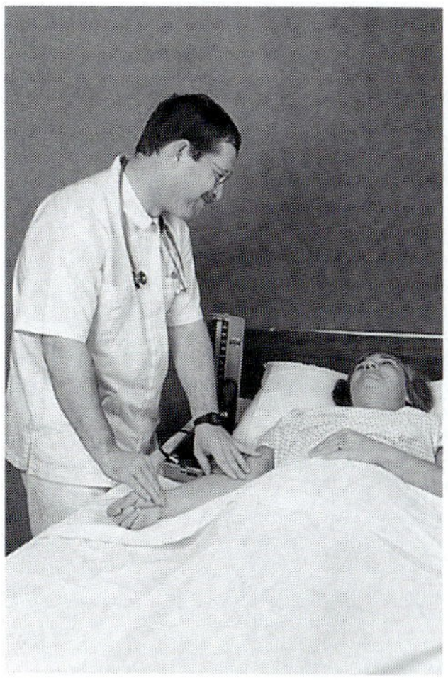

Step 2 Client's forearm supported on bed.

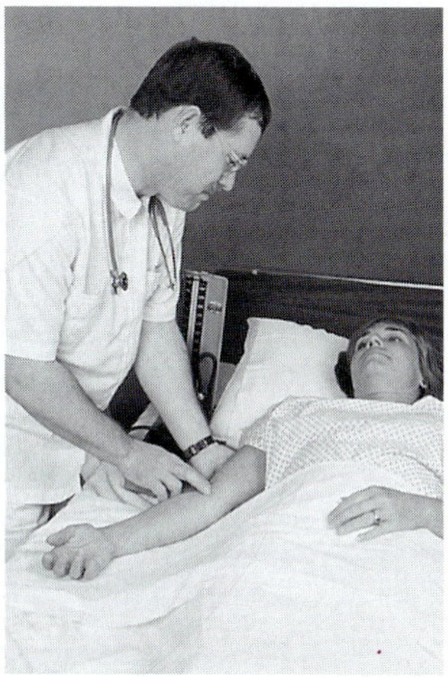

Step 4(1) Nurse palpating client's brachial artery.

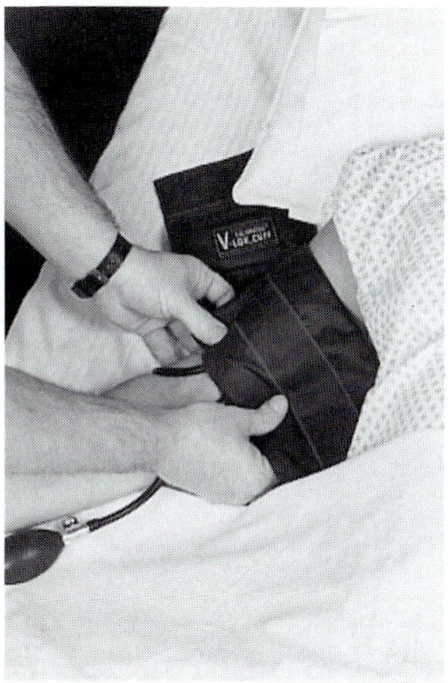

Step 4(2) Center bladder of cuff above artery.

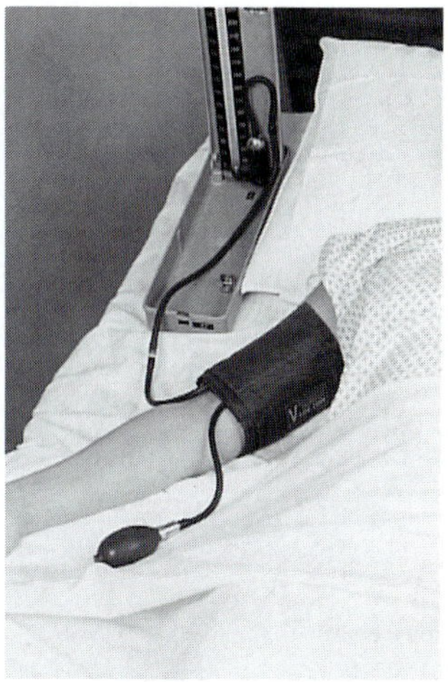

Step 4(3) BP cuff wrapped around upper arm.

STEPS	RATIONALE
5. Position manometer vertically at eye level. Observer should be no farther than 1 m (approximately 1 yard) away.	Accurate readings are obtained by looking at the meniscus of the mercury at eye level. The meniscus is the point where the crescent-shaped top of the mercury column aligns with the manometer scale. Looking up or down at the mercury results in distorted readings.
6. Palpate brachial or radial artery with fingertips of one hand while inflating cuff rapidly to pressure 30 mm Hg above point at which pulse disappears. Slowly deflate cuff and note point when pulse reappears.	Identifies approximate systolic pressure and determines maximal inflation point for accurate reading. Prevents auscultatory gap. If unable to palpate artery because of weakened pulse, an ultrasonic stethoscope can be used (see Chapter 11).
7. Deflate cuff fully and wait 30 seconds.	Prevents venous congestion and false high readings.
8. Place stethoscope earpieces in ears and be sure sounds are clear, not muffled.	Each earpiece should follow angle of ear canal to facilitate hearing.
9. Relocate brachial artery and place bell or diaphragm chestpiece of stethoscope over it. Do not allow chestpiece to touch cuff or clothing (see illustration).	Proper stethoscope placement ensures optimal sound reception. Stethoscope improperly positioned causes muffled sounds that often result in false low systolic and false high diastolic readings.
10. Close valve of pressure bulb clockwise until tight.	Tightening of valve prevents air leak during inflation.
11. Inflate cuff to 30 mm Hg above palpated systolic pressure (see illustration).	Ensures accurate measurement of systolic pressure.
12. Slowly release valve and allow mercury to fall at rate of 2 to 3 mm Hg/sec.	Too rapid or slow a decline in mercury level can cause inaccurate readings.
13. Note point on manometer when first clear sound is heard.	First Korotkoff sound indicates systolic pressure.
14. Continue to deflate cuff gradually, noting point at which sound disappears in adults. Note pressure to nearest 2 mm Hg.	Beginning of the fifth Korotkoff sound is recommended by American Heart Association as indication of diastolic pressure in adults. Fourth Korotkoff sound involves distinct muffling of sounds and is recommended by the American Heart Association as indication of diastolic pressure in children.
15. Deflate cuff rapidly and completely. Remove cuff from client's arm unless measurement must be repeated.	Continuous cuff inflation causes arterial occlusion, resulting in numbness and tingling of client's arm.
16. If this is first assessment of client, repeat procedure on other arm.	Comparison of BP in both arms detects circulatory problems. (Normal difference of 5 to 10 mm Hg exists between arms.)

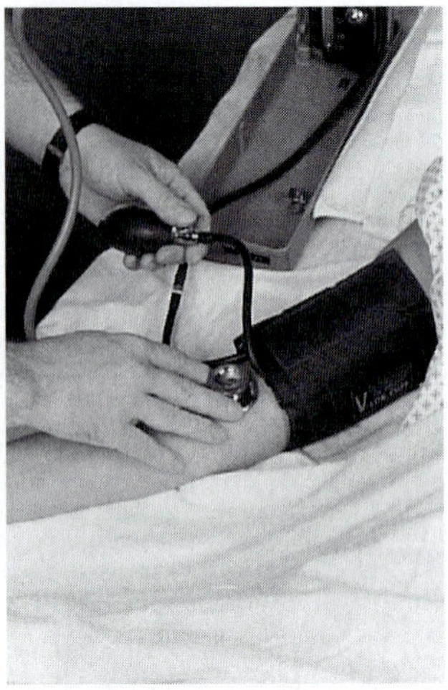

Step 9 Stethoscope over brachial artery to measure BP.

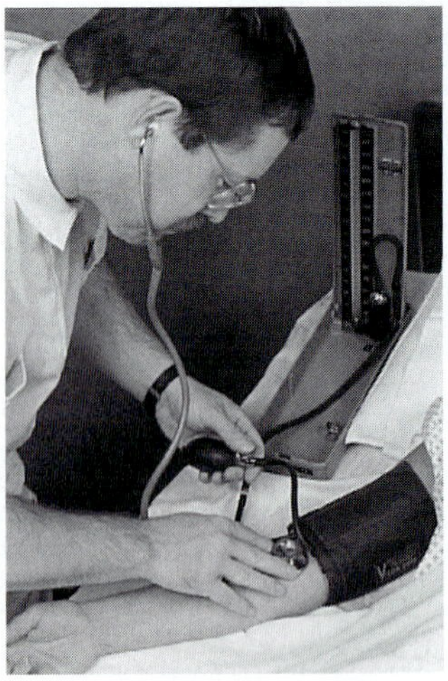

Step 11 Inflating BP cuff.

STEPS	RATIONALE
17. Assist client in returning to comfortable position and cover upper arm if previously clothed.	Restores comfort and provides sense of well-being.
18. Discuss findings with client as needed.	Promotes participation in care and understanding of health status. Makes client accountable for follow-up assessment.
19. Wash hands.	Reduces transmission of microorganisms.
20. Clean earpieces and diaphragm of stethoscope with alcohol swab as needed (optional).	Controls transmission of microorganisms when nurses share stethoscope.

ASSESSING BLOOD PRESSURE BY AUSCULTATION—LOWER EXTREMITIES

STEPS	RATIONALE
1. Wash hands.	Reduces transmission of microorganisms.
2. Assist client to prone position.	Prone position provides best access to popliteal artery.
CRITICAL DECISION POINT **If unable to assume position, assist client to supine position with knee slightly flexed.**	
3. Move aside bed linen and any constrictive clothing from leg.	Ensures proper cuff application.
4. Locate popliteal artery behind knee.	Artery palpation site lies just below client's thigh, in back of knee in popliteal space.
5. Apply large leg cuff 2.5 cm (1 inch) above artery around posterior aspect of middle thigh. Center arrows marked on cuff over artery.	Proper cuff size is necessary for accurate reading. Cuff must be wide and long enough to allow for larger girth of the thigh. Narrow cuff causes false high readings.
6. Using popliteal artery, follow Steps 5 through 15 for auscultation of upper extremity.	
7. If this is first assessment of client, repeat procedure on other leg.	Comparison of BP in both legs detects circulatory problems.
8. Assist client in returning to comfortable position and cover leg if previously clothed.	Restores comfort and promotes sense of well-being.
9. Discuss findings with client as needed.	Promotes participation in care and understanding of health status. Makes client accountable for follow-up assessment.
10. Wash hands.	Reduces transmission of microorganisms.
11. Clean earpieces and diaphragm of stethoscope with alcohol swab as needed (optional).	Controls transmission of microorganisms when nurses share stethoscope.

ASSESSING BLOOD PRESSURE BY PALPATION

STEPS	RATIONALE
1. Follow Steps 1 to 5 of auscultation method for upper extremity.	
2. Palpate brachial, radial, or popliteal artery with fingertips of one hand. Inflate cuff to a pressure 30 mm Hg above point at which pulse disappears.	Ensures accurate detection of true systolic pressure once pressure valve is released.

CRITICAL DECISION POINT **If unable to palpate artery because of weakened pulse, a Doppler ultrasonic stethoscope can also be used (see illustration).**

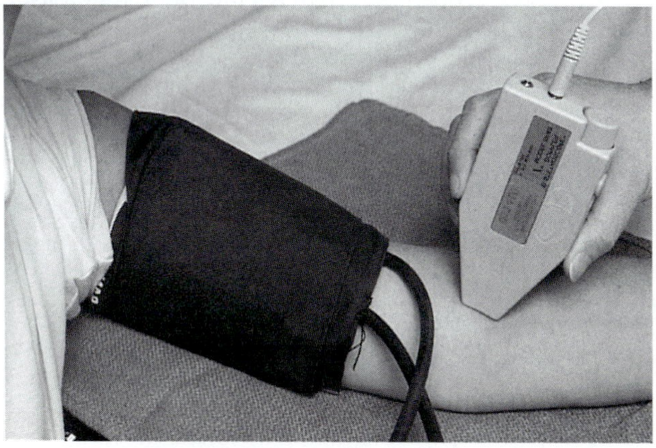

Step 2 Doppler stethoscope over brachial artery to measure BP.

STEPS	RATIONALE
3. Slowly release valve and deflate cuff, allowing mercury to fall at rate of 2 to 3 mm Hg/sec.	Too rapid or slow a decline in mercury level can result in inaccurate readings.
4. Note point on manometer when pulse is again palpable.	Palpation can identify the systolic pressure only.
5. Deflate cuff rapidly and completely. Remove cuff from client's extremity unless measurement must be repeated.	Continuous cuff inflation causes arterial occlusion, resulting in numbness and tingling of client's arm.
6. Assist client in returning to comfortable position and cover upper arm if previously clothed.	Restores comfort and promotes sense of well-being.
7. Discuss findings with client as needed.	Promotes participation in care and understanding of health status.
8. Wash hands.	Reduces transmission of microorganisms.

EVALUATION

1. If BP is assessed for the first time, establish BP as baseline if it is within normal range.	Used to compare future BP measurements.
2. Compare BP reading with client's previous baseline and normal BP for client's age.	Allows nurse to assess for change in condition. Provides comparison with future BP measurements.
3. **Unexpected outcomes** that may occur include:	
➤ Blood pressure is above or below expected normal range for client's age.	Indicates potential for alterations in vascular resistance, blood volume, and cardiac function (e.g., circulatory shock).
➤ Blood pressure is inaudible or difficult to obtain.	Repeat assessment in 1 to 2 minutes. Attempt alternative sites and methods that can provide accurate measurements.
➤ A difference of more than 10 mm Hg between BP measurements on upper extremities.	Indicates potential alteration in peripheral vascular anatomy.

RECORDING AND REPORTING

1. Record BP and site assessed on vital sign flowsheet (Fig. 10-7, p. 251) or nurses' notes. Also record any signs or symptoms of BP alterations.	Vital sign measurements should be recorded promptly on flowsheets to avoid omissions from client's record.
2. Report abnormal findings to nurse in charge or physician.	Abnormalities may require immediate implementation of therapy. Measurement of BP after administration of specific therapies should be documented in narrative form in nurses' notes.

FOLLOW-UP ACTIVITIES

1. Client with hypertension may have various therapies ordered by physician (e.g., antihypertensives, control of or reduction in IV fluid infusion, or administration of diuretics).
2. For the client with orthostatic hypotension:
   a. Place the client in a supine position.
   b. Restrict activity that may drop BP further.
3. Client with hypotension may have various therapies ordered by physician (e.g., increased infusion of IV fluids or vasopressor medications).

Special Considerations

- Systolic BP in legs may be 10 to 40 mm Hg higher than in upper extremities because of pressure needed for blood to reach periphery. Diastolic BP may be the same or lower.
- As long as cuff is inflated, client feels numbness or tingling in arm because of reduced blood flow.
- Pressures should be recorded to near 2 mm Hg.
- If a digital or aneroid sphygmomanometer is used, it should be calibrated to a mercury sphygmomanometer on an annual basis.
- Auscultation in lower extremities is used in clients with certain BP abnormalities so that nurse can compare BP in arms and legs.
- Average leg cuff for adult is 18 cm (7.2 inches) wide and 36 cm (14.4 inches) long.
- Average upper extremity cuff used with obese clients is 15 to 16 cm (6 to 6.4 inches) wide and 30 cm (12 inches) long.
- Orthostatic BP measurements are obtained for clients prone to postural hypotension. **Orthostatic** or **postural hypotension** is a sudden drop in BP that occurs when a client changes from lying to sitting or standing position. The signs and symptoms of postural hypotension include lightheadedness or dizziness when changing position. In severe cases, loss of consciousness may occur. Postural hypotension is commonly observed in clients who are on extended bed rest, or taking vasodilators, antihypertensives, or tricyclic antidepressants. To obtain orthostatic measurements take three BP measurements consecutively with client supine; at edge of bed, legs dangling; and standing. Record each measurement along with subjective reports of dizziness, loss of balance, or other sensations. A drop of systolic BP more than 20 between measurements or a standing BP less than 100 systolic is reportable (Wong, 1995). The nurse takes safety precautions to avoid falls during orthostatic measurements.

Teaching Considerations

- Educate client about risks for hypertension. Persons with family history of hypertension are at significant risk. Obesity, cigarette smoking, heavy alcohol consumption, high blood cholesterol and triglyceride levels, and continued exposure to stress are factors linked to hypertension (Joint National Committee on Detection, Evaluation, and Treatment of High Blood Pressure, 1993).
- Clients with hypertension should learn about BP values, long-term follow-up care and therapy, the usual lack of symptoms, therapy's ability to control but not cure, and benefits of a consistently followed treatment plan.
- Instruct primary care giver to take BP at same time each day and after client has had a brief rest. Take BP sitting or lying down; use same position and arm each time pressure is taken.
- Instruct primary care giver that if the pressure is difficult to hear, it may be that the cuff is too loose, not big enough, or too narrow; the stethoscope is not over arterial pulse; cuff was deflated too quickly or too slowly; or cuff was not pumped high enough for systolic readings.

Pediatric Considerations

- Blood pressure is not a routine part of assessment in children under 3 years.
- Blood pressure measurement can frighten children. Prepare child for squeezing feeling of inflated BP cuff by comparing sensation to elastic band on finger.
- Obtain BP in child before anxiety-producing tests or procedures are performed. At times it may be unrealistic to wait 5 minutes to assess BP. In emergency situations, do not wait.
- Average width of cuff bladder for infant is 2.4 to 3.2 inches; average length of cuff bladder for child is 4.8 to 5.4 inches.
- When a child reaches adolescence, BP varies by body size. Normal range for 13- to 18-year-olds at the 90th percentile is 124 to 136/77 to 84 for boys and 124 to 127/63 to 74 for girls.

Gerontologic Considerations

- Older adults, especially the frail elderly, have lost upper arm mass requiring special attention to selection of BP cuff size.
- An older adult's BP range is normally 140 to 160/80 to 90.
- Older adults have an increase in systolic pressure related to decreased vessel elasticity.
- Older adults often experience a fall in BP after eating.
- Older adults are instructed to change position slowly and wait after each change to avoid postural hypotension and to prevent injuries.

Home Care Considerations

- Assess home noise level to determine the room that will provide the quietest environment for assessing BP.
- Assess family's financial ability to afford a sphygmomanometer for performing BP evaluations on a regular basis.
- Consider an electronic BP cuff for home if client has hearing difficulties.

SKILL 10-5 Assessing Respirations

The mechanism of respiration exchanges O_2 and CO_2 between cells of the body and the atmosphere. Three processes are involved in respiration: *ventilation,* mechanical movement of gases into and out of the lungs; *diffusion,* movement of O_2 and CO_2 between the alveoli and the red blood cells; and *perfusion,* distribution of red blood cells to and from the pulmonary capillaries.

The nurse directly assesses ventilation by observing the rate, depth, and rhythm of respiratory movements. Accurate assessment of respiration depends on recognizing normal thoracic and abdominal movements. Normal breathing is active and passive. On inspiration the thin-walled diaphragm contracts, causing abdominal organs to move downward and forward thereby increasing the vertical size of the chest cavity. At the same time, the ribs lift upward and outward and the sternum lifts outward to aid the transverse expansion of the lungs. On expiration the diaphragm relaxes upward, the ribs and sternum return to their relaxed position, and the abdominal organs return to their original position (Fig. 10-11). During quiet breathing the chest wall gently rises and falls. More energy is required during inspiration than during expiration. Little energy is needed to expire air out of the lungs. Expiration is an active process only during exercise, voluntary hyperventilation, and certain disease states.

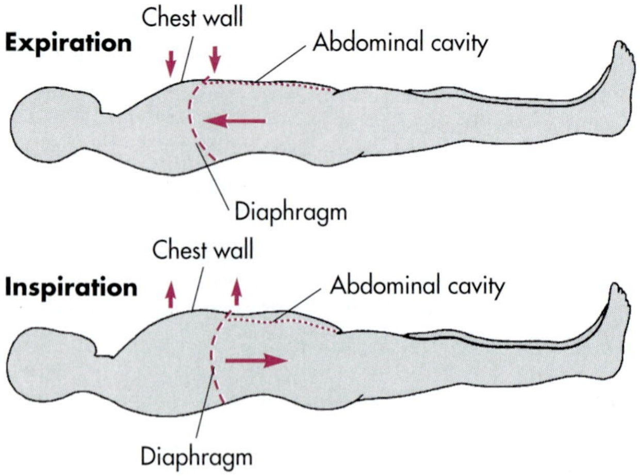

Fig. 10-11 Illustration of diaphragmatic and chest wall movement during inspiration and expiration.

EQUIPMENT

- **Wristwatch with second hand or digital display**
- **Pen, pencil, vital sign flowsheet or record form**

DELEGATION CONSIDERATIONS

The skill of respiration measurement can be delegated to unlicensed assistive personnel.

- Inform care provider of appropriate client position when obtaining respirations.
- Inform care provider of appropriate duration of respiratory rate count.
- Inform care providers if client is at risk for increased or decreased respiratory rate and inform nurse of any changes.

STEPS	RATIONALE
ASSESSMENT	
1. Determine need to assess client's respirations:	
a. Note risk factors for respiratory alterations.	Certain conditions place client at risk for alterations in ventilation detected by changes in respiratory rate, depth, and rhythm. Fever, pain and anxiety, diseases of chest wall or muscles, constrictive chest or abdominal dressings, gastric distention, chronic pulmonary disease (emphysema, bronchitis, asthma), traumatic injury to chest wall with or without collapse of underlying lung tissue, presence of a chest tube, respiratory infection (pneumonia, acute bronchitis), pulmonary edema and emboli, head injury with damage to brainstem, and anemia can result in respiratory alteration.

STEPS	RATIONALE
b. Assess for signs and symptoms of respiratory alterations such as bluish or cyanotic appearance of nail beds, lips, mucous membranes, and skin; restlessness, irritability, confusion, reduced level of consciousness; pain during inspiration; labored or difficult breathing; adventitious breath sounds (Chapter 11), inability to breathe spontaneously; thick, frothy, blood-tinged, or copious sputum produced on coughing.	Physical signs and symptoms may indicate alterations in respiratory status related to ventilation.
2. Assess for factors that normally influence character of respirations:	Allows nurse to accurately assess for presence and significance of respiratory alterations.
a. Exercise.	Respirations increase in rate and depth to meet the need for additional oxygen.
b. Anxiety.	Respirations increase in rate and depth as a result of stimulation by the sympathetic nervous system.
c. Acute pain.	Pain alters rate and rhythm of respirations; breaths become shallow.
d. Smoking.	Chronic smoking changes pulmonary airways resulting in an increased rate.
e. Medications.	Narcotic analgesics, general anesthetics, and sedative hypnotics depress rate and depth; amphetamines and cocaine may increase rate and depth; bronchodilators cause dilation of airways that ultimately can slow respiratory rate.
f. Postural changes.	Standing or sitting erect promotes full ventilatory movement and lung expansion; stooped or slumped posture impairs ventilatory movement; lying flat prevents full chest expansion.
g. Neurological injury.	Damage to the brainstem impairs the respiratory center and inhibits rate and rhythm.
h. Anemia.	Decreased hemoglobin levels lower the amount of oxygen carried in the blood, which results in increased respiratory rate to increase oxygen delivery.
3. Assess pertinent laboratory values:	
a. Arterial blood gases (ABGs): normal ABGs (values may vary slightly within institutions): pH 7.35-7.45 $PaCO_2$ 35-45 PaO_2 80-100 SaO_2 94%-98%	Arterial blood gases measure arterial blood pH, partial pressure of O_2 and CO_2, and arterial O_2 saturation, which reflects client's oxygenation status.
b. Pulse oximetry (SpO_2): normal SpO_2 90%-100%: 85%-89% may be acceptable for certain chronic disease conditions; less than 85% is abnormal (Skill 10-7).	SpO_2 less than 85% is often accompanied by changes in respiratory rate, depth, and rhythm.
c. Complete blood count (CBC): normal CBC for adults (values may vary within institutions): (1) Hemoglobin: 14 to 18 g/100 mL, males; 12 to 16 g/100 ml, females. (2) Hematocrit: 40% to 54%, males; 38% to 47%, females. (3) Red blood cell count: 4.6 to 6.2 million µl, males; 4.2 to 5.4 million µl, females (see Chapter 43).	Complete blood count measures red blood cell count, volume of red blood cells, and concentration of hemoglobin, which reflects client's capacity to carry O_2.
4. Determine previous baseline respiratory rate (if available) from client's record.	Allows nurse to assess for change in condition. Provides comparison with future respiratory measurements.

STEPS	RATIONALE

NURSING DIAGNOSIS

Clustering of defining characteristics from the assessment data may reveal the following nursing diagnoses for clients requiring this skill.

- Risk for activity intolerance
- Impaired gas exchange
- Inability to sustain spontaneous ventilation
- Ineffective airway clearance
- Ineffective breathing pattern

Related factors are individualized based on client's condition or needs.

PLANNING

STEPS	RATIONALE
1. **Expected outcomes** following completion of procedure:	
➤ Respiratory rate is within normal range.	Adults average 12 to 20 respirations per minute.
➤ Respirations are regular and of normal depth.	Respiratory status is stable.
2. If client has been active, wait 5 to 10 minutes before assessing respirations.	Exercise increases respiratory rate and depth. Respirations should be assessed at rest to allow for objective comparison of values.
3. Assess respirations after pulse measurement in adult.	Inconspicuous assessment of respirations immediately after pulse assessment prevents client from consciously or unintentionally altering rate and depth of breathing.
4. Be sure client is in comfortable position, preferably sitting or lying with the head of the bed elevated 45 to 60 degrees.	Sitting erect promotes full ventilatory movement.

CRITICAL DECISION POINT Clients with difficulty breathing **(dypsnea)** such as those with congestive heart failure or abdominal ascites or in late stages of pregnancy should be assessed in the position of greatest comfort. Repositioning may increase the work of breathing, which will increase respiratory rate.

CRITICAL DECISION POINT Position of discomfort may cause client to breathe more rapidly.

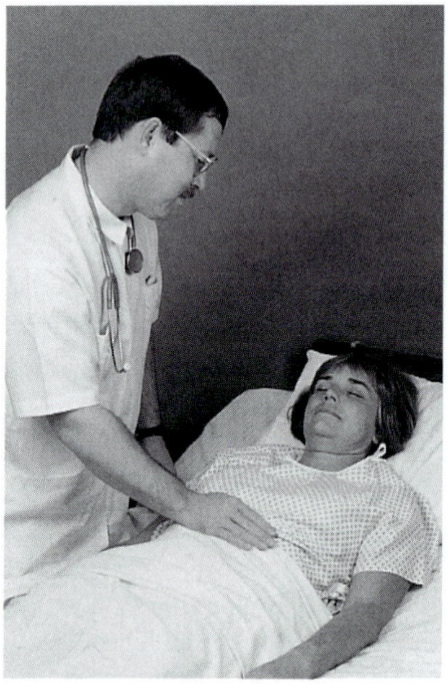

Step 3 Nurse's hand over client's abdomen to check respiration.

IMPLEMENTATION

STEPS	RATIONALE
1. Draw curtain around bed and/or close door. Wash hands.	Maintains privacy. Prevents transmission of microorganisms.
2. Be sure client's chest is visible. If necessary, move bed linen or gown.	Ensures clear view of chest wall and abdominal movements.
3. Place client's arm in relaxed position across the abdomen or lower chest, or place nurse's hand directly over client's upper abdomen (see illustration).	A similar position used during pulse assessment allows respiratory rate assessment to be inconspicuous. Client's or nurse's hand rises and falls during respiratory cycle.
4. Observe complete respiratory cycle (one inspiration and one expiration).	Rate is accurately determined only after nurse has viewed respiratory cycle.

STEPS	RATIONALE
5. After cycle is observed, look at watch's second hand and begin to count rate: when sweep hand hits number on dial, begin time frame, counting one with first full respiratory cycle.	Timing begins with count of one. Respirations occur more slowly than pulse; thus timing does not begin with zero.
6. If rhythm is regular, count number of respirations in 30 seconds and multiply by 2. If rhythm is irregular, less than 12, or greater than 20, count for 1 full minute.	Respiratory rate is equivalent to number of respirations per minute. Suspected irregularities require assessment for at least 1 minute.
CRITICAL DECISION POINT **Respiratory rate less than 12 or greater than 20 requires further assessment (Chapter 11) and may require immediate intervention.**	
7. Note depth of respirations, subjectively assessed by observing degree of chest wall movement while counting rate. Nurse can also objectively assess depth by palpating chest wall excursion (Chapter 11) after rate has been counted. Depth is shallow, normal, or deep.	Character of ventilatory movement may reveal specific disease state restricting volume of air from moving into and out of the lungs.
CRITICAL DECISION POINT **Shallow and slow respirations (hypoventilation) may require immediate intervention.**	
CRITICAL DECISION POINT **Kussmaul respirations, abnormally deep but regular respirations, are a sign of diabetic ketoacidosis that requires immediate intervention.**	
8. Note rhythm of ventilatory cycle. Normal breathing is regular and uninterrupted. Sighing should not be confused with abnormal rhythm. Periodically people unconsciously take single deep breaths or sighs to expand small airways prone to collapse.	Character of ventilations can reveal specific types of alterations.
CRITICAL DECISION POINT **Occasional periods of apnea, the cessation of respiration for several seconds, is a symptom of underlying disease and must be reported to physician or nurse in charge.**	
CRITICAL DECISION POINT **Cheyne-Stokes respiration, characterized by alternating periods of apnea and hyperventilation, is a symptom of underlying disease and must be reported to physician or nurse in charge.**	
9. Replace bed linen and client's gown.	Restores comfort and promotes sense of well-being.
10. Wash hands.	Reduces transmission of microorganisms.
11. Discuss findings with client as needed.	Promotes participation in care and understanding of health status.

EVALUATION

STEPS	RATIONALE
1. If respirations are assessed for the first time, establish rate, rhythm, and depth as baseline if within normal range.	Used to compare future respiratory assessment.
2. Compare respirations with client's previous baseline and normal rate, rhythm, and depth.	Allows nurse to assess for changes in client's condition and for presence of respiratory alterations.

STEPS	RATIONALE
3. Unexpected outcomes that may occur include: ➤ Respiratory rate is below 12 **(bradypnea)** or above 20 **(tachypnea).** ➤ Rhythm may be irregular (Table 10-6). ➤ Depth of respirations may be increased or decreased.	May indicate ventilatory or respiratory problems caused by pain, chest trauma, pulmonary or heart disease, medication side effects, neurological disease. May result from pathological conditions or client's position.

Recording and Reporting

1. Record respiratory rate on vital sign flowsheet (see Fig. 10-7) or nurses' notes. Record abnormal depth and rhythm in narrative form in nurses' notes.	Vital sign measurement should be recorded promptly on flowsheet to avoid omissions from record.
2. Report abnormal findings to nurse in charge or physician.	Abnormalities may require immediate implementation of therapy. Measurement of respiratory rate, depth, and rhythm after administration of specific therapies should be documented in narrative form in nurses' notes.
3. Correlate respiratory rate, depth and rhythm with data obtained from pulse oximetry and arterial blood gas measurements if available.	Assessment of ventilation, perfusion, and diffusion are interrelated.

Follow-up Activities

1. If respiratory rate, depth or rhythm is abnormal, the nurse acts by:
   a. Assisting client to semi-Fowler's or high-Fowler's position (unless contraindicated).
   b. Verifying appropriate route and amount of oxygen delivery if client receiving oxygen therapy (Chapter 12).
   c. Providing oxygen as ordered by the physician (Chapter 12) if client exhibits signs or symptoms of respiratory distress.
   d. Maintaining patency of artificial airway (Chapter 14) to allow adequate airflow.
2. If abnormalities are present, physician may order chest x-ray or arterial blood gas measurement (Chapter 43) to determine cause or nature of abnormality.

• • • • •

Table 10-6 Alterations in Breathing Pattern

Alteration	Description	Alteration	Description
Bradypnea	Rate of breathing is regular but abnormally slow (less than 12 breaths per minute).	Cheyne-Stokes respiration	Respiratory rate and depth are irregular, characterized by alternating periods of apnea and hyperventilation. Respiratory cycle begins with slow, shallow breaths that gradually increase to abnormal rate and depth. The pattern reverses, breathing slows and becomes shallow, climaxing in apnea before respiration resumes.
Tachypnea	Rate of breathing is regular but abnormally rapid (greater than 20 breaths per minute).		
Hyperpnea	Respirations are increased in depth. Occurs normally during exercise.		
Apnea	Respirations cease for several seconds. Persistent cessation results in respiratory arrest.		
Hyperventilation	Rate and depth of respirations increase. Hypocarbia may occur.	Kussmaul respiration	Respirations are abnormally deep but regular.
Hypoventilation	Respiratory rate is abnormally low, and depth of ventilation may be depressed. Hypercarbia may occur.	Biot's respiration	Respirations are abnormally shallow for two to three breaths followed by irregular period of apnea.

Special Considerations

- Clients with chest or abdominal pain frequently splint chest wall or abdomen movement to minimize discomfort, thus decreasing depth of breathing.
- Normal respiratory rate for given age is best basis for comparison if client's baseline rate has been abnormal.
- *Do not* administer high concentrations of O_2 to client with chronic lung disease. This may depress respirations.

Teaching Considerations

- Clients who demonstrate decreased ventilation may benefit from being taught deep-breathing and coughing exercises (Chapter 35).
- Instruct family member to contact home care nurse or physician if unusual fluctuations in respiratory rate occur.

Pediatric Considerations

- Normal average respiratory rate for newborns is 35 to 40; infant (6 months) is 30 to 50; toddler (2 years) is 25 to 32; and child is 20 to 30.
- Infant's respirations are primarily diaphragmatic and thus observed by abdominal movement.
- Infants tend to breathe less regularly.
- Nurse can simply observe infant or young child while chest and abdomen are exposed.
- The young child may breathe slowly for a few seconds and then suddenly breathe more rapidly.
- Apnea monitors may be used for infants or newborns who are at risk for respiratory compromise or arrest.

Gerontologic Considerations

- Aging causes ossification of costal cartilage and downward slant of ribs, resulting in more rigid rib cage, which reduces chest wall expansion. Kyphosis and scoliosis that can occur in older adults may also restrict chest expansion.
- Depth of respirations tend to decrease with aging.
- Older adults may depend more on accessory abdominal muscles during respiration than weakened thoracic muscles.

Home Care Considerations

- Assess for environmental factors in the home that may influence client's respiratory rate such as second-hand smoke, poor ventilation, or gas fumes.

SKILL 10-6 Measuring Oxygen Saturation (Pulse Oximetry)

Pulse **oximetry** is the noninvasive measurement of oxygen saturation. A pulse oximeter is a probe with a light-emitting diode (LED) connected by cable to an oximeter (Fig. 10-12). Light waves emitted by the LED are absorbed and then reflected back by oxygenated and deoxygenated hemoglobin molecules. The reflected light is processed by the oximeter, which calculates pulse oxygen saturation (SpO_2). SpO_2 is a reliable estimate of arterial oxygen saturation (SaO_2). In adults, the oximeter probe can be applied to the earlobe, finger, toe, or bridge of the nose.

The measurement of SpO_2 is simple, painless, and has few of the risks associated with more invasive measurements of SaO_2 such as arterial blood gas sampling. However, the measurement of SpO_2 is affected by factors that affect light transmission such as outside light sources or client motion. Light reflection from hemoglobin molecules can be influenced by carbon monoxide in the blood, jaundice, and intravascular dyes. Conditions that decrease arterial blood flow such as peripheral vascular disease, hypothermia, pharmacological vasoconstrictors, **hypotension,** or peripheral edema affect accurate determination of SpO_2.

Because light reflected from hemoglobin molecules is processed to determine SpO_2, any abnormality in the type or amount of hemoglobin affects oxygen saturation and SpO_2 values. The more hemoglobin that is saturated by oxygen, the higher the **oxygen saturation.** Normal SpO_2 is greater than 90%. Pulse oximetry is clinically indicated in clients who have an unstable oxygen status or in those who are at risk for alterations in oxygenation.

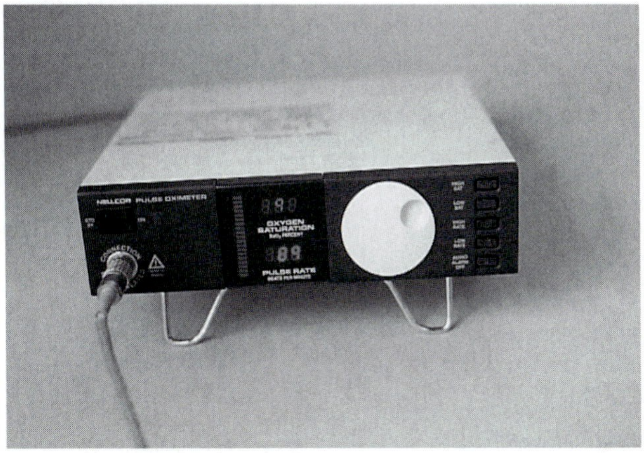

Fig. 10-12 Oximeter.

EQUIPMENT

- Oximeter
- Oximeter probe appropriate for client and recommended by manufacturer
- Acetone or nail polish remover
- Pen, pencil, vital sign flowsheet or record form

DELEGATION CONSIDERATIONS

The skill of oxygen saturation measurement can be delegated to unlicensed assistive personnel.

- Inform care provider of appropriate sensor site for measurement of oxygen saturation.

STEPS	RATIONALE
ASSESSMENT	
1. Determine need to measure client's oxygen saturation:	
a. Note risk factors for alteration of oxygen saturation.	Certain conditions place clients at risk for decreased oxygen saturation: acute or chronic compromised respiratory function, recovery from general anesthesia or conscious sedation, or traumatic injury to chest wall with or without collapse of underlying lung tissue.
b. Assess for signs and symptoms of alterations in oxygen saturation such as altered respiratory rate, depth, or rhythm; adventitious breath sounds (Chapter 11); cyanotic appearance of nail beds, lips, mucous membranes, and skin; restlessness, irritability, confusion; reduced level of consciousness; labored or difficulty breathing.	Physical signs and symptoms may indicate abnormal oxygen saturation.
2. Assess for factors that normally influence measurement of SpO_2 such as oxygen therapy, hemoglobin level, and temperature.	Allows nurse to accurately assess oxygen saturation variations. Peripheral vasoconstriction related to hypothermia can interfere with SpO_2 determination.
3. Consult agency's policy or review client's medical record for physician's order for pulse oximetry.	Medical order may be required to assess oxygen saturation with pulse oximetry.
4. Assess site most appropriate for sensor probe placement (e.g., bridge of nose, ear, fingernail bed). Site must have adequate local circulation and be free of moisture.	Sensor requires pulsating vascular bed to identify hemoglobin molecules that absorb emitted light. Changes in SpO_2 are reflected in the circulation of finger capillary bed within 30 seconds and the capillary bed of earlobe within 5 to 10 seconds. Moisture impedes ability of sensor to detect SpO_2 levels.
5. Determine previous baseline SpO_2 (if available) from client's record.	Allows nurse to assess for change in condition. Provides comparison with future temperature measurements.

NURSING DIAGNOSIS

Clustering of defining characteristics from the assessment data may reveal the following nursing diagnoses for clients requiring this skill.

- Dysfunctional ventilatory weaning response
- Risk for activity intolerance
- Impaired gas exchange
- Inability to sustain spontaneous ventilation
- Ineffective airway clearance
- Ineffective breathing pattern

Related factors are individualized based on client's condition or needs.

PLANNING

STEPS	RATIONALE
1. **Expected outcomes** following completion of procedure:	
➤ Client's SpO_2 remains between 90% and 100%.	Indicates adequate oxygenation.
➤ Client's oxygenation therapies are adjusted without invasive measures.	
2. Obtain appropriate equipment and place at bedside.	Mixing probes from different manufacturers can result in burn injury to client. Clip-on ear probes are convenient, quicker to apply, but more susceptible to movement interference.

STEPS	RATIONALE
3. Explain purpose of procedure to client and how oxygen saturation will be measured.	Promotes client cooperation and increases compliance.

IMPLEMENTATION

STEPS	RATIONALE
1. Wash hands.	Reduces transmission of microorganisms.
2. Position client comfortably. If finger is chosen as monitoring site, support lower arm.	Ensures probe positioning and decreases motion interference with signal.
3. Instruct client to breathe normally.	Prevents large fluctuations in respiratory rate and depth and possible changes in SpO_2.
4. If finger is to be used, remove fingernail polish with acetone from digit to be assessed.	Ensures accurate readings. Opaque coatings decrease light transmission; nail polish containing blue pigment can absorb light emissions and falsely alter saturation.
5. Attach sensor probe to finger, ear, or bridge of nose (see illustration).	Select sensor site based on peripheral circulation and extremity temperature. Peripheral vasoconstriction can alter SpO_2.

CRITICAL DECISION POINT Do not attach probe to finger, ear, or bridge of nose if area is edematous or skin integrity is compromised. Do not attach probe to fingers that are hypothermic. Select ear or bridge of nose if client has a history of peripheral vascular disease.

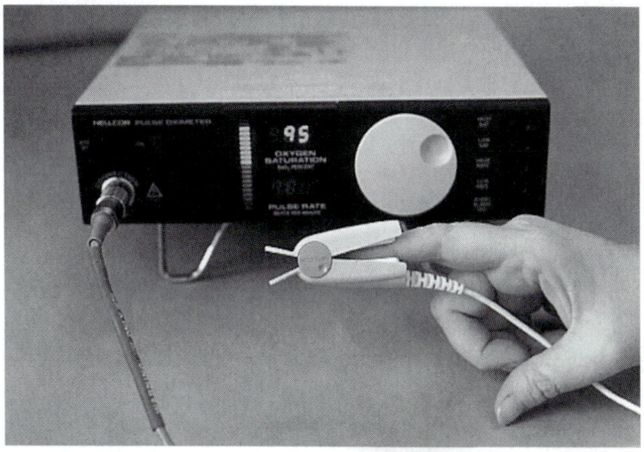

Step 5 Oximeter probe that attaches to ear or finger.

STEPS	RATIONALE
6. Turn on oximeter by activating power. Observe pulse waveform/intensity display and audible beep. Correlate oximeter pulse rate with client's radial pulse.	Pulse waveform/intensity display enables detection of valid pulse or presence of interfering signal. Pitch of audible beep is proportional to SpO_2 value. Double checking pulse rate ensures oximeter accuracy.

CRITICAL DECISION POINT Oximeter pulse rate, client's radial pulse, and apical pulse should be equivalent. Differences requires reevaluation of oximeter probe placement and may require reassessment of pulse rates.

STEPS	RATIONALE
7. Leave probe in place until oximeter readout reaches constant value and pulse display reaches full strength during each cardiac cycle. Read SpO_2 on digital display.	Reading may take 10 to 30 seconds depending on site selected.
8. Discuss findings with client as needed.	Promotes participation in care and understanding of health status.
9. Remove probe and turn oximeter power off.	Batteries can be depleted if oximeter left on.
10. Assist client in returning to comfortable position.	Restores comfort and promotes sense of well-being.
11. Wash hands.	Reduces transmission of microorganisms.

STEPS	RATIONALE
EVALUATION	
1. If oxygen saturation is assessed for the first time, establish SpO_2 as baseline if it is within normal range.	Used to compare future assessments of oxygen saturation.
2. Compare SpO_2 with clients's previous baseline and normal SpO_2. Note use of oxygen therapy.	Allows nurse to assess for change in client's condition and presence of respiratory alteration.
3. **Unexpected outcomes** that may occur include:	
➤ Client's SaO_2 is less than 90%.	Client may demonstrate signs and symptoms of hypoxemia and require immediate medical intervention to increase SpO_2.
➤ Pulse waveform/intensity display is weak.	Client may have compromised cardiac status or decreased peripheral blood flow. Locate different peripheral vascular bed, and reposition pulse oximeter probe. Assess apical and radial pulse to evaluate cardiovascular status.
RECORDING AND REPORTING	
1. Record SpO_2 on vital sign flowsheet or nurses' notes, indicating type and amount of oxygen therapy used by client during assessment. Also record any signs and symptoms of oxygen desaturation in narrative form in nurses' notes.	Vital sign measurement should be recorded promptly on flowsheet to avoid omissions from record. Oxygen therapy affects SpO_2.
2. Report abnormal findings to nurse in charge or physician.	Abnormalities may require immediate implementation of therapy. Assessment of oxygen saturation after administration of specific therapies should be documented in narrative form in nurses' notes.
3. Correlate SpO_2 with SaO_2 obtained from arterial blood gas measurements if available.	Documents reliability of noninvasive assessment.
4. Record in nurses' notes client's use of continuous or intermittent pulse oximetry.	Documents use of equipment for third-party payors.

FOLLOW-UP ACTIVITIES

1. For oxygen saturation below normal expected range, the nurse acts by:
   a. Assisting the client to semi-Fowler's or high-Fowler's position (unless contraindicated).
   b. Verifying appropriate route and amount of oxygen delivery if client receiving oxygen therapy.
   c. Implementing measures to reduce client's energy consumption by avoiding unnecessary activity, anxiety, and emotional stress.
2. Evaluate client's SpO_2 when awake and asleep, since oxygen desaturation frequently occurs in the sleeping compromised client.
3. Periodic arterial blood gases may be needed to validate oximetry reading.
4. Keep oximeter plugged in to keep battery pack charged in the event of portable use.
5. If SpO_2 is abnormal or intensity display weak, repeat measurement on alternative site or use another sensor.

• • • • •

Special Considerations

- Clients who smoke cigarettes or use nicotine gum may have reduced peripheral circulation, which can make monitoring difficult and reduce accuracy of pulse oximetry monitor.
- For clients who have peripheral vascular disease or Raynaud's syndrome or who simply have cold hands, the nurse may have difficulty in obtaining oximetry readings; an alternative site should be considered.
- Decreased pH, increased temperature, and increased $PaCO_2$ cause oxyhemoglobin curve to shift to right, resulting in lower saturation for the same PaO_2. Conversely, elevated pH, low temperature, decreased 2,3-diphosphoglycerate (DPG), and decreased $PaCO_2$ shift curve to left, resulting in higher saturation at lower PaO_2 (Schnapp and Cohen, 1990).
- Skin under oximetry probes during continuous pulse oximetry monitoring should be inspected routinely for alterations in skin integrity.

Teaching Considerations

- Teach client significance of monitoring oxygen saturation.
- Teach client signs and symptoms of hypoxemia: headache, somnolence, confusion, dusky color, shortness of breath, dyspnea.
- Teach client effect of high-risk behaviors, such as cigarette smoking, on oxygen saturation.

Pediatric Considerations

- Infant and toddler sensors attached to adhesive sensor pads are available and conform to digits, palm of hand, and sole of foot.
- Earlobe and bridge-of-nose sensors are not used for infants and toddlers.

Gerontologic Considerations

- Identifying an acceptable pulse oximeter probe site may be difficult on older adults because of likelihood of peripheral vascular disease, decreased CO_2, cold-induced vasoconstriction, and anemia.

Home Care Considerations

- Pulse oximetry is used in home care to noninvasively monitor oxygen therapy or changes in oxygen therapy.

CRITICAL THINKING EXERCISES

1. An unlicensed assistive care giver obtains routine vital signs and reports a BP of 94/70 and a right radial pulse of 114 which "skips around." What actions should the nurse take when receiving this report?
2. A 78-year-old postoperative client complains of dizziness. Vital signs are: BP 100/70, apical pulse 98 with 6 beat pulse deficit, RR 20, tympanic temperature of 99.6° F, and CVP of 4 cm H_2O. List the nursing diagnoses for this client in priority order. What medical and nursing interventions should the nurse anticipate?
3. A client arrives at the ambulatory clinic complaining of flulike symptoms. A nursing history reveals a two-pack-per-day smoking habit. Physical assessment reveals adventitious breath sounds and cyanotic nail beds. What vital signs will be affected and what abnormal values should the nurse expect?
4. A 21-year-old client with history of epilepsy is admitted to the ambulatory surgical unit following hemorrhoidectomy. An IV is in place in the right antecubital fossa. How should vital signs be obtained during the admission assessment?
5. A nursing assistant obtains a BP of 150/100 on an African-American man with a history of renal insufficiency. The nurse reevaluates the BP and obtains 138/86. What could explain the difference in the two measurements? What actions should the nurse take?

REFERENCES

American Heart Association: *Recommendations for human blood pressure determination by sphygmomanometers,* Dallas, 1988, The Association.

Joint National Committee on Detection, Evaluation, and Treatment of High Blood Pressure: The fifth report of the Joint National Committee on Detection, Evaluation, and Treatment of High Blood Pressure, *Arch Intern Med* 153:154-183, January 1993.

Banasik J, Broderson M: The effect of lateral position on CVP, *Heart Lung* 23:296, 1991.

Burke MB, Walsh MB: *Gerontologic nursing,* St Louis, 1992, Mosby.

Eoff M, Joyce B: Temperature measurments in children, *Amer J Nurs* 81(12):1010, 1981.

Fulmer T, Degutis LC: Elderly patients in the emergency department, *Clin Issues Crit Care Nurs* 3(1):89, 1992.

Graves RD, Markarian MF: Three-minute time interval when using an oral mercury-in-glass thermometer with or without J-temp sheaths, *Nurs Res* 29:323, 1980.

Hollerbach AD, et al.: Accuracy of radial pulse assessment by length of counting interval, *Heart Lung* 19:258, May 1990.

Holtzclaw B: The febrile response in critical care: State of the science, *Heart Lung* 21(5):482, 1992.

Mountcastle VB: *Medical physiology,* vol 2, ed 14, St Louis, 1980, Mosby.

Neff J et al: Effect of respiratory rate, respiratory depth and open versus closed mouth breathing on sublingual temperature, *Res Nurs Health,* 12:195, 1992.

Pontious S, et al: Accuracy and reliability of temperature measurement by instrument and site, *J Pediat Nurs* 9(2):114-123, 1994.

Schnapp LM, Cohen NH: Pulse oximetry: Uses and abuses, *Chest* 98:1244, 1990.

Stephen SB, Sexton PR: Neonatal axillary temperatures: Increases in readings over time. *Neonatal Network* 5(6):25-28, 1987.

Thomas SA, et al: Nursing blood pressure research, 1980-1990: A bio-psycho-social perspective, *Image: J of Nurs Scholarship* 25(2):157-164, 1993.

Urden LD, Lough ME, Stacy KM: Priorities in critical care nursing, ed 2, St Louis, 1995, Mosby.

Wong DL: *Whaley and Wong's nursing care of infants and children,* ed 5, St Louis, 1995, Mosby.

Wold G: *Basic geriatric nursing,* St Louis, 1993, Mosby.

CHAPTER 11

Physical Examination and Health Assessment

OBJECTIVES

Mastery of content in this chapter will enable the nurse to:

- Define key terms.
- Discuss purposes of physical assessment.
- Describe the techniques used with each physical assessment skill.
- Describe the proper position for the client during each phase of the examination.
- Discuss the importance of understanding cultural diversity when assessing clients.
- List techniques used to promote the client's physical and psychological comfort during an examination.
- Make environmental preparations before an examination.
- Identify information to collect from the nursing history before an examination.
- Discuss normal physical findings in a young and middle-age adult compared with those for an older adult.
- Discuss ways to incorporate health teaching into an examination.
- Identify self-screening examinations commonly performed by clients.
- Successfully complete a physical examination of each major body system.
- Document assessment findings on a physical examination form.

KEY TERMS

Accommodation reflex
Alopecia
Anemia
Atrophy
Auscultation
Bronchophony
Bruit
Buccal
Carcinoma
Cardiac
Cerumen
Conjunctiva
Consensual light reflex
Costovertebral angle (CVA) tenderness
Crackles
Cyanosis
Dorsum
Echophony
Edema

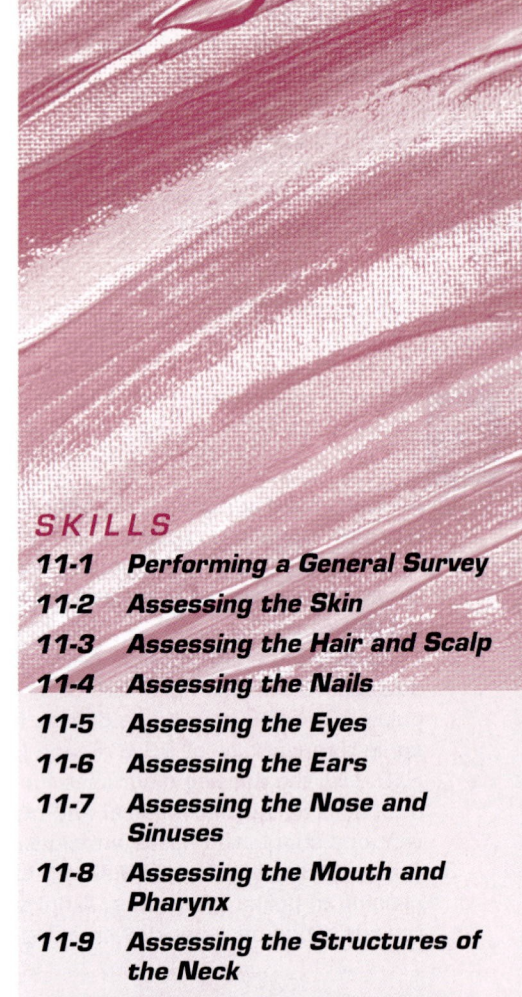

SKILLS

11-1 Performing a General Survey
11-2 Assessing the Skin
11-3 Assessing the Hair and Scalp
11-4 Assessing the Nails
11-5 Assessing the Eyes
11-6 Assessing the Ears
11-7 Assessing the Nose and Sinuses
11-8 Assessing the Mouth and Pharynx
11-9 Assessing the Structures of the Neck
11-10 Assessing the Thorax and Lungs
11-11 Assessing the Heart and Vascular System
11-12 Assessing the Breasts
11-13 Assessing the Abdomen
11-14 Assessing the Female Genitalia
11-15 Assessing the Male Genitalia
11-16 Assessing the Rectum and Anus
11-17 Assessing the Musculoskeletal System
11-18 Assessing the Neurological System

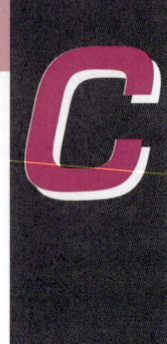

Erythema
Exophthalmos
Friction rub
Gait
Heave
Hirsutism
Hyperpigmentation
Inspection
Integument
Intercostal spaces
Introitus
Lunula
Melanin
Mucopurulent
Nares
Ocular
Olfaction
Orthostatic hypotension
Otitis media
Ototoxic
Pallor
Palpation
Palpebral
Percussion
PERRLA
Pleura
Point of maximal impulse (PMI)
Pruritus
Sebaceous glands
Speculum
Thrill
Thrombophlebitis
Tinnitus
Tuberculosis
Valgus
Varus
Whispered pectoriloquy

Nurses are most often the first to detect changes in clients' conditions, regardless of the setting. For this reason the ability to think critically and interpret the meaning of client behaviors and presenting physiological changes is very important. The skills of physical assessment and examination are powerful tools with which to detect subtle as well as obvious changes in a client's health.

A complete health assessment involves a detailed review of a client's condition, with the nurse collecting a nursing history and performing a behavioral and physical examination. The health history is a lengthy interview with a client to gather subjective data about any presenting conditions. A physical examination is a head-to-toe review of each body system that offers objective information about the client. The client's condition and response affect the extent of the examination. Accuracy of a physical assessment improves clinical judgments (Table 11-1). Once data are gathered, the nurse groups significant findings into patterns of data that reveal actual or potential nursing diagnoses. Each abnormal finding directs the nurse to gather additional data. Information gathered during an initial assessment and examination provides the baseline for a client's functional abilities and serves as a comparison for future assessment findings. In addition, the information helps the nurse select the best nursing measures to manage the client's health problems.

Inspection, palpation, percussion, auscultation, and olfaction are examination techniques that enable the nurse to collect a broad range of physical data about clients. **Inspection** is the process of observation. It is a visual examination of body parts to detect normal characteristics or significant physical signs. An experienced nurse learns to make several observations, almost simultaneously, while becoming very perceptive of early warnings of abnormalities. The secret is to always pay attention to the client. Watch all movements and look carefully at any body part being inspected. It is important to recognize normal physical characteristics of clients of all ages before trying to distinguish abnormal findings. Experience is needed to recognize normal variations among clients, as well as ranges of normal in an individual. An examiner methodically takes the time necessary to carefully inspect body parts. Inspection is the easiest assessment skill to perform, but if an examiner becomes hurried, significant signs may be overlooked and incorrect conclusions may be made about a client's condition. Good lighting and full exposure of body parts are essential for inspection. Each area is inspected for size, shape, color, symmetry, position, and the presence of abnormalities. If possible, each area inspected is compared with the same area on the opposite side of the body. When necessary, use additional light, such as a penlight, to inspect body cavities such as the mouth and throat. *Do not hurry. Pay attention to detail.*

Table 11-1 Development of Individualized Nursing Diagnoses

Assessment Method	Findings	Patterns	Nursing Diagnosis
Inspection of skin	Skin along sacral area is intact. There is 3 cm area of redness around coccyx; skin blanches on palpation. No skin lesions are observed.	There is pressure area around coccyx.	Risk for impaired skin integrity
Palpation of skin	Skin is moist from diaphoresis. There is tenderness to palpation around sacral area. There is good skin turgor.	Skin moisture promotes maceration.	
Historical data	Client suffered fractured left leg. Client is immobilized due to left leg traction.	Continued pressure is exerted over sacrum.	

Palpation involves use of the sense of touch. Through palpation the hands can make delicate and sensitive measurements of specific physical signs, including resistance, resilience, roughness, texture, temperature, and mobility. Palpation is often used with or after visual inspection. The nurse uses different parts of the hand to detect specific characteristics. For example, the dorsum (back) of the hand is sensitive to temperature variations. The pads of the fingertips detect subtle changes in texture, shape, size, consistency, and pulsatility of body parts. The palm of the hand is especially sensitive to vibration. The nurse measures position, consistency, and turgor by lightly grasping the body part with the fingertips.

The client should be relaxed and positioned comfortably because muscle tension during palpation impairs the ability to palpate correctly. Asking the client to take slow, deep breaths enhances muscle relaxation. Tender areas are palpated last. The nurse asks the client to point out more sensitive areas and notes any nonverbal signs of discomfort. Clients appreciate warm hands, short fingernails, and a gentle approach. Palpation may be either light or deep and is controlled by the amount of pressure applied with the fingers or hand (Fig. 11-1). Light palpation always precedes deep palpation. The nurse must not palpate without considering the client's condition, the area being palpated, and the reason for using palpation. For example, a client admitted to the emergency room following an automobile accident will be examined for obvious external as well as potential internal injury. The nurse should consider the factors surrounding the client's injury and inspect the chest wall carefully before performing any palpation around the area of the ribs.

The nurse applies tactile pressure slowly, gently, and deliberately. The nurse's hand is placed on the part to be examined and depressed about 1 cm (½ inch). Tender areas are examined further. The sensation of touch is best preserved with light intermittent pressure. After light palpation, deeper palpation may be used to examine the condition of organs. The nurse depresses the area being examined approximately 2 cm (1 inch). Caution is the rule. Bimanual palpation involves one hand placed over the other while pressure is applied. The upper hand exerts downward pressure as the other hand feels the subtle characteristics of underlying organs and masses. A student nurse should not attempt deep palpation without the assistance of a qualified instructor to ensure that the client does not suffer internal injury.

Percussion involves tapping the body with the fingertips to evaluate the size, borders, and consistency of body organs and to discover fluid in body cavities. It requires much skill. In combination with other assessment findings, percussion denotes location, size, and density of underlying structures. The nurse strikes the body's surface with a finger to create a vibration that travels through body tissues. Sound waves are heard as percussion tones arising from vibrations 4 to 6 cm deep in body tissues (Seidel et al., 1995). The character of sound depends on the density of underlying tissues. For example, the normal lung transmits sounds with high intensity and low pitch, whereas the solid liver transmits a high-pitched sound of soft intensity.

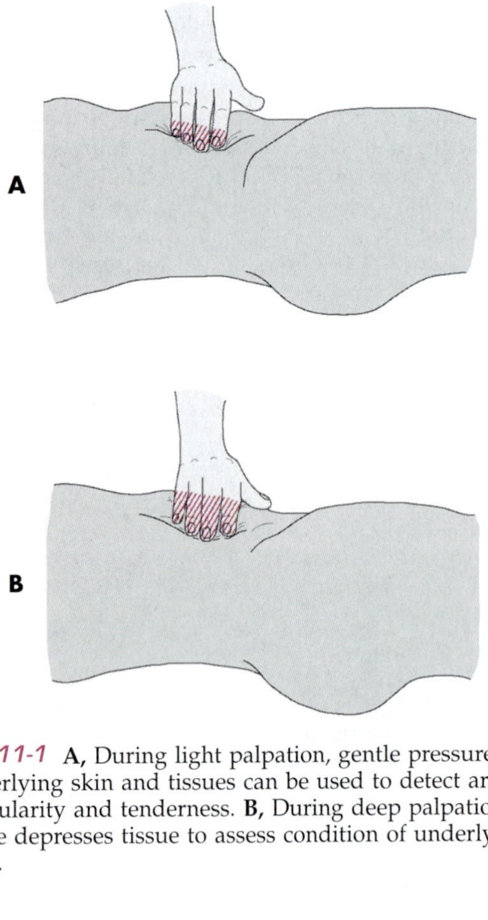

Fig. 11-1 **A,** During light palpation, gentle pressure against underlying skin and tissues can be used to detect areas of irregularity and tenderness. **B,** During deep palpation, nurse depresses tissue to assess condition of underlying organs.

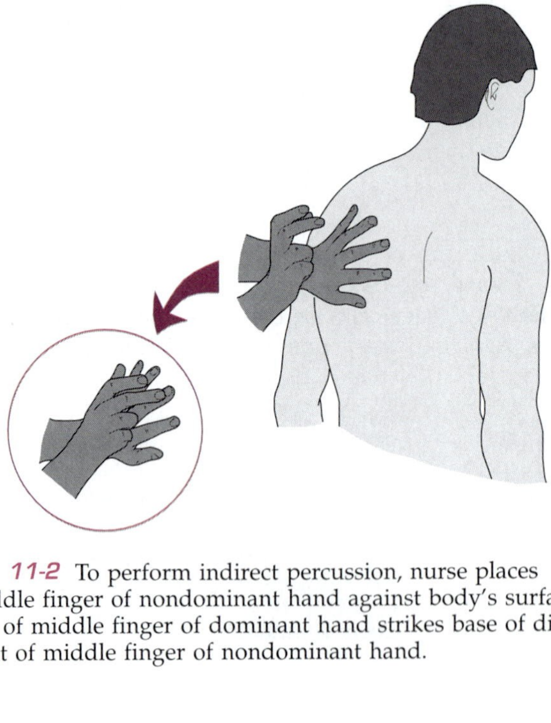

Fig. 11-2 To perform indirect percussion, nurse places middle finger of nondominant hand against body's surface. Tip of middle finger of dominant hand strikes base of distal joint of middle finger of nondominant hand.

Table 11-2 Sounds Produced by Percussion

Sound	Intensity	Pitch	Duration	Quality	Common Location
Tympany	Loud	High	Moderate	Drumlike	Enclosed, air-containing space; gastric air bubble, puffed-out cheek
Resonance	Moderate to loud	Low	Long	Hollow	Normal lung
Hyperresonance	Very loud	Very low	Longer than resonance	Booming	Emphysematous lung
Dullness	Soft to moderate	High	Moderate	Thudlike	Liver, spleen, gallbladder
Flatness	Soft	High	Short	Flat	Muscle

There are two methods of percussion: direct and indirect. The direct method involves striking the body surface directly with one or two fingers. The indirect technique is performed by placing the middle finger of the examiner's nondominant hand (pleximeter hand) firmly against the body surface. With palm and fingers remaining off the skin, the tip of the middle finger of the dominant hand (plexor hand) strikes the base of the distal joint of the pleximeter (Fig. 11-2). The examiner uses a quick, sharp stroke with the plexor finger, keeping the forearm stationary. The wrist remains relaxed to deliver the proper blow. Once the finger has struck, the wrist snaps back. If the blow is not sharp, if the pleximeter hand is held loosely, or if the palm rests on the body surface, the sound is dampened or softened and the nurse cannot detect the presence of underlying structures. A light, quick blow produces the clearest sounds. Table 11-2 describes the five different percussion sounds.

Auscultation is listening to sounds produced by the body. Some sounds can be heard with the unaided ear, although most sounds are heard only with a stethoscope. To auscultate correctly, listen in a quiet environment. Listen for the presence of sound as well as its characteristics. It is important for a student to recognize normal sounds, such as the passage of blood through an artery, heart sounds, and movement of air through the lungs, to detect abnormal sounds. The nurse is more successful in auscultation after knowing what type of sounds arise from each body structure and the location in which they can most easily be heard. Likewise, the nurse becomes familiar with areas that normally do not emit sounds.

To auscultate correctly, the nurse needs good hearing acuity, a good stethoscope, and knowledge of how to use the stethoscope properly. Nurses with hearing disorders should purchase stethoscopes with greater sound amplification or ask colleagues to check findings through auscultation, or both. Always place the stethoscope directly on client's naked skin because clothing obscures and changes sound.

Through auscultation the nurse notes the following characteristics of sound:

Frequency—Number of sound wave cycles generated per second by a vibrating object. The higher the frequency, the higher the pitch of a sound and vice versa.

Loudness—Amplitude of a sound wave. Auscultated sounds are described as *loud* or *soft*.

Quality—Sounds of similar frequency and loudness from different sources. Terms such as *blowing* or *gurgling* describe quality of sound.

Duration—Length of time that sound vibrations last. Duration of sound is short, medium, or long. Layers of soft tissue dampen the duration of sounds from deep internal organs.

A nurse cannot be successful at auscultation without knowing how to use a stethoscope properly. Chapter 10 describes the parts of the acoustic stethoscope and use of

EXERCISES TO INCREASE FAMILIARITY WITH STETHOSCOPE

1. Place earpieces in both ears with tips of earpieces turned toward the face. *Lightly* blow into the stethoscope's diaphragm. Again place earpieces in both ears, this time with ends turned toward the back of the head. *Lightly* blow into the stethoscope's diaphragm. The earpiece should follow the contour of the ear canal. After learning the right fit for the loudest sound, wear the stethoscope the same way each time.
2. Put the stethoscope on and *lightly blow* into the diaphragm. If sound is barely audible, *lightly* blow into the bell. Sound is carried through only one part of the chestpiece at a time. If sound is greatly amplified through the diaphragm, the diaphragm is in position for use. If sound is barely audible through the diaphragm, the bell is in position for use.
3. Listen while moving the diaphragm lightly over the hair on your arm. The bristling sound created by rubbing of hair against the diaphragm mimics a sound heard in the lungs. Also, always be sure to keep the diaphragm stationary and firm to reduce extraneous sounds.
4. Place the stethoscope on and gently tap tubing. The sound can distract from being able to hear sounds created by body organs. Always avoid stretching or moving the tubing; it should hang freely.

Table 11-3 Assessment of Characteristic Odors

Odor	Site or Source	Potential Causes
Alcohol	Oral cavity	Ingestion of alcohol; diabetes
Ammonia	Urine	Urinary tract infection
Body odor	Skin, particularly in areas where body parts rub together (e.g., under arms, breasts)	Poor hygiene, excess perspiration (hyperhidrosis), foul-smelling perspiration (bromidrosis)
Feces	Wound site	Wound abscess
	Vomitus	Bowel obstruction
	Rectal area	Fecal incontinence
Foul-smelling stools in infant	Stool	Malabsorption syndrome
Halitosis	Oral cavity	Poor dental and oral hygiene, gum disease
Sweet, fruity ketones	Oral cavity	Diabetic acidosis
Stale urine	Skin	Uremic acidosis
Sweet, heavy, thick odor	Draining wound	*Pseudomonas* (bacterial) infection
Musty odor	Casted body part	Infection inside cast
Fetid, sweet odor	Tracheostomy or mucous secretions	Infection of bronchial tree (*Pseudomonas* bacteria)

the bell and diaphragm. Useful exercises for the nurse to practice to become more familiar with a stethoscope are described in the box on p. 283.

The final skill a nurse may use during assessment is **olfaction.** Certain alterations in body function create characteristic body odors (Table 11-3). The sense of smell can detect abnormalities that go unrecognized by any other means.

This chapter discusses physical assessment techniques for each body system. A head-to-toe organizational format is presented to provide guidelines for the nurse wishing to perform a total physical examination. Skills for assessing each body system describe step-by-step assessment procedures, equipment necessary for examiniation, methods for preparing clients, normal findings, potential signs and symptoms of system alterations, and nursing diagnoses resulting from the nurse's findings. Because the skills of physical assessment involve collecting assessment data, nursing diagnoses for each skill follow the evaluation.

PREEXAMINATION PREPARATIONS

Proper preparation of the environment, equipment, and client ensures a smooth physical examination with few interruptions. A disorganized approach when preparing for a physical examination can cause errors and incomplete findings.

Preparing the Environment

To promote client comfort and ensure an efficient examination, the examination room should have the following features: privacy for the client (a separate examination room; curtains or dividers to enclose the client's bed; in the home, a bedroom can be used); a warm, comfortable temperature; proper examination clothing for the client; adequate direct lighting without distortion from shadows; control of outside noises; precautions to prevent interruptions by visitors or other health care personnel; and a bed or table set at examiner's waist level.

Preparing the Equipment

The nurse uses a variety of equipment for a physical examination (see box on p. 285). To facilitate the examination, the equipment should be readily accessible, in proper working order (check batteries and light of ophthalmoscope), and warmed (if possible, run warm water over speculum blades and rub diaphragm of stethoscope briskly between hands before applying to client's skin).

Preparing the Client

To ensure an accurate assessment and physical examination, the client must be properly prepared physically and psychologically. A tense, anxious client will not be able to go through many of the physical maneuvers required during an examination or to cooperate with the nurse's instructions. To prepare the client properly, the nurse:

1. Provides for client's physical comfort by allowing the opportunity to empty the bowel or bladder (a good time to collect needed specimens).
2. Provides privacy while the client changes into a gown (allows for accessibility of body parts) and gives the client time to undress, assisting if necessary. If the examination is limited to certain body systems (e.g., head and neck), it may be unnecessary for the client to undress.
3. Drapes body parts that need not be exposed.
4. Eliminates drafts, controls room temperature, and provides warm blankets.
5. Helps the client assume proper positions during the examination so that body parts are accessible and the client stays comfortable (Table 11-4). The nurse adjusts drapes accordingly. A client's ability to assume positions will depend on physical strength and degree of wellness. Some positions are embar-

EQUIPMENT AND SUPPLIES FOR PHYSICAL EXAMINATION

- Cotton applicators
- Cytobrush
- Disposable pad
- Drapes
- Eye chart (e.g., Snellen chart)
- Flashlight and spotlight
- Forms (e.g., physical, laboratory)
- Gloves (clean)
- Goniometer
- Gown for client
- Water-soluble lubricant
- Ophthalmoscope
- Otoscope
- Glass microscope slides and slip covers
- Paper towels
- Percussion hammer
- Ruler (regular and centimeter)
- Safety pin
- Scale with height measurement rod
- Specimen containers
- Sphygmomanometer and cuff
- Stethoscope
- Swabs or sponge forceps
- Tape measure
- Thermometer
- Tissues
- Tongue depressor
- Tuning fork
- Vaginal speculum
- Wristwatch with second hand or digital display

rassing; keep a client in position no longer than is necessary.

6. Minimizes client's anxiety and fear by conveying an open, receptive, and professional approach. The nurse thoroughly explains what will be done, what the client should expect to feel, and how the client can cooperate.
7. Uses simple terms when describing steps of the examination.
8. Uses relaxed voice tone and facial expressions to put client at ease.
9. Encourages the client to ask questions and mention discomfort felt during the examination.
10. Has a third person of the client's gender in the examination room during examination of genitalia. Third person ensures that the examiner will behave ethically.
11. Paces or times examination process according to the client's physical and emotional tolerance.

It is difficult to examine clients in beds or on stretchers. Special examination tables make clients easily accessible and help them assume special positions. The tables are high and narrow, so the nurse must carefully assist clients so that they do not fall while getting on and off the tables. A confused, combative, or uncooperative client should not be left on an examination table without supervision. A client can be made more comfortable by raising the head of the table 30 degrees and by offering a small pillow.

PHYSICAL ASSESSMENT OF VARIOUS AGE-GROUPS

The nurse uses different interview styles and approaches for examining and interviewing clients of different age-groups. The following tips will assist in data collection during physical examination:

Children and Adolescents

1. Routine examinations of children have a focus on health promotion and illness prevention, particularly for care of well children with competent parenting and no serious health problems (Wong, 1995). The focus is on growth and development, sensory screening, dental examination, and behavioral assessment.
2. Children who are chronically ill, disabled, in foster care, or foreign-born adopted may require additional examination visits.
3. When obtaining histories of infants and children, gather all or part of information from parents or guardians.
4. Parents may think they are being tested by the examiner. Offer support during examination and do not pass judgment.
5. Call children by their first name, and address parents as "Mr. and Mrs. Brown" rather than by first names.
6. Open-ended questions often allow parents to share more information and to describe more of the child's problems.
7. Interviewing older children allows the nurse to observe parent-child interactions.
8. Older children often can provide details about their health history and severity of symptoms.
9. Adolescents tend to respond best when treated as adults and individuals.
10. The adolescent has a right to confidentiality. After talking with parents about historical information, the nurse speaks alone with the adolescent.

Older Adults

11. Do not stereotype aging clients. Most are able to adapt to change and learn about their health.
12. Be patient, relaxed, and unhurried with older adults.
13. Provide adequate space for an examination, particularly if the client uses a mobility aid.
14. Plan the history and examination; taking into account the older adult's energy level, physical limitations, pace, and adaptability. More than one session may be needed to complete the assessment (Lueckenotte, 1996).
15. Measure performance under the most favorable of

Table 11-4 Positions for Examination

Position	Areas Assessed	Rationale	Limitations
Sitting 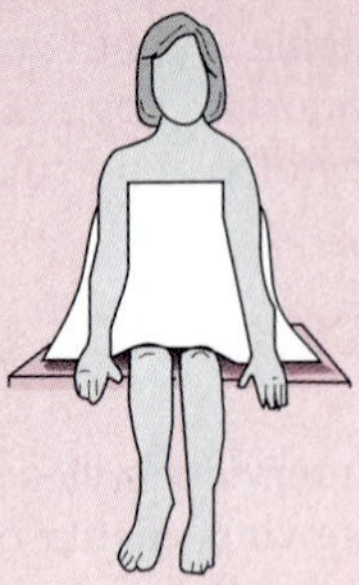	Head and neck, back, posterior thorax and lungs, anterior thorax and lungs, breasts, axillae, heart, vital signs, and upper extremities	Sitting upright provides full expansion of lungs and provides better visualization of symmetry of upper body parts.	Physically weakened client may be unable to sit. Examiner should use supine position with head of bed elevated instead.
Supine 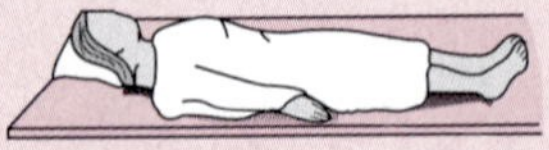	Head and neck, anterior thorax and lungs, breasts, axillae, heart, abdomen, extremities, pulses	This is most normally relaxed position. It provides easy access to pulse sites.	If client becomes short of breath easily, examiner may need to raise head of bed.
Dorsal recumbent 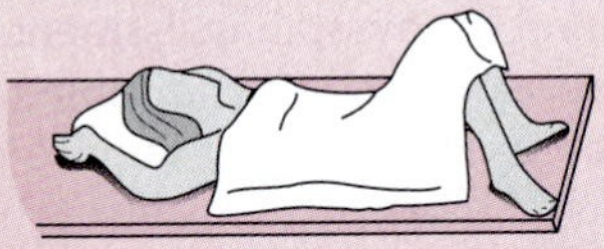	Head and neck, anterior thorax and lungs, breasts, axillae, heart, abdomen	Position is used for abdominal assessment because it promotes relaxation of abdominal muscles.	Clients with painful disorders are more comfortable with knees flexed.
Lithotomy* 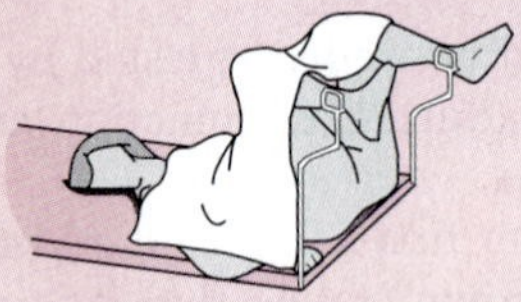	Female genitalia and genital tract	This position provides maximal exposure of genitalia and facilitates insertion of vaginal speculum.	Lithotomy position is embarrassing and uncomfortable, so examiner minimizes time that client spends in it. Client is kept well draped.
Sims' 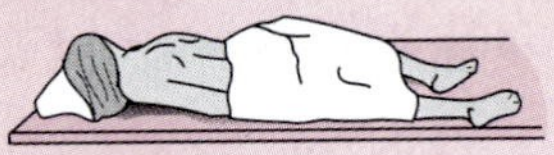	Rectum and vagina	Flexion of hip and knee improves exposure of rectal area.	Joint deformities may hinder client's ability to bend hip and knee.
Prone 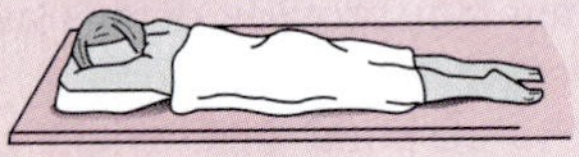	Musculoskeletal system	This position is used only to assess extension of hip joint.	This position is poorly tolerated in clients with respiratory difficulties.
Lateral recumbent 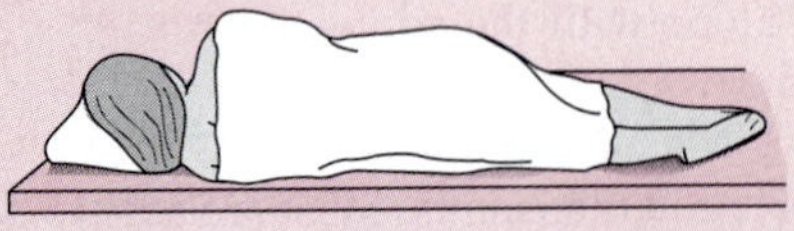	Heart	This position aids in detecting murmurs.	This position is poorly tolerated in clients with respiratory difficulties.
Knee-chest* 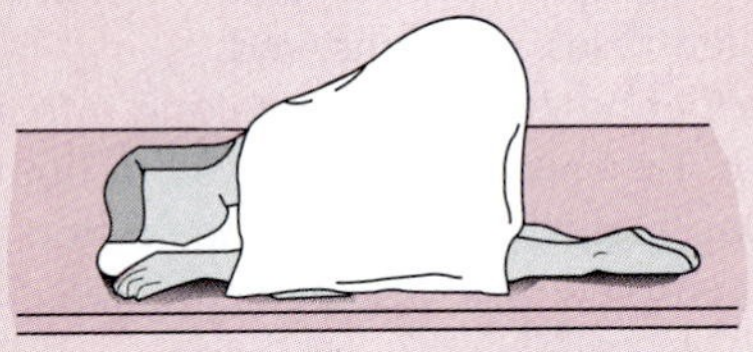	Rectum	This position provides maximal exposure of rectal area.	This position is embarrassing and uncomfortable.

*Clients with arthritis or other joint deformities may be unable to assume this position.

conditions. Take advantage of natural opportunities for assessment (e.g., during bathing, grooming, and mealtime) (Lueckenotte, 1996).

16. Sequence an examination to keep position changes to a minimum. Be efficient throughout the examination to limit client movement.
17. Be sure an examination of an older adult includes review of mental status.

GUIDELINES

1. Set priorities for assessment procedures based on a client's presenting signs and symptoms or health care needs. For example, a client who develops sudden shortness of breath should first undergo an assessment of the lungs and thorax. If a client is acutely ill, the nurse may choose to assess only the involved body systems. The nurse's judgment is needed to ensure that an examination is relevant and inclusive.
2. Use a systematic process when performing an examination so that important assessments are not deleted. A head-to-toe approach includes all body systems, beginning with the head and neck structures and ending with assessment of musculoskeletal and neurological function. Follow the sequence of inspection, palpation, percussion, and auscultation (except for abdominal assessment). This sequence ensures a comprehensive assessment and improves accuracy of findings.
3. Allow the client to be an active participant. Clients are usually knowledgeable about their physical condition. Often the client can let the nurse know when certain findings are normal or when actual changes have occurred.
4. Follow standard precautions for infection control. Examination techniques cause the nurse to have contact with body fluids and discharge. When there are breaks in the skin, lesions, or wounds, gloves should be worn during palpation and percussion to reduce contact with microorganisms. If a client has excessive drainage from a wound, the examiner should wear a gown.
5. Organize the examination. Compare both sides of the body for symmetry. If a client becomes fatigued, offer rest periods. Perform painful procedures near the end of the examination.
6. Record quick notes during the examination to avoid keeping the client waiting.
7. Consider client's race, gender, and age. These are three important variables that influence assessment findings and techniques to use.
8. Integrate physical assessment into routine nursing care measures. The nurse learns to use all physical assessment skills during activities such as bathing, administration of medications, or other therapies or while conversing with a client.
9. Respect the cultural differences of clients. A client's health beliefs, use of alternative therapies, nutritional habits, relationships with family, and comfort with close physical contact during an examination must be considered (see box above).
10. Integrate health education into physical assessment activities. Throughout the examination there are "teachable moments" when the nurse can share findings and educate clients about health promotion.
11. Record summary of the examination in specific anatomical and scientific terms and in the sequence that findings are gathered. Use commonly accepted medical abbreviations to keep notes brief and concise.

CULTURAL AWARENESS OF TOUCH DURING PHYSICAL EXAMINATION

Physical contact with a client can convey a variety of meanings, depending on the client's cultural background. Consider these guidelines, but remember that each client is an individual and may respond differently.

Hispanics
- Highly tactile
- Very modest (men and women)
- May ask for health care provider of same gender
- Women may refuse to be examined by male health care provider

Asians/Pacific Islanders
- Avoid touching (patting head is strictly taboo)
- Touching during an argument equals loss of control (shame)
- Public display of affection toward members of same gender is permissible (but not toward members of opposite gender)

African-Americans
- May not like to be touched without permission
- May exercise level of distrust or caution initially in care provider

Native Americans
- Shake hands lightly
- May not like to be touched without permission
- Nonverbal communication is important

Modified from Lueckenotte A: *Gerontologic nursing*, St Louis, 1996, Mosby; Seidel HM et al: *Mosby's guide to physical examination*, ed 3, St Louis, 1995, Mosby.

SKILL 11-1 Performing a General Survey

The general survey begins a review of the client's primary health problems. It includes assessment of the client's vital signs, height and weight, general behavior, and appearance. Data for the survey are initially obtained as the nurse collects the nursing history. The survey provides information about characteristics of an illness, a client's hygiene and body image, emotional state, recent changes in weight, and developmental status. If abnormalities or signs of problems are found, the nurse can direct attention to specific body systems later in the examination. The survey can reveal important information about the client's behavior that can influence how the nurse communicates instructions to the client and conducts portions of the examination.

EQUIPMENT

- Stethoscope
- Sphygmomanometer and cuff
- Thermometer
- Standing platform scale or stretcher scale
- Table model or basket scale (infants only)
- Digital watch or wristwatch with second hand
- Tape measure

DELEGATION CONSIDERATIONS

The general survey requires problem solving and knowledge application unique to a professional nurse. Unlicensed assistive personnel may monitor assessment data (e.g., measure height and weight, I&O, and vital signs) and report a client's subjective signs and symptoms. All monitoring data must be reported to an RN.

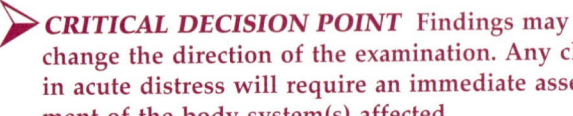

STEPS	RATIONALE
ASSESSMENT	
1. Note if client is in any acute distress: difficulty breathing, pain, anxiety. If such signs are present, defer general survey until later.	Signs establish priorities regarding what part of the examination to conduct first.
CRITICAL DECISION POINT Findings may change the direction of the examination. Any client in acute distress will require an immediate assessment of the body system(s) affected.	
2. Determine client's primary language.	May require assistance from interpreter or family member.
3. Reconfirm (after reviewing history) primary reason client has sought health care.	Keeps examination focused on client to ensure that client's expectations are addressed.
4. Ask if client knows own normal pulse rate and blood pressure at rest.	Provides means to compare nurse's assessment findings to detect change.
5. Consider factors or conditions that may normally alter reading of vital signs.	See Chapter 10.
6. Ask what client's normal height and weight are.	Client's response may reveal degree of satisfaction with weight and size.
7. Determine if sudden gain or loss in weight has occurred, amount of weight change, and period of time in which it occurred.	Sudden loss in weight can indicate presence of serious disease or significant change in dietary habits and exercise.
8. Review client's past fluid intake and output (I&O) records.	Fluid and electrolyte balance maintains health and function in all body systems. Intake includes all liquids taken orally, by feeding tube, and parenterally. Liquid output includes urine, diarrheal stool, vomitus, drainage from gastric suction, and drainage from postsurgical tubes, such as chest tubes or Jackson-Pratt drains.
9. Assess if client has recently been dieting or following exercise program.	Regular strenuous exercise and changes in dietary habits promote weight loss.

STEPS	RATIONALE
10. Determine client's type of diet and who in family does cooking.	Certain diets can result in serious nutrient losses. Client may require assistance from family member or friend as a result of illness.
11. Assess client's general perceptions about personal health.	Nurse's assessment of client's general appearance coupled with client's own perceptions may reveal specific problem areas.

PLANNING

STEPS	RATIONALE
1. **Expected outcomes** following completion of procedure:	
➤ Client's general level of wellness will be determined.	General survey is a quick overview that often reveals signs and symptoms of potential problems. It helps the nurse adapt the examination to client's needs.
➤ Client's expectations for health care visit and examination are met.	Reason client seeks health care is incorporated into nurse's approach to ensure that all questions are answered and client is prepared as much as possible to accept and understand results and implications of examination.
➤ Client's vital signs will be within average normal range for clients of same age (Chapter 10).	Vital signs are stable.
➤ Client's height and weight will be within desired range for height and weight of client of same age.	Body size is normal.
➤ Client's skinfold thickness will be within normal desired value (50th percentile) for client of same age and size.	Nutritional status is normal.
➤ Client's behaviors or appearance will not demonstrate signs of physical or emotional stress (e.g., unkempt appearance, inappropriate affect, poor posture).	Emotional status is normal.
➤ Client stands upright with parallel alignment of hips and shoulders.	
➤ Client sits with some degree of rounding of shoulders.	
➤ Client walks with arms swinging freely at sides, head and face lead the body. Body movements are purposeful.	Normal posture, gait, and movement are evident.
➤ Client is dressed properly for activity and weather; there is no unpleasant body odor; hair is groomed; skin and nails are clean.	Dress and grooming are appropriate.
➤ Client has no obvious physical injuries or trauma; behavior and self-report demonstrate good eating and sleeping habits and positive self-esteem; client denies use of alcohol or illegal drugs.	No overt clinical indications of abuse.
2. Prepare client:	
a. Explain procedure to client, noting that vital sign and height and weight measurements require individual to assume certain positions.	Understanding promotes client's cooperation.
b. Be sure client removes shoes and any heavy clothing.	Ensures accurate weight measurement.

IMPLEMENTATION

STEPS	RATIONALE
1. Assess temperature, pulse, respiration, and blood pressure.	See Chapter 10.
2. Calibrate scale by setting weight at zero and noting if balance beam registers in middle of mark. Electronic scale with digital display should read "zero" before use.	Calibrated scales ensure accurate measurements.

STEPS	RATIONALE
3. Weigh client (client is able to bear weight):	
a. Ask client to stand on platform facing scale and to remain still (see illustration).	Client's movement causes balance beam to oscillate and may result in inaccurate reading. Electronic scale registers weight once client stops movement.
b. Slowly adjust scale weight until balance beam registers in middle of mark or until digital scale shows a display.	Scale weight used to balance beam is equal to client's weight.
4. Measure height (client is able to bear weight):	
a. Have client remain standing on scale platform, facing toward or away from scale.	
(1) Raise metal rod on back of scale and swing rod over top of client's head. Be sure rod is parallel to floor.	Height is measured by placing smooth, flat surface against crown or vertex of head. Client's position encourages keeping head erect. Erect posture ensures accurate reading.
(2) Instruct client to stand erect, exercising good posture (see illustration). Read height in in/cm (inches/centimeters) as recorded on height scale.	
b. Alternative for measuring height of child in home: attach metal or paper measuring tape perpendicular against wall; have child stand against wall, adjacent to tape; place 1-inch thick book on child's head so that end of book forms right angle with wall; note point of juncture of tape measure and underside of book.	
5. Weigh client (client is unable to bear weight):	
a. Prepare stretcher scale by placing light cloth or paper covering over stretcher platform.	Reduces transmission of microorganisms.
b. Calibrate scale to zero with covering in place.	Covering adds to weight measured on scale.
c. Raise height of client's bed to level of stretcher scale. With one or two assistants, transfer client to scale using proper body mechanics and transfer techniques (Chapters 28 and 29).	Prevents muscular strain on nurse and client during transfer. Prevents client from accidentally falling.
d. Instruct client to be still while weight is measured.	Movement can cause inaccurate reading.

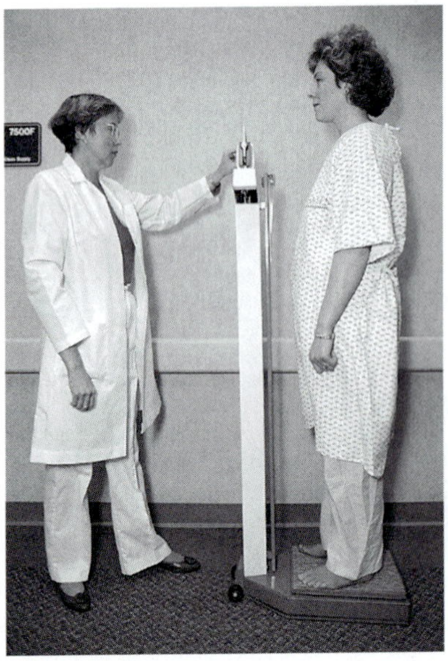

Step 3a Client stands on scale as nurse adjusts balance.

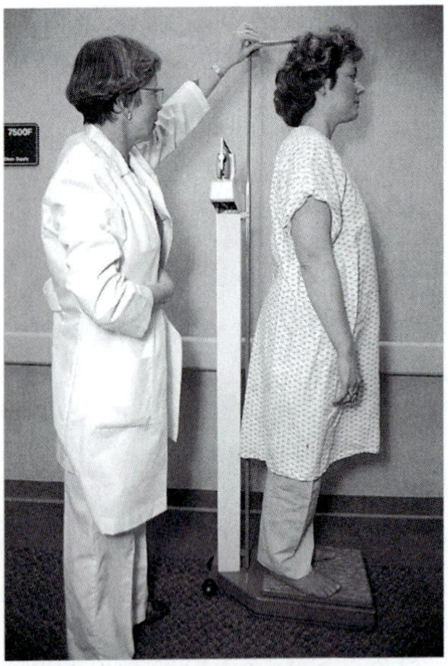

Step 4a[2] Client stands erect during measurement of height.

STEPS	RATIONALE
6. Measure height (client is unable to bear weight):	
a. Position client supine in bed with legs extended and soles of feet supported upright.	
b. With tape measure, determine height from soles of feet to vertex of head.	Height is measurement from vertex of head to soles of feet.
7. Weigh and measure height of infant:	
a. Be sure room temperature is warm.	Infants are weighed nude and are susceptible to temperature fluctuations because of immature thermoregulation.
b. Place light cloth or paper covering on basket or platform.	Reduces transmission of microorganisms.
c. Place unclothed infant in basket or on platform. Hold hand lightly above infant during measurement (see illustration).	Nurse's hand prevents accidental fall from scale without adding extra weight.
d. Note weight in grams (pounds and ounces).	Standard for measurement.
e. Measure infant's length. Place infant supine on paper-covered table. Hold head in midline. Gently grasp knees and extend fully against table. Keep feet in normal flexed position with toes pointed to ceiling. Mark the paper at top of head and heel of feet. Measure between the two points on the paper.	Accurate measurement requires full extension of infant's legs and upright position of head and feet.

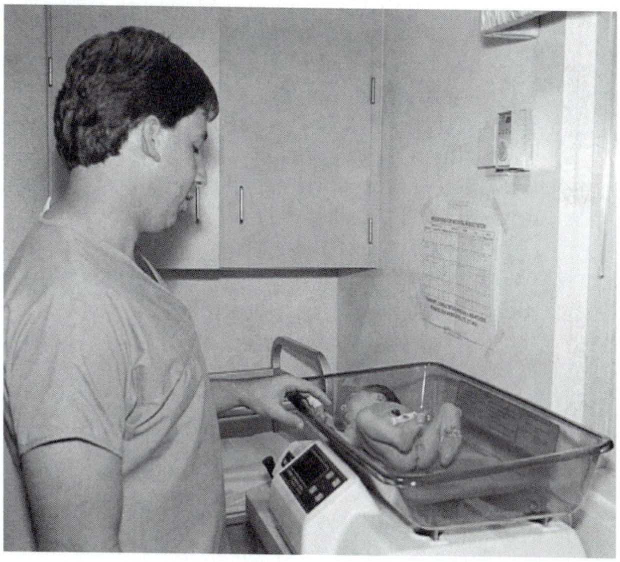

Step 7c Nurse places hand over scale as infant is weighed.

STEPS	RATIONALE
8. Throughout assessment note client's verbal and nonverbal behaviors.	Behaviors may reflect specific physical abnormalities.
9. Assess the following aspects of behavior and appearance:	
a. Gender and race. Note the client's physical features.	Gender influences type of examination performed and manner in which assessments are made. Different physical characteristics and predisposition to illnesses are related to gender and race.
b. Age.	Influences the normal features or characteristics to observe during the examination.
c. Body type (trim and muscular, obese, excessively thin).	Can reflect level of health, age, and lifestyle.
d. Posture. Note alignment of shoulders and hips while client stands and sits. Observe whether the client has a slumped, erect, or bent posture.	May reveal musculoskeletal problem, mood, or presence of pain.
e. Body movements. Are they purposeful? Are there tremors of the extremities? Are any body parts immobile?	May indicate neurological or muscular problem or emotional stress.

STEPS	RATIONALE
f. Gait. Observe **gait** when client walks into room or is at bedside (if ambulatory). Note if movements are coordinated or uncoordinated.	
g. Hygiene and grooming. Note appearance of hair, skin, and nails. Are the client's clothes clean? Note amount and type of cosmetics used.	Grooming may reflect activity level prior to examination, resources available to purchase grooming supplies, client's mood, and self-care practices.
h. Dress. Appropriate for temperature and weather conditions?	May reflect culture, lifestyle, economic status, and personal preferences.
i. Body odor.	May result from physical exercise, poor hygiene, or certain physical ailments. Poor oral hygiene may cause bad breath.
j. Affect and mood. Note if verbal expressions match nonverbal behavior. Note appropriateness to situation.	Reflect client's feelings and emotional status.
k. Speech. Is it understandable and moderately paced? Is there an association with the person's thoughts?	May reflect neurological impairment, injury or impairment of mouth, or differences in dialect and language.
l. Client abuse. Observe client interaction with spouse or partner, older adult child, or care giver. Be alert for indications of fear, hesitancy to report health status, or willingness to let care giver control assessment interview. Does partner or care giver have a history of violence, alcoholism, or drug abuse? Is the person unemployed, ill, or frustrated with caring for client? Note if client has any obvious physical injuries.	Abuse is often first suspected in clients who have suffered obvious physical injury or neglect, show signs of malnutrition, or have bruises on the extremities or trunk. Partners or care givers often have history of abusive or addictive behaviors.
(1) If there is high suspicion of abuse, interview the client in private.	Client is more likely to reveal problems when suspected abuser is absent from room.
CRITICAL DECISION POINT **Nurse must be discrete in how interview is handled. It may be necessary to defer the assessment to a later time, when the partner or care giver is not present. Asking a partner or care giver to leave during an assessment may create an awkward situation.**	
(2) Note the following in a child: blood on underclothing, pain in genital area, difficulty sitting or walking.	These signs may be indicative of child sexual abuse.
(3) Note the following in a female client: injury or trauma inconsistent with reported cause, obvious injuries to face or neck (black eyes, broken nose, lip lacerations, broken teeth, strangulation marks or burns).	These signs may indicate domestic abuse.
(4) Note the following in an older adult: injury or trauma inconsistent with reported cause, bruises on extremities, chafing or excoriation on wrist or legs (restraints), burns, dried blood, prolonged interval between injury and time medical care was sought (Haviland, 1989).	Signs indicative of older adult abuse or neglect are usually first seen by health care providers since clients often fail to report the problem to family or friends.
CRITICAL DECISION POINT **A pattern of findings indicating abuse usually mandates a report to a social service center (refer to own state guidelines). Nurse should obtain immediate consultation with physician, social worker, and other support staff to ensure that client will be able to return to a safer environment.**	

STEPS	RATIONALE
m. Substance abuse. Consider characteristics common to those who abuse alcohol, prescribed medications, or illegal drugs (see the box below). Use a caring and nonjudgmental approach, asking the following questions: Have you ever felt the need to **C**UT DOWN on your drinking or drug use? Have people **A**NNOYED you by criticizing your drinking or drug use? Have you ever felt bad or **G**UILTY about drinking or drug use? Have you ever used or had a drink first thing in the morning as an **E**YE-OPENER to steady your nerves or make you feel normal?	Substance abuse involves emotional and life-style issues. If two or more of the CAGE (acronym) questions are positive, suspect substance abuse.

➤ *CRITICAL DECISION POINT* Single visit to a health care agency may not reveal an abuse problem. Nurse must look for a pattern and then gather a well-focused history. Nurse may need to refer client to drug or alcohol treatment program. Consider family or significant other support resources.

RED FLAGS FOR SUSPICION OF SUBSTANCE ABUSE

- Clients who frequently miss appointments
- Clients who frequently request written excuses for work
- Clients who have chief complaints of insomnia, "bad nerves," or pain that does not fit a particular pattern
- Clients who often report lost prescriptions (e.g., tranquilizers or pain medications) or ask for frequent refills
- Clients who make frequent emergency room visits
- Clients who have a history of changing doctors or who bring in medication bottles prescribed by several different providers
- Clients with histories of gastrointestinal bleeding, peptic ulcers, pancreatitis, cellulitis, or frequent pulmonary infections
- Clients with frequent sexually transmitted diseases, complicated pregnancies, multiple abortions, or sexual dysfunction
- Clients who complain of chest pains or palpitations or who have histories of admissions to rule out myocardial infarction
- Clients who give histories of activities that place them at risk for human immunodeficiency virus (HIV) infections (multiple sexual partners, multiple rapes)
- Clients with family history of addiction; history of childhood sexual, physical, or emotional abuse; social and financial or marital problems

Modified from Master S, Terpstra JK: Recognition and diagnosis. In Schnoll SH, Horvatich PK, Terpstra JK: *Prescribing drugs with abuse liability*, Richmond, Va, 1992, DSAM, MCV-VCU.

EVALUATION

STEPS	RATIONALE
1. Ask client if expectations for visit and examination were met.	Measures client's level of satisfaction with health care provider. This can be a factor in long-term compliance with treatment recommendations.
2. Compare client's vital signs with baseline or normal range for client's age (Chapter 10).	Determines baseline physiological status and presence of alterations.
3. Compare client's height and weight with normal standards on height and weight chart (Table 11-5).	Determines client's size in relation to desirable height and weight for age and size.
4. Compare client's skinfold thickness with 50th percentile for men and women.	Reveals general nutritional status by presence or absence of body fat.
5. Compare client's appearance and behaviors with those typified as normal.	Behaviors can be individualistic. Nurse observes for behavioral signs indicative of emotional illness, such as excessive emotional displays, apathy or underactivity, reported delusions, and rambling speech.

Table 11-5 Height and Weight Table: Weights for Persons 29 to 59 Years According to Build*

Men					Women				
Height†					Height†				
Feet	Inches	Small Frame	Medium Frame	Large Frame	Feet	Inches	Small Frame	Medium Frame	Large Frame
5	2	128-134	131-141	138-150	4	10	102-111	109-121	118-131
5	3	130-136	133-143	140-153	4	11	103-113	111-123	120-134
5	4	132-138	135-145	142-156	5	0	104-115	113-126	122-137
5	5	134-140	137-148	144-160	5	1	106-118	115-129	125-140
5	6	136-142	139-151	146-164	5	2	108-121	118-132	128-143
5	7	138-145	142-154	149-168	5	3	111-124	121-135	131-147
5	8	140-148	145-157	152-172	5	4	114-127	124-138	134-151
5	9	142-151	148-160	155-176	5	5	117-130	124-141	137-155
5	10	144-154	151-163	158-180	5	6	120-133	130-144	140-159
5	11	146-157	154-166	161-184	5	7	123-136	133-147	143-163
6	0	149-160	157-170	164-188	5	8	126-139	133-150	146-167
6	1	152-164	160-174	168-192	5	9	129-142	139-153	149-170
6	2	155-168	164-178	172-197	5	10	132-145	142-156	152-173
6	3	158-172	167-182	176-202	5	11	135-148	145-159	155-176
6	4	162-176	171-187	181-207	6	0	138-151	148-162	158-179

Source of basic data: *Build study*, Society of Actuaries and Association of Life Insurance Medical Directors of America, 1980. Copyright 1983 Metropolitan Life Insurance Company.
*Indoor clothing weighing 5 pounds for men and 3 pounds for women.
†Shoes with 1-inch heels.

STEPS	RATIONALE
6. Over repeated visits or contacts, compare client's appearance and behaviors with those characteristic of either an abusive relationship or substance abuse pattern.	Behaviors can be subtle.
7. Unexpected outcomes that may occur include:	
➤ Client displays signs of distress, such as shortness of breath, acute pain, anxiety.	Physical distress indicates acute problems requiring immediate attention.
➤ Client verbalizes dissatisfaction with purpose of examination and nurse's lack of interest in client's real concerns.	More time may be necessary to deescalate client's anxiety or anger (Chapter 2) and to make client a willing partner in the physical examination.
➤ Client's vital signs are above or below normal expected range for client of same age.	Vital sign alterations can be result of a number of pathological conditions.
➤ Client's height is above or below normal desired range for person of same age.	Characteristic of growth disorder (e.g., dwarfism or gigantism).
➤ Client's weight is above or below normal desired range for person of same age and height.	Nutritional problems may be attributed to changes in eating habits, sources of nutrients, or pathological conditions.
➤ Client shows clear pattern of physical injury and behavioral indicators for physical abuse.	Client at risk in relationship with spouse, partner, parent, or child.
➤ Client acknowledges abuse of alcohol and/or drugs.	May indicate that client is receptive to referral to a treatment program.

NURSING DIAGNOSIS

Clustering of defining characteristics from the assessment data may reveal the following nursing diagnoses for clients requiring this skill. (Confirmation of any one diagnosis will usually require more data gathering during actual examination.)

- ➤ Altered nutrition: less than body requirements
- ➤ Altered nutrition: more than body requirements
- ➤ Fluid volume deficit (or Risk for fluid volume deficit)
- ➤ Fluid volume excess

- Altered nutrition: risk for more than body requirements
- Anxiety
- Fear
- Bathing/hygiene, self-care deficit
- Impaired physical mobility
- Ineffective breathing pattern
- Pain
- Altered family processes: alcoholism
- Care giver role strain

Related factors are individualized based on the client's condition or needs.

RECORDING AND REPORTING

1. Record client's vital signs on vital sign flow sheet.	Provides graphic representation of changes in vital sign values.
2. Record height and weight in nurses' notes or flow sheet.	Repeated weight measurements are entered in flow sheet for comparison.
3. Record description of client's general appearance and skinfold thickness in nurses' notes.	Provides means for determining changes in client's condition over time.
4. Describe client's behaviors using objective terminology. Include client's self-report of signs and symptoms.	Used to compare subsequent behavioral responses.
5. Report abnormalities in vital signs or any acute symptoms to nurse in charge or physician.	May require immediate therapy.

• • • • •

Special Considerations

- Before contacting an interpreter, determine the language spoken by the client at home; it may be different from the language spoken publicly. It is best to have an interpreter of the same gender as the client and one who is older and more mature as an interpreter. Have the interpreter translate as closely to verbatim as possible.
- Normally, person's weight can fluctuate daily because of fluid loss or retention (1 L of water weighs 1 kg or 2.2 pounds).
- Client should be weighed on same scale, at same time, with same clothing each day.
- When client is unresponsive, nurse may need assistance to maintain plantar flexion of feet to determine supine client's height correctly. In critically ill clients height becomes important measure to determine body surface area; measurement is used to compute hemodynamic factors.
- Body fat can be estimated from height and weight results compared with standardized height and weight charts. Generally, weight of 15% to 20% above standard indicates excess body fat; however, fluid retention is one factor that must be ruled out.
- A more detailed assessment of a client's nutritional status can be made by measuring triceps skinfold thickness. Consult with a dietitian about how to perform this measurement accurately.

Teaching Considerations

- During general survey, inform client about normal range of vital signs for age and physical condition and normal weight for height and body frame.
- Explain that it is best to weigh self in the morning after voiding and before food or drink is taken.
- If client is on established diet, discuss any problems client has in diet preparation or food selection. The best form of weight reduction is to achieve gradual weight loss by increasing exercise and decreasing caloric intake. Refer to clinical dietitian for specific information.
- Treatment for substance abuse requires a long-term commitment. Simply teaching the "rights and wrongs" of substance abuse will likely have little effect and may make client less receptive to treatment. Be sure client receives experienced counselor for support.

Pediatric Considerations

- Measurement of physical growth is a key element in evaluation of a child's health status. Children may also require measurement of head circumference. Growth charts are available from the National Center for Health Statistics.
- Infants are weighed nude. Children may be weighed in light underclothes or gown.
- A child's interactions with parents provide valuable information regarding the child's behavior.

Gerontologic Considerations

- An older adult's presenting signs and symptoms can be deceiving. An older adult has a diminished physiological reserve that often causes the client to not always exhibit the expected, or "classic," signs and symptoms of a disease. The characteristic presentation of illness in older adults is more commonly one of blunted or atypical signs and symptoms (Lueckenotte, 1996).

- Nutritional problems are frequently noted in older adults. Skipping meals is a common practice. The amount of food eaten diminishes, and the adequacy of nutrition becomes questionable. The following factors pose risks for malnutrition in older adults: limited income, loneliness, abuse of alcohol and other central nervous system depressants, forgetfulness, inability to feed self, reduced strength and mobility, and decreased vision (Ebersole and Hess, 1994).

Home Care Considerations

- The focus and extent of a physical examination will vary by setting. In the home the focus may be on the client's musculoskeletal system to determine ability to perform basic self-care tasks. Clients in the home have been recently seen in a health care agency. The nurse should ensure that the home assessment builds on any problem areas identified in a previous setting.
- Many clients will not have a scale at home. Transport of small portable scale may be required.
- Consult referring physician as to the assessment findings and proposed plan of care.

SKILL 11-2 Assessing the Skin

The skin provides the body's external protection, regulates body temperature, and acts as a sensory organ for pain, temperature, and touch. Assessment can reveal a variety of conditions, including changes in oxygenation, circulation, nutrition, local tissue damage, and hydration.

In a hospital setting clients are at risk for skin breakdown and lesions resulting from trauma to the skin while receiving care, exposure to pressure during immobilization, or reaction to medications used in treatment. In nursing homes and extended care facilities, frail and immobile clients are at risk for pressure ulcers. The nurse may initially inspect all skin surfaces or may assess the skin gradually while other body systems are examined. Assessment of the skin can reveal presence of lesions but findings also help to determine the type of hygiene required by a client. Assessment of the skin involves inspection, palpation, and olfaction.

EQUIPMENT

- **Gooseneck or high-intensity lamp**
- **Disposable gloves**
- **Clear plastic centimeter ruler**

DELEGATION CONSIDERATIONS

Unlicensed assistive personnel often provide routine hygiene to a client and assist with self-care activities. For this reason the staff member must know what changes in the skin are indicative of problems to report. Unlicensed assistive personnel should know signs of pressure developing on the skin as well as the significance of new lesions, draining lesions, and lesions that change in appearance over time. All findings should be reported to the RN for assessment.

STEPS	RATIONALE
ASSESSMENT	
1. Ask if client has noted any changes in the skin **(integument),** especially a change in the size or color of a mole or other darkly pigmented growth or spot. Note any dryness, **pruritus,** oozing, bleeding, or change in the appearance of a bump or nodule; the spread of pigmentation beyond its borders; a change in sensation; itchiness, tenderness, or pain.	Client is best judge to determine skin change. Skin cancer may first be noticed as localized change in color.
2. Determine if client works or spends excess time outside. If so, is a sunscreen worn?	Exposed areas such as face and arms will be more pigmented than rest of body. Sunscreen reduces risk of skin **carcinoma** (cancer) if used in conjunction with decreased sun exposure (American Cancer Society, 1995).
3. Determine if client has history of exposure to ultraviolet radiation (natural and artificial), fair complexion, occupational exposure to coal tar, pitch, creosote, arsenic compounds or radium, and a family history of skin cancer.	These characteristics are risk factors for skin cancer (American Cancer Society, 1996).

STEPS	RATIONALE
4. Question client about frequency of bathing and type of soap used.	Excessive bathing and use of certain harsh soaps contribute to dry skin.
5. Ask if client has had recent trauma to skin.	Traumatic injury can cause bruising and changes in skin texture.
6. Ask if client has history of allergies.	Skin rashes commonly occur from allergies.
7. Ask if client uses topical medications or home remedies on the skin.	Incorrect use of topical agents may cause inflammation or irritation.
8. Ask if client uses sunlamp or tanning pills or goes to tanning salon.	Overexposure of skin to tanning irritants can cause skin cancer.
9. Ask if client has family history of serious skin disorders (psoriasis).	Family history can predispose client to skin disorders.

PLANNING

STEPS	RATIONALE
1. **Expected outcomes** following completion of procedure:	
➤ Client remains comfortable.	Various position changes are needed to inspect all skin surfaces.
➤ Skin color is uniform over body, ranging in tone from ivory or light pink to ruddy pink in white skin; light to deep brown or olive in dark skin. Sun-darkened skin may be found around knees and elbows and on face and hands. Palms, soles of feet, and nail beds are lighter in color.	These are normal findings on inspection.
➤ The skin is smooth, soft, dry, and warm. Texture is not uniform throughout (palms of hands and soles of feet are thicker).	These are normal findings on palpation.
➤ Skin lifts easily and snaps back immediately, is resilient on release.	Normal turgor is evident.
➤ Client is able to discuss hygiene practices and skin care appropriate to need.	Nurse's instruction is individualized to client's learning needs within sociocultural norms.
➤ Client is able to identify factors that increase risk of skin cancer while demonstrating self-examination of the skin.	Important in disease prevention.
2. Prepare equipment.	
3. Prepare client:	
a. Client may sit initially.	Position allows nurse to inspect head and neck, upper trunk anteriorly and posteriorly, and upper and lower extremities.
b. Ask client to lie supine and turn to side during examination.	Position allows visualization of buttocks and genital area.
c. Explain to client that it is necessary to inspect all skin surfaces to ensure normal skin integrity. If lesions are found, explain need to palpate lesions gently.	Client may become embarrassed because skin condition is often associated with hygiene.
d. Expose only single body part to be inspected at one time.	Minimizing exposure of body parts reduces client anxiety.
e. Nurse may request client to clean skin with soap and water or remove cosmetics.	Makeup, body secretions, or soil may cover areas of skin requiring inspection and mask determining characteristics such as skin color or presence of lesions.

IMPLEMENTATION

STEPS	RATIONALE
1. Wash hands. If client has moist or open lesions, apply gloves.	Reduces transmission of infection.
2. Begin with a brief but careful overall visual sweep of the entire body; then observe each body part during the examination.	Gives a good idea of the distribution and extent of any lesions and overall symmetry in skin color.

STEPS	RATIONALE
3. Inspect color of skin surfaces, comparing color of symmetrical body parts. Look first at areas unexposed to sun.	Skin color varies from body part to body part. Changes in color can be indicative of pathological alterations (Table 11-6).
CRITICAL DECISION POINT **Be alert for basal cell carcinomas, commonly seen in sun-exposed areas and frequently occurring in a background of sun-damaged skin.**	
4. Carefully inspect color of face, oral mucosa, lips, conjunctiva, sclera, and nail beds.	Nurse can more readily identify abnormalities in areas of body where **melanin** production is lowest.
5. Look for any patches or areas of skin color variation (e.g., hyperpigmentation).	Localized skin changes may indicate circulatory changes.
CRITICAL DECISION POINT **When assessing the skin of a client with bandages, cast, restraints, or other restrictive devices, note areas of** pallor **and decreased temperature, which may indicate arterial occlusion. Release of pressure from the restrictive device may be necessary.**	
6. Use ungloved fingertips to palpate skin surfaces to feel moisture of skin.	Moisture is directly related to degree of hydration and condition of outer lipid layer of the skin surface (DeWitt, 1990).
7. With gloved hands, inspect character of any secretions; note color, odor, amount, and consistency (e.g., thin and watery or thick and oily).	Character of secretions from skin lesions helps to indicate type of lesion.
8. Using **dorsum** (back) of hand, palpate for temperature of skin surfaces (nurse may remove a glove temporarily if worn). Compare symmetrical body parts. Compare upper and lower body parts. Note distinct temperature differences. Note localized areas of warmth.	Increased or decreased skin temperature reflects increase or decrease in blood flow. Skin on dorsum of hand is thin, which allows detection of subtle temperature changes. A stage I pressure ulcer may cause warmth and **erythema** (redness) of an area.

Table 11-6 Skin Color Variations

Color	Condition	Causes	Assessment Locations
Bluish (cyanosis)	Increased amount of deoxygenated hemoglobin (associated with hypoxia)	Heart or lung disease, cold environment	Nail beds, lips, mouth, skin (severe cases)
Pallor (decrease in color)	Reduced amount of oxyhemoglobin	Anemia	Face, conjunctivae, nail beds, palms of hands
	Reduced visibility of oxyhemoglobin resulting from decreased blood flow	Shock	Skin, nail beds, conjunctivae, lips
Loss of pigmentation	Vitiligo	Congenital or autoimmune condition causing lack of pigment	Patchy areas on skin over face, hands, arms
Yellow-orange (jaundice)	Increased deposit of bilirubin in tissues	Liver disease, destruction of red blood cells	Sclera, mucous membranes, skin
Red (erythema)	Increased visibility of oxyhemoglobin caused by dilation or increased blood flow	Fever, direct trauma, blushing, alcohol intake	Face, area of trauma, sacrum, shoulders, other common sites for pressure ulcers
Tan-brown	Increased amount of melanin	Suntan, pregnancy	Areas exposed to sun: face, arms; areolae, nipples

STEPS	RATIONALE
9. Stroke skin surfaces lightly with fingertips to detect texture of skin's surface. Note whether skin is smooth or rough, thick or thin, tight or supple and if localized areas of hardness or lesions are present.	Localized texture changes result from trauma, surgical wounds, or lesions.
10. Palpate deeply any areas that appear irregular in texture.	Deep palpation allows nurse to detect localized areas of hardness and/or tenderness within subcutaneous skin layers.

CRITICAL DECISION POINT **Localized areas of hardness from repeated injections may be found over injection sites. Such areas are common in clients who receive insulin, heparin, or regular vitamin B_{12} injections. Develop a plan to rotate injection sites more carefully.**

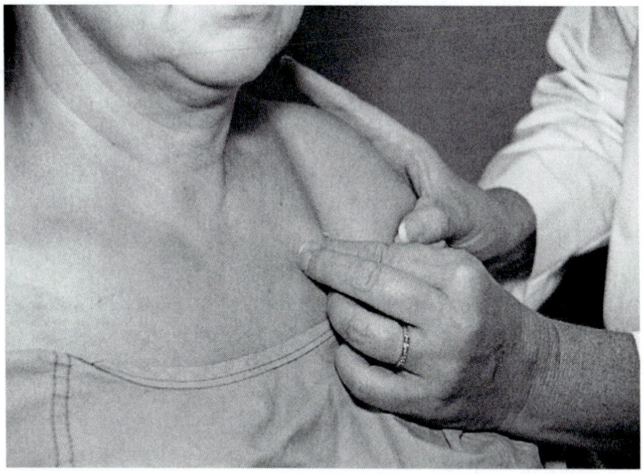

Step 11 Assessment of skin turgor.

STEPS	RATIONALE
11. Assess skin turgor by first grasping fold of skin on back of client's forearm or sternal area with the fingertips. Release skinfold and note ease and speed with which skin returns to place (see illustration).	Turgor is measure of skin's elasticity.
12. Assess condition of skin, paying particular attention to regions of pressure (e.g., sacrum, greater trochanter, heels, occipital area, and clavicles). If areas of redness are noted, place fingertip over area and apply gentle pressure, then release.	Normal reactive hyperemia (redness) is visible effect of localized vasodilation, body's normal response to lack of blood flow to underlying tissue. Affected area of skin will blanch with fingertip pressure.

CRITICAL DECISION POINT **Evidence of normal reactive hyperemia should result in repositioning of client and development of turning schedule if client is dependent.**

STEPS	RATIONALE
13. When lesion is detected, inspect color, location, texture, size, shape, type (see box on p. 300). Note also grouping (e.g., clustered or linear) and distribution (localized or generalized). Be sure skin is well illuminated.	Certain skin lesions can be identified by a characteristic pattern of features.
14. Gently palpate any lesion to determine mobility, contour (flat, raised, or depressed), and consistency (soft or hard). If lesion is moist or draining, apply disposable gloves before palpation.	Gentle palpation prevents accidental rupture of underlying cysts. Gloves reduce transmission of microorganisms.
15. Note if client complains of tenderness during palpation.	Tenderness may be indicative of inflammation or pressure on body part.
16. Measure size of lesion (height, width, depth) with centimeter ruler.	Provides for baseline to assess changes in lesion over time.
17. Inspect areas of skin for **edema** (swelling), paying particular attention to dependent body parts such as feet and ankles, sacrum, and scapular areas. Note color, location, and shape of area.	Edema is result of accumulation of fluid in tissues. Poor venous return causes edema in dependent body parts. Direct trauma causes localized edema.

TYPES OF PRIMARY SKIN LESIONS

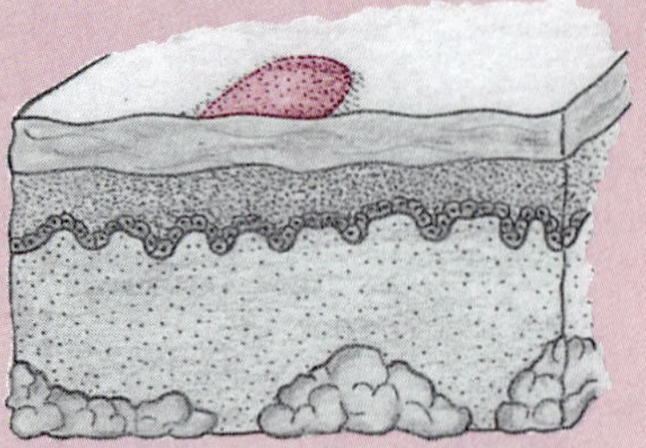

Macule: flat, nonpalpable change in skin color, smaller than 1 cm (e.g., freckle, petechia)

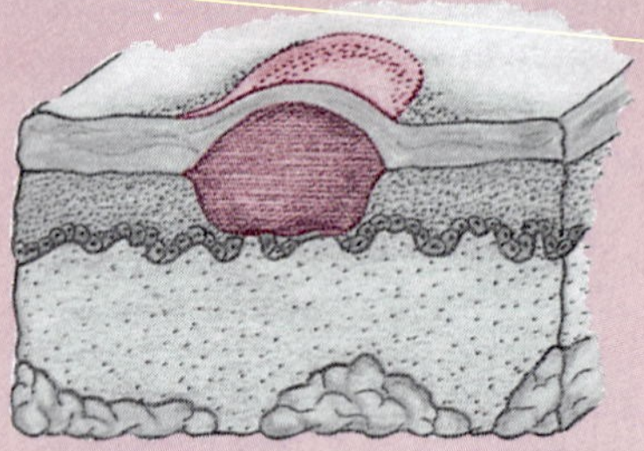

Papule: palpable, circumscribed, solid elevation in skin, smaller than 0.5 cm (e.g., elevated nevus)

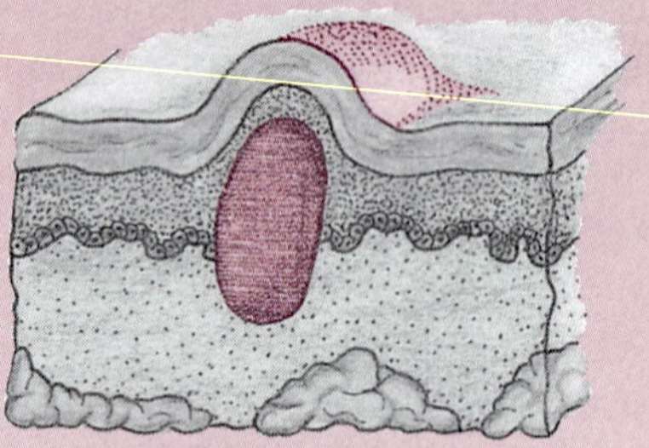

Nodule: elevated solid mass, deeper and firmer than papule, 0.5-2.0 cm (e.g., wart)

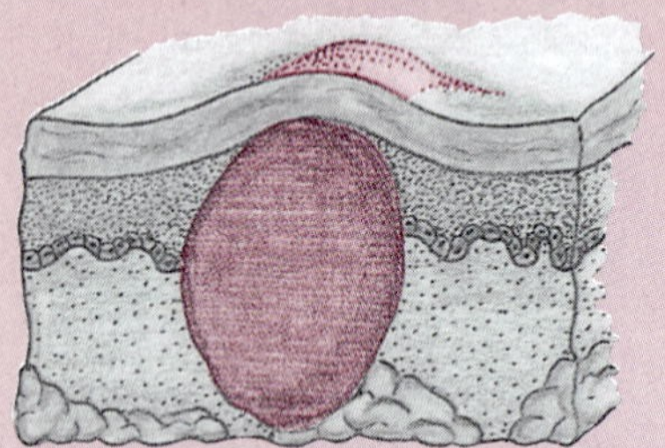

Tumor: solid mass that may extend deep through subcutaneous tissue, larger than 1-2 cm (e.g., epithelioma)

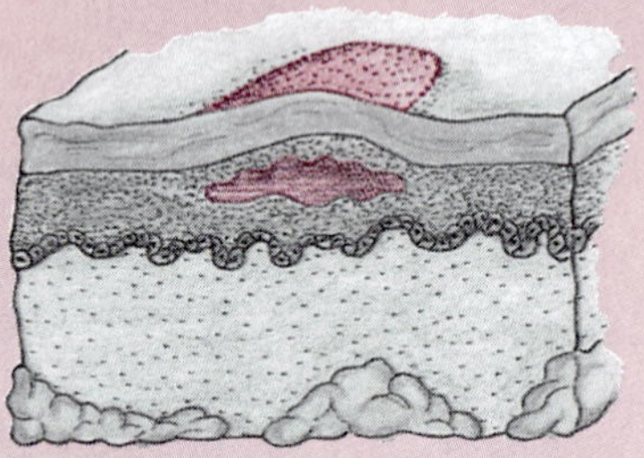

Wheal: irregularly shaped, elevated area or superficial localized edema, varies in size (e.g., hive, mosquito bite)

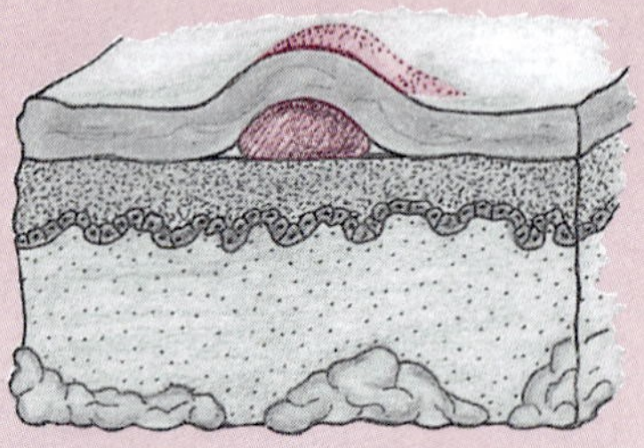

Vesicle: circumscribed elevation of skin filled with serous fluid, smaller than 0.5 cm (e.g., herpes simplex, chickenpox)

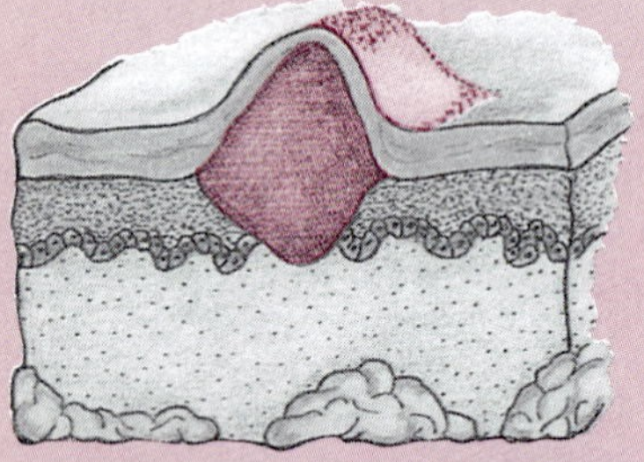

Pustule: circumscribed elevation of skin similar to vesicle but filled with pus, varies in size (e.g., acne, staphylococcal infection)

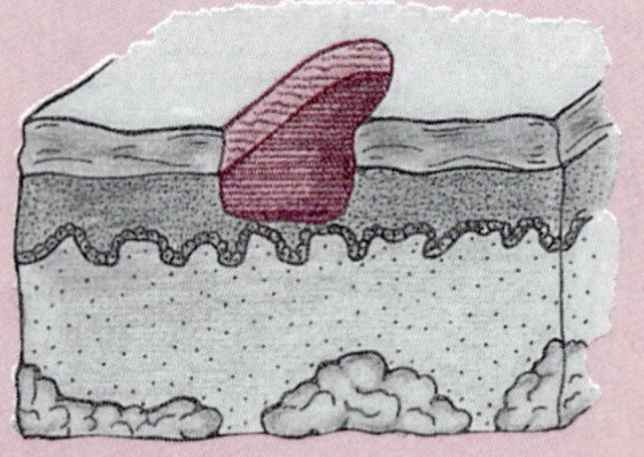

Ulcer: deep loss of skin surface that may extend to dermis and frequently bleeds and scars, varies in size (e.g., venous stasis ulcer)

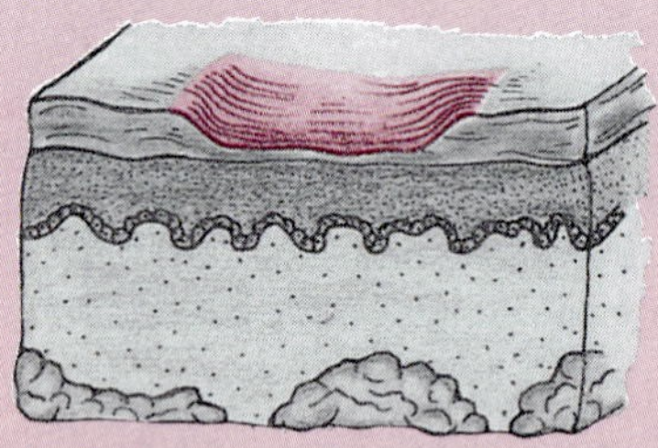

Atrophy: thinning of skin with loss of normal skin furrow with skin appearing shiny and translucent, varies in size (e.g., arterial insufficiency)

STEPS	RATIONALE
18. Palpate edematous areas, noting mobility, consistency, and tenderness.	Assists in determining extent of edema.
19. Assess for pitting edema by pressing edematous area firmly with thumb for 5 seconds, then releasing. Note depth of pitting in millimeters. 2 mm indentation = 1+ edema 4 mm indentation = 2+ edema 6 mm indentation = 3+ edema 8 mm indentation = 4+ edema	
20. At end of examination, remove and dispose of gloves and wash hands.	Reduces transmission of infection.

STEPS	RATIONALE
EVALUATION	
1. Compare assessment findings with previous observations of skin and normal skin characteristics.	Detects change in client's condition and determines skin integrity.
2. Have client describe the American Cancer Society warning signals for cancerous skin lesions.	
3. **Unexpected outcomes** that may occur include:	
➤ Client's skin demonstrates abnormal coloring.	Abnormalities may result from factors such as cancerous lesions, other primary lesions (some common with aging), trauma, fever, or circulatory alterations.
➤ Client's skin reveals erythema.	Prolonged pressure, usually over bony prominences, has been unrelieved.
➤ Client's skin is dry with reduced turgor.	Findings are a result of dehydration, inadequate hygiene measures, and/or aging.
➤ Client's skin is warm throughout.	Indicates fever.
➤ Client's skin has localized areas of warmth or cold.	May indicate localized area of infection (warm) or circulatory alteration (cool).
➤ Areas of edema, redness, and warmth noted along arms and legs.	Common pattern among intravenous drug users indicating recent injections.
➤ Skin lesions are present.	Lesions may result from trauma, allergic reaction, or a variety of pathological conditions.

NURSING DIAGNOSIS

Clustering of defining characteristics from the assessment data may reveal the following nursing diagnoses for clients requiring this skill:

- Altered peripheral tissue perfusion
- Risk for impaired skin integrity
- Impaired skin integrity

Related factors are individualized based on the client's condition or needs.

RECORDING AND REPORTING

1. Describe condition of client's skin in nurses' notes.	Provides means to assess changes in client's condition and provides data to evaluate effect of nursing therapies.
2. Report abnormalities in skin (e.g., pressure ulcer, draining lesion, or wound) to nurse in charge or physician.	May require initiation of medical therapy.

• • • • •

Special Considerations

- Well-lit room may be satisfactory, but examination light allows nurse to see less accessible areas more clearly.
- Dry skin may indicate dehydration, use of harsh soaps, too-frequent bathing, or lack of humidity in room.
- "Winter itch" is common in climates with low humidity during winter months.
- With reduced turgor, skin remains suspended or "tented" for few seconds before slowly returning to place. Clients with reduced turgor require special consideration in prevention of pressure ulcers.
- Incidence of melanoma, an aggressive form of skin cancer, has increased about 4% annually since 1973, with incidence rate more than 40 times higher among whites than blacks (American Cancer Society, 1996). The cancer can spread to other parts of the body quickly. Quick detection and prompt cure are critical.
- Skin texture of adult is normally not uniform throughout. Irregularities in texture may be result of scarring from recent trauma.
- Petechiae are tiny (pinpoint-size) red or purple spots on the skin caused by small hemorrhages in the skin layers. May indicate serious blood clotting disorder, drug reaction, or liver disease.

Teaching Considerations

- Teach client to conduct a monthly self-examination of the skin, noting moles, blemishes, and birthmarks. Tell client to inspect all skin surfaces. Cancerous melanomas start as small molelike growths that increase in size, change color, become ulcerated, and bleed. A simple ABCD rule outlines warning signals (American Cancer Society, 1996):

A is for asymmetry
B is for border irregularity, ragged or notched edges
C is for color; pigmentation is not uniform
D is for diameter; greater than 6 mm

- Tell client to report to a physician or primary care provider any change in skin lesions or a sore that does not heal.
- Instruct client to prevent skin cancer by avoiding overexposure to the sun. Protective clothing (e.g., wide-brimmed hats and long sleeves) and sunscreen should be worn. Apply sunscreen with SPF (sun protection factor) greater than or equal to 15 approximately 15 minutes before going into the sun and after swimming or perspiring. Avoid exposure to the sun's ultraviolet rays at midday (10 AM to 3 PM), when the rays are the strongest. Do not use indoor sunlamps or tanning salons. Medications such as oral contraceptives and antibiotics can make skin more sensitive to sun.
- To treat "winter itch," tell client to avoid hot water, harsh soaps, and drying agents such as rubbing alcohol (see Chapter 6).
- Tell client to apply lotion and moisturizers to the skin regularly to reduce itching and drying and wear cotton clothing (Hardy, 1990).

Pediatric Considerations

- Because of the possible link between severe sunburns in childhood and greatly increased risk of melanoma in later life, children in particular should be protected from the sun (American Cancer Society, 1996).
- Skin changes that commonly occur in children: infants develop rashes from food allergies; adolescents develop acne.
- Infants should be kept covered as much as possible during the examination to prevent temperature changes.

Gerontologic Considerations

- Specifically instruct older adults who tend to have delayed wound healing about reporting changes in skin lesions.
- Skin changes common with aging include wrinkling, reduced elasticity, spotty pigmentation ("liver spots") in areas exposed to sun, and excessive dryness. Commonly occurring lesions include seborrheic keratosis (pigmented macular-papular lesion that can be warty, scaly, or greasy in appearance); senile ectasis or cherry angioma (bright, ruby-red or purplish papular lesion); acrochordons or skin tags (soft pinkish-tan to light-brown pedunculated lesions); and senile lentigines (gray-brown irregular macular lesions on sun-exposed areas) (Lueckenotte, 1994).

SKILL 11-3 Assessing the Hair and Scalp

The nurse assesses the condition and distribution of the two types of body hair—terminal and vellus. Terminal hair is long, coarse, thick hair that is easily visible on the scalp, axillae, and pubic areas. Vellus hairs are soft, tiny hairs covering the entire body except for palms and soles. As in skin assessment, the nurse may inspect body hair all at one time or at different points during the examination. For example, the nurse can inspect hair on the scalp while assessing all head and neck structures and inspect pubic hair during the genital examination. This approach minimizes any embarrassment the client might experience.

EQUIPMENT

- Examination light
- Disposable gloves

DELEGATION CONSIDERATIONS

Unlicensed assistive personnel often provide routine hygiene to a client and assist with self-care activities. For this reason the staff member must know what changes in the client's hair and scalp are indicative of problems. All findings should be reported to the RN for assessment.

STEPS	RATIONALE
ASSESSMENT	
1. Ask if client is wearing a wig or a hairpiece and request that it be removed.	Interferes with complete inspection of hair and scalp. (Client may defer this part of examination.)
2. Determine if client has noted change in growth or loss of hair or lesions of scalp.	Changes may occur subtly over time.

STEPS	RATIONALE
3. Identify type of shampoo, other hair care products, and curling irons used for grooming.	Excessive use of shampoo or other chemical agents and burning by curling iron may cause drying or brittleness.
4. Determine if client has experienced recent trauma to scalp.	Trauma may be cause of bruising or localized lesions.
5. Ask if client is undergoing chemotherapy (if hair loss is noted) or vasodilator drugs (minoxidil) (if hair growth is noted).	Chemotherapeutic agents kill cells that multiply rapidly, such as tumor cells and normal hair cells. Minoxidil causes excessive hair growth.
6. Note if client recently spent time outdoors, such as camping.	Risk of ticks attaching to skin or scalp.
7. Review diet history recorded previously.	Nutrition can influence condition of hair.

PLANNING

STEPS	RATIONALE
1. **Expected outcomes** following completion of procedure:	
➤ Client maintains a positive body image.	
➤ Hair will be evenly distributed over scalp and pubic areas.	
➤ Scalp hair may be coarse or fine, curly or straight, and should be shiny, smooth, and pliant. Color varies from very light blond to black to gray and may show alterations from rinses or dyes.	
➤ Scalp will be smooth and inelastic, with even coloration, without lesions or presence of vermin.	Skin integrity is maintained.
➤ Vellus hair is evenly distributed over symmetrical body parts.	
➤ Client discusses proper hair care practices.	
2. Prepare client:	
a. Client may sit initially.	Position allows nurse to inspect scalp thoroughly.
b. Client may be asked to lie supine.	Allows for inspection of distribution of body hair.
3. Explain to client that inspection of hair and scalp requires separation of hair shafts. If lesions or lice are expected, explain need to wear gloves.	Client may be sensitive about personal appearance. Embarrassment may occur because condition of hair reflects client's overall hygiene.

IMPLEMENTATION

STEPS	RATIONALE
1. Wash hands and apply gloves if lice or lesions are expected.	Reduces transmission of infection.
2. Observe the color, distribution, quantity, thickness, texture, and lubrication of hair.	Changes in hair distribution may reflect hormonal changes, changes from aging, poor nutrition, or use of certain hair care products.
3. Focus inspection on areas of baldness or thinning of hair.	**Alopecia** (baldness) may be related to genetic tendency or may be caused by skin disorders such as tinea capitis (ringworm).
4. Inspect scalp for cleanliness and presence of lesions by carefully separating shafts of hair. Inspect each lesion using same guidelines described in Skill 11-2. Ask if client has noted anything unusual.	Pulling of hair can cause client discomfort. Lesions can easily go unnoticed with thick hair growth. Lumps may result from localized trauma.
5. Inspect scalp contour and palpate for unusual masses or prominences. In newborns fontanels should feel flat, firm, and well demarcated against skull's bony edges. In newborns change in contour results from overlapping of cranial bones that have not yet fused.	
6. If hair is in poor condition, inspect hair follicles to determine presence of lice. Stand away from client during inspection.	Head and crab lice attach their eggs to hair shafts and follicles, are difficult to see, and can easily attach to clothing and be transmitted to other persons.

STEPS	RATIONALE
7. Inspect for bites or pustular eruptions in areas where skin surfaces meet (i.e., behind ears). Look for grayish or brown oval ticks.	Lice gather in areas of body where exposure is limited. Ticks are also commonly found on the head.
8. Inspect hair over perineal area for crab lice (pediculosis pubis).	Site where lice develop after contact with infested clothing or people.
9. Remove gloves and dispose in appropriate container. Wash hands.	Reduces transmission of microorganisms and vermin.
10. Inspect hair distribution over lower extremities.	Change can indicate circulatory alterations.

EVALUATION

1. Compare findings with previous observations and normal characteristics of hair.	Detects change in condition or presence of abnormalities.
2. **Unexpected outcomes** that may occur include:	
➤ Terminal scalp hair may be dry, brittle, discolored, coarse, or stringy. There may be localized areas of baldness.	May result from poor hygiene, nutritional deficiencies, hormonal changes, or alterations from chemotherapy.
➤ Scalp will be scaly or have lesions or vermin present.	Result of poor hygiene or trauma.
➤ Hair shafts appear to have oval particles of dandruff.	"Dandruff" could actually be eggs of head or crab lice.
➤ Hair follicles have bites or pustular eruptions.	Symptoms of lice infestation are evident.
➤ Vellus hair is absent or unevenly distributed over symmetrical body parts.	May result from local arterial insufficiency.
➤ Client is unable to recall proper methods to perform hair care. Review variables affecting client's interest and responsiveness.	Reinstruction may be necessary.

NURSING DIAGNOSIS

Clustering of defining characteristics from the assessment data may reveal the following nursing diagnoses for clients requiring this skill:

- Altered peripheral tissue perfusion
- Body-image disturbance
- Impaired skin integrity
- Bathing/hygiene self-care deficit

Related factors are individualized based on the client's condition or needs.

RECORDING AND REPORTING

1. Describe condition of hair and scalp in nurses' notes.	Documents changes in condition of hair and scalp. Provides means of evaluating results of hygiene care and other therapies.

FOLLOW-UP ACTIVITIES

1. Following the examination, be sure to provide equipment for client to comb and/or brush hair.

• • • • •

Special Considerations

- Excessive dryness, coarseness, or brittleness may result from aging, poor nutrition, or use of certain hair care products.
- Disturbances in body function such as febrile illness or exposure to general anesthesia can cause hair loss.
- If hair is in obviously good condition, it is not necessary to inspect entire scalp. Client is often best guide in locating lesions.
- With onset of puberty, change in amount and distribution of hair growth occurs. Women with **hirsutism,** a hormonal disorder, have hair growth on upper lip, chin, and cheeks, with coarse body hair.
- Scaling or dryness of scalp may be caused by dandruff or psoriasis.

Teaching Considerations

- Warn client that certain hair care products or lubricants can clog sebaceous glands and promote scalp infections.

- Instruct client about basic hygiene practices for care of the hair and scalp (Chapter 6).
- Instruct client who has head lice to shampoo thoroughly with pediculicide (shampoo available at drugstores) in cold water, comb thoroughly with fine-tooth comb (following product directions), and discard comb. Some preparations are applied to wet hair as a shampoo; others are applied to dry hair. An extrafine-tooth comb is used to remove dead lice and remaining eggs. A dilute vinegar rinse may aid in removal of eggs.
- Instruct client about ways to reduce transmission of lice:
  - Do not share personal care items with others.
  - Vacuum rugs, car seats, pillows, furniture, and flooring thoroughly and discard vacuum bag.
  - Seal nonwashable items in plastic bags for 14 days if family is unable to afford dry-cleaning and does not have vacuum cleaner.
  - Wash hands thoroughly.
  - Launder all clothing, linen, and bedding in soap and hot water and dry in hot dryer for at least 20 minutes. Dry-clean nonwashable items (Wong, 1995).
- Instruct client that sexual partner must be notified if lice were sexually transmitted.

Pediatric Considerations

- Newborns have anterior and posterior fontanels (spaces of unossified tissue where cranial bones have not closed), which can be felt under scalp.
- Head lice are common parasites in school-age children.

Gerontologic Considerations

- In older adults hair becomes dull gray, white, or yellow as well as dry and brittle.
- Older men lose facial hair, whereas older women may develop hair on the chin and upper lip.

Home Care Considerations

- The incidence of pediculosis in the schools has been increasing. Parents should be encouraged to notify others if a child becomes infected. Children should not reenter school until completely free of lice and eggs.

SKILL 11-4 Assessing the Nails

The nails can reflect an individual's general state of health, nutritional status, occupation, and level of self-care. Even a person's psychological state may be revealed by evidence of nail biting. The most visible portion of the nails is the nail plate, the transparent layer of epithelial cells covering the nail bed (Fig. 11-3). The vascularity of the nail bed creates the nail's underlying color. The semilunar whitish area at the base of the nail bed is called the **lunula,** from which the nail plate develops. The condition of the nails can reveal systemic or local disease. The nurse inspects the nail and palpates for abnormalities.

DELEGATION CONSIDERATIONS

Unlicensed assistive personnel commonly provide routine hygiene to a client and assist with self-care activities. For this reason the staff member must know what changes in the nails are indicative of problems to report. The staff member also should know not to cut or trim nails. All findings should be reported to the RN for assessment.

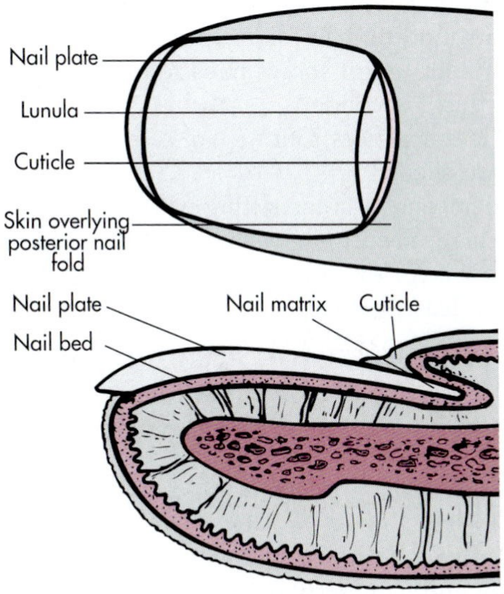

Fig. 11-3 Components of nail unit. (From Thompson JM et al: *Mosby's manual of clinical nursing,* ed 2, St Louis, 1989, Mosby.)

STEPS	RATIONALE
ASSESSMENT	
1. Ask if client has experienced any recent or continuous trauma or changes in the fingernails or toenails (splitting, discoloration).	Trauma may change shape and growth of nail, with potential loss of all or portion of nail. Repeated trauma may occur from repetitive action such as use of computer keyboard. Systemic conditions can change color, growth, and shape of nail.
2. Has the client had symptoms of pain, swelling, presence of systemic disease with fever, psychological or physical stress?	Can indicate if changes are due to local or systemic problem.
3. Question client's nail care practices and use of nail polish remover.	Chemical agents can cause excessive drying of nails. Improper nail care can damage nails and cuticles.
4. Determine risks for nail or foot problems:	
a. Diabetes	Vascular changes of diabetes reduce blood flow to peripheral tissues; foot lesions and thickened nails are common.
b. Obesity	Overweight clients have difficulty bending over to inspect toenails.
c. Older adults	Older adults have difficulty performing foot care because of reduced vision, lack of coordination, or difficulty bending over. There are changes in nail consistency, making nails thick, brittle, and difficult to cut.
PLANNING	
1. Expected outcomes following completion of procedure:	
➤ Nails are transparent, smooth, well rounded, and convex with a nail bed angle of 160 degrees. Edges underneath are clean. Surrounding cuticles are smooth, intact, noninflamed.	Nail is normal and without trauma.
➤ In light-skinned individuals nail beds are pink with translucent tips. Dark-skinned individuals have more deeply pigmented nail beds; brown or black pigmentation is normally present in longitudinal streaks.	Color varies among different races.
➤ Nail base is firm on palpation.	
➤ Surrounding nail folds are smooth and intact.	
➤ Capillary refill shows nails returning to pink color within 3 seconds.	Nails have normal circulation.
➤ Client practices routine nail care.	Client learns importance of regular nail care.
2. Prepare client:	
a. Client may assume sitting or lying position.	Promotes client comfort.
b. Explain need to inspect nails and cuticles.	Promotes client relaxation.
3. To view color of nails, ask client to remove polish from at least one nail.	Allows full visualization of nail features.
CRITICAL DECISION POINT **Determine if client has artificial nails. Color cannot be assessed without removal of artificial nail or coating.**	
IMPLEMENTATION	
1. Inspect nails for color, shape, thickness, cleanliness, length, and symmetry (toenails and fingernails).	Color of nails indicates status of blood oxygenation. Cleanliness reflects status of hygiene or possibly nature of occupation. Nail shape varies among individuals. Changes in shape and curvature of nails can indicate systemic disease.

STEPS	RATIONALE
2. Note the angle between the nail and the nail bed. Have client place together the nail (dorsal) surfaces of the fingertips of corresponding fingers of the right and left hands. If nails are clubbed, the diamond-shaped window at the base of the nails disappears and the angle between the distal tips increases.	Angle of nail bed may change because of chronic lack of oxygen (see box below).
3. Inspect the lateral and proximal nail folds around the nail. Are they bitten to the quick?	Tissues may be damaged from biting or repeated trauma.
4. Inspect the nail plate. Look for ridging, grooves, depressions, and pitting.	Longitudinal ridging and beading are common. Variations can be due to repeated trauma, chronic inflammation, or systemic disease.
5. Palpate the nail bed for firmness by gently squeezing the nail between your thumb and the pad of your finger. Does nail adhere to nail bed?	Clubbing causes softening of nail bed and flattening of nail. Separation of nail plate from the bed is common with local infections and trauma.
6. Palpate nail by grasping client's finger; note color of nail bed. Next, apply gentle, firm pressure with the thumb to the nail bed. Release thumb quickly. Watch for color change.	Nail bed appears white or blanched as pressure obstructs circulation. On release of pressure, circulation is restored and nail returns to pink color immediately.

EVALUATION

1. Compare condition of nails with normal nail characteristics.	Determines presence of abnormalities.
2. Ask client to describe nail care practices.	Demonstrates learning.

ABNORMALITIES OF NAIL BED

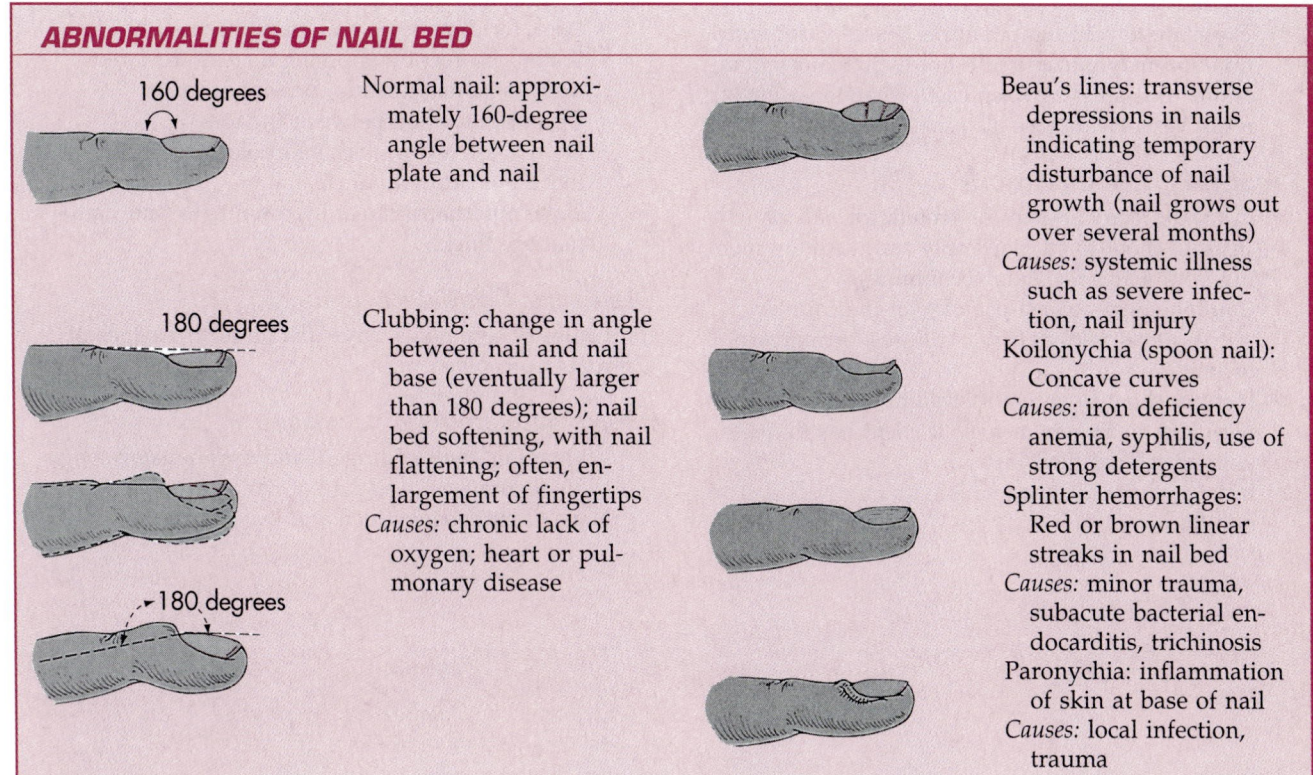

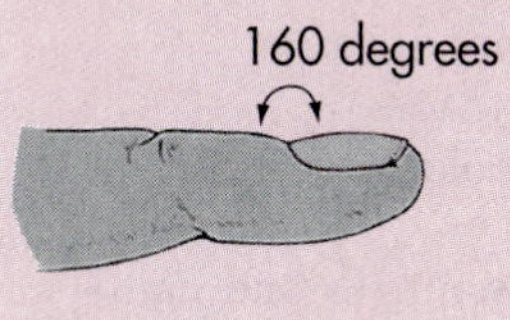

Normal nail: approximately 160-degree angle between nail plate and nail

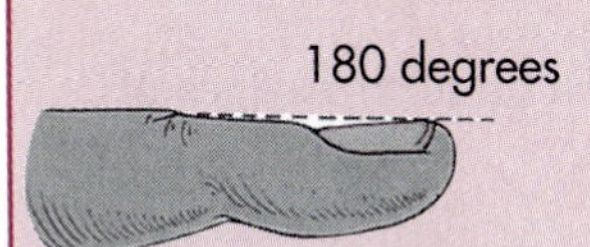

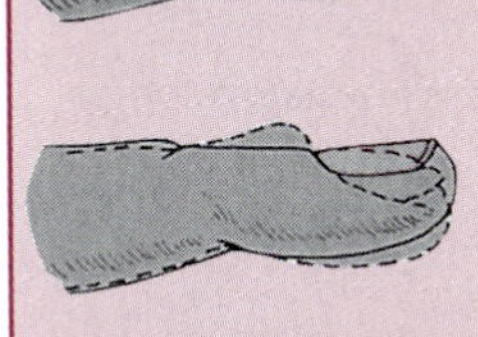

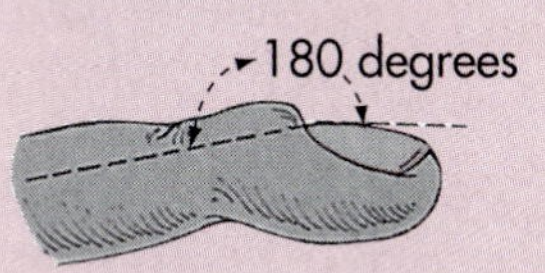

Clubbing: change in angle between nail and nail base (eventually larger than 180 degrees); nail bed softening, with nail flattening; often, enlargement of fingertips
Causes: chronic lack of oxygen; heart or pulmonary disease

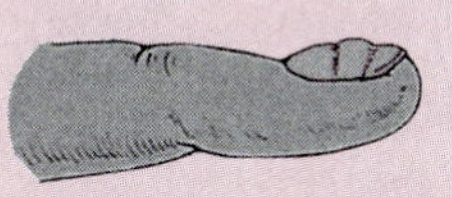

Beau's lines: transverse depressions in nails indicating temporary disturbance of nail growth (nail grows out over several months)
Causes: systemic illness such as severe infection, nail injury

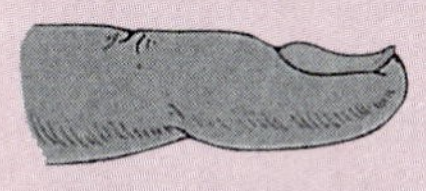

Koilonychia (spoon nail): Concave curves
Causes: iron deficiency anemia, syphilis, use of strong detergents

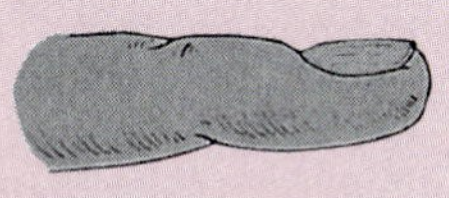

Splinter hemorrhages: Red or brown linear streaks in nail bed
Causes: minor trauma, subacute bacterial endocarditis, trichinosis

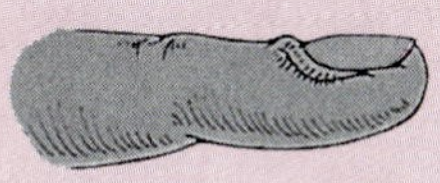

Paronychia: inflammation of skin at base of nail
Causes: local infection, trauma

STEPS	RATIONALE
3. **Unexpected outcomes** that may occur include:	
➤ Nails have abnormal color:	
Bluish or purplish cast.	Sign of **cyanosis,** caused by excess of deoxygenated hemoglobin in the blood.
White cast or pallor.	Sign of **anemia,** reduced red blood cell count.
➤ Nails are thin.	Result of reduced circulation or nutritional deficiency.
➤ Nail folds are dry, inflamed, rough; nails are short, ragged.	Result of nail biting.
➤ Edges of fingers or toes are thickened.	Result of callus formation.
➤ Nail beds reveal abnormalities (see box on p. 307).	Result of systemic disease or trauma.
➤ Dirt is found underneath nail edges.	Result of poor hygiene and/or repetitive work in soil, solutions, debris that lodges under nails.
➤ Nail plate separates from the bed.	Result of psoriasis, trauma, candidal or *Pseudomonas* infection.

NURSING DIAGNOSIS

Clustering of defining characteristics from the assessment data may reveal the following nursing diagnoses for clients requiring this skill:

- Altered peripheral tissue perfusion
- Bathing/hygiene self-care deficit
- Dressing/grooming self-care deficit
- Impaired gas exchange
- Impaired tissue integrity

Related factors are individualized based on the client's condition or needs.

RECORDING AND REPORTING

1. Describe condition of nails in nurses' notes.	Data are used for future comparison and to document response to hygienic measures.

• • • • •

Special Considerations

- Jagged, bitten, or broken nail edges or cuticles can predispose a client to localized infection.
- Exposure to cold temperatures causes vasoconstriction and may impair refill. Local circulatory alterations (i.e., pressure from cast or bandage) impair refill. Vascular disease also may impair refill.

Teaching Considerations

- Discuss dietary sources of protein for nail growth.
- Instruct client to cut nails only after soaking them in warm water for about 10 minutes.
- Caution client against use of over-the-counter preparations to treat corns, calluses, or ingrown toenails.
- Instruct client to cut nails straight across and even with tops of fingers or toes. If client has diabetes, nails should be filed instead.
- Instruct client to shape nails with emery board or nail file.
- If client is diabetic:
  - Wash feet daily in warm water.
  - Inspect feet daily in a place with good lighting.
  - Look for dry places and cracks in the skin.
  - Soften dry feet by applying a cream or lotion such as Nivea, Eucerin, or Alpha Keri.
  - Do not put lotion between the toes.
  - Do not use sharp objects to poke or dig under toenail or around cuticle.
  - Have a podiatrist treat ingrown nails and nails that are thick.

Pediatric Considerations

- Children commonly have dirt under the edges of nails from play.

Gerontologic Considerations

- With aging, nails of fingers and toes develop longitudinal striations, and rate of nail growth slows. Nails often become thick and brittle.

SKILL 11-5 Assessing the Eyes

The ability to see clearly is often taken for granted. Vision is vital to performing activities of daily living, communicating effectively with others, and analyzing and learning about events that occur within our world daily. The nurse often cares for clients with preexisting visual alterations and clients undergoing diagnostic or therapeutic procedures that may impair vision. The nurse must be familiar with the typical symptoms of eye disease. Assessment of visual symptoms may lead to identification of specific eye disorders and determination of the level of assistance clients require in self-care.

Examination of the eye includes skills for assessing visual acuity, visual fields, extraocular movements, and external and internal eye structures. Fig. 11-4 shows a cross section of the eye.

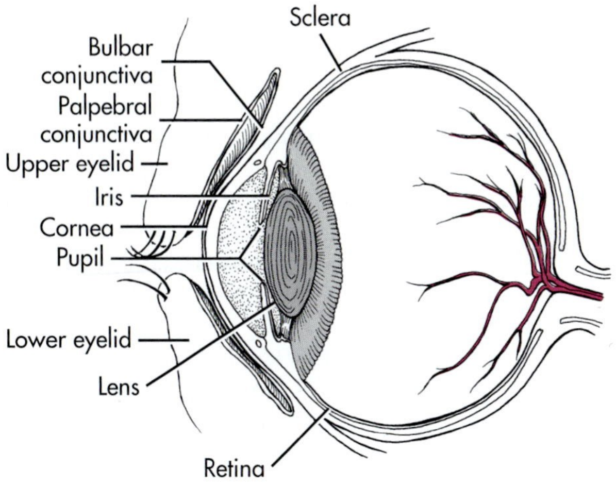

Fig. 11-4 Cross section of eye.

EQUIPMENT

- Newspaper or magazine
- Snellen chart (paper chart or projection screen)
- Opaque index card or plastic eye shield
- Cotton-tipped applicator
- Penlight or flashlight
- Ophthalmoscope
- Disposable gloves (optional)

DELEGATION CONSIDERATIONS

Unlicensed assistive personnel may be able to determine a problem with a client's visual acuity while the client reads a menu, newspaper, or other printed material. Findings should be reported to the RN for assessment. Otherwise this skill requires problem solving and knowledge application unique to a professional nurse.

STEPS	RATIONALE
ASSESSMENT	
1. Question if client has history of **ocular** (eye) disease, eye trauma, diabetes, hypertension, or eye surgery.	Some diseases or trauma can cause risk for partial or complete visual loss. Surgery may have been performed for a visual disorder.
2. Ask if client has experienced eye pain, photophobia (sensitivity to light), burning, itching, excess tearing or crusting, diplopia (double vision), blurred vision, awareness of spots or floaters, flashing lights, halos around lights.	Identification of common symptoms of eye disease may indicate need for physician referral or use of preventive health care practices.
3. Determine if there is a family history of eye disorders or diseases.	Certain eye problems such as glaucoma are inherited.
4. Assess client's occupational history and recreational hobbies. Are safety glasses worn?	Clients who perform close, intricate work often experience eye fatigue. Working with computers may cause eye strain. Certain occupational tasks (e.g., working with chemicals) and recreational activities (e.g., fencing or motorcycle riding) place persons at risk for eye injury unless precautions are taken.
5. Glasses or contacts should be worn during certain portions of the examination for accurate assessment. Misuse of contact lens wear can cause client's ocular symptoms.	

STEPS	RATIONALE
6. Ask if client has visited an ophthalmologist or optometrist recently.	Date of last examination reveals level of preventive care taken by client.
7. Assess medications that client is currently taking, including eye drops or ointment.	Determines need to assess client's knowledge of medications. Certain medications can cause visual symptoms.

PLANNING

STEPS	RATIONALE
1. **Expected outcomes** following completion of procedure:	
➤ Client denies pain throughout examination except during ophthalmoscopic examination (sensitivity to light is common, causing sense of discomfort).	
➤ Client has normal visual acuity (20/20) with or without correction.	Eye structures are intact and functioning.
➤ Client has full visual fields and parallel eye movement in each of the six directions of gaze.	No neurological or muscular disorder.
➤ Eyes are aligned.	
➤ Position of eyes, eyelids, and eyebrows is normal.	
➤ Eyebrows are symmetrical.	
➤ Clarity noted in sclera with conjunctiva clear and pink.	
➤ *P*upils are *E*qual and *R*ound, *R*eact briskly to *L*ight and *A*ccommodation **(PERRLA).**	Optic nerve is intact.
➤ Corneal light reflex is equal.	
➤ Internal eye structures are normal in color, size, and shape. Optic disk is without pathological conditions.	
➤ Client describes signs and symptoms of eye disease.	Information allows client to recognize visual problems early.
2. Prepare client:	
a. Client may sit or stand during assessment of visual acuity. Client stands prescribed distance from Snellen chart to test visual acuity. Client may sit when Snellen projection screen is used.	
b. During remainder of examination client may sit.	Promotes client's comfort and improves nurse's access to eye structures being examined.
c. Explain to client each portion of examination. When examining external eye structures, explain how nurse's hands and equipment will be positioned.	Client may be apprehensive during eye examination, particularly if there are symptoms of alterations. Fear of loss of sight causes anxiety.
d. Use confident but gentle approach. Ask client to inform nurse if there is discomfort.	Minimizes client anxiety.

IMPLEMENTATION

STEPS	RATIONALE
1. Test visual acuity:	
a. If client wears glasses or contact lenses, ask client to read print from newspaper or magazine while wearing lenses or glasses. Be sure lighting is adequate.	Assessment of visual acuity, the ability to see small details, tests central vision.

➤ ***CRITICAL DECISION POINT*** **Be sure client is able to read. Asking client to read aloud can help determine literacy.**

STEPS	RATIONALE
b. If client is unable to see print clearly, test visual acuity by using the Snellen chart or screen for each eye. Screen consists of a mirror into which a slide of the chart is projected.	

STEPS	RATIONALE
(1) Test vision first without client wearing corrective lenses.	
(2) Position client 20 feet (6.1 m) away from chart or the adjusted distance from the screen.	Allows for standardization of findings.
(3) Instruct client to read smallest line of print possible three times: once with both eyes and then with each eye separately, alternating by covering each eye with opaque card or eye shield (see illustration).	

CRITICAL DECISION POINT Do not let client apply pressure to the eyes.

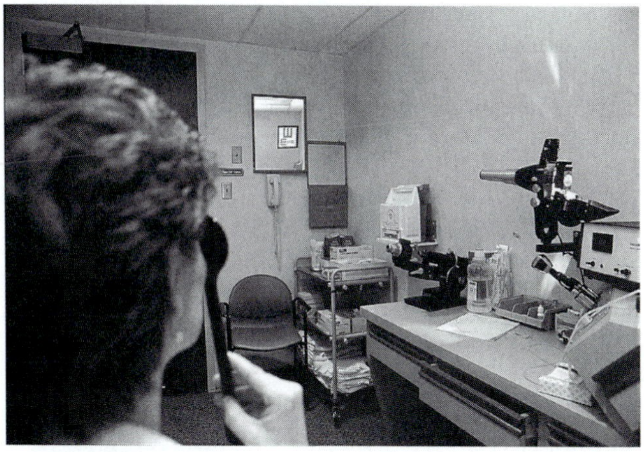

Step 1b[3] Assessment of visual acuity using projection screen with E chart.

STEPS	RATIONALE
(4) Note the smallest line in which the client can read all the letters correctly; record the visual acuity for that line.	Normal visual acuity indicates that central vision (macular function) is intact.
(5) Repeat test with client wearing glasses (but not if glasses are intended only for reading).	Reading glasses are prescribed only for distances of 12 to 14 inches.
(6) If client is unable to read, use an E chart or one with pictures. With E chart, ask client to point in direction each E is pointing. Ask children to identify images on chart.	
c. If client cannot read largest letters or figures of Snellen chart:	Tests for low vision is indicated.
(1) Hold a hand 30 cm (1 foot) from client's face. Have client count upraised fingers.	Tests for object discrimination.
(2) Shine penlight into the eye, then turn light off. Ask if client sees light turned on or off.	Assesses for light perception.
2. Test visual fields:	
a. Ask client to stand or sit 1 meter (approximately 3 feet) away, facing nurse at eye level.	
b. Ask client to gently close or cover the right eye while nurse covers left eye so the open eyes are directly opposite each other. Both nurse and client should look at each other's eye.	Field of vision is superimposed on that of client.
c. Nurse fully extends arm midway between client and self, then moves it centrally with fingers moving.	
d. Ask client to state when movement of fingers is first seen. Compare client's response to the time nurse first noted the fingers moving. Procedure is repeated for all directional fields.	Point at which finger can first be viewed indicates farthest limit of visual field for that direction.

CRITICAL DECISION POINT Visual fields test can be imprecise. Any obvious abnormalities should be reported.

STEPS	RATIONALE
3. Test extraocular movements:	
a. Instruct client to remain in position and look straight ahead toward nurse, keeping head motionless throughout examination.	Assessment tests for parallel eye movement. Movement of head interferes with accurate assessment.
b. Nurse holds finger a comfortable distance (6 to 12 inches [15 to 30 cm]) in front of client's eyes.	Keeping finger comfortable distance from client prevents blurring and eye strain.
c. Nurse asks client to follow movement of finger with eyes, keeping head still. Nurse moves finger slowly through each of six directional gazes (see illustration).	Assesses movement of each of six pairs of extraocular muscles—to right, left, and up, down, on each diagonal.
d. Nurse keeps finger within normal field of vision.	Forcing client to look beyond visual field may cause nystagmus (rhythmic oscillation of eyes).
e. Nurse observes parallel eye movement, position of upper eyelid in relation to iris, and presence of nystagmus (see illustrations).	Eyes move together in parallel. Upper eyelid should cover iris only slightly. Eyelid does not cover pupil.

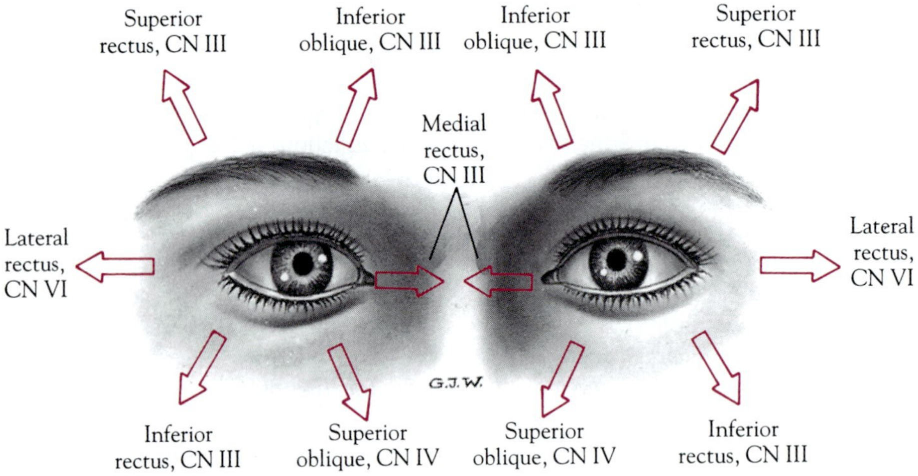

Step 3c Six directions of gaze. (From Seidel HM et al: *Mosby's guide to physical examination,* ed 3, St Louis, 1995, Mosby.)

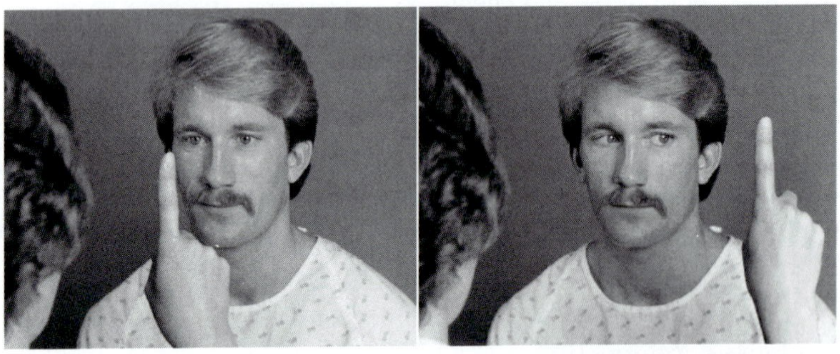

Step 3e Testing client's directions of gaze.

STEPS	RATIONALE
4. Test eye alignment:	
a. Instruct client to look straight ahead toward nurse.	
b. Darken room lights.	Makes penlight visible.
c. Flash a penlight onto the bridge of the client's nose from 60 to 90 cm (2 to 3 feet) away.	Light will reflect onto surface of eye.
d. Look for the spot on both corneas where the light shines.	Light will normally reflect on the cornea in the same spot on both eyes.
5. Assess external eye structures:	
a. Wash hands and apply disposable gloves.	Prevents contact with infectious drainage, especially while inspecting conjunctivae.
b. If client wears contact lenses, request their removal.	Examination of eye structures (e.g., lacrimal gland and conjunctiva) with lens in place during examination could injure eye.
c. Stand or sit directly in front of client at eye level. Instruct client to look at nurse's face.	Allows nurse to clearly inspect position and alignment of eyes in addition to characteristics of all external eye structures.
d. Inspect position of eyes in relation to each other. Note any protrusion or bulging.	Assesses parallel alignment of eyes. May indicate genetic, neurological, or metabolic alterations.
e. If abnormal placement is suspected, measure distance between two pupils by placing small ruler at bridge of nose and asking client to gaze straight ahead.	Large spacing between eyes (hypertelorism) may indicate mental retardation. Normal distance between pupils is 4.5 to 5.5 cm (1¾ to 2¼ inches).
f. Observe eyebrows for size, extension, texture of hair, alignment, and movement. Ask client to raise and lower brows.	Eyebrows are normally symmetrical with equal distribution of hair growth. Client should be able to move eyebrows easily. Inability to move eyebrows indicates paralysis of facial nerve.
g. If flaking of skin is seen around eyebrows, ask if client has experienced eye irritation.	Form of dandruff may affect eyebrows, with particles of skin entering eyes and irritating eyelids or conjunctivae.
h. Ask client to keep eyes open in a normal position. Inspect eyelids for position, color, condition of surface, and condition and direction of eyelashes.	Normally eyelids do not cover pupil, and sclera cannot be seen above iris. Lids are close to eyeball. Eyelashes are normally distributed evenly and curved outward from eye.
i. Note if any portion of lower conjunctiva is visible.	With eyelids open or closed, no palpebral conjunctiva should be visible. Malposition of lid margins may lead to conjunctival irritation.
j. Ask client to close eyes and inspect eyelid positions.	Eyelids should close completely and symmetrically. Failure to close exposes cornea to dryness and irritation.

CRITICAL DECISION POINT **Clients who have incomplete closure of the eyelids (e.g., following stroke, facial nerve paralysis, localized trauma) are at risk for corneal exposure and drying. Frequent lubrication of cornea and possible application of protective eye patch will be necessary to prevent corneal injury.**

STEPS	RATIONALE
k. Have client keep both eyes closed. Raise both eyebrows gently with the thumb and index finger to stretch the skin. Look for color, edema, and presence of lesions. If inflammation or lesion is present, ask if client is experiencing any discomfort.	Normally lids are smooth and same color as client's skin. There should be no inflammation, drainage, edema, or lesions. Lids close symmetrically.
l. Inspect lower lids by having client open the eyes. Note blink reflex.	Person blinks involuntarily and bilaterally as many as 20 times per minute.

STEPS	RATIONALE
m. Inspect lacrimal apparatus (see illustration). Note presence of edema or inflammation at upper outer wall of anterior part of each orbit.	Anterior surface of eye is moistened by tears secreted from lacrimal gland. Gland can be site of tumors or infections.
n. Palpate area of gland gently to detect tenderness.	Normally lacrimal gland cannot be seen or palpated.
o. Inspect for excess tearing of eyes and edema of inner canthus.	Obstruction of nasolacrimal duct causes blockage to flow of tears.
p. If tearing is noted, gently palpate lower eyelid just inside lower orbital rim.	Palpation will cause regurgitation of tears if duct is blocked.
q. Inspect **conjunctiva.** Gently retract lower lid by pressing the thumb or index finger against the lower bony orbit (see illustration). Have the client look up, down, and side to side. Inspect color of conjunctiva and note any edema or lesions. Note color of underlying sclera.	Retraction provides full exposure. Normal **palpebral** conjunctiva lining the lids is light pink in color. Sclera is seen under bulbar conjunctiva; normally it is color of white porcelain in whites and light yellow in blacks.

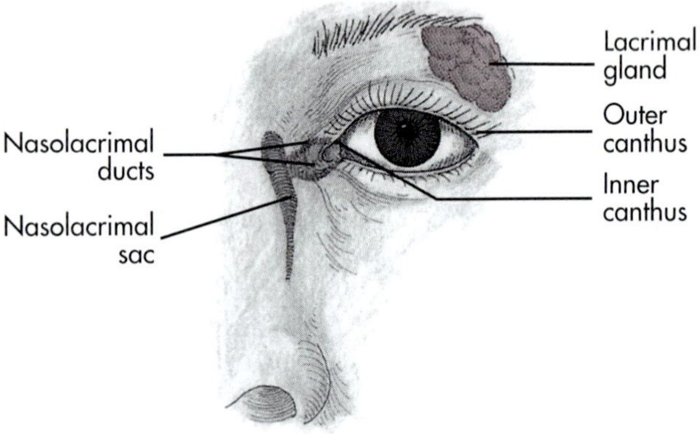

Step 5m Lacrimal apparatus secretes and drains tears, which moisten and lubricate eye structures.

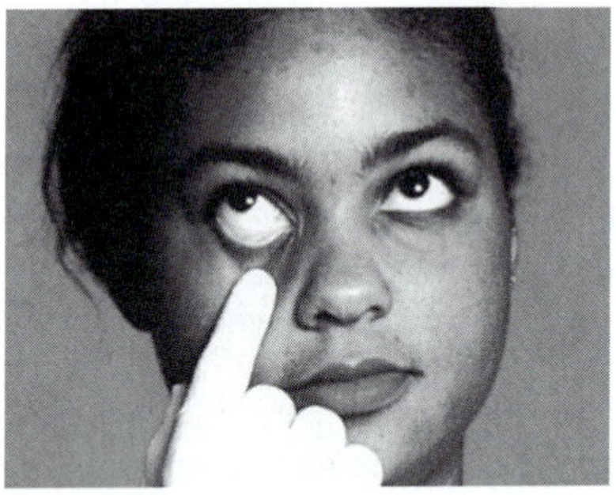

Step 5q Technique for retracting lower eyelid. (From Barkauskas VH: *Health and physical assessment,* St Louis, 1994, Mosby.)

CRITICAL DECISION POINT Do not apply direct pressure to the eye. Pressure can cause ocular injury.

STEPS	RATIONALE
r. Inspect upper conjunctiva only when a foreign body is suspected. To retract upper eyelid, ask client to look down, relax eyes, and avoid any sudden movement. Gently grasp upper lid, pulling it down and forward. Place end of cotton-tipped applicator 1 cm (½ inch) above lid margin. Push down on eyelid with applicator, turning lash inside out (see illustration). Light grasp of lashes keeps lid inverted.	Maneuver breaks suction between lid and globe.

CRITICAL DECISION POINT Carefully inspect and remove foreign object. If object seems embedded in eye tissue, have ophthalmologist examine client as soon as possible.

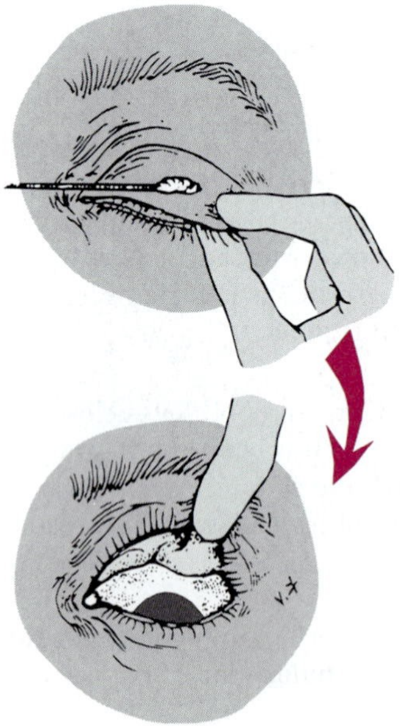

Step 5r Technique for inspecting upper palpebral conjunctiva.

STEPS	RATIONALE
s. After inspection, pull eyelashes gently forward and instruct client to look up. Eyelid returns to normal position. Repeat for other eye.	Exposure of upper palpebral conjunctiva allows inspection for foreign bodies. Client's ability to relax prevents accidental trauma during use of applicator.
t. Stand at the client's side and have the client look straight ahead. Shine a penlight obliquely across the cornea's entire surface. Look for clarity and texture. Repeat for other eye.	Illumination should show a shiny, transparent, and smooth cornea.

CRITICAL DECISION POINT **Report any irregularity in the surface, indicating a tear or abrasion, to an ophthalmologist immediately.**

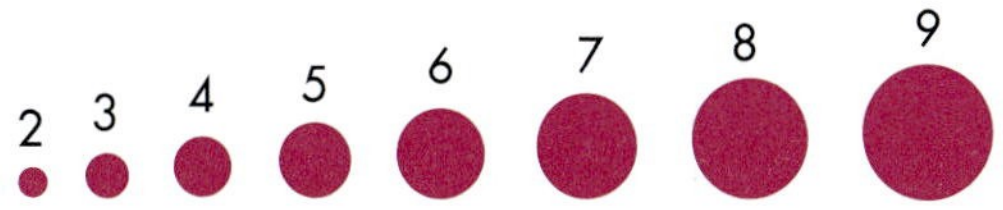

Step 5v Chart depicting pupillary size in millimeters.

STEPS	RATIONALE
u. Remove gloves and wash hands thoroughly.	Drainage from conjunctival infection can be highly contagious. Prevents contamination of examination equipment to be used in subsequent assessment.
v. Inspect pupils for size, shape, and equality (see illustration).	Normal pupils are round, clear, and equal in size and shape.
w. Inspect surrounding iris for symmetry of shape.	Normal iris is clearly visible. Defects along inner margins of iris may be result of surgical correction for glaucoma.
x. Test pupillary reflexes. To test reaction to light, dim room lights. Nurse should still be able to see client's pupils. As client looks straight ahead, move penlight from side of client's face and direct light on pupil. Observe pupillary response of both eyes (see illustrations), noting briskness and equality of reflex.	Darkened room normally ensures brisk response of pupils to light. Pupil that is illuminated constricts (direct light reaction). Pupil in other eye should constrict equally **(consensual light reflex).** Pupils should constrict briskly.

CRITICAL DECISION POINT **Do not have client look at the light; this causes false reaction to accommodation.**

STEPS	RATIONALE
y. Test **accommodation reflex** by first asking client to look at a distant object (far wall) and then at a test object (finger or pencil) held by nurse approximately 10 cm (4 inches) from bridge of client's nose. Watch for pupil movement.	When focusing on near object, pupils of both eyes should converge and accommodate by constricting.

A

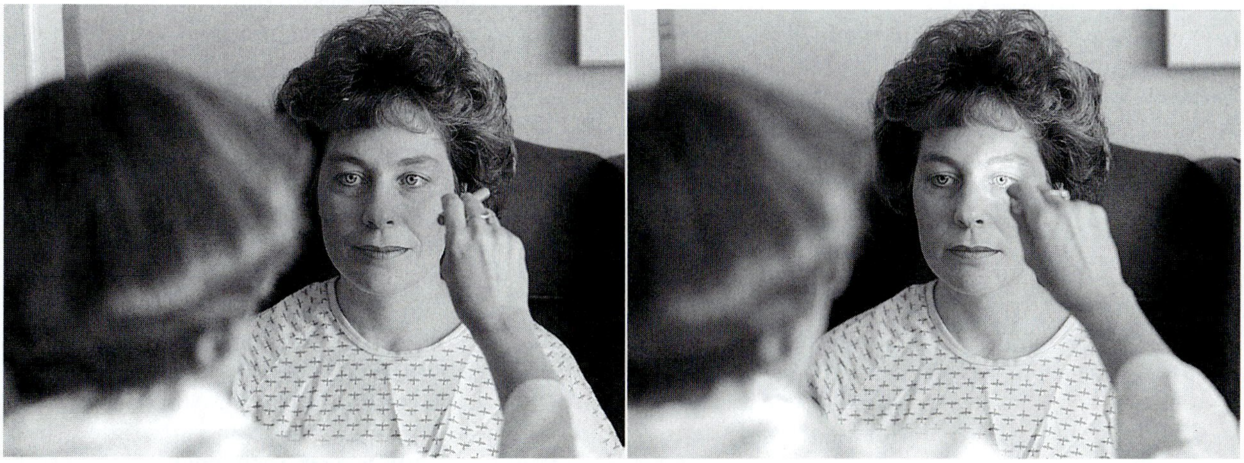

B

Step 5x **A,** To check pupil reflexes, nurse first holds penlight to side of client's face. **B,** Illumination of pupil causes pupillary constriction.

STEPS	RATIONALE
6. Perform ophthalmoscopic examination:	
a. Practice holding ophthalmoscope (see illustration). Use index finger to rotate lens dial at top of battery tube. This changes the light image. The dial at top of the viewer rotates clockwise for selection of a lens that adjusts focus for the examiner. Reading the newspaper with the ophthalmoscope is useful practice. Keep both eyes open when looking through the keyhole.	

CRITICAL DECISION POINT **Examination is usually performed routinely only by nurses in advanced practice.**

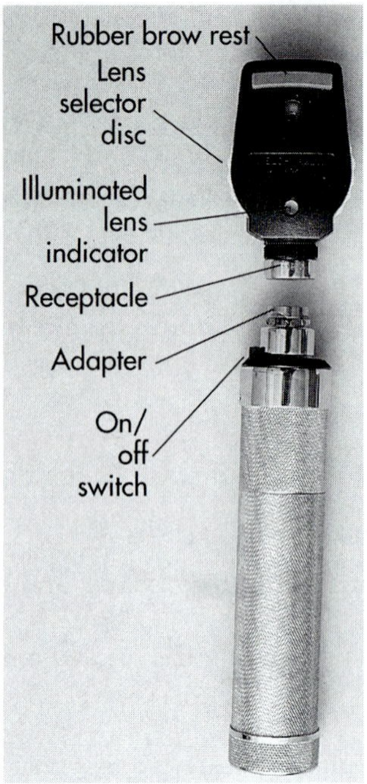

Step 6a Ophthalmoscope. (From Seidel HM et al: *Mosby's guide to physical examination*, ed 3, St Louis, 1995, Mosby.)

STEPS	RATIONALE
b. Have client sit in front of nurse with eyes at same height as nurse's.	Provides nurse easy access to illuminate eye structures.
c. Darken room.	Promotes pupil dilation, allowing more light from ophthalmoscope to enter eye.
d. Have client remove eyeglasses, but contact lenses may be left in place.	
e. Turn ophthalmoscope light on and rotate lens to clear adjustment. Keep index finger on lens dial to refocus during examination.	Lens settings depend on whether examiner or client has errors in refraction (nearsightedness or farsightedness). Setting of 0 is good starting point but may require adjustment for examiner to see eye structures clearly.
f. Ask client to keep both eyes open during examination and to focus on distant object behind nurse.	Nurse's ability to visualize eye structures requires that client keep eyelids open and head still.
g. Nurse examines client's right eye by holding ophthalmoscope in right hand against right eye. Reverse for left eye.	Permits easiest access to illuminate pupil and view structures.
h. Nurse rests ophthalmoscope comfortably against face over right eye and keeps both eyes open. Index finger remains on lens disk. At distance of 25 cm (10 inches) from client and 25 degrees lateral to central line of vision, focus light on pupil. Bright orange glow ("red reflex") can be seen in pupil.	Red reflex indicates light is directed onto pupil and internal structures are illuminated. Orange color is same as that of retina. Focusing light from distance allows nurse to aim ophthalmoscope accurately.
i. Nurse keeps light focused on red reflex and slowly brings head and ophthalmoscope toward client's face from side at 15-degree angle and not directly toward eye (see illustration). As light approaches pupil, nurse begins to see structures of fundus. Rotation of lens disk brings structures into focus. Nurse systematically scans fundus in	Visualization of internal structures requires clear focusing and proper illumination. At any one time examiner sees only small portion of retina. Accurate inspection requires nurse to view each part of fundus separately. Optic disk is most prominent structure and serves as point from which inspection begins.

STEPS | **RATIONALE**

detail, beginning with optic disk and moving outward toward blood vessels and periphery (see illustrations A and B).

Normal fundus: clear, creamy pink, or yellow optic nerve disk; reddish pink retina (whites) or darkened retina (African Americans); light-red arteries and dark-red veins; 3:2 vein-to-artery ratio in size proportion; avascular macula (site of central vision) is two disk diameters temporal to optic disk, is yellow dot and avascular.

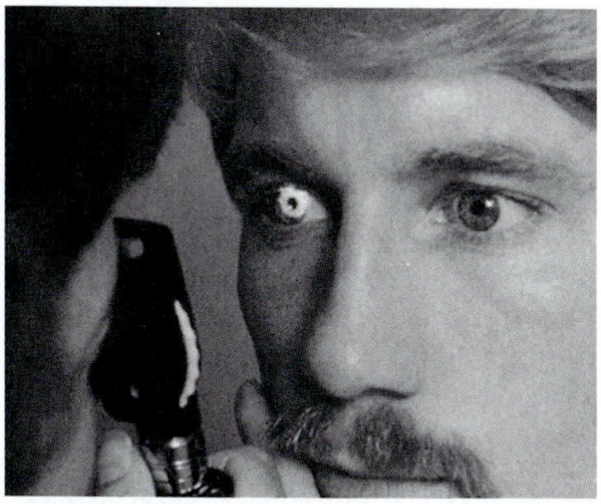

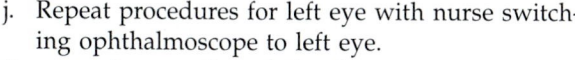

Step 6i(1) Position for visualizing internal eye structures with ophthalmoscope.

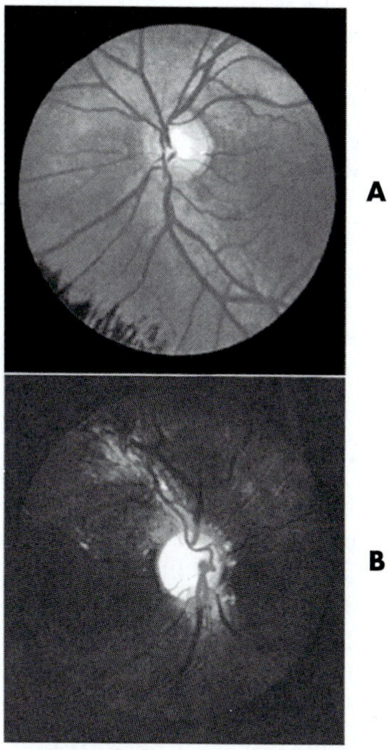

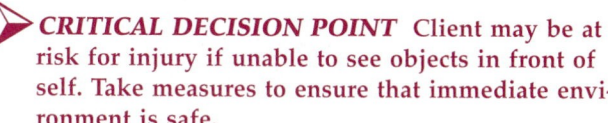

Step 6i(2) Normal fundus. **A,** White adult. **B,** African-American. (From Selected Topics in Ophthalmology, *Medcom clinical lecture guides,* Garden Grove, Calif, 1973, Medcom.)

j. Repeat procedures for left eye with nurse switching ophthalmoscope to left eye.

7. Remove gloves and wash hands.

Prevents transmission of infection.

EVALUATION

1. Compare findings with normal assessment characteristics of eye.

Determines presence of abnormalities.

2. Ask client to identify common symptoms of eye problems.

Demonstrates learning of warning signs.

3. **Unexpected outcomes** that may occur include:
   - Visual acuity is reduced; client is unable to see objects or perceive light. Has difficulty with self-care activities.

     May be caused by either an acute or a long-term problem. If acute, refer to ophthalmologist immediately.
   - Nurse sees finger before client does during visual field testing. Client's visual fields are narrowed.

     Indicates optic nerve problem.

CRITICAL DECISION POINT Client may be at risk for injury if unable to see objects in front of self. Take measures to ensure that immediate environment is safe.

   - Eye movements are unequal in all or specific gazes.

     May be caused by alteration in neurological or muscular function.
   - Light reflects on different spot on each eye.

     Eyes are misaligned.

STEPS	RATIONALE
➤ Both eyes bulge.	**Exophthalmos,** a thyroid disorder, is the cause.
➤ Common forms of inflammation of eyelid: • *Hordeolum* or *stye:* small sebaceous glands near eyelashes become inflamed; localized painful, reddened area is present, usually on lower lid. • *Chalazion:* cyst of internal sebaceous glands; usually localized, nontender, and firm with freely movable skin. • *Marginal blepharitis:* inflammation of eyelid margin; lids become inflamed, scaly, and crusted.	These are common eyelid disorders.
➤ Ptosis of eyelids is noted (eyelid covers upper part of iris).	Drooping of lid is due to edema or possibly nerve paralysis.
➤ Conjunctivae may be inflamed with exudate or pale in color. Crusty drainage is evident on lid margins.	Infectious conjunctivitis results in inflammation and exudate; can be highly contagious. Anemia causes pale conjunctivae.
➤ Pupils may be unequal in size or shape, sluggish to respond to light.	Usually indicates intracranial alteration, glaucoma, or effects of eye medications.
➤ Pupils appear cloudy.	Indicative of cataracts.
➤ Dilated pupils can result from glaucoma, trauma, neurological disorders, eye medications (e.g., atropine), and withdrawal from opioids. Constricted pupils may be caused by inflammation of iris or use of drugs (e.g., pilocarpine, morphine, or cocaine). Pinpoint pupils are common sign of opioid intoxication (Caulker-Burnett, 1994).	
➤ Abnormalities (e.g., hemorrhages, edema of optic nerve disk, cupping of disk with interruption of vascular supply) noted in retinal examination.	Requires follow-up by ophthalmologist; common problems are hypertension, diabetes, glaucoma.
➤ Client is unable to identify warning signs of eye problems.	Reinstruction is necessary.

NURSING DIAGNOSIS

Clustering of defining characteristics from the assessment data may reveal the following nursing diagnoses for clients requiring this skill:

- ➤ Bathing/hygiene self-care deficit
- ➤ Feeding self-care deficit
- ➤ Risk for injury
- ➤ Sensory/perceptual alteration: visual
- ➤ Pain
- ➤ Knowledge deficit regarding visual health

Related factors are individualized based on the client's condition and needs.

RECORDING AND REPORTING

1. Record standardized numbers at end of line on Snellen test read by client. Note *sc* (without correction) or *cc* (with correction).	Documents status of acuity with or without corrective lenses.
2. Record observations made of eye structures and results of functional assessments.	Provides data for comparison with subsequent assessments. Abbreviations: *OD,* right eye; *OS,* left eye; *OU;* both eyes.
3. Report serious abnormalities to nurse in charge or physician.	Immediate medical attention may be required.

FOLLOW-UP ACTIVITIES

1. Refer client to ophthalmologist or optometrist for further testing of visual acuity, treatment of intraocular injury, or further assessment of internal eye condition.
2. If client has visual acuity or visual field loss, make adjustments to support self-care measures (e.g., feeding, bathing and hygiene, dressing).

STEPS **RATIONALE**

3. If client's vision is severely impaired, obtain information about community resources for visually impaired clients. Conduct an assessment of safety factors within home environment (see Chapter 41).
4. If client has foreign body in eye, apply an eye patch loosely over eye. This keeps eyelid closed, reducing constant irritation from lid rubbing against foreign body.

• • • • •

Special Considerations

- Presence of foreign object or corneal abrasion is very painful. Client may have difficulty relaxing.
- Normally, only portion of eye examination that may cause some discomfort is ophthalmoscopic examination (bright light focused on fovea centralis can be uncomfortable).
- *Xanthoma palpebrarum,* deposits of fat (lipid) on eyelids is associated with clients who have hyperlipidemia.

Teaching Considerations

- Clients younger than age 40 should have complete eye examinations every 3 to 5 years (or more often if family history reveals risks such as diabetes or hypertension).
- Clients older than age 40 should have eye examinations every 2 years to screen for glaucoma.
- Clients older than age 65 should have yearly eye examinations.
- Review with client typical symptoms of eye disease (see client history).
- Any client with eyelid inflammation should be cautioned against rubbing eyes because of risk of spreading inflammation or infection to uninvolved eye.
- Client with visual acuity or visual field problems needs to learn how to make the home safer (e.g., removing obstacles; having color contrasts; keeping rooms, stairwells, and walkways well lit) (see Chapter 41).

Pediatric Considerations

- Show child ophthalmoscope and demonstrate how light operates.
- A variety of letter or symbol vision tests are available for children: Home Eye Test for Preschoolers, Blackbird Storybook Home Eye Test, Faye Symbol Chart (Wong, 1995).

Gerontologic Considerations

- Instruct older adult client to take the following precautions because of normal visual changes: avoid driving at night, increase lighting in home to reduce risk of falls, paint first and last steps of a staircase and edge of each step in between a bright color to aid depth perception.
- Common visual changes with aging include reduced acuity (presbyopia), loss of or reduction in peripheral vision, reduced tearing, sensitivity to glare or bright lights, fading of iris, and loss of outer third of eyebrows.
- Arcus senilis, a halo around cornea, is common in older adults but is abnormal in anyone younger than age 40.

Home Care Considerations

- Measurement of visual acuity and visual fields helps nurse determine level of assistance client requires with daily living activities and ability of client to safely ambulate and function independently within home. Client and family may need to make adjustments in how rooms are arranged at home and in obtaining self-help aids (see Chapter 41). Safety precautions (see Teaching Considerations) should also be a part of nurse's plan.
- Examination assesses client's ability to read educational materials. Client may require large-print reading materials or use of magnifying glass.

SKILL 11-6 Assessing the Ears

The nurse assesses the condition of the structures of the ear (Fig. 11-5) by inspecting and palpating external ear structures, inspecting middle ear structures with an otoscope, and testing the inner ear by measuring hearing acuity. Ears are easy to examine because of their accessibility. However, care must be taken in use of the otoscope to minimize risk of injury to the eardrum and other internal structures. Generally the client experiences only minor discomfort during the assessment unless preexisting inflammatory conditions of outer ear structures are present.

Understanding the mechanisms for sound transmission helps the nurse identify the nature of hearing disorders. Sound travels through the ear by air and bone conduction. The following sequence explains the components of hearing: (1) sound waves in the air enter the external ear, passing through the outer ear canal; (2) sound waves reach the

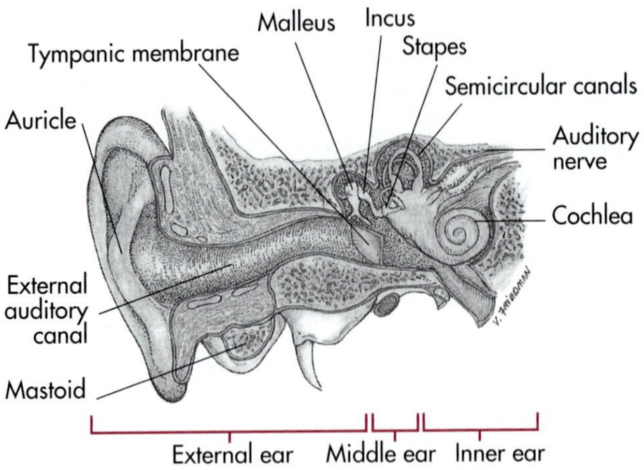

Fig. 11-5 Structures of external, middle, and inner ear.

tympanic membrane, causing it to vibrate; (3) vibrations are transmitted through the middle ear by the bony ossicular chain to the oval window at the opening of the inner ear; (4) cochlea receives the sound vibration; (5) nerve impulses from the cochlea travel to the auditory (eighth cranial) nerve and the cerebral cortex.

Hearing disorders are caused by several types of problems, including mechanical dysfunction (blockage of external ear by cerumen or a foreign body), trauma (foreign bodies or excess noise exposure), neurological disorders (auditory nerve damage), acute illnesses (viral infection), and toxic effects of certain medications.

EQUIPMENT

- **Otoscope (speculums for otoscope come in various sizes to conform to ear canal; choose largest one that fits comfortably)**
- **Tuning fork**
- **Disposable gloves (optional; necessary only if ear has discharge)**

DELEGATION CONSIDERATIONS

Unlicensed assistive personnel should know how to recognize clients with obvious hearing impairments. Review for the staff member how to communicate most effectively with the client. All assessment requires problem solving and knowledge application unique to a professional nurse. For this skill, delegation is inappropriate.

STEPS	RATIONALE
ASSESSMENT	
1. Ask if client has experienced ear pain, itching, discharge, **tinnitus** (ringing in ears), or change in hearing ability.	Signs and symptoms indicate infection or hearing loss.
2. Assess risks for hearing problems: *Infants and children*—hypoxia at birth, meningitis, birth weight less than 1500 g (3.28 pounds), family history of hearing loss, congenital anomalies of skull or face, nonbacterial intrauterine fetal infections (rubella, herpes, syphilis), frequent ear infections, maternal drug use, hyperbilirubinemia, and head trauma. *Adults*—Exposure to industrial or recreational noise, genetic disease (Meniere's disease), neurodegenerative disorders.	These factors can increase risk of permanent hearing loss caused by associated hypoxia, injury, or congenital predisposition.
3. Assess client's occupation in terms of exposure to loud noises and availability of protective devices.	Prolonged noise exposure can cause temporary and permanent hearing loss.
4. Note behavior during earlier assessments that may indicate hearing problem: failure to respond when spoken to; requests to repeat comments; leaning forward to hear; and child's inattentiveness or use of monotonous voice tone.	Clients with hearing loss cope with sensory deficit through a variety of behavioral cues.
5. Determine if client takes large doses of aspirin or other **ototoxic** drugs (e.g., aminoglycosides, furosemide, streptomycin, cisplatin, ethacrynic acid).	Medications have side effects of hearing loss.
6. Determine whether client uses a hearing aid.	Determination allows nurse to assess client's ability to care for device and permits nurse to adjust voice tone to communicate with client.

STEPS	RATIONALE
7. If client has had a recent hearing problem, note onset, contributing factors, affected ear(s), and effect on activities of daily living.	Determines nature and severity of hearing problem.
8. Assess if client has repeated history of cerumen buildup in ear.	Cerumen impaction is common cause of conduction deafness.

PLANNING

1. **Expected outcomes** following completion of procedure:
   - ➤ Client denies discomfort during otoscope insertion.
   - ➤ Auricle and external ear canal are clear and smooth; color is same as face. Cerumen is present in canal in small amounts. — Small amount of cerumen is normal.
   - ➤ Eardrum is translucent, shiny, and pearly gray; light reflex is present. Membrane is free of tears or breaks. — Eardrum is intact.
   - ➤ Client responds to nurse's questions without excess requests to have nurse repeat questions. — Hearing acuity is normal; client can identify spoken word.
   - ➤ Tuning fork tests are normal.
   - ➤ Client identifies risks for hearing loss. — Information enables client to take steps to avoid exposure to risks.
2. Prepare equipment.
3. Prepare client:
   a. Explain steps of procedure, particularly when otoscope is inserted, and assure client that procedure usually is painless. — Introduction of otoscope is painless unless ear canal is inflamed.
   b. Have adult client sit during examination. — Sitting offers easy access to ear structures.
   c. Allow infant or young child to sit on parent's lap. If necessary, restrain child in side-lying position for otoscopic examination. — Restraining child prevents accidental injury to internal ear structures during procedure.

IMPLEMENTATION

EXTERNAL EAR

1. Wash hands. Apply gloves if client has discharge from ear. — Reduces transmission of infection.
2. Inspect size, shape, symmetry, position, and landmarks of auricle (see illustration). Auricles are normally level with each other, and upper point of attachment to head is in straight line with lateral outer canthus (corner of eye). Position of auricle should also be almost vertical. — Abnormal placement of ears may result from mental retardation or other congenital anomalies.

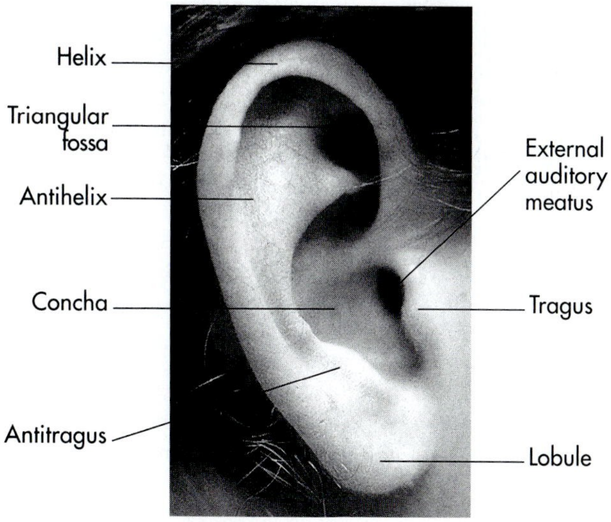

Step 2 Anatomical structures of auricle. (From Seidel HM et al: *Mosby's guide to physical examination*, ed 3, St Louis, 1995, Mosby.)

STEPS	RATIONALE
3. Note color of auricles and presence of any moles, cysts, or nodules.	Color can be affected by external temperature or infectious process. Moles can be cancerous.
4. Palpate auricle for texture and tenderness. If client complains of pain, gently pull auricle and press on tragus and behind the ear over the mastoid bone.	Localizes sites of inflammation.
CRITICAL DECISION POINT **If palpation of external ear increases the pain, external ear infection is likely. If palpation does not increase pain, infection may involve middle ear. Tenderness can indicate infection requiring immediate medical treatment.**	
5. Inspect skin around and behind auricle for scratches, inflammation, lesions, or swelling. In children, note small openings or sinuses. Palpate any lesions gently.	Scratches or lesions may predispose to infection. Sinus or opening may reveal fistula that drains into area of ear or neck.
6. Observe opening of ear canal for size, discharge, foreign bodies, or inflammation.	Narrowing of ear canal by obstruction reduces client's hearing acuity. Skin of ear canal rests closely against underlying cartilage and thus is extremely tender when inflamed. Yellow waxy substance called **cerumen** is common.
CRITICAL DECISION POINT **Discharge may be accompanied by an odor.**	
7. Inspect canal for buildup of cerumen. If canal is clear, ask how client usually cleans ears.	Allows nurse to assess client's hygiene practices. Small amount of cerumen normally should be in ears. Absence of cerumen indicates that client uses special method for cleaning canal.
EAR CANAL AND EARDRUM	
1. Be sure canal is clear of foreign objects.	If foreign object is present, inserting otoscope can embed object deeper into canal.
2. Instruct client about importance of holding head still during insertion of otoscope. Turn on light by rotating disk at top of battery tube. Young child or infant can be restrained by having child sit sideways in parent's lap with one arm hugging parent and other at child's side. Parent holds child by restraining arm with one hand and holding child's head against parent's shoulder with other. Child also can be restrained in side-lying position, with arms at sides and head turned with ear pointed toward ceiling.	Sudden movement by client can damage canal or eardrum.
3. Ask adult client to tip head slightly toward shoulder opposite ear being examined. Hold the handle of the otoscope in the space between the thumb and index finger, supported on the middle finger (see illustration).	This technique leaves the ulnar side of the hand to rest against the client's head, stabilizing the otoscope as it is inserted into the ear canal.

STEPS	RATIONALE
4. Use one of two grips: (1) hold battery tube along the client's neck with the fingers against the neck or (2) brace the inverted otoscope lightly against the side of the client's head or cheek.	Grip stabilizes the otoscope and prevents accidental movement deep into the ear canal.
5. Pull auricle gently to insert otoscope: a. *Adults or older children*—Pull auricle gently up, back, and slightly outward. b. *Infants*—Pull auricle back and down.	Pulling auricle straightens ear canal for proper insertion of otoscope.
6. Insert speculum slightly downward and forward (1.0 to 1.5 cm [½ inch]) into the ear canal, taking care not to abrade lining of canal (see illustration).	Lining of the ear canal has little subcutaneous fat between it and underlying bone, making it highly sensitive to minor trauma.

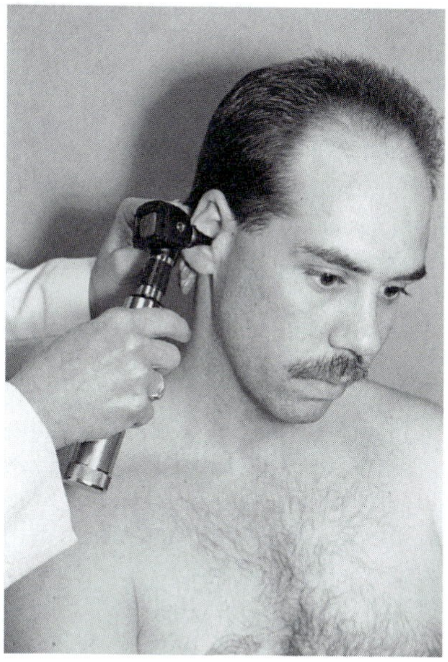

Step 3

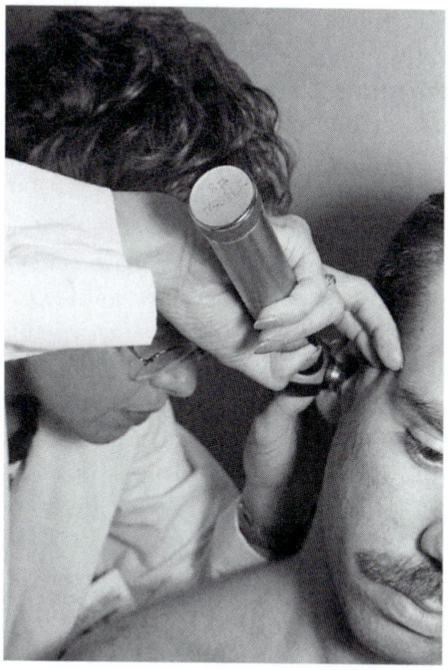

Step 6 Position of otoscope during examination of external auditory canal.

STEPS	RATIONALE
7. Inspect inner canal for color, discharge, scaling, lesions, foreign bodies, and cerumen.	Disorder of inner canal interferes with sound conduction.
8. Inspect eardrum by observing one quadrant at a time. Move otoscope slightly to see entire tympanic membrane and its periphery. Observe for cone of light (light reflex), ring of fibrous cartilage surrounding oval membrane, and umbo of malleus near center of membrane (see illustration). Look carefully for any tears or breaks.	Normal eardrum is translucent, shiny, and pearly gray. Eardrum angles away from ear canal, causing cone of light. Absence of light reflex indicates bulging of membrane.

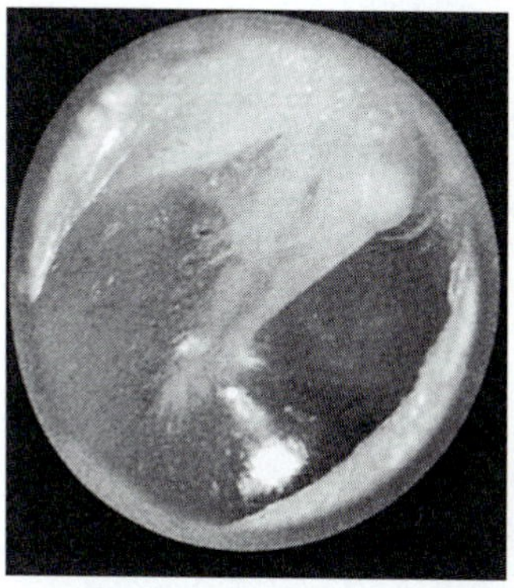

Step 8 Normal right tympanic membrane. (Courtesy Richard A. Buckingham, M.D., Abraham Lincoln School of Medicine, University of Illinois, Chicago; from Malasanos L et al: *Health assessment*, ed 4, St Louis, 1990, Mosby.)

STEPS	RATIONALE
9. Dispose of gloves and wash hands.	Prevents transmission of infection.

STEPS	RATIONALE
HEARING ACUITY	
1. Ask client to remove any hearing aid that is worn.	
2. Note the client's response to questions. If hearing loss is suspected, check the client's response to the whispered voice *(whispered pertoriloquy)*. Test one ear at a time while client occludes the other ear. Have client gently move finger up and down during test. While standing 1 to 2 feet (30 to 60 cm) away from ear being tested, cover the mouth so client cannot read your lips. After exhaling fully, softly whisper random numbers with two equally accented syllables (e.g., *nine four*). Ask the client to repeat what was heard.	Determines if client can identify voice tones. Seidel et al. (1995) report that clients normally hear numbers clearly when whispered, responding correctly at least 50% of the time.
3. Repeat by gradually increasing voice intensity until client correctly repeats numbers.	Reflects hearing deficit.
4. Test other ear and compare results.	
5. If hearing loss is suspected, perform a tuning fork test.	Checks for lateralization of sound. Vibrating tuning fork transmits sound through bone directly to inner ear structures, bypassing external and middle ear.
a. *Weber's test:* Hold fork at its base and tap it lightly against heel of palm. Place base of vibrating fork on midline vertex of client's head or middle of forehead (see illustration). Ask client if sound is heard equally in both ears or better in one ear.	Client with normal hearing hears sound equally in both ears or in midline of head. In conduction deafness, sound is heard in impaired ear. In unilateral sensorineural hearing loss, sound is heard only in normal ear.
b. *Rinne test:* Place stem of vibrating tuning fork against client's mastoid process (see illustration). Begin counting interval with your watch. Ask client to tell you when sound is no longer heard; note number of seconds. Quickly place still vibrating tines 1 to 2 cm (½ to 1 inch) from ear canal, and ask client to tell you when sound is no longer heard (see illustration). Continue counting the time the sound is heard by air conduction. Compare number of seconds for bone conduction versus air conduction.	Air-conducted sound should be heard twice as long as bone-conducted sound. In conduction deafness, bone-conducted sound can be heard longer. In sensorineural loss, sound is not as loud and is heard longer through air.

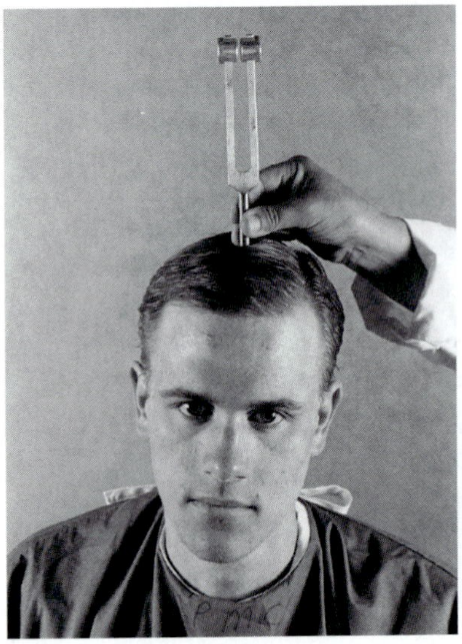

Step 5a Weber test.

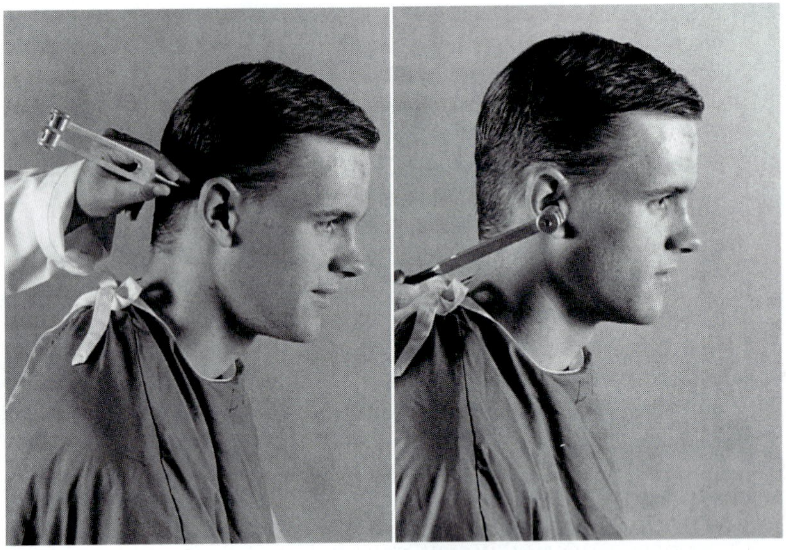

Step 5b Rinne test.

STEPS	RATIONALE
EVALUATION	
1. Compare findings with normal assessment characteristics of ears.	Determines presence of abnormalities.
2. Ask client to describe risks for hearing loss.	Demonstrates learning.
3. **Unexpected outcomes** that may occur include:	
➤ Auricle or ear canal is swollen, inflamed, and tender to palpation. Drainage or lesions may be detected.	Usually indicates infection.
➤ Ears are set lower, below line with lateral canthus.	This is a sign of a congenital abnormality such as Down's syndrome.
➤ Tympanic membrane is pink, red, and bulging.	Indicates inflammation, possibly **otitis media.**
➤ Hearing acuity is reduced; client cannot identify spoken word.	Indicates conduction or nerve deafness.
➤ Tuning fork tests reveal hearing loss.	Indicates conduction or nerve deafness.
➤ Client is unaware of hearing risks.	Reinstruction is necessary.

NURSING DIAGNOSIS

Clustering of defining characteristics from the assessment data may reveal the following nursing diagnoses for clients requiring this skill:

- Risk for injury
- Pain
- Sensory/perceptual alteration: auditory
- Knowledge deficit regarding hygiene

Related factors are individualized based on the client's condition and needs.

RECORDING AND REPORTING

1. Record observations from examination in nurses' notes. Record presence of hearing deficit in plan of care.	Documentation of assessment data provides baseline for future assessments and records client's response to specific therapies. Nursing measures should be planned to adapt to client's communication needs.
2. Record results of Weber's test and note if Rinne test is positive or negative.	Allows nurse to plan for consistently effective communication techniques if hearing loss is present.
3. Report sudden hearing loss to charge nurse or physician.	Hearing loss may require further assessment.

FOLLOW-UP ACTIVITIES

1. Obtain information for client about community resources for the hearing impaired.
2. Client believed to have a hearing deficit should be referred for audiometry.

• • • • •

Special Considerations

- For client with obvious hearing impairment, nurse should speak clearly and concisely, stand so that client can see face, stand toward client's good ear, speak in low pitch, and not yell.
- Teachers of children may be good resource to report unusual behaviors in classroom.

Teaching Considerations

- Instruct client about the proper way to clean outer ear (see Chapter 9).
- Tell client to avoid inserting pointed objects into ear canal.
- Encourage clients older than age 65 to have regular hearing checks. Explain that a reduction in hearing is a normal part of aging but can be successfully reduced with use of a hearing aid.
- If client wears a hearing aid, instruct on proper care and maintenance (see Chapter 9).
- Instruct family members of client with hearing losses to avoid shouting, to speak in low tones, and to be sure client can see speaker's face.

Pediatric Considerations

- In newborns hearing can be determined by eliciting startle reflex and by observing infant's response to loud noises.
- Foreign bodies in ear are not uncommon in children. Pencil erasers and beans are frequent examples. Symptoms include pain, discharge, and impaired hearing.

Gerontologic Considerations

- Older adults experience an inability to hear high-frequency sounds and consonants (e.g., s, z, t, and g). Deterioration of cochlea and thickening of tympanic membrane cause older adults to gradually lose hearing acuity.

Home Care Considerations

- Clients with hearing deficits should install necessary safety alarms with lights in the home to ensure ability to "see" a flashing light when telephone rings, smoke alarm sounds, or oven timer rings.

SKILL 11-7 Assessing the Nose and Sinuses

Assessment of a client's nose and sinuses takes little time, and procedures are relatively simple. If the client has a nasogastric or nasotracheal tube inserted, however, the nurse should take care to inspect the nasal mucosa extra thoroughly. Such tubes can cause considerable trauma and discomfort. The nurse uses inspection and palpation to assess the nose and sinuses. A more detailed examination requires use of a nasal speculum to visualize the nasal turbinates. Care should be taken in use of the speculum to avoid injury to nasal tissues.

DELEGATION CONSIDERATIONS

Unlicensed assistive personnel should know how to monitor for the presence of irritation or breakdown in mucosa, due to irritation from nasogastric or nasointestinal tubes. Findings should be reported to the RN for further assessment. All assessment skills require problem solving and knowledge application unique to a professional nurse. For this skill, delegation is inappropriate.

EQUIPMENT

- **Penlight**
- **Nasal speculum (optional)**
- **Sinus transilluminator (optional)**
- **Disposable gloves (optional)**

STEPS	RATIONALE
ASSESSMENT	
1. Determine if client has experienced any trauma to nose.	Can cause septal deviation and asymmetry of external nose.
2. Assess if client has history of allergies, nasal discharge, epistaxis (nosebleeds), or postnasal drip.	Useful in determining source or nature of nasal and sinus drainage.
3. If client has a history of nasal discharge, assess character, amount, odor, duration, and associated symptoms (e.g., sneezing, nasal congestion, obstruction, or mouth breathing).	Can help to rule out presence of infection, allergy, or drug use (snorting of drugs causes nasal discharge).
4. Assess for history of nosebleeds, including site, frequency, amount of bleeding, treatment, and difficulty in stopping bleeding.	Characteristics may reveal trauma, medication use, or excessive dryness as causative factors.
5. Ask if client uses nasal spray or drops; have client explain regimen.	Overuse of over-the-counter nasal preparations can cause physical change in mucosa.
6. Ask if client snores at night or has difficulty breathing.	Difficulty in breathing or snoring may indicate septal deviation or obstruction.
PLANNING	
1. **Expected outcomes** following completion of procedure:	
➤ Client experiences minimal discomfort.	Nasal mucosa can become very sensitive when inflamed.
➤ Nose is aligned, symmetrical, firm, without obvious lesions, and nontender.	Skin is same color as face.
➤ Nasal mucosa is pink and moist without lesions.	
➤ Air passes freely through nose as client breathes.	
➤ Septum is in midline.	Deviated septum is relatively common.
➤ Sinuses are nontender.	Absence of local irritation.
➤ Sinuses glow when illuminated.	Reveals normal air in sinuses.
➤ Client explains precautions for using nasal spray.	Demonstrates learning.

STEPS	RATIONALE
2. Prepare client:	
a. Explain steps of procedure and assure client that examination will not be painful or interfere with breathing.	Minimizes client's anxiety.
b. Have client assume sitting position with head tilted backward.	Provides for visualization of internal nasal structures.

IMPLEMENTATION

STEPS	RATIONALE
1. Wash hands. Apply gloves if client has drainage or bleeding from nose.	Reduces transmission of infection.
2. Inspect nose externally for shape, skin color, alignment, and presence of deformity or inflammation.	Recent trauma may cause edema and discoloration.
3. If swelling or deformities exist, gently palpate the ridge and soft tissue of the nose by placing one finger on each side of the nasal arch and gently moving fingers from the nasal bridge to the tip. Note tenderness, masses, and underlying deviations.	Assesses extent of deformity. Asymmetry may indicate trauma.
4. Place a finger on the side of the client's nose and occlude one naris. Ask client to breathe with mouth closed. Repeat for other naris.	Assesses patency of **nares** (nostrils).
5. Illuminate anterior nares with penlight and inspect nasal mucosa. Note color of mucosa and any lesions, discharge, swelling, or presence of bleeding.	Character of discharge and inflammation indicate allergy or infection.

CRITICAL DECISION POINT **Perforation and erosion of the septum and puffiness and/or increased vascularity of the mucosa can indicate habitual use of intranasal cocaine and opioids. Client may require appropriate support and counseling intervention.**

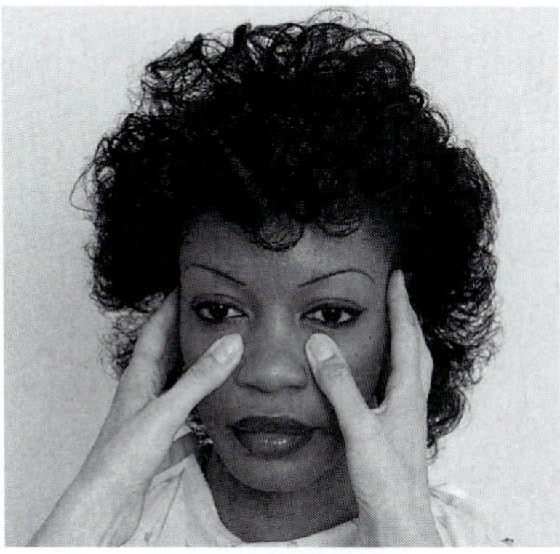

Step 10 Palpation of maxillary sinuses. (From Wilson SF, Thompson JM: *Respiratory disorders,* Mosby's Clinical Series, St Louis, 1990, Mosby.)

STEPS	RATIONALE
6. In clients with a nasogastric, nasointestinal, or nasotracheal tube, inspect nares for excoriation, inflammation, or sloughing of skin.	Swallowing or coughing reflex causes movement of tubes against nares. Failure to anchor tube properly causes pressure against nares and mucosa.

CRITICAL DECISION POINT **Serious inflammation and/or sloughing may require repositioning of tube at nares or even reinsertion into opposite naris. Consult physician if reinsertion is questioned.**

STEPS	RATIONALE
7. Ask client to tip head back slightly. Inspect septum for alignment, perforation, or bleeding.	Position provides clear view of septum and turbinates. Normal septum is close to midline and thicker anteriorly.
8. Option: Insert nasal speculum into each naris and advance approximately 1 cm (½ inch). Hold handle at 90-degree angle to side of nose.	Provides clear view of septum and turbinates.
9. Palpate frontal sinus by placing thumb up and under the client's eyebrow, using gentle pressure.	Pressure elicits tenderness if sinus is swollen or inflamed.

CRITICAL DECISION POINT **Do not apply pressure to the eyes.**

STEPS	RATIONALE
10. Palpate maxillary sinuses by placing thumbs over maxillary sinus, just to each side of nose, and apply gentle upward pressure (see illustration).	Elicits tenderness in presence of inflammation.

STEPS	RATIONALE
11. If sinus tenderness is present or infection is suspected, transillumination should be performed: a. Darken room. b. View maxillary sinus by placing the transilluminator light lateral to the client's nose, just beneath the medial aspect of the eye (see illustration A). c. Have client open mouth. Check to see if hard palate is illuminated. d. View frontal sinus by placing the light against the medial aspect of each supraorbital rim (see illustration B). A dim red glow of light should be seen just above the eyebrow.	Transillumination detects air or fluid in the sinuses. Absence of glow indicates that sinus contains secretions.

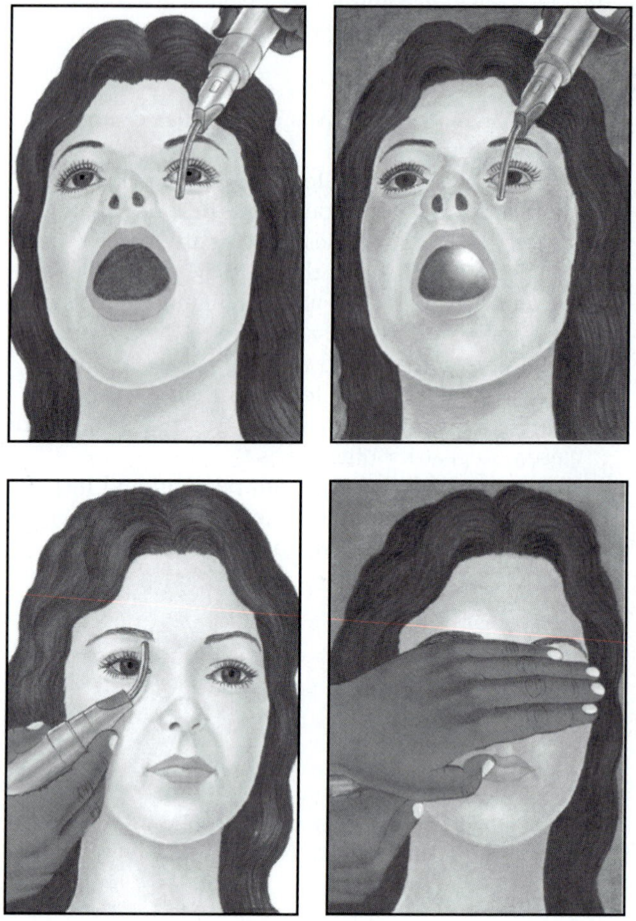

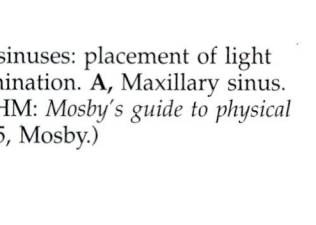

Step 11 Transillumination of sinuses: placement of light and expected area of transillumination. **A,** Maxillary sinus. **B,** Frontal sinus. (From Seidel HM: *Mosby's guide to physical examination,* ed 3, St Louis, 1995, Mosby.)

STEPS	RATIONALE
12. Remove gloves, wash hands, and dispose of supplies in proper receptacle.	Reduces transmission of infection.

EVALUATION

1. Compare findings with normal assessment characteristics of nose and sinuses.	Determines presence of abnormalities.
2. Have client report on use of nasal spray.	Demonstrates level of compliance with therapy.
3. **Unexpected outcomes** that may occur include:	
➤ Nose is asymmetrical.	Frequently results from trauma.
➤ Nasal mucosa is inflamed and swollen, with yellowish or green drainage.	Indicates local irritation or infection.
➤ Mucosa is pale with clear, watery discharge.	This is a result of allergy.
➤ Mucoid discharge is present.	Indicates rhinitis.
➤ Nasal airway is obstructed by lesions, swelling, deviated septum, or drainage.	Alters client's ease in breathing.
➤ Septum is perforated.	Result of repeated use of intranasal cocaine.
➤ Sinuses are tender.	Indicates infection or allergy.
➤ Sinuses illuminate with areas of dark color.	Indicates presence of fluid in sinuses.
➤ Client overuses nasal spray.	Reinstruction is necessary.

STEPS	RATIONALE

NURSING DIAGNOSIS

Clustering of defining characteristics from the assessment data may reveal the following nursing diagnoses for clients requiring this skill:

- Ineffective breathing pattern
- Impaired tissue integrity
- Pain
- Knowledge deficit regarding use of nasal spray

Related factors are individualized based on the client's condition or needs.

RECORDING AND REPORTING

STEPS	RATIONALE
1. Record observations in nurses' notes.	Documents baseline findings and changes in client's condition.
2. Report abnormalities to nurse in charge or physician.	Client may require specific therapies.

• • • • •

Teaching Considerations

- Caution client against overuse of over-the-counter nasal sprays. Overuse of such sprays can cause a rebound effect and essentially worsens nasal irritation.
- Instruct parents on care of children with nosebleeds: Have child sit up and lean forward to avoid aspiration of blood; apply pressure to anterior of nose with thumb and forefinger as child breathes through mouth; apply ice or a cold cloth to bridge of nose if pressure fails to stop bleeding.

Pediatric Considerations

- Nasal flaring in children may indicate respiratory difficulty.
- If child has been crying, a watery discharge from nose is normal.
- Discharge from one nostril may be caused by a foreign body in nares.

Gerontologic Considerations

- Older adults may report problems with sense of smell during examination. Instruct them in importance of installing smoke detectors throughout home and to always check dated food labels for possible spoilage.

SKILL 11-8 Assessing the Mouth and Pharynx

The condition of the oral cavity can reveal significant information about a client's overall health, such as state of hydration and nutritional status, hygiene practices, and any specific pathological conditions. Too frequently the nurse hurries through an assessment of the mouth and pharynx; it is important to perform the procedure thoroughly. The nurse can easily miss a lesion or local area of inflammation under or around the tongue and along the mucosal surfaces. A convenient time to perform the assessment is while administering oral hygiene.

EQUIPMENT

- **Tongue depressor**
- **Penlight**
- **Disposable gloves**
- **Gauze square**

DELEGATION CONSIDERATIONS

Unlicensed assistive personnel frequently administer oral hygiene to clients and should learn to report to the RN any findings made during hygiene care. Staff members may be the first to see a change in hydration or appearance of a mucosal lesion, for example. The skill of assessment requires problem solving and knowledge application unique to a professional nurse. For this skill, delegation is inappropriate.

STEPS	RATIONALE
ASSESSMENT	
1. Determine if client wears dentures or retainers and if they are comfortable.	Dentures must be removed to visualize and palpate gums. Ill-fitting dentures and retainers chronically irritate mucosa and gums and may pose risk for mouth cancer.
2. Determine if client has had recent change in appetite or weight.	Symptoms may result from painful conditions of mouth or poor oral hygiene.
3. Assess if client has pain from chewing or difficulty in swallowing or moving tongue or jaws. If so, ask if mouth lesions are present and how long they have been noticed.	May be associated with broken tooth, tooth grinding, or temporomandibular joint problems. Difficulty chewing, swallowing, or moving tongue or jaw are also late symptoms of oral cancer (American Cancer Society, 1996).
4. Assess client's dental hygiene practices, including use of fluoride toothpaste, frequency of brushing and flossing, and frequency of dental visits.	Provides nurse opportunity for health education during examination. Assessment may also reveal need for financial support.
5. Determine if client smokes or chews tobacco.	Tobacco users have greater risk for mouth and throat cancers than nonusers (American Cancer Society, 1996).
6. Review history of alcohol consumption.	Heavy drinkers appear to have increased risk for oral cancer. Effects of alcohol are independent of tobacco use (Franco, 1991).
PLANNING	
1. **Expected outcomes** following completion of procedure:	
➤ Client remains comfortable.	Oral mucosa can become sensitive when inflamed.
➤ Mucosal surfaces are glistening, pink or light red, soft, moist, and smooth.	
➤ Lips are pink, moist, symmetrical, and smooth.	
➤ Upper molars rest directly on lower molars, with upper incisors slightly overriding the lower incisors.	
➤ Normal adult has 32 teeth.	
➤ Teeth are white, smooth, and shiny.	Indicates that good hygiene is performed regularly.
➤ Mucosal surfaces are glistening pink or light red, soft, moist, and smooth.	
➤ Gums are pink, moist, smooth, and firm, with a tight margin at each tooth.	Indicates adequate hydration and nutrition.
➤ Tongue is medium or dull red, moist, slightly rough on top surface, smooth along lateral margins, and mobile.	No lesions or neurological impairments are found.
➤ Palate and pharynx are pink to red, well hydrated, and smooth. (Hard palate is rough.)	
➤ Gums and buccal mucosa are hyperpigmented.	This hyperpigmentation is normal in 10% of light-skinned individuals and in as many as 90% of dark-skinned individuals older than age 50.
➤ Uvula and soft palate rise when client says "ah."	Normal innervation by vagus (tenth cranial) nerve.
➤ Client follows oral hygiene practices.	Understanding benefits of improved hygiene motivates behavior change.
➤ Client knows warning signs and risk factors for oral cancer.	Enables client to assume preventive health care habits.
2. Prepare client:	
a. Have client sit facing nurse at eye level.	Allows nurse to visualize internal structures easily.
b. Explain need to open mouth fully during examination.	Client's cooperation reduces examination time, improves visibility of mouth structures, and eliminates need to use tongue depressor.

STEPS	RATIONALE
IMPLEMENTATION	
1. Wash hands and apply gloves.	Reduces transmission of infection.
2. Have client close mouth normally. Inspect lips from end to end (see illustration). (Have female client remove lipstick beforehand.) Inspect lips for color, texture, hydration, contour, symmetry, and lesions.	Provides full view of lips. Asymmetry may be caused by facial nerve paralysis.
3. Ask the client to clench the teeth and smile. Look for position of upper molars and incisors in relation to lower teeth.	Allows for assessment of teeth occlusion and symmetry of smile.
4. Have the client remove any dental appliances before proceeding with the examination.	Provides for full view of gums and mucosa.
5. Inspect and count the teeth, noting position, wear, presence of caries and alignment. View posterior surface of teeth by having client open mouth and relax lips. Use a tongue depressor to retract the lips and cheeks to view back molars. Inspect base of teeth for tartar and note any dental caries or extraction sites.	Allows for assessment of quality of dental hygiene or evidence of trauma.
6. View inner oral mucosa by asking client to open and relax mouth slightly. Retract client's lower lip away from the teeth (see illustration); repeat for upper lip. Note color, texture, hydration, and lesions such as ulcers, abrasions, or cysts.	Client's ability to relax and open mouth prevents pulling or tension on mucosa. Child may participate by retracting lips for nurse to examine mucosa.
CRITICAL DECISION POINT **If small, yellow-white raised lesions are noted on the lips or mucosa, these are probably Fordyce's spots (ectopic sebaceous glands).**	
7. If lesions are present, palpate with hand for tenderness, size, and consistency.	Allows discrimination between solid mass, ulceration, and cyst.

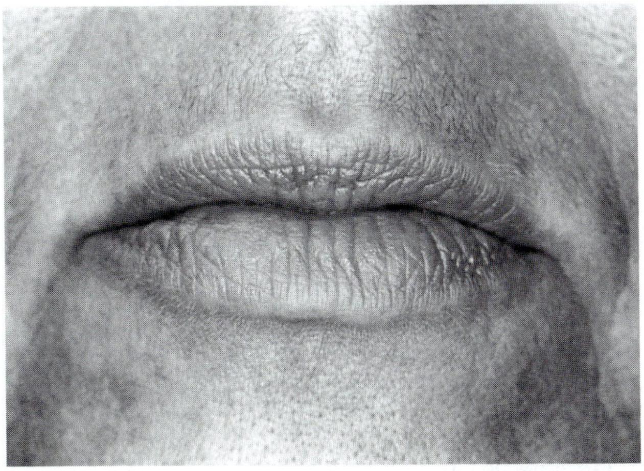

Step 2 Inspect lips.

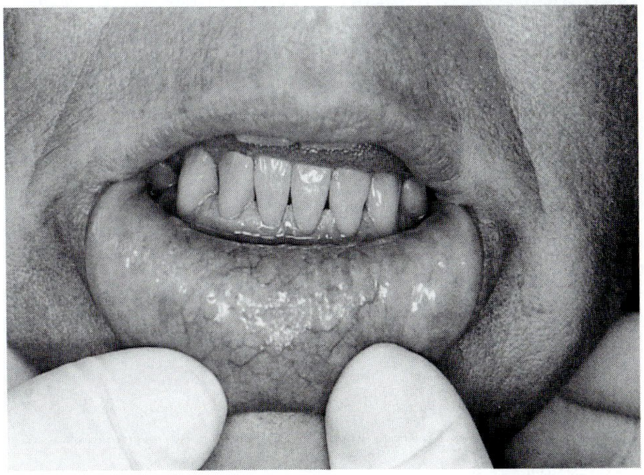

Step 6 Inspection of inner oral mucosa of lower lip.

STEPS	RATIONALE
8. Ask client to open mouth. Inspect **buccal** mucosa (lining of cheeks) by gently retracting cheeks with tongue depressor (see illustration) or gloved finger covered with gauze. Use penlight to view more posterior mucosa. View surface of mucosa from right to left and top to bottom. Observe for color, texture, and hydration.	Full retraction is needed to see all mucosal surfaces.
CRITICAL DECISION POINT This is a good site to inspect for jaundice and pallor.	
9. Palpate cheek with one finger along the inner mucosa and the thumb along the outside cheek.	Assesses for deep-seated lumps or ulcerations.
10. While retracting cheeks, inspect gums for color, edema, retraction, bleeding, and lesions. Ask client if areas of tenderness exist. Be sure to view back molar area.	Gingivitis (inflammation of gums) is a common periodontal disease of adults. Back gums are difficult areas to reach during hygiene.
11. Palpate gums gently with a gloved finger; note resistance. Observe for any thickening or masses and presence of any lesions.	Determines firmness. Periodontal disease causes spongy gums that bleed easily.
CRITICAL DECISION POINT Periodontal disease may indicate vitamin C deficiency, requiring a more detailed dietary history.	
12. Inspect tongue by asking client to relax mouth and protrude tongue halfway. Illuminate with penlight while inspecting all sides of tongue. Note color, size, position, and texture of tongue and any coatings or lesions. Also look for any deviation, tremor, or limitation in movement.	If client is forced to protrude tongue too far, gag reflex is elicited. Positioning of tongue also tests for hypoglossal nerve function.
13. Continue examination by asking client to lift the tongue and place its tip on the palate, behind the upper incisors (see illustration). Carefully inspect the floor of the mouth.	Oral cancer frequently develops in floor of mouth. The ventral surface of the tongue is pink and smooth with large veins between the frenulum folds.
CRITICAL DECISION POINT Presence of any nodules or cysts should be reported immediately.	

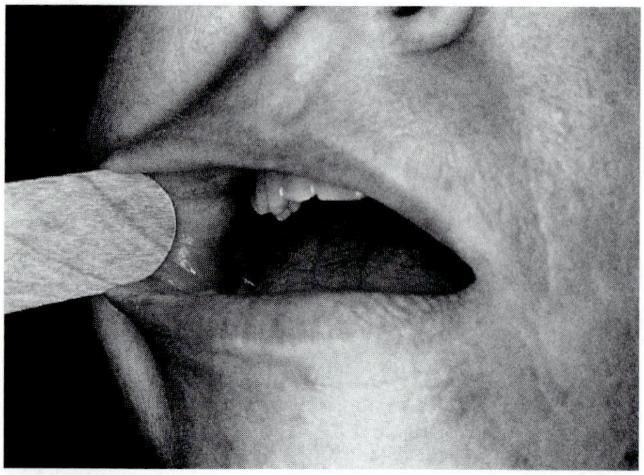

Step 8 Retraction of buccal mucosa allows for clear visualization.

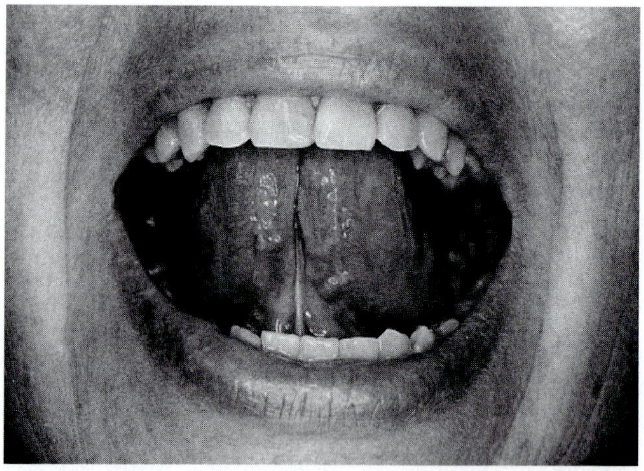

Step 13 Undersurface of tongue is highly vascular.

STEPS	RATIONALE
14. Ask client to raise the tongue up and move it from side to side. Look for symmetry.	Tongue mobility and function are essential for normal swallowing, chewing, and taste.
15. Before palpating tongue, explain procedure. Ask client to extend tongue. Grasp tip with gauze square, and gently retract to one side. Palpate full length of tongue and base for areas of hardening or ulceration. Repeat on other side.	Client may fear sensation of being unable to swallow. Detects areas of hardening, which can be a sign of a malignant lesion.
16. With client extending head backward and holding mouth open, inspect hard and soft palates (see illustration). Penlight may be needed. Note color, shape, texture, and extra bony prominences or defects.	Hard palate is located anteriorly and is dome shaped. Soft palate extends toward pharynx.
17. Ask client to say "ah." Place tongue blade on middle third of tongue, taking care not to press the lower lip against the teeth. With penlight, view the uvula and soft palate. Both should rise centrally (see illustration).	Tongue depressor placed anteriorly may cause posterior tongue to mound and obstruct view. Tongue depressor placed posteriorly may elicit gag reflex. Assesses tenth cranial (vagus) nerve function. Uvula and soft palate should rise.
18. With penlight, inspect posterior pharynx, including anterior and posterior tonsillar pillars. Observe color, hydration, drainage, and any lesions. Note the tonsils in the cavity between pillars.	These are common sites for infection or inflammation.
19. Throughout examination, notice whether client has halitosis (bad breath).	Can be indicative of poor oral hygiene, ingestion of alcohol, certain foods, or metabolic disturbances such as diabetes.

CRITICAL DECISION POINT Be respectful to client before exploring ways to control or reduce halitosis.

20. Remove gloves. Wash hands and dispose of supplies in receptacle.	Reduces transmission of infection.

EVALUATION

1. Compare findings with normal assessment characteristics of mouth and pharynx.	Determines presence of abnormalities. Findings document client's response to hygiene measures.
2. Have client describe routine used for home oral care.	Demonstrates application of knowledge.

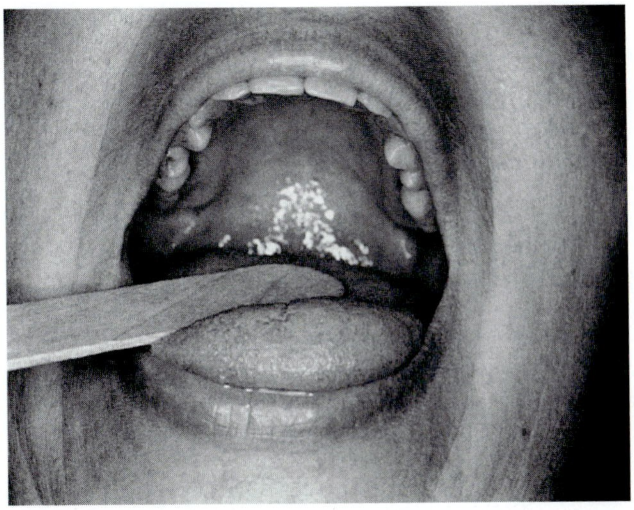

Step 16 Hard palate is located anteriorly in roof of mouth.

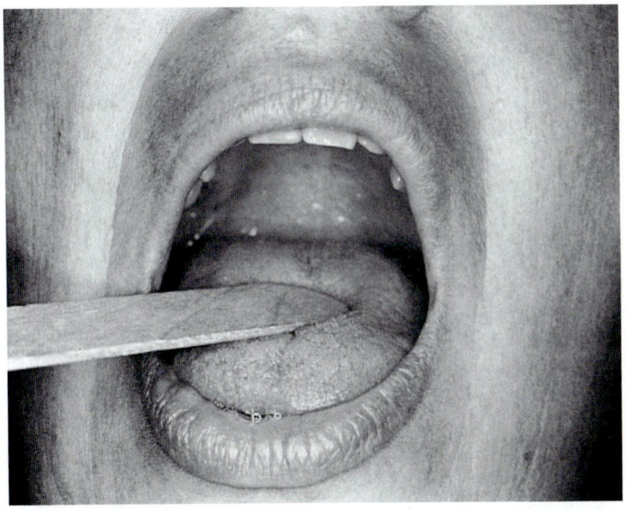

Step 17

STEPS	RATIONALE
3. Have client describe warning signs of oral cancer and any risk factors to which client is exposed.	
4. **Unexpected outcomes** that may occur include:	
➤ Vesicular eruptions, singular or multiple, are found on lips. Common "cold sores" are caused by herpes simplex virus.	
➤ Lips are dry, cracked, and tender.	Can result from dehydration, constant licking, mouth breathing, or exposure to cold.
➤ Upper or lower incisors protrude. Upper incisors do not overlap with lower incisors.	Indicates malocclusion.
➤ Mucosa has thick white patches. Patches may be difficult to remove.	Thick white coating indicates poor hygiene. Leukoplakia results from excessive drinking and smoking; these lesions are precursors to cancer.
➤ Mucosa is dry and inflamed and has ulcerations or excoriations.	This is a result of dehydration, trauma, or possibly infection.
➤ Teeth are chalky white with black or brown discolorations. Dental caries form along gum lines and between teeth, where food particles accumulate.	Change in color indicates dental caries.
➤ Client complains of oral pain.	Pain may result from dentures rubbing against gums or an actual lesion.
➤ Tongue is coated and edematous.	This is caused by dehydration, poor hygiene, or nutrition.
➤ Gums are inflamed, tender, bleed easily, and separate from base of teeth.	These findings indicate gingivitis.
➤ Client exhibits reddened and edematous uvula and tonsils with yellow exudate.	Sore throat from bacterial or viral infection is indicated.
➤ Client reports failure to follow hygiene practices.	Reinstruction or further discussion regarding client's health practices is needed.
➤ Client is unable to recall warning signs of oral cancer.	May require further discussion.

NURSING DIAGNOSIS

Clustering of defining characteristics from the assessment data may reveal the following nursing diagnoses for clients requiring this skill:

- Altered oral mucous membrane
- Bathing/hygiene self-care deficit
- Knowledge deficit regarding oral hygiene
- Pain
- Impaired swallowing

Related factors are individualized based on the client's condition or needs.

RECORDING AND REPORTING

1. Record condition of oral cavity structures in nurses' notes or assessment flow sheet.	Establishes baseline data for future comparisons after therapies.
2. Report any lesions or bleeding to nurse in charge or physician.	Conditions indicate need for follow-up care.

FOLLOW-UP ACTIVITIES

1. If client has dental caries or denture irritation, refer to dentist.
2. After an examination is a good time to have the client perform dental hygiene and to observe technique.

• • • • •

Special Considerations

- Malocclusion can interfere with chewing.
- Dark surface stains on teeth may be caused by tea, coffee, or tobacco.
- The use of smokeless tobacco (plug, leaf, and snuff) is on the increase in the United States. The 1993 Youth Risk Behavior Survey by the Centers for Disease Control and Prevention (CDC) reported that 20% of male high-school students used smokeless tobacco (American Cancer Society, 1996). The excess risk of cancer of the cheek and gum may reach 50-fold among long-term snuff users.
- Ill-fitting dentures cause inflammation of gums.

Teaching Considerations

- Discuss proper techniques for oral hygiene, including brushing and flossing.
- Explain early warning signs of oral cancer, including a sore that bleeds easily and does not heal, a lump or thickening, and a persistent red or white patch on mucosa. Difficulty chewing or swallowing are late changes.
- Encourage children and adults to have dental examinations every 6 months.

Pediatric Considerations

- A helpful rule in estimating the number of temporary teeth for children who are 2 years old or younger (Wong, 1995):

  Expected number = Child's age in months − 6

  Full set of teeth is 20 in child and 32 in adult.
- Child may benefit from parent demonstrating how to say "ah." Most older children can be examined without tongue blade. Since infants and toddlers usually resist keeping mouth open, nurse may perform assessment near end of examination.
- Determine if client's dentist uses dental sealants. Rozier and Beck (1991) report a significant decline in oral caries related to use of sealants.

Gerontologic Considerations

- In older adults gum recession occurs from loss of tissue elasticity or periodontal tissue.
- Loose or missing teeth are common because bone resorption increases.
- Yellow or darkened teeth are also common in the older adult because of the general wear and tear that exposes the darker underlying dentin.
- An older adult's teeth often feel rough when tooth enamel calcifies.
- The mucosa is normally dry because of reduced salivation.
- Varicosities (swollen veins) under the tongue are common in the older adult.
- Older adults may need to eat soft foods and cut food into small pieces because of difficulty in chewing and changes in the teeth.

SKILL 11-9 Assessing the Structures of the Neck

Primary structures within the neck that the nurse assesses include the neck muscles, lymph node chains, carotid arteries and jugular veins, thyroid gland, and trachea. The nurse usually defers assessment of carotid arteries and jugular veins until the cardiovascular assessment (see Skill 11-11). Thorough assessment of the lymphatic system eventually requires examination of all regions—head and neck, breasts, genitalia, and extremities. Generally the nurse assesses for similar characteristics of all neck structures, including symmetry, size, shape, and any lesions. The assessment techniques are normally painless, involving inspection, palpation, and auscultation.

EQUIPMENT

- Stethoscope
- Glass of water

DELEGATION CONSIDERATIONS

This skill requires problem solving and knowledge application unique to a professional nurse. For this skill, delegation is inappropriate.

STEPS	RATIONALE
ASSESSMENT	
1. Ask if client has had recent infection or cold.	This can cause temporary or permanent lymph node enlargement.
2. If client reports presence of an enlarged lymph node, focus history on whether client has had a recent infection. Nurse may also choose to review client's history to consider possibility of HIV infection.	Enlarged lymph node can be normal but can also indicate local or systemic infection and presence of malignancy.
3. Determine if client has history of thyroid problem or takes thyroid medications.	Disease or medications may influence tissue growth of thyroid gland.
4. Ask if client has had change in temperature preference (more or less clothing); swelling in neck; change in texture of hair, skin, or nails; fatigue; or change in emotional stability (e.g., depression).	Symptoms indicative of thyroid disease.
5. Ask if client has had a history of neck pain with restriction in movement.	Neck pain may indicate muscle strain, head injury, local nerve injury, or an enlarged or swollen lymph node.
6. Review client's medical history for pneumothorax (collapsed lung) or bronchial tumor.	These preexisting conditions place client at increased risk for tracheal displacement.
PLANNING	
1. **Expected outcomes** following completion of procedure:	
➤ Neck moves freely, without discomfort or dizziness and with full range of motion.	
➤ Lymph nodes are nonpalpable and not visible.	Normal findings with no evidence of infection.
➤ Lymph nodes identified in examination are small, mobile, and nontender.	This is a common finding after a serious infection.
➤ Thyroid gland is not visible. If palpable, the gland is small, smooth, and free of nodules.	
➤ Trachea is in midline.	
➤ Client describes signs of lymph node or thyroid gland abnormalities.	
2. Prepare client:	
a. Have client sit.	Provides easy access. Nurse examines all neck structures from behind, to side, and in front of client.
b. Explain that client will not experience choking sensation while trachea is palpated.	Client may be anxious about palpation of airway.
IMPLEMENTATION	
1. Inspect the neck in the usual anatomical position, with slight hyperextension. Look for symmetry of neck muscles (see illustration).	Normal bilateral symmetry should be noted.

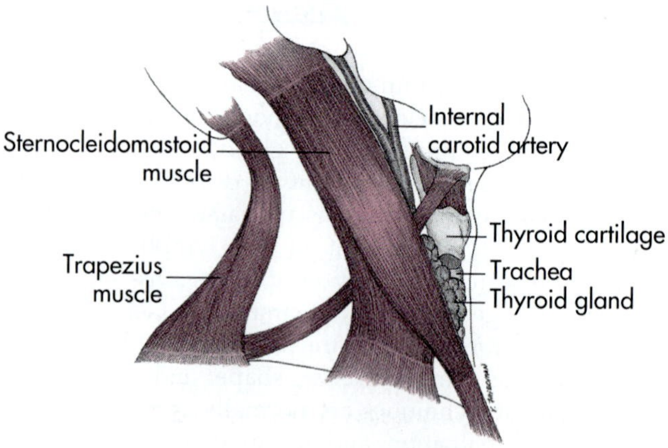

Step 1 Anatomical position of major neck structures. Note triangles formed by sternocleidomastoid muscle, lower jaw, and anterior neck (anteriorly) and sternocleidomastoid muscle, trapezius muscle, and lower neck (posteriorly).

STEPS	RATIONALE
2. Ask client to flex the neck with chin to the chest. Then have client hyperextend neck backward. Last, have client move head sideways so that ear moves toward shoulder.	Tests for function of sternocleidomastoid, trapezius, and, again, sternocleidomastoid muscles.
3. Ask client to raise chin and tilt head slightly, without tensing neck muscles. Inspect area where lymph nodes are distributed; compare both sides for symmetry, edema or masses, and erythema or red streaks (see illustration).	Position stretches skin slightly over any possible enlarged nodes. Tensing interferes with eventual palpation of nodes. Normally nodes are not visible.
4. Have client relax with the neck flexed slightly forward and, if needed, toward the nurse. Stand to the side of the client. With the pads of the middle three fingers, palpate gently in a rotary motion for superficial lymph nodes (see illustration). Check each node methodically in the following sequence: Occipital nodes at base of skull Postauricular nodes over mastoid Preauricular nodes just in front of ear Retropharyngeal nodes at angle of mandible Submaxillary nodes Submental nodes in midline behind mandibular tip	Maneuver relaxes tissues and muscles.

CRITICAL DECISION POINT Avoid vigorous palpation as this may obliterate small nodes and cause stimulation of carotid sinus.

STEPS	RATIONALE
5. Palpate and compare both sides of the neck for enlargement of nodes, noting location, size, shape, surface characteristics, consistency, mobility, tenderness, and warmth of nodes.	Character of mass aids in determining likelihood of mass being a benign lesion, a malignant lesion, or hypertrophic tissue.

CRITICAL DECISION POINT Nodes that are large, fixed, inflamed, or tender indicate a problem that should be reported.

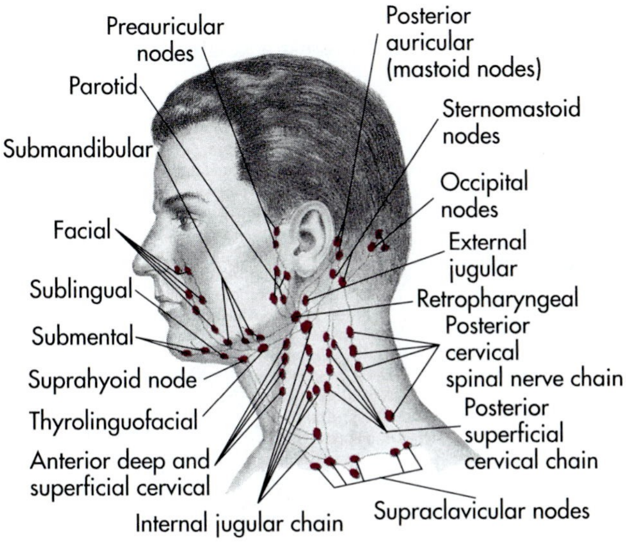

Step 3 Head and neck lymphatic chain. (From Seidel HM et al: *Mosby's guide to physical examination,* ed 3, St Louis, 1995, Mosby.)

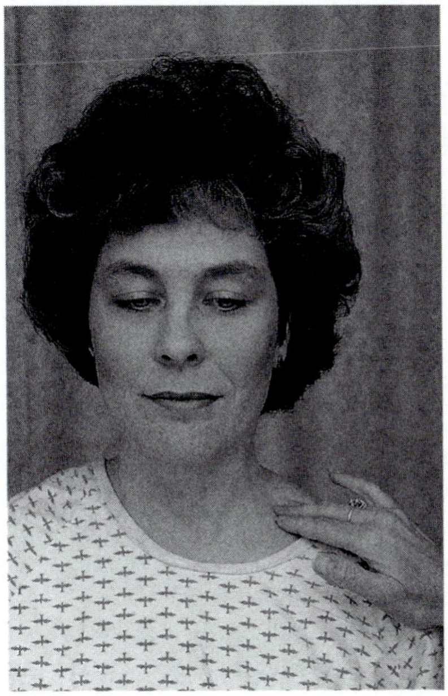

Step 4 Palpation of supraclavicular lymph nodes.

STEPS	RATIONALE
6. If the skin is mobile, move the skin over the area of the nodes.	Ensures detection of any enlargement.

CRITICAL DECISION POINT **Do not simply move the fingers over the skin; this prevents detection of smaller nodes. Also, do not apply excessive pressure because small nodes can be missed and palpable nodes obliterated.**

STEPS	RATIONALE
7. Have client bend the head forward and relax the shoulders. Palpate supraclavicular nodes by hooking the index and third finger over the clavicle, lateral to the sternocleidomastoid muscle.	Position allows for palpation of deep cervical nodes.
8. If an enlarged node is found, explore adjacent areas and regions drained by the nodes for signs of infection (e.g., inflammation, tenderness, warmth), or malignancy (enlargement of multiple nodes that are nontender, hard, and discrete).	
9. Stand in front of client and inspect area of lower neck overlying thyroid gland for symmetry, visible masses, and any subtle fullness at the base of the neck (see illustration).	Gross inspection may reveal area of gland enlargement.

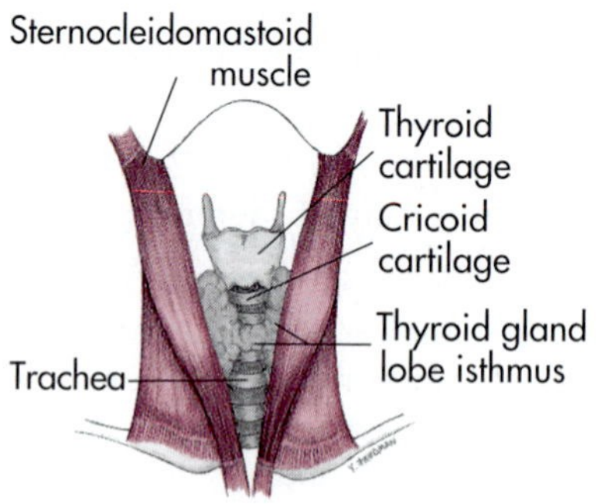

Step 9 Anatomical position of thyroid gland.

STEPS	RATIONALE
10. Provide the client a glass of water. Ask client to extend neck slightly and take a swallow of water; note any bulging of the thyroid gland.	Hyperextension helps to tighten the skin for better visualization. Swallow causes an enlarged gland to bulge.
11. To palpate thyroid gland, nurse stands in front of or behind the client. Use light, gentle palpation, allowing fingers to drift over the gland.	Technique allows hand to sense any abnormalities.

CRITICAL DECISION POINT **Excessive pressure over thyroid from palpation may prevent examiner from detecting nodules.**

STEPS	RATIONALE
12. Have client flex the neck slightly forward and laterally toward the side being examined. Give client cup of water and instruct to sip and swallow when directed.	Position relaxes the sternocleidomastoid muscle.
13. Posterior approach:	
a. Place both hands around the client's neck, with two fingers of each hand on the sides of the trachea just beneath the cricoid cartilage.	
b. Palpate the gland for size, shape, configuration, consistency, tenderness, and presence of nodules.	
c. As the client swallows, feel for movement of the thyroid isthmus. Note any enlargement of the isthmus.	The thyroid should move beneath the fingers when the client swallows.

STEPS	RATIONALE
d. To examine each lobe, have the client swallow and displace the trachea, first to the right and then to the left, until all lobes are examined; during examination of the right lobe, move the fingers of the left hand between the trachea and the right sternocleidomastoid muscle (see illustration). Then place fingers of the right hand behind the right sternocleidomastoid muscle, and gently press the hands together to palpate the lobe. Repeat approach for left lobe with hands in reverse positions.	Normal thyroid is small, smooth, and free of nodules.
14. Anterior approach:	
a. While standing at client's side, use the pads of the index and middle fingers to palpate the left lobe with the right hand and the right lobe with the left hand. Do this as the client swallows.	
b. Move the skin medially over the sternocleidomastoid muscle, and reach under its anterior borders while the fingers stay beneath the cricoid cartilage.	Gentle displacement of trachea allows palpation of main body of each thyroid gland.
15. If gland appears enlarged, place the diaphragm of the stethoscope over the thyroid.	Blood flow through the thyroid arteries increases and causes a fine vibration in an enlarged gland. Will be heard as a soft, rushing sound **(bruit).**
16. Defer carotid and jugular vein examination until assessment of cardiovascular system.	
17. With client lying or sitting, place thumb and index finger on each side of trachea, just above suprasternal notch (see illustration). Trachea is normally in midline above suprasternal notch. Avoid forceful pressure.	Gentle palpation prevents eliciting cough reflex.

CRITICAL DECISION POINT **Lateral displacement may be result of pneumothorax, a medical emergency. Consider client's history and notify physician.**

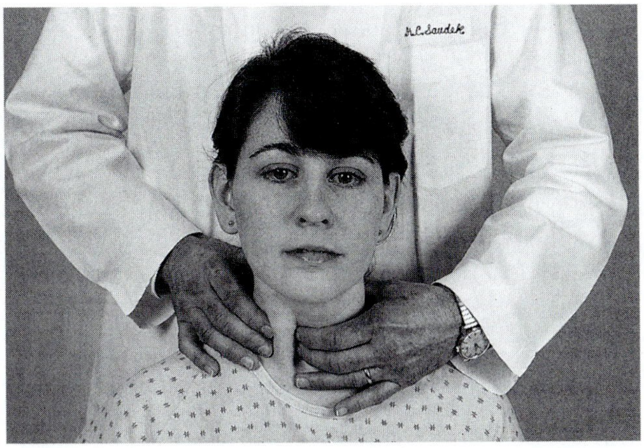

Step 13d Palpation of right thyroid lobe from behind client. (From Seidel HM et al: *Mosby's guide to physical examination,* ed 3, St Louis, 1995, Mosby.)

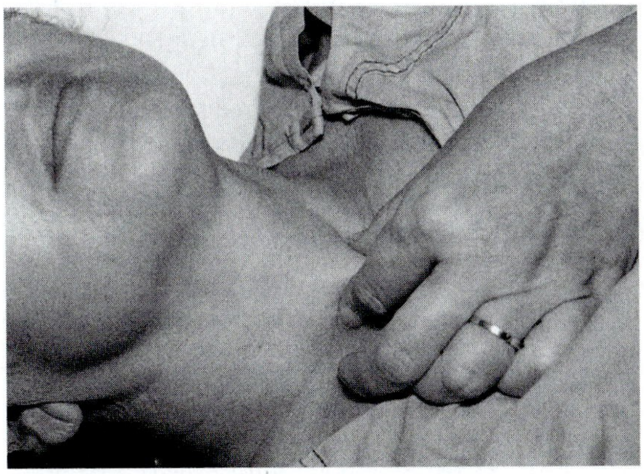

Step 17 Palpation of trachea.

STEPS	RATIONALE
EVALUATION	
1. Compare findings with normal assessment characteristics of neck structures.	Determines presence of abnormalities.
2. **Unexpected outcomes** that may occur include:	
➤ Lymph nodes are palpable, nontender, fixed, and hard.	May indicate a malignant lesion.
➤ Lymph nodes are palpable, tender, large, and mobile.	Indicates inflammation, infection, or both.
➤ Thyroid gland is palpable and has nodules.	Indicates enlargement from hypothyroidism or hyperthyroidism or reveals benign or malignant lesions.
➤ Trachea is deviated to right or left.	Bronchial mass or pneumothorax is probable cause.
➤ Client is unable to describe characteristics of neck mass.	Reinstruction necessary.

NURSING DIAGNOSIS

Clustering of defining characteristics from the assessment data may reveal the following nursing diagnoses for clients requiring this skill:

- Pain
- Risk for infection

Related factors are individualized based on the client's condition or needs.

RECORDING AND REPORTING

1. Record observations in nurses' notes or assessment flow sheet. Be specific in describing lymph node chain involved and location of any mass.	Provides baseline findings for comparison.
2. If any palpable mass is present in neck, report to physician immediately.	Potential nature of problems may necessitate further diagnosis or treatment.

FOLLOW-UP ACTIVITIES

1. Tracheal deviation may indicate need for chest x-ray examination.

• • • • •

Special Considerations

- Goiter involving the thyroid gland is relatively rare. However, client may benefit from education about normal dietary sources of iodine, such as green leafy vegetables or seafood.
- Noting which lymph nodes are enlarged may indicate a site of infection. For example, ear infections usually drain to preauricular or deep cervical nodes.
- Right lobe of thyroid is normally larger than left. Enlarged gland results from thyroid dysfunction. Masses or nodules may indicate cancerous lesions.

Teaching Considerations

- For clients with thyroid disease, stress importance of regular compliance with medication schedule.
- Instruct client to call physician when an enlarged lump or mass is noted in the neck.
- Instruct client about the lymph nodes and how infection can commonly cause node tenderness.

Pediatric Considerations

- In children, small, nontender immovable nodes are normal.
- Cervical and postauricular nodes can quickly enlarge in response to any mild stimulus from infection or inflammation.

Gerontologic Considerations

- Number of lymph nodes declines, and size of nodes may decrease with advancing age.

SKILL 11-10 Assessing the Thorax and Lungs

Physical assessment of the thorax and lungs requires a review of ventilatory and respiratory functions of the lungs. Any alteration in pulmonary function usually affects other body systems. For example, reduced oxygenation can cause changes in mental alertness because of the brain's sensitivity to lowered oxygen levels. Thus the nurse must carefully assess findings from all body systems when determining the nature of pulmonary problems.

To perform an assessment accurately, the nurse should be familiar with the anatomical landmarks of the chest wall (Fig. 11-6). This assists in identifying findings in relation to the location of the lobes of the lung (Fig. 11-7, *A-C*) and the position of each rib. The apex of each lung is at the top, and the base is at the bottom. To locate the position of each rib, the nurse begins by finding the Angle of Louis at the manubriosternal junction. The angle is a vis-

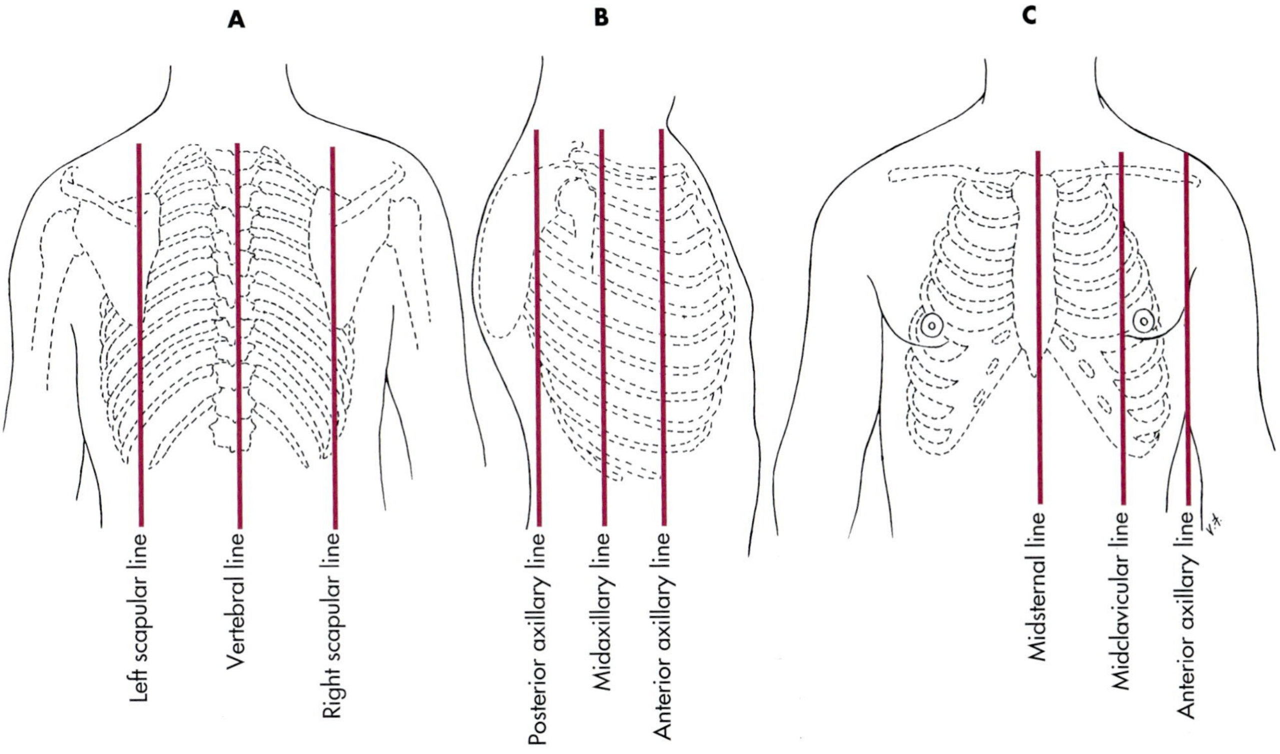

Fig. 11-6 Anatomical landmarks of chest wall. **A,** Posterior view. **B,** Lateral view. **C,** Anterior view.

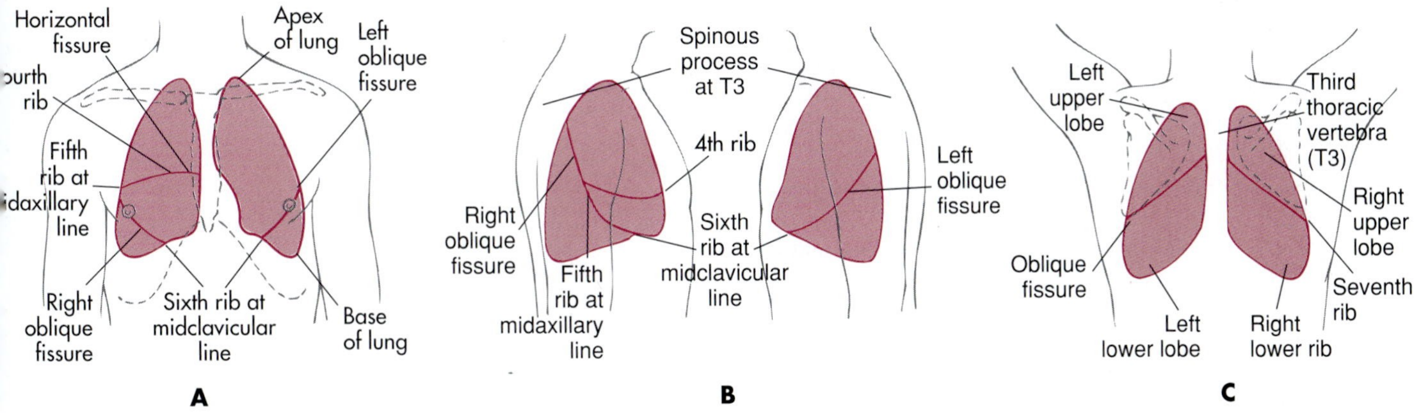

Fig. 11-7 Position of lung lobes in relation to anatomical landmarks. **A,** Anterior. **B,** Lateral. **C,** Posterior.

ible and palpable angulation of the sternum and the point at which the second rib articulates with the sternum. The nurse counts the ribs and intercostal spaces from this point. The number of each intercostal space corresponds to that of the rib just above it.

Examination of the lungs and thorax requires the client to be undressed to the waist. A female client may keep a gown draped loosely over her chest while the posterior chest is examined. Good lighting is essential. The nurse should assess clients at risk for pulmonary problems, such as the client confined to bed rest or the client with chest pain who cannot fully expand the lungs. The examination begins with the client sitting for assessment of the posterior and lateral chest. The client may sit or lie down for examination of the anterior chest.

EQUIPMENT

- **Stethoscope**
- **Disposable gloves (optional: if handling a sputum specimen)**

DELEGATION CONSIDERATIONS

Unlicensed assistive personnel should learn to monitor status of client's respirations and report changes in rate and depth. All other assessment skills of the lung and thorax require problem solving and knowledge application unique to a professional nurse. For these skills, delegation is inappropriate.

STEPS	RATIONALE
ASSESSMENT	
1. Assess history of tobacco or marijuana use, including type of tobacco, duration and amount in pack years (Pack years = Number of years smoking × Number of packs per day), age started, and efforts to quit.	Smoking is a risk factor linked with incidence of lung cancer, heart disease, and chronic lung disease (emphysema, bronchitis). Cigarette smoking is responsible for 90% of lung cancers among men and 79% among women (American Cancer Society, 1996).
2. Ask if client experiences any of the following: *persistent cough* (productive or nonproductive), *sputum production, chest pain,* shortness of breath, orthopnea, dyspnea during exertion, poor activity tolerance, and *recurrent attacks of pneumonia or bronchitis.*	Symptoms indicative of respiratory alterations may help nurse localize any objective findings. (Warning signals for lung cancer are in *italic* type.)
3. Determine if client works in environment containing pollutants such as asbestos, coal dust, or chemical irritants. Does client have exposure to second hand cigarette smoke?	Environmental pollutants are risk factors for various lung diseases.
4. Review history for known or suspected HIV infection, substance abuse, low income, and residence in nursing home (American Thoracic Society, 1992).	Known risk factors for exposure to and/or development of **tuberculosis.**
5. Ask if client has history of cough, hemoptysis, weight loss, fatigue, night sweats, and/or fever.	Signs and symptoms for both tuberculosis and HIV infection.
6. Assess for history of allergies to pollen, dust, or other airborne irritants, as well as to any foods, drugs, or chemical substances.	Symptoms client demonstrates may be caused by allergic response to allergen: choking feeling, bronchospasm with respiratory stridor, wheezing on auscultation, dyspnea, cyanosis, and diaphoresis.
7. Review family history for cancer, tuberculosis, allergies, or chronic obstructive pulmonary disease (COPD).	Conditions increase client's risk for lung disease.
PLANNING	
1. Expected outcomes following completion of procedure: ➤ Chest contour is symmetrical, with anteroposterior diameter ⅓ to ½ of the transverse (side-to-side) diameter. ➤ Scapulas are symmetrical and closely attached to thoracic wall. The normal spine is straight, without lateral deviation. ➤ Posteriorly, the ribs slope across and downward. No bulging is evident in intercostal spaces.	

STEPS	RATIONALE
➤ Respirations are passive, diaphragmatic or costal, and regular (12 to 20 per minute in adult).	
➤ Chest wall is not tender.	
➤ Chest excursion is symmetrical, with 3 to 5 cm (1½ to 2 inches) expansion.	Full ventilatory movement is occurring.
➤ Symmetry of tactile fremitus over all lung fields is evident.	Sound passes evenly through lung tissue.
➤ Lung is resonant to percussion.	Normal sound indicates lung is filled with air.
➤ **Echophony**—spoken voice sound "eee" is muffled.	Lung is air-filled.
➤ Normal breath sounds clear to auscultation bilaterally.	Air flows without interference or obstruction.
➤ Client is able to describe factors that predispose to lung disease.	Awareness of risks can improve compliance with healthful behavior.
➤ Client assumes appropriate posture for best ventilation.	Client can learn about benefits of good posture as examination maneuvers are performed.
2. Prepare client:	
a. Have client sit upright. For bedridden client, elevate head of bed 45 to 90 degrees.	Promotes full lung expansion during examination.

CRITICAL DECISION POINT **Be sure client's position in bed does not impede full expansion of the lung.**

STEPS	RATIONALE
b. Allow client to lie supine or in Sims' position, with position changes necessary during examination.	These positions are used for clients who cannot tolerate sitting.
c. Remove gown or drape first from posterior chest, keeping legs covered. As examination progresses, remove gown from area being examined.	Avoids unnecessary exposure and provides full visibility of thorax.
d. Explain all steps of procedure, encouraging client to relax and breathe normally.	Anxiety may increase client's respiratory rate, thus interfering with analysis of findings.

IMPLEMENTATION

POSTERIOR THORAX

STEPS	RATIONALE
1. Standing at midline position behind client, inspect thorax for shape, deformities, position of the spine, slope of the ribs, retraction of **intercostal spaces** during inspiration, and bulging of intercostal spaces during expiration.	Allows for identification of any factors that may impair chest expansion and any symptoms of respiratory distress. (In child, shape of chest is almost circular, with anteroposterior diameter in 1:1 ratio. In adult, chest is twice as wide as deep, with 1:2 anteroposterior diameter. Chronic lung disease results in 1:1 ratio.) Clients with breathing problems assume postures that improve ventilation.

CRITICAL DECISION POINT **If client holds chest wall during breathing, this may be symptomatic of localized chest pain. Assess nature of pain further.**

STEPS	RATIONALE
2. Determine the rate and rhythm of breathing (see Chapter 10).	This is a good time to measure respirations, with client relaxed and unaware of inspection.
3. Palpate posterior chest wall, costal spaces, and intercostal spaces, noting any masses, pulsations, unusual movement, or areas of localized tenderness. If suspicious mass or swollen area is detected, palpate for size, shape, and typical qualities of lesion (see Skill 11-2).	Palpation assesses further characteristics and confirms or supplements findings from assessment. Localized swelling or tenderness may indicate trauma to ribs or underlying cartilage.

STEPS	RATIONALE

CRITICAL DECISION POINT **If client notes pain, do not palpate deeply. A fractured rib fragment could be displaced.**

4. Standing behind client, place thumbs along the spinal processes at the tenth rib, with the palms lightly contacting the posterolateral surfaces (see illustration). The nurse's thumbs should be about 2 inches (5 cm) apart, with the thumbs pointing toward the spine and the fingers pointing laterally. Press hands toward client's spine to form small skinfold between thumbs. After exhalation, client takes deep breath. Note movement of thumbs (see illustration). Normally thumbs separate 3 to 5 cm (1½ to 2 inches) during chest excursion.

Palpation of chest excursion assesses depth of client's breathing. Technique is good measure to evaluate client's ability to perform deep-breathing exercises (see Chapter 35).

CRITICAL DECISION POINT **Do not slide the hands over the skin. This will give a false measure of excursion.**

A 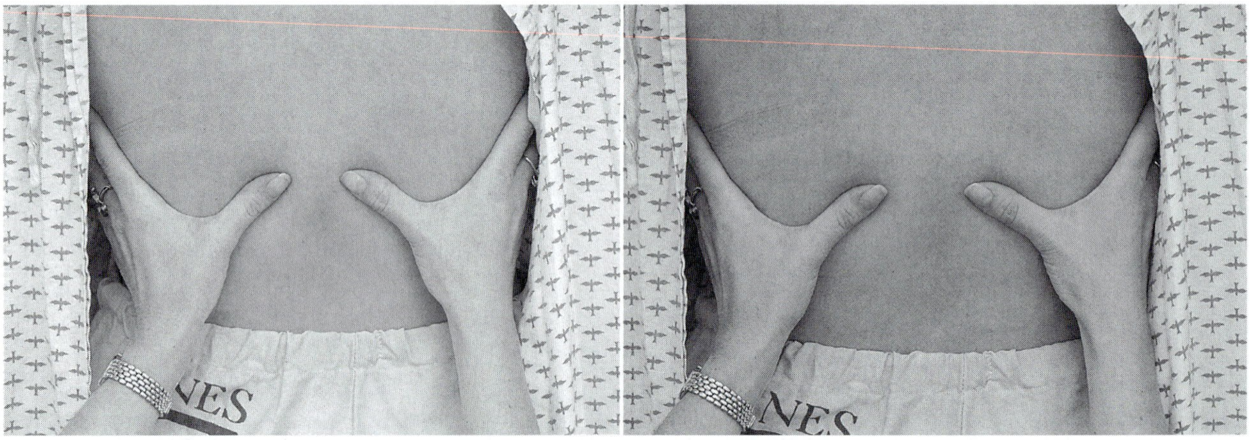 B

Step 4 **A,** Position of nurse's hands for palpation of posterior thorax excursion. **B,** As client inhales, movement of chest excursion separates nurse's thumbs.

5. While palpating chest excursion, note symmetry of chest wall movement.

Assesses equality of underlying lung expansion. Limited movement on one side may indicate that client is voluntarily splinting during ventilation because of pain.

6. Place ball or lower palm of dominant hand over symmetrical intercostal spaces, beginning at the lung apex and moving downward. Use a firm, light touch. Ask the client to repeat the words "ninety-nine" or "one-one-one" in a voice of uniform intensity. Feel for a faint vibration as the client speaks (see illustration).

Palpation of posterior chest wall reveals vocal or tactile fremitus. Vibrations created by movement of vocal cords travel through lung tissue to chest wall. Failure to palpate vibration indicates airway obstruction caused by mucous plug, tumor, or collapsed lung tissue. Palm of hand is most sensitive to vibrations. Symmetrical placement of hands allows for comparison of fremitus on both sides of thorax, top to bottom.

CRITICAL DECISION POINT **If fremitus is faint, have client speak in a louder or lower tone of voice.**

STEPS	RATIONALE
7. Moving from side to side and top to bottom, percuss posterior chest wall. Follow same pattern as with palpation (see Step 6). Ask client to fold arms forward across chest. Using indirect percussion, percuss intercostal spaces over symmetrical areas of the lungs. Compare percussion notes for all lung lobes.	Determines density of underlying lung tissue. Position separates scapulas to expose more lung tissue to assessment. Normal lung is air filled.
8. Auscultate breath sounds. Have client fold arms in front of the chest and keep the head bent forward while taking slow deep breaths with the mouth slightly open. For adult, place diaphragm of stethoscope firmly on chest wall over intercostal spaces (see illustration). Listen to entire inspiration and expiration at each stethoscope position. Systematically compare breath sounds over right and left sides (see Step 6). If sounds are faint, ask client to breathe harder and faster temporarily (Table 11-7).	Assesses movement of air through tracheobronchial tree. Nurse's recognition of normal airflow sounds allows detection of sounds caused by mucus or airway obstruction. Sounds are characterized by length of inspiratory and expiratory phases.

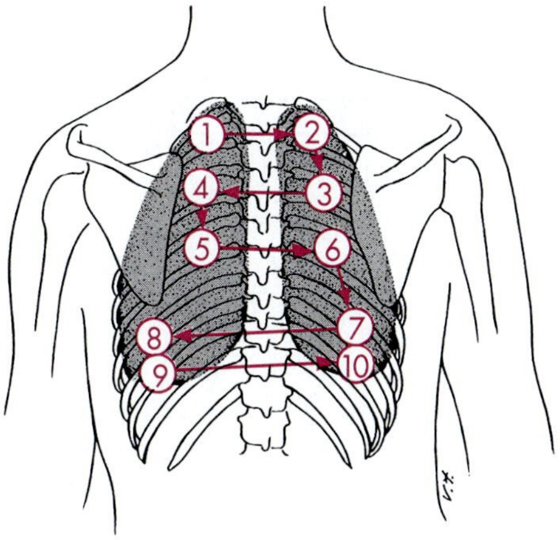

Step 6 Nurse follows systematic pattern when comparing fremitus, percussion notes, and auscultation posteriorly.

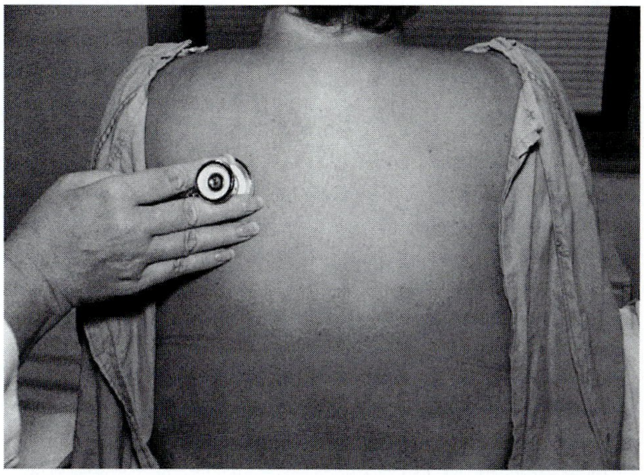

Step 8 Use of diaphragm of stethoscope to auscultate breath sounds.

Table 11-7 **Normal Breath Sounds**

Description	Location	Origin
Vesicular		
Vesicular sounds are soft, breezy, and low pitched. Inspiratory phase is 3 times longer than expiratory phase.	Best heard over lung's periphery (except over scapula)	Created by air moving through smaller airways
Bronchovesicular		
Bronchovesicular sounds are medium-pitched and blowing sounds of medium intensity. Inspiratory phase is equal to expiratory phase.	Best heard posteriorly between scapulae and anteriorly over bronchioles lateral to sternum at first and second intercostal spaces	Created by air moving through large airways
Bronchial		
Bronchial sounds are loud and high pitched with hollow quality. Expiration lasts longer than inspiration (3:2 ratio).	Best heard over trachea	Created by air moving through trachea close to chest wall

STEPS	RATIONALE
9. If tactile fremitus, percussion, or auscultation are abnormal, place diaphragm of stethoscope over intercostal spaces systematically. Ask client to say "ninety-nine" or "eee" in a normal voice tone. Auscultate lobes of the lung.	Tests for spoken or whispered voice sounds **(whispered pectoriloquy)** may further indicate nature of abnormalities (normally sounds are muffled).
10. Ask the client to whisper "ninety-nine" while lobes are again auscultated.	Voice sounds normally travel through lung and chest wall to create a faint, indistinct sound.

LATERAL THORAX

1. Instruct client to raise arms straight into air; inspect chest wall for same characteristics as reviewed for posterior chest.	Improves access to lateral thoracic structures.
2. Extend palpation, percussion, and auscultation of posterior thorax to lateral sides of chest, except for excursion measurement (see illustration).	Allows for location of abnormalities in lateral lung fields.

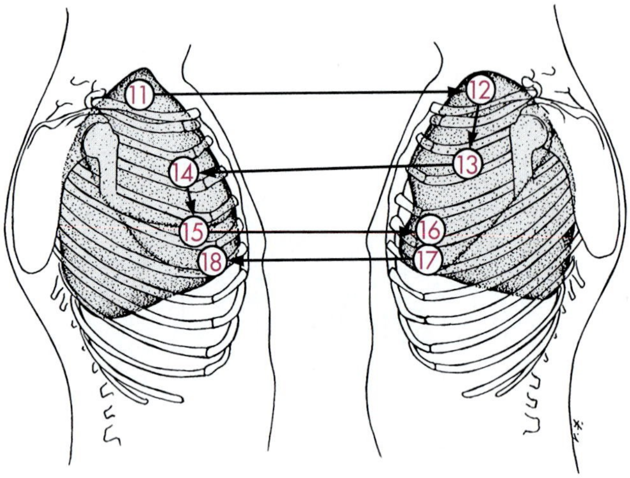

Step 2 Nurse follows systematic pattern for assessment laterally.

CRITICAL DECISION POINT You cannot assess excursion laterally.

ANTERIOR THORAX

1. Inspect accessory muscles of breathing: sternocleidomastoid, trapezius, and abdominal muscles. Note effort to breathe.	Extent to which accessory muscles are used reveals degree of effort to breathe.
2. Inspect width or spread of angle made by costal margins and tip of sternum. Angle is usually larger than 90 degrees between margins.	Indicates congenital, acquired, or traumatic alterations that may influence client's chest expansion.
3. Observe the client's breathing pattern, observing symmetry and degree of chest wall and abdominal movement. Respiratory rate and rhythm are more often assessed anteriorly.	Assesses client's effort to breathe; symmetrical, passive movement indicates no respiratory distress.
4. Palpate anterior thoracic muscles and skeleton for lumps, masses, tenderness, or unusual movement.	Localized swelling or tenderness may indicate trauma to underlying ribs or cartilage.
5. Palpate anterior chest excursion. Place hands over each lateral rib cage, with thumbs approximately 5 cm (2 inches) apart and angled along each costal margin. Thumbs are pushed toward client's midline to create skinfold between thumbs. As client inhales deeply, thumbs should normally separate approximately 3 to 5 cm (1½ to 2 inches), with each side expanding equally.	Assesses depth of client's breathing and ability to perform deep-breathing exercises.

STEPS	RATIONALE
6. With palm of hand, palpate systematically over anterior chest for tactile fremitus (see illustration). In a female, retract breasts gently to palpate chest wall.	Reduced or absent fremitus indicates airway obstruction by mucus, tumor, or collapsed tissue. Sounds will not transmit through breast tissue.

➤ *CRITICAL DECISION POINT* Fremitus is best felt next to the sternum at the second intercostal space, at the level of bronchial bifurcation. If the client's breasts are large, this portion of the examination may be omitted.

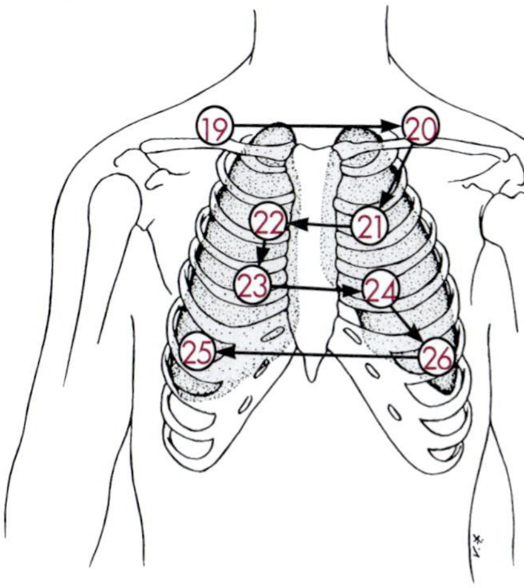

Step 6

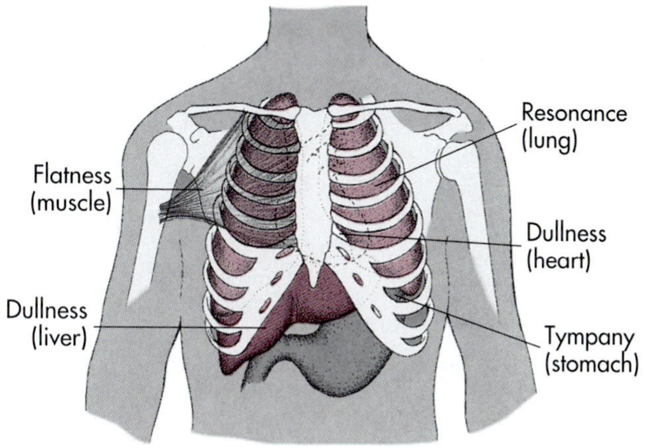

Step 7 Variations in percussion notes in normal thorax and upper abdomen.

STEPS	RATIONALE
7. Percuss thorax between intercostal spaces with client lying or sitting (procedure is easier if client lies down). Begin above clavicles; move across and then down as during palpation for fremitus.	Lying position facilitates ability to deliver sharp blow to chest wall to elicit clear sound. Percussion over anterior thorax enables nurse to locate position of liver, heart, and lung. Normal lung is resonant. Underlying liver, heart, and stomach create percussion notes different from that of lung (see illustration).
8. With client sitting, auscultate anterior thorax following same pattern as for percussion. If adventitious sounds are auscultated, have client cough. Listen with stethoscope to determine if sound has disappeared (Table 11-8).	Sitting position maximizes chest expansion and airflow through tracheobronchial tree. Expiration lasts longer than inspiration (3:2 ratio). Coughing can clear airways and remove adventitious sounds.

EVALUATION

STEPS	RATIONALE
1. Compare findings with normal assessment characteristics for thorax and lungs.	Determines presence of abnormalities.
2. Have client identify factors leading to lung disease.	Demonstrates learning.
3. **Unexpected outcomes** that may occur include:	
➤ Chest contour is abnormal, with anteroposterior diameter in 1:1 ratio.	Barrel-shaped chest is caused by aging and chronic lung disease.
➤ Posturing is observed, with client leaning over table or splinting side of chest with hand.	Indicates breathing difficulties (chronic lung disease and pain, respectively).
➤ Bulging of intercostal spaces is seen.	Results from client's exerting great effort to breathe.
➤ Respirations are rapid or slow and irregular (see Chapter 10).	Specific respiratory problems will alter rate and rhythm of respirations.

Table 11-8 Adventitious Sounds

Sound	Site Auscultated	Cause	Character
Crackles (previously called *rales*) 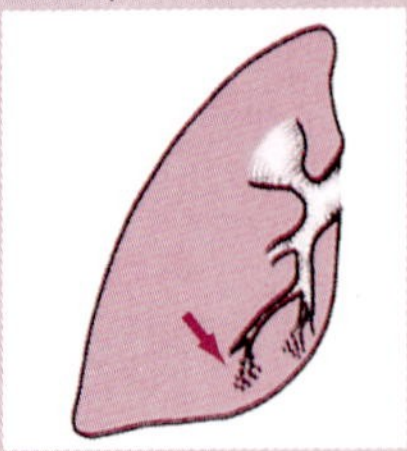	Most commonly heard in dependent lobes: right and left lung bases	Random, sudden reinflation of groups of alveoli; also related to increase in fluid in small airways*	Fine crackles are high-pitched fine, short, interrupted crackling sounds heard during end of inspiration, usually not cleared with coughing* Moist crackles are lower, more moist sounds heard during middle of inspiration; not cleared with coughing
Rhonchi 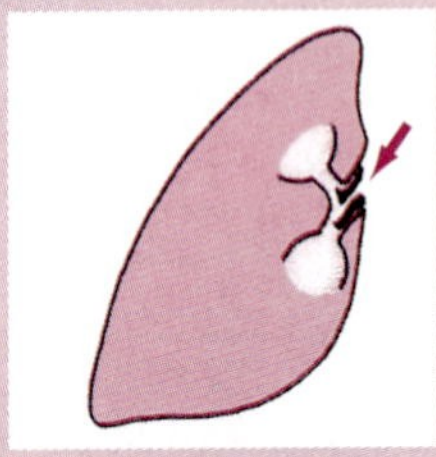	Primarily heard over trachea and bronchi; if loud enough, can be heard over most lung fields	Muscular spasm, fluid, or mucus in larger airways, causing turbulence	Loud, low-pitched, rumbling coarse sounds heard most often during inspiration or expiration; may be cleared by coughing
Wheezes 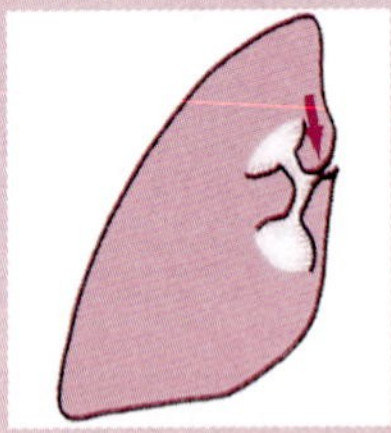	Can be heard over all lung fields	High-velocity air flow through severely narrowed bronchus	High-pitched, continuous musical sounds like a squeak heard continuously during inspiration or expiration; usually louder on expiration; do not clear with coughing†
Pleural friction rub 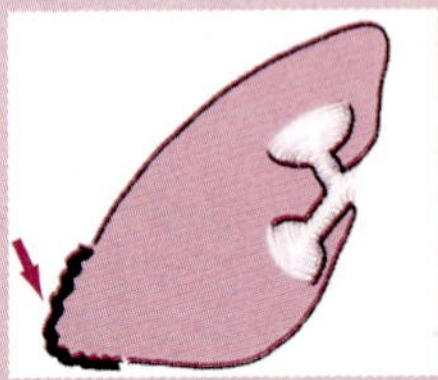	Heard over anterior lateral lung field (if client is sitting upright)	Inflamed pleura, parietal pleura rubbing against visceral pleura	Dry, grating quality heard best during inspiration; does not clear with coughing; heard loudest over lower lateral anterior surface

*Data from Forgacs P: *Chest* 73:399, 1978.
†Data from Wilkins RL, Hodgkin JE, Lopez B: *Lung sounds: a practical guide*, St Louis, 1988, Mosby.

STEPS	RATIONALE
➤ Chest excursion is reduced.	Depth of breathing is reduced by pain, postural deformity or fatigue.
➤ Nurse is unable to palpate tactile fremitus.	Mucus, collapse of lung tissue, or lung lesions block sound vibration.
➤ Percussion note is dull or flat over lung tissue.	Dullness occurs over the scapula, ribs, sternum, or spine. Dullness over lung tissue may be created by presence of fluid. Flat percussion note is created by underlying lung mass.
➤ Abnormal breath sounds (adventitious sounds) are auscultated over one or both lobes.	Location and character indicate abnormality.
➤ **Bronchophony** is present, with spoken voice sounds becoming clear during auscultation.	If fluid compresses lung tissue, vibrations from the client's voice are transmitted to chest wall and become clear.
➤ Whispered pectoriloquy is evident; whispered voice sounds become clear and distinct.	Consolidation of the lungs causes sound to become clear.

STEPS	RATIONALE
➤ Client is unfamiliar with risks for lung disease.	Reinstruction is necessary.
➤ Client fails to assume preferred posture for optimal ventilation.	This is difficult to change quickly; may require exercise and further discussion.

NURSING DIAGNOSIS

Clustering of defining characteristics from the assessment data may reveal the following nursing diagnoses for clients requiring this skill:

- ➤ Impaired gas exchange
- ➤ Ineffective airway clearance
- ➤ Ineffective breathing pattern
- ➤ Knowledge deficit regarding risks for lung disease
- ➤ Pain
- ➤ Fatigue
- ➤ Risk for infection

Related factors are individualized based on the client's condition or needs.

RECORDING AND REPORTING

1. Record observations and findings in nurses' notes or assessment flow sheet.	Documents baseline findings. Data provide means to evaluate client's ongoing status and response to therapies.
2. Record respiratory rate and character on vital signs flow sheet.	Provides simple means to compare trends and changes.
3. Report abnormalities to nurse in charge or physician.	Findings may indicate need for therapy.

FOLLOW-UP ACTIVITIES

1. If client has a productive cough and mucus is purulent, obtaining a specimen is appropriate. Record amount, color, and odor of mucus.

• • • • •

Special Considerations

- ➤ Clients with asthma have symptoms aggravated by change in temperature and humidity, irritating fumes or smoke, emotional stress, and physical exertion.
- ➤ Clients with chronic respiratory disease will likely need to sit up throughout the examination due to potential shortness of breath.
- ➤ Fremitus is normally symmetrical but decreased over heart and breast tissue.
- ➤ The most common symptom of pulmonary tuberculosis is a cough. Initially cough is nonproductive. If untreated, it becomes productive with mucoid or **mucopurulent** sputum. Other symptoms include night sweats and weight loss. The condition may be diagnosed by chest x-ray examination, sputum for acid-fast bacillus, and sputum for culture and sensitivity.

Teaching Considerations

- ➤ Explain risk factors for chronic lung disease and lung cancer, including cigarette smoking; history of smoking for more than 20 years; exposure to industrial substances (e.g., arsenic and asbestos, particularly for persons who smoke); exposure to radiation from occupational, medical, and environmental sources; air pollution; tuberculosis; exposure to radon, especially in cigarette smokers; and environmental tobacco smoke in nonsmokers (American Cancer Society, 1996).
- ➤ Discuss warning signs of lung cancer such as a persistent cough, sputum streaked with blood, chest pains, and recurrent attacks of pneumonia or bronchitis.

Pediatric Considerations

- ➤ Children younger than age 6 exhibit noticeable abdominal or diaphragmatic movement. Older children and adults exhibit more costal or thoracic movement. Men may have more diaphragmatic movement than women.
- ➤ Use bell to auscultate breath sounds in children. Breath sounds are louder in children because of their thin chest walls.

Gerontologic Considerations

- ➤ Older adults have a costal angle (anteriorly) of slightly less than 90 degrees. The anteroposterior diameter may be increased from kyphosis.
- ➤ In older adults chest expansion is reduced because of calcification of rib cartilage and partial contraction of inspiratory muscles.
- ➤ Older adults should be vaccinated against the flu in the early fall. It is impossible to get the flu from a flu shot. Side effects to the vaccine, including low-grade fever and redness/tenderness at the injection site, may occur (Lueckenotte, 1994).

SKILL 11-11 Assessing the Heart and Vascular System

The heart and the vascular system can be assessed together because the two systems work in unison to deliver blood to organs, tissues, and cells. An alteration in cardiac function may be detected by changes in the vascular system and vice versa. A client who presents signs or symptoms of heart **(cardiac)** problems, such as chest pain, may be suffering a life-threatening condition requiring immediate attention. In this situation the nurse acts quickly and decides on the portions of the examination that are absolutely necessary. When a client's condition is stable, a more thorough assessment can reveal baseline heart and vascular function and any risks for heart disease. Clients tend to seek information about heart disease because it remains a leading cause of death in the United States.

The nurse may begin assessment of the heart after examining the thorax because the client is already in a suitable position with the chest exposed. Assessment then proceeds to the vascular system. The nurse uses inspection, palpation, auscultation, and percussion during the examination.

DELEGATION CONSIDERATIONS

Unlicensed assistive personnel can be trained to assess apical pulse and peripheral pulses correctly. Assessment of peripheral pulses is important for all staff to know, particularly in specialty areas such as vascular surgery and orthopedics, where the skill is performed frequently.

- Familiarize the staff member with the importance of assessing peripheral pulses in specific clients.
- Instruct the unlicensed assistive personnel to recognize temperature and color changes along with changes in peripheral pulses.

Comprehensive heart and vascular assessment requires problem solving and knowledge application unique to a professional nurse. For this skill, delegation is inappropriate.

EQUIPMENT

- Stethoscope
- Doppler stethoscope (optional)
- Conducting gel
- Two rulers, one regular and one centimeter

STEPS	RATIONALE
ASSESSMENT	
1. Assess client for history of smoking, alcohol intake, caffeine intake (coffee, tea, soft drinks, chocolate), use of "recreational" drugs, exercise habits, and dietary patterns and intake.	Smoking, alcohol ingestion, cocaine use, lack of regular exercise, high intake of caffeine, and intake of foods high in carbohydrates, fats, and cholesterol are risk factors for cardiovascular disease.
2. Determine if client is taking medications for cardiovascular function (e.g., antidysrhythmics, antihypertensives) and if client knows their purpose, dosage, and side effects.	Allows nurse to assess client's compliance with and understanding of drug therapies. Medications for cardiovascular function cannot be taken intermittently.
3. Ask if client has experienced dyspnea, chest pain or discomfort, palpitations, excess fatigue, cough, leg pain or cramps, edema of the feet, cyanosis, fainting, and orthopnea. Ask if symptoms occur at rest or during exercise.	These are the cardinal symptoms of heart disease. Cardiovascular function may be adequate during rest but not during exercise.
4. If client reports chest pain, determine if it is cardiac in nature. Anginal pain is usually a deep pressure or ache that is substernal and diffuse, radiating to one or both arms, neck, or jaw.	Determines if immediate care is necessary.
5. Determine if client has a stressful lifestyle.	Repeated exposure to stress may increase risk for heart disease.
6. Assess family history for heart disease, diabetes, high cholesterol levels, hypertension, stroke, or rheumatic heart disease.	Family history of heart problems increases risk for heart and vascular disease, as do these other factors.

STEPS	RATIONALE
7. Ask client about a history of heart trouble (e.g., congestive heart failure, congenital heart disease, coronary artery disease, dysrhythmias, murmurs) or vascular disease (hypertension, phlebitis, varicose veins).	Knowledge reveals client's level of understanding of condition. A preexisting condition influences examination techniques used by nurse and expected findings.
8. Determine if client has history of obesity. Note current height and weight measures (see Skill 11-1).	Obesity may alter cardiac and vascular function.
9. Ask if client has experienced leg cramps, numbness or tingling in extremities, sensation of cold hands or feet, pain in the legs, or swelling or cyanosis of the feet, ankles, or hand.	These are common signs and symptoms of peripheral vascular disease.
10. If client experiences pain or cramping in the lower extremities, ask if it is relieved or aggravated by walking or standing for long periods or during sleep.	Relationship of symptoms to exercise can clarify whether problem is vascular or musculoskeletal. Pain caused by vascular condition tends to increase with activity. Musculoskeletal pain is not usually relieved when exercise ends.
11. Ask female clients if they wear tight-fitting garters or hosiery and sit or lie in bed with legs crossed.	Tight clothing around lower extremities can impair venous return.

PLANNING

1. **Expected outcomes** following completion of procedure:

HEART

➤ There are no visible or palpable pulsations or lifts (exception: point of maximal impulse or epigastric area may show a pulsation in thin clients).	Rules out valvular problems or major vessel disorders.
➤ Abdominal aorta is palpable.	Major vessel is patent.
➤ Heart is in normal sinus rhythm with rate from 60 to 100 beats per minute (adolescent through adult).	
➤ Heart sounds S_1 and S_2 are normal, without extra sounds or murmurs.	
➤ **Point of maximal impulse (PMI)** is palpable at fifth intercostal space at left midclavicular line in adult. PMI is at third or fourth intercostal space at left midclavicular line in infant or child.	
➤ Client describes changes in own behavior that may improve cardiovascular function.	Information may improve client's health care habits.
➤ Client lists risks for heart disease.	
➤ Client describes schedule, dosage, purpose, and benefits of medications being taken for cardiovascular function.	Information related to health benefits may improve compliance with therapy.

VASCULAR

➤ Blood pressure is normal (see Chapter 10).	
➤ Carotid pulse is localized, strong, elastic, and equal bilaterally. No change occurs during inspiration or expiration.	Rules out atherosclerotic changes in vessels.
➤ No carotid bruit is present.	Vessel is patent.
➤ Jugular veins distend when client lies supine and flatten when client is in sitting position.	Venous pressure is normal.
➤ Extremities are warm and pink, with normal hair growth and nail thickness.	These are indicators of good tissue perfusion.
➤ All peripheral pulses are equal, elastic, and 2+.	Normal pulse characteristics.

STEPS	RATIONALE
2. Prepare client:	
a. Be sure that client is relaxed and comfortable.	An anxious or uncomfortable client can have mild tachycardia that may lead the nurse to misinterpret the findings.
b. Have client assume semi-Fowler's or supine position.	Provides adequate visibility and access to left thorax and mediastinum. Client with heart disease often experiences shortness of breath while lying flat.
c. Explain procedure. Avoid facial gestures reflecting concern.	Client with previously normal cardiac history may become anxious if nurse shows concern.
d. Be sure that room is quiet.	Subtle, low-pitched heart sounds are difficult to hear.

IMPLEMENTATION

HEART

STEPS	RATIONALE
1. Form a mental image of the exact location of the heart (see illustration). In an adult the heart is in the center of the chest (precordium), behind and to the left of the sternum, with a small section of the right atrium extending to the right of the sternum. The base of the heart is the upper portion, and the apex is the bottom tip. The surface of the right ventricle composes most of the heart's anterior surface.	Technique improves ability to assess findings accurately and determine possible source of abnormalities.
2. Be familiar with cardiac landmarks (see illustration). Find the Angle of Louis just below the suprasternal notch and between the sternal body and manubrium. It can be felt as a ridge in the sternum approximately 2 inches below the notch. Slip fingers down each side of angle to feel adjacent ribs. The intercostal spaces are just below each rib. Find the second intercostal space: space on client's right is (1) *aortic area;* space on left is (2) *pulmonic area.* Carefully move fingers down left side of sternum to the third intercostal space, (3) *second pulmonic area.* The *tricuspid area* (4) is located at the fourth left intercostal space along the sternum. Move fingers laterally to client's left to locate fifth intercostal space at left midclavicular line, the (5) *mitral area.* The *epigastric area* (6) is at the tip of the sternum.	Familiarity with landmarks allows nurse to describe findings more clearly and ultimately may improve assessment.

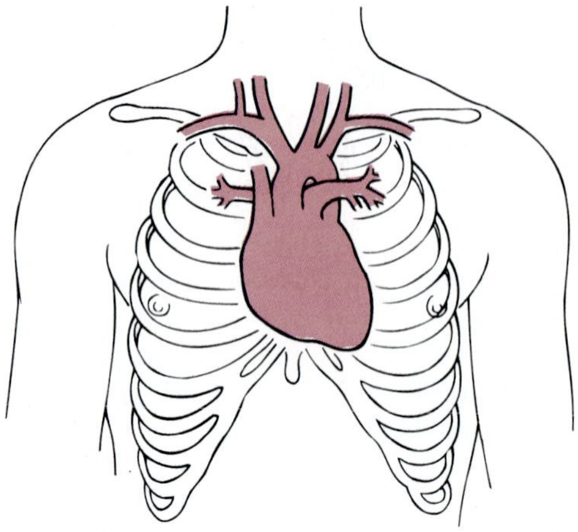

Step 1 Anatomical position of heart.

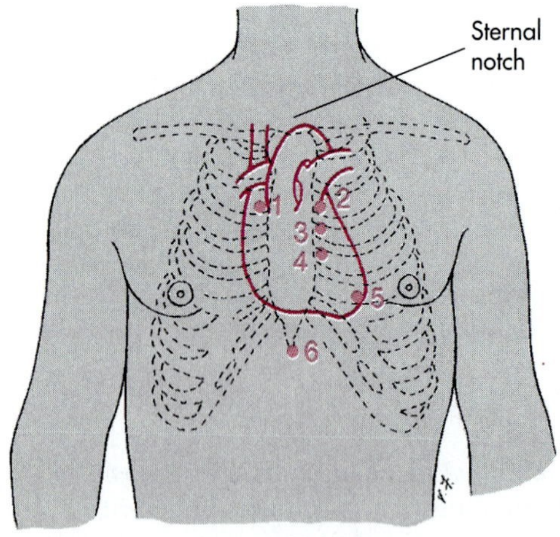

Step 2 Areas for examination of heart.

STEPS	RATIONALE
3. Stand to the client's right and look first at the precordium with the client supine. Note any visible pulsations and more exaggerated lifts. Look closely at the area of the apex. a. The apical impulse may become visible only when the client sits up, bringing the heart closer to the anterior wall. It is easily obscured by obesity.	May reveal size and symmetry of the heart. The apical impulse should be visible at the midclavicular line in the fifth intercostal space.
4. Be sure that your hands are warm. With the client remaining supine, palpate systematically over the six anatomical landmarks: palpate each site with the proximal halves of the four fingers held gently together or with the whole hand. Touch gently and allow the movements to rise to your hand. Note any **thrill**—a fine, palpable rushing vibration—felt best over the base of the heart near the right or left second intercostal space.	Position improves likelihood of detecting pulsations. The surface of the fingers will sense any vibrations.

CRITICAL DECISION POINT Presence of a thrill is not normal and may indicate a disruption of blood flow caused by a defect in closure of a heart valve or atrial septal defect.

STEPS	RATIONALE
5. If pulsations or vibrations are palpated, time their occurrence in relation to systole or diastole by either auscultating heart sounds simultaneously or palpating the carotid artery.	Carotid impulse and first heart sound (S_1) occur almost at the same time. Helps to reveal cause of abnormality.
6. Locate the PMI by palpating with fingertips along fifth intercostal space in midclavicular line (see illustration). Note a light, brief pulsation in an area 1 to 2 cm (½ to 1 inch) in diameter at the apex.	In the presence of serious heart disease, the PMI will be located to the left of the midclavicular line.

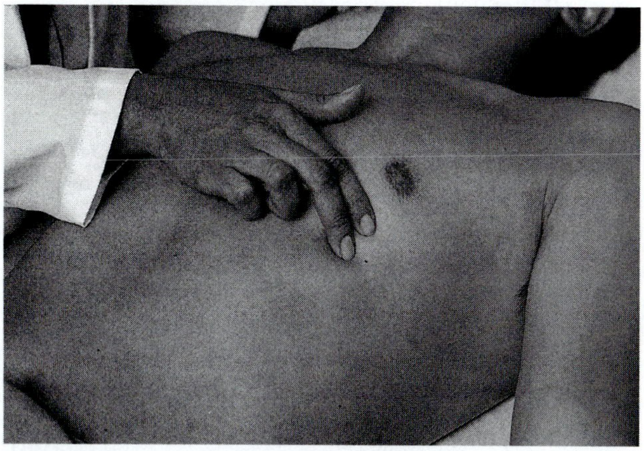

Step 6 Palpation of point of maximal impulse at fifth intercostal space along midclavicular line. (From Canobbio MM: *Cardiovascular disorders,* St Louis, 1990, Mosby.)

CRITICAL DECISION POINT A stronger than expected impulse may be a heave *or lift,* which may indicate increased cardiac output or left ventricular hypertrophy.

STEPS	RATIONALE
7. If palpating PMI is difficult, turn client onto left side.	Maneuver moves the heart closer to the chest wall.
8. Inspect the epigastric area and palpate the abdominal aorta. Note a localized strong beat.	Rules out reduced blood flow or diffuse pulse, which may indicate a number of abnormalities.

STEPS

RATIONALE

9. Auscultate heart sounds. Begin by having client sit up and lean slightly forward; then have client lie supine; and end the examination with client in a left lateral recumbent position (see illustrations).

Different positions help to clarify type of sounds heard. Sitting position is best to hear high-pitched murmurs (if present). Supine is common position to hear all sounds. Left lateral recumbent is best position to hear low-pitched sounds.

> ***CRITICAL DECISION POINT*** **In a female client it may be necessary to lift the left breast to listen better to the chest wall.**

10. While auscultating sounds, ask client not to speak but to breathe comfortably. Begin with the diaphragm of the stethoscope; then alternate with the bell. Do not press bell too firmly against chest wall because transmission of sound will be destroyed.

a. Begin at the apex or PMI; then move systematically to the tricuspid area, second pulmonic area, and pulmonic and aortic areas. (NOTE: Some examiners use reverse sequence.) At normal slow rates S_1 is high pitched and dull in quality and sounds like a "lub." This sound precedes the systolic phase of heart contraction. S_1 is best heard at the apex.

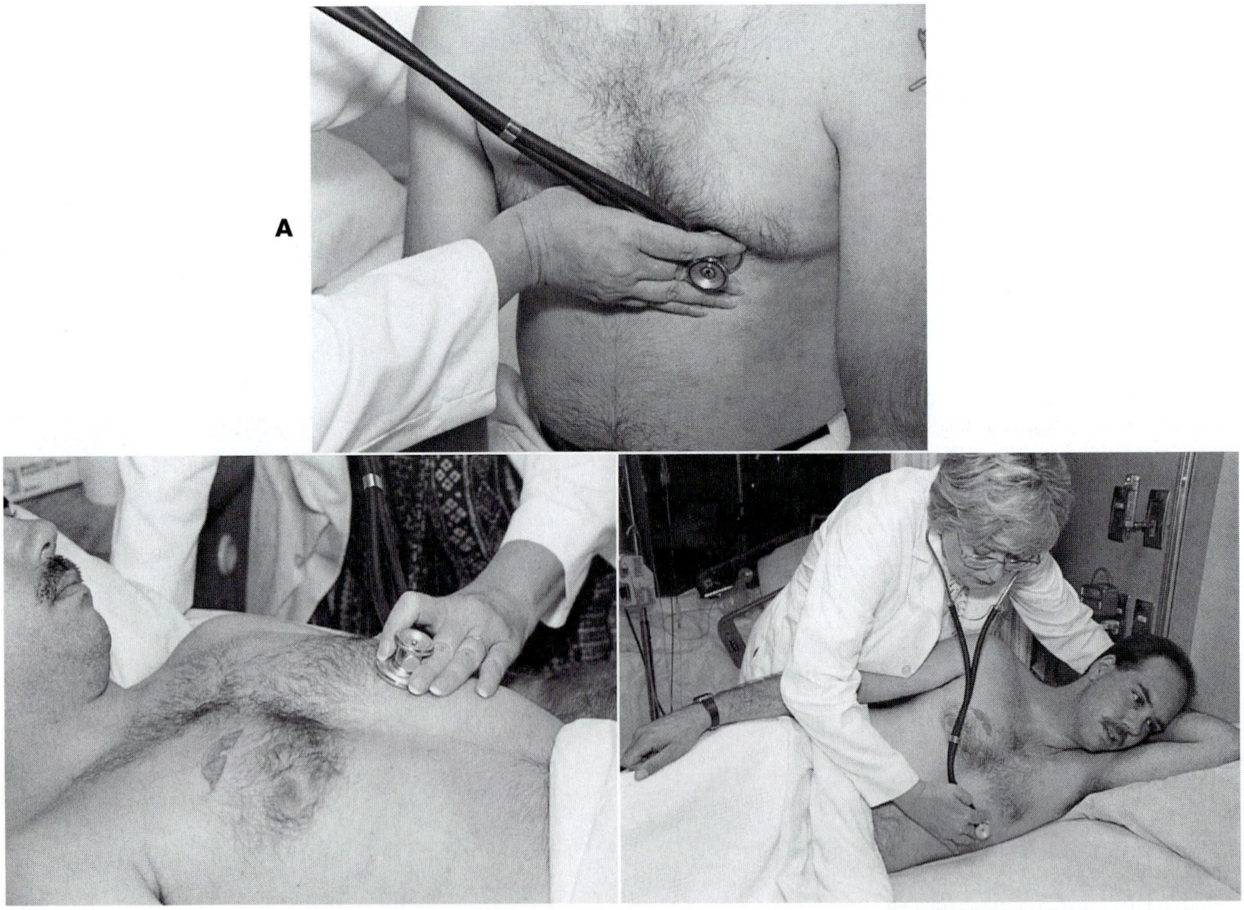

Step 9 Client positions for auscultation of heart sounds. **A,** Sitting. **B,** Supine. **C,** Left lateral.

STEPS	RATIONALE
CRITICAL DECISION POINT **Inch the stethoscope along; do not jump from one area to another.**	
b. Listen for S_2 at each site. It precedes the diastolic phase and sounds like "dub." This sound is best heard at the aortic area. Heart sounds will vary by pitch, loudness, and duration, depending on the auscultatory site (Table 11-9).	Normal sounds S_1 and S_2 are high pitched and best heard with diaphragm. Examiner must become familiar with these sounds.
c. After both sounds are heard clearly as "lub-dub," count each combination of S_1 and S_2 as one heart beat. Count the number of beats for 1 minute.	Determines apical pulse rate.
CRITICAL DECISION POINT **Do not try to hear all heart sounds at once. Isolate each sound carefully. Listen to each pause in the cycle. Take time to tune in and listen carefully for any unusual sounds.**	
d. Assess heart rhythm by noting the time between S_1 and S_2 (systole) and then the time between S_2 and the next S_1 (diastole). Listen to the full cycle at each auscultation area. Note regular intervals between each sequence of beats. There should be a distinct pause between S_1 and S_2.	Alterations in rhythm indicate abnormalities. Failure of heart to beat at regular intervals is a dysrhythmia, which interferes with heart's ability to pump effectively.

Table 11-9 Heart Sounds According to Auscultatory Area

	Aortic	Pulmonic	Second Pulmonic	Mitral	Tricuspid
Pitch	$S_1 < S_2$	$S_1 < S_2$	$S_1 < S_2$	$S_1 < S_2$	$S_1 < S_2$
Loudness	$S_1 < S_2$	$S_1 < S_2$	$S_1 < S_2$*	$S_1 > S_2$†	$S_1 > S_2$
Duration	$S_1 > S_2$	$S_1 > S_2$	$S_1 > S_2$	$S_1 > S_2$	$S_1 > S_2$

Modified from Seidel, HM et al: *Mosby's guide to physical examination,* 3 ed, St Louis, 1995, Mosby.
*S_1 is relatively louder in second pulmonic area than in aortic area.
†S_1 may be louder in mitral area than in tricuspid area.

Table 11-10 Common Types of Dysrhythmias

Definition	Cause
Sinus dysrhythmia: Pulse rate changes during respiration, increasing at peak of inspiration and declining during expiration.	Blood is momentarily trapped in lungs during inspiration, causing fall in heart's stroke volume.
Sinus tachycardia: Pulse rhythm is regular, but rate is accelerated to more than 100 beats/min.	Exercise, emotional stress, and caffeine or alcohol ingestion are common factors that cause increased firing of sinoatrial node.
Sinus bradycardia: Pulse rhythm is regular, but rate is slower than normal at 40 to 60 beats/min.	Sinoatrial node fires less frequently. This is common in well-conditioned athletes and with use of antidysrhythmic medications.
Premature ventricular contraction: Premature beat occurs before regularly expected heart contraction.	Ventricle contracts prematurely because of electrical impulse bypassing normal conduction pathway. It may occur so early that it is difficult to detect as second beat. It may be followed by a pause.
Atrial fibrillation: Rapid, random contractions of atria cause irregular ventricular beats at 130 to 150 beats/min.	Atria discharge very rapidly, with some impulses not reaching ventricles. This condition occurs in rheumatic heart disease and mitral stenosis. It causes reduced cardiac output.

STEPS	RATIONALE
e. When heart rate is irregular, compare apical and radial pulses (Table 11-10). Auscultate the apical pulse and then immediately palpate the radial pulse. A colleague can assess the radial pulse while the nurse assesses the apical.	Determines if a pulse deficit (radial pulse is slower than apical) exists. Deficit indicates that ineffective contractions of the heart fail to send pulse waves to the periphery.
11. Continue to auscultate for extra heart sounds at each auscultatory site.	
a. Use the bell of the stethoscope and listen for low-pitched extra heart sounds such as S_3 and S_4 gallops, clicks, and rubs. S_3, or a ventricular gallop, occurs just after S_2 at the end of ventricular diastole. It may sound like "lub-dub-ee" or "Ken-tuc-ky." S_4, or an atrial gallop, occurs just before S_1 or ventricular systole. It sounds like "dee-lub-dub" or "Ten-nes-see."	Gallops may be caused by premature rushes of blood into a ventricle that is stiff or dilated or an atrial contraction pushing against a ventricle that is not accepting blood.
b. Listen for clicks as short high-pitched extra sounds.	Clicks are caused by abnormalities such as mitral valve prolapse or prosthetic valves.
c. Listen for **friction rubs** as squeaky or rubbing sounds.	Rubs are a result of inflamed visceral and parietal layers of the pericardium rubbing against one another.
12. Auscultate for heart murmurs over each of the auscultation sites.	Murmurs are sustained swishing or blowing sounds heard at the beginning, middle, or end of systole or diastole. They are caused by increased blood flow through a normal valve, forward flow through a stenotic valve or into a dilated vessel or chamber, or backward flow through a valve that fails to close.
a. When a murmur is detected, determine if it occurs between S_1 and S_2 (systolic murmur) or between S_2 and the next S_1 (diastolic murmur).	
b. Listen carefully to note where the murmur can be heard best.	Certain murmurs are heard best at select anatomical sites.
c. Assess for radiation by listening for a murmur over areas in addition to where it is heard best. Murmurs can sometimes be heard over the neck or back.	
d. Note the intensity of the murmur: Grade 1: barely audible. Grade 2: audible immediately but faint. Grade 3: loud, without thrust or thrill. Grade 4: loud, with thrust or thrill. Grade 5: very loud, with thrust or thrill; audible with stethoscope only partially applied. Grade 6: louder; may be heard without stethoscope.	Related to rate of blood flow through the heart or the amount of blood regurgitated. A thrill is a continuous palpable sensation like the purring of a cat. A thrust is the upward lift felt when palpating the chest wall.
e. Note if the murmur is low, medium, or high in pitch. Use the bell for low-pitched sounds.	Pitch depends on velocity of blood flow through the valves.

VASCULAR SYSTEM

1. With the client sitting, auscultate the blood pressure at the brachial artery site in both arms (Chapter 10).	Abnormalities may suggest atherosclerosis or diseases of the aorta.

CRITICAL DECISION POINT **Readings between the arms may vary by as much as 10 mm Hg and tend to be higher in the right arm (Seidel, 1995).**

STEPS	RATIONALE
2. Compare sitting blood pressure with blood pressures measured while client is in lying and standing positions.	Comparing pressure readings with client in different positions rules out presence of orthostatic hypotension.

CRITICAL DECISION POINT **A fall in systolic blood pressure greater than 20 mm Hg and a fall in diastolic pressure signify** orthostatic **hypotension. Client may become dizzy and lightheaded.**

3. Assess Carotid Arteries:

STEPS	RATIONALE
a. Have client remain in sitting position.	Allows easier mobility of neck to expose artery for inspection and palpation.
b. Inspect neck on both sides for obvious pulsations of artery. Ask client to turn head slightly away from artery being examined. Sometimes pulse wave can be seen.	Carotids are only sites to assess quality of pulse wave (see illustration). Experience is required to evaluate wave in relation to events of cardiac cycle.

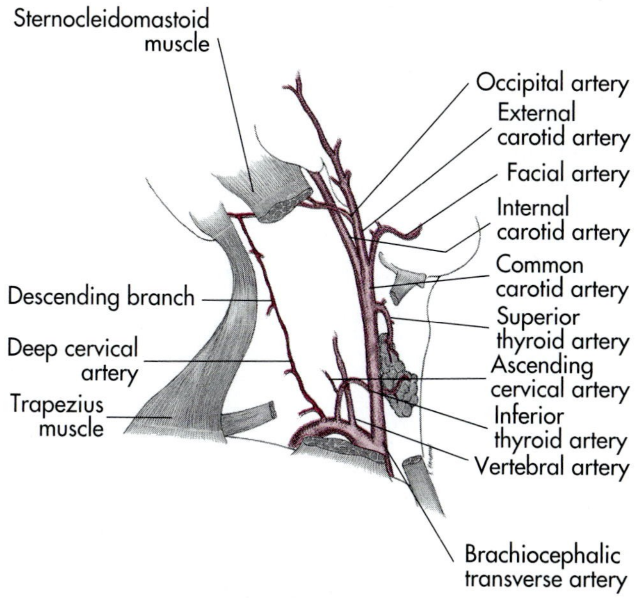

Step 3b Anatomical position of carotid artery.

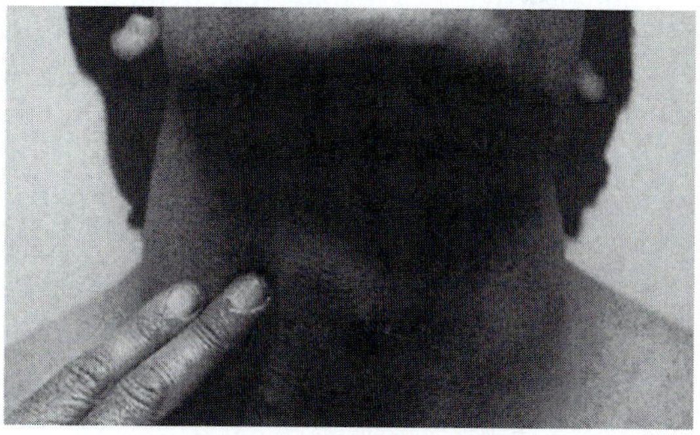

Step 3c Palpation of internal carotid artery along margin of sternocleidomastoid muscle. (Seidel HM et al: *Mosby's guide to physical examination*, ed 3, St Louis, 1995, Mosby.)

STEPS	RATIONALE
c. Palpate each carotid artery separately. Slide index and middle fingers around medial edge of sternocleidomastoid muscle. Ask client to raise chin slightly, keeping the head straight (see illustration). Note rate and rhythm, strength, and elasticity of artery. Also note if pulse changes as client inspires and expires.	If both arteries were occluded simultaneously, client could lose consciousness from reduced circulation to brain. Turning head improves access to artery. Change may indicate a sinus dysrhythmia.

CRITICAL DECISION POINT **Do not vigorously palpate or massage the artery. Stimulation of carotid sinus may cause a reflex drop in heart rate and blood pressure.**

STEPS	RATIONALE
d. Place bell of stethoscope over each carotid artery, auscultating for blowing sound (bruit) (see illustration).	Narrowing of carotid artery's lumen by arteriosclerotic plaques causes disturbance in blood flow. Blood passing through narrowed section creates turbulence and emits blowing or swishing sound.

4. Assess Right Internal Jugular Vein:

Vein follows more direct anatomical path to the right atrium of heart to assess venous pressure.

STEPS	RATIONALE
a. Ask client to first lie in a supine position.	Position makes external jugular easily visible for examination. Vessels distend, reflecting pressure in right atrium of heart.
b. Next, have client sit and gradually lower head of bed to 30 to 45 degrees. Keep neck and upper thorax exposed (see illustration).	Vein is usually not evident with client sitting up. As client slowly leans back, level of pulsations begins to rise above level of manubrium as much as 1 or 2 cm as client reaches 45-degree angle. Position prevents kinking or stretching of vein.

CRITICAL DECISION POINT Avoid neck hyperextension or flexion to ensure that vein is not stretched or kinked.

STEPS	RATIONALE
c. Measure the highest visible point of the internal jugular vein by using two rulers. Line up the bottom edge of a regular ruler with the top of the area of pulsation in the vein. Then align a centimeter ruler perpendicular to the first ruler at the level of the sternal angle. Measure in centimeters the distance between the second ruler and the sternal angle (see illustration on p. 359).	Height of jugular vein resembles a manometer, reflecting venous pressure. Pressure is influenced by blood volume, the capacity of the right atrium to receive blood and pump it to the right ventricle, and the ability of the right ventricle to contract and force blood into the pulmonary artery.
d. Repeat measurement on the other side. Note bilateral pressures higher than 3 cm (1.2 inches).	This is an indication of elevated central venous pressure.

CRITICAL DECISION POINT Clinically, observing a client in the Fowler's position with an obvious visible jugular pulsation suggests need for immediate treatment.

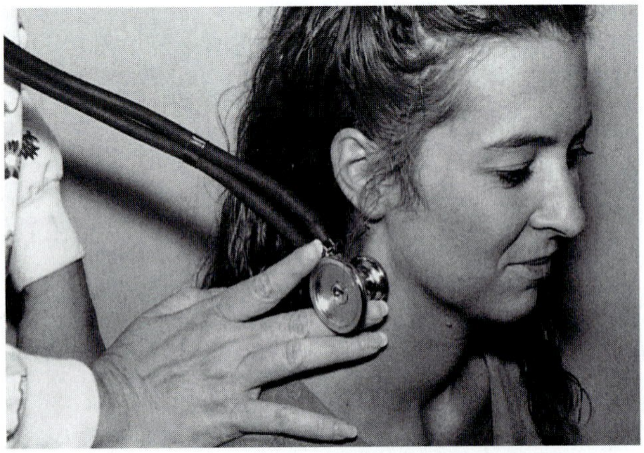

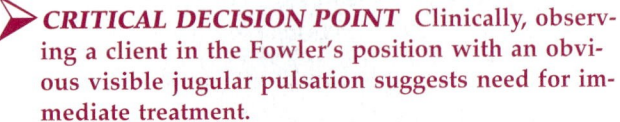

Step 3d Auscultation for carotid artery bruit.

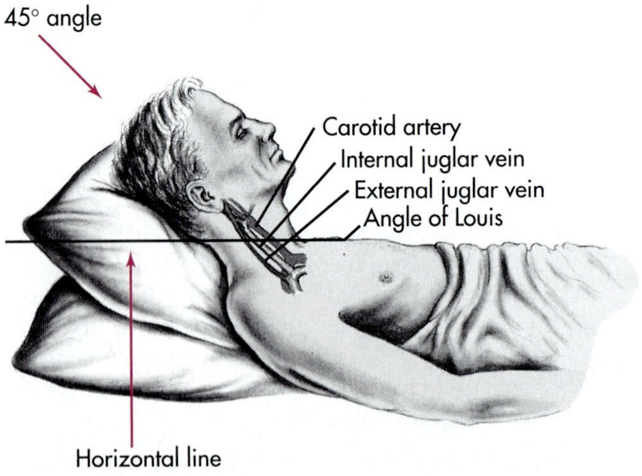

Step 4b Position of client to assess jugular vein distention. (From Thompson JM et al: *Mosby's manual of clinical nursing*, ed 2, St Louis, 1989, Mosby.)

STEPS	RATIONALE

5. Assess Integrity of Vascular System:

a. Inspect color of client's skin and mucous membranes (data may have been gathered previously during assessment of oral cavity and integument). Focus on face and upper extremities, looking at the color of the skin, mucosa, and nail beds.

Color of skin or mucous membranes reveals status of blood flow and arterial oxygen saturation.

➤ ***CRITICAL DECISION POINT*** **If cyanosis is seen (bluish discoloration of lips, mouth, conjunctiva, nail beds), refer to available lab data on oxygen saturation.**

Table 11-11 Signs of Venous and Arterial Insufficiency

Assessment Criterion	Venous	Arterial
Color	Normal or cyanotic	Pale; worsened by elevation of extremity; dusky-red when extremity is lowered
Temperature	Normal	Cool (blood flow blocked to extremity)
Pulse	Normal	Decreased or absent
Edema	Often marked	Absent or mild
Skin changes	Brown pigmentation around ankles	Thin, shiny skin; decreased hair growth; thickened nails

b. Inspect lower extremities for changes in color and condition of the skin (Table 11-11). Also note skin and nail texture, hair distribution, venous patterns, edema, and scars or ulcers.

Determines if venous or arterial insufficiency is present.

➤ ***CRITICAL DECISION POINT*** **Good time to ask client about history of leg pain.**

c. Have client raise both legs about 60 degrees. Ask client to alternately flex and extend feet for about 1 minute. Then have client sit up with legs dangling down.

Assesses for arterial insufficiency. There is slight pallor as client moves feet; normal color returns in about 10 seconds. Veins in feet and ankles fill in about 15 seconds.

d. Have client return to lying position with head elevated. With client's knee slightly flexed, acutely dorsiflex client's foot. Ask if pain is felt in the calf (see illustration).

Test is called Homan's sign; it can reveal pain on flexion, which is a sign of venous thrombosis or **thrombophlebitis**.

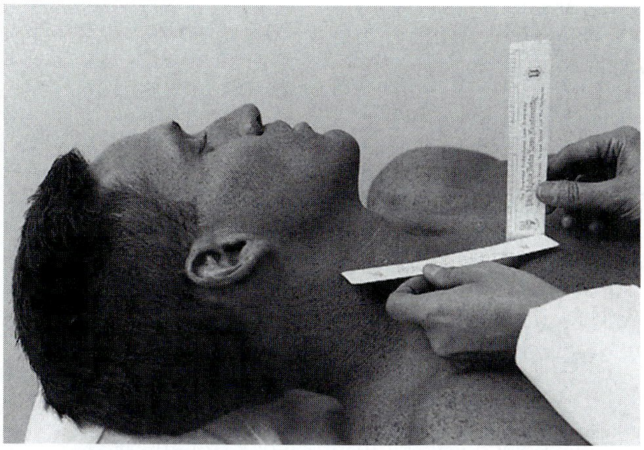

Step 4c Measurement of jugular vein distention. (From Seidel HM et al: *Mosby's guide to physical examination,* ed 3, St Louis, 1995, Mosby.)

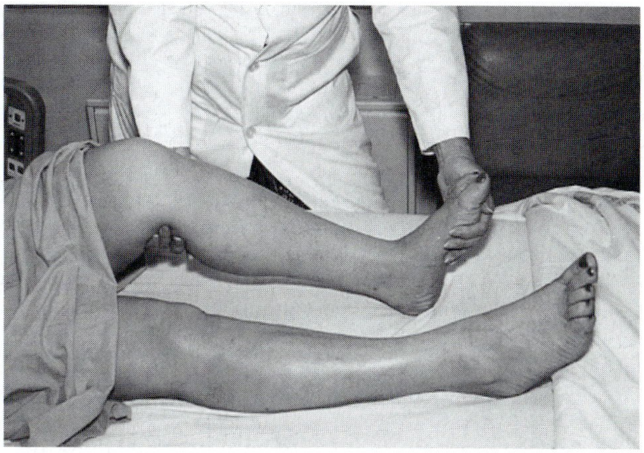

Step 5d Dorsiflexion to test for Homan's sign.

STEPS	RATIONALE
e. Inspect lower extremity further, looking for redness, thickening, or tenderness along superficial veins.	
f. If edema is present in extremities, assess for pitting by gently pressing index finger over bony prominence of tibia for 5 seconds and note depression. Edema is measured by the 1+ to 4+ scale (see Skill 11-2).	Normally there is no depression or the depression fills rapidly. Depth of pitting determines degree of edema (see illustration).

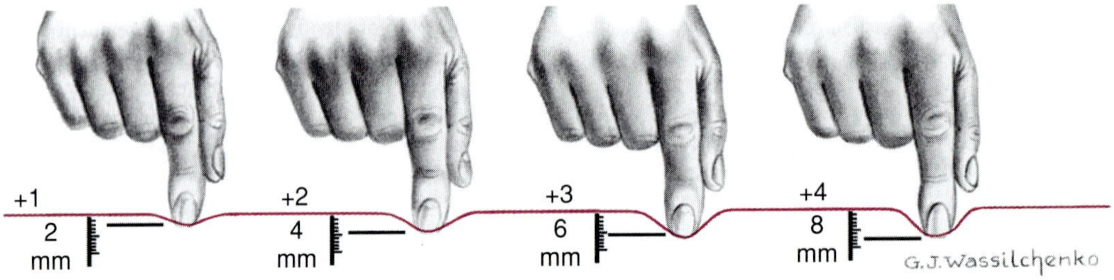

Step 5f Assessing for pitting edema. (From Seidel HM et al: *Mosby's guide to physical examination,* ed 3, St Louis, 1995, Mosby.)

STEPS	RATIONALE
g. Palpate temperature of extremities with dorsum (back) of hand.	Temperature measures degree of blood flow to body part.
6. Assess Each Peripheral Artery for Following Characteristics:	Palpation of peripheral arteries determines adequacy of blood flow to extremities.
a. Elasticity of vessel wall. (Depress and release artery, noting ease with which it springs back to shape.)	Determines integrity of vessel. Artery should be easily palpable and should return to shape after pressure is released.
b. Rate and rhythm of pulse. (Measure rate for 1 minute.)	Radial pulse is chosen to assess heart rate. Other peripheral pulses are assessed only to determine condition of local blood flow.
c. Strength of pulse.	Measure of force ejecting blood against arterial wall. Rating scale for strength: 0 Absent, not palpable. 1+ Pulse is diminished, barely palpable, easy to obliterate. 2+ Easily palpable, normal pulse. 3+ Full pulse, increased. 4+ Strong bounding pulse; cannot be obliterated.
d. Type of pulse.	Useful in describing nature of pulse wave; requires experience.
e. Measure equality of pulses by comparing, for example, left radial with that of right. Measure symmetry by comparing left brachial with left radial and so on.	Comparison of both arteries allows nurse to determine any localized obstruction or disturbance in blood flow.
7. Palpate radial pulse by lightly placing tips of first and second fingers in groove formed along radial side of forearm, lateral to flexor tendon of wrist (see illustration).	Pulse is relatively superficial and should not require deep palpation.
8. Palpate ulnar pulse by placing fingertips along ulnar side of forearm (see illustration).	Palpated when arterial insufficiency to hand is expected or when nurse assesses effects that radial occlusion (e.g., during arterial blood gas sampling) might have on circulation to hand (Chapter 43).

STEPS	RATIONALE
9. Palpate brachial pulse by locating groove between biceps and triceps muscles above elbow at antecubital fossa (see illustration). Place tips of first two fingers in muscle groove.	Artery runs along medial side of extended arm, requiring moderate palpation.
10. With client supine, palpate femoral pulse by placing first two fingers over inguinal area below inguinal ligament, midway between pubic symphysis and anterosuperior iliac spine (see illustration).	Supine position prevents flexion in groin area, which interferes with artery access.
11. Palpate popliteal pulse by having client slightly flex knee with foot resting on table or bed. Instruct client to keep leg muscles relaxed. Palpate deeply into popliteal fossa with fingers of both hands placed just lateral to midline. Client may also lie prone to achieve exposure of artery (see illustration).	Flexion of knee and muscle relaxation improve accessibility of artery. Popliteal pulse is one of the more difficult pulses to palpate.
12. Have client lie supine with feet relaxed, and palpate dorsalis pedis pulse. Gently place fingertips between great and first toe; slowly move fingers along groove between extensor tendons of great and first toe until pulse is palpable (see illustration).	Artery lies superficially and does not require deep palpation. Pulse may be congenitally absent.

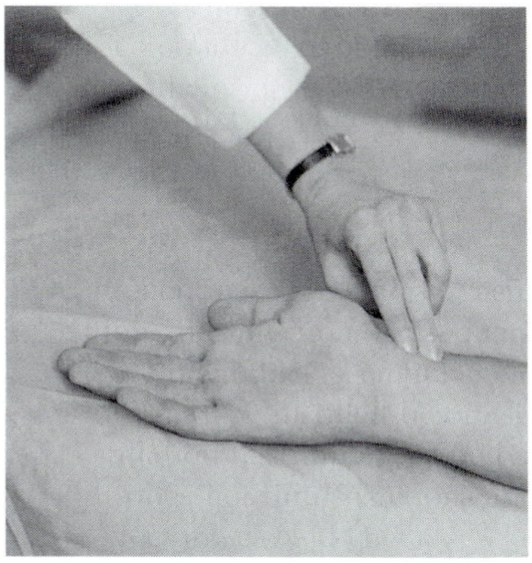

Step 7 Palpation of radial pulse.

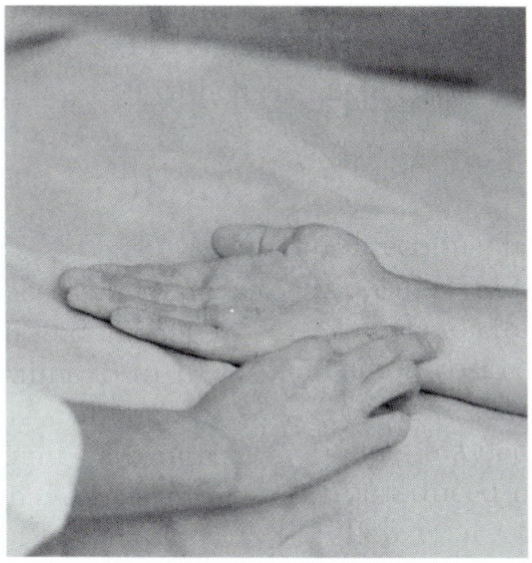

Step 8 Palpation of ulnar pulse.

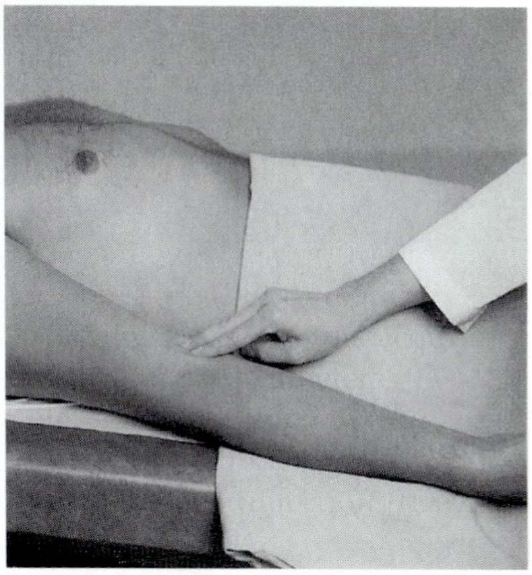

Step 9 Palpation of brachial pulse.

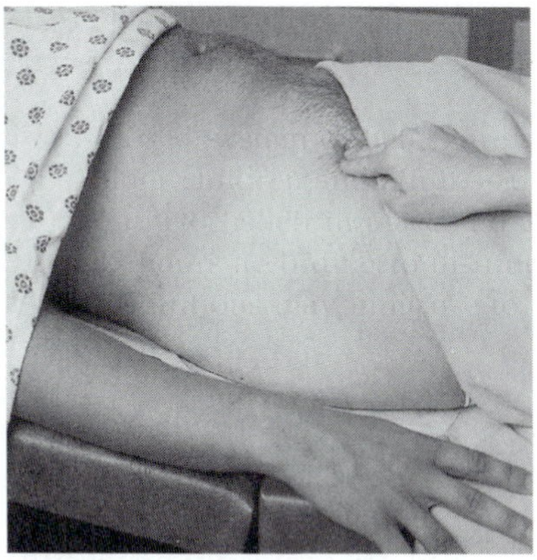

Step 10 Palpation of femoral pulse.

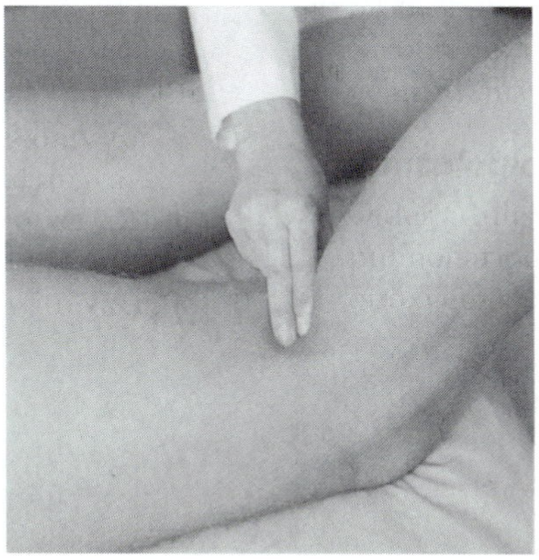

Step 11 Palpation of popliteal pulse.

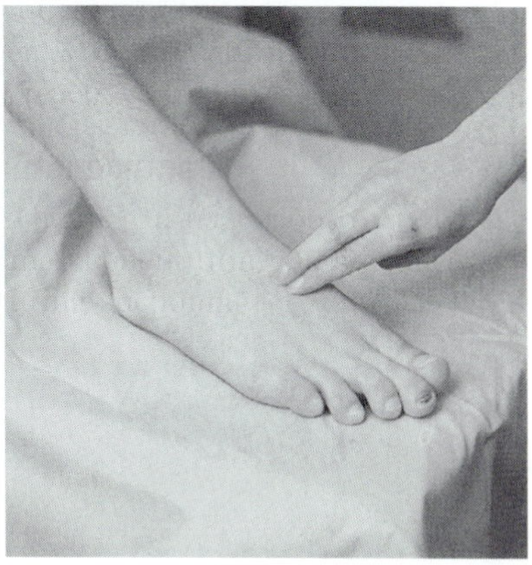

Step 12 Palpation of dorsalis pedis pulse.

STEPS	RATIONALE
13. Palpate posterior tibial pulse by having client relax and slightly extend feet. Place fingertips behind and below medial malleolus (ankle bone) (see illustration).	Artery is easily palpable with foot relaxed.

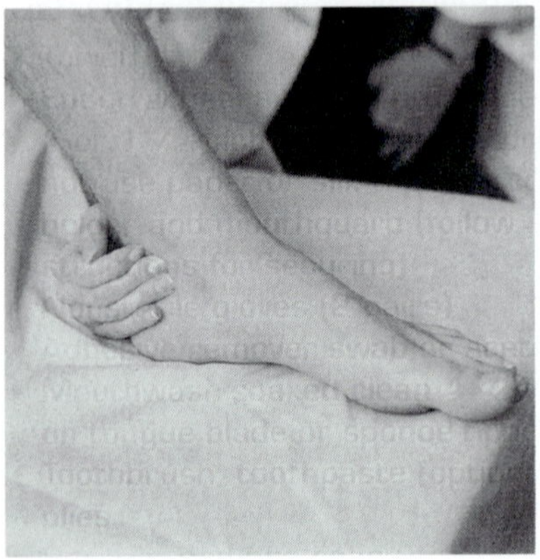

Step 13 Palpation of posterior tibial pulse.

STEPS	RATIONALE
14. If it is difficult to palpate a pulse or the pulse is not palpable, use an ultrasound stethoscope over the pulse site:	
a. Connect the stethoscope headset to the ultrasound probe.	Ultrasound stethoscope amplifies sounds, allowing nurse to hear low-velocity blood flow through peripheral arteries.
b. Apply conducting gel to the client's skin over the pulse site or onto transducer tip of probe.	Gel creates airtight seal for sound transmission.
c. Turn on volume control of stethoscope.	
d. Gently apply ultrasound probe at a 45- to 90-degree angle on the skin at the pulse site (see illustration). Turn volume up as needed.	Excess pressure can obliterate pulse.
15. Assess the lymphatic system by palpating the area of the client's groin, moving down toward the inner thigh (see illustration). The vertical chain of nodes lies close to the upper portion of the great saphenous vein. The horizontal nodes are just below the inguinal ligament. Use firm but gentle pressure. Note size, tenderness, mobility, and location.	Enlargement of superficial inguinal lymph nodes can indicate infection or malignancy in abdominal cavity, as well as systemic infection.

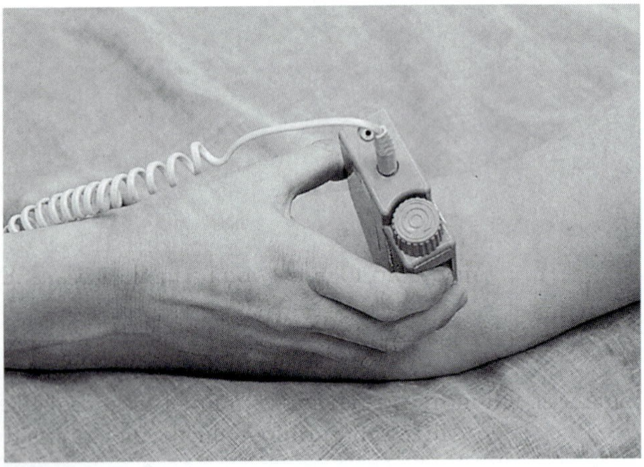

Step 14d Ultrasound stethoscope in position on brachial artery.

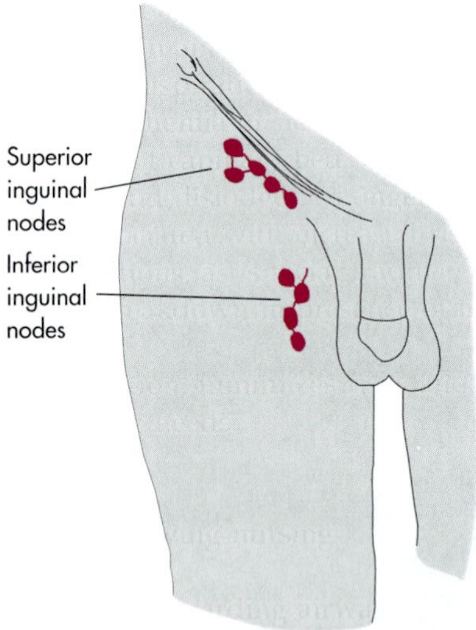

Step 15 Inguinal lymph nodes.

STEPS	RATIONALE
EVALUATION	
1. Compare findings with normal assessment characteristics of heart and vascular system.	Determines presence of abnormalities.
2. If heart sounds are not audible or if pulses are not palpable, ask another nurse to validate assessment.	Abnormal assessment findings can be caused by examiner's error.
3. Ask client to describe behaviors that increase risk for heart and vascular disease.	Demonstrates learning.
4. **Unexpected outcomes** that may occur include:	
➤ Pulsations, vibrations, or both are palpable.	These are result of valvular problem, murmur, or both.
➤ PMI is found to left of midclavicular line.	Result of cardiomegaly.
➤ Heart rate is irregular, with rate less than 60 beats per minute or more than 100 beats per minute.	Dysrhythmia may indicate inadequate cardiac output.
➤ Pulse deficit is noted.	There is risk for inadequate cardiac output.
➤ Extra heart sounds S_3 or S_4 are auscultated.	Extra sounds indicate atrial or ventricular gallop.
➤ Murmur is auscultated.	Impaired blood flow through heart may indicate need for immediate medical attention.
➤ Client is unable to explain risks for heart or vascular disease.	Reinstruction is necessary.
➤ Client demonstrates hypertension or hypotension (see Chapter 10).	These may be a result of arteriosclerosis, renal or heart disease, reaction to medications, and a variety of other medical conditions.
➤ Absent carotid pulse wave.	Arterial occlusion or stenosis may be present.
➤ A bruit is auscultated over the carotid pulse.	
➤ Jugular venous pressure is elevated.	This is a sign of right-sided heart failure.
➤ Skin is pale, cool, thin, and shiny, with reduced hair growth and nail thickening.	These signs are results of chronic arterial insufficiency.
➤ Skin is warm but cyanotic; dependent edema is present in ankles; brown pigmentation is noted.	Signs of venous stasis are evident.
➤ Peripheral pulses are 0 to 1+.	Arterial blood flow to tissues is inadequate.
➤ Positive Homan's sign is noted, with pain in calf during dorsiflexion.	Risk exists for clot in client's deep leg veins.
➤ Lymph nodes are enlarged, hardened, and tender.	This may be indication of infection or metastatic disease.

NURSING DIAGNOSIS

Clustering of defining characteristics from the assessment data may reveal the following nursing diagnoses for clients requiring this skill:

- Activity intolerance
- Altered peripheral tissue perfusion
- Risk for impaired skin integrity
- Decreased cardiac output
- Pain
- Knowledge deficit regarding risks for heart disease

Related factors are individualized based on the client's condition or needs.

RECORDING AND REPORTING

1. Record all findings for heart and vascular assessment in nurses' notes or flow sheet.	Documents baseline findings. Data also measure client's response to various therapies.
2. Record any instruction provided to client and client's response.	Documentation provides for continuity of care.
3. Report immediately to physician any irregularities in heart function and indications of impaired arterial blood flow.	Any abnormalities can threaten client's health.

FOLLOW-UP ACTIVITIES

1. Clients with dysrhythmias or pulse deficits may require an electrocardiogram or Holter monitor per physician's order.

2. Clients with venous thrombosis should not have lower leg massaged because of risk of dislodging a clot. Warning should be placed in care plan or Kardex.

• • • • •

Special Considerations

- Clients with heart disease may have shortness of breath and may benefit from elevating upper body during most of examination.
- Central cyanosis is evident from bluish discoloration of mucosa at base of tongue. This indicates poor oxygen saturation, seen in lung disease and congenital heart defects of children.
- Peripheral cyanosis is evident from bluish discoloration of lips, appendages, and nail beds. This condition results from low cardiac output or local vasoconstriction.
- Increased cardiac output (e.g., after fever, exercise) results in strong pulse.
- Varicosities (superficial veins that become dilated) are common in people who must stand for prolonged periods.

Teaching Considerations

- Explain risk factors for heart disease: high dietary intake of saturated fat or cholesterol, lack of regular aerobic exercise, smoking, excess weight, stressful lifestyle, hypertension, and family history of heart disease.
- Refer client (if appropriate) to resources available for controlling or reducing risks (e.g., nutritional counseling, exercise class, and stress-reduction programs).
- Explain that research shows clinical benefit from reducing dietary intake of cholesterol and saturated fats. Tell client that about 70% to 75% of saturated fatty acids come from meats, poultry, fish, and dairy products and that the one-step diet recommended by the National Institutes of Health includes an intake of total fat less than 30% of calories, saturated fatty acids less than 10% of calories, and cholesterol less than 300 mg/100 ml (Ernst, 1989).
- Encourage client to have regular measurement of total blood cholesterol levels and triglycerides. More than one cholesterol measurement is needed to assess the blood cholesterol level accurately. Low-density lipoprotein (LDL) cholesterol is the major component of atherosclerotic plaques. Separate measurement of LDL cholesterol is wise in a client with high total blood cholesterol levels. An LDL cholesterol level of 160 mg/dl or higher indicates high risk.
- Tell client blood pressure reading. Explain normal reading for client's age. Discuss implications of abnormalities.
- Instruct clients with risk or evidence of vascular insufficiency in the lower extremities to avoid wearing tight clothing over the lower body or legs, to avoid sitting or standing for long periods, to walk regularly, and to elevate feet when sitting.
- Older adults with hypertension may benefit from regular monitoring of blood pressure (daily, weekly, or monthly). Home monitoring kits are available. Teach client how to use them.
- Advise client to avoid cigarette smoking because nicotine causes vasoconstriction.

Pediatric Considerations

- Perform cardiac assessment on infant or toddler while quiet, before more uncomfortable procedures.
- It is not uncommon for children to have third heart sounds (S_3).
- Sinus dysrhythmia occurs normally in many children.
- Children have louder, higher-pitched heart sounds because of their thin chest walls.

Gerontologic Considerations

- PMI may be difficult to find in an older adult because anteroposterior diameter of the chest deepens.
- Accidental massage of the carotid sinus during palpation of the carotid artery can be a particular problem for older adults, causing a sudden drop in heart rate from vagal nerve stimulation.
- Varicosities are common in the older adult because the veins normally fibrose, dilate, and stretch.
- The older adult should be carefully assessed for carotid bruits.

SKILL 11-12 Assessing the Breasts

It is important to examine the breasts of female and male clients. A small amount of glandular tissue, a potential site for the growth of cancer cells, is located in the male breast. In contrast, most of the female breast is glandular tissue. The client remains comfortable during the examination.

Breast cancer affects one out of every nine women in the United States (American Cancer Society, 1996). It is second only to lung cancer as the leading cause of death in women. Early detection is the key to cure.

Fibrocystic breast disease is a benign condition involving a variety of breast changes observed in premenopausal women: cysts, adenosis, fibrosis, and fibroadenoma (Hockenberger, 1993). Incidence of fibrocystic breast disease is high.

Examination of the breasts should be a routine part of any female client's health screening. A major responsibility for the nurse is to teach clients health behaviors such as breast self-examination (BSE). The American Cancer Society (1996) has noted a decline in breast cancer mortality and attributes improvements to increases in breast cancer awareness and screening and improved cancer treatments. Most breast masses are discovered by clients themselves. The American Cancer Society recommends the following screening guidelines for early detection of breast cancer (see box at left).

AMERICAN CANCER SOCIETY'S SCREENING GUIDELINES FOR BREAST CANCER DETECTION IN ASYMPTOMATIC WOMEN

Age 20-39
Monthly breast self-exam, clinical breast exam every 3 years

Age 40-49
Monthly breast self-exam, annual clinical breast exam, mammography annually, baseline mammogram by age 40

Age 50+
Monthly breast self-exam, annual clinical breast exam, annual mammography

American Cancer Society: *Breast Cancer Facts and Figures* 1997, Atlanta, 1997, The Society.

EQUIPMENT

- **Disposable gloves (only when open sores exist or client has drainage from nipples)**

DELEGATION CONSIDERATIONS

An unlicensed assistive personnel member can learn to reinforce to female clients the importance of breast self-examination. However, the RN is responsible for providing the health education necessary for the client to understand fully the personal risks for breast cancer and how to perform the examination correctly. Breast assessment requires problem solving and knowledge application unique to a professional nurse. For this skill, delegation is inappropriate.

STEPS	RATIONALE
ASSESSMENT	
1. Determine if female client is older than age 40, has a personal or family history of breast cancer, had early-onset menarche (before age 12) or late-age menopause (after age 50), has never had children or gave birth to first child after age 30, or has not breast fed child.	Risk factors for occurrence of breast cancer.
2. Ask if client (either sex) has noticed pain, lump, thickening, or tenderness of breast; discharge, distortion, retraction, or scaling of nipple; or change in size of breast.	These are all potential signs and symptoms of breast cancer. Allows nurse to focus on specific areas of breast during assessment.
CRITICAL DECISION POINT Have client point out any lumps.	
3. Ask if female client performs monthly BSE. If so, ask what time of month examination is performed in relation to menstrual cycle. Have client describe or demonstrate method used.	One of primary roles of nurse during assessment of breast is to educate client about breast cancer and technique for BSE. Early detection of cancerous lesion increases possibility of cure.

STEPS	RATIONALE
CRITICAL DECISION POINT **If client denies performing BSE, try to learn factors influencing client's behavior.**	
4. Assess if client is taking oral contraceptives, digitalis, diuretics, steroids, or estrogen hormones. Determine client's caffeine intake.	Medications may cause nipple discharge. Hormones and caffeine may cause fibrocystic changes in the breast.
5. Determine history of fibrocystic breast.	Prepares nurse for finding lumps in breast.
6. If client reports a breast mass, ask about length of time since lump was first noted, whether lump comes and goes or is always present, whether there have been changes in the lump (e.g., size, relationship to menses), and whether there are associated symptoms.	Helps to determine nature of mass.
PLANNING	
1. **Expected outcomes** following completion of procedure:	
➤ Breasts usually extend from the third to the sixth ribs, with nipple at level of fourth intercostal space. One breast is commonly larger than the other.	
➤ Young to middle-age adult: breasts are smooth, symmetrical, without retraction or flattening. Tissue is firm, elastic, with presence of soft, lobular underlying tissue. Areolas are smooth and round or oval, nearly equal bilaterally. Nipples point in symmetrical directions; they are everted and without drainage.	These are normal findings.
➤ Older adult: breasts are smaller than in middle age, evidenced by shrunken, wrinkled appearance of skin. Breasts sag. Tissue may feel stringy and nodular. Nipples point downward.	Changes in elasticity of tissue occur. Changes in estrogen level reduce size of glandular tissue.
➤ Lymph nodes are nonpalpable.	
➤ Client is able to perform BSE correctly.	Learning of a skill is best measured through demonstration feedback.
➤ Client denies having felt anxious during examination.	
➤ Client is able to list signs and symptoms of breast cancer.	Demonstrates cognitive learning.
2. Prepare equipment.	
3. Prepare client for examination:	
a. Have client remove top of gown or expose breasts fully.	Allows simultaneous viewing of both breasts.
b. Client initially assumes standing or sitting position, with arms hanging loosely at her sides.	Inspection is performed with breasts in normal position.
c. If mirror is available, place it in front of client during examination.	Client can learn normal appearance of breasts and what to look for when performing self-examination.
d. Explain (1) each step of examination clearly, describing what signs or features to observe for; (2) normal findings and deviations; and (3) proper techniques for thorough assessment.	During examination nurse's explanations serve to educate client about how to perform self-examination and what to observe for. To recognize abnormalities, client must be familiar with normal appearance of breasts.
e. Allow client opportunities to ask questions and discuss concerns.	Breasts are linked to female's reproductive capacity and sexuality. Threat of abnormalities can cause severe anxiety.

STEPS	RATIONALE

IMPLEMENTATION

FEMALE CLIENT

1. Describe observations or findings made during examination in relation to imaginary lines that divide breast into four quadrants and tail (see illustration).

   Location of finding by common reference point helps successive examiners to confirm findings and locate abnormalities.

2. Inspect both breasts for size and symmetry. Note position of breasts and nipples in relation to underlying intercostal space. Observe area of chest over which breast extends.

   Change in size or shape may indicate underlying mass or presence of inflammation.

3. Observe contour or shape of breast, noting any masses, flattening, retraction, or dimpling. If retraction is suspected, ask client to assume three positions: raise arms above the head, press hands against the hips, and extend arms straight ahead while sitting and leaning forward.

   Underlying mass, swelling, or inflammation may cause bulging or retraction of breast tissue. Maneuvers cause contraction of pectoral muscles, which accentuates presence of retraction.

4. Inspect overlying skin for color and venous pattern. If breasts are large, carefully lift breasts to inspect underlying skin surfaces. Normal breasts are same color as surrounding skin surfaces.

   Vascular changes, edema, or inflammation may cause skin color changes. Undersurface of breast is common site for redness and excoriation caused by rubbing of breast against chest wall.

5. Inspect areolas and nipples for color, size, shape, and discharge. Note direction in which nipples point and presence of rashes or ulcerations. If there is discharge from nipple, note its color.

   Hormonal changes cause changes in color and size of areolas and nipples throughout woman's life span. Presence of underlying lesions may cause change in size, shape, and position of nipples. Underlying lesions may extend to skin's surface, causing ulcerations. Lesions or infection may cause discharge from nipples to range from bloody red to green or brown.

   Be sure to know if client recently gave birth to a child. Clear yellow discharge 2 days after childbirth is common.

➤ *CRITICAL DECISION POINT* This can be a time to explain to the client how to examine the nipples. Caution client against squeezing the nipples too hard because this may cause tissue injury.

6. Palpate lymph nodes (see illustration).
   a. Have client sit with arms at sides and muscles relaxed. Face the client, stand on the side being examined, and support client's arm in slightly flexed position while abducting that arm from the chest wall.

      This position allows easy palpation of axillary lymph nodes.

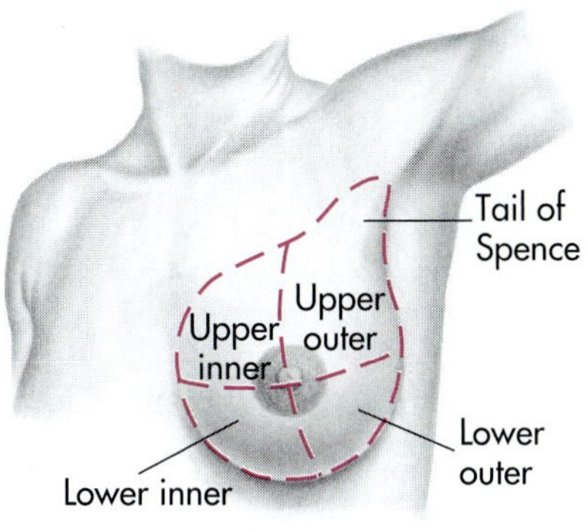

Step 1 Quadrants of left breast and axillary tail of Spence. (From Seidel HM et al: *Mosby's guide to physical examination*, ed 3, St Louis, 1995, Mosby.)

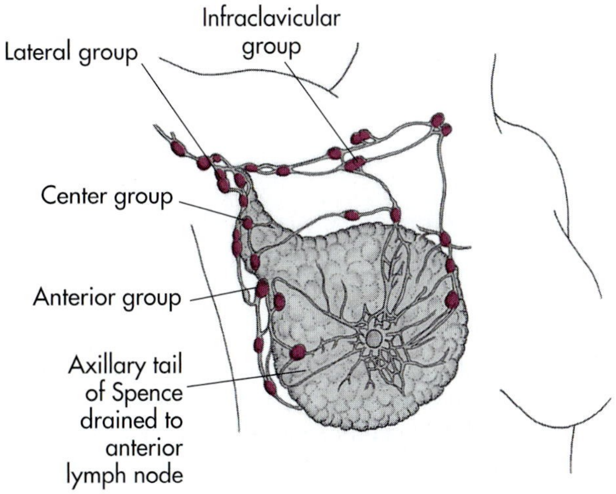

Step 6 Anatomical location of axillary and clavicular lymph nodes.

STEPS	RATIONALE
b. Place the free hand against the client's chest wall and high in the axillary hollow. With the fingertips, press gently down over the surface of the ribs and muscles (see illustration).	Breast cancer can metastasize to lymph nodes.
c. Palpate the following areas: edge of the pectoralis major muscle along anterior axillary line; chest wall in midaxilla; upper part of humerus; anterior edge of latissimus dorsi muscle along posterior axillary line.	
d. Palpate along the upper and lower clavicular ridges.	Location of supraclavicular and infraclavicular nodes.
e. Note number, location, consistency, movability, and size of nodes. If enlarged node is present, ask client if it is tender.	Characteristics of node help to determine cause of enlargement.
f. Reverse procedure for the other breast.	

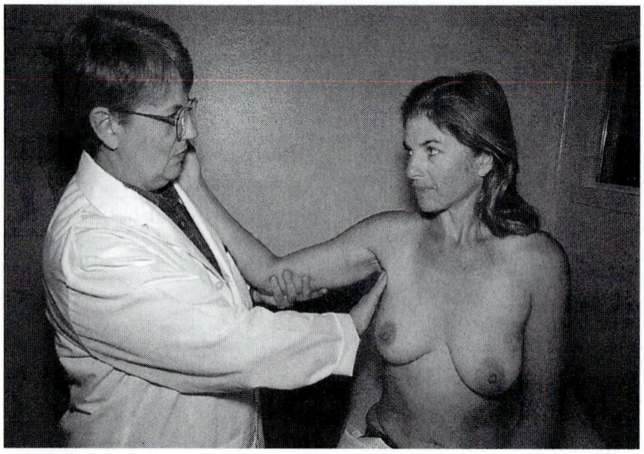

Step 6b Nurse supports client's arm and palpates axillary lymph nodes.

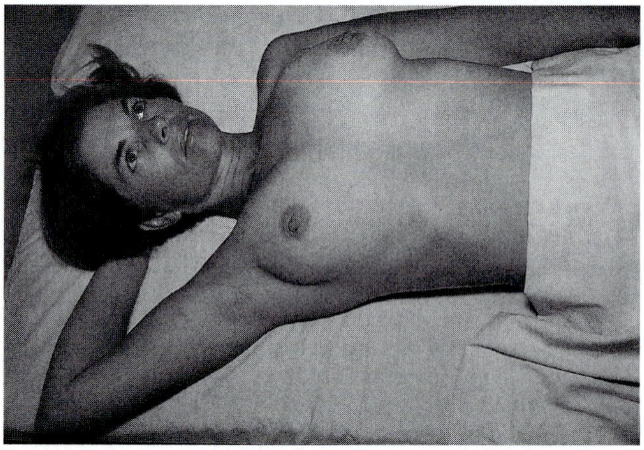

Step 7 Client lies flat with right arm abducted and hand under head to flatten breast tissue.

CRITICAL DECISION POINT **It can be hard for client to learn to palpate lymph nodes. Lying down with arm abducted makes area more accessible. Client uses left hand for right axilla and vice versa.**

STEPS	RATIONALE
7. Have client lie supine with right arm abducted and hand placed under head (see illustration). A small pillow or towel can be placed under client's right shoulder blade.	Position allows breast tissue to flatten evenly against client's chest wall.
8. During this portion of the examination, review the steps of BSE with the client.	Client is prepared for routine self-examination.
9. If client complains of lump or mass, examine opposite breast first.	Objective comparison of normal and abnormal tissue is ensured.

STEPS | **RATIONALE**

10. Stand at client's right side. Gently compress breast tissue against the chest wall using the pads of the first three fingers (see illustration).
Use a systematic approach in one of two ways:
a. A back-and-forth technique with the fingers moving up and down each quadrant (see illustration).
b. Clockwise or counterclockwise, forming small circles with the fingers along each quadrant and the tail.

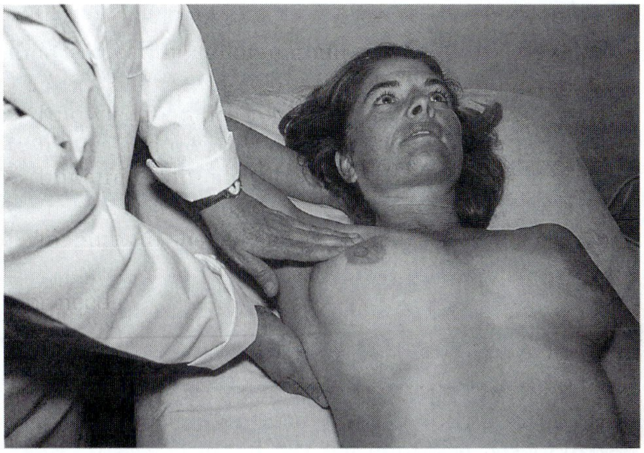

Step 10 Nurse palpates breast tissue.

Cover entire breast and tail, directing attention to any areas of tenderness.

Entire breast tissue must be thoroughly palpated to rule out presence of mass.

11. While palpating breasts, take client's fingertips and move them gently over breast tissue. Lobular feel of glandular tissue is normal. Lower edge of each breast may feel firm and hard.

Consistency of underlying tissue changes with age, pathological conditions, and hormonal variations. Client must learn to feel normal variations of own breast tissue to be able to recognize abnormal masses. Lower edge is inframammary ridge.

➤*CRITICAL DECISION POINT* If client feels an area that is fibrous but normal, validate finding with client. Fibrocystic breast tissue feels lumpy, but it is present bilaterally.

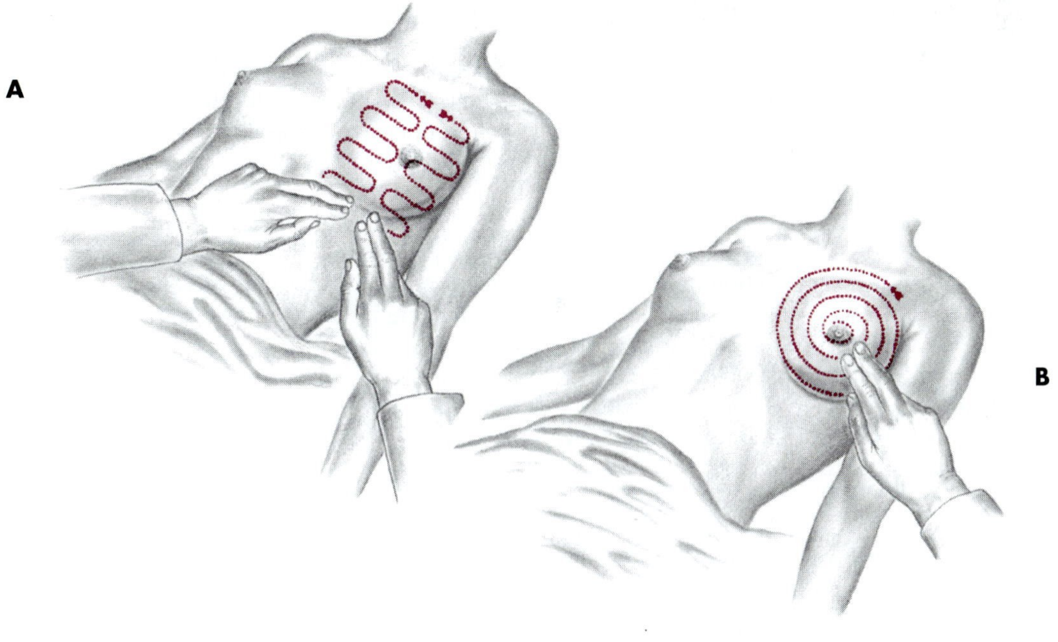

Step 10a Methods for breast palpation. **A,** Back and forth. **B,** Concentric circles. (From Seidel HM et al: *Mosby's guide to physical examination,* ed 3, St Louis, 1995, Mosby.)

STEPS	RATIONALE
12. If an unusual mass is found, palpate for the following characteristics: location in relation to quadrants, diameter in centimeters, shape (e.g., round or discoid), consistency (soft, firm, or hard), tenderness, mobility, discreteness (are boundaries of mass easily detected?).	Data may facilitate identification of type of mass.
13. Use finger to gently compress the areola. Then with thumb and index finger gently compress nipple, observing for discharge.	Involvement of glandular tissue may cause discharge from nipple.
➤ ***CRITICAL DECISION POINT*** **Caution client again against squeezing the nipple.**	
14. Repeat procedure for opposite breast.	
15. After palpation is completed, have client demonstrate self-palpation.	Return demonstration provides feedback to measure client's learning and to determine need for further instruction.

MALE CLIENT

1. Inspect nipple and areola of male client for nodules, edema, and ulceration. Note any swelling of breasts. Palpate breast tissue in same systematic pattern as for females.	Signs of breast cancer are same as for female client.

EVALUATION

1. Compare findings with normal assessment characteristics.	Determines presence of abnormalities.
2. Have female client perform self-examination.	Feedback demonstrates that client knows to observe for relevant signs.
3. Have client describe actual findings of self-examination in relation to normal findings.	Evaluates application of knowledge regarding normal findings and abnormalities.
4. **Unexpected outcomes** that may occur include:	
➤ Breasts are lumpy and painful, with occasional nipple discharge. Symptoms are more apparent during menstrual period. Lumps are soft, well-differentiated, movable, and bilateral.	These are common signs of fibrocystic disease.
➤ Breasts are smooth and symmetrical, without retraction or flattening. Localized mass is palpable on one side. Mass may be hard or soft, tender or nontender, mobile or fixed, and well differentiated. There is no discharge from nipples. Lymph nodes are nonpalpable. Client is unable to detect mass.	Symptoms indicate small, discrete breast mass. Client should be referred to physician immediately. Repeated experience is necessary for client to become familiar with own breasts.
➤ Breast reveals dimpling or retraction unilaterally. Skin over area is inflamed with increased vascularity. Contour of involved breast is irregular; nipple is distorted with serous or bloody discharge. Palpable mass is hard, fixed, nontender, and irregular in shape. Lymph nodes are palpable.	Symptoms indicate more advanced invasive lesion. Immediate referral to physician is required.
➤ Client demonstrates BSE incorrectly.	Further instruction is necessary.

NURSING DIAGNOSIS

Clustering of defining characteristics from the assessment data may reveal the following nursing diagnoses for clients requiring this skill:

- ➤ Anxiety
- ➤ Body-image disturbance
- ➤ Fear
- ➤ Knowledge deficit regarding preventive health care
- ➤ Pain

Related factors are individualized based on the client's condition and needs.

STEPS	RATIONALE
RECORDING AND REPORTING	
1. Record all findings and client education in nurses' notes.	Documents abnormalities or changes. Provides baseline data and ensures continuity of care.
2. Report abnormalities to nurse in charge or physician.	Further diagnosis will be required.

• • • • •

Special Considerations

- Pregnancy causes breasts to enlarge two to three times previous size; nipples enlarge and may become erect; areola darkens; and superficial veins become prominent. Menopause causes breasts to shrink and tissue to become soft.
- Male breast cancer is rare. Routine self-examinations are unnecessary. Swelling of male breasts may result from obesity or glandular enlargement.
- Venous patterns are more easily seen in thin clients or pregnant women.
- In light-skinned women the areola turns brown during pregnancy and remains dark. In dark-skinned women the areola is brown before pregnancy (Seidel et al., 1995).
- For larger pendulous breasts, nurse may use bimanual palpation. Support inferior portion of breast in one hand while palpating breast tissue against supporting hand.
- A tumor of one breast may also involve lymph nodes on the opposite side.
- Between 1989 and 1992, mortality rates for breast cancer declined among whites but increased among African-American women. Nurse should consider if client has limited access to medical care or if social or cultural factors influence client's interest in screening.

Teaching Considerations

- Best time for self-examination is last day of menstrual period, when breasts are no longer swollen or tender. Postmenopausal women should examine breasts same time each month. Pregnant women should examine breasts routinely each month.
- Instruct client on BSE (see the box on p. 372).
- Women with fibrocystic breast disease must become familiar with character of cystic masses. It is recommended that these women avoid caffeine and theophylline intake (although findings are controversial).
- If client finds a mass during self-examination, caution client against rubbing or touching area excessively. Pressure against cancerous or infected mass can disrupt cells and cause spread.
- Discuss signs and symptoms of breast cancer and fibrocystic breast disease with client.

Gerontologic Considerations

- In older adults ligaments supporting breast tissue weaken, causing breasts to sag and nipples to lower. Actual breast tissue feels stringy and nodular. Older women may ignore BSE, assuming that changes are a result of aging. These changes mimic breast cancer.
- Many older women fail to perform regular BSE or seek routine medical screening because of limited fixed income. The nurse should help find access to free screening programs.
- Musculoskeletal limitations, diminished peripheral sensation, reduced eyesight, and changes in joint range of motion can limit an older woman's ability to palpate and inspect the breasts. A friend or family member may need to learn how to perform a breast examination.

BREAST SELF-EXAMINATION

Instruct client on BSE. All women 20 years and older should perform this self-examination monthly using the following steps:

- Stand before a mirror. Look at both breasts for anything unusual, such as discharge from the nipples, puckering, dimpling, or scaling of the skin.
- To note changes in the shape of the breasts, perform the following measures (see illustration):
  - Watch in the mirror while raising the arms above the head.
  - Press hands firmly on the hips and bow slightly toward the mirror when pulling the shoulders and elbows forward.

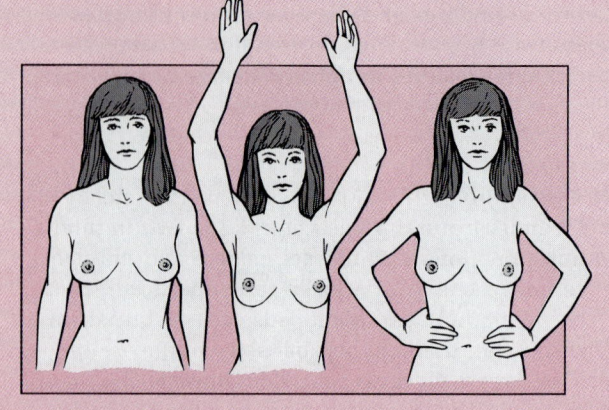

- In the shower or in front of a mirror, palpate each breast. Raise the right arm and use three or four fingers of the left hand to explore the breast carefully (see illustration). Then start at the outer edge, pressing the flat part of the fingers in small circles, moving the circles slowly around the breast, gradually working toward the nipple (see illustration). Pay close attention to the area between the breast and armpit and feel for unusual lumps or masses. Repeat the process for the left breast.

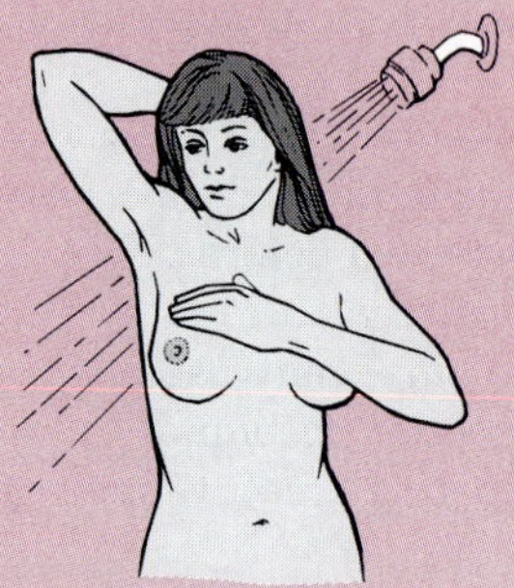

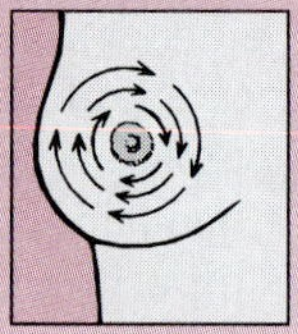

- Gently palpate each nipple, looking for discharge (see illustration). Caution against pinching.

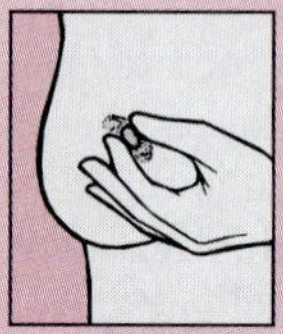

- Repeat the third and fourth steps lying down. Lie flat on the back with the right arm over the head and a small pillow under the right shoulder. Palpate the right breast (see illustration). Repeat the process on the left breast.
- Call your physician if you find a lump.

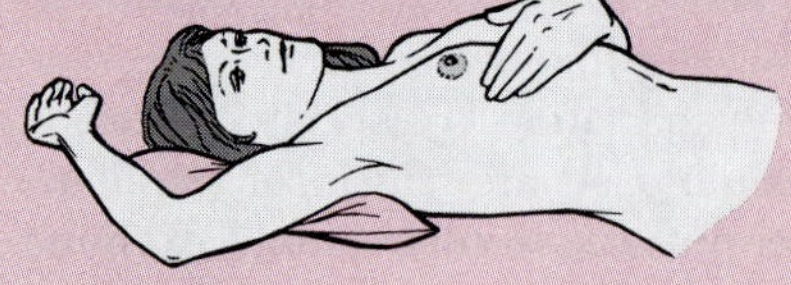

Illustrations from Payne WA, Hahn DB: *Understanding your health,* ed 2, St Louis, 1989, Mosby.

SKILL 11-13 Assessing the Abdomen

The abdominal examination can be complex because of the multiple organs located within and near the abdominal cavity. A thorough assessment is necessary to interpret all findings accurately. For example, if the client has abdominal pain, the symptom could be caused by alterations in organs such as the stomach, gallbladder, or intestines; or the pain may be the result of spinal or muscular injury. Abdominal pain is one of the most common symptoms clients report when seeking medical care. An accurate assessment requires matching the client's history with a careful assessment of the location of physical symptoms.

When performing the assessment, the nurse should maintain a mental image of the anatomical location of each organ. This practice ensures that the nurse is using assessment skills correctly. The nurse should remember to include assessment of organs that lie posteriorly, such as the kidneys.

An abdominal assessment is routine after abdominal surgery and for any client who has undergone invasive diagnostic tests of the gastrointestinal tract (Chapter 44). The order of an abdominal assessment differs from that of other assessments. The nurse begins with inspection and follows with auscultation. It is important to auscultate before palpation and percussion; otherwise, these later maneuvers may alter the frequency and character of bowel sounds.

EQUIPMENT

- Stethoscope
- Tape measure
- Examination light
- Marking pen

DELEGATION CONSIDERATIONS

This skill requires problem solving and knowledge application unique to a professional nurse. For this skill, delegation is inappropriate. However, assistive personnel should know to report to the RN any changes in the client's bowel habits or dietary intake and the development of abdominal pain.

STEPS	RATIONALE
ASSESSMENT	
1. If client has abdominal or low back pain, assess the character of pain in detail (location, onset, frequency, precipitating factors, aggravating factors, type of pain, severity, course).	Knowing pattern of characteristics of pain helps determine its source.
2. Carefully observe client's movement and position, such as:	
a. Lying still with knees drawn up. b. Moving restlessly to find a comfortable position. c. Lying on one side or sitting with knees drawn up to chest.	Positions assumed by the client may reveal nature and source of pain (e.g., peritonitis, renal stone, and pancreatitis).
CRITICAL DECISION POINT **These observations often can be made during routine care activities.**	
3. Assess client's normal bowel habits: frequency of stools; character of stools; recent changes in character of stools; measures used to promote elimination, such as laxatives, enemas, dietary intake; and eating and drinking habits.	These data, compared with information from physical assessment, may help to identify cause and nature of elimination problems.
4. Determine if client has had abdominal surgery, trauma, or diagnostic tests of the gastrointestinal tract.	Surgical or traumatic alterations of abdominal organs may cause changes in expected findings (e.g., position of underlying organs). Diagnostic tests may change character of stool.
5. Assess if client has had any recent changes in weight or intolerance to diet (e.g., nausea, vomiting, or cramping), especially in last 24 hours.	Changes may indicate alterations in upper gastrointestinal tract (e.g., stomach or gallbladder) or lower colon.

STEPS	RATIONALE
6. Assess for difficulty in swallowing, belching, flatulence, bloody emesis (hematemesis), black or tarry stools (melena), heartburn, diarrhea, or constipation.	Characteristic signs and symptoms are indicative of gastrointestinal alterations.
7. Ask if client takes antiinflammatory medications (e.g., aspirin, steroids, and nonsteroidal antiinflammatory drugs), or antibiotics.	Pharmacological agents may cause gastrointestinal upset or bleeding.
8. Inquire about family history of cancer, kidney disease, alcoholism, hypertension, or heart disease.	Data may reveal risk for alterations identifiable during examination.
9. Determine if female client is pregnant.	Pregnancy causes changes in abdominal shape and contour.
10. Assess client's usual intake of alcohol.	Chronic alcohol ingestion can cause gastrointestinal and liver problems.
11. Review client's history for health care occupation, hemodialysis, intravenous drug use, household or sexual contact with hepatitis B virus (HBV) carrier, sexually active (heterosexual person more than one sex partner in previous 6 months), sexually active homosexual or bisexual man, international traveler in area of high HBV prevalence.	These are risk factors for HBV exposure (Reece, 1993).

PLANNING

1. Expected outcomes following completion of procedure:	
➤ Umbilicus is flat or concave, positioned midway between xiphoid process and symphysis pubis. Color is same as surrounding skin. No discharge is present.	
➤ Abdomen is soft and symmetrical with smooth and even contour. No mass or tenderness is palpable.	
➤ In obese clients rolls of adipose tissue are often present along the flanks, and client denies tightness in the abdomen.	
➤ Peristaltic movement or aortic pulsation may be seen across the abdomen.	
➤ Bowel sounds are active and audible in all four quadrants.	Peristalsis is normal.
➤ Abdomen is tympanic on percussion.	Normal air is found in intestines.
➤ No **costovertebral angle (CVA) tenderness** is present.	
➤ Liver is nonpalpable. Location of borders is normal.	
➤ Spleen is nontender and nonpalpable.	
➤ Consecutive measurements reveal no change in abdominal girth.	Rules out distention.
➤ Aortic pulsation is transmitted forward.	
➤ Client denies discomfort or worsening of existing discomfort following examination.	
➤ Client is able to list warning signs of colon cancer.	Demonstrates learning.
2. Prepare client:	
a. Ask if client needs to empty bladder.	Palpation of full bladder can cause discomfort and feeling of urgency and make it difficult for client to relax.
b. Keep upper chest and legs draped. Be sure that room is warm. Expose area from just above the xiphoid process down to the symphysis pubis.	Maintains client's comfort during examination, promoting relaxation.

STEPS	RATIONALE
c. Have client lie supine or in a dorsal recumbent position with arms down at sides and knees slightly bent. A small pillow may be placed under client's knees.	Position promotes optimal relaxation of abdominal muscles. Tightening of muscles prevents adequate palpation.

CRITICAL DECISION POINT **Do not let client place the arms under the head because this can cause the abdominal muscles to tighten.**

STEPS	RATIONALE
d. Maintain conversation during assessment except during auscultation. Explain steps calmly and slowly.	Client's ability to relax during assessment improves accuracy of findings.
e. Ask client to locate tender areas.	Painful areas are assessed last. Manipulation of body part can increase client's pain and anxiety and make remainder of assessment difficult to complete.

IMPLEMENTATION

STEPS	RATIONALE
1. Describe observations or findings in relation to system of landmarks that divides abdominal region into quadrants; line extending from tip of xiphoid process to symphysis pubis crosses line intersecting umbilicus, dividing abdomen into four equal sections (see illustration). Some clinicians may also divide the abdomen into nine equal sections for the abdominal examination (see illustration).	Location of findings by common reference point helps successive examiners to confirm findings and locate abnormalities.
2. While inspecting client's abdomen, stand on client's right side and look from above the abdomen. Direct the examination light over abdomen.	Position helps to detect shadows and movement.
3. Sit down and look across abdomen.	Sitting position allows examiner to assess contour.
4. Inspect skin of abdomen's surface for color, scars, venous patterns, rashes, lesions, silvery white striae (stretch marks), and artificial openings. Observe lesions for characteristics described in Skill 11-2.	Scars reveal evidence that client has had past trauma or surgery. Striae indicate stretching of tissue from growth, obesity, pregnancy, ascites, or edema. Venous patterns may reflect liver disease (portal hypertension). Artificial openings indicate bowel or urinary diversion (Chapter 27).
5. If bruising is noted, ask if client self-administers injections (e.g., heparin or insulin).	Frequent injections can cause bruising and hardening of underlying tissues.

CRITICAL DECISION POINT **Bruising may also indicate physical abuse, accidental injury, or bleeding disorders.**

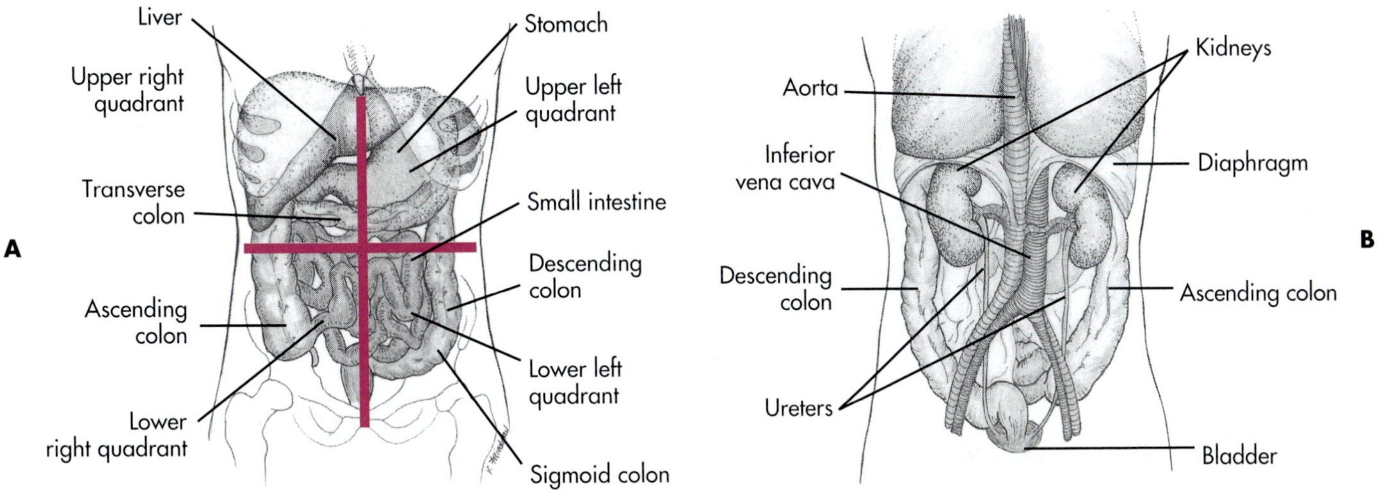

Step 1 **A,** Division of abdomen into quadrants. **B,** Posterior view of abdominal sections.

STEPS	RATIONALE
6. Inspect the position, shape, and color of the umbilicus. Note inflammation, discoloration, discharge, or protruding masses.	An everted (pouch extends outward) umbilicus usually indicates distention. A hernia can also cause the umbilicus to protrude upward.
7. Inspect the contour, symmetry, and surface motion of the abdomen. Note any masses, bulging, or distention. (Flat abdomen forms a horizontal plane from xiphoid process to symphysis pubis. Round abdomen protrudes in convex sphere from horizontal plane. Concave abdomen sinks into muscular wall. All are normal.)	Changes in symmetry or contour may reveal underlying masses, fluid collection, or gaseous distention.
8. If abdomen appears distended, note if distention is generalized. Look at the flanks on each side.	Distention may be caused by the six *F*s (fat, flatus, feces, fluids, fibroid, and fetus). If gas causes distention, flanks do not bulge. If fluid causes distention, flanks bulge. Tumor may cause a more unilateral bulging or distention. Pregnancy causes symmetrical bulge in lower abdomen.
9. If distention is present, have client roll onto one side. Look for a protuberance on the dependent side.	Results from fluid that is causing distention.
10. Ask client if abdomen feels unusually tight.	Continued sensation of fullness helps to detect distention. Feeling of fullness after a heavy meal causes only temporary distention. Tightness is not felt with obesity.
11. If distention is suspected, measure size of abdominal girth by placing tape measure around abdomen at level of umbilicus. Use the marking pen to indicate where tape measure was applied.	Consecutive measurements will show any increase or decrease in abdominal distention.
12. Observe abdominal contour while asking client to take a deep breath and hold it. Look for bulges.	Maneuver forces diaphragm downward and reduces the size of abdominal cavity. Any enlarged organs in upper abdominal cavity (e.g., liver or spleen) may descend below ribs to cause a bulge.
13. Ask client to raise head. Again note any bulges.	Position causes superficial abdominal wall masses, hernias, and muscle separations to become apparent.
14. Observe for movement or pulsations of abdominal surface by looking across abdomen from side. Observe for 1 to 2 minutes. Also inspect epigastric area, midline above umbilicus for aortic pulsation.	Presence of aortic pulsation, respiratory or peristaltic movements, and any muscular contraction can be visible on the abdominal surface.
➤ *CRITICAL DECISION POINT* Aortic pulsation will coincide with each systolic beat.	
15. Ask client not to talk. If nasogastric or intestinal tube is connected to suction, turn off momentarily.	Sound obscures bowel sounds.
16. Place diaphragm of stethoscope lightly over each of the four abdominal quadrants. Listen until repeated gurgling or bubbling sounds are heard in each quadrant (minimum of 5 to 20 seconds). Describe sounds as normal or audible, absent, hyperactive, or hypoactive. Listen 3 to 5 minutes over each quadrant before deciding that bowel sounds are absent.	Determines presence or absence of peristalsis. Normally sounds occur irregularly every 5 to 20 seconds. Absent sounds indicate cessation of gastric motility.
➤ *CRITICAL DECISION POINT* Best time to auscultate is between meals.	
17. Place bell of stethoscope over the epigastric region of the abdomen and each quadrant. Auscultate for vascular sounds.	Determines presence of turbulent blood flow (bruit) through thoracic or abdominal aorta.

STEPS	RATIONALE
CRITICAL DECISION POINT If aortic bruit is auscultated, stop assessment and notify physician immediately.	Percussion or palpation over abdominal bruit can cause damage if bruit is result of an abdominal aneurysm. Palpation can cause rupture of already weakened vessel wall.
18. Place the bell of the stethoscope over each upper quadrant anteriorly or the costovertebral angle posteriorly (with client sitting).	Determines presence of renal artery bruit.
19. Have client return to supine position. Gently percuss each of four abdominal quadrants systematically. Note areas of tympany and dullness.	Reveals presence of air or fluid in stomach and intestines. Normal percussion is tympanic because of swallowed air in gastrointestinal tract. Presence of fluid or underlying masses is revealed by dull percussion.
20. To locate lower border of liver, start percussion at the right iliac crest and move upward along the right midclavicular line. Slowly inch pleximeter finger until note becomes dull. Mark point on skin where sounds change.	Detects position of lower border of liver. Percussion note changes from tympanic to dull at lower border, usually found at right costal margin.
CRITICAL DECISION POINT Report any extension beyond the right costal margin.	
21. Percuss down from the clavicle along intercostal spaces at the right midclavicular line. Slowly inch pleximeter finger downward toward right costal margin until note becomes dull. Be sure pleximeter finger is in intercostal space during percussion (see illustration). Using a measuring tape, measure distance between upper and lower border of liver; 6 to 12 cm (2½ to 5 inches) is normal.	Detects position of upper border of liver. Percussion note changes from resonant to dull at upper border, usually found in fifth, sixth, or seventh intercostal space. Diseases such as cirrhosis, hepatitis, and cancer enlarge the liver.
22. Ask client to sit. Gently but firmly percuss over each costovertebral angle along scapular lines. Use ulnar surface of fist to percuss *directly* against client's skin or *indirectly* by placing nondominant hand flat against costovertebral angle and percussing hand with dominant hand (see illustration). Note if client experiences pain.	Determines presence of kidney inflammation.

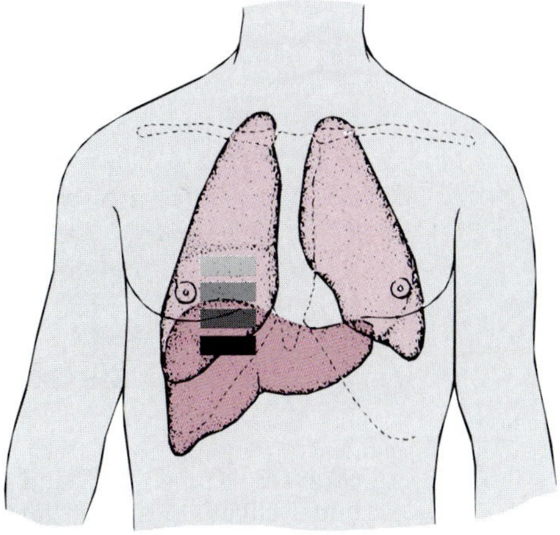

Step 21 To locate liver's upper border, nurse percusses downward, noting change in sound from resonance (lung) to dullness (liver).

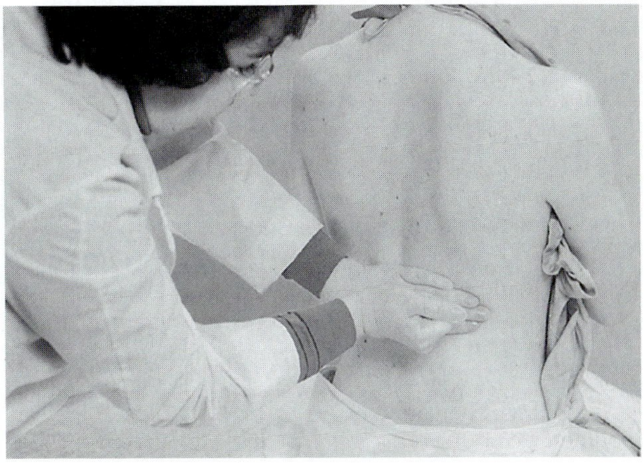

Step 22 Indirect percussion for tenderness at costovertebral angle. (From Seidel HM et al. *Mosby's guide to physical examination,* ed 3, St Louis, 1995, Mosby.)

STEPS	RATIONALE
➤ *CRITICAL DECISION POINT* To avoid tickling, place the client's hand on the abdomen with the nurse's hand on the client's.	
23. Lightly palpate over each abdominal quadrant, laying the palm of the hand with fingers extended and approximated lightly on the abdomen. Keep the palm and forearm horizontal. The pads of the fingertips depress the skin approximately 1 cm (½ inch) in a gentle dipping motion (see illustration). a. Note muscular resistance, distention, tenderness, and superficial masses or organs. b. Observe client's face for signs of discomfort. c. Note if abdomen is firm or soft to touch.	Detects areas of localized tenderness, degree of tenderness, and presence and character of underlying masses. Palpation of sensitive area causes guarding (voluntary tightening of underlying abdominal muscles). Client's verbal and nonverbal cues may indicate discomfort from tenderness. Firm abdomen may indicate active obstruction with fluid or gas building up. Soft abdomen is normal or reveals that obstruction is resolving.
➤ *CRITICAL DECISION POINT* Remember, palpate painful areas last. Avoid quick jabs.	
➤ *CRITICAL DECISION POINT* If client remains relaxed and no apparent abnormalities have been noted, this is a good time to discuss signs and symptoms of colon cancer from a preventive perspective.	
24. Just below umbilicus and above symphysis pubis, palpate for a smooth, rounded mass. While applying light pressure, ask if client has sensation of need to void.	Detects presence of dome of distended bladder.

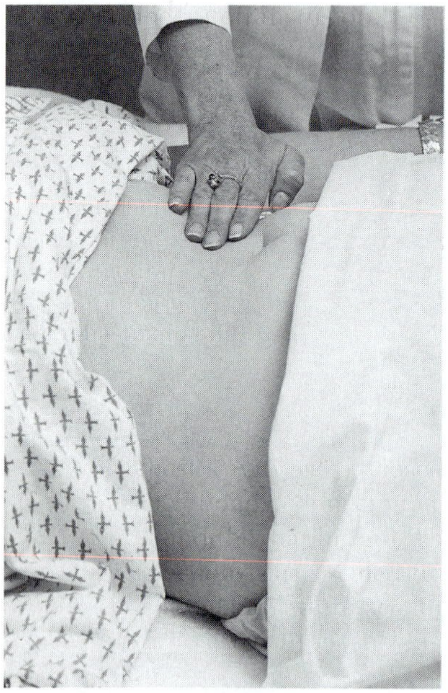

Step 23 Light palpation of abdomen.

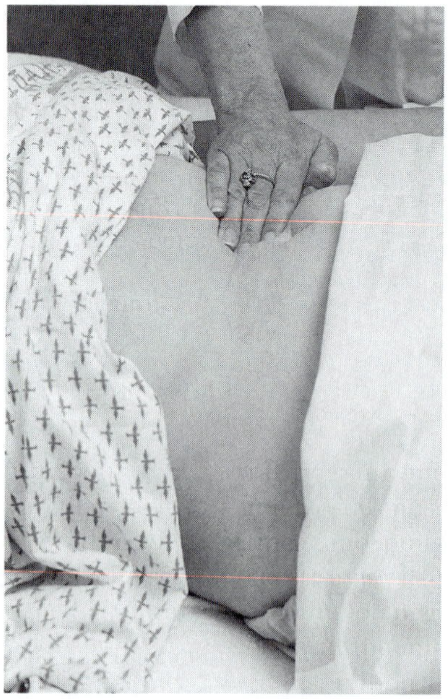

Step 27 Deep palpation of abdomen.

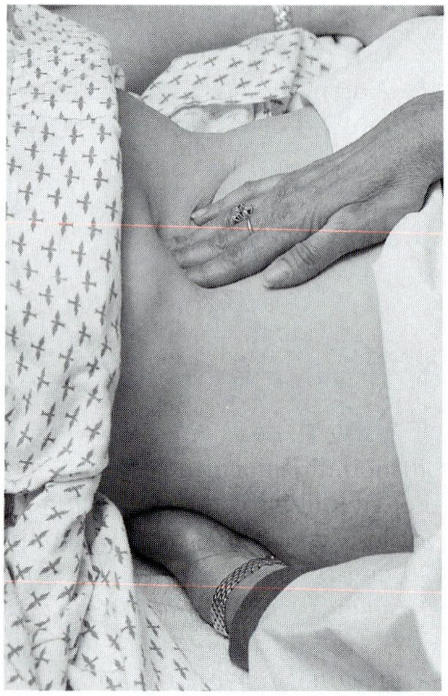

Step 28 Nurse's left hand is placed under client's posterior thorax at eleventh and twelfth ribs. Nurse's right hand palpates inward and upward to feel liver's edge as client inhales.

STEPS	RATIONALE
➤ ***CRITICAL DECISION POINT*** **Routinely check for distended bladder if client has been unable to void, client has been incontinent, or an indwelling Foley catheter is not draining well.**	
25. If masses are palpated, note size, location, shape, consistency, tenderness, mobility, and texture.	Characteristics help to reveal type of mass.
26. When tenderness is present, press one hand slowly and deeply into the involved area and then let go quickly. Note if pain is aggravated.	Tests for rebound tenderness. Results are positive if pain increases.
27. Perform deep palpation, being sure the client is relaxed. Depress the palm and fingers approximately 2.5 to 7.5 cm (1 to 3 in) into the abdomen (see illustration).	Detects less obvious masses and delineates abdominal organs.
➤ ***CRITICAL DECISION POINT*** **Never use deep palpation over a surgical incision or extremely tender organs.**	
28. Locate lower border of liver by placing left hand under client's right posterior thorax at the eleventh and twelfth ribs (just under small of back). Apply gentle upward pressure with left hand. With fingers of the right hand pointing toward client's right costal margin, place the hand on the right upper quadrant well below the costal margin (or lower border of liver). Ask client to take a deep breath, and gently palpate inward and upward with right hand. As client inhales, edge of liver may be felt (see illustration) as it descends.	Allows for location of liver and determination if organ is enlarged or disease is present. Upward pressure of left hand along with deep-breathing maneuver causes liver to descend and be entrapped briefly for palpation. Edge of liver cannot usually be palpated in normal adult. Normal liver is nontender and has regular contour and sharp edge.
29. Palpate the spleen by standing at the client's right side and placing the right hand over the client's left anterior costal margin. Place the left hand under the client's left costovertebral angle. Ask the client to inhale while pressing upward with the left hand and inward with the fingertips of the right hand.	Technique allows for palpation of an enlarged spleen.
30. Assess aortic pulsation by using the thumb and forefinger of one hand to palpate deeply into the upper abdomen, just left of the midline. Feel for a pulsation transmitted forward.	Can detect presence of aortic enlargement.
➤ ***CRITICAL DECISION POINT*** **Do not palpate aortic pulsation if aneurysm is suspected.**	
EVALUATION	
1. Compare assessment findings with normal assessment characteristics of abdomen.	Determines presence of abnormalities.
2. Ask client to describe signs and symptoms of colon cancer.	
3. **Unexpected outcomes** that may occur include:	
➤ Abdomen is asymmetrical, with palpable mass, and dull to percussion.	Findings may indicate enlarged liver, spleen, or tumor.
➤ Abdomen protrudes symmetrically, with skin taut. Client complains of tightness.	These are results of gaseous distention.
➤ Bowel sounds are absent.	Gastrointestinal motility has ceased.

STEPS	RATIONALE
➤ Hyperactive bowel sounds are evident.	Sounds are result of increase in gastrointestinal motility. Commonly they result from anxiety, diarrhea, overuse of laxatives, inflammation of the bowel, or reaction of the intestines to certain foods.
➤ Rebound abdominal tenderness is found.	Results from peritoneal irritation (e.g., appendicitis or pancreatitis).
➤ Bladder is palpable over symphysis pubis.	Bladder is distended.
➤ Liver is tender and/or enlarged.	Tenderness is indicative of hepatitis. Enlargement may be due to cancerous involvement or cirrhosis.
➤ Spleen is palpable.	
➤ Aortic pulsation expands laterally.	Result of enlarged aorta is possibly due to an aneurysm (dilation of vessel wall).
➤ Abdominal girth is increased.	Fluid has built up within peritoneal cavity.
➤ Client is unable to describe signs and symptoms of colon cancer.	Reinstruction is necessary.

NURSING DIAGNOSIS

Clustering of defining characteristics from the assessment data may reveal the following nursing diagnoses for clients requiring this skill:

- ➤ Altered nutrition: less than body requirements
- ➤ Constipation
- ➤ Diarrhea
- ➤ Pain
- ➤ Anxiety

Related factors are individualized based on the client's condition or needs.

RECORDING AND REPORTING

1. Record results of assessment in nurses' notes or flow sheet.	Documents baseline data and any change in client's condition. Also serves to document tolerance to any diagnostic testing.
2. Record content of any client instruction.	Ensures continuity of client education.
3. Report serious abnormalities, such as absent bowel sounds, presence of mass, or acute pain, to nurse in charge and physician.	Signs and symptoms indicate potentially serious alterations requiring further diagnosis or treatment.

• • • • •

Special Considerations

- ➤ Normal venous patterns are faint except in very thin clients.
- ➤ All subsequent measurements of abdominal girth should be taken at same level of umbilicus to provide objective means to evaluate changes. Nurse may use water-based pen to make a mark on abdomen for subsequent measurements.
- ➤ Normal ventilation involves rhythmic movement of abdomen as diaphragm descends and rises. Normally a slight pulsation of aorta occurs with each beat of systole.
- ➤ If abnormal percussion notes are assessed, it may be helpful to perform thorough palpation of affected area immediately to ensure an accurate examination.

Teaching Considerations

- ➤ Long-term progressive weight loss (late symptom), change in bowel habits, and blood in stools are signs of colon cancer. (See Skill 11-16 for screening recommendations.)
- ➤ Explain that factors such as diet, regular exercise, limited use of over-the-counter drugs causing constipation, establishment of regular elimination schedule, and good fluid intake promote normal bowel elimination (see Chapter 26).
- ➤ Caution client about dangers of excessive use of laxatives or enemas.
- ➤ If client has acute pain, explain activities or positions to avoid.
- ➤ Explain to client the need to have a controlled weight reduction program when attempting to lose weight.
- ➤ If client is a health care worker or has contact with blood or body fluids of affected persons, encourage client to receive series of three hepatitis B vaccine doses.

Pediatric Considerations

- Most common palpable mass in child is feces, usually felt in right lower quadrant.
- Have a child stand erect and then lie supine during inspection of abdominal surface. Normal abdomen of infants and young children is cylindrical in erect position and flat in supine position.
- In infants and children skin is usually taut and without wrinkles or creases.

Gerontologic Considerations

- Older adult often lacks abdominal tone; underlying organs are more easily palpable.
- A weakened intestinal musculature and decreased peristalsis affect the large intestine. Constipation along with nausea, flatulence, and heartburn are common.
- Stress to older adults importance of adequate fluid intake, regular exercise, and a diet with at least 4 servings daily of fresh fruit and vegetables and high-fiber foods to promote normal defecation.

SKILL 11-14 Assessing the Female Genitalia

An examination of the female genitalia includes an assessment of external genitalia and a vaginal examination. The external examination is relatively simple, but the vaginal examination requires the skills of an expert practitioner. A beginning nurse does not perform the vaginal examination but is expected to assist either the physician or an advanced practice nurse with the procedure. Both examinations should be a part of each woman's preventive health care because uterine and vaginal cancer have high incidence rates. In addition, adolescents and young adults should have regular gynecological examinations to screen for sexually transmitted diseases (STDs). The average age of menarche among young girls has declined, and the majority of male and female teenagers are sexually active by age 19 (Wong, 1995).

Typically, the client feels anxious during the examination. It is one of the most difficult experiences for adolescents. A person's cultural background can further add to apprehension. To avoid embarrassing the client, the nurse uses a calm, reassuring, and attentive approach. Comfort is established through correct positioning and draping. Each portion of the examination is explained so that the client can anticipate the nurse's actions.

EQUIPMENT

- **Examination table with stirrups and cover**
- **Disposable gloves (2 pairs)**
- **Vaginal speculum**
- **K-Y Jelly**
- **Adjustable light**
- **Glass microscopic slides and cover slips**
- **Sponge forceps or swabs**
- **Plastic spatulas and/or cytobrush**
- **Specimen bottles with fixative spray**

DELEGATION CONSIDERATIONS

Unlicensed assistive personnel are trained to perform routine hygiene for a client, including catheter care. This gives the staff member the opportunity to observe the condition of the client's genitalia frequently. The nurse should be sure that unlicensed assistive personnel:

- Know to report any unusual discharge, client complaint of tenderness, or presence of any obvious lesions or masses.
- Explain thoroughly to a client the purpose of perineal hygiene and catheter care (Chapters 6 and 25).
- Avoid any attempt to manipulate or inspect the client's genitalia other than that required for hygiene.

The physical examination of a client's genitalia requires problem solving and knowledge application unique to a professional nurse. Any observations should be reported to the RN. Delegation of an examination is inappropriate.

STEPS	RATIONALE
ASSESSMENT	
1. Determine if client had previous illness or surgery involving reproductive organs, including history of STD.	Can influence appearance and position of organs being examined.
2. Review client's menstrual history, including age at menarche; frequency and duration of menstrual cycle; character of flow, such as amount and presence of clots; presence of dysmenorrhea (painful menstruation); pelvic pain; and dates of last two menstrual periods.	Information helps to reveal level of woman's reproductive health, including normalcy of menstrual cycle.
3. Ask client to describe obstetrical history, including description of each pregnancy, delivery, and history of abortions or miscarriages.	Physical findings made during assessment of genitalia and reproductive organs vary depending on client's history of pregnancy.
4. Ask client to describe current and past contraceptive practices and problems experienced. Determine whether client uses safe sex practices. Discuss risks of contracting HIV and STDs.	Use of certain types of contraceptives may influence reproductive health. Sexual history reveals risks for STDs.
5. Determine if client has symptoms or history of genitourinary problems. Symptoms might include burning during urination, frequency, urgency, nocturia, hematuria, incontinence, or stress incontinence.	Urinary problems may be associated with gynecological disorders, including STDs.
6. Ask if client has had signs of bleeding outside normal menstrual period or after menopause or has had unusual vaginal discharge.	These are warning signs for cervical and endometrial cancer.
7. Determine if client is between ages 40 and 50 and has history of chlamydia, herpes simplex, or cervical dysplasia; has multiple sex partners; smokes; has had multiple pregnancies; or had first sexual intercourse at young age.	Risk factors for cervical cancer.
8. Determine if client is between ages of 40 and 60; has a history of ovarian dysfunction, cancer of the breast or endometrium, irradiation of pelvic organs, or endometriosis; has a family history of ovarian or breast cancer; or has a history of infertility or nulliparity.	Risk factors for ovarian cancer.
9. Determine if client is postmenopausal, obese, or infertile; had early menarche (before age 12); had late menopause (after age 50); has history of hypertension, diabetes, or liver disease; or has family history of endometrial, breast, or colon cancer.	Risk factors for endometrial cancer.
PLANNING	
1. Expected outcomes following completion of procedure:	
➤ Pubic hair of adult forms a triangle over perineum and along medial surfaces of thighs. Underlying skin is free of inflammation, irritation, or lesions.	No hormonal abnormalities.
➤ Skin of perineum is smooth, clean, and slightly darker than other skin. Mucous membranes appear dark pink and moist.	
➤ Labia majora are symmetrical; they appear either dry or moist and are without inflammation, edema, discharge, lesions, or lacerations.	No infection present.
➤ Labia minora are thinner than labia majora; one side may be larger than the other.	
➤ Clitoris is pink, without lesions.	

STEPS	RATIONALE
➤ Urethral orifice is intact and without exudate or inflammation. Meatus is anterior to vaginal orifice and pink in color.	
➤ Vaginal orifice is moist and without inflammation, discoloration, lesions, or edema. It is symmetrical and without prolapse of tissue.	No infection or signs of sexual abuse.
➤ Bartholin's and Skene's glands are nonpalpable and without discharge.	Glands are free of infection.
➤ Muscle tone in vaginal introitus is good.	
➤ *Vaginal examination.* Cervix is pink, smooth, and round. Its diameter is about 1 inch (2.5 cm) in a young woman and smaller in an older adult. The cervix is in midline and without lesions or discharge. Vaginal walls are pink, moist, smooth and without discharge or lesions. Pap smear is negative.	
➤ Client denies discomfort during examination.	
➤ Client carries on conversation during examination without nonverbal signs of discomfort.	
➤ Client is able to discuss importance of routine vaginal examinations and perform genital self-examination.	Demonstrates knowledge of preventive health care.
➤ Client describes common signs and symptoms of gynecological cancer and STDs.	Provides knowledge base to eliminate risk factors in lifestyle.
2. Prepare client for examination:	
a. Ask client to empty bladder.	Frequently physician wishes to collect urine specimen. Prevents urine from being accidentally expelled during examination.
b. Assist client to lithotomy position:	
(1) Client lies supine on bed or examination table, flexes knees perpendicular to bed, relaxes thighs, and allows each leg to abduct to the side.	Position is used to examine only external genitalia.
(2) Elevate client's head on pillow.	Provides comfort.
(3) Client lies supine with knees flexed, legs abducted, and feet in stirrups. Have client stabilize each foot in stirrup and then slide buttocks down to edge of examination table.	Position allows full visualization and access to genital area for speculum examination.

➤ ***CRITICAL DECISION POINT*** **Client who suffers pain or deformity of the joints may be unable to assume a lithotomy position. Have client abduct only one leg or lie on side with upper thigh and knee drawn up to the chest (see illustration).**

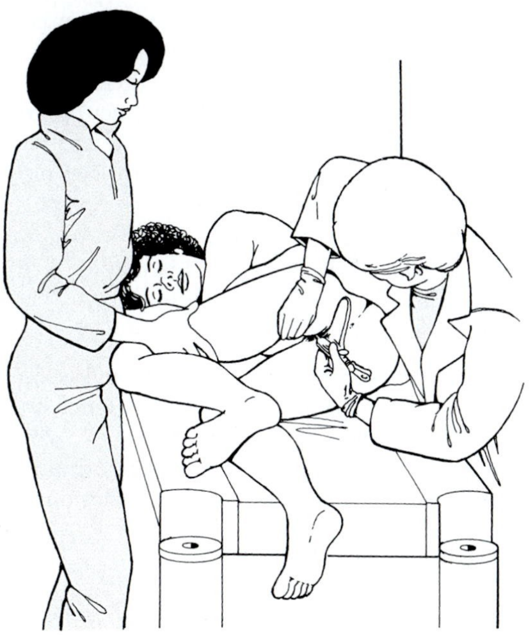

Alternate knee chest position for gynecological examination. (From Seidel HM et al: *Mosby's guide to physical examination*, ed 3, St Louis, 1995, Mosby.)

STEPS	RATIONALE
(4) Have client place arms at sides or fold arms across chest.	Prevents tightening of abdominal muscles.
c. Place rectangular sheet with corner of drape over sternum; adjacent corners fall over each knee, and fourth corner covers perineum.	Prevents unnecessary exposure of body parts. Clients often are embarrassed by exposure of external genitalia.
d. Explain each step of procedure thoroughly to client.	Genital examination can cause anticipatory anxiety. Thorough explanation relieves client's fears and promotes cooperation.
3. Have a female colleague in attendance during the examination.	Provides client with feeling of security during examination. Legally protects examiner.

IMPLEMENTATION

EXTERNAL GENITALIA

STEPS	RATIONALE
1. Wash hands and apply disposable gloves.	Reduces transmission of infection. Gloves make it easier to manipulate perineal structures and prevent spread of infection.
2. Start the examination by touching the thigh first before advancing to the perineum.	Prevents sudden, unexpected stimulation of perineum.
CRITICAL DECISION POINT **Perineum is very sensitive and tender.**	
3. With perineum well illuminated, inspect quantity and distribution of hair growth and condition of underlying skin, noting color and presence of lesions or inflammation. Also inspect skin of pubic area for lice, inflammation, or lesions.	Hair quantity and distribution reveal hormonal status and sexual maturity. Pubic area may be site for pediculosis pubis, which develops after contact with lice-infested clothing or after contact with a human carrier.
CRITICAL DECISION POINT **Lice are highly contagious. Educate client as to how the infestation can be transmitted and the measures necessary to eliminate them. (See Skill 11-2.)**	
4. Inspect the surface characteristics of the labia majora. Note the contour and any areas of inflammation, edema, lacerations, lesions, or discharge. If structures appear distorted or if vaginal orifice is asymmetrical, palpate tissues later in examination.	Assesses for gross abnormalities. Hormonal alterations can cause changes in pattern of hair growth. Irregularities may be result of lesions, scars, or inflammation of underlying tissue.
5. Explain that the next phase of the examination is to inspect deeper perineal structures.	Respects client's sensitivity to the examination.
6. With nondominant hand, gently place thumb and index finger inside labia minora and retract tissues outward (see illustration). Be sure to have firm hold during retraction. Inspect labia minora for symmetry, size, color, lesions, and discharge.	Retraction allows for inspection of structures and tissues within the labial folds. Firm hold prevents repeated retractions against sensitive tissues. Labia can be enlarged because of infection, underlying lesions, or trauma. Labia may also be site for venereal lesions.
CRITICAL DECISION POINT **This may be a good time to begin discussion of genital self-examination (see Teaching Considerations).**	
7. Use other hand to palpate the labia minora between the thumb and second finger. Note consistency and presence of tenderness or lesions.	Tissue should feel soft on palpation and without tenderness.
8. Inspect clitoris for size and color. Note any drainage, inflammation, edema, ulcerations, or lesions.	Assesses for presence of malignant lesions (clitoris is common site in older women) or syphilitic lesions (common site in younger women). Inflammation causes clitoris to become bright red. Syphilitic chancres are small open ulcers that drain serous fluid.

STEPS	RATIONALE
CRITICAL DECISION POINT **Any lesions that raise suspicion of an STD should be reported to physician immediately.**	
9. Inspect vaginal opening or orifice. Note condition of hymen just inside orifice. Hymen is thin strip of tissue that may restrict opening of vagina in virgin. Inspect tissue for inflammation, edema, discoloration, discharge, and lesions.	Determines symmetry of opening. Can be site for infection and venereal lesions.
10. Note the color and position of the urethral meatus. Look just anterior to the vaginal orifice for a pink slit or pinhole opening.	Can be site of polyps or fistulas. Irritation or inflammation may be the result of repeated urinary tract infections.
CRITICAL DECISION POINT **Urethral meatus may be difficult to locate, especially in women who have had multiple childbirths. May be close to or slightly within vaginal introitus.**	
11. With the labia still retracted, examine the Skene's glands: a. Tell client that you are going to insert one finger into the vagina and that she will feel pressure. b. With palm facing upward, insert index finger of the examining hand, as far as the second joint, into the vagina. c. Exert upward pressure to milk the Skene's glands while moving the finger outward. d. Do the examination on both sides of the urethra and then directly on the urethra (see illustration). Look for color, odor, and consistency of discharge.	Skene's glands can be a site of infection; gonococcal infection is common (Seidel et al., 1995).

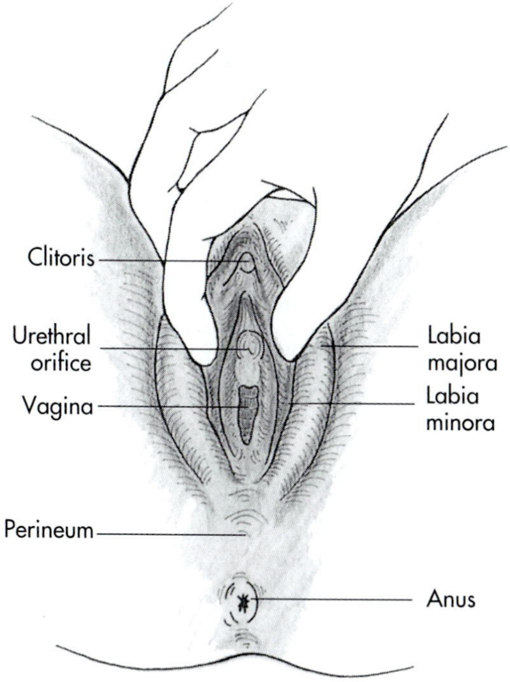

Step 6 Female external genitalia.

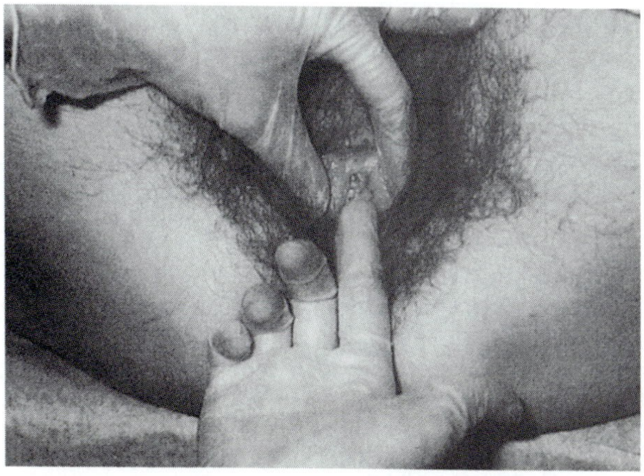

Step 11d Milking urethra and paraurethral glands.

STEPS	RATIONALE
12. Keeping the labia retracted, tell the client that you will press around the entrance to the vagina. Palpate the lateral tissue between your index finger and thumb. Focus on the posterior end of the vaginal orifice, the location of Bartholin's glands. Note any swelling, tenderness, warmth, or masses. Palpate and observe bilaterally; each gland is separate.	Determines if glands are infected, indicated by swelling or discharge.

CRITICAL DECISION POINT **Any discharge from Skene's or Bartholin's glands should be cultured and sent to the laboratory for analysis.**

13. If discharge has been found, remove gloves and dispose. Reapply a new pair of disposable gloves.

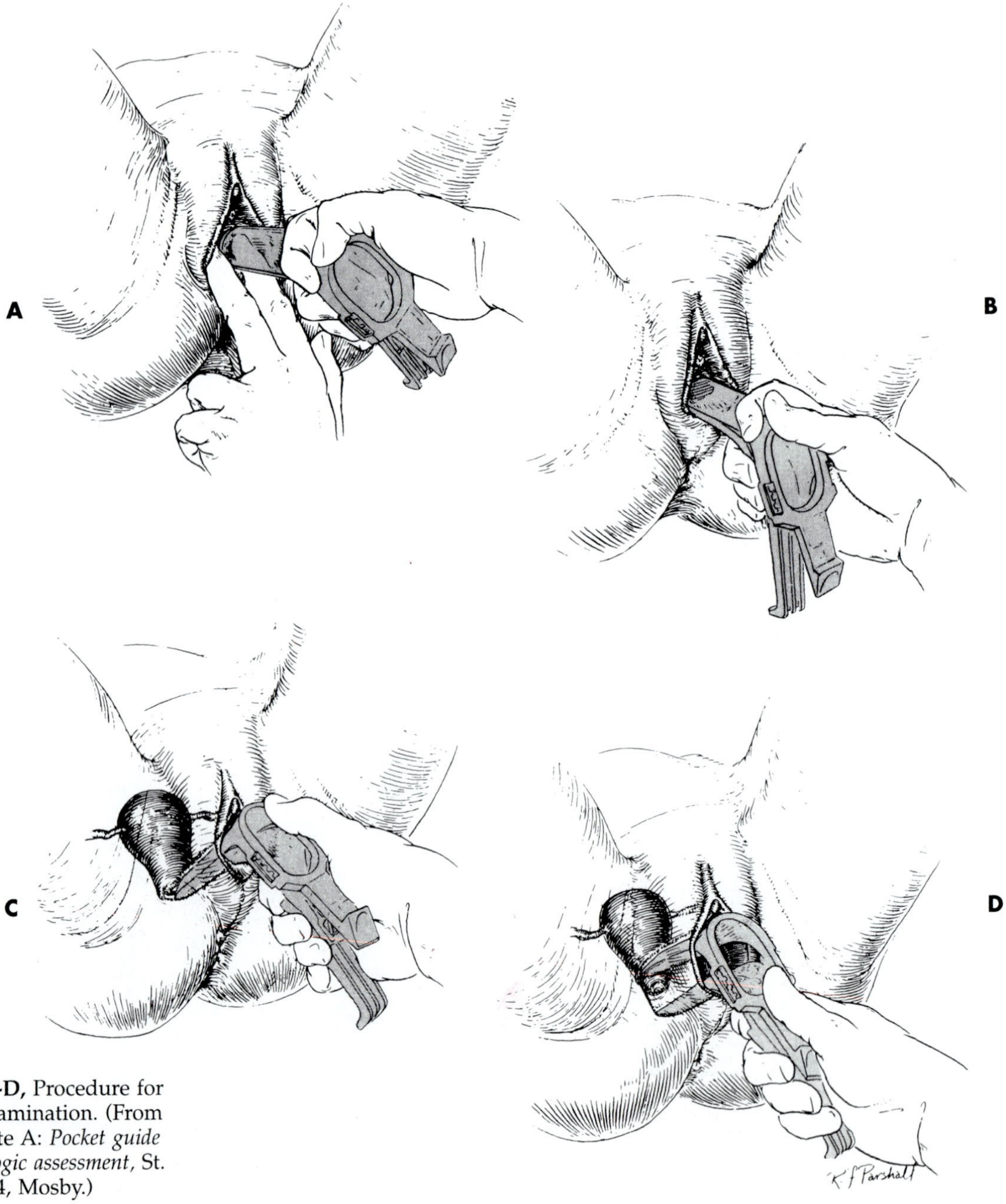

Step 4 **A-D,** Procedure for vaginal examination. (From Lueckenotte A: *Pocket guide to gerontologic assessment,* St. Louis, 1994, Mosby.)

STEPS	RATIONALE
14. With gloved index and middle fingers in the vaginal orifice, ask client to strain downward as if voiding. Note any bulging of vaginal walls. Feel for normal tension in muscles.	Assesses degree of muscular wall support.
15. Nurse may also examine the anus at this time (Skill 11-16).	
16. If only an external examination is to be performed, offer client perineal hygiene; then remove gloves and wash hands.	Reduces infection transmission. Perineal hygiene provides for client's comfort.

INTERNAL GENITALIA

STEPS	RATIONALE
1. Assist examiner in selecting proper size of **speculum.** Smallest size fits a virgin. Sexually active woman may require medium size. Woman who has had multiple children requires medium to large size.	Improper size of speculum can cause trauma to vaginal wall.
2. Place speculum under warm running water. Lubricant can be used if no Pap smear is to be collected.	Water is ideal lubricant. Warm temperature causes less discomfort. Lubricant interferes with Pap test results.
3. As examiner positions self on a stool facing client's perineum, adjust light over the examiner's shoulder, directed toward vaginal opening.	Illumination is required to properly view internal genitalia.
4. Talk with client or explain procedure as examiner begins to insert speculum. Two fingers are gently inserted into the vagina. Then the examiner presses down on the perineal body just inside the **introitus.** With speculum blades closed, the examiner introduces the speculum obliquely (rotated 50 degrees counterclockwise from the vertical position) past the fingers. Then the speculum is inserted downward at a 45-degree angle toward the examination table. Once the wide portions of the blades pass the orifice, fingers are removed and speculum is rotated so that blades are horizontal. The blades are opened slowly after full insertion (see illustration).	Insertion technique avoids trauma to the urethra because maneuver corresponds with normal downward slope of vaginal canal. Distraction may help to relieve client's anxiety. Explanation helps client to anticipate sensations.
5. Warn client that a stretching sensation may be felt as blades are opened and then locked into position.	Locked position allows examiner to have full view of cervix, which is at posterior end of vaginal canal.
6. Nurse remains at examiner's side as cervix is inspected. The cervix and its opening (os) are examined for diameter, color, appearance, position, surface characteristics, lesions, and discharge (see illustration).	Bluish cervix is early sign of pregnancy. Cervix is a common site for cancer and chronic yeast infection.

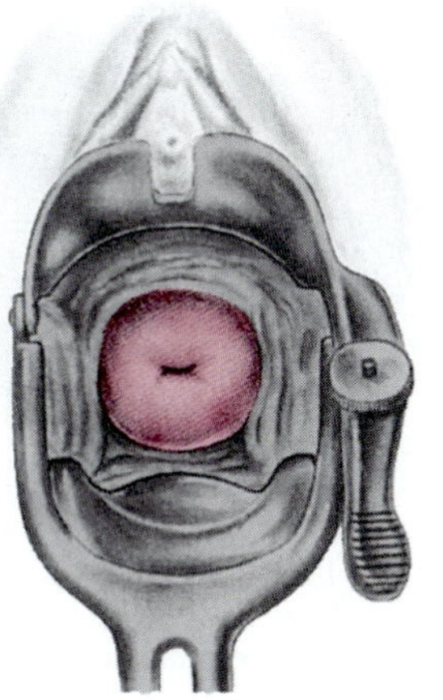

Step 6 Appearance of cervix through vaginal speculum.

STEPS	RATIONALE
7. Assist examiner in obtaining a Pap smear: a. Hand the examiner the cytobrush or a cotton-tipped swab (examiner's preference). The examiner gently inserts brush or applicator through os and rotates it 360 degrees (see illustration).	Pap smear is a painless screening test for cervical cancer. Collects columnar cells that normally line the passageway leading into the central cavity of the uterus.
CRITICAL DECISION POINT **Do not use cytobrush for pregnant clients.**	
b. With the brush or swab, apply cells to the glass slide by rolling or twisting the brush or swab across the glass surface.	Ensures proper specimen collection for cell identification.
c. Spray fixative solution on the slide and label the slide.	
d. Hand examiner the spatula. Examiner places the tip of the longer arm in os and rotates spatula 360 degrees to scrape outer surface of cervix (see illustration).	Collects squamous cells that line surface of cervix.
e. Apply cells on tip of spatula to glass slide. Spray slide with fixative solution. Label slide.	Proper labeling ensures accurate diagnosis for correct client.
8. Stand by examiner's side as examination is completed. Let client know that speculum is about to be withdrawn. (Examiner inspects for cervical bleeding and observes integrity of vaginal walls.)	Speculum withdrawal may cause minimal pulling of tissue.
9. Assist client to lower legs from stirrups or straighten legs from abducted position. Help client return to supine position.	Assuming lithotomy position for a prolonged time can be uncomfortable.
10. Offer perineal hygiene. Once examination is completed, remove gloves and wash hands.	Reduces transmission of microorganisms.

E VALUATION

1. Compare findings with normal assessment characteristics for genitalia.	Determines presence of abnormalities.
2. Evaluate client's emotional response toward examination. Note voice tone, facial expression, body position, or movement.	Nonverbal behaviors may reflect client's level of anxiety.

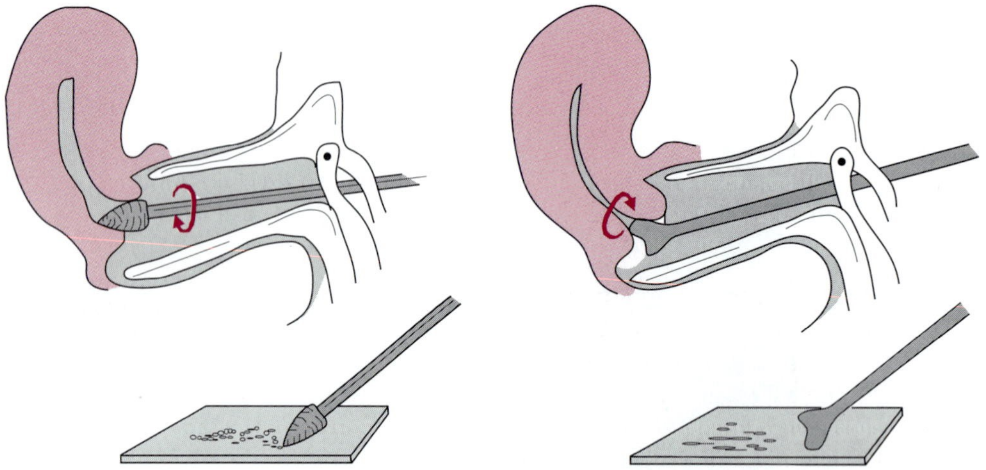

Step 7 Methods for obtaining Pap smear. *Left,* Cytobrush collects cells of endocervix. *Right,* Spatula collects cells of outer cervix.

STEPS	RATIONALE
3. Ask client to discuss importance of routine vaginal examinations and method of performing genital self-examination.	Measures understanding of risks related to vaginal and uterine cancer.
4. **Unexpected outcomes** that may occur include:	
➤ White, chalky, malodorous discharge is noted within labial folds and over clitoris.	Poor hygiene is indicated.
➤ Clitoris is inflamed. Bartholin's and Skene's glands are palpable and tender. Discharge is expressed on palpation.	Infection of genitalia and/or lower urinary tract is expected.
➤ Urethral meatus is inflamed, irritated, and tender.	Sign of repeated urinary tract infections.
➤ Portion of vaginal wall prolapses or falls into orifice during straining.	Result of vaginal prolapse.
➤ Portion of rectum causes bulging of the posterior vaginal wall.	Sign of rectal prolapse.
➤ Client complains of abdominal or pelvic discomfort, pain or burning on urination, bleeding between menstruation, vaginal discharge, and an itchy rash around vagina.	Symptoms of STD.
➤ Ulcers are present involving genitalia, cervix, and vaginal walls.	Indicative of a form of STD.
➤ Vaginal discharge and cervical bleeding are evident. Positive Pap smear indicates cancer.	Cervical cancer is indicated.
➤ Client is unable to explain importance of regular vaginal examinations.	Reinstruction may be needed.
➤ Client is unable to perform genital self-examination or explain warning signs of STD.	Reinstruction may be needed.

NURSING DIAGNOSIS

Clustering of defining characteristics from the assessment data may reveal the following nursing diagnoses for clients requiring this skill:

- Anxiety
- Body-image disturbance
- Fear
- Risk for infection
- Knowledge deficit regarding perineal care, risks for cancer, or STDs
- Pain
- Sexual dysfunction

Related factors are individualized based on the client's condition or needs.

RECORDING AND REPORTING

1. Record all assessment findings and describe client's reaction to examination.	Documents baseline data and any change in client's condition. Evaluates response to procedure.
2. Record extent of client instruction and client's response.	Documentation provides for improved continuity of care.
3. Record time and date of obtaining specimen and transport to laboratory.	
4. Record size of speculum used.	This is helpful information if further examinations are to be done.
5. Report any abnormalities observed to nurse in charge or physician.	Abnormalities may indicate need for further diagnostic study or treatment.

FOLLOW-UP ACTIVITIES

1. If an STD is expected, client will require a thorough abdominal and oral examination to detect evidence of systemic disease and oropharyngeal infection.
2. Client suspected of having STD will require ongoing appointments to monitor progress of infection, reduce chance of reinfection, and detect signs of relapse.
3. Cases of STD must be reported to the local health department.

• • • • •

Special Considerations

- A woman with any of the following conditions may be unable to assume the lithotomy position: lower extremity amputation, arthritis, neurological injury or disorder, muscular disease, scoliosis, and short stature. These conditions predispose the client to joint pain, paralysis, joint stiffness, lack of muscle control, spasticity, and contractures (Seidel et al., 1995). Let the client make the decision as to the best position for her to assume.
- It will take several days for results of the Pap smear to be available.
- Best time to collect a Pap smear is 5 days after menstruation.

Teaching Considerations

- Instruct client about purpose and recommended frequency of Pap smears and gynecological examinations:
  - Perform Pap smear annually with a pelvic examination in women who are, or have been, sexually active, and in women who have reached the age of 18.
  - After three or more consecutive annual examinations with normal findings, the Pap test may be done less often at the discretion of the physician. However, most physicians encourage annual examinations.
  - Women at high risk for cervical cancer and those older than 40 require an annual examination and Pap smear.
- Instruct on genital self-examination:
  - Using a mirror, position self to examine the area covered by the pubic hair.
  - Spread the hair apart, looking for bumps, sores, or blisters.
  - Look for any warts, which may appear as small, bumpy spots and then enlarge to fleshy, cauliflower-like lesions.
  - Spread the outer vaginal lips apart, and look at the clitoris for bumps, blisters, sores, or warts.
  - Look at both sides of the inner vaginal lips. The area around the urinary and vaginal opening should be inspected for bumps, blisters, sores, or warts.
- Explain these warning signs of an STD: pain or burning on urination, pain in pelvic area, bleeding between menstruation, itchy rash around vagina, and vaginal discharge (different from usual).
- Teach measures to prevent STDs:
  - Reduce number of people with whom one has sexual contact.
  - Avoid sexual partners who have had multiple partners.
  - Avoid sexual partners known to have an infection of the genitalia.
  - Male partner should use a condom.
- Excessive douching should be avoided to maintain normal bacterial balance in the vagina.
- Instruct client on importance of and techniques for perineal hygiene (see Chapter 6).

Pediatric Considerations

- Extent of examination depends on child's age and complaints. Normally an examination of the external genitalia is all that is needed in a well child. Perform the internal examination only for specific problems such as bleeding, discharge, trauma, or suspected sexual abuse.
- An adolescent requires the same examination and positioning as an adult. The first examination is critical in establishing a client's trust and comfort. A bad experience may cause the adolescent not to pursue preventive health care.
- Signs and symptoms of sexual abuse in children and adolescents include evidence of general abuse or neglect; evidence of trauma to genital or anal areas; unusual skin color or pigmentation in genital or anal area; presence of STD; anorectal itching, bleeding, or pain; fecal incontinence; genitourinary problems, including rash or sores, vaginal odor, pain, itching, bleeding, discharge, dysuria, and urinary tract infections; and behavioral changes (Koop, 1988).
- Evaluation of external genitalia in preschoolers, school-age girls, and adolescents causes anxiety because of modesty and concern for privacy.

Gerontologic Considerations

- An older client may require more time and assistance to assume the lithotomy position.
- With menopause the labia majora become thin, and with advancing age they atrophy. The pubic hair thins and the vaginal introitus constricts.
- Because of hormonal and structural changes, the older woman is predisposed to vaginitis, painful intercourse (dyspareunia), bleeding, and uterine prolapse (Lueckenotte, 1994).
- Older women may have scarring of perineum caused by lacerations or episiotomies from childbirth.
- Older women may have malignant changes that result in dry, scaly nodular lesions of the clitoris.

SKILL 11-15 Assessing the Male Genitalia

An examination of the male genitalia includes assessment of the external genitalia (Fig. 11-8) and the inguinal ring and canal. As with the female genital examination, assessment can be embarrassing for the client. Adolescents and men are often fearful of having an erection during the examination. The nurse examining the client should learn to relax during the examination because anxiety can heighten embarrassment for both the nurse and client. In addition, it is important to "know the language"; a client may refer to his genitals with terms that the nurse is not familiar with (Seidel et al., 1995). Use of the common language may help the client relax and feel accepted. Most important, do not joke or use inappropriate nonverbal expressions. Always act professionally. Also be sure to make the client an active decision maker during the examination. In addition, the nurse should have a male colleague in attendance when possible.

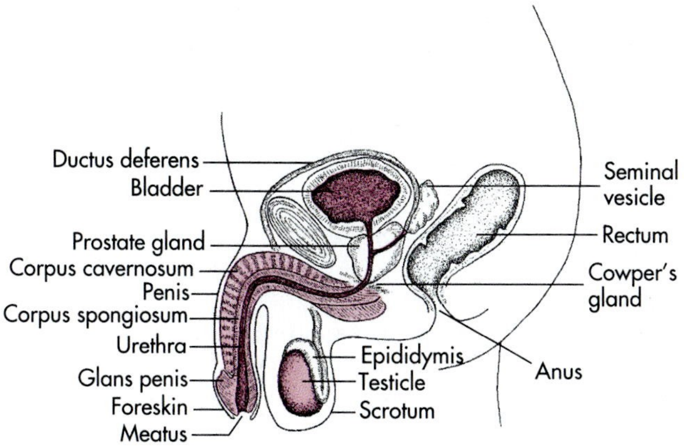

Fig. 11-8 External and internal male genitalia.

Because the incidence of STD in adolescents and young adults is high, an assessment of the genitalia should be a routine part of any health maintenance examination for this age-group. If the genital assessment is the only one to be performed, the nurse must be sure to collect a thorough nursing history.

EQUIPMENT

- **Disposable gloves**
- **Culture swab (optional)**
- **Drapes**

DELEGATION CONSIDERATIONS

Unlicensed assistive personnel will be trained to provide routine hygiene and catheter care to clients. It is important for staff to know how to observe for unusual discharge, color changes, or the presence of lesions. Training should ensure that unlicensed assistive personnel:

- Know to explain to the client the purposes and steps for perineal hygiene and catheter care.
- Report any changes in the condition of the genitalia to the RN.
- Do not attempt to manipulate the genitalia more than is required for routine hygiene.

The examination of the male genitalia is a skill that requires problem solving and knowledge application unique to a professional nurse. For this skill, delegation is inappropriate.

STEPS	RATIONALE
ASSESSMENT	
1. Review client's normal urinary elimination pattern: frequency of voiding; history of nocturia; character and volume of urine; daily fluid intake; symptoms of burning, urgency, or frequency; difficulty starting stream; and hematuria.	Urinary problems can be directly associated with reproductive problems, particularly because of the anatomy of the male reproductive and urinary systems.
2. Assess client's sexual history and use of safe sex habits (e.g., number of partners, use of condom).	Reveals client's risk for and understanding of STD.
3. Determine if client has had previous surgery or illness involving urinary or reproductive organs, including STD.	Alterations resulting from disease or surgery may be responsible for client's presenting symptoms and changes in organ structure or function.
4. Ask if client has noted penile pain or swelling, lesions of the genitalia, or urethral discharge.	These signs and symptoms are commonly associated with STDs.
5. Determine if client has noticed heaviness or painless enlargement of testis or irregular lumps.	Signs and symptoms are early warning signs for testicular cancer.

STEPS	RATIONALE
6. If client reports an enlargement in the inguinal area, assess if it is intermittent or constant, associated with straining or lifting, or painful (is pain affected by coughing, lifting, or straining at stool?).	Signs and symptoms of potential inguinal hernia.
7. Assess client's knowledge of testicular self-examination.	

PLANNING

STEPS	RATIONALE
1. Expected outcomes following completion of procedure:	
➤ Client denies discomfort during examination and shows no nonverbal signs of anxiety.	
➤ Foreskin retracts easily.	
➤ Glans penis is pink and smooth, with urethral meatus positioned on the ventral surface just millimeters from the tip.	
➤ Small amount of white secretion is present between glans and foreskin.	Amount varies depending on level of hygiene.
➤ Opening of urethral meatus is glistening and pink.	
➤ Shaft is without swelling or lesions.	Infection is absent.
➤ Scrotum hangs freely with both testes descended (left testis is lower than right).	
➤ Scrotal skin is loose and without lesions.	
➤ Testes are smooth, ovoid, and nontender.	Normal development is evident.
➤ Epididymis and vas deferens are smooth and discrete, without lumps or tenderness.	
➤ Spermatic cord is palpable without tenderness.	
➤ No bulging or protrusion is observed or palpated in scrotal or inguinal area.	Absence of hernia is observed.
➤ Lymph nodes are nonpalpable.	No systemic infection is found.
➤ Client performs testicular self-examination correctly.	Demonstrates client's understanding.
➤ Client describes symptoms of STD.	Demonstrates learning.
2. Prepare client:	
a. Explain each step of assessment procedure before examining the client, and review results of findings.	Reduces client's apprehension, and promotes cooperation and understanding.
b. Ask client to empty bladder.	Promotes relaxation during procedure.
c. Have adult client lie supine with chest, abdomen, and lower legs draped, or allow client to stand with upper body covered with a gown.	Prevents unnecessary exposure of body parts.
d. Throughout examination, manipulate genitalia gently and move through assessment as quickly as possible.	Minimizes client's discomfort and preserves modesty.

➤ ***CRITICAL DECISION POINT*** **Excessive manipulation can cause an erection.**

IMPLEMENTATION

STEPS	RATIONALE
1. Wash hands and apply disposable gloves.	Reduces transmission of microorganisms.
2. Observe the size and shape of the penis and testes, color and texture of scrotal skin, and character and distribution of pubic hair. The adult client will have pubic hair extending from base of penis over the symphysis pubis; hair will be coarse and curly. Scrotal skin is wrinkled and darker than surrounding skin.	Reveals sexual maturity of client.

STEPS	RATIONALE
3. Inspect skin covering genitalia for lice, rashes, excoriations, or lesions.	*Pediculus pubis* (crab lice) may attach eggs to pubic hair. Spread by sexual contact, the infestation results in the lice biting, which causes intense itching. Scratching may cause secondary infection.
4. If lice are present, dispose of gloves and apply new pair.	

CRITICAL DECISION POINT **Lice are highly contagious. Educate client about how lice are contracted and the appropriate measures to eliminate them.**

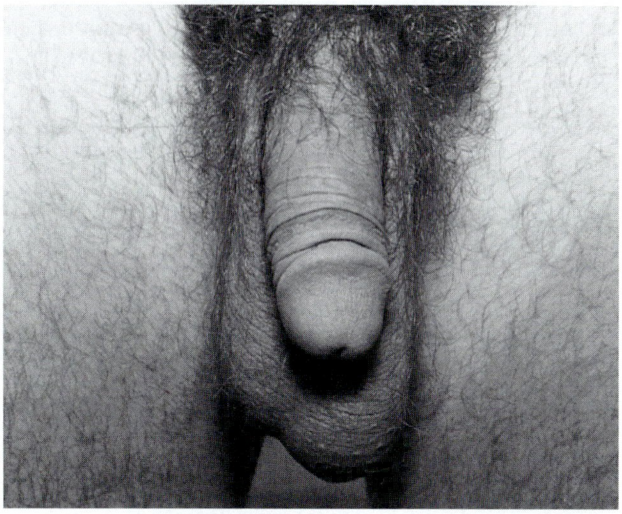

Step 5 Normal male genitalia (circumcised).

STEPS	RATIONALE
5. Inspect structures of penis (see illustration).	
a. Note the dorsal vein.	Normally apparent along shaft.
b. In uncircumcised males, retract foreskin to reveal glans and urethral meatus. Note position of meatus and observe for discharge, edema, inflammation, and lesions of glans.	Assesses for presence of infection, congenital anomalies, or lesions.
c. If abnormal discharge from meatus is present, obtain specimen by gently milking penis from base to urethra. Brush culture swab across meatus.	Obtain for culture to determine if discharge is infectious and type of causative organism (Chapter 43).
d. Compress the glans gently between the thumb and index finger. Observe the opening of urethral meatus, and note any discharge.	Maneuver opens meatus for inspection.
e. Check entire circumference of glans for lesions.	Lesions may develop along undersurface.
f. Carefully inspect area between foreskin and glans.	Common site for venereal lesions. Small amount of thick, white secretion between glans and foreskin is normal.
g. Palpate any lesions for tenderness, size, consistency, and shape.	Character of lesion indicates type of lesion.
h. Inspect entire shaft of penis. Note color of skin and presence of lesions, scars, or areas of edema.	Abnormalities may develop at any point along shaft. Clients who have been lying in bed for prolonged period may develop edema.

CRITICAL DECISION POINT **Do not forget to inspect undersurface.**

STEPS	RATIONALE
i. Palpate shaft between thumb and first two fingers. Note areas of hardness and tenderness.	Can be indicative of an infectious mass or malignant growth.
j. After inspection of penis, pull foreskin down to original position.	Foreskin may act as a constricting band around penis, reducing blood flow and causing edema and pain.

CRITICAL DECISION POINT **This is good time to begin discussion of genital self-examination.**

STEPS	RATIONALE
6. Inspect scrotum's size, shape, symmetry, and presence of lesions or edema. Scrotum should hang freely from perineum behind penis.	Allows nurse to rule out presence of infection, lesions, and structural abnormalities.
CRITICAL DECISION POINT **Be very cautious. Scrotum is highly sensitive.**	
7. Gently lift scrotal sac to view posterior surface.	Structures within scrotal sac are very sensitive.
8. As client retracts penis upward, gently palpate each testis and epididymis with thumb and first two fingers. Palpate organs for size, shape, and consistency. Ask client if sensation of tenderness is noted. In infants, determine if testes have descended into scrotal sac.	Reveals presence of infection and benign or malignant masses.
9. Continue to palpate the vas deferens separately as it follows the spermatic cord through the inguinal ring.	Assesses for inflammatory changes as may be caused by diabetes.
10. Ask client to stand. Inspect both inguinal areas for signs of obvious bulging. Ask client to hold breath and bear down.	Assesses for presence of hernia through inguinal wall or canal.
11. Palpate inguinal ring and canal (see illustration) by taking left index finger and gently invaginating loose scrotal tissue on left side. Start at a point low on scrotum so finger moves freely. Follow spermatic cord up to inguinal ring. Tip of finger may enter inguinal canal, but do not force it. Once finger reaches farthest point, have client again bear down.	Technique allows nurse to palpate hernia high within inguinal ring. Excess stretching of scrotal tissue can cause client discomfort.

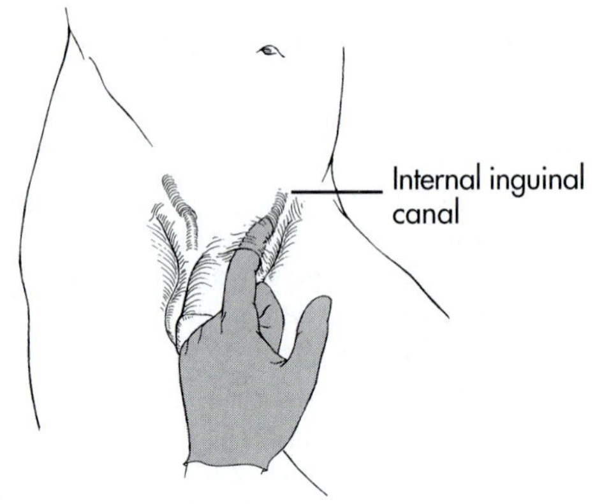

Step 11 Palpation of internal inguinal canal.

STEPS	RATIONALE
12. Repeat procedure, using right finger to examine left side.	
13. Palpate lymph nodes in inguinal area for size, shape, consistency, and tenderness.	Indicates presence of local or systemic infection or metastatic disease.
14. Remove gloves and wash hands.	Reduces transmission of infection.

EVALUATION

STEPS	RATIONALE
1. Compare findings with normal assessment characteristics for genitalia.	Determines presence of abnormalities.
2. Evaluate client's level of anxiety after examination, noting tone of voice, facial expression, and behaviors.	Client's response to examination may require further discussion with nurse to relieve anxiety.
3. Have client perform genital self-examination independently.	Demonstration is most effective way to evaluate learning of a skill.
4. Have client explain symptoms of STD and testicular cancer.	Explanation provides cognitive feedback.

STEPS	RATIONALE
5. **Unexpected outcomes** that may occur include:	
➤ Purulent discharge from urethra is present, with swelling along penile shaft. Epididymis is very tender to palpation, with swelling of scrotal sac. Papular lesions or ulcers may be present on glans, shaft, or scrotum.	Signs and symptoms indicative of sexually transmitted infection.
➤ Inguinal lymph nodes are enlarged and tender to palpation.	Signs of infection or metastatic disease.
➤ Pea-sized testicular lumps are palpable; client denies pain.	Indicates testicular tumor.
➤ Severe pain, tenderness, and swelling of scrotum. Skin of scrotum feels warm to touch. Discharge from urethra may be present. Lymph nodes are enlarged.	Symptoms reveal infection of epididymis or testis.
➤ Excessive secretions are present between glans and foreskin.	May indicate poor perineal hygiene.
➤ Client incorrectly demonstrates self-examination.	Reinstruction or further practice is needed.
➤ Client is unable to describe signs and symptoms of STD and testicular cancer.	Reinstruction is necessary.

NURSING DIAGNOSIS

Clustering of defining characteristics from the examination data may reveal the following nursing diagnoses:

- ➤ Anxiety
- ➤ Risk for infection
- ➤ Knowledge deficit regarding preventive health care
- ➤ Pain
- ➤ Sexual dysfunction

Related factors are individualized based on the client's condition or needs.

RECORDING AND REPORTING

1. Describe all assessment findings in nurses' notes or flow sheet. Note client's reaction to examination.	Documents baseline data and any change in client's condition.
2. Record any instruction provided and client's response.	Documentation provides for continuity in education.
3. Report abnormalities to nurse in charge or physician.	May indicate that further diagnosis or treatment is necessary.
4. Report and record date and time cultures were sent to laboratory.	Provides means for follow-up.

FOLLOW-UP ACTIVITIES

1. Results of a culture of the urethral discharge require a few days.

• • • • •

Special Considerations

- ➤ If manipulation of the genitalia causes an erection, the examination should be deferred until later.
- ➤ Phimosis is a condition in which the foreskin cannot be retracted. This may interfere with hygiene and increases the risk of cancer.
- ➤ Herpes lesion begins as single or multiple reddish papules that eventually become clear, fluid-filled vesicles. Later, large ulcers form.

Teaching Considerations

- ➤ All men who are 15 years and older should perform a genital self-examination on a monthly basis.
- ➤ Explain steps of genital examination:
  - Perform examination after a warm bath or shower, when the scrotal sac is relaxed.
  - Stand naked in front of a mirror. Hold the penis in your hand, and examine the head. If you are uncircumcised, pull back the foreskin.
  - Inspect and palpate the entire head of the penis in a clockwise motion, looking carefully for any bumps, sores, or blisters. Also look for bumpy warts (Fig. 11-9).
  - Look at opening of penis for discharge.
  - Look along entire shaft of the penis for the same signs.

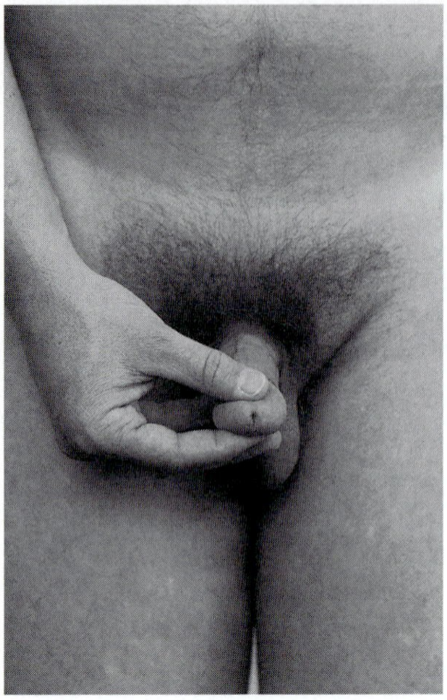

Fig. 11-9 Male genital examination. (From Seidel HM et al: *Mosby's guide to physical examination,* ed 3, St Louis, 1995, Mosby.)

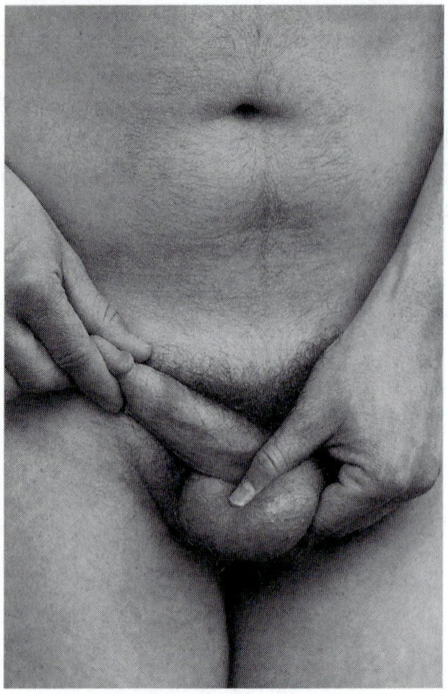

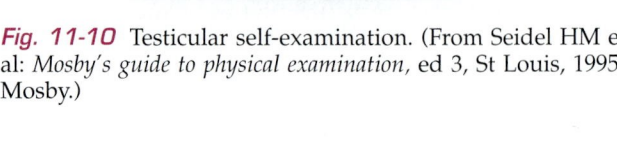

Fig. 11-10 Testicular self-examination. (From Seidel HM et al: *Mosby's guide to physical examination,* ed 3, St Louis, 1995, Mosby.)

- Be sure to separate pubic hair at the base of the penis and carefully examine skin underneath.

➤ Explain steps of testicular examination:
- Perform examination after bath or shower.
- Stand naked in front of mirror. Look for swelling or lumps in skin of scrotum.
- Use both hands, placing the index and middle fingers under the testicles and thumbs on top (Fig. 11-10).
- Gently roll the testicle, feeling for lumps, thickening, or a change in consistency (hardening).
- Find the epididymis (cordlike structure on top and back of testicles; it is not a lump).
- Feel for small pea-sized lumps on front and side of testicle. Lumps are usually painless and are abnormal. Lumps are symptomatic of cancer.
- Call physician if client finds a lump.

➤ Counsel client with an STD about diagnosis, treatment, and measures to prevent spread of the disease.

➤ Tell client with STD that sexual partners must be informed of need to have an examination.

Pediatric Considerations

➤ In infants, do not try to retract foreskin until child is several months old. Skin is usually too tight.

➤ The first sign of male puberty involves an increase in the size of the testes, usually beginning between ages 9½ and 13½ years.

➤ Normally the left testicle is lower than the right.

Gerontologic Considerations

➤ With aging the testes decrease in size and firmness.

➤ The scrotum becomes more pendulous.

SKILL 11-16 Assessing the Rectum and Anus

An examination of the rectum and anus is conducted as a separate procedure or as a continuation of the examination of the genitalia and reproductive organs. The examination is important because findings may detect colorectal cancer in its early stages. In male clients the examiner can also detect prostatic tumors. The examination is usually not performed in young children or adolescents. Since the examination can be uncomfortable and embarrassing, the nurse uses a calm, gentle approach.

EQUIPMENT

- Disposable gloves
- Lubricant
- Examination light

DELEGATION CONSIDERATIONS

This skill requires problem solving and knowledge application unique to a professional nurse. For this skill, delegation is inappropriate.

STEPS	RATIONALE
ASSESSMENT	
1. Determine if client has experienced change in bowel function: character of stool, onset and duration, accompanying symptoms (e.g., pain, flatus, cramping), anal pain or discomfort, or rectal bleeding (color, relation to defecation, amount).	These are warning signs of colorectal cancer or other gastrointestinal alterations.
2. Determine if client has personal or family history of colorectal cancer, polyps, Gardner's syndrome, or inflammatory bowel disease. Note if client is older than 40.	These are risk factors for colorectal cancer.
3. Is client's diet high in beef and animal fats and low in fiber content?	Bowel cancer may be linked to dietary intake of fat or insufficient fiber intake.
4. Determine if client has undergone screening for colorectal cancer (digital examination, stool blood slide test, proctoscopy).	Undergoing this screening reflects understanding and compliance with preventive health care measures.
5. Assess medication history for use of laxatives or cathartics.	Repeated use can cause diarrhea and eventual loss of intestinal muscle tone.
6. Assess for use of codeine or iron preparations.	Codeine causes constipation. Iron turns feces black and tarry.
7. Ask male client if he has noted weak or interrupted urine flow, inability to urinate, difficulty starting or stopping urine flow, polyuria, nocturia, hematuria, or dysuria. Does client have continuing pain in lower back, pelvis, or upper thighs?	These are warning signs of prostatic cancer, or they may indicate infection.
PLANNING	
1. **Expected outcomes** following completion of procedure:	
➤ Client denies discomfort during examination.	
➤ Perianal skin is smooth and uninterrupted.	
➤ Anal area is clear, normal color, without lesions or irregularities.	
➤ Anal sphincter muscle tone is normal.	
➤ Rectal walls are even and smooth and without nodules.	
➤ No evidence of rectal bleeding is present.	Mucosa is intact without lesions.
➤ Prostate gland is normal size, firm, without bogginess, tenderness, or nodules.	
➤ Client explains risks and symptoms of colon and prostatic cancer.	Demonstrates learning.

STEPS	RATIONALE
2. Prepare client:	
a. Explain steps of procedure, giving client chance to ask questions.	Minimizes client's anxiety and promotes relaxation.
b. Following genital examination, female client may remain in dorsal recumbent position for the rectal examination. Otherwise, left lateral side-lying position is preferred.	
c. Have male client stand and bend over forward with hips flexed and upper body resting across examination table.	
d. Nonambulatory male client can be examined in side-lying position.	
e. Drape client to expose only the anal area.	Minimizes embarrassment.

IMPLEMENTATION

STEPS	RATIONALE
1. Wash hands and apply gloves.	Reduces transmission of infection.
2. For pediatric client, inspect symmetry of gluteal folds.	Asymmetry may indicate dislocation of hip.
3. For pediatric client, gently scratch skin around anus and note response.	Assesses for presence of anal reflex.
CRITICAL DECISION POINT **No further examination is usually required of pediatric client.**	
4. Use nondominant hand and gently retract the buttocks. Inspect the perianal and sacrococcygeal areas.	Technique provides better view of perianal and sacrococcygeal areas.
5. Inspect condition of perianal tissues, noting color of skin, closure of anal sphincter, presence of lesions, hemorrhoids, ulcers, inflammation, rashes, or discoloration.	Voluntary external muscle sphincter keeps anus closed. Perianal area is more pigmented and coarser than skin overlying buttocks. Fungal infection may cause irritation.
6. Ask client to bear down as though having a bowel movement.	Maneuver causes any hemorrhoids or fissures within anal canal to appear.
7. Apply lubricant to gloved index finger of dominant hand.	Minimizes friction during palpation of rectal walls.
8. Ask client to bear down gently as though having a bowel movement as nurse presses pad of finger against anal opening (see illustration).	Relaxes external anal sphincter.

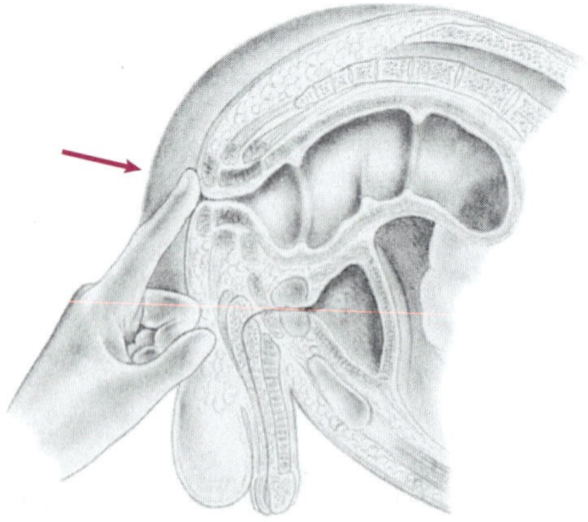

Step 8 Correct procedure for inserting finger into rectum. (From Seidel HM et al: *Mosby's guide to physical examination,* ed 3, St Louis, 1995, Mosby.)

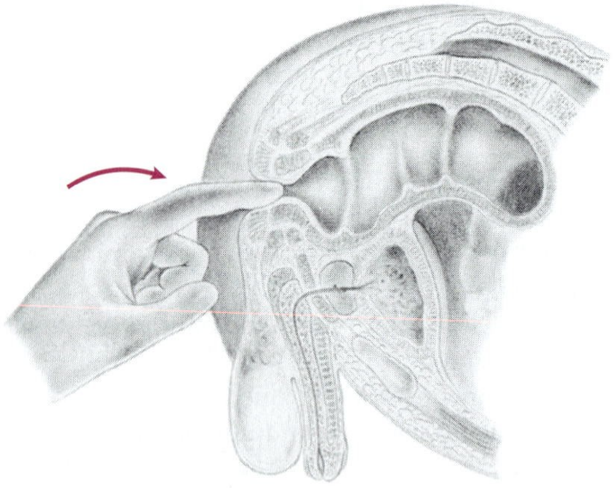

Step 10 As external sphincter relaxes, slip finger into anal canal. (From Seidel HM et al: *Mosby's guide to physical examination,* ed 3, St Louis, 1995, Mosby.)

STEPS	RATIONALE
9. Warn client that it is normal to have sensation of having bowel movement during palpation.	Insertion of examiner's finger causes rectal fullness that normally elicits defecation.
10. As anal sphincter relaxes, slip fingertip gently into anus and direct it along rectal canal toward client's umbilicus (see illustration).	Angle toward umbilicus follows contour of rectum.

➤ *CRITICAL DECISION POINT* Never force digital insertion; this prevents tissue injury and vagal nerve stimulation.

11. Note initial tone of anal sphincter; then ask client to tighten sphincter around the finger.	Muscle should close snugly and evenly around nurse's finger without discomfort. Weak sphincter may indicate a neurological problem.

➤ *CRITICAL DECISION POINT* An anal fissure or fistula can be extremely tender, preventing examination from being completed.

12. Rotate finger to examine the muscular anal ring.	Ensures palpation to all tissues. Ring should feel smooth and exert even pressure around finger.
13. As finger passes anal canal, the rectum balloons out and turns posteriorly. Advance finger and palpate lateral and posterior rectal walls for tenderness, irregularities, polyps, masses, or nodules.	Rectal wall is a site for tumors.

➤ *CRITICAL DECISION POINT* Inability to advance finger may be due to fecal impaction.

14. Once finger is advanced fully, ask client to bear down again. Feel for a mass pushing against fingertip.	Any high lesions within the rectum will descend against fingertip.
15. In male clients, turn the hand so that the finger palpates the anterior rectal wall. Feel for prostate, a rounded, heart-shaped structure about 2½ to 4 cm (1 to 1½ inches) in diameter with less than 1 cm (½ inch) protrusion into the rectum (see illustration). Note size, shape, and consistency of prostate.	Maneuver allows for palpation of prostate gland.

➤ *CRITICAL DECISION POINT* Warn client that maneuver may create feeling of urge to urinate but explain that he will not.

➤ *CRITICAL DECISION POINT* Once completed, review signs and symptoms of prostate cancer.

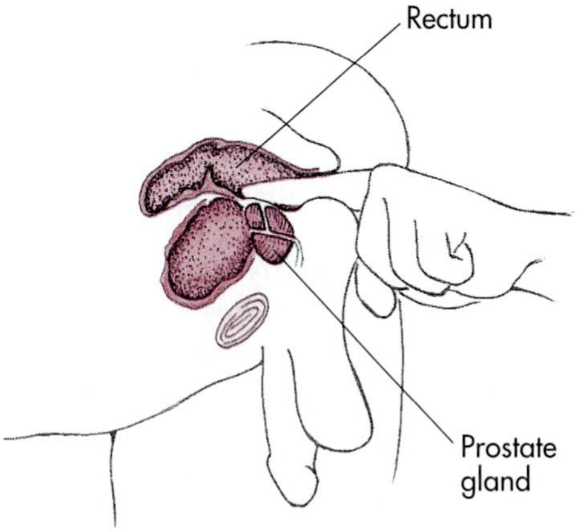

Step 15 Palpation of prostate gland.

16. For all clients, gently withdraw finger and observe it for feces.	Character of stool may reveal blood, mucus, or black, tarry stool.

➤ *CRITICAL DECISION POINT* This may be good time to discuss signs and symptoms of and risk factors for colorectal cancer.

STEPS	RATIONALE
17. Test any abnormal-appearing stool for microscopic evidence of blood (Chapter 43).	Lesions located high in colon or rectum may cause erosion of rectal wall that results in blood loss of small proportions. Blood can be identified through laboratory analysis.
18. Clean any moisture or drainage from rectal area and assist client to sitting position. Drape lower torso.	Restores client's comfort and prepares client for next examination.
19. Dispose of gloves and wash hands.	Reduces transmission of infection.

EVALUATION

1. Compare findings with normal assessment characteristics for the rectum.	Determines presence of abnormalities.
2. During examination, note client's facial expression and tone of voice. Ask if pain is felt during rectal palpation.	Determines if technique used during examination is painful.
3. Ask client to describe risks for and signs of colorectal or prostate cancer.	Determines level of learning.
4. **Unexpected outcomes** that may occur include:	
➤ Anal area is tender, with hemorrhoids visible. Visible oozing of bloody drainage may occur.	Symptomatic of external hemorrhoids.
➤ Anal sphincter is weakened.	May place client at risk for bowel incontinence.
➤ Client experiences acute rectal pain.	Indicates local disease (e.g., fissure, thrombosed hemorrhoid) or rock-hard constipation.
➤ Lesion or irregularity in mucosa is palpated along rectal wall.	Symptoms may indicate rectal tumor.
➤ Prostate gland may be enlarged, with presence of hard nodule.	Symptoms of prostate cancer.
➤ Stool for microscopic blood (guaiac) tests positive.	Evidence of bleeding in gastrointestinal tract.
➤ Hardened stool is noted in rectal and anal canal.	Indicates constipation.
➤ Client is unable to describe signs or risks for colorectal or prostate cancer.	Additional instruction is required.

NURSING DIAGNOSIS

Clustering of defining characteristics from examination data may reveal the following nursing diagnoses:

- ➤ Anxiety
- ➤ Constipation
- ➤ Knowledge deficit regarding cancer risk factors
- ➤ Pain

Related factors are individualized based on the client's condition or needs.

RECORDING AND REPORTING

1. Describe all assessment findings in nurses' notes or flow sheet. Note client's reaction to examination.	Documents baseline data and any change in client's condition.
2. Record all instructions and client's response.	Documentation of client education improves continuity of care.
3. Report abnormalities, such as palpable mass or blood in stool, to nurse in charge or physician.	May require further diagnosis or treatment.
4. Report and record date and time specimens were sent to laboratory.	Provides means for follow-up.

FOLLOW-UP ACTIVITIES

1. If client has abnormal mass or bleeding, a proctosigmoidoscopy will probably be ordered by physician to examine higher colonic tissues.

Special Considerations

- Some institutions do not permit nurses to perform digital examinations. When policy permits, have a qualified examiner present to assist a student.
- A false-positive guaiac test result can occur in relation to ingestion of certain foods and medications (see Chapter 43).
- Prostate cancer incidence rates are 37% higher for African Americans than for European Americans (American Cancer Society, 1996).

Teaching Considerations

- Discuss the American Cancer Society's guidelines for early detection of colorectal cancer:
  - Digital rectal examination yearly after age 40.
  - Stool blood test (guaiac test) yearly after age 50.
  - Proctosigmoidoscopy (visual inspection of rectum and lower colon with a hollow, lighted, flexible tube) performed by a physician every 3 to 5 years after age 50 or on physician's advice.
- Review warning signs of colorectal cancer.
- Discuss diet planning to reduce fat and increase fiber content.
- Warn client against problems caused by overuse of laxatives, cathartic medications, codeine, or enemas.
- Discuss with male client the American Cancer Society's guidelines for early detection of prostate cancer:
  - Digital rectal examination performed annually after age 40.
  - Annual prostate-specific antigen blood test after age 50.
  - If either of preceding tests proves suspicious, prostate ultrasound testing may be conducted for men at high risk.
- Review signs of prostatic cancer.

Pediatric Considerations

- Examination is performed only when there are any symptoms of problems, such as intraabdominal or pelvic mass, tenderness, bladder distention, or bowel abnormalities.
- Children's rectal walls are not palpated because of danger of causing trauma.

Gerontologic Considerations

- External anal sphincter may be slightly lax.
- Constipation is common in older adults; fecal mass may be palpated.

SKILL 11-17 Assessing the Musculoskeletal System

The nurse's assessment of the musculoskeletal system includes a general inspection of gait, posture, and body position, as well as a more thorough assessment of major bone, joint, and muscle groups. Much of the assessment can be performed while the nurse examines other body systems; for example, while assessing neck structures, the nurse can also assess neck range of motion (ROM). It is easy for the nurse to integrate musculoskeletal assessment into routine activities of care, for example, while bathing or positioning the client. Assessment is especially important when the client reports pain or loss of joint or muscle function.

Frequently muscular disorders are manifestations of neurological disease. Therefore a neurological assessment is often conducted at the same time.

Information from the assessment can be valuable in determining a client's ability to perform activities of daily living or to tolerate exercise. The client's condition often may require use of assistive devices to maintain mobility and self-care function. The examination uses inspection and palpation.

EQUIPMENT

- Goniometer
- Tape measure

DELEGATION CONSIDERATIONS

Unlicensed assistive personnel will often assist clients with ambulation, transfer, and positioning. As a result, the staff member should be trained in recognizing problems with gait and ROM. The nurse should be responsible for informing unlicensed assistive personnel about the following:

- Clients at risk for gait problems
- Importance of never moving or forcing a joint beyond the client's current range of motion.
- Clients with muscular weakness will require special assistance with transfer and ambulation.
- Need to report any problems noted in range of motion, appearance of a joint, or muscle strength.

Physical examination of musculoskeletal function is a skill that requires problem solving and knowledge application unique to a professional nurse. For this skill, delegation is inappropriate.

STEPS	RATIONALE
ASSESSMENT	
1. Determine if client is involved in competitive sports (particularly one involving collision and contact), fails to warm up adequately, is in poor physical condition, or has had a rapid growth spurt (adolescents).	These are risk factors for sports injury.
2. Review client history (particularly with female clients) for heavy alcohol use, cigarette smoking, constant dieting, calcium intake less than 500 mg daily, thin and light body frame, nulliparous state, occurrence of menopause before age 45, postmenopausal state, bilateral oophorectomy (ovary removal), family history of osteoporosis, or European American, Asian, or Native American race.	These are risk factors for osteoporosis.
3. Ask client to describe history of alteration in bone, muscle, or joint function (e.g., recent fall, trauma, lifting heavy objects, bone or joint disease with sudden or gradual onset) and location of alteration.	Assists in assessing nature of musculoskeletal problem.
4. Assess nature and extent of client's pain: location, duration, severity, predisposing and aggravating factors, relieving factors, and type of pain.	Alterations in bone, joints, or muscle are frequently accompanied by pain, which has implications not only for comfort but also ability to perform activities of daily living.
5. Determine how client's alteration influences ability to perform activities of daily living (e.g., bathing, feeding, dressing, toileting, and ambulating) and social functions (e.g., household chores, work, recreation, sexual activities).	Level of nursing care is determined by extent to which client can perform self-care. Type and degree of restriction in continuing social activities influence topics for client education.
6. Assess height decrease of woman older than 50 by subtracting current height from recall of maximum adult height (Reed and Birge, 1988).	Measurement screens for osteoporosis. Study by Reed and Birge (1988) found that 75% of clients who had lost 2 inches or more in height were later found to have osteoporosis on x-ray examination.
PLANNING	
1. **Expected outcomes** following completion of procedure:	
➤ Client denies discomfort or worsening of existing pain following examination.	
➤ Gait is normal, with arms swinging freely at side. Head and face lead body, and balance is good.	
➤ Posture is erect. Head is held erect, with hips and shoulders aligned in parallel. There is an even contour of shoulder, level scapulae and iliac crests, with alignment of head over gluteal folds.	
➤ Normal cervical, thoracic, and lumbar curves are present.	
➤ Bilateral symmetry of extremities in length, circumference, alignment, position, and skin folds (Seidel et al., 1995).	Absence of deformities or injury.
➤ Muscles are firm, without tenderness.	
➤ Full active ROM is present in all joints with good muscle tone. ROM is equal between contralateral joints.	Absence of contractures, spasticity, or muscular weakness.
➤ No deformities or crepitus found.	
➤ Muscle groups are strong, without atrophy.	
➤ Client demonstrates ROM exercises.	Demonstrates learning.

STEPS	RATIONALE
2. Prepare client:	
a. Integrate musculoskeletal assessment during other portions of physical assessment or during nursing care.	As in assessment of integument, nurse can conduct assessment of musculoskeletal system as client moves in bed, rises from chair, walks, or goes through movements required during complete physical examination. Integration saves time for both nurse and client.
b. Plan time for short rest periods during assessment.	Movement of body parts and various maneuvers may fatigue client.

CRITICAL DECISION POINT Especially important to consider rest periods with older adult.

STEPS	RATIONALE
c. Instruct client on proper position for each portion of assessment—sitting, supine, prone, or standing.	Muscles and joints should be exposed and free to move to allow for accurate measurement. Each joint or muscle group may require different position for measurement.
d. Explain steps of procedures.	Elicits client's cooperation.

IMPLEMENTATION

STEPS	RATIONALE
1. Inspect **gait** as client walks into examination room and stands. Observe for foot dragging, shuffling or limping, balance, presence of obvious deformity in lower extremities, and position of the trunk in relation to the legs.	Gait is more natural if client is unaware of nurse's observation. Nature of gait may indicate type of alteration. Ambulation can accentuate presence of deformity.
2. Stand behind client and observe postural alignment (position of hips relative to shoulders). Look sideways at cervical, thoracic, and lumbar curves (see illustration).	Postural changes may indicate muscular, bone, or joint deformity; pain; or muscular fatigue. Head should be held erect. Abnormal curves of posture include lordosis (swayback, increased lumbar curvature), kyphosis (hunchback, exaggerated posterior curvature of thoracic spine), and scoliosis (lateral spinal curvature) (see illustration).
3. Ask client to walk in straight line and return to original standing position.	Allows more formal assessment of gait and balance.

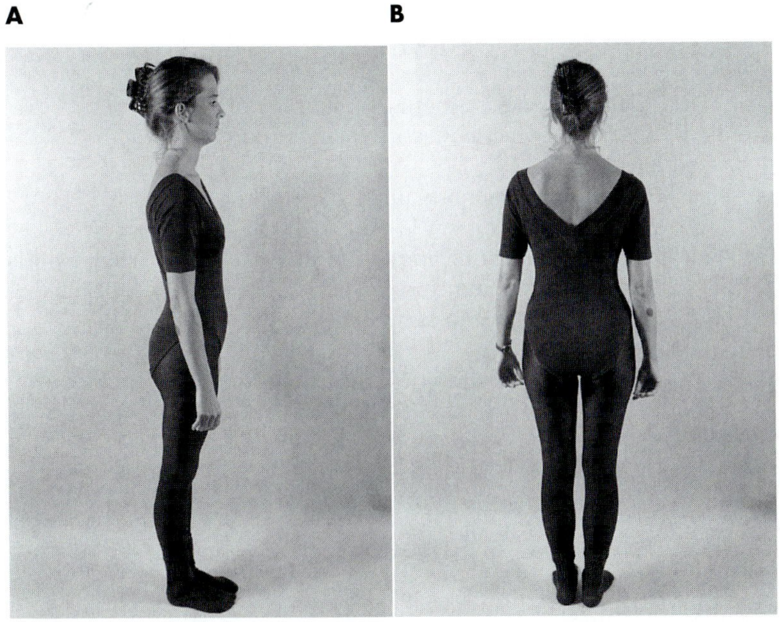

Step 2 Posture. **A,** Side view. **B,** Posterior view.

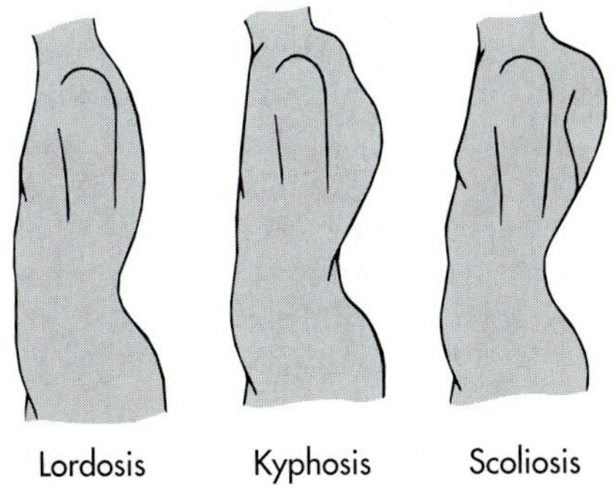

Step 2 Common postural abnormalities.

STEPS	RATIONALE
4. Make a general observation of the extremities. Look at overall size, gross deformity, bony enlargement, alignment, and symmetry.	General review helps to pinpoint areas requiring in-depth assessment.
5. Gently palpate all bones, joints, and surrounding muscles in a complete examination. In a focused assessment, palpate only an involved area. Note any heat, tenderness, edema, or resistance to pressure.	May reveal changes resulting from trauma or chronic disease.
6. Assist client in putting each major joint through its full ROM (Table 11-12). Observe equality of motion in same body parts:	
a. Give client adequate space to move each muscle group.	
b. Active motion: Instruct client in moving each joint through its normal range.	Client needs no support or assistance and is able to move joint independently.
c. Passive motion: Have client relax and move the same joints passively until the end of the range is felt. Support extremity at joint.	Detects presence of deformities, reduced mobility, or fixation of joints. Assessment of client's normal ROM provides baseline for assessing later changes after surgery or inactivity.

CRITICAL DECISION POINT Do not force the joint if there is pain or muscle spasm.

7. If a joint appears to have increased or limited ROM, measure precise degree of motion with goniometer (if available):

CRITICAL DECISION POINT Goniometer may be obtainable from the physical therapy department.

a. Position center of protractor at center of joint being measured (see illustration).

b. Extend each arm of goniometer along body parts extending from joint.

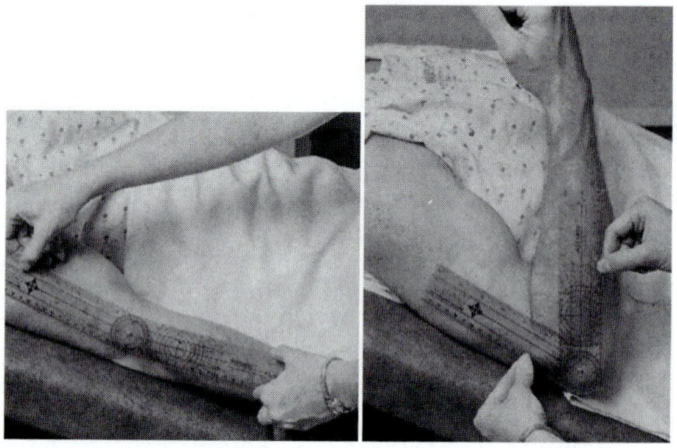

Step 7a Measurement of joint range of motion using goniometer.

STEPS	RATIONALE
c. Measure joint angle before moving joint.	Obtains precise measurement of joint extension.
d. Take joint through its full ROM, and measure angle again (see illustration).	Obtains precise measurement of joint flexion.
e. Compare reading with normal degree of joint movement.	Determines abnormalities.
8. While measuring ROM, note any instability of joint:	Crepitus is crunching or grating that occurs when joint is moved. It indicates pathological condition of joint.
a. Palpate for unusual movement of joint during its movement. Note any deformity.	Signs of injury to supportive tissues.
b. Palpate joint for swelling, stiffness, tenderness, and heat; note any redness. For example: • Palpate each joint in the hand and wrist. Palpate interphalangeal joints with thumb and index finger. • Palpate the popliteal space, then the tibiofemoral joint. • Use the thumb and fingers of both hands to compress the forefoot, palpating each metatarsophalangeal joint.	Reveals joint abnormalities or presence of cyst or bony overgrowths.

Table 11-12 Terminology for Normal Range of Motion Positions

Term	Range of Motion	Examples of Joints
Flexion	Movement decreasing angle between two adjoining bones; bending of limb	Elbow, fingers, knee
Extension	Movement increasing angle between two adjoining bones	Elbow, knee, fingers
Hyperextension	Movement of body part beyond its normal resting extended position	Head
Pronation	Movement of body part so that front or ventral surface faces downward	Hand, forearm
Supination	Movement of body part so that front or ventral surface faces upward	Hand, forearm
Abduction	Movement of extremity away from midline of body	Leg, arm, fingers
Adduction	Movement of extremity toward midline of body	Leg, arm, fingers
Internal rotation	Rotation of joint inward	Knee, hip
External rotation	Rotation of joint outward	Knee, hip
Eversion	Turning of body part away from midline	Foot
Inversion	Turning of body part toward midline	Foot
Dorsiflexion	Flexion of toes and foot upward	Foot
Plantar flexion	Bending of toes and foot downward	Foot

STEPS / RATIONALE

9. While assessing ROM, ask client to allow extremity to relax or hang limp. Support extremity and move limb through ROM to detect muscular resistance. It may be helpful to palpate muscle mass being tested also.

Rationale: Detects muscle tone in major muscle groups. Normal tone causes mild, even resistance to movement through entire ROM. If muscle has increased tone (hypertonicity), any sudden movement of joint is met with considerable resistance. Hypotonic muscle moves without resistance. Muscle feels flabby.

10. Assess muscle strength. Be sure client is in stable position, one that will allow active contraction of muscle groups. Assess muscle strength by applying gradual increase in pressure to muscle group. Have client resist pressure applied by attempting to move against resistance (e.g., flex elbow). Have client maintain resistance until told to stop. Compare symmetrical muscle groups. For example:

a. Attempt to open client's eyelids as client keeps lids tightly closed (ocular muscles).
b. Place hand on client's upper jaw as client turns head laterally against resistance (neck muscles) (see illustration).
c. Place hands over client's deltoid muscles with client's arms abducted to 90 degrees; have client hold position against resistance (deltoid muscles).
d. Place hand over client's slightly raised and extended leg as client tries to hold it up against resistance (hip musculature).
e. Place hand on dorsal surface of client's neutrally positioned foot as client attempts to bend foot up (ankle and foot).

Rationale: Assesses strength of major muscle groups. Client's position should not be one that would easily cause a loss of balance or a fall.

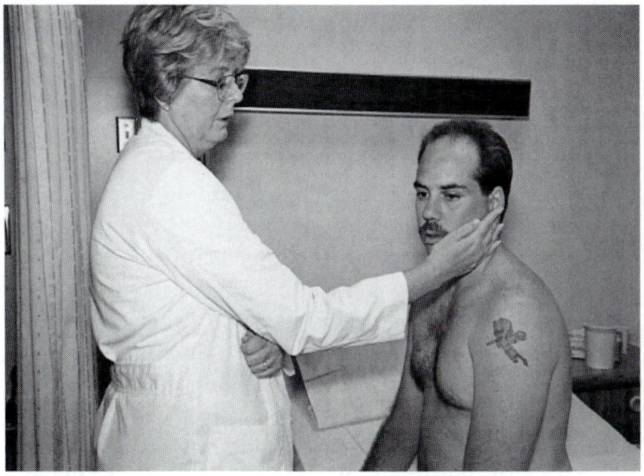

Step 10b Testing muscle strength.

11. Rate muscle strength on scale of 0 to 5:

	Grade
No voluntary contraction	0
Slight contractility, no movement	1
Full range of motion, passive	2
Full range of motion, active	3
Full range of motion against gravity, some resistance	4
Full range of motion against gravity, full resistance	5

STEPS	RATIONALE
12. If muscle weakness is identified, measure muscle size with tape measure placed around body of muscle. Compare with same muscle on opposite side of body.	Indicates degree of atrophy.

EVALUATION

1. Compare findings with normal assessment characteristics of musculoskeletal structures.	Determines presence of abnormalities.
2. Evaluate level of client's discomfort following procedure.	Determines if manipulation of musculoskeletal structures aggravated client's discomfort.
3. **Unexpected outcomes** that may occur include:	
➤ Joints are prominent, swollen, and tender with nodules or overgrowth of bone in distal joints.	Signs of arthritis.
➤ Reduced ROM in one or more major joints—shoulder, elbow, wrist, fingers, knee, hip. Client may have pain during movement, with joint unstable, stiff, painful, or swollen or with obvious deformity.	Signs and symptoms of muscle or joint alterations.
➤ Client demonstrates weakness in one or more major muscle groups, or gait demonstrates poor balance with shuffling or stumbling of feet.	Problem can be musculoskeletal or neurological in origin.
➤ Postural abnormalities such as lordosis, kyphosis, or scoliosis are noted. Reduced ROM in spine is observed.	Alteration is caused by congenital or traumatic conditions.

NURSING DIAGNOSIS

Clustering of defining characteristics from the assessment data may reveal the following nursing diagnoses for clients requiring this skill:

- ➤ Body-image disturbance
- ➤ Risk for injury
- ➤ Impaired physical mobility
- ➤ Pain

Related factors are individualized based on the client's condition or needs.

RECORDING AND REPORTING

1. Record all findings in nurses' notes.	Documents baseline status and any change in client's condition.
2. Report acute pain or sudden muscle weakness to nurse in charge or physician.	May be indicative of condition requiring immediate treatment.

• • • • •

Special Considerations

- ➤ Neurological assessment is often conducted simultaneously because muscles may be weakened as result of nerve innervation loss.
- ➤ Always use caution when examining a sports injury.
- ➤ Never attempt to move joint when fracture is suspected. Clients weakened by illness usually require passive motion assessment. With aging, ROM decreases in all joints because of reduction in muscle fiber size and tightening of joints.
- ➤ Clients who have been immobilized for several days and those who have bone or joint disease, surgical correction of joint or bone, or pain are at risk for reduced ROM. Joint that cannot be moved beyond a certain point within its range has a contracture.
- ➤ Upper and lower extremity on client's dominant side is normally stronger than that on nondominant side.
- ➤ Pain, rather than weakness, may cause reduced muscle strength. Likewise, long-term pain can lead to muscle weakening.

Teaching Considerations

- ➤ Instruct client about correct postural alignment. Consult with physical therapist to provide client with exercises for improving posture.
- ➤ To reduce bone demineralization, instruct older adult client on a proper weight-bearing exercise

program (e.g., walking, low-impact aerobics) to be followed three or more times a week. Also encourage intake of calcium to meet recommended daily allowance. Increased vitamin D aids calcium absorption. In women, recommended calcium supplements are 1000 mg before menopause and 1500 mg after menopause. Encourage female client to consult with physician regarding use of estrogen replacement.

- Explain to clients with low back pain that they can benefit from modification of work factors (e.g., lifting heavy weights, use of protective equipment), regular aerobic exercise, and exercises that strengthen the back and increase trunk flexibility.
- Instruct older adults about fall prevention. Modifications can be made in the home environment to reduce the risk of falls (see Chapter 41).
- When client is unable to perform self-care easily, instruct on use of assistive devices (e.g., zippers on clothing instead of buttons and elevation of chairs to minimize bending of knees and hips).
- Instruct older adult client to pace activities to compensate for loss in muscle strength.

Pediatric Considerations

- Infants must be carefully examined for musculoskeletal anomalies resulting from genetic or fetal insults. An examination includes review of posture, generalized movement, symmetry and skin creases of the extremities, muscle strength, and hip alignment.
- Normally the back of a newborn is rounded or C-shaped from the thoracic and pelvic curves.
- Scoliosis, lateral curvature of the spine, is an important childhood problem, especially in females. (For closer examination, have child stand erect, wearing only underclothes. Observe from behind, looking for asymmetry of shoulders and hips.) The disorder becomes apparent at puberty, especially in girls, who note uneven dress hems.
- The shape of bones may vary in children. Most conditions are benign, for example, valgus of the lower legs (lateral bowing of tibia), which is common in toddlers until they have well-developed lower back and leg muscles; **varus** of the knee (opposite of **valgus**) is normal in children from age 2 to 7 years (Wong, 1995). If either of these conditions is excessive, further evaluation is needed.
- Watching a child during play can reveal information about musculoskeletal function.

Gerontologic Considerations

- Older adult's gait normally has smaller steps and a wider base of support.
- Older adults tend to assume a stooped, forward-bent posture, with hips and knees somewhat flexed and arms bent at the elbows and the level of the arms raised (Ebersole and Hess, 1994).
- In older adults joints often become swollen and stiff, with reduced ROM resulting from cartilage erosion and fibrosis of synovial membranes.
- Older adults may develop kyphosis because of osteoporosis.

SKILL 11-18 Assessing the Neurological System

The neurological system is responsible for many functions, including initiation and coordination of movement, reception and perception of sensory stimuli, organization of thought processes, control of speech, and storage of memory. Numerous factors have the potential for influencing a client's neurological status. Medications, fatigue, metabolic disturbances, and alterations in oxygenation are just a few examples. Thus an assessment of neurological function can be complex, depending on a client's condition and the signs and symptoms.

An efficient nurse integrates neurological measurements with other parts of the physical examination. For example, mental and emotional status is observed as the nursing history is collected. The nurse might measure coordination while assessing musculoskeletal function.

Many variables are considered when deciding the extent of an examination. A client's level of consciousness influences the ability to follow directions and participate in a complete examination. If a client is physically disabled, it becomes necessary to defer assessment of motor function. A client's chief complaint often determines whether a neurological assessment is necessary. If a client has a headache, a neurological assessment is important. However, if the client has abdominal pain, the neurological review is not as critical.

EQUIPMENT

- Cotton applicator or cotton ball
- Tongue blades (2)
- Test tubes (2), one filled with hot water, other filled with cold
- Reflex hammer
- Vials containing coffee or vanilla extract
- Vials containing sugar and salt
- Familiar objects (coin or paper clip)
- Penlight
- Snellen chart
- Tuning fork
- Reading material

DELEGATION CONSIDERATIONS

Unlicensed assistive personnel should know to inform the nurse of any changes in a client's behavior or level of consciousness. Some neurological conditions can be life threatening. The physical examination of the neurological system requires problem solving and knowledge application unique to a professional nurse. For this skill, delegation is inappropriate.

STEPS	RATIONALE
ASSESSMENT	
1. Determine if client is taking analgesics, sedatives, hypnotics, antipsychotics, antidepressants, or nervous system stimulants as medication.	These forms of drugs can alter level of consciousness or cause behavioral changes.
2. Assess client's use of alcohol or sedative-hypnotics.	Abuse can cause tremors, ataxia, and changes in peripheral nerve function.
3. Determine if client has recent history of seizures/convulsions. Clarify sequence of events (aura, fall to ground, motor activity, loss of consciousness), character of any symptoms, and relationship of seizure to time of day, fatigue, or emotional stress.	Seizure activity often originates from central nervous system alteration. Characteristics of seizure help determine its origin.
4. Screen client for headache, tremors, dizziness, vertigo, numbness or tingling of body part, visual changes, weakness, pain, or changes in speech.	Symptoms frequently originate from alterations in central nervous system or peripheral nervous system function. Identification of specific patterns of these symptoms may aid in diagnosis of pathological condition.
5. Discuss with spouse, family members, or friends any recent changes in client's behavior, for example, increased irritability, mood swings, or memory loss.	Behavioral changes may result from intracranial pathological states.
6. Assess client for history of change in vision, hearing, smell, taste, or touch.	Major sensory nerves originate from the brainstem. These symptoms may help to localize nature of the problem.
7. If an older adult client displays sudden acute confusion (delirium), review history for drug toxicity (anticholinergics, diuretics, digoxin, cimetidine, sedatives, antihypertensives, antiarrhythmics), serious infections, metabolic disturbances, heart failure, and severe anemia.	Delirium is one of the most common mental disorders in older persons. Acute condition is always potentially reversible.
8. Review client's history for head or spinal cord injury, hypertension, or psychiatric disorders.	Factors may cause neurological symptoms or behavioral changes to develop, focusing assessment on possible cause.
PLANNING	
1. **Expected outcomes** following completion of procedure:	
➤ Client incurs no injury during examination.	Clients who are confused or have poor coordination must be protected from injury.
➤ Client is alert, oriented, and responds appropriately to all questions.	Client is alert to surroundings and cognitively aware.
➤ Client maintains eye contact and shows interest in the examination.	
➤ Appearance is well kept.	

STEPS	RATIONALE
➤ Speech is fluent with proper inflections.	
➤ Client demonstrates immediate recall of recent and past events.	Memory is intact.
➤ Client is able to interpret abstract ideas and make associations of related concepts.	Thought processes are normal.
➤ Sensation is intact for pain, temperature, light touch, and position.	Sensation is normal.
➤ Cranial nerves are intact.	
➤ Gait is even and balance is steady.	Normal coordination and brainstem function are found.
➤ Muscle strength is normal and symmetrical.	
➤ Reflexes are symmetrical and 2+.	Spinal cord pathways are intact.
2. Prepare client:	
a. Explain procedure to client.	Minimizes client's anxiety.
b. Integrate portions of neurological assessment with other parts of examination: cranial nerve function with survey of head and neck, mental and emotional status during nursing history, and reflexes while assessing musculoskeletal system.	Saves time and prevents client's fatigue.
c. Client may sit, lie down, or stand, depending on portion of assessment.	Sitting or lying down provides position of comfort during mental and emotional assessment. Cranial nerve, cerebellar, sensory, and reflex function are assessed with client sitting. Nurse assesses balance with client standing.
d. Screen neurological function when client presents no major symptom complex or has no recent history of head or spinal cord injury or disease. (Nurse assesses level of consciousness, orientation, pupillary reflexes, movement of extremities, and sensations).	Eliminates need for complete neurological examination, which can be time consuming.

Table 11-13 Glasgow Coma Scale

Action	Response	Score
Eyes open	Spontaneously	④
	To speech	3
	To pain	2
	None	1
Best verbal response	Oriented	⑤
	Confused	4
	Inappropriate words	3
	Incomprehensible sounds	2
	None	1
Best motor response	Obeys commands	⑥
	Localized pain	5
	Flexion withdrawal	4
	Abnormal flexion	3
	Abnormal extension	2
	Flaccid	1
	TOTAL SCORE	⑮

IMPLEMENTATION

MENTAL AND EMOTIONAL STATUS

STEPS	RATIONALE
1. For clients who are alert and responsive to conversation, conduct a mental status examination. Kahn's mental status questionnaire (MSQ) and Folstein's Mini-Mental State (MMS) (see box on p. 410) are two good tools.	Measure orientation and cognitive function. MMS maximum score is 30; 21 or less indicates cognitive impairment.
2. If client's alertness is questioned, assess client's level of consciousness by directing questions and giving instructions that require response. Be sure client is as fully awake as possible before testing alertness. Note appropriateness of emotions, responses, and ideas expressed.	Alteration in mental status may result from brain disorders, drug effects, or electrolyte and metabolic changes. Nurse can assess client's optimal level of alertness only by being assured that client is fully responsive before testing.
a. Use the Glasgow Coma Scale (GCS) to measure consciousness objectively (Table 11-13).	Scale is used to evaluate neurological status over time. The higher the score, the more normal the level of function.

FOLSTEIN'S MINI-MENTAL STATE EXAMINATION

Maximum Score	Score	
Orientation		
5	( )	What is the (year) (season) (date) (day) (month)?
5	( )	Where are we: (state) (county) (town) (hospital) (floor)?
Registration		
3	( )	Name 3 objects: 1 second to say each. Then ask the patient all 3 after you have said them. Give 1 point for each correct answer. Then repeat them until he learns all 3. Count trials and record.
Attention and Calculation		
5	( )	Serial 7's. 1 point for each correct. Stop after 5 answers. Alternatively spell "world" backwards.
Recall		
3	( )	Ask for the 3 objects repeated above. Give 1 point for each correct.
Language		
9	( )	Name a pencil, and watch (2 points) Repeat the following: "No ifs, ands or buts" (1 point) Follow a 3-stage command: "Take a paper in your right hand, fold it in half, and put it on the floor" (3 points) Read and obey the following:

Close Your Eyes (1 point)

Write a sentence (1 point)

Copy design (1 point)

____________ Total score

ASSESS level of consciousness along a continuum

____

Alert   Drowsy   Stupor   Coma

Instructions for Administration of Mini-Mental State Examination

Orientation

(1) Ask for the date. Then ask specifically for parts omitted, e.g., "Can you also tell me what season it is?" One point for each correct.

(2) Ask in turn "Can you tell me the name of this hospital?" (town, county, etc.). One point for each correct.

Registration

Ask the patient if you may test his memory. Then say the names of 3 unrelated objects, clearly and slowly, about one second for each. After you have said all 3, ask him to repeat them. This first repetition determines his score (0-3) but keep saying them until he can repeat all 3, up to 6 trials. If he does not eventually learn all 3, recall cannot be meaningfully tested.

Attention and Calculation

Ask the patient to begin with 100 and count backwards by 7. Stop after 5 subtractions (93, 86, 79, 72, 65). Score the total number of correct answers.

If the patient cannot or will not perform this task, ask him to spell the word "world" backwards. The score is the number of letters in correct order, e.g., dlrow = 5, dlorw = 3.

Recall

Ask the patient if he can recall the 3 words you previously asked him to remember. Score 0-3.

Language

Naming: Show the patient a wrist watch and ask him what it is. Repeat for pencil. Score 0-2.

Repetition: Ask the patient to repeat the sentence after you. Allow only one trial. Score 0 or 1.

3-Stage command: Give the patient a piece of plain blank paper and repeat the command. Score 1 point for each part correctly executed.

Reading: On a blank piece of paper print the sentence "Close your eyes" in letters large enough for the patient to see clearly. Ask him to read it and do what it says. Score 1 point only if he actually closes his eyes.

Writing: Give the patient a blank piece of paper and ask him to write a sentence for you. Do not dictate a sentence, it is to be written spontaneously. It must contain a subject and verb and be sensible. Correct grammar and punctuation are not necessary.

Copying: On a clean sheet of paper, draw intersecting pentagons, each side about 1 in., and ask him to copy it exactly as it is. All 10 angles must be present and 2 must intersect to score 1 point. Tremor and rotation are ignored.

Estimate the patient's level of sensorium along a continuum, from alert on the left to coma on the right.

From Folstein MF, Folstein S, McHugh PR: Mini-Mental State; a practical method for grading the cognitive state of patients for the clinician, *J Psychiatric Res* 12:189, 1975.

STEPS	RATIONALE
CRITICAL DECISION POINT Caution use of scale with clients who have sensory losses. These clients may be responsive but are unable to sense painful stimuli over certain areas of the body.	
3. Rephrase or ask similar question if it is uncertain whether client understands.	Client's inappropriate response may be caused by a communication or language problem rather than deterioration of mental status.
4. If client's responses are inappropriate, ask short, to-the-point questions regarding information the client knows, for example: "Tell me your name." "Tell me who I am." "What is the name of this place?" "Tell me where you live." "What day is this?" "What month is this?"	Measures client's orientation to person, place, and time within environment.
5. If client is unable to respond to questions of orientation, offer simple commands, for example, "Squeeze my fingers" or "Move your toes."	Levels of consciousness exist along a continuum from full alertness and responsiveness to inability to consciously initiate meaningful behaviors to unresponsiveness to external stimuli.
6. When client fails to respond to verbal command, test response to painful stimuli.	The more reduced the level of consciousness, the greater the impairment of cerebral function.
a. Apply firm pressure with thumb over root of client's fingernail.	Client should withdraw from pain.
CRITICAL DECISION POINT Avoid pinching skin to elicit response because this can cause bruising and disfigurement.	
BEHAVIOR AND APPEARANCE	
1. During general survey and throughout assessment, observe client's mannerisms and actions, noting verbal and nonverbal behavior. Note if client responds appropriately to directions and what type of mood client displays. Does client participate cooperatively with examination?	Client's mood or behavioral responses may indicate specific disease process. Client normally is anxious or concerned about findings during physical examination. Euphoria or lack of concern is inappropriate in presence of threatening events.
2. Observe client's appearance: personal hygiene, cleanliness, fit and state of repair of clothes, choice of clothing and appropriateness to setting and type of weather, and use and appropriateness of makeup.	Appearance can reflect client's self-image. An unkempt appearance may result from poor self-image, inability to attend to process of grooming, emergency, or inability to keep clothing clean.
LANGUAGE FUNCTION	
1. Observe manner of client's speech. Note voice inflection, tone, and volume.	Manner of speech may reveal client's mood and behavioral status.
2. If communication with client is unclear:	
a. Ask client to name a familiar object to which the nurse points.	
b. Ask client to respond to simple verbal or written commands such as "Sit up."	
c. Ask client to read simple sentences (such as on menu) out loud.	Assesses ability of client to understand spoken or written words and to express self, a test for aphasia.
INTELLECTUAL FUNCTION	
1. Ask client to repeat a short series of numbers forward and then backward (e.g., 7, 3, 1 and 1, 3, 7). Gradually increase the number of digits until client fails to repeat digits correctly.	Assesses immediate recall. Normally a person can repeat a series of five to eight digits forward and four to six backward.

STEPS	RATIONALE
2. Refer to Mini-Mental Status examination for test of short-term memory (see box on p. 410).	
3. Have client recall events occurring during the same day, such as what was eaten for breakfast or what form of transport was used to arrive at the clinic or hospital.	Assesses recent memory.
CRITICAL DECISION POINT Validate accuracy with family member.	
4. Ask client to recall previous medical history or family history of illness. You may also ask when client's birthday or a special day in history is.	Assesses past memory.
5. Ask what client knows about illness or reason for hospitalization.	Assesses client's knowledge level and ability to learn and understand.
6. Have client explain meaning of simple proverb, for example, "A stitch in time saves nine" or "Don't count your chickens before they're hatched." Note if explanations are literal or abstract.	Determines ability to interpret abstract ideas or concepts. Higher level of intellectual functioning is needed for abstract thinking. Client with altered mentation interprets phrase literally or merely rephrases words.

Table 11-14 Cranial Nerve Function and Assessment

Number	Name	Type	Function	Method
I	Olfactory	Sensory	Sense of smell	Ask client to identify different nonirritating aromas such as coffee and vanilla.
II	Optic	Sensory	Visual acuity	Use Snellen chart or ask client to read printed material while wearing glasses.
III	Oculomotor	Motor	Extraocular eye movement	Assess directions of gaze.
			Pupil constriction and dilation	Measure pupil reaction to light reflex and accommodation.
IV	Trochlear	Motor	Upward and downward movement of eyeball	Assess directions of gaze.
V	Trigeminal	Sensory and motor	Sensory nerve to skin of face	Lightly touch cornea with wisp of cotton. Assess corneal reflex. Measure sensation of light pain and touch across skin of face.
			Motor nerve to muscles of jaw	Palpate temples as client clenches teeth.
VI	Abducens	Motor	Lateral movement of eyeballs	Assess directions of gaze.
VII	Facial	Sensory and motor	Facial expression	As client smiles, frowns, puffs out cheeks, and raises and lowers eyebrows, look for asymmetry.
			Taste	Have client identify salty or sweet taste on front of tongue.
VIII	Auditory	Sensory	Hearing	Assess ability to hear spoken word.
IX	Glossopharyngeal	Sensory and motor	Taste	Ask client to identify sour or sweet taste on back of tongue.
			Ability to swallow	Use tongue blade to elicit gag reflex.
X	Vagus	Sensory and motor	Sensation of pharynx	Ask client to say "ah." Observe palate and pharynx movement.
			Movement of vocal cords	Assess speech for hoarseness.
XI	Spinal accessory	Motor	Movement of head and shoulders	Ask client to shrug shoulders and turn head against passive resistance.
XII	Hypoglossal	Motor	Position of tongue	Ask client to stick out tongue to midline and move it from side to side.

STEPS	RATIONALE
7. Ask client to identify similarities or associations between terms or simple concepts; for example, "A dog is to a beagle as a cat is to a ________," or "What do a tree and a rose have in common?"	Association is a higher intellectual function.
8. Ask client why he or she decided to seek health care or how client would react if he or she suddenly became ill when alone at home.	Measures client's judgment and ability to make logical decisions.
CRANIAL NERVE FUNCTION	
1. Assess function of each of the 12 cranial nerves (Table 11-14).	Detects presence of motor and sensory impairment of nerves whose pathways extend from various intracranial sites.
CRITICAL DECISION POINT **Some of the cranial nerve tests may be performed during other parts of the physical examination: e.g., directions of gaze during eye examination and ability to hear spoken word during ear examination.**	
SENSORY FUNCTION	
1. Perform all sensory testing with client's eyes closed.	Client should not be able to see when or where stimulus strikes skin.
CRITICAL DECISION POINT **Quick screening of sensory function is usually sufficient unless client has symptoms of reduced sensation, motor impairment, or paralysis.**	
2. When testing, apply minimal stimulation initially. Increase gradually until client becomes aware of it.	Prevents injury to client.
CRITICAL DECISION POINT **Stronger stimulation is needed over back, buttocks, and areas of skin that are heavily cornified.**	
3. Assess client's sensation to pain, temperature, light touch, vibration, position, and two-point discrimination (Table 11-15). Determine if client can discriminate side of body tested.	Testing can indicate alteration along sensory pathways from periphery through spinal cord to brain. Each type of sensation follows different nerve pathway.
4. Apply sensory stimuli in random, unpredictable order. Note anatomical area where sensation is reduced.	Maintains client's attention. Orderly sequence of stimulation makes it easy for client to outguess examiner and anticipate where stimulus is, even though client's sensation may be reduced.
5. Compare symmetrical areas of body while applying stimuli to face, arms, legs, and trunk.	Sensations along body's surface are felt equally on both sides.
6. Ask client to say when a particular stimulus is perceived.	Validates actual perception of sensation. Altered area of sensation allows examiner to pinpoint sensory nerve or affected spinal cord segment.
7. Test client's cognitive ability to interpret sensations by placing a coin or other familiar object in client's hand while eyes are closed. Ask client to identify object.	Identification of familiar object by touch indicates function of sensory cerebral cortex.
MOTOR FUNCTION	
1. Assess gait, stance, and muscle strength and tone following procedures described in musculoskeletal assessment (Skill 11-17). Changes in gait may indicate specific neurological disease.	Assessment of muscle strength can reveal presence of partial or complete motor paralysis. Extent of muscle involvement indicates whether lesion involves peripheral motor nerves, spinal cord, or cerebral cortex.

Table 11-15 Assessment of Sensory Nerve Function

Function	Equipment	Method	Precautions
Pain	Broken tongue blade or wooden end of cotton applicator 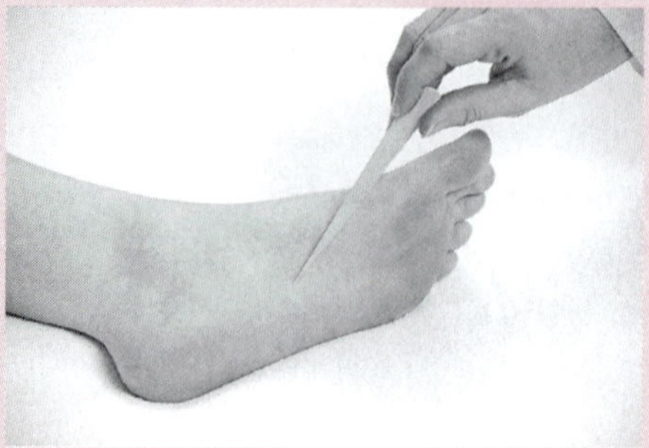	Ask client to voice when dull or sharp sensation is felt. Alternately apply sharp and blunt ends of tongue blade to skin's surface. Note areas of numbness or increased sensitivity.	Remember that areas where skin is thickened, such as heel or sole of foot, may be less sensitive to pain.
Temperature	Two test tubes, one filled with hot water and other with cold	Touch skin with tube. Ask client to identify hot or cold sensation.	Omit test if pain sensation is normal.
Light touch	Cotton ball or cotton-tip applicator 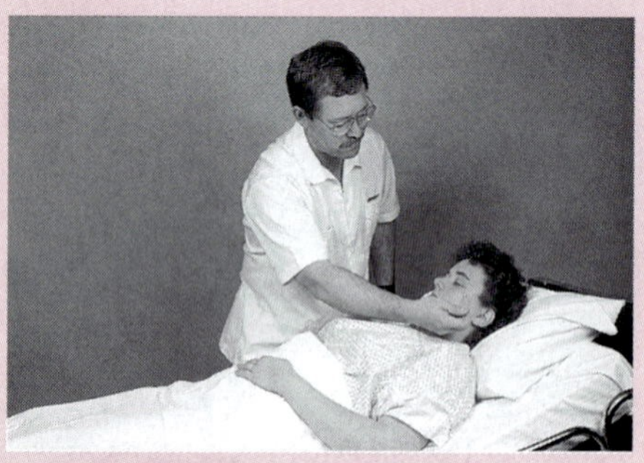	Apply light wisp of cotton to different points along skin's surface. Ask client to voice when sensation is felt.	Apply at areas where skin is thin or more sensitive (e.g., face, neck, inner aspect of arms, top of feet and hands).
Vibration	Tuning fork	Apply stem of vibrating fork to distal interphalangeal joint of fingers and interphalangeal joint of great toe, elbow, and wrist. Have client voice when vibration is first felt and when vibration stops. Dampen tines of fork at different times.	Be sure client feels vibration and not merely pressure.
Position		Grasp finger or toe, holding it by its sides with thumb and index finger. Alternate moving finger or toe up and down. Ask client to state when finger is up or down. Repeat with toes.	Avoid rubbing adjacent appendages as finger or toe is moved. Do not move joint laterally; return to neutral position before moving again.
Two-point discrimination	Two broken tongue blades	Lightly apply one or both tongue blade tips simultaneously to skin's surface. Ask client if one or two pricks are felt. Find distance at which client can no longer distinguish two points.	Apply blade tips to same anatomical site (e.g., fingertips, palm of hand, or upper arms). Minimum distance at which client can discriminate two points varies (2 to 8 mm on fingertips).

STEPS	RATIONALE
2. Ask client to sit. Demonstrate for client method for rapidly striking thigh with palm of hand, evenly, without hesitation. Then have client repeat maneuver. Note smoothness of movement.	Assesses client's coordination of upper extremity in performing rapid, rhythmical movement.
CRITICAL DECISION POINT **Coordination tests can be confusing. Demonstration is appropriate because the test is for motor function, not cognitive assessment.**	
3. Demonstrate and have client alternately strike thigh with hand supinated and then pronated. Note speed and symmetry of movement.	Ability to perform skilled motor act is disturbed by cerebellar dysfunction.
4. Stand in front of client, holding your index finger stationary 2 feet in front of client's face. Ask client to touch your finger with index finger and then to touch own nose alternately (see illustration). Client moves finger back and forth repeatedly. Observe for tremor of hand or awkward movement.	Point-to-point test assesses upper extremity coordination.

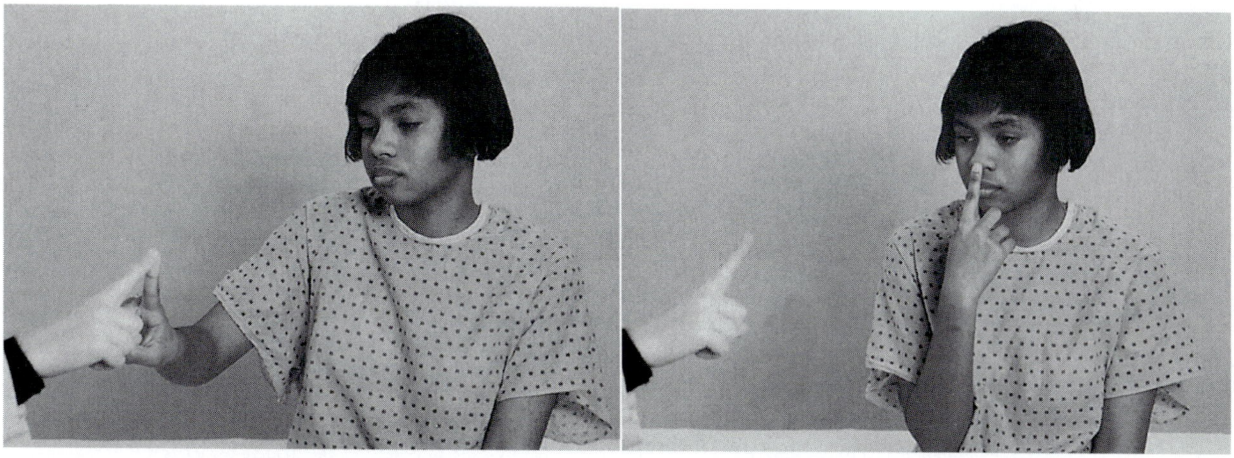

Step 4 Fine motor coordination. (From Seidel HM et al: *Mosby's guide to physical examination*, ed 3, St Louis, 1995, Mosby.)

STEPS	RATIONALE
5. Have client lie supine. Place your hand at ball of client's foot. Ask client to tap hand with foot as quickly as possible. Note speed and smoothness of movement.	Assesses lower extremity coordination.
6. Ask client to sit with eyes closed and to place heel of one foot just below knee of opposite leg. Then instruct client to slide heel down shin toward foot.	Presence of involuntary movements or difficulty in controlling heel may indicate cerebellar problem. Normally maneuver is performed evenly, without heel sliding off leg.
7. Have client stand with feet close together, eyes closed. Note presence of swaying.	Romberg's test assesses balance. Cerebellar disease causes imbalance even with eyes open.
8. Ask client to close eyes and stand on one foot and then the other.	This is an additional test for balance.

STEPS	RATIONALE
REFLEXES	
1. Assess deep tendon reflexes (Table 11-16). Reflexes should be symmetrical on both sides of body. Reflexes are graded on scale: 0 No response. 1+ Low normal with slight muscle contraction. 2+ Normal, visible muscle twitch and movement of arm or leg. 3+ Brisker than normal but may not indicate disease. 4+ Hyperactive, very brisk. Spinal cord disorder suspected.	Assesses integrity of sensory and motor pathways along reflex arc and specific spinal cord segments.
a. Ask client to relax extremity to be tested.	Prevents voluntary movement or muscle tensing that interferes with reflex response.
b. Position limb to stretch slightly muscle being tested.	Improves ability to initiate reflex.
c. Hold reflex hammer loosely between thumb and fingers.	Reflex hammer should swing freely to tap tendon briskly to elicit clean response.
d. Tap tendon briskly (see illustration).	
e. Compare symmetry of reflex from one side of body to other.	Asymmetry of reflex response indicates alteration in reflex pathway.
EVALUATION	
1. Compare findings with normal assessment characteristics.	Determines presence of abnormalities.
2. Unexpected outcomes that may occur include: ➤ Client scores low on the Mini-Mental State test. ➤ Client is confused, at times difficult to arouse by verbal stimulus.	Reveals alteration in consciousness and thought processes.

Table 11-16 Assessment of Common Reflexes

Type	Procedure	Normal Reflex
Deep tendon reflexes		
Biceps	Flex client's arm up to 45 degrees at elbow with palms down. Place your thumb in antecubital fossa at base of biceps tendon and your fingers over the biceps muscle. Strike triceps tendon with reflex hammer.	Flexion of arm at elbow
Triceps	Flex client's arm at elbow, holding arm across chest, or hold upper arm horizontally and allow lower arm to go limp. Strike triceps tendon just above elbow.	Extension at elbow
Patellar	Have client sit with legs hanging freely over side of table or chair or have client lie supine and support knee in a flexed 90-degree position. Briskly tap patellar tendon just below patella.	Extension of lower leg
Achilles	Have client assume same position as for patellar reflex. Slightly dorsiflex client's ankle by grasping toes in palm of your hand. Strike Achilles tendon just above heel at ankle malleolus.	Plantar flexion of foot
Cutaneous reflexes		
Gluteal	Have client assume side-lying position. Spread buttocks apart and lightly stimulate perineal area with cotton applicator.	Contraction of anal sphincter
Abdominal	Have client stand or lie supine. Stroke abdominal skin with base of cotton applicator over lateral borders of rectus abdominis muscle toward midline. Repeat test in each abdominal quadrant.	Contraction of rectus abdominis muscle with pulling of umbilicus toward stimulated side
Plantar	Have client lie supine with legs straight and feet relaxed. Take handle end of reflex hammer and stroke lateral aspect of sole from heel to ball of foot, curving across ball of foot toward big toe.	Bending of toes downward

STEPS	RATIONALE
➤ Client is not consistently oriented to person, place, time, or event. ➤ Speech is slow and slurred. ➤ Client is able to recall past events but unable to repeat series of five numbers. ➤ Client is unable to interpret proverbs or associate related concepts. ➤ Sensory and motor function are intact, except client is slow to respond to instructions.	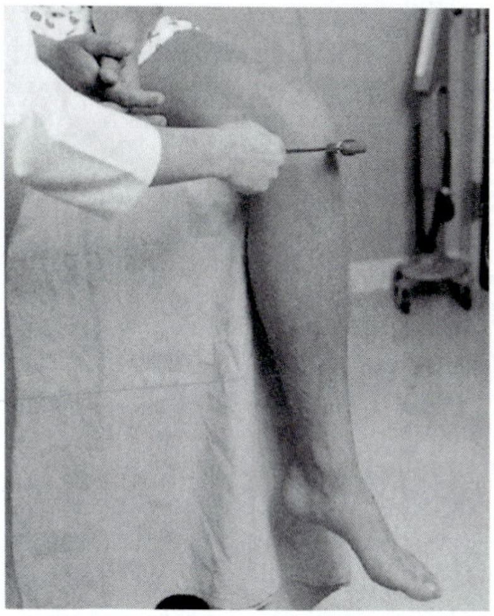 *Step 1d* Position for eliciting patellar tendon reflex. Lower leg normally extends.
➤ Client has reduced sensation to temperature, touch, and painful stimuli.	May be caused by peripheral nerve or spinal cord injury.
➤ Cranial nerve function is abnormal.	Lesion or inflammation is present along nerve distribution.
➤ Client has unsteady gait, dragging of foot.	May indicate cerebellar problem or disturbance of motor tract.
➤ Client is unable to perform rapidly alternating movements.	Indicates cerebellar problem.
➤ Reflexes test 0 to 1+ or 3+ to 4+.	Pathological condition exists along spinal cord tract or reflex arc.

NURSING DIAGNOSIS

Clustering of defining characteristics from the examination data may reveal the following nursing diagnoses for clients requiring this skill:

- ➤ Altered thought processes
- ➤ Risk for impaired skin integrity
- ➤ Risk for injury
- ➤ Impaired physical mobility
- ➤ Impaired swallowing
- ➤ Impaired verbal communication
- ➤ Self-care deficit (specify type)
- ➤ Sensory/perceptual alterations: vision, hearing, and/or touch
- ➤ Unilateral neglect

Related factors are individualized based on the client's condition or needs.

RECORDING AND REPORTING

1. Record all assessment findings in nurses' notes. Record Glasgow Coma Scale score. Record reflexes using stick figure.	Documents baseline data and change in client's condition.
2. Report abnormalities to nurse in charge or physician.	Further diagnosis or treatment may be required.

• • • • •

Special Considerations

- Client's mental and emotional function can be assessed easily as nurse poses questions and gives instructions throughout examination.
- Fully conscious client responds to questions quickly and perceives events occurring. As consciousness deteriorates, client may demonstrate irritability, shortened attention span, reduced perception of environment, and unwillingness to cooperate.
- Comatose state is one in which client fails to respond to verbal and painful stimuli. Fever and pain commonly cause confusion, disorientation, and irritability, depending on severity.
- Unkempt hair, dirty body, and broken and dirty fingernails are good indicators of grooming habits. Poorly fitting clothes may be a symptom of poverty rather than inappropriate apparel.
- Cerebellar disease causes wide-based, staggering gait. Parkinson's disease causes slow, shuffling gait, but as client walks there is increased rapidity or propulsive nature to gait as though person is about to fall. Paraplegia is paralysis of lower extremities. Quadriplegia is paralysis of upper and lower extremities. Hemiplegia is paralysis of one half of body (arm and leg).

Teaching Considerations

- Client's cultural and educational background influence ability to answer test questions. Do not ask questions related to concepts or ideas with which client is unfamiliar.
- Explain to family or friends the implications of any behavioral or mental impairment shown by client.
- If client has sensory or motor impairments, explain measures to ensure safety (e.g., use of ambulation aids or use of safety bars in bathrooms or stairways).
- Teach older adult clients to plan enough time to complete tasks because reaction time is slowed.
- Teach older adult clients and diabetics to observe skin surfaces for areas of trauma because their perception of pain is reduced.

Pediatric Considerations

- In children there is no special testing for behavior. Instead, nurse's assessment is overall impression of child's personality, affect, level of activity, social interaction, and attention span (Wong, 1995).
- Cognitive perceptual development is best assessed using a formal screening test such as the Denver Developmental Screening Test (DDST).

Gerontologic Considerations

- Older adults have decreased ability to respond to multiple stimuli.
- Older adult has reduced number of taste buds and reduced ability to discriminate odors.
- Sense of touch and pain may be diminished.
- Deep tendon and superficial reflexes are present but may also be slightly decreased.
- Older adults are at risk for acute confusion, resulting from an adverse or unwanted effect of a diagnostic or therapeutic intervention. Anticholinergic drugs (e.g., thioridazine, amitriptyline, atropine, and theophylline), histamine$_2$-blocking agents (e.g., cimetidine, ranitidine), analgesics (e.g., meperidine, NSAIDs), sedative hypnotics (e.g., triazolam and benzodiazepines), and cardiovascular drugs (e.g., nifedipine and beta blockers) pose risk. The condition is characterized by reduced ability to focus and to sustain or shift attention; change in cognitive status; or perceptual disturbance that develops over a short time. Client can also have memory impairment and illusions or hallucinations. True acute confusion tends to last 3 to 4 days (Foreman and Zane, 1996).

COMPLETING THE EXAMINATION

The nurse may record findings from the physical assessment during the examination or at the end. Most institutions have special forms for easy recording of data. The nurse checks to be sure that assessment recording is complete. The nurse reviews all findings before assisting clients with dressing in case there is a need to validate information. Findings from physical assessment are integrated into the client's care plan.

After completing the assessment, the nurse helps the client dress and assume a comfortable position either in bed or in a chair. When the client is comfortable, the nurse shares a summary of assessment findings. This is an excellent time to reinforce client teaching and to request feedback from the client to evaluate understanding of information shared. If the assessment findings have revealed serious abnormalities, the client's physician is consulted before any findings are revealed. It is the physician's responsibility to make definitive medical diagnoses. The nurse can explain the type of abnormality found and the need for the physician to conduct an additional examination.

The nurse can have assistive personnel make sure the examination area is cleaned. Within an institution it is important to be sure that supplies of equipment are restocked. Infection control practices are used in removing materials or instruments soiled with potentially infectious wastes. Afterward, the staff member washes hands. If the client's bedside was the examination site, the staff member clears away soiled items from the table and makes sure the bed linen is dry and clean. The client may appreciate a clean gown and the opportunity to wash face and hands.

The client often needs several ancillary examinations, such as x-ray or laboratory testing, after a physical examination. These tests provide additional information to rule out the presence of abnormalities and help diagnose specific conditions.

Throughout the physical assessment the nurse makes insightful clinical decisions that contribute to the client's health care management. As a result of more thorough data gathering, the nurse is able to make nursing diagnoses more accurately. Therefore the nursing care plan becomes more individualized and comprehensive. Physical assessment findings also reveal whether specific nursing measures were successful in managing client problems.

CRITICAL THINKING EXERCISES

1. Mr. Rozier enters the community clinic and presents the following history: smoker for 22 years, has a productive cough, and complains of shortness of breath on exertion. What physical examination priorities can be made for Mr. Rozier? What further information might you want to know?
2. If Mrs. Lockhart has difficulty lying flat in the supine position, what examination(s) will be most difficult to perform?
3. Ms. Alou is visited in her home as follow-up to repair of a fractured hip. As the nurse assigned to Ms. Alou, you are to visit her soon. What will likely be your priorities when you examine Ms. Alou for the first time?
4. As you administer morning hygiene to Mr. Phillips, hospitalized for an acute myocardial infarction, what portions of the physical examination lend themselves to being incorporated into hygiene activities?

REFERENCES

American Cancer Society: *1996 Cancer facts and figures,* Atlanta, 1996, The Society.

American Cancer Society: *1997 Cancer facts and figures,* Atlanta, 1996, The Society.

American Thoracic Society: Control of tuberculosis in the United States, *Am Rev Respir Dis* 146(6):1623, 1992.

Caulker-Burnett I: Primary care screening for substance abuse, *Nurse Pract* 19(6):42, 1994.

DeWitt S: Nursing assessment of the skin and dermatologic lesions, *Nurs Clin North Am* 25(1):235, 1990.

Ebersole P, Hess P: *Toward healthy aging: human needs and nursing response,* ed 4, St Louis, 1994, Mosby.

Ernst ND: The national cholesterol education program's recommendations for treatment of high blood cholesterol, *Fam Community Health* 12(1):23, 1989.

Foreman MD, Zane D: Nursing strategies for acute confusion in elders, *Am J Nurs* 96(4):44, 1996.

Franco EL: Multiple cancers of the upper aero-digestive tract: the challenge of risk factor identification, *Cancer Lett* 60:1, 1991.

Hardy MA: A pilot study of the diagnosis and treatment of impaired skin integrity: dry skin in older persons, *Nurs Diagnosis* 1(2):57, 1990.

Haviland S, O'Brien J: Physical abuse and neglect of the elderly: assessment and intervention, *Orthop Nurs* 8(4):11, 1989.

Hockenberger SJ: Fibrocystic breast disease: every woman is at risk, *Plast Surg Nurs* 13(1):37, 1993.

Koop CE: The Surgeon General's letter on child sexual abuse, Rockville, Md, 1988, US Department of Health and Human Services, Public Health Service.

Lueckenotte A: *Gerontologic nursing,* St Louis, 1996, Mosby.

Lueckenotte A: *Pocket guide to gerontologic assessment,* St Louis, 1994, Mosby.

Master S, Terpstra JK: Recognition and diagnosis. In Schnoll SH, Horvatich PK, Terpstra JK: *Prescribing drugs with abuse liability,* Richmond, Va, 1992, DSAM, MCV-VCU.

Reece SM: Immunization strategies for the elimination of hepatitis B, *Nurs Pract* 18:2, 1993.

Reed AT, Birge SJ: Screening for osteoporosis, *J Gerontol Nurs* 14(7):18, 1988.

Rozier RG, Beck JD: Epidemiology of oral diseases, *Curr Opin Dentistry* 1:308, 1991.

Seidel HM et al: *Mosby's guide to physical examination,* ed 3, St Louis, 1995, Mosby.

Wong DL: *Whaley & Wong's nursing care of infants and children,* ed 5, St Louis, 1995, Mosby.

ADDITIONAL READING

Barger SE: The delivery of early and periodic screening, diagnosis and treatment programs by NPs in a nursing center, *Nurs Pract* 18(6):65, 1993.

Carlson KJ et al: Screening for ovarian cancer: recommendations and rationale, *Ann Intern Med* 121(2):141, 1994.

Catalona WJ et al: Comparison of digital rectal examination and serum prostate specific antigen in the early detection of prostate cancer: results of a multicenter clinical trial of 6,630 men, *J Urol* 151:1283, 1994.

Forgacs P: The functional basis of pulmonary sounds, *Chest* 73:399, 1978.

Haid M et al: Digital rectal examination, serum prostate specific antigen, and prostatic ultrasound: how effective is this diagnostic triad? *J Surg Oncol* 56:32, 1994.

Lierman L et al: Predicting breast self-examination using the theory of reasoned action, *Nurs Res* 39(2):97, 1990.

McConnell E: Auscultating bowel sounds, *Nursing 90* 20:106, 1990.

McHugh J, McHugh W: How to assess deep tendon reflexes, *Nursing 90* 20:62, 1990.

Nokes KM et al: Development of an HIV assessment tool, *Image J Nurs Sch* 26(2):133, 1994.

UNIT V

Oxygenation

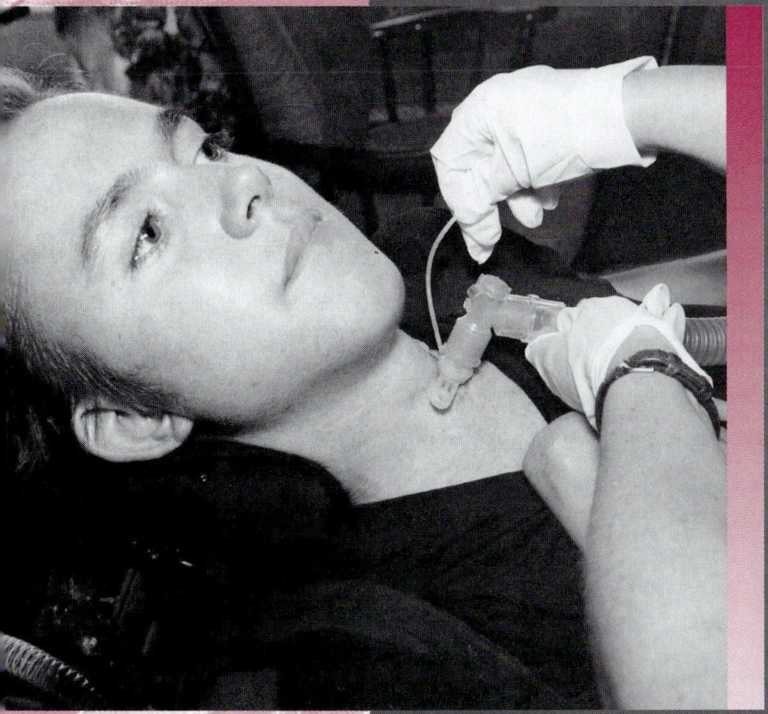

CHAPTER 12

Oxygen Therapy

OBJECTIVES

Mastery of content in this chapter will enable the nurse to:

- Define key terms.
- Discuss indications for oxygen therapy.
- Discuss methods of oxygen therapy.
- Demonstrate applying a nasal cannula and an oxygen mask.
- Demonstrate administering oxygen therapy to a client with an artificial airway.
- Demonstrate proper use of incentive spirometry.
- Demonstrate using continuous positive airway pressure (CPAP).
- Demonstrate administering mechanical ventilation.
- Demonstrate how to measure a peak expiratory flow rate (PEFR).

KEY TERMS

Cyanosis
Hypercapnia
Hypoxemia
Hypoxia
Incentive spirometry
Nasal cannula
Negative pressure ventilation
Oxygen mask
Oxygen therapy
Oxygen toxicity
Peak expiratory flow rate
Positive pressure ventilation
Pressure-cycled ventilation
T tube
Tidal volume
Tracheostomy collar
Volume-cycled ventilation

SKILLS

12-1 ***Applying a Nasal Cannula or Oxygen Mask***
12-2 ***Administering Oxygen Therapy to a Client with an Artificial Airway***
12-3 ***Using Incentive Spirometry***
12-4 ***Administering Mechanical Ventilation***
12-5 ***Measuring Peak Expiratory Flow Rates***

Oxygen therapy is the administration of supplemental oxygen to a client to prevent or reduce **hypoxia,** a condition in which there is insufficient oxygen to meet the metabolic demands of the tissues and cells. Hypoxia results from **hypoxemia,** a deficiency of arterial blood oxygen.

Various disease states require the use of oxygen therapy to correct impaired gas exchange and the resultant hypoxia. An example of such a disease state is the client with pneumonia. Pneumonia results in impaired gas exchange due to fluid and secretions in the lung, causing a decrease in oxygen diffusion from the lungs to the arterial blood supply. A client with chronic bronchitis, a chronic obstructive pulmonary disease (COPD), may have normal arterial oxygen levels during the day but may experience oxygen desaturation, a reduction in the arterial oxygen level during sleep, requiring oxygen at night to prevent hypoxia. A client with emphysema, another type of COPD, may experience low oxygen levels all the time or associated with increased activity, exercise-induced hypoxia. Clients with COPD and carbon dioxide (CO_2) retention are at risk for developing CO_2 narcosis induced by administration of too high levels of oxygen. The normal drive for respiration, a rising CO_2 level, is not sensitive to changes in CO_2 in clients with COPD and CO_2 retention due to the chronic elevation of CO_2. Therefore in these clients changes in the oxygen level stimulate changes in ventilation. If high levels of oxygen are administered to them,

COMPLICATIONS OF OXYGEN THERAPY

- Oxygen toxicity
  - Adult respiratory distress syndrome
  - Noncardiogenic pulmonary edema
- Increased CO_2 retention
  - Confusion
  - Headache
  - Decreased level of consciousness
  - Somnolence
- CO_2 narcosis
- Respiratory arrest

their stimulus to breathe is extinguished. Administration of oxygen therapy is not without possible complications (see box above).

The nursing assessment of a client requiring supplemental oxygen therapy may reveal many findings associated with hypoxia. Presenting symptoms depend on the client's age, level of health, present disease process, and the presence of chronic illnesses. Anxiety, confusion, and restlessness are early signs of hypoxia. Other assessment findings include changes in blood pressure, cardiac dysrhythmias, such as premature ventricular contractions (PVCs), tachypnea, dyspnea, drowsiness, headaches, disorientation, forgetfulness, and nausea.

Cyanosis, a bluish discoloration of the skin and mucous membranes, is a late sign of hypoxia. Cyanosis is caused by vasoconstriction of the peripheral blood vessels or decreased oxyhemoglobin. It can be seen in clients who are very cold or have decreased peripheral circulation due to vascular disease and in those with a decreased level of circulating oxyhemoglobin. The nurse never assumes a lack of cyanosis means adequate oxygenation. Cyanosis caused by hypoxia is assessed in the oral mucosa, the conjunctiva of the eye, and around the lips, known as circumoral cyanosis.

OXYGEN SYSTEMS

The oxygen delivery system selected depends on the level of oxygen support the client needs based on the severity of the hypoxia and the disease process. Other factors considered include the client's age, level of health and orientation level, the presence of an artificial airway, whether the setting is in the hospital or the home, the type of home environment, and the type of support and care given after discharge.

Oxygen is available in a number of systems. Oxygen provided in a hospital or institutional setting is a bulk liquid oxygen system designed to store the oxygen at −34° C (−29° F) and deliver it as a gas at wall outlets in the client's room. An oxygen flowmeter is required to regulate the flow rate in liters of oxygen delivered (Fig. 12-1).

Compressed oxygen is available in gas cylinders and exists as a nonliquefied gas at 1800 to 2400 pounds per square inch (psi) at 21° C (70° F). Oxygen cylinders used in hospitals include the large "H" size, holding about 6600 L of oxygen and the small "E" size, holding 625 L of oxygen. An oxygen regulator/flowmeter controls the flow rate of oxygen delivered from the cylinder. The H size is used as a main source, as the tank is not easily portable. The E size is smaller and allows portability (Fig. 12-2).

Skills presented in this chapter focus on administration of oxygen therapy and respiratory maneuvers to improve oxygenation and promotion of lung expansion. The nursing care measures used are based on specific assessment findings.

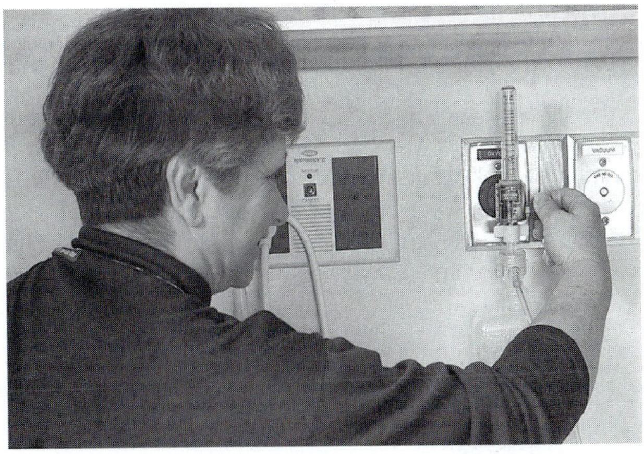

Fig. 12-1 Flow meter attached to oxygen source.

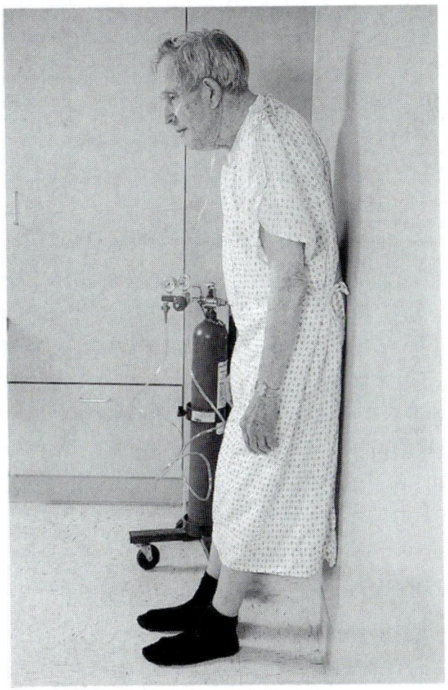

Fig. 12-2 Smaller E-tank for portability.

GUIDELINES

1. Know the client's normal range of vital signs. Hypoxia can affect the client's vital signs. Pulse may become rapid and irregular because of cardiac dysrhythmias. Initially blood pressure is elevated. If hypoxia remains uncorrected, hypotension may develop. Respiratory rate and depth are increased.
2. Know the client's usual behavioral pattern. The nurse, friends, and family may notice behavioral changes such as restlessness, agitation, anxiety, apprehension, and inability to concentrate. As hypoxia worsens, the client's activity tolerance decreases, and the client may become confused, with loss of short-term memory. Worsening of a hypoxic state may lead to a decreased level of consciousness and coma.
3. Know the client's medical history. It is important to be aware of the client with COPD who is a carbon dioxide retainer. High inspired oxygen concentrations may result in severe side effects such as respiratory depression. Clients with cardiovascular disease, such as left ventricular failure, may not be able to supply oxygen to the tissues due to decreased cardiac output. Supplemental oxygen helps decrease the work of the left ventricle and increase oxygen delivery to the tissues.
4. Be aware of environmental conditions. These can affect the client's level of oxygenation or safety if oxygen therapy is administered. Clients with chronic respiratory diseases have difficulty maintaining optimal oxygen levels in polluted environments. If a client is to receive home oxygen therapy, an environmental assessment is completed to determine respiratory hazards in the home such as the use of gas stoves or kerosene space heaters or the presence of smokers in the home.
5. Assess for a temporary or permanent abnormal chest wall configuration. Temporary abnormalities that can affect oxygenation include obesity, pregnancy, and trauma. Congenital musculoskeletal abnormalities such as kyphosis affect oxygenation because of decreased full lung expansion.
6. Document the client's smoking history. Smoking damages the lungs' mucociliary clearance mechanism and paralyzes the ciliary action, resulting in a decreased ability to clear mucus from the airways. Mucus pools in the airways create an environment for the development of infections. Accumulation of mucus may lead to the development of chronic bronchitis. Long-term chronic bronchitis ultimately results in hypoxia.
7. Know the client's most recent hemoglobin values. Hemoglobin carries oxygen and CO_2 to and from the cells. The presence of decreased hemoglobin levels reduces the amount of oxygen transported to the cells and CO_2 transported away from the cells.
8. Know the client's past and current arterial blood gas (ABG) values. A state of acidemia increases the ability of hemoglobin to release oxygen to the tissue. Alkalemia prevents the hemoglobin from easily releasing oxygen to the tissues (Dickson, 1995).
9. Know the client's cardiac output. Estimate the cardiac output by the blood pressure. If the client is hypotensive, the cardiac output is low or inadequate, and oxygen delivery to the tissues will be reduced. Oxygen is regarded as a medication. Increasing the oxygen liter flow rate for shortness of breath is similar to doubling heart medication. It is important that the client receiving oxygen therapy understands proper use of the equipment.

Safety measures for oxygen use are very important (see box at left). These measures are taught to the client and care givers to ensure proper use. In the hospital setting, signage is used to alert care givers and visitors that oxygen is in use (Fig. 12-3).

OXYGEN SAFETY GUIDELINES

- Oxygen is a medication and should not be adjusted without a physician's order.
- An "Oxygen in Use" sign must be placed on the client's door and in the client's room. If oxygen is used at home, a sign is placed on the door of the house.
- Oxygen delivery systems must be kept 10 feet from any open flames.
- Oxygen supports combustion; however, it will not explode.
- No smoking should be allowed on the premises.
- A "No Smoking" sign is placed on the client's door and in the client's home. If oxygen is used at home, a sign is placed on the door of the house.
- When oxygen cylinders are used, they must be secured so that they will not fall over. Oxygen cylinders are stored upright, chained, or in appropriate holders.

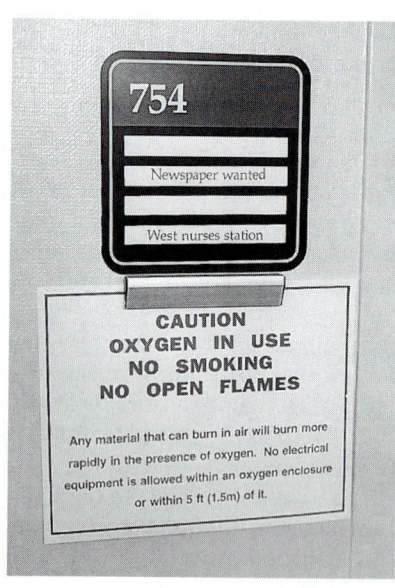

Fig. 12-3 Proper display for oxygen in use sign.

SKILL 12-1 Applying a Nasal Cannula or Oxygen Mask

NASAL CANNULA

A **nasal cannula** is a simple, comfortable device for delivering oxygen to a client (Fig. 12-4). The two tips of the cannula, about 1.5 cm (½ inch) long, protrude from the center of a disposable tube and are inserted into the nostrils. Oxygen is delivered via the cannula at a flow rate from 0.5 to 6 L/min. Higher flow rates dry airway mucosa and do not increase the inspired oxygen concentration (F_IO_2). Approximate F_IO_2 can be estimated by the flow rate (Table 12-1). The delivered oxygen percentage will vary, depending on the rate and depth of the client's breathing.

A nasal cannula is an effective mechanism for oxygen delivery. It allows the client to breathe through the mouth or nose, is available for all age-groups, and is adequate for short-term or long-term use. Cannulas are inexpensive, disposable, generally comfortable, and easily accepted by most clients.

OXYGEN MASK

An **oxygen mask** is shaped to fit snugly over the client's mouth and nose and is secured in place with a strap. The two primary types of masks are those delivering a low F_IO_2 and those delivering a high F_IO_2.

A simple face mask is a flexible, cone-shaped device with a metal strip to mold the mask to the nose, an adjustable head strap, and multiple exhalation ports (Fig. 12-5). The mask is contraindicated for clients who retain CO_2. The percentage of oxygen that can be delivered with a simple face mask ranges from 40% to 60% (Table 12-1).

Table 12-1 Flow Rate and Approximate F_IO_2

Flow (L/min)	F_IO_2
Nasal cannula	
1	21%-24%
2	24%-28%
3	28%-32%
4	32%-36%
5	36%-40%
6	40%-44%
Face mask	
5-6	40%
6-7	50%
7-10	60%

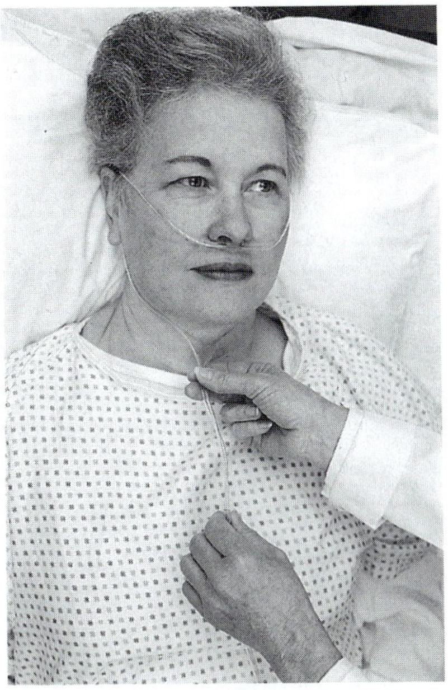

Fig. 12-4 Nasal cannula is useful for low oxygen concentration (2 L/min) for clients with chronic lung disease.

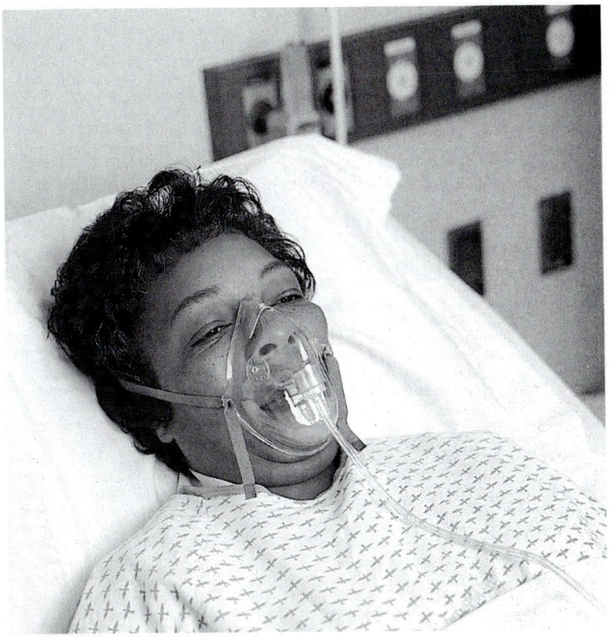

Fig. 12-5 Simple face mask can deliver concentrations of 35% to 50% using flow rates of 6 to 10 L/min.

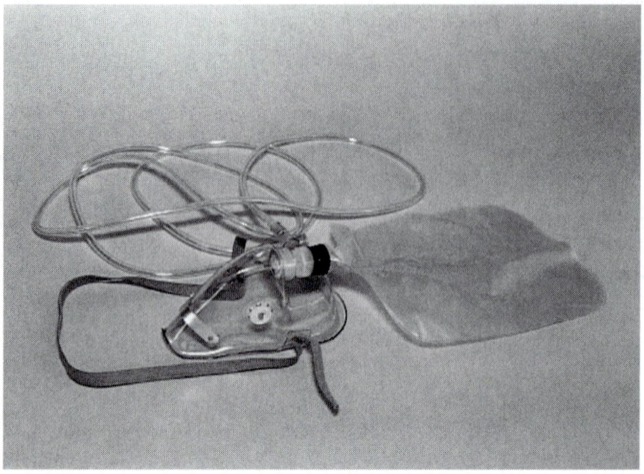

Fig. 12-6 Non-rebreathing mask.

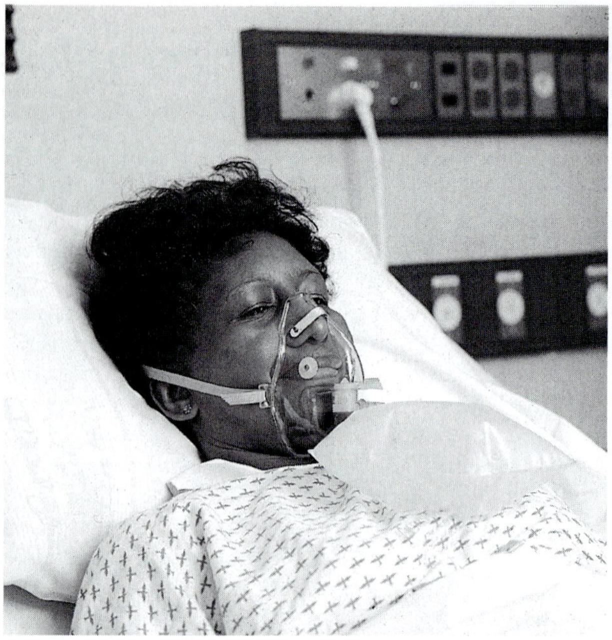

Fig. 12-7 Partial rebreather mask can deliver concentrations of 60% to 90% using flow rates of 6 to 10 L/min.

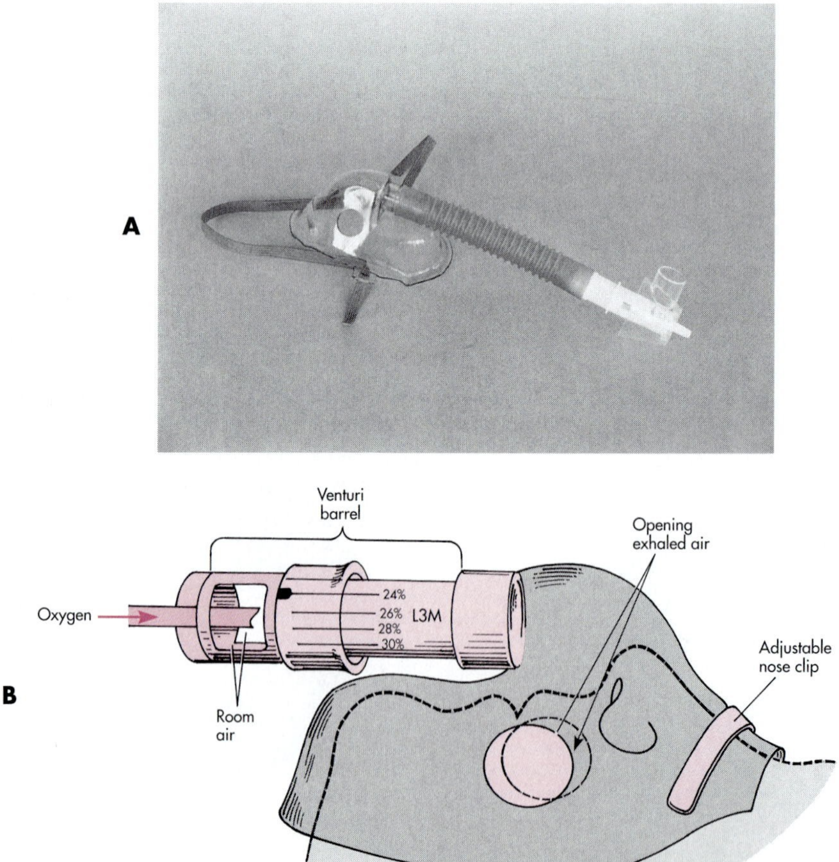

Fig. 12-8 **A,** Venturi mask; **B,** Turning venturi barrel sets percentage of oxygen delivered from 24% to 50% at preset intervals.

A nonrebreathing mask is a flexible, cone-shaped device with a reservoir bag attached. A one-way flap valve is between the bag and mask to allow for inhalation of oxygen and prevent accumulation of expired CO_2. A one-way flap valve covers the exhalation ports to prevent dilution of oxygen with entrained room air (Fig. 12-6). A nonrebreathing mask is used for severe hypoxia; flow rates of 10 L/min can produce an F_IO_2 of 80% to 95%, depending on the client's respiratory rate and depth. To ensure the client's inspiratory demands are being met, observe the reservoir bag; it should not collapse during inspiration.

A partial rebreathing mask is a flexible, cone-shaped device with a reservoir bag attached (Fig. 12-7). This mask differs from the nonrebreathing mask as there are no one-way flap valves between the bag and the exhalation ports. The partial rebreathing bag is indicated for clients with severe hypoxia and delivers an F_IO_2 of 60% to 90%.

A Venturi mask is a cone-shaped device with entrainment ports of various sizes at the base of the mask (Fig. 12-8). The entrainment ports are adjustable to permit regulation of F_IO_2 from 24% to 50%. This mask is useful because it delivers a more precise concentration of oxygen to the client (Table 12-2).

The face tent is a shieldlike device that fits under the client's chin and sweeps around the face (Fig. 12-9). Oxygen concentrations of 21% to 50% may be delivered. A concentration of 21% is delivered if the device is used with compressed air for aerosol purposes only, since atmospheric air contains 21% oxygen. When higher oxygen concentrations are desired, the flow rate is set at 10 L/min. The actual concentration of oxygen delivered will be affected by the rate and depth of the client's respirations.

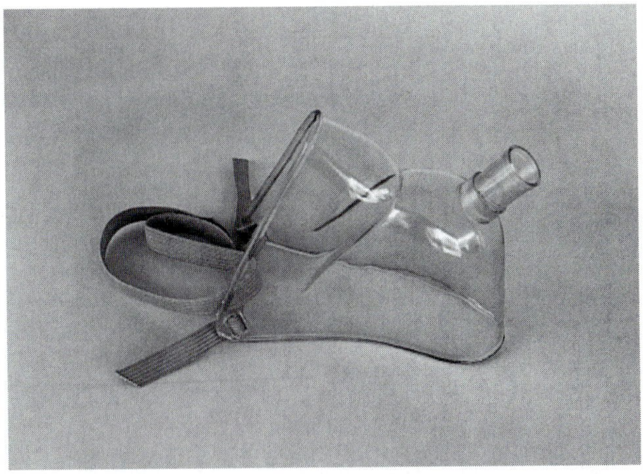

Fig. 12-9 Face tent for oxgen delivery.

Table 12-2 Venturi Mask Systems

F_IO_2 Setting	Minimal O_2 Flow Rate (L/min)
24%	4
28%	4
31%	6
35%	8
40%	8
50%	10

EQUIPMENT

- Nasal cannula or oxygen mask
- Oxygen tubing
- Humidifier, if indicated
- Sterile water for humidifier
- Oxygen source
- Oxygen flowmeter
- Appropriate room signs

DELEGATION CONSIDERATIONS

The skills of setting up and applying a nasal cannula or an oxygen mask can be delegated to appropriately trained unlicensed assistive personnel. The nurse assesses and checks device setup and client.

- Inform and assist care provider in proper way to set up and apply the oxygen delivery device.
- Instruct care provider regarding any unexpected outcomes associated with the oxygen delivery device and the need to inform nurse if any occur.

STEPS	RATIONALE
ASSESSMENT	
1. Observe for signs and symptoms associated with hypoxia.	Assessment provides the nurse with baseline data.
a. Acute changes: apprehension, anxiety, decreased level of consciousness (LOC), increased pulse rate, increased rate and depth of respiration, decreased lung sounds, elevated blood pressure, dyspnea, use of accessory muscles of respiration, and cardiac dysrhythmias.	

STEPS	RATIONALE
b. Insidious changes: pallor, increased fatigue, decreased ability to concentrate, dizziness, behavioral changes, cyanosis, clubbing, and adventitious lung sounds.	
CRITICAL DECISION POINT Clients with sudden changes in their vital signs, level of consciousness (LOC), or behavior may be experiencing profound hypoxia.	
CRITICAL DECISION POINT Clients who demonstrate changes over time may have a worsening of a chronic or an existing condition or a new medical problem. Clients with a decreased hemoglobin level may have decreased oxygenation because the hemoglobin cannot carry enough oxygen to meet physiological needs.	
2. Observe for patent airway and remove airway secretions.	Secretions can plug the airway, decreasing the amount of oxygen that is available for gas exchange in the lung.
3. If available, note client's most recent ABG results.	ABG levels objectively document the client's pH, arterial oxygen, arterial CO_2, and arterial oxygen saturation (Nelson, 1993).
CRITICAL DECISION POINT Note if the current oxygen therapy has been meeting the client's oxygenation needs. Determine what factors have changed, resulting in the new assessment findings.	
4. Review client's medical record for the medical order for oxygen, noting delivery method, flow rate, and duration of oxygen therapy.	
5. Complete respiratory system assessment (Chapter 11).	Determines presence of respiratory abnormalities impeding oxygenation.

NURSING DIAGNOSIS

Clustering of defining characteristics from the assessment data may reveal the following diagnoses for clients requiring this skill:

- Impaired gas exchange
- Ineffective breathing pattern

Related factors are individualized based on client's condition or needs.

PLANNING

STEPS	RATIONALE
1. **Expected outcomes** following completion of procedure: ➤ Client's vital signs will return to baseline. ➤ Client's work of breathing will decrease. ➤ Client will experience increased lung expansion. ➤ Client's LOC will return to baseline. ➤ ABG values or pulse oximetry measurements will return to normal or baseline. ➤ Client's nares and nasal mucosa remain intact.	Client will experience improved oxygenation.
2. Explain the procedure to client and family.	

STEPS	RATIONALE
IMPLEMENTATION	
1. Wash hands.	Reduces transmission of microorganisms.
2. Attach nasal cannula or oxygen mask to oxygen tubing.	Humidification is not used for rates less than 4 L/min. At flow rates greater than 4 L/min humidification helps prevent drying of nasal and oral mucous membranes.
3. Adjust oxygen flow rate to prescribed dosage, usually between 1 and 6 L/min.	
4. Apply oxygen delivery device and adjust elastic headband or plastic slide until it fits snugly and comfortably (see Fig. 12-4). Allow sufficient slack on oxygen tubing and secure to client's clothes.	Directs flow of oxygen into client's upper respiratory tract. Client is more likely to keep apparatus in place if it fits comfortably.
5. Observe for proper function of oxygen delivery device: a. Nasal cannula: cannula is positioned properly in the nares. b. Nonrebreathing mask: reservoir bag should fill on exhalation and not collapse on inhalation. c. Partial rebreathing mask: reservoir should fill on exhalation and not collapse on inhalation. d. Venturi mask: percentage of F_IO_2 should correlate with flow rate (see Table 12-2). e. Face tent: mist should always be present. Ensures patency of delivery device and accuracy of oxygen flow rate. f. Assess flowmeter and oxygen source for proper setup and prescribed flow rate.	
6. Monitor changes in the oxygen flow rate with pulse oximetry (see Chapter 10).	Monitoring with pulse oximetry allows for noninvasive, cost-effective trending of the client's arterial oxygen saturation and pulse rate (Hess, 1993).
CRITICAL DECISION POINT **Encourage physician to obtain ABG levels 10 to 15 minutes after initiating oxygen therapy, if indicated. ABG levels provide objective data regarding blood oxygenation and effectiveness of therapy (Chapter 43).**	
7. Wash hands.	Reduces transmission of microorganisms.
EVALUATION	
1. Observe for decreased anxiety, improved level of consciousness and cognitive abilities, decreased fatigue, absence of dizziness, decreased pulse with regular rhythm, decreased respiratory rate, return to normal blood pressure, improved color, and return to client's vital signs and level of oxygenation baseline measures.	Provides assessment of effectiveness of interventions.
2. Monitor arterial blood gas levels or observe pulse oximetry for oxygen saturation.	Documents client's level of oxygenation.
3. Assess adequacy of oxygen flow each shift.	Ensures patency of the oxygen delivery device.
4. Observe client's nares and nasal mucous membranes for evidence of skin breakdown.	Oxygen therapy can cause drying of nasal mucosa and skin breakdown where the delivery device comes in contact with the face, neck, and ears.

STEPS	RATIONALE
5. **Unexpected outcomes** that may occur include:	
➤ Client experiences skin breakdown, irritation, drying of nasal mucosa, sinus pain, or epistaxis.	One or more of these signs indicates adverse response to *method* of oxygen delivery.
➤ Client experiences continued hypoxia.	Uncorrected hypoxia can result in cardiac dysrhythmias, unconsciousness, and death.

Recording and Reporting

1. Record the respiratory assessment findings; method of oxygen delivery, flow rate, client's response; any adverse reactions or side effects; change in physician's orders.	Documents client's response to therapy and oxygen delivery method.

Follow-up Activities

1. Obtain physician's orders for follow-up pulse oximetry monitoring or ABG determinations.
2. Implement measures to maintain skin integrity (see Chapter 8).
3. Notify the physician about the continued hypoxia.

• • • • •

Special Considerations

- Clients who retain CO_2 may experience a depressed respiratory drive when oxygen flow rates greater than 2 L/min are used. Chronic **hypercapnia** reduces the body's ability to sense an elevated CO_2 level as a stimulus to increase respiration.
- Physician may order warm humidification, which increases relative humidity of inspired air to 100% at body temperature. This may increase mobilization of pulmonary secretions.
- If skin redness is observed, reduce pressure by loosening the elastic strap, changing the position of the mask, or adding padding behind the ear. If skin breakdown occurs, begin interventions to promote healing.

Teaching Considerations

- Begin discharge teaching if client is to continue oxygen therapy after discharge.
- Teach the client and family the importance of and rationale for oxygen therapy.
- Discuss safety precautions for oxygen usage (see the box on p. 424) with the client and family.
- Discuss signs of oxygen toxicity and CO_2 retention (e.g., confusion, headache, decreased LOC, somnolence, CO_2 narcosis, or respiratory arrest) (see the box on p. 423).

Gerontologic Considerations

- The arterial oxygen level falls 4 mm Hg per decade of life. A 70 year old will have a normal arterial PO_2 between 75 and 80 mm Hg (Weilitz, 1996).
- The older adult has a reduced oxygen carrying capacity (Hgb $\times$ 1.34, the amount in cubic centimeters of oxygen each hemoglobin molecule can carry) due to a decreased hemoglobin level.

Home Care Considerations

- The client and family must know how to use the oxygen delivery system (e.g., cylinders, concentration, or liquid oxygen) and delivery device.
- Teach family members what changes the client may demonstrate that indicate worsening hypoxia.
- Oxygen tubings in the home setting are available in lengths of 15 m (50 feet).

SKILL 12-2 Administering Oxygen Therapy to a Client with an Artificial Airway

Clients with an artificial airway require constant humidification to the airway. An artificial airway bypasses the normal filtering and humidification process of the nose and mouth. The two devices that supply humidified gas to an artificial airway are a T tube and a tracheostomy collar.

The **T tube,** also called a Briggs adaptor, is a T-shaped device with a 15 mm (3⁄5 inch) connection which connects an oxygen source to an artificial airway, e.g., endotracheal (ET) tube or tracheostomy (Fig. 12-10). The recommended flow rate is 10 L/min with a nebulizer set to the appropriate F_IO_2.

A **tracheostomy collar** is a curved device with an adjustable strap that fits around the client's neck (Fig. 12-11). There are two ports: an exhalation port that remains patent at all times and the port that connects to the oxygen source with large-bore tubing. The flow rate is set at 10 L/min with a nebulizer set to the appropriate F_IO_2 that provides humidification to the lower airways via the tracheostomy tube opening.

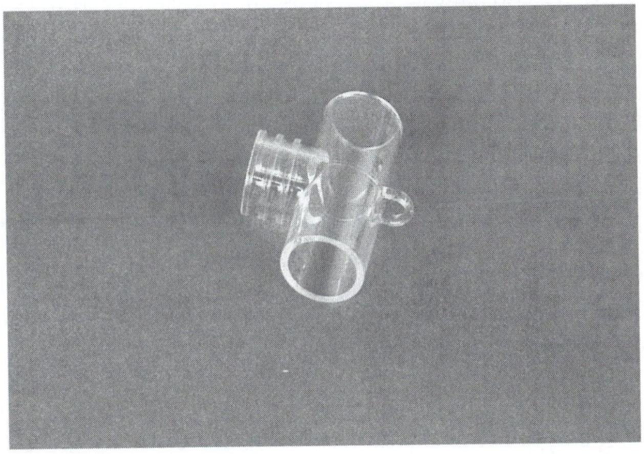

Fig. 12-10 T tube.

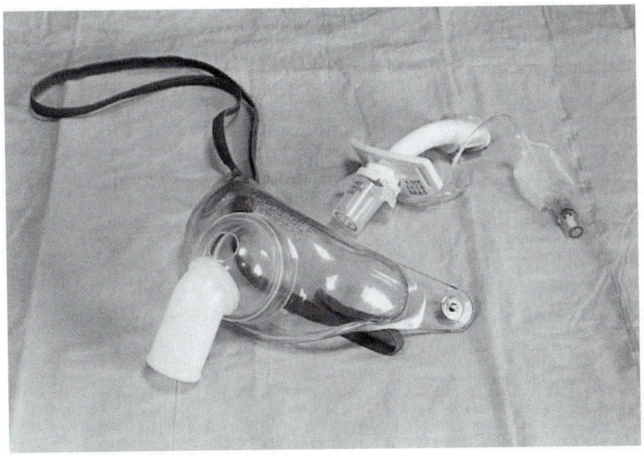

Fig. 12-11 Tracheostomy collar.

EQUIPMENT

- **T tube or tracheostomy collar**
- **Large-bore oxygen tubing**
- **Nebulizer**
- **Sterile water for nebulizer**
- **Oxygen or gas source**
- **Gloves**
- **Flowmeter**
- **"Oxygen in use" sign**

DELEGATION CONSIDERATIONS

The skills of setting up and applying a T tube or a tracheostomy collar to a client with an artificial airway can be delegated to appropriately trained unlicensed assistive personnel. The nurse assesses and checks the device setup and the client.

- Inform and assist care provider in proper way to set up and apply T tube or tracheostomy collar.
- Instruct care provider regarding any unexpected outcomes associated with the oxygen delivery device and the need to inform nurse if any occur.

STEPS	RATIONALE
ASSESSMENT	
1. Observe for signs and symptoms associated with hypoxia.	Assessment provides the nurse with baseline data.
a. Acute changes: apprehension, anxiety, decreased LOC, increased pulse rate, increased rate and depth of respiration, decreased lung sounds, elevated blood pressure, dyspnea, use of accessory muscles of respiration, and cardiac dysrhythmias.	Clients with sudden changes in their vital signs, LOC, or behavior may be experiencing profound hypoxia.
b. Insidious changes: pallor, increased fatigue, decreased ability to concentrate, dizziness, behavioral changes, cyanosis, clubbing, and adventitious lung sounds.	Clients who demonstrate changes over time may have a worsening of a chronic or an existing condition or a new medical problem.
➤ **CRITICAL DECISION POINT** Clients with a decreased hemoglobin level may have decreased oxygenation because the hemoglobin cannot carry enough oxygen to meet physiological needs.	
2. Observe for patent airway and remove airway secretions.	Secretions can plug the airway, decreasing the amount of oxygen that is available for gas exchange in the lung. Secretions can also occlude the T tube or tracheostomy collar, impeding oxygen delivery to the client (see Chapter 14).
3. If available, note client's most recent ABG results.	ABG levels objectively document the client's pH, arterial oxygen, arterial CO_2, and arterial oxygen saturation.
➤ **CRITICAL DECISION POINT** Note if the current oxygen therapy has been meeting the client's oxygenation needs. Determine what factors have changed, resulting in the new assessment findings.	
4. Review client's medical record for the medical order for oxygen, noting delivery method, flow rate, and duration of oxygen therapy.	
5. Complete total respiratory system assessment (Chapter 11).	Determines presence of respiratory abnormalities impeding oxygenation.

NURSING DIAGNOSIS

Clustering of defining characteristics from the assessment data may reveal the following diagnoses for clients requiring this skill:

- ➤ Impaired gas exchange
- ➤ Ineffective breathing pattern
- ➤ Ineffective airway clearance

Related factors are individualized based on client's condition or needs.

PLANNING

STEPS	RATIONALE
1. **Expected outcomes** following completion of procedure: ➤ Client's vital signs will return to baseline. ➤ Client's work of breathing will decrease. ➤ Client will experience increased lung expansion. ➤ Client's LOC will return to baseline. ➤ ABG values or pulse oximetry measurements will return to normal or baseline.	Client will experience improved oxygenation.
2. Explain the purpose of the T tube or tracheostomy collar to the client and family.	Explanation decreases the client's anxiety and reduces oxygen consumption.

STEPS	RATIONALE
IMPLEMENTATION	
1. Wash hands, apply gloves, and apply goggles.	Reduces transmission of microorganisms and prevents contact with pulmonary secretions.
CRITICAL DECISION POINT Clients with excessive secretions or forceful productive coughs place the care giver at risk for contact with pulmonary secretions.	
2. Attach T tube or tracheostomy collar to large-bore oxygen tubing and to humidified room air or oxygen source, if indicated.	Provides supplemental humidification to avoid drying of the airway.
3. If oxygen is ordered, adjust flow rate to 10 L/min or as ordered, adjust nebulizer to proper F_IO_2 setting, and attach T tube or tracheostomy collar to endotracheal or tracheostomy tube.	Flow rate ensures humidification; nebulizer regulates F_IO_2.
4. Monitor changes in the oxygen flow rate with pulse oximetry (see Chapter 10).	Monitoring with pulse oximetry allows for noninvasive, cost-effective trending of the client's arterial oxygen saturation and pulse rate.
CRITICAL DECISION POINT Encourage physician to obtain ABG values 10 to 15 minutes after initiating oxygen therapy. ABG values provide objective data regarding blood oxygenation and effectiveness of therapy (Chapter 43).	
5. Observe that T tube does not pull on endotracheal or tracheostomy tube. Observe for secretions within T tube or tracheostomy collar and suction as necessary (Chapter 14).	Pulling effect can increase client's discomfort and cause pressure to side of client's mouth or tracheal stoma. Maintains patent airway.
6. Observe oxygen tubing frequently for accumulation of fluid. If fluid is present, drain tube away from client and discard fluid in proper receptacle.	Excess water is medium for bacterial growth. Draining contaminated water into proper receptacle prevents contamination of entire humidifying unit.
7. Set up suction equipment at client's bedside.	Client may experience increased airway secretions due to humidification.
8. Remove gloves and goggles; wash hands.	Reduces transmission of microorganisms and contamination with pulmonary secretions.
EVALUATION	
1. Observe for decreased anxiety, improved LOC and cognitive abilities, decreased fatigue, absence of dizziness, decreased pulse with regular rhythm, decreased respiratory rate, return to normal blood pressure, improved color, and return to client's vital signs and level of oxygenation baseline measures.	Provides assessment of effectiveness of interventions.
2. Observe the position of the oxygen delivery device to ensure that it is not pulling on the artificial airway.	Pulling on the artificial airway may result in damage to the oral cavity or stoma.
3. Monitor arterial blood gas levels or observe pulse oximetry.	Documents client's level of oxygenation.
4. **Unexpected outcomes** that may occur include:	
➤ Client experiences stoma irritation; thick, tenacious secretions; pressure areas on neck or near stoma site.	One or more of these indicates adverse response to *method* of oxygen delivery.
➤ Client experiences continued hypoxia.	Uncorrected hypoxia can result in cardiac dysrhythmias, coma, and death.

STEPS	RATIONALE
➤ ***CRITICAL DECISION POINT*** **Determine if the cause of the continued hypoxia is the oxygen delivery device, plugging of the airway, the oxygen flow rate, or a new clinical problem.**	

RECORDING AND REPORTING

1. Record the respiratory assessment findings; method of oxygen delivery, flow rate, client's response; any adverse reactions or side effects; change in physician's orders.	Documents method of oxygen therapy and client's response.

FOLLOW-UP ACTIVITIES

1. Suction secretions from artificial airway and lungs as indicated.
2. Begin discharge planning if client is to receive oxygen therapy after discharge.
3. Implement measures to maintain skin integrity (see Chapter 8).
4. Notify the physician about the continued hypoxia.

• • • • •

Special Considerations

- ➤ Make sure oxygen tubing is long enough to provide for client's mobility needs.
- ➤ Humidified air is frequently warmed to increase relative humidity of inspired air to 100% at body temperature.
- ➤ Humidification of airway secretions reduces irritation of the mucosa and may increase ease of secretion removal.
- ➤ Excessive accumulation of water in oxygen tubing occurs more frequently at higher humidities.
- ➤ The T tube is designed to fit a 15 mm tracheostomy tube. Adapters are used to connect a smaller tracheostomy tube to the T tube.

Teaching Considerations

- ➤ Teach the client and family alternative communication techniques (Chapter 2) to enhance communication with care givers and to reduce frustration.
- ➤ Teach the client and family the importance of and rationale for the oxygen therapy.
- ➤ Teach the client and family safety precautions for oxygen use (see box on p. 424).
- ➤ Teach the client and family signs and symptoms of oxygen toxicity and CO_2 retention (e.g., confusion, headache, decreased LOC, or somnolence) (see box on p. 423).

Home Care Considerations

- ➤ The client with an artificial airway who is at home may have a permanent tracheostomy, as well as a T tube or a tracheostomy collar.
- ➤ The client or care giver should be able to perform tracheostomy care and suctioning techniques (Chapter 14).

SKILL 12-3 *Using Incentive Spirometry*

Incentive spirometry assists the client in deep breathing. An incentive spirometer (IS) is most often used following abdominal or thoracic surgery to help reduce the incidence of postoperative complications (Wall, 1995). Postoperative deep breathing and coughing have been shown to be as effective as using an incentive spirometer (Bell, 1993) when performed frequently. The advantage of the IS is the visual feedback to clients about the depth of their breaths. The two types of spirometers are flow oriented and volume oriented.

Flow-oriented ISs have one or more plastic chambers with freely movable, colored balls. As the client inhales slowly, the balls are elevated to a premarked area (Fig. 12-12). The goal is to keep the balls elevated for as long as possible to ensure maximal sustained inhalation, not to snap the balls to the top of the chamber with a rapid, very brief, low-volume breath. Even if a very slow inspiration does not elevate the balls, this pattern may achieve greater lung expansion. The advantage of a flow-oriented IS is the slow, steady expansion of the lung.

Volume-oriented ISs have a bellows that the client must raise to a predetermined volume by inhaling slowly (Fig.

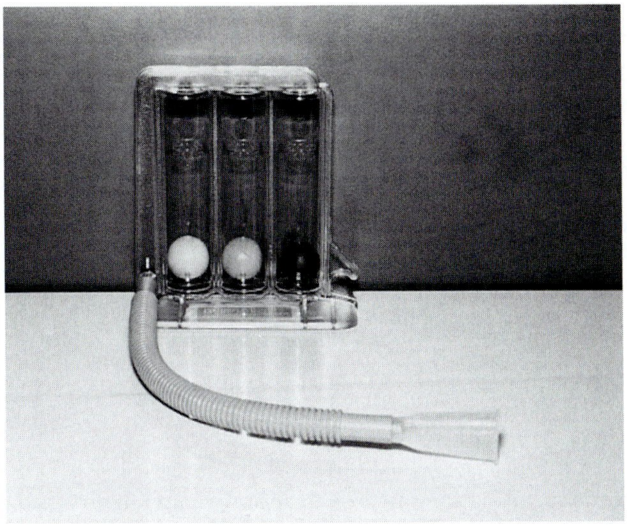

Fig. 12-12 Flow-oriented incentive spirometer.

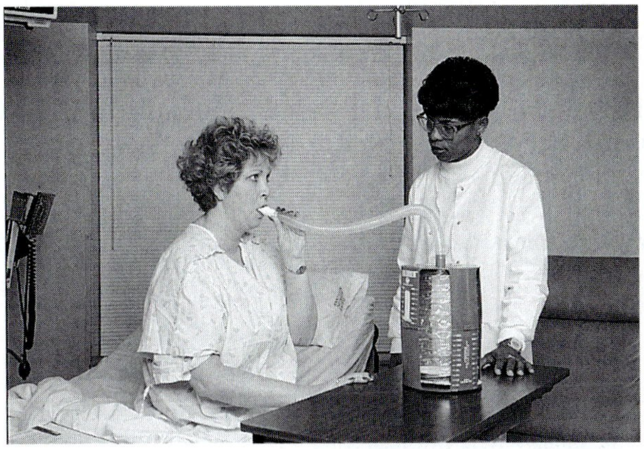

Fig. 12-13 Volume-oriented incentive spirometer.

12-13). An achievement light or counter is used to provide feedback to the client. Some devices have a marker that moves up as the client inhales. The advantage of the volume-oriented IS is that a known inspiratory volume can be achieved and measured with each breath.

The use of the IS encourages clients to breathe deeply and achieve their normal inspiratory capacity. Incentive spirometry is used most often with postoperative clients. It is helpful to determine the client's baseline preoperative inspiratory capacity. An inspiratory volume one half to three quarters of baseline is an acceptable postoperative volume. Clients benefiting from incentive spirometry include those using it preoperatively, especially before abdominal, cardiac, or orthopedic surgery; clients with a history of smoking, pneumonia, or chronic respiratory disease; and clients with atelectasis.

EQUIPMENT

- **Flow-oriented IS or volume-oriented IS**

DELEGATION CONSIDERATIONS

The skill of assisting a client with incentive spirometry can be delegated to appropriately trained unlicensed assistive personnel. The nurse assesses and checks the device setup and the client following implementation.

- Inform and assist the care provider in the proper way to set up and use the IS.
- Inform the care provider of client's target goal for spirometry.

STEPS	RATIONALE
ASSESSMENT	
1. Identify clients who would benefit from incentive spirometry (e.g., postoperative clients, clients recovering from chest trauma, or clients with pneumonia or atelectasis).	Alerts health care personnel to those clients at risk for respiratory complications during illness or postoperatively.
2. Assess client's respiratory status, including symmetry of chest wall expansion, respiratory rate and depth, sputum production, and lung sounds (Chapter 11).	Decreased chest wall movement, crackles or decreased lung sounds, increased respiratory rate, or increased sputum production can indicate a need for incentive spirometry or other respiratory maneuvers to improve lung expansion.
3. Review the physician's order for incentive spirometry.	Health care institutions frequently require a medical order for incentive spirometry in order to receive third-party reimbursement for the spirometer.

STEPS	RATIONALE

NURSING DIAGNOSIS

Clustering of defining characteristics from the assessment data may reveal the following nursing diagnoses for clients requiring this skill:

- Impaired gas exchange
- Ineffective breathing pattern
- Ineffective airway clearance

Related factors are individualized based on client's condition or needs.

PLANNING

1. **Expected outcomes** following completion of procedure:
   - Client will demonstrate correct use of the IS.
   - Client will demonstrate increased lung expansion.
   - Client achieves target volume.
   - Client has normal breath sounds.
2. Explain the procedure to the client and family.
   Rationale: Understanding the purpose of incentive spirometry and its proper use will improve compliance with use.

IMPLEMENTATION

1. Wash hands.
   Rationale: Reduces transmission of microorganisms.
2. Instruct client to assume semi-Fowler's or high Fowler's position.
   Rationale: Promotes optimal lung expansion during respiratory maneuver.
3. Demonstrate how to place lips to completely cover mouthpiece.
   Rationale: Demonstration is a reliable technique for teaching psychomotor skill and enables client to ask questions.
4. Instruct client to inhale slowly and maintain a constant flow, like pulling through a straw. When maximal inspiration is reached, client should hold breath for 2 to 3 seconds and then exhale slowly.
   Rationale: Maintains maximal inspiration; reduces risk of progressive collapse of individual alveoli.

> ***CRITICAL DECISION POINT*** **Clients should rest between IS breaths to prevent hyperventilation and fatigue.**

5. Have client repeat the maneuver until goals are achieved.
   Rationale: Ensures correct use of the spirometer and client's understanding of use.
6. Wash hands.
   Rationale: Reduces transmission of microorganisms.

EVALUATION

1. Observe client's ability to use incentive spirometry by return demonstration.
   Rationale: Determines client's ability to perform breathing exercise correctly.
2. Assess if the client is able to achieve the target volume or frequency.
   Rationale: Measures compliance with therapy.
3. Auscultate chest during respiratory cycle.
   Rationale: Documents chest wall expansion and identifies any abnormal lung sounds.
4. **Unexpected outcomes** that may occur include:
   - Client is unable to achieve incentive spirometry target volumes and frequency independently.
   - Client has decreased lung expansion.
     Rationale: At risk for retained pulmonary secretions.
   - Client has abnormal breath sounds.
     Rationale: Indicates atelectasis and/or retained secretions.

RECORDING AND REPORTING

1. Record the lung sounds before and after incentive spirometry, the frequency of use, the volumes achieved, and any adverse effects.
   Rationale: Documents treatment received; may be used for third-party reimbursements.

FOLLOW-UP ACTIVITIES

1. After IS exercises, clients should practice cough control techniques (Chapter 13).
2. Provide assistance with suctioning if clients cannot effectively cough up their secretions.

• • • • •

Special Considerations

- Clients with flail chest require other respiratory maneuvers to correct asymmetrical chest wall motion.
- Clients who may experience difficulty with incentive spirometry include those who are confused, malnourished, or cognitively impaired and those who lack necessary motor skills.
- Use a nose clip if client is unable to breathe through the mouthpiece.

Teaching Considerations

- Teach client to examine sputum for consistency, amount, and color changes.
- Identify learning objectives for preparing client to use the IS: correctly places the mouthpiece; achieves satisfactory maximal inspiration; repeats the maneuver the required number of times; and understands the rationale for performing incentive spirometry.

Gerontologic Considerations

- Older adults may have difficulty coordinating the use of the IS. They may require additional time to learn the procedure; however, once they understand and learn the procedure, they will be very capable of continuing with the plan.
- The older adult has an increased respiratory rate, between 16 and 25 breaths per minute. Observe closely for hyperventilation and fatigue.

Home Care Considerations

- Have client return demonstrate correct procedure for use before discharge.

SKILL 12-4 Administering Mechanical Ventilation

Clients requiring mechanical ventilation need support for ventilation and/or oxygenation. Clinical problems such as respiratory failure, exacerbation of chronic obstructive lung disease, status asthmaticus, Guillain-Barré syndrome, spinal cord trauma, respiratory muscle paralysis, and pneumonia may require mechanical ventilation support. Clients requiring acute mechanical ventilation are most often cared for in an intensive care unit. An endotracheal tube (ETT) or a tracheostomy tube will need to be placed to attach the ventilator.

There are two types of mechanical ventilation: positive pressure and negative pressure. Positive pressure ventilation is the usual method of ventilation. **Positive pressure ventilation** delivers a positive pressure to inflate the lungs. The increased positive intrathoracic pressure may impede venous return to the right side of the heart, resulting in a decreased cardiac output, tachycardia, and hypotension. The nurse must be alert for these side effects.

Negative pressure ventilation is used for clients with primary neuromuscular illnesses that interfere with normal respiratory muscle function, such as multiple sclerosis, muscular dystrophy, and early stages of COPD. The client is fitted with a poncho or shell that is connected to the ventilator. Air is removed from between the client's chest wall and the interior wall of the poncho or shell, causing the client to inhale. The client using negative pressure ventilation does not need an artificial airway.

Many types of mechanical ventilators are available for acute care use. Mechanical ventilators are available in pressure-cycled and volume-cycled machines. **Pressure-cycled ventilation** delivers a specified pressure to the client, achieving a **tidal volume,** or amount of air, in milliters, per breath (Fig. 12-14). **Volume-cycled ventilation** delivers a specified tidal volume. Volume-cycled ventilators are most often used in the clinical setting. Clients using pressure-cycled ventilators are at higher risk for development of pneumothorax, hypotension, and decreased cardiac output as a result of the ventilator's achieving the prescribed pressure without regard for lung compliance. Volume-cycled ventilators achieve tidal volume with preset pressure limits and are more sensitive to lung compliance. Time-cycled ventilators provide an inspiratory phase until a preset time is reached. This often results in varying tidal volumes.

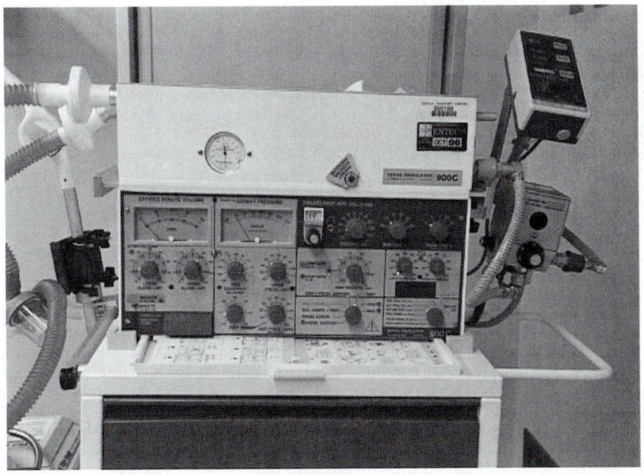

Fig. 12-14 Pressure-cycled mechanical ventilation.

MODES OF VENTILATION

There are many different modes of mechanical ventilation to support different conditions and physiological processes. Modes of ventilation include control mode (CM), continuous mandatory ventilation (CMV), synchronized intermittent mandatory ventilation (SIMV), and pressure support ventilation (PSV). CMV, SIMV and PSV are the more frequently used modes of ventilation. They support oxygenation and provide varying levels of ventilatory support that can be adjusted to meet the client's needs (Table 12-3). CMV provides continuous ventilation to the client, maintaining the respiratory rate and tidal volume. SIMV attempts to synchronize the ventilator breaths with the client's spontaneous breathing. This reduces competition between the ventilator and the client.

PSV is actually a spontaneous breathing mode, because the ventilator does not deliver a preset tidal volume or rate. PSV provides a preset pressure to augment the inspiratory process and help overcome the initial work of breathing. It is used both for ventilation and to assist in weaning the client. Clients on PSV need to be assessed frequently for respiratory muscle fatigue and potential periods of apnea.

Positive end-expiratory pressure (PEEP) and CPAP are adjuncts to ventilation used to increase oxygenation. PEEP is positive airway pressure maintained at the end of exhalation. This allows more time for gas exchange and opens small airways and closed alveolar units, thus improving oxygenation. CPAP is the maintenance of a positive airway pressure above atmospheric pressure during inspiration and expiration in the spontaneously breathing client. CPAP improves oxygenation in the same manner as PEEP.

ALARMS AND SETTINGS

The mechanical ventilator has a number of settings to adjust the amount of oxygen delivered, the amount of tidal volume, the time for inspiration and expiration, and the pressure at which each breath is delivered. The tidal volume, the amount of air per breath, is usually set at 10 to 15 ml/kg body weight. The respiratory rate is usually set at 10 to 16 breaths per minute. Initially the oxygen may be set at 100% if the reason for intubation and ventilation was cardiopulmonary arrest. The goal of providing oxygenation is to maintain an arterial PO_2 of greater than or equal to 60 mm Hg using an FiO_2 of 50% or less. Table 12-4 lists the ventilator parameters the nurse must become familiar with to care for a client on mechanical ventilation.

There are a number of alarms on the ventilator to ensure client safety. Each ventilator is a little different; however, the basic alarms are similar. Alarms common to all ventilators include high pressure, low pressure, low exhaled volume, and oxygen alarms (Table 12-5). The nurse must know how to respond to the ventilator alarms and what nursing actions may be required to preserve the client's respiratory status. The two most frequent alarms are the high pressure and low pressure alarms. The high pres-

Table 12-3 Modes of Mechanical Ventilation

Mode	Definition	Indications	Comments
Control mode (CM)	Preset tidal volume and preset rate delivered to the client regardless of the client's respiratory effort. Client cannot initiate breaths or change the ventilatory pattern.	Neuromuscular disease Drug overdose Reduction of work of breathing	Client may require sedation to reduce competition with the ventilator. Rarely used.
Continuous mandatory ventilation (CMV)	Preset tidal volume at preset rate is delivered to the client. The client can initiate breaths that are delivered at the preset tidal volume.	Reduction of work of breathing Respiratory muscle fatigue COPD Postanesthesia	Client may need sedation to reduce spontaneous breaths.
Synchronized intermittent mandatory ventilation (SIMV)	Preset tidal volume at preset rate is synchronized with the client's spontaneous breathing to reduce competition between machine-delivered and client-spontaneous breaths.	Primary ventilatory mode Used to wean clients from mechanical ventilation	Client synchrony with the ventilator is improved. Rates ≤6 can result in increased work of breathing.
Pressure support ventilation (PSV)	Provides positive pressure during the inspiratory cycle of a spontaneous inspiratory effort (Weilitz, 1996).	Weaning clients with COPD Primary ventilatory mode in higher pressures	There is no preset respiratory rate. The nurse must assess for respiratory muscle fatigue and periods of apnea. Decreases work of breathing by overcoming resistance of airway and ventilatory circuit.

Table 12-4 Ventilator Parameters

Parameter	Definition	Ventilator Setting
Tidal volume (V_T)	Amount of air inspired and expired with each breath	10 to 15 ml/kg of body weight
Respiratory rate (R or RR)	Number of breaths delivered per minute	10 to 16 breaths per minute
Fraction of inspired oxygen (FIO_2)	Amount of oxygen the client receives	21% to 100% to maintain PaO_2 60 to 80 torr
PEEP	Positive pressure applied at end expiration to improve oxygenation	+3 to 5 cm H_2O may be used to approximate physiological PEEP* May require higher levels (>5 cm H_2O) in respiratory failure (e.g., ARDS)
Sigh	Larger than normal breath to provide hyperinflation; helps prevent atelectasis	Usually twice the tidal volume breath; about 10 to 15 ml/kg Rate is usually set at 10 to 15 times per hour
Sensitivity	Determines the inspiratory effort required to trigger the ventilator	Set to respond to an inspired volume of less than 1% of the client's tidal volume
Peak airway pressure	The maximal pressure level required to deliver the desired tidal volume	<40 cm H_2O
I:E ratio	Comparison of inspiratory (I) to expiratory (E) time	Normally set 1:1, 1:2, or 1:3 Example: inspiration 2 seconds, expiration 4 seconds; then I:E = 1:2
Exhaled minute ventilation (V_E)	Measures the exhaled minute ventilations in liters	Alarm set at 15% greater than client's average V_E

*Some clinicians believe that the ETT with inflated cuff creates a closed system with the ventilator and does not require 3 to 5 cm of PEEP.

Table 12-5 Troubleshooting Mechanical Ventilation

Ventilator Alarm	Possible Cause	Nursing Interventions
Sudden increase in peak airway pressure (high pressure alarm)	Coughing Airway plugging	Clear secretions by suctioning
	Changes in client position	Reposition client
	Pneumothorax	Assess breath sounds and chest wall movement
	Incorrect ETT position	Verify placement of ETT Assess breath sounds Verify cm level of ETT
	Kinked ventilator circuit	Check circuit; unkink tubing
	Excessive water in ventilator circuit	Drain ventilator tubing
Gradual increase in peak airway pressure	Decreasing lung compliance	Evaluate breath sounds; suction
	Exacerbation of acute process	Check for reversible causes: airway plugging, bronchospasm
Sudden decrease in peak airway pressure (low pressure alarm)	Client disconnected from ventilator	Check for disconnection
	Leak in ventilator circuit	Evaluate circuit connections; tighten loose connections
Change in minute ventilation or tidal volume	Leak in ETT cuff	Check cuff seal
Decrease	Airway secretions	Suction excessive secretions
	System leak	Check circuit connections
	Increased respiratory rate	Evaluate respiratory rate
Increase	Hypoxia	Evaluate for signs of hypoxia. Evaluate need to obtain ABG sample or monitor pulse oximetry
Change in respiratory rate	Client anxiety	Reassure client
	Increased metabolic demand	Evaluate body temperature, heart rate, and rhythm
	Hypoxia	Obtain ABG levels or monitor pulse oximetry

sure alarm is usually set at 10 to 15 cm greater than the peak airway pressure. When this alarm sounds, it indicates the ventilator has met resistance to delivering the tidal volume and requires more pressure to inflate the lungs. The client may have coughed during the inspiratory cycle, may need suctioning, or may have changed position. More acute problems that require immediate nursing intervention include the development of a pneumothorax or displacement of the ETT or tracheostomy tube. The low pressure alarm sounds when the ventilator has no resistance to inflating the lung. The client may be disconnected from the ventilator, or a leak has developed in the ventilator circuit.

Once the condition for which the client required mechanical ventilation is corrected, the weaning process is initiated. Weaning from mechanical ventilation is the gradual reduction of ventilation and oxygenation support until the client is breathing spontaneously and can be oxygenated with a low-flow oxygen device. Many clients who are unable to wean from the mechanical ventilator may be transferred to subacute nursing care for continued care or in preparation for home mechanical ventilation. Generally these clients are hemodynamically stable; however, they require continual ventilatory support.

The mechanical ventilator also has settings to regulate the temperature of the water in the humidifier, known as the cascade. The temperature of the heater in the cascade is set at or just below normal body temperature. This provides warm, moistened air for delivery to the airway. The cascade is a potential source of contamination of the ventilator circuit if the water that collects in the ventilator tubing is drained back into the cascade unit.

HOME MECHANICAL VENTILATION

The client on mechanical ventilation can be successfully managed in the home. Neuromuscular disease such as amyotrophic lateral sclerosis (ALS), muscular dystrophy, brain and spinal cord diseases, chest wall disease, central hypoventilation syndrome, and advanced COPD are just a few of the diseases for which clients are managed at home on mechanical ventilators. Many factors determine if a client and family are candidates for home ventilation. Assessment criteria include the desire of the client and family, the client's acceptance of ventilator dependence, the client's and family's ability to understand and perform daily care procedures, the home environment, personnel resources, monetary resources, and resources and technologies for support in the community.

The goals of long-term ventilator care should include extension of life, enhancement of the quality of life, provision of an environment that enhances individual potential, reduction of morbidity, improvement of physical and physiological function, and cost-effectiveness. Clients and families who are candidates for home mechanical ventilation should be prepared for discharge by a multidisciplinary team including representatives of nursing, medicine, dietary service, social service, the home health nurse, and the home care durable medical equipment company. The nurse in the hospital must be familiar with the home ventilator to assist the client with discharge planning and education.

EQUIPMENT

- **Appropriate mechanical ventilator**
- **50 psi oxygen source**
- **Ventilator circuit**
- **Humidification source**
- **Heated passover system**
- **Artificial nose**
- **Heated wire system**
- **Ambu-bag with oxygen connecting tubing and flowmeter**
- **Gloves**

DELEGATION CONSIDERATIONS

The skill of administering mechanical ventilation requires problem solving and knowledge application unique to a professional nurse. For this skill delegation is inappropriate.

STEPS	RATIONALE
ASSESSMENT	
1. Observe for signs and symptoms associated with hypoxia.	Assessment provides the nurse with baseline data.
a. Acute changes: apprehension, anxiety, decreased LOC, increased pulse rate, increased rate and depth of respiration, decreased lung sounds, elevated blood pressure, dyspnea, use of accessory muscles of respiration, and cardiac dysrhythmias.	Clients with sudden changes in their vital signs, LOC, or behavior may be experiencing profound hypoxia.
b. Insidious changes: pallor, increased fatigue, decreased ability to concentrate, dizziness, behavioral changes, cyanosis, clubbing, and adventitious lung sounds.	Clients who demonstrate changes over time may have a worsening of a chronic or an existing condition or a new medical problem.

STEPS	RATIONALE
2. Observe for patent airway and remove airway secretions.	Secretions can plug the airway, decreasing the amount of oxygen that is available for gas exchange in the lung. Secretions can also occlude the T tube or tracheostomy collar, impeding oxygen delivery to the client.
3. If available, note client's most recent ABG results.	ABG values objectively document the client's pH, arterial oxygen, arterial CO_2, and arterial oxygen saturation.

➤ *CRITICAL DECISION POINT* **Note if the current ventilation therapy is meeting the client's oxygenation and ventilation needs. Determine what factors have changed, resulting in the new assessment findings.**

STEPS	RATIONALE
4. Review client's medical record for the medical order for mechanical ventilation, noting mode of ventilation, respiratory rate, oxygen setting, and tidal volume.	
5. Complete total respiratory system assessment (Chapter 11).	Determines presence of respiratory abnormalities impeding oxygenation and ventilation.

NURSING DIAGNOSIS

Clustering of defining characteristics from the assessment data may reveal the following nursing diagnoses for clients requiring this skill:

- Impaired gas exchange
- Ineffective breathing pattern
- Ineffective airway clearance
- Inability to sustain spontaneous ventilation
- Dysfunctional ventilatory weaning response
- Risk for infection

Related factors are individualized based on client's condition or needs.

PLANNING

STEPS	RATIONALE
1. Expected outcomes following completion of procedure: ➤ Client will have increased lung expansion. ➤ Client will maintain ABG levels and pulse oximetry measurements within normal range or at baseline. ➤ Client experiences reduction in feelings of dyspnea and work of breathing. ➤ Client uses communication board, paper and pencil, or computer to state needs.	Client experiences improved oxygenation and ventilation.
2. Explain to client and family the purpose and reasons for initiation of mechanical ventilation.	

IMPLEMENTATION

STEPS	RATIONALE
1. Wash hands; apply gloves and goggles.	Reduces transmission of microorganisms and exposure to pulmonary secretions.
2. Attach mechanical ventilator to ETT or tracheostomy tube. Observe for proper functioning of mechanical ventilator.	Ensures client is receiving proper mechanical ventilation.

➤ *CRITICAL DECISION POINT* **The mechanical ventilator requires programming of accurate settings before attaching to the client. This is most often the responsibility of the respiratory therapist; however, it may also be a collaborative responsibility of the nurse.**

STEPS	RATIONALE
➤ ***CRITICAL DECISION POINT*** **Verify that the ETT or tracheostomy tube is properly positioned by listening to both lungs and assessing chest wall symmetry.**	
3. Observe client for synchronization with mechanical ventilation and response to therapy.	Ensures client is comfortable using ventilator and has not experienced any adverse hemodynamic effects.
➤ ***CRITICAL DECISION POINT*** **Monitor heart rate, blood pressure, respiratory rate, and cardiac rhythm. Implementation of mechanical ventilation can result in decreased venous return and associated hemodynamic changes.**	
4. Secure ventilator tubing to reduce pull on tracheostomy or ET tube.	Prevents accidental dislodging of artificial airway.
➤ ***CRITICAL DECISION POINT*** **Note the level of the ETT at the lips or nares to provide a baseline for depth of tube placement.**	
5. Set up suction equipment.	Need to provide airway care and suctioning as needed of ET or tracheostomy tube to prevent plugging of the airway and to reduce the risk of infection.
➤ ***CRITICAL DECISION POINT*** **Determine if the client will need an oral suction setup as well as endotracheal suctioning.**	
6. Collaborate with the physician frequently about the status of the client and the response to therapy.	
➤ ***CRITICAL DECISION POINT*** **Encourage the physician to obtain ABG levels 10 to 15 minutes after initiation of therapy or a change in ventilator setting. ABG levels provide objective data regarding oxygenation and ventilation.**	
7. Remove gloves and goggles; wash hands.	Reduces transmission of microorganisms and exposure to pulmonary secretions.

EVALUATION

1. Evaluate client's response to mechanical ventilation. Observe for decreased anxiety; improved LOC and cognitive abilities; decreased fatigue; absence of dizziness; decreased pulse, regular rhythm; decreased respiratory rate and work of breathing; return to normal blood pressure; improved color.	Hypoxia and hypercapnea are reduced or corrected.
2. Monitor ABG levels—observe pulse oximetry.	Documents client's level of oxygenation.
3. Observe integrity of client ventilator system.	Ensures adequate delivery of mechanical ventilation.
4. Observe client's communication with staff, family, and friends.	Documents the effectiveness and efficiency of communication measures.
5. **Unexpected outcomes** that may occur include:	
➤ Client experiences stiff, noncompliant lung; alveolar edema; pulmonary congestion; chest pain; intraalveolar hemorrhage; substernal chest pain; pneumothorax; continued decrease in blood pressure related to use of positive pressure.	Signs and symptoms of **oxygen toxicity.** Physician should be notified at once.
➤ Hypoxia.	Continued hypoxia can result in anxiety, ineffective breathing patterns, decreased LOC, decreased cardiac output, cardiac dysrhythmias, and death.

STEPS	RATIONALE
➤ Hypercapnia.	Continued hypercapnia can result in decreased level of consciousness, cardiac dysrhythmias, respiratory arrest, and death.

RECORDING AND REPORTING

1. Record the respiratory assessment findings, mode of mechanical ventilation, oxygen level, actual client tidal volume, ordered tidal volume, actual client respiratory rate, ordered respiratory rate, peak airway pressure, client's response to mechanical ventilation, level of the ETT, any adverse reactions or side effects, and change in the physician's orders.	Documents therapy received and the client's response.

FOLLOW-UP ACTIVITIES

1. Provide ETT care/tracheostomy care (Skills 14-3 through 14-8).
2. Monitor client's response to therapy by reviewing pulse oximetry measurements, chest x-ray films, and arterial blood gas levels.

• • • • •

Special Considerations

- Clients need a period of adjustment to be comfortable on mechanical ventilation.
- Frequent visits by the nurse and quick responses to call bells will help alleviate fears.
- Frequent airway care is necessary to prevent clogging of artificial airway with secretions.
- Frequent oral care is necessary to prevent infection and subsequent contamination of the airway.
- Before turning client, empty water that has accumulated in the ventilator tubing to prevent accidental dumping of water into airway. Empty water away from the ventilator cascade.

Teaching Considerations

- The client and family are taught about the rationale for mechanical ventilation.
- Teach the client and family about the alarms and what they mean.
- Teach the client and family alternative communication techniques to reduce frustration and fear.

Home Care Considerations

- Clients requiring home mechanical ventilation need to be taught complete care of the mechanical ventilator system, suctioning, and artificial airway care. Skills include assembling the ventilator circuit, cleaning the circuit, and daily equipment maintenance (Rice, 1995).
- The client and family should have a thorough knowledge of the operation of the home ventilator, the knobs and settings, and the power sources.
- Use a checklist for ensuring consistency of care for the client on a ventilator.
- Evaluate the following areas during each visit: oxygen flow, alarm system, inspiratory pressure, high pressure alarm, tidal volume setting, humidifier, respiratory rate, tubing, temperature, resuscitation bag, tracheostomy care, breath sounds, suctioning, and tubing changes.
- The durable medical equipment provider, the home health nurse, and the primary care nurse should develop a teaching plan to ensure that the client and family have a complete working knowledge of the ventilator before discharge.
- Instruct the client and primary care giver about what to do in case of respiratory distress or power failure. Check to determine availability of emergency batteries.
- Instruct the family on use of the Ambu-bag.

SKILL 12-5 Measuring Peak Expiratory Flow Rates

Pulmonary function studies are essential for diagnosis of pulmonary disease. For clients with chronic airflow obstruction such as asthma, measurement of the **peak expiratory flow rate** (PEFR) gives objective data about the severity of the airway obstruction. The PEFR is the maximum flow rate, in liters, that can be generated during a forced expiratory maneuver using a peak flowmeter.

Benefits to measuring the PEFR are that it is simple, quantitative, reproducible, and inexpensive, and it correlates well with forced expiratory volume at 1 second (FEV_1). The PEFR is a more objective measure of severity than symptoms such as wheezing and shortness of breath. PEFR measures are used to assess asthma severity, monitor response to therapy, both acutely and chronically, diagnose exercise-induced asthma, detect asymptomatic deterioration in lung function, and assess the degree of airflow obstruction during health care visits.

A plan of action is developed with the client and the physician to address changes in the PEFR. When the PEFR drops, the client has a specific plan of action that includes changes in medication, when to notify the physician, and changes in the medical therapy. It is important that the client and care giver know and understand the specific plan, the expected change in the PEFR, and when to notify the physician or go to the emergency room (Walsh, 1992).

The disadvantage of PEFR is that it is effort dependent. The client must be willing and cooperative with the procedure to obtain accurate and reliable measurements. Because PEFR measures only large airway function, clients with mild asthma may be underdiagnosed.

EQUIPMENT

- Peak flowmeter

DELEGATION CONSIDERATIONS

The skill of measuring peak expiratory flow rates requires problem solving and knowledge application unique to a professional nurse. For this skill delegation is inappropriate.

STEPS	RATIONALE
ASSESSMENT	
1. Observe for signs of airway obstruction: shortness of breath, wheezing, use of accessory muscles of respiration, cyanosis, and nasal flaring.	Indicates client is in distress. Airway obstruction can be life threatening and demands immediate intervention.
2. Observe for patent airway and the need for removal of any secretions.	Secretions increase airway resistance and may plug the airway.
3. Complete respiratory assessment.	Provides objective baseline data.
4. Review client's medical record for the order to measure PEFR and expected rate to be achieved by the client.	Provides client outcome measure when treatment is at effective levels.

NURSING DIAGNOSIS

Clustering of defining characteristics from the assessment data may reveal the following nursing diagnoses for clients requiring this skill:

- ➤ Impaired gas exchange
- ➤ Ineffective breathing pattern
- ➤ Knowledge deficit regarding measuring PEFR

Related factors are individualized based on client's condition or needs.

PLANNING

STEPS	RATIONALE
1. **Expected outcomes** following completion of procedure:	
➤ Client's PEFR will remain within 20% of personal best.	PEFR less than 80% of personal best indicates the need for more aggressive therapy and continual daily monitoring.
➤ Client correctly uses PEFR.	Correct use of PEFR is essential to determine adequacy of expiratory airflow in clients with airway reactivity.
2. Explain the procedure to the client and family.	Promotes client and family cooperation.

STEPS	RATIONALE
IMPLEMENTATION	
1. Place indicator at base of the numbered scale (see illustration).	Starts reading from zero.
2. Have client stand up.	Increases lung expansion and promotes deep breathing.
➤ **CRITICAL DECISION POINT** **If clients are unable to stand, have them sit on a chair or on the edge of the bed or in high Fowler's position.**	
3. Have client take a deep breath.	Maximal effort is required for an accurate reading.
4. Have client place the meter in the mouth and close the lips around the mouthpiece (see illustration).	Increases the accuracy of measurement, and the exhalation will be directed through the peak flowmeter.
5. Have client blow out as hard and as fast as possible.	Maximal effort is required for an accurate reading.
6. Have client repeat steps 1 through 5 two more times, noting the highest number achieved.	Demonstrates the best effort.

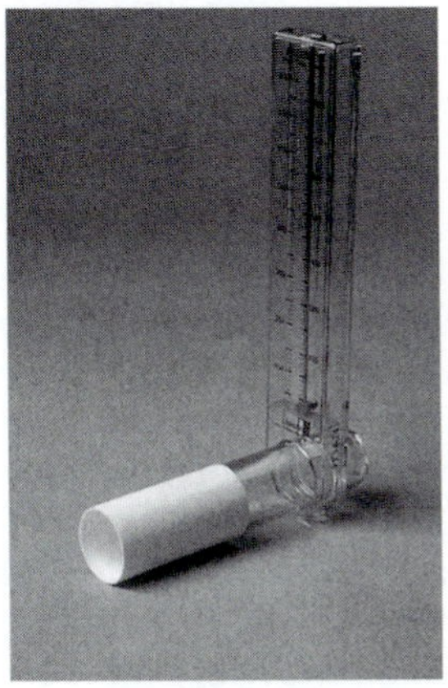

Step 1

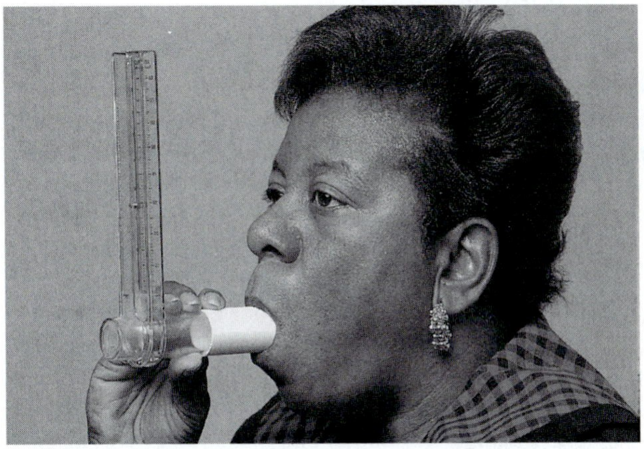

Step 4

STEPS	RATIONALE
EVALUATION	
1. Determine the client's PEFR and compare with the client's personal best.	Provides objective measure of client's symptoms. The personal best PEFR is obtained after the client is receiving effective therapy and has been determined to be maximally bronchodilated.
2. Reassess client for improvement in symptoms if bronchodilator therapy has been initiated.	PEFR is frequently measured following bronchodilator therapy to measure the client's response.
3. Observe client performing PEFR.	Documents learning and correct use of PEFR.
4. **Unexpected outcomes** that may occur include:	
➤ Client is unable to perform PEFR measurement.	Indicates client is in distress and requires intervention such as bronchodilator therapy.
➤ Client's PEFR measurement is less than 80% of personal best.	May indicate a poor effort by the client or severe airway obstruction.
RECORDING AND REPORTING	
1. Record the PEFR measurement, the client's ability to use the peak flowmeter, any symptoms the client may be experiencing, and any therapy the client may have received as a result of the PEFR measurement.	Documents PEFR and the client's response to therapy.

STEPS **RATIONALE**

FOLLOW-UP ACTIVITIES

1. Determine frequency of PEFR measurement if the client has experienced symptoms of airway obstruction.

• • • • •

Special Considerations

- Be sure the client does not become light headed while performing the PEFR measurement. If this occurs, allow more time between measurements.
- Instruct the client in the care of the peak flowmeter.

Teaching Considerations

- Begin teaching the client how to measure PEFR independently and record the measurements.
- Teach the client how to recognize and record the best reading.
- Review the plan of action and when to notify the physician when there are changes in the PEFR to ensure understanding and ability to implement the plan.

Home Care Considerations

- Review the plan for notification of the physician when there are changes in the PEFR.
- Have the client demonstrate use of the peak expiratory flowmeter to demonstrate the client's ability to follow directions and use the flowmeter correctly.

CRITICAL THINKING EXERCISES

1. Your client with asthma will be monitored with a peak expiratory flowmeter. What are the key concepts the client and family need to be taught?
2. The peak airway pressure for your client on mechanical ventilation rises suddenly. What are the nursing interventions necessary to ensure that the client has adequate ventilation? What are the possible causes of the increased peak airway pressure?
3. Your client is receiving oxygen therapy via nasal cannula at 3 L/min. The client has a respiratory rate of 12 and a large depth of respiration (tidal volume of 700 ml/breath). Can you accurately determine the client's fraction of inspired oxygen? Why?
4. During discharge instructions, your client comments to you that increasing the oxygen flow rate will help when the client feels breathless. How will you respond?

REFERENCES

Bell DA: Do incentive spirometers reduce the rate of postoperative pulmonary complications? *Perspectives in Resp Nurs* 4(3):1, 1993.

Dickson AL: Understanding the oxyhemoglobin dissociation curve, *Crit Care Nurse* 15(5):54, 1995.

Hess D, Kacmarek RM: Techniques and devices for monitoring oxygenation, *Resp Care* 38(6):646, 1993.

Nelson LD: Assessment of oxygenation: oxygenation indices, *Resp Care* 38(6):631, 1993.

Potter PA, Perry AG: *Fundamentals of nursing: concepts, process, and practice,* ed 4, St Louis, 1997, Mosby.

Rice R: *Home health nursing practice: concepts and application,* ed 2, St Louis, 1995, Mosby.

Wall MP: Postoperative respiratory complications, *Perspect Respir Nurs* 6(4):1, 1995.

Walsh M: Peak expiratory flow-rate monitoring, *Perspect Respir Nurs* 3(1):1, 1992.

Weilitz PB: Respiratory system. In Leuckenotte AG: *Gerontologic Nursing,* St Louis, 1996, Mosby.

ADDITIONAL READING

Anderson JM: Management of four arterial blood gas problems in adult mechanical ventilation: decision-making algorithms and rationale for their use, *Crit Care Nurse* 16(3):62, 1996.

Brooks-Brunn JA: Postoperative atelectasis and pneumonia: risk factors, *American Journal of Critical Care* 4(3):340, 1995.

Gift AG, Moore T, Soeken K: Relaxation to reduce dyspnea and anxiety in COPD patients, *Nurs Res* 41(4):242, 1992.

Hardy KA: A review of airway clearance: new techniques, indications, and recommendations, *Resp Care* 39(5):440, 1994.

Kim MJ, McFarland GK, McLane AM: *Pocket guide to nursing diagnoses,* ed 6, St Louis, 1995, Mosby.

Lewis SM, Collier IC: *Medical-surgical nursing assessment and management of clinical problems,* ed 4, St Louis, 1995, Mosby.

Lueckenotte AG: *Gerontologic assessment,* ed 2, St Louis, 1994, Mosby.

McCance KL, Huether SE: *Pathophysiology: the biologic basis for disease in adults and children,* ed 2, St Louis, 1994, Mosby.

Misasi RS, Keyes JL: Matching and mismatching ventilation and perfusion in the lung, *Crit Care Nurs* 16(3):23, 1996.

Palmer CLK, Grove S: Developing the nursing diagnosis of impaired oxygenation: abnormally low SvO_2 value, *Crit Care Nurse* 16(1), 1996.

Rice R: *Manual of home health nursing procedures,* St Louis, 1995, Mosby.

CHAPTER 13

Performing Chest Physiotherapy

OBJECTIVES

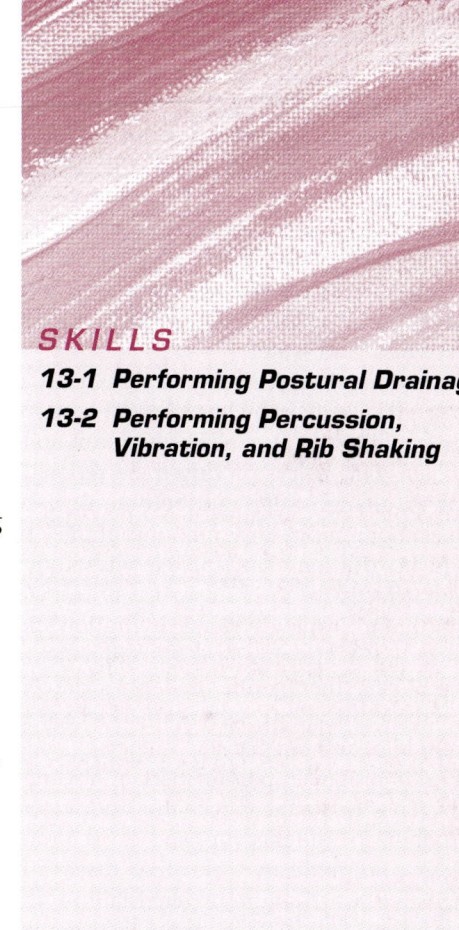

Mastery of content in this chapter will enable the nurse to:

- Define key terms.
- Assess the need to perform chest physiotherapy (CPT) maneuvers, including indications and physical assessment.
- Assess the need to modify or discontinue CPT maneuvers, including contraindications and individual variations.
- Explain how to prepare the client, the family, the nurse, and the therapist for the performance of each CPT maneuver.
- Identify goals for performing each CPT maneuver.
- Perform in a step-by-step method the outlined CPT maneuvers, including standard and modified versions.
- Describe expected and unexpected outcomes of each CPT maneuver.
- Describe discharge teaching and planning related to the use of each CPT maneuver in the home setting.

KEY TERMS

Chest physiotherapy
Cough
Mucociliary transport
Percussion
Postural drainage
Rib shaking
Vibration

SKILLS

13-1 Performing Postural Drainage
13-2 Performing Percussion, Vibration, and Rib Shaking

Chest physiotherapy (CPT) consists of physical maneuvers such as cough, chest wall percussion (P), vibration (V), rib shaking (RS), and postural drainage (PD). These maneuvers improve airway clearance of mucus in clients with retained tracheobronchial secretions. Diseases associated with accumulation of excessive mucus in the tracheobronchial tree include atelectasis, bronchitis, asthma, cystic fibrosis, and bronchiectasis. CPT is often used with other therapeutic modalities, including antibiotic therapy, avoidance of specific airway irritants, smoking cessation, bronchodilator treatment, aerosol therapy, and systemic hydration, to reduce mucus production and facilitate airway clearance. The goal is to reduce and prevent further airway obstruction and ventilatory dysfunction.

The precise mechanism by which CPT maneuvers enhance clearance of airway secretions is not fully understood. In general, they are designed to facilitate movement of secretions from smaller peripheral airways into larger central airways, where cough and suctioning are effective in removing them. Postural drainage involves placing the client in different positions to use gravitational forces for moving mucus from specific bronchi into the trachea. Exactly how externally applied forces of P, V, and RS are transmitted to the airways to move secretions toward the head is unclear. **Cough** is a natural lung clearance mechanism that aids in removal of mobilized secretions. Coughing forcefully exhales air, providing clearance of mucus primarily from the large central airways, including the trachea and mainstem bronchus.

When disease causes excessive sputum production, therapeutic interventions are needed to help natural airway clearance mechanisms (cough and mucociliary transport) clear the airways of obstructing mucus. In the normal lung the **mucociliary transport** system is able to keep the airways clear of excessive mucus and inhaled particles. This system lines the internal lumen of the entire tracheobronchial tree and consists of a thin layer of mucus that is constantly being propelled toward the larynx by cells that have hairlike projections called cilia. Inhaled particles are trapped on the mucus, and the cilia act as a conveyor belt to sweep the mucus toward the throat, where it can be swallowed or removed by coughing. In this way, airways normally remain clear and mucus is constantly being cleared almost as fast as it is made. Normal mucus remains thin, white, and watery.

In various disease states, mucus clearance slows down or the cilia are overwhelmed by production of excessively large quantities of mucus. The lung can no longer clear the mucus as fast as it is produced. Secretions stagnate in the airways, change color, and become thick and sticky. The cilia cannot remove large amounts of thick mucus from the lungs. In addition, many people with lung disease cannot cough effectively to clear airways. Therefore it becomes important to employ systemic hydration and other maneuvers to aid in clearing lung secretions as fast as they are made. These therapeutic modalities prevent mucus from stagnating and allow secretions to return to their normal thin, white, and watery consistency.

Fluids are an important part of a lung clearance program. They make the mucus thin and watery so that it can be mobilized, coughed up, and expectorated more easily. Unless contraindicated by other disease states, such as congestive heart failure or renal failure, fluids should be given along with CPT in order to make mucus thin and watery. During an acute exacerbation, it often takes three or four CPT treatments a day and 3 to 4 L of fluid a day to mobilize and thin secretions. During more stable states, one to two CPT treatments and 2 to 4 L of fluid a day can often keep secretions thin and watery, thereby preventing stagnation of mucus, which can lead to airway infection, airway obstruction, shortness of breath, increased work of breathing, and abnormal gas exchange.

This chapter presents two CPT skills as they are implemented in the clinical and home setting. Although they are separate skills, they must be thought of as different components of CPT. All must be mastered if treatment is to be effective.

GUIDELINES

The nurse plans the client's care and subsequent selection of CPT skills based on specific assessment findings. The following guidelines help the nurse in physical assessment and subsequent decision making:

1. Know the client's normal range of vital signs. Conditions such as atelectasis and pneumonia requiring CPT can affect a client's vital signs. The degree of change is related to the level of hypoxia, overall cardiopulmonary status, and tolerance to activity.
2. Know the client's present medications. Certain medications, particularly diuretics and antihypertensives, cause fluid and hemodynamic changes. These changes may decrease the client's tolerance of the positional changes of postural drainage. Steroid medications increase the client's risk of pathological rib fractures and often contraindicate RS.
3. Know the client's medical and surgical history. Certain conditions, such as increased intracranial pressure, spinal cord injuries, or abdominal aneurysm resection, contraindicate the positional changes of postural drainage. Thoracic trauma may contraindicate P, V, and RS.
4. Know the client's level of cognitive function. Participation in controlled cough techniques requires the client to understand and to follow instructions. Congenital or acquired cognitive limitations may alter the client's ability to learn and to participate in these techniques.
5. Be aware of the client's exercise tolerance. CPT maneuvers are fatiguing. When the client is not used to physical activity, initial tolerance of the maneuvers may be decreased. However, with gradual increases in activity and planned CPT, the client's tolerance of the procedure improves.

DELEGATION CONSIDERATIONS

The skills in this chapter can be delegated to respiratory and physical therapy and appropriately trained assistive personnel.

- Assess the client's chest x-ray films and examine the client's chest to determine the proper positions to use.
- Provide the therapists specific instruction on the proper postures and positions to use.

SKILL 13-1 Performing Postural Drainage

In health, several factors provide for normal clearance of tracheobronchial secretions: normal functioning of the mucociliary escalator; adequate systemic hydration; absence of airway disease or infection; normal cough reflex; and normal ability to deep breathe, exercise moderately, and carry out activities of daily living. Loss of or alterations in one or several of these factors can interfere with normal clearance of tracheobronchial secretions. A good example is the client with severe bronchitis who gets an airway infection, becomes dehydrated because of anorexia, and stays in bed for several days. These circumstances can lead to stagnation of mucus in the airways. A postoperative client who is maintaining bed rest and cannot take deep breaths because of pain is also predisposed to abnormal clearance of tracheobronchial secretions.

Postural drainage is the gravitational clearance of airway secretions from specific bronchial segments by using one or more of 10 different body positions. Each position drains a specific corresponding section of the tracheobronchial tree, either from the upper, middle, or lower lung field, into the trachea. Coughing or suctioning can then remove secretions from the trachea. Fig. 13-1 shows the upper, middle, and lower lobe bronchi. The figures in Table 13-1 show the bronchial lobes and their corresponding body postures for drainage.

Various pathophysiological conditions predispose the client to abnormal airway clearance and subsequent retention of lung secretions in peripheral airways. These retained secretions may be localized or diffuse. For example, clients with tuberculosis frequently have involvement of their upper lung fields, and posturing would be performed to drain only these specific upper lobe areas. In contrast, clients with bronchiectasis, asthma, bronchitis, or cystic fibrosis frequently have more diffuse involvement of many lung fields, which may require postural drainage of several areas. Clients maintaining bed rest who cannot turn may be placed in several or all drainage positions for several times throughout the day to prevent atelectasis and stasis of lung secretions. Areas are selected for drainage based on (1) knowledge of the client's condition and disease process, (2) physical assessment of the chest, (3) chest x-ray examination results, and (4) the extent of pathology and lobe involvement based on the physical examination and chest x-ray findings.

EQUIPMENT

- Trendelenburg's hospital bed or tilt table
- Water pitcher and glass
- Chair (for draining upper lobes)
- One to four pillows
- Tissues and paper bag
- Clear graduated screw-top container

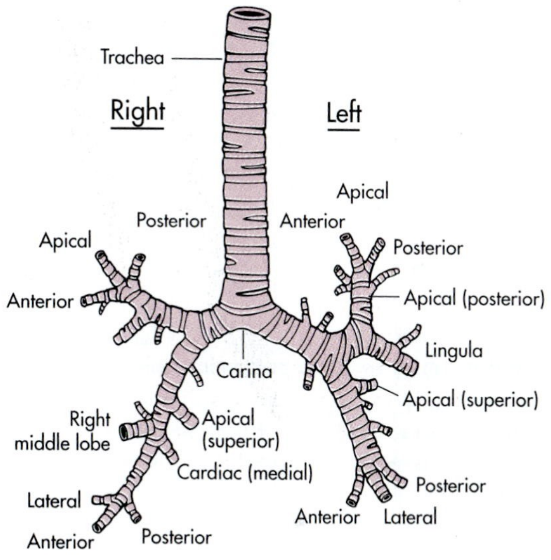

Fig. 13-1 Tracheobronchial tree. (Modified from Frownfelter DL, Dean E: *Principles and practice of cardiopulmonary therapy*, ed. 3, St Louis, 1996, Mosby.)

Table 13-1 Positions and Procedures for Drainage, Percussion, and Vibration

Area and Procedure	Percussion	Vibration
Left and right upper lobe anterior apical bronchi Have client sit in chair, leaning back. Percuss and vibrate with heel of hands at shoulders and fingers over collarbones (clavicles) in front; can do both sides at same time. Note body posture and arm position of nurse. Nurse's back is kept straight, and elbows and knees are slightly flexed. 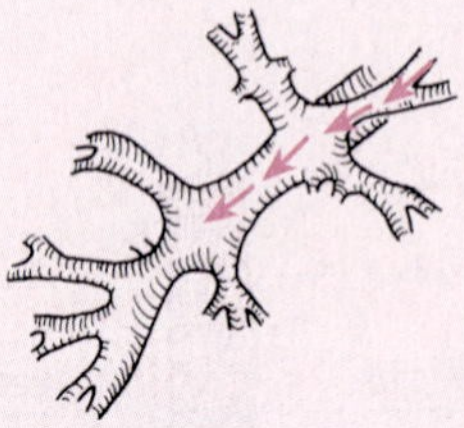	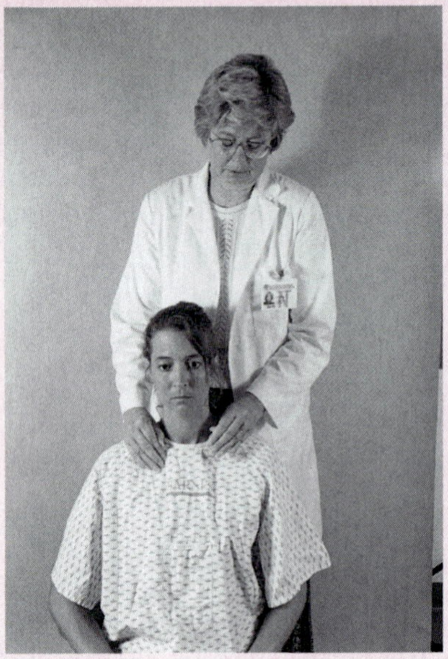	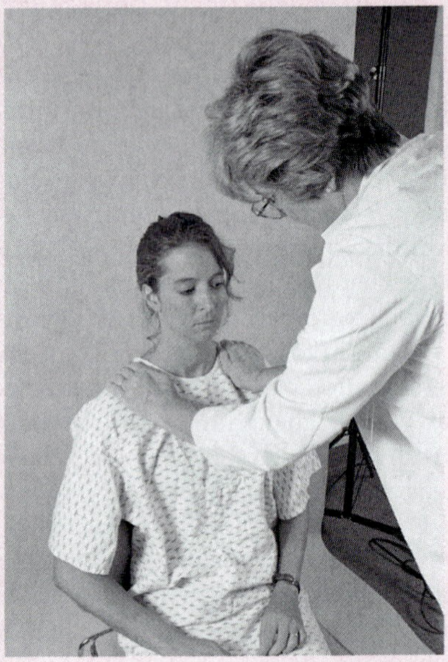
Left and right upper lobe posterior apical bronchi Have client sit in chair, leaning forward on pillow or table. Percuss and vibrate with hands on either side of upper spine. Can do both sides at same time. 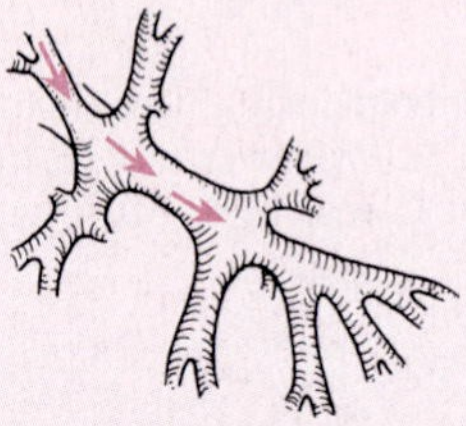	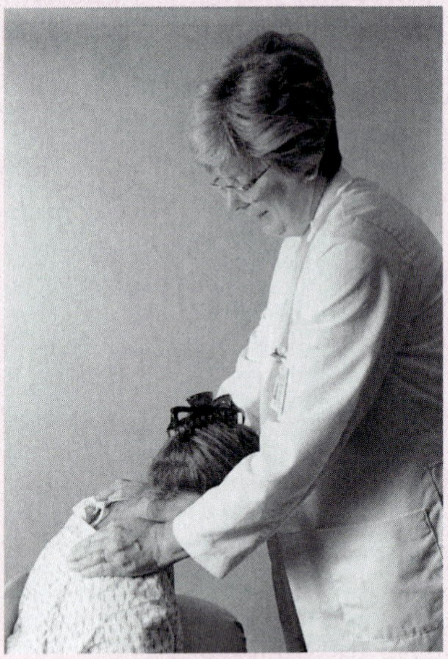	

Table 13-1 Positions and Procedures for Drainage, Percussion, and Vibration—cont'd

Area and Procedure	Percussion	Vibration
Right and left anterior upper lobe bronchi Have client lie flat on back with small pillow under knees. Percuss and vibrate just below clavicle on either side of sternum.	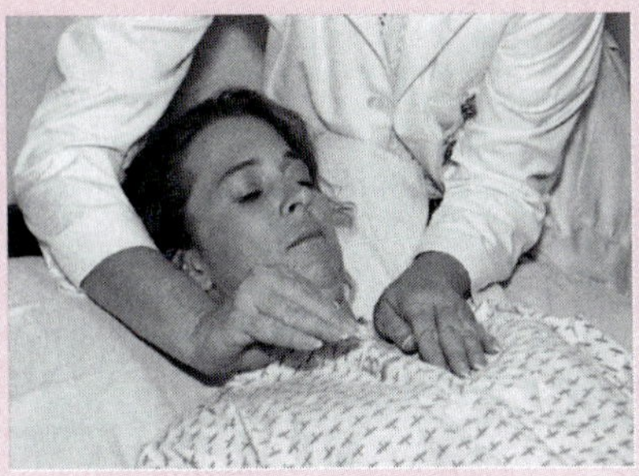	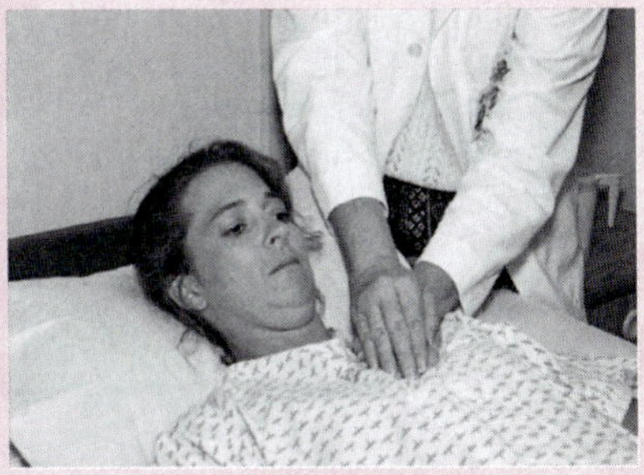 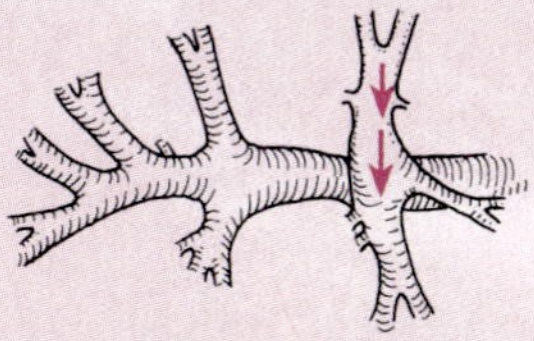
Left upper lobe lingular bronchus Have client lie on right side with arm over head in Trendelenburg's position, with foot of bed raised 30 cm (12 in). Place pillow behind back, and roll client one-quarter turn onto pillow. Percuss and vibrate lateral to left nipple below axilla.	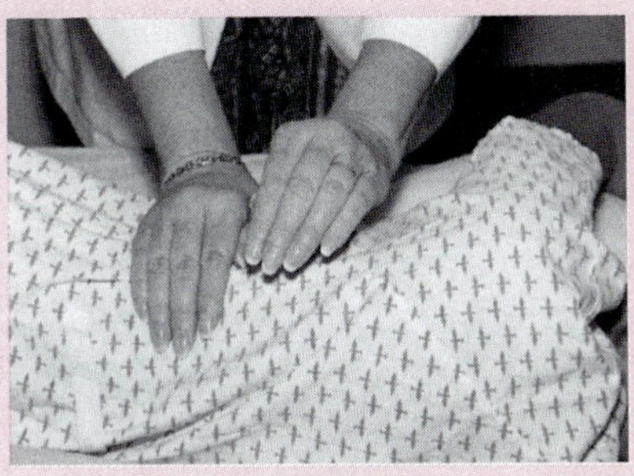	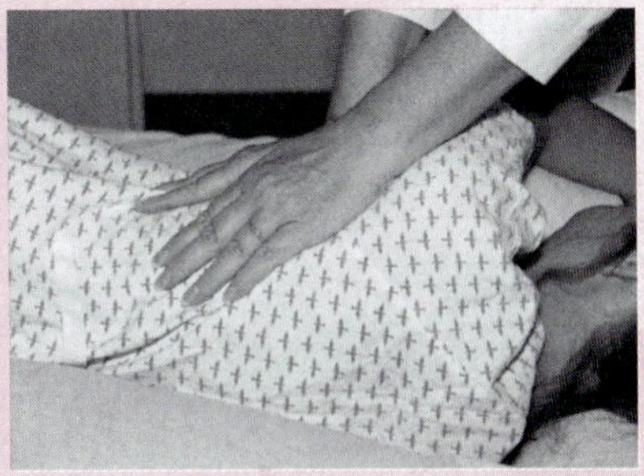 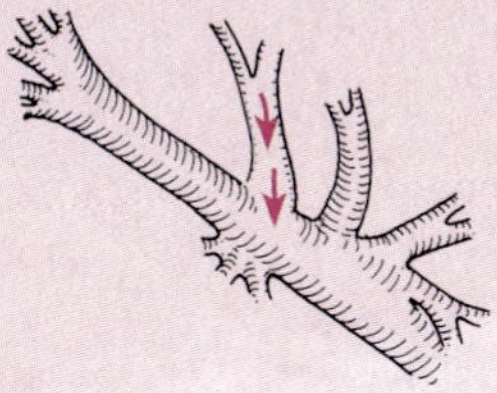
Right middle lobe bronchus Have client lie on left side; raise foot of bed 30 cm (12 in). Place pillow behind back and roll client one-quarter turn onto pillow. Percuss and vibrate to right nipple below axilla.	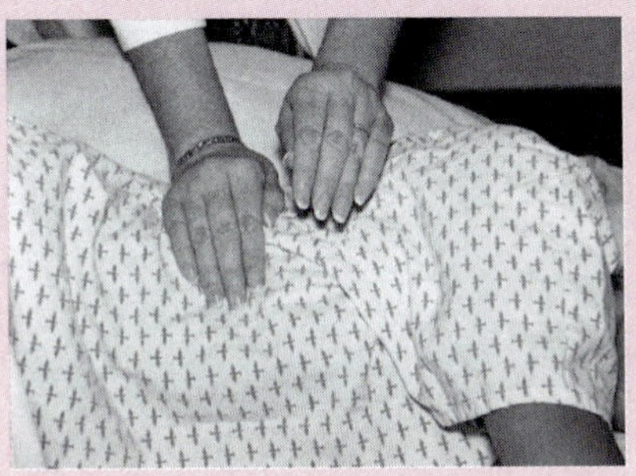	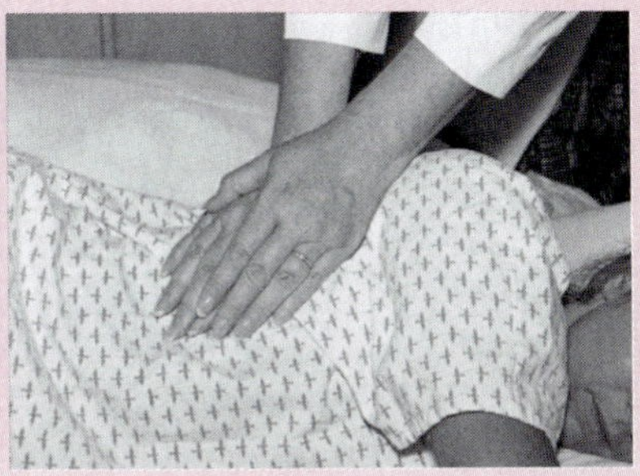 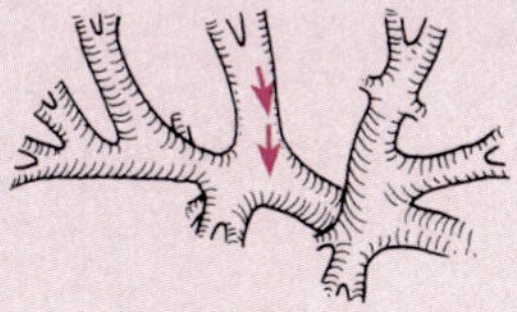

Continued.

Table 13-1 Positions and Procedures for Drainage, Percussion, and Vibration—cont'd

Area and Procedure	Percussion	Vibration
Left and right anterior lower lobe bronchi Have client lie on back in Trendelenburg's position, with foot of bed elevated 45 to 50 cm (18 to 20 in). Have knees bent on pillow. Percuss and vibrate over lower anterior ribs on both sides.	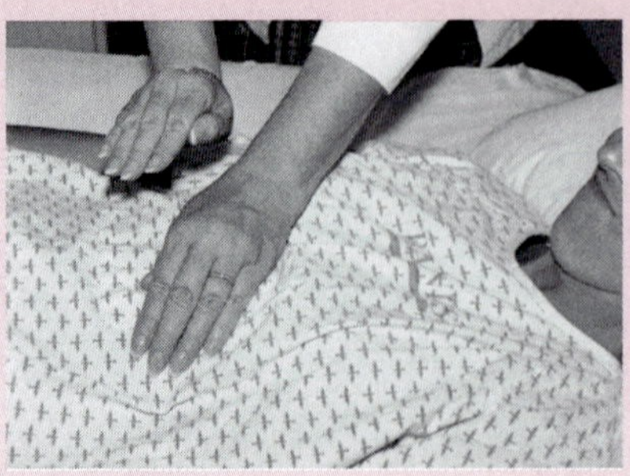	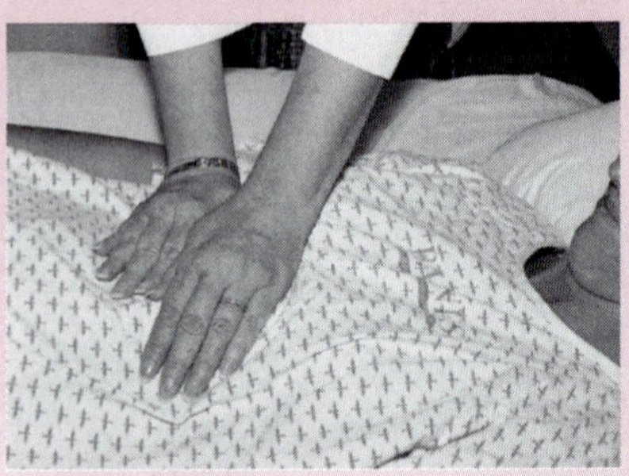 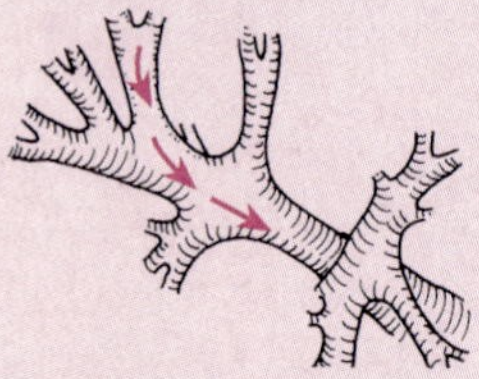
Right lower lobe lateral bronchus Have client lie on left side in Trendelenburg's position with foot of bed raised 45 to 50 cm (18 to 20 in). Percuss and vibrate on right side of chest below shoulder blades (scapulas) posterior to midaxillary line.	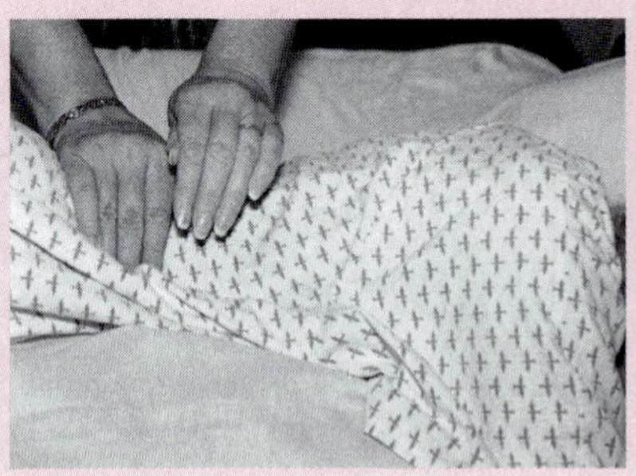	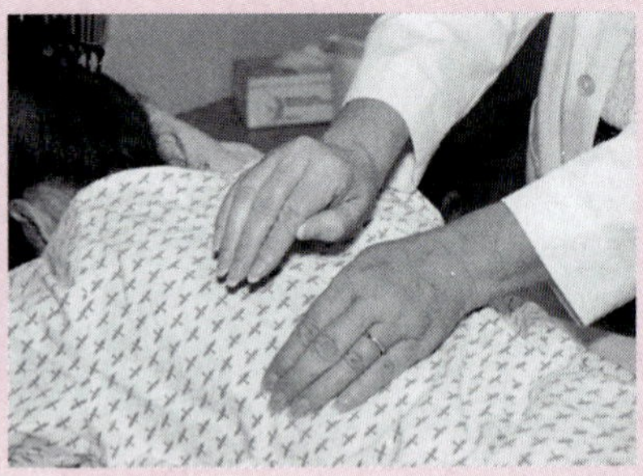 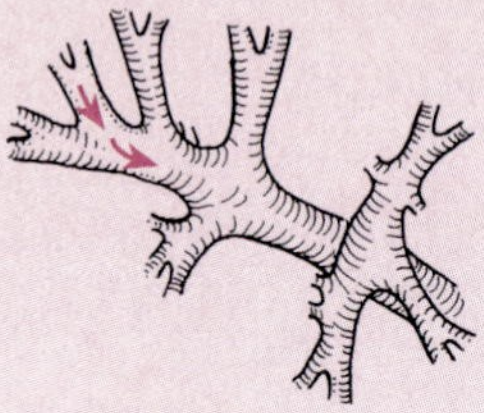
Left lower lobe lateral bronchus Have client lie on right side in Trendelenburg's position with foot of bed raised 45 to 50 cm (18 to 20 in). Percuss and vibrate on left side of chest below scapulas posterior to midaxillary line.	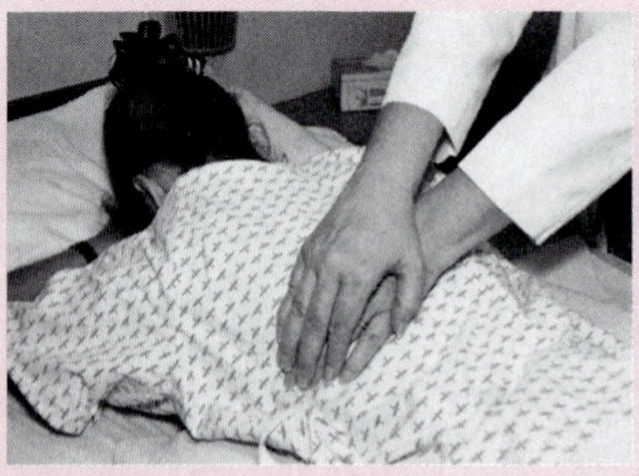	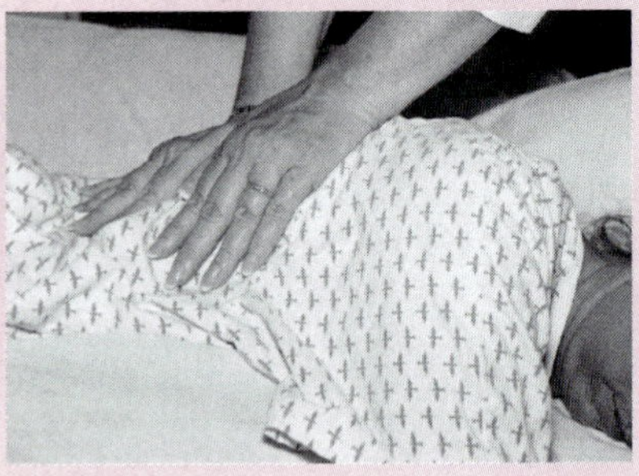 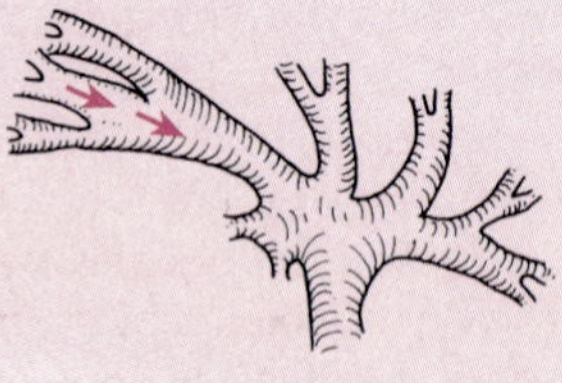

Table 13-1 Positions and Procedures for Drainage, Percussion, and Vibration—cont'd

Area and Procedure	Percussion	Vibration
Right and left lower lobe superior bronchi Have client lie flat on stomach with pillow under stomach. Percuss and vibrate below scapulas on either side of spine.	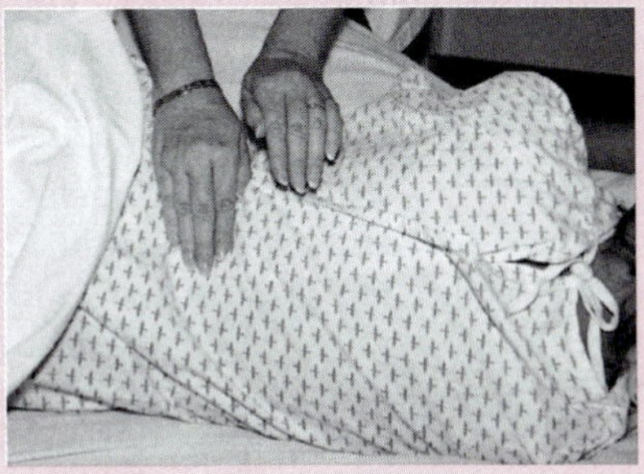	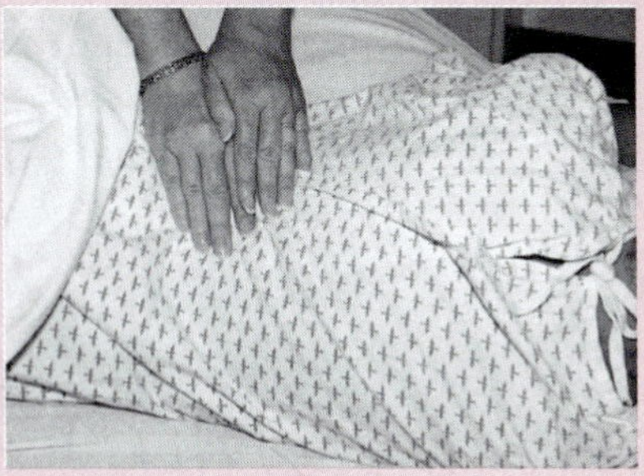 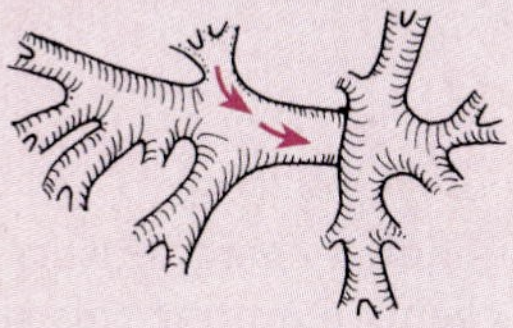
Left and right posterior basal bronchi Have client lie on stomach in Trendelenburg's position with foot of bed elevated 45 to 50 cm (18 to 20 in). Percuss and vibrate over lower posterior ribs on either side of spine.	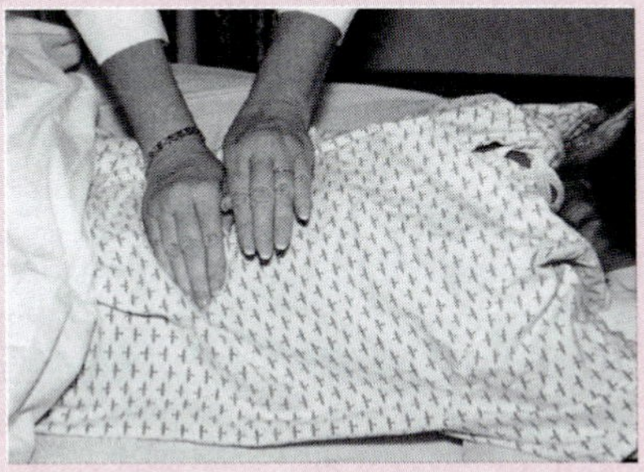	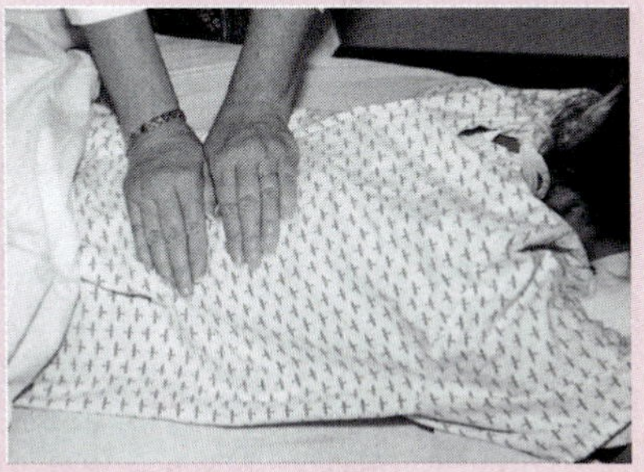 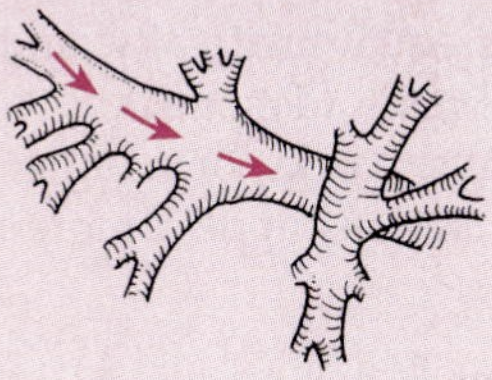

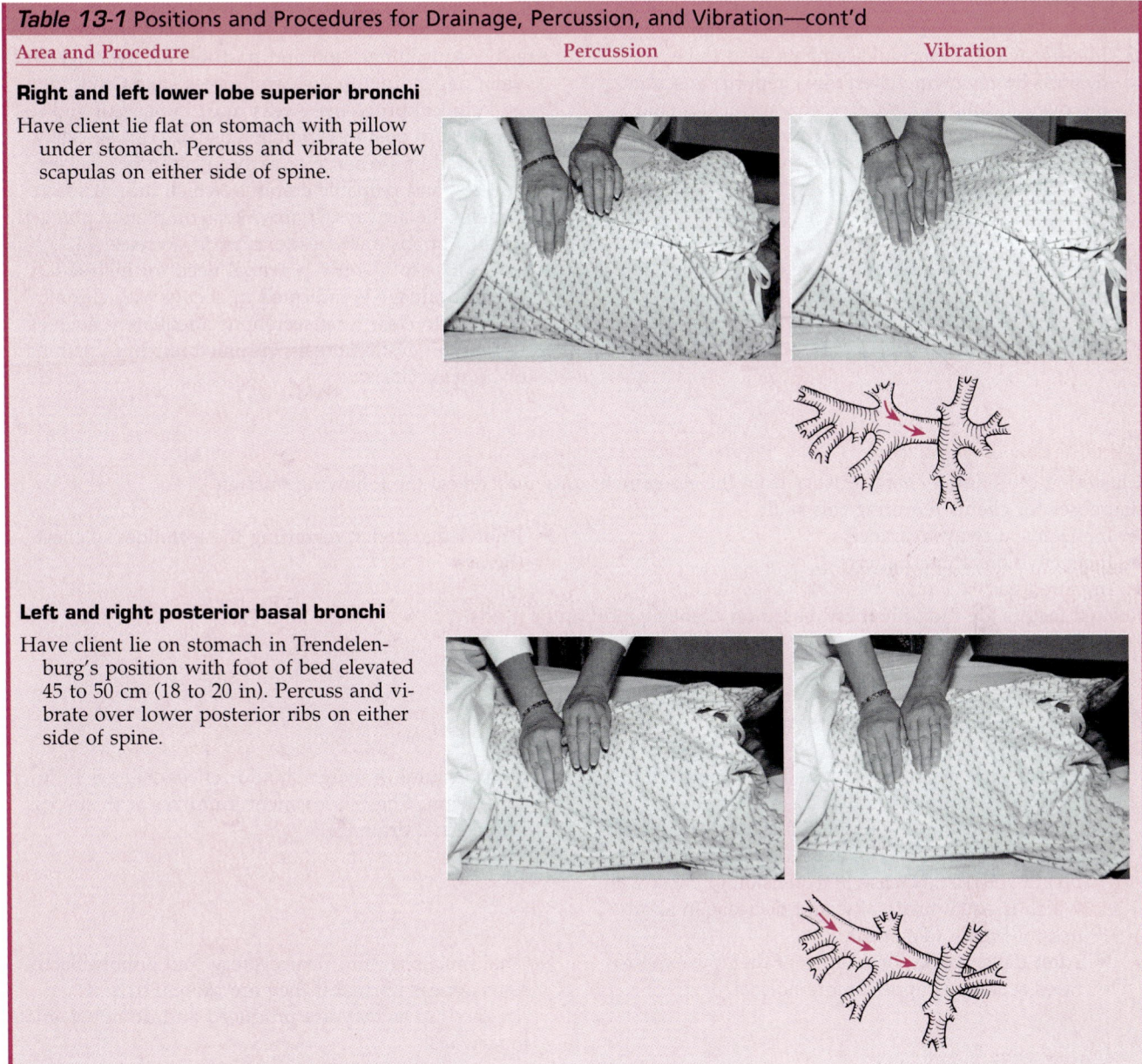

STEPS / RATIONALE

ASSESSMENT

1. Assess for possible impairment of airway clearance.

   Rationale: Certain circumstances, disease processes, and conditions place client at risk for impaired airway clearance.

2. Identify signs and symptoms that indicate the need to perform postural drainage: x-ray film changes consistent with atelectasis, pneumonia, or bronchiectasis; ineffective coughing; thick, sticky, tenacious, and discolored secretions that are difficult to cough up; abnormal breath sounds, such as wheezing, crackling, and gurgling; palpable crepitus; increased vocal fremitus; complete loss or decrease in fremitus and breath sounds.

   Rationale: X-ray film data and signs and symptoms indicate accumulation of pulmonary secretions.

STEPS	RATIONALE
3. Identify which bronchial segments need to be drained by reviewing chest x-ray reports; auscultating over all lung fields for wheezes, crackles, and gurgles (Chapter 11); palpating over all lung fields for crepitus, fremitus, and chest expansion.	Areas of lung congestion and postures for drainage will vary, depending on disease process, client condition, and clinical problems. Areas most in need of and responsive to postural drainage usually can be easily identified by presence of early inspiratory crackles, gurgles, and palpable crepitus, which indicate secretions in the airways. If airway is completely plugged, breath sounds and chest excursion decrease.
4. Determine client's understanding of and ability to perform home postural drainage.	Allows nurse to identify potential need for instruction. Home drainage is indicated in clients with chronic inability to clear lung secretions adequately, such as those with cystic fibrosis, chronic bronchitis, asthma, or bronchiectasis.

NURSING DIAGNOSIS

Clustering of defining characteristics from the assessment data may reveal the following nursing diagnoses for clients requiring this skill:

- Ineffective airway clearance
- Ineffective breathing pattern
- Impaired gas exchange
- Knowledge deficit regarding the techniqes of chest therapy

Related factors are individualized based on client's condition or needs.

PLANNING

1. Expected outcomes following completion of procedures:

STEPS	RATIONALE
➤ Airways are cleared of retained secretions. Signs include absent or diminished early inspiratory crackles and gurgles; absent or diminished palpable crepitus; return of absent or diminished breath sounds; increase in expansion of chest wall, which is equal bilaterally; and decrease in shortness of breath (dyspnea).	Careful postural drainage should reflect changes in lung congestion. Chest assessment improves with successful postural drainage.
➤ After days, weeks, or months of therapy, expectorated secretions appear more normal.	Normal mucus is thin, clear, watery, and bubbly. Secretions appear normal if they are mobilized and coughed up as they are produced and do not stagnate in airways.
➤ Sputum is coughed up more easily with one or two coughs.	Secretions are easier to cough up if they are thin and watery and have been mobilized into trachea with drainage.
➤ Client subjectively notices less dyspnea, especially after several days of therapy, and can breathe more deeply and more easily.	Removal of mucus relieves airway obstruction and decreases work of breathing.
➤ Clients who comply with long-term chest therapy for chronic lung disease usually notice decrease in frequency and severity of lung infections and exacerbations.	Retained secretions are excellent media for bacterial growth. If secretions are cleared regularly, airway infection is less likely to occur.
➤ Body temperature, white blood cell count, and chest x-ray films are normal.	Changes are often seen in clients with lung infection such as postoperative atelectasis or with pneumonia caused by mucus plugging that has been successfully reversed with aggressive chest therapy.
➤ Results of pulmonary function and blood gas studies improve.	Relief of mucosal obstruction can result in improved lung volumes and flows and improved blood gas levels.

STEPS	RATIONALE
2. Prepare client:	
a. Explain purpose and rationale for procedure. Explain how it will be done, how long it will take, and any discomforts or side effects.	Helps promote cooperation. Well-prepared client is usually more relaxed and comfortable, which is essential for effective drainage.
b. Encourage high fluid intake program if not contraindicated by other diseases and if physician approves. Keep record of client's fluid intake.	Fluids thin secretions and make them easier to cough up. Clients need close monitoring and encouragement when first starting high fluid intake program.
➤ ***CRITICAL DECISION POINT*** **Contraindications to high fluid intake are congestive heart failure and renal failure. When forcing fluids, build up daily intake gradually and strive toward 8 to 12 8-oz glasses or until mucus is thin, white, and watery.**	
c. Plan treatments so they do not overlap with meals or tube feeding. Avoid postural drainage for 1 to 2 hours after meals. Stop all gastric tube feedings for 30 to 45 minutes before postural drainage. Check for residual feeding in client's stomach; if greater than 100 ml, hold treatment.	Postural drainage should be done when client's stomach is empty to avoid reflux or vomiting and aspiration of stomach contents.
d. Schedule treatments at appropriate times during day.	Postural drainage should be scheduled to obtain best results and should not conflict with other activities.
e. Have client remove any tight or restrictive clothing.	Helps client relax and allows deep breathing.
IMPLEMENTATION	
1. Wash hands.	Reduces transmission of microorganisms.
2. Select congested areas to be drained based on assessment of all lung fields, clinical data, and chest x-ray data.	To be effective, treatment must be individualized to treat specific areas involved.
3. Place client in position to drain congested areas; first area selected may vary from client to client. (Refer to Table 13-1, p. 450 for correct positioning to drain upper, middle, and lower lobe bronchi.) Help client assume position as needed. Teach client correct posture and arm and leg positioning. Place pillows for support and comfort.	Specific positions are selected to drain each area involved.
4. Have client maintain posture for 10 to 15 minutes.	In adults, draining each area takes time.
5. During 10 to 15 minutes of drainage in each posture, perform chest P, V, or RS (Skill 13-2) over area being drained. Table 13-1 shows all postures and hand placement for P, V, and RS.	These maneuvers provide mechanical forces that aid in mobilization of airway secretions.
➤ ***CRITICAL DECISION POINT*** **After 10 to 15 minutes of drainage in first posture, have client sit up and cough. Save expectorated secretions in a clear container. If client cannot cough, suctioning may need to be performed.**	Any secretions mobilized into central airways should be removed by cough or suctioning before placing client into next drainage position. Coughing is most effective when client is sitting up and leaning forward.
6. Have client rest briefly if necessary.	Short rest periods between postures can prevent fatigue and help client better tolerate therapy.
7. Have client take sips of water.	Keeping mouth moist aids in expectoration of secretions.
8. Repeat Steps 3 through 7 until all congested areas selected have been drained. Each treatment should not exceed 30 to 60 minutes.	Postural drainage is used only to drain areas involved and is based on individual assessment.
9. Wash hands.	Reduces transmission of microorganisms.

STEPS	RATIONALE
EVALUATION	
1. Evaluate changes in chest assessment after drainage.	Clearance of secretions usually relieves gurgling, early inspiratory crackles, and palpable crepitus.
2. Inspect character and amount of sputum.	Determines if secretions are adequately thinned.
3. Review diagnostic reports including tests, chest x-ray films, and blood gas levels.	Provides objective data on improvements in lung function.
4. Have client explain purpose and procedure for postural drainage.	Evaluates client's understanding of procedure.
5. **Unexpected outcomes** that may occur include:	
➤ Client experiences severe dyspnea with bronchospasm, hypoxemia, and hypercarbia (hypercapnia).	In seriously ill clients with severe respiratory insufficiency, mobilization of secretions into large central airways can precipitate bronchospasm and increased work of breathing. These changes can worsen gas exchange and increase dyspnea. Clients at risk include those with (1) status asthmaticus and (2) severe exacerbation of bronchitis who are debilitated and tired and whose blood gas levels are consistent with severe hypoxemia and hypercarbia. Chest therapy may have to be discontinued or modified for these clients. They may tolerate only 3 to 5 minutes of drainage per hour. Bronchodilator inhalation should be scheduled before postural drainage.
➤ Hemoptysis occurs.	This may be caused by infection, erosion of blood vessels, or other causes.
➤ No secretions are obtained.	There may be a lack of secretions, or secretions may be too thick to mobilize. Continue therapy for several days to 1 week in well-hydrated client before deciding on its efficacy.
➤ There is no change in crackles and gurgles; crepitus is present; shortness of breath occurs; chest wall does not expand.	These may result from excessive secretions or secretions being too thick to mobilize on one treatment. Continue therapy.
➤ Client is unable to explain purpose of postural drainage.	Further instruction is required.
RECORDING AND REPORTING	
1. Record in nurses' notes pretherapy and posttherapy assessment of chest; frequency and duration of treatment; postures used and bronchial segments drained; cough effectiveness; need for suctioning; color, amount, and consistency of sputum; hemoptysis or other unexpected outcomes; client's tolerance and reactions.	Helps evaluate outcomes and need for changes in therapy.
2. If client and family receive instruction in home care, chart instructions given; understanding of therapy; demonstration of skill; reactions to need for home care; barriers to learning and implementation; referral for follow-up, that is, home care, rehabilitation, or pulmonary nurse specialist.	Provides continuity of client education among nursing staff.
3. Immediately report severe dyspnea, hemoptysis, severe bronchospasm, or hypotension to physician.	

FOLLOW-UP ACTIVITIES

1. Use inhaled bronchodilators 20 minutes before postural drainage for client at risk for bronchospasm.
2. In severe hemoptysis, stop therapy, call physician, remain calm, stay with client, request assistance, and keep client comfortable, warm, and quiet.

• • • • •

Special Considerations

- Contraindications to therapy may include problems that preclude use of Trendelenburg's position or other postures, such as severe hypertension, severe hypoxemia, severe shortness of breath, head injuries, increased intracranial pressure, recent severe myocardial failure, lung hemorrhage, certain surgical procedures, pain, or traction.
- Have fluids available according to client's diet, likes, and dislikes. Teach client kinds and quantities of fluid to drink at home. Have client keep track of exact amount of fluid intake.
- Some clients are very sensitive and self-conscious about coughing up secretions. Be careful and nonjudgmental when observing their mucus.
- Discomforts and side effects are usually mild but may include increased shortness of breath; increased cough during and for 45 to 60 minutes after treatment; and when in Trendelenburg's position, nasal congestion and feeling of fullness in head, which subsides once client is upright. Offer reassurance that client can sit up and rest at any time if necessary.
- Review Table 13-1 for ideas on how to place pillows in each position. Note that in all flat and Trendelenburg's positions, pillow can be placed under head to promote comfort. Rib cage remains slanted as long as pillow is not under shoulder or upper back. To drain lingula and right middle lobe, as shown, roll client one-quarter turn back from side-lying position and place pillow behind back for comfort and support.
- Best times for treatments are (1) in morning before breakfast, when client can clear secretions that accumulate overnight; and (2) about 1 hour before bedtime, so that lungs are clear before sleeping and client has time after treatment to cough up any mobilized secretions. Frequency depends on need and client's tolerance and may vary from once daily to every 2 to 4 hours in an acute situation. When client's condition is acute, short (10-minute), frequent treatments are tolerated best. As condition stabilizes, one to four 30- to 45-minute treatments work best. If client is receiving inhaled bronchodilators or aerosol treatment, postural drainage should be done 20 minutes after such therapy. Plan for rest period after postural drainage. Do not schedule major activities (such as exercise or bath) right after chest therapy treatment, especially in clients with severe obstructive lung disease.
- Sometimes client may experience transient dyspnea and fatigue because of irritation and bronchospasm from mobilizing secretions. Dyspnea usually subsides after sputum is coughed up.
- Small amounts of blood-streaked sputum usually clear with good drainage. Notify physician. If sputum is pure blood, stop all therapy and notify physician immediately. Keep client calm.
- Secretions are not always mobilized and coughed up after each posture. If, after two or three coughs, nothing is expectorated, proceed with next posture. Often secretions are coughed up 30 to 60 minutes after postural drainage.
- Postural drainage after various types of chest surgery has developed into a speciality. If specific posturing guidelines are used, they can be very effective in preventing and treating atelectasis and pneumonia.

Teaching Considerations

- Instruct client's family or primary care giver to recognize when the client's respiratory status requires breathing exercises or postural drainage.
- Encourage primary care giver or family member to encourage the client to participate in physical activities that will increase respiratory efficiency.
- Teach client and significant others how to assume postures at home. Some postures may need to be modified to meet individual needs, for example, side-lying Trendelenburg's position to drain lateral lower lobes may have to be done with client lying flat on side or in side-lying semi-Fowler's position if client is very short of breath.

Gerontologic Considerations

- Postural drainage in the elderly should be done while taking extra care and assessment. Change positions more slowly and closely assess for any changes in oxygen saturation or vital signs with position changes.

Home Care Considerations

- Assess home environment for ventilation. Determine client's access to clean, fresh air. Assess the home for air conditioning and client's reaction to air conditioning.
- Discuss need for home postural drainage with family. Assess if they perceive need for home care and if any barriers exist to learning and implementing home program. If specialized home or outpatient follow-up is needed, refer client to pulmonary nurse specialist, pulmonary rehabilitation team, or home health care personnel.

➤ In home setting, the Trendelenburg's position can be achieved in several ways. Select the most comfortable and practical method that best suits client:
- First choice is Trendelenburg's hospital bed if client has insurance coverage or can afford it. Some clients, however, do not like hospital equipment in their home.
- Twin bed can be propped up at the foot with 30- to 45-cm (12- to 18-inch) blocks or bricks.
- Client can purchase slant board or make one out of old door or tabletop. Surface can be padded with foam or blankets.
- Client's hips can be elevated with stack of old newspapers and pillows or foam wedge. These props tend to be uncomfortable and often flatten out because of client's body weight.
- Wedge or stack of papers can be placed under bed board.

SKILL 13-2 Performing Percussion, Vibration, and Rib Shaking

During postural drainage, physical maneuvers (P, V, and RS) can be performed on the rib cage by a trained nurse, therapist, or family member. The techniques are done on specific parts of the rib cage over each area being drained. Normally the mucociliary escalator and cough transport can effectively clear airway secretions. When airway clearance is impaired in certain disease states, however, these techniques are combined with postural drainage to help clear mucus. Exactly why these physical maneuvers enhance clearance of mucus is not known.

These techniques are defined and explained in detail in this skill. **Percussion** involves clapping the chest wall with cupped hands. If done correctly, it painlessly sets up vibrations in the chest to dislodge retained secretions. **Vibration** is a downward vibrating pressure done only during exhalation with the flat part of the palm over the area being drained. **Rib shaking** is a constant downward rocking motion on the rib cage done with the flat part of the hand during exhalation. These last two maneuvers are performed only during prolonged exhalation through pursed lips. They augment the natural movement of the rib cage during exhalation.

The natural expiratory movement of the chest wall involves (1) a decrease in the lateral and anteroposterior diameter of the lower ribs as they move downward and closer together and (2) a decrease in the anteroposterior diameter of the upper chest as the sternum, the clavicles, and the upper rib cage move downward. Pressure during V and RS is always directed toward these natural expiratory movements of the rib cage. They become even more effective if the client can relax the rib cage muscles during exhalation and blow out using abdominal muscles. This relaxation during V and RS enhances the rocking motion of the rib cage, makes V optimal, and assists in dislodging mucus plugs.

In diseases associated with mucus plugging, the rib cage frequently becomes hyperinflated because air is trapped behind obstructed airways. The ribs can become somewhat fixed in their upward and outward position and lose their excursion and flexibility; RS and V can improve both. They can also help to reduce air trapping by augmenting prolonged exhalation and relaxation of the chest wall muscles.

Before attempting to master these techniques, the nurse must know that each posture is associated with a general area of the rib cage to be percussed and vibrated. These postures and the specific areas are shown in Table 13-1. Generally, for any given posture, the area to be percussed and vibrated can be thought of as that portion of the rib cage at the greatest vertical height. Areas that are never percussed or vibrated regardless of their vertical height include the clavicles, breast tissue, sternum, spine, waist, and abdomen; the action must always stay over the ribs.

EQUIPMENT

- Hospital bed or tilt table placed in Trendelenburg's position
- Chair (for upper lobes)
- One to four pillows
- Water pitcher and glass
- Tissues and paper bag
- Clear graduated screw-top container
- Mechanical vibrator or percussor (optional)
- Single layer of clothing

STEPS	RATIONALE
ASSESSMENT	
1. Assess breathing pattern, including muscles used for breathing, respiratory rate and depth, extent of excursion, and chest wall movement.	Certain disease states place client at risk of developing an ineffective breathing pattern. Rapid, shallow breathing with client using accessory muscles is seen in chronic obstructive lung disease, asthma, pain, hypoxemia, pneumonia, and atelectasis.
2. Identify signs and symptoms and conditions that indicate need to perform these skills, such as use of postural drainage (Skill 13-1, Assessment); abnormal chest assessment indicating bronchial congestion; abnormal breathing pattern.	When tolerated and not contraindicated, these techniques are done during postural drainage.
3. Identify and assess rib cage over bronchial segment being drained for pain, tenderness, abnormal configuration, abnormal excursion or chest wall movement during breathing, muscle tension.	Chest wall areas to be assessed and to receive P, V, and RS vary with each postural drainage position (Table 13-1). When rib fracture or osteoporosis is present, P, V, and RS are contraindicated.
4. Assess client's understanding and ability to cooperate with therapy, both in hospital and at home.	Allows nurse to identify potential need for instruction of client, family, or significant others.
PLANNING	
1. Expected outcomes following completion of procedure:	
➤ Airways are cleared of retained secretions. Signs include absent or diminished early inspiratory crackles and gurgles; absent or diminished palpable crepitus; return of absent or diminished breath sounds; increase in expansion of chest wall, which is equal bilaterally; decrease in shortness of breath (dyspnea).	Careful postural drainage should reflect changes in lung congestion. Chest assessment improves with successful postural drainage.
➤ After days, weeks, or months of therapy, expectorated secretions appear more normal:	Normal mucus is thin, clear, watery, and bubbly.
Sputum in jar settles into two layers (clear, serous layer with bubbly layer on top) instead of four layers (tiny plugs at bottom, cloudy discolored serous layer, large plugs, and bubbles at top).	Secretions appear normal if they are mobilized and coughed up as they are produced and do not stagnate in airways.
➤ Sputum is coughed up more easily with one or two coughs.	Secretions are easier to cough up if they are thin and watery and have been mobilized into trachea with drainage.
➤ Client subjectively reports less dyspnea, especially after several days of therapy, and can breathe more deeply and more easily.	Removal of mucus relieves airway obstruction and decreases work of breathing.
➤ Clients who comply with long-term chest therapy for chronic lung disease usually notice decrease in frequency and severity of lung infections and exacerbations.	Retained secretions are excellent media for bacterial growth. If secretions are cleared regularly, airway infection is less likely to occur.
➤ Body temperature, white blood cell count, and chest x-ray films are normal.	Changes are often seen in clients with lung infection such as postoperative atelectasis or with pneumonia caused by mucus plugging that has been successfully reversed with aggressive chest therapy.
➤ Results of pulmonary function and blood gas studies improve.	Relief of mucosal obstruction can result in improved lung volumes and flows and improved blood gas levels.
➤ Client demonstrates decreased respiratory rate, increased depth of breathing, ability to exhale longer through pursed lips, ability to relax chest muscles and exhale using only abdominal muscles, increased relaxation and mobility of rib cage, improved excursion of rib cage.	Signs of improved breathing pattern.

STEPS	RATIONALE
2. Prepare client:	
a. Explain procedure in detail: how it will be done, how long it will take, and any discomforts or side effects.	P, V, and RS cannot be done effectively without client's cooperation.
b. Encourage and help client to relax and deep breathe during P, V, and RS. Have client practice exhaling slowly through pursed lips while relaxing chest wall muscles. Client should blow out using abdominal muscles, not rib cage muscles.	P, V, and RS are most effective if client breathes properly and works well with therapist. If done properly these techniques should not cause pain or discomfort.
IMPLEMENTATION	
1. With client placed in appropriate drainage position (Skill 13-1, Implementation, Steps 1 through 3), assess and identify chest wall area to be percussed and vibrated (Table 13-1).	In general, for any given posture, rib cage area to be percussed and vibrated is in highest vertical position. Careful assessment of rib cage movement guides nurse in following natural movement during V and RS.
2. Instruct client to relax, take slow, deep breaths, and exhale using abdominal, diaphragmatic, pursed-lip breathing.	Client should not lie passively, but should relax and take deep breaths.
3. Use good body mechanics when clapping: elevate bed to comfortable working height and stand close to bed with arms directly in front and knees slightly bent. Avoid bending over.	Avoids undue strain on therapist's back and legs.
4. Begin P on appropriate part of chest wall over draining area (Table 13-1). Perform P for 5 minutes in each posture as tolerated. Always ask if client is experiencing any discomfort, such as undue pressure or stinging of the skin.	P helps clear mucus and should be painless, since air in hand acts as cushion.
a. Place hands side by side on chest wall over area to be drained. Hands should be cupped with fingers and thumbs held tightly together. Make sure that entire outer portion of hand makes contact with chest wall to avoid air leaks (Table 13-1).	This hand position creates an air pocket that sends vibrations through the chest wall but is not painful.
b. When clapping, most of arm movement should come from the elbow and shoulder joint. Cupping can be done for 5 minutes without stopping or 2 to 3 minutes, alternating with V and RS.	Using the larger muscles of the arms and shoulders improves endurance.
c. Alternately clap chest with cupped hands to create rhythmic popping sound resembling galloping horse. Clapping can be done at moderate or fast speed, whichever is most comfortable and effective.	The popping sound comes from the air pocket that is formed between the hand and the chest wall.
5. Perform chest wall V over each area being drained. See Table 13-1 for correct hand position to use in each posture. Vs are usually done in sets of three followed by coughing so that any mobilized mucus can be expectorated.	Vs during slow exhalation and coughing help to clear mucus.
a. To perform V, gently place hands over area being drained, and have client take slow, deep breath through nose.	Slow inhalation helps relaxation.
b. Gently resist chest wall as it rises during inhalation.	Slight resistance on inhalation aids in expansion of rib cage.
c. Have client hold breath and then exhale through pursed lips, while contracting abdominal muscles and relaxing chest wall muscles. Chest wall should relax and fall.	Pursed-lip breathing makes exhalation easier. Relaxation of the chest wall makes V more effective.

STEPS	RATIONALE
d. While client is exhaling, gently push down and vibrate with flat part of hand.	Vibrate only during exhalation so as to follow the natural downward movement of the rib cage.
e. Repeat V three times, then have client cascade cough by taking deep breath and doing series of small coughs until end of breath. Client should not inhale between coughs. Vibrate chest wall as client coughs. When applying pressure to ribs, always follow natural movement of rib cage. As client becomes comfortable and learns to relax rib cage during exhalation, chest wall movement and flexibility will increase. Allow client to sit up and cough as needed between Vs.	Coughing with V aids in clearing mucus.
6. Assess client's tolerance of V and ability to relax chest wall and breathe properly as instructed.	Client's poor tolerance may necessitate discontinuing procedure.
7. If client is able to achieve proper breathing and relaxation, perform RS, which is usually done with V.	RS helps clear mucus.
a. Place flat part of hand over area being drained (Table 13-1). Maintain good body mechanics: lower bed so client is about at nurse's hip level; work with arms directly in front; maintain good leverage; do not lean over or strain back.	Proper positioning of therapist prevents strain on back muscles.
b. Have client inhale slowly through nose.	
c. During inhalation, apply light pressure on ribs and stretch skin so it is tight.	
d. Have client hold breath for 2 seconds.	
e. As client exhales, increase pressure. Maintain pressure while applying intermittent rocking motion on ribs. Pressure is directed toward following natural expiratory rib cage movement.	RS helps to dislodge mucus.
f. Client must exhale through pursed lips and relax chest wall muscles as much as possible.	If rib cage is relaxed, ribs can be rocked more vigorously in direction they naturally move.
g. Repeat RS three times, have client inhale deeply, and then do rib shaking during cascade cough.	Coughing helps to clear mobilized secretions.
h. Perform a total of three or four sets of three Vs with RS and coughing in each posture as tolerated. Strength and frequency of V and RS will vary: V requires all muscles in arm and shoulder to contract and tremble; RS requires applying controlled pressure from shoulders and back while slightly leaning on chest; rocking motion is created by flexing and extending elbows using triceps.	
i. Suction if client is unable to cough up mucus.	
8. In each posture, complete Vs and/or RS.	
9. If long-term therapy is needed, teach client and significant others P, V, and RS for home use. If they cannot learn or use, refer for outpatient or home health follow-up.	Long-term use of these techniques can optimize airway clearance, reduce symptoms and infection, and improve chest mobility.

EVALUATION

1. Evaluate changes in chest assessment after P, V, and RS.	These maneuvers usually relieve signs of congestion, slow respiratory rate, and improve chest mobility and expansion.
2. Inspect character of mucus.	Determines if mucus is adequately thinned.
3. Review diagnostic test results for pulmonary function.	Determines airway clearance and oxygenation status.

STEPS	RATIONALE
4. Observe care giver during P, V, and RS.	Return demonstration is an effective means to measure learning.
5. **Unexpected outcomes** that may occur include:	
➤ Client experiences severe dyspnea with bronchospasm, hypoxemia, and hypercarbia (hypercapnia).	In seriously ill clients with severe respiratory insufficiency, mobilization of secretions into large central airways can precipitate bronchospasm and increase work of breathing. These changes can worsen gas exchange and increase dyspnea.
➤ Hemoptysis occurs.	Hemoptysis may be caused by infection, erosion of blood vessels, or other causes.
➤ No secretions are obtained.	This may be the result of a lack of secretions or secretions being too thick to mobilize.
➤ No change is noted in crackles and gurgles; crepitus is present; shortness of breath occurs; chest wall does not expand.	This may be the result of lobar atelectasis with mucus plugging. Call physician and obtain chest x-ray examination.
➤ Client experiences rib fracture, rib pain, or tenderness of chest wall.	If techniques are not done properly, rib pain and fractures can occur.

Reporting and Recording

1. For treatment given, along with postural drainage, record in nurses' notes pretherapy and posttherapy assessment of chest mobility; client's cooperation with and tolerance of P, V, and RS; client's ability to relax and breathe properly; duration of percussion; number of V and RS series; cough effectiveness; suctioning.	Documents in client's record specific procedures and lung lobes involved. In addition, documentation is needed for third-party reimbursement.
2. If client and significant others receive instruction in home use of P, V, and RS, chart instructions given; understanding of theory and skills; demonstration of P, V, and RS techniques; referral for follow-up.	Documentation of client teaching notes specifically what information client should know and what was taught.

Follow-up Activities

1. Use inhaled bronchodilators 20 minutes before P, V, and RS in clients at risk for bronchospasm.
2. In severe hemoptysis, stop therapy, remain calm, stay with client, request assistance, and keep client comfortable, warm, and quiet.
3. If rib fracture is suspected, notify physician, obtain chest x-ray film, and curtail P, V, and RS.

• • • • •

Special Considerations

- ➤ P, V, and RS may be contraindicated in certain situations, including rib fracture, fracture of other rib cage structures such as clavicle or sternum, pain, severe dyspnea, and severe osteoporosis, so nurse should obtain physician's order.
- ➤ Do not perform if client is uncooperative or if client has broken back or rib, rib pain or tenderness, bleeding in the lung, chest or back pain, upset stomach, or serious heart disease.
- ➤ After chest surgery, P and RS are done more gently because they may increase pain and splinting and lead to more problems with atelectasis. Gentle vibration, deep breathing, and coughing are preferred, along with postural drainage. Small mechanical vibrators used well above or well below the client's thoracotomy incision are effective and well tolerated.
- ➤ Never use P, V, or RS over spine, breast tissue, sternum, or shoulder blades. Always stay over rib cage.
- ➤ If client is unresponsive, on mechanical ventilation, or is uncooperative, the breathing pattern usually cannot be altered. Vibrate during the exhalation phase between machine breaths.
- ➤ Students should learn RS under the guidance of a trained therapist.
- ➤ Sometimes client may experience transient dyspnea and fatigue because of irritation and bronchospasm from mobilizing secretions. Dyspnea usually subsides after sputum is coughed up.
- ➤ Clients at risk include those with (1) status asthmaticus and (2) severe exacerbation of bronchitis who are debilitated and tired and whose blood gas levels are consistent with severe hypoxemia and hypercarbia. Chest therapy may have to be discon-

tinued or modified for these clients. They may tolerate only 3 to 5 minutes of drainage per hour. Bronchodilator inhalation should be scheduled before postural drainage.

- Small amounts of blood-streaked sputum usually clear with good drainage. Notify physician. If sputum is pure blood, stop all therapy and notify physician immediately. Keep client calm.
- Continue therapy for several days to 1 week in well-hydrated client before deciding on its efficacy.
- Thin, frail clients with osteoporosis are most susceptible to injury and should be taught other secretion control measures; e.g., forceful coughing, humidification, etc.

Teaching Considerations

- Instruct client to use frequent mouthwashes.
- Instruct client to use tissues in expectorating and to assess sputum for blood, color, consistency, amount, and odor.
- Teach family members carefully and observe them closely as they demonstrate techniques for P, V, and RS.

Gerontologic Considerations

- P, V, and RS usually have to be done more gently in the elderly. In the frail elderly use a mechanical vibrator on low speed instead of manual P, V, and RS.

Home Care Considerations

- Mechanical devices are sometimes used (1) at home if a trained therapist is not available or (2) if client does not tolerate manual therapy. They are available through most home equipment companies.
- If home therapy is needed, instruct a family member in techniques of P, V, and RS. Assess willingness to learn and follow through in home setting.

CRITICAL THINKING EXERCISES

1. **Describe three pathophysiological mechanisms responsible for development of ineffective airway clearance.**
2. **Describe the position that should be used and identify where on the chest wall percussion and vibration should be done for drainage of the lingula.**
3. **Describe special considerations when using CPT techniques in clients with the following problems:**
   a. **Status asthmaticus**
   b. **Postthoracotomy pain**
   c. **Bronchiectasis**
   d. **Steroid dependency**
4. **Describe controlled cascade coughing and the physiological theory that provides the reason for its effectiveness.**

REFERENCES

Dean E: Oxygen transport: a physiologically-based framework for the practice of cardiopulmonary physiotherapy, *Physiotherapy* 80:347, 1994.

Potter PA, Perry AG: *Fundamentals of nursing,* ed 4, St Louis, 1997, Mosby.

Silverberg R, et al: A survey of the prevalence and application of chest physical therapy in US burn centers, *J Burn Care and Rehab* 16:154, 1995.

Thompson J, et al: *Mosby's manual of clinical nursing,* ed 2, St Louis, 1992, Mosby.

Thoren L: Post-operative pulmonary complications: Observations on their prevention by means of physiotherapy, *Acta Chir Scand* 107:193, 1954.

ADDITIONAL READING

Johnson D, Kelm C: Postoperative physical therapy after coronary artery bypass surgery, *Am J Respir Crit Care Med* 152:953, 1995.

Patton MD, Schaerf R: Thoracotomy, critical pathway, and clinical outcomes, *Cancer-Practice: A multidisciplinary journal of cancer care* 3(5):286, 1995.

Williams MT: Chest physiotherapy and cystic fibrosis, *Chest* 106(6):1872, 1994.

CHAPTER 14

Airway Maintenance

OBJECTIVES

Mastery of content in this chapter will enable the nurse to:

- Define key terms.
- Identify guidelines used in managing the airway.
- Describe the methods of airway management for anatomical and artificial airways, respectively.
- Discuss the indications for airway suctioning.
- Discuss the indications for tracheostomy care.
- Suction the client's mouth of excess secretions.
- Suction the client's posterior pharynx or trachea through the nose.
- Suction the client's airway through an endotracheal tube.
- Suction the client's airway through a tracheostomy tube.
- Safely secure an endotracheal tube to the client's face.
- Safely secure a tracheostomy tube around the neck.
- Cleanse and dress the tracheostomy site.
- Correctly inflate the cuff on an endotracheal or tracheostomy tube.
- Change a tracheostomy tube in selected clients.

SKILLS

14-1 Performing Oral Pharyngeal (Yankauer) Suctioning

14-2 Performing Nasal Pharyngeal and Nasal Tracheal Suctioning

14-3 Performing Endotracheal or Tracheostomy Tube Suctioning

14-4 Performing Endotracheal or Tracheostomy Tube Suctioning Using a Closed System (In-Line) Catheter

14-5 Performing Endotracheal Tube Care

14-6 Performing Tracheostomy Care

14-7 Inflating the Cuff on an Endotracheal or Tracheostomy Tube

KEY TERMS

Artificial airway
Atelectasis
Bronchospasm
Bronchus
Closed system suction catheter
Cuff
Endotracheal (ET) tubes
Fenestration
Hypercapnia
Hypoxemia
Hypoxia
In-line suction catheter
Intubation
Laryngospasm
Lower airway respiratory system
Nasal airway
Obturator
Oral airway
Outer cannula
Oxygen therapy
Patent
Pharynx
Respiratory distress
Sputum
Suction
Suction catheter
Tracheal stenosis
Tracheoesophageal fistula
Tracheomalacia
Tracheostomy
Upper airway
Yankauer suction

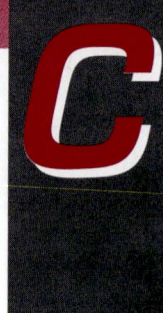

Many courses of action are available to promote an open or **patent** airway, which has the potential to become obstructed by mucus or a foreign body. These actions may not require a physician's order, depending on the situation. The physician should be consulted if there is any concern about the appropriateness of the intervention or if the obstruction does not respond to treatment. The nurse must consider maintaining the patency of the nose and **upper airway** as well as the trachea and **lower airway respiratory systems.** Based on continual assessment of the client, the nurse can include in the plan of care measures that aid in maintaining patency of the upper and lower airway. Hydration, nutrition, chest therapy airway clearance techniques, "flutter" mucous clearance device therapy, deep breathing, coughing, humidity, and aerosol therapy are noninvasive techniques that are helpful in maintaining a patent airway. For selected clients, medications such as antibiotics, bronchodilators, steroids, decongestants, antihistamines, and expectorants are adjuncts to these therapies.

In some clients use of the above techniques and medications is not sufficient to maintain a patent airway, and the client is at risk for development of **respiratory distress.** More invasive measures directed at maintaining airway patency may be necessary, especially in the critically ill client. This chapter focuses on nonemergent techniques designed to maintain patency of the anatomical and **artificial airways.** Techniques discussed include suctioning the anatomical and artificial airways (endotracheal tube, **tracheostomy** tube), caring for clients with an endotracheal tube or a tracheostomy tube, and properly inflating the **cuff** on an artificial airway.

GUIDELINES

1. Know client's normal range of vital signs. Baseline vital signs serve as a means to identify individual abnormalities and to recognize onset of illness or disease. Normal vital signs for one client may be abnormal for another client.
2. Know client's medical history. Certain disorders such as chronic obstructive pulmonary diseases (including asthma and cystic fibrosis, pneumonia, thoracic surgery, chest trauma, and abdominal surgery) place the client at increased risk for an obstructed airway. Other conditions that may increase the client's risk for aspiration of gastric contents into the lung and resulting airway obstruction include the presence of enteral feeding tubes or other nasal or oral gastric tubes, a decreased level of consciousness, and a decreased swallowing ability. Clients with a history of nasal problems, such as nasal trauma, deviated nasal septum, or chronic sinus problems causing mucosal swelling, may have narrow nasal passages, which can affect the nurse's ability to easily pass a **suction catheter.**
3. Know client's baseline respiratory assessment. Baseline assessment has two meanings. First, know what is historically normal for the client regarding pulmonary signs and symptoms, including chest assessment and **sputum** production. Second, know what the client's condition has been for the past 4, 8, 12, 16, or 24 hours. These are relative baseline measurements that assist the nurse in distinguishing between gradual and acute changes in the client's status.
4. Perform a systematic respiratory assessment (see Chapter 11) of upper and lower airways, including identifying respiratory rate, respiratory pattern, respiratory muscles used, breath sounds, ability to cough effectively, integrity of the rib cage, and the characteristics of sputum production (Chapter 11).
5. Determine the type and frequency of intervention, based on assessment findings. Care that is appropriate for one day or shift can change, resulting in an increase or decrease in frequency of care or alterations in the type of intervention.
6. Identify and become familiar with the application of equipment available at the institution. Many types of artificial airways, suction catheters, and suction machines are available. Knowing how to operate the equipment before it is needed benefits both the nurse and the client.
7. Test all equipment before use. Have adequate supplies on hand at the bedside. Equipment must work properly to provide safe nursing care. Determining that the suction machine is generating inadequate negative suction pressure or that there are no suction catheters at the bedside when the client has a mucous plug or overwhelming secretions is not safe, competent nursing practice.
8. Know client's home care plan. Absence or interruption of certain therapies such as bronchodilators can place the client at risk for an obstructed airway during the hospitalization or after discharge from the hospital.
9. Know the side effects of medications and other therapies. Some medications such as beta blockers have the side effect of **bronchospasm.** An adverse effect of narcotics and sedatives is respiratory depression. Similarly, too much oxygen can reduce the drive to breathe in clients with **hypercapnia** (elevated carbon dioxide tension). Position changes may affect the client adversely. For example, in clients with impaired spinal cord innervation of the respiratory muscles, supine positions place the diaphragm at a mechanical disadvantage and increase the risk of aspiration.

SKILL 14-1 Performing Oral Pharyngeal (Yankauer) Suctioning

Nurses use a Yankauer, or tonsillar tip, **suction** device to perform oral pharyngeal suctioning (Fig. 14-1). A **Yankauer suction** catheter is made of rigid, minimally flexible plastic. The tip of this suction catheter usually has one large and several small eyelets through which the mucus enters with application of negative pressure. The Yankauer suction catheter is angled to facilitate removal of pharyngeal secretions through the mouth. This catheter is used instead of a standard suction catheter when oral secretions are extremely copious and thick because it can

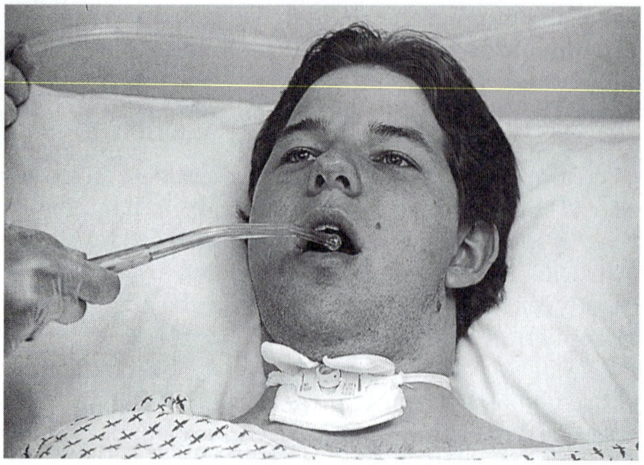

Fig. 14-1 Oropharyngeal suctioning.

handle large volumes of secretions better than a standard suction catheter. The Yankauer suction catheter is not used to suction the nares because of its size.

The Yankauer suction device is useful in the removal of secretions from the mouth in clients after oral and maxillofacial surgery, trauma to the mouth, or neurovascular injury and cerebrovascular accident causing hemiparesis and drooling or impaired swallowing. Clients with artificial airways and impaired swallowing ability may require use of the Yankauer suction device to promote oral hygiene. Alert clients or unlicensed assistive care givers of the client can be easily taught how to use this apparatus and control the oral secretions.

DELEGATION CONSIDERATIONS

The skill of performing oral pharyngeal (Yankauer) suctioning can be delegated to unlicensed assistive personnel and sometimes to the client and family.

- Educate and assist client and care provider until competent in proper technique to apply, clean, and store Yankauer suction device.
- Teach client and care provider appropriate suction limits for oral pharyngeal suctioning and risks of applying excessive or inadequate suction pressure.
- Caution client and care provider to avoid mouth sutures and to avoid applying suction against sensitive tissues.
- Caution client and care provider to avoid dislodging tubings in the client's nose or mouth.

EQUIPMENT

- **Towel, cloth, or disposable paper**
- **Nonsterile gloves**
- **Yankauer or tonsillar tip suction catheter**
- **Face shield or mask**
- **Disposable cup or nonsterile basin**
- **Tap water (about 100 ml)**
- **Portable or wall suction machine**
- **Connecting tubing (6 feet)**
- **Oral airway (if indicated)**
- **Washcloth (if indicated)**

STEPS — **RATIONALE**

ASSESSMENT

1. Observe for signs and symptoms associated with upper airway obstruction requiring oral pharyngeal suctioning: gurgling on inspiration or expiration, restlessness, obvious excess oral secretions, drooling, gastric secretions or vomitus in mouth, coughing without clearing secretions from upper airway.

Physical signs and symptoms may indicate need to perform this procedure. Worsening status may result in total airway obstruction and hypoxia. The risk of aspiration of gastric contents and airway obstruction is increased in clients with vomiting, delayed gastric emptying, impaired esophageal sphincter control, hiatal hernia, impaired cough, or impaired gag reflex.

CRITICAL DECISION POINT **Signs and symptoms associated with** hypoxia **(low oxygen utilization at the cellular or tissue level),** hypoxemia **(low oxygen tension in the blood), or hypercapnia (elevated carbon dioxide tension in the blood) may also be present: apprehension, anxiety, decreased ability to concentrate, lethargy, decreased level of consciousness (especially acute) increased fatigue and dizziness, behavioral changes (especially irritability), increased pulse rate, increased rate of breathing, decreased depth of breathing, elevated blood pressure, cardiac dysrhythmias, pallor, cyanosis, dyspnea, and use of accessory muscles for breathing.**

Table 14-1 Suction Catheters and Vacuum Setting

Age	Size of Catheter (Fr)
Newborn	6-8
Infant-18 mo	6-8
18 mo	8-10
24 mo	10
2-4 yr	10-12
4-7 yr	12
7-10 yr	12-14
10-12 yr	12-14
Adult	12-16

Vacuum Setting	Wall Suction	Portable Suction
Infants	60-100 mm Hg	3-5 mm Hg
Children	100-120 mm Hg	5-10 mm Hg
Adults	120-150 mm Hg	7-15 mm Hg

STEPS	RATIONALE
2. Assess client's knowledge about use of the catheter.	Reveals need for client instruction.
3. Assess for risk factors such as impaired cough, gag reflex, or swallowing or decreased level of consciousness.	Risk factors may prevent client from protecting the airway from aspiration or from clearing secretions safely.

NURSING DIAGNOSIS

Clustering of defining characteristics from the assessment data may reveal the following nursing diagnoses for clients requiring this skill:

- Ineffective airway clearance
- Risk for aspiration
- Ineffective breathing pattern
- Impaired gas exchange
- Risk for infection
- Knowledge deficit regarding airway clearance techniques and devices
- Impaired swallowing

Related factors are individualized based on a client's condition or needs.

PLANNING

STEPS	RATIONALE
1. **Expected outcomes** following completion of procedure:	
➤ Upper airway (oral **pharynx**) is cleared of secretions.	Upper airway is normally free of excess secretions.
➤ No gurgling is heard in pharynx on inspiration and expiration.	Presence of secretions in large upper airway produces noisy respirations.
➤ Oral secretions are diminished or absent.	Excessive drooling indicates that client is unable to handle oral secretions.
➤ Vomitus and gastric secretions are absent from mouth.	Gastric secretions retained in oral cavity increase client's risk for aspiration pneumonia.
2. Explain to client how the procedure will help clear airway secretions and relieve some breathing problems. Explain that coughing, gagging, or (less commonly) sneezing is normal and lasts only a few seconds. Encourage client to cough out secretions during procedure. Practice, if able. Splint surgical incisions, if necessary.	Gagging or coughing will only occur when the posterior pharynx is deeply suctioned or as a result of excess secretions. Coughing secretions out of lower airway or posterior pharynx will decrease the amount of suctioning required. Encourages cooperation and minimizes risks and associated anxiety.
3. Position client and place towel across client's chest.	Promotes client comfort and removal of airway secretions. Towel protects client's gown and bed linen from contamination by secretions.

IMPLEMENTATION

STEPS	RATIONALE
1. Wash hands and apply gloves. Apply mask or face shield.	Reduces transmission of microorganisms.
2. Fill cup or basin with approximately 100 ml of water.	For cleansing catheter after suctioning.
3. Turn suction device on; set regulator to appropriate negative pressure (Table 14-1).	Elevated pressure settings increase risk of trauma to the oral mucosa.
4. Connect one end of connecting tubing to suction machine and other to Yankauer suction catheter. Check that equipment is functioning properly by suctioning small amount of water from cup or basin.	Prepares suction apparatus. Ensures equipment function and lubricates catheter.
5. Remove client's oxygen mask, if present. Nasal cannula may remain in place. Keep oxygen near client's face. Try removing the straps from around the client's head that hold the mask in place and leaving the mask in place until ready to suction client.	Allows access to mouth.

➤ **CRITICAL DECISION POINT** Be prepared to quickly reapply supplemental oxygen if respiratory distress develops and at end of suctioning.

STEPS	RATIONALE
6. Insert catheter into mouth along gum line to pharynx. Move catheter around mouth until secretions are cleared. Encourage client to cough. Replace oxygen mask.	Catheter provides continuous suction. Take care not to allow suction tip to invaginate oral mucosal surfaces. Coughing moves secretions from lower airway into mouth and upper airway.
➤ ***CRITICAL DECISION POINT*** **Be careful not to dislodge any oral tubing or tubing in posterior pharynx, such as nasogastric tubes.**	
7. Rinse catheter with water in cup or basin until connecting tubing is cleared of secretions. Turn off suction. May need to wash face if secretions are present on client's skin.	Rinses catheter and reduces probability of transmission of microorganisms. Clean suction tubing enhances delivery of set suction pressure. Prevents skin breakdown.
8. Reassess respiratory status. Repeat procedure, if indicated. May need to use standard suction catheter to reach into trachea if respiratory status not improved.	Directs nurse to continue or cease intervention or to choose another intervention.
9. Remove towel, and place in trash or in laundry if soiled. Reposition client; Sims' position encourages drainage and should be used if client has decreased level of consciousness.	Reduces transmission of microorganisms. Facilitates drainage of oral secretions.
10. Discard remainder of water into appropriate receptacle. Rinse basin in warm soapy water and dry with paper towels. Discard disposable cup into appropriate receptacle. Place catheter in clean dry area.	Reduces transmission of microorganisms and maintains medical asepsis. Moist environment encourages microorganism growth.
➤ ***CRITICAL DECISION POINT*** **Catheter should be kept in non-airtight container such as brown paper or plastic bag attached to bed rail or in suction canister area. It should not be stored where it will come in contact with secretions or excretions or will contaminate clean supplies. Closure in an airtight container promotes bacterial growth.**	
11. Remove gloves and mask or face shield and dispose in appropriate receptacle. Wash hands.	Reduces transmission of microorganisms to other clients. Clean equipment should not be handled with contaminated gloves.

EVALUATION

1. Compare assessment findings before and after procedure.	Identifies physiological response to the suction procedure.
2. Auscultate chest and airways for adventitious sounds.	
3. Observe client perform Yankauer suctioning and document description of performance of skill.	Documents client's or unlicensed care giver's ability to perform procedure correctly.
4. **Unexpected outcomes** that may occur include:	
➤ Client becomes cyanotic, tachycardic or bradycardic, more restless, or exhibits other signs of hypoxemia or hypercapnia.	Client may have aspirated or cardiopulmonary compromise may have developed as result of tissue hypoxia.
➤ Bloody secretions are suctioned.	Bloody secretions can result from trauma to oral or pharyngeal mucosa; excessively high suction pressures may have been used.

STEPS	RATIONALE
RECORDING AND REPORTING	
1. Record in nurses' notes respiratory assessments before and after suctioning; use of Yankauer suction catheter; duration of suctioning period (if unusual, as in nearly continuous secretions); secretions obtained—odor, amount, color, consistency; frequency of suctioning; client's tolerance of procedure; amount of negative suction pressure used (unless standardized in institution or deviation from usual). Record instruction to care givers and ability to correctly perform procedure.	Documents cardiopulmonary status, nursing care, expected and unexpected outcomes, and provides baseline for future assessments. Documents teaching and competency of care giver.

FOLLOW-UP ACTIVITIES

1. Worsening respiratory distress
   a. Evaluate need for nasal, oral pharyngeal, or tracheal suctioning.
   b. Evaluate need for other means to protect airway (e.g., oral intubation, airway, positioning).
   c. Evaluate need for supplemental oxygen (Chapter 12).
   d. Evaluate need for manual breathing assistance after suctioning.
2. Return of bloody secretions
   a. Evaluate amount of suction pressure used.
   b. Evaluate possibility of mucosal trauma from catheter tip.
   c. Check laboratory clotting indicators or medication interactions that may predispose client to bleeding.

• • • • •

Special Considerations

- For portable suction machines, as the secretion collection jar fills, the efficiency of the suction decreases. The collection container should be emptied with use of splash precautions when half full.
- Clients with the following conditions are at risk for accumulation of oral secretions: decreased level of consciousness, impaired gag reflex, impaired swallowing, nasogastric tubes that decrease or irritate esophageal lumen, impaired cough, heavy sedation, oral surgery, oral trauma, head injury, spine injury.
- Clients at risk for bloody secretions include those with hemophilia or blood dyscrasias or those receiving chemotherapy, anticoagulant therapy, and other medications with antiplatelet activity, including some antibiotics. Lower suction pressure should be applied.
- Clients who bite the catheter, preventing thorough suctioning, may require insertion of an **oral airway.**
- If trauma to oral mucosa repeatedly occurs, incorporate frequent oral hygiene into nursing plan (Chapter 6). Nurse must also evaluate whether procedure was correctly performed.
- A Yankauer suction device is frequently used in clients with swallowing problems such as occur after stroke, **intubation,** or ear, nose, or throat surgery. Observe client to be sure that sutures, tubes, traumatized tissue, and dressings are undisturbed.
- If indicated, the nurse can leave a small disposable cup of tap water at the bedside for client rinsing. If the client is unable to independently rinse the suction device, the nurse should periodically rinse secretions from the tubing. Suction ability is reduced when secretions accumulate in the tubing, and secretions remaining in the tubing may increase risk of infection.
- Yankauer suction devices can be soaked in hydrogen peroxide and rinsed thoroughly to remove encrusted secretions and then reused. Mouthwash mixed with hydrogen peroxide results in a fresher smell and taste.
- Do not allow suction equipment to fall to the floor or become contaminated by excrement, including nasogastric tube drainage.

Home Care Considerations

- In the home the secretion collection container is cleaned and disinfected or changed every 24 hours according to home care or institutional protocol. In many institutions the disposable secretion collection canister is sealed and disposed of in its entirety as biohazardous material.
- Assess knowledge level of the client, family, and primary care giver to determine the amount of instruction required and the frequency of visits necessary to reach the goals.
- Assess home for the presence of respiratory irritants, including cigarette smoke, dust, pollen, or chemicals.

SKILL 14-2 Performing Nasal Pharyngeal and Nasal Tracheal Suctioning

Nasal pharyngeal and nasal tracheal suctioning maintain a patent airway by removing secretions from the pharynx or throat and the trachea. This type of suctioning is used when suctioning with a Yankauer device is ineffective or inappropriate or when the lower airway requires removal of secretions. It involves inserting a small rubber or plastic tube into the naris to the pharynx or trachea and then applying negative pressure to withdraw mucus.

The major differences between pharyngeal and tracheal suctioning are the depth suctioned and the potential for complications. Pharyngeal suctioning only removes secretions from the back of the throat and requires clean technique. Tracheal suctioning extends into the lower airway and necessitates aseptic technique. The nurse assesses the client to determine frequency and depth of suctioning. Some clients may require suctioning every hour or two, whereas others need to be suctioned only once or twice a day. How far to insert the suction catheter for tracheal suctioning depends on the size of the client, especially children. Infants and young children can accept insertion of a catheter 8 to 14 cm (3 to 5.5 in), whereas the older child to adolescent can allow insertion of the catheter to a depth of 14 to 20 cm (5.5 to 8 in). These lengths vary with each child; children who are small for their age have shorter airways that require less deep suctioning. The nurse can verify the correct catheter length by measuring the distance from nose (or mouth) to ear and nose (or mouth) to sternal notch for nasal (or oral) tracheal suctioning.

The nurse uses these techniques of suctioning primarily to remove accumulated nasal pharyngeal and tracheal secretions in the absence of an artificial airway. If the secretions are only in the nose and mouth, then only the pharynx requires suctioning, although in most instances the nurse will suction both the pharynx and the trachea. Secretions should be suctioned from the pharynx as often as necessary. Secretions that are not removed are more likely to be aspirated into the lungs, increasing the risk for potential infection and respiratory failure. In addition, the nurse may need to remove other body fluids, primarily blood and gastric contents, from the oral and posterior pharynx to prevent their aspiration as well.

The carina, located at the bifurcation of the mainstem bronchi, has many cough receptors. Many times the nurse will be able to stimulate a client's decreased cough reflex by passing a suction catheter to the carina. Once the client coughs, clearing of the lower airway is more effective.

Suctioning has many risks associated with performing the procedure. The most serious ones relate to hypoxemia, often resulting in cardiac dysrhythmias, although nasal trauma and bleeding can develop as well as mucosal injury from the suction catheter.

DELEGATION CONSIDERATIONS

This skill requires problem solving and knowledge application unique to a professional nurse. For this skill, delegation is inappropriate.

EQUIPMENT

- **Appropriate-size suction catheter (smallest diameter that will remove secretions effectively) (see Table 14-1)**
- **Small Y-adapter (if catheter does not have a suction control port)**
- **Water-soluble lubricant**
- **Two sterile gloves or one sterile and one nonsterile glove**
- **Sterile basin**
- **Sterile normal saline solution or water (about 100 ml)**
- **Clean towel or paper drape**
- **Portable or wall suction**
- **Connecting tubing (6 feet)**
- **Nasal or oral airway (if indicated)**
- **Mask or face shield**

STEPS	RATIONALE
ASSESSMENT	
1. Assess signs and symptoms of upper and lower airway obstruction requiring nasal or oral tracheal suctioning, including wheezes, crackles, or gurgling on inspiration or expiration; restlessness; ineffective coughing; unilateral or lobar absent or diminished breath sounds (in absence of pneumonectomy or lobectomy); tachypnea; hypertension or hypotension;	Physical signs and symptoms result from decreased oxygen to tissues as well as pooling of secretions in upper and lower airways.

STEPS	RATIONALE
cyanosis; decreased level of consciousness, especially acutely; excess nasal secretions, drooling, gastric secretions or vomitus in mouth. Signs and symptoms associated with hypoxia (low oxygen utilization at cellular or tissue level), hypoxemia (low oxygen tension in blood), or hypercapnia (elevated carbon dioxide tension in blood) may also be present: apprehension, anxiety, decreased ability to concentrate, lethargy, decreased level of consciousness (especially acute), increased fatigue, dizziness, behavioral changes (especially irritability), increased pulse rate, increased rate of breathing, decreased depth of breathing, elevated blood pressure, cardiac dysrhythmias, pallor, cyanosis, dyspnea, use of accessory muscles for breathing.	
CRITICAL DECISION POINT **Risk factors for upper or lower airway obstruction include obstructive lung disease; pulmonary infections; impaired mobility; sedation; decreased level of consciousness; seizures; presence of feeding tube; decreased gag or cough reflex; decreased swallowing ability; allergies; sinus drainage; head, neck, or chest tumors.**	
2. Determine factors that normally influence upper or lower airway functioning	
a. Fluid status	Fluid overload may increase amount of secretions. Dehydration promotes thicker secretions.
b. Lack of humidity	The environment influences secretion formation and gas exchange necessitating airway suctioning when the client cannot clear secretions effectively.
c. Infection	Clients with respiratory infections are prone to increased secretions that are thicker and sometimes more difficult to expectorate.
d. Anatomy	Abnormal anatomy can impair normal drainage of secretions. For example, nasal swelling, deviated septum, or facial fractures may impair nasal drainage. Tumors in or around the lower airway may impair secretion removal by occluding or externally compressing the lumen of the airway.
3. Assess client's understanding of procedure.	Reveals need for client instruction and encourages cooperation.
4. Obtain physician's order if indicated by agency policy.	Some institutions require a physician's order for tracheal suctioning.

NURSING DIAGNOSIS

Clustering of defining characteristics from the assessment data may reveal the following nursing diagnoses for clients requiring this skill:

- Ineffective airway clearance
- Risk for aspiration
- Ineffective breathing pattern
- Impaired gas exchange
- Risk for infection
- Knowledge deficit regarding airway clearance techniques and devices
- Impaired swallowing
- Inability to sustain spontaneous ventilation

Related factors are individualized based on a client's condition or needs.

STEPS	RATIONALE
PLANNING	
1. **Expected outcomes** following completion of procedure: ➤ Lower and upper airways are cleared of secretions as evidenced by absent or diminished crackles, wheezes, and gurgles on inspiration and expiration; return of absent or diminished breath sounds; normalization of heart rate, blood pressure, respiratory rate and effort; absence of drooling, gastric secretions or vomitus in mouth, and nasal secretions. ➤ Client verbalizes easier breathing.	Airways are cleared of secretions. In the presence of infection more secretions are produced; as infection improves, the amount of secretions and the need for suctioning diminish.
2. Explain to client how procedure will help clear airway and relieve breathing problems. Explain that temporary coughing, sneezing, gagging, or shortness of breath is normal during the procedure. Encourage client to cough out secretions. Practice coughing, if able. Splint surgical incisions, if necessary.	Encourages cooperation and minimizes risks, anxiety, and pain.
3. Explain importance of and encourage coughing during procedure.	Facilitates secretion removal and may reduce frequency of future suctioning.
4. Assist client to assume position comfortable for nurse and client (usually semi-Fowler's or sitting upright with head hyperextended, unless contraindicated).	Reduces stimulation of gag reflex, promotes client comfort and secretion drainage, prevents aspiration and nurse strain. Hyperextension facilitates insertion of catheter into trachea.
5. Place towel across client's chest.	Reduces transmission of microorganisms by protecting gown from secretions.
IMPLEMENTATION	
1. Wash hands and apply face shield if splashing is likely.	Reduces transmission of microorganisms.
2. Connect one end of connecting tubing to suction machine; and place other end in convenient location near client. Turn suction device on and set vacuum regulator to appropriate negative pressure (Table 14-1, p. 466).	Excessive negative pressure damages nasal pharyngeal and tracheal mucosa and can induce greater hypoxia.
3. If indicated, increase supplemental **oxygen therapy** to 100% or as ordered by physician. Encourage client deep breathing.	These measures reduce suction-induced hypoxemia.
➤ ***CRITICAL DECISION POINT*** **Oxygen must be readjusted as ordered by physician after procedure to avoid increased risk of oxygen toxicity and absorption atelectasis from prolonged administration of high concentrations of oxygen. Many mechanical ventilators have a button that increases inspired oxygen to 100% for short time and then returns it to previous level.**	
4. Prepare suction catheter: a. Open suction kit or catheter with use of aseptic technique. If sterile drape is available, place it across client's chest or on the over-bed table. Do not allow the suction catheter to touch any nonsterile surfaces.	Maintains asepsis and reduces transmission of microorganisms.

STEPS	RATIONALE
b. Unwrap or open sterile basin and place on bedside table. Be careful not to touch inside of basin. Fill with about 100 ml sterile normal saline solution or water.	Saline or water is used to clean tubing after each suction pass.
c. Open lubricant. Squeeze small amount onto open sterile catheter package without touching package.	Prepares lubricant while maintaining sterility. Water-soluble lubricant is used to avoid lipoid aspiration pneumonia.
5. Apply sterile glove to each hand, or apply nonsterile glove to nondominant hand and sterile glove to dominant hand.	Reduces transmission of microorganisms and allows nurse to maintain sterility of suction catheter.
6. Pick up suction catheter with dominant hand without touching nonsterile surfaces. Pick up connecting tubing with nondominant hand. Secure catheter to tubing (see illustration).	Maintains catheter sterility. Connects catheter to suction.

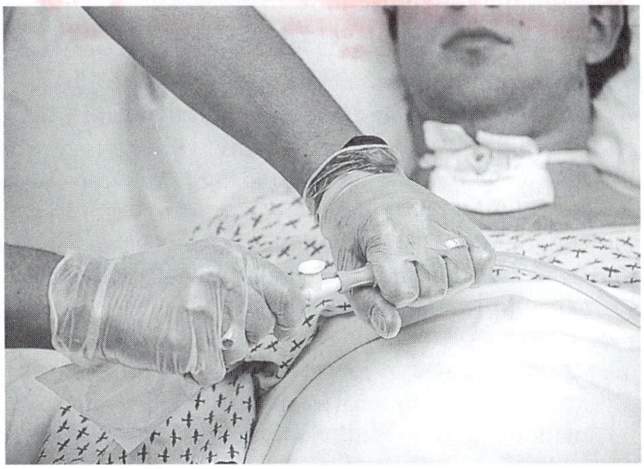

Step 6

STEPS	RATIONALE
7. Check that equipment is functioning properly by suctioning small amount of normal saline solution from basin.	Ensures equipment function. Lubricates internal catheter and tubing.
8. Coat distal 6 to 8 cm (2 to 3 in) of catheter with water-soluble lubricant.	Lubricates catheter for easier insertion.
9. Remove oxygen delivery device, if applicable, with nondominant hand. Without applying suction and using dominant thumb and forefinger, gently but quickly insert catheter into naris during inhalation with slight downward slant or through mouth. Do not force through naris (see illustration).	

CRITICAL DECISION POINT **Be sure to insert catheter during client inhalation, especially if inserting catheter into trachea, because epiglottis is open. Do not insert during swallowing or catheter will most likely enter esophagus. *Never* apply suction during insertion.**

a. Pharyngeal suctioning: in adults, insert catheter about 16 cm; in older children, 8 to 12 cm (3 to 5 in); in infants and young children, 4 to 8 cm (2 to 3 in). Rule of thumb is to insert catheter distance from tip of nose (or mouth) to base of ear lobe.

b. Tracheal suctioning: in adults, insert catheter about 20 cm; in older children, 14 to 20 cm (5.5 to 8 in); and in young children and infants, 8 to 14 cm (3 to 5.5 in).

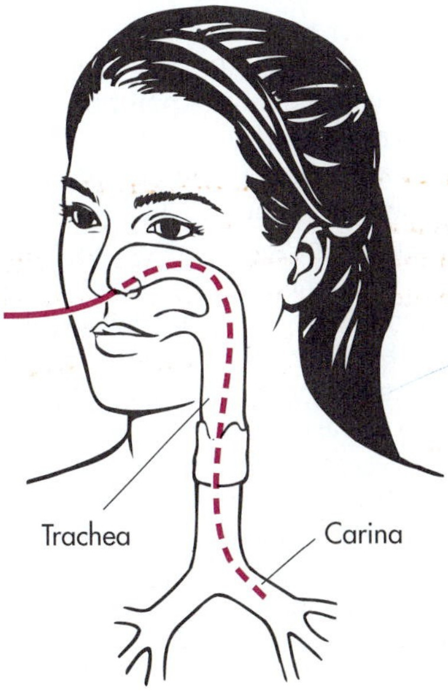

Step 9

STEPS	RATIONALE
c. Positioning: in some instances turning client's head to right helps nurse suction left mainstem bronchus; turning head to left helps nurse suction right mainstem bronchus. If resistance is felt after insertion of catheter for maximum recommended distance, catheter has probably hit carina. Pull catheter back 1 cm before applying suction.	Application of suction pressure while introducing catheter into trachea increases risk of damage to mucosa and increases risk of hypoxia because of removal of entrained oxygen present in airways. Epiglottis is open on inspiration and facilitates insertion into trachea. Client should cough. If client gags or becomes nauseated, catheter is most likely in esophagus and must be removed.
CRITICAL DECISION POINT **Use the nasal approach and perform tracheal suctioning before pharyngeal suctioning whenever possible. The mouth and pharynx contain more bacteria than the trachea does. If copious oral secretions are present before beginning the procedure, suction mouth with Yankauer suction device.**	
10. Apply intermittent suction for up to 10 to 15 seconds by placing and releasing nondominant thumb over vent of catheter and slowly withdrawing catheter while rotating it back and forth between dominant thumb and forefinger. Encourage client to cough. Replace oxygen device, if applicable.	Intermittent suction and rotation of catheter prevents injury to mucosa. If catheter "grabs" mucosa, remove thumb to release suction. Suctioning longer than 10 seconds can cause cardiopulmonary compromise, usually from hypoxemia or vagal overload.
11. Rinse catheter and connecting tubing with normal saline or water until cleared.	Removes secretions from catheter. Secretions that remain in suction catheter or connecting tubing decrease suctioning efficiency.
12. Assess for need to repeat suctioning procedure. Allow adequate time between suction passes for ventilation and oxygenation. Ask client to deep breathe and cough.	Observe for alterations in cardiopulmonary status. Suctioning can induce hypoxemia, dysrhythmias, laryngospasm, and bronchospasm. Deep breathing reventilates and reoxygenates alveoli. Repeated passes clear the airway of excessive secretions but can also remove oxygen and may induce **laryngospasm.**
13. When pharynx and trachea are sufficiently cleared of secretions, perform oral pharyngeal suctioning to clear mouth of secretions. Do not suction nose again after suctioning mouth.	Removes upper airway secretions. More microorganisms are generally present in mouth.
14. When suctioning is completed, roll catheter around fingers of dominant hand. Pull glove off inside out so that catheter remains coiled in glove. Pull off other glove over first glove in same way to seal in contaminants. Discard in appropriate receptacle. Turn off suction device.	Reduces transmission of microorganisms.
15. Remove towel, place in laundry or appropriate receptacle, and reposition client. (Nurse may need to wear clean gloves for personal care.)	Reduces transmission of microorganisms. Promotes comfort.
16. If indicated, readjust oxygen to original level because client's blood oxygen level should have returned to baseline.	Prevents absorption **atelectasis** and oxygen toxicity while allowing client time to reoxygenate blood.
17. Discard remainder of normal saline into appropriate receptacle. If basin is disposable, discard into appropriate receptacle. If basin is reusable, rinse it out and place it in soiled utility room.	Reduces transmission of microorganisms.
18. Remove face shield and discard into appropriate receptacle. Wash hands.	Reduces transmission of microorganisms.
19. Place unopened suction kit on suction machine table or at head of bed.	Provides immediate access to suction catheter.

STEPS	RATIONALE
EVALUATION	
1. Compare client's respiratory assessments before and after suctioning.	Determines airway clearing and patency.
2. Ask client if breathing is easier.	Provides subjective data about client's perception of effect of suctioning.
3. **Unexpected outcomes** that may occur include:	
➤ Client becomes cyanotic, tachycardic, bradycardic, more restless, less alert; has cardiac arrest; dysrhythmias develop.	Effect of prolonged hypoxemia on client's cardiopulmonary and cerebral circulation. Client may have aspirated gastric secretions.
➤ Returned secretions are bloody.	Suctioning denuded cilia and mucosal lining. Bloody secretion may also indicate presence of infection.
➤ Nurse is unable to pass suction catheter through first naris attempted.	Obstruction is present or catheter is misplaced.
➤ Client has spasmodic episode of coughing.	Suctioning irritates trachea. Bronchospasm may occur. Prolonged coughing episodes can disrupt ventilation and interfere with venous return to heart.
➤ No secretions are obtained.	When client is poorly hydrated and is not receiving humidified oxygen or room air, pulmonary secretions can consolidate in airways. Secretions may not be in proximal airways but in distal airways where they cannot be suctioned.
➤ Suction catheter cannot be removed easily.	Rarely, repeated suctioning may cause laryngospasm.
RECORDING AND REPORTING	
1. Chart in nurses' notes respiratory assessments before and after suctioning; size of suction catheter used; duration of suctioning period, if unusual; route(s) used to suction; secretions obtained; odor, amount, color, consistency of secretions; frequency of suctioning; client's tolerance of procedure; amount of negative suction pressure used (unless standardized in institution or deviation from usual).	Documents cardiopulmonary status, nursing care, and outcomes and provides baseline for future assessment.

FOLLOW-UP ACTIVITIES

1. Worsening respiratory assessment:
   a. Limit length of suctioning.
   b. Determine need for more frequent suctioning, possibly of shorter duration.
   c. Determine need for supplemental oxygen. Supply oxygen between suctioning passes.
   d. Determine need for manual assistance with breathing after suctioning.
   e. Initiate resuscitation measures.
   f. Notify physician.
2. Return of bloody secretions:
   a. Determine amount of suction pressure used. May need to be decreased.
   b. Determine nurse's use of intermittent suction and catheter rotation.
   c. Evaluate suctioning frequency.
   d. Evaluate use of medications affecting blood clotting and laboratory blood clotting studies.
3. If unable to pass suction catheter through first naris attempted:
   a. Try other naris or oral route.
   b. Insert **nasal airway,** especially if suctioning through client naris frequently.
   c. Follow naris floor to avoid turbinates.
   d. If obstruction is mucus, apply suction to relieve obstruction, but do not apply suction to mucosa. If obstruction is felt to be a blood clot, consult with physician.
   e. Increase lubrication.

STEPS **RATIONALE**

4. Period of spasmodic coughing:
   a. Allow client to use supplemental oxygen.
   b. Unless emergent situation occurs, allow period of spasmodic coughing to subside before second catheter pass.
   c. Administer bronchodilator as prescribed by physician.
   d. Instill topical anesthetic such as lidocaine, as prescribed by physician.
5. No secretions obtained:
   a. Evaluate fluid status.
   b. Evaluate infection status.
   c. Evaluate humidity source for supplemental oxygen.
   d. Evaluate need for physical measures to move secretions from distal to proximal airways.
6. Unable to remove suction catheter (critical situation):
   a. Disconnect suction source from catheter, but leave catheter in trachea.
   b. Connect oxygen source to catheter.
   c. Notify physician immediately.
   d. Anticipate physician's order for inhaled bronchodilator such as racemic epinephrine.
   e. Prepare for emergency resuscitation.

• • • • •

Special Considerations

- For portable suction machines, as the secretion collection jar fills, the efficiency of the suction decreases. The collection container should be emptied when half full.
- Clients with the following conditions are at greater risk for retained secretions: sinusitis; recent surgery; rib fractures; decreased level of consciousness; increased intracranial pressure; impaired gag reflex; impaired or absent cough; heavy sedation; neuromuscular diseases, including spinal cord injury; pneumonia; chronic obstructive pulmonary diseases (COPD), including cystic fibrosis and asthma, congestive heart failure, and pulmonary edema. Certain physical injuries contraindicate use of nasal pharyngeal suctioning: skull fractures, especially basilar, and nasal fractures.
- Fluid and nutrition: inadequately hydrated clients may have thick secretions; inadequately nourished clients have impaired total lung function and ability to fight infection.
- Nasal structure: septal deviations impair secretion drainage and catheter passage. Clients with history of deviated septum or facial trauma may require placement of nasal airway before pharyngeal suctioning is attempted (see Chapter 15). Clients in some geographical areas have tendency toward swollen nasal mucosa from allergies or other conditions. Consult with the physician about topical or systemic decongestants.
- Face shield reduces risk of droplet contamination of nurse's face and eyes.
- Positioning: Sims' position encourages drainage of oral and nasal secretions and should be used in clients who are comatose or semialert.
- Clients with repeated nasal pharyngeal suctioning are at risk for return of bloody secretions and may require insertion of nasal airway.
- In many institutions the disposable secretion collection canister is sealed and discarded in its entirety as biohazardous material.

Pediatric Considerations

- Infants and young children have a smaller-diameter airway than adults do and proportionally larger tongue. Glottis is higher; thorax is smaller, with more horizontal ribs in soft rib cage. Diaphragm is higher and often impaired by abdominal size.
- Bulb suctioning is often used in infants and young children.

Gerontologic Considerations

- Older adults have lost some properties of elastic recoil and gas exchange.
- Capillaries of older adults are often fragile, predisposing client to bleeding problems.
- Older clients may have coronary artery disease, which places them at increased risk for cardiopulmonary compromise. In addition, older adults may be taking blood-thinning medications such as aspirin for the prevention of coronary or cerebral artery occlusion.

Home Care Considerations

- Although most clients with airway clearance problems at home have a tracheostomy, some also require nasal pharyngeal suctioning. Catheters are often used for a 24-hour period and then cleaned and disinfected; or catheters are cleaned with soapy water after each use and discarded after 24 hours.
- In the home the secretion collection container is cleaned and disinfected or changed every 24 hours according to home care or institutional protocol.

CARE OF THE CLIENT WITH AN ARTIFICIAL AIRWAY: THE FOLLOWING MATERIAL APPLIES TO SKILLS 14-3 THROUGH 14-7

Endotracheal (ET) tubes and tracheostomy ("trach") tubes are artificial airways inserted to relieve mechanical airway obstruction, provide a route for mechanical ventilation, permit easy access for secretion removal, and protect the airway from gross aspiration in clients with impaired cough or gag reflexes.

ET intubation is a procedure performed by a physician or specially trained personnel (e.g., nurse, respiratory therapist, or rescue personnel). An ET tube is inserted through the naris (nasal ET tube) or the mouth (oral ET tube) past the epiglottis and vocal cords into the trachea.

ET tubes are usually left in place for as long as 4 weeks, after which time a tracheostomy tube is inserted directly into the trachea through a small incision made in the client's neck by the physician. Although ET tubes are temporary, a tracheostomy tube can be temporary or permanent depending on the client's condition. One advantage of tracheostomy tubes in clients receiving mechanical ventilation is that they are shorter and decrease dead space ventilation. In selected clients decreasing dead space enhances the ability to wean from a mechanical ventilator, making the tracheostomy tube a temporary need. In other clients removal of critical airway structures with radical neck surgical procedures dictates the need for a permanent tracheostomy tube.

ET tubes are usually made of plastic or rubber; tracheostomy tubes are made of several different materials, including various polyvinylchloride- or silicone-based plastics and stainless steel or metallic compounds. Metal tracheostomy tubes are thermal sensitive and must be protected from extreme heat and cold to prevent tissue injury in the client. Some metal and plastic tracheostomy tubes contain an inner cannula that can be temporarily withdrawn for cleaning airway-occluding mucus without removing the entire tracheostomy tube. In critical care areas or acute care situations, an inner cannula is not always needed in clients being suctioned routinely; however, an inner cannula is essential in clients who are not suctioned and who cannot consistently expectorate sputum from the tracheostomy tube.

Adult, but not pediatric, sizes of ET tubes have a cuff molded onto the **outer cannula** to (1) prevent the aspiration of oral secretions or gastric contents into the lung or (2) obstruct the escape of air from mechanical ventilator breaths through the upper airway. Although pediatric tracheostomy tubes do not contain a cuff because of the small airway diameter of the child, adult sizes are available cuffed or noncuffed. A cuff on a tracheostomy tube serves the same purpose as one on an ET tube. Cuffs are made of a balloonlike inflatable plastic; usually they are manually inflated with air by the nurse or respiratory therapist. Plastic-covered foam cuffs are self–air inflating if the inflation port is left open to the atmosphere. Before the development of plastic tracheostomy tubes, cuffs were manually attached to the outer cannula of metal tracheostomy tubes, but the cuffs became displaced and occluded the airway, creating a safety hazard. Therefore nonpermanent cuffs are rarely used today.

Tracheostomy tubes are available as either fenestrated or nonfenestrated. (A fenestration is a small hole.) In tracheostomy tubes the **fenestration** is usually on the outer, or greater, curve of the outer cannula of a tracheostomy tube; the inner cannula does not usually contain a fenestration. (ET tubes are not fenestrated primarily because of the risk of aspiration and also because of associated injury to the vocal cords with speech.) When the cuff is deflated and the inner cannula is removed, a fenestrated tracheostomy tube permits the client to talk because exhaled air passes over the vocal cords. Phonation is optimized when the outer cannula is plugged, forcing all inhaled and exhaled air to travel by normal nasal and oral routes. A fenestrated tracheostomy tube usually allows the client to talk only in the absence of mechanical ventilation. (NOTE: Clients can also talk if there is no cuff or if the cuff is deflated when a nonfenestrated tracheostomy tube is used.) Newer types of cuffed tracheostomy tubes allow the client to talk during mechanical ventilation with the use of a narrow fenestrated catheter molded to the external surface of the outer cannula. This catheter is connected to an independent air source that blows air over the vocal cords, permitting phonation that ranges from an audible whisper to a clear voice.

Although nursing care is fairly standardized for all types of ET tubes, tracheostomy care must be individualized to the client and the type of tube in place. For example, caring for a client with a tracheostomy tube with an inner cannula is different from caring for one without this device. Care of a client with stomatitis differs from care of a client with a noninflamed or noninfected stoma site. These considerations must be addressed when planning nursing care.

After insertion of an ET or tracheostomy tube, the cuff (when present and medically indicated) is inflated. Preventing cuff-related problems is a critical component of nursing care and depends on securing the tube and inflating the cuff properly. In many institutions these functions are shared by nursing and respiratory therapy staff. An inadequately secured ET or tracheostomy tube moves up and down the tracheobronchial tree. Allowing an ET tube to slip too far down into the lungs can prevent ventilation of a lung, usually the left lung (and sometimes the right upper lobe also) because of anatomical differences. Allowing an ET tube to slide too far up the tracheobronchial tree can allow air to escape through or damage the vocal cords and epiglottis or permit aspiration of upper airway secretions. Properly securing the ET or tracheostomy tube prevents incidental extubation from coughing or pulling on the tube. In addition, movement of an ET or tracheostomy tube can cause development of granulation tissue on the vocal cords, epiglottis, or trachea. Additional risks of movement of an artificial airway are **tracheal stenosis, tracheomalacia,** erosion of the innominate artery, and **tracheoesophageal fistula,** particularly when the cuff is overinflated. Risks for each of these complications can be reduced with proper nursing care.

The goals of correctly inflating the cuff on an artificial airway are to promote lung inflation for mechanical ventilation, to prevent aspiration of gastric contents, and at the same time to allow drainage of secretions that accumulate between the epiglottis and the cuff (see the box below). The amount of air inserted in the cuff is based on several factors; the two most important factors are the size of the client's trachea and the external diameter of the artificial airway. If two clients of approximately the same size are intubated—one with a size 6 and one with a size 8—the client with the larger tube (size 8) will require less air in the cuff. This is because the larger tube occludes more of the airway than the smaller tube does. There are several techniques to inflate a cuff. The one presented in this chapter, minimal-leak technique, meets the goals of cuff inflation (see Skill 14-7).

After the tube is inserted and secured and the cuff is inflated, the chief concern of the nurse is to maintain patency of the ET or tracheostomy tube. In clients who cannot clear the airway of secretions, patency is achieved primarily through periodic suctioning of the artificial airway. Some clients with a tracheostomy tube are able to cough secretions out of the tracheostomy tube completely, whereas others are able only to cough secretions up into the tracheostomy tube. The latter clients may not require suctioning when an inner cannula is present because it can be safely removed, cleaned, and reinserted.

INDICATIONS FOR CUFF INFLATION

Mechanical Ventilation
- Continuous airway pressure
- Positive end-expiratory pressure (PEEP)
- Inability to meet ventilatory requirements with cuff down
- Inability to meet oxygen requirements with cuff down

Risk of Aspirating Gastric Contents
- Feeding tube, especially large bore, in stomach
- Gastroesophageal reflux disease
- Hiatal hernia

During and After Meals
- Impaired emptying
- Decreased gag reflex
- Impaired swallowing

Applying the laws of physics allows the nurse to understand the effects of secretions in the airway. Increasing the diameter of a tube (or artificial airway) decreases airway resistance. Decreasing the diameter of a tube increases airway resistance and therefore the work of breathing. Removing secretions from the artificial airway maintains patency, increases the diameter of the tube, and decreases the work of breathing. In addition, as stated before, a cough can be stimulated by suctioning; an effective cough reduces or eliminates the need for suctioning. The client helps maintain airway patency with facilitation of the natural cough reflex.

Usually suctioning is performed with the same kind of suction catheter as that used in nasal tracheal suctioning (see Table 14-1). However, this skill is easier to perform than nasal tracheal suctioning because there is already direct access to the lower airway. Systemic complications associated with ET or tracheostomy tube suctioning are similar to those related to nasal or oral tracheal tube suctioning, but the client who requires an artificial airway may have more physiological compromise and may be at greater risk for development of complications. Some institutions use a **closed system suction catheter** or **in-line suction catheter** device, especially in critically ill or highly contagious clients (see Skill 14-4).

A comprehensive plan and execution of care include properly securing the tube, inflating the cuff, maintaining patency by suctioning, and encouraging communication and oral hygiene, skills that are not included in this chapter. The intubated client is unable to speak because placement of the ET and tracheostomy tube prevents normal airflow over and vibration of the vocal cords. When caring for an intubated client, the nurse is encouraged to use verbal and nonverbal communication skills to converse (Albarran, 1991). Alphabet charts, pen and paper, slates or chalk boards, or magnetic pen doodle boards are some commonly used communication tools. There are many more simple to sophisticated communication devices that can be used. A speech therapist can assist the nurse to establish effective communication.

Placement of an oral ET tube impedes performance of oral hygiene measures. Excessive manipulation of the tube can dislodge it; toothbrushing and mouth rinsing are difficult to perform because there is always the risk of fluid aspiration around the ET tube because the epiglottis is held open by the tube. The nurse promotes oral hygiene through the use of various techniques. One technique is to rotate the ET tube from one side of the mouth to the other on alternate days, thereby reducing pressure on the sides of the client's mouth and allowing improved visualization and cleaning of one side of the client's mouth. The use of a special toothbrush with a vacuum port also may be helpful in cleaning teeth and oral mucous membranes.

SKILL 14-3 Performing Endotracheal or Tracheostomy Tube Suctioning

EQUIPMENT

- Bedside table
- Suction catheter of appropriate size (see Table 14-1)
- Water-soluble lubricant, if indicated
- Two sterile gloves or one sterile and one nonsterile glove
- Sterile basin
- Approximately 100 ml of sterile normal saline solution or water
- Clean towel or sterile drape
- Portable or wall suction apparatus
- 6 feet of connecting tubing
- Face shield

DELEGATION CONSIDERATIONS

The skill of performing ET tube suctioning requires problem solving and knowledge application unique to a professional nurse. For this skill, delegation is inappropriate.

The skill of performing tracheostomy tube suctioning can be delegated to unlicensed assistive personnel and sometimes to the client in special situations. These situations include clients with permanent tracheostomy tubes after head and neck surgery and clients receiving mechanical ventilation at home.

- Educate and assist client and care provider until competent in proper technique to suction, clean, and store catheter and suction machine.
- Teach client and care provider appropriate suction limits for suctioning tracheostomy tube and risks of applying excessive or inadequate suction pressure.
- Teach client and care giver signs and symptoms of hypoxemia and methods to prevent and treat hypoxemia.

STEPS	RATIONALE
ASSESSMENT	
1. Observe for signs and symptoms of lower airway obstruction possibly causing hypoxemia or hypercapnia requiring ET or tracheostomy tube suctioning: apprehension, anxiety, decreased ability to concentrate, lethargy or other neurological or behavioral symptoms; coughing; secretions in artificial airway; wheezes, crackles, or gurgles on inspiration or expiration; restlessness or irritability; ineffective cough; unilateral (in absence of pneumonectomy or lobectomy) or bilateral absent or diminished breath sounds; abnormal vital signs including tachypnea, acutely shallow respirations, tachycardia or bradycardia, hypertension or hypotension; cyanosis; decreased level of consciousness (especially acute); decreased oxygen saturation by pulse oximetry.	Physical signs and symptoms result from lower airway obstruction and tissue hypoxia.
2. Determine factors that influence normal airway function: impaired cough reflex, recent surgery, decreased level of consciousness, ineffective or absent cough, chemical neuromuscular blockade, heavy sedation, neuromuscular diseases, pneumonia, COPD (including asthma and cystic fibrosis), congestive heart failure, pulmonary edema, adult respiratory distress syndrome, hyaline membrane disease, diaphragmatic weakness or paralysis.	Allows nurse to identify clients at risk for airway obstruction needing ET or tracheostomy tube suctioning.

STEPS	RATIONALE
3. Examine sputum microbiology data.	Certain bacteria are more easily transmitted or require isolation because of virulence or antibiotic resistance.
4. Assess client's understanding of procedure and feeling of lower airway congestion needing suctioning.	Identifies need for client teaching and validates other assessments that indicate need to perform procedure.

NURSING DIAGNOSIS

Clustering of defining characteristics from the assessment data may reveal the following nursing diagnoses for clients requiring this skill:

- Ineffective airway clearance
- Risk for aspiration
- Ineffective breathing pattern
- Impaired gas exchange
- Risk for infection
- Knowledge deficit regarding airway clearance techniques and devices
- Impaired swallowing
- Inability to sustain spontaneous ventilation

Related factors are individualized based on a client's condition or needs.

PLANNING

STEPS	RATIONALE
1. **Expected outcomes** following completion of procedure:	
➤ Absent or diminished crackles, wheezes, and gurgles in large airways on inspiration and expiration, normalization of heart rate, normalization of respiratory rate, increased depth of respiration, normalization of blood pressure, absence of cyanosis, increased oxygen saturation by pulse oximetry. Client verbalizes easier breathing and decreased congestion.	Lower and upper airways are cleared of secretions.
➤ Decreased, thinner, and normal-colored secretions are evident, with resolution of infection. Secretions should return to client's baseline sputum characteristics.	Exudate and cellular debris lessen as infection resolves, producing thinner, decreased, and normal-colored secretions.
2. Explain procedure and client's participation. Encourage coughing secretions out during procedure. Practice coughing, if able. Splint surgical incisions, if necessary.	Encourages cooperation, minimizes risks, reduces anxiety. Facilitates secretion removal and may reduce frequency of future suctioning.
3. Assist client to assume position comfortable for nurse and client, usually semi-Fowler's or Fowler's.	Promotes client comfort; prevents nurse muscle strain. Promotes maximal lung expansion and deep breathing. Also reduces risk of aspiration.
4. Place towel across client's chest.	Reduces transmission of microorganisms. Prevents soiling of client's bed linens and clothes.

IMPLEMENTATION

STEPS	RATIONALE
1. Wash hands and apply face shield.	Reduces transmission of microorganisms.
2. Connect one end of connecting tubing to suction machine and place other end in convenient location. Turn suction device on and set vacuum regulator to appropriate negative pressure (see Table 14-1).	Excessive negative pressure damages tracheal mucosa and can induce greater hypoxia.
3. Prepare suction catheter:	
a. Aseptically open suction catheter package. If sterile drape is available, place it across client's chest. Do not allow suction catheter to touch any nonsterile surface.	Prevents contamination of clothing and provides a sterile surface on which to lay suction catheter between passes, if needed. Prepares catheter and prevents transmission of microorganisms.
b. Unwrap or open sterile basin and place on bedside table. Be careful not to touch inside of basin. Fill with about 100 ml of sterile normal saline.	Normal saline is used to rinse catheter after suctioning.
4. If indicated, open lubricant. Squeeze onto sterile catheter package without touching package.	Prepares lubricant for use while maintaining sterility. Lubricant facilitates insertion, especially in narrow tubes.

STEPS	RATIONALE
CRITICAL DECISION POINT Clients with copious secretions and clients coughing secretions into ET tube may not require catheter lubrication.	
5. Apply one sterile glove to each hand, or apply nonsterile glove to nondominant hand and sterile glove to dominant hand.	Reduces transmission of microorganisms and allows nurse to maintain sterility of suction catheter.
6. Pick up suction catheter with dominant hand without touching nonsterile surfaces. Pick up connecting tubing with nondominant hand. Secure catheter to tubing.	Maintains catheter sterility.
CRITICAL DECISION POINT Be sure to keep the hand that is touching the catheter sterile. Do not switch the catheter from hand to hand.	
7. Check that equipment is functioning properly by suctioning small amount of saline from basin.	Ensures equipment function; lubricates catheter and tubing.
8. Coat distal 6 to 8 cm (2 to 3 in) of catheter with water-soluble lubricant. In some situations catheter is lubricated only with normal saline. Nursing assessment determines need for lubrication.	Promotes easier catheter insertion. If lubricant is needed, it must be water soluble to prevent petroleum-based aspiration pneumonia.
CRITICAL DECISION POINT Be careful to not overlubricate suction catheter. Excessive lubricant can adhere to artificial airway, causing obstruction, especially if allowed to dry.	
9. Hyperinflate and/or hyperoxygenate client before suctioning, using manual resuscitation Ambu-bag connected to oxygen source (Chapter 15) or sigh mechanism on mechanical ventilator. Some mechanical ventilators have a button that when pushed delivers 100% oxygen for a few minutes and then resets to the previous value.	Hyperinflation decreases atelectasis caused by negative pressure of suctioning. Preoxygenation converts large proportion of resident lung gas to 100% oxygen to offset amount used in metabolic consumption while ventilator or oxygenation is interrupted, as well as to offset volume lost during suction procedure.
CRITICAL DECISION POINT Be careful not to allow client to remain on high fraction of inspired oxygen (F_IO_2), such as 100%, too long. Atelectasis can develop from all of nitrogen washing out of lung. Long-term administration of high oxygen concentrations can predispose client to oxygen toxicity or absorption atelectasis.	
10. Open swivel adapter or if necessary remove oxygen or humidity delivery device with nondominant hand.	Exposes artificial airway.
11. Without applying suction, gently but quickly insert catheter using dominant thumb and forefinger into artificial airway (best to time catheter insertion with inspiration) until resistance is met or client coughs, then pull back 1 cm.	Application of suction pressure while introducing catheter into trachea increases risk of damage to tracheal mucosa, as well as increased hypoxia related to removal of entrained oxygen present in airways. Pulling back stimulates cough and removes catheter from mucosal wall.
CRITICAL DECISION POINT If unable to insert catheter past the end of the ET tube, the catheter is probably caught in the Murphy eye (i.e., side hole at distal end of ET tube that allows for collateral air flow in event of mainstem intubation). If this happens, rotate the catheter to reposition it away	

STEPS	RATIONALE
from the Murphy eye, or withdraw it slightly and reinsert with the next inhalation. Usually the catheter meets resistance at the carina. One indication that the catheter is at the carina is acute onset of coughing because the carina contains many cough receptors.	
12. Apply intermittent suction by placing and releasing nondominant thumb over vent of catheter; slowly withdraw catheter while rotating it back and forth between dominant thumb and forefinger. Encourage client to cough. Watch for respiratory distress.	Intermittent suction and rotation of catheter prevents injury to tracheal mucosal lining. If catheter "grabs" mucosa, remove thumb to release suction.
➤ ***CRITICAL DECISION POINT*** **If the client develops respiratory distress during the suction procedure, immediately withdraw the catheter and supply additional oxygen and breaths as needed. Oxygen can be administered directly through the catheter in an emergency. Disconnect suction and attach oxygen at prescribed flow rate through the catheter.**	
13. Close swivel adapter or replace oxygen delivery device. Encourage client to deep breathe, if able. Some clients respond well to several manual breaths from the mechanical ventilator or Ambu-bag.	Reoxygenates and reexpands alveoli. Suctioning can cause hypoxemia and atelectasis.
14. Rinse catheter and connecting tubing with normal saline until clear. Use continuous suction.	Removes catheter secretions. Secretions left in tubing decrease suction and provide environment for microorganism growth. Secretions left in connecting tube decrease suctioning efficiency.
15. Assess client's cardiopulmonary status for secretion clearance and complications. Repeat steps 1 through 15 once or twice more to clear secretions. Allow adequate time (at least 1 full minute) between suction passes for ventilation and reoxygenation.	Suctioning can induce dysrhythmias, hypoxia, and bronchospasm and impair cerebral circulation or adversely affect hemodynamics (Clark et al., 1990; Crosby and Parsons, 1992; Dam, Wild, and Baun, 1994; Kerr et al., 1993; Rudy et al., 1991). Repeated passes with suction catheter clear airway of excessive secretions and promote improved oxygenation.
16. Perform nasal and oral pharyngeal suctioning. After nasal and oral pharyngeal suctioning are performed, catheter is contaminated; do not reinsert into ET or tracheostomy tube.	Removes upper airway secretions.
➤ ***CRITICAL DECISION POINT*** **Upper airway is considered "clean," and lower airway is considered "sterile." Therefore same catheter can be used to suction from sterile to clean areas, but not from clean to sterile areas.**	
17. Disconnect catheter from connecting tubing. Roll catheter around fingers of dominant hand. Pull glove off inside out so that catheter remains in glove. Pull off other glove over first glove in same way to contain contaminants. Discard into appropriate receptacle. Turn off suction device.	Reduces transmission of microorganisms. Clean equipment should not be touched with contaminated gloves.
18. Remove towel and place in laundry, or remove drape and discard in appropriate receptacle.	

STEPS	RATIONALE
19. Reposition client as indicated by condition. Nurse may need to reapply clean gloves for client's personal care.	Promotes comfort. Sims' position encourages drainage and reduces risk of aspiration.
20. Discard remainder of normal saline into appropriate receptacle. If basin is disposable, discard into appropriate receptacle. If basin is reusable, rinse and place in soiled utility room.	
21. Remove and discard face shield and wash hands.	Reduces transmission of microorganisms.
22. Place unopened suction kit on suction machine or at head of bed according to institution preference.	Provides immediate access to suction catheter.

➤ ***CRITICAL DECISION POINT*** **Always remember to restock suction catheter supply, especially if catheters must be ordered from central service and are not available on floor stock, so there is no delay when client needs to be suctioned again.**

EVALUATION

1. Compare client's respiratory assessments before and after suctioning.	Identifies physiological effects of suction procedure to restore airway patency.
2. Ask client if breathing is easier and if congestion is decreased.	Provides subjective confirmation that airway obstruction is relieved with suctioning procedure.
3. Observe airway secretions.	Provides data to document presence or absence of respiratory tract infection.
4. **Unexpected outcomes** that may occur include:	
➤ Client becomes cyanotic, tachycardic, bradycardic, more restless, has cardiac arrest, dysrhythmias develop.	Suctioning-induced cardiopulmonary or cerebral compromise has occurred. Suctioning removes oxygen in addition to tracheobronchial secretions. As a result, hypoxemia leads to tissue hypoxia. Client may have aspirated secretions.
➤ Bloody secretions are returned.	Suctioning denuded cilia and mucosal lining. Bloody secretions can also indicate presence of infection. Clients with abnormal coagulation studies may bleed. Clients may be receiving medications that impede normal coagulation.
➤ Client has paroxysms of coughing.	Suctioning procedure induced airway spasm. Prolonged coughing episodes can disrupt ventilation and interfere with venous return to heart.
➤ No secretions are obtained.	When client is poorly hydrated or is not receiving humidified oxygen or room air, pulmonary secretions can consolidate in airways. Secretions may be located too distally to be suctioned.

RECORDING AND REPORTING

1. Chart in nurses' notes: respiratory assessments before and after suctioning; size of suction catheter used; amount of negative suction pressure used; duration of suctioning period, if unusual; route(s) used to suction; secretions obtained and odor, amount, color, consistency; frequency of suctioning; client's tolerance of procedure (unless standardized in institution or deviation from usual).	Documents cardiopulmonary status, nursing care given, and outcomes, and provides baseline for future assessments.

FOLLOW-UP ACTIVITIES

1. Worsening respiratory status:
   a. See Follow-Up Activities for Skill 14-2 (p. 478).

  b. Evaluate need for supplemental oxygen. Supply oxygen between catheter passes.
  c. Evaluate length of time between catheter insertion and removal of catheter.
  d. Evaluate size of suction catheter used to determine if it occluded lumen of tube by more than one half of tube diameter.
  e. Evaluate need for closed system (in-line) suction catheter.

2. Bloody secretions:
  a. Evaluate amount of suction pressure used. May need to be decreased.
  b. Evaluate use of intermittent suction and catheter rotation. Continuous suction and lack of rotation of catheter cause pulling of mucosal tissue.
  c. Evaluate need for suctioning frequency. Consider decreasing frequency.
  d. Evaluate blood coagulation studies. Client may require administration of blood products or medications to establish normal blood clotting.
  e. Determine presence of infection.
  f. Evaluate use of humidity. Lack of humidity can cause dry mucous membranes.
3. Paroxysms of coughing:
  a. Administer supplemental oxygen.
  b. Allow client to rest between passes of suction catheter.
  c. Consult with physician regarding need for inhaled bronchodilators or topical anesthetics.
4. No secretions were obtained (see Skill 14-2, Follow-Up Activities, p. 475).

• • • • •

Special Considerations

- With ET or trach tube, there is loss of upper airway functions, including warming, filtering, and humidifying. Clients with artificial airway need supplemental humidity.
- If client has thick, sticky secretions, assess hydration and infection. Inadequately hydrated clients may have thick secretions. Normal saline (5 to 10 ml) may be instilled before suctioning, followed by two or three deep breaths or manual breaths through the mechanical ventilator. Instillation of saline has limited value, but it usually stimulates a cough that moves secretions from distal to proximal airways. Saline instillation helps lubricate the airway making it easier to move the secretions, but it does not affect the consistency of secretions (Ackerman, 1993).
- The suction catheter should occlude less than 50% of the internal diameter of the artificial airway. An easy rule to follow is to limit the catheter size (Fr) to double the airway size. A size 8 ET tube should be suctioned with a size 16 Fr or smaller suction catheter. However, the suction catheter should be large enough to quickly and effectively remove airway secretions. Taking longer to remove secretions with a smaller diameter catheter may not be most effective and safest for the client.
- Conditions increasing risk for adverse effects of suctioning include prematurity, low oxygen tension or saturation, shock, myocardial infarction, congestive heart failure, respiratory failure, sepsis, and hepatic failure.
- Spasmodic coughing may occur more frequently in clients with asthma, cystic fibrosis, COPD, congestive heart failure, or toxic inhalation.
- Face shield protects nurse's eyes and mucous membranes from droplet contamination.

Pediatric Considerations

- Small-diameter suction catheters required in pediatrics are very flexible and may be more difficult to manipulate.
- Because of small diameter of suction catheter, thick secretions may be more difficult to remove.
- Infant airways have less cartilage and may collapse easily, especially in premature infants or those with reactive airways.

Home Care Considerations

In the home setting stress the importance of brief intervals of applying suction pressure. Those performing suctioning should hold their breath during the application of negative suction pressure to help them remember to not suction too long.

SKILL 14-4 Performing Endotracheal or Tracheostomy Tube Suctioning Using a Closed System (In-Line) Catheter

See introductory text for Skill 14-3, pp. 477 to 478.

Use of a closed system catheter (in-line) allows quicker lower airway suctioning without applying gloves or a mask and does not interrupt ventilation and oxygenation in critically ill clients. In addition, the nurse is protected from contamination by the client's secretions (Noll, Hix, and Scott, 1990; Witmer, Hess, and Simmons, 1991).

The introductory material for Skill 14-3 provides additional information regarding the suctioning of artificial airways.

EQUIPMENT

- **Closed system or in-line suction catheter**
- **10 ml of normal saline solution in syringe or vials**
- **Portable or wall suction apparatus**
- **6 feet of connecting tubing**
- **Two clean gloves (optional)**

DELEGATION CONSIDERATIONS

The skill of ET tube suctioning with a closed system (in-line) catheter requires problem solving and knowledge application unique to a professional nurse. For this skill, delegation is inappropriate.

The skill of performing tracheostomy tube suctioning with a closed system catheter can be delegated to unlicensed assistive personnel or the client in special situations (e.g., when a client has a permanent tracheostomy tube and may be receiving mechanical ventilation in the home or extended care facility).

- Educate and assist client and care provider until competent in proper technique to apply and care for closed system (in-line) catheter.
- Teach client and care provider appropriate suction limits for suctioning and risks of applying excessive or inadequate suction pressure.
- Teach client and care giver risks of inappropriate or incorrect application of closed system (in-line) suction catheter.

STEPS	RATIONALE
ASSESSMENT	
1. Observe for signs and symptoms of lower airway obstruction possibly causing hypoxemia or hypercapnia requiring ET or tracheostomy tube suctioning: secretions in artificial airway; coughing, wheezes, or crackles on inspiration and/or expiration; restlessness; ineffective cough; unilateral (in absence of lobectomy or pneumonectomy) or bilateral absent or diminished breath sounds; tachypnea; acute shallow respirations; acute tachycardia or bradycardia; acute hypotension or hypertension; cyanosis; decreased oxygen saturation by pulse oximetry; decreased level of consciousness especially acute; acute atelectasis or collapse of segment or lobe on chest x-ray films.	Physical signs and symptoms result from lower airway obstruction and tissue hypoxia. Mucous plug obstructs airflow into the lung, resulting in atelectasis or collapse.
2. Determine factors that influence normal airway function: impaired cough or gag reflex, decreased level of consciousness, ineffective or absent cough reflex, heavy sedation, neuromuscular diseases affecting chest or abdominal muscles, pneumonia or bronchitis, COPD, congestive heart failure, pulmonary edema, adult respiratory distress syndrome, hyaline membrane disease, diaphragmatic paralysis.	Allows nurse to accurately evaluate need to perform ET or tracheostomy tube suctioning. Client's inability to protect airway or clear secretions effectively indicates need for suctioning.
3. Examine sputum microbiology data.	Certain bacteria are more easily transmitted or require isolation because of virulence or antibiotic resistance.
4. Assess client's understanding of procedure and feeling that lower airway congestion needs suctioning.	Identifies need for client teaching and validates other assessments, indicating need to perform skill.

STEPS	RATIONALE

NURSING DIAGNOSIS

Clustering of defining characteristics from the assessment data may reveal the following nursing diagnoses for clients requiring this skill:

- Ineffective airway clearance
- Risk for aspiration
- Ineffective breathing pattern
- Impaired gas exchange
- Risk for infection
- Knowledge deficit regarding airway clearance techniques and devices
- Impaired skin integrity
- Impaired swallowing
- Inability to sustain spontaneous ventilation

Related factors are individualized based on a client's condition or needs.

PLANNING

1. **Expected outcomes** following completion of procedure:
   - Client does not develop lower respiratory tract infection from retained secretions or cross-contamination. Also, client does not cross-contaminate nurse or another client with infected secretions.

     Rationale: Removal of airway secretions reduces risk of pulmonary infection. Containment of secretions reduces risk of droplet transmission to nurse or other client.
   - Absent or diminished crackles and wheezes in large airways on inspiration and expiration, normalization of heart rate, normalization of respiratory rate, increased depth of respiration, normalization of blood pressure, normalization of oxygen saturation by pulse oximetry, absence of cyanosis, decreased or absent coughing are evident.
   - Signs of infection (fever, chills, night sweats, yellow-green sputum, elevated white blood cell count) are absent.

     Rationale: Lower and upper airways are cleared of secretions.
2. Explain procedure and client's participation. Explain that temporary coughing, sneezing, gagging, or shortness of breath is normal during the procedure. Encourage client to cough secretions out during procedure. Practice coughing, if able. Splint surgical incisions, if necessary.

   Rationale: Encourages cooperation, minimizes risks, reduces anxiety. Coughing facilitates secretion removal and may reduce frequency of future suctioning. Splinting reduces client pain and results in more effective cough effort.
3. Assist client to assume position comfortable for nurse and client, usually semi-Fowler's or Fowler's. If client is unconscious, place in side-lying position.

   Rationale: Promotes client and nurse comfort, reducing nurse's back muscle strain. Promotes maximal lung expansion and deep breathing. Also reduces risk of aspiration.
4. Place towel across client's chest.

   Rationale: Reduces transmission of organisms by protecting client's gown from secretions.

IMPLEMENTATION

1. Wash hands. Optional: apply clean gloves.

   Rationale: Reduces cross-transmission of microorganisms.
2. Attach suction:
   a. In many institutions the catheter is attached to the mechanical ventilator circuit by a respiratory therapist. If catheter is not already in place, open suction catheter package using aseptic technique, attach closed suction catheter to ventilator circuit by removing swivel adapter and placing closed suction catheter apparatus on ET or tracheostomy tube, and connect Y on mechanical ventilator circuit to closed suction catheter with flex tubing (see illustrations). The catheter becomes part of the circuit and is often changed by respiratory therapist with each circuit change or every 24 hours.

STEPS	RATIONALE
b. Connect one end of connecting tubing to suction machine and connect other to end of closed system or in-line suction catheter, if not already done. Turn suction device on and set vacuum regulator to appropriate negative pressure (see Table 14-1). Many closed system suction catheters require slightly higher suction pressures; consult manufacturer's guidelines (Connelly and Stone, 1991).	Prepares suction apparatus. Excessive negative pressure damages tracheal mucosa and can induce greater hypoxia. Inadequate suction pressure reduces effectiveness of suctioning, necessitating more passes or longer suctioning time.
3. Hyperinflate and/or hyperoxygenate client with Ambu-bag or manual breathing mechanism on mechanical ventilator according to institution protocol and clinical status (usually 100% oxygen).	Decreases atelectasis caused by negative pressure and increases oxygen available to tissues during suctioning.
4. Unlock suction control mechanism if required by manufacturer. Open saline port and attach saline syringe or vial.	Prepares suction apparatus.
5. Pick up suction catheter enclosed in plastic sleeve with dominant hand. If client requires normal saline to stimulate cough, advance catheter 2 to 3 cm (1 to 1.5 in) and squeeze vial or push syringe with other hand to release 5 to 10 ml of normal saline during inspiratory cycle.	Saline travels down suction catheter and into airway. Timing delivery of the saline with inhalation allows saline to be delivered into the lung rather than blown into ventilator circuit.
6. Wait until client inhales normal saline or mechanical ventilator delivers a breath to disperse saline and then quickly but gently insert catheter on next inhalation. To insert catheter, use a repeating maneuver of pushing catheter and sliding (or pulling) plastic sleeve back between thumb and forefinger until resistance is felt or client coughs.	
CRITICAL DECISION POINT **Some catheters contain depth markings that are useful in positioning catheter.**	Catheter sterility and secretion containment are provided by plastic sheath. Mechanical ventilator breaths, oxygen, and positive end-expiratory pressure (PEEP) are not interrupted during suctioning. Catheter slides within the plastic sheath. Coughing occurs or resistance is felt when the catheter touches the carina.

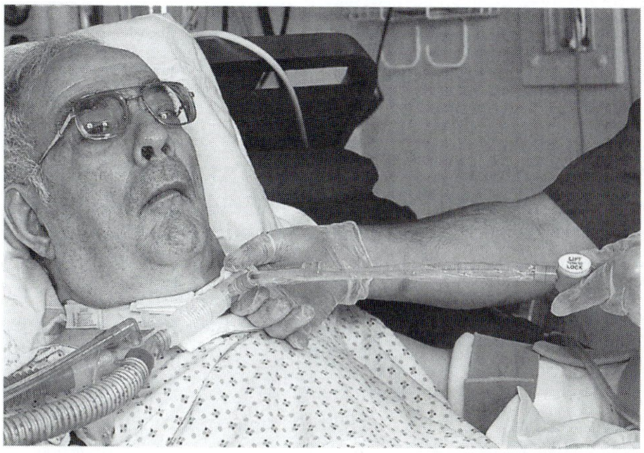

Step 2a(1)

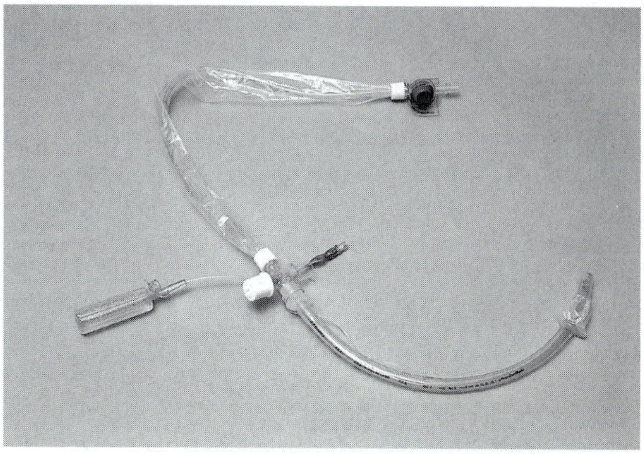

Step 2a(2) Closed system suction catheter attached to endotracheal tube.

STEPS	RATIONALE
7. Encourage client to cough and apply suction by squeezing on suction control mechanism while withdrawing catheter. It is difficult to apply intermittent pulses of suction and nearly impossible to rotate the catheter compared with a standard catheter. Be sure to withdraw catheter completely into plastic sheath so it does not obstruct airflow.	Removes secretions from airway. Plastic sheath limits rotational movement of catheter. Catheter left in ET or tracheostomy tube limits airflow.
8. Reassess cardiopulmonary status, including pulse oximetry, to determine need for subsequent suctioning or complications. Repeat steps 5 through 8 one to two more times to clear secretions. Allow adequate time (at least 1 full minute) between suction passes for ventilation and reoxygenation.	Repeated passes clear airway of secretions to promote ventilation and oxygenation. Suctioning can cause complications such as dysrhythmias, hypoxia, and bronchospasm.
9. When airway is clear, withdraw catheter completely into sheath. Be sure that colored indicator line on catheter is visible in the sheath. Squeeze vial or push syringe while applying suction to rinse inner lumen of catheter. Use at least 5 to 10 ml of saline. Lock suction mechanism, if applicable, and turn off suction.	Black line is reference point to determine correct position of catheter when not in use. Inability to see black line suggests catheter is in airway and may be impeding airflow. Interior of catheter must be rinsed to prevent bacterial growth inside catheter. Failure to lock mechanism can result in inadvertent continuous suction and serious complications.
10. If client requires oral or nasal suctioning, perform Skill 14-1 or 14-2 with separate standard suction catheter.	Catheter is continuously connected to ET or tracheostomy tube. Separate suction catheter is necessary for oral or nasal suctioning.
11. Reposition client.	Promotes comfort and drainage of secretions and prevents pressure areas.
12. Remove gloves and discard into appropriate receptacle and wash hands.	Reduces transmission of microorganisms.
13. Turn off suction device.	Clean equipment should not be touched with contaminated gloves or hands.

➤ ***CRITICAL DECISION POINT*** **Most in-line suction catheters have safety features that do not require the suction to be turned off. Use care to make sure that the suction control valve cannot be inadvertently compressed, causing continuous suction.**

EVALUATION

STEPS	RATIONALE
1. Compare client's respiratory assessments before and after suctioning.	Identifies objective measures for benefit of suctioning.
2. Observe airway secretions.	Documents presence or absence of respiratory tract infection.
3. Ask client if breathing is easier.	Provides subjective data about client's perception of effect of suctioning.
4. **Unexpected outcomes** that may occur include:	
➤ Client becomes cyanotic, tachycardic, bradycardic, or more restless; has cardiac arrest; dysrhythmias develop.	Suctioning induced cardiopulmonary compromise. Suctioning removes oxygen in addition to tracheobronchial secretions. Hypoxia results.
➤ Bloody secretions are returned.	Suctioning denuded cilia and mucosal lining. Bloody secretions can also indicate presence of infection.
➤ Client has paroxysms of coughing.	Suctioning induced airway spasm. Prolonged coughing episodes can disrupt ventilation and interfere with venous return to heart.
➤ No secretions are obtained.	When client is poorly hydrated or is not receiving humidified oxygen or room air, pulmonary secretions can consolidate in airways. Also, secretions may be too distal to suction from proximal airways.

STEPS	RATIONALE
RECORDING AND REPORTING	
1. Chart in nurses' notes: respiratory assessments before and after suctioning; size of suction catheter used; amount of negative suction pressure used (unless standardized in institution or deviation from usual); duration of suctioning period, if unusual; route(s) used to suction; secretions obtained and odor, amount, color, consistency; frequency of suctioning; client's tolerance of procedure.	Documents cardiopulmonary status, nursing care given, and outcomes and provides baseline for future assessments.

FOLLOW-UP ACTIVITIES

1. Worsening respiratory status:
   a. See Follow-Up Activities for Skills 14-2 and 14-3 (pp. 475 and 483-484).
   b. Evaluate size of suction catheter used to determine if it occluded lumen of tube by more than one half of tube diameter.
2. Bloody secretions:
   a. Evaluate amount of suction pressure used. May need to be decreased.
   b. Evaluate coagulation (blood clotting) studies and medications affecting coagulation.
   c. Evaluate length of time between catheter insertion and removal of catheter.
   d. Evaluate need for suctioning frequency.
3. Paroxysms of coughing:
   a. Consult physician about need for inhaled bronchodilators or topical anesthetic.
   b. Allow client to rest between passes of suction catheter.
4. No secretions were obtained (see Skills 14-2 and 14-3, Follow-Up Activities). Consider using standard catheter once to determine if closed system catheter is ineffective.

• • • • •

Special Considerations

- If client has thick, sticky secretions, assess hydration and infection. Inadequately hydrated clients may have thick secretions. Normal saline (5 to 10 ml) may be instilled before suctioning. Saline instillation has limited value but stimulates a cough. It does not thin secretions and may have a harmful effect in selected clients (Ackerman, 1993; Hagler and Traver, 1994; Raymond, 1995).
- Conditions increasing risk for adverse effects of suctioning include prematurity, increased oxygen needs, shock, myocardial infarction, respiratory failure, and sepsis.
- Spasmodic coughing may occur more frequently in clients with asthma, COPD, and congestive heart failure.
- Closed system catheters are available only for older children and adult-size artificial airways.
- Catheter is left in place and changed every 24 to 48 hours according to institution protocol.
- Institutions may limit use to clients with specific infections, fraction of inspired oxygen (FiO_2) or positive end-expiratory pressure (PEEP) requirements, or frequent suctioning because of its acquisition cost compared with standard catheters. Some research suggests that in-line suction catheters may actually be more cost-effective because of reduced nursing time and client infections (DePew et al., 1994; Johnson et al., 1994).

Pediatric Considerations

- Weight of closed system catheters may displace ET tube more easily in child than adult because of short distance of trachea.
- Bronchospasm may develop more readily during suctioning in children with prematurity, underdeveloped airways, or reactive airways diseases.

Gerontologic Considerations

- Older adults with ischemic cardiac or obstructive pulmonary disease may benefit from maintenance of oxygen supply during suctioning.

SKILL 14-5 Performing Endotracheal Tube Care

See introductory text for Skill 14-3, pp. 477-478.

DELEGATION CONSIDERATIONS

This skill requires problem solving and knowledge application unique to a professional nurse. For this skill, delegation is inappropriate.

EQUIPMENT

- Towel
- Endotracheal and oral pharyngeal suction equipment
- 1 or $1^1/_2$-inch wide adhesive or waterproof tape (do not use paper or silk tape) or commercial ET tube holder and mouthguard (follow manufacturer's instructions for securing)
- Nonsterile gloves (2 pairs)
- Adhesive remover swab or acetone on cottonball
- Mouthwash-soaked clean 4 × 4–inch gauze secured on tongue blade or sponge-tipped applicators
- Toothbrush, toothpaste (optional), and shaving supplies
- One wet and one soapy washcloth or paper towels
- Clean 2 × 2–inch gauze
- Tincture of benzoin, liquid adhesive, or skin prep pads
- Tongue blade (optional)
- Face shield, if indicated

STEPS	RATIONALE
ASSESSMENT	
1. Observe for signs and symptoms of need to perform ET tube care: soiled or loose tape; pressure sore on naris, lips, or corner of mouth; excess nasal or oral secretions; client moving tube with tongue, biting tube or tongue; tube repositioned by physician or other specially trained personnel; foul-smelling mouth.	Presence of ET tube impairs ability of client to swallow oral secretions. Client is also at increased risk for development of pressure areas from impaired circulation as tube is pulled or pressed against nasal or oral mucosa.
2. Observe for factors that increase risk of complications from ET tube: type and size of tube, movement of tube up and down trachea (in and out), duration of tube placement, cuff overinflation or underinflation, presence of facial trauma, malnutrition, and neck or thoracic radiation.	Nasal tube cannot be rotated from side to side like oral tube. Pressure sores are more likely. Tube moving up and down trachea predisposes client to develop tracheoesophageal fistula or tracheomalacia, can become dislodged from the lower airway (incidental extubation), or can enter mainstem **bronchus.** Cuff underinflation may allow aspiration, whereas cuff overinflation may cause ischemia or necrosis of tracheal tissue from obstruction of capillary bed. Client can "tongue" oral tube easily and dislodge it. Longer duration of intubation is associated with increased risk of lower airway complications, as is facial trauma. Tissue is more prone to breakdown in presence of malnutrition and radiation.
3. Assess client's knowledge of procedure.	Encourages cooperation; minimizes risks and anxiety. Identifies teaching needs.

NURSING DIAGNOSIS

Clustering of defining characteristics from the assessment data may reveal the following nursing diagnoses for clients requiring this skill:

- Ineffective airway clearance
- Risk for aspiration
- Ineffective breathing pattern
- Knowledge deficit regarding airway clearance techniques and devices
- Impaired skin integrity

STEPS	RATIONALE

➤ Impaired gas exchange
➤ Risk for infection
➤ Impaired swallowing
➤ Inability to sustain spontaneous ventilation

Related factors are individualized based on a client's condition or needs.

PLANNING

1. **Expected outcomes** following completion of procedure:
   - ➤ ET tube is maintained in correct position in client's trachea.

     Complications of lower airway and vocal cords may result when ET tube moves up or down trachea. If tube depth is too shallow, vocal cord injury or incidental extubation may occur. If tube depth is too deep, one bronchus and lung may be occluded from airflow and opposite lung may become hyperinflated.
   - ➤ Client's skin around mouth and oral mucous membranes does not have pressure areas or other injury from biting: tube is repositioned on opposite side of mouth or center of mouth at least every 24 to 48 hours according to institution protocol (oral ET tube only); oral airway, if used, is cleaned and reinserted to prevent biting of tongue or inner cheeks.

     ET tube does not place undue pressure against corners of mouth causing pressure area. Client is not able to bite inner cheeks or tongue. Tube may exert pressure against capillaries, impede blood flow, and cause breakdown (Fig. 14-2).
   - ➤ ET tube is resecured at proper depth as evidenced by the following: clean tape is firmly secured to cheeks, upper lip or top of nose, and tube only; depth of tube is same as when started or as ordered (same centimeter marking at gums or lips); bilateral breath sounds are equal.

     ET tube care prevents movement of tube out of airway or into mainstem bronchus.
2. Obtain another nurse's assistance in this procedure.

   Reduces risk of incidental extubation of ET tube.
3. Explain procedure and client's participation, including importance of the following: not biting or moving ET tube with tongue; trying not to cough when tape is off ET tube; keeping hands down and not pulling on tubing; removal of tape from face can be uncomfortable.

   Reduces anxiety, encourages cooperation, and reduces risks.

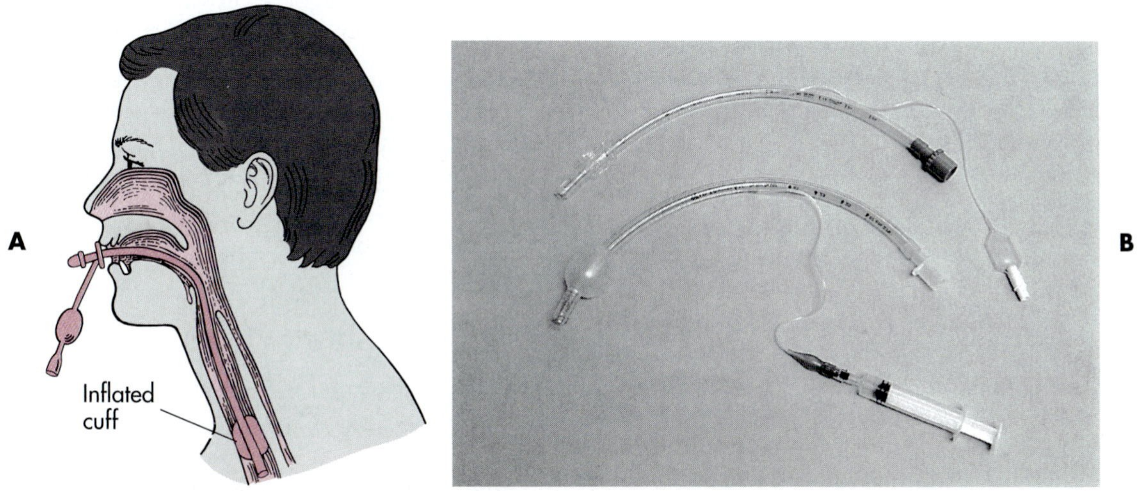

Fig. 14-2 **A,** Endotracheal (ET) tube with inflated cuff. **B,** ET tubes with uninflated and inflated cuffs and syringe for inflation.

STEPS	RATIONALE
4. Assist client to assume position comfortable for both nurse and client (usually supine or semi-Fowler's).	Promotes client comfort; prevents nurse muscle strain.
5. Place towel across chest.	Reduces transmission of organisms and protects bed clothes and linens from contamination.

IMPLEMENTATION

STEPS	RATIONALE
1. Wash hands. Apply face shield if indicated.	Reduces transmission of microorganisms.
2. Administer endotracheal, nasal, and oral pharyngeal suction.	Removes secretions. Diminishes client's need to cough during procedure.
CRITICAL DECISION POINT **If possible, also perform this procedure 1 hour after inhaled bronchodilator therapy, when airway is less irritable.**	
3. Connect Yankauer suction catheter to suction source (see Skill 14-1).	Prepares client for oral pharyngeal suctioning.
4. Prepare tape. Cut a piece of tape long enough to go completely around client's head from naris to naris plus 6 inches: adult 24 to 48 cm (1 to 2 feet). Lay tape adhesive side up on bedside table. Cut and lay 8 to 16 cm (3 to 6 inches) of tape, adhesive sides together, in center of long strip to prevent tape from sticking to hair. Smaller strip of tape should cover area between ears around back of head.	Preparing tape ahead allows nurse to have one hand positioned on ET tube throughout procedure. Adhesive tape must encircle head below ears with sufficient tape to wrap around tube.
5. Apply gloves. Instruct helper to apply pair of gloves and hold ET tube firmly at client's lips or naris. Note the number marking on the ET tube at the gum line.	Reduces transmission of microorganisms. Maintains proper tube position and prevents incidental extubation.
CRITICAL DECISION POINT **Do not allow helper to hold the tube away from the lips or naris. Doing so allows too much "play" in the tube and increases the risk of tube movement and incidental extubation. Never let go of the ET tube, even for a moment. Client could move or cough and the tube could become dislodged.**	
6. Carefully remove tape from ET tube and client's face. If tape is difficult to remove, moisten with (soapy) wet washcloth, water, or adhesive tape remover. Discard tape in appropriate receptacle if nearby.	Provides nurse with access to skin under tape for assessment and hygiene. Reduces transmission of microorganisms.
7. Use adhesive remover swab to remove excess adhesive left on face after tape removal. Wash adhesive remover from face.	Promotes hygiene. Unremoved adhesive can cause damage to skin and prevent poor adhesion of new tape.
8. Remove oral airway or bite block, if present, and place on towel.	Provides access to and complete observation of client's oral cavity.
CRITICAL DECISION POINT **Do not remove oral airway if client is actively biting ET tube. Wait until tape is partially or completely secured to ET tube.**	
9. Clean mouth, gums, and teeth opposite ET tube with mouthwash solution and 4 × 4–inch gauze, sponge-tipped applicators, or saline swabs. Brush teeth as indicated. If necessary, administer oral pharyngeal suctioning with Yankauer suction catheter.	Promotes hygiene and reduces risk of infection to teeth and gums.

STEPS	RATIONALE
10. *Oral ET tube only:* Remembering "cm" ET tube marking at lips or gums, with help of assistant move ET tube to opposite side or center of mouth. Do not change tube depth.	Prevents formation of pressure sores at sides of client's mouth. Ensures correct position of tube.
11. Repeat oral cleaning as in Step 9 on opposite side of mouth.	Removes secretions from mouth and oral pharynx.
12. Clean face and neck with soapy washcloth, rinse, and dry. Shave male client as necessary (see Chapter 6).	Moisture and beard growth prevent adhesive tape adherence.
13. Pour small amount of skin protectant or liquid adhesive on clean 2 × 2–inch gauze and dot on upper lip (oral ET tube) or across nose (nasal ET tube) and cheeks to ear. Allow to dry completely.	Protects skin from tape burns and makes more adherent.
14. Slip tape under client's head and neck, adhesive side up. Take care not to twist tape or catch hair. Do not allow tape to stick to itself. It helps to gently stick tape to tongue blade, which serves as a guide. Then slide tongue blade under client's neck. Center tape so that double-faced tape extends around back of neck from ear to ear.	Positions tape to secure ET tube in proper position.
15. On one side of face, secure tape from ear to naris (nasal ET tube) or edge of mouth (oral ET tube). Tear remaining tape in half lengthwise, forming two pieces that are ½ to ¾ inches wide. Secure bottom half of tape across upper lip (oral ET tube) or across top of nose (nasal ET tube) (see illustration a). Wrap top half of tape around tube and up from bottom (see illustration b). Tape should encircle tube at least two times for security.	Secures tape to face. Using top tape to wrap prevents downward drag on ET tube.

➤ *CRITICAL DECISION POINT* Do not tear tape past edge of mouth or naris. Tearing tape back to the cheek or ear reduces the holding power of the tape and allows greater tube movement.

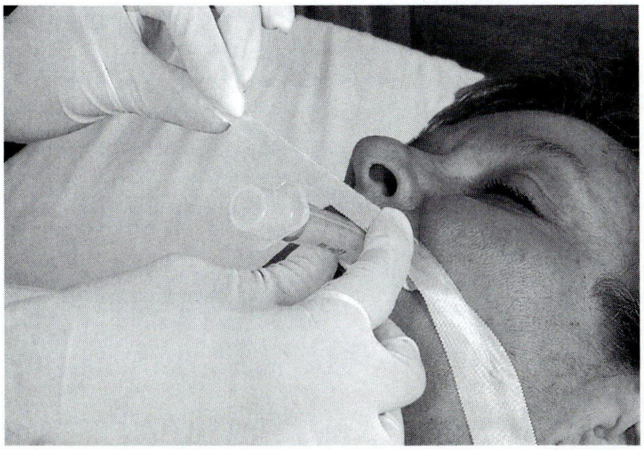

Step 15(a)

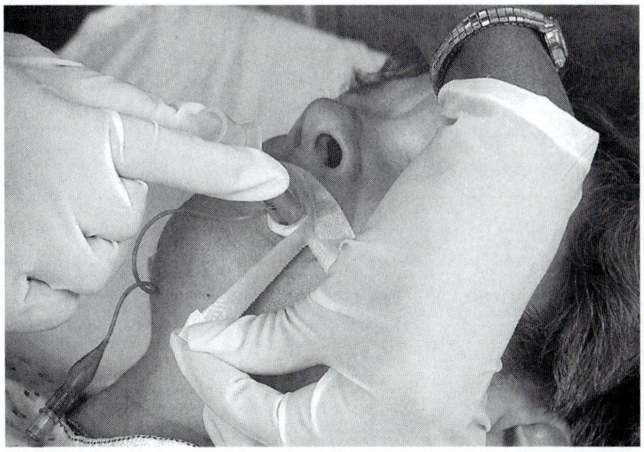

Step 15(b)

STEPS	RATIONALE
16. Gently pull other side of tape firmly to pick up slack and secure to opposite side of face and ET tube the same as the first piece. NOTE: ET tube is secured. Assistant can release hold (nurse may want assistant to help reinsert oral airway).	Secures tape to face and tube. ET tube should be at same depth at the lips (see illustration). Check earlier assessment for verification of tube depth in centimeters.

CRITICAL DECISION POINT **Do not pull tape so tight as to decrease blood flow through neck veins and arteries, especially in clients with head injury.**

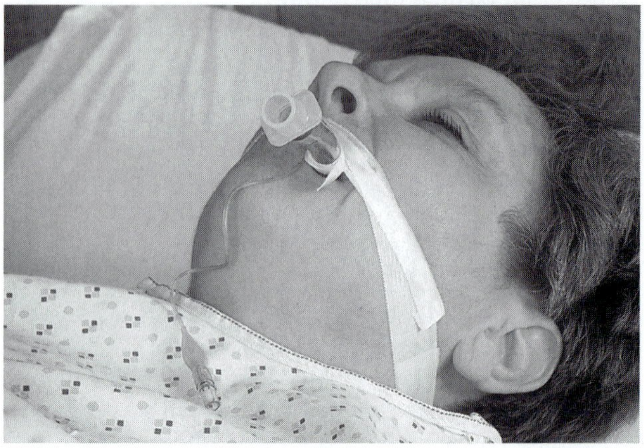

Step 16

STEPS	RATIONALE
17. If not already done, remove and clean oral airway in warm soapy water and rinse well. Hydrogen peroxide can aid in removal of crusted secretions. A mouthwash rinse will freshen client's mouth. Shake excess water from oral airway.	Promotes hygiene. Reduces transmission of microorganisms.
18. Reinsert oral airway without pushing tongue into oropharynx (Chapter 15).	Prevents client from biting ET tube and allows access for oral pharyngeal suctioning.

CRITICAL DECISION POINT **Secure oral airway with tape, if indicated.**

STEPS	RATIONALE
19. Discard soiled items in appropriate receptacle. Remove towel and place in laundry.	Reduces transmission of microorganisms.
20. Reposition client.	Promotes comfort.
21. Remove gloves and face shield and wash hands. Assistant is also to remove gloves and wash hands before leaving client's room. Place clean items (e.g., tincture of benzoin, mouthwash, excess swabs) in place of storage.	Reduces transmission of microorganisms. Contaminated gloves and hands should not touch clean items.

EVALUATION

STEPS	RATIONALE
1. Compare respiratory assessments before and after ET tube care.	Identifies any changes in presence and quality of breath sounds after procedure.
2. Observe depth and position of ET tube according to physician recommendation.	ET tube position should not be altered.
3. Assess security of tape by gently tugging at tube.	Tape should remain attached to face. Client may cough.
4. Assess skin around mouth and oral mucous membranes for intactness and pressure areas.	Tape should not tear skin. Pressure areas should be absent.
5. **Unexpected outcomes** that may occur include:	
➤ Tape is loose; ET tube is moving in or out.	Tube is improperly secured by taping method.
➤ Breath sounds are unequal.	Tube may have slipped into right mainstem bronchus if only right lung has adequate breath sounds.
➤ Pressure areas are present at corner of mouth or inner naris.	Pressure of tube impairs blood flow to skin and mucous membrane.
➤ Skin tears are present on cheeks, upper lip, or top of nose.	Presence of injured skin.
➤ Client is able to speak or audible air escapes from mouth.	ET tube may have been moved from original position to larger portion of airway, usually higher in trachea, and air is escaping around cuff.

STEPS	RATIONALE
RECORDING AND REPORTING	
1. Chart in Kardex with pencil: appropriate depth of ET tube, frequency of ET tube care, pressure sore care needed, and designated intervals. In some institutions this information is also placed on an index card and kept at the bedside for immediate referral.	Provides continuity of care and documents that oral hygiene was completed.
2. Chart in nurses' notes: assessments before and after care, supplies used, client's tolerance of procedure, frequency and extent of ET tube care.	Documents cardiopulmonary status, nursing care delivered, and client's response.

FOLLOW-UP ACTIVITIES

1. ET tube is moving in and out:
   a. Repeat taping procedure.
   b. If client is very active or if there are other reasons (e.g., excessive oral secretions or facial injury that impairs ability to apply tape effectively) and self-extubation is a concern, consider using a commercial mouth guard for holding ET tube. These devices generally secure with straps.
   c. In very active clients without facial injury who are at risk for self-extubation, consider applying a second piece of tape around the back of the head but going *over* the ears. This method of taping makes an X across the face and is more secure than a single piece of tape; however, the client may be at increased risk for skin injury with double the amount of tape.
2. Unequal breath sounds:
   a. Evaluate ET tube for proper depth before and after ET tube care. If ET tube is deeper or shallower, reposition tube only if allowed by institution and nurse has received appropriate instructions.
   b. Notify physician, who may order chest x-ray film to verify placement, and then reposition ET tube.
   c. Evaluate client for possible mucous plug.
3. Pressure areas from tube:
   a. Increase frequency of ET tube care. Apply antimicrobial ointment per institutional protocol.
   b. *Nasal ET tube only:* if tube is very painful for client, soak clean 2 × 2–inch gauze in anesthetic solution (e.g., xylocaine solution or xylocaine jelly). Open soaked 2 × 2–inch gauze and fold lengthwise one or two times (resulting in piece that is ½ by 4 inches [1 cm to 10 cm]) and wrap around tube to center ET tube in naris and away from pressure area. Obtain physician's order, if necessary.
   c. Align oxygen and humidity supply tubings so that they do not pull ET tube, creating pressure areas.
   d. Monitor for infection.
   e. If skin tear is present on cheeks or over nose or upper lip, apply protective barrier such as Stomahesive patch or hydrocolloid dressing and apply tape to this. Change dressing according to institution protocol or manufacturer's recommendations.
4. Air escaping around tube (see Skill 14-7).
   a. Verify correct position of tube.
   b. If tube position is correct, assess proper cuff inflation.
   c. If tube position is incorrect, reposition according to protocol or notify physician.

• • • • •

Special Considerations

➤ When ET tube is first placed, initial verification of its position in trachea is made by auscultation of bilateral breath sounds. Final position verification is confirmed by chest x-ray examination. The tip of the ET tube should be 2 to 3 cm above the carina. Documentation of depth of tube (in centimeters) at the lips, teeth, or gum line should be noted. If tube is not at designated position, perform respiratory assessment, notify physician, and follow physician's orders. If tube is at proper level, continue with procedure.

➤ Face shield protects nurse's eyes and mucous membranes from droplet contamination.

➤ If client has beard, it should be trimmed (with family or physician consent) to allow for proper securing of ET tube. If client has beard and tape cannot be used, consider applying commercial ET tube holder with straps to secure the ET tube extending around the back of the head.

- To aid in tape removal, fold last ½ inch of tape wrapping ET tube back on itself, adhesive sides together.
- Clients who have had ET tube in place for 3 or more days may have reddened, tender skin.

Teaching Considerations

- Qualified family members may serve as the assistant, but they are not usually able to perform the procedure without nursing supervision.

Pediatric Considerations

- Neonatal and pediatric procedures for securing ET tubes and suctioning airways may vary (McLean et al., 1992; Warnock and Porpora, 1994).
- Infant skin may be more prone to tearing when tape is removed.

Gerontologic Considerations

- Older adult skin may be more prone to tearing when tape is removed.
- Older adults with tendency toward inadequate nutrition may be more prone to complications.

SKILL 14-6 Performing Tracheostomy Care

See introductory text for Skill 14-3, pp. 477-478.

DELEGATION CONSIDERATIONS

The skill of performing tracheostomy care can be delegated to unlicensed assistive personnel and to the client under most situations. Clients with permanent tracheostomy tubes must learn this skill. In critically ill clients receiving mechanical ventilation, this skill usually should not be delegated to the client or family.

- Educate and assist client and care provider until competent in proper technique to clean around the tracheostomy tube and to change the tracheostomy tube ties.
- Teach client and care provider emergency procedures in event tracheostomy tube inadvertently becomes dislodged when ties are changed.

EQUIPMENT

- Bedside table
- Towel
- Tracheostomy suction supplies
- Sterile tracheostomy care kit, if available (be sure to collect supplies listed that are not available in kit)
- Three sterile 4 × 4–inch gauze pads
- Hydrogen peroxide
- Normal saline solution
- Sterile cotton-tipped swabs
- Sterile tracheostomy dressing (precut and sewn surgical dressing)
- Sterile basin
- Small sterile brush
- Roll of twill tape, tracheostomy ties, or Velcro tracheostomy ties
- Scissors
- Sterile gloves (2)
- Face shield

STEPS	RATIONALE
ASSESSMENT	
1. Observe for signs and symptoms of need to perform tracheostomy care: excess peristomal secretions, excess intratracheal secretions, soiled or damp tracheostomy ties, soiled or damp tracheostomy dressing, diminished airflow through tracheostomy tube, signs and symptoms of airway obstruction requiring tracheostomy tube suctioning (see Skill 14-3).	Signs and symptoms are related to presence of secretions at stoma site or within tracheostomy tube. The accompanying illustrations show a partially inflated cuff on an outer cannula, syringe used for cuff inflation, and an **obturator** that is used to insert outer cannula (see illustrations a and b).
2. Observe for factors (e.g., hydration, humidity, infection, nutrition, and ability to cough) that normally influence tracheostomy airway functioning.	Allows nurse to accurately assess need to perform tracheostomy care.
3. Assess client's understanding of and ability to perform own tracheostomy care.	Allows nurse to identify potential need for instruction.
4. Check when tracheostomy care was last performed.	Tracheostomy care is provided at least every 8 to 12 hours and more often if indicated.

STEPS	RATIONALE

NURSING DIAGNOSIS

Clustering of defining characteristics from the assessment data may reveal the following nursing diagnoses for clients requiring this skill:

- Ineffective airway clearance
- Risk for aspiration
- Ineffective breathing pattern
- Impaired verbal communication
- Impaired gas exchange
- Risk for infection
- Knowledge deficit regarding airway clearance techniques and devices
- Impaired skin integrity
- Impaired swallowing
- Inability to sustain spontaneous ventilation

Related factors are individualized based on a client's condition or needs.

PLANNING

STEPS	RATIONALE
1. **Expected outcomes** following completion of procedure:	
➤ Inner cannula and outer cannula of trach tube are free of secretions; ties are clean, secured snugly, and tied in double square knot.	Trach tube is patent and secure. Tracheostomy tube that is clear and free of secretions optimizes the amount of oxygen delivered to client and limits risk of infection from retained secretions.
➤ Stoma site is pink, does not bleed, and is free of secretions.	Indicates absence of infection at stoma site. Dry, intact tracheostomy stoma reduces risk of subsequent systemic infection.
2. Have another nurse or family member assist in this procedure.	Prevents accidental extubation of tracheostomy tube.
3. Explain procedure and client's participation.	Encourages cooperation, minimizes risks, and reduces anxiety.
4. Assist client to position comfortable for both nurse and client (usually supine or semi-Fowler's).	Promotes client comfort and prevents nurse muscle strain.
5. Place towel across client's chest.	Reduces transmission of microorganisms.

IMPLEMENTATION

STEPS	RATIONALE
1. Wash hands and apply gloves and face shield if applicable.	Reduces transmission of microorganisms.

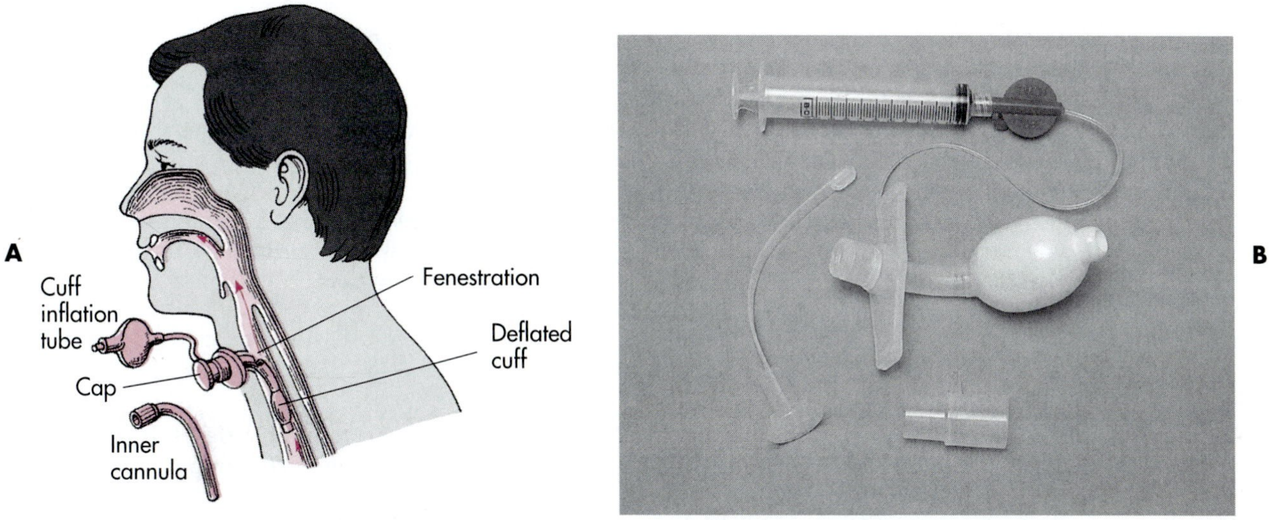

Step 1 **A,** Tracheostomy tube (fenestrated) with inner cannula removed and cap in place to allow speech (Lewis and Collier, 1992). Tubes without opening interfere with speech. **B,** Tracheostomy tube with obturator for insertion and syringe for inflation of cuff.

STEPS	RATIONALE
2. Suction tracheostomy (see Skill 14-3 or 14-4). Before removing gloves, remove soiled tracheostomy dressing and discard in glove with coiled catheter.	Removes secretions to avoid occluding outer cannula while inner cannula is removed. Reduces need for client to cough.
3. While client is replenishing oxygen stores, prepare equipment on bedside table. Open sterile tracheostomy kit. Open three 4 × 4–inch gauze packages using aseptic technique and pour normal saline on one package and hydrogen peroxide on another. Leave third package dry. Open two cotton-tipped swab packages, and pour normal saline on one package and hydrogen peroxide on the other. Open sterile tracheostomy dressing package. Unwrap sterile basin and pour about 0.5 to 2 cm (¾ inch) hydrogen peroxide into it. Open small sterile brush package and place aseptically into sterile basin. If using large roll of twill tape, cut appropriate length of tape (see Step 13) and lay aside in dry area. Do not recap hydrogen peroxide and normal saline.	Prepares equipment and allows for smooth, organized completion of tracheostomy care.
4. Apply gloves. Keep dominant hand sterile throughout procedure. (For tracheostomy tube with inner cannula, complete Steps 5 through 17. For tracheostomy tube with no inner cannula or Kistner button, complete Steps 9 through 17).	Reduces transmission of microorganisms.
5. Remove oxygen source and then inner cannula with nondominant hand. Drop inner cannula into hydrogen peroxide basin.	Removes inner cannula for cleaning. Hydrogen peroxide loosens secretions from inner cannula.
6. Place tracheostomy collar, T-tube or ventilator oxygen source over outer cannula.	Maintains supply of oxygen to client.
CRITICAL DECISION POINT **T-tube and ventilator oxygen devices cannot be attached to all outer cannulas when the inner cannula is removed.**	
7. To prevent oxygen desaturation in affected clients, quickly pick up inner cannula and use small brush to remove secretions inside and outside inner cannula.	Tracheostomy brush provides mechanical force to remove thick or dried secretions.
8. Hold inner cannula over basin and rinse with normal saline, using nondominant hand to pour normal saline.	Removes secretions and hydrogen peroxide from inner cannula.
9. Replace inner cannula and secure "locking" mechanism, if applicable. Reapply trach collar, T-tube (Briggs), or ventilator oxygen source.	Secures inner cannula and reestablishes oxygen supply.
10. With hydrogen peroxide–saturated cotton-tipped swabs and 4 × 4–inch gauze, clean exposed outer cannula surfaces and stoma under faceplate extending 5 to 10 cm (2 to 4 inches) in all directions from stoma. Clean in circular motion from stoma site outward using dominant hand to handle sterile supplies.	Aseptically removes secretions from stoma site. Moving in outward circle pulls mucus and other contaminants from stoma to periphery.
11. With normal saline–saturated cotton-tipped swabs and 4 × 4–inch gauze, rinse hydrogen peroxide from tracheostomy tube and skin surfaces.	Rinses hydrogen peroxide from surfaces. If not removed from skin, hydrogen peroxide can promote tissue injury.
12. With dry 4 × 4–inch gauze, pat lightly at skin and exposed outer cannula surfaces.	Dry surfaces prohibit formation of moist environment for microorganism growth and skin excoriation.

STEPS	RATIONALE
13. Instruct assistant, if available, to apply gloves and securely hold tracheostomy tube in place. With assistant holding tracheostomy tube, cut ties. (Follow manufacturer's guidelines for Velcro ties. Be sure to cut off excess ties, if applicable.)	Promotes hygiene and reduces transmission of microorganisms. Secures trach tube. Reduces risk of incidental extubation.

CRITICAL DECISION POINT Assistant must *not* release hold on tracheostomy tube until new ties are firmly tied. If working without an assistant, do not cut old ties until new ties are in place and securely tied.

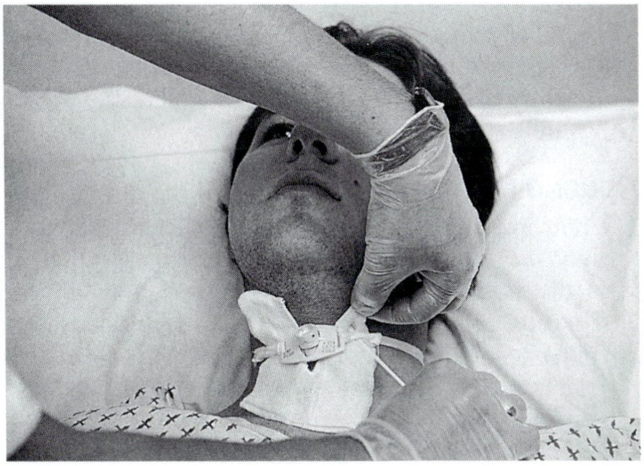

Step 14

STEPS	RATIONALE
a. Cut a length of twill tape long enough to go around client's neck two times (about 24 to 30 inches for an adult); cut ends on diagonal.	Cutting ends of tie on diagonal aids in inserting tie through eyelet.
b. Insert one end of tie through faceplate eyelet and pull ends even.	
c. Slide both ends of tie behind head and around neck to other eyelet and insert one tie through second eyelet.	
d. Pull snugly.	
e. Tie ends securely in double square knot, allowing space for only one loose or two snug finger(s) in tie.	One finger-length of slack prevents ties from being too tight when tracheostomy dressing is in place and also prevents movement of trach tube in lower airway.
14. Insert fresh tracheostomy dressing under clean ties and faceplate (see illustration).	Absorbs drainage. Dressing prevents pressure on clavicle heads.
15. Position client comfortably and assess respiratory status.	Promotes comfort. Some clients may require posttracheostomy care suctioning.
16. Remove gloves and face shield and discard in appropriate receptacle.	Reduces transmission of microorganisms. Contaminated gloves should not touch clean supplies.
17. Replace cap on hydrogen peroxide and normal saline bottles. Store reusable liquids and unused supplies in appropriate place.	Once opened, normal saline can be considered free of bacteria for 24 hours, after which it should be discarded.
18. Wash hands.	Reduces transmission of microorganisms among clients.

EVALUATION

1. Compare assessments before and after tracheostomy care.	Determines effectiveness of tracheostomy care.
2. Assess comfort of new tracheostomy ties.	Tracheostomy ties are uncomfortable and place client at risk for injury when they are too loose or too tight.
3. Observe inner and outer cannulas for secretions.	Presence of secretions on cannulas indicates the need for more vigorous tracheostomy care.
4. Assess stoma for signs of infection or skin breakdown.	Broken skin places client at risk for infection. Stomal infection necessitates change in tracheostomy skin care plan.

STEPS	RATIONALE
5. Unexpected outcomes that may occur include:	
➤ Ties are looser than one finger snug.	Ties improperly secured.
➤ Stoma site is hard and reddened with or without excessive or foul-smelling secretions.	Stomatitis is present.
➤ Pressure sore from faceplate or ties is present.	Pressure from faceplate or ties impairs blood flow to tissues.
➤ Client coughed out tracheostomy tube.	Improper technique used to change ties.
➤ Portion of inner cannula is exposed.	Inner cannula is not secured properly in outer cannula.
➤ Respiratory distress caused by mucus plug in cannula.	Inability to clear secretions through tracheostomy tube may result in mucus plug.

Recording and Reporting

1. Chart in Kardex: type and size of tracheostomy tube, frequency of tracheostomy care, special care in event of stomatitis.	Provides continuity of care.
2. Chart in nurses' notes: assessments, supplies used, frequency and extent of tracheostomy care, client's tolerance of procedure.	Documents cardiopulmonary and tracheostomy site status, nursing care, and client's response to procedure.

Follow-up Activities

1. Excessively loose or tight tracheostomy ties:
   a. Adjust ties or apply new ties.
2. Stomatitis:
   a. Increase frequency of tracheostomy care.
   b. Consider intermittent application of heat to increase blood flow and promote healing.
   c. Consider applying topical antibacterial solution and allowing it to dry and provide bacterial barrier.
   d. Consider applying hydrocolloid or transparent dressing just under stoma to protect skin from breakdown.
   e. Consult with skin care specialist.
3. Pressure sores:
   a. Increase frequency of tracheostomy care and keep dressing under faceplate at all times.
   b. Consider using double dressing or applying hydrocolloid or Stomahesive dressing around stoma.
4. Accidental extubation:
   a. Call for assistance.
   b. Replace old tracheostomy tube with new tube. Some experienced nurses or respiratory therapists may be able to quickly reinsert tracheostomy tube. Be sure to keep spare tracheostomy tube of same size and kind at bedside in event of emergency replacement. Same-size ET tube can be inserted in stoma in an emergency.
   c. Be prepared to manually ventilate clients in whom respiratory distress develops.
   d. Notify physician.
5. Respiratory distress from mucous plug of cannula:
   a. Remove inner cannula, if applicable, for cleaning, or cannula can be suctioned.
   b. Notify physician or specially trained personnel if tracheostomy tube requires replacement.

• • • • •

Special Considerations

- Some institutions use disposable (sterile) inner cannulas. They are removed and discarded every 8 to 12 hours, and new ones are inserted. Tracheostomy care tray may not be needed, but swabs, normal saline, and hydrogen peroxide are still used to clean stoma.
- Face shield protects nurse's eyes and mucous membranes from droplet contamination.
- Yeast infections can form under moist dressings or tracheostomy ties.
- Clients with the following have a greater need for tracheostomy care: tracheal stomatitis, pneumonia,

bronchitis, tracheitis, excessive perspiration or diaphoresis, short and fat neck.

- There are alternate methods to apply tracheostomy ties. The one presented is considered the safest and easiest to master. Commercial products that use Velcro and similar fastening devices are available in some institutions.
- Clients with new tracheostomy frequently have bloody secretions for 2 to 3 days after procedure or for 24 hours after each tracheostomy tube change. In most institutions the tracheostomy ties are not changed for 24 hours after initial surgical placement.
- Tracheostomy obturator should be attached to head of bed of client with fresh tracheostomy. Obturators of different brands and sizes of tracheostomy tubes are not interchangeable. The obturator facilitates reinsertion of the outer cannula if it is accidentally dislodged. In addition, the same size and kind of sterile tracheostomy tube should be kept at the bedside for emergent replacement, especially in clients with cuffed tracheostomy tubes.
- Manual resuscitation bag with mask should be kept at bedside of clients with new tracheostomies in event tracheostomy tube becomes dislodged and client requires breathing assistance.
- Do not cut 4 × 4–inch gauze for tracheostomy dressing. Loose strings enter stoma and can cause infection and irritation.
- If long-term placement of tracheostomy tube is anticipated, nurse should plan to teach client and family tracheostomy care.
- *Hydration:* inadequate hydration can cause thicker secretions. *Humidity:* inadequate inspired humidity predisposes client to drying, crusted secretions, and dry infected mucous membranes. *Infection:* secretions increase in quantity in infected areas. *Nutrition:* inadequate nutrition predisposes client to poor healing and greater risk of infection. *Ability to cough:* coughing effectively removes airway secretions. Weak coughing ability promotes secretion accumulation. Coughing ability is altered in tracheostomy clients.
- Thin individuals are more prone to development of pressure areas at clavicular heads.

Teaching Considerations

- Different types of tracheostomy tubes have different faceplates. Some are rigid; others are not. Instruct care givers not to lift up on rigid faceplates or they may dislodge tube.
- Some commercial tracheostomy tube holders require removal of excess tie material to fit properly.

Pediatric Considerations

- Children generally have shorter necks, so stoma may be more difficult to clean.
- Pediatric tracheostomy tubes (smaller than size 4) do not contain an inner cannula.

Gerontologic Considerations

- Older adults may have more fragile skin and may be more prone to skin breakdown from secretions or pressure.
- Older adults with impaired nutrition may not heal well.

SKILL 14-7 Inflating the Cuff on an Endotracheal or Tracheostomy Tube

See introductory text for Skill 14-3, pp. 477-478.

EQUIPMENT

- Endotracheal/tracheostomy suction apparatus (Skill 14-3 or 14-4)
- Stethoscope
- 5 or 10 ml syringe
- Alcohol wipe
- Face shield, if indicated
- Gloves, if indicated

DELEGATION CONSIDERATIONS

This skill requires problem solving and knowledge application unique to a professional nurse except in rare instances involving clients receiving home mechanical ventilation. For this skill, delegation is inappropriate.

STEPS	RATIONALE

ASSESSMENT

1. Observe for signs and symptoms of need to perform care, including gurgling on expiration, decreased exhaled tidal volume (mechanically ventilated client), spasmodic coughing, tense test balloon on tube, flaccid test balloon on tube, and unexpected phonation.
   Partially deflated cuff allows secretions to enter trachea and permits vocalization. High cuff pressure can result in necrosis, tracheomalacia, or tracheoesophageal fistula. Overinflated cuff may cause client to cough.
2. If client is discharged with a cuffed tracheostomy tube, determine care giver's understanding of procedure.
   Identifies teaching needs.

NURSING DIAGNOSIS

Clustering of defining characteristics from the assessment data may reveal the following nursing diagnoses for clients requiring this skill:

- Ineffective airway clearance
- Risk for aspiration
- Ineffective breathing pattern
- Impaired verbal communication
- Impaired gas exchange
- Risk for infection
- Knowledge deficit regarding airway clearance techniques and devices
- Impaired skin integrity
- Impaired swallowing
- Inability to sustain spontaneous ventilation

Related factors are individualized based on a client's condition or needs.

PLANNING

1. **Expected outcomes** following completion of procedure:
   - Mechanically ventilated clients receive prescribed tidal volume.
     Proper inflation of cuff ensures client receives tidal volume.
   - Minimal leak is auscultated at end inspiration.
     Allows drainage of secretions during inhalation when airway is at widest, but prevents gross aspiration during exhalation when airway is narrower. Prevents continuous contact of tracheal mucosa with cuff.
   - No evidence of excessive phonation, aspiration of gastric or mouth contents, tracheoesophageal fistula, or tracheomalacia is found.
     Proper level of cuff inflation is consistently maintained. Aspiration and phonation can occur when cuff is underinflated. Tracheoesophageal fistula and tracheomalacia can occur when the cuff is overinflated.
2. Explain procedure and client's participation. Explain that some coughing during procedure is normal.
   Encourages cooperation, minimizes risks, and reduces anxiety.
3. Assist client to position comfortable for nurse and client (usually semi-Fowler's).
   Promotes client comfort, prevents nurse muscle strain, and facilitates drainage.

IMPLEMENTATION

1. Wash hands, and apply gloves and face shield, if indicated.
   Reduces transmission of microorganisms.
2. Suction secretions through ET or tracheostomy tube and also mouth (see Skill 14-1, 14-3, or 14-4).
   Ensures patent airway and facilitates hearing airflow with stethoscope. Prevents aspiration of oral secretions when cuff is deflated.
3. Connect syringe to pilot balloon.
   Allows immediate access to equipment for adjusting cuff pressure.
4. Place stethoscope in sternal notch or above tracheostomy tube and listen for minimal amount of air leak at end of inspiration (see illustration).
   Assesses proper cuff inflation.

Step 4

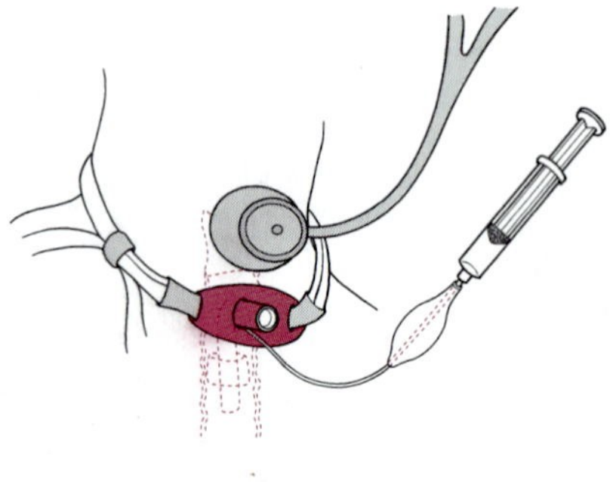

STEPS	RATIONALE
5. If no air leak is heard, remove all air from cuff.	Releases excessive cuff pressure, which reduces capillary blood flow and increases risk of tissue necrosis.
6. Slowly inflate cuff by adding 0.5 to 1 ml of air at a time while listening with stethoscope. At point where no air leak is heard, stop instilling air and very slowly withdraw up to 0.5 ml of air until point where air leak is audible with stethoscope only at end of inspiration.	Inflates cuff to minimal leak. If air leak is audible with ear, air leak is too large. If no air leak is heard, cuff is overinflated.
7. If excessive air leak is heard, slowly add air as in Step 6.	Air leak may prevent adequate lung expansion and increase risk of aspiration.
8. Remove stethoscope and wipe diaphragm with alcohol wipe.	Reduces transmission of microorganisms.
9. Remove syringe and discard into appropriate receptacle or store per policy. Do not leave attached to pilot balloon valve.	Reduces transmission of microorganisms.

CRITICAL DECISION POINT **Leaving syringe in pilot balloon can cause valve to break or "stick open." When syringe is removed, air is lost from cuff.**

10. Reposition client.	Promotes comfort.
11. Remove gloves and face shield. Discard into appropriate receptacle. Wash hands.	Reduces transmission of microorganisms.

EVALUATION

1. Compare respiratory assessments before and after cuff care.	Determines effectiveness of cuff care procedure.
2. Observe exhaled tidal volume from mechanical ventilator.	Exhaled tidal volume should be not less than 50 ml of delivered tidal volume.
3. Auscultate for audible air leak.	Air leak should only be heard with stethoscope.
4. Observe for excessive phonation, presence of gastric secretions in airway secretions, tracheoesophageal fistula.	Occurs with inadequate or excessive cuff inflation.
5. **Unexpected outcomes** that may occur include:	
➤ No air leak is auscultated at end inspiration.	Improper cuff inflation.
➤ Excessive air leak is heard through inspiration and expiration.	Cuff may have ruptured.
➤ Intratracheal bleeding (bright red) is noted.	Erosion of blood vessel is probably caused by high cuff pressure.
➤ Air leaks from cuff after syringe is removed from pilot balloon.	Pilot balloon valve may be broken or "stuck open," allowing air to escape from cuff.
➤ Client coughs excessively.	Cuff is overinflated or secretions are drained from above cuff into lower airway.
➤ Cuff requires increased amounts of air to maintain minimal leak.	Cuff has leak in cuff system or client has tracheomalacia.

RECORDING AND REPORTING

1. Chart in nurses' notes: presence of minimal leak at end inspiration, volume of air injected into cuff, secretions obtained when suctioning, and frequency of cuff care. Documents safe cuff pressure levels.

FOLLOW-UP ACTIVITIES

1. Excessive cuff pressure:
   a. Remove air from cuff and reassess minimal leak.
2. Excessive volume required to inflate cuff:
   a. Notify physician.
   b. Consider client may need insertion of larger tube.

STEPS **RATIONALE**

3. Intratracheal bleeding:
   a. Notify physician.
   b. Hyperinflate cuff with several additional milliliters of air to tamponade bleeding.
   c. Evaluate laboratory blood clotting studies and medications that may impede coagulation or promote bleeding.
4. Broken or open pilot balloon valve:
   a. Insert two- or three-way stopcock into valve and turn off valve after cuff is properly inflated.
   b. Clamp tubing between pilot balloon valve and ET tube or trach tube as close to balloon as possible.
   c. Prepare for reinsertion of tube by trained personnel or physician.
5. Excessive air leak:
   a. Reposition client or tubing.
   b. Reinflate cuff if needed.
   c. Prepare for insertion of new tube by physician or trained personnel if cuff ruptures.
   d. Prepare to manually ventilate client if needed.
6. Cuff requires increased amounts of air to maintain minimal leak.
   a. Reassess position of tube. ET tube cuff may be higher in trachea (where airway is wider) than previously.
   b. Withdraw all air from cuff so pilot balloon is completely deflated (flat). Remove syringe from pilot balloon. Watch to see if air reenters pilot balloon (cuff). If so, there is leak in cuff and tube requires replacement.
   c. Fill cuff appropriately. Apply gauze-padded clamps to pilot balloon tubing. (Do not use clamps with teeth, which will damage tubing.) If leak does not recur, pilot balloon valve may be broken. Institutional policy varies on how to correct this problem. Most tubes require replacement. Some institutions insert a blunt needle and stopcock in place of the broken valve. If leak recurs, cuff has a leak. Tube must be replaced if client's cardiopulmonary status is compromised.

• • • • •

Special Considerations

- Gloves are worn when caring for clients with communicable diseases or contaminated secretions.
- In some institutions cuff pressure is measured with a manometer. Cuff pressure should not exceed 20 to 25 cm H_2O or 14 to 17 mm Hg to maintain adequate capillary blood flow. Cuff pressure monitoring can be misleading if tube is much smaller or larger than size of airway. Cuffs can be properly inflated with pressures well below these values. When elevated cuff pressures are necessary to ventilate a client, the cuff should be temporarily deflated every 2 to 4 hours to reestablish capillary blood flow and drain secretions.
- Clients with ET tubes do not commonly ingest food or medications orally.
- Clients who are alert and do not require mechanical ventilation may need inflation of the cuff while eating, 30 to 60 minutes after meals, and after administration of medication to reduce risk of aspiration.

Teaching Considerations

- When foam-cuffed tracheostomy tube is used, there is no valve in the pilot balloon. Red air port is left open to atmosphere and regulates the amount of air necessary to seal the cuff without exerting excessive pressure against capillaries and mucosal surfaces.
- The volume of air required to properly inflate a cuff is dependent on size of the airway and size of the tube. If a large and a small tube are placed in clients with similar-size airways, the client with the larger tube will need less air in the cuff than the client with the smaller tube.
- Minimal leak technique allows secretions between the epiglottis and top of cuff to drain. In contrast, occlusive techniques allow secretions to collect in the subglottic area, which can result in conditions such as epiglottitis, pharyngitis, and tracheal stenosis.

Pediatric Considerations

- Pediatric tracheostomy tubes do not have cuffs.
- Neonatal and many pediatric ET tubes do not contain cuffs.

CRITICAL THINKING EXERCISES

1. The Kardex indicates that correct placement for the ET tube is 24 cm at the lips. During assessment you observe that the loose tape is at 26 cm; however, the tube is at 20 cm at the lips and the client is starting to lose tidal volume. What should you do?
2. The client develops a bloody nose after nasotracheal suctioning. What actions should you take?
3. The tracheostomy site is draining green purulent material, but you suction white material from the lungs. What actions are needed for this problem?
4. When removing tape from the client's face, skin is also removed (tape burn). How can you prevent or treat this?

REFERENCES

Ackerman MH: The effect of saline lavage prior to suctioning, *Am J Crit Care* 2(4):326, 1993.

Albarran AW: A review of communication with intubated patients and those with tracheostomies within an intensive care environment, *Intensive Care Nurs* 7(3):179, 1991.

Clark AP et al: Effects of endotracheal suctioning on mixed venous oxygen saturation and heart rate in critically ill adults, *Heart Lung* 19(suppl):552, 1990.

Connelly M, Stone K: Descriptive determination of negative airway pressure with closed system suctioning, *Heart Lung* 20(3):298, 1991.

Crosby LJ, Parsons LC: Cerebrovascular response of closed head-injured patients to a standardized endotracheal tube suctioning and manual hyperventilation procedure, *J Neurosci Nurs* 24(1):40, 1992.

Dam V, Wild MC, Baun MM: Effect of oxygen insufflation during endotracheal suctioning on arterial pressure and oxygenation in coronary artery bypass graft patients, *Am J Crit Care* 3(3):191, 1994.

DePew CL et al: Open vs closed-system endotracheal suctioning: a cost comparison, *Crit Care Nurse* 14(1):94, 1994.

Hagler DA, Traver GA: Endotracheal saline and suction catheters: sources of lower airway contamination, *Am J Crit Care* 3(6):444, 1994.

Johnson KL et al: Closed versus open endotracheal suctioning: costs and physiological consequences, *Crit Care Med* 22(4):658, 1994.

Kerr ME et al: Head-injured adults: recommendations for endotracheal suctioning, *J Neurosci Nurs* 255(2):86, 1993.

McLean S et al: Three methods of securing endotracheal tubes in neonates: a comparison, *Neonatal Network* 11(3):17, 1992.

Noll ML, Hix CD, Scott G: Closed tracheal suction systems: effectiveness and nursing implications, *AACN Clin Issues Crit Care Nurs* 1(2):318, 1990.

Raymond SJ: Normal saline instillation before suctioning: helpful or harmful? A review of the literature, *Am J Crit Care* 4(4):267, 1995.

Rudy EB et al: Endotracheal suctioning in adults with head injury, *Heart Lung* 20(6):667, 1991.

Warnock C, Porpora K: A pediatric trach card: transforming research into practice . . . iatrogenic complications of deep suctioning are avoided, *Pediatr Nurs* 20(2):186, 1994.

Witmer MT, Hess D, Simmons M: An evaluation of the effectiveness of secretion removal with the Ballard closed-circuit suction catheter, *Respir Care* 36(8):844, 1991.

ADDITIONAL READING

AARC clinical practice guideline: endotracheal suctioning of mechanically ventilated adults and children with artificial airways, *Respir Care* 38(5):500, 1993.

Anderson CE, Savignac AC: Nasoendotracheal tube obstruction secondary to inferior turbinate impaction, *AANA J* 59(6):538, 1991.

Ashurst S: Suction therapy in the critically ill patient, *Br J Nurs* 1(10):485, 1992.

Bell S et al: Implementing a research-based protocol: an interactive approach, *AACN Clin Issues* 55(2):147, 1994.

Clark L: A critical event in tracheostomy care, *Br J Nurs* 4(12):676, 1995.

Copnell B, Fergusson D: Endotracheal suctioning: time-worn ritual or timely intervention? *Am J Crit Care* 4(2):100, 1995.

Crimlisk JT et al: The closed tracheal suction system: implications for critical care nursing, *DCCN* 13(6):292, 1994.

Czarnik RE et al: Differential effects of continuous versus intermittent suction on tracheal tissue, *Heart Lung* 20(2):144, 1991.

DePew CL, Noll ML: Inline closed-system suctioning: a research analysis, *DCCN* 13(2):73, 1994.

Dettenmeier PA: *Pulmonary nursing care*, St Louis, 1992, Mosby.

Fowler S, Knapp-Spooner C, Donohue D: The ABC's of tracheostomy care, *J Pract Nurs* 45(1):44, 1995.

Gallagher TJ: Endotracheal intubation, *Crit Care Clin* 8(4):6655, 1992.

Glass C et al: Nurses' ability to achieve hyperinflation and hyperoxygenation with a manual resuscitation bag during endotracheal suctioning, *Heart Lung* 22(2):1558, 1993.

Gunderson LP, Stone KS, Hamlin RL: Endotracheal suctioning–induced heart rate alterations, *Nurs Res* 40(3):139, 1991.

Knipper JS: Minimizing the complications of tracheal suctioning, *Focus Crit Care* 13(4):23, 1986.

Knox AM: Performing endotracheal suction on children: a literature review and implications for nursing practice, *Intens Crit Care Nurs* 9(1):488, 1993.

Kovac AL: Upper airway trauma and obstruction: a review of causes, evaluation, management, *Respir Care* 38(4):351, 1993.

Macmillan C: Nasopharyngeal suction study reveals knowledge deficit, *Nurs Times*, 91(50):28, 1995.

Odell A et al: Endotracheal suction for adult, non-head-injured patients: a review of the literature, *Intens Crit Care Nurs* 9(4):274, 1993.

Redlick EL: Closed-system, in-line endotracheal suctioning, *Crit Care Nurse* 13(4):47, 1993.

Runton N: Suctioning artificial airways in children: appropriate technique, *Pediatr Nurs* 18(2):115, 1992.

Stone DJ, Bogdonoff DL: Airway considerations in the management of patients requiring long-term endotracheal intubation, *Anesth Analg* 74(2):276, 1992.

Taft AA et al: A comparison of two methods of preoxygenation during endotracheal suctioning, *Respir Care* 36(11):1195, 1991.

Weilitz PB, Dettenmeier PA: Test your knowledge of tracheostomy tubes, *AJN* 94(2):46, 1994.

CHAPTER 15

Closed Chest Drainage Systems

OBJECTIVES

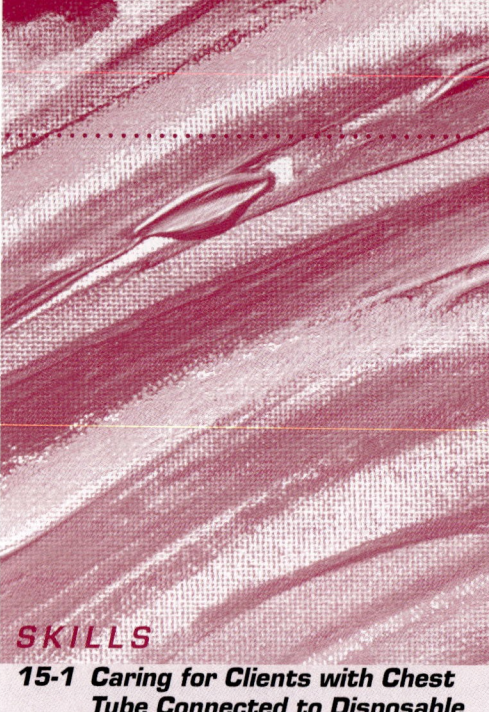

Mastery of content in this chapter will enable the nurse to:

- Define key terms.
- Explain the physiology of normal respiration.
- List three common sites for chest tube placement.
- List three conditions requiring chest tube insertion.
- Describe two closed chest drainage systems: water-seal and waterless systems.
- Describe chest tube suction.
- Describe methods of troubleshooting chest tube systems.
- Discuss the care of clients with chest tubes.
- Describe autotransfusion.

KEY TERMS

Atmospheric pressure
Chest tube
Client-centered air leak
Hemopneumothorax
Hemothorax
Intrapleural
Intrapulmonic
Mediastinal shift
Negative pressure
Parietal pleura
Pneumothorax
Positive pressure
Subcutaneous emphysema
Tidaling
Visceral pleura

SKILLS

The chest cavity is a closed structure bound by muscle, bone, connective tissue, vascular structures, and the diaphragm. This cavity has three distinct sections, each sealed from the others: one section for each lung and a third section for the mediastinum, which surrounds structures such as the heart, esophagus, trachea, and aorta.

The lungs are covered with a membrane called the **visceral pleura.** The interior chest wall is lined with another membrane, called the **parietal pleura.** The potential space between the visceral and parietal pleura is filled with approximately 4 ml of lubricating fluid and is called the **intrapleural** space. To expand the lungs, negative intrapleural pressure must be maintained. During inspiration the intercostal muscles pull outward and the diaphragm contracts and pulls down, thereby increasing the size of the chest cavity. This increase in size causes an increase in the amount of **negative pressure** (vacuum effect) being exerted in the intrapleural space.

Inspiration occurs when the increased negative pressure pulls the lungs against the enlarged chest cavity, expanding their size. The expanding lungs cause the **intrapulmonic** pressure to fall lower than **atmospheric pressure.** This increase in negative pressure within the lungs causes air to rush into the lungs until the intrapulmonic pressure is equal to the pressure in the atmosphere. When

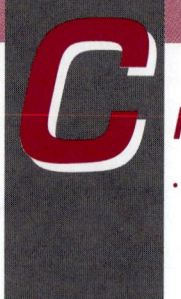

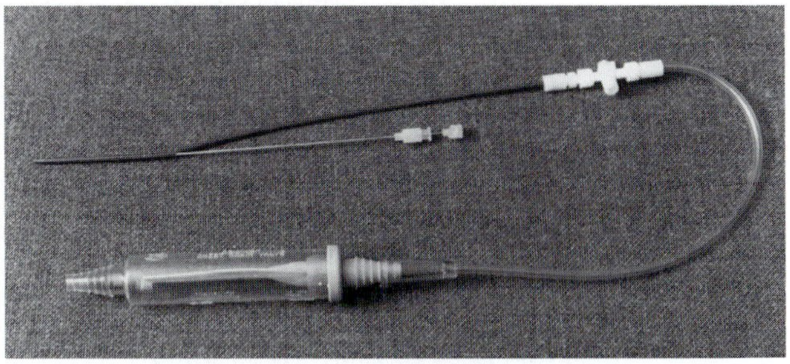

Fig. 15-1 The one-way valve.

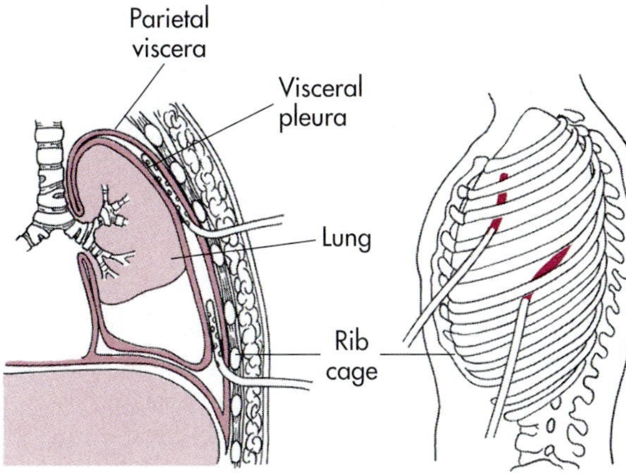

Fig. 15-2

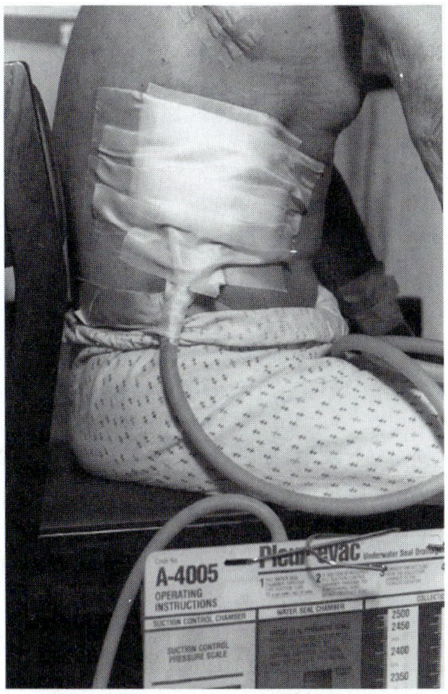

Fig. 15-3

the chest cavity stops expanding and the lungs are full of air, the respiratory muscles and diaphragm relax, returning the chest cavity to its resting stage. At this time the intrapulmonic pressure is the same as the atmospheric pressure. During expiration a passive relaxation of the respiratory muscles causes the chest cavity space to decrease. This decrease in space causes the intrapulmonic pressure to increase, which forces the air from the lungs back into the atmosphere.

Trauma, disease, or surgery can result in air or fluid leaking into the intrapleural space. Small leaks are absorbed spontaneously. Occasionally, in emergency situations, a one-way valve (Heimlich valve) is inserted through the chest wall to treat air leaks (Connor, 1987) (Fig. 15-1). This one-way valve allows air to exit from the intrapleural space on expiration but prevents air from reentry during inspiration (Lewis, Collier, and Heitkemper, 1996). No drainage chamber is used with this simple device.

A **chest tube** is inserted after chest trauma or open chest surgery or in the case of a large intrapleural leak. A closed chest drainage system and possibly suction are attached to the chest tube to promote drainage of air and fluid. Lung reexpansion occurs as the fluid or air is removed.

The location of the chest tube indicates the type of drainage expected. Apical and anterior chest tube placement promotes removal of air, which is necessary in the case of a **pneumothorax.** Because air rises, these chest tubes are placed high, allowing evacuation of air from the intrapleural space and allowing the lung to reexpand (Fig. 15-2). The air is discharged into the atmosphere; therefore little or no drainage is in the collection chamber.

Chest tubes are placed low and posterior or lateral to drain fluid (Figs. 15-2 and 15-3). Fluid in the intrapleural space is affected by gravity and localizes in the lower portion of the lung cavity. Tubes placed in these positions drain blood and fluid. Frequently this drainage is assisted by applying suction. Fluid drainage is expected after open chest surgery and with some chest trauma.

A mediastinal chest tube is placed just below the sternum (Fig. 15-4) and is connected to a drainage system. This tube drains blood or fluid, preventing its accumulation around the heart. A mediastinal tube is commonly used after open heart surgery. There is no **tidaling** (rocking) in mediastinal drainage because the tube is not placed in a lung cavity.

A variety of disposable commercial chest drainage systems is available. The single-chamber system is used primarily in the treatment of pneumothorax. It allows air from the pneumothorax to bubble out of the water seal and escape through the air outlet while preventing air from reentering the intrapleural space. This system is used in emergency situations. However, it is not recommended for the evacuation of fluid because drainage would raise the level of the water-seal liquid. An increased height of fluid in the water seal increases the resistance to drainage on expiration and eventually stops the drainage entirely (Phipps et al., 1995).

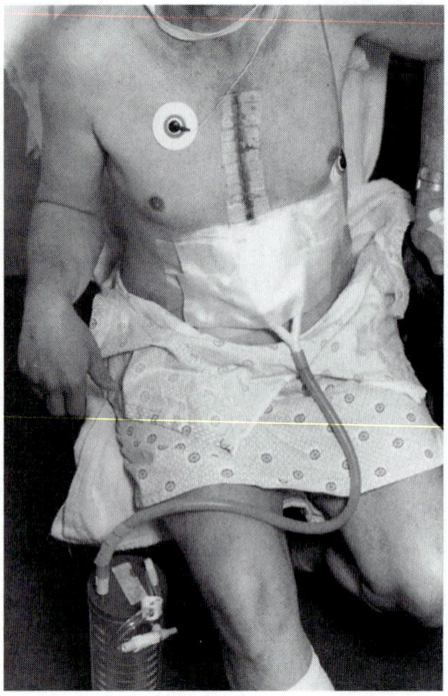

Fig. 15-4

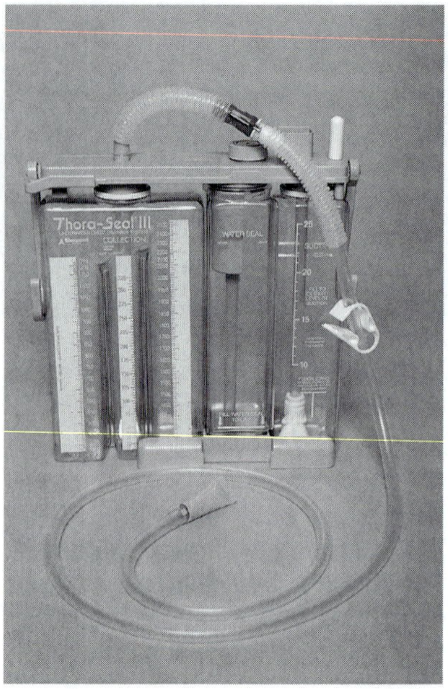

Fig. 15-5

One-chamber commercial systems are available; however, most practitioners prefer a two- or three-chamber system because it drains both a **hemothorax** and a pneumothorax effectively and removes the possibility of using a one-chamber system on a hemothorax (Fig. 15-5). Water-seal or the newer waterless chest drainage systems can be purchased. Both systems are presented in this text. In both systems the first chamber provides a compartment for fluid or blood drainage and a second compartment for either a water seal or a one-way valve. The third compartment is for suction control, which may or may not be used.

TWO-CHAMBER WATER-SEAL SYSTEM

On expiration, fluid or air is forced out of the intrapleural space. Gravity or suction is pulled down the chest tube into the drainage collection chamber. On entering the drainage collection chamber, this fluid or air displaces the air present in the chamber by pushing it through the water seal and out of the system into the atmosphere.

THREE-CHAMBER WATER-SEAL SYSTEM

If suction is to be used, the two-chamber water-seal system (Fig. 15-5) is set up with the suction control chamber added. A prescribed amount of sterile fluid is poured into the suction control chamber, which is then attached to a suction source by tubing. The suction is turned up until the water in the suction control bottle exhibits a continuous, gentle bubbling. This provides the prescribed amount of suction (negative pressure).

If the suction source delivers more negative pressure than the suction control chamber water level allows, there is no danger because atmospheric air is pulled into the suction control chamber through an inlet, causing the excess suction to dissipate. The extra air pulled into the chamber causes vigorous bubbling. If this occurs, the suction source setting needs to be lowered to reduce noise and evaporation of the fluid. The absence of bubbling indicates that no suction is being exerted in the system. The suction setting should be raised to restore gentle bubbling.

TWO-CHAMBER WATERLESS SYSTEM

The waterless system's principles are similar to those of the water-seal system except that fluid is not required for setup. Since water is not used, accidentally tipping over the system does not compromise the client's condition.

The water seal is replaced by a one-way valve (Fig. 15-6) located near the top of the system. Most of the container is the drainage chamber. The suction chamber does not depend on water. It contains a float ball, which is set by a suction control dial after the suction source is turned on. A diagnostic air-leak indicator is located on the face of the unit. It does require 15 ml of fluid for visualization. The indicator's function is to identify one of the following:

1. That the lung is expanding normally. This is indicated by a gentle tidaling of the fluid in the water seal or diagnostic indicator.
2. The lung is probably reexpanded if after 2 or 3 days the tidaling has stopped.
3. An air leak is in the system if, while facing the system, the observer sees the fluid bubbling left to right. The source of the air leak must be located and remedied.

THREE-CHAMBER WATERLESS SYSTEM

If suction is ordered, attach the suction chamber port to the suction source by tubing, turn the suction on, and set

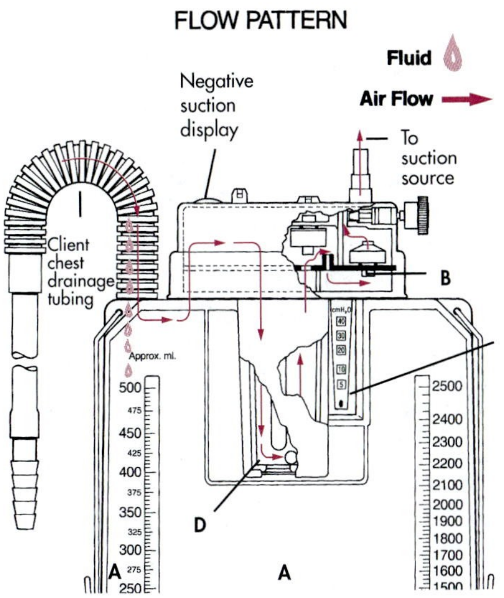

Fig. 15-6 Disposable waterless chest drainage system with suction.

the float ball at the prescribed setting. If the float ball will not rise to the prescribed level, increase the suction source setting until it does. The system is now functioning with suction.

Both commercial systems have two suction settings: one at either the suction control chamber or at the float ball setting and the other at the suction source. The chamber or float ball setting is a safety factor to reduce the possibility that the intrapleural tissues will receive too much suction, causing injury.

GUIDELINES

1. Document client's baseline vital signs, lung sounds, and respiratory status. Changes in the vital signs or respiratory status can indicate a malfunction of the chest drainage system.
2. For the water-seal system, observe the water seal for intermittent bubbling from its U-tube or a rise and fall of fluid that is synchronous with respirations.
   a. Constant bubbling in the water seal or a sudden, unexpected stoppage of water-seal activity is considered abnormal and requires immediate attention.
   b. Unexpected stoppage of activity may indicate a blockage.

   In these situations immediate attention and correction are indicated. After 2 to 3 days, tidaling or bubbling on expiration is expected to stop, indicating that the lung has reexpanded.
3. In the waterless system, look for a rise and fall of fluid in the diagnostic air-leak indicator synchronous with respirations. Constant left-to-right bubbling (when facing the indicator) or violent rocking is considered abnormal and may indicate an air leak.
4. Know the type and amount of expected chest tube drainage.
   a. A sudden decrease in the amount of chest tube drainage can indicate a possible clot or obstruction in the chest tube.
   b. A sudden increase of more than 100 ml of drainage can indicate fresh bleeding from the thorax.
   c. Any drainage from a pneumothorax is limited to the fluid caused by chest tube insertion trauma.
5. Know the expected color of the drainage. Drainage from recent open chest surgery is initially bright red and gradually becomes serous as the postoperative course continues. Pleural effusions usually drain straw-colored fluid.
6. In the water-seal system, observe for constant, gentle bubbling in the suction control chamber when it is connected to suction. In the waterless system a designated amount of suction is maintained by setting the suction source and dialing the prescribed suction level in the float ball column.
7. Assess both types of systems for air leaks. If an air leak exists, determine whether the air leak is within the client **(client-centered air leak)** or within the chest tube system (system-centered air leak). To determine this, place a rubber-tipped hemostat on the tubing near the chest wall. (Leave this clamp in place no longer than 10 seconds) (Beare and Myers, 1994). If the air leak that was occurring stops, the air leak is within the client. If this is a new finding, the physician must be notified. If the air leak continues despite the clamped chest tube, the air leak is within the system. Ensure that all tubing connections are tight (Carroll, 1991).
8. Note the color and amount of chest tube drainage on a regular basis. Make a mark to indicate the fluid level on the side of the drainage collection chamber at the end of the shift. Note the drainage amount as output.

DELEGATION CONSIDERATIONS

The skills in this chapter require problem solving and knowledge application unique to a professional nurse. For these skills, delegation is inappropriate.

- The nurse should inform all staff how to properly position clients with chest tubes in place.

SKILL 15-1 Caring for Clients with Chest Tube Connected to Disposable Drainage Systems

There are two types of commercial systems: the water-seal and the waterless systems.

EQUIPMENT

- Prescribed drainage system
- Water-seal system and:
  - Sterile water or normal saline (NS) solution to cover lower 2.5 cm (1 inch) of water-seal U-tube
  - Sterile water or NS to pour into the suction control chamber if suction is to be used
- Waterless system and:
  - Vial of 30 ml injectable sodium chloride or water
  - 20-ml syringe
  - 21-gauge needle
  - Antiseptic swab
- Chest tube tray (all items are sterile)
  - Knife handle (1)
  - Chest tube clamp
  - Small sponge forceps
  - Needle holder
  - Knife blade No. 10
  - 3-0 Silk sutures
  - Tray liner (sterile field)
  - Curved 8-inch Kelly clamps (2)
  - 4 × 4–inch sponges (10)
  - Suture scissors
  - Hand towels (3)
- Dressings
  - Petrolatum gauze
  - Several 4 × 4–inch gauze dressings
  - Large dressings (2)
  - 4-Inch tape or elastic bandage (Elastoplast)
- Head cover
- Face mask/face shield
- Sterile gloves
- Rubber-tipped hemostats for each chest tube (2)
- 1-Inch adhesive tape for taping connections

STEPS	RATIONALE
ASSESSMENT	
1. Obtain baseline vital signs and O_2 saturation.	Baseline vital signs are essential for any invasive procedure. Clients requiring chest tube insertion frequently have respiratory distress and vital signs are taken serially. A decreased blood pressure and increased heart rate may indicate a tension pneumothorax.
2. Observe for changes in heart rate, oxygen saturation (O_2 sat), blood pressure, respiratory pattern, increased apprehension, and chest pain.	Changes in these parameters may indicate worsening of the initial condition.
3. Assess client for known allergies.	Povidone-iodine is an antiseptic used to cleanse the skin. Lidocaine is a local anesthetic administered to reduce pain. The chest tube will be held in place with tape. Iodine, lidocaine, and tape are common allergens.
4. Review client's medication record for anticoagulant therapy.	Anticoagulation therapy such as aspirin, coumarin, or heparin can increase procedure-related blood loss.

NURSING DIAGNOSIS

Clustering of defining characteristics from the assessment data may reveal the following nursing diagnoses for clients requiring this skill:

- ➤ Anxiety
- ➤ Impaired gas exchange
- ➤ Pain

Related factors are individualized based on client's condition or needs.

PLANNING

STEPS	RATIONALE
1. **Expected outcomes** following completion of procedure: ➤ Client is oriented and more relaxed. ➤ Vital signs are stable. ➤ Client reports no chest pain.	Decreased hypoxia reduces anxiety. Reexpansion of the lung reduces chest pain.

STEPS	RATIONALE
➤ Breath sounds are auscultated in all lobes. Lung expansion is symmetrical, hypoxia is absent, and respirations are nonlabored.	Reexpansion of the lung promotes normal respirations.
➤ Chest tube remains in place and chest drainage system remains airtight.	Ensures patency of the system.
➤ Gentle tidaling (rocking) is evident in water seal or diagnostic indicator.	Indicates system is functioning normally.
2. Check agency policy and determine whether informed consent is needed.	Most institutions require informed, written permission for chest tube insertion.
3. Review physician's role and responsibilities for chest tube placement (Table 15-1).	Helps differentiate physician and nurse roles so that the nurse can function more effectively.
4. Explain procedure to client.	Reduces anxiety and promotes client cooperation.
5. Wash hands.	Reduces transmission of microorganisms.
6. Set up the prescribed drainage system.	
a. Water-Seal System:	
(1) Obtain a water-seal chest drainage system. Remove wrappers and prepare to set up the system.	Maintains sterility of the system. The system is packaged in this manner so it can be used under sterile operating room conditions (Carroll, 1986).

Table 15-1 **Physician's Role and Responsibility in Chest Tube Placement**

Role	Responsibility
Explain purpose, procedure, and possible complications to the client and have client sign consent form.	Provides informed consent.
Wash hands. Cleanse chest wall with antiseptic.	Reduces transmission of microorganisms.
Don mask and gloves.	Maintains surgical asepsis.
Drape area of chest tube insertion with sterile towels.	Maintains surgical asepsis.
Inject local anesthetic and allow time to take effect.	Decreases pain during procedure.
Use blunt or sharp dissection to create incision in the skin and chest wall.	Opens chest for insertion of chest tube. A trocar is outdated and increases risk of tissue damage.
Thread a clamped chest tube through the incision. Physician clamps chest tube until system is connected to water seal.	Inserts chest tube into the intrapleural space. Clamping prevents entry of atmospheric air into the chest and worsening of the pneumothorax.
Suture chest tube in place, if suturing is policy or physician preference.	Secures chest tube in place.
Cover the chest insertion site with sterile petrolatum gauze, 4 × 4-inch gauze, and large dressings to form an occlusive dressing supported with an elastic bandage (Elastoplast).	Holds chest tube in place and occludes site around chest tube. Helps stabilize chest tube and holds dressing tightly in place. Helps prevent bacteria entry.
Water-seal system: Remove connector cover from client's end of chest drainage tubing with sterile technique. Secure drainage tubing to the chest tube and drainage system.	Physician is responsible for making certain that the system is set up properly, the proper amount of water is in the water seal, the dressing is secure, and the chest tube is securely connected to the drainage system.
Water seal suction: Connect system to suction or supervise a nurse connecting it to suction, if suction is to be used.	The physician is responsible for determining and checking the amount of fluid that is to be added to the suction control chamber and prescribing the suction setting.
Waterless system: Remove connector cover from client's end of chest drainage tubing with sterile technique. Secure drainage tubing to the chest tube and drainage system.	Physician is responsible for making certain that the system is set up properly and the chest tube is securely connected to the drainage system.
Waterless suction: Turn on suction source. Set float ball level to prescribed setting.	Physician is responsible for prescribing level of float ball and prescribing the suction setting.
The physician or nurse adds sterile water or NS to diagnostic indicator.	Allows quick assurance that the system is functioning properly.
Unclamp the chest tube.	Connects chest tube to drainage.
In both systems the physician orders and reviews chest x-ray studies.	Verifies correct chest tube placement.

STEPS	RATIONALE
(2) Can be set up as a two- or three-chamber system.	
(3) While maintaining sterility of the drainage tubing, stand the system upright and add sterile water or NS to the appropriate compartments.	Reduces possibility of contamination.
(4) For a two-chamber system (without suction), add sterile solution to the water-seal chamber (second chamber), bringing fluid to the required level as indicated.	Maintains water seal.
(5) For a three-chamber system (with suction), add sterile solution to the water-seal chamber (second chamber). Add amount of sterile solution prescribed by physician to the suction control (third chamber), usually 20 cm (8 inches). Connect tubing from suction control chamber to suction source.	Depth of rod below fluid level dictates the highest amount of negative pressure that can be present within the system. For example, 20 cm of water is approximately −20 cm of water pressure. Any additional negative pressure applied to the system is vented into the atmosphere through the suction control vent. This safety device prevents damage to pleural tissues from an unexpected surge of negative pressure from the suction source.
b. Waterless System:	
(1) Obtain a waterless system. Remove sterile wrappers and prepare to set up equipment.	Maintains sterility of the system. The system is packaged in this manner so it can be used under sterile operating room conditions (Carroll, 1986).
(2) For a two-chamber system (without suction) nothing is added or needs to be done to the system.	The waterless two-chamber system is ready for connecting to the client's chest tube after opening the wrappers.
(3) For a three-chamber waterless system with suction: connect tubing from suction control chamber to the suction source.	The suction source provides additional negative pressure to the system.
(4) Instill 15 ml of sterile water or NS into the diagnostic indicator injection port located on top of the system.	This step is not necessary for mediastinal drainage because there will be no tidaling. Also, in an emergency it is not necessary because the system does not require water for setup.
7. Tape all connections in a spiral fashion with 1-inch adhesive tape. Then:	Prevents atmospheric air from leaking into the system and the client's intrapleural space.
a. Check both systems for patency by:	
(1) Clamping the drainage tubing that will connect the client to the system.	
(2) Connecting tubing from the float ball chamber to the suction source.	
(3) Turning on the suction to the prescribed level.	Provides a chance to ensure an airtight system before connecting it to the client. Allows correction or replacement of system if it is defective before connecting it to the client. NOTE: Bubbling will be seen at first because there is air in the tubing and system initially. This should stop after a few minutes unless there are other sources of air entering the system.
CRITICAL DECISION POINT **If bubbling continues, check connections and locate source of the air leak, as described in Table 15-2.**	
8. Turn off suction source and unclamp drainage tubing before connecting client to the system.	Having the client connected to suction when it is initiated could damage pleural tissues from sudden increase in negative pressure. The suction source is turned on again after the client is connected to the three-chamber system.

Table 15-2 Problem-Solving with Chest Tubes

Problem	Solution
Air leak in water-seal system	Locate leak.
Continuous bubbling in the water-seal chamber, indicating leak between client and the water seal.	Tighten loose connections between client and water seal. Loose connections cause air to enter the system. Leaks are corrected when constant bubbling stops.
Bubbling continues, indicating the air leak has not been corrected.	Cross-clamp chest tube close to client's chest. If bubbling stops, the air leak is inside the client's thorax (client centered) or at the chest tube insertion site (Palau and Jones, 1986). *Unclamp tube and notify physician immediately.* Reinforce chest dressing. Leaving chest tube clamped with a client-centered leak can cause collapse of the lung, mediastinal shift, and eventual collapse of the other lung from the buildup of air pressure within the pleural cavity.
Bubbling continues, indicating leak is not client centered.	In an alternating fashion, gradually move clamps down the drainage tubing away from the client and toward the suction control chamber, moving one clamp at a time. When bubbling stops, leak is in the section of tubing or connection that is in between the two clamps. Replace tubing or secure connection and release clamps.
Bubbling continues, indicating leak is not in the tubing.	Leak is in the drainage system. Change drainage system (Palau and Jones, 1986).
Water-seal is disconnected.	Connect water seal and tape connection.
Water-seal U-tube is no longer submerged in sterile fluid.	Add sterile solution to the water-seal bottle until the distal tip is 2 cm under surface level *or* set the water-seal bottle upright so that the tip is submerged.
Air leak in the waterless system	Locate leak.
Continuous left-to-right bubbling in the diagnostic air-leak indicator.	Tighten loose connections between client and water seal. Loose connections allow air to enter the system. Recheck for source of air leak if bubbling continues.
Negative pressure display ceases to display "yes" on inspiration (Davol Inc.).	
Bubbling and lack of display "yes" continues, indicating leak is not in connections.	Cross-clamp chest tube close to client's chest. If bubbling stops, the air leak is inside the client's thorax (client centered) or at the chest tube insertion site (Palau and Jones, 1986). *Unclamp tube and notify physician immediately.* Reinforce chest dressing. Leaving chest tube clamped with a client-centered leak can cause collapse of the lung, mediastinal shift, and eventual collapse of the other lung from the buildup of air pressure within the pleural cavity.
Bubbling continues, indicating the leak is not client centered.	In an alternating fashion, gradually move clamps down the drainage tubing away from the client and toward the suction control chamber, moving one clamp at a time. When bubbling stops, leak is in the section of tubing or connection that is in between the two clamps. Replace tubing or secure connection and release clamps.
Bubbling continues, indicating leak is not in the tubing.	Leak is in the drainage system. Change drainage system (Palau and Jones, 1986).
In both systems air leaks can lead to:	
Tension pneumothorax Severe respiratory distress Chest pain	Determine that chest tubes are not clamped, kinked, or occluded. Obstructed chest tubes trap air in the intrapleural space when there is a client-centered leak.
Absence of breath sounds on affected side	Notify physician immediately.
Hyperresonance on affected side	Prepare immediately for another chest tube insertion; obtain a one-way valve or large-gauge needle for short-term emergency release of air in the intrapleural space; have emergency equipment such as oxygen and code cart near the client.
Mediastinal shift to unaffected side Hypotension Tachycardia Supraclavicular bulging on affected side	
Trapping of fluid in dependent loops of drainage tubing	Drain tubing contents into drainage bottle. Coil excess tubing on mattress and secure in place.

STEPS	RATIONALE
9. Position the client: During the chest tube insertion, the client will need to be positioned so the side in which the tube will be placed is accessible to the physician. After the tube is placed, the client will be positioned in:	Permits optimal drainage of fluid and/or air.
a. Semi-Fowler's to high Fowler's position to evacuate air (pneumothorax).	Air rises to the highest point in the chest. Pneumothorax tubes are usually placed on the anterior aspect at the midclavicular line, second or third intercostal space (Carroll, 1986).
b. High Fowler's position to drain fluid (hemothorax).	Permits optimal drainage of fluid. Posterior tubes are placed on the midaxillary line, eighth or ninth intercostal space.

IMPLEMENTATION

STEPS	RATIONALE
1. Wash hands and put on gloves.	Reduces transmission of microorganisms.
2. Administer parenteral premedications, such as sedatives or analgesics, as ordered.	

➤ *CRITICAL DECISION POINT* Many sedatives and analgesics suppress respirations. Monitor the client closely to determine that the respiratory status is not worsened by the analgesics. Reduces client anxiety and pain during procedure.

STEPS	RATIONALE
3. Assist physician in providing psychological support to the client. (See physician's responsibilities in Table 15-1.)	
a. Reinforce preprocedure explanation.	Reduces client anxiety and assists in efficient completion of procedure.
b. Instruct client throughout procedure.	
4. Show anesthetic to physician.	Allows physician to read label of drug before administering it to client.
5. Hold anesthetic solution bottle upside down with label facing physician. Physician will withdraw solution.	Allows physician to withdraw solution properly while maintaining surgical asepsis.
a. Physician places chest tube. (A standard procedure is detailed in Table 15-1.)	
6. Help physician attach drainage tube to chest tube.	Connects drainage system and suction (if ordered) to the chest tube.
7. Tape the tube connection between the chest and drainage tubes.	Secures chest tube to drainage system and reduces risk of air leaks causing breaks in the airtight system.
8. Check patency of air vents in system:	
a. Water-seal vent must not be occluded.	Permits the displaced air to pass into the atmosphere.
b. Suction control chamber vent must not be occluded when suction is used.	Provides safety factor of releasing excess negative pressure into the atmosphere.
c. Waterless systems have relief valves without caps.	
9. Coil excess tubing on mattress next to the client. Secure with a rubber band and safety pin or the system's clamp.	Prevents excess tubing from hanging over the edge of the mattress in a dependent loop. Drainage could collect in the loop and occlude the drainage system.
10. Adjust tubing to hang in a straight line from top of the mattress to the drainage chamber.	Promotes drainage.
11. If the chest tube is draining fluid, indicate the date and time (e.g., 0900) that drainage was begun on the drainage chamber's write-on surface.	Provides a baseline for continuous assessment of the type and quantity of drainage.

STEPS	RATIONALE
a. Postoperative assessment is done every 15 minutes for the first 2 hours. This assessment interval then changes *on the basis of client's status.* Mark the time and level of drainage on the calibrated write-on strip periodically.	Permits timely and efficient account of the amount of drainage from the chest tube. Drainage is marked at specified periods of time and documented on the nurses' notes and intake and output (I&O) sheet. Ensures early detection of complications.
12. Strip or milk chest tube only if indicated (this means compressing the tube to encourage clots to pass through the tube):	
CRITICAL DECISION POINT **Check your institutional policy before stripping or milking chest tubes. This practice is being discontinued at some institutions because it is believed that stripping the tube greatly increases intrapleural pressure, which could damage the pleural tissue.**	
a. Postoperative mediastinal chest tubes are manipulated if nursing assessment indicates an obstruction of drainage resulting from clots or debris in the tubing.	Stripping is controversial and should be performed only if hospital policy permits and there is a physician's order (Johanson, Wells, and Dungea, 1988; Phipps et al., 1995). Stripping creates a high degree of negative pressure and has potential of pulling lung tissue or pleura into drainage holes of the chest tube (Carroll, 1991).
13. Provide two rubber-tipped hemostats for each chest tube. Rubber-tipped hemostats are usually attached to the top of the client's bed with adhesive tape or clamped to client's clothing during ambulation.	Chest tubes are double clamped under specific circumstances: a. To assess for an air leak (see Table 15-2). b. To empty or change the collection bottle or chamber (Gross, 1993). c. To change disposable systems. Have the new system ready to be connected before clamping the tube, so that transfer can be rapid and the drainage system reestablished. d. To assess if client is ready to have chest tube removed. This is done by physician's order (Gross, 1993). In this situation nurse must monitor client for the re-creation of a pneumothorax (see Table 15-2).
14. Assist client to a comfortable position.	Reduces client anxiety and promotes cooperation.
15. Remove gloves and dispose of used, soiled equipment.	Prevents accidents involving contaminated equipment.
16. Wash hands.	Reduces spread of microorganisms.

EVALUATION

1. Monitor vital signs, oxygen saturation, amount and type of drainage, and insertion site every 15 minutes for the first 2 hours.	Provides immediate information about procedure-related complications such as respiratory distress.
2. After first 2 hours, assess client's physical and psychological status as indicated.	Detects early signs and symptoms of complications: Apprehension—increase in client anxiety, restlessness, inability to concentrate. Respiratory distress—alteration in rate and/or depth of respirations, difficulty breathing, breath sounds. **Subcutaneous emphysema**—air that is being trapped in the subcutaneous tissue.
3. Assess client in activities of daily living related to care of the drainage system.	Reveals client's emotional response to procedure. Detects educational needs and reinforces activities of care for the system.

STEPS	RATIONALE
4. Observe:	
a. Chest tube dressing.	Ensure that dressing is occlusive and note any drainage.
➤ ***CRITICAL DECISION POINT*** **Check the dressing carefully. It can come loose from the skin, although this may not be readily apparent.**	
b. Tubing should be free of kinks and dependent loops.	This will ensure proper drainage.
c. The chest drainage system should be upright and below level of tube insertion. Note presence of clots or debris in tubing.	System must be in this position to function properly.
➤ ***CRITICAL DECISION POINT*** **Monitor the position of the system relative to the chest tube carefully, especially during client transport.**	
d. Water seal for fluctuations with client's inspiration and expiration.	
(1) Waterless system: Diagnostic indicator for fluctuations with client's inspirations and expirations.	Fluid should rise in the water seal or diagnostic indicator with inspiration and fall with expiration. This indicates that the system is functioning properly (Lewis, Collier, and Heitkemper, 1996).
(2) Water-seal system: Constant bubbling in the water-seal chamber (see Table 15-2).	When system is initially connected to the client, bubbles are expected from the chamber. These are from air that was present in the system and in the client's intrapleural space. After a short time, the bubbling stops. Fluid continues to fluctuate in the water seal on inspiration and expiration until the lung is reexpanded or the system becomes occluded.
e. Waterless system: Left-to-right bubbling in diagnostic indicator.	
f. Type and amount of fluid drainage: Nurse should note color and amount of drainage, client's vital signs, and skin color. What is the normal amount of drainage?	
(1) Less than 50 to 200 ml/hr immediately postoperative in a mediastinal chest tube (Johanson, Wells, Dungea, 1988); approximately 500 ml in the first 24 hours (Duncan et al, 1987). Dark-red drainage is expected early in the postoperative period, turning serous with time (Lewis, Collier, and Heitkemper, 1996).	
(2) Between 100 and 300 ml of fluid may drain in a posterior chest tube during the first 2 hours after insertion. This rate decreases after 2 hours; 500 to 1000 ml can be expected in the first 24 hours. Drainage is grossly bloody during the first several hours after surgery and then changes to serous (Lewis, Collier, and Heitkemper, 1996). Remember that a sudden gush of drainage may be retained blood and not active bleeding. This increase in drainage can result from client position change.	Reexpansion of lungs forces drainage into the tube. Coughing can also cause large gushes of drainage. Excessive amounts and/or the continued presence of frank bloody drainage the first several hours after surgery should be reported to the physician, along with client's vital signs and respiratory status.
g. Water-seal system: Bubbling in the suction control chamber (when suction is being used) (see Table 15-2).	Suction control chamber has constant, gentle bubbling. Tubing to the suction source should be free of obstruction and the suction source should be turned to the appropriate setting.

STEPS	RATIONALE
h. Waterless system: The suction control (float ball) indicates the amount of suction the client's intrapleural space is receiving.	The suction float ball dictates the amount of suction in the system. The float ball allows no more suction than dictated by its setting. If the suction source is set too low, the suction float ball cannot reach the prescribed setting. In this case the suction must be increased for the float ball to reach the prescribed setting (Davol, Inc.).
5. Assess client for decreased respiratory distress and chest pain, breath sounds over affected lung area, and stable vital signs.	Increase in respiratory distress and/or chest pain, decrease in breath sounds over the affected and nonaffected lungs, marked cyanosis, asymmetrical chest movements, presence of subcutaneous emphysema around tube insertion site or neck, hypotension, tachycardia, and/or **mediastinal shift** are critical and indicate a severe change in client status, such as excessive blood loss or tension pneumothorax. Notify physician immediately.
6. **Unexpected outcomes** that may occur include:	
➤ Water-seal system: Constant bubbling in water-seal chamber is unrelated to respirations.	Indicates air leak, either client centered or in the system (see Table 15-2).
➤ Waterless system: When facing the chamber, left-to-right bubbling in diagnostic chamber. Absence of "yes" in negative pressure display.	Never clamp a client-centered air leak. Instead, reinforce dressing to occlude air leak.
➤ Substantial increase in bright-red drainage with tachycardia and hypotension.	Indicates client is actively bleeding.
➤ Water-seal system: No drainage from hemothorax and/or no fluctuation in water seal within first 48 hours after tube insertion.	Indicates that tubing is occluded. Clots or kinks may have occluded the tubing, or the internal end of the chest tube may be against the pleural lining.
➤ Waterless system: No drainage from hemothorax. No tidaling in diagnostic indicator.	Indicates that the tubing is occluded.
➤ Water-seal system: No bubbling in suction control chamber when suction is being used.	Indicates tubing to suction source is obstructed, kinked, or leaking or the suction source is too low or off.
➤ Waterless system: Suction level control ball is falling from prescribed level or is not functioning.	Increase suction source setting to prescribed level. Adjust the float ball level to the prescribed amount.
➤ Water-seal system: Noisy and excessive bubbling in suction control chamber.	Indicates suction source is delivering too much negative pressure to the system. Suction should be turned lower to maintain gentle bubbling.
➤ Waterless system: No change in the system. Suction control ball level controls amount of suction the client receives even if source is turned too high.	Systems continue to function normally although suction source may be delivering more suction than needed. Suction source can be turned down so long as float ball remains at the prescribed setting.
➤ Water-seal system U-tube not submerged in water.	Indicates the water seal is not being maintained and air can reenter the intrapleural space. Sterile water or NS must be added to the water seal chamber.
➤ Waterless system: Not a concern because there is no water seal.	
➤ Water-seal system: Drainage system turned on its side.	Indicates the water seal is not being maintained and air can reenter the intrapleural space.
➤ Waterless system: Not a concern because there is no water seal.	
➤ Waterless system: Violent rocking or tidaling in diagnostic chamber.	May indicate extreme intrapleural pressure changes (Davol, Inc.).

STEPS	RATIONALE
RECORDING AND REPORTING	
1. Record and report stated allergies or anticoagulant medications the client is taking.	Reduces possibility of procedural complications.
2. Record baseline vital signs, including oxygen saturation.	Provides comparison to postoperative vital signs and oxygen saturation levels.
3. Record vital signs and O_2 saturation every 15 minutes for at least 2 hours postoperatively.	Documentation of vital signs postoperatively is a record of client's eventful or uneventful recovery.
4. Check chest tube insertion site and dressings at least every 15 minutes for 2 hours postoperatively and thereafter as client status indicates.	Provides documentation that chest tube remains in proper position whether or not subcutaneous emphysema exists. Observe dressing for dryness and note if intact.
5. Record chest drainage output hourly for at least 2 hours and then record as client status indicates.	
CRITICAL DECISION POINT **Document time, type, and amount of drainage. Look at the fluid in the collection tubing, not just the fluid in the collection chamber. Is the drainage bright red, dark red or pink? Is it opaque or can you see through it?**	
6. Record water-seal or air-leak indicator activity frequently for proper tidaling or improper bubbling.	Documents proper or improper functioning of system.
7. If suction is used, record the amount of bubbling in the water-seal suction control chamber or verify proper float ball setting in the waterless system at least once each shift.	Documents that the client is receiving the prescribed amount of suction.
8. Record and report air leaks and what was done to fix them.	Documents proper maintenance of system.
9. Record client compliance to coughing, deep breathing, and activity.	Documents cooperation in postoperative activities that reduce time for lung reexpansion.
10. Mediastinal drainage requires the following documentation: time, amount, and type of drainage every 15 minutes for 2 hours postoperatively, then as client status indicates.	Tidaling does not occur because the tube is not in a pleural cavity.

FOLLOW-UP ACTIVITIES

1. Locate the source of external air leak; correct situation if it is in the chest drainage system; notify physician and document. A client-centered leak is an emergency situation requiring physician notification and intervention. The nurse should immediately reinforce the dressing to make it as occlusive as possible.
2. Notify physician. Immediate intervention is needed to prevent hypovolemic shock. Monitor vital signs and mark drainage in write-on column at least every 15 to 30 minutes.
3. Correct any visible occlusions caused by kinks and document. Milk or strip tubing to remove visible clots if approved and ordered and document. Notify physician if no visible kinks or clots are found and tidaling does not begin.
4. Correct kink occlusions or leaks in tubing, remove occlusion to air vent, or increase suction at the suction source and document.
5. Reduce suction to prescribed setting.
6. Set water-seal or disposable system upright. The system can be placed in a stand or hung on the side of the bed. If you use the stand, be sure to place it in a location so that it won't be kicked or knocked over. Encourage client to cough and deep breathe. Document.
7. Assess the waterless system for air leaks; possibly chest tube pulled loose. Assess vital signs. Notify physician.

• • • • •

Special Considerations

- Client with a hemothorax who is also receiving anticoagulants may need to have anticoagulant therapy reduced or discontinued until the hemothorax is resolved or controlled. Monitor these clients carefully for bleeding at the insertion site and for increased amounts of drainage.
- Only chest tube clamps or rubber-tipped hemostats should be used to clamp chest tubes. Other types of tools might create holes in the tubing, causing an air leak.
- Make sure that the client is not lying on the drainage tubing and that it is not depressed or kinked. If the tubing is kinked, it will not drain properly.

SKILL 15-2 Removing Chest Tubes

Actual removal of a chest tube is the function of physicians and advanced practice nurses (APNs). An APN is a nurse with a master's degree in a specialized area of nursing. If nurses are to remove a chest tube, this procedure should be a written component of the agency's policy and procedures standards.

The nurse (1) prepares the client for chest tube removal by assessing the need for preremoval analgesia and obtaining the required medication orders and (2) instructs the client about the process and what will be requested of the client. During removal of the chest tube, it is important that the client take a deep breath and hold it until the physician has removed the tube. This maneuver prevents air from being sucked into the chest as the tube is pulled out and before an occlusive dressing is applied.

This skill details for the nurse the actual nursing responsibilities and physician action for chest tube removal.

EQUIPMENT

- Suture set
  - Sterile scissors
  - Sterile forceps
- Sterile gloves
- Face mask/face shield
- Prepared sterile dressing
  - Petrolatum on top
  - 4 × 4-inch gauze dressings
  - Large dressings
- 4-inch adhesive tape or elastic bandage (Elastoplast) cut into strips

STEPS	RATIONALE
ASSESSMENT	
1. Lung reexpansion is complete when:	
a. Chest x-ray film reveals total lung reexpansion.	
b. Water-seal fluctuation has stopped for 24 hours.	Pleura of the expanded lung seals the holes on the internal tip of the chest tube, halting fluctuation in the water seal. This can be expected 2 to 3 days after chest tube insertion.
c. Drainage is decreased to less than 50 ml/day.	Drainage has been removed, allowing the lung to reexpand.
d. Percussion reveals tympany.	Normal percussion occurs with reexpansion.
e. Auscultation of lungs reveals breath sounds are present throughout the chest cavity.	Normal breath sounds are heard with reexpansion.
2. Clamp chest tube 12 to 24 hours before removal, or as ordered by the physician. Assess for changes in vital signs, chest pain, and level of apprehension.	Physician orders tube clamping before removal to assess client's tolerance.
CRITICAL DECISION POINT **If the client develops respiratory distress when the tube is clamped, assess the client, unclamp the tube, and call the physician.**	

NURSING DIAGNOSIS

Clustering of defining characteristics from the assessment data may reveal the following nursing diagnoses for clients requiring this skill:

- Risk for impaired gas exchange

Related factors are individualized based on a client's condition or needs.

STEPS	RATIONALE
PLANNING	
1. **Expected outcomes** following completion of procedure:	
➤ Lung reexpansion occurs within 3 days.	This is a normal reexpansion time.
➤ Client does not experience discomfort.	
➤ Spontaneous healing of chest tube insertion site occurs after removal of tube without infection or other complications.	Large nonporous occlusive dressing at puncture site promotes uncomplicated healing.
2. Explain procedure to client.	Reduces anxiety and promotes client cooperation.
IMPLEMENTATION	
1. Administer prescribed medication for pain relief about 30 minutes before procedure.	Reduces discomfort and relaxes client.
2. Assist client to sit on edge of bed or to lie on the side without chest tubes.	Physician prescribes client's position to facilitate tube removal.
3. Support client physically and emotionally while physician or APN removes dressing and clips sutures.	Reduces anxiety and promotes cooperation.
4. Physician or APN prepares an occlusive dressing of petroleum gauze on a pressure dressing and sets it aside on a sterile field.	Essential to prepare in advance for quick application to the wound on tube withdrawal.
5. Physician or APN asks the client to take a deep breath and hold it or exhale completely and hold it.	Prevents air from being sucked into the chest as the tube is removed.
6. Wash hands and apply gloves.	Reduces transmission of microorganisms.
7. Physician or APN quickly pulls out the chest tube.	Prevents entry of air through the chest wound.
8. Physician or APN quickly and aseptically applies sterile prepared dressing over the wound and firmly secures it in position with elastic bandage (Elastoplast) or wide tape. Sometimes skin clips or pursestring sutures are used to hold the wound together before dressing is applied.	Keeps wound aseptic. Prevents entry of air into the chest. Wound closure occurs spontaneously. Clips or sutures aid in skin closure.
9. Assist client to a comfortable position.	Ensures that client is comfortable.
10. While wearing gloves, remove used equipment from bedside. Place it in appropriate area for medical waste products.	Prevents spread of microorganisms.
11. Remove gloves and wash hands.	Reduces transmission of microorganisms.
EVALUATION	
1. Assess lung sounds and observe client for subcutaneous emphysema or respiratory distress during the first few hours after removal.	Provides for early notification of physician if adverse symptoms occur. Chest tubes may need reinsertion.
2. Assess client's vital signs, oxygen saturation, and psychological status.	Detects early signs and symptoms of complications.
3. Ask about the client's level of pain or comfort. Observe for nonverbal cues of pain.	Could be signs that wound has not closed well. Ascertains client's tolerance of procedure.
4. Check chest dressing for drainage and patency. When changing dressing, note wound for signs of healing.	Ensures occlusion and proper healing of chest wound.
5. **Unexpected outcomes** that may occur include:	
➤ Client has dyspnea, chest pain, labored respirations.	These are signs of recurrence of pneumothorax or hemothorax.
RECORDING AND REPORTING	
1. Record removal of tube, the amount of drainage in the collection bottle, appearance of wound and dressing, and client's response. Client's response should also include vital signs and respiratory assessment.	Documents procedure, status of wound and dressing, and client's response.

STEPS | **RATIONALE**

FOLLOW-UP ACTIVITIES

1. Notify physician immediately of respiratory distress, unstable vital signs, symptoms of subcutaneous emphysema, client-centered air leaks, or decreasing oxygen saturation levels.
2. Prepare for chest tube reinsertion if indicated.

• • • • •

Special Considerations

- When viewing chest x-ray film immediately after tube removal, the chest tube tract may still be visible.
- Clients may still have a small pneumothorax, which will be spontaneously absorbed.

SKILL 15-3 Postoperative Autotransfusion

Autotransfusion has become more widely used since the public has become aware of the risks associated with blood transfusions. When autotransfusion is linked with chest drainage, it becomes a relatively risk-free, inexpensive, and easy method of replacing mediastinal blood previously lost to allow for lung reexpansion after open heart or thoracic surgery. (See Chapter 23 for skills related to transfusions.) Clients requiring this skill must also have an intravenous line in place (see Chapter 20).

EQUIPMENT

- **Pleur-evac adult/pediatric single-use chest drainage and autotransfusion unit**
- **Pleur-evac A-1500 replacement bag (Fig. 15-7)**

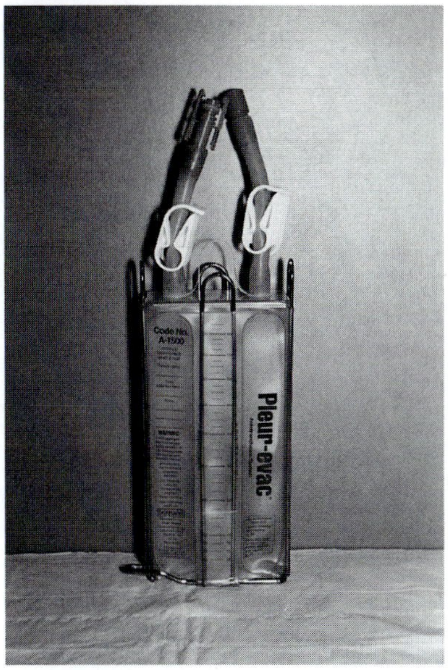

Fig. 15-7

STEPS | **RATIONALE**

ASSESSMENT

1. See Assessment for Skill 15-1, p. 510.

The addition of the autotransfusion unit to the closed chest drainage unit requires no additional assessments.

NURSING DIAGNOSIS

Clustering of defining characteristics from the assessment data may reveal the following nursing diagnoses for clients requiring this skill:

- Risk for infection
- Risk for injury

Related factors are individualized based on a client's condition or needs.

STEPS	RATIONALE
PLANNING	
1. **Expected outcomes** following completion of procedure:	
➤ Vital signs, hematocrit, and hemoglobin will stabilize.	Reinfusion prevents the loss of blood usually associated with closed chest drainage.
➤ The drainage system will function correctly and the lung will reexpand in 48 to 72 hours.	Negative pressure will have been reestablished in the intrapleural space.
➤ The IV line will remain patent.	A patent IV is necessary for reinfusion of cleansed mediastinal tube drainage.
➤ Explain procedure to client.	Reduces anxiety and promotes client cooperation.
IMPLEMENTATION	
1. System setup	
a. Set up the Pleur-evac autotransfusion system according to technique that maintains the sterility of the unit and following the three steps printed on the front of the unit (Deknatel, Inc.) (Fig. 15-8).	Contamination of the unit provides a ready source of infection to the client.

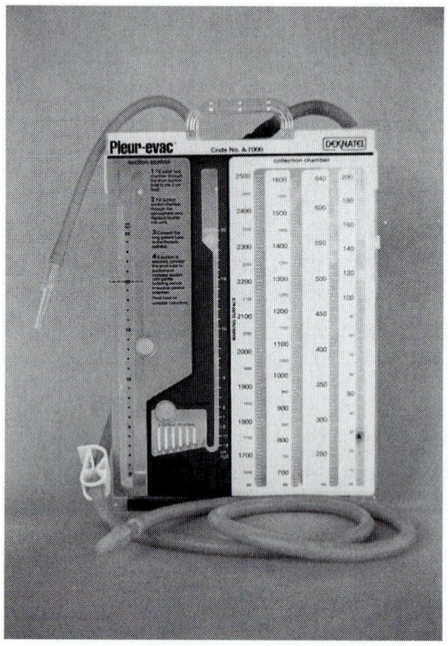

Fig. 15-8

STEPS	RATIONALE
b. Make certain all connections are tight and all clamps are open.	Tight connections ensure an airtight system and open clamps allow chest drainage to enter the autotransfusion system (ATS) bag.
c. A 200 μm double-sided mesh filter is located in the ATS bag to filter the drainage.	Filtering the drainage removes extraneous materials and microemboli.
d. The ATS collection bag has a capacity of 1000 ml marked in increments of 25 ml and an area for marking times and amounts.	See Skill 15-1, Evaluation, Step 4f(1) (p. 516) for expected drainage amounts.
2. Wash hands and apply gloves.	Reduces transmission of microorganisms.
3. Continued collection:	
a. Open a Pleur-evac A-1500 replacement bag using proper technique and close the two white clamps.	Contamination of the unit provides a ready source of contamination to the client. The closed clamps maintain a closed system during replacement.
b. Use the high-negativity relief valve to reduce excessive negativity.	This eases the removal of the initial collection bag from the metal support stand.
c. Bag transfer:	
(1) Close clamp on chest drainage tubing.	Prevents air from entering the chest cavity through the tube and collapsing the lung.

STEPS	RATIONALE
(2) Close the two white clamps on the top of the initial ATS collection bag.	Maintains a closed system for the reinfusion, preventing contamination of the blood.
(3) Connect the chest drainage tube to the new ATS bag with the red connectors.	Establishes a new autotransfusion system.
(4) Make certain that all connections are tight.	Ensures an airtight system.
(5) Open all clamps on chest drainage tube and replacement bag.	Reestablishes an autotransfusion collection system.
d. Connect the red and blue connectors on top of the initial collection bag and remove it by lifting it from the side hook and then from the foot hook.	Maintains a closed system within the bag and removes it for use in autotransfusion.
e. Secure the replacement bag by connecting the foot hook, replacing the metal frame into the side hook of the Pleur-evac unit, and pushing down to secure the frame onto the hook.	Provides safe attachment of the replacement bag to the Pleur-evac unit.
f. The replacement bag is removed by placing the thumbs on the top of the metal frame and pushing up with the fingers to slide the bag out.	
4. Pleur-evac autotransfusion reinfusion:	
a. Use a new microaggregate filter to reinfuse each autotransfusion bag.	Prevents the infusion of microemboli and provides maximal filtration for each bag.
b. Access the bag by inverting it and spiking the bag through the spike port with the microaggregate filter and twisting.	Connects the autotransfusion bag to the transfusion tubing.
c. With the bag upside down, gently squeeze the bag to remove the air and prime the filter with blood.	Gentle pressure is used to prevent hemolysis.
d. Hang the bag on an intravenous (IV) pole and continue to prime the tubing until all air is gone. Clamp the tubing, attach it to the client's IV access, and adjust the clamp to deliver the reinfusion at the appropriate rate.	Removes all air from the transfusion tubing and establishes the reinfusion. Gravity, a blood cuff (not to exceed 150 mm Hg pressure), or a blood-compatible IV pump may be used (see Chapter 21).
e. If ordered, anticoagulants (citrate phosphate dextrose or heparin) can be added to the reinfusion through the self-sealing port in the autotransfusion connector.	Prevents clotting in the autotransfusion.
5. Discontinuing autotransfusion	
a. Clamp the chest drainage tube and connect it directly to the Pleur-evac unit with the red and blue connectors.	Prevents air from entering the chest cavity through the tube and collapsing the lung.
b. Open the chest drainage tube clamp.	All drainage will be collected directly in the Pleur-evac unit and must be appropriately discarded.
6. Discard used supplies and wash hands.	Reduces transmission of microorganisms.

EVALUATION

1. Monitor vital signs, hematocrit, and hemoglobin.	Helps determine the effects of the treatment.
2. Monitor the chest drainage system and the client's lung sounds.	Helps determine the proper functioning of the system and its effectiveness.
3. Assess the IV infusion site for infiltration and phlebitis.	A patent IV infusion site must be maintained.
4. **Unexpected outcomes** that may occur include:	
➤ Chest tube becomes displaced. ➤ Air embolism occurs. ➤ Pneumothorax occurs. ➤ Infection is evident.	A tight seal around the tube must be maintained at all times, and tension on the tubing between the client and the drainage system must be avoided. Absence of a tight seal permits atmospheric air to enter the pleural space, increasing the risk of unexpected outcomes.

STEPS	RATIONALE
RECORDING AND REPORTING	
1. Record drainage, reinfusion with times, and amounts of each.	Drainage and reinfusion amounts are extremely important in maintaining optimum condition of these clients. The total time for drainage and reinfusion of the drainage is to be no longer than 4 hours.
2. Describe the condition of the IV infusion site.	Documents site check.
3. Report unusual findings and client responses to nurse in charge or physician.	May require a change in therapy.

FOLLOW-UP ACTIVITIES

1. Continuous client teaching maximizes compliance with client's activity limitations and alerts the nurse to unusual events.

• • • • •

Special Considerations

➤ Clients with massive blood loss before the implementation of the autotransfusion may require additional transfusions or plasma expanders to reestablish a normal circulating volume.

CRITICAL THINKING EXERCISES

1. Why is it important to check vital signs, check for air leaks, and note the amount of chest drainage every 15 to 30 minutes for at least 2 hours after the insertion of a chest tube?
2. Describe the assessment required for a stable client with a chest tube.
3. You are providing care for a client with a chest tube. You note bubbling in the water-seal chamber. What is the significance of this bubbling?
4. You notice that your client's chest tube dressing is loose and away from his chest in several areas. What effect could this loose dressing have on the client's condition?
5. Your client is in respiratory distress. You notice that the water-seal chamber of the chest tube collection bottle is empty. What is the connection between the respiratory distress and the empty water-seal chamber?

REFERENCES

Beare P, Myers JL: *Adult health nursing,* ed 2, St Louis, 1994, Mosby.
Carroll PF: The ins and outs of chest drainage systems, Nursing 86 16(12):26, 1986.
Carroll PF: What's new in chest-tube management, RN 54(5):34, 1991.
Connor PA: When and how do you use a Heimlich flutter valve? Am J Nurs 87:288, 1987.
Davol, Inc. (Subsidiary of CR Bard, Inc.): Thora-Klex chest drainage system quick reference guide, Warwick, RI, Davol.
Deknatel, Inc: Pleur-evac adult/pediatric chest drainage and autotransfusion: unit package insert, Fall River, Mass, Deknatel.
Duncan C, Erickson R, Weigel RM: Effect of chest tube management on drainage after cardiac surgery, Heart Lung 16(1):1, 1987.
Gross S: Current challenges, concepts, and controversies in chest-tube management, AACN *Clin Iss Crit Care Nurs* 4(2):260, 1993.
Johanson BC, Wells SJ, Dungea CU: *Standards for critical care,* ed 3, St Louis, 1988, Mosby.
Lewis ML, Collier IC, Heitkemper M: *Medical-surgical nursing: assessment and management of clinical problems,* ed 4, St Louis, 1996, Mosby.
Palau D, Jones S: Test your skill at trouble shooting chest tubes, RN October, 1986.
Phipps WJ, et al, editors: Medical-surgical nursing: concepts and clinical practice, ed 4, St Louis, 1995, Mosby.

ADDITIONAL READING

Carson MM, Barton DM, Morrison CC: Managing pain during mediastinal chest tube removal, *Heart Lung,* 23(6):500, 1994.
Erickson RS: Mastering the ins and outs of chest drainage, I. *Nursing 89* 19(5):36, 1989.
Erickson RS: Mastering the ins and outs of chest drainage, II. Nursing 89 19(6):46, 1989.
Farley J: About chest tubes, Nursing 88 18(6):16, 1988.
Gift AG, Bolgiano CS, Cunningham J: Sensations during chest tube removal, Heart Lung 20(2):131, 1991.
Iberti TJ, Stern PM: Chest tube thoracostomy, *Crit Care Med* 8(4):879, 1992.
Tarver RD, Conces DJ: The misplaced tube. Emerg Med, 25(2):61, 1993.

CHAPTER 16

Emergency Measures for Life Support

OBJECTIVES

Mastery of content in this chapter will enable the nurse to:

- Define key terms.
- Describe the factors that place individuals at risk for foreign body airway obstruction.
- State signs and symptoms associated with foreign body airway obstruction.
- Discuss indications for a nasal airway.
- Discuss indications for an oral airway.
- Discuss indications for an Ambu-bag.
- State indications for cardiopulmonary resuscitation (CPR).
- State the goals for CPR.
- Demonstrate in a laboratory or clinical situation: removal of foreign body airway obstruction, insertion of a nasal airway and an oral airway, use of an Ambu-bag, CPR.

KEY TERMS

Airway obstruction
Ambu-bag
Aspiration
Cardiac output
Cardiopulmonary arrest
Cardiopulmonary resuscitation (CPR)
Foreign body airway obstruction maneuver (FBAOM)
Heimlich maneuver
Head tilt-chin lift
Minute ventilation
Nasal airway
Oral airway
Perfusion
Respiratory arrest
Ventilation

SKILLS

16-1 Removing a Foreign Body Airway Obstruction
16-2 Inserting a Nasal Airway
16-3 Inserting an Oropharyngeal Airway
16-4 Using an Ambu-bag
16-5 Performing Cardiopulmonary Resuscitation

The oxygen transport system consists of the lungs and cardiovascular system. Adequacy of oxygen delivery depends on the amount of oxygen entering the lungs **(ventilation),** the blood flow to the lungs and to the body tissues **(perfusion),** the adequacy of diffusion of respiratory gases, the pumping ability of the heart, and the capacity of the blood to carry oxygen.

The blood's capacity to carry oxygen is influenced by the amount of dissolved oxygen in the plasma, the amount and type of hemoglobin, and the affinity of hemoglobin for oxygen. Also critical in the process of gas exchange is the ability of the heart to pump blood between the lungs and peripheral tissue.

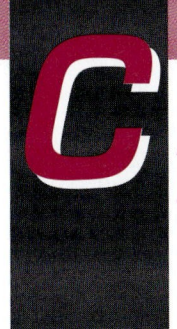

Respiratory gases are exchanged in the alveoli and in the tissues. Oxygen is transferred from the lungs to the blood, and carbon dioxide is transferred from the blood to the lungs to be exhaled as a waste product. At the capillary level, oxygen is transferred from the blood to the tissues, and carbon dioxide is transferred from the tissues to the blood to return to the lungs and be exhaled. This transfer depends on the process of diffusion.

The hemoglobin molecule is the carrier for both oxygen and carbon dioxide; it combines with oxygen to form oxyhemoglobin. Whenever the concentration of inspired oxygen declines, there is less oxygen available for the tissues. Decreases in inspired oxygen concentration (FiO_2) can be caused by an upper or lower airway obstruction, decreased environmental oxygen (as occurs at high altitudes), or absence of breathing, as in respiratory or cardiac arrest.

An acute **airway obstruction** reduces the amount of inspired oxygen delivered to the alveoli. As a result the amount of oxygen available for diffusion into the blood is decreased.

A respiratory or cardiac arrest is an emergency situation that can occur at any time. Inability to exchange waste air for fresh air or lack of heart contraction to deliver blood to tissues impairs cellular oxygenation. Clients at risk for either type of arrest include those with airway obstruction, cardiopulmonary illnesses, severe fluid and electrolyte disturbances, and excessive ingestion of chemical substances.

Cardiopulmonary resuscitation should be performed only when true cessation of breathing and/or pulselessness has occurred. It is intended for clients who are expected to live. It should not be used in clients in the terminal stages of illness.

GUIDELINES

1. Maintenance of a safe environment for the child under two is essential. This age group is at greatest risk for foreign body aspiration of objects from their surroundings. Children frequently put coins, buttons, or small objects from the floor or tabletop into their mouths. This risk is increased due to the added mobility of this age group. Also, table foods that are not cut into an appropriate size pose a risk to the child's airway.
2. Counsel clients not to talk or laugh with food in their mouths. The inspiratory effort to initiate talking or laughing can cause aspiration of food and thus airway obstruction. Drinking liquids, especially alcohol, while chewing food can also cause choking and precipitate aspiration.
3. Know the client's baseline vital signs, noting any irregularities in cardiac rhythm. Dysrhythmias can precipitate a cardiopulmonary arrest. Cardiovascular conditions that place the client at risk for dysrhythmias include coronary artery disease, myocardial infarction, and open heart surgeries.
4. Know the most recent serum electrolyte values. Electrolyte imbalances (e.g., those involving potassium and calcium) can precipitate cardiopulmonary arrest.
5. When an overdose of a chemical substance is present, know the type and amount of the substance ingested. Certain chemicals, such as alcohol, tranquilizers, and depressants, depress the respiratory center and can result in a respiratory arrest. Overdoses of some drugs, such as heroin, can cause ventricular dysrhythmias and cardiopulmonary arrest.
6. Know the physician orders and client's wishes regarding life-sustaining activities. Advance directives and living wills are a portion of the client's chart. Health care agencies have written policies and procedures for staff concerning the implementation of these decisions.

DELEGATION CONSIDERATIONS

The skill of removing a foreign body can be performed by trained assistive personnel.

- Caution the care provider to allow clients experiencing foreign body obstruction to clear the airway themselves, if at all possible.

SKILL 16-1 Removing a Foreign Body Airway Obstruction

An airway obstructed by a foreign body threatens life. In adults partially chewed food, especially meats and raw vegetables, and in children small toys or game pieces are the types of foreign bodies that most often result in partial or complete airway obstruction.

Inability to remove a foreign body impairs gas exchange and can result in unconsciousness and, possibly, cardiopulmonary arrest. Should arrest occur, CPR must be initiated at once. However, CPR is ineffective if the foreign body remains in the airway. Efforts must continue to remove the obstruction. Often, full cardiac arrest can be prevented if the obstruction can be removed immediately. Prevention of foreign body aspiration is equally important.

In the adult and child, aspiration of a foreign body can be frequently prevented by (1) chewing pieces of food slowly and thoroughly, (2) avoiding excessive alcohol intake at mealtime, (3) choosing age-appropriate toys and foods and restricting their use accordingly, (4) keeping children from placing small toys or game pieces in their mouths or noses, and (5) avoiding excessive laughing, talking, and drinking during chewing and swallowing.

In the unconscious client the tongue and other soft palate structures, as well as dentures and other nonpermanent dental work, can become dislodged and obstruct the airway. In addition, it is not uncommon for an unconscious client or others with diminished or absent cough and gag reflexes (e.g., stroke victims) to vomit and then aspirate stomach contents.

In the unconscious client, aspiration of a foreign body can frequently be prevented by (1) removing all nonpermanent dental work, (2) inserting an oral airway (Skill 16-3) to maintain tongue position, (3) inserting a nasogastric tube (Chapter 24) to drain stomach contents, (4) placing the client in a side-lying position to prevent aspiration, and (5) when appropriate, inserting an endotracheal tube (this procedure is done by a physician or health care provider who is experienced and licensed to perform this skill) to maintain a patent airway and prevent aspiration.

The keys to successful management of foreign body airway obstruction are (1) early recognition that an obstructed airway exists and (2) recognition of the extent to which the airway is obstructed. If the client is able to breathe and/or speak without difficulty and cough forcefully, no immediate intervention is necessary.

The client who has difficulty breathing or is not breathing, is cyanotic, or is unable to speak, cough, or cough forcefully needs immediate assistance. In addition a client may indicate complete airway obstruction by clutching the neck.

EQUIPMENT

Hospital Setting

- Emergency cart
- Suction equipment
- Face shield and gloves (if indicated and time permits)

Home Setting

- None; however, bulb syringe or kitchen baster may be useful in clearing oral secretions in an emergency. Any protective devices (e.g., mouth shield or gloves) should be utilized if they are available.

STEPS | **RATIONALE**

ASSESSMENT

1. Identify signs and symptoms of foreign body airway obstruction needing immediate intervention:

   The client must not be left alone.

   a. Cardiac: irregular pulse, rapid or slow pulse, cyanosis.

   b. Respiratory: irregular breathing pattern, choking, gagging, rapid or slow shallow breathing, apneic breathing periods, high-pitched inspiratory noises ("crowing" type), stridor, wheezing, inability to forcefully cough, inability to cough at all, inability to speak, use of accessory breathing muscles.

   c. Oral: blood or vomitus in mouth or on face, partially chewed food in mouth, freely floating dentures or nonpermanent dental work in mouth, tongue in posterior oropharynx.

CRITICAL DECISION POINT **Clients postoperative from oral surgery may experience more intense oral mucosal swelling or have their jaws wired together, thus requiring special attention to detailed assessment.**

   d. Signs and symptoms of foreign body airway obstruction *not needing immediate intervention* include ability to speak, cough forcefully, or breathe in and out; stable vital signs; alertness; wheezing between coughs.

CRITICAL DECISION POINT **Tachypnea places the child at risk for aspiration.**

   e. The universal sign is the client clutching the neck with thumb and fingers. Physical signs and symptoms may indicate need to perform FBAOM. Foreign body airway obstruction commonly occurs during eating and may be complete or partial.

STEPS	RATIONALE
➤ ***CRITICAL DECISION POINT*** **Do not leave clients who are experiencing a possible choking episode alone at any time. Intervention must be immediate if the client's condition worsens.**	
2. Assess for factors such as obesity or the late stages of pregnancy and characteristics of the foreign body.	Such factors can influence the outcome of the FBAOM or require modification in intervention techniques.
3. Assess client's and family's understanding of FBAOMs and anticipated outcomes.	Allows nurse to identify potential for teaching needs and determine if family is incapable of assessment and intervention.
➤ ***CRITICAL DECISION POINT*** **Must be done quickly and in some situations the nurse omits this step.**	

NURSING DIAGNOSIS

Clustering of defining characteristics from the assessment data may reveal the following nursing diagnoses for clients requiring this skill:

- Ineffective airway clearance
- Risk for aspiration
- Ineffective breathing pattern
- Impaired gas exchange
- Risk for altered respiratory function
- Altered cardiopulmonary tissue perfusion

Related factors are individualized based on a client's condition or needs.

PLANNING

1. Expected outcomes following completion of procedure:	
➤ Foreign body is dislodged and removed.	Airway cleared of obstruction.
➤ Nurse is able to identify clients and families needing instruction in FBAOM. If possible, explain FBAOMs to client and emphasize importance of relaxation during maneuvers.	Families need to know how to perform FBAOMs.
➤ Clients are very anxious. Tense chest, arms, and abdominal muscles can limit effectiveness of maneuvers.	
2. Help client take position that allows nurse to perform maneuvers easily. Unconscious clients should be placed on the floor. Alert clients may be seated in chair or allowed to stand.	Protects client and nurse from injury.
3. Remove dentures or other nonpermanent dental work.	Prevents further airway obstruction.
4. Activate emergency medical services.	Additional help may be necessary.

IMPLEMENTATION

HEIMLICH MANEUVER

The Heimlich maneuver can be utilized in most adults and children. For clients who are in the late stages of pregnancy or are markedly obese, chest thrusts should be administered. In infants, back blows and chest thrusts should be utilized.

Conscious Client, Sitting or Standing

1. Stand behind client and wrap arms around client's waist.	Allows access to client's chest and provides support.
2. Keep elbows bent.	Prevents squeezing client's ribs and ensures that force is applied directly under the diaphragm.
3. Make a fist with one hand; place the thumb side against the client's abdomen in the midline slightly above the navel and well below the tip of the xiphoid process.	Fist provides force without injury from fingers.

STEPS	RATIONALE
4. Grasp the fist with the other hand and press it into the client's abdomen with a quick upward thrust (see illustration).	Subdiaphragmatic thrust elevates diaphragm, forcing air from lungs.
5. Repeat the abdominal thrusts up to five times or as many as needed to dislodge obstruction.	Foreign body may not be removed on first attempt.
6. Periodically stop and assess the client for progress.	Partial dislodgement may have occurred.
7. Continue if the client is still conscious and still obstructed.	
Supine Client	
1. Position client face up, and kneel astride the victim's thighs.	Allows access to client's chest.
2. Place the heel of one hand against the client's abdomen in the midline slightly above the navel and well below the xiphoid process.	Correct hand position provides force for thrust without injury to internal body structures.
3. Place the second hand directly on top of the first and lock fingers if desired.	Locking fingers prevents client injury and stabilizes heels of the nurse's hands.
4. Press into the client's abdomen with a quick upward thrust. Subdiaphragmatic thrust elevates diaphragm, forcing air from lungs.	
5. Repeat up to five times.	Foreign body may not be removed on first attempt.
CHEST THRUSTS	
Sitting or Standing Client	
1. Stand behind client and encircle the client's chest with both arms under the client's armpits. Allow client's body to rest against nurse's (see illustration).	Allows easy access to client's chest and provides support for delivering thrusts.
2. Place the thumb side of one fist on the middle of the client's breastbone, taking care to avoid the xiphoid process and rib cage margin.	Correct hand position prevents injury to internal body structures.
3. Grab the fist with the other hand and perform backward thrusts.	Provides force to dislodge foreign body.
4. Repeat up to five times.	Foreign body may not be removed on first attempt.

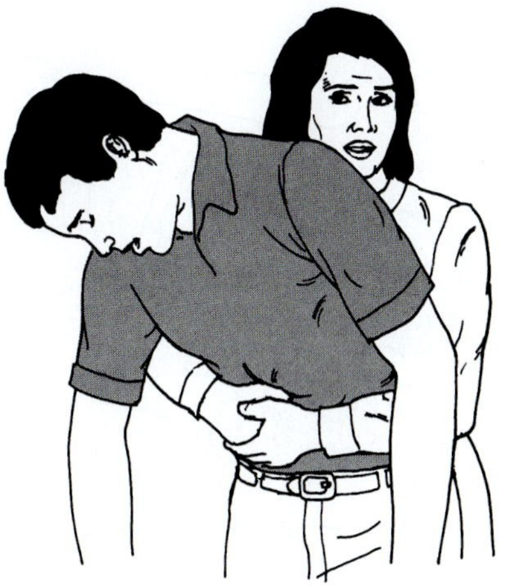

Step 4 Heimlich maneuver.

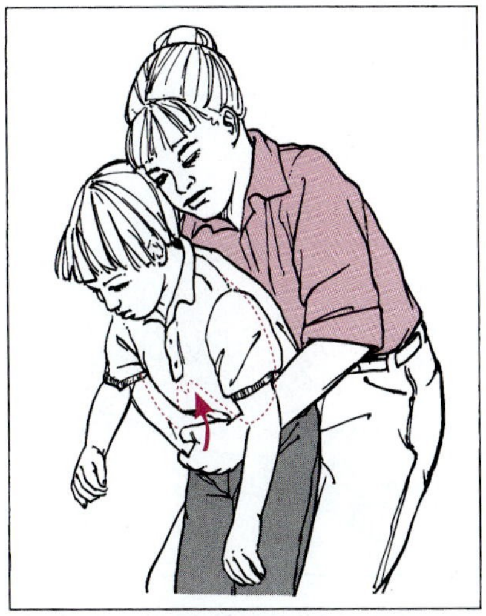

Step 1 Heimlich maneuver with child standing. (From Textbook of Basic Life Support for Healthcare Providers, 1994, American Heart Association, Dallas.)

STEPS	RATIONALE
Supine Client	
1. Place the client face up, and kneel close to the client's side (see left illustration).	Allows easy access to client's chest.
2. Place the heel of the hand on the lower sternum (similar to cardiac compressions).	Correct hand position prevents injury to internal body structures.
3. Press inward slowly and distinctly 1½ to 2 inches in adults as for CPR.	Increases intrathoracic pressure and forces exhalation to expel foreign body.
4. Repeat up to five times.	Foreign body may not be removed with first attempt.
BACK BLOWS AND CHEST THRUSTS FOR INFANTS	
1. Hold infant prone, resting on nurse's forearm, with the infant's head lower than the trunk, making certain to support the head. (This can be performed standing or sitting. With larger infants the nurse should sit and rest the forearm on the thigh for support.) (See right illustration.)	Provides access to client's back and provides support for back blows. Head must be lower to encourage outward movement of foreign body.
2. Using the heel of the hand deliver up to five back blows forcefully between the shoulder blades.	Increases intrathoracic pressure and forces exhalation to cough out foreign body.
CRITICAL DECISION POINT **Careful placement of back blows is imperative as lower placement on the back can result in internal organ damage.**	
3. Place the free hand flat on the infant's back supporting the head, and in such a way that the infant is sandwiched between the two arms. Turn the infant supine. Drape the infant over the thigh with the infant's head lower than the trunk, while continuing to support the infant's head.	Repositions the infant for chest thrusts.
4. Provide up to five downward thrusts over the lower third of the sternum (as in CPR, Skill 16-5; see p. 543).	Increases intrathoracic pressure and forces exhalation to cough out foreign body.
FINGER SWEEP	
1. Wash hands and apply gloves and face shield, if possible.	Reduces transmission of microorganisms.
2. Open client's mouth, grasping tongue and lower jaw with thumb and index finger and lift up.	Opens client's airway. Draws tongue away from back of throat.

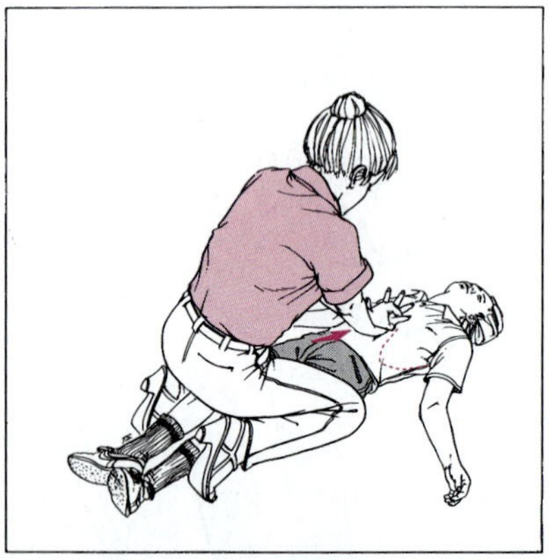

Step 1 Heimlich maneuver with child lying. (From Textbook of Basic Life Support for Healthcare Providers, 1994, American Heart Association, Dallas.)

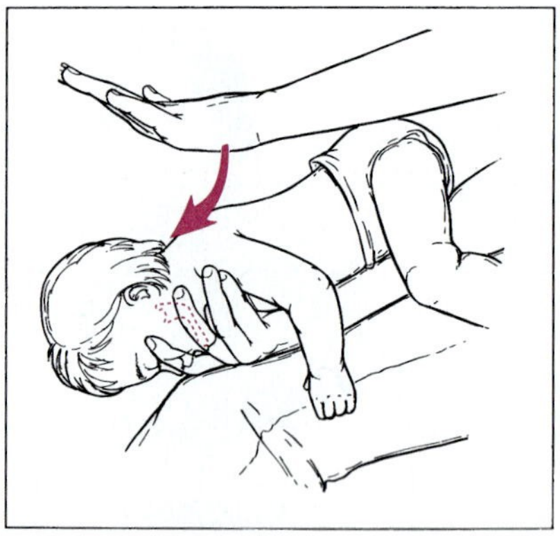

Step 1 Back blows in infant. (From Textbook of Basic Life Support for Healthcare Providers, 1994, American Heart Association, Dallas.)

STEPS	RATIONALE
➤ ***CRITICAL DECISION POINT*** **In clients with a cervical spine injury pull tongue up and out of mouth and lower jaw slightly but do not move neck. If unable to open client's mouth easily, place thumb and index finger of one hand on upper and lower gum line and push teeth apart.**	
3. Insert index finger of other hand along cheek to posterior pharynx and using a sweeping or hooking motion, dislodge foreign body and pull it up into and out of mouth (American Heart Association, 1994).	Removes foreign body.
➤ ***CRITICAL DECISION POINT*** **Be careful not to force foreign body deeper into client's airway. Finger sweep is performed on infants only if the foreign body is visualized.** **Thumb can be used to help remove foreign body once located. In addition, pushing foreign body against side of pharynx is often helpful to help maneuver it up and out.**	
4. Take pulse and respiration measurements. If absent, begin cardiopulmonary resuscitation (Skill 16-5). In unconscious adults attempt rescue breathing (Skill 16-5). In children, attempt ventilation, if unsuccessful, perform abdominal thrusts before attempting rescue breathing. In infants, perform back blows and chest thrusts.	Determines cardiopulmonary status. Inability to ventilate unconscious victim suggests presence of foreign body.
➤ ***CRITICAL DECISION POINT*** **In children, only abdominal thrusts are done.**	
5. Repeat sequence of finger sweep and thrust maneuver as long as necessary.	Repeated attempts are often needed to clear foreign body.
6. Remove and dispose of gloves and face shield into appropriate receptacle. Wash hands.	Reduces transmission of microorganisms.

EVALUATION

STEPS	RATIONALE
1. Observe that foreign body is removed. Compare client's respiratory status before and after FBAOM, if possible.	Provides information concerning changes in client's vital signs.
➤ ***CRITICAL DECISION POINT*** **The presence of wheezing or rhonchi could indicate aspiration.**	
2. If teaching care givers, evaluate technique.	Practicing skills and demonstrating competence increases ability to perform in emergent situation.
3. **Unexpected outcomes** that may occur include:	
➤ Foreign body is not dislodged or is partially dislodged but not removed.	
• Call for immediate medical or surgical assistance.	Foreign body continues to obstruct airway.
➤ Client vomits.	
• Prevent aspiration. Suction if appropriate.	
➤ Foreign body is dislodged but enters the lung.	Needs care beyond scope of nursing practice.
• Repeat one or all maneuvers and stay with client.	Help is coming. Second attempt may be successful.
• Monitor pulse and respiratory status. Begin CPR if client arrests (Skill 16-5).	Maintains cardiopulmonary function.

STEPS	RATIONALE
RECORDING AND REPORTING	
1. Record nursing progress notes, including:	
a. Precipitating event, if known.	Alerts nurses to problem area (e.g., types of foods or toys that must be monitored closely).
b. Vital signs, if taken, and other assessments (skin color, ability to speak, breathe, talk) before and after FBAOMs.	Determines level of cardiopulmonary function.
c. Maneuver(s) performed.	Documents care given.
d. Result of maneuver(s) performed.	Documents effect of care given.
e. Any additional assistance requested or received and scope of assistance.	Documents additional care given and by whom (e.g., tracheostomy physician).

FOLLOW-UP ACTIVITIES

1. Assess pulse, respirations, and blood pressure.
2. Reassess client and family and remain with client.
3. After implementation of maneuvers, if foreign body is removed:
   a. Instruct client and family in maneuvers should obstruction occur again. Obstruction can be relieved before hospitalization.
   b. Recommend that client seek medical advice as soon as possible. Nonvisible internal injury may have occurred.
4. *After* implementation of maneuver if foreign body is not removed:
   a. State that additional help is needed but that nurse will remain with client. Client will be reassured to know additional help is coming.

• • • • •

Special Considerations

- Clients at greater risk of foreign body aspiration include those with the following conditions: neuromuscular diseases such as myasthenia gravis and amyotrophic lateral sclerosis; cerebral vascular accident (stroke) with hemiparesis; cleft palate; lesions of head, neck, esophagus, upper airway; seizure disorders; unconsciousness; heavy sedative or narcotic use; diminished or absent cough and gag reflexes.
- Nurse should not strain muscles to reach around client and perform maneuvers. Positioning for child depends on its age. Infant, up to 1 year of age, is placed over rescuer's arm with head lower than trunk. Children, usually ages 1 to 8, can be draped across rescuer's thighs with rescuer kneeling on the floor or held from behind with the nurse's arms wrapped around the abdomen (Wong, 1995) or placed on the floor with the rescuer in a straddle position (Wong, 1995).
- If airway remains obstructed after performing FBAOM, nurse should be prepared with equipment for physician to perform intubation or tracheostomy. In event of cardiopulmonary arrest, nurse must be prepared to initiate basic life support CPR (Skill 16-5).
- Combination of three maneuvers to remove a foreign body airway obstruction is more effective than each single maneuver. The back blows and manual thrust maneuvers work by increasing intrathoracic pressure, forcing the client to "cough" and expel foreign body.
- Each maneuver should be delivered as if it were the only one needed to dislodge foreign body. According to the American Heart Association, back blows only are recommended for the infant.
- While performing chest thrusts: if hands are too low, xiphoid process can be fractured. If hands are too high, intrathoracic pressure will not be sufficiently increased to expel foreign body. If client is supine, this is same position used when performing CPR. Placing hands over xiphoid process or over ribs can cause fractures and internal injuries.
- Meat is the most common cause of obstruction in adults, whereas many foods, toys, coins, and other foreign bodies cause obstruction in children.

Teaching Considerations

- Instruct client and family on how to avoid obstruction by removing, modifying, or avoiding offending agent; instruct client and family in maneuvers should obstruction occur again.
- Ask client and family to state signs and symptoms of foreign body obstruction.
- Have client and family perform techniques on doll or dummy. Observe for correct technique.

Pediatric Considerations

- Not every child who gags or coughs while eating is truly choking. A child in distress cannot speak, becomes cyanotic, and collapses (Wong, 1995). If the distress is manifested by wheezing, difficulty breathing, drooling or a croupy cough, the obstruction is most likely due to swelling in the airway or epiglottis and not a foreign body. This is an emergency situation, and the infant or child needs immediate medical attention.
- In all children and infants (and occasionally adults) be careful when using finger sweep not to force foreign body deeper into throat. Blind finger sweep is not recommended in infants and children.
- Back blows only are recommended for infants according to the AHA (1994).

Gerontologic Considerations

- Chest walls of older adults are less compliant. Improper technique of FBAOM may result in fractured rib(s) or xiphoid process or internal injury.
- Older adults often cannot chew food as well. They may also have impaired swallowing because of illness, such as stroke or Parkinson's disease, and as a result their risk for choking increases.

SKILL 16-2 Inserting a Nasal Airway

A nasal airway is a flexible curved piece of rubber or plastic with one wide or trumpet-like end flange and one narrow end that, once inserted, extends from the nares (remains external to the nose) past the sinuses to the pharynx (Fig. 16-1A).

The nasal airway varies in length (measured in centimeters or inches) and diameter (measured in millimeters). Some companies indicate nasal airway size by number (e.g., 5, 6, 7, 8, 9, 10), others by grouping two or more numeric sizes into one nasal airway (e.g., small, medium, large). In general, a small nasal airway corresponds to a 5 or 6 mm diameter nasal airway, a medium nasal airway corresponds to a 7 or 8 mm diameter nasal airway, and a large nasal airway corresponds to a 9 or 10 mm diameter nasal airway.

The nurse chooses the size of a nasal airway based on the size (ideal body weight), nasal structure, sex, and age of the client. To determine the correct length, measure from the tragus of the ear to the nostril and add 1 inch. The largest airway possible should be utilized.

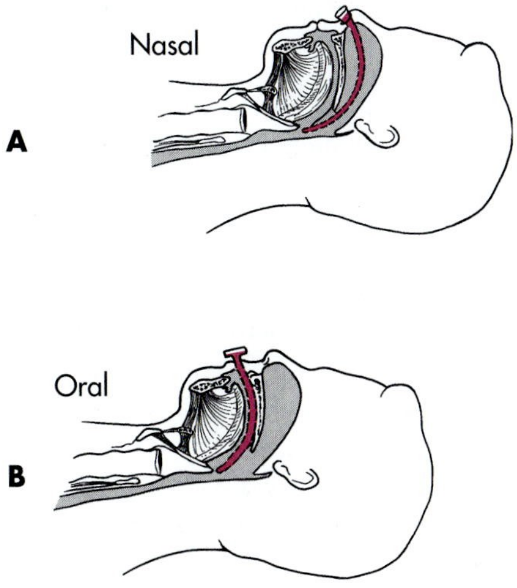

Fig. 16-1 Placement of airways; **A,** Nasal **B,** Oral.

EQUIPMENT

- **Appropriate size nasal airway**
- **Nonsterile gloves**
- **Water-soluble lubricant**
- **Tissues**
- **Tape**
- **Appropriate suction equipment, if needed**
- **Face shield, if indicated**

DELEGATION CONSIDERATIONS

The skill of insertion of a nasal airway requires problem solving and knowledge application unique to the professional nurse. For this skill, delegation is inappropriate.

STEPS	RATIONALE
ASSESSMENT	
1. Identify signs and symptoms of need to insert a nasal airway: frequent nasopharyngeal or nasotracheal suctioning, edematous nasal mucosa, bleeding of nasal mucosa secondary to irritation from suctioning.	Certain conditions require a nasal airway to be in place.
2. Determine size of nasal airway to use: a. Weight: <100 lb: 5,6, or small <150 lb: 7,8, or medium >150 lb: 9,10, or large b. Gender: Males may use next larger size.	Proper size ensures a patent airway and minimizes trauma to client.
3. Assess client's knowledge of procedure.	Identifies learning needs and can facilitate client's cooperation.

NURSING DIAGNOSIS

Clustering of defining characteristics from the assessment data may reveal the following nursing diagnoses for clients requiring this skill:

- Ineffective airway clearance
- Impaired gas exchange
- Risk for infection
- Risk for impaired skin integrity
- Ineffective breathing pattern

Related factors are individualized based on a client's condition or needs.

STEPS	RATIONALE
PLANNING	
1. Expected outcomes following completion of procedure:	
➤ Suctioning-induced nasal edema decreases and bleeding diminishes immediately and ultimately stops.	Limited irritation results from insertion of nasal airway.
➤ Nasal air passage is patent.	Artificial airway maintains patency.
➤ Client is more cooperative to nasopharyngeal or nasotracheal suctioning.	Client is more comfortable because of decreased pain in nares from repeated suctioning; promotes ability to breathe more easily.
➤ No pressure area is evident on nares.	Prolonged use of nasal airway can result in pressure area around nares.
2. Explain reasons for insertion of airway and client's participation.	Relieves anxiety and encourages cooperation.
3. Help client assume comfortable position, usually semi-Fowler's.	Promotes client comfort.
IMPLEMENTATION	
1. Wash hands, put on gloves and face shield.	Reduces transmission of microorganisms.
2. Prepare nasal airway. Use principles of medical asepsis:	
a. Remove nasal airway from package, check for smooth edges.	Prevents insertion of damaged product that could produce further trauma.
b. Open lubricant package, squeeze 10 to 15 cc of lubricant on nasal airway package or tissue.	Provides large surface area of lubricant with which to coat nasal airway.
c. Lubricate entire nasal airway, making sure narrow end is generously coated with lubricant.	Provides "slick" surface for insertion and prevents friction against dry mucous membranes, which causes trauma.
3. Clean excess secretions from client's nares with tissues. Assess appropriate naris for insertion by alternately occluding each naris and asking client to inhale. If necessary, suction secretions (Chapter 14).	Provides largest possible diameter airway for ease of insertion.
4. Holding nasal airway by wide end, insert it into naris using gentle inward and downward pressure until the "trumpet-like" end is at the naris.	Prevents trauma by following natural course of nasal structures.

STEPS	RATIONALE
CRITICAL DECISION POINT Have the client take slow deep breaths to ease insertion. If client gags, the airway may be too large and a different size should be selected.	
5. Clean excess lubricant from client's face and nares.	Excess lubricant dries and acts as obstruction if not removed.
6. Secure airway if necessary (see Chapter 14 for taping endotracheal tube).	Prevents accidental removal and deeper penetration into nasal and pharyngeal structures.
7. Place client in comfortable position.	Promotes client comfort.
8. Remove gloves and face shield and discard in appropriate receptacle. Wash hands.	Reduces transmission of microorganisms.
9. At least daily, remove nasal airway, clean in warm soapy water, and reinsert. Hydrogen peroxide can be used to remove crusts. Small brush is helpful to clean inner core of nasal airway. After cleansing rinse nasal airway thoroughly.	Removes accumulated secretions and microorganisms. Nasal airway can obstruct drainage from sinuses; failure to remove and allow drainage can precipitate sinusitis.
CRITICAL DECISION POINT Some institutions may require more frequent removal and alternating between nostrils.	
10. Assess pressure points at end of phalange.	Promotes early identification of impaired skin integrity.
11. Auscultate breath sounds.	Determines airway placement and effectiveness.
EVALUATION	
1. Observe nares to determine that previous edema and bleeding are diminished.	
2. Observe for patency of nasal airway.	
3. Assess client's respiratory status and observe color, odor, consistency, and quantity of secretions.	Identifies client's response to insertion of nasal airway and/or removal of airway secretions.
4. Observe nares for signs of pressure from airway.	
5. **Unexpected outcomes** that may occur include:	
➤ Nurse is unable to insert nasal airway.	
• Attempt to insert into other naris.	
➤ Excessive edema or obstruction may be present.	
• Attempt to insert a smaller sized airway.	
➤ Airway may be smaller than anticipated.	
➤ Client begins to have nasal bleeding.	Airway insertion causes irritation or bleeding.
• Apply pressure over nasal pressure points for at least 5 to 10 minutes. Allows blood clotting system to form clot.	
• If bleeding continues, notify physician and follow instructions.	Notify physician. Care exceeds scope of nursing practice.
• Monitor vital signs.	Excessive bleeding predisposes client to further airway distress due to the presence of blood in the trachea.
➤ Client complains of severe pain in ear and has fever.	Otitis media can result from impaired sinus drainage secondary to nasal airway.
➤ Client complains of headache (over sinuses) with or without fever. Nasal drainage becomes purulent.	Sinusitis may be present.
RECORDING AND REPORTING	
1. Record in nurses' progress notes:	
a. Assessment finding for inserting nasal airway.	Documents degree and potential cause of obstruction.
b. Size and site (right/left nares) of airway inserted.	Documents size for other care givers.
c. Airway is in the correct position.	Documents placement.

STEPS	RATIONALE
d. Client's tolerance of procedure.	Documents outcomes.
e. Secretions suctioned.	Documents nursing care and provides assessment parameters for future.
f. Method of securing (if done).	Documents nursing care.

Follow-up Activities

1. Report uncontrolled bleeding to physician.
2. Report presence of severe ear pain and any adverse change in color, odor, consistency, or quantity of nasal secretions; report headaches; monitor fever.

Special Considerations

- Clients with the following conditions are at greater risk for complication when nasal airway is inserted: chronic sinus infections or drainage, nasal fractures, spontaneous intranasal bleeding, deviated septum, postoperative reconstructive nasal and facial surgery.
- Excessive epistaxis is dangerous in clients with hemophilia, active leukemia, aplastic anemia, or those on anticoagulant therapy.
- Petroleum-based lubricants (e.g., petrolatum) should not be used because of dangers of chemical aspiration pneumonia.

Pediatric Considerations

- Nasopharyngeal airways are more frequently used in young children and infants.

Gerontologic Considerations

- In the older client mucosal membrane tissues are fragile and bleed easily. Gentle insertion is a must.

SKILL 16-3 Inserting an Oropharyngeal Airway

An oropharyngeal airway is a minimally flexible curved piece of hard plastic (Fig. 16-2). When inserted, it extends from just outside the lips, over the tongue, and to the pharynx (see Fig. 16-1, p. 533). Oral airways enable the nurse to suction through a central core, facilitate resuscitation, and maintain airway patency in the unconscious client. The airways facilitating resuscitation and maintaining airway patency in the unconscious client do not have a central core for suctioning.

The oral airway is sized for adults and children, varying in length and width. Pediatric sizes are 000, 00, 0, 1, 2, and 3. Adult sizes are 4 through 10 or small, medium, and large. The nurse chooses the size of an oral airway based on the client's age and the width and length of the client's mouth. Size is correct if, when the flange is held parallel to the front teeth with the airway against the client's cheek, the end of the curve reaches the angle of the jaw. General size guidelines for choosing an oral airway for children are provided in Table 16-1.

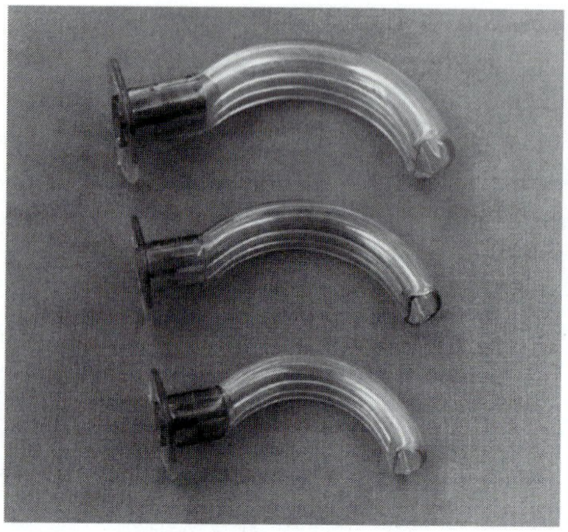

Fig. 16-2 Oral airways.

Table 16-1 Oral Airway Guidelines for Size by Age

Size	Age
000	Premature neonates
00	Newborn
0	Newborn to 1 yr
1	1 to 2 yr
2	2 to 6 yr
3	6 to 18 yr
4 and larger	≥18 yr

EQUIPMENT

- Appropriate-size oral airway
- Nonsterile gloves
- Tissues or washcloths
- Suction equipment, if indicated
- Tape (optional)
- Face shield, if indicated

DELEGATION CONSIDERATIONS

The skill of insertion of an oral airway requires problem solving and knowledge application unique to the professional nurse. For this skill delegation is inappropriate.

STEPS	RATIONALE
ASSESSMENT	
1. Identify need to insert an oral airway. Signs and symptoms include upper airway "gurgling" with respiratory cycle, increased oral secretions or excretions, excessive drooling, grinding teeth, clenched teeth, biting of oral tracheal or gastric tubes, labored respirations, and increased respiratory rate.	Certain conditions place clients at risk for obstruction of upper airway.
2. Determine factors that normally influence upper airway functioning, such as age (children have a proportionally larger tongue), presence of nasal and oral airway, and drainage tubes (swallowing is more difficult with tubes in place).	Allows nurse to accurately assess need for an oral airway.
3. Assess for presence of gag reflex.	Provides guide as to when oral airway can be safely removed in postoperative client.
➤ **CRITICAL DECISION POINT** **Never insert an oropharyngeal airway in an unconscious client.**	
4. Assess client's knowledge of procedure.	Identifies learning needs and facilitates client's cooperation with procedure.

NURSING DIAGNOSIS

Clustering of defining characteristics from the assessment data may reveal the following nursing diagnoses for clients requiring this skill:

- ➤ Ineffective airway clearance
- ➤ Risk for aspiration
- ➤ Ineffective breathing pattern
- ➤ Impaired gas exchange
- ➤ Risk for infection
- ➤ Inability to sustain spontaneous ventilation

Related factors are individualized based on a client's condition or needs.

STEPS	RATIONALE
PLANNING	
1. **Expected outcomes** following completion of procedure:	
➤ Client's respiratory status improves, as evidenced by easier respirations with a normal rate, easier removal of secretions, and lack of gurgling noise in throat with respirations.	Airway is cleared of secretions.
➤ Client is not able to grind teeth or bite tubes.	Oral airway prevents tooth contact with other teeth or with tubes.
➤ Client does not swallow tongue or otherwise obstruct airway.	Oral airway maintains tooth and tongue position.
2. Position client; semi-Fowler's position is preferred.	Promotes client comfort and provides easy access to oral cavity.
IMPLEMENTATION	
1. Wash hands and apply nonsterile gloves and face shield.	Reduces transmission of microorganisms.

STEPS	RATIONALE
2. Whenever possible use a padded tongue blade to open the client's mouth, if necessary use the thumb and forefinger of nondominant hand to pry jaws and teeth apart.	Provides access to oral cavity.
3. Insert oral airway:	
a. Hold oral airway with curved end up, insert distal until the airway reaches the back of the throat, then turn airway over 180 degrees and follow natural curve of tongue. The outer phalange should be just outside the client's lips.	Provides patent airway and prevents displacement of client's tongue into posterior oropharynx.
➤ ***CRITICAL DECISION POINT*** **In some clients it may be possible to depress the tongue with a tongue blade and inset the airway with the tip pointing down, sliding it over the tongue.**	
4. Secure with tape if the client attempts to push out with tongue.	Prevents expulsion of airway.
➤ ***CRITICAL DECISION POINT*** **Taping an airway in place can limit the client's ability to expel vomitus.**	
5. Suction secretions, if needed.	Removes secretions; maintains patent airway.
6. Reassess client's respiratory status.	Directs nurse to initiate intervention.
7. Clean client's face with soft tissue or washcloth.	Promotes hygiene.
8. Discard tissue into appropriate receptacle, place washcloth in dirty or soiled linen bag, remove gloves and face shield, and discard in appropriate receptacle; wash hands.	
9. Administer mouth care frequently.	Increases client comfort and removes debris. It also provides moisture to oral mucosal tissues.
➤ ***CRITICAL DECISION POINT*** **Do not use lemon glycerine swabs for oral care as they are drying to mucosal tissues and promote bacterial growth.**	

EVALUATION

1. Observe client's respiratory status and compare respiratory assessments before and after insertion of oral airway.	Identifies client's response to insertion of airway.
2. Assess that airway is patent, that client does not occlude airway by biting tube, and that client's tongue does not obstruct airway.	
3. **Unexpected outcomes** that may occur include:	
➤ Client continually coughs and gags when airway inserted.	Airway may be too large or long.
➤ Client pushes airway out of place or out of mouth.	Airway not secured.
➤ Nurse is unable to insert oral airway in client; client may be combative or the nurse may be unable to pry mouth open.	One nurse performing procedure is insufficient to protect nurse or client; obtain additional assistance.

RECORDING AND REPORTING

1. Record in nurses' progress notes:	
a. Assessment finding for inserting an oral airway.	Documents respiratory status and need for intervention.
b. Size of oral airway.	Documents size for other care givers.
c. Placement.	Documents correct placement.

STEPS	RATIONALE
d. Other procedures performed at same time, especially positioning, secretions obtained.	Documents nursing care.
e. Client's tolerance of procedure.	Documents outcomes.

FOLLOW-UP ACTIVITIES

1. If client continually gags, remove oral airway and turn client on side. Attempt to replace with smaller sized oral airway.
2. If client continues to push oral airway out of mouth, this indicates that airway is not secured or that client is able to maintain patent airway without presence of artificial airway.
3. Assess need for airway.
4. Obtain additional assistance if unable to insert oral airway.
5. Remove oral airway at least one or two times daily; clean in warm soapy water, rinse thoroughly, and reinsert. Hydrogen peroxide and small brush can be used to remove crusted secretions. Wear gloves.
6. Administer mouth care every 2 to 4 hours.

• • • • •

Special Considerations

- Clients at greater risk for upper airway obstruction are infants, children, and adults with cold and flu, loss of consciousness, seizure disorders, neuromuscular diseases, increased oral secretions or excretions, facial trauma.
- If airway obstruction is not relieved and respiratory status is not improved or declines, obtain immediate assistance.
- Avoid causing trauma to gums or hard palate. Keep airway in midline. Client may cough initially. If this lasts more than few minutes or if client is gagging, airway may be too long. Try next smaller size. Some airways can be cut shorter; however, ends are usually rough. Cutting an oral airway is not recommended. Consider insertion of nasal airway if gagging or coughing continues.

Teaching Considerations

- Instruct family members in proper cleaning techniques. Observe their technique for adequacy.

Pediatric Considerations

- Oral airways are seldom utilized in the treatment of airway obstruction in children and infants. Due to the narrowness of a child's airway, oral airways are often more occlusive than beneficial.

SKILL 16-4 Using an Ambu-bag

"Ambu" stands for "air mask bag unit" (Fig. 16-3). Many health professionals think of an Ambu-bag as being used only in emergency situations such as cardiopulmonary arrest, but it has many other uses. The Ambu-bag is important in providing manual hyperinflation of the lungs prior to and following suctioning secretions from the respiratory tract. Its use is also necessary in the transportation of ventilator-dependent clients between hospital areas.

An Ambu-bag has the following components: a mask, an endotracheal or tracheostomy tube adapter, a large reservoir or "bag," an oxygen adapter and sometimes reservoir tubing to increase oxygen concentration, and a valve or spring system to control air flow. Bags are available in infant, child, and adult models to deliver inhaled volumes of 240 to 2000 ml per breath, depending on the manufacturer.

Ambu-bags are not difficult to use. The mask is firmly placed over the client's nose and mouth or is connected to the endotracheal or tracheostomy tube with the adapter.

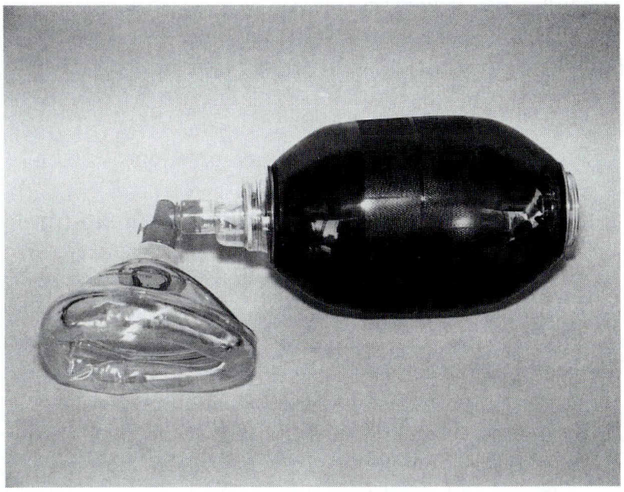

Fig. 16-3 Ambu-bag.

The reservoir is compressed with one or both hands, forcing air into the airways. Larger volumes are attained when using two hands. When the bag is released, it self-inflates, ready for the next breath. If necessary, the bag can deliver supplemental oxygen.

EQUIPMENT

- **Two nonsterile gloves**
- **Ambu-bag with mask for nonintubated client or Ambu-bag with ET or tracheal tube adapter for intubated clients**
- **Oxygen supply tubing and oxygen source, if needed**
- **Oral, nasotracheal, endotracheal, or tracheostomy suctioning apparatus**
- **Face shield, if indicated**

DELEGATION CONSIDERATIONS

The skilled use of an Ambu-bag requires problem solving skills and knowledge application unique to the professional nurse. For this skill delegation is inappropriate.

STEPS	RATIONALE
ASSESSMENT	
1. Identify need to use Ambu-bag manual ventilator. Signs and symptoms of need for manual ventilatory assistance include diminished respirations or pulse; apneic periods; cyanosis; acutely elevated $PaCO_2$; acutely decreased PaO_2, "bucking" or fighting mechanical ventilator; elevated intracranial pressure; thick, tenacious sputum; suctioning mucous plugs; cardiopulmonary arrest.	Certain conditions place client at risk for needing Ambu-bag manual ventilatory assistance.
2. Factors that affect respiratory drive include level of consciousness (LOC), neurological injury or central nervous system tumor, poor gas exchange (metabolic or respiratory alkalosis or acidosis), direct pulmonary injury, metabolic rate, psychosocial factors.	Nurse is able to accurately assess need to provide Ambu-bag manual ventilation.
3. In alert client, determine knowledge of procedure or determine care giver knowledge of procedure (for home administration).	Identifies learning needs and opportunity for teaching.

NURSING DIAGNOSIS

Clustering of defining characteristics from the assessment data may reveal the following nursing diagnoses for clients requiring this skill:

- ➤ Ineffective airway clearance
- ➤ Ineffective breathing pattern
- ➤ Impaired gas exchange
- ➤ Inability to sustain spontaneous ventilation

Related factors are individualized based on a client's condition or needs.

PLANNING

STEPS	RATIONALE
1. Expected outcomes following completion of procedure:	
➤ Improved vital signs and, when appropriate, intracranial pressure is decreased as evidenced by pressure waves and digital readout.	Ambu-bag manual ventilatory assistance was successful.
➤ Secretions are loosened and easier to remove as evidenced by improved respiratory rate, secretions or mucous plugs suctioned from large airways, clearing breath sounds, decrease in restlessness.	Ambu-bag manual ventilatory assistance was successful.
➤ Arterial blood gases are improved in cardiopulmonary arrest, during transportation, after seizures and apneic episodes.	Ambu-bag manual ventilatory assistance was successful.

STEPS	RATIONALE
2. Explain procedure and client's participation.	Encourages cooperation and minimizes risks.
3. Position client comfortably.	Promotes client comfort, prevents strain on nurse.
IMPLEMENTATION	
1. If not emergency situation (e.g., cardiopulmonary arrest), wash hands and apply gloves and face shield.	Reduces transmission of microorganisms.
2. Prepare suction apparatus, if needed.	Readies equipment for use.
3. Connect oxygen supply tubing to Ambu-bag and oxygen flowmeter. Adjust oxygen flowmeter to ordered F_IO_2 or 100% F_IO_2, if indicated.	Provides supplemental oxygen.
4. If client is intubated and normal saline lavage is ordered to facilitate secretion removal:	
a. Remove oxygen delivery device.	Prepares artificial airway for hyperinflation with Ambu-bag.
b. Instill 5 to 10 ml sterile normal saline during inspiration.	Normal saline stimulates cough, which loosens secretions.
c. Connect Ambu-bag to artificial airway and administer one breath every 3 to 5 seconds to hyperventilate by compressing Ambu-bag with two hands.	Increases PaO_2 and decreases $PaCO_2$ before suctioning.
d. Suction client. Repeat the preceding step as needed.	Removes secretions.
5. If client is unconscious and not intubated:	
a. Insert an oropharyngeal airway.	Helps maintain airway patency.
b. If not contraindicated, tilt the head using a chin lift maneuver.	Opens the airway, facilitates ventilation, and reduces the amount of air entering the client's stomach.
c. Place Ambu-bag mask over client's nose and mouth. Maintain head in a tilted position with the last two fingers of the nondominant hand. Apply pressure with remaining fingers and thumb to seal mask in place.	Correct placement of mask forms an occlusive seal for proper ventilation.
d. Compress the bag with the dominant hand. Administer breaths according to CPR protocol.	Avoids hypocapnia (low $PaCO_2$) and hypercapnia (elevated $PaCO_2$). Provides adequate ventilation.
CRITICAL DECISION POINT **If the chest fails to rise, reposition the mask, make a firm seal, and compress the bag again.**	
e. Be prepared to suction client as indicated. Client may need nasogastric tube insertion.	Pulmonary secretions may be loosened. Client may vomit if too much air is swallowed.
6. Assess client throughout procedure. Continue to "bag" client until assessment indicates it is no longer necessary, such as:	Provides supplemental ventilation and oxygenation. Assesses cardiopulmonary and neurological status.
a. Increased blood pressure; improved color, vital signs, and level of consciousness; decreased coughing.	
b. Presence of spontaneous respirations.	
c. Decreased intracranial pressure (ICP).	
7. Repeat Steps 4 through 6 as needed. Then remove bag and replace oxygen delivery device.	Restores supplemental oxygen.
8. Turn off oxygen flow to Ambu-bag. Disconnect bag from oxygen tubing, if indicated. Some institutions leave bag connected to oxygen source at all times.	Discontinues oxygen supply to bag.
9. Reposition client.	Promotes comfort.

STEPS	RATIONALE
10. Remove "elbow" that connects bag to ET tube, tracheostomy tube, or mask, if able, and wash in warm soapy water. Shake off excess water and allow to dry. (Use of a towel to dry may leave unwanted particles.) When dry, reconnect mask or elbow to Ambu-bag.	Reduces transmission of microorganisms.
11. Remove gloves and face shield and dispose of in proper receptacle. Wash hands.	Reduces transmission of microorganisms.

EVALUATION

1. Monitor vital signs, O_2 saturation, and other physiological parameters, and compare assessments before and after Ambu-bag use. Documents client's response to Ambu-bag procedure.	
2. Observe the amount, quality, and consistency of suctioned secretions.	
3. If instructing care givers, provide for return demonstration of technique.	Correctly performing technique independently is a reliable method to evaluate learning.

4. **Unexpected outcomes** that may occur include:
- ➤ Client becomes acidotic/hypercapnic:
  - Intubation and continuous ventilation needed.
  - Ventilator rate/tidal volume must be increased.
  - Client needs additional supplemental breathing.
- ➤ Client becomes alkalotic/hypocapnic:
  - Decrease volume/rate of bagging.

RECORDING AND REPORTING

1. Chart in nurses' progress notes: a. Assessments before and after bagging. b. Rate and volume of bagging. c. Amount of normal saline lavage, if used. d. Amount of supplemental oxygen used. e. Client's tolerance of procedure. f. Secretions suctioned (quality and quantity).	Documents cardiopulmonary status.

FOLLOW-UP ACTIVITIES

1. Inform physician of client's response to Ambu-bag ventilatory assistance.
2. Observe for rebound hypoventilation.

• • • • •

Special Considerations

- ➤ Clients at greater risk of needing Ambu-bag are those with pneumonia, seizure or sleep apnea disorders, multiple trauma, cardiopulmonary arrest, sudden infant death syndrome, drug overdose, neurological injury. Also at risk is ventilator-dependent client needing transportation to another hospital area.
- ➤ 15 mm Ambu-bag adapter must be obtained for most metal and silastic tracheostomy tubes. Lavage is most effective if cuff is inflated throughout procedure.

Teaching Considerations

- ➤ Demonstrate techniques of bagging to care givers. Allow time for practice on dummy or client. Assess for proper technique in administering procedure and cleaning equipment.

Pediatric Considerations

- ➤ Infant and pediatric Ambu-bags are designed to provide a tight seal and to deliver appropriate air volumes. Use of an adult bag for an infant or child is inappropriate.

Gerontologic Considerations

- ➤ For older clients who are edentulous a tight seal may be difficult to obtain and sustain. For such clients the use of two care givers, one to maintain a seal and a second to compress the bag, is desirable.

SKILL 16-5 Performing Cardiopulmonary Resuscitation

Cardiopulmonary arrest can occur at any time. It is characterized by an absence of pulse or respirations (respiratory arrest is the more common in children). If the nurse determines that the client has experienced cardiac arrest, CPR must be initiated. Cardiopulmonary resuscitation is a basic emergency procedure for life support, consisting of artificial respiration and manual external cardiac massage. Cardiopulmonary resuscitation has three main goals, called the ABCs of cardiopulmonary resuscitation: establish an *A*irway, initiate *B*reathing, and maintain *C*irculation. When an arrest occurs, oxygen is not delivered to the tissues, carbon dioxide is not transported from the tissues, tissue metabolism becomes anaerobic, and metabolic and respiratory acidosis occurs. Tissue damage, including permanent heart and brain damage, occurs within 6 minutes. In a respiratory arrest, cessation of respirations occurs; the pulse often remains present for up to approximately 6 minutes.

Once it is determined that a respiratory or cardiac arrest has occurred, the nurse must quickly provide a patent airway by removing any obvious foreign body obstruction (Skill 16-1), removing airway secretions (Chapter 14), inserting an oral airway (Skill 16-3), or hyperextending the neck as detailed in this skill.

The initiation of breathing is achieved by one of two methods. First, if immediately available, the nurse can use an Ambu-bag manual ventilator (Skill 16-4). Second, the nurse can initiate mouth-to-mouth artificial ventilation as described in this skill. Cardiopulmonary resuscitation barrier devices or pocket mouth-to-mouth ventilation masks are available to protect the nurse from the client's secretions during mouth-to-mouth breathing. These devices also promote more effective respirations by maintaining a better seal.

The maintenance of circulation is achieved by external cardiac compression. Three elements must be present to ensure safe and efficient cardiac massage. First, the client's spine must be supported during compression by placing the client on a hard surface such as a board or the floor. Second, sternal pressure must be forceful but not traumatic (Lewis, 1996). Third, to be safe and efficient, the nurse must have proper hand placement for compression.

EQUIPMENT

- **Ambu-bag, if available**
- **CPR pocket mask or barrier device, if available**
- **Chest compression board, if available**
- **Gloves, if available**
- **Resuscitation cart, if available**
- **Face shield, if available**

DELEGATION CONSIDERATIONS

The skill of cardiopulmonary resuscitation can be performed by assistive personnel.

- Caution the care provider to make certain the client is indeed pulseless before initiating chest compressions.
- Review the procedures for opening the airway if the client has any risk for cervical neck trauma.
- Caution the provider regarding the differences between infants, children, and adults.

STEPS	RATIONALE
ASSESSMENT	
1. Determine if client is unconscious by shaking client and shouting "Are you OK?"	Confirms that client is unconscious as opposed to intoxicated, sleeping, or hearing impaired.
2. Activate emergency medical services.	The majority of adult victims are in ventricular fibrillation and need defibrillation and antiarrhythmic drugs as soon as possible.
3. Determine breathlessness and carotid or brachial (use with infants) pulse.	Presence of pulse and respirations contraindicates initiation of CPR.

NURSING DIAGNOSIS

Clustering of defining characteristics from the assessment data may reveal the following nursing diagnoses for clients requiring this skill:

- ➤ Ineffective breathing pattern
- ➤ Decreased cardiac output
- ➤ Impaired gas exchange
- ➤ Inability to sustain spontaneous ventilation

Related factors are individualized based on a client's condition or needs.

STEPS	RATIONALE
PLANNING	
1. Call for assistance, seek help from passersby, call for additional nurses.	One person cannot maintain CPR indefinitely. Without relief, rescuer fatigues, chest compressions are ineffective, and volume of air ventilated into victim's lungs decreases.
2. **Expected outcomes** following completion of procedure:	
➤ Client regains pulse and respirations.	CPR was successful.
• Physician may terminate CPR in event of irreversible brain or cardiac damage or may have knowledge of advance directive.	
IMPLEMENTATION	
1. Place victim on hard surface such as floor, ground, or backboard. Victim must be flat. If necessary, logroll victim to flat, supine position using spine precautions.	External compression of heart is facilitated. Heart is compressed between sternum and spinal vertebrae, which must be on a hard and firm surface.
2. Assume correct and comfortable position.	Nurse may be administering CPR for extended period, particularly in community setting. Correct, comfortable position decreases skeletal muscle fatigue and promotes more effective compressions.
a. One-Person Rescuer:	
(1) Position to face victim, on knees, parallel to victim's sternum.	Allows rescuer to quickly move back and forth from victim's mouth to sternum.
b. Two-Person Rescuer:	
(1) One person faces victim, kneeling parallel to victim's head. Second person moves to opposite side and faces victim, kneels parallel to victim's sternum.	Allows one rescuer to maintain breathing while other maintains circulation, without getting in each other's way.
3. If available, apply gloves and face shield.	Reduces transmission of microorganisms.
4. Open airway:	
a. If no head or neck trauma, use *head tilt–chin lift* method (AHA, 1994) (see illustration).	The tongue is the most common cause of airway obstruction in the unconscious client. Airway obstruction from tongue is relieved. If necessary, remove foreign body (see Skill 16-1).
b. Jaw thrust maneuver (see illustration) can be used by health professionals but is not taught to general public. Grasp angles of victim's lower jaw and lift with both hands, displacing the mandible forward while tilting the head backward.	When head and/or neck trauma is suspected, this maneuver opens the airway while maintaining proper head and neck alignment, thus reducing the risk of further damage to the neck.

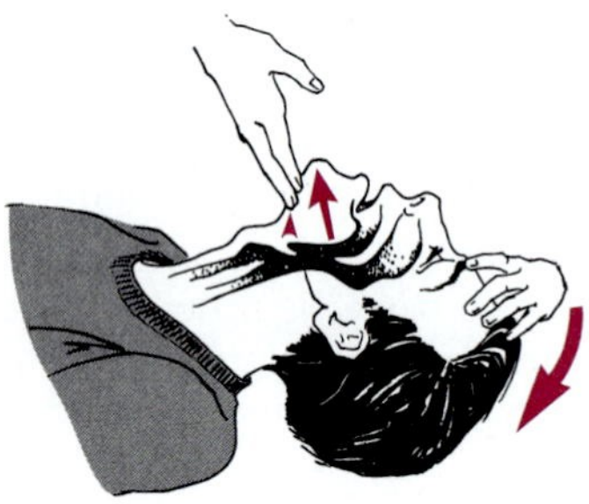

Step 4a

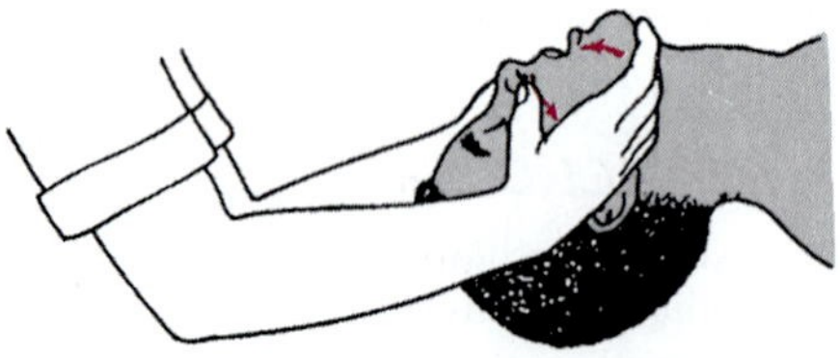

Step 4b

STEPS	RATIONALE
5. If readily available insert oral airway (Skill 16-3).	Maintains tongue on anterior floor of mouth and prevents obstruction of posterior airway by tongue.
6. If the victim does not resume breathing, administer artificial respiration:	Airtight seal is formed and air is prevented from escaping through nose.

a. MOUTH-TO-MOUTH:

Adult:

(1) Pinch victim's nose with the thumb and index fingers and occlude mouth with nurse's mouth or use CPR pocket mask. Maintain head tilt, chin lift while administering breaths so air enters lungs and not stomach. Blow two slow full breaths into victim's mouth (each breath should take 0.5 to 2 seconds); allow victim to exhale between breaths. Continue giving 12 breaths per minute (AHA, 1994).

Rationale: Hyperventilation is promoted and assists in maintaining adequate blood oxygen levels. In most adults this volume is 800 to 1200 ml and is sufficient to make the chest rise.

CRITICAL DECISION POINT **An excess of air volume and fast inspiratory flow rates are likely to cause pharyngeal pressures that exceed esophageal opening pressures, allowing air to enter the stomach and result in gastric distention, thereby increasing the risk of vomiting and compromised respiration.**

Child:

Place nurse's mouth over child's mouth (see illustration) or use CPR pocket mask. For mouth-to-mouth resuscitation of child, administer two slow breaths lasting 1 to 1½ seconds with a pause between. Continue giving 20 breaths per minute (AHA, 1994).

Rationale: Airtight seal is formed and air is prevented from escaping from nose.

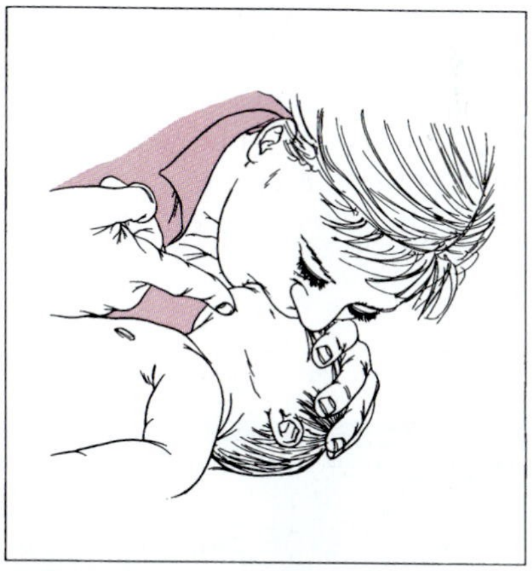

Step 6a Mouth to mouth and nose seal. (From Textbook for Healthcare Providers, 1994, American Heart Association, Dallas.)

Infant:

(1) Because an infant's air passages are smaller and resistance to flow is quite high, making recommendations about the force or volume of the rescue breaths is difficult. Place nurse's mouth over infants's nose and mouth. However, three factors should be remembered: (1) rescue breaths are the single most important maneuver in assisting a nonbreathing child, (2) an appropriate volume is one that makes the chest rise and fall, and (3) slow breaths provide an adequate volume at the lowest possible pressure, thereby reducing the risk of gastric distention.

b. MOUTH-TO-NOSE:

Keep the victim's head tilted with one hand on the forehead. Use the other hand to lift the jaw and close the mouth. Seal rescuer's lips around the victim's nose and blow. Allow passive exhalation.

Rationale: In some victims (those whose mouth cannot be opened or whose jaws or mouth is seriously injured) mouth to nose can be a more effective method of ventilation.

STEPS	RATIONALE
CRITICAL DECISION POINT It may be necessary to open the victim's mouth on occasion to allow trapped exhaled air to escape.	
c. **AMBU-BAG: Adult and Child:**	
(1) For Ambu-bag resuscitation use proper size face mask and apply it under chin, up and over victim's mouth and nose (see illustration).	Airtight seal is formed; as bag is compressed, oxygen enters client.
(2) Observe for rise and fall of chest wall with each respiration (see illustration). Listen for air escaping during exhalation and feel for flow of air. If lungs do not inflate, reposition head and neck and check for visible airway obstruction, such as vomitus.	Repositioning ensures airway is properly opened and that artificial respirations are entering lungs.
7. Suction secretions if necessary or turn victim's head to one side, unless contraindicated.	Suctioning prevents airway obstruction. Turning client's head to one side allows gravity to drain secretions.
8. Check for presence of carotid (adults) or brachial (infants) pulse after restoring breathing.	Carotid artery pulse is the most easily accessible and persists when other peripheral pulses are no longer palpable.

CRITICAL DECISION POINT Make certain the assessment is long enough to thoroughly assess absence of pulse. Following respiratory arrest the pulse may be very slow and weak.

CRITICAL DECISION POINT Performing external cardiac compressions on a victim who has a pulse may result in serious medical complications.

CRITICAL DECISION POINT In the nonintubated victim in an acute care setting it may be possible to utilize two rescue breathers with the Ambu-bag. In this case one rescuer maintains the seal, and the other utilizes two hands to compress the bag, thus delivering greater volumes.

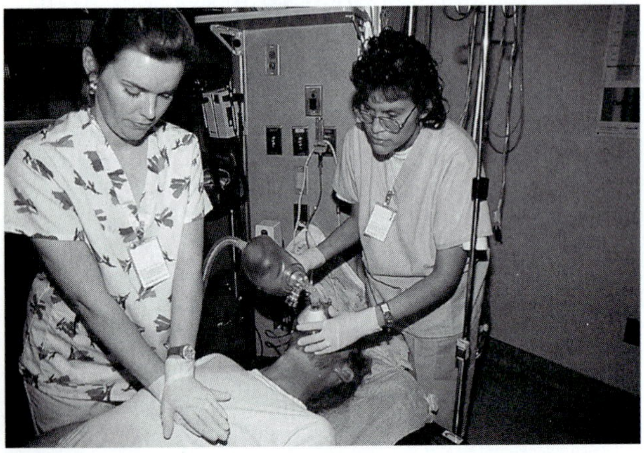

Step 6c(1)

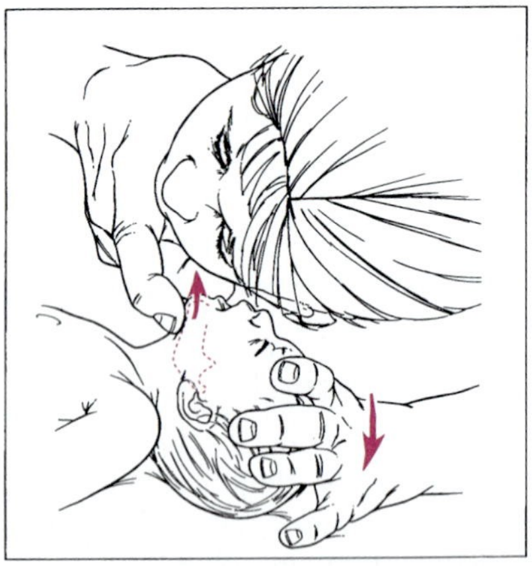

Step 6c(2) (From Textbook of Basic Life Support for Healthcare Providers, 1994, American Heart Association, Dallas.)

STEPS	RATIONALE

9. If pulse is absent, initiate chest compressions:

a. Assume correct hand position:

Places hands and fingers over heart in proper position. Prevents xiphoid process and rib fracture, which can further compromise cardiopulmonary status.

Adult:

(1) Place hands 1 to 2 cm above xiphoid process on sternum. Keep hands parallel to chest and fingers above chest. Interlocking fingers is helpful. Keep fingers off of the chest wall. Extend arms and lock elbows. Maintain arms straight and shoulders directly over victim's sternum (see illustration).

CRITICAL DECISION POINT **It is critical to keep the hands off of the xiphoid process by marking that area with two fingers of one hand and then placing the heel of the other hand next to them. The hand marking the xiphoid process can then be moved and placed on top of the other hand.**

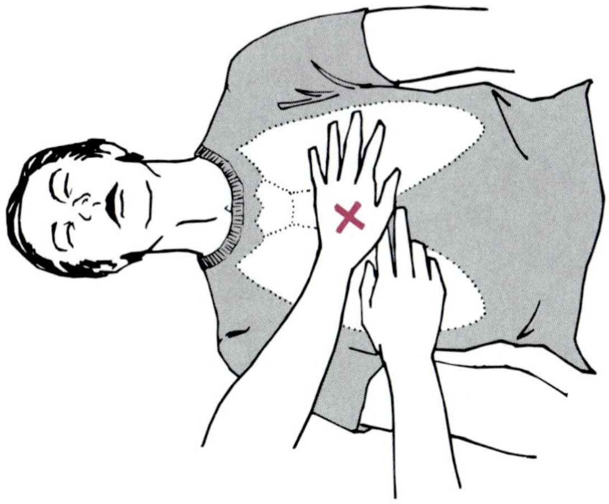

Step 9a(1) Adult.

Child:

(1) Place heel of one hand 1 to 2 cm above xiphoid process (see illustration). Maintain head tilt with other hand, if possible, to maintain patent airway.

Infant:

(1) Place index and middle fingers of one hand on sternum above xiphoid process. Fingers should be 1 cm below nipple line and perpendicular to sternum and not slanted (see illustration).

CRITICAL DECISION POINT **Ensure fingers are off the ribs.**

b. Compress sternum to proper depth from shoulders and then release pressure, maintaining contact with skin to ensure ongoing proper placement of hands. Do not rock, but transmit weight vertically down.

Compression occurs only on sternum and is meant to squeeze the heart between the sternum and spine. Pressure necessary for external compression is created by nurse's upper arm muscle strength and upper body. When the compression is released, the heart fills.

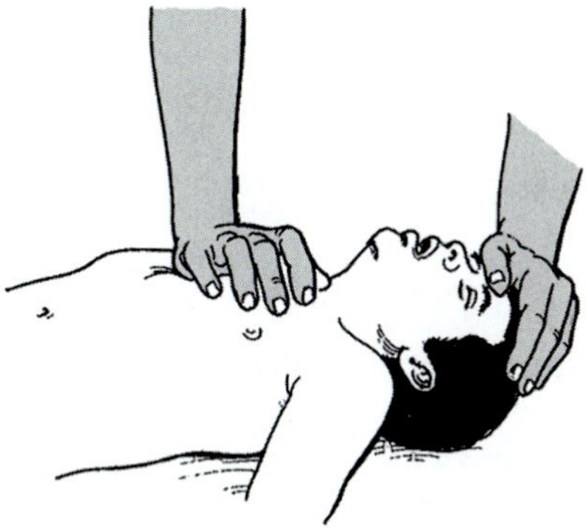

Step 9a(1a) Child.

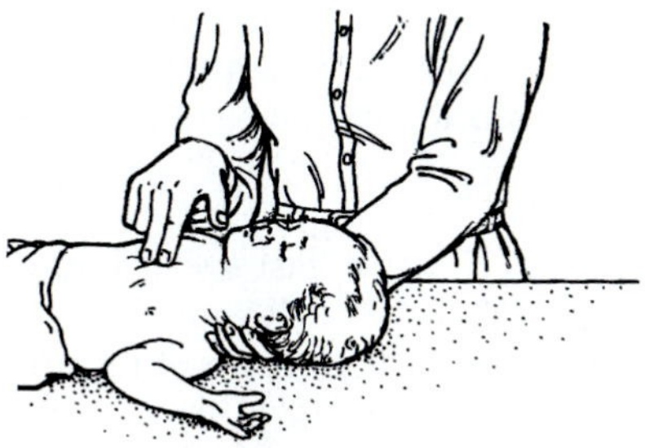

Step 9a(1b) Infant.

STEPS	RATIONALE
(1) *Adult and adolescent:* 4 to 5 cm (1½ to 2 inches) (see illustration). (2) *Older child:* 3 to 4 cm (1 to 1½ inches). (3) *Toddler and preschooler:* 2 to 4 cm (¾ to 1½ inches). (4) *Infant:* 1 to 2 cm (½ to 1 inch).	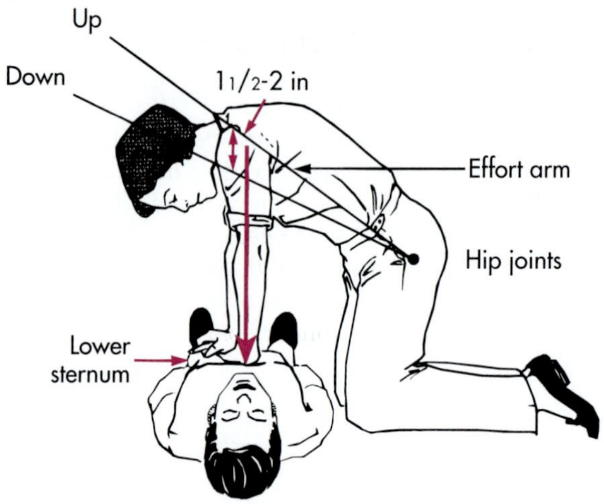*Step 9b (1)* Compression occurs only on sternum. Pressure necessary for external compressin is created by nurse's upper arm muscle strength.
c. Maintain proper rate of compression: (1) Adult and adolescent: 80 to 100 per minute (count "one 1000; two 1000"). (2) Older child: 100 per minute. (3) Child: 100 per minute. (4) Infant: at least 100 per minute.	Proper number of compressions per minute should be delivered to ensure adequate cardiac output.

CRITICAL DECISION POINT **Ratio of compressions to breaths for two rescuers is 5 to 1; for one rescuer, the ratio is 15 to 2.**

d. Continue mouth-to-mouth or Ambu-bag ventilations. (1) Adult and adolescent: every 5 seconds (12 per minute). (2) Older child: every 4 seconds (15 per minute). (3) Child: every 3 seconds (20 per minute). (4) Infant and toddler: every 3 seconds (20 per minute).	Promotes adequate ventilations to excrete waste gas and supply oxygen.
10. Palpate for carotid or brachial pulse with each external chest compression for first full minute (2 person rescue). If carotid pulse is not palpable, compressions are not strong enough or hand position is incorrect.	Assessment of pulse validates that adequate stroke volume is achieved with each compression.
11. Continue CPR until relieved, until victim regains spontaneous pulse and respirations, until the rescuer is exhausted and unable to perform CPR effectively, or until physician discontinues CPR.	Artificial cardiopulmonary function is maintained.
12. Remove and discard into appropriate receptacle: gloves, face shield, and pocket mask.	Reduces transmission of microorganisms.

EVALUATION

1. Palpate carotid pulse at least every 5 minutes after first minute of CPR.	Documents adequacy of external cardiac compressions.
2. Observe for spontaneous return of respirations or heart rate.	Performance of CPR on a client with a pulse is dangerous.
3. Cardiopulmonary resuscitation is not interrupted for more than 5 seconds.	Maintains adequacy of oxygenation and circulation.

STEPS	RATIONALE
4. **Unexpected outcomes** that may occur include:	
➤ Client develops skeletal injury such as fractured ribs or sternum, or internal organ injury such as lacerated lung or liver.	Improper technique causes injury or client is predisposed to injury secondary to aging or medical problems, such as osteoporosis.
➤ Rescuer is unassisted, tires, and is unable to continue.	CPR is ineffective.

Recording and Reporting

1. Immediately report arrest indicating exact location of victim. a. In hospital setting, follow hospital policy. b. In community setting, dial 911 or other emergency number.	Obtains immediate expert assistance for victim.
2. Record in nurses' notes onset of arrest, medication given, procedures performed, and victim's response.	Documents medical care delivered.

Follow-up Activities

1. Notify victim's family and provide support:
   a. Contact chaplain services.
   b. Contact social worker.
2. Reassure successfully resuscitated victim:
   a. Educate regarding presence of any equipment.
   b. Help client work through fears of rearrest.
3. Complete postmortem care on victims for whom CPR was unsuccessful (Chapter 45).

• • • • •

Special Considerations

- Oral airways are readily available in hospital and extended care and outpatient settings. Cardiopulmonary resuscitation pocket masks with one-way valves are available as required by OSHA guidelines (Occupational Health and Safety Act, 1992). However, they are not available in all community settings. *Cardiopulmonary resuscitation can effectively be accomplished without an oral airway or CPR pocket mask.* However, the rescuer must take appropriate measures to reduce the transmission of infectious agents (e.g., hepatitis B, HIV, herpes virus, tuberculosis) as proposed by the Centers for Disease Control and Prevention (1989).
- Spinal cord injury should be suspected with motor vehicle accident, falls, face or head injury or laceration, diving accident, or football or other contact sports injury.
- Unconsciousness can be caused by substance abuse, hypoglycemia, ketoacidosis, shock. If unconscious person has adequate respirations and pulse, remain until further assistance is present. Place the victim in the recovery position. Continue to determine presence of pulse and respiration because respiratory or cardiopulmonary arrest is still possible.
- "Code status" should be determined on clients by the physician and documented in the client record. The rule in most institutions is to "code" all clients unless ordered otherwise.
- Lay learners are taught one-person CPR. With one-person CPR the ratio of compressions to ventilations in infants and children up to 8 years is 5:1; 8 years to adult, 15:2.
- Cricoid pressure can be used by health professionals to prevent regurgitation. With excessive pressures, the trachea can collapse, leading to airway obstruction.
- Pupillary responses do not consistently reflect effectiveness of CPR and client's condition.
- Cardiopulmonary resuscitation is interrupted when changing CPR personnel, during defibrillation, or when transporting the victim. During intubation, CPR may be interrupted for more than 5 seconds but should not exceed 30 seconds. Nurse should remind rescue team of number of seconds elapsing during intubation.

Teaching Considerations

- If a client is at risk for cardiopulmonary arrest, the family or care givers should be instructed and certified in CPR by certified instructor from the institution, the American Red Cross, or the American Heart Association.
- The client and family should keep emergency numbers taped to the phone. These numbers may

include fire department, ambulance, hospital, and physician. Instruct client and family whom to call. The family may also need to know what to do when a client is found "deceased."

- It is extremely helpful if the family has a list of medications the client is presently taking.

Pediatric Considerations

- All persons involved in administering CPR must understand the different breathing/compression ratios, hand (fingers) placement and depth of compression in children and infants as compared to adults.
- Infants and children experience only respiratory arrest much more frequently than full cardiopulmonary arrest.

Gerontologic Considerations

- In the older adult compressions often result in rib or cartilage fractures. Cardiopulmonary resuscitation should be continued.

Home Care Considerations

- In the community setting, instruct someone to call for emergency medical service. Dial 0 or 911, depending on community resources. Tell operator or dispatcher exact location of victim; in hospital setting, instruct someone to call a CODE by following agency procedure. Do not hang up (enhanced 911 can find location).
- Soft surface such as mattress, car seat, or grassy surface decreases efficiency of external cardiac compressions.

CRITICAL THINKING EXERCISES

1. While using an Ambu-bag on a client, you observe that it is getting more difficult to blow air into the client's lungs. What could be wrong? What assessments should be made?
2. You are the first person on the scene of a choking victim. The individual runs to the rest room. What should be your response?
3. The nasal airway was not secured. It is accidentally pushed down into the client's nasal passage during suctioning. What should you do?
4. How would you modify CPR or FBAOM for a pregnant client?
5. You are performing CPR in an isolated location; help is unavailable. How long should you continue CPR?

REFERENCES

American Heart Association, Basic Life Support for Healthcare Providers, Dallas, 1994, American Heart Association.

Centers for Disease Control: Guidelines for prevention of transmission of human immunodeficiency virus and hepatitis B virus to health-care and public safety workers, *MMWR* 38(suppl 6):1, 1989.

Elkin MK, Perry AG, Potter PA: Nursing interventions & clinical skills. St Louis, 1996, Mosby.

Lewis SM, Collier IC, Heitkemper MM: *Medical-surgical nursing,* ed 4, St Louis, 1996, Mosby.

Occupational Health and Safety Act, 1992 *Occupational exposure to blood borne pathogens,* OSHA 3127, 1992.

Wong DL: *Whaley and Wong's Nursing care of infants and children,* ed 4, St Louis, 1995, Mosby.

ADDITIONAL READING

Bishop M: Practice guidelines for airway care during resuscitation, *Resp Care* 40(4):393, 1995.

Brandon D, Johannigman JA: Ventilatory support during cardiopulmonary resuscitation, *Resp Care* 40(5):479, 1995.

Derkay CS, Lefebvree SM, George MR: Retrieving foreign bodies from upper aerodigestive tracts of children, *AORN* 60(1):53, 1994.

Kain ZN, O'Connor TZ, Berde CB: Management of tracheobronchial and esophageal foreign bodies in children: A survey study, *J Clin Anesthes* 6(1,2):28, 1994.

Kharasch M, Graff J: Emergency management of the airway, *Crit Care Clin* 11(1), 1995.

Lurie K: Active compression-decompression CPR: a progress report, *Resuscitation* 28:115, 1994.

McConnell E: Clinical do's & don'ts: Inserting an oropharyngeal airway properly: *Nursing 94* (12):20, 1994.

Pardee D: Basic life support and advanced cardiac life support changes, *Prog Cardiovasc Nurs* 8(2):3, 1993.

Sanders AB: The development of AHA guidelines for emergency cardiac care, *Resp Care* 40(4):338, 1995.

Sheehy S, Jimmerson C: *Manual of clinical trauma care* ed 2, St Louis, 1994, Mosby.

Tietjen PA, Kaner RJ, Quinn CE: Aspiration emergencies, *Resp Emer* 15(1):117, 1994.

Willens JS: Strengthen your life-support skills, *Nursing 93* (4):54, 1993.

Wong MJ, Lenihan KM: Advances in cardiopulmonary resuscitation, *Crit Care Nurs Clin N Amer* 7(2):227, 1995.

UNIT VI

Medications

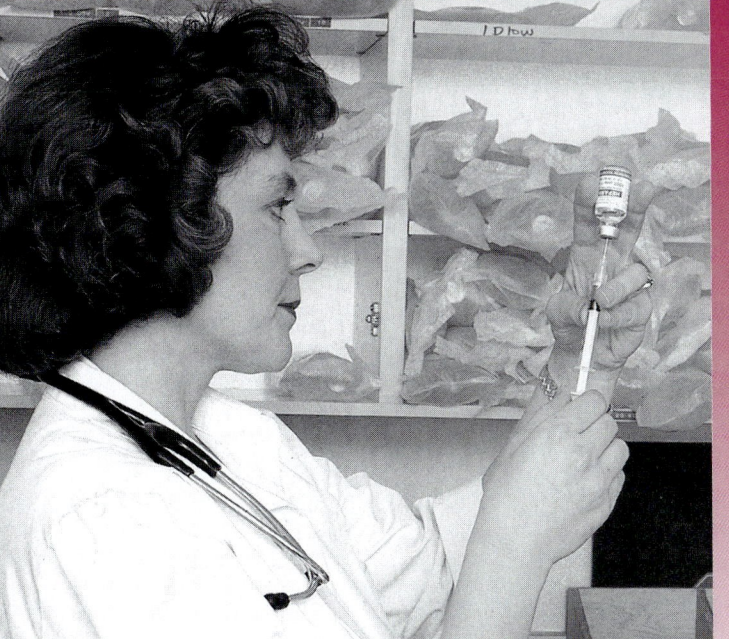

CHAPTER 17

Preparing for Medication Administration

OBJECTIVES

Mastery of content in this chapter will enable the nurse to:

- Define key terms.
- Identify guidelines for safe administration of medications.
- Identify aseptic techniques used in preparing and administering oral medications.
- Discuss common types of drug actions.
- Identify the system of measurement for a given prescribed drug.
- Calculate drug dosages using the fractional equation method.
- Describe two methods for delivering medications to the nursing unit.
- Describe the five rights of drug administration.

KEY TERMS

Anaphylaxis
Aspiration
Compliance
Drug dependence
Drug plateau
Duration of action
Enteric coated
Floor stock
Idiosyncratic reaction
NPO
Onset of action
Over-the-counter drug
Peak action
Plateau
Side effect
Synergistic reaction
Telephone order
Unit dose system
Verbal order

Safe and accurate administration of medications is one of the nurse's most important responsibilities when caring for clients. The nurse's judgment is critical for safe drug administration. The nurse must understand a drug's action and side effects, administer it correctly, and monitor the client's response to the drug.

DRUG FORMS

Drugs are available in a variety of forms or preparations. The form of the drug determines its route of administration. The composition of a drug is designed to enhance its absorption and metabolism within the body. Drugs are available in several forms (Table 17-1) such as solid, liquid, and powder.

DRUG ACTIONS

When administering medications the nurse should be aware that a drug, because of its chemical makeup and physiological action, can produce more than one effect.

Therapeutic Effects

The therapeutic effect is the intended or predicted physiological response a drug causes. Each drug has a desired

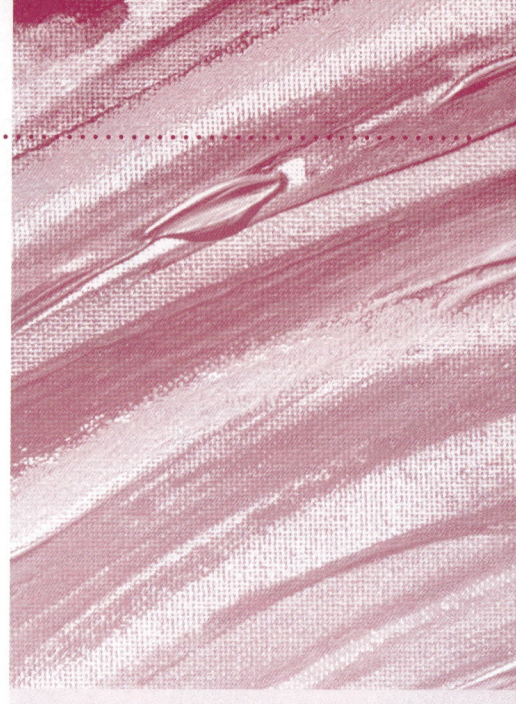

Table 17-1 Forms of Medication by Route of Administration

Medication Forms Commonly Prepared for Administration by Oral Route	
Solid forms	
Capsules	Medication encased in a gelatin shell
Tablets	Powdered medication compressed into hard disk or cylinders
Liquid forms	
Elixir	Clear fluid containing water and alcohol
Extract	Concentrated drug form made by removing the active portion of a drug from its other components
Solution	One or more substances dissolved in water
Suspension	Finely dissolved particles in a liquid medium
Syrup	Medication dissolved in a concentrated sugar solution
Other oral forms and terms associated with oral preparations	
Troche (lozenge)	Medication that dissolves in mouth, not meant for ingestion
Aerosol	Aqueous medication sprayed and absorbed in the mouth and upper airway, not meant for ingestion
Enteric coated	Tablet that is coated so that it does not dissolve in stomach, meant for intestinal absorption
Sustained release	Tablet or capsule that contains small particles of a drug coated with material that requires a varying amount of time to dissolve
Medication forms commonly prepared for administration by topical route	
Aqueous	One or more substances dissolved in water
Creams	Nongreasy, semisolid preparation
Liniment	Oily liquid
Lotion	Emollient liquid that can be clear solution, suspension, or emulsion
Paste	Medication preparation that is thick and has poor skin penetration
Transdermal patch	Disk or patch embedded with a drug that is absorbed through the skin over a designated period of time
Medication forms commonly prepared for administration by parenteral route	
Solution	Preparation that contains water with one or more dissolved compounds; the solution must be sterile
Powder	Particles of drug that are reconstituted with water, dissolved and administered parenterally; the solution must be sterile
Medication forms commonly prepared for instillation into body cavities	
Suppository	Drugs mixed with gelatin and shaped for insertion into a body cavity. The drug is meant to dissolve releasing the drug
Intraocular disk	Disk (similar to a contact lens) embedded with a drug that is inserted into the client's eye. The drug is absorbed over a designated period of time.

or therapeutic effect for which it is prescribed. For example, the nurse administers codeine phosphate to relieve a client's pain. A single medication may have many therapeutic effects. For example, aspirin creates analgesia and reduces inflammation of arthritis.

Side Effects

Predictably, a drug causes unintended secondary effects. **Side effects** may be harmless or injurious. In the example of codeine phosphate, a client may experience constipation. If the side effects are serious enough to outweigh the beneficial effects of a drug's therapeutic action, the prescriber may discontinue the drug. Clients may stop taking medications because of side effects.

Toxic Effects. After prolonged intake of high doses of medication, ingestion of drugs intended for external application, or when a drug accumulates in the blood because of impaired metabolism or excretion, a toxic effect may develop. Toxic effects may be lethal, depending on the drug's action. For example, morphine, a narcotic analgesic, relieves pain by depressing the central nervous system. However, toxic levels of morphine cause severe respiratory depression and death.

Idiosyncratic Reactions. Medications may cause unpredictable effects, such as an **idiosyncratic reaction** in which a client overreacts or underreacts to a drug or has a reaction different from normal. Predicting which clients will have an idiosyncratic response is impossible. For example, *Ativan*, an antianxiety medication when given to the older adult may cause agitation and delirium.

Allergic Reactions. Allergic reaction is another unpredictable response to a drug. Exposure to an initial dose of a medication may cause an immunological response.

Table 17-2 Mild Allergic Reactions

Symptom	Description
Urticaria (hives)	Raised, irregularly shaped skin eruptions with varying sizes and shapes; eruptions have reddened margins and pale centers.
Eczema (rash)	Small, raised vesicles that are usually reddened; often distributed over the entire body.
Pruritus	Itching of the skin; accompanies most rashes.
Rhinitis	Inflammation of mucous membranes lining the nose, causing swelling and a clear watery discharge.
Wheezing	Constriction of smooth muscles surrounding bronchioles that decreases diameter of airways; occurs primarily on inspiration because of severely narrowed airways; development of edema in pharynx and larynx further obstructs airflow.

The drug acts as an antigen, which causes antibodies to be produced. With repeated administration the client develops an allergic response to the drug, its chemical preservatives, or a metabolite of it.

An allergic reaction may be mild or severe. Allergic symptoms vary, depending on the client and the drug. Among the different classes of drugs, antibiotics cause a high incidence of allergic reactions. Common, mild allergy symptoms are summarized in Table 17-2. Severe or **anaphylactic** reactions are characterized by sudden constriction of bronchiolar muscles, edema of the pharynx and larynx, and severe wheezing and shortness of breath. The client may become severely hypotensive, necessitating emergency resuscitation measures.

It is common practice for clients who are hospitalized and have a known drug allergy to have this information recorded in a clearly identifiable place so that it is easily seen by all those involved in the client's care. In many institutions this information is often recorded on the front of the client's medical record on an eye-catching sticker. Client allergies should always be recorded on the client's medication administration record. Clients cared for in other settings (e.g., home) and who have a known history of an allergy to a medication should be encouraged to wear an identification bracelet or medal, which alerts all health care providers to the allergies in case the client is unconscious when receiving medical care.

Drug Tolerance and Dependence

Drug tolerance occurs when clients receive the same drug for long periods of time and require higher doses to produce the same effect. Clients who are taking various pain medications may develop tolerance over time.

Generally, clients hospitalized for acute episodes of illness do not develop tolerance. It may take a month or even longer for this phenomenon to occur (McCaffery and Ferrell, 1994). Drug tolerance is not the same as drug dependence. Two types of **drug dependence** exist: psychological (or addiction) and physical. In psychological dependence the client desires the medication for some benefit other than the intended effect. Physical dependence implies that a client will suffer some ill effect if the medication is not given. When clients receive medications for a short term (such as for postoperative pain), dependence is rare (McCaffery and Ferrell, 1994).

Drug Interactions

When one drug modifies the action of another drug, a drug interaction occurs. Drug interactions are common in individuals taking many medications. A drug may potentiate or diminish the action of other drugs and may alter the way in which another drug is absorbed, metabolized, or eliminated from the body.

When two drugs are given simultaneously, they can have a synergistic or additive effect. With a **synergistic reaction** the physiological action of the two drugs in combination is greater than the effect of the drugs when given separately. Alcohol is a central nervous system depressant that has a synergistic effect on antihistamines, antidepressants, and narcotic analgesics.

A drug interaction is not always undesirable. Often a physician orders combination drug therapy to create a drug interaction for therapeutic benefit. For example, a client with moderate hypertension typically receives several drugs, such as diuretics and vasodilators, that act together to keep blood pressure at a desirable level.

Drug Dose Responses

After the nurse administers a drug, it undergoes absorption, distribution, metabolism, and excretion. These processes determine how much of the administered dose reaches the site of action. These processes are influenced by many things such as body surface area, body water content, body fat content, and protein stores.

When certain medications such as antibiotics are prescribed, the goal is to achieve a constant drug blood level within a safe therapeutic range. The client and nurse must follow regular dosage schedules and administer prescribed doses at correct intervals. Knowledge of the following time intervals of drug action also helps to anticipate a drug's effect:

1. **Onset of drug action**—Period of time it takes after a drug is administered for it to produce a response.
2. **Peak action**—Time it takes for a drug to reach its highest effective concentration.
3. **Duration of action**—Length of time during which the drug is present in a concentration great enough to produce a response.
4. **Plateau**—Blood serum concentration reached and maintained after repeated, fixed doses.

Table 17-3 Factors Influencing Choice of Administration Routes

Route	Disadvantages/Contraindications
Oral, buccal, sublingual	
Easy and comfortable to administer, economical, may produce local or systemic effects.	Avoid giving to clients with alterations in gastrointestinal function (e.g., nausea and vomiting), reduced motility (after general anesthesia or inflammation of bowel), and surgical resection of portion of gastrointestinal tract. Some drugs are destroyed by gastric secretions. Oral administration is contraindicated in clients unable to swallow (e.g., clients with neuromuscular disorders, esophageal strictures, and lesions of the mouth). Oral medications cannot be given when client has gastric suction and are contraindicated in clients before some tests or surgery. An unconscious or confused client may be unable or unwilling to swallow or hold medication under the tongue. Oral medications may irritate the lining of the gastrointestinal tract, discolor teeth, or have an unpleasant taste.
SQ, IM, IV, intradermal routes	
Routes provide means of administration when oral drugs are contraindicated. More rapid absorption occurs than with topical or oral routes. IV infusion provides drug delivery when client is critically ill. If peripheral perfusion is poor, IV route is preferred over injections.	Risk of introducing infection, drugs are expensive, and these routes are avoided in clients with bleeding tendencies. Risk of tissue damage with SQ injections. IM and IV routes are dangerous because of rapid absorption. These routes cause considerable anxiety in many clients, especially children.
Skin	
Topical	
Topical skin applications provide primarily local effect. Route is painless. Limited side effects occur.	Extensive applications may be bulky and cause difficulty in maneuvering. Clients with skin abrasions are at risk for rapid drug absorption and systemic effects.
Transdermal	
Transdermal applications provide prolonged systemic effects, with limited side effects.	Application leaves oily or pasty substance on skin and may soil clothing.
Mucous membranes*	
Therapeutic effects are provided by local application to involved sites. Aqueous solutions are readily absorbed and capable of causing systemic effects. Mucous membranes provide route of administration when oral drugs are contraindicated.	Mucous membranes are highly sensitive to some drug concentrations. Insertion of rectal and vaginal medication often causes embarrassment. Rectal suppositories are contraindicated if clients have had rectal surgery or if active rectal bleeding is present.
Inhalation	
Inhalation provides rapid relief for local respiratory problems. Route provides easy access for introduction of general anesthetic gases.	Some local agents can cause serious systemic effects.
Intraocular Disk	
Route is advantageous in that it does not require frequent administration like eyedrops. The client can also wear disk when sleeping or swimming. Dry eyes do not affect drug delivery.	Local reactions can occur such as tearing, itchiness, or redness of the eye. Client must be taught how to insert disk into and remove from the eye. Client may be anxious about doing this. Medication can be expensive. Medication is contraindicated in clients with infections of the eye.

*Includes eyes, ears, nose, and vaginal, rectal, buccal, and sublingual routes.

Routes of Administration

The route chosen for administering a drug depends on its properties and desired effect and on the client's physical and mental condition. The nurse is often the best person to judge the route most desirable for a client. Table 17-3 summarizes the routes of drug administration and the factors influencing the choice of those routes.

SYSTEMS OF DRUG MEASUREMENT

The proper administration of medication depends on the nurse's ability to compute drug dosages accurately and measure medications correctly. A careless mistake in placing a decimal point or adding a zero to a dosage can lead to a fatal error. The prescriber and client depend on the nurse to check the dosage before administering a drug. The most common system used in the measurement of medications is the metric system. The apothecary and household systems can also be used.

Metric System

As a decimal system, the metric system is the most logically organized of the measurement systems. Metric units can be easily converted and computed through simple multiplication and division. Each basic unit of measure is organized into units of 10. Multiplying or dividing by 10 forms secondary units. In multiplication, the decimal point moves to the right; in division, the decimal moves to the left.

The basic units of measure in the metric system are the meter (length), the liter (volume), and the gram (weight). For drug calculations the nurse uses primarily volume and weight units. In the metric system small or large letters are used to designate the basic units:

Gram = g or Gm
Liter = l or L

Small letters are abbreviations for subdivisions of major units:

Milligram = mg
Milliliter = ml

A system of Latin prefixes designates subdivision of the basic units: deci- (1/10 or 0.1), centi- (1/100 or 0.01), and milli- (1/1000 or 0.001). Greek prefixes designate multiples of the basic units: deka- (10), hecto- (100), and kilo- (1000). When writing drug dosages in metric units, physicians and nurses use either fractions or multiples of a unit. Fractions are always in decimal form, and a zero is always placed in front of the decimal to prevent error.

Apothecary System

The apothecary system of measurement is familiar to most people in the United States. The standards for measurement can be easily seen in the home: milk is bottled in pints and quarts, a yardstick has inches and feet, and a bathroom scale weighs in pounds.

Very few, if any, liquid or solid drug dosages are ordered in the apothecary system today. Use of the apothecary system increases the risk of administration errors. Conversion errors can occur because small letters or symbols are used in this system. These symbols for measurement units can be confused with whole numbers. For example; 1℥ can be confused with the number 13, the apothecary "gr" symbol for grain can be confused with the metric system symbol "g" for gram.

Household Measurements

Household measures are familiar to most people and are used when more accurate systems of measure are unnecessary. Included in household measures are drops, teaspoons, tablespoons, cups, and glasses for volume; and ounces and pounds for weight. Although pints and quarts are considered household measures, they are used in the apothecary system.

PREPARING FOR MEDICATION ADMINISTRATION

Prior to the actual administration of medication, the nurse may need to carry out several steps, namely, conversion of units within a system or between systems, and calculation of drug dosages.

CRITICAL DECISION POINT **Drugs ordered in** units **and** milliequivalents **are not convertible to metric, apothecary, or household measurements**

Conversions

Drugs are not always dispensed in the unit of measure in which they are ordered. Drug companies package and bottle certain standard equivalents. The nurse often must convert available units of volume and weight to desired dosages or vice versa. The nurse must know approximate equivalents in all of the measurement systems or make use of conversion tables. See Tables 17-4 and 17-5. An example follows:

The nurse receives an order: vancomycin 1 gram IV
The pharmacy supplies: vancomycin in 500 mg vials
Since the drug dose on the drug label is in milligrams, conversion should be from grams to milligrams
To convert gram to milligrams, move the decimal point three spaces to the right.

$$1.0 \text{ g} = 1.000 \text{ mg}$$

Once this information is known the nurse can move to the next step: dosage calculations.

Dosage Calculations

Dosages can be calculated in more than one way. A simple formula that can be applied when preparing solid or liquid forms of medications is the fractional equation method:

$$\frac{\text{Dose strength}}{\text{Quantity available}} = \frac{\text{Desired dosage}}{\text{Amount to administer}}$$

Table 17-4 Volume Equivalents of Measurement

Metric	Apothecary	Household
1 ml	15 minims (m) or 16 (m)	15 drops (gtt)
4-5 ml	1 fluidram (f)	1 teaspoon (tsp)
15 ml	4 fluidrams (f)	1 tablespoon (tbsp)
30 ml	1 fluid ounce (f)	2 tablespoons (tbsp)
240 ml	8 fluid ounces (f)	1 cup (c)
480 ml (approximately 500 ml)	1 pint (pt)	1 pint (pt)
960 ml (approximately 1 L)	1 quart (qt)	1 quart (qt)
3840 ml (approximately 4000 ml)	1 gallon (gal)	1 gallon (gal)

Table 17-5 Weight Equivalents of Measurement

Metric	Apothecary	Household
1 mg	1/60 gr	—
60 mg	1 gr	—
1 g	15 gr	—
4 g	ʒ	—
30 g	1 oz(℥)	1 oz
500 g	1.1 lb	1 lb
1000 g (1 kg)	2.2 lb	2 lb

The dose strength available is the weight or volume of drug available in units supplied by the pharmacy (the dose strength available may be listed on the drug label as the contents of a tablet or capsule or the amount of drug dissolved per unit volume of liquid). The quantity available is the basic unit or quantity of the drug containing the dose strength available (for solid drugs the quantity available may be one tablet or capsule). The desired dosage is the amount of pure drug the provider prescribes for a client. The amount to administer is the unknown amount to give. When calculated it represents the actual amount of available medication the nurse will give to the client (always expressed in the same unit as the quantity available). Continuing with our example above:

$$\frac{500 \text{ mg}}{1 \text{ vial}} = \frac{1000 \text{ mg}}{\times \text{ (Amount to administer)}}$$

$$500x = 1000 \text{ mg}$$

$$x = 2 \text{ vials}$$

To administer the proper dosage (1000 mg), the nurse would administer 2 vials of vancomycin.

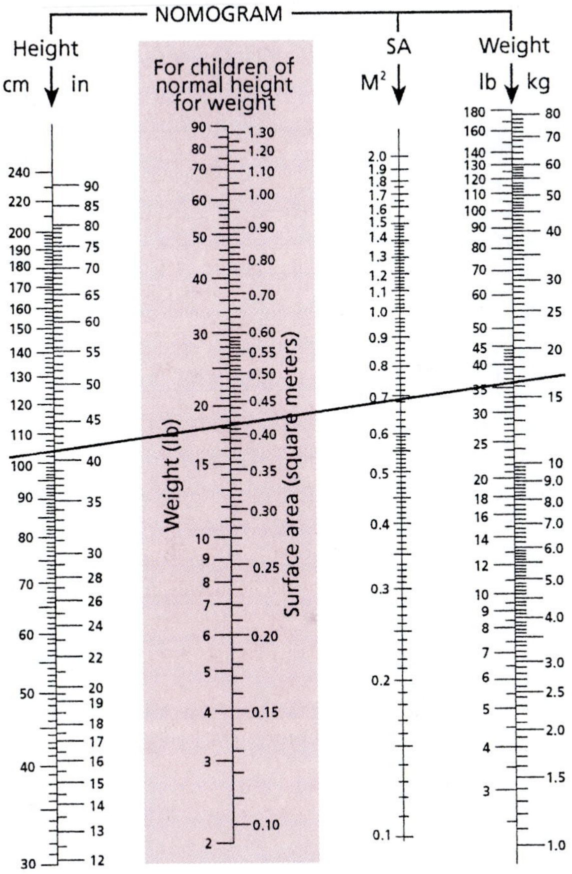

Fig. 17-1 West Nomogram (for estimation of surface body areas). Surface area is indicated where a straight line connecting height and weight intersects surface area (SA) column or, if patient is approximately of normal proportion, from weight alone (enclosed area). (From Behrman RE, Vaughan VC, editors: *Nelson textbook of pediatrics,* ed 14, Philadelphia, 1992, WB Saunders; modified from data of E. Boyd by CD West.)

Pediatric Dosages

Few drugs are packaged in pediatric dosages. Children metabolize and excrete drugs differently than the average adult body. Therefore various formulas involving age, weight, and body surface have been devised to determine children's dosages from adult dosages. The nurse reviews institutional policy for the method used in determining pediatric dosages. The most common method is to use a nomogram that relates the height and weight of a child in terms of body surface area. To do this the nurse uses the *West Nomogram* (Fig. 17-1) for estimation of body surface area (BSA). Once BSA has been determined it is used in the formula below to determine the pediatric dosage of a drug. Always double-check pediatric calculations with another nurse.

$$\text{Child's dose} = \text{BSA of child } (m^2)/1.7 \text{ } m^2 \times \text{Adult dose}$$

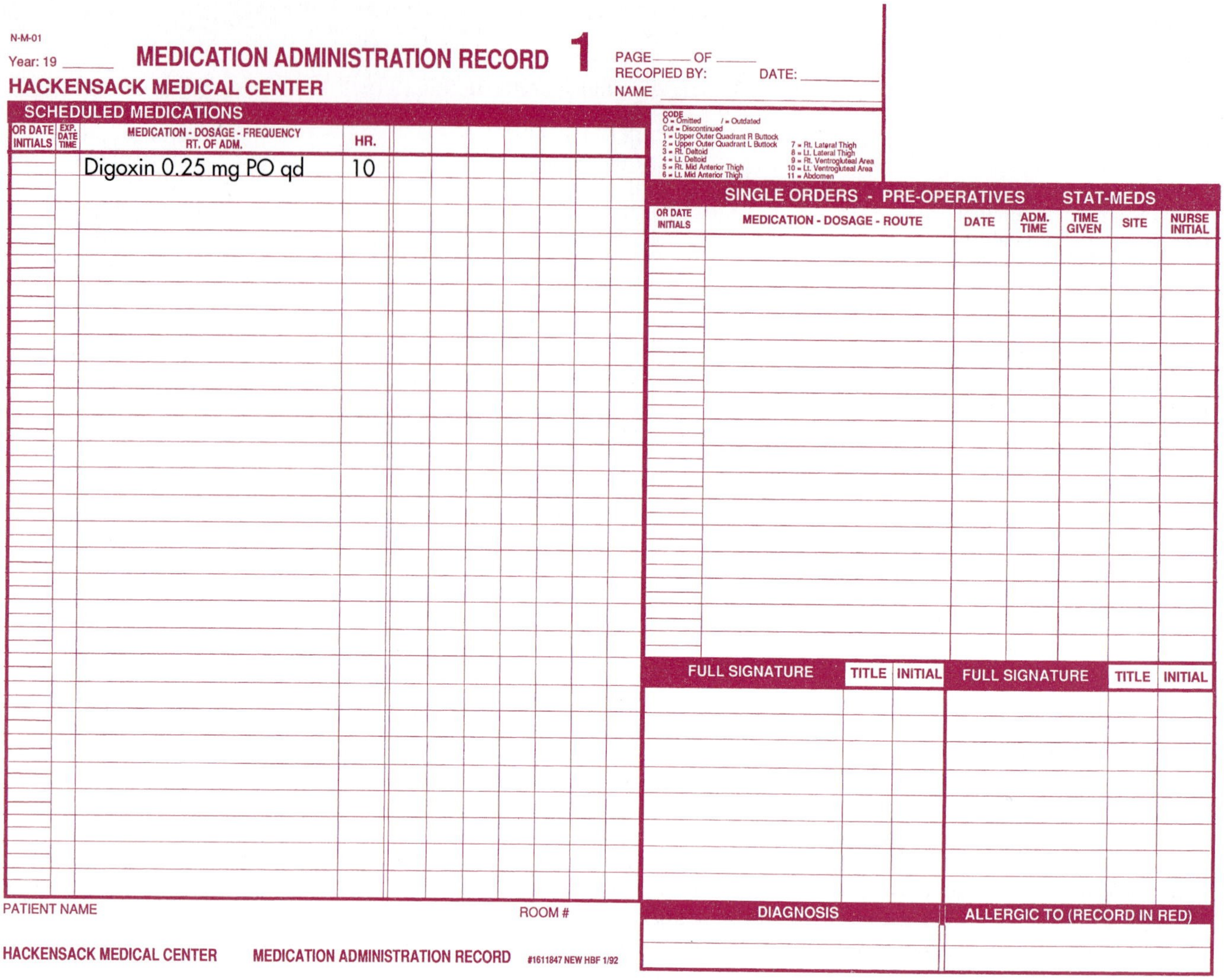

N-M-01

Year: 19 ____ **MEDICATION ADMINISTRATION RECORD 1**

PAGE ____ OF ____
RECOPIED BY: DATE: ____
NAME ____

HACKENSACK MEDICAL CENTER

SCHEDULED MEDICATIONS

OR DATE INITIALS	EXP. DATE TIME	MEDICATION - DOSAGE - FREQUENCY RT. OF ADM.	HR.
		Digoxin 0.25 mg PO qd	10

CODE
O = Omitted / = Outdated
Cut = Discontinued
1 = Upper Outer Quadrant R Buttock
2 = Upper Outer Quadrant L Buttock
3 = Rt. Deltoid
4 = Lt. Deltoid
5 = Rt. Mid Anterior Thigh
6 = Lt. Mid Anterior Thigh
7 = Rt. Lateral Thigh
8 = Lt. Lateral Thigh
9 = Rt. Ventrogluteal Area
10 = Lt. Ventrogluteal Area
11 = Abdomen

SINGLE ORDERS - PRE-OPERATIVES STAT-MEDS

OR DATE INITIALS	MEDICATION - DOSAGE - ROUTE	DATE	ADM. TIME	TIME GIVEN	SITE	NURSE INITIAL

FULL SIGNATURE	TITLE	INITIAL	FULL SIGNATURE	TITLE	INITIAL

PATIENT NAME ROOM #

DIAGNOSIS

ALLERGIC TO (RECORD IN RED)

HACKENSACK MEDICAL CENTER MEDICATION ADMINISTRATION RECORD #1611847 NEW HBF 1/92

Fig. 17-2 Medication Administration Record. (Courtesy of Hackensack University Medical Center, Hackensack, NJ.)

Older Adult Dosages

As yet no special formulas for calculating drug dosages for older adults exist. Most drug references do not list recommended older adult dosages. Because of changes in older adults' metabolism and excretion of drugs, the nurse should be cautious when dosages are ordered on the high end of an adult dosage range. Consultation with the prescriber may help to ensure safe dosage administration.

DRUG DISTRIBUTION

Drug distribution is the responsibility of the institution or community pharmacist. In a hospital a variety of systems may be used to distribute medications to a nursing unit. The standard for drug distribution is the **unit dose system.** In this system, each client on the nursing unit has a medication drawer that contains enough of the client's current medications, usually, for a 24-hour period. The advantage to unit dose dispensing of medications is that it reduces drug cost for institutions and also reduces medication errors.

Some drugs may be distributed as floor stock. **Floor stock** are medications that are distributed to the nursing unit in bulk (either individually wrapped or in bottles). Generally, medications that are appropriate for floor stock are those that are routinely prescribed or prescribed on a PRN basis. Examples of these medications are stool softeners, antacids, and antipyretics. Newer medication dispensing systems, such as computer-assisted or electronic devices, are variations of unit dose and floor stock systems. For example, the Pyxis Corporation designs the MedStation. This system can carry a variety of medications, housed in individual compartments that are accessed by the nurse after requesting the medication from a computerized screen. Medications that are frequently used, such as floor stock medications and narcotics, are often housed in the MedStation. All medications retrieved

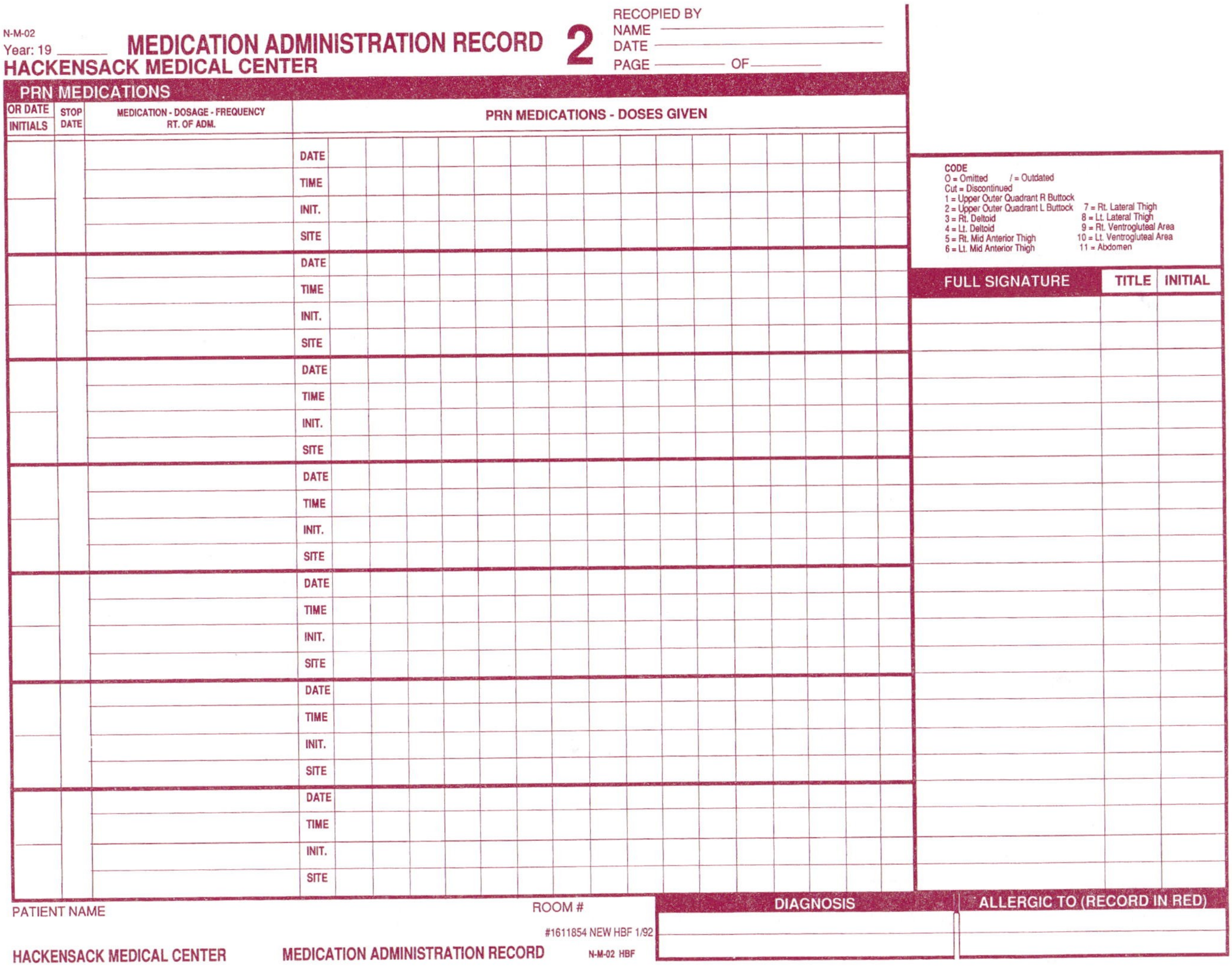
N-M-02
Year: 19 ______
MEDICATION ADMINISTRATION RECORD 2
HACKENSACK MEDICAL CENTER
RECOPIED BY
NAME
DATE
PAGE ______ OF ______
PRN MEDICATIONS
OR DATE INITIALS | STOP DATE | MEDICATION - DOSAGE - FREQUENCY RT. OF ADM. | PRN MEDICATIONS - DOSES GIVEN
DATE
TIME
INIT.
SITE
CODE
O = Omitted / = Outdated
Cut = Discontinued
1 = Upper Outer Quadrant R Buttock
2 = Upper Outer Quadrant L Buttock
3 = Rt. Deltoid
4 = Lt. Deltoid
5 = Rt. Mid Anterior Thigh
6 = Lt. Mid Anterior Thigh
7 = Rt. Lateral Thigh
8 = Lt. Lateral Thigh
9 = Rt. Ventrogluteal Area
10 = Lt. Ventrogluteal Area
11 = Abdomen
FULL SIGNATURE | TITLE | INITIAL
PATIENT NAME
ROOM #
DIAGNOSIS
ALLERGIC TO (RECORD IN RED)
#1611854 NEW HBF 1/92
HACKENSACK MEDICAL CENTER
MEDICATION ADMINISTRATION RECORD
N-M-02 HBF

Fig. 17-2, cont'd Medication Administration Record

from the MedStation are recorded in the system's computer. Baxter Healthcare Corporation manufactures the Sure-Med Unit Dose Center, which provides single doses of floor stock medications.

MEDICATION ADMINISTRATION

Preparing and administering medications requires accuracy by the nurse. The nurse must pay full attention to the procedure and try not to do other tasks simultaneously. Accuracy is greatest when the nurse observes the "five rights" of drug administration:

1. The *right* drug.
2. The *right* dose.
3. The *right* client.
4. The *right* route.
5. The *right* time.

Correct Transcription and Communication of Orders

The nurse or a designated unit secretary writes the prescriber's complete order on the appropriate medication administration record (MAR) (Fig. 17-2). The transcribed order includes the client's full name, room, and bed number; date the order is written; date the drug order expires; drug name and dosage; and time and route of administration. Each time a drug dose is prepared the nurse refers to the MAR. With unit dose systems, only one transcription is necessary, limiting the opportunity for errors. When transcribing orders, the nurse should be sure names, dosages, and symbols are legible. A registered nurse is responsible for checking and initialing all transcribed orders.

In some institutions a computer printout lists all currently ordered medications with dosage information (Fig. 17-3). Orders are entered directly into the computer, preventing the need for transcription of orders. The same printout may be used to record medications given.

```
6900A-3277     THE BARNES-JEWISH HOSPITAL OF ST. LOUIS
          12:00 NN SCHEDULED MEDICATIONS DUE 6900A        03/26/00
                                          ISSUED 10:15 AM 03/26

6901-1
                                                               GIV NGIV

HEPARIN SODIUM HEPARIN (FOR IV CATHETER IRRIGATION), (10
UNITS/ML) 30ML VIAL, 1ML, IV PUSH, Q6H (12-6), (03/22/00
06PM-..)
                                                               --- ---

6903-1
                                                               GIV NGIV

CEFOTAN CEFOTETAN DISODIUM INJ 1GM/10ML,    IV PIGGYBACK,
Q12H (12-12), (03/25/00 12MN-..)
                                                               --- ---

HEPARIN SODIUM HEPARIN (FOR IV CATHETER IRRIGATION), (10
UNITS/ML) 30ML VIAL, 3ML, IV PUSH, Q6H (12-6), (03/26/00
06AM-..)
                                                               --- ---

6905-1
                                                               GIV NGIV

LACRILUBE OPHTHALMIC OINTMENT BOTH EYES(OU), Q4H (4-8-12-4-8-
12), (03/16/00 12MN-..)
                                                               --- ---

6907-1
                                                               GIV NGIV

REGLAN METOCLOPRAMIDE TAB, 10MG,, PO, Q6H (12-6), (03/26/00
12MN-..)
                                                               --- ---
```

Fig. 17-3 Computer list of ordered medications. (Courtesy of Barnes-Jewish Hospital, St Louis.)

A registered nurse checks all transcribed orders against the original order for accuracy and thoroughness. If an order seems incorrect or inappropriate, the nurse consults the prescriber. The nurse who gives the wrong medication or an incorrect dosage is legally responsible for the error.

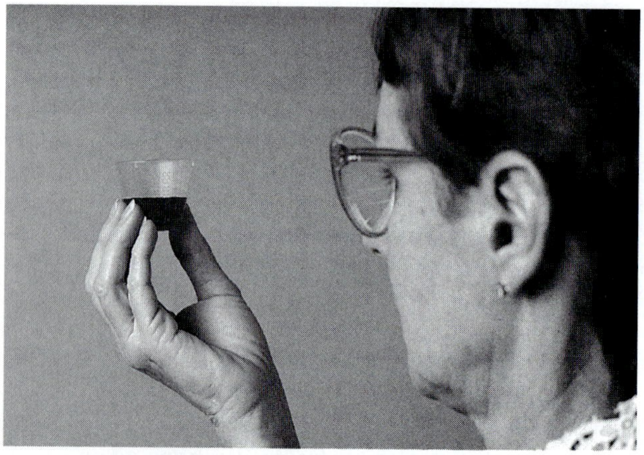

Fig. 17-4 Reading fluid at the meniscus.

Accurate Dose Measurement

When measuring liquid drugs, the nurse uses standard measuring receptacles such as a medicine cup or a syringe. Several key principles are important for the nurse to observe when using measuring receptacles.

1. Drugs poured into medication cups should be done so at eye level. This allows the nurse to accurately see the desired amount. This amount should be even with the base of the meniscus (Fig. 17-4).
2. Drugs drawn into syringes should be done slowly so as to prevent bubbles from entering the syringe. Air displaces medications and may lead to inaccurate measurement of doses.

Correct Administration

To administer medications safely the following guidelines are applied.

Receiving Medication Orders

1. A medication order is required for any drug to be administered by the nurse. The nurse should be aware of institutional policy regarding which providers, other than physicians, may prescribe medications. Many

states now allow advance practice nurses as well as physician assistants to prescribe medications.

2. Check all transcribed orders carefully against the prescriber's order. Any smudged or illegible transcriptions must be rewritten.
3. Ensure that the medication order contains the following elements: the date the order was written, the name of the drug to be administered, the dosage of the drug to be administered, the route of administration, and the signature of the prescriber.
4. Assess the client's history of allergies. If the medication is contraindicated, notify the prescriber.
5. Be informed about each drug ordered, including drug action and purpose, normal dosage and route, time interval for action, side effects, and nursing implications for administration and monitoring.
6. Give medications within 30 minutes of the time ordered to ensure that therapeutic blood levels are maintained. STAT medications should be given immediately. Prescribers commonly order a NOW dose of a medication and follow this order with a timed order. NOW medication orders should be given as soon as the medication becomes available but generally should be given within 60 minutes. Preoperative medications should be given at the specified time. Insulin should be given at a precise interval before a meal.
7. A **verbal order** is a medication or treatment order received by the nurse in the presence of the prescriber. Verbal orders are entered into the client's medical record by the nurse and transcribed the same way as if the prescriber wrote the order. (Fig. 17-5). The name of the prescriber is written next to that of the nurse. **Telephone orders** are medication or treatment orders given to the nurse by the prescriber, generally after the nurse updates the prescriber about a change in the client's condition. The nurse follows institutional policy regarding the receiving, recording, and transcription of verbal and telephone orders. Generally, verbal and telephone orders must be signed by the provider within 24 hours.

Administering Medications from the MAR

1. Ensure the medication order has not expired. Follow institution's policy for renewal of medication orders.
2. Gather or review assessment data that may influence drug administration. This may include, but is not limited to, the client's vital signs, laboratory data, or behavior. If data contraindicate medication administration or the client no longer requires the drug, withhold medication and notify prescriber.
3. When preparing a dose always check the label on the drug against the MAR. Prior to entering the client's room, the nurse should recheck all medications gathered against the MAR.
4. Take time to calculate drug doses accurately. Standard measuring receptacles should be used in preparing liquid medications. Calculate doses while preparing the drug.

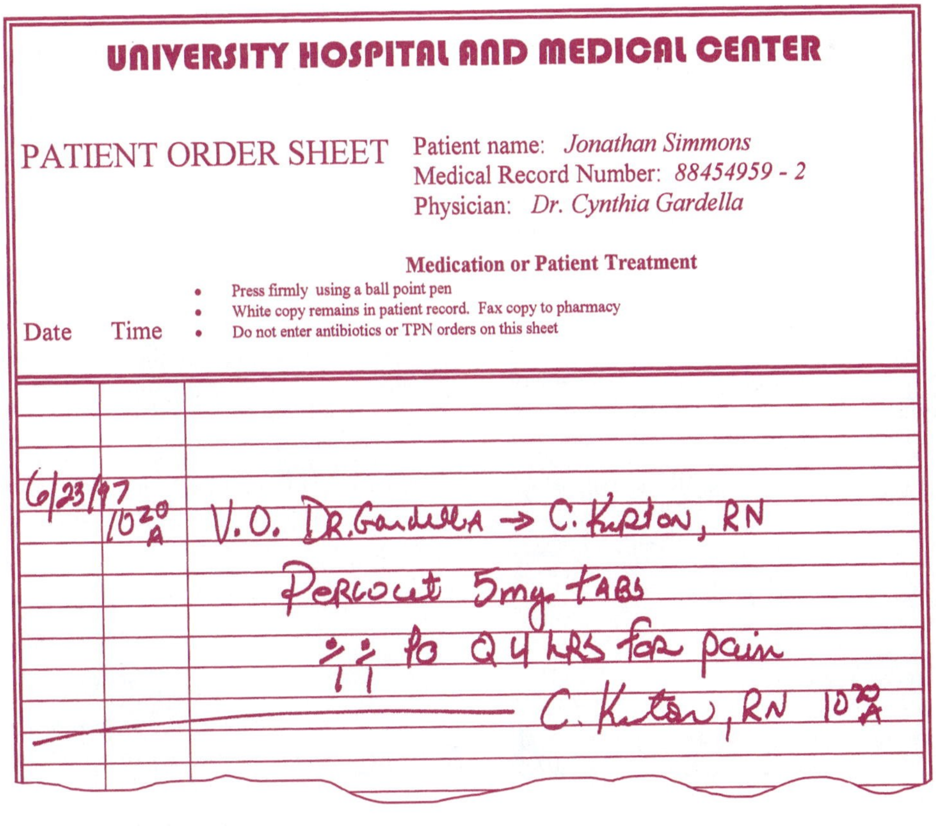
UNIVERSITY HOSPITAL AND MEDICAL CENTER

PATIENT ORDER SHEET

Patient name: Jonathan Simmons
Medical Record Number: 88454959 - 2
Physician: Dr. Cynthia Gardella

Medication or Patient Treatment

- Press firmly using a ball point pen
- White copy remains in patient record. Fax copy to pharmacy
- Do not enter antibiotics or TPN orders on this sheet

Date	Time	Medication or Patient Treatment
6/23/97	10 20 A	V.O. Dr. Gardella → C. Kurton, RN
		Percocet 5mg tabs
		ii po Q 4 hrs for pain
		C. Kurton, RN 10 20 A

Fig. 17-5 Example of a verbal order.

5. When administering nonparenteral medications, clean technique is acceptable. In clean technique wash hands with soap and water or an antiseptic solution (Chapter 33). When an antiseptic is used, the technique can be considered aseptic. The nurse avoids touching tablets, capsules, and liquids. When parenteral medications are administered, strict aseptic technique (see Chapter 34) is used when handling syringes and intravenous equipment.
6. Administer only personally prepared medications. Never administer a drug prepared by another nurse.
7. To avoid common errors, do not give medications from containers with labels that are unmarked or illegible; do not give medications that have changed from clear to cloudy or have changed color; discard a liquid medication if sediment can be seen in the bottom of the medication container, unless the medication is a suspension; and always check the expiration date of a drug.
8. Tablets and capsules should be maintained in their wrappers and opened at the client's bedside. This allows the nurse to review, with the client, each drug that is administered. Clients may also refuse one or more medications. The nurse may then remove the refused medication and proceed with the administration of all other medications.

Administering Medications to Clients

1. Clients must be correctly identified by checking the name on the MAR with the client's identification band worn on the wrist (Fig. 17-6). Replace any smudged or illegible bracelets. The nurse also asks the client to "Please state your name." When administering medications to children, parents should be used to identify the child.
2. With each drug inform the client of the drug's name, purpose, action, and potential undesired effects.
3. Respect a client's right to refuse a medication. If a client refuses a medication, never return unwrapped medication to a container; discard it. If the medication wrapper remains intact, the medication may be returned to the client's unit dose drawer. When scored tablets are broken in half, do not save parts of tablets to be used later; discard portion not used.
4. As you are administering medications, review, with the client, each of the medications before being taken or before disposing of the medication packet (wrapper). Evaluate the client's understanding of the purpose of the medication. If the medication is new to the client, take this opportunity to teach the client about the medication.
5. Remain with the client as the client takes the medication. Provide assistance if necessary (e.g., for the client who is weak and unable to administer eye drops). Do not leave medications at a client's bedside without a prescriber's order.

Administering Medications to Children. When administering medications to a child, the parents can be a valuable resource to the nurse. Parents may have administered medications to the child at home. The nurse can ask the parents about the child's usual reaction to medication. Based upon this information, the nurse modifies the activity to ensure that the medication is taken by the child. If not contraindicated by institutional policy, the child may willingly accept oral, topical, optic, otic, nasal, or rectal medications when administered by the parent under nursing supervision. When giving medication by injection, safety of the child, nurse, and parent is paramount. The nurse involves the parent in comforting the child during this task.

Postadministration Activities

1. After administering a drug, the nurse records it immediately in the appropriate form. Information that is often recorded includes:
   - Drug name
   - Dosage
   - Route of administration

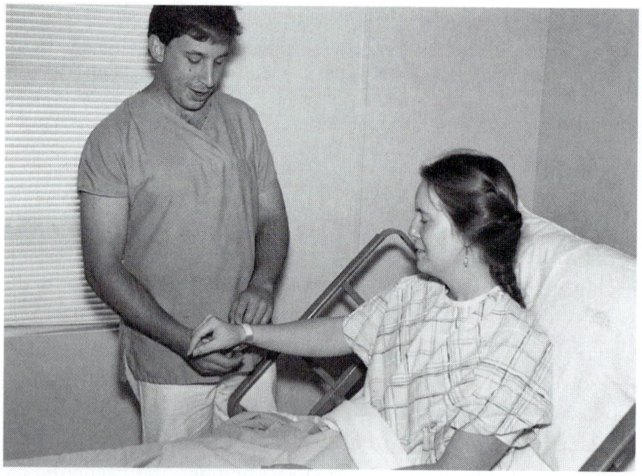

Fig. 17-6 Before administering any medication, nurse checks clients identification bracelet.

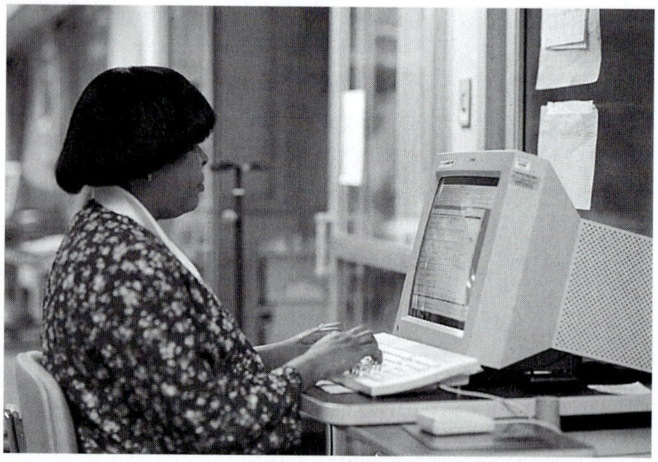

Fig. 17-7 Nurse using computer to chart administration of medication.

- Time of administration
- Signature and title of nurse administering drug

Usually this information is recorded on a special medication flow sheet or MAR (see Fig. 17-2 and Fig. 17-3). Many institutions have a computerized MAR. The nurse records information using an electronic signature assigned by the institution (Fig. 17-7).

2. Any data pertinent to the client's response or assessment data collected at the time of administration should be recorded either on the nurses' notes or appropriate flow sheets.
3. If the client refuses a medication, the reason for refusal is recorded in the nurse's notes. The MAR may require a special symbol that indicates that the client refused the medication. The prescriber should be notified of the client's refusal.
4. Monitor the client during the period after drug administration for any serious side effects.

SPECIAL HANDLING OF MEDICATIONS

Controlled Substances

Any medication that has the potential for abuse is handled in a manner differently than other drugs. These medications are called controlled substances and are often referred to as narcotics. Narcotics delivered to the nursing unit are kept in a locked cabinet. At the beginning of each nursing shift, two registered nurses must count all of the narcotics in the locked cabinet and record this information on a narcotic information record. Computerized or electronic distribution systems may make counting narcotics unnecessary by automatically counting and recording the nurse's electronic signature as the dose is dispensed.

CRITICAL DECISION POINT Any narcotics unaccounted for must be reported to the nurse manager or nurse supervisor immediately.

When administering narcotics to a client, the nurse follows these general guidelines:

1. Prior to obtaining the desired narcotic, check the narcotic administration record for the number of narcotics left for the narcotic you will be administering to the client. Compare this number with the supply available. If it is correct, obtain desired dosage of narcotic. If incorrect notify nurse manager and follow institutional policy for missing narcotics.
2. Count the remaining supply. The following information is often recorded on the narcotic administration sheet after removal of your dose:
   - Client's name
   - Prescribing physician
   - Client's medical record number
   - Dosage of the drug ordered
   - Number of tablets (or injectables) remaining
   - Nurse's signature
3. Administer the narcotic according to agency policy.
4. If the narcotic cannot be given to the client (e.g., client refuses, medication contaminated, change in vital signs), the medication must be "wasted." Narcotic wasting often requires that another nurse witness the administering nurse discard the medication according to the hospital's policy. When narcotics are wasted, this information is recorded on the narcotic administration form or another designated form. The witnessing nurse must record on that form a signature indicating the medication has been discarded in the proper manner.

Investigational Medications

Drugs used in investigational therapies may or may not be administered by a nurse. The nurse reviews agency policy that indicates if nursing personnel may participate in the administration of experimental drugs.

When administering experimental therapies, the nurse follows these general guidelines:

1. Review agency policy on the administration of experimental therapies by the nurse.
2. Prior to administration of experimental therapies the nurse reviews the client record to ensure that the client's informed consent was obtained.
3. The nurse reviews the experimental protocol for special handling, or administration instructions. The nurse monitors the client according to experimental protocol.

MEDICATION ERRORS

A medication error is any event that could cause or lead to a client receiving an inappropriate drug therapy or failing to receive appropriate drug therapy (Edgar, 1994). Medication errors, made by nurses, occur when the nurse fails to follow routine procedures such as checking dosage calculations, deciphering illegible handwriting, properly identifying a client, or administering drugs with which the nurse is unfamiliar. When an error occurs it should be acknowledged immediately and reported to the appropriate hospital personnel (e.g., nurse manager and physician). Measures to counteract the effects of the error may be necessary. The nurse is also responsible for completing an incident report describing the nature of the incident. Incident reports assist administrative personnel in identifying hospital system problems that contribute to medication errors.

CLIENT AND FAMILY TEACHING

A properly informed client is more likely to take medications correctly. The nurse provides information about the purpose of medications, their actions, side effects, dosage schedules, and actions to take in case side or toxic effects develop. Special instructional booklets or leaflets are often available as teaching aids. When teaching clients about their medications it is best to include persons identified as being significant to the client's recovery. This may include family members, partners, or home care providers.

Teaching Clients About Side Effects

All medications have side effects. The nurse teaches the client and family members about side effects associated with each medication prescribed. Because medications can have many side effects, teaching the client about all of them can overwhelm the client and impede learning; remember, client learning is a continual process. When beginning to teach a client about a new medication, evaluate each of the side effects and teach the client about the ones that are the *most likely* to occur and occur early after administration. For example, some antibiotics cause hypersensitivity reactions, hepatoxicity, nephrotoxicity, and platelet dysfunction. Hypersensitivity reactions are likely to occur shortly after taking a few doses of an antibiotic. The other side effects tend to occur after long-term antibiotic administration. Teach clients about side effects in terms of things that they can see, feel, touch, or hear. For example, thrombocytopenia, a reduction in the number of platelets in the blood, can be a side effect of a drug. The client cannot see, feel, touch, or hear thrombocytopenia. However, thrombocytopenia can cause bleeding. The nurse teaches the client how to *look for* evidence of bleeding. Be sure to teach the client what to do about side effects when they are discovered.

Medications and the Client's Activities of Daily Living

The nurse evaluates the client's activities of daily living and the effect they will have on the client's ability to comply with medication schedules. When medications are initiated in the acute care setting they are often administered around the clock. In the community, it may not be reasonable to think clients can administer medications according to this schedule. In collaboration with the prescriber or the pharmacist, the nurse teaches the client and family members how to adjust medication schedules that are consistent with the client's lifestyle, including what to do if doses are missed.

Client activities can affect administration and absorption of certain drugs, as is the case with insulin. Insulin, a hormone used to treat diabetes mellitus, is administered by injection into the client's subcutaneous tissue. Exercise, an essential component in the treatment of diabetes, affects insulin absorption. The nurse modifies insulin teaching based on the level of exercise performed by the client.

Clients and Drug Safety

Evaluating the effectiveness of teaching ensures that the client can administer drugs in a safe manner. One method to evaluate client understanding is to create medication cards with the name of the drug on the front of the card and all pertinent drug information on the back of the card. The nurse flashes the card in front of the client and asks the client to read the name of the medication (this also ensures that the client can read the names of the medication). If the client correctly identifies the name of the medication, ask the client the following questions:

- Why are you taking this medication?
- How often do you take this medication?
- What side effects can occur with this medication?
- If this side effect occurs, what are you going to do about it?

It may be helpful to have actual labeled medication bottles with the drug name. Drug bottles often have fine print and may not be easily read by the client with impaired visual acuity.

Be sure to evaluate the client's sensory, motor, and cognitive functions which, when impaired, may affect the client's ability to safely self-administer medications. When impairments are assessed, family members, friends, or home health aides may be available to assist with medication administration. Many self-help devices are also available for purchase (e.g. pill boxes with times displayed, and electronic dispensers).

CRITICAL THINKING EXERCISES

1. You are admitting Matthew Smathers to your unit. He refuses to wear an identification bracelet. Explain what you would say to Mr. Smathers so that he understands why he must wear the identification bracelet. How would you intervene if he continues to refuse to wear the identification bracelet?
2. You are administering a drug that you have not administered before. You calculate the dosage and receive 250 mg as the appropriate dose. You always recheck your math. When you calculate the dosage again you obtain a dose of 375 mg. What would you do next?
3. The nurse administers a drug to a client and 15 minutes later the client becomes nauseous and vomits. After ensuring client comfort, what is the next appropriate action by the nurse?

REFERENCES

Edgar TA, Lee DS, Cousins DD: Experience with a national medication error reporting program, *Amer J Hosp Pharm* 51:1335-8, 1994.

McCaffery M, Ferrell B: Understanding opiodes & addiction, *Nursing 94* 24(8):56-9, 1994.

ADDITIONAL READING

Brown M, Mulholand JL: *Drug calculations: process and problems for clinical practice,* St Louis, 1995, Mosby.

Cohen MR: Do we still need the apothecary system?, *Nursing 93* 23:2, 1993.

Lilley LL, Guanci R: Applying systems theory, *Am J Nurs* 95:11, 1995.

McKenry LM, Salerno, E: *Mosby's Pharmacology in Nursing,* ed 19, St Louis, 1995, Mosby.

Potter PA, Perry AG: *Fundamentals of Nursing: concepts, process, and practice,* ed 4, St Louis, 1997, Mosby.

CHAPTER 18

Oral and Topical Medications

OBJECTIVES

Mastery of content in this chapter will enable the nurse to:

- Define key terms.
- Correctly administer a medication by oral, nasogastric, topical, ophthalmic, and otic routes.
- Correctly administer medications for irrigation and instillation.
- Identify guidelines for administering oral, nasogastric, topical, ophthalmic, and otic medications.
- Describe factors to assess before administering medications.
- Differentiate types of topical administrations that require sterile technique and those that require clean medical aseptic technique.
- Instruct clients in proper use of metered-dose inhalers (MDIs).
- Identify conditions contraindicating the administration of medications.
- Prepare a teaching plan regarding medication usage for a select client.

SKILLS

18-1 Administering Oral Medications
18-2 Administering Medications by Nasogastric Tube
18-3 Administering Skin Applications
18-4 Administering Eye Medications
18-5 Administering Ear Drops
18-6 Administering Ear Irrigations
18-7 Administering Nasal Instillations
18-8 Using Metered-Dose Inhalers
18-9 Administering Vaginal Instillations
18-10 Administering Rectal Suppositories

KEY TERMS

Adrenergic drug
Anaphylaxis
Anesthetics
Antianginal
Cerumen
Cycloplegic
Dermatitis
Dermatological
Eczema
Glaucoma
Lotion
Nares
Nasal
Nitroglycerin
O.D.
Ointment
Ophthalmic
Orifice
O.S.
Otic
O.U.
Overdose
Pillating device
Pruritus
Suppository
Suspension
Sympathomimetic
Topical
Transdermal
Vertigo

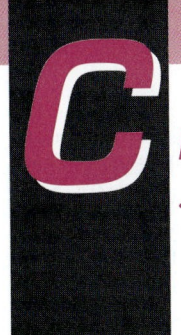

The easiest and most desirable way to administer medications is by mouth. Clients usually are able to ingest or self-administer oral drugs with a minimum of problems. Situations, however, may arise that contraindicate the client's receiving medications by mouth. The primary contraindications to giving oral medications include the presence of gastrointestinal alterations, the inability of a client to swallow food or fluids, and the use of gastric suction. An important precaution to take when administering any oral preparation is to protect clients from aspiration. Aspiration occurs when food, fluid, or medication intended for gastrointestinal administration inadvertently is administered into the respiratory tract. The nurse protects the client from aspiration by evaluat-

PROTECTING THE CLIENT FROM ASPIRATION

Evaluating the Client's Ability to Swallow

Ask the client to repeat certain sounds that require the same muscle movements as swallowing: "me-me-me" (for the lips); "la-la-la" (for the tongue); "ga-ga-ga" (for the soft palate and pharynx).

Assess the swallowing reflex by having the client slide his tongue backward along the palate.

Position your thumb and index finger on your client's larynx, ask the client to swallow. Normally the larynx elevates.

Evaluating the Client's Cough

See Chapter 35 on proper techniques of coughing.

Evaluating the Client's Gag Reflex

Assess the gag reflex by stroking the posterior pharyngeal wall with a tongue blade.

Never check the gag reflex in a client who does not exhibit an intact cough or swallow reflex. To protect the airway check that the client has all three: a positive cough, gag, and swallow reflex.

Modified from: Gauqitz DG: How to protect the dysphagic stroke patient, *Amer J Nurs*, 95:34, 1995.

ing the client's ability to safely swallow oral medications (see the box above). Properly positioning the client is also essential in preventing aspiration. Unless contraindicated, the nurse positions the client in a seated position when administering oral medications. The lateral position can also be used when the client's swallow, gag, and cough are intact. A client who has difficulty swallowing should be evaluated by appropriate personnel (e.g., speech therapist) prior to receiving oral preparations.

Topical administration of medications involves applying drugs locally to skin, mucous membranes, or tissue membranes. The nurse applies medications to the skin by painting, spraying, or spreading medication over an area, applying moist dressings, soaking body parts in solution, or giving medicated baths. Adhesive-backed medicated disks can also be applied to the skin to provide a continuous release of medication over several hours or days. Systemic effects from topical agents can occur if the skin is thin, if the drug concentration is high, or if contact with the skin is prolonged.

Topical administration avoids puncturing skin and lessens the risk of infection and tissue injury that may occur with injections. Gastrointestinal disturbances are encountered less frequently than with oral administration. The risk of serious side effects is generally low, but serious systemic effects can occur.

Drugs applied to membranes such as the cornea of the eye or rectal mucosa are absorbed quickly because of the membrane's vascularity. When drug concentrations are high, systemic effects can occur. For example, bradycardia may occur following atropine instillation to the eye. Mucous and other tissue membranes differ in their sensitivity to medications. The cornea of the eye, for example, is extremely sensitive to chemicals. Clients commonly experience burning sensations during administration of eye and nose drops. Medications are generally less irritating to vaginal or rectal mucosa.

Medications for topical use can be administered in the following ways:

1. Direct application of liquid—eye drops, gargling, swabbing the throat.
2. Inserting drug into body cavity—**suppository** insertion into rectum or vagina or creams and foams inserted into the vagina.
3. Instillation of fluid into body cavity (fluid is retained)—ear drops, nose drops, bladder and rectal instillation.
4. Irrigation of body cavity (fluid is not retained)—flushing eye, ear, vagina, bladder, or rectum with medicated fluid.
5. Spraying—instillation into nose or throat.
6. Inhalation of medicated aerosol spray—distributes medication throughout the **nasal** passages and tracheobronchial airway.
7. Direct application to skin or mucosa—**lotion, ointments,** creams, patches, and disk.

GUIDELINES

1. Assess client's sensory function, including sight, hearing, touch, and physical coordination. Sensory and coordination deficits may impair client's ability to see medications, open prescription bottles, and read labels at home.
2. Clients often receive more than one oral medication at a time. The nurse evaluates each medication for potential drug-drug or drug-food interactions. Always consult with pharmacist when in doubt.
3. Evaluate whether medication can be taken with food. Some drugs require an empty stomach to enhance absorption. Other drugs can irritate the stomach lining and should always be taken with food.
4. For all medications administered orally or topically, gather information pertinent to the drug(s) ordered: action, purpose, normal dosage and route, common side effects, time of onset and peak action, nursing implications.
5. For all medications administered orally or topically, review prescriber's order for client's name, name of drug, strength, time of administration, and site of application.
6. Before applying topical medication, bathe any surface that may be contaminated with blood, body fluids, secretions, or excretions.
7. Use clean disposable gloves when applying topical medications to prevent absorption of the medication into nurse's skin.

8. Some topical medications are poorly absorbed on peripheral extremities. Follow manufacturer's recommendation for proper application of medication.
9. Check for client allergies prior to administration, particularly to preservatives or fragrances in topical drugs.
10. Know potential local and systemic effects of all topically applied medications.
11. If clients are mentally and physically able, prepare the client for discharge by instructing them on self-administration techniques.

DELEGATION CONSIDERATIONS

The skills in this chapter require problem solving and professional knowledge application unique to a professional nurse. Delegation of these skills is inappropriate. The RN should inform unlicensed care providers about potential side effects of medications and to report their occurrence.

SKILL 18-1 Administering Oral Medications

The easiest and most desirable way to administer medications is by mouth. The majority of medications the nurse administers are given by this route. The nurse usually prepares the medications for the client to self-administer, and prepares oral medications in an area designed for medication preparation or at the unit dose cart.

EQUIPMENT

- Medication cart or tray
- Disposable medication cups
- Glass of water, juice, or preferred liquid
- Drinking straw
- Pill-crushing or pillating device (optional)
- Paper towels
- Medication administration record (MAR) or computer printout

STEPS	RATIONALE
ASSESSMENT	
1. Assess for any contraindications to client receiving oral medication: Is client able to swallow? Is client suffering from nausea/vomiting? Is client diagnosed as having bowel inflammation or reduced peristalsis? Has client had recent gastrointestinal surgery? Does client have gastric suction?	Alterations in gastrointestinal function interfere with drug distribution, absorption, and excretion. Clients with gastrointestinal suction might not receive benefit from the medication because it may be suctioned from gastrointestinal tract before it can be absorbed.
2. Assess client's medical history, history of allergies, medication history, and diet history.	These factors can influence how certain drugs act. Information also reflects client's need for medications.
CRITICAL DECISION POINT Drug allergies should be listed on *each* page of the MAR and prominently displayed on the client's medical record.	
3. Gather and review assessment and laboratory data that may influence drug administration.	Physical examination or laboratory data may contraindicate drug administration.
CRITICAL DECISION POINT If contraindications exist, withhold medication and inform prescriber.	
4. Assess client's knowledge regarding health and medication usage.	Determines client's need for drug education. Also assists in identifying client's adherence to drug therapy at home. Assessment may reveal drug use problems such as drug tolerance. This occurs when a client desires more and more medication to achieve the desired effect. Other drug use problems are noncompliance, abuse, addiction, or dependence.
CRITICAL DECISION POINT If drug abuse, addiction, or dependence is suspected refer client to the appropriate health care professional.	

STEPS	RATIONALE
5. Assess client's preferences for fluids.	Offering fluids during drug administration is an excellent way to increase client's fluid intake. Fluids ease swallowing and facilitate absorption from the gastrointestinal tract. However, fluid restrictions must be maintained.

CRITICAL DECISION POINT Evaluate whether drug can be administered with the preferred fluid. For example, some drugs may not be administered with dairy products.

NURSING DIAGNOSIS

Clustering of defining characteristics from the assessment data may reveal the following nursing diagnoses for clients requiring this skill:

- Impaired swallowing
- Knowledge deficit regarding drug therapy
- Noncompliance (regarding drug regimen)

Related factors are individualized based on a client's condition or needs.

PLANNING

STEPS	RATIONALE
1. Expected outcomes following completion of procedure:	
➤ Client experiences desired medication effect within period of onset of medication.	Drug has exerted its therapeutic action.
➤ Client denies any gastrointestinal discomfort or symptoms of alterations.	Oral medications can irritate gastrointestinal mucosa.
➤ Client explains purpose of medication and drug dose schedule.	Demonstrates understanding of drug therapy.
2. Check accuracy and completeness of each MAR or computer printout with prescriber's written medication order. Check client's name, drug name and dosage, route of administration, and time for administration.	The order sheet is the most reliable source and only legal record of drugs client is to receive.

CRITICAL DECISION POINT Incomplete orders should be clarified with the prescriber prior to implementation.

STEPS	RATIONALE
3. Recopy or reprint any portion of the MAR that is illegible.	Soiled or illegible MAR forms or computer printouts can be a source of drug error.

IMPLEMENTATION

STEPS	RATIONALE
1. Prepare medications:	
a. Wash hands.	Reduces transfer of microorganisms.
b. Arrange medication tray and cups in medication preparation area or move medication cart to position outside client's room.	Organization of equipment saves time and reduces error.
c. Unlock medicine drawer or cart.	Medications are safeguarded when locked in cabinet or cart.
d. Prepare medications for one client at a time. Keep all pages of MARs or computer printouts for one client together.	Prevents preparation errors.
e. Select correct drug from stock supply or unit dose drawer. Compare label of medication with MAR or computer printout (see illustration).	Reading label and comparing it against transcribed order reduces errors.
f. Calculate drug dose as necessary. Double-check calculation.	Double-checking reduces risk of error.

STEPS	RATIONALE
g. To prepare tablets or capsules from a floorstock bottle, pour required number into bottle cap and transfer medication to medication cup. Do not touch medication with fingers. Extra tablets or capsules may be returned to bottle. Medications that need to be broken in order to administer half the dosage can be broken, using a gloved hand or cut with a **pillating device** (see illustration). Tablets that are to be broken in half must be prescored. Prescored tablets are identified by a manufactured line that transverses the center of the tablet.	Drugs are very expensive; avoid waste.

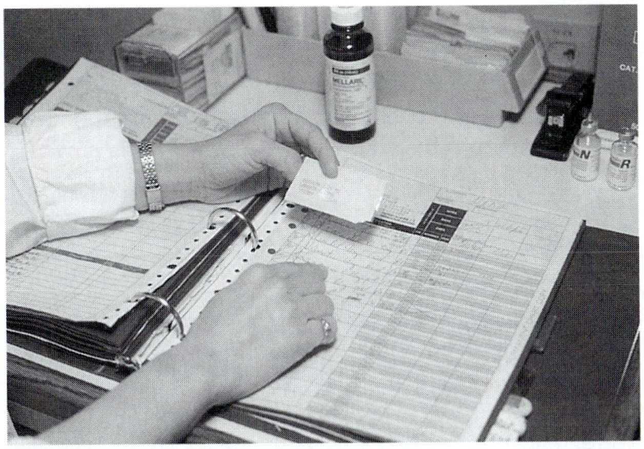

Step 1e The nurse checks the label of the medication with the transcribed medication order.

STEPS	RATIONALE
h. To prepare unit dose tablets or capsules, place packaged tablet or capsule directly into medicine cup. (Do not remove wrapper.)	Wrapper maintains cleanliness of medications and identifies drug name and dosage.
i. All tablets or capsules to be given to client at same time may be placed in one medicine cup except for those requiring preadministration assessments (e.g., pulse rate or blood pressure).	Keeping medications that require preadministration assessments separate from others makes it easier for the nurse to withhold drugs as necessary.
j. If client has difficulty swallowing, use pill-crushing device such as a mortar and pestle to grind pills (see illustration). If a pill-crushing device is not available, place tablet between two medication cups and grind with a blunt instrument. Mix ground tablet in small amount of soft food (custard or applesauce.)	Large tablets can be difficult to swallow. Ground tablet mixed with palatable soft food is usually easier to swallow.

CRITICAL DECISION POINT Not all drugs can be crushed (e.g., capsules and enteric-coated drugs). Consult with pharmacist when in doubt.

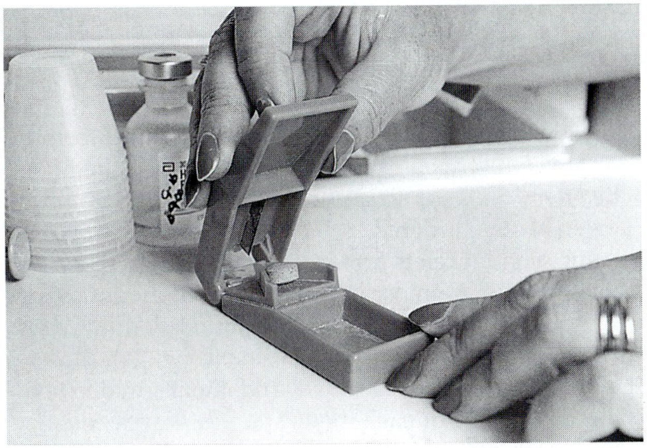

Step 1g

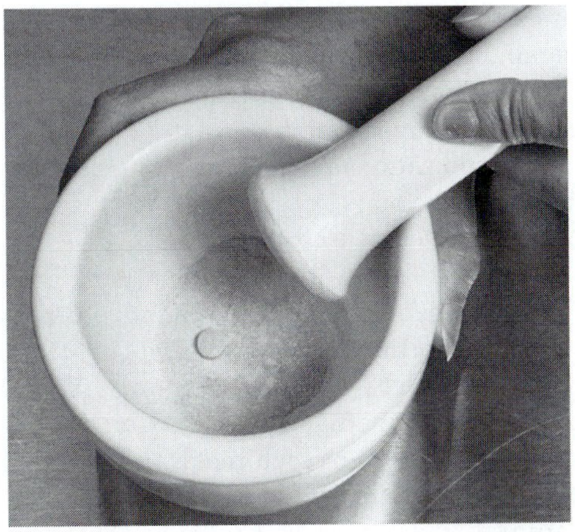

Step 1j

STEPS	RATIONALE
k. Prepare liquids:	
(1) Remove bottle cap from container and place cap upside down.	Prevents contamination of inside of cap.
(2) Hold bottle with label against palm of hand while pouring.	Spilled liquid will not soil or fade label.
(3) Hold medication cup at eye level and fill to desired level on scale (see illustration a). Scale should be even with fluid level at its surface or base of meniscus, not edges (see illustration b).	Ensures accuracy of measurement.

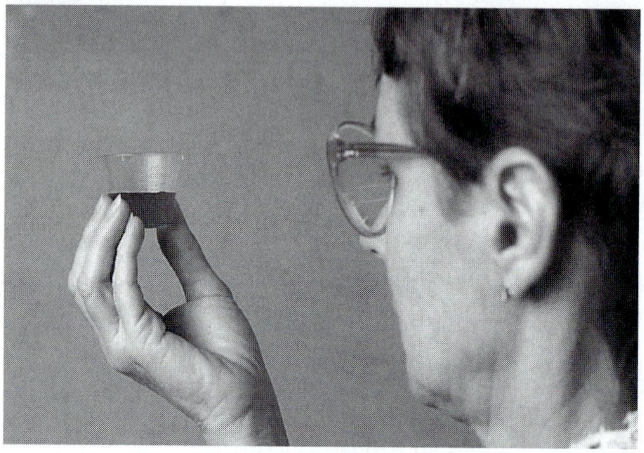

Step 1k(3)a Reading fluid at the meniscus.

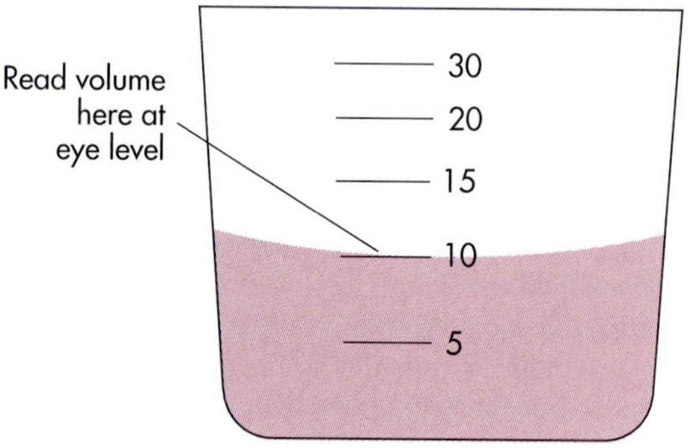

Step 1k(3)b

STEPS	RATIONALE
(4) Discard any excess liquid into sink. Wipe lip and neck of bottle with paper towel.	Prevents contamination of bottle's contents and prevents bottle cap from sticking.
l. When preparing narcotics, check narcotic record for previous drug count and compare with supply available.	Controlled substance laws require careful monitoring of dispensed narcotics.
m. Check expiration date on all medications.	Medications used past expiration date may be inactive or harmful to client.
n. Compare MAR or computer printout with prepared drug and container.	Reading label second time reduces error.
o. Return stock containers or unused unit dose medications to shelf or drawer and read label again.	Third check of label reduces administration errors.
p. Do not leave drugs unattended.	Nurse is responsible for safekeeping of drugs.
2. Administering medications:	
a. Take medications to client at correct time.	Medications are administered within 30 minutes before or after prescribed time to ensure intended therapeutic effect. STAT or single-order medications should be given at time ordered.
b. Identify client by comparing name on MAR or computer printout with name on client's identification bracelet (see illustration on p. 571). Ask client to state name.	Identification bracelets are made at time of client's admission and are most reliable source of identification. Replace any missing or faded identification bracelets.
c. Explain purpose of each medication and its action to client. Allow client to ask any questions about drugs.	Client has right to be informed, and client's understanding of purpose of each medication improves compliance with drug therapy.

STEPS	RATIONALE

CRITICAL DECISION POINT If client refuses medication, withhold medication and notify prescriber.

d. Assist client to sitting or side-lying position if sitting is contraindicated by client's condition.

Sitting position decreases risk of aspiration during swallowing.

CRITICAL DECISION POINT Check the client's swallow, and cough and gag reflexes (see box on p. 566) if in doubt about client's ability to manage oral medications. Withhold medication if swallow, cough, or gag is impaired and notify MD.

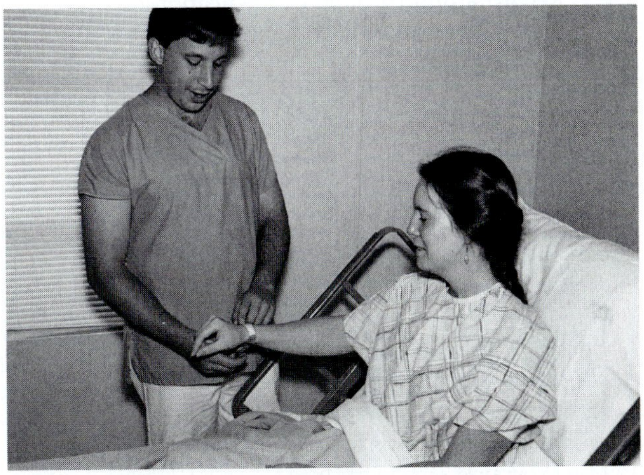

Step 2b Nurse idenditifies client by comparing name on MAR with client's identification bracelet.

e. Administer drugs properly:

(1) Client may wish to hold solid medications in hand or cup before placing in mouth.

Client can become familiar with medications by seeing each drug.

(2) Offer water or juice to help client swallow medications. Give cold carbonated water if available and not contraindicated.

Choice of fluid promotes client's comfort and can improve fluid intake. Carbonated water helps passage of tablet through esophagus.

(3) For sublingual-administered drugs, have client place medication under tongue and allow it to dissolve completely. Caution client against swallowing tablet.

Drug is absorbed through blood vessels of undersurface of tongue. If swallowed, drug is destroyed by gastric juices or so rapidly detoxified by liver that therapeutic blood levels are not attained.

(4) For buccal-administered drugs, have client place medication in mouth against mucous membranes of the cheek until it dissolves.

Buccal medications act locally on mucosa or systemically as they are swallowed in saliva.

CRITICAL DECISION POINT Avoid administering liquids until buccal medication has dissolved.

(5) Mix powdered medications with liquids at bedside and give to client to drink.

When prepared in advance, powdered drugs may thicken and even harden, making swallowing difficult.

(6) Caution client against chewing or swallowing lozenges.

Drug acts through slow absorption through oral mucosa, not gastric mucosa.

(7) Give effervescent powders and tablets immediately after dissolving.

Effervescence improves unpleasant taste of drug and often relieves gastrointestinal problems.

f. If client is unable to hold medications, place medication cup to the lips and gently introduce each drug into the mouth, one at a time. Do not rush.

Administering single tablet or capsule eases swallowing and decreases risk of aspiration.

g. If tablet or capsule falls to the floor, discard it and repeat preparation.

Drug is contaminated when it touches floor.

STEPS	RATIONALE
h. Stay until client has completely swallowed each medication. Ask client to open mouth if uncertain whether medication has been swallowed.	Nurse is responsible for ensuring that client receives ordered dosage. If left unattended, client may not take dose or may save drugs, causing risk to health.
i. For highly acidic medications (e.g., aspirin), offer client nonfat snack (e.g., crackers) if not contraindicated by client's condition.	Reduces gastric irritation.
j. Assist client in returning to comfortable position.	Maintains client's comfort.
k. Dispose of soiled supplies and wash hands.	Reduces transmission of microorganisms.
l. Record administration of medication on MAR, with nurse's initials or signature.	Timely recording reduces medication errors. The nurse's signature establishes accountability for administering drug.
m. Return MAR or computer printouts to appropriate file for next administration time.	MAR or computer printouts are used as reference for when next dosage is due. Loss can lead to administration error.
n. Replenish stock such as cups and straws, return cart to medicine room, and clean work area.	Clean working space assists other staff in completing duties efficiently.

EVALUATION

1. Return within 30 minutes to evaluate client's response to medications.	Evaluates drug's therapeutic benefit and can detect onset of side effects or allergic reactions.
2. Ask client or family member to identify drug name and explain purpose, action, dosage schedule, and potential side effects of drug.	Determines level of knowledge gained by client and family.
3. **Unexpected outcomes** that may occur include:	
➤ Client exhibits side effects common to medication.	Drugs cause secondary effects that can be harmful.
➤ Client exhibits toxic drug effects.	Toxic effects are the result of prolonged intake of high doses of medications.
➤ Client exhibits allergic reaction to drug with symptoms such as urticaria, rash, **pruritus,** rhinitis, and wheezing.	Client sensitizes immunologically to constituents of drug.
➤ Client is unable to explain drug information.	Reinstruction is necessary.

RECORDING AND REPORTING

1. Record actual time each drug was administered on the MAR or computer printout. Include initials or signature (see illustration, p. 557).	Prompt documentation prevents errors such as repeated doses. Nurse's signature establishes accountability for administering the drug.
2. If drug is withheld, record reason in nurses' notes. Circle time the drug normally would have been given on the MAR or computer printout.	Provides documented explanation for why routinely ordered medication was not administered.
3. Report adverse effects/client response to nurse in charge or MD.	Aids in determining if further treatment needed.

➤ *CRITICAL DECISION POINT* Depending on medication, immediate prescriber notification may be required.

FOLLOW-UP ACTIVITIES

1. Always notify prescriber when the client exhibits a toxic effect or allergic reaction, or with the onset of side effects. Withhold further doses.
2. Further assess the client's or family member's knowledge of medications and guidelines for drug safety.

Special Considerations

- Clients with neuromuscular disorders, esophageal strictures, lesions of the mouth, and those who are unresponsive or comatose and cannot swallow should not receive medications by the oral route. The nurse should request that the prescriber order the medication by an alternate route (e.g., intravenously).
- Clients with drug allergies should wear special identification bracelet that is color-coded and lists drugs to which client is allergic.
- Liquid medications packaged in single-dose cups need not be poured into medicine cups. They can be administered directly from the single-dose cup.
- An accurate measuring technique for small doses of liquid is drawing liquids into a syringe (with needle removed).
- Enteric-coated pills must not be crushed. The enteric coating delays absorption to prevent irritation to the stomach.

Teaching Considerations

- Instruct client on specific information pertaining to drug regimen (purpose, action, dosage, dosage intervals, side effects, foods to avoid or take with drugs).
- All clients should learn the basic guidelines for drug safety (see Chapter 41).

Pediatric Considerations

- Liquid forms of medication are safer to swallow to avoid aspiration of small pills.
- Bitter or distasteful oral preparation will be rejected by the child. The taste of these medications can be disguised by specially made preparations (e.g. jam, honey). The nurse can also offer the child juice or an ice pop after medication administration.
- Measure small amount of liquid medications using a plastic calibrated syringe.

Gerontologic Considerations

- Physiological changes of aging influence how oral medications are distributed, absorbed, and excreted. Common changes include loss of elasticity in oral mucosa; reduction in parotid gland secretion causing dry mouth; delayed esophageal clearance, impaired swallowing; reduction in gastric acidity and stomach peristalsis, increased susceptibility to highly acidic drugs; and reduced colon motility, slowing drug excretion.
- Rinse the client's oral cavity frequently with tepid water, floss daily, and brush gently.
- Administer a full glass of water (unless restricted) with medications to aid passage of the drug. Give the client time to swallow.
- Taking medications with a nonfat snack reduces gastric distress.
- The gag reflex in older client may be diminished due to continually inserting and removing dentures (Gauqitz, 1995).

Home Care Considerations

- See Skill 41-3, Medication and Medical Device Safety and Skill 42-4, Helping Clients with Self-Medication.

SKILL 18-2 Administering Medications by Nasogastric Tube

Clients with nasogastric tubes often receive nothing by mouth. Oral medications that need to be administered to these clients can be given by the nasogastric tube. To administer medications by a nasogastric tube, the nurse modifies the form of a tablet to be administered by crushing and dissolving it. Medications may also be available in liquid form. Generally, sustained-release, chewable, long-acting, or enteric-coated tablets and capsules are not administered by gastric tubes. Consult with the hospital pharmacy when in doubt.

EQUIPMENT

- 60 ml syringe
  - Cone tip for large-bore tubes (Asepto syringe or Toomey syringe)
  - Luer lock tip for small-bore tubes
- Stethoscope
- Graduate container
- Water
- Medication to be administered
- Pill crusher if medication in tablet form
- Medication administration record (MAR) or computer printout
- Disposable gloves

STEPS	RATIONALE

ASSESSMENT

1. Assess for any contraindications to client receiving oral medication: Has the client been diagnosed as having bowel inflammation or reduced peristalsis? Has client had recent gastrointestinal surgery? Does client have gastric suction? Can the suction be temporarily turned off?
   - *Rationale:* Alterations in gastrointestinal function interfere with drug distribution, absorption, and excretion. Clients with gastrointestinal suction might not receive benefit from the medication because it may be suctioned from gastrointestinal tract before it can be absorbed.

➤ **CRITICAL DECISION POINT** **Always review client's postoperative orders for gastric tube care. Manipulation and irrigation of tube, or instillation of medication may be contraindicated.**

2. Assess client's medical history, history of allergies, medication history, and diet history.
   - *Rationale:* These factors can influence how certain drugs act. Information also reflects client's need for medications.
3. Gather and review assessment and laboratory data that may influence drug administration.
   - *Rationale:* Physical examination or laboratory data may contraindicate drug administration.

➤ **CRITICAL DECISION POINT** **Withhold medication and inform the prescriber of your findings.**

4. Prior to the administration of medications verify placement of the gastric tube (see Chapter 23).

NURSING DIAGNOSIS

Clustering of defining characteristics from the assessment data may reveal the following nursing diagnoses for clients requiring this skill:

- Impaired swallowing
- Feeding self-care deficit
- Altered nutrition: less than body requirements

Related factors are individualized based on a client's condition or needs.

PLANNING

1. **Expected outcomes** following completion of procedure:
   - Client experiences desired medication effect within period of onset of medication.
     - *Rationale:* Drug has exerted its therapeutic action.
   - Client's feeding tube remains patent after administration of medication.
     - *Rationale:* A patent nasogastric tube indicates passage of medication into stomach, ensuring proper absorption. A blocked tube can later interfere with irrigation and fluid instillation.
2. Compare MAR or computer printout with label of medication.
   - *Rationale:* Ensures client receives correct medication.
3. Check client's identification bracelet and ask name.
   - *Rationale:* Ensures correct client receives medication.
4. Explain procedure to client, including description of medication to be instilled into nasogastric tube.
   - *Rationale:* Makes client a participant in care and minimizes anxiety. Begins client teaching regarding medications.

IMPLEMENTATION

1. Wash hands.
   - *Rationale:* Reduces transfer of microorganisms.
2. Prepare medications for instillation into feeding tube. Whenever possible, medications should be in liquid form to prevent particles from adhering to the internal lumen of the tube (Shuster, 1994). Prepare graduated container by pouring 50 to 100 ml of water into it.
   - *Rationale:* Adequate preparation saves nursing time.

➤ **CRITICAL DECISION POINT** **Nasogastric/intestinal tubes for decompression should not have medications administered into them.**

STEPS	RATIONALE
a. Crush tablets using a pill-crushing device such as a mortar and pestle to grind pills into a fine powder. If a pill-crushing device is not available, place tablet between two medication cups and grind with a blunt instrument. Dissolve in at least 30 ml of warm water.	
b. Capsules: Ensure that contents of capsule (granules or gelatin) can be expressed from its covering (consult with pharmacist). Open capsule or pierce gelcap with needle and empty contents into 30 ml of warm water. Gelcaps can also be dissolved in warm water.	Ensures contents of tablets or capsules are a fine powder or solution so as not to occlude nasogastric tube.
3. Prepare client by placing client in a high-Fowler's position.	Reduces risk of aspiration.
CRITICAL DECISION POINT **Ensure high-Fowler's position is not contraindicated by client's medical condition.**	
4. Apply clean gloves.	Reduces transfer of microorganisms.
5. Verify placement of client's nasogastric tube (see Skill 23-3 or Skill 23-4).	Reduces risk of aspiration of medication.
6. Aspirate stomach contents (see illustration). Note volume. Return aspirate to client.	
CRITICAL DECISION POINT **If large volume aspirate is found (e.g., 100 ml or more), return aspirate to client, withhold medication, and notify client's health care provider.**	Large volume aspirates (e.g., 100 ml) can contribute to gastric distention, esophageal reflux, and vomiting; all of which place the client at risk for aspiration (Shuster, 1994). Returning aspirate to client prevents loss of electrolytes and hydrochloric acid.
7. Pinch nasogastric tube and remove syringe. Remove bulb or plunger and reinsert tip of syringe into nasogastric tube.	Pinching nasogastric tube prevents leakage or spillage of stomach contents. Removal of bulb or plunger prepares syringe for delivery of medications.
8. Using a graduated container, instill 10 ml of water into nasogastric tube. Unpinch tube, allow water to flow by gravity. Administer first dose of medication (see illustration). Follow medication with 10 ml of water.	Ensures instillation of each medication. Maintains patency of nasogastric tube.

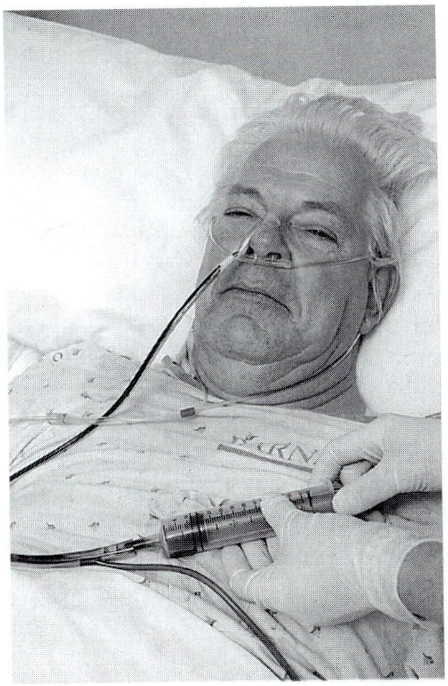

Step 6

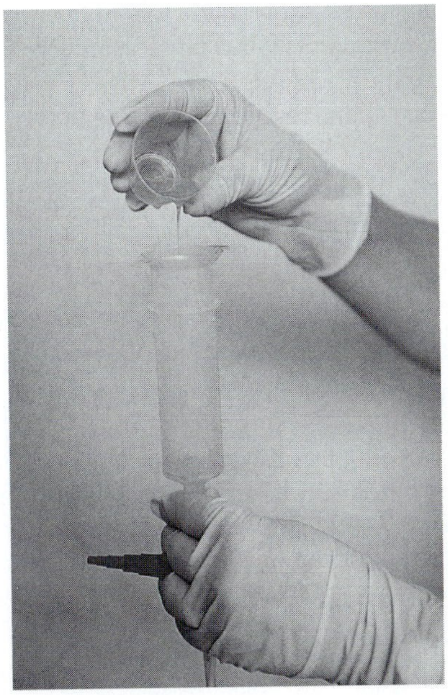

Step 8

STEPS	RATIONALE
➤ *CRITICAL DECISION POINT* If water or medication does not flow freely a *gentle* push with bulb of asepto syringe or plunger of Toomey syringe may facilitate flow of fluid.	
9. Follow last dose of medication with 30 to 60 ml of water.	Maintains patency of nasogastric tube. Ensures passage of medication into stomach.
a. When tube feeding is not being administered, clamp the proximal end of the feeding tube and cap end of tube.	Prevents air from entering the stomach between medication administration.
b. When continuous tube feeding is being administered by an infusion pump:	
(1) Following medication administration the feeding is stopped for 1 hour (check agency policy).	Allows for adequate absorption of medication.
10. Remove gloves, dispose of soiled supplies, rinse graduated container and syringe with tap water. Wash hands.	Reduces transmission of microorganisms.

EVALUATION

1. Return within 30 minutes to evaluate client's response to medications.	By monitoring client's response, nurse assesses drug's therapeutic benefit and can detect onset of side effects or allergic reactions.
2. **Unexpected outcomes** that may occur include:	
➤ Client does not receive medication as prescribed because of a blocked nasogastric tube.	Requires interventions to unclog tube to ensure drug delivery (see box below).

RECORDING AND REPORTING

1. Record in nurses' notes method used to check placement of nasogastric tube, volume of stomach aspirate, and if indicated pH of stomach aspirate (see Chapter 23).	Prompt documentation prevents errors such as repeated doses. Nurse's signature establishes accountability for administering the drug.
2. Record actual time each drug was administered on the MAR or computer printout. Include initials or signature (see illustration, p. 558).	
3. If drug is withheld, record reason in nurses' notes. Circle time the drug normally would have been given on the MAR or computer printout.	Provides documented explanation for why routine ordered medication was not administered.
4. Report adverse effects/client response to nurse in charge or MD.	Aids in determining if further treatment needed.

UNCLOGGING A BLOCKED FEEDING TUBE

- Prevent tube from becoming blocked by rinsing it with warm water before and after administering each dose of medication.
- Do not use cranberry juice or soda to flush or unblock the feeding tube. They only make the tube sticky.
- If tube is blocked get an order for a pancrelipase tablet (such as Viokase Tablets) and a sodium bicarbonate tablet (to help balance the pH). Crush these tablets together and mix them to form a slurry. Attempt to deliver the mixture to the site of blockage by inserting a smaller tube into the feeding tube, if necessary. Keep the mixture in your client's feeding tube for 15 to 30 minutes and then irrigate.

Modified from: Klang, M: Medicating tube-fed patients, *Nursing 96* 26:18, 1996.

STEPS	RATIONALE

FOLLOW-UP ACTIVITIES

1. Always notify prescriber when the client exhibits a toxic effect or allergic reaction, or with the onset of side effects. Withhold further doses.
2. Clients with continuous tube feeding should have tubes flushed with at least 50 ml of water every 4 to 8 hours to maintain patency. Check agency policy.

• • • • •

Special Considerations

- Drugs in syrup form, such as iron elixirs, are acidic. Often these drugs clump, clogging feeding tubes when they come in contact with enteral formulas. Be sure to rinse tube thoroughly with warm water before and after giving medications (Klang, 1996).
- Concentrated medications need to be thoroughly diluted. Dilution is particularly important when the feeding tube extends beyond the pylorus, where residual volume is insufficient to dilute medications and avoid cramping (Klang, 1996).
- Medication compatibility with enteral products has not been well studied. The nurse should suspect incompatibility when the desired effect of medications is not achieved.

Pediatric Considerations

- Volumes for instillation of medications or for irrigation of nasogastric tubes may be smaller. Check agency policy.

SKILL 18-3 Administering Skin Applications

Many locally applied drugs such as lotions, patches, pastes, and ointments can create systemic and local effects if absorbed through the skin. To protect the nurse from accidental exposure, the nurse should apply these drugs using gloves and applicators. If the client's skin is intact, the nurse uses clean technique when applying lotions, patches, ointments, etc. If the client has an open wound, sterile technique is important.

Skin encrustations and dead tissues harbor microorganisms and block contact of medications with the tissues to be treated. Simply applying new medications over previously applied drugs does little to prevent infection or offer therapeutic benefit. The nurse cleans the skin thoroughly before applying medications by washing the area gently with soap and water, soaking an involved site, or locally debriding tissue.

Each type of medication, whether an ointment, lotion, powder, or patch, should be applied in a specific way to ensure proper penetration and absorption. For example, the nurse applies lotions and creams by spreading them lightly onto the skin's surface, whereas powders are dusted lightly over affected areas.

EQUIPMENT

- **Clean gloves (for intact skin) or sterile gloves (nonintact skin)**
- **Ordered agent (powder, cream, ointment, spray, patch)**
- **Cotton-tipped applicators or tongue blades (optional)**
- **Basin of warm water, washcloth, towel, nondrying soap**
- **Sterile dressing, tape**
- **Medication administration record (MAR) or computer printout**

STEPS	RATIONALE
ASSESSMENT	
1. Assess condition of client's skin. (If topical agent is present, first wash site with mild, nondrying soap and warm water.) Assess for symptoms of skin irritation such as pruritus or burning. Cleanse site thoroughly so the nurse can obtain a proper assessment of skin surface.	Assessment provides baseline to determine change in condition of skin after therapy. Application of certain topical agents can lessen or aggravate these symptoms.
2. Carefully inspect the condition of the skin or membranes over which medications are to be applied before administration. Do not administer topical medications to skin whose integrity is altered, unless indicated.	

STEPS	RATIONALE
3. Determine whether client has known allergy to topical agent. Ask if client has had reaction to a cream or lotion applied to the skin.	Allergic contact **dermatitis** is relatively common and can worsen **dermatological** condition.
4. Determine amount of topical agent required for application by assessing affected area, reviewing prescriber's order, and reading application directions carefully (a thin, even layer is usually adequate).	An excessive amount of topical agent can cause chemical irritation of skin, negate drug's effectiveness, and/or cause adverse systemic effects, such as decreased white cell counts.
5. Assess client's knowledge of action and purpose of medication being given and interest in treating health problem.	Reveals client's level of understanding and whether instruction is necessary.
6. Determine if client is physically able to apply medication by assessing fine grasp, hand strength, reach, coordination.	Necessary if client is to self-administer drug in the home.

NURSING DIAGNOSIS

Clustering of defining characteristics from the assessment data may reveal the following nursing diagnoses for clients requiring this skill:

- Impaired skin integrity
- Ineffective management of therapeutic regimen (individual)
- Knowledge deficit regarding medication application
- Pain

Related factors are individualized based on a client's condition or needs.

PLANNING

STEPS	RATIONALE
1. Expected outcomes following completion of procedure:	
➤ Client is able to identify drug and describe action, purpose, dosage, side effects, and schedule of medication.	Demonstrates learning.
➤ Client is able to apply medication without assistance on prescribed schedule.	Demonstrates learning and compliance.
➤ With repeated applications, skin becomes clear, without inflammation or drainage from lesions.	Existing lesions heal and/or disappear.
2. Compare MAR or computer printout with label of medication.	Ensures client receives correct medication.
3. Check client's identification bracelet and ask name.	Ensures correct client receives medication.
4. Explain procedure to client, including description of skin area to be treated.	Makes client a participant in care and minimizes anxiety.

IMPLEMENTATION

STEPS	RATIONALE
1. Wash hands, arrange supplies at bedside, and apply clean gloves.	Reduces transmission of infection. Topical agents are not usually premeasured in medication room.
CRITICAL DECISION POINT If skin is broken (e.g., wound) use sterile gloves, not clean gloves.	
2. Close room curtain or door and position client comfortably. Remove gown or bed linen, keeping unaffected skin areas draped.	Provides client privacy and easy access to area being treated. Promotes client's comfort.
3. Wash affected area, removing all debris, crustations, and previous medication.	Removal of debris enhances penetration of topical drug through skin. Cleansing removes microorganisms resident in remaining debris.
4. Pat skin dry or allow area to air dry.	Excess moisture can interfere with even application of topical agent.
5. If skin is excessively dry and flaking, apply topical agent while skin is still damp.	Retains moisture within skin layers.
6. Remove gloves, and apply new clean gloves.	Sterile gloves are used when applying agents to open, noninfectious skin lesions. Disposable gloves prevent cross-contamination of infected or contagious lesions, and protect nurse from drug effects.

STEPS	RATIONALE
7. Apply topical agent.	
a. Technique for applying creams, ointments, and oil-based lotions:	
(1) Place approximately 1 to 2 teaspoons of medication in palm of gloved hand and soften by rubbing briskly between hands.	Softening of topical agent makes it easier to spread on skin.
(2) Once medication is thin and smooth, spread it evenly over skin surface, using long, even strokes that follow direction of hair growth.	Ensures even distribution of medication. Technique prevents irritation of hair follicles.
(3) Explain to client that skin may feel greasy after application.	Ointments often contain oils.
b. Technique for applying **nitroglycerin** (an **antianginal**) ointment:	
(1) Apply desired number of inches of ointment over paper measuring guide (see illustration).	Ensures correct dosage of medication.
(2) Antianginal medication may be applied to the chest area, back, upper arm, or legs. Do not apply on hairy surfaces or over scar tissue.	If client complains of headaches, apply ointment farther from head. Application on hairy surfaces or scar tissue may interfere with absorption.
(3) Apply ointment to skin surface by holding edge or back of the paper wrapper and placing ointment and wrapper directly on the skin (see illustration). Do not rub or massage ointment into skin.	Minimizes chance of ointment covering gloves and later touching nurse's hands. Medication is designed to absorb slowly over several hours and should not be massaged.
CRITICAL DECISION POINT **Rotate site when applying nitroglycerin pastes.**	
(4) Date and initial paper and note time.	Prevents missing doses.
(5) Secure ointment and paper with a strip of tape (optional).	Prevents tape from becoming loose.
(6) Remove previous dosage paper. Wipe off residual medication with tissue.	Prevents **overdose** that can occur with multiple dosage papers left in place.
c. Technique for applying a **transdermal** patch:	
(1) Choose a clean, dry area of the body that is free of hair.	Increases absorption.

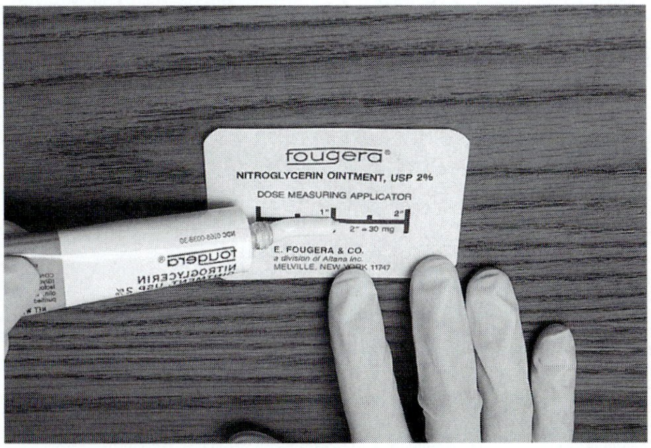

Step 7b(1)

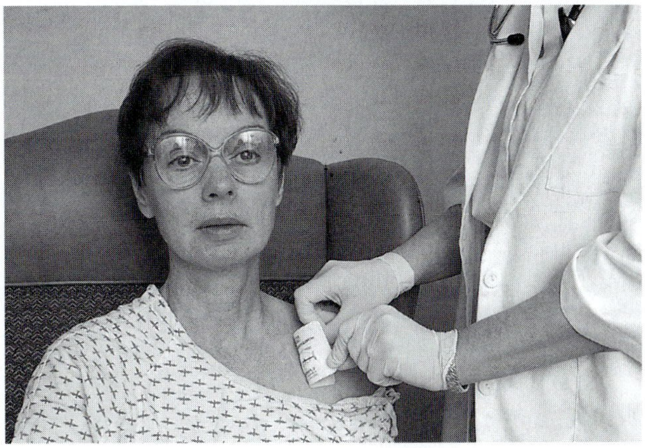

Step 7b(3)

STEPS	RATIONALE
CRITICAL DECISION POINT **Do not attempt to apply the patch on skin that is oily, burned, broken out, cut, or irritated in any way.**	
(2) Carefully remove the patch from its protective covering. Hold the patch by the edge; do not touch the adhesive edges.	Touching only the edges assures that the patch will adhere and that the medication dosage has not been changed.
(3) Immediately apply the patch, pressing firmly with the palm of one hand for 10 seconds. Make sure it sticks well, especially around the edges.	
(4) Date and initial patch and note time.	Visual reminder prevents missing or extra doses.
(5) After 24 hours (for most patches) remove the patch and choose a different site. Do not apply to previously used sites for at least 1 week.	
(6) Dispose of patches by folding in half with sticky sides together. Throw the patch in the trash away from children and pets.	
d. Technique for applying aerosolized medication (spray):	
(1) Shake container vigorously.	Mixes contents and propellant to ensure distribution of fine, even spray.
(2) Read container's label for distance recommended to hold spray away from area (usually 6 to 12 inches, 15 to 30 cm).	Proper distance ensures fine spray hits skin surface. Holding container too close results in thin, watery distribution.
(3) If neck or upper chest is to be sprayed, ask client to turn face away from spray or briefly cover face with towel.	Prevents inhalation of spray.
(4) Spray medication evenly over affected site (in some cases spray is timed for select period of seconds).	Entire affected area of skin should be covered with thin spray.
e. Technique for applying a **suspension**-based lotion:	
(1) Shake container vigorously.	Mixes powder throughout liquid to form well-mixed suspension.
(2) Apply small amount of lotion to small gauze dressing or pad and apply to skin by stroking evenly in direction of hair growth.	Method of application leaves protective film of powder on skin after water base of suspension dries. Technique prevents irritation to hair follicles.
(3) Explain to client that area will feel cool and dry.	Water evaporates to leave thin layer of powder.
f. Technique for applying a powder:	
(1) Be sure skin surface is thoroughly dry.	Minimizes caking and crusting of powder.
(2) Fully spread apart any skin folds such as between toes or under axilla.	Fully exposes skin surface for application.
(3) Dust skin site lightly with dispenser so that area is covered with fine, thin layer of powder.	Thin layer of powder is more absorbent and reduces friction by increasing area of moisture evaporation (Anders, 1982).
8. Cover skin area with dressing if ordered by physician.	May help prevent agent from being rubbed off skin. Protects clothing from being stained.
9. Assist client to comfortable position, reapply gown, and cover with bed linen as desired.	Provides for client's sense of well-being.
10. Remove gloves, dispose of soiled supplies in receptacle especially designated for such articles, and wash hands.	Keeps client's environment neat and reduces transmission of infection and/or residual medication to children, pets, or others.

STEPS	RATIONALE
EVALUATION	
1. Ask the client or significant other to name the medication and its action, purpose, dosage, schedule, and side effects.	Evaluates learning.
2. Have client keep a diary of dosages taken.	Confirm compliance with prescribed therapy.
3. Observe client apply lotion, ointment, or patch.	Return demonstration measures learning.
4. Inspect condition of skin between applications.	Determines if skin condition improves.
5. **Unexpected outcomes** that may occur include:	
➤ Skin site may appear inflamed and edematous with blistering and oozing of fluid from lesions.	Signs indicative of subacute inflammation or **eczema** that can develop from worsening of skin lesions.
➤ Client continues to complain of pruritus and tenderness.	Indicates slow or impaired healing; alternate therapies may be needed.
➤ Client is unable to explain information about drug.	Reinstruction is necessary, or client is unable to learn.
➤ Client fails to administer drug as ordered.	Indicates need to reexplore client's health beliefs.
RECORDING AND REPORTING	
1. Describe condition of skin before topical agent application in nurses' notes.	Documents client's condition and helps evaluate progress and response to therapy.
2. Record type of agent applied, strength, and site of application in nurses' notes and on MAR.	Prompt documentation prevents medication errors.
3. Report any abnormalities in condition of skin to nurse in charge or physician.	May indicate change in type of agent used or method of treatment.

FOLLOW-UP ACTIVITIES

1. Offer client or family member opportunity to apply topical agent during next application and to ask questions.

• • • • •

Special Considerations

➤ Antianginal (nitroglycerin) ointments are usually ordered in inches and can be measured on small sheets of paper marked off in ½-inch markings. Unit dose packages are available. (**Warning:** one package equals 1 inch; smaller amount should not be measured from this package.)

➤ Clients should be cautioned about using alternative forms of medications or drugs if using patches. For example, clients should not smoke while using a nicotine patch. Clients should not apply nitroglycerine ointment in addition to the patch unless specifically ordered to do so by their physician.

➤ If skin is inflamed, use only warm water rinse without soap for cleansing.

➤ When applying creams or ointments do not pat or rub skin. This may cause irritation.

Teaching Considerations

➤ A family member or friend may have to learn skill of topical application.

➤ When instructing client, be sure lighting is adequate and area to be treated is well exposed.

Gerontologic Considerations

➤ Many changes occur in the skin of the older adult client. The nurse should be aware of these changes when applying topical medications so that proper application can occur. For example, the older adult client's skin is often subject to increased capillary fragility, which can lead to bruising. The nurse handles the skin gently when applying an ointment. Table 18-1 lists common age-related skin changes and assessment findings.

Home Care Considerations

➤ Instruct client to dispose of applicators, patches, and similar materials into cardboard or plastic disposable containers. Careful disposal is necessary to ensure the safety of the client, other adults, pets, and children.

Table 18-1 Effect of Aging on the Integumentary System

Changes	Assessment Findings
Decreased subcutaneous fat, muscle laxity, degeneration of elastic fibers, collagen stiffening	Increased wrinkling, sagging breast and abdomen, redundant flesh around eyes, slowness of skin to flatten when pinched together (tenting)
Decreased extracellular water, surface lipids, and sebaceous gland activity	Dry flaking skin with possible signs of excoriation caused by pruritis
Increased capillary fragility and permeability	Evidence of bruising
Increased melanocytes in basal layer with pigment accumulation	Senile lentingines on face and back of hands
Diminished blood supply	Decrease in rosy appearance of skin and mucous membranes; cool to touch; diminished awareness of pain, touch, temperature and peripheral vibration
Decrease in proliferative capacity	Diminished rate of wound healing

Modified from: Lewis SM, Collier IC, Heitkemper MM, Assessment and management of clinical problems, *Medical surgical nursing*, ed 4, St Louis, 1996, Mosby.

SKILL 18-4 Administering Eye Medications

Common eye **(ophthalmic)** medications used by clients are drops and ointments, including over-the-counter preparations such as artificial tears and vasoconstrictors (e.g., *Visine* and *Murine*). However, many clients receive prescribed ophthalmic drugs for eye conditions such as **glaucoma,** infections, and postcataract extraction. Recently, a third type of medication is being used, intraocular disks. Medications delivered this way resemble a contact lens. The disk is placed into the conjunctival sac where it remains in place for up to one week.

The eye is the most sensitive organ to which the nurse applies medications. The cornea is richly supplied with sensitive nerve fibers. Care must be taken to prevent instilling medication directly onto the cornea. The conjunctival sac is much less sensitive and thus a more appropriate site for medication instillation.

Any client receiving topical eye medications should learn correct self-administration of the medication, especially clients with glaucoma, who must often undergo lifelong medication administration for control of their disease. Donnelly (1987) recommends instructing clients by breaking down the procedure for drop instillation into a series of steps so that if problems occur their exact nature can be determined. Nurses can easily instruct clients while administering medications. At times it may become necessary for family members to learn how to administer eye medications. This is particularly true immediately after eye surgery when a client's vision is so impaired that it is difficult to assemble needed supplies and handle applicators correctly.

Eye medications come in a variety of concentrations. Instilling the wrong concentration may cause local irritation to eyes, as well as systemic effects. Certain eye medications, such as mydriatics and **cycloplegics,** temporarily blur a client's vision. Use of the wrong drug concentration can prolong these undesirable effects.

EQUIPMENT

- Medication bottle with sterile eye dropper or ointment tube
- Medicated intraocular disk
- Cotton ball or tissue
- Washbasin filled with warm water and washcloth
- Eye patch and tape (optional)
- Clean gloves
- Medication administration record (MAR) or computer printout

STEPS	RATIONALE
ASSESSMENT	
1. Review prescriber's medication order for number of drops (if a liquid), and eye (right = **O.D.**; left = **O.S.**; both = **O.U.**) to receive medication.	Ensures correct administration of medication.
2. Assess condition of external eye structures (Skill 11-5). (May also be done just before drug instillation.)	Provides baseline to later determine if local response to medications occurs. Also indicates need to clean eye before drug application.
3. Determine whether client has any known allergies to eye medications. Also ask if client has allergy to latex.	Protects client from risk of allergic drug response. Will require use of nonlatex gloves.
4. Determine whether client has any symptoms of visual alterations.	Certain eye medications act to either lessen or increase these symptoms. Nurse must be able to recognize change in client's condition.
5. Assess client's level of consciousness and ability to follow directions.	If client becomes restless or combative during procedure, a greater risk of accidental eye injury exists.
6. Assess client's knowledge regarding drug therapy and desire to self-administer medication.	Client's level of understanding may indicate need for health teaching. Motivation influences teaching approach.
7. Assess client's ability to manipulate and hold dropper.	Reflects client's ability to learn to self-administer drug.

NURSING DIAGNOSIS

Clustering of defining characteristics from the assessment data may reveal the following nursing diagnoses for clients requiring this skill:

- Health-seeking behaviors or desire for high-level wellness (self-care)
- Risk for injury
- Impaired physical mobility
- Knowledge deficit (regarding drug actions and purpose)
- Pain
- Sensory perceptual alteration (visual)

Related factors are individualized based on a client's condition or needs.

STEPS	RATIONALE
PLANNING	
1. **Expected outcomes** following completion of procedure:	
➤ Client experiences desired effect of medication.	
➤ Client denies discomfort.	Drug is administered correctly without injury to client.
➤ Client experiences no side effects, and symptoms (e.g., irritation) are relieved.	Drug is distributed and absorbed properly.
➤ Client is able to discuss information about medication and technique correctly.	Demonstrates learning.
➤ Client demonstrates self-instillation of eye drops.	Demonstrates learning.
2. Compare MAR or computer printout with label of eye medication.	Ensures right drug is administered.
3. Check client's identification bracelet and ask name.	Ensures correct client receives medication.
4. Explain procedure to client.	Relieves anxiety about medication being instilled into eye.
IMPLEMENTATION	
1. Wash hands and arrange supplies at bedside; apply clean gloves.	Reduces transmission of microorganisms; ensures a smooth, orderly procedure.
2. Ask client to lie supine or sit back in chair with head slightly hyperextended.	Position provides easy access to eye for medication instillation and minimizes drainage of medication through tear duct.

CRITICAL DECISION POINT Do not hyperextend the neck of a client with cervical spine injury.

STEPS	RATIONALE
3. If crusts or drainage are present along eyelid margins or inner canthus, gently wash away. Soak any crusts that are dried and difficult to remove by applying damp washcloth or cotton ball over eye for a few minutes. Always wipe clean from inner to outer canthus (see illustration).	Crusts or drainage harbors microorganisms. Soaking allows easy removal and prevents pressure from being applied directly over eye. Cleansing from inner to outer canthus avoids entrance of microorganisms into lacrimal duct.
4. Hold cotton ball or clean tissue in nondominant hand on client's cheekbone just below lower eyelid.	Cotton or tissue absorbs medication that escapes eye.
5. With tissue or cotton resting below lower lid, gently press downward with thumb or forefinger against bony orbit (see illustration).	Technique exposes lower conjunctival sac. Retraction against bony orbit prevents pressure and trauma to eyeball and prevents fingers from touching eye.
6. Ask client to look at ceiling.	Action retracts sensitive cornea up and away from conjunctival sac and reduces stimulation of blink reflex.
7. Instill eye drops while explaining steps to client:	
a. With dominant hand resting on client's forehead, hold filled medication eye dropper approximately 1 to 2 cm (½ to ¾ inch) above conjunctival sac (see illustration).	Helps prevent accidental contact of eyedropper with eye structures, thus reducing risk of injury to eye and transfer of infection to dropper. Ophthalmic medications are sterile.

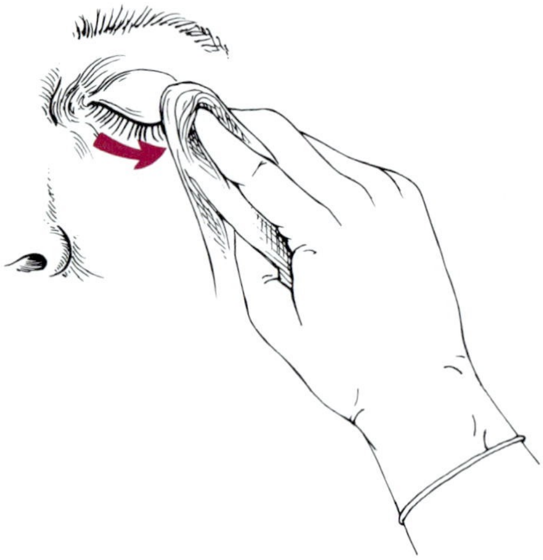

Step 3

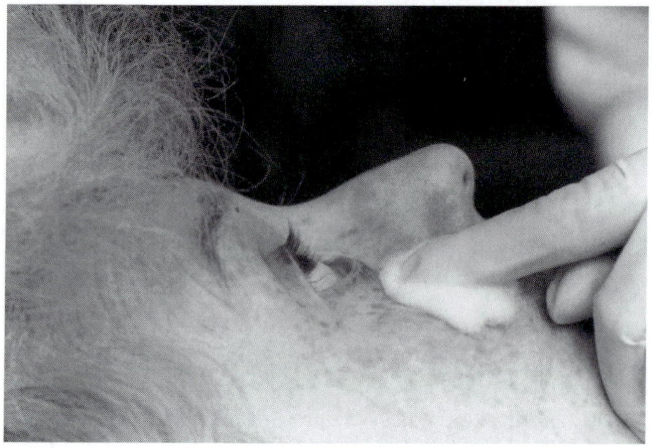

Step 5

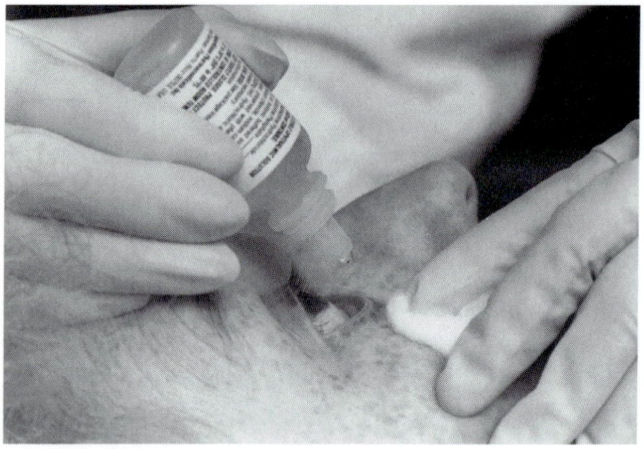

Step 7a

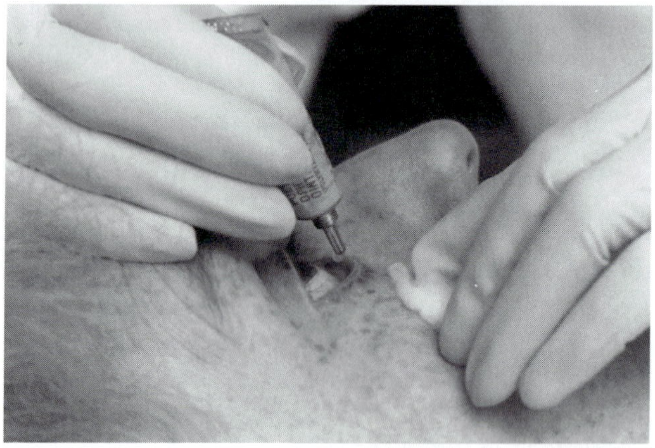

Step 8b

STEPS	RATIONALE
b. Drop prescribed number of medication drops into conjunctival sac.	Conjunctival sac normally holds 1 or 2 drops. Provides even distribution of medication across eye.
c. If client blinks or closes eye or if drops land on outer lid margins, repeat procedure.	Therapeutic effect of drug is obtained only when drops enter conjunctival sac.
d. When administering drugs that cause systemic effects; with a clean tissue apply gentle pressure to client's nasolacrimal duct for 30 to 60 seconds.	Prevents overflow of medication into nasal and pharyngeal passages. Prevents absorption into systemic circulation.
e. After instilling drops, ask client to close eye gently.	Helps to distribute medication. Squinting or squeezing of eyelids forces medication from conjunctival sac.
8. Instill eye ointment:	
a. Ask client to look at ceiling.	Action retracts sensitive cornea up and away from conjunctival sac and reduces stimulation of blink reflex.
b. Holding ointment applicator above lower lid margin, apply thin stream of ointment evenly along inner edge of lower eyelid on conjunctiva (see illustration) from the inner canthus to outer canthus.	Distributes medication evenly across eye and lid margin.
c. Have client close eye and rub lid lightly in circular motion with cotton ball, if rubbing is not contraindicated.	Further distributes medication without traumatizing eye.
9. Intraocular disk	
a. Application:	
(1) Open package containing the disk. Gently press your fingertip against the disk so that it adheres to your finger. Position the convex side of the disk on your fingertip.	Allows nurse to inspect disk for damage or deformity.
(2) With your other hand, gently pull the client's lower eyelid away from his eye. Ask client to look up.	Prepares conjunctival sac for receiving medicated disk.
(3) Place the disk in the conjunctival sac, so that it floats on the sclera between the iris and lower eyelid.	Ensures delivery of medication.
(4) Pull the client's lower eyelid out and over the disk.	Ensures accurate medication delivery.
CRITICAL DECISION POINT You should not be able to see the disk at this time. Repeat step 4 if you can see the disk.	
b. Removal:	
(1) Wash hands and don gloves.	
(2) Explain procedure to client.	
(3) Gently pull on the client's lower eyelid to expose the disk.	
(4) Using your forefinger and thumb of your opposite hand, pinch the disk and lift it out of the client's eye.	
10. If excess medication is on eyelid, gently wipe it from inner to outer canthus.	Promotes comfort and prevents trauma to eye.
11. If client had eye patch, apply clean one by placing it over affected eye so entire eye is covered. Tape securely without applying pressure to eye.	Clean eye patch reduces chance of infection.
12. Remove gloves, dispose of soiled supplies in proper receptacle, and wash hands.	Maintains neat environment at bedside and reduces transmission of microorganisms.

STEPS	RATIONALE
E VALUATION	
1. Note client's response to instillation; ask if any discomfort was felt.	Determines if procedure was performed correctly and safely.
2. Observe response to medication by assessing visual changes and noting any side effects.	Evaluates effects of medication.
3. Ask client to discuss drug's purpose, action, side effects, and technique of administration.	Determines client's level of understanding.
4. Have client demonstrate self-administration of next dose.	Provides feedback regarding competency with skill.
5. **Unexpected outcomes** that may occur include:	
➤ Client complains of burning or pain.	Eye drops instilled onto cornea or dropper touched surface of eye.
➤ Client experiences local side effects (e.g., headache, bloodshot eyes, local eye irritation).	Drug concentration and client's sensitivity both influence chances of side effects developing.
➤ Client experiences systemic effects from drops (e.g., increased heart rate and blood pressure from epinephrine, decreased heart rate and blood pressure from timolol).	Systemic absorption through tear duct can cause potentially dangerous effects.
CRITICAL DECISION POINT Notify prescriber immediately. Remain with client. Withhold further doses.	
➤ Client is unable to discuss information about medication correctly.	Reinstruction is needed, or client is unable to learn.
➤ Client is unable to instill eye drops.	Further practice is necessary.

Recording and Reporting

1. Record drug, concentration, number of drops, time of administration, and eye (left, right, or both) that received medication on MAR.	Timely documentation prevents drug errors (e.g., repeated or missed doses).
2. Record appearance of eye in nurses' notes.	Documents status or condition of eye.
3. Record and report any undesirable side effects to nurse in charge or physician.	Nature of client's reaction may require additional therapy.

Follow-up Activities

1. Clients who will be administering drugs at home should demonstrate instillation until performed correctly. Otherwise instruct family member.

• • • • •

Special Considerations

- ➤ Ophthalmic **anesthetics** and antibiotics may cause the same type of adverse reactions as systemically administered drugs (e.g., **anaphylaxis**).
- ➤ If eye drops are stored in refrigerator, rewarm to room temperature before administering.
- ➤ Clients experienced in self-instillation may be allowed to give drops under nurse's supervision (check agency policy).
- ➤ Never press directly against client's eyeball.
- ➤ Warn clients receiving mydriatics that vision will be temporarily blurred. Wearing sunglasses will reduce photophobia.
- ➤ Clients who receive medications that paralyze the ciliary muscles of the eye (e.g., Scopolamine; *Isopto Hyoscine,* Atropine; *Isopto Atropine* and cycloplegics) should temporarily not drive nor attempt to perform any activity that requires acute vision.

Teaching Considerations

- ➤ Many clients lack confidence in their ability to instill drops without supervision. Others are unable to manipulate the dropper or are unable to see. The nurse teaches others, such as a family member, to instill drops into the client's eye.

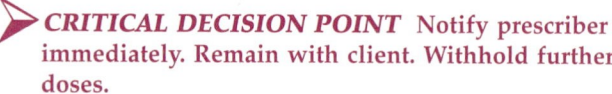

Pediatric Considerations

- When instilling drops in an infant or young child, have parent gently restrain child's head with child in parent's lap.
- Infants often clench the eyes tightly to avoid eye drops. To administer drops in an uncooperative infant, with the head gently restrained, place the drops at the nasal corner where the lids meet. When the child opens the eye the medication will flow into the eye.
- Eye ointments are easily placed into the sleeping child's eye.

Gerontologic Considerations

- The nurse carefully reviews the client's medical history for eye medications that should be given with caution. Eye medications, such as beta-blockers, can be systemically absorbed and cause complications.
- Prior to discharging the older client, the nurse evaluates the client's ability to perform all the necessary steps for the administration of eye drops and ointments.
- The nurse teaches family members of clients unable to perform the necessary skills. Clients without this type of assistance should be evaluated for home health nursing.

Home Care Considerations

- When using over-the-counter eye drops, clients should not share medications with other family members. Risk of infection transmission is high.
- Clients with chronic health care problems should consult with their health care provider prior to using over-the-counter eye medications.

SKILL 18-5 Administering Ear Drops

When administering ear **(otic)** medications the nurse should be aware of certain safety precautions. Internal ear structures are very sensitive to temperature extremes. Failure to instill a solution at room temperature can cause **vertigo** (severe dizziness) or nausea and debilitate a client for several minutes. Although structures of the outer ear are not sterile, use sterile drops and solutions in case the eardrum is ruptured. Entrance of nonsterile solutions into the middle ear can cause serious infection. A final precaution is to avoid forcing any solution into the ear. The nurse must not occlude the ear canal with a medicine dropper, because this can cause pressure within the canal during instillation and subsequent injury to the eardrum. If these precautions are followed, instillation of ear drops is a safe and effective therapy.

EQUIPMENT

- Medication bottle with dropper
- Cotton-tipped applicator
- Cotton ball (optional)
- Clean gloves (optional, only if client has drainage)
- Medication administration record (MAR) or computer printout

STEPS	RATIONALE
ASSESSMENT	
1. Review prescriber's medication order for number of drops to instill, and ear (right, left, or both) to receive medication.	Ensures safe and correct administration of medication.
2. Assess condition of external ear structures and canal (Skill 11-6).	Provides baseline to later determine if local response to medication occurs, whether client's condition improves, or whether it will be necessary to clean ear before instilling medication.
3. Determine whether client has symptoms of discomfort and/or hearing impairment.	Disorders of external ear can be painful. Occlusion of external ear canal by swelling, drainage, or **cerumen** can impair hearing acuity. These conditions may change after drug instillation and require ongoing monitoring.
4. Assess client's level of consciousness and ability to follow instructions.	Client must lie still during drug administration. Sudden movements can cause injury from ear dropper.

STEPS	RATIONALE
5. Assess client's level of knowledge regarding drug therapy and motivation to self-administer medication.	Client's knowledge level determines whether health teaching is required. Motivation influences teaching approach.
6. Assess client's ability to grasp and manipulate dropper.	Determines client's ability to self-administer drug.

NURSING DIAGNOSIS

Clustering of defining characteristics from the assessment data may reveal the following nursing diagnoses for clients requiring this skill:

- Health-seeking behaviors or desire for high-level wellness (self-care)
- Risk for injury
- Impaired physical mobility
- Knowledge deficit regarding drug actions and purpose
- Pain
- Sensory perceptual alteration (auditory)

Related factors are individualized based on a client's condition or needs.

PLANNING

STEPS	RATIONALE
1. Expected outcomes following completion of procedure:	
➤ Client denies discomfort during administration.	Procedure is performed correctly without injury to client.
➤ Ear canal becomes clear, without drainage, excess cerumen, or inflammation, as medication is repeatedly instilled.	Drug action is effective.
➤ Client's hearing acuity improves.	This response occurs only if hearing loss was caused by obstruction in external ear canal.
➤ Client is able to explain steps for instilling eardrops and demonstrates technique for administration.	Cognitive and psychomotor learning occurs.
2. Compare MAR and computer printout with label of medication.	Ensures right drug is administered.
3. Check client's identification bracelet and ask name.	Ensures right client receives drug.
4. Explain each step of procedure to client, allowing for questions.	Reduces client anxiety; timing of instruction enhances learning.

IMPLEMENTATION

STEPS	RATIONALE
1. Wash hands and arrange supplies at bedside. Apply clean gloves (if drainage is present).	Reduces transmission of microorganisms; helps nurse perform procedure smoothly.
2. Have client assume side-lying position (if not contraindicated by client's condition) with ear to be treated facing up, or client may sit in chair or at the bedside.	Position provides easy access to ear for instillation of medication. Ear canal is in position to receive medication.
3. Straighten ear canal by pulling auricle backward and outward.	Straightening of ear canal provides direct access to deeper external ear structures.
4. If cerumen or drainage occludes outermost portion of ear canal, wipe out gently with cotton-tipped applicator (see illustration).	Cerumen and drainage harbor microorganisms and can block distribution of medication.
➤ ***CRITICAL DECISION POINT*** **Do not force wax inward to block or occlude canal. Occlusion of canal interferes with normal sound conditions.**	
5. Instill prescribed drops holding dropper 1 cm (½ inch) above ear canal (see illustration).	Instilling drops into occluded canal can cause injury to eardrum.
6. Remove gloves, dispose of soiled supplies, and wash hands.	Reduces transmission of microorganisms.
7. Ask client to remain in side-lying position for 2 to 3 minutes. Apply gentle massage or pressure to tragus of ear with finger (see illustration).	Allows complete distribution of medication. Pressure and massage moves medication inward.

STEPS	RATIONALE
8. At times the prescriber orders insertion of portion of cotton ball into outermost part of canal. Do not press cotton into canal.	Inserting cotton into outer canal prevents escape of medication when client sits or stands. Cotton should not block canal to impair hearing.
9. Remove cotton after 15 minutes.	Time period promotes drug distribution and absorption.
10. Dispose of soiled supplies and wash hands.	Reduces transmission of microorganisms.
11. Assist client to comfortable position after drops are absorbed.	Restores comfort.

EVALUATION

STEPS	RATIONALE
1. Ask client if any discomfort is felt during instillation.	Determines if procedure is performed correctly and reveals severity of symptoms.
2. Evaluate condition of external ear between drug instillations.	Determines response to medication.
3. Evaluate client's hearing acuity.	Hearing may change after drug administration.
4. Ask client to explain technique for instilling ear drops and purpose of medication.	Evaluates degree of learning.
5. Have client demonstrate self-administration of next dose.	Provides feedback regarding competency with skill.
6. **Unexpected outcomes** that may occur include:	
➤ Ear canal is inflamed, swollen, tender to palpation. Drainage is present.	Symptoms of continuing ear infection are present.
➤ Ear canal is occluded by cerumen.	Wax has become impacted in canal.
➤ Client is unable to explain drug information and steps for drug instillation.	Nurse must repeat instructions, or client is unable to learn.
➤ Client's hearing acuity continues to be reduced.	Obstruction within ear canal is unrelieved.
➤ Client has difficulty self-administering ear drops.	Reinstruction is needed.

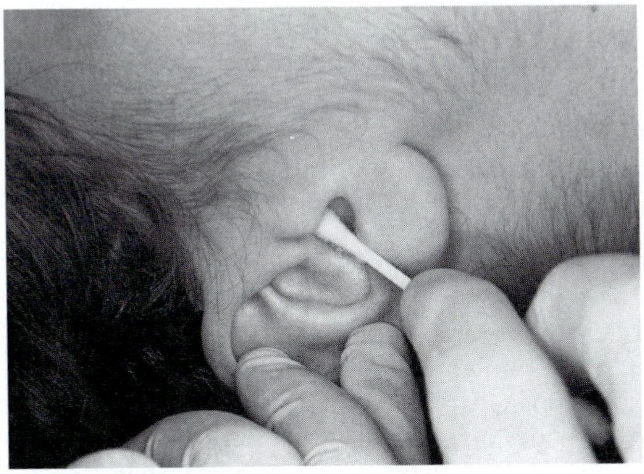

Step 4

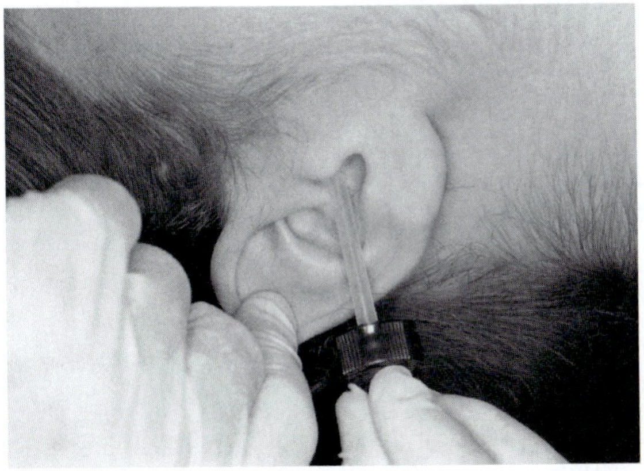

Step 5

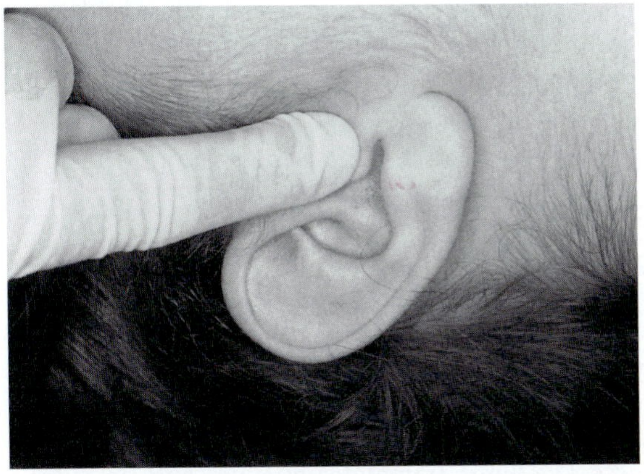

Step 7

STEPS	RATIONALE
RECORDING AND REPORTING	
1. Record drug, concentration, number of drops, time administered, and ear into which drops instilled on MAR.	Timely documentation prevents drug errors, such as repeated doses.
2. Record condition of ear canal in nurses' notes.	Documents client's status and response to therapy.
3. Report any sudden change in client's hearing acuity.	May require further medical care.

FOLLOW-UP ACTIVITIES

1. Have client demonstrate instillation of ear drops until performed correctly.

• • • • •

Special Considerations

- If client suffers hearing loss, use communication techniques such as enunciating words, getting client's attention, speaking in normal tone of voice, talking toward client's best ear.
- Ear drops should be warmed to room temperature. Hold bottle in hands or place in warm water.

Teaching Considerations

- This procedure is simple to teach clients and family members.
- Instruct client in proper way to cleanse ears, avoiding use of sharp objects in ear canal.
- Teach the signs of hearing loss and the need for frequent follow-up care to parents with children who have chronic otitis media.

Pediatric Considerations

- For children younger than 3 years of age gently pull the pinna of the ear downward and straight back.
- Infants or young children should be restrained in the supine position with the head turned to expose the affected ear. Hold the child in this position until the drug has time to be absorbed.

Gerontologic Considerations

- Some older adults experience excessive accumulation of cerumen in the ear. This should be removed before administration of medication.

SKILL 18-6 Administering Ear Irrigations

Medications used to irrigate or wash out a body cavity such as the ear (otic) are delivered through a stream of solution. The common indications for irrigation of the external ear are presence of a foreign body, local inflammation of the canal, and accumulation of cerumen. Irrigations should be done with liquid warmed to body temperature to avoid vertigo (dizziness) or nausea in clients (Fry, 1992).

The greatest danger during administration of an ear irrigation is rupture of the tympanic membrane. Fluids must not be instilled under pressure or with the ear canal occluded by the irrigating device.

EQUIPMENT

- Clean disposable gloves
- Otoscope (optional)
- Irrigation syringe
- Basin
- Towel
- Cotton balls
- Mineral oil or over-the-counter softener (optional)
- Medication administration record (MAR) or computer printout

STEPS	RATIONALE
ASSESSMENT	
1. Review prescriber's order including solution to be instilled and the affected ear(s).	Ensures safe and correct administration of medication.
2. Review medical record for history of ruptured tympanic membrane or visualize client's tympanic membrane using an otoscope (see Skill 11-6).	Contraindicates irrigation.
3. Inspect the pinna and external auditory meatus for redness, swelling, drainage, abrasions, and presence of cerumen or foreign objects. (If indicated, use an otoscope to inspect deeper portions of the auditory canal.) (See Skill 11-6).	Findings provide baseline to monitor effects of medication or solution.

STEPS	RATIONALE
4. Ask if client is experiencing discomfort. Note client's ability to hear clearly.	Pain is symptomatic of external ear infection or inflammation. Occlusion of auditory canal by cerumen or foreign object can impair hearing.
5. Review client's knowledge of purpose for irrigation and of normal care of the ears.	May indicate need for instruction regarding hygiene.

NURSING DIAGNOSIS

Clustering of defining characteristics from the assessment data may reveal the following nursing diagnoses for clients requiring this skill:

- Risk for injury
- Knowledge deficit (regarding irrigation purpose)
- Pain
- Sensory perceptual alterations (auditory)
- Risk for infection

Related factors are individualized based on a client's condition or needs.

PLANNING

STEPS	RATIONALE
1. **Expected outcomes** following completion of procedure:	
➤ Client denies pain during instillation.	Fluid is properly instilled.
➤ Client hears conversation clearly.	Obstruction in ear canal is resolved.
➤ Client is able to discuss purpose of irrigation and describe correct ear care techniques.	Feedback reflects client's learning.
➤ Skin overlying meatus and canal becomes clear, without redness, swelling, tenderness, or discharge. Canal is clear of cerumen and foreign material.	Inflammation, irritation, and occlusion of canal are relieved.
2. If client is found to have impacted cerumen, instill 1 to 2 drops of mineral oil or over-the-counter softener into ear twice a day for 2 to 3 days before irrigation.	Loosens cerumen and ensures easier removal during irrigation.
3. Check client's identification by reading identification bracelet and asking name.	Ensures correct client receives irrigation.
4. Explain procedure. Warn that the irrigation may cause sensation of dizziness, ear fullness, and warmth.	Prepares client to anticipate effects of irrigation and promotes cooperation.

IMPLEMENTATION

STEPS	RATIONALE
1. Wash hands, arrange supplies at bedside, and apply gloves.	Reduces transfer of microorganisms; helps nurse to perform procedure smoothly.
2. Close curtain or room door.	Maintains privacy.
3. Assist client to a sitting or lying position with head turned toward the affected ear (see illustration). Place towel under client's head and shoulder and have client hold basin under affected ear.	Position minimizes leakage of fluids around neck and facial area. Solution will flow from ear canal to basin.

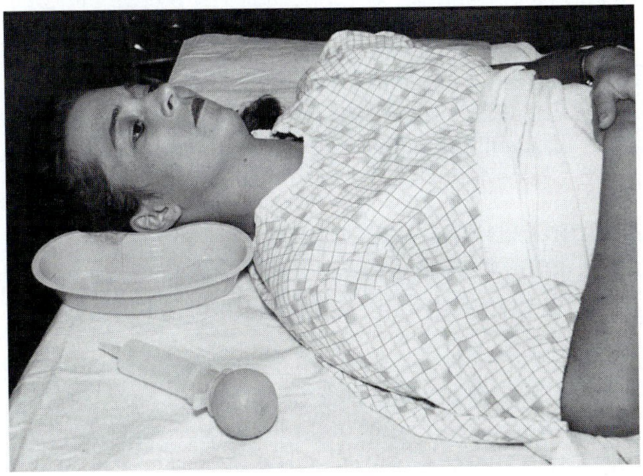

Step 3

STEPS	RATIONALE
4. Pour irrigating solution into sterile round basin.	
5. Gently clean auricle and outer ear canal with moistened cotton applicator. Do *not* force drainage or cerumen into the ear canal.	Prevents infected material from reentering ear canal.
6. Fill irrigating syringe with solution (approximately 50 ml).	Enough fluid is needed to provide a steady irrigating stream.
7. Gently grasp the auricle of the ear and straighten the ear canal by pulling it backward and outward.	Allows fluid to flow through length of the canal.
8. Slowly instill irrigating solution by holding the tip of the syringe 1 cm (½ inch) above the opening to the ear canal. The fluid should be directed toward the superior aspect of the ear canal. Allow fluid to drain out during instillation. Continue until canal is cleansed or solution is used (see illustration).	Slow instillation prevents buildup of pressure in the ear canal and ensures contact of the solution with all canal surfaces.

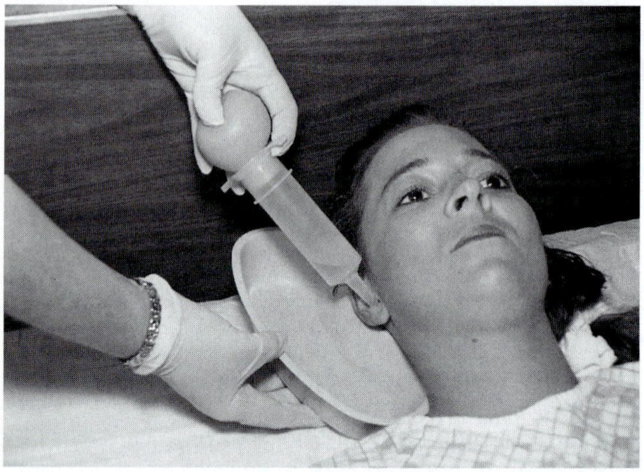

Step 8

STEPS	RATIONALE
9. Do *not* occlude the canal with the tip of the syringe.	Buildup of fluid in canal under forced pressure could cause rupture of the tympanic membrane.
10. Dry outer ear canal with cotton ball. Leave cotton loosely in place for 5 to 10 minutes.	Maintains comfort. Absorbs excess moisture in ear canal.
11. Assist client to a sitting position.	Maintains comfort.
12. Wash hands, remove gloves, and dispose of supplies.	Reduces transmission of infection.

EVALUATION

1. Ask client if discomfort is noted during instillation of solution.	Fluid instilled improperly under pressure causes discomfort.
2. Reinspect condition of meatus and canal.	Determines if solution relieves symptoms and removes foreign materials.
3. Measure client's hearing acuity.	Determines if conduction deafness is relieved.
4. Ask client to describe purpose of irrigation and proper techniques for ear care.	Reflects client's understanding of procedure and proper hygiene.
5. **Unexpected outcomes** that may occur include:	
➤ Client experiences increased ear pain.	Rupture of eardrum may have occurred.
➤ Ear canal remains occluded with cerumen.	Repeat irrigation is required.
➤ Client is unable to explain ear care practices.	Reinstruction is necessary.

RECORDING AND REPORTING

1. Record in nurses' notes and/or MAR, procedure, amount of solution instilled, time of administration, and ear receiving irrigation.	Timely documentation prevents treatment errors.
2. Record appearance of external ear and client's hearing acuity in nurses' notes.	Documents condition of ear and hearing status.
3. Record and report any undesirable side effects to nurse in charge or physician.	Nature of client's reaction may require additional therapy.

• • • • •

Special Considerations

- Always attempt to remove foreign objects in the ear by first simply straightening the ear canal. This may cause the object to fall out.
- If vegetable matter is occluded in the canal never irrigate the ear. The material can swell on contact with water.
- Refer clients to an otolaryngologist if a foreign object remains after irrigation.

Pediatric Considerations

- When cleansing the ear of a small child be certain the child's head is immobilized to prevent puncturing the ear drum. It may be necessary to have the child's parent participate in this procedure.

Teaching Considerations

- Instruct client that cerumen has an antibacterial effect that maintains an acid pH in the auditory canal.
- Instruct clients to clean ears daily with a washcloth, soap, and warm water.
- Warn clients against placing objects (including cotton swabs) in the ears.

Home Care Considerations

- Clients with increased cerumen production can use diluted vinegar warmed to body temperature as an irrigant 1 to 2 times per week for an effective, safe, and economical means of cerumen removal (Fry, 1992).
- Instruct the client to use a clean bulb syringe for irrigation.

SKILL 18-7 Administering Nasal Instillations

Clients with nasal sinus alterations may receive drugs by spray, drops, or tampons. The most commonly administered form of nasal instillation is a decongestant spray or drops used to relieve sinus congestion and cold symptoms. Many over-the-counter nose drops contain **sympathomimetic** drugs (such as *Afrin* or *Neo-Synephrine*). These drugs are relatively safe when administered nasally because only small doses are needed. However, the drugs can enter the systemic circulation by way of the nasal mucosa or gastrointestinal tract if an excess amount is swallowed. Repeated use of sprays can worsen nasal congestion because of a rebound effect. It is easy for a client to self-administer sprays. The client can be placed in a seated position with the head in a slightly hyperextended position.

Nasal drops (prescribed) often contain antibiotics for the treatment of sinus infections. Proper positioning of clients during instillation of drops is essential for medication to reach the affected sinus. The client should be instructed to lay in the supine position with head tilted back.

EQUIPMENT

- **Prepared medication with clean dropper or spray container**
- **Facial tissue**
- **Small pillow (optional)**
- **Washcloth (optional)**
- **Gloves (optional, only if client has extensive nasal drainage)**
- **Medication administration record (MAR) or computer printout**

STEPS	RATIONALE
ASSESSMENT	
1. For nasal drops, determine which sinus is affected by referring to medical record.	Affects client's position during drug instillation.
2. Assess client's history of hypertension, heart disease, diabetes, and hyperthyroidism.	These conditions can contraindicate use of decongestants that stimulate central nervous system. Side effects of transient hypertension, tachycardia, palpitations, and headache may occur.
3. Inspect condition of nose and sinuses (see Chapter 11-7). Palpate sinuses for tenderness.	Provides baseline to monitor effects of medication. Presence of discharge interferes with drug absorption.
4. Assess client's knowledge regarding use of nasal instillations and technique for instillation and willingness to learn self-administration.	May necessitate health teaching regarding use of drugs. Motivation influences teaching approach.

STEPS	RATIONALE

NURSING DIAGNOSIS

Clustering of defining characteristics from the assessment data may reveal the following nursing diagnoses for clients requiring this skill:

- Health-seeking behaviors or desire for high-level wellness (self-care)
- Risk for injury
- Knowledge deficit (regarding drug action and purpose)
- Pain

Related factors are individualized based on a client's condition or needs.

PLANNING

STEPS	RATIONALE
1. **Expected outcomes** following completion of procedure:	
➤ Client is able to breathe with ease through nose.	Nasal congestion has been relieved.
➤ Client's nasal sinuses become clear, moist, pink, without drainage after repeated instillations (applies to antiinfective medications).	Inflammation of mucosa has been relieved.
➤ Client is able to explain medication's purpose and administers nasal instillations correctly.	Feedback reflects client's learning.
2. Compare MAR or computer printout with label of nasal medication.	Ensures right drug is administered.
3. Check client's identification bracelet and ask name.	Ensures right client receives drug.
4. Explain procedure to client regarding positioning and sensations to expect, such as burning or stinging of mucosa, or choking sensation as medication trickles into throat.	Helps client anticipate experience of procedure to reduce anxiety.

IMPLEMENTATION

STEPS	RATIONALE
1. Wash hands. Arrange supplies and medications at bedside.	Reduces transmission of microorganisms; ensures smooth, orderly procedure.
2. Instruct client to clear or blow nose gently unless contraindicated (e.g., risk of increased intracranial pressure or nosebleeds).	Removes mucus and secretions that can block distribution of medication.
3. Administer nasal drops:	
a. Assist client to supine position.	Position provides access to nasal passages.

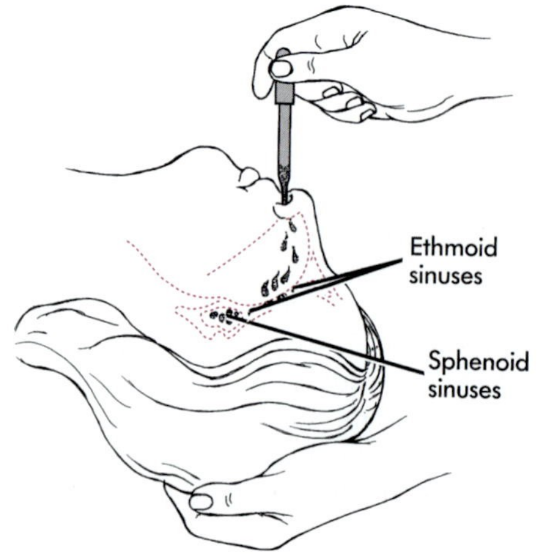

Step 3b(2)

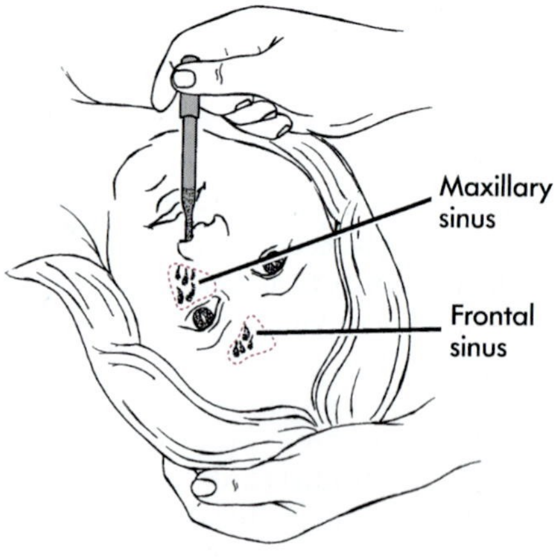

Step 3b(3)

STEPS	RATIONALE
b. Position head properly:	
(1) For access to posterior pharynx, tilt client's head backward.	
(2) For access to ethmoid or sphenoid sinus, tilt head back over edge of bed or place small pillow under client's shoulder and tilt head back (see illustration on p. 594).	
(3) For access to frontal and maxillary sinus, tilt head back over edge of bed or pillow with head turned toward side to be treated (see illustration on p. 594).	Position allows medication to drain into affected sinus.
c. Support client's head with nondominant hand.	Prevents straining of neck muscles.
d. Instruct client to breathe through mouth.	Mouth breathing reduces chance of aspirating nasal drops into trachea and lungs.
e. Hold dropper 1 cm (½ inch) above **nares** and instill prescribed number of drops toward midline of ethmoid bone.	Avoids contamination of dropper. Instilling toward ethmoid bone facilitates distribution of medication over nasal mucosa.
f. Have client remain in supine position 5 minutes.	Prevents premature loss of medication through nares.
g. Offer facial tissue to blot runny nose, but caution client against blowing nose for several minutes.	Allows maximal amount of medication to be absorbed.
4. Assist client to a comfortable position after drug is absorbed.	Restores comfort.
5. Dispose of soiled supplies in proper container and wash hands.	Maintains neat, orderly environment. Reduces spread of microorganisms.

EVALUATION

1. Observe client for onset of side effects 15 to 30 minutes after administration.	Drugs absorbed through mucosa can cause systemic reaction.
2. Ask if client is able to breathe through nose after decongestant administration. May be necessary to have client occlude one nostril at a time and breathe deeply.	Determines effectiveness of decongestant medication.
3. Reinspect condition of nasal passages between instillations.	Condition of mucosa reveals response to medication.
4. Ask client to review risks of overuse of decongestants and methods for administration.	Feedback ensures that client can self-administer drugs properly.
5. Have client demonstrate self-medication.	Feedback demonstrates learning.
6. **Unexpected outcomes** that may occur include:	
➤ Client is unable to breathe easily through nasal passages. Mucosa appears swollen.	Congestion is unrelieved. Client may be experiencing rebound effect.
➤ Nasal mucosa remains inflamed and tender with discharge from nares.	Inflammatory or infective process remains.
➤ Client complains of sinus headache.	Sinuses remain congested.
➤ Client is unable to explain technique and risks of drug therapy.	Further explanation is required.
➤ Client is unable to self-administer medication.	Reinstruction is necessary.

RECORDING AND REPORTING

1. Record medication administration including drug name, concentration, number of drops; nostril into which drug was instilled; and time of administration.	Timely documentation prevents drug errors.
2. Record client's response in nurses' notes.	Documents response to therapy.
3. Report any unusual systemic effects to nurse in charge or physician.	Response may require further treatment or monitoring.

• • • • •

Special Considerations

- Clear nasal discharge indicates sinus problem. Yellow or greenish discharge indicates infection.
- Use over-the-counter nasal sprays or nose drops for only one illness; bottles become easily contaminated with bacteria.

Pediatric Considerations

- When administering nasal medications to children positioning the child with the head extended over the edge of the bed or pillow facilitates smooth instillation of nasal drops. Instruct the child or parent to remain in this position for at least 1 minute to ensure that drops come into contact with affected tissue.

Teaching Considerations

- Instruct clients that each family member should have a different dropper or spray applicator. Applicators should be washed or rinsed after each use.
- Caution clients against overuse of nasal spray decongestants as can cause rebound effect; worsening of mucosal swelling. Risk increases as more drug is used.

SKILL 18-8 Using Metered-Dose Inhalers

Metered-dose inhalers (MDI) are hand-held inhalers that disperse medications through an aerosol spray, mist, or fine powder to penetrate lung airways (Fig. 18-1). The deeper passages of the respiratory tract provide a large surface area for drug absorption. The alveolar-capillary network absorbs medication rapidly.

Inhaled medications are usually designed to produce local effects; for example, bronchodilators open narrowed bronchioles, and mucolytic agents liquefy thick mucous secretions. However, since these medications are absorbed rapidly through the pulmonary circulation, some have the potential for producing systemic side effects (e.g., Isoproterenol *[Isuprel]* dilates bronchioles but can also cause cardiac dysrhythmias).

Clients who receive drugs by inhalation frequently suffer from chronic respiratory disease. Drugs administered by inhalation provide control of airway hyperreactivity or constriction. Because clients depend on these medications for disease control, they must learn about the medication and how to administer them safely.

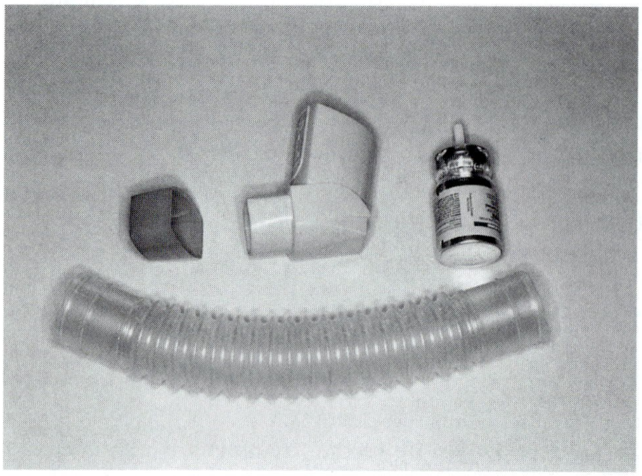

Fig. 18-1 Example of a metered dose inhaler (MDI) with spacer.

Drugs can be administered by MDIs in high concentrations with few side effects. A MDI delivers a measured dose of the drug with each push of a canister. Approximately 5 to 10 pounds of pressure must be used to activate the aerosol. This may be a problem for older age clients because hand strength diminishes with age. Because use of a metered-dose inhaler requires coordination during the breathing cycle, many clients spray only the back of their throats and fail to receive a full dose. The inhaler must be depressed to expel medication just as the client

COMMON PROBLEMS IN USING AN INHALER

1. Not taking the medication as *prescribed*, but taking either too much or too little.
2. Incorrect activation. This usually occurs through pressing the canister *before* taking a breath. Both should be done simultaneously so that the drug can be carried down to the lungs with the breath.
3. Forgetting to shake the inhaler. The drug is in a suspension, and therefore particles may settle. If the inhaler is not shaken, it may not deliver the correct dosage of the drug.
4. Not waiting long enough between puffs. The whole process should be repeated to take the second puff, otherwise an incorrect dosage may occur, or the drug may not penetrate into the lungs.
5. Failure to clean the valve. Particles may jam up the valve in the mouthpiece unless it is cleaned occasionally. This is a frequent cause of failure to get 200 puffs from one inhaler.
6. Failure to observe whether the inhaler is actually releasing a spray. If it is not, this should be checked with the pharmacist.

inhales. This ensures the medication reaches the lower airways. Poor coordination can be solved by the use of spacer devices *(Aerochamber, Inspirease)* or the use of a breath-activated MDI *(Maxair Autoinhaler)* (Weilitz and Van Sciver, 1996).

EQUIPMENT

- **Metered-dose inhaler with medication canister**
- **Aerochamber (optional)**
- **Facial tissues (optional)**
- **Wash basin or sink with warm water**
- **Paper towel**
- **Medication administration record (MAR) or computer printout**

STEPS	RATIONALE
ASSESSMENT	
1. Assess client's ability to hold, manipulate, and depress canister and inhaler.	Any impairment of grasp or presence of hand tremors interferes with client's ability to depress canister within inhaler.
2. Assess client's readiness to learn: client asks questions about medication, disease, or complications; requests education in use of inhaler; is mentally alert; participates in own care.	Affects client's ability to understand explanations and actively participate in teaching process.
3. Assess client's ability to learn: client should not be fatigued, in pain, or in respiratory distress; assess level of understanding of technical vocabulary terms.	Mental or physical limitations affect client's ability to learn and methods nurse uses for instruction.
4. Assess client's knowledge and understanding of disease and purpose and action of prescribed medications.	Knowledge of disease is essential for client to realistically understand use of inhaler.
5. Assess drug schedule and number of inhalations prescribed for each dose.	Influences explanations nurse provides for use of inhaler.
6. If previously instructed in self-administration of inhaled medicine, assess client's technique in using an inhaler.	Nurse's instruction may require only simple reinforcement depending on client's level of dexterity.

NURSING DIAGNOSIS

Clustering of defining characteristics from the assessment data may reveal the following nursing diagnoses for clients requiring this skill:

- ➤ Health-seeking behaviors or desire for high-level wellness (self-care)
- ➤ Risk for injury
- ➤ Ineffective management of therapeutic regimen
- ➤ Knowledge deficit regarding use of MDI

Related factors are individualized based on a client's condition or needs.

STEPS	RATIONALE
PLANNING	
1. **Expected outcomes** following completion of procedure:	
➤ Client describes techniques for use of MDI.	Ensures compliance with therapeutic regimen.
➤ Client correctly self-administers metered dose.	Demonstrates learning.
➤ Client's breathing patterns are effective.	Demonstrates proper administration of medication.
➤ Client's gas exchange is adequate.	Demonstrates proper administration of medication.
2. Instruct client in comfortable environment by sitting in chair in hospital room or sitting at kitchen table in home.	Client will be more likely to remain receptive of nurse's explanations.
3. Provide adequate time for teaching session.	Prevents interruptions. Instruction should occur when client is receptive.
IMPLEMENTATION	
1. Wash hands and arrange equipment needed.	Reduces transfer of microorganisms and saves time.
2. Allow client opportunity to manipulate inhaler, canister, and spacer device (aerochamber [Fig. 18-1]). Explain and demonstrate how canister fits into inhaler.	Client must be familiar with how to use equipment.

STEPS	RATIONALE
3. Explain what metered dose is, and warn client about overuse of inhaler, including drug side effects.	Client must not arbitrarily administer excessive inhalations because of risk of serious side effects. If drug is given in recommended doses, side effects are uncommon.
4. Explain steps for administering inhaled dose of medication (demonstrate steps when possible):	Use of simple, step-by-step explanations allows client to ask questions at any point during procedure.
a. Remove mouthpiece cover from inhaler.	
b. Shake inhaler well.	Ensures fine particles are aerosolized.
c. Have client take a deep breath and exhale.	Prepares the client's airway to receive the medication.
d. Instruct the client to position the inhaler in one of two ways.	
(1) Open lips and place inhaler in mouth with opening toward back of throat (see illustration).	
(2) Position the device 1 to 2 inches from the mouth (see illustration).	Directs aerosol spray toward airway. Positioning the mouthpiece 1 to 2 inches from the mouth is considered the best way to deliver the medication.
e. With the inhaler properly positioned, have client hold inhaler with thumb at the mouthpiece and the index finger and middle finger at the top. This is called a three-point or lateral hand position.	Metered-dose inhalers work best when clients use a three-point or lateral hand position to activate canisters (Statz, 1984).
f. Instruct client to tilt head back slightly, inhale slowly and deeply through mouth, depress medication canister fully.	Medication is distributed to airways during inhalation. Inhalation through mouth rather than nose draws medication more effectively into airways.
g. Hold breath for approximately 10 seconds.	Allows tiny drops of aerosol spray to reach deeper branches of airways.
h. Exhale through pursed lips.	Keeps small airways open during exhalation.
5. Explain steps to administer inhaled dose of medication using a spacer such as an aerochamber (demonstrate when possible):	
a. Remove mouthpiece cover from metered-dose inhaler and mouthpiece of aerochamber.	Inhaler fits into end of aerochamber.

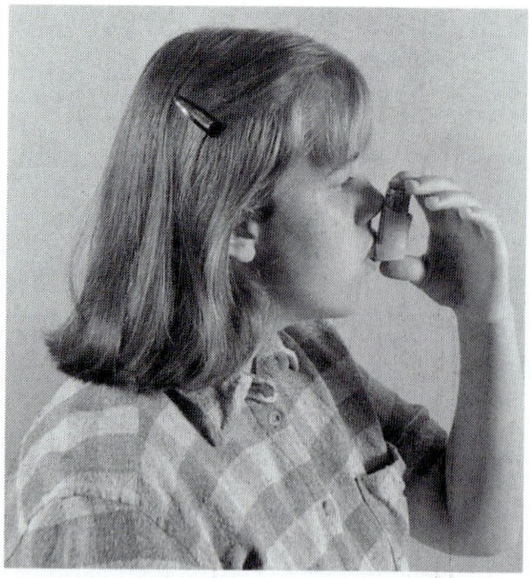

Step 4d(1) One technique for use of the inhaler. The client opens lips and places inhaler in mouth with opening toward back of throat.

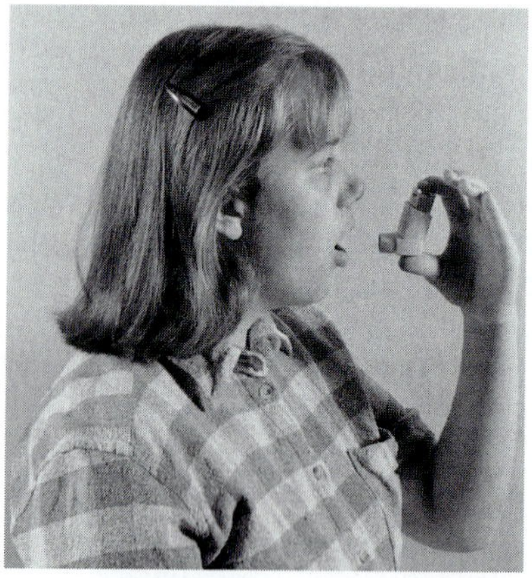

Step 4d(2) One technique for use of the inhaler. The client positions the mouthpiece 1 to 2 inches from the mouth. This is considered the best way to deliver the medication.

STEPS	RATIONALE
b. Insert MDI into end of aerochamber (see illustration).	Aerochamber is a spacer that traps medication released from the MDI; the client then inhales the drug from the device. These devices deposit up to 80% more medication in the lungs rather than the oropharynx (Weilitz, 1994).
c. Shake inhaler well.	Ensures fine particles are aerosolized.
d. Place aerochamber mouthpiece in mouth and close lips. Do not insert beyond raised lip on mouthpiece. Avoid covering small exhalation slots with the lips.	Medication should not escape through mouth.
e. Breathe normally through aerochamber mouthpiece.	Allows client to relax before delivering medication.
f. Depress medication canister, spraying one puff into aerochamber.	Emits spray that allows finer particles to be inhaled. Large droplets are retained in aerochamber.
g. Breathe in slowly and fully (for 5 seconds).	Ensures particles of medication are distributed to deeper airways.
h. Hold full breath for 5 to 10 seconds.	Ensures full drug distribution.
6. Instruct client to wait 2 to 5 minutes between inhalations or as ordered by prescriber.	Drugs must be inhaled sequentially. First inhalation opens airways and reduces inflammation. Second or third inhalations penetrate deeper airways.
7. Instruct client against repeating inhalations before next scheduled dose (see the box on p. 596).	Drugs are prescribed at intervals during day to provide constant drug levels and minimize side effects. Beta-**adrenergic** MDIs are used either on an "as needed" basis or regularly every 4 to 6 hours.
8. Explain that client may feel gagging sensation in throat caused by droplets of medication on pharynx or tongue.	Results when inhalant is sprayed and inhaled incorrectly.
9. Instruct client in removing medication canister and cleaning inhaler in warm water.	Accumulation of spray around mouthpiece can interfere with proper distribution during use.
10. Ask if client has any questions.	Clarifies misconceptions or misunderstanding.

EVALUATION

1. Have client explain and demonstrate steps in use of inhaler.	Return demonstration provides feedback for measuring client's learning.
2. Ask client to explain drug schedule.	Improves likelihood of compliance with therapy.

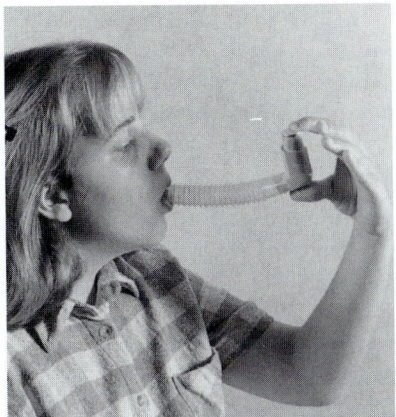

Step 5b Spacer (aerochamber) for metered-dose inhaler.

STEPS	RATIONALE
3. Ask client to describe side effects of medication and criteria for calling physician.	Allows client to recognize signs of overuse and need to seek medical support when drugs are ineffective.
4. After medication instillation, assess client's respirations and auscultate lungs.	Determines status of breathing pattern and adequacy of ventilation.
5. **Unexpected outcomes** that may occur include:	
➤ Client's breathing pattern is ineffective; respirations are rapid and shallow.	May need to reassess type of medication or delivery method.
➤ Client experiences paroxysms of coughing.	Aerosolized particles irritate posterior pharynx.
➤ Client experiences cardiac dysrhythmias.	Client may experience side effects from medication.
➤ Client may not be able to self-administer medication properly.	Alternative delivery routes or methods may need to be explored.
➤ Client is unable to explain technique and risks of drug therapy.	Further teaching may be required.

Recording and Reporting

1. Document in nurses' notes what skills were taught and client's ability to perform skills.	Information provides continuity to teaching plan so other members of nursing staff will not teach same material.
2. Record time when client used the inhaler and the amount (puffs).	Timely documentation prevents errors and overuse.
3. Report any undesirable effects from medication.	Client's response to medical regimen is necessary to progress toward goals.

Follow-up Activities

1. Client may need supervised practice for several different steps of procedure before being able to perform each skill independently.
2. If client experiences cardiac dysrhythmias from medication administration it may be necessary to place the client on telemetry monitoring to document the type of dysrhythmias. If the client experiences symptoms with the dysrhythmias (e.g., lightheadedness, syncope) withhold all further doses of medication. Discuss with prescriber.

• • • • •

Special Considerations

➤ Signs and symptoms of overuse of xanthines and sympathomimetic drugs include tachycardia, palpitations, headache, restlessness, and insomnia.
➤ Client may gag or swallow medication if unable to inhale while spray is administered.
➤ Client's need for a bronchodilator more than every 4 hours can signal respiratory problems.

Teaching Considerations

➤ Teach client how to determine fullness of canisters, using displacement in water (Fig. 18-2).
➤ Do not try to teach a client how to use an inhaler during an episode of shortness of breath. Client's attention span will be very poor.

Pediatric Considerations

➤ Educate child and parent about the need to use inhaler during school hours. Help family find resources within the school or day care facility.

Gerontologic Considerations

➤ Elderly client may be unable to depress medication canister because of weakened grasp.

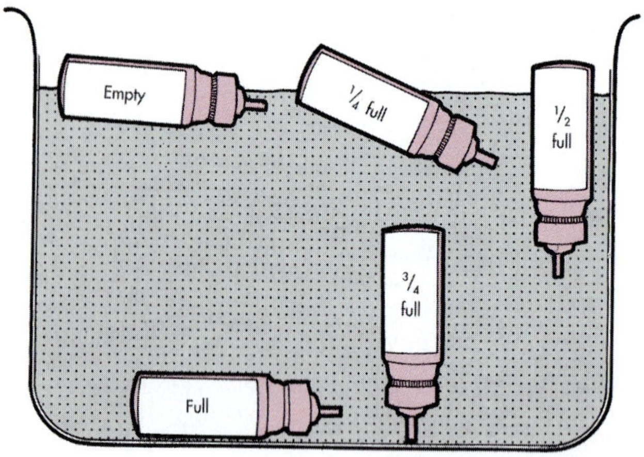

Fig. 18-2 A simple method of estimating amount left in the inhalant canister is to place it in a container filled with water. The position the canister takes in the water determines the amount of inhalant remaining.

SKILL 18-9 Administering Vaginal Instillations

Female clients can often develop vaginal infections requiring topical application of antiinfective agents. Vaginal medications are available in foam, jelly, cream, or suppository form. Medicated irrigations or douches can also be given. However, their excessive use can lead to vaginal irritation.

Vaginal suppositories are oval shaped and come individually packaged in foil wrappers. Storage in a refrigerator prevents the solid suppositories from melting. A suppository is inserted into the vagina with a gloved hand or applicator. After insertion, body temperature causes the suppository to melt and be distributed. Foam, jellies, and creams are administered with an inserter or applicator. Clients often prefer administering their own vaginal medications and should be given privacy to do so. After instillation of the drug, a client may wish to wear a perineal pad to collect excess drainage. Because vaginal medications are frequently given to treat infection, any discharge may be foul smelling. Good aseptic technique should be followed, and the client should be offered frequent opportunities to maintain perineal hygiene (see Skill 6-2).

EQUIPMENT

- Vaginal creams, foam, jelly, or suppositories, or irrigating solutions
- Applicators
- Disposable gloves
- Tissues
- Paper towel
- Perineal pad
- Drape
- Water-soluble lubricants
- Bedpan
- Irrigation or douche container
- Medication administration record (MAR) or computer printout

STEPS	RATIONALE
ASSESSMENT	
1. Review prescriber's order including client's name, drug name, form (cream or suppository), route, dosage, and time of administration.	Ensures safe and correct administration of medication.
CRITICAL DECISION POINT Caution: Rectal and vaginal suppositories may be stored together in a refrigerator. Vaginal suppositories are larger and more oval.	
2. Review pertinent information related to medication, including action, purpose, side effects, and nursing implications.	Allows nurse to administer drug properly and to monitor client's response.
3. Inspect condition of external genitalia and vaginal canal (Skill 11-14). (May be done just before insertion.)	Findings provide baseline to monitor effect of medication.
4. Ask if client is experiencing any symptoms of pruritus, burning, or discomfort.	Assesses for symptoms of vaginal irritation.
5. Assess client's ability to manipulate applicator or suppository and to properly position self to insert medication. (May be done just before insertion.)	Mobility restriction indicates level of assistance required from nurse.
6. Review client's knowledge of purpose of drug therapy and interest in self-administering medication.	May indicate need for health teaching. Understanding influences compliance with therapy.

NURSING DIAGNOSIS

Clustering of defining characteristics from the assessment data may reveal the following nursing diagnoses for clients requiring this skill:

- Health-seeking behaviors or desire for high-level wellness (self-care)
- Risk for noncompliance (with drug therapy)
- Impaired physical mobility
- Knowledge deficit regarding vaginal medication administration
- Pain
- Sexual dysfunction

Related factors are individualized based on a client's condition or needs.

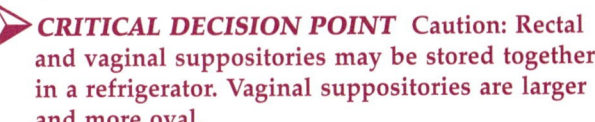

STEPS	RATIONALE
PLANNING	
1. **Expected outcomes** following completion of procedure:	
➤ Vaginal tissues are pink and smooth. Genitalia are clear and without discharge.	Tissues take on normal characteristics.
➤ Client denies symptoms of discomfort.	Inflammation has resolved.
➤ A small amount of discharge may be seen that is the color of medication exiting from vaginal canal.	When suppository or cream becomes distributed, small amount may escape from **orifice.**
➤ Client is able to discuss information about prescribed drug.	Feedback reflects client's learning.
➤ Client self-administers suppository or medication.	Demonstrates learning.
2. Compare MAR or computer printout with label of medication.	Ensures right medication is administered.
3. Check client's identification bracelet and ask name.	Ensures correct client receives medication.
4. Explain procedure to client. Be specific if client plans on self-administering medication.	Promotes client's understanding. Enables client to self-administer drug if physically able.
IMPLEMENTATION	
1. Wash hands, arrange supplies at bedside, and don clean gloves.	Reduces transfer of microorganisms; helps nurse perform procedure smoothly.
2. Close room curtain or door.	Provides privacy.
3. Check client's identification by reading identification bracelet and asking name.	Ensures the correct client receives medication.
4. Assist client to lie in dorsal recumbent position.	Position provides easy access to and good exposure of vaginal canal. Dependent position also allows suppository to dissolve in vagina without escaping.
5. Keep abdomen and lower extremities draped.	Minimizes client's embarrassment.
6. Be sure vaginal orifice is well-illuminated by room light.	Proper insertion requires visualization of external genitalia if not self-administered.
7. Inspect condition of external genitalia and vaginal canal (Skill 11-14).	Provides baseline to monitor effect of medication.
8. For suppository insertion:	
a. Remove suppository from wrapper and apply liberal amount of petroleum jelly to smooth or rounded end (see illustration). Lubricate gloved index finger of dominant hand.	Lubrication reduces friction against mucosal surfaces during insertion.
b. With nondominant gloved hand, gently separate labial folds.	Exposes vaginal orifice.

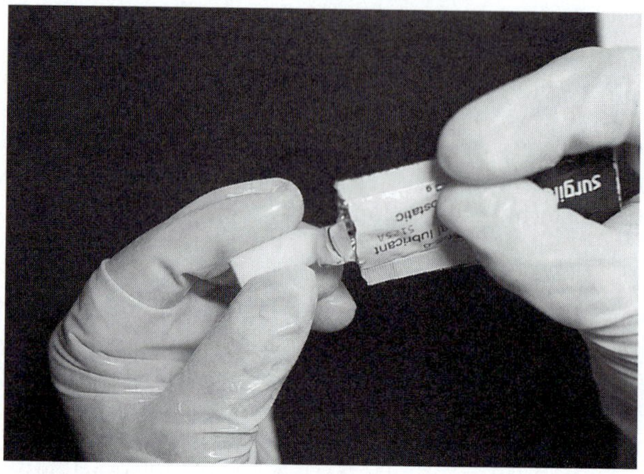

Step 8a

STEPS	RATIONALE
c. Insert rounded end of suppository along posterior wall of vaginal canal entire length of finger (7.5 to 10 cm or 3 to 4 in) (see illustration).	Proper placement of suppository ensures equal distribution of medication along walls of vaginal cavity.
d. Withdraw finger and wipe away remaining lubricant from around orifice and labia.	Maintains comfort.
9. For application of cream or foam:	
a. Fill cream or foam applicator following package directions.	Dose is instilled based on volume in applicator.
b. With nondominant gloved hand, gently separate labial folds.	Exposes vaginal orifice.
c. With dominant gloved hand, insert applicator approximately 5 to 7.5 cm (2 to 3 inches). Push applicator plunger to deposit medication into vagina (see illustration).	Allows equal distribution of medication along vaginal walls.
d. Withdraw applicator and place on paper towel. Wipe off residual cream from labia or vaginal orifice.	Residual cream on applicator may contain microorganisms.
10. For irrigation and douche:	
a. Place client on bedpan with absorbent pad underneath.	Allows hips to be higher than shoulders and solution reaches posterior wall of the vagina. Bedpan collects solution.
b. Be sure fluid is at body temperature. Run fluid through container nozzle (priming the tubing).	Body temperature promotes client comfort. Priming tubing removes air and moistens the nozzle tip.
c. Gently separate labial folds and direct nozzle toward the sacrum, following the floor of the vagina.	Correct angle allows nozzle access into the vagina.
d. Raise the container approximately 30 to 50 cm (12 to 20 inches) above level of vagina. Insert the nozzle 7 to 10 cm (3 to 4 inches). Allow the solution to flow while rotating the nozzle. Administer all the irrigating solution.	Rotating the nozzle allows irrigation of all areas in the vagina.
e. Withdraw the nozzle and assist the client to a comfortable sitting position.	Remaining solution drains by gravity.
f. Allow client to remain on bedpan for a few minutes. Cleanse perineum with soap and water.	Ensures all solution drains from vagina. Provides comfort for the client.
11. Instruct client who received suppository or cream to remain on her back for at least 10 minutes.	Medication will be distributed and absorbed evenly throughout vaginal cavity and not be lost through orifice.

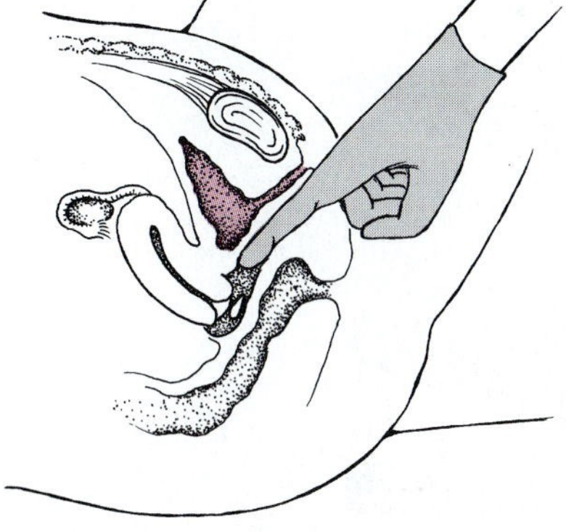

Step 8c

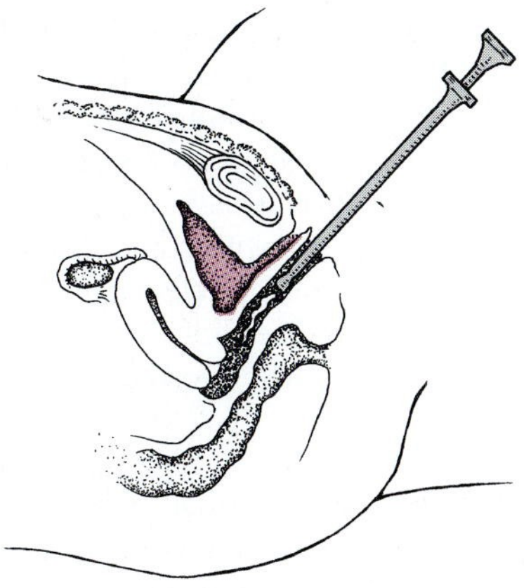

Step 9c

STEPS	RATIONALE
12. If applicator is used, wash with soap and warm water, rinse, and store for future use.	Vaginal cavity is not sterile. Soap and water assist in removal of bacteria and residual cream.
13. Offer perineal pad when client resumes ambulation.	Provides client comfort.
14. Remove and dispose of gloves and other soiled equipment; wash hands.	Reduces transmission of microorganisms.
EVALUATION	
1. Inspect condition of vaginal canal and external genitalia between applications.	Determines whether vaginal medication effectively reduced irritation or inflammation of tissues.
2. Question client regarding continued pruritus, burning, or discomfort.	Determines whether symptoms are relieved.
3. Ask client to discuss purpose, action, side effects of medication.	Reflects client's understanding of drug therapy.
4. Have client demonstrate administration of next dose.	Reflects learning of technique.
5. **Unexpected outcomes** that may occur include:	
➤ A thick, white, patchy, curdlike discharge is clinging to vaginal walls. Vaginal walls appear bright pink or inflamed.	Signs of yeast infection, a common female disorder.
➤ Client reports localized pruritus and burning.	Result of infection or inflammation.
➤ Client is unable to discuss drug therapy correctly.	Requires repeated instruction, or client is unable to learn.
➤ Client is unable to self-administer medication.	Reinstruction is necessary.
RECORDING AND REPORTING	
1. Record appearance of vaginal canal and genitalia in nurses' notes and report any unusual findings.	Documented description provides guidelines to determine change in client's condition and records client's response to therapy.
2. Record drug name, dosage, time administered, and route on MAR.	

Special Considerations

- ➤ Be sure perineal structures are well visualized during assessment and administration of medication.
- ➤ Clients with restricted mobility in knees or hips may lie supine with legs abducted.

Teaching Considerations

- ➤ Teach client value of and technique for regular perineal hygiene.

SKILL 18-10 Administering Rectal Suppositories

A variety of medications may be given rectally. Drugs administered rectally exert either a local effect on gastrointestinal mucosa, such as promoting defecation, or systemic effects, such as relieving nausea or providing analgesia. The rectal route is not as reliable as oral or parenteral routes in terms of drug absorption and distribution. However, the medications are relatively safe, since they rarely cause local irritation or side effects. Rectal medications are contraindicated in clients with rectal surgery or active rectal bleeding.

Rectal suppositories differ in shape from vaginal suppositories, being thinner and bullet shaped (Fig. 18-3). The rounded end prevents anal trauma during insertion. When the nurse administers the suppository, placing it past the internal anal sphincter and against the rectal mucosa is important. Improper placement can result in expulsion of the

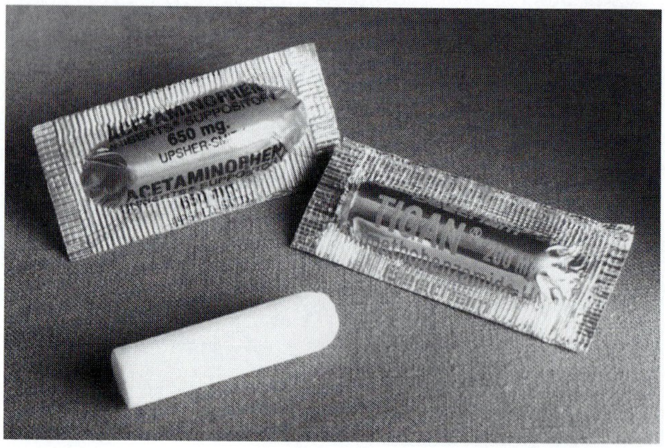

Fig. 18-3

suppository before the medication dissolves and is absorbed into the mucosa. Never force a suppository into a mass of fecal material. It may be necessary to administer a small cleansing enema before a suppository can be inserted. If a client prefers to self-administer a suppository, the nurse should give specific instructions so that the medication is deposited correctly.

EQUIPMENT

- **Rectal suppository**
- **Lubricating jelly (water soluble)**
- **Clean gloves**
- **Tissue**
- **Drape**
- **Medication administration record (MAR) or computer printout**

STEPS	RATIONALE
ASSESSMENT	
1. Review prescriber's order, including client's name, drug name, form, route, and time of administration.	Ensures safe and correct administration of medication.
2. Review pertinent information related to medication, including action, purpose, side effects, and nursing implications.	Allows nurse to administer drug properly and to monitor client's response.
3. Review medical record for history of rectal surgery or bleeding.	Conditions contraindicate use of suppository.
4. Review any presenting signs and symptoms of gastrointestinal alterations (e.g., constipation or diarrhea).	Conditions may indicate use of suppository.
5. Assess client's ability to hold suppository and to position self to insert medication.	Mobility restriction indicates need for nurse to assist with drug administration.
6. Review client's knowledge of purpose of drug therapy and interest in self-administering suppository.	May indicate need for health teaching. Level of motivation influences teaching approach.

NURSING DIAGNOSIS

Clustering of defining characteristics from the assessment data may reveal the following nursing diagnoses for clients requiring this skill:

- Constipation
- Health-seeking behaviors or desire for high-level wellness (self-care)
- Impaired physical mobility
- Knowledge deficit regarding suppository administration
- Pain

Related factors are individualized based on a client's condition or needs.

STEPS	RATIONALE
PLANNING	
1. **Expected outcomes** following completion of the procedure:	
➤ Client reports relief or reduction in symptoms for which medication is prescribed.	Drug acts effectively.
➤ Client describes purpose of medication.	Feedback reflects client's learning.
➤ Client self-administers suppository.	Demonstrates learning.
2. Compare MAR or computer printout with label of medication.	Ensures right medication is administered.
3. Check client's identification bracelet and ask name.	Ensures correct client receives medication.
4. Explain procedure to client. Be specific if client wishes to self-administer drug.	Promotes client's understanding and cooperation. Enables client to self-administer drug if physically able.
IMPLEMENTATION	
1. Wash hands, arrange supplies at bedside, and apply gloves.	Reduces transfer of microorganisms, helps nurse perform procedure smoothly.
2. Close room curtain or door.	Maintains privacy and minimizes embarrassment.
3. Assist client in assuming a left side-lying Sims' position with upper leg flexed upward.	Position exposes anus and helps client to relax external anal sphincter. Left side lessens the likelihood of the suppository or feces being expelled.
4. Keep client draped with only anal area exposed.	Maintains privacy and facilitates relaxation.

STEPS	RATIONALE
5. Examine condition of anus externally and palpate rectal walls as needed (see Skill 11-16). Dispose of gloves by turning them inside out and placing them in proper receptacle if they become soiled.	Determines presence of active rectal bleeding. Palpation determines whether rectum is filled with feces, which may interfere with suppository placement. Reduces transmission of infection.

➤ ***CRITICAL DECISION POINT*** **Generally, rectal suppository is contraindicated in the presence of active rectal bleeding. Unless suppository is for constipation, placing medication in a rectum filled with feces may be poorly absorbed or prematurely expelled with defecation.**

STEPS	RATIONALE
6. Apply new pair of disposable gloves (if previous gloves were soiled and discarded).	Minimizes contact with fecal material to reduce transmission of infection.
7. Remove suppository from foil wrapper and lubricate rounded end with jelly. Lubricate gloved index finger of dominant hand.	Lubrication reduces friction as suppository enters rectal canal.
8. Ask client to take slow deep breaths through mouth and to relax anal sphincter.	Forcing suppository through constricted sphincter causes pain.
9. Retract client's buttocks with nondominant hand. With gloved index finger of dominant hand, insert suppository gently through anus, past internal sphincter, and against rectal wall, 10 cm (4 inches) (see illustration).	Suppository must be placed against rectal mucosa for eventual absorption and therapeutic action.

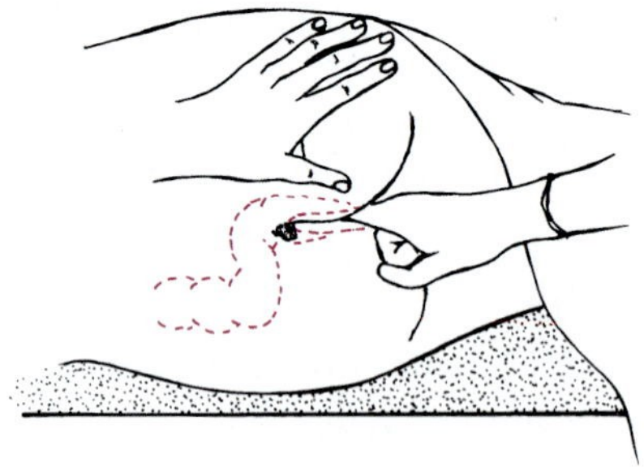

Step 9

STEPS	RATIONALE
10. Withdraw finger and wipe client's anal area.	Provides comfort.
11. Discard gloves by turning them inside out, and dispose in appropriate receptacle.	Reduces transfer of microorganisms.
12. Ask client to remain flat or on side for 5 minutes.	Prevents expulsion of suppository.
13. If suppository contains laxative or fecal softener, place call light within reach so client can obtain assistance to reach bedpan or toilet.	Ability to call for assistance provides client with sense of control over elimination.
14. Wash hands and dispose of gloves and other equipment.	Reduces risk of transfer of infection.

EVALUATION

1. Return within 5 minutes to determine if suppository was expelled.	Determines if drug is properly distributed. Reinsertion may be necessary.
2. Ask if client experienced localized anal or rectal discomfort during insertion.	Determines whether insertion of suppository was irritating.
3. Evaluate client for relief of symptoms for which medication was prescribed to relieve or eliminate. (Within time expected action of drug occurs.)	Determines medication's effectiveness.
4. Ask client to explain purpose of medication.	Reflects client's understanding of drug therapy.
5. Have client demonstrate administration of next dose of medication.	Demonstration measures learning.
6. **Unexpected outcomes** that may occur include:	
➤ Side effects of specific medication develop. Symptoms previously reported are unrelieved.	Dependent on type of drug administered. May require alternate therapy.

STEPS	RATIONALE
➤ Client reports rectal pain during insertion.	Suppository may need to be better lubricated, or rectal route may be contraindicated.
➤ Client is unable to explain purpose of drug therapy.	Reinstruction is necessary, or client is unwilling or unable to learn.
➤ Client is unable to self-administer medication.	Reinstruction is necessary.

Recording and Reporting

1. Record drug name, dosage, route, and time of administration on medication record.	Timely recording prevents drug errors.
2. Record and report client's response to medication, including any unusual reactions.	Documents effect of medication.

• • • • •

Special Considerations

- ➤ Do not palpate client's rectum if client has had rectal surgery.
- ➤ If client has hemorrhoids, use liberal amount of lubricant and handle area gently.
- ➤ With experience nurse is able to feel internal sphincter relax around finger after suppository passes up into rectum.

Teaching Considerations

- ➤ If client chooses to self-administer suppositories, teach principles and techniques of infection control to prevent contact with and spread of fecal material.

Gerontologic Considerations

- ➤ Elderly clients with loss of sphincter control may have difficulty retaining suppository.

Critical Thinking Exercises

1. You observe your client, a 76-year-old man, whom you have just instructed in how to utilize a metered-dose inhaler (MDI), unable to inhale the medication. How would you intervene?
2. You have mistaken the abbreviations for right eye and left eye and have given the eye drops incorrectly. Having discovered your error, what steps must you take?
3. What would you tell a client and the client's family about donning gloves before instilling eye drops?
4. Your client has a 20% body surface area, partial-thickness burn of the lower abdomen and left thigh. He has been applying Silvadene q 8 hr to the wound at home for the last 3 days. You discover upon your home visit that he has used almost 8 ounces of ointment, which should have lasted approximately 2 weeks, and that it is caked on the wound. How would you teach the client appropriate application of Silvadene to his burns?
5. You see a nurse crushing an enteric-coated medication to give to a client. How would you intervene?

References

Anders JE: Topical, a welter of options calls for refined applications techniques, *RN* 45:33, 1982.

Donnelly D: Instilling eye drops: Difficulties experienced by patients following cataract surgery, *J Advanc Nurs* 12:2335, 1987.

Fry TL: Earwax. In Dorbrand L, Hoole AJ, Pickard CG, editors: *Manual of clinical problems in adult ambulatory care,* Boston, 1992, Little, Brown and Company.

Gauqitz DG: How to protect the dysphagic stroke patient, *Amer J N* 95:34, 1995.

Klang, M: Medicating tube-fed patients, *Nursing 96,* 26:18, 1996.

Lewis SM, Collier IC, Heitkemper MM: Assessment and management of clinical problems, In *Medical Surgical Nursing,* ed 4, St Louis, 1996, Mosby.

Shuster MH: Enteral feeding of the critically ill. In Ackerman M, editor, *AACN Clin Issues in Crit Care Nurs* 5 (4):459, 1994.

Statz E: Hand strength and metered dose inhalers, *Amer J Nurs* 84:8000, 1984.

Weilitz PB, Van Sciver T: Obstructive pulmonary disease. In Lewis SM, Collier IC, Heitkemper MM, editors: *Medical surgical nursing: Assessment and management of clinical problems,* ed 4, St Louis, 1996, Mosby.

Weixleer D: Correcting metered-dose inhaler misuse, *Nursing 94* 24(7):62-64, 1994.

CHAPTER 19

Parenteral Medications

OBJECTIVES

Mastery of content in this chapter will enable the nurse to:

- Define key terms.
- Identify advantages and disadvantages of administering medications by each injection route.
- Discuss factors to consider when selecting injection sites.
- Explain the importance of selecting the proper size syringe and needle for an injection.
- Discuss ways to promote client comfort while administering an injection.
- Explain risks associated with administering injections.
- Correctly prepare an injectable medication from a vial and an ampule.
- Correctly administer a subcutaneous, intramuscular, and intradermal injection.
- Correctly administer an intravenous infusion by intravenous bolus, piggyback, or large-volume infusion.
- Compare the risks of three different intravenous routes.

SKILLS

19-1 Preparing Injections from Ampules and Vials

19-2 Mixing Medications from Two Vials

19-3 Administering Intradermal Injections

19-4 Administering Subcutaneous Injections

19-5 Administering Intramuscular Injections

19-6 Adding Medications to Intravenous Fluid Containers

19-7 Administering Intravenous Medications by Intermittent Infusion Sets and Miniinfusion Pumps

19-8 Administering Medications by Intravenous Bolus

KEY TERMS

Air embolus
Ampules
Anaphylactic reaction
Aqueous
Aspirate
Bolus
Compatibility
Diluent
Heparin lock
Incompatibility
Induration
Infiltration
Infusion
Injection
Intradermal injection
Intramuscular (IM) injection
Intravenous (IV) injection
Parenteral
Phlebitis
Piggyback infusion
Subcutaneous (SC, SQ) injection
Vial
Z-track method

Parenteral injections are used to instill medications into body tissues. The procedures are invasive and thus pose greater risk than that associated with administering oral medications. Injected drugs act more quickly than oral medications, and thus the client's condition can change rapidly. The nurse must monitor the client's response closely and be aware of potential side effects or allergic reactions and the risk of infection that occurs once a needle pierces the skin. The nurse uses strict aseptic technique whenever preparing and administering injections. Infection can originate from a variety of sources (Table 19-1).

Parenteral drug administration can be done by four different routes:

1. **Subcutaneous (SC, SQ) injection**—injection into tissues just below the dermis of the skin
2. **Intramuscular (IM) injection**—injection into the body of a muscle

Table 19-1 Preventing Infection During an Injection

Principle	Technique
Prevent contamination of solution	Add date, time, and initials to vials when opened. Swab opened multidose vials with alcohol before piercing.
Prevent needle contamination	Avoid letting needle touch contaminated surface: outer edges of ampule or vial, outer surface of needle cap, nurse's hands, countertop, or table surface.
Prevent syringe contamination	Avoid touching length of plunger or inner part of barrel. Keep tip of syringe covered with cap or needle.
Prepare skin	Wash grossly contaminated sites with soap and water. Before giving an injection, use an alcohol swab to clean site; swab from center of site and move outward approximately 5 cm from center (2 inches).
Prior to handling any equipment, handwashing is essential to reduce the transfer of microorganisms.	

3. **Intradermal injection**—injection into the dermis just under the epidermis
4. **Intravenous (IV) injection**—injection into a vein

Each type of **injection** requires a certain set of skills to make certain that the medication reaches the proper location. Failure to inject a medication correctly can result in complications such as a drug response that is too rapid, nerve injury with associated pain, localized bleeding, tissue necrosis, and sterile abscess.

Parenteral medication is delivered to a client by using a needle and syringe. Needles and syringes come in a variety of sizes. The nurse determines the appropriate size of syringe and length of needle based on the type of medication to be delivered, the volume of solution to be delivered, and the medication route. A variety of electronic devices also can be used to deliver parenteral medications. Electronic devices ensure a constant delivery of medication. They are often used when vasoactive substances are delivered. Vasoactive medications can produce rapid, dramatic physiological changes. Use of electronic devices ensures a more controlled administration of set doses.

SYRINGES

A syringe consists of a cylindrical barrel, a tip designed to fit the hub of a hypodermic needle, and a close-fitting plunger (Fig. 19-1). Syringes are single-use and disposable. They are packaged separately, with or without a sterile needle, in a paper wrapper or rigid plastic container. Syringes, in general, are classified as non–Luer-lok or Luer-lok. This nomenclature is based on the design of the syringe's tip. *Non–Luer-lok* syringes use needles that slip onto the tip. *Luer-lok* syringes (Fig. 19-2, A) require special needles that are twisted onto the tip and lock themselves in place. The Luer-lok design prevents the inadvertent removal of the needle from the syringe.

Syringes come in various sizes, ranging from 1 to 60 ml in capacity (Fig. 19-2). The nurse, using knowledge about the type of syringes, determines which is the most appropriate to use. The nurse uses large syringes to administer certain IV drugs and to add medications to IV solutions. It is unusual to use a syringe larger than 5 ml for an injection. A 2 to 3 ml syringe is adequate for IM and SC injections. Some syringes have two scales along the barrel. One

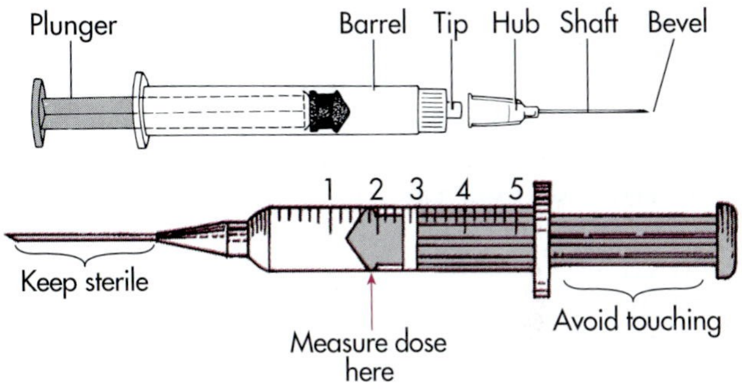

Fig. 19-1 Parts of a syringe.

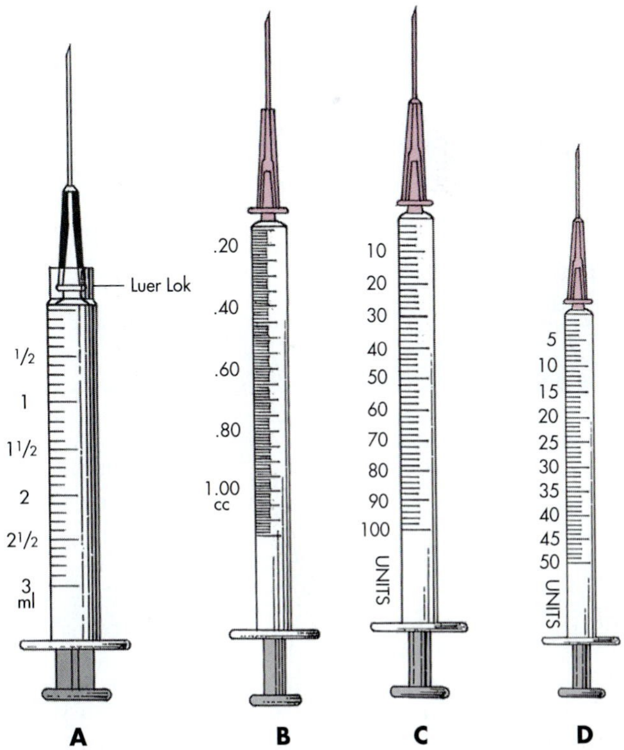

Fig. 19-2 Types of syringes. **A,** Syringe with 3 ml capacity is marked in 0.1 (tenths); **B,** tuberculin syringe is marked in 0.01 (hundreths) for doses of less than 1 ml. Insulin syringes marked in units in two sizes: **C,** 100 U; or **D,** 50 U (lo-dose).

scale is divided into minims and the other into tenths of a milliliter. Before use, the nurse carefully examines the syringe to ensure that the current scale is being used. The tuberculin syringe (Fig. 19-2, *B*) has a long, thin barrel with a preattached thin needle. The syringe, calibrated in sixteenths of a minim and hundredths of a milliliter, has a capacity of 1 ml. The nurse uses a tuberculin syringe to prepare small amounts of medication such as small, precise doses for infants or young children. Insulin syringes (Fig. 19-2, *C* and *D*) hold 0.5 to 1 ml and are calibrated in units. Insulin syringes that hold 0.5 ml are known as low-dose syringes (50 units per 0.5 ml) and are easier to read. Insulin syringes in the United States and Canada are U-100s, designed for use with U-100–strength insulin. Each milliliter of solution contains 100 units of insulin.

NEEDLES

Needles come packaged in individual sheaths to allow flexibility in choosing the right needle for a client. Some needles are preattached to standard size syringes.

A needle has three parts: the hub, which fits onto the tip of a syringe; the shaft, which connects to the hub; and the bevel, or slanted tip (see Fig. 19-1). The needle hub, shaft, and bevel must remain sterile at all times. To prevent contamination, the nurse places the needle onto the syringe with the cap intact, using gentle force (Fig. 19-3).

A

B

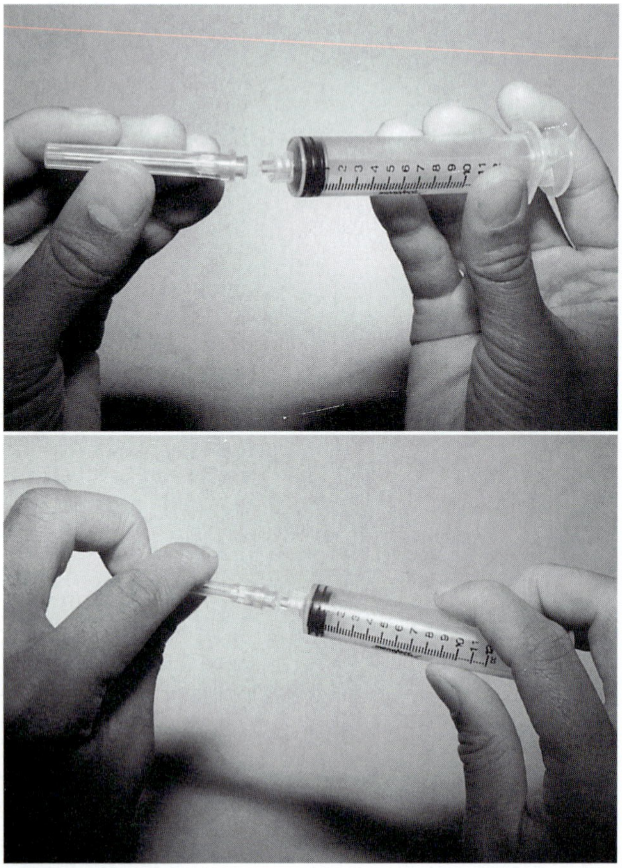

Fig. 19-3

Needle Features

The tip of a needle, or the bevel, is always slanted. The bevel creates a narrow slit when injected into tissue; it quickly closes when the needle is removed to prevent leakage of medication, blood, or serum. A short beveled tip is best for IV injections because it is not easily occluded against the inside of a blood vessel wall. Long beveled tips are sharper and narrower, which minimizes discomfort when tissue is entered for an SC or IM injection.

Needles vary in length from ¼ inch to 3 inches (Fig. 19-4). The nurse chooses the needle length according to the client's size and weight and the type of tissue into which the drug is to be injected. A child or slender adult generally requires a shorter needle. The nurse uses a longer needle (1 inch to 1½ inches) for IM injections and a shorter needle (⅜ to ⅝ inch) for SC injections.

The smaller the needle gauge, the larger the needle diameter. The selection of a gauge depends on the viscosity of fluid to be injected or infused. The rationale for needle selection is included in each skill.

DISPOSABLE INJECTION UNITS

Disposable single-dose prefilled syringes are available for some medications. With these syringes the nurse does not need to prepare medication doses, except perhaps to expel portions of unneeded medication.

The Tubex and Carpujet injection systems include reusable plastic syringes that hold disposable, prefilled sterile-cartridge-needle units (Fig. 19-5). The nurse slips the cartridge into the syringe, secures it (following package directions), and checks for air bubbles in the syringe.

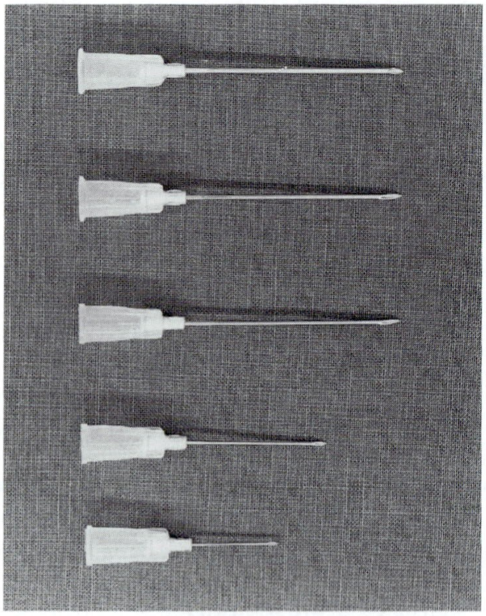

Fig 19-4 Hypodermic needles arranged in order of gauge. *Top to bottom:* 19-gauge, 20-gauge, 21-gauge, 23-gauge, and 25-gauge.

A

B

C

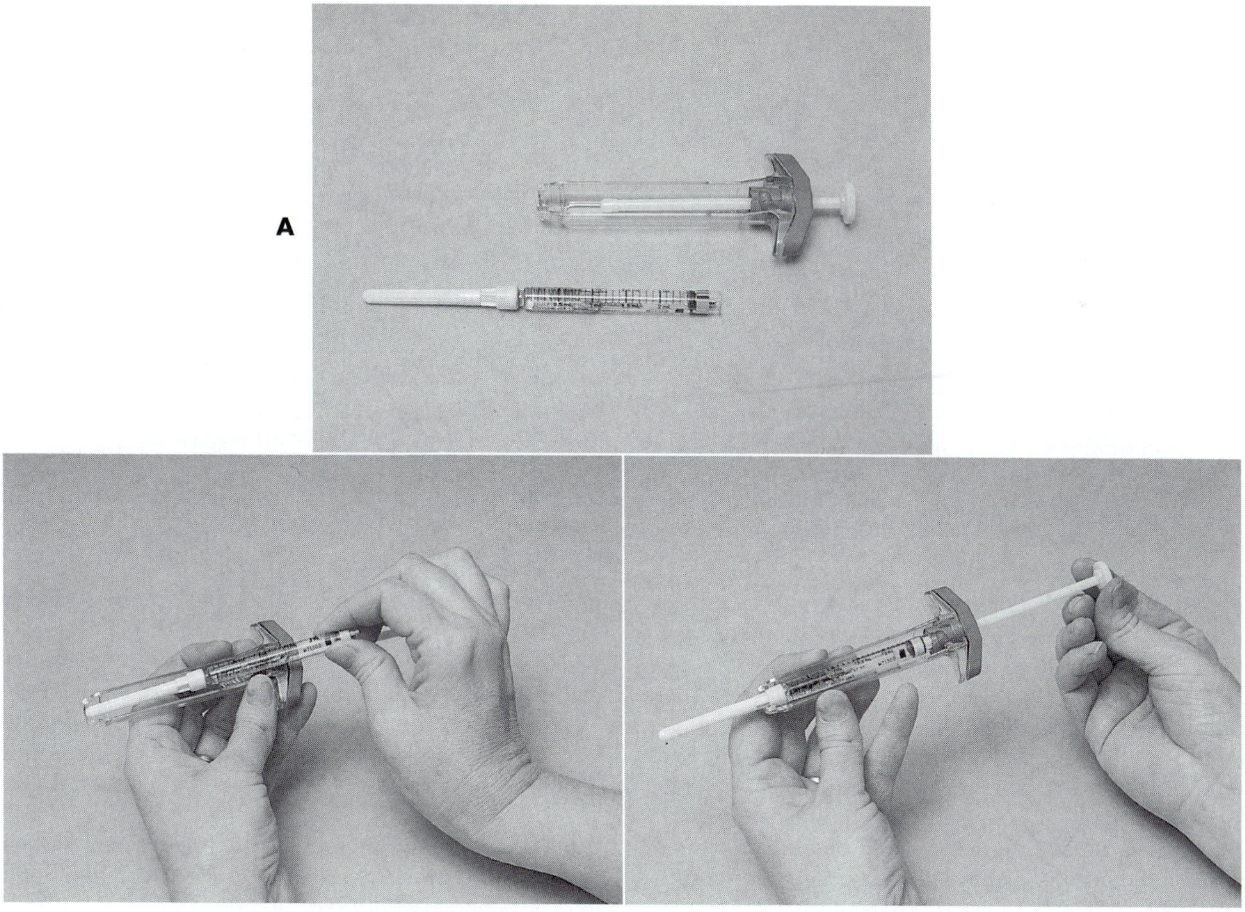

Fig. 19-5 **A,** Carpujet syringe and prefilled sterile cartridge with needle. **B,** Assembling the Carpujet. **C,** The cartridge slides into the syringe barrel, turns, and locks at the needle end. The plunger then screws into the cartridge end.

The nurse advances the plunger to expel excess medication, as with a regular syringe. Another type of injection system involves screwing a plungerlike device into the end of a prefilled vial containing a needle. After the medication is given, the entire unit is disposed of in a receptacle. This design reduces the risk of needle-stick injury.

PROTECTING YOURSELF FROM NEEDLE-STICK INJURY

The most frequent route of exposure to bloodborne disease is from needle-stick injuries (Bohony, 1993). To reduce the frequency of needle-stick injury, many institutions now supply "safety devices" for the nurse to use when handling sharp objects. One example is the safety syringe, which is equipped with a plastic guard or shield that slips over the needle as it is withdrawn from the skin. Another example is a shielded needleless device (Skill 19-7). Additional measures are summarized in number nine in the guidelines that follow.

GUIDELINES

1. Use strict aseptic technique during all steps of preparation and administration.
2. To prepare medication for administration, fill a syringe by aspirating the fluid. Pull the plunger outward from the barrel while keeping the attached needle tip immersed in the medication solution. To prevent contamination and maintain sterility, hold only the outside of the syringe barrel and the handle on the plunger. Avoid touching the tip of the needle, the inside of the barrel, the shaft of the plunger, or the needle with an unsterile object.
3. Know the volume and characteristics of the medication to be administered. Injecting too large a volume of medication can cause extreme pain and local tissue damage.
4. Identify the bony prominences and anatomical structures that outline the chosen injection sites. Correct

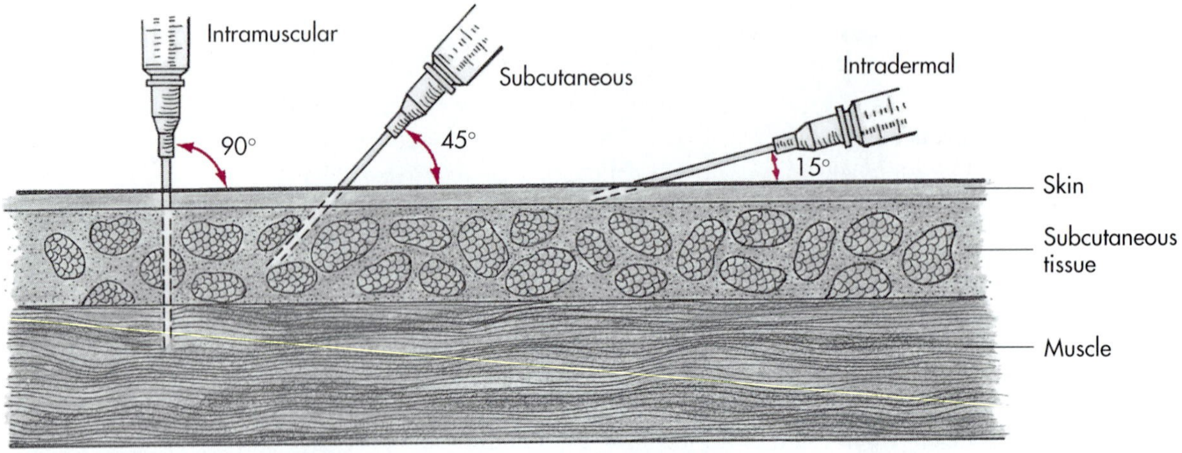

Fig. 19-6 Comparison of the angles of insertion of IM (90 degrees), SQ (45 degrees) in thin to average size clients, and ID (15 degrees) injections.

identification of the specific muscle mass will prevent injury to major nerves and blood vessels located near the injection site.

5. Insert the needle at the proper angle to deliver medication into the correct tissue (Fig. 19-6).
6. Before injecting the medication, aspirate by pulling back on the plunger to ensure that the needle has not pierced a vein or artery. Injection directly into a blood vessel can cause a rapid drug response. If blood is aspirated, remove the needle, dispose of the syringe and medication, and prepare a new dose of medication.*
7. Attempt to minimize the client's discomfort when giving an injection by observing the following guidelines:
   a. Use sharp beveled needles in the shortest length and smallest gauge possible.
   b. Change the needle if liquid medication has coated the shaft of the needle. This prevents tracking of medication through the client's SC tissue.
   c. Position and flex limbs appropriately to reduce muscular tension.
   d. Divert the client's attention from the injection procedure.
   e. Insert the needle smoothly and quickly. Do not hesitate, and slowly push the needle into tissue.
   f. Inject the medication slowly but smoothly to reduce pain.
   g. Hold the syringe steady once the needle is in the tissue to prevent tissue damage.
   h. Withdraw the needle smoothly at the same angle used for insertion.
   i. Gently apply an antiseptic pad (e.g., alcohol) to the site. However, alcohol can cause discomfort at the injection site. Some advocate the use of a dry, sterile gauze pad to be placed firmly against the skin after the needle has been removed (Beyea and Nicoll, 1996).
   j. Apply gentle pressure at the injection site. Massaging the injected area is no longer recommended (Beyea and Nicoll, 1996).
   k. Rotate injection sites to prevent the formation of **indurations** and abscesses.
8. Use the guidelines for administering medications listed in Chapter 17.
9. After administering injections, do not recap needles before disposal. Recapping a needle may predispose the nurse to an accidental needle-stick injury. Dispose of needles in an appropriate puncture-proof and leak-proof container (Centers for Disease Control and Prevention [CDC], 1988).

Exception: Do not aspirate SC heparin.

DELEGATION CONSIDERATIONS

The skill of medication administration requires problem solving and knowledge application unique to a professional nurse. Delegation of any of the skills covered in this chapter is inappropriate. Be sure unlicensed care providers know to report any unexpected drug reactions to an RN ASAP.

SKILL 19-1 Preparing Injections from Ampules and Vials

Ampules contain single doses of injectable medication in a liquid form. They are available in sizes from 1 to 10 ml or more (Fig. 19-7). An ampule is made of glass with a constricted neck that must be snapped off to allow access to the medication. A colored ring around the neck indicates where the ampule is prescored to be broken easily. Medications are easily withdrawn from the ampule by aspirating the fluid with a needle (filter needle optional) and syringe. The fluid enters the syringe because pulling on the plunger creates a vacuum in the syringe barrel.

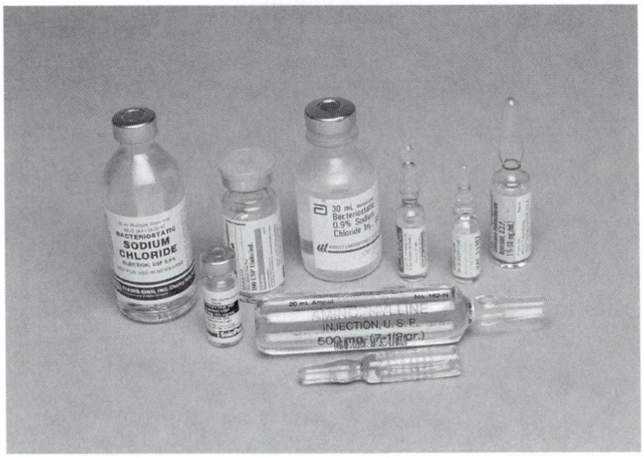

Fig. 19-7 Assorted ampules and vials.

A **vial** is a plastic or glass container with a rubber seal at the top (Fig. 19-7). A vial that is entered and then discarded, regardless of the amount of medication used, is called a single-dose vial. A vial that can be entered into several times and contains several doses of medication is called a multidose vial. A metal cap protects the rubber seal. It is removed when the nurse is first preparing the vial for use. Vials contain liquid or dry forms of medications; drugs that are unstable in solution are packaged in a dry powder form. The vial label specifies the amount of diluent to be used to dissolve the powdered drug to prepare a desired drug concentration. Unlike the ampule, the vial is a closed system, and air must be injected into the container to permit easy withdrawal of the solution.

EQUIPMENT

Medication in an ampule
- Syringe and two needles (filter needle optional)
- Small gauze pad or alcohol swab

Medication in a vial
- Syringe and two needles (filter needle optional)
- Small gauze pad or alcohol swab
- Diluent, for example, normal saline or sterile water (optional)

Both
- Medication administration record or computer printout

STEPS	RATIONALE
ASSESSMENT	
1. If medication is to be injected, assess the client's body build, muscle size, and weight.	Determines type and size of syringe and needles to be used for injection.
PLANNING	
1. Check medication administration record or computer printout.	Verifies orders.
2. **Expected outcome** following completion of procedure:	
➤ Proper dose is prepared. No air bubbles are present within syringe barrel.	Air bubbles displace medication. Elimination of air ensures medication is prepared correctly.
IMPLEMENTATION	
1. Wash hands.	Reduces transmission of microorganisms.
2. Assemble supplies at work area in medicine room.	Makes procedure orderly. Organization saves nursing time and demonstrates organization skills.
3. Check medication order, medication administration record, or printout against label on the ampule or vial.	Ensures right drug and dose to prepare.

STEPS	RATIONALE
4. AMPULE PREPARATION:	
a. Tap top of ampule lightly and quickly with finger until fluid moves from neck of ampule. (See illustration.)	Dislodges any fluid that collects above neck of ampule. All solution moves into lower chamber.
b. Place small gauze pad around neck of ampule.	Placing pad around neck of ampule protects nurse's fingers from trauma as glass tip is broken off.
c. Snap neck of ampule quickly and firmly away from hands (see illustration).	Protects nurse's fingers and face from shattering glass.
d. Draw up medication quickly.	System is open to airborne contaminants.
e. Hold ampule upside down, or set it on a flat surface. Insert syringe or filter needle (see agency policy) into center of ampule opening. Do not allow needle tip or shaft to touch rim of ampule.	Broken rim of ampule is considered contaminated. When ampule is inverted, solution does dribble out if needle tip or shaft touches rim of ampule.
f. Aspirate medication into syringe by gently pulling back on plunger (see illustration).	Withdrawal of plunger creates negative pressure within syringe barrel, which pulls fluid into syringe.
g. Keep needle tip under surface of liquid. Tip ampule to bring all fluid within reach of the needle.	Prevents aspiration of air bubbles.
h. If air bubbles are aspirated, do not expel air into ampule.	Air pressure may force fluid out of ampule and medication will be lost.
i. To expel excess air bubbles, remove needle from ampule. Hold syringe with needle pointing up. Tap side of syringe to cause bubbles to rise toward needle. Draw back slightly on plunger, and then push plunger upward to eject air.	Withdrawing plunger too far will remove it from barrel. Holding syringe vertically allows fluid to settle in bottom of barrel. Pulling back on plunger allows fluid within needle to enter barrel so fluid is not expelled. Air at top of barrel and within needle is then expelled.
CRITICAL DECISION POINT **When trying to expel excess air bubbles, do not eject fluid.**	
j. If syringe contains excess fluid, use sink for disposal. Hold syringe vertically with needle tip up and slanted slightly toward sink. Slowly eject excess fluid into sink. Recheck fluid level in syringe by holding it vertically.	Medication is safely dispersed into sink. Position of needle allows medication to be expelled without it flowing down needle shaft. Rechecking fluid level ensures proper dose.
k. Cover needle with its safety sheath or cap. Change needle on syringe or use filter needle if suspect medication is on needle shaft.	Prevents contamination of needle. New needle prevents tracking medication through skin and subcutaneous tissues.

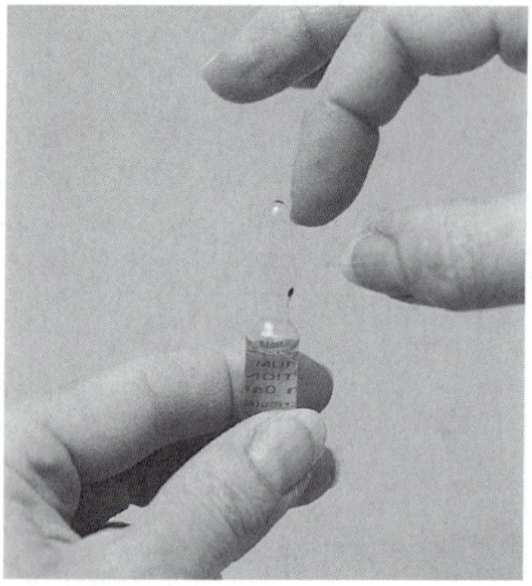
Step 4a

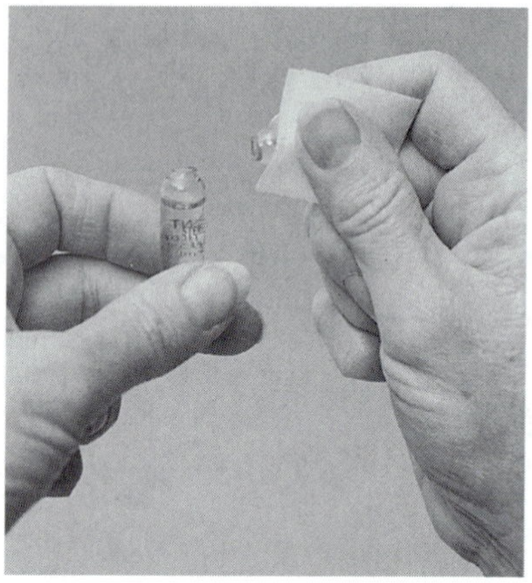
Step 4c

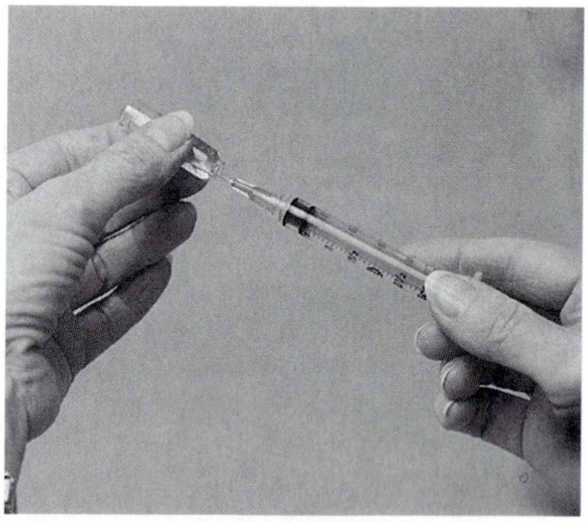
Step 4f

STEPS	RATIONALE
5. *Vial containing a solution:*	
a. Remove cap covering top of unused vial to expose sterile rubber seal, keeping rubber seal sterile. If a multidose vial that has been used before is being used again, firmly and briskly wipe surface of rubber seal with alcohol swab and allow it to dry.	Vial comes packaged with cap to prevent contamination of rubber seal. Cap cannot be replaced after seal removal. Allowing alcohol to dry prevents needle from being coated with alcohol and mixing with medication.
b. Pick up syringe and remove needle cap. Pull back on plunger to draw amount of air into syringe equivalent to volume of medication to be aspirated from vial.	Air must first be injected into vial to prevent buildup of negative pressure in vial when aspirating medication.
c. With vial on flat surface, insert tip of needle with beveled tip entering first through center of rubber seal (see illustration). Apply pressure to tip of needle during insertion.	Center of seal is thinner and easier to penetrate. Injecting beveled tip first and using firm pressure prevent coring of rubber seal, which could enter vial or needle.
d. Inject air into the vial's airspace, holding on to plunger.	Air must be injected before aspirating fluid. Injecting into vial's airspace prevents formation of bubbles and inaccuracy in dosage.
CRITICAL DECISION POINT Hold plunger with firm pressure; plunger may be forced backward by air pressure within the vial.	
e. Invert vial while keeping firm hold on syringe and plunger (see illustration). Hold vial between thumb and middle fingers of nondominant hand. Grasp end of syringe barrel and plunger with thumb and forefinger of dominant hand to counteract pressure in vial.	Inverting vial allows fluid to settle in lower half of container. Position of hands prevents forceful movement of plunger and permits easy manipulation of syringe.
f. Keep tip of needle below fluid level.	Prevents aspiration of air.
g. Allow air pressure from the vial to fill syringe gradually with medication. If necessary, pull back slightly on plunger to obtain correct amount of solution.	Positive pressure within vial forces fluid into syringe.

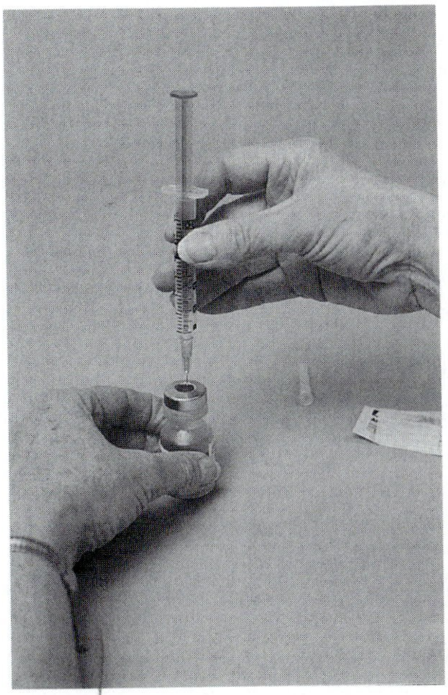

Step 5c

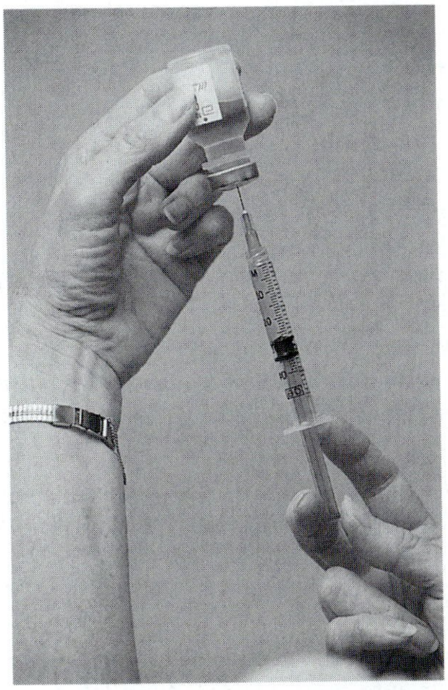

Step 5e

STEPS	RATIONALE
h. When desired volume has been obtained, position needle into vial's airspace; tap side of syringe barrel carefully to dislodge any air bubbles. Eject any air remaining at top of syringe into vial.	Forcefully striking barrel while needle is inserted in vial may bend needle. Accumulation of air displaces medication and causes dosage errors.
i. Remove needle from vial by pulling back on barrel of syringe.	Pulling plunger rather than barrel causes plunger to separate from barrel, resulting in loss of medication.
j. Hold syringe at eye level, at 90-degree angle, to ensure correct volume and absence of air bubbles. Remove any remaining air by tapping barrel to dislodge any air bubbles (see illustration). Draw back slightly on plunger; then push plunger upward to eject air. Do not eject fluid.	Holding syringe vertically allows fluid to settle in bottom of barrel. Pulling back on plunger allows fluid within needle to enter barrel so fluid is not expelled. Air at top of barrel and within needle is then expelled.

Step 5j

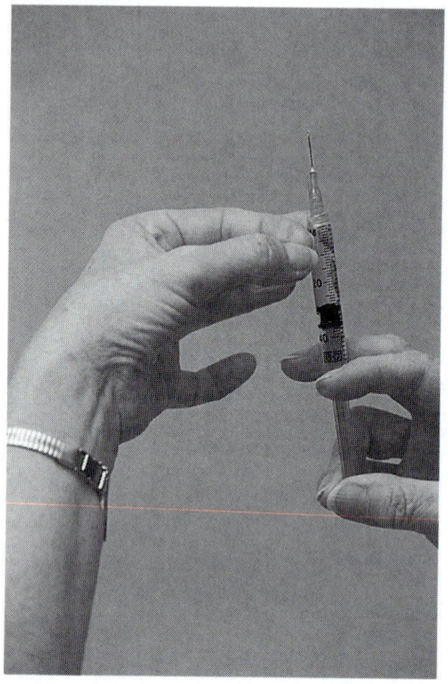

STEPS	RATIONALE
k. If medication is to be injected into client's tissue, change needle to appropriate gauge and length according to route of medication.	Inserting needle through a rubber stopper may dull beveled tip. New needle is sharper. Because no fluid is along shaft, needle will not track medication through tissues.
l. For multidose vial, make label that includes date of mixing, concentration of drug per milliliter, and nurse's initials.	Ensures that future doses will be prepared correctly. Some drugs must be discarded after certain number of days after mixing of vial.
6. Vial containing a powder (reconstituting medications):	
a. Remove cap covering vial of powdered medication and cap covering vial of proper **diluent.**	Cap prevents contamination of rubber seal.
b. Draw up diluent into syringe following Step 5b through j.	Prepares diluent for injection into vial containing powdered medication.
c. Insert tip of needle through center of rubber seal of vial of powdered medication. Inject diluent into vial. Remove needle.	Diluent begins to dissolve and reconstitute medication.
d. Mix medication thoroughly. Roll in palms. Do not shake.	Ensures proper dispersal of medication throughout solution.
e. Reconstituted medication in vial is ready to be drawn into new syringe. Read label carefully to determine dose after reconstitution.	Once diluent has been added, concentration of medication (mg/ml) determines dose to be given.

STEPS	RATIONALE
7. Dispose of soiled supplies. Place broken ampule and/or used vials and used needle in puncture-proof and leak-proof container. Clean work area and wash hands.	Proper disposal of glass and needle prevents accidental injury to staff. Controls transmission of infection.
E VALUATION	
1. Compare dose in syringe with desired dose.	Ensures that accurate dose has been prepared.
2. **Unexpected outcomes** that may occur include:	
➤ Air bubbles remain within syringe barrel.	Creates risk of incorrect dose.
➤ Excess or insufficient volume of medication is prepared.	Incorrect dose may be delivered.

Special Considerations

- Be sure to select needle long enough to reach bottom of ampule. If needle is longer than needed to administer medication, choose new needle just before injection.
- Never use wet alcohol swab to wrap around top of ampule because alcohol may leak into ampule.
- If you suspect that glass fragments may be in ampule, discard it and begin again. Special filter needles are available to aspirate medication from ampule to syringe.
- Dry powdered drugs usually dissolve easily. It may be necessary to withdraw needle from vial and then mix contents thoroughly. Mix by gently shaking or rolling vial between hands.
- When preparing medication from single-dose vial, do not assume that volume listed on label is total volume in vial. Some manufacturers provide small amount of extra liquid, expecting loss during preparation. Be sure to draw up only desired volume.

Home Care Considerations

- See Skills 41-3 and 42-5.

SKILL 19-2 Mixing Medications from Two Vials

Occasionally the nurse must mix medications from two vials or from a vial and an ampule. This avoids the need to give a client more than one injection at a time. It is essential that any medications to be mixed are compatible. When mixing medications, the nurse must remember the differences in how to aspirate fluid correctly from each type of container. When using multidose vials, the nurse must not contaminate the vial's contents with medication from another vial or ampule.

Mixing medications from a vial and ampule is simple because adding air to withdraw medication from an ampule is unnecessary. The nurse prepares medications from the vial first and then, using the same syringe and needle, withdraws medication from the ampule. Mixing medications from two vials is somewhat more complicated because air must be added to both vials.

Special consideration must be given to the proper preparation of insulin, which comes in vials. Insulin is the hormone used to treat diabetes. Often clients with diabetes receive a combination of different types of insulin to control their blood sugar levels. Regular insulin is a clear solution that can be given subcutaneously or intravenously. The other types of insulin contain the addition of a protein that slows absorption. Cloudy insulin preparations cannot be given intravenously.

There are simple guidelines for mixing two kinds of insulin in the same syringe:

1. Regular insulin can be mixed with any other type of insulin. It should always be drawn into the syringe *first*.
2. NPH (Neutral Protamine Hagedorn) insulin can be mixed only with regular insulin.
3. Lente insulins can be mixed with each other and with regular insulin, but they should not be mixed with any other types of insulin.

EQUIPMENT

- **Single-dose or multidose vials and ampules containing medications**
- **Syringe with needle**
- **Extra needles**
- **Alcohol swab**
- **Container for disposing of syringes, needles, and glass**
- **Medication administration record or computer printout**

STEPS	RATIONALE
ASSESSMENT	
1. Assess client's body build, muscle size, and weight.	Determines type and size of syringe and needles for injection.
2. Consider medications to be mixed and type of injection.	Determines order of drawing up medications and size of syringe.
PLANNING	
1. **Expected outcomes** following completion of procedure:	
➤ Combined medications equal correct dose. No air bubbles are present in syringe barrel.	Indicates medication is prepared correctly.
2. Check medication administration record or computer printout.	Verifies orders.
IMPLEMENTATION	
1. Wash hands.	Reduces transmission of microorganisms.
2. Assemble supplies at work area in medication preparation area.	Makes procedure orderly.
MIXING MEDICATIONS FROM VIALS	
1. Take syringe and **aspirate** volume of air equivalent to first dose of medication (vial A).	Air must be introduced into vial to create positive pressure needed to withdraw solution.
2. Inject air into vial A, making sure needle does not touch solution (see Fig. 19-8, *A*).	Prevents cross-contamination.
3. Holding on to plunger, withdraw needle and syringe from vial A. Aspirate air equivalent to second dose of medication (vial B).	Air is injected into vial B to create positive pressure needed to withdraw desired dose.
4. Insert needle into vial B, inject air, and then fill syringe with proper volume of medication from vial (Fig. 19-8, *B*).	First portion of dose has been prepared.
5. Withdraw needle and syringe from vial B. Ensure that proper volume has been obtained.	Ensures correct dose is prepared.
6. Determine at which point on syringe scale combined volume of medications should measure.	Prevents accidental withdrawal of too much medication from second vial.
7. Insert needle into vial A, being careful not to push plunger and expel medication into vial. Invert vial and carefully withdraw desired amount of medication into syringe (Fig. 19-8, *C*).	Positive pressure within vial A allows fluid to fill syringe without need to aspirate.

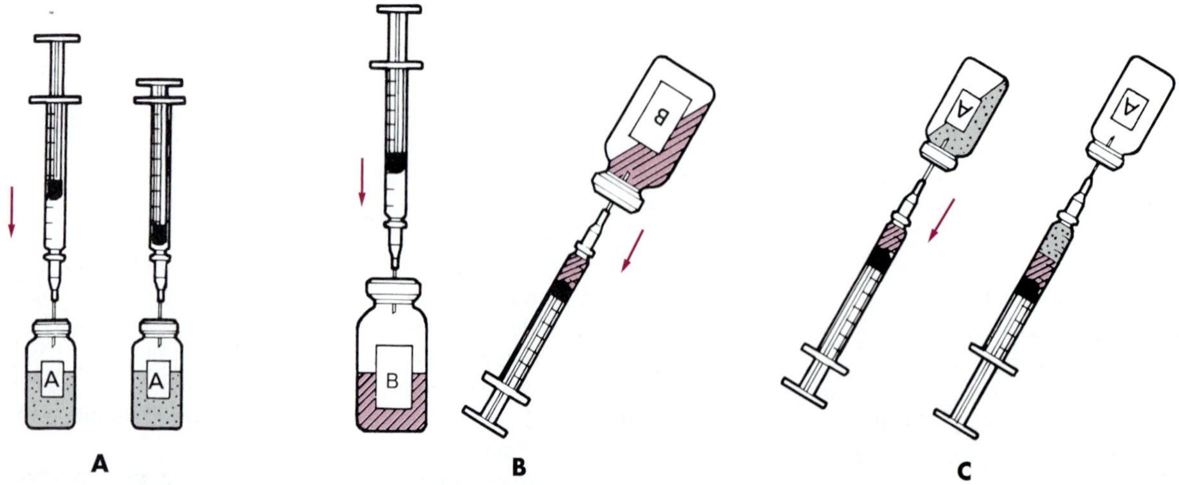

Fig. 19-8 **A,** Injecting air into vial A. **B,** Injecting air into vial B and withdrawing dose. **C,** Withdrawing medication from vial A; medications are now mixed.

STEPS	RATIONALE
8. Withdraw needle and expel any excess air or fluid from syringe.	Air bubbles should not be injected into tissues. Excess fluid causes incorrect dose.
➤ *CRITICAL DECISION POINT* If too much medication is withdrawn from second vial, discard syringe and start over. Do not push medication back into vial.	
9. Change needle to appropriate needle gauge and length according to route of medication. Keep needle sheathed or capped until administration time.	New needle prevents tracking of medication into tissues. Cover or cap maintains needle sterility.
10. Dispose of soiled needle and supplies in proper receptacles.	Controls spread of infection and prevents accidents.
11. Wash hands.	Reduces transmission of infection.

MIXING INSULIN

STEPS	RATIONALE
1. Take insulin syringe and aspirate volume of air equivalent to dose to be withdrawn from modified insulin (cloudy vial) (see illustration).	Air must be introduced into vial to create pressure needed to withdraw solution.
2. Inject air into vial of modified insulin (cloudy vial). Be sure that needle does not touch solution.	Prevents cross-contamination.
3. Withdraw needle and syringe from vial and aspirate air equivalent to dose to be withdrawn from unmodified regular insulin (clear vial).	Air is injected into vial to withdraw desired dose.
4. Insert needle into vial of unmodified regular insulin (clear vial), inject air, and then fill syringe with proper regular insulin dose (see illustration).	First portion of dose has been prepared. Always fill syringe with unmodified (regular) insulin first to prevent contamination of the regular insulin bottle with NPH or Lente insulin. The immediate effect required from short-acting regular insulin can be modified if contaminated by longer-acting insulin.
5. Withdraw needle and syringe from vial by pulling on barrel; check dose.	Prevents accidental pulling of plunger, which may cause loss of medication. Ensures correct dose prepared.
6. Determine at which point on syringe scale combined units of insulin should measure.	Prevents accidental withdrawal of too much insulin from second vial.
7. Insert needle into vial of modified insulin (cloudy vial). Be careful not to push plunger and expel medication into vial. Invert vial and carefully withdraw desired amount of insulin into syringe (see illustration).	Positive pressure within vial of modified insulin allows fluid to fill syringe without need to aspirate.

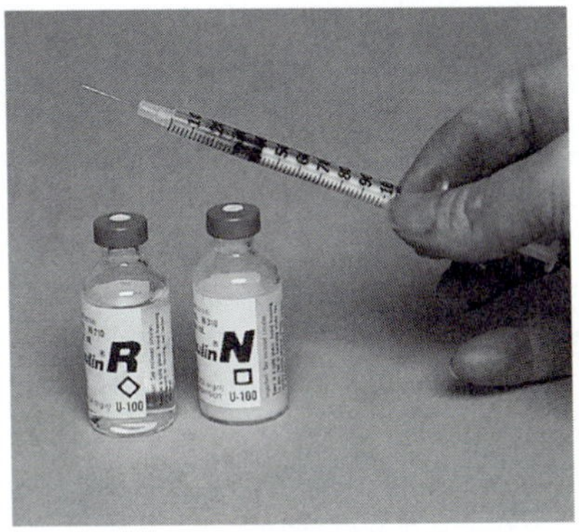

Step 1

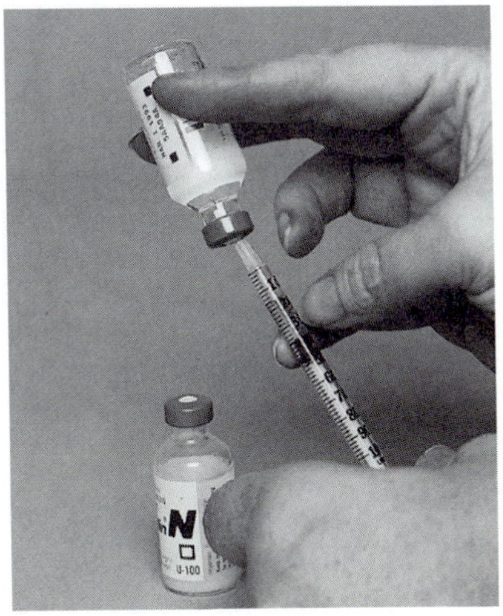

Step 4

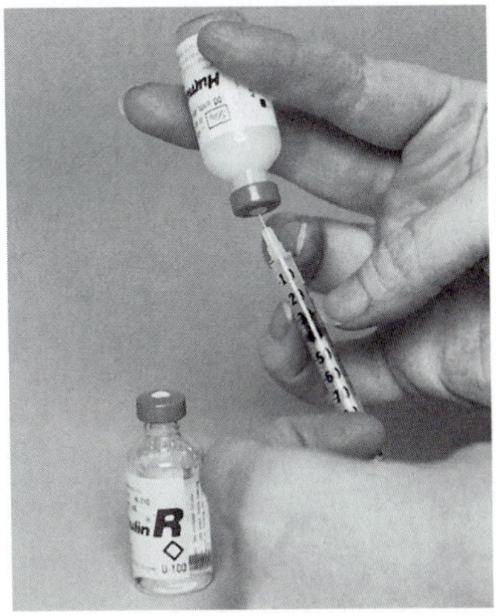

Step 7

STEPS	RATIONALE
8. Withdraw needle and check fluid level in syringe. Keep needle of prepared syringe sheathed or capped.	Ensures accurate dose. Insulin can cause serious hypoglycemia.
➤ ***CRITICAL DECISION POINT*** **Medication safety tip: Check dosage with another licensed professional.**	
9. Dispose of soiled supplies in proper receptacle.	Controls spread of infection.
10. Wash hands.	Reduces transmission of infection.

EVALUATION

1. Check syringe carefully for total combined dose of medications.	Accurate dose ensures safe medication administration.
2. **Unexpected outcomes** that may occur include:	
➤ Air bubbles remain in syringe barrel.	Creates risk of incorrect dose.
➤ Excess or insufficient volume of medication is prepared.	

FOLLOW-UP ACTIVITIES

1. Administer mixture of insulins within 5 minutes of preparation. Regular insulin binds with neutral protamine Hagedorn (NPH) and the action of regular insulin is reduced.

• • • • •

Special Considerations

- If two modified forms of insulin are mixed, it makes no difference which vial is prepared first.

Teaching Considerations

- Because insulin is essential to life, clients must be able to prepare and inject insulin at least once per day (see Chapter 42).
- Assess client's ability to mix insulins. Insulins can be prescribed in premixed formulations. Clients unable to perform this task should discuss options with their health care provider.

Pediatric Considerations

- Children of about 8 or 9 years should be able to prepare and administer their own insulin.
- Younger children may need participation/supervision of a parent.
- The nurse assesses the pediatric client's physical readiness, psychological readiness, and development in activities of daily living before teaching a client how to self-administer insulin injection.
- Family education is essential to successful diabetes management in the pediatric client.

Gerontologic Considerations

- Physiological changes in the older adult, such as decreased peripheral vision, presbyopia, and reduction in the power of skeletal and voluntary muscle contractions, may make it difficult for clients to self-administer injections.
- The nurse assesses the older client's physical readiness, psychological readiness as well as development in activities of daily living before teaching a client how to self-administer insulin.
- Clients unable to perform the task may be assisted by family members, a visiting nurse, or home health attendants.

Home Care Considerations

- Some clients may prefer to use their syringe more than once. Insulin preparations have bacteriostatic additives that inhibit growth of bacteria commonly found on the skin. Many studies have shown that it is both safe and practical for the syringe to be used more than once if the client desires (Valentine, 1996).

SKILL 19-3 Administering Intradermal Injections

The nurse typically gives intradermal injections for skin testing, for example, in tuberculin screening and allergy tests. Because these medications are potent, they are injected into the dermis, where blood supply is reduced and drug absorption occurs slowly. A client may have an **anaphylactic reaction** if the medications enter the client's circulation too rapidly. For clients with a history of numerous allergies, the physician often performs skin testing.

Skin testing often requires the nurse to visually inspect the test site; therefore intradermal sites should be free of lesions and relatively hairless. The inner forearm and upper back are ideal locations.

To administer an injection intradermally, the nurse uses a tuberculin or small syringe with a short (¼ to ½ inch), fine-gauge (26 or 27) needle. The angle of insertion for an intradermal injection is 5 to 15 degrees (see Fig. 19-6, p. 612). Only small amounts of medication (0.01-0.1 ml) are injected intradermally. If a bleb does not appear or if the site bleeds after needle withdrawal, the medication may have entered SC tissues. In this situation skin test results will not be valid.

EQUIPMENT

- **1 ml tuberculin syringe with preattached 26- or 27-gauge needle**
- **Small gauze pad and/or alcohol swab**
- **Vial or ampule of skin test solution**
- **Disposable gloves**
- **Medication administration record or computer printout**
- **Skin pencil**

STEPS	RATIONALE
ASSESSMENT	
1. Review physician's medication order for client's name, drug name, dose, time, and route of administration.	Ensures safe and correct administration of medication.
2. Know information regarding expected reaction when testing skin with specific allergen or medication.	Type of reaction depends on client's ability to mount a cell-mediated response.
3. Assess client's history of allergies, type of substance, and normal allergic reaction.	Nurse should not administer any substance to which client is known to be allergic.
4. Check date of expiration for medication vial or ampule.	Drug potency may increase or decrease when outdated.
5. Assess client's knowledge of purpose and reactions of skin testing.	Reveals need for client instruction.

NURSING DIAGNOSIS

Clustering of defining characteristics from the assessment data may reveal the following nursing diagnoses for clients requiring this skill:

- ➤ Anxiety
- ➤ Knowledge deficit regarding skin testing
- ➤ Pain
- ➤ Risk for impaired skin integrity
- ➤ Risk for injury

Related factors are individualized based on a client's condition or needs.

STEPS	RATIONALE
PLANNING	
1. **Expected outcomes** following completion of procedure:	
➤ Client experiences very mild burning sensation during injection but no discomfort after injection.	Normal reaction to medication deposited in dermis.
➤ Small light-colored bleb approximately 6 mm (¼ inch) in diameter forms at site and gradually disappears. Minimal bruising may be present.	Medication is in dermis and is eventually absorbed. Bruising is result of minor bleeding from capillaries.
➤ Client is able to identify signs of a skin reaction and their significance.	Demonstrates learning.
2. Prepare correct dose from vial or ampule (see Skill 19-1). Check dose carefully.	Ensures that medication is sterile and dose is accurate.

STEPS	RATIONALE
3. Identify client by checking identification armband and asking client's name. Compare with medication administration record.	Ensures that correct client receives ordered drug.
4. Explain steps of procedure, and tell client that injection will cause a slight burning or sting.	Helps minimize client's anxiety.

IMPLEMENTATION

STEPS	RATIONALE
1. Close room curtain or door.	Provides privacy.
2. Wash hands thoroughly.	Reduces transfer of microorganisms.
3. Select appropriate injection site. Inspect skin surface over sites for bruises, inflammation, or edema. Note lesions or discolorations of forearm. Select site three to four fingerwidths below antecubital space and one handwidth above wrist.	Injection sites should be free of abnormalities that may interfere with drug absorption. An intradermal site should be clear so that results of skin test can be seen and interpreted correctly.
4. Assist client to comfortable position with elbow and forearm extended and supported on flat surface.	Stabilizes injection site for easiest accessibility.
5. Apply disposable gloves.	Follow CDC recommendations to prevent accidental exposure to blood and body fluids (Centers for Disease Control and Prevention, 1988).
6. Cleanse site with an antiseptic swab. Apply swab at center of the site and rotate outward in a circular direction for about 5 cm (2 inches).	Mechanical action of swab removes secretions containing microorganisms.
7. Hold swab or square of sterile gauze between third and fourth fingers of nondominant hand.	Gauze or swab remains readily accessible when needle is withdrawn.
8. Remove needle cap or sheath from needle by pulling it straight off.	Keeping needle from touching sides of cap prevents contamination.
9. Hold syringe between thumb and forefinger of dominant hand with bevel of needle pointing up.	Smooth injection requires proper manipulation of syringe parts. With bevel up, medication is less likely to be deposited into tissues below dermis.
10. With nondominant hand, stretch skin over site with forefinger or thumb.	Needle pierces tight skin more easily.
11. With needle almost against client's skin, insert it slowly at 5- to 15-degree angle until resistance is felt. Then advance needle through epidermis to approximately 3 mm (1/8 inch) below skin surface. Needle tip can be seen through skin (see illustration).	Ensures that needle tip is in dermis.

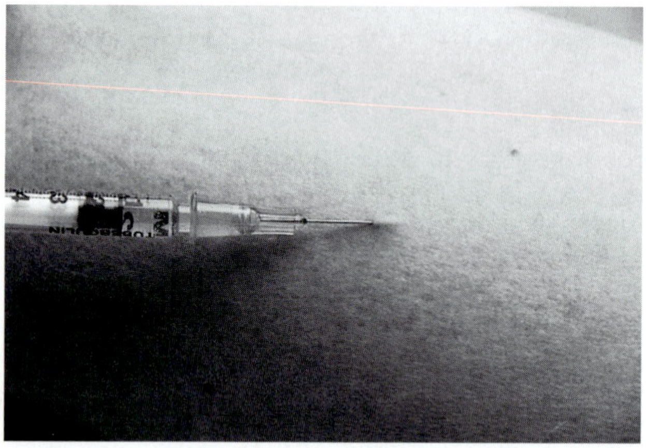

Step 11

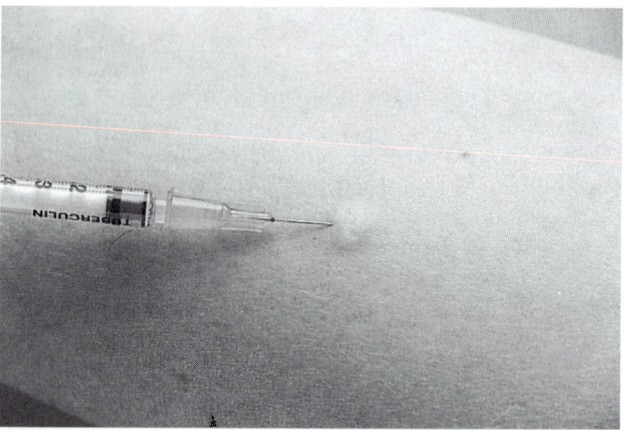

Step 13

STEPS	RATIONALE
12. Inject medication slowly. Normally, resistance is felt. If not, needle is too deep; remove and begin again.	Slow injection minimizes discomfort at site. Dermal layer is tight and does not expand easily when solution is injected.

CRITICAL DECISION POINT It is not necessary to aspirate because dermis is relatively avascular.

STEPS	RATIONALE
13. While injecting medication, notice that small bleb resembling mosquito bite appears on skin's surface (see illustration).	Bleb indicates that medication is deposited in dermis.
14. Withdraw needle while applying alcohol swab or gauze gently over site.	Support of tissue around injection site minimizes discomfort during needle withdrawal. Some advocate use of dry gauze to minimize client discomfort associated with alcohol on nonintact skin.
15. Do not massage site.	Massage may disperse medication into underlying tissue layers and alter test results.
16. Assist client to comfortable position.	Gives client sense of well-being.
17. Discard uncapped needle or needle enclosed in safety shield and attached syringe in puncture-proof and leak-proof receptacles.	Prevents injury to clients and health care personnel. Capping of needles places the health care worker at risk for a needle-stick injury. Special safety shields protect against needle sticks.
18. Remove gloves and wash hands.	Reduces transmission of microorganisms.

EVALUATION

STEPS	RATIONALE
1. Stay with client and observe for any allergic reactions.	Severe anaphylactic reaction is characterized by dyspnea, wheezing, and circulatory collapse.
2. Inspect bleb. Use skin pencil to draw circle around perimeter of injection site.	Site must be read at various intervals to determine test results. Pencil mark makes site easy to find.
3. Ask client to discuss implications of skin testing and signs of hypersensitivity.	Client's ability to recognize signs of skin testing helps to ensure timely reporting of results.
4. **Unexpected outcomes** that may occur include:	
➤ Raised, reddened, or hard zone forms around test site **(induration).**	Indicates sensitivity to injected allergen (positive test for tuberculin skin testing).
➤ Onset of allergic reaction develops within minutes.	Allergen is absorbed into bloodstream, causing allergic reaction.
➤ Client is unable to explain purpose or signs of skin testing.	Client requires further instruction or is unable to learn at this time.

FOLLOW-UP ACTIVITIES

1. Read site within 48 to 72 hours of injection.

RECORDING AND REPORTING

STEPS	RATIONALE
1. Record amount and type of testing substance and date and time on medication record (see illustration, p. 557).	Timely documentation prevents future administration errors.
2. Record area of injection and appearance of skin on nurses' notes.	
3. Report any undesirable effects from medication to nurse in charge or physician.	Client's response may indicate additional medical therapy.

• • • • •

Special Considerations

Tuberculin Skin Testing

➤ Nurse must use caution when testing clients with low concentration of medication. Negative skin test does not mean that client is not allergic to larger therapeutic dose.

➤ Client should wear allergy identification band listing all substances to which client is allergic.

➤ Caution client not to wash off markings around injection site.

➤ Positive tuberculin reaction is indicated by induration (hardening) of skin around injection site of 10

mm or more in immunocompetent clients and 5 mm or more in immunocompromised clients. Read at 48 to 72 hours. Induration of 5 to 9 mm is doubtful unless known exposure has occurred.
- Positive tuberculin test indicates exposure, not active disease.

Teaching Considerations

- When clients are tested in a clinic or other outpatient setting, have them call in results of skin tests if a follow-up appointment is not made.
- Explain to client how to observe for skin reactions.

SKILL 19-4 Administering Subcutaneous Injections

A SC injection involves depositing medication into the loose connective tissue underlying the dermis. SC tissue is not as richly supplied with blood vessels as muscles; thus drugs are not absorbed as quickly as those given intramuscularly. One exception is heparin, which is absorbed quickly by both SC and IM routes. Anything affecting local blood flow to tissues, such as physical exercise or the local application of hot or cold compresses, influences the rate of drug absorption. Conditions such as circulatory shock or occlusive vascular disease impair client's blood flow and thus contraindicate SC injections.

Drugs given subcutaneously are isotonic, nonirritating, nonviscous, and water soluble. Examples of drugs given by this route are epinephrine, insulin, tetanus toxoid, allergy medications, narcotics, and heparin. Only small doses of medications (0.5 to 1 ml) should be given subcutaneously. The tissue is sensitive to irritating solutions and large volumes of medications. Medications collecting within the tissues can cause sterile abscesses, which appear as hardened, painful lumps.

The best sites for SC injections include vascular areas around the outer aspect of the upper arms, the abdomen from below the costal margins to the iliac crests, and the anterior aspect of the thighs. These areas are easily accessible, especially for clients who must self-administer insulin.

The site most frequently recommended for insulin and heparin injections is the abdominal wall. Other sites include the scapular areas of the upper back and the upper ventral or dorsal gluteal areas (Fig. 19-9). Injection sites should be free of infection, skin lesions, scars, bony prominences, and large underlying muscles or nerves. Rotation of injection from major site to major site, once a common practice, is no longer necessary when clients use human insulins. Human insulins are almost exclusively prescribed for clients. Clients can choose one site (e.g., the abdomen), but then be sure to systematically rotate sites within that region.

The amount of adipose tissue on the client's body influences the nurse's choice of needle length and angle of needle insertion. Generally a 25-gauge ⅝-inch needle with a medium bevel inserted at a 45-degree angle (see Fig. 19-6, p. 612) deposits medication into the SC tissue of a normal-size client. If a client is obese, the nurse often pinches the tissue and uses a needle long enough to insert through the fatty tissue at the base of the skinfold. The preferred needle length is one half the width of the skinfold. A ⅞-inch needle is the longest needle for SC use. For injection in obese clients, the angle of insertion is 90 degrees. Cachectic clients may have insufficient tissue for subcutaneous injections. Insulin is injected into the abdomen usually at a 90-degree angle. To ensure that the medication reaches SC tissue, follow this rule: if 2 inches of tissue can be grasped, the needle should be inserted at a 90-degree angle; if 1 inch of tissue can be grasped, the needle should be inserted at a 45-degree angle. The upper abdomen is the best injection site for clients with little peripheral subcutaneous tissue.

EQUIPMENT

- **Syringe (1-3 ml)**
- **Needle (27-25 gauge, ⅜-⅝ inch)**
- **Small gauze pad and/or alcohol swab**
- **Medication ampule or vial**
- **Disposable gloves**
- **Medication administration record or computer printout**

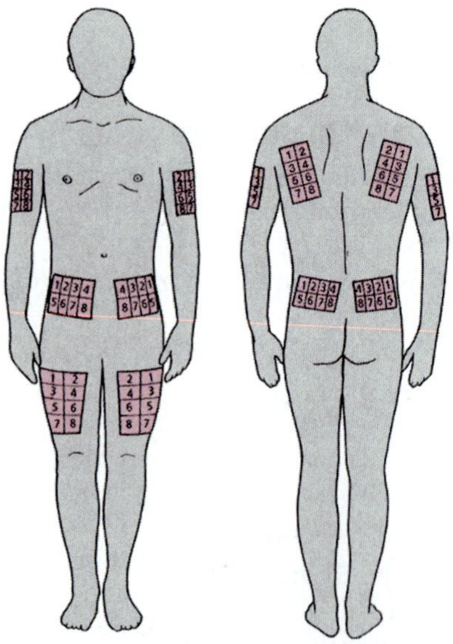

Fig. 19-9 Common sites for subcutaneous injections.

STEPS	RATIONALE
ASSESSMENT	
1. Review physician's medication order for client's name, drug name, dose, time, and route of administration.	Ensures safe and correct administration of medication.
2. Gather information pertinent to drug(s) ordered: action, purpose, time of onset and peak action, normal dosage, common side effects, nursing implications.	Nurse must be able to anticipate drug's effects and observe client's response. Allows nurse to judge appropriateness of therapy as client's condition changes.
3. Assess for factors that may contraindicate SC injections, such as circulatory shock or reduced local tissue perfusion.	Reduced tissue perfusion interferes with drug absorption and distribution.
4. Assess indications for SC injections: unconscious or confused client; client who is unable to swallow or has gastrointestinal disturbances; presence of gastric suction.	Contraindicates use of oral medications; parenteral route thus is more desirable.
5. Assess client's medical history, history of allergies, and medication history.	May influence how certain drug acts. Information also indicates client's need for medication.
6. Assess adequacy of client's adipose tissue.	Physiological changes of aging or client illness may influence amount of SC tissue a client possesses. This influences methods for administering injections.
7. Assess client's knowledge regarding medication to be received.	Information may pose implications for client education. Assessment may also reveal drug use problems at home.
8. Observe client's verbal and nonverbal responses toward injection.	Injections can be painful. Clients may experience considerable anxiety, which can increase pain.

NURSING DIAGNOSIS

Clustering of defining characteristics from the assessment data may reveal the following nursing diagnoses for clients requiring this skill:

- Anxiety
- Knowledge deficit regarding drug therapy
- Pain
- Risk for impaired skin integrity
- Risk for injury

Related factors are individualized based on a client's condition or needs.

STEPS	RATIONALE
PLANNING	
1. **Expected outcomes** following completion of procedure:	
➤ Client experiences mild burning at injection site.	SC medications are nonirritating to tissues, but displacement of tissues causes mild burning.
➤ No allergies or undesired effects of medication occur.	Drug action is normal.
➤ Client explains purpose, dosage, and effects of medication.	Demonstrates learning.
2. Check medication administration record or computer printout.	Verifies order.
3. Prepare correct medication dose from ampule or vial (see Skill 19-1). Check dose carefully.	Ensures that medication is sterile. Preparation techniques differ for ampule and vial.
4. Identify client by checking identification armband and asking client's name. Compare with medication administration record.	Ensures that correct client is receiving medication.
5. Explain procedure to client and proceed in calm, confident manner.	Helps client anticipate nurse's actions. Calm approach minimizes client's anxiety.
IMPLEMENTATION	
1. Close room curtains or door.	Provides privacy.
2. Wash hands and apply disposable gloves.	Reduces transmission of microorganisms.

STEPS	RATIONALE
3. Keep sheet or gown draped over body parts not requiring exposure.	Proper selection of injection site may require exposure of body parts.
4. Select appropriate injection site. Inspect skin's surface over sites for bruises, inflammation, or edema. Palpate site for masses, edema, or tenderness. NOTE: When administering heparin subcutaneously, use abdominal injection sites.	Injection site should be free of lesions that might interfere with drug absorption. NOTE: Anticoagulant may cause local bleeding and bruising when injected into areas such as arms and legs, which are involved in muscular activity.
5. Be sure that needle size is correct by grasping skinfold at site with thumb and forefinger. Measure skinfold from top to bottom; be sure that needle is approximately one half this length.	Ensures that needle will be injected into SC tissue.
6. Assist client to comfortable position. Instruct client to relax arm, leg, or abdomen, depending on site chosen for injection. Talk with client about subject of interest.	Relaxation of area minimizes discomfort during injection. Promoting client's comfort through positioning and distraction helps reduce anxiety.
7. Re-locate site using anatomical landmarks.	Accurate injection of medication requires insertion in correct site to avoid injury to underlying nerves, bone, or blood vessels.
8. Cleanse site with antiseptic swab (see illustration). Apply swab at center of site and rotate outward in circular direction for about 5 cm (2 inches).	Mechanical action of swab removes secretions containing microorganisms.
9. Hold swab or square of sterile gauze between third and fourth fingers of nondominant hand.	Swab or gauze remains readily accessible for when needle is withdrawn.
10. Remove needle cap or sheath from needle by pulling it straight off.	Preventing needle from touching sides of cap prevents contamination.
11. Hold syringe between thumb and forefinger of dominant hand as if grasping a dart, or hold syringe across tops of fingertips (see illustration).	Quick, smooth injection requires proper manipulation of syringe parts.
12. Administer injection:	
a. For average-size client, spread skin tightly across injection site or pinch skin with nondominant hand.	Needle penetrates tight skin easier than loose skin. Pinching skin elevates SC tissue.

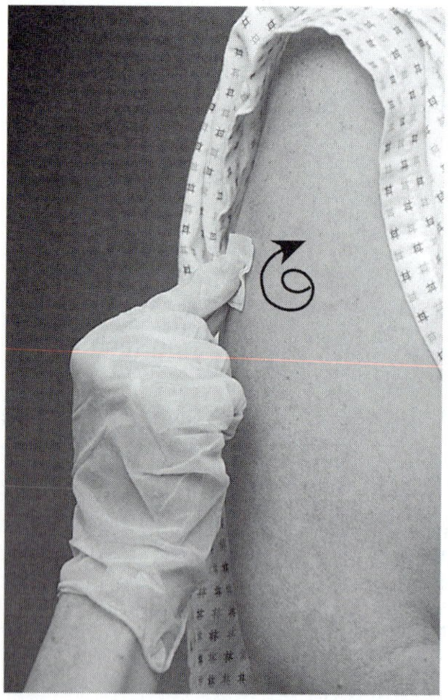

Step 8 Cleansing site with circular motion.

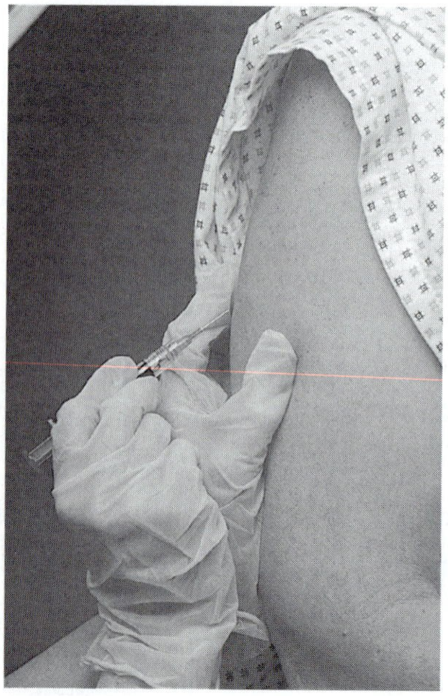

Step 11 Holding syringe as if grasping a dart.

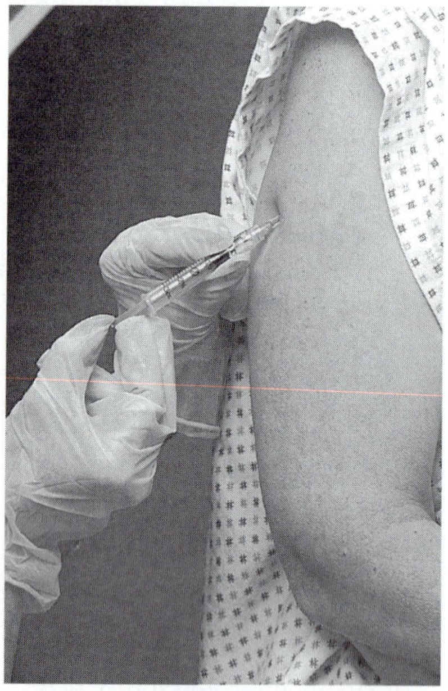

Step 14 Pull back on plunger to aspirate.

STEPS	RATIONALE
b. Inject needle quickly and firmly at 45- to 90-degree angle. (Then release skin, if pinched.)	Quick, firm insertion minimizes discomfort. (Injecting medication into compressed tissue irritates nerve fibers.)
c. For obese client, pinch skin at site and inject needle at 90-degree angle below tissue fold.	Obese clients have fatty layer of tissue above SC layer.
13. After needle enters site, grasp lower end of syringe barrel with nondominant hand. Move dominant hand to end of plunger. Avoid moving syringe.	Properly performed injection requires smooth manipulation of syringe parts. Movement of syringe may displace needle and cause discomfort.
14. Slowly pull back on plunger and aspirate medication for 5 seconds (see illustration) (Beyea and Nicoll, 1995). If blood appears in syringe, withdraw needle, discard medication and syringe properly, and repeat procedure. If no blood appears, inject medication slowly. NOTE: Some institutional policies recommend not aspirating SC heparin injections.	Aspiration of blood into syringe indicates IV placement of needle. SC medications are generally not intended for IV absorption. Slow injection reduces pain and trauma.
15. Withdraw needle quickly while placing antiseptic swab or sterile gauze gently above or over site.	Supporting tissues around injection site minimizes discomfort during needle withdrawal. Some advocate use of dry gauze to minimize client discomfort associated with alcohol on nonintact skin.
16. Apply gentle pressure to site. (If heparin is given, press alcohol swab or gauze to site for a few seconds.)	Aids absorption.
17. Assist client to comfortable position.	Gives client sense of well-being.
18. Discard uncapped needle or needle enclosed in safety shield (see illustrations A and B) and attached syringe in puncture-proof and leak-proof receptacle	Prevents injury to client and health care personnel. The CDC (Centers for Disease Control and Prevention, 1988) warns that capping needles increases risk of needle-stick injury.
19. Dispose of used supplies, remove gloves, and wash hands.	Reduces transmission of microorganisms.

EVALUATION

STEPS	RATIONALE
1. Return to room and ask if client feels any acute pain, burning, numbness, or tingling at injection site.	Continued discomfort may indicate injury to underlying bones or nerves.
2. Observe client's response to medication 30 minutes after injection.	Determines efficacy of drug and allows evaluation of undesirable side effects.
3. Ask client to explain purpose and effects of medication.	Evaluates client's understanding of information taught.

A

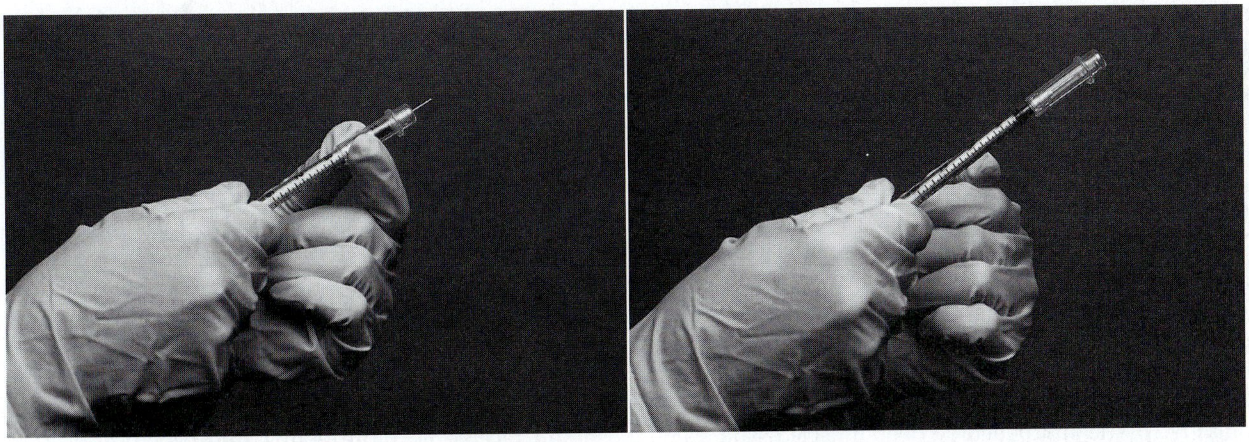

B

Step 18 Needle with plastic guard to prevent needle sticks. **A,** Position of guard before injection. **B,** After injection the guard locks in place, covering the needle.

STEPS	RATIONALE
4. **Unexpected outcomes** that may occur include:	
➤ Client complains of localized pain or continued burning at injection site.	Indicates potential injury to nerve or tissues.
➤ Client displays signs of urticaria, eczema, pruritus, wheezing, and dyspnea.	Indicates allergic response to drug.
➤ Client is unable to discuss information regarding medication.	Reinstruction is necessary, or client is unable to learn at this time.

FOLLOW-UP ACTIVITIES

1. Assess client over several hours for possible allergic reactions especially when a first time drug is given.

RECORDING AND REPORTING

1. Immediately after administration, chart medication dose, route, site, time, and date given in medication record. Correctly sign according to institutional policy (see illustration, p. 557).	Timely documentation prevents future drug administration errors.
2. Report any undesirable effects from medication to nurse in charge or physician.	Client's response may indicate need for additional medical therapy.
3. Record client's response to pain medications or similar drugs in nurses' notes.	Documents client's response to care.

Special Considerations

- ➤ Be sure client wears allergy bracelet indicating medications and substances to which client is allergic.
- ➤ Well-illuminated area is necessary to inspect injection site thoroughly.
- ➤ Keeping syringe and needle out of client's line of vision often minimizes anxiety.

Teaching Considerations

- ➤ Clients who require daily injections will need to learn techniques of self-administration (see Skills 42-5 and 42-6). A family member or a significant other should also be taught injection techniques.
- ➤ Clients with hypertrophy of skin due to repeated insulin injections (common with beef or pork formulations) should be taught to avoid site until problem resolves.

Gerontologic Considerations

- ➤ Aging clients have reduced subcutaneous skinfold thickness. Skin is less elastic than that of younger clients.

Home Care Considerations

- ➤ Clients can be taught that disposable syringes can be reused for several insulin injections at home.

SKILL 19-5 Administering Intramuscular Injections

An injection given by the IM route deposits medication into deep muscle tissue. The vascularity of muscle tissue results in fast drug absorption. An **aqueous** solution is absorbed in 10 to 30 minutes, as opposed to at least 30 minutes when given subcutaneously (McConnell, 1982). However, an increased risk of injecting drugs directly into blood vessels exists. As with SC injections, any factor that interferes with local tissue blood flow affects the rate and extent of drug absorption.

A nurse uses a longer and heavier-gauge needle to pass through SC tissue and penetrate deep muscle tissue. Generally, for the average adult, a 21- to 23-gauge 1½-inch needle inserted at a 90-degree angle will pass through SC tissue and enter deep muscle (see Fig. 19-6, p. 612). An older adult or cachectic client may require a shorter, smaller-gauge needle because of muscle atrophy. For well-developed children a 1-inch needle will penetrate deep muscle. Emaciated muscles absorb medication poorly and should be avoided when possible.

Muscle is less sensitive to irritating and viscous drugs. A normal, well-developed adult client can safely tolerate as much as 4 ml of medication in larger muscles such as the gluteus medius (Beyea and Nicoll, 1995). Older infants and children under the age of 2 receiving IM injection should receive no more than 1 ml of medication (Wong, 1995).

The Z-track technique is recommended for IM injections. The Z- track technique, pulling the skin either downward or laterally before injection, reduces leakage of medication into subcutaneous tissue and minimizes pain (Beyea and Nicoll, 1995).

The nurse selects an IM site, preferably in a large, deep muscle such as the ventrogluteal. It is important to apply a new needle to the syringe after preparing the drug so that no solution remains on the outside needle shaft. The nurse pulls the overlying skin and SC tissues approximately 2.5 to 3.5 cm (1 to 1½ inches) down or laterally to the side. Then the area is cleansed with an antiseptic swab. Holding the skin taut with the nondominant hand, the nurse injects the needle deep into the muscle. With practice the nurse learns to hold the syringe and aspirate with one hand. The nurse injects the drug slowly if there is no blood return on aspiration. The needle remains inserted for 10 seconds to allow the medication to disperse evenly. The nurse releases the skin after withdrawing the needle, which leaves a zigzag path that seals the needle track wherever tissue planes slide across each other (Fig. 19-14, A-*B*). The drug is less likely to escape from the muscle tissue.

VENTROGLUTEAL MUSCLE

The ventrogluteal muscle involves the gluteus medius and minimus. It is situated deep and away from major nerves and blood vessels and is a safe site for all clients. Research has shown that injuries such as fibrosis, nerve damage, abscess, tissue necrosis, muscle contraction, gangrene, and pain have been associated with all the common IM sites except the ventrogluteal site. *The ventrogluteal site is the preferred injection site for adults and anyone over 7 months old* (Beyea and Nicoll, 1995).

The nurse locates the muscle by placing the heel of the hand over the greater trochanter of the client's hip with the wrist almost perpendicular to the femur. The right hand is used for the left hip, and the left hand is used for the right hip. The nurse points the thumb toward the client's groin and the fingers toward the client's head, points the index finger to the anterosuperior iliac spine, and extends the middle finger back along the iliac crest toward the buttock. The index finger, the middle finger, and the iliac crest form a V-shaped triangle, and the injection site is the center of the triangle (Fig. 19-10).

A

B

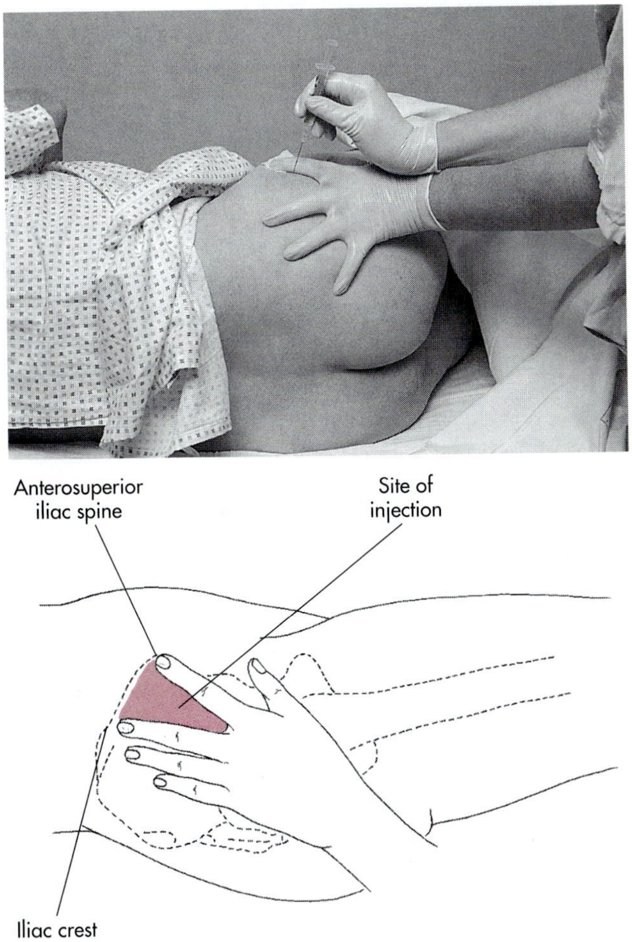

Fig 19-10 **A,** Injection site for ventrogluteal muscle avoids major nerves and blood vessels. **B,** Anatomic view of ventrogluteal muscle injection site.

A

B

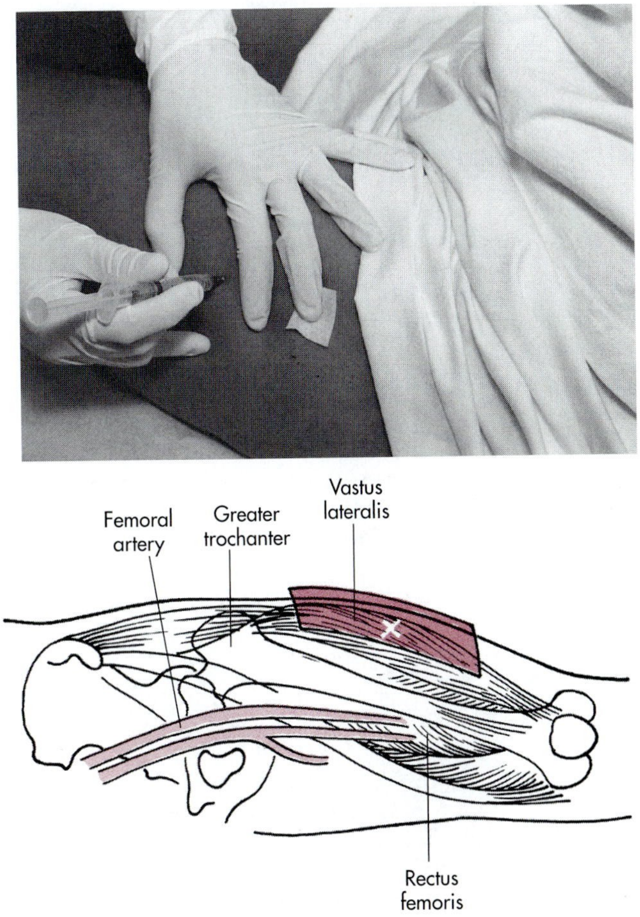

Fig 19-11 **A,** Giving IM injection in vastus lateralis site. **B,** Landmarks for vastus lateralis site.

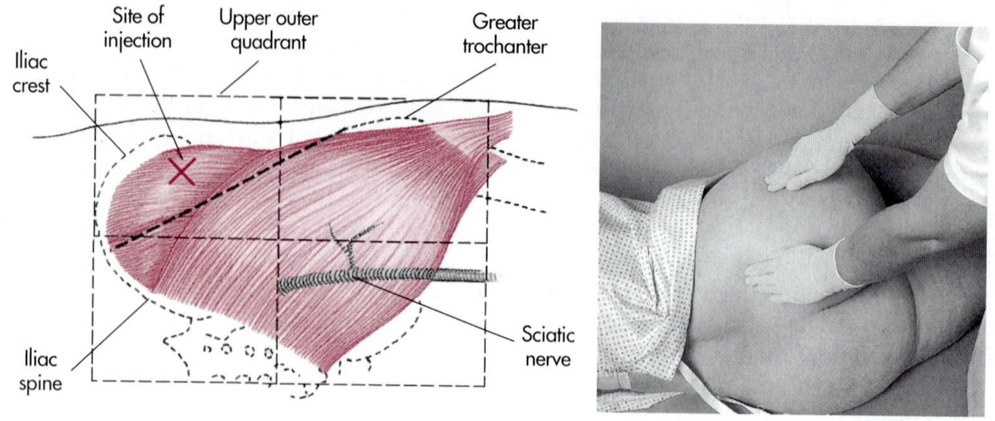

Fig. 19-12 **A,** Landmarks for dorsogluteal site. **B,** Locating right dorsogluteal site (client is on left side).

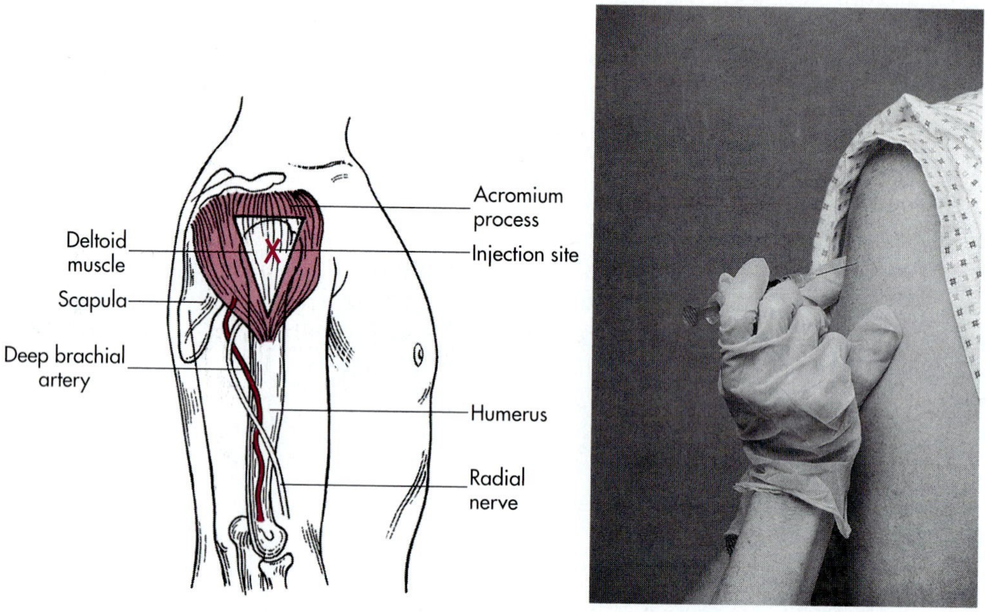

Fig. 19-13 **A,** Landmarks for deltoid site. **B,** Giving IM injection in deltoid site.

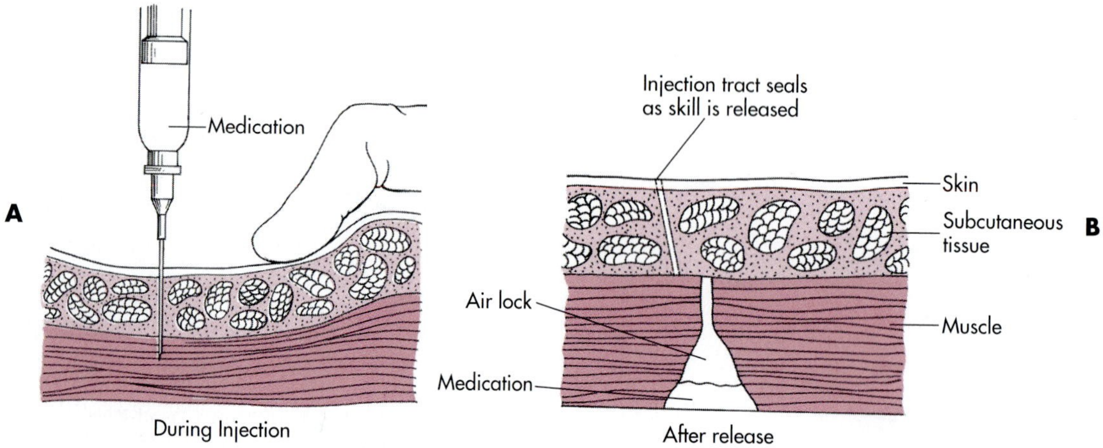

Fig. 19-14 **A,** Pull on overlying skin during IM injection moves tissues to prevent later tracking. **B,** The Z-track left after injection prevents the deposit of medication through sensitive tissue.

VASTUS LATERALIS MUSCLE

The vastus lateralis muscle is another injection site used in the adult client and for infants under 7 months of age (Beyea and Nicoll, 1995). The muscle is thick and well developed. It is located on the anterior lateral aspect of the thigh; in an adult it extends from a handbreadth above the knee to a handbreadth below the greater trochanter of the femur (Fig. 19-11). The middle third of the muscle is the suggested site for injection. The width of the muscle usually extends from the midline of the thigh and the midline of the thigh's outer side.

DORSOGLUTEAL MUSCLE

The dorsogluteal muscle has been a traditional site for IM injections; however, a risk exists of striking the underlying sciatic nerve or major blood vessels. Insertion of a needle into the sciatic nerve can cause permanent or partial paralysis of the involved leg. In clients with flabby, sagging tissues, the site is difficult to locate. It is described here only as a last choice for an injection.

The dorsogluteal site is located in the upper outer quadrant of the buttock, approximately 5 to 8 cm (2 to 3 inches) below the iliac crest (Fig. 19-12, *A*). Clients may lie prone with toes turned medially or in a side-lying position with the upper leg flexed at hip and knee. The best method for locating the dorsogluteal site is:

1. Locate the posterior superior iliac spine and the greater trochanter of the femur. Draw an imaginary line between the two anatomical landmarks. The sciatic nerve runs parallel to and below the line. The injection site is above and lateral to the line (Fig. 19-12, *B*).

DELTOID MUSCLE

Although the deltoid site is easily accessible, the muscle is not well developed in many adults. The radial and ulnar nerves and the brachial artery lie within the upper arm along the humerus (Fig. 19-13, *A*). The nurse should use this site only for small medication volumes (0.5 to 1.0 ml) or when other sites are inaccessible because of dressings or casts.

To locate the deltoid muscle, the nurse fully exposes the client's upper arm and shoulder. A tight-fitting sleeve should not be rolled up. The nurse instructs the client to relax the arm at the side and flex the elbow. The client may sit, stand, or lie down (Fig. 19-13, *B*). The nurse palpates the lower edge of the acromion process, which forms the base of a triangle in line with the midpoint of the lateral aspect of the upper arm. The injection site is in the center of the triangle, about 2.5 to 5 cm (1 to 2 inches) below the acromion process (see Fig. 19-13, *A*). The nurse may also locate the site by placing four fingers across the deltoid muscle, with the top finger along the acromion process. The injection site is then three fingerwidths below the acromion process.

EQUIPMENT

- **Syringe: 2-3 ml for adult; 0.5-1 ml for infants and small children**
- **Needles (2): 21-23 gauge, 1-1 1/2 inches for adults; 1 inch for children**
- **Small gauze pad and/or alcohol swab**
- **Medication ampule or vial**
- **Disposable gloves**
- **Medication administration record or computer printout**

STEPS	RATIONALE
ASSESSMENT	
1. Review physician's medication order for client's name, drug name, dose, time, and route of administration.	Ensures safe and correct administration of medication.
2. Gather information pertinent to drug(s) ordered: action, purpose, time of onset and peak action, normal dose, common side effects, nursing implications.	Nurse must be able to anticipate drug's effects and observe client's response. Allows nurse to judge appropriateness of therapy as client's condition changes.
3. Consider factors that may contraindicate IM injection, for example, muscle atrophy, reduced blood flow, or circulatory shock.	Atrophied muscle absorbs medication poorly. Factors interfering with blood flow to muscles impair drug absorption.
CRITICAL DECISION POINT Consider calling prescriber for alternate route of medication administration.	
4. Assess client's medical history, history of allergies, and medication history.	May influence action of certain drugs. Information also indicates client's need for medication.
5. Assess client's knowledge regarding medication and dosage schedule.	Information may pose implications for client education. Assessment may also reveal drug use problems at home.

STEPS	RATIONALE
6. Observe client's verbal and nonverbal responses toward receiving injection.	Injections can be painful. Clients may experience considerable anxiety, which can increase pain.

NURSING DIAGNOSIS

Clustering of defining characteristics from the assessment data may reveal the following nursing diagnoses for clients requiring this skill:

- Anxiety
- Pain
- Risk for impaired skin integrity
- Risk for injury

Related factors are individualized based on a client's condition or needs.

PLANNING

STEPS	RATIONALE
1. **Expected outcomes** following completion of procedure:	
➤ Client experiences temporary mild burning at injection site.	Displacement of tissues during injection causes discomfort.
➤ No allergies or undesired effects occur.	Drug action is normal.
➤ Client explains purpose and effects of medication.	Demonstrates learning.
➤ Client demonstrates no behaviors reflecting anxiety.	Anticipatory guidance relieves anxiety.
2. For adults, select a 1.5 in needle. For children, select a 1 in needle.	Needle must be long enough to reach muscle. Adipose tissue layer over the ventral gluteal muscle is less than 3.75 cm (1.47 in) in depth (Beyea and Nicoll, 1995).
3. Prepare correct dose from ampule or vial (see Skill 19-1). Check dose carefully.	Ensures that medication is sterile and dose is accurate.
4. Change needle on syringe.	Prevents tracking of irritating substances as needle passes into muscle.
5. Identify client by checking identification armband and asking client's name. Compare with medication ticket.	Ensures that correct client is receiving medication.
6. Explain procedure, location of injection site, and how positioning lessens discomfort (see box). Proceed in calm manner.	Allows client to anticipate injection so as to lessen anxiety.

IMPLEMENTATION

STEPS	RATIONALE
1. Close room curtains or door.	Provides client privacy.
2. Wash hands and apply gloves.	Reduces transmission of microorganisms.
3. Keep sheet or gown draped over body parts not requiring exposure.	Proper selection of injection site may require exposure of body parts.
4. Select appropriate injection site by assessing size and integrity of muscle. Palpate for areas of tenderness or hardness. Note presence of bruising or area of infection.	Muscle should be soft when relaxed and firm when tense; indicates healthy tissue.

➤ **CRITICAL DECISION POINT** When choosing an injection site, do not use an area that is bruised or has signs associated with infection.

POSITIONING CLIENT FOR COMFORT WITH INTRAMUSCULAR INJECTION

- Giving an injection to a client in the side-lying position: Have the client flex the knee, then pivot the leg forward from the hip approximately 20 degrees so it can rest on the bed.
- Giving an injection to a client in the supine position: Have the client flex the knee on the side where the injection is to be administered.
- Giving an injection to a client in the prone position: Have the client "toe in" to rotate the femur internally.

Modified from Beyea SC, Nicoll LH: Back to basics: administering IM injections the right way, *Am J Nurs* 96(1), 1996.

STEPS	RATIONALE
5. Assist client to comfortable position, depending on site chosen: ventrogluteal—client lies on side or back, flexes knee and hip on side to be injected; vastus lateralis—client lies flat, supine, with knee slightly flexed; dorsogluteal—client lies prone with feet turned inward or lies on side with upper knee and hip flexed and placed in front of lower leg; deltoid—client may sit or lie flat with lower arm flexed but relaxed across abdomen or lap.	Position that reduces strain on muscle minimizes discomfort of injection.
CRITICAL DECISION POINT **Ensure that client's position is not contraindicated by medical condition.**	
6. Relocate site using anatomical landmarks.	Injection into correct anatomical site prevents injury to nerves, bones, and blood vessels.
7. Position nondominant hand and pull the skin down to administer in a Z-track.	Reduces discomfort and incidence of lesions.
8. Cleanse site with antiseptic swab. Apply swab to center of site and rotate outward in circular direction for about 5 cm (2 inches).	Mechanical action of swab removes secretions containing microorganisms.
9. Hold swab or square of sterile gauze between third and fourth fingers of nondominant hand.	Swab or gauze remains readily accessible for when needle is withdrawn.
10. Remove needle cap or sheath from needle by pulling it straight off.	Preventing needle from touching sides of cap prevents contamination.
11. Hold syringe between thumb and forefinger of dominant hand as if holding a dart. Hold it with palm down at 90-degree angle.	Quick, smooth injection requires proper manipulation of syringe. Needle must be injected at 90-degree angle to enter muscle.
12. Administer injection:	
a. Inject needle quickly at 90-degree angle into muscle (see illustration).	Ensures that medication reaches muscle mass.
b. If client's muscle mass is small, grasp body of muscle between thumb and fingers.	Ensures that medication reaches muscle mass.

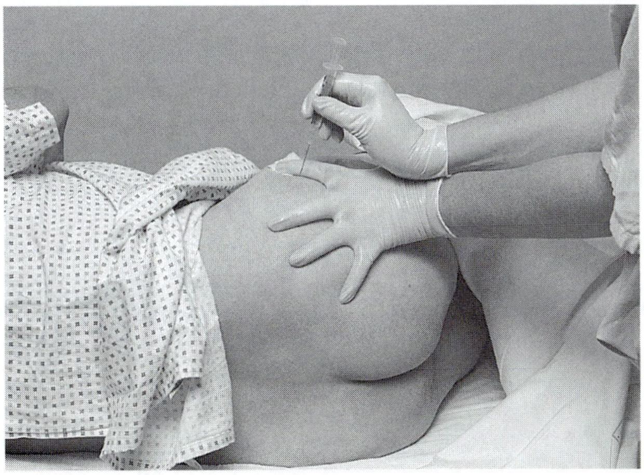

Step 12a

STEPS	RATIONALE
13. After needle enters site, grasp lower end of syringe barrel with nondominant hand to stabilize syringe. Continue to hold skin tightly with nondominant hand. Move dominant hand to end of plunger. Avoid moving syringe.	Smooth manipulation of syringe parts reduces discomfort from needle movement. Skin must remain pulled until after drug is injected.
14. Slowly pull back on plunger 5 to 10 seconds. If no blood appears, inject medication slowly at a rate of 10 sec/ml.	Aspiration of blood into syringe indicates IV placement of needle. IM medications are not for IV use. Slow injection reduces pain and tissue trauma (Beyea and Nicoll, 1995).

➤ ***CRITICAL DECISION POINT*** **If blood appears in syringe, remove needle and dispose of medication and syringe properly. Repeat preparation procedure.**

STEPS	RATIONALE
15. Wait ten seconds, then smoothly and steadily withdraw needle while placing antiseptic swab or dry gauze gently above or over injection.	Support of tissues around injection site minimizes discomfort during needle withdrawal. Some advocate use of dry gauze to minimize client discomfort associated with alcohol on nonintact skin.
16. Apply gentle pressure. Do not massage site.	Massage can damage underlying tissue.
17. For ventrogluteal and vastus lateralis sites, encourage leg exercises.	Promotes drug absorption.
18. Discard uncapped needle or needle enclosed in safety shield and attached syringe into puncture-proof and leak-proof receptacle.	Prevents injury to clients and health care personnel. The CDC (Centers for Disease Control and Prevention, 1988) recommends that needles not be recapped before disposal. New safety shields prevent needle-stick injuries.
19. Dispose of soiled supplies, remove gloves, and wash hands.	Reduces transmission of microorganisms.

EVALUATION

1. Return to room and ask if client feels any acute pain, burning, numbness, or tingling at injection site.	Continued discomfort may indicate injury to underlying bones or nerves.
2. Inspect site, note any bruising or induration.	Bruising or induration indicates complication associated with injection. Notify nurse in charge or health care provider. Apply warm compress to site.
3. Return to evaluate client's response to medication in 10 to 30 minutes.	IM medications are absorbed quickly; undesired effects may also develop rapidly. Nurse's observations determine efficacy of drug action.
4. Ask client to explain purpose and effects of medication.	Evaluates client's understanding of information taught.
5. **Unexpected outcomes** that may occur include:	
➤ Client continues to complain of localized pain, numbness, or tingling.	Indicates injury to nerves or tissues.
➤ Client develops signs and symptoms of allergy or side effects.	Extent of symptoms depends on client's sensitivity to drug and dose of drug.
➤ Client is unable to explain purpose or effects of medication.	Client requires reinstruction, or client is unable to learn at this time.

STEPS	RATIONALE
RECORDING AND REPORTING	
1. Immediately chart medication, dosage, route, site, time, and date given in medication administration record. Correctly sign according to institutional policy (see illustration, p. 557).	Timely documentation prevents future drug administration errors.
2. Report any undesirable effects from medication to nurse in charge or physician.	Client's response may indicate additional medical therapy.
3. Record client's response to pain medications or similar drugs in nurses' notes.	Documents client's response to care.

FOLLOW-UP ACTIVITIES

1. Assess client over several hours for possible allergic reactions especially when a first time drug is given.

• • • • •

Special Considerations

- Clients who have had a cerebrovascular accident (stroke) or spinal cord injury often have muscle atrophy.
- Use good illumination when assessing injection site.

Teaching Considerations

- Clients requiring regular injections, for example, vitamin B_{12}, should learn importance of rotating sites. Injections may be given by family members, client, or home health nurse.
- Instruct client and primary care giver to maintain sterile technique.
- Instruct client and primary care giver to observe injection sites for complications.
- Instruct client and primary care giver to observe for medication side effects.
- Allow for several return demonstrations by client on drawing up medications from vial or ampule and on injection technique.
- Teach proper methods of disposal of needles and equipment.

Pediatric Considerations

- The dorsogluteal and deltoid muscles are no longer recommended as injection sites in children.

Home Care Considerations

- See Skills 41-3 and 42-5.

SKILL 19-6 Adding Medications to Intravenous Fluid Containers

Of all the methods for drug administration, the IV route poses the greatest risks for a client. Through IV **infusion** medications enter the venous circulation directly and thus can cause rapid effects. The nurse must observe the client closely for symptoms of adverse reactions. Special attention is given to dose calculation and drug preparation. The nurse carefully checks the "five rights" of safe drug administration and is aware of the desired action and potential side effects of each medication.

Mixing drugs in large volumes of fluids is relatively safe and easy. The nurse or pharmacist dilutes IV medications in volumes of 50 to 1000 ml of compatible IV fluids such as normal saline, dextrose and water, or lactated Ringer's solution. In many hospital settings the pharmacy adds drugs to primary containers of IV solutions to ensure asepsis. Because a drug in an IV solution is not in a concentrated form, the risk of side effects or fatal reactions is minimal. Vitamins and potassium chloride are two types of drugs commonly added to IV fluids.

Many parenteral medications are highly alkaline and irritating to muscle and SC tissue. Thus the IV route is best to minimize client discomfort. The nurse administers drugs intravenously by five methods:

1. As mixtures within large volumes of IV fluids.
2. By **piggyback infusion** of a solution containing the prescribed medication and a small volume of fluid (50 ml, 100 ml) through an adjoining container or existing IV line (see Skill 19-7).

3. By Volutrol infusion in which a small container, holding 50 to 150 ml of fluid, is attached below the primary infusion bag (see Skill 19-7).
4. By various electronic infusion devices (see Skill 19-7).
5. By injection of a bolus or small volume of medication through an existing IV infusion line or heparin or saline IV lock (see Skill 19-8).

In all the methods the client has either an existing IV infusion line or an IV access site in the form of a **heparin lock** or a saline lock. In most institutions and settings there are policies that identify the medications that nurses are allowed to inject directly into a client's veins through venipuncture.

EQUIPMENT

- Vial or ampule of prescribed medication
- Syringe of appropriate size (5-20 ml)
- Sterile needle (1-1½ inch, 19-21 gauge) with special filters (optional)
- Correct diluent (e.g., sterile water or normal saline)
- Sterile IV fluid container (bag or bottle, 50-1000 ml in volume)
- Alcohol or antiseptic swab
- Label to attach to IV bag or bottle
- Medication administration form or computer printout

STEPS	RATIONALE
ASSESSMENT	
1. Check physician's order to determine type of IV solution to use and type of medication and dosage.	Client's overall physical condition dictates type of IV solution used. Ensures safe and accurate drug administration.
2. Collect information necessary to administer drug safely, including action, purpose, side effects, normal dose, time of peak onset, nursing implications.	Allows nurse to give drug safely and to monitor client's response to therapy.
3. When more than one medication is to be added to IV solution, assess for **compatibility** of medications.	Drug **incompatibility** often becomes apparent when drugs are mixed together. Chemical reactions that occur result in clouding or crystallization of IV fluids. Check hospital policy for drug compatibility list.
4. Assess client's systemic fluid balance, as reflected by skin hydration and turgor, body weight, pulse, and blood pressure.	Danger of continuous IV infusions is that fluids may infuse too rapidly, causing circulatory overload.
5. Assess client's history of drug allergies.	IV administration of drugs causes rapid effects. Allergic response can be immediate.
6. Assess IV insertion site for signs of **infiltration** or **phlebitis** (Chapter 20).	An intact, properly functioning site ensures that medication is given safely.
7. Assess client's understanding of purpose of drug therapy.	May reveal need for education.

NURSING DIAGNOSIS

Clustering of defining characteristics from the assessment data may reveal the following nursing diagnoses for clients requiring this skill:

- Knowledge deficit regarding drug therapy
- Risk for fluid volume excess
- Risk for impaired skin integrity
- Risk for injury

Related factors are individualized based on a client's condition or needs.

PLANNING

STEPS	RATIONALE
1. **Expected outcomes** following completion of procedure:	
➤ Client experiences no medication side effects or adverse reactions.	Drugs were given safely.
➤ Client develops no signs or symptoms of fluid volume excess.	IV rate is monitored correctly.
➤ IV site remains free of swelling or inflammation.	Fluid was delivered intravenously.
➤ Client will explain purpose and side effects of medication.	Demonstrates learning.
2. Assemble supplies in medication room.	Ensures orderly procedure with less chance of supply contamination.

STEPS	RATIONALE
3. Prepare prescribed medication from vial or ampule. (If filter needle is used, replace it with regular needle before injecting medication into IV fluid container.)	Different techniques are used for each type of container.
4. Identify client by reading identification band and asking name. Compare with medication ticket.	Ensures that correct client receives ordered medication.
5. Prepare client by explaining that medication is to be given through existing IV line or one to be started. Explain that no discomfort should be felt during drug infusion. Encourage client to report symptoms of discomfort.	Most IV medications do not cause discomfort when diluted. However, potassium chloride can be irritating. Pain at insertion site may be early indication of infiltration.

IMPLEMENTATION

STEPS	RATIONALE
1. Wash hands thoroughly.	Reduces transfer of microorganisms.
2. Add medication to new container:	
a. Solutions in a bag. Locate medication injection port on plastic IV solution bag. Port has small rubber stopper at end. Do not select port for IV tubing insertion or air vent.	Medication injection port is self-sealing to prevent introduction of microorganisms after repeated use.
b. Solutions in bottles. Locate injection site on IV solution bottle, which is often covered by a metal or plastic cap.	Accidental injection of medication through main tubing port or air vent can alter pressure within bottle and cause fluid leaks through air vent. Cap seals bottle to maintain its sterility.
c. Wipe off port or injection site with alcohol or antiseptic swab (see illustration).	Reduces risk of introducing microorganisms into bag during needle insertion.
d. Remove needle cap or sheath from syringe and insert needle of syringe through center of injection port or site; inject medication (see illustration).	Injection of needle into sides of port may produce leak and lead to fluid contamination.

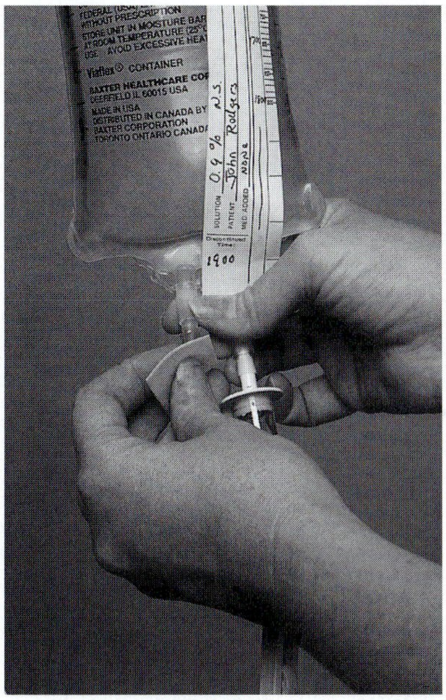

Step 2c

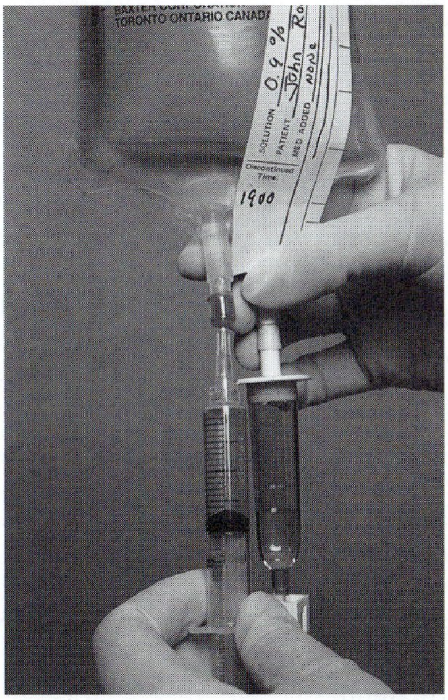

Step 2d

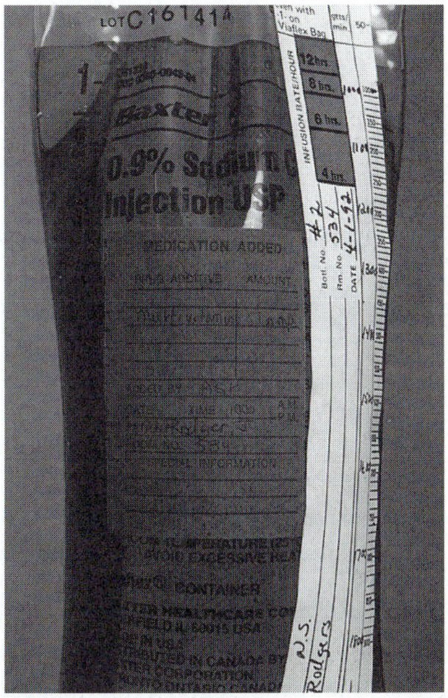

Step 2g

STEPS	RATIONALE
e. Withdraw syringe from bag or bottle.	Open tubing port in bottle provides direct route for microorganisms to enter solution. Bags have self-sealing port.
f. Mix medication and IV solution by holding bag or bottle and turning it gently end to end.	Allows even distribution of medication.
g. Complete medication label with name and dose of medication, date, time, and nurse's initials. Stick it on bottle or bag. *Optional* (check institution's policy): Apply a flow strip that identifies the time that the solution was hung and intervals indicating fluid levels (see illustration).	Label can be easily read during infusion of solution. Informs nurses and physicians of contents of bag or bottle.
➤ *CRITICAL DECISION POINT* Do not use felt-tip markers on plastic surfaces. The ink can penetrate the plastic and leak into the IV solution.	
h. Spike bag or bottle with IV tubing and hang (see Chapter 20). Regulate infusion at ordered rate.	Prevents rapid infusion of fluid.
3. Add medication to existing container:	
a. Prepare vented IV bottle or plastic bag:	
(1) Check volume of solution remaining in bottle or bag.	Proper minimal volume (see drug insert) is needed to dilute medication adequately.
(2) Close off IV infusion clamp.	Prevents medication from directly entering circulation as it is injected into bag or bottle.
(3) Wipe off medication port with an alcohol or antiseptic swab.	Mechanically removes microorganisms that could enter container during needle insertion.
(4) Insert syringe needle through injection port and inject medication.	Injection port is self-sealing and prevents fluid leaks.
(5) Lower bag or bottle from IV pole and gently mix. Rehang bag.	Ensures medication is evenly distributed.
b. Complete medication label and stick it to bag or bottle.	Informs nurses and physicians of contents of bag or bottle.
c. Open infusion clamp and regulate infusion to desired rate.	Prevents rapid infusion of fluid.
4. Properly dispose of equipment and supplies. Do not cap needle of syringe. Specially sheathed needles are discarded as a unit with needle covered.	Proper disposal of needle prevents injury to nurse and client. Capping of needles increases risk of needlestick injuries.
5. Wash hands.	Reduces transmission of microorganisms.
EVALUATION	
1. Observe client for signs or symptoms of drug reaction.	IV medications can cause rapid effects.
2. Observe for signs and symptoms of fluid volume excess.	Rapid uncontrolled infusion can cause circulatory overload.
3. Periodically return to client's room to assess IV insertion site and rate of infusion.	Over time IV site may become infiltrated or needle may become malpositioned. Flow rate may change according to client's position or volume left in container.
4. Observe for signs or symptoms of IV infiltration.	Infiltrated drugs can injure tissue.
5. Have client explain purpose and effects of drug therapy.	
6. **Unexpected outcomes** that may occur include:	
➤ Client has undesired reaction to medication.	Response depends on client's sensitivity and drug's action.
➤ Client develops signs of fluid volume excess, for example, abnormal breath sounds (crackles), blood pressure changes, jugular venous distention, edema, shortness of breath, intake greater than output.	Excess fluid intake can compromise circulatory regulation.

STEPS	RATIONALE
➤ IV site becomes swollen, warm, reddened, and tender to touch (see Chapter 20).	Indicates signs of phlebitis.
➤ IV site becomes cool, pale, and swollen (Chapter 20).	Indicates signs of infiltration.
➤ Client is unable to explain purpose, side effects of medication.	Reinstruction is necessary or client is unable to learn at this time.

Recording and Reporting

1. Record solution and medication added to parenteral fluid on appropriate form (Fig. 19-15).	Information is used to monitor type of solutions client receives and fluid intake over 24 hours.
2. Report any side effects to nurse in charge or physician.	Reaction may require therapeutic intervention.

Follow-up Activities

1. Monitor status of IV on an ongoing basis, looking for signs of infiltration and/or phlebitis.

• • • • •

Special Considerations

- Check with pharmacist or consult drug literature for drug compatibility.
- For monitoring of IV fluid infusion, note that vitamins, minerals, and most electrolytes are relatively safe. Potassium chloride, if allowed to infuse too quickly, can cause cardiac dysrhythmias.
- Pharmacies use special plastic caps to seal bottles previously mixed.
- When adding medication to a glass bottle with a vented administration set, be sure there is sufficient fluid in the bottle or bag. After closing the IV flow clamp, detach the air vent cap while keeping the end sterile. Remove needle from the medication syringe, and insert the tip of the syringe into the air vent port. Instill medication and reattach the air vent.

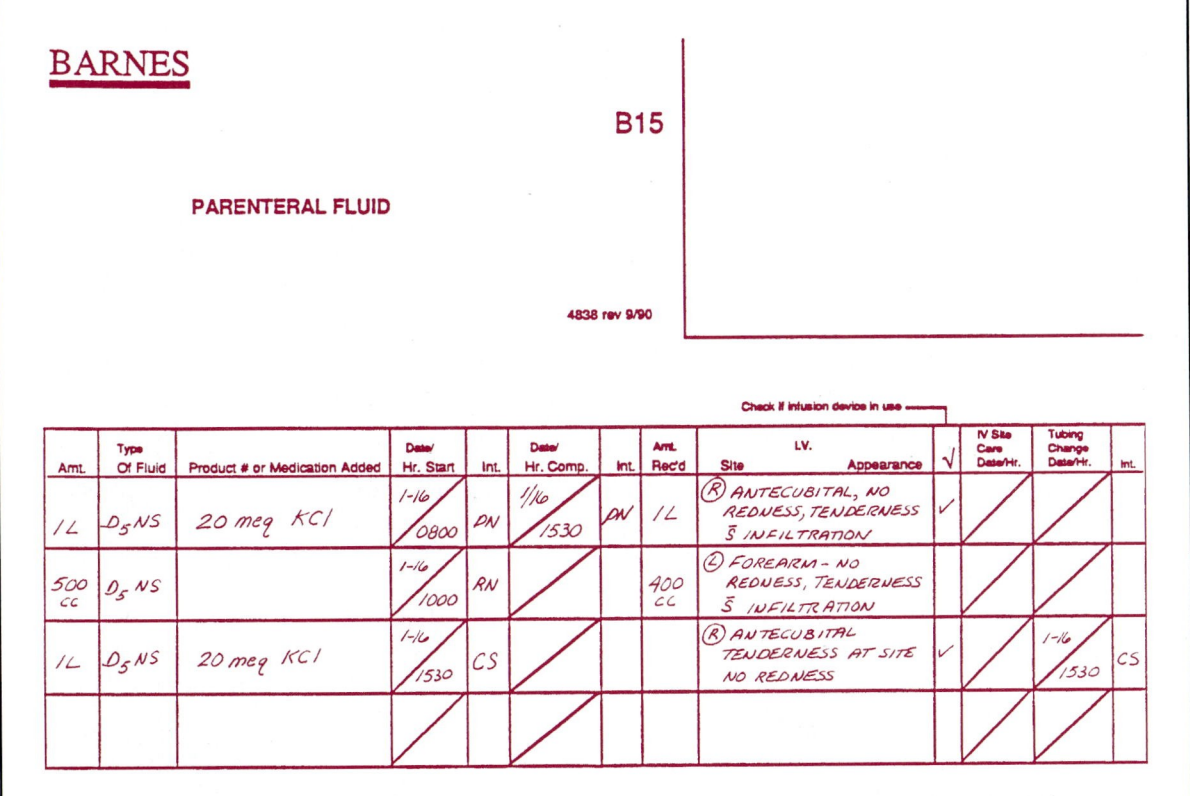

BARNES

B15

PARENTERAL FLUID

4838 rev 9/90

Check if infusion device in use

Amt.	Type Of Fluid	Product # or Medication Added	Date/ Hr. Start	Int.	Date/ Hr. Comp.	Int.	Amt. Rec'd	I.V. Site Appearance	√	IV Site Care Date/Hr.	Tubing Change Date/Hr.	Int.
1L	D_5NS	20 meq KCl	1-16 / 0800	DN	1/16 / 1530	DN	1L	(R) ANTECUBITAL, NO REDNESS, TENDERNESS S̄ INFILTRATION	✓			
500 cc	D_5 NS		1-16 / 1000	RN			400 cc	(L) FOREARM - NO REDNESS, TENDERNESS S̄ INFILTRATION				
1L	D_5NS	20 meq KCl	1-16 / 1530	CS				(R) ANTECUBITAL TENDERNESS AT SITE NO REDNESS	✓		1-16 / 1530	CS

Fig. 19-15

SKILL 19-7 Administering Intravenous Medications by Intermittent Infusion Sets and Miniinfusion Pumps

Administering drugs by intermittent infusion is a method in which the nurse dilutes IV medications in small volumes of solution and administers them over a short period. Administering drugs by this method reduces the risk of rapid drug-dose infusion and provides greater comfort and independence for the client. Clients receiving drugs by intermittent infusion have an established IV line that is kept patent by intermittent flushes of normal saline.

Intermittent infusion of drugs can be administered in several ways:

1. *Piggyback.* A piggyback is a small (25 to 100 ml) IV bag or bottle connected to short tubing lines that connect to the *upper* Y port of a primary infusion line or to an intermittent venous access (Fig. 19-16, *A*). The piggyback tubing is a microdrip or macrodrip system (see Chapter 20). The set is called a "piggyback" because the small bag or bottle is set higher than the primary infusion bag or bottle. In the piggyback setup the main line does not infuse when the piggybacked medication is infusing. The port of the primary IV line contains a back check valve that automatically stops the flow of the primary infusion once the piggyback infusion flows. After the piggyback solution infuses and the solution within the tubing falls below the level of the primary infusion drip chamber, the back-check valve opens and the primary infusion again flows.
2. *Tandem.* A tandem setup is a small (25 to 100 ml) IV bag or bottle connected to a short tubing line to the *lower* Y port of a primary infusion line or to an intermittent venous access (Fig. 19-16, *B*). The tandem set is placed at the same height as the primary infusion bag or bottle. In the tandem setup the tandem and the main line infuse simultaneously. The nurse must monitor the tandem setup closely. If the tandem setup is not immediately clamped when the medication is infused, the IV solution from the primary line will back up into the tandem line.
3. *Volume-control administration.* Volume-control administration (e.g., Volutrol, Buretrol, Pediatrol) sets are small (50 to 150 ml) containers that attach just below the primary infusion bag or bottle. The set is attached and filled in a manner similar to that used with a regular IV infusion. However, the priming filling of the set is different, depending on the type of filter (floating valve or membrane) within the set. Follow the package directions for priming sets.
4. *Miniinfusion pump.* The miniinfuser pump is battery operated. It allows medications to be given in very small amounts of fluid (5 to 60 ml) within controlled infusion times using standard syringes (Fig. 19-17).

The CDC and Occupational Safety and Health Administration (OSHA) have made very strong recommendations that all intermittent infusion methods be needleless. This can be achieved by using stopcocks to attach medication tubings to the main line. Needleless or shielded needle devices for infusion lines are manufactured by various companies for this purpose (Fig. 19-18). The needleless infusion lines have blunt-ended cannulas or recessed

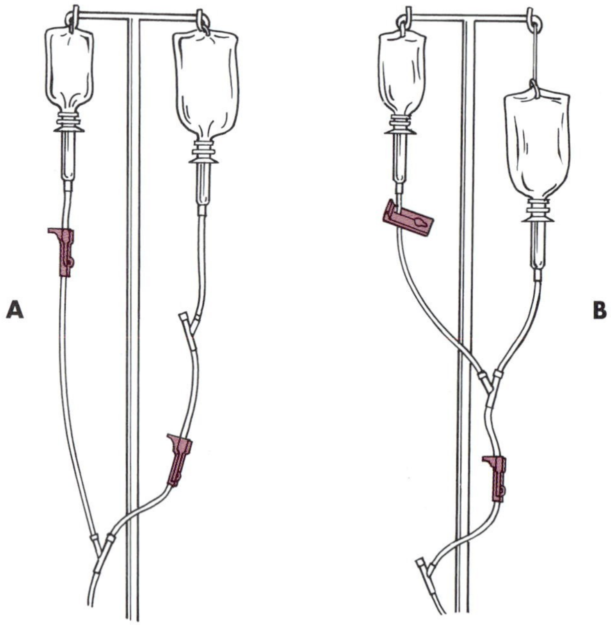

Fig 19-16 Intermittent infusion sets. **A,** Piggyback set. **B,** Tandem set.

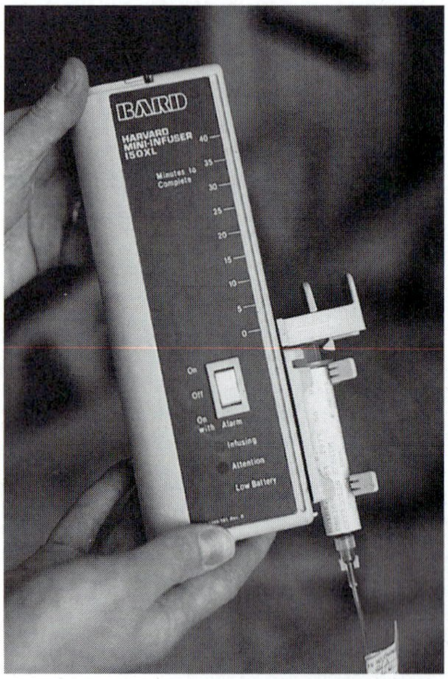

Fig. 19-17

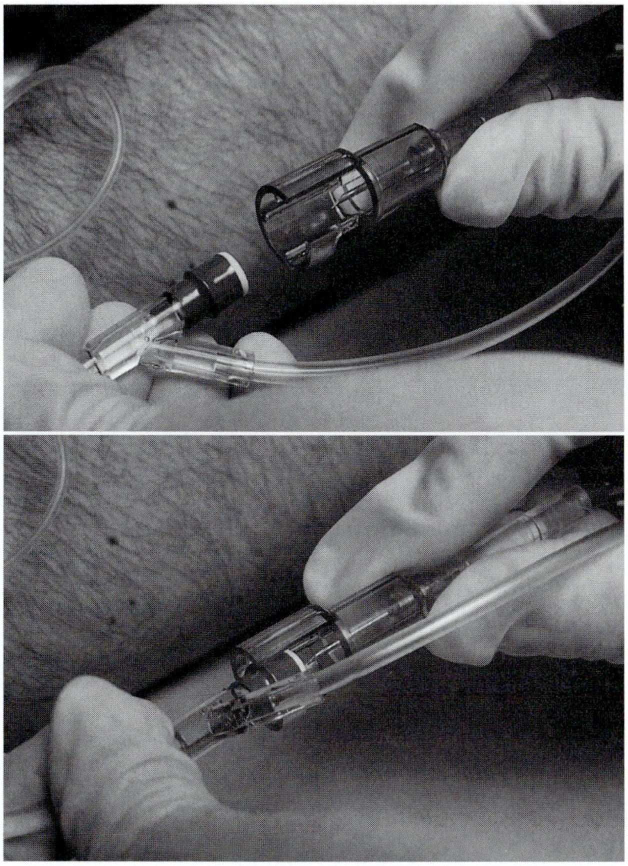

Fig. 19-18 Example of needleless device.

connection ports, eliminating the risk of exposure to an IV needle.

EQUIPMENT

Piggyback, Tandem, or Miniinfuser Pump

- Gloves (for connecting IV tubing)
- Medication prepared in 5-150 ml labeled infusion bag or syringe
- Short microdrip or macrodrip tubing set for piggyback (may have needleless system attachment)
- Needleless device
- Miniinfusion pump
- Adhesive tape (optional)
- Antiseptic swab
- IV pole or rack
- Medication administration record or computer printout

Volume-Control Administration Set

- Gloves (for connecting IV tubing)
- Volutrol or Burette
- Infusion tubing (may have needleless system attachment)
- Syringe (5-20 ml)
- Vial or ampule of ordered medication
- Medication label
- Medication administration record or computer printout

STEPS	RATIONALE
ASSESSMENT	
1. Check physician's order to determine type of IV solution to be used, type of medication, dose, and route and time of administration.	Client's overall physical condition dictates type of IV solution used. Ensures safe and accurate drug administration.
2. Collect information necessary to administer drug safely, including action, purpose, side effects, normal dose, time of peak onset, nursing implications.	Allows nurse to give drug safely and to monitor client's response to therapy.
3. Assess patency of client's existing IV infusion line (see Chapter 20) by noting infusion rate of main IV line.	IV line must be patent and fluids must infuse easily for medication to reach venous circulation effectively.
4. Assess IV insertion site for signs of infiltration or phlebitis: redness, pallor, swelling, tenderness on palpation.	Confirmation of placement of IV needle or catheter and integrity of surrounding tissues ensures that medication is administered safely.
5. Assess client's history of drug allergies.	Effects of medications can develop rapidly after IV infusion. Nurse should be aware of clients at risk.
6. Assess client's understanding of purpose of drug therapy.	May reveal need for education.

NURSING DIAGNOSIS

Clustering of defining characteristics from the assessment data may reveal the following nursing diagnoses for clients requiring this skill:

- ➤ Knowledge deficit regarding drug therapy
- ➤ Risk for injury
- ➤ Risk for impaired skin integrity

Related factors are individualized based on a client's condition or needs.

STEPS	RATIONALE
PLANNING	
1. **Expected outcomes** following completion of procedure:	
➤ Drug infuses without adverse reactions.	Drug was given safely with desired therapeutic effect.
➤ Medication infuses within desired period.	IV line remains patent.
➤ IV site remains intact without signs of swelling or inflammation or symptoms of tenderness at site.	Fluid infuses into vein rather than tissues.
➤ Client is able to explain drug purpose, action, side effects, and dosage.	Demonstrates learning.
2. Assemble supplies at bedside.	Drug preparation usually is not required. Nurse may assemble infusion tubing and bag of medication in medication room or client's room.
IMPLEMENTATION	
1. Wash hands and apply gloves.	Reduces transmission of microorganisms. During handling of IV tubing there is some risk of blood exposure.
2. Check client's identification by looking at armband and asking client's name.	Ensures drug is administered to correct client.
3. Explain purpose of medication and side effects to client. Explain that medication is to be given through existing IV line. Encourage client to report symptoms of discomfort at site.	Keeps client informed of planned therapies.
4. Piggyback or Tandem Infusion	
a. Connect infusion tubing to medication bag (see Chapter 20). Allow solution to fill tubing by opening regulator flow clamp. Recover end of tubing.	Infusion tubing should be filled with solution and free of air bubbles to prevent **air embolus.**
b. Hang piggyback medication bag above level of primary fluid bag. (Hook may be used to lower main bag.) Hang tandem infusion at same level as primary fluid bag.	Height of fluid bag affects rate of flow to client.
c. Connect tubing of piggyback or tandem infusion to appropriate connector on primary infusion line:	
(1) *Stopcock:* Wipe off stopcock port with alcohol swab and connect tubing. Turn stopcock to open position.	Stopcock eliminates need for needle.
(2) *Needleless system:* Wipe off needleless port, and insert tip of piggyback or tandem infusion tubing.	The CDC strongly recommends needleless connections to prevent accidental needle-stick injuries (Association for Practitioners in Infection Control, 1993). Establishes route for IV medication to enter main IV line.
(3) *Tubing Port:* Connect sterile needle to end of piggyback or tandem infusion tubing, remove cap, cleanse injection port on main IV line, and insert needle through center of port.	Prevents introduction of microorganisms during needle insertion.
d. Regulate flow rate of medication solution by adjusting regulator clamp. (Usually medication should infuse within 20 to 90 minutes.)	Provides slow, intermittent infusion of medication in 20 to 90 minutes, maintains therapeutic blood levels.
e. After medication has infused, check flow regulator on primary infusion. Back-check valve on piggyback stops flow of the primary infusion until second medication infuses. The tandem and primary infusions flow together until the tandem set empties. The primary infusion should automatically begin to flow after the piggyback or tandem solution is empty.	Valve prevents backup of medication into main infusion line. Checking flow rate ensures proper administration of IV fluids.

STEPS	RATIONALE
f. Regulate main infusion line to desired rate, if necessary.	Infusion of piggyback may interfere with main line infusion rate.
g. Leave secondary bag and tubing in place for future drug administration, or discard in appropriate containers.	Establishment of secondary line produces route for microorganisms to enter main line. Repeated changes in tubing increase risk of infection transmission (check agency policy).
5. Miniinfusion Administration:	
a. Connect prefilled syringe to miniinfusion tubing.	Special tubing designed to fit syringe delivers medication to main IV line.
b. Carefully apply pressure to syringe plunger, allowing tubing to fill with medication.	Ensures that tubing is free of air bubbles to prevent air embolus.
c. Place syringe into miniinfusion pump (follow product directions). Be sure that syringe is secure.	
d. Connect miniinfusion tubing to main IV line.	
(1) *Stopcock:* Wipe off stopcock port with alcohol swab and connect tubing. Turn stopcock to open position.	Stopcock reduces risk of needle-stick injuries.
(2) *Needleless system:* Wipe off needleless port, and insert tip of miniinfuser tubing (see illustration).	Needleless system reduces risk of needle-stick injuries.
(3) *Tubing port:* Connect sterile needle to miniinfuser tubing, remove cap, cleanse injection port on main IV line, and insert needle through center of port.	Cleansing reduces transmission of microorganisms.
e. Hang infusion pump with syringe on IV pole alongside main IV bag. Press button on pump to begin infusion (see illustration). *Optional:* Set alarm.	Pump automatically delivers medication at safe, constant rate based on volume in syringe. (Alarm is used if medication is delivered into heparin/saline lock.)

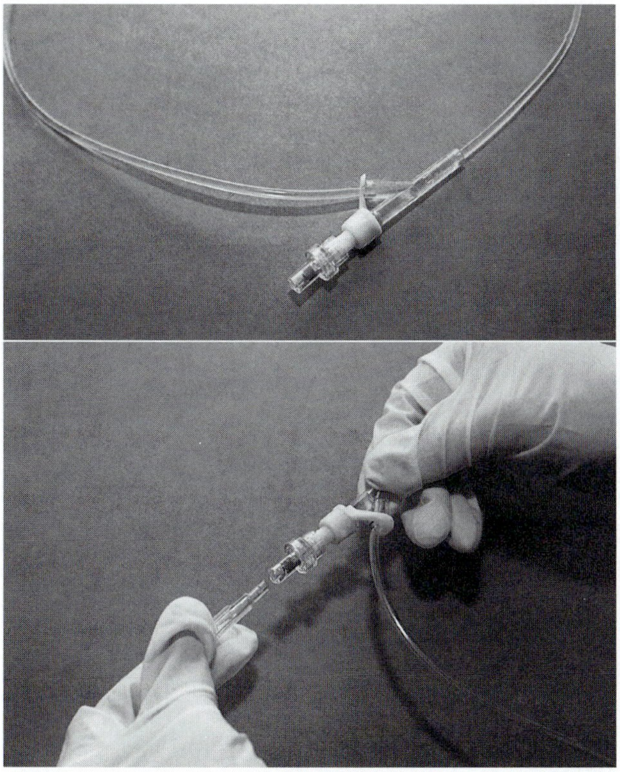

Step 5d(2) Example of needleless device using valve-like system.

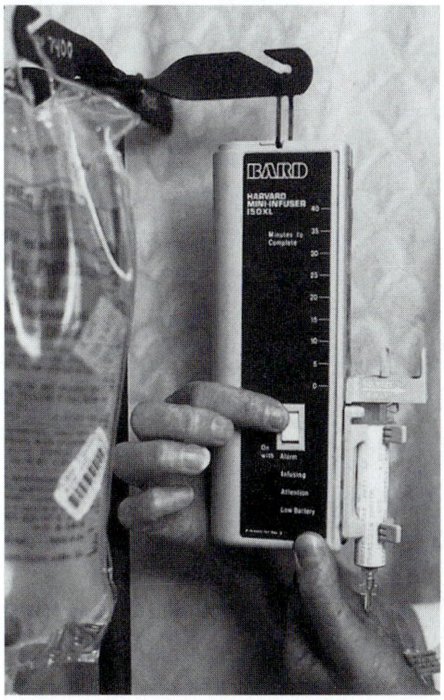

Step 5e

STEPS	RATIONALE
f. After medication has infused, check flow regulator on primary infusion. Infusion should automatically begin to flow once pump stops. Regulate main infusion line to desired rate as needed. NOTE: If stopcock is used, turn off miniinfusion line.	Maintains patency of primary IV line.
6. Volume-Control Administration Set (e.g., Volutrol):	
a. Assemble supplies in medication room.	Controls risk of contaminating IV solution.
b. Prepare medication from vial or ampule (see Skill 19-1).	Ensures that medication is sterile.
c. Check client's identification by looking at armband and asking name. Compare with medication ticket.	Ensures that drug is administered to correct client.
d. Explain procedure to client. Encourage client to report symptoms of discomfort at site.	Keeps client informed of planned therapies.
e. Fill Volutrol with desired amount of fluid (50 to 100 ml) by opening clamp between Volutrol and main IV bag (see illustration).	Small volume of fluid dilutes IV medication and reduces risk of too-rapid infusion.
f. Close clamp. Check to be sure clamp on air vent of Volutrol chamber is open.	Prevents additional leakage of fluid into Volutrol. Air vent allows fluid in Volutrol to exit at regulated rate.
g. Clean injection port on top of Volutrol with antiseptic swab.	Prevents introduction of microorganisms during needle insertion.
h. Remove needle cap or sheath, insert syringe needle through port, and then inject medication (see illustration). Gently rotate Volutrol between hands.	Rotating mixes medication with solution in Volutrol to ensure equal distribution.
i. Regulate IV infusion rate to allow medication to infuse in 30 to 90 minutes.	For optimal therapeutic effect, drug should infuse in prescribed time interval.

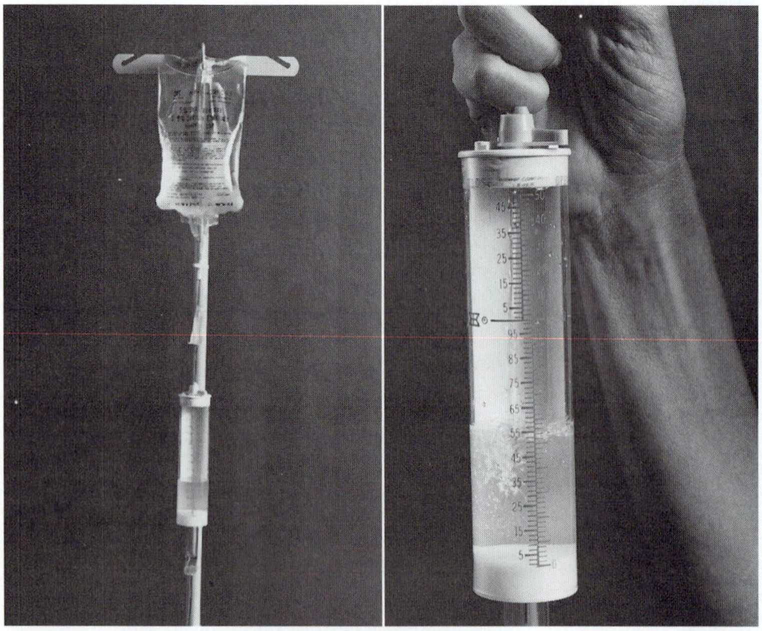

Step 6e

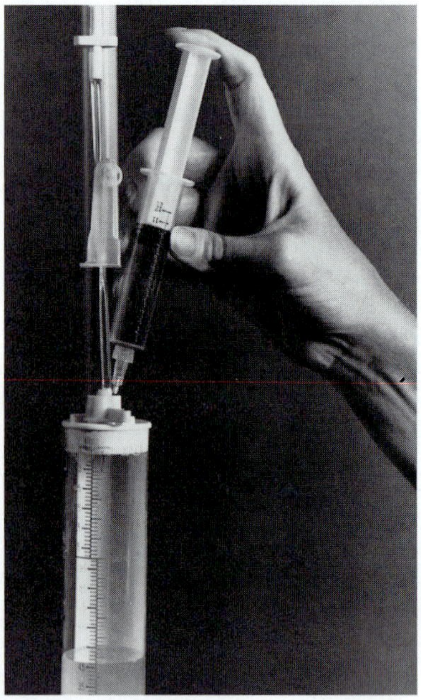

Step 6h

STEPS	RATIONALE
j. Label Volutrol with name of drug, dosage, total volume (including diluent), and time of administration.	Alerts nurses to drug being infused. Prevents other medications from being added to Volutrol.
k. Dispose of uncapped needle or needle enclosed in safety shield and syringe in proper container.	Prevents accidental needle sticks.
7. Remove disposable gloves. Wash hands.	Reduces transmission of microorganisms.

EVALUATION

1. Observe client for signs of adverse reactions.	IV medications act rapidly.
2. During 20 to 90 minutes of infusion, periodically check infusion rate and condition of IV site.	IV line must remain patent for proper drug administration. Development of infiltration necessitates discontinuing infusion.
3. Ask client to explain purpose and side effects of medication.	Evaluates client's understanding of instruction.
4. **Unexpected outcomes** that may occur include:	
➤ Client develops adverse drug reaction.	Nature of reaction depends on drug, dose, and client's sensitivity. Stop medication infusion immediately.
➤ Medication does not infuse over desired period.	Can result from improper calculation of flow rate, malpositioning of IV needle at insertion site, or infiltration.
➤ Client develops signs and symptoms of phlebitis or infiltration.	Fluid infuses into tissues. Vein is inflamed.
➤ Client is unable to explain medication purpose or side effects.	Reinstruction is required.

RECORDING AND REPORTING

1. Record drug, dose, route, and time administered on medication administration record or computer printout (see Fig. 17-1).	Timely documentation prevents medication errors, for example, repeated doses.
2. Record volume of fluid in medication bag or Volutrol on intake and output (I&O) form.	Fluid balance is regulated and monitored on basis of total fluid intake.
3. Report any adverse reactions to nurse in charge or physician.	Reaction may require therapeutic intervention.

FOLLOW-UP ACTIVITIES

1. After drug infuses, be sure to add IV solution to Volutrol.
2. IV can run dry unless solution is added to Volutrol for continuous infusion.

Special Considerations

- ➤ Never give IV medications via blood products.
- ➤ IV medication should never be given when site is swollen and tender to palpation or when infusion flows slowly when regulating clamp is wide open.
- ➤ For piggybacking an IV line, a 21- or 23-gauge needle ensures that drug will infuse easily into main IV line.
- ➤ Secondary line tubing can be used again by adding a new piggyback or tandem container. Check agency policy to determine how long lines are considered usable.

Home Care Considerations

- ➤ See Skill 41-3.

SKILL 19-8 Administering Medications by Intravenous Bolus

An IV **bolus** involves introducing a concentrated dose of a drug directly into the systemic circulation. An IV bolus may be given directly into a vein, into an existing IV line through an injection port, or through a saline or heparin lock. A saline lock consists of an indwelling needle or catheter attached to a plastic tube with a sealed injection port on the end. Institutional policy dictates which medications the nurse may give by IV push.

The IV bolus is the most dangerous method for drug administration because it allows no time to correct errors. In addition, a bolus may cause direct irritation to the lining of blood vessels.

Thus the nurse must be sure that the IV catheter or needle is correctly positioned in the client's vein. An IV bolus should never be given if the insertion site appears puffy or edematous or if the fluid from a connecting IV line cannot flow at the proper rate. Accidental injection of a medication into tissues surrounding a vein can cause pain, necrotic sloughing of tissues, and abscesses.

EQUIPMENT

IV Push (Existing Line)

- Disposable gloves
- Medication in vial or ampule
- Syringe (3-5 ml)
- Needles (21 and 25 gauge) (optional)
- Antiseptic swab
- Watch with second hand or digital readout
- Medication administration record or computer printout

IV Push (IV Lock)

- Disposable gloves
- Medication in vial or ampule
- Syringe (1-5 ml)
- Vial of appropriate flush solution (saline most common, but heparin may also be used; if heparin is used, most common concentration is 10 to 100 units; check agency policy)
- Needleless device or sterile needles (21 and 25 gauge)
- Antiseptic swab
- Watch with second hand or digital readout
- Medication administration record or computer printout

STEPS	RATIONALE
ASSESSMENT	
1. Check physician's order for type of medication, dosage, time, and route of administration.	Ensures safe and accurate drug administration.
2. Collect information necessary to administer drug safely, including action, purpose, side effects, normal dose, time of peak onset, nursing implications.	Allows nurse to give drug safely and to monitor client's response to therapy.
3. If drug is to be given through existing IV line, determine compatibility and type of additives within IV solution.	IV medication may not be compatible with additives.
4. Assess condition of needle insertion site (IV line or saline lock) for signs of infiltration or phlebitis.	Drug should not be administered if site is edematous or inflamed.
5. Check client's history of drug allergies.	IV bolus delivers drug rapidly. Allergic reaction could prove fatal.
6. Assess client's understanding of purpose of drug therapy.	May reveal need for education.

NURSING DIAGNOSIS

Clustering of defining characteristics from the assessment data may reveal the following nursing diagnoses for clients requiring this skill:

- ➤ Knowledge deficit regarding drug therapy
- ➤ Risk for impaired skin integrity
- ➤ Risk for injury

Related factors are individualized based on a client's condition or needs.

STEPS	RATIONALE
PLANNING	
1. **Expected outcomes** following completion of procedure:	
➤ Drug infuses without adverse reactions occurring.	Drug is given safely.
➤ IV site remains clear, without swelling.	Fluid infuses into vein.
➤ Client will explain purpose and side effects of medication.	Demonstrates learning.
2. Assemble supplies in medication room.	Ensures sterile preparation of medications.
IMPLEMENTATION	
1. Wash hands and apply gloves.	Reduces transmission of microorganisms. IV push method carries risk of contacting blood.
2. Prepare medication from vial or ampule (see Skill 19-1).	Ensures that medication is sterile.
3. Check client's identification by looking at armband and asking name. Compare with medication ticket.	Ensures that drug is administered to correct client.
4. Explain procedure to client. Encourage client to report symptoms of discomfort at IV site.	Informs client of planned therapies.
5. IV Push (Existing Line):	
a. Select injection port of IV tubing closest to client. Whenever possible, injection port should be a stopcock or other needleless component.	CDC and OSHA strongly recommend that all IV injection sites be needleless to prevent needle-stick injuries (Association for Practitioners in Infection Control, 1993).
b. Connect syringe to IV line:	
(1) Needleless system: Remove cap of needleless injection port and clean with antiseptic. Insert tip of syringe containing medication.	Ensures sterility.
(2) Needle system: Select port indicating site for needle insertion. Clean port with antiseptic swab. Insert small-gauge needle of syringe containing drug through center of port.	Prevents introduction of microorganisms. Prevents damage to port diaphragm.
c. Occlude IV line by pinching tubing just above injection port. Pull back gently on syringe's plunger to aspirate for blood return (see illustration).	Final check ensures that medication is being delivered into bloodstream.

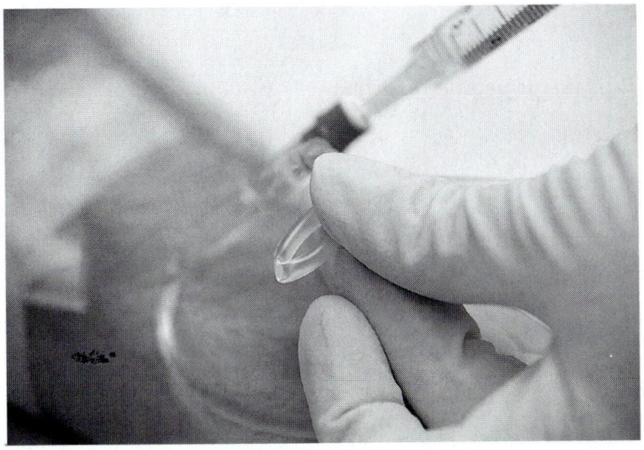

Step 5c

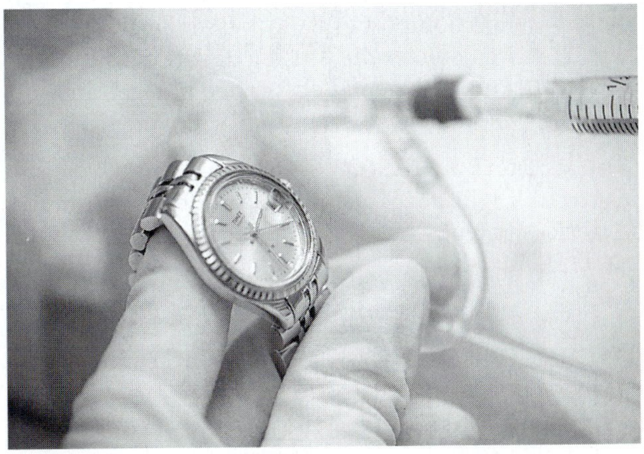

Step 5d

STEPS	RATIONALE
d. After noting blood return, inject medication slowly over several minutes (see illustration). Use a watch to time administrations. (Read directions on drug package.)	Ensures safe drug infusion. Rapid injection of IV drug can be fatal.
e. After injecting medication, release tubing, withdraw syringe, and recheck fluid infusion rate.	Injection of bolus may alter rate of fluid infusion. Rapid fluid infusion can cause circulatory fluid overload.

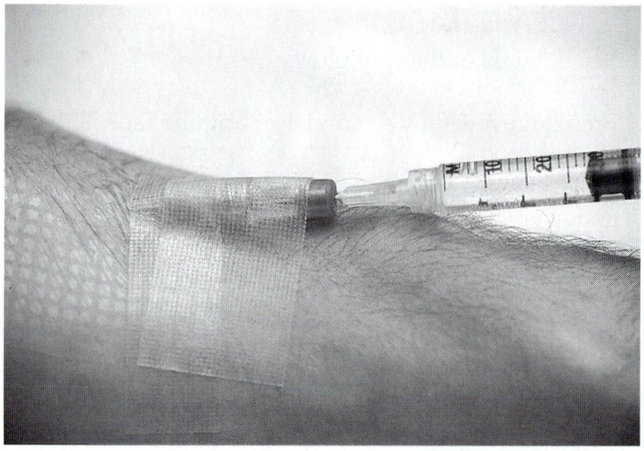

Step 6b(2)

6. IV Push (IV Lock):

STEPS	RATIONALE
a. Prepare flush solutions according to hospital policy.	
(1) Saline flush method (preferred method):	
• Prepare 2 to 3, 1 ml syringes with 1 ml of normal saline 0.9%.	Normal saline has been found to be effective in keeping IV locks patent.
• Attach 25-gauge needle to syringes (optional if needleless system is used).	
(2) Heparin flush method (traditional method):	
• Prepare 1 syringe with 1 ml of heparin flush solution.	Used to assess for blood return in heparin lock. Flush solution keeps saline lock patent after drug is administered.
• Prepare 2 syringes with 1 ml of normal saline.	
• Attach 25-gauge needle to syringes (optional if needleless system is used).	
b. Administer drug:	
(1) Clean lock's injection port with the antiseptic swab.	Cleaning prevents introduction of microorganisms during needle insertion.
(2) Insert syringe of normal saline 0.9% through injection port of IV lock (see illustration). Remove needle if using needleless system.	
(3) Pull back gently on syringe plunger and check for blood return.	Indicates if needle or catheter is in vein.

CRITICAL DECISION POINT At times a heparin lock will not yield a blood return even though lock is patent.

STEPS	RATIONALE
(4) Flush reservoir with 1 ml normal saline by pushing slowly on plunger.	Cleans needle and reservoir of blood.

CRITICAL DECISION POINT Observe closely the area of skin above the IV catheter. Note any puffiness or swelling as the reservoir is flushed, which could indicate infiltration into the vein, requiring removal of catheter.

STEPS	RATIONALE
(5) Remove needle and saline-filled syringe.	
(6) Clean lock's injection port with antiseptic swab.	Prevents transmission of infection.
(7) Insert or attach syringe containing prepared medication through center of diaphragm or end cap.	
(8) Inject medication bolus slowly over several minutes. (Each medication has recommended rate for bolus administration. Check package directions.) Use watch to time administration.	Rapid injection of IV drug can cause death.
(9) After administering bolus, withdraw syringe.	
(10) Recleanse lock's diaphragm or cap with antiseptic swab.	Prevents transmission of infection.
(11) Attach syringe with 1 ml normal saline. Inject normal saline flush.	Irrigation with saline prevents occlusion of IV access device and ensures all medication delivered.
(12) *Option:* Heparin flush After instilling saline, attach syringe containing 1 ml diluted heparin flush. Inject heparin slowly and then remove syringe.	Maintains patency of IV needle by inhibiting clot formation. Diluted heparin avoids anticoagulation. SASH method: *S*aline, *A*dministration of medication, *S*aline, *H*eparin.
7. Dispose of uncapped needles and syringes in puncture-proof and leak-proof container.	Prevents accidental needle-stick injuries.
8. Remove gloves and wash hands.	Reduces transmission of microorganisms.

EVALUATION

1. Observe client closely for adverse reactions during administration and for several minutes thereafter.	IV medications act rapidly.
2. Observe IV site during injection for sudden swelling.	Determines development of infiltration into tissues surrounding vein.
3. Ask client to explain drug's purpose and side effects.	Evaluates learning.
4. **Unexpected outcomes** that may occur include:	
➤ Client develops adverse reaction to medication.	Drug's potency may cause maximal responses or side effects.
➤ IV site becomes puffy.	Infiltration indicates immediate discontinuation of injection.
➤ Client is unable to explain medication information.	Requires reinstruction or client is unable to learn at this time.

RECORDING AND REPORTING

1. Record drug, dose, route, and time on medication form.	Timely documentation prevents medication errors.
2. Report any adverse reactions to nurse in charge or physician.	Adverse response to IV bolus drug may necessitate emergency measures.

FOLLOW-UP ACTIVITIES

1. Bolus medications can cause rapid changes in client's physiological status. Some drugs (e.g., vasopressor and antiarrythmics) will require blood pressure and heart rate monitoring.

• • • • •

Special Consideration

➤ Be sure to loosen tape or dressing over IV site to see it clearly before administering drug.

CRITICAL THINKING EXERCISES

1. You are working with a critical care nurse who has been "floated" to your unit. You observe this nurse drawing up 0.25 mg of digoxin into a 3 ml syringe. The nurse does not dilute the medication and is preparing to give this medication by IV bolus. You tell her that neither you nor any other nurse has given digoxin IV bolus. She tells you that she does so almost every day. Would you intervene in this situation? What rationale would you use to justify your position?
2. Fifteen minutes after you have hung an IV antibiotic, the client is itching and clawing at her skin and hair. You determine that the client may be having an allergic reaction to the antibiotic. What steps would you take immediately? Why?
3. You have prepared an IM injection for your client. You did not assess the client before preparing the medication. You draw the medication up in a syringe with a 1 1/2-inch 21-gauge needle. When you arrive to give the injection, you find that the client is cachectic and has very little muscle mass. How would you proceed with your assessment and intervention? Give your rationale.
4. Your client is receiving insulin at home and has run out of syringes. You have some 1 ml tuberculin syringes and subcutaneous needles on hand. The client needs to receive 18 units of NPH insulin and 4 units of regular insulin. How would you draw this up? How many tenths of a ml of each type of insulin would you draw up?

REFERENCES

Association for Practitioners in Infection Control: APIC position paper: prevention of device-mediated blood-borne infections to health care workers, *Am J Infect Control* 21(2):76, 1993.

Beyea SC, Nicoll LH: Administration of medications via the intramuscular route: an integrative review of the literature and research-based protocol for the procedure, *Appl Nurse Res 8(1):23, 1995.*

Beyea SC, Nicoll LH: Back to basics: administering IM injections the right way, *Am J Nurs* 96(1):34, 1996.

Bohony J: Fighting the needlestick battle without needles, *Medsurg Nurs* 2(6):469, 1993.

Centers for Disease Control and Prevention: Update: universal precautions for prevention of transmission of HIV, hepatitis B virus and other bloodborne pathogens in health care settings, *MMWR* 37:377, 1988.

Lewis SM, Collier IC, Heitkemper MM: *Medical-surgical nursing: assessment and management of clinical problems,* ed 4, St Louis, 1996, Mosby.

McConnell EA: The subtle art of really good injections, *RN* 45:24, 1982.

Valentine V: Nursing role in management of patient with diabetes. In Lewis SM, Collier IC, Heitkemper MM, editors: *Medical-surgical nursing: assessment and management of clinical problems,* ed 4, St Louis, 1996, Mosby.

Wong D: *Whaley & Wong's nursing care of infants and children,* ed 5, St Louis, 1995, Mosby.

ADDITIONAL READING

Beecroft PC, Kongelbeck RS: How safe are intramuscular injections? *AACN Clin Issues* 5:207, 1994.

Blodget JB: Managing injection reactions, *Nursing 95* 29(9):46, 1995.

Cantrell SA: American Society of Health-Systems Pharmacists: Understanding infusion devices, *Nursing 95* 29(9):32J, 1995.

Centers of Disease Control, Public Health Service, US Department of Health and Human Services: Guidelines for isolation precautions in hospitals. II. Recommendations for isolation precautions in hospitals, *Am J Infect Control* 24:32, 1996.

Clark JB, Queener SF, Karb VB: *Pharmacologic basis of nursing practice,* ed 5, St Louis, 1997, Mosby.

Gahart BL: *Intravenous medications,* ed 13, St Louis, 1996, Mosby.

Garner JS et al: Guidelines for isolation precautions in hospitals. I. Evolution of isolation practices, *Am J Infect Control* 24:24, 1996.

Whitman M: The push is on: delivering medications safely by I.V. bolus, *Nursing 95* 29(8):52, 1995.

UNIT VII

Fluid Balance

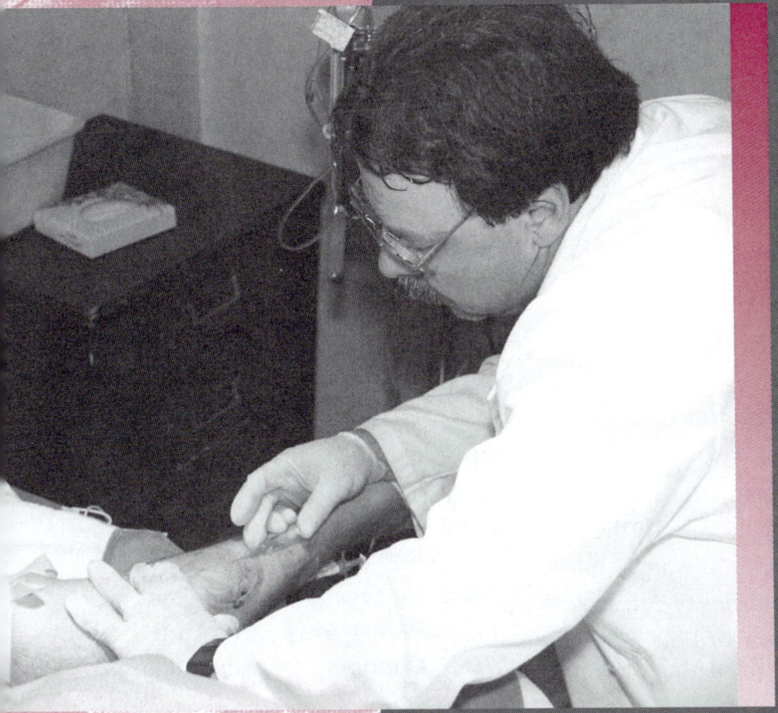

CHAPTER 20

Intravenous and Vascular Access Therapy

OBJECTIVES

Mastery of content in this chapter will enable the nurse to:

- Define key terms.
- Discuss conditions requiring intravenous (IV) therapy.
- Identify potential nursing diagnoses for clients requiring IV therapy.
- Explain how to prepare the client and family for IV therapy.
- Identify individualized outcomes for clients requiring IV therapy.
- Demonstrate initiation of IV therapy, regulation of IV flow rate, changing of IV solutions, changing of IV tubing, changing of IV dressings, and discontinuing a peripheral IV.
- Identify common types of vascular access devices (VADs) and describe their care and maintenance.
- Identify the educational needs of clients with VADs.

SKILLS

20-1 Initiating Intravenous Therapy

20-2 Inserting a Peripherally Inserted Central Catheter

20-3 Regulating Intravenous Flow Rate

20-4 Changing Intravenous Solutions

20-5 Changing Infusion Tubing

20-6 Changing a Peripheral Intravenous Dressing

20-7 Caring for Vascular Access Devices

20-8 Discontinuing Peripheral Intravenous Access

KEY TERMS

Cannula
Central venous catheter (CVC)
Drop factor
Effective osmolality
Electrolyte
Electronic infusion device (EID)
Embolus
Exit site
Fluid volume deficit (FVD)
Fluid volume excess (FVE)
Heparin lock
Hypertonic
Hypokalemia
Hypomagnesemia
Hyponatremia
Hypoosmolar
Hypophosphatemia
Hypotonic
Implanted infusion port
Infiltration
Infusion pump
Injection cap
Isotonic
IV Plug
Noncoring Huber needle
Over-the-needle catheter (ONC)
Percutaneous
Peripherally inserted central catheter (PICC)
Phlebitis
Saline lock
Sharps container
Solute solution
Subcutaneous tunnel
Vascular access device (VAD)
Venipuncture

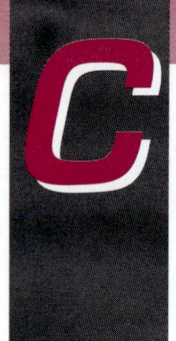

PARENTERAL REPLACEMENT OF FLUIDS

Fluids may be infused directly into the circulating blood volume in order to supplement or replace enteral fluids. Parenteral fluid replacement includes intravenous (IV) fluid and electrolyte therapy, blood therapy (Chapter 21), and total parenteral nutrition (TPN) (Chapter 24). The goal of IV fluid administration is to correct or prevent fluid and electrolyte imbalances or to provide IV medication therapy. When IV therapy is necessary, the nurse must know the correct solution and equipment needed and how to initiate an infusion, regulate the fluid infusion rate, care for and maintain the system, identify and correct problems, and discontinue the infusion.

Intravenous Solutions

Prepared IV solutions fall into three general categories: isotonic, hypotonic, and hypertonic (Table 20-1). An **isotonic** solution has a total electrolyte content of approximately 310 mEq/L. A **hypotonic** solution has a total electrolyte content of less than 250 mEq/L. A **hypertonic** solution has a total electrolyte content of 375 mEq/L or greater (Metheny, 1992). All IV fluids should be carefully given, especially hypertonic solutions, because these solutions pull fluid into the vascular space by osmosis, resulting in an increased vascular volume that can result in pulmonary edema, particularly in clients with cardiac or renal diseases. The type and amount of IV solution ordered by the physician are determined by serum electrolyte values and fluid volume balance. The nurse must understand the rationale for IV fluid administration and the type of IV solution ordered. Because the names of IV solutions are often abbreviated or shortened, the nurse must be careful to give the correct solution (see box below).

In addition to the specific IV fluid ordered, the physician often includes additives such as vitamins or potassium. Clients with properly functioning kidneys who are NPO (nothing by mouth) should have potassium added to the IV solution. Prepared bags of IV fluids with potassium already added should be used if available. This decreases the chance of fluid contamination. If the physician's order does not include potassium, the nurse should double-check the order. Kidneys routinely excrete potassium, and if there is no potassium intake orally or parenterally, **hypokalemia** can develop.

Intravenous Catheters

The majority of peripheral venous catheters in the United States are made of Teflon or polyurethane. These catheters are associated with fewer infectious complications than others on the market. Metal needles are used infrequently because of the complication of IV fluid infiltration (Tully et al, 1981). The trend is to eliminate a needle device left in place. Many companies make a short catheter with a removable needle that looks just like a butterfly minus the needle. Pediatrics use the same small bore catheters instead of needles. Needles have a high rate of infiltration. Commonly used over-the-needle flexible catheters comprise a metal stylet, which is used to pierce the skin, and a Teflon, polyurethane, or silicone catheter, which is threaded into a vein and remains there for the instillation of fluid. These flexible catheters do not dislodge from the vein as easily as butterfly needles. In addition, large volumes of fluids and medications can be quickly administered through the catheter without a high risk of infiltration. A 20- to 22-gauge flexible catheter is used in most situations for adults, while a 22- to 24-gauge catheter can be used for pediatric and elderly clients or for any other client with small or fragile veins. Stable venous access is more reliably achieved with plastic or Teflon catheters than with needles, so these are the usual choice for venipunc-

Table 20-1 Concentration of Select Intravenous Solutions

Isotonic	Hypotonic	Hypertonic
0.9% sodium chloride*	0.45% sodium chloride	3% to 5% sodium chloride
Lactated Ringer's	0.3% sodium chloride	5% dextrose in lactated Ringer's
5% dextrose in water†	2.5% dextrose in 0.45% sodium chloride	≥10% dextrose in water†

*Solution has 154 mEq of sodium and 154 mEq of chloride and expands the plasma volume (Metheny, 1992).
†Dextrose is metabolized, leaving free water to be distributed evenly in all fluid compartments (Horne, Heitz, and Swearingen, 1991).

COMMON NAMES FOR INTRAVENOUS SOLUTIONS

Solution	Other Names
0.9% sodium chloride	Normal saline 0.9% NaCl 0.9% NS NS
0.45% sodium chloride	One-half-strength normal saline 0.45% NaCl 0.45% NS ½ NaCl ½ NS
Dextrose 5% in 0.9% sodium chloride	D_5 normal saline D_5 0.9% NaCl D_5 0.9% NS D_5 NS
Dextrose 5% in 0.45% sodium chloride	D_5 One-half-strength normal saline D_5 0.45% NaCl D_5 0.45% NS D_5 ½ NaCl D_5 ½ NS
Lactated Ringer's	LR
Dextrose 5% in lactated Ringer's	D^5 LR

ture, especially if irritating medications are to be given. In general, use the smallest catheter that will deliver the needed fluids at the appropriate rate. If the administration of large volumes of IV fluids or blood or blood products is anticipated, a size 20-gauge or 18-gauge angiocatheter is necessary to allow rapid infusion of IV fluids or viscous blood product solutions.

Health care workers experience approximately 800,000 accidental needle sticks and sharp injuries each year (Association for Practitioners in Infection Control, 1993). Common causes of accidental needle-stick injuries include recapping incidents, assembling or accessing IV tubing devices, disposing of contaminated sharps, using alternative methods to cover used needles on IV needle assemblies, and intentionally detaching IV lines. IV catheters and butterfly or winged catheters are devices commonly associated with a high risk for injuries. In order to help prevent accidental injury, needles should not be recapped and are disposed of in puncture-proof containers, referred to as **sharps containers.** In emergencies a one-handed "scoop" technique may be used to cover needles (OSHA, 1991) (Fig. 20-1 A-C). More health care agencies are using protected needle devices that allow a needle to remain covered during and after use or the agencies are eliminating the use of needles altogether. These "needleless" systems come in a variety of needle, catheter, and tubing products.

A B C

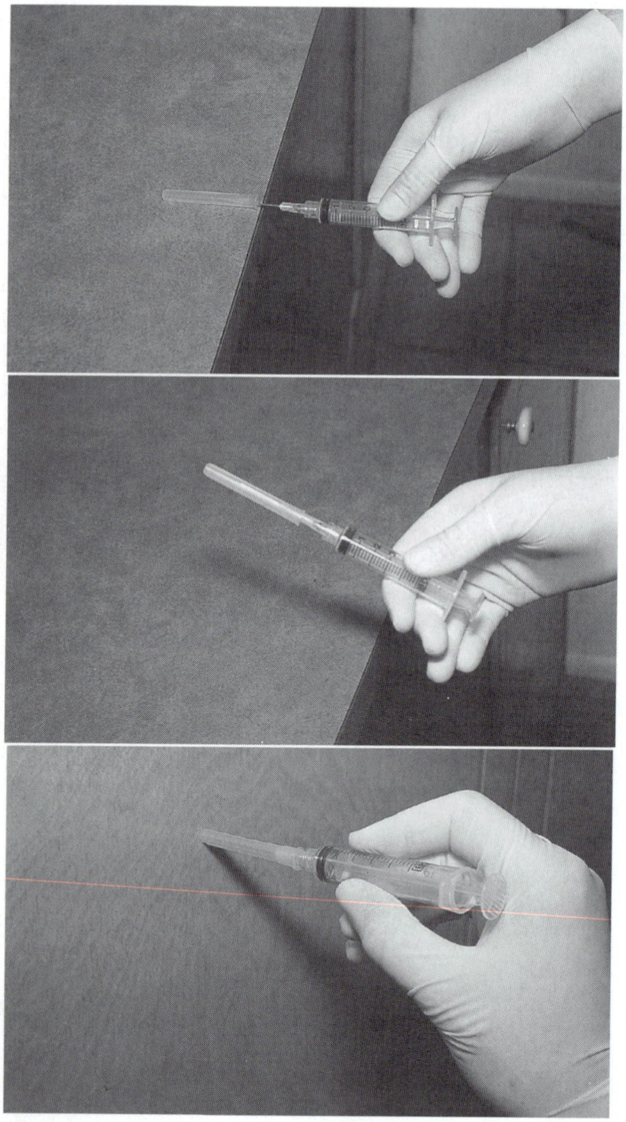

Fig. 20-1 **A,** Insert contaminated needle into cap using one hand. **B,** Have cap slip fully over needle. **C,** Push cap against firm surface.

GUIDELINES

1. Know the client's normal range of vital signs. Altered fluid or electrolyte imbalances can affect vital signs. Dehydration can produce hypotension and tachycardia. Fluid overload can result in hypertension and a bounding pulse. Disturbances in serum potassium can result in an irregular pulse.
2. Know the client's developmental stage. The proportion of total body water to body mass changes from infancy to the older adult years.
3. Know the client's weight. Body size affects total body water. Fat contains no water; the obese client thus has proportionately less body water.
4. Know the client's medical history and present medications or therapies. Certain drugs such as diuretics or steroids affect fluid and electrolyte balance. Likewise, a client may be on a specific diet, such as a low-sodium diet for water retention. Determine whether the client has had IV therapy before.
5. Beware of prolonged environmental conditions that can affect the client's fluid status. Prolonged exposure to hot, humid weather can lead to fluid and electrolyte imbalances, particularly in the infant, the older adult, and the chronically ill client.
6. Know if the client is right- or left-handed. When possible, place an IV into the nondominant arm.
7. Determine that the present IV system is intact. A system in which none of the connections have separated ensures that the sterility of the system has been maintained. If the nurse suspects that the infusion tubing has separated from the IV catheter or needle, sterility is no longer assumed, and a new system, including sterile tubing, solution, and catheter or needle must be reestablished.
8. Note when the last IV tubing and dressing change occurred.
9. Maintain sterility of a patent IV system using the Centers for Disease Control (CDC, 1996) recommendations (see box on p. 655).
10. Know the standard precautions for infection control and the Occupational Safety and Health Administration (OSHA) standards for occupational exposure to blood-borne pathogens (see box on p. 655).

CDC GUIDELINES TO DECREASE INTRAVASCULAR INFECTION RELATED TO IV THERAPY

- Palpate catheter insertion site for tenderness daily through the intact dressing.
- Visually inspect a catheter site if client develops tenderness at site, fever without obvious source, or symptoms of local or bloodstream infection.
- Wash hands before and after palpating, inserting, replacing, or dressing any intravascular device.
- Cleanse skin site before venipuncture with an appropriate antiseptic, including 70% alcohol, 10% povidone-iodine.
- Do not palpate insertion site after skin has been cleansed with antiseptic.
- Use sterile gauze or transparent dressing to cover a catheter site.
- Replace IV tubing, including piggyback tubing and stopcocks, no more frequently than at 72 hour intervals unless clinically indicated.
- Replace tubing used to administer blood, blood products, or lipid emulsions within 24 hours of initiating infusion.
- There are no recommendations for the hang time of IV fluids.
- Replace dressing over peripheral venous catheters when catheter is replaced or when dressing becomes damp, loosened, or soiled.
- Clean injection ports with 70% alcohol or povidone-iodine before accessing system.
- Do not use in line filters routinely for infection control.
- In adults, replace short, peripheral venous catheters and rotate sites every 48 to 72 hours.
- In adults, replace heparin locks every 96 hours.
- Do not routinely apply topical antimicrobial ointment to the insertion site of peripheral venous catheters or central venous catheter-insertion sites.
- No recommendation for the frequency of replacement of PICC catheter.

Adapted from Centers for Disease Control and Prevention: Guideline for Prevention of Intravascular Device-Related Infections, Infect Control Hosp Epidemiol, 17(7):438-472, 1996.

OSHA STANDARDS FOR REDUCING OCCUPATIONAL EXPOSURE TO BLOOD-BORNE PATHOGENS

1. Gloves must be worn when there is a reasonable expectation that the employee may contact blood, for example, during venipuncture or while changing IV administration sets.
2. Contaminated needles and other sharps must be placed in puncture-resistant containers properly labeled as a biohazard; when the containers are full, they are to be sealed and disposed of properly.
3. Contaminated needles should not be bent, sheared, recapped, or removed from the syringe after use.
4. Reports to OSHA of needle-stick injuries are required, and the health care agency must provide medical evaluation and follow-up.
5. Hepatitis B vaccination is to be made available to all employees who have occupational exposure.
6. Training and education must be offered to high-risk workers, such as nurses who initiate IV therapy, concerning precautions for prevention of exposure and use of personal protective equipment.
7. Each facility must have an infection control plan, including methods for reduction of the health care worker's exposure to biohazardous wastes.
8. Facilities must have engineering and work practice controls to eliminate or minimize employee exposure. Controls may include sharps disposal containers and self-sheathing needles.

From Occupational Safety and Health Act: Bloodborne pathogens, *Federal Register* 56(235):64, 175, Dec 6, 1991.

SKILL 20-1 Initiating Intravenous Therapy

The goal of IV fluid administration is correction or prevention of fluid and electrolyte disturbances in clients who are or may become acutely ill. For example, a client with third-degree burns over 40% of the body is critically ill and has severe fluid and electrolyte imbalances. Fluid therapy must be continuously regulated in a burn client because of continual changes in fluid and electrolyte balance. A client who is NPO after surgery receives IV fluid replacement to prevent fluid and electrolyte imbalances; the infusion is usually discontinued when the client resumes oral intake.

Another reason to perform a venipuncture is to provide IV access for intermittent or emergency medication administration. This administration route is often accomplished through the use of a heparin or normal saline lock, which is an IV catheter attached to a rubber plug or injection cap to maintain a closed system. Sometimes a short piece of extension tubing is used. This administration setup is flushed with a heparin or normal saline solution (refered to as a **heparin** or normal **saline lock**) every 8 hours or before and after each administration of medication to maintain patency of the IV catheter (see Chapter 19). Peripheral IV access is not to be used for administration of medications that are irritants or vesicants (i.e., chemotherapy, TPN). These types of medications should be administered through a central venous access site whenever possible.

Concern for the personal safety of nurses who work with IV therapy products has gained importance in recent years because of the possibility of transmission of organisms such as hepatitis B virus (HBV) and human immunodeficiency virus (HIV). The most common cause of exposure of nurses to blood during IV therapy is by needle stick. To prevent this, new products are being developed that decrease the chance of an accidental needle stick. Products that allow the connection of multiple tubings for IV solution or medication administration without the use of needles (needleless systems) are available. Other products with recessed needles or needle protectors can be used to prevent contact with exposed needles.

DELEGATION CONSIDERATIONS

The skills in this chapter require problem solving and knowledge application unique to a professional nurse. For these skills, delegation is inappropriate. For peripherally inserted central catheter (PICC) line insertion, only nurses who have completed a specialized PICC course, consisting of didactic and practical instruction, and have demonstrated competency in PICC line insertion are qualified to insert PICC lines. (Some state nursing practice acts do not allow nurses to insert PICCs.)

EQUIPMENT

- Correct IV solution (with time tape attached)
- Proper catheter for venipuncture (will vary with client's body size and reason for IV fluid administration; Fig. 20-2,*A*)

For IV fluid infusion

- Administration set (choice depends on type of solution and rate of administration; infants and children require microdrip tubing, which provides 60 gtt/ml)
- 0.22 μmm filter (if required by agency policy or if particulate matter is likely)
- Extension tubing (used when a longer IV line is necessary)

A

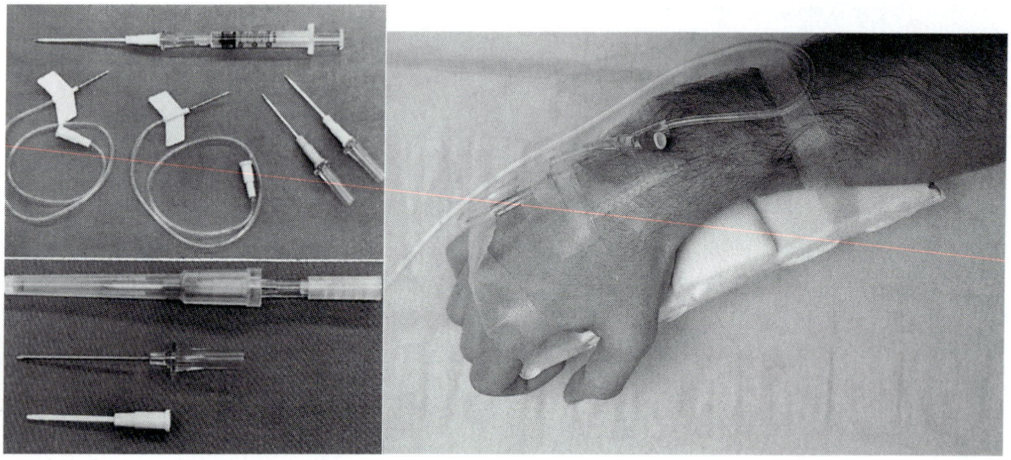

B

Fig. 20-2 **A,** IV catheters. **B,** Arm on armboard.

For heparin or normal saline lock
- Injection cap (also called IV plug)
- IV loop or short piece of extension tubing, if necessary
- 1 to 3 ml of normal saline or heparin flush (10 to 100 U/ml as ordered)
- Syringes and 25-gauge needles
- Alcohol and povidone-iodine cleansing swabs or sticks
- Disposable gloves
- Tourniquet (can be a source of contamination; use a single-use product)
- Arm board, if needed (used to maintain wrist or elbow joint position when ONC is placed close to or over a joint [Fig. 20-2, *B*]; will help prevent infiltration of IV)
- Non-allergenic tape
- Towel (to place under client's hand or arm); some agencies use an IV start kit, which contains a sterile drape to place under the client's arm, cleansing and antiseptic preparations, dressings, and a small roll of sterile, precut tape.
- IV pole, rolling or ceiling mounted
- Special gown with snaps at shoulder seams (makes removal with IV tubing easier), if available
- Needle disposal container (also called sharps container)

Gauze dressing only
- 2 × 2 or 4 × 4 sterile gauze sponge (follow agency policy)

Transparent dressing only
- Transparent dressing

STEPS	RATIONALE
ASSESSMENT	
1. Review client's medical record for physician's order stating type and amount of IV fluid and rate of fluid administration. In addition, nurse follows "five rights" for administration of medications (see Chapter 17).	An order requesting the initiation of a peripheral IV access and administration of an IV solution must be made by a physician prior to the implementation of this procedure.
CRITICAL DECISION POINT **In most medical facilities, physicians do not write an order to "initiate peripheral access" or "perform venipuncture." "Start IV" may be written followed by the exact IV therapy order. The order to perform the venipuncture is implied. If the order is confusing or in question, clarify with the physician before proceeding.**	
2. Identify the client whose potential for fluid and electrolyte imbalance may require IV fluid therapy. Observe for signs and symptoms indicating fluid or electrolyte imbalances.	
a. Edema Edema can be rated for severity by assessing pitting over bony prominences. 1+ indicates barely detectable edema to 4+ for deep persistent pitting (see Chapter 11).	Indicates expanded interstitial volume. This is usually most evident in dependent areas (i.e., feet and ankles).
CRITICAL DECISION POINT **The presence of periorbital edema suggests significant fluid retention.**	
b. Greater than 2% increase or decrease in body weight	Daily weights document fluid retention or loss. Change in body weight of 1 kg corresponds to 1 L of fluid retention or loss (Horne and Swearingen, 1997).
c. Dry skin and mucous membranes	May signal fluid volume deficit.
d. Distended neck veins	Suggests fluid volume excess.
e. Blood pressure changes	Elevated blood pressure may indicate volume excess due to increase in stroke volume. Decreased blood pressure may indicate fluid volume deficit due to a decrease in stroke volume.

STEPS	RATIONALE
f. Irregular pulse rhythm	May occur with potassium, calcium, and/or magnesium abnormalities.
g. Auscultation of crackles or rhonchi in lungs	May signal fluid buildup in the lungs due to fluid volume excess.
h. Inelastic skin turgor (after pinching, fails to return to normal position within 3 seconds)	With fluid volume deficit, the pinched skin stays elevated for several seconds.
➤ *CRITICAL DECISION POINT* This is a less reliable indicator for older adults since their skin has lost elasticity naturally due to aging.	
i. Anorexia, nausea, and vomiting	May occur with acute fluid volume deficit or fluid volume excess.
j. Thirst	Symptomatic of fluid volume deficit.
k. Decreased urine output	Monitoring urinary output is one method of assessing fluid balance. During dehydration, kidney attempts to restore fluid balance by reducing urine production. Average daily adult urine output is 1500 ml; urine output of less than 400 ml/24 hr (oliguria) signals the retention of metabolic wastes (Horne and Swearingen 1997).
l. Behavioral changes	Restlessness and confusion may occur with fluid volume deficit or acid-base imbalance.
3. Obtain information from drug reference books or pharmacist about composition of IV fluids, purposes for administration, potential incompatibilities, and side effects to monitor for.	This allows detection of an inadvisable IV fluid order and helps to determine priority assessments.
4. Determine client's understanding of the reason for IV fluids, what to expect during the venipuncture, and the client's psychological readiness for venipuncture and IV therapy.	Determines teaching needs. Indicates the need for special or intensive psychological support.
5. Assess for the following factors: Child or older adult; presence of heart failure or renal failure, skin lesions, infection or low platelet count.	Persons at extremes in age develop fluid imbalances more rapidly because they have a proportionately larger extracellular fluid volume; persons with heart failure cannot adapt to sudden increases in vascular volume, and persons with renal failure cannot eliminate excess extracellular fluid.

NURSING DIAGNOSIS

Clustering of defining characteristics from the assessment data may reveal the following nursing diagnoses for clients requiring this skill:

- Fluid volume deficit
- Risk for fluid volume deficit
- Risk for infection

Related factors are individualized based on a client's condition or needs.

PLANNING

1. Expected outcomes following completion of procedure:	
➤ Fluid and electrolyte balances return to normal; vital signs and other abnormal assessment parameters stabilize and return to normal.	Indicates correction of fluid and electrolyte imbalances and circulatory system's response to fluid and electrolyte replacement.
➤ IV line is patent.	Ensures free instillation of IV fluids without infiltration.
➤ Infiltration is absent with no swelling and pallor at venipuncture site.	Infiltration results from dislodging of catheter or needle into subcutaneous space.

STEPS	RATIONALE
➤ Inflammation is absent.	Inflammation results from irritation of vein by catheter, IV solution, additives, or bacteria.
➤ Client will understand purpose and risks of IV therapy.	
2. Prepare client and family by explaining the procedure, its purpose, and what is expected of client.	Decreases anxiety and promotes cooperation.
3. Identify accessible vein for placement of IV needle or catheter by inspection; this will most likely require application of a tourniquet. The most appropriate veins to utilize are cephalic, basilic, and median cubital for adults (see illustration). For infants, the most appropriate veins include scalp and foot veins. The CDC (1996) reports that the site at which a catheter is placed influences subsequent risk of catheter-related infection.	

➤ ***CRITICAL DECISION POINT*** **Never use foot veins in adults unless physician specifically orders you to do so.**

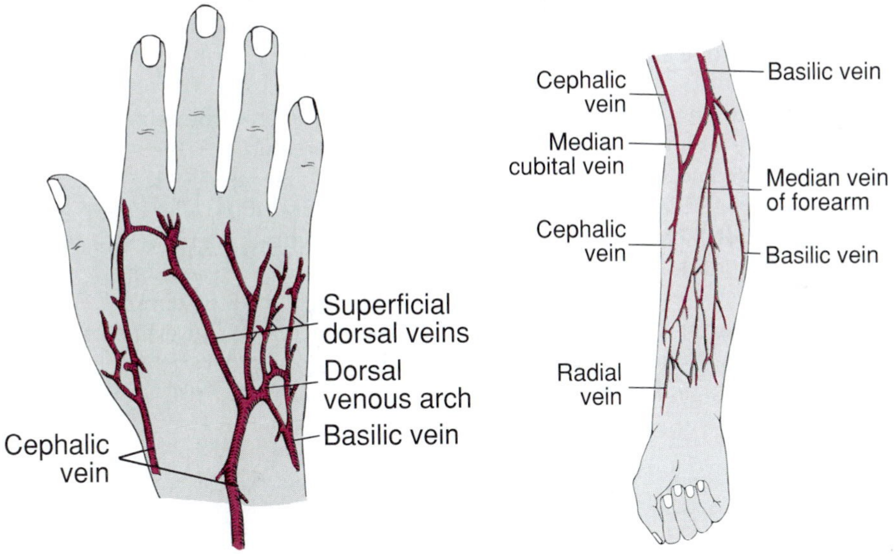

Step 3 Anatomic drawing of IV sites in hand *(left)* and forearm *(right)*.

a. Avoid bony prominences.	Selection of appropriate vein promotes ease and placement of IV needle or catheter.
b. Use most distal portion of vein first.	If damage to the vein occurs, the proximal site of the same vein is still usable.
c. Avoid placing IV catheter near client's wrist or antecubital fossa, if possible.	Frequent bending of the wrist or arm increases the likelihood of infiltration and phlebitis and has a high potential to affect the IV flow rate.
d. For peripheral catheters, upper extremity insertions pose less of a risk of phlebitis than lower extremity insertions. In adults, hand veins have a lower risk of phlebitis than upper arm or wrist veins (CDC, 1996).	
e. Avoid placing IV in client's dominant arm, if possible.	Allows greater freedom of movement.

STEPS	RATIONALE
f. Avoid using an extremity where sensation is decreased, such as one affected by hemiparesis experienced after a stroke.	Ability to perceive pain helps in early detection of complications.
g. Avoid inserting IV through an infection, rash, or any break in the skin.	Increases the risk for IV-related bacteremia.
h. Avoid previously accessed veins, injured veins, or sclerotic veins. Insert proximal to injured areas.	

IMPLEMENTATION

STEPS	RATIONALE
1. Wash hands.	Reduces transmission of microorganisms.
2. Organize equipment on clean clutter-free bedside stand or clean overbed table.	Reduces risk of contamination and accidents.
3. Change client's gown to the more easily removed gown with snaps at the shoulder, if available.	Use of a special IV gown facilitates safe removal of the gown.
4. Open sterile packages using sterile aseptic technique (see Chapter 34).	Maintains sterility of equipment and reduces spread of microorganisms.
5. Prepare IV infusion tubing.	
a. Check solution, using "five rights" of drug administration (see Chapter 17). Make sure prescribed additives, such as potassium and vitamins, have been added. Check solution for color, clarity, and expiration date. Check bag for leaks, which is best if done before reaching the bedside.	IV solutions are medications and should be carefully checked to reduce risk of error. Solutions that are discolored, contain particles, or are expired are not to be used. Leaky bags present an opportunity for infection and must not be used.
b. Open infusion set, maintaining sterility of both ends of tubing. Many sets allow for priming of tubing without removal of end cap.	Prevents bacteria from entering infusion equipment and bloodstream.
c. Place roller clamp (see illustration) about 2 to 4 cm (1 to 2 inches) below drip chamber and move roller clamp to "off" position (see illustration).	Close proximity of roller clamp to drip chamber allows more accurate regulation of flow rate. Moving clamp to "off" prevents accidental spillage of IV fluid on client, nurse, bed, or floor.
d. Remove protective sheath over IV tubing port on plastic IV solution bag. For bottled IV solution, remove metal cap and metal and rubber disks beneath cap (see illustration).	Provides access for insertion of infusion tubing into solution.

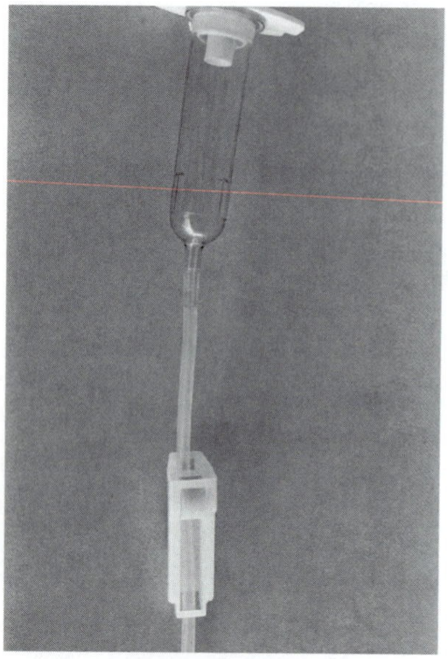

Step 5c(a) Roller camp, open.

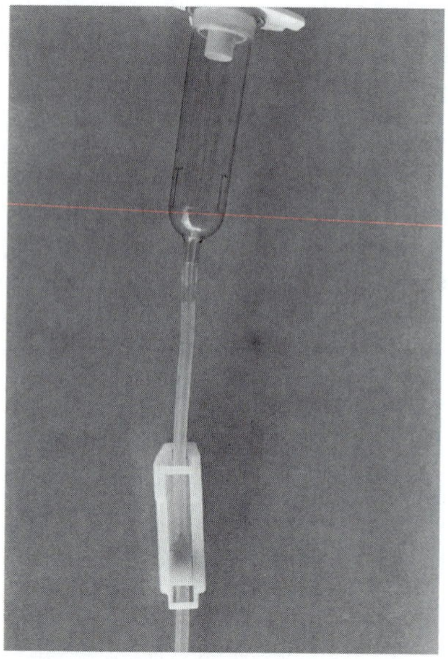

Step 5c(b) Roller clamp, closed.

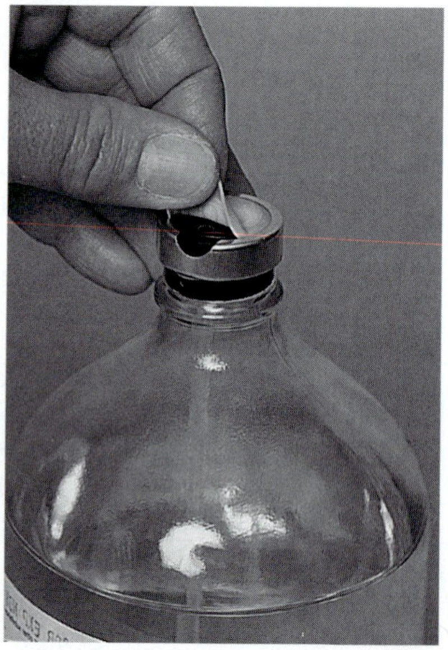

Step 5d Removing cap from IV bottle.

STEPS | **RATIONALE**

A

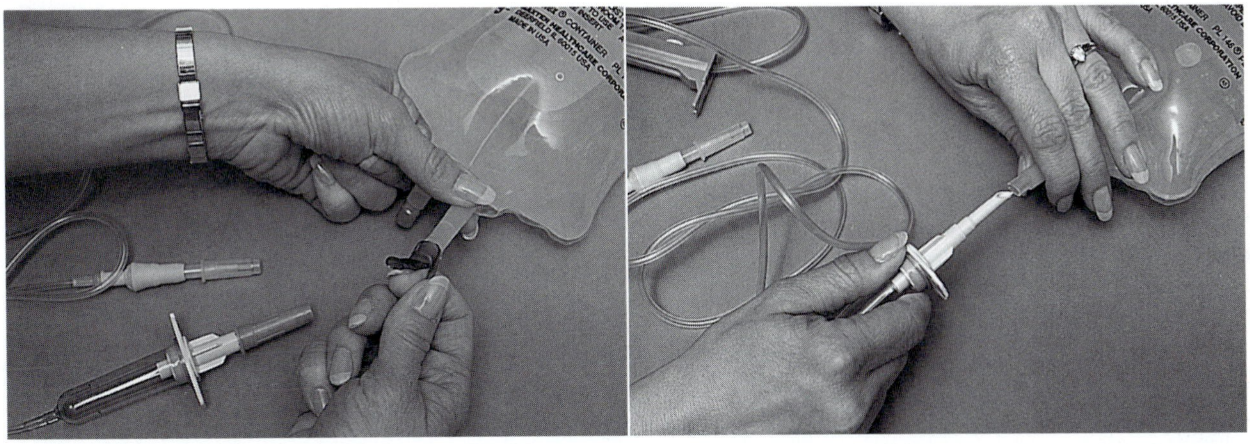

B

Step 5e **A,** Removing protective covering on IV bag **B,** Inserting spike into IV bag.

e. Insert infusion set into fluid bag or bottle. Remove protector cap from tubing insertion spike, not touching spike (see illustration A), and insert spike into opening of IV bag (see illustration B). Cleanse rubber stopper on bottled solution with antiseptic and insert spike into black rubber stopper of IV bottle.

Prevents contamination of solution from contaminated insertion spike.

➤ *CRITICAL DECISION POINT* Do not touch spike because it is sterile. If contamination occurs, (e.g., spike is accidently dropped on the floor), then discard that IV tubing and obtain a new one.

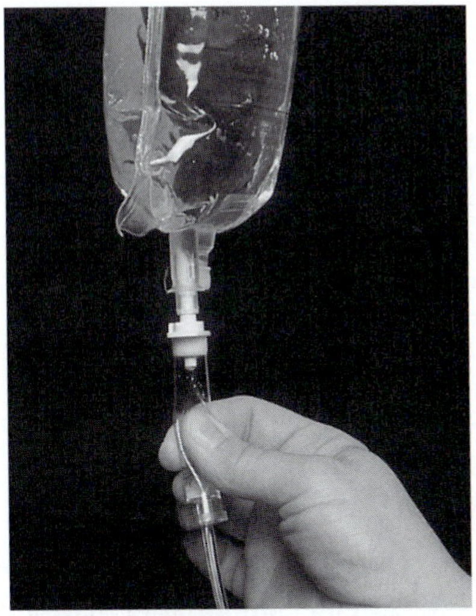

Step 5f Squeezing drip chamber to fill with fluid.

f. Prime infusion tubing by filling with IV solution:
   ➤ Compress drip chamber and release, allowing it to fill one-third to one-half full (see illustration).

Creates suction effect; fluid enters drip chamber to prevent air from entering tubing.

g. Remove tubing protector cap (some tubing can be primed without removal) and slowly release roller clamp to allow fluid to travel from drip chamber through tubing to needle adapter. Return roller clamp to off position after tubing is primed (filled with IV fluid).

Slow fill of tubing decreases turbulence and chance of bubble formation. Removes air from tubing and permits tubing to fill with solution. Closing the clamp prevents accidental loss of fluid.

h. Be certain tubing is clear of air and air bubbles. To remove small air bubbles, firmly tap IV tubing where air bubbles are located. Check entire length of tubing to ensure that all air bubbles are removed.

Large air bubbles can act as emboli.

i. Replace tubing cap protector on end of tubing.

Maintains system sterility.

STEPS	RATIONALE
6. Prepare heparin or normal saline lock for infusion:	
a. If a loop or short extension tubing is needed because of an awkward IV site placement, use sterile technique to connect the IV plug to the loop or short extension tubing. Inject 1 to 3 ml normal saline through the plug and through the loop or short extension tubing.	Removes air to prevent introduction into the vein. Do the same with the saline plug.
7. Select appropriate IV needle or ONC.	Necessary to puncture vein and instill IV fluid.
8. Select most distal site of vein to be used.	If sclerosing or damage to vein occurs, a more proximal site of same vein is still usable.
9. If large amount of body hair is present at needle insertion site, clip it.	Reduces risk of contamination from bacteria on hair. Also assists in maintaining an intact dressing and makes removal of tape less painful.
CRITICAL DECISION POINT **Do not shave area. Shaving may cause microabrasions and predispose client to infection.**	
10. If possible, place extremity in dependent position.	Permits venous dilation and visibility.
11. Place tourniquet 10 to 12 cm (4 to 5 inches) above insertion site. Tourniquet should obstruct venous, not arterial, flow (see illustration). Check presence of distal pulse.	Diminished arterial flow prevents venous filling. The pressure of the tourniquet should cause the vein to dilate. Further methods for vein dilation are listed in Step 14.
12. Apply disposable gloves. Eye protection and mask may be worn (see agency policy).	Decreases exposure to HIV, hepatitis, and other bloodborne organisms (Centers for Disease Control, 1987) and prevents spraying of blood on nurse's mucous membranes.
13. Place needle adapter end of infusion set nearby on sterile gauze or sterile towel.	Permits smooth, quick connection of infusion to IV needle once vein is punctured.
14. Select well-dilated vein. Methods to foster vein dilation include:	
a. Stroking the extremity from distal to proximal below the proposed venipuncture site.	Increases the volume of blood in the vein at the venipuncture site.
b. Opening and closing the fist.	Muscle contraction increases the amount of blood in the extremity.
c. Light tapping over the vein.	Fosters venous dilation.
d. Applying warmth to the extremity for several minutes, for example, with a warm washcloth.	Increases blood supply and fosters venous dilation.
15. (If area of insertion appears to need cleansing, use soap and water first.) Then cleanse insertion site using firm, circular motion (middle to outward) with povidone-iodine solution; refrain from touching the cleansed site; allow the site to dry for at	Povidone-iodine is a topical antiinfective that reduces skin surface bacteria; touching the cleansed area would introduce organisms from the nurse's hand to the site. Povidone-iodine must dry to be effective in reducing microbial counts (Baranowski, 1993).

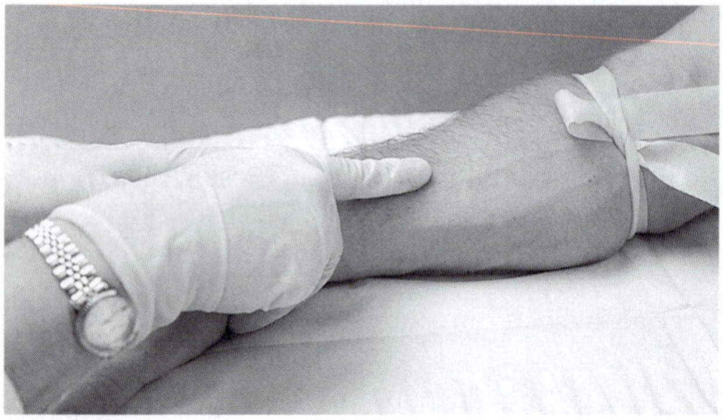

Step 11 Selection of vein with tourniquet applied.

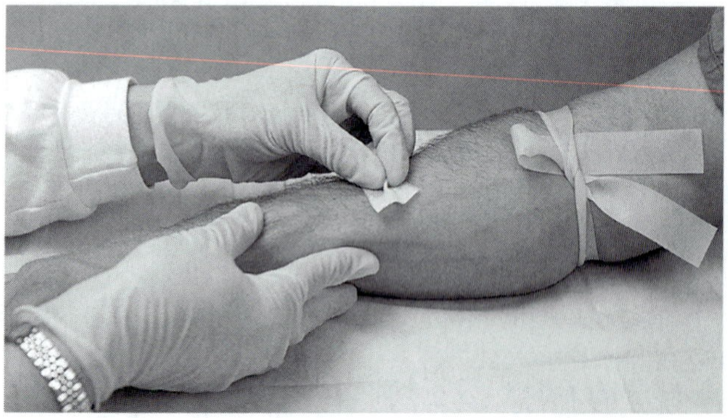

Step 15 Cleanse insertion site with antiseptic prep.

STEPS | **RATIONALE**

least 2 minutes. If the client is allergic to iodine, use 70% alcohol and allow to dry for 60 seconds (see illustration).

16. Perform **venipuncture.** Anchor vein by placing thumb over vein and by stretching the skin against the direction of insertion 2 to 3 inches distal to the site.

Butterfly needle: Hold needle at 20- to 30-degree angle with bevel up slightly distal to actual site of venipuncture.

ONC: Insert with bevel up at 20- to 30-degree angle slightly distal to actual site of venipuncture in the direction of the vein (see illustrations).

IV catheter safety device: Insert using same position as for ONC.

Places needle parallel to vein. When vein is punctured, risk of puncturing posterior vein wall is reduced.

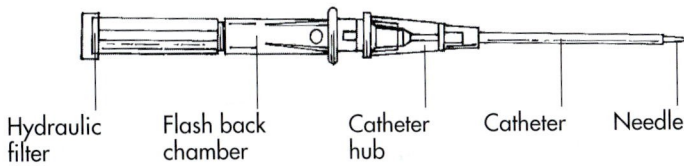

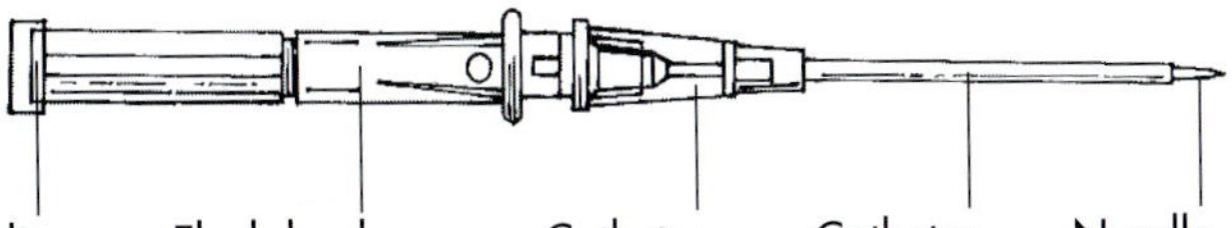

Step 16(a) Illustration of ONC—over-the-needle catheter.

CRITICAL DECISION POINT **Only *one* needle/catheter should be utilized for each attempt at insertion.**

CRITICAL DECISION POINT **No more than three attempts at initiating the IV access should be made by a single nurse.**

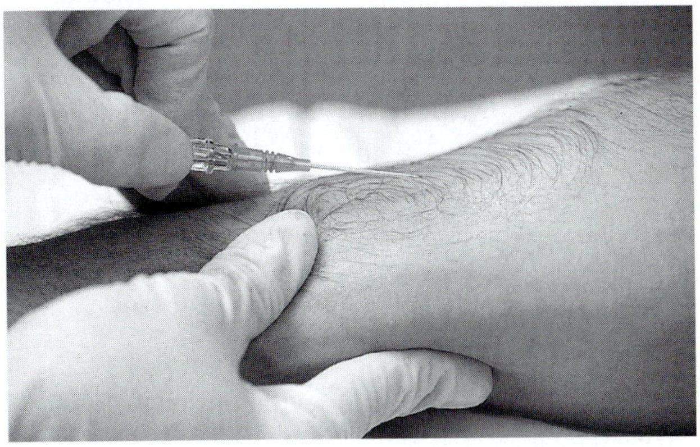

Step 16(b) Puncturing of skin with ONC catheter.

17. Look for blood return through tubing of butterfly needle or flashback chamber of ONC, indicating that needle has entered vein. Lower needle until almost flush with skin. Advance butterfly needle until hub rests at venipuncture site. Advance ONC catheter ¼ inch into vein and then loosen stylet (see illustrations). Advance catheter into vein until hub rests at venipuncture site. Do not reinsert the stylet once it is loosened. (If available, advance the safety device by using push-off tab to thread the catheter.)

Increased venous pressure from tourniquet increases backflow of blood into catheter or tubing. Reinsertion of the stylet can cause catheter breakage in the vein.

A

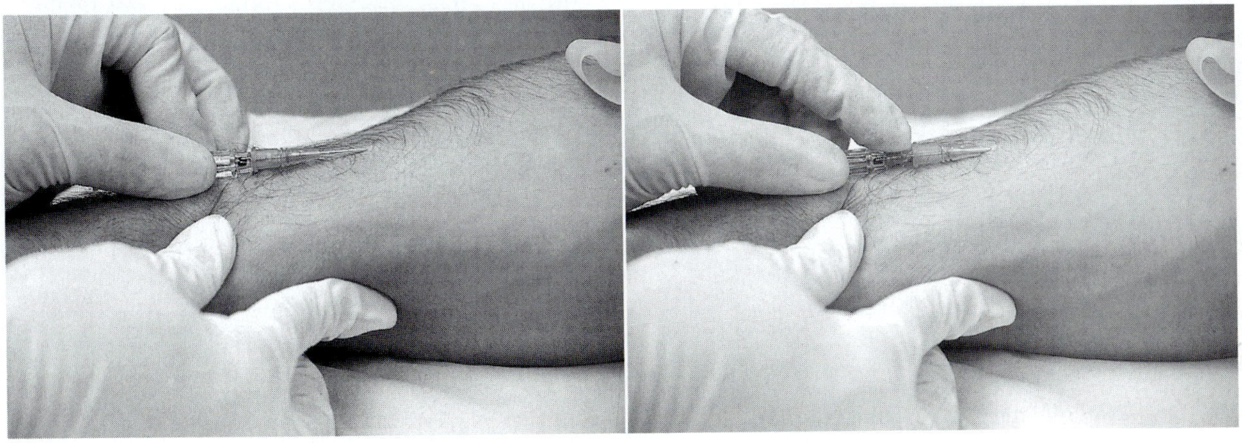

B

Step 17 A & B **A,** Entering vein with bevel up. **B,** Advance catheter off stylet using one handed technique.

STEPS	RATIONALE
18. Stabilize the catheter with one hand by placing pressure on the hub or on the vein above the insertion site. Release tourniquet and remove stylet from ONC. Do not recap the stylet. For a safety device, slide the catheter off the stylet while gliding the protective guard over the stylet. A click indicates the device is locked over the stylet.	Permits venous flow, reduces backflow of blood, and allows connection with administration set.
19. Quickly connect needle adapter of administration set or heparin lock to hub of ONC or butterfly tubing. Do not touch point of entry of needle adaptor.	Prompt connection of infusion set maintains patency of vein. Maintains sterility.
20. Bloodless method: Hold pressure over tip of inserted catheter with your thumb; with your index finger and thumb remove cap and attach tubing to catheter hub (see illustration).	Prevents risk of exposure to blood.
21. Release roller clamp slowly to begin infusion at a rate to maintain patency of IV line (not necessary with a heparin lock).	Permits venous flow and prevents clotting of vein and obstruction of flow of IV solution.

➤ *CRITICAL DECISION POINT* Be sure to calculate rate so as not to infuse IV solution too rapidly or too slowly.

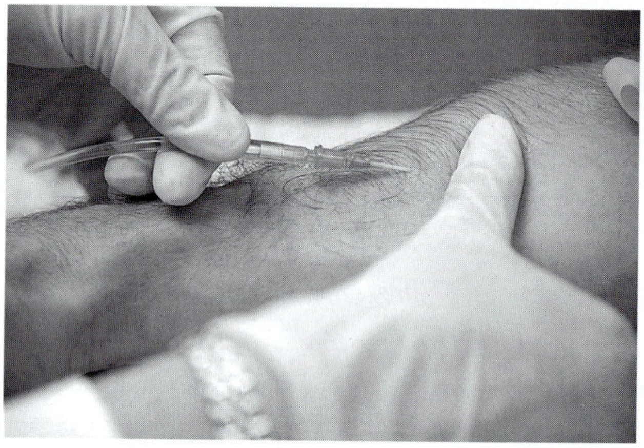

Step 20 Connecting IV tubing to ONC catheter.

STEPS	RATIONALE
22. Secure IV catheter or needle. (Procedures can differ; follow agency policy): a. Gauze dressing: (1) Place narrow piece (½ inch) of tape under catheter hub with sticky side up and cross tape over catheter (see illustration).	Prevents accidental removal of catheter from vein. Prevents back-and-forth motion, which can irritate the vein and introduce bacteria on the skin into the vein.

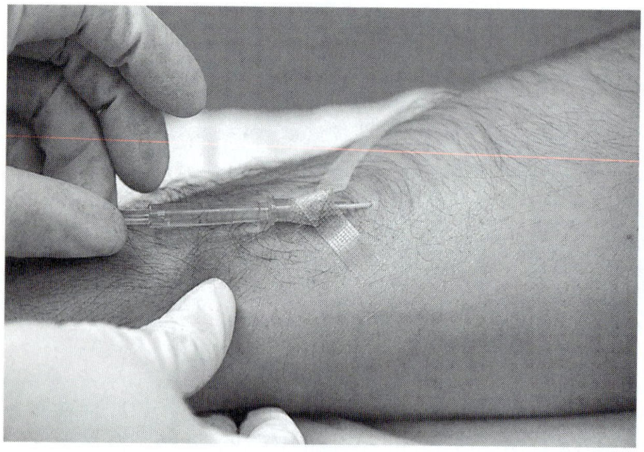

Step 22a(1) Taping ONC catheter to skin.

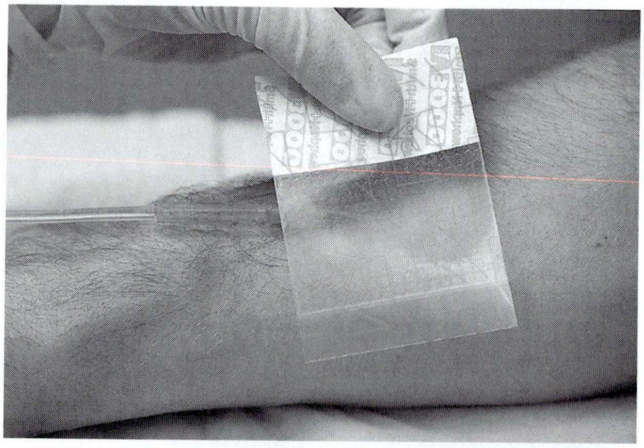

Step 22b(1) Apply transparent dressing over IV site and catheter.

STEPS	RATIONALE
(2) Place second piece of narrow tape directly across hub of catheter.	Further prevents displacement of catheter.
(3) Place 2 × 2 or 4 × 4 gauze sponge over insertion site and catheter hub and secure completely with 1-inch piece of tape. Do not cover connection between IV tubing and catheter hub.	Occlusive dressing protects site from bacterial contamination. Connection between administration set and hub needs to be uncovered to facilitate changing the tubing if necessary. CDC (1996) no longer recommends application of antimicrobial ointment to catheter site.
b. Transparent dressing:	
(1) Apply dressing to site first (no tape)(see illustration). Dressing is molded around catheter hub to secure catheter from movement.	
(2) Apply one piece of tape across edge of dressing closest to the hub. Proceed to use two ½-inch pieces of tape around connection and catheter. Apply 1-inch piece of tape over hub for security.	
23. Secure loop. Secure a loop of infusion tubing to dressing with piece of 1-inch tape. Place tape on tape, not on dressing (reduces the action of the transparent film if placed on top of it).	Stabilizes connection of administration set to catheter. Prevents weight of tubing from pulling catheter or needle out of venipuncture site.
24. For *IV fluid administration* adjust flow rate to correct drops per minute (Skill 20-3).	Maintains correct rate of flow for IV solution. Flow can fluctuate so it must be checked at intervals for accuracy.
a. For *heparin lock* flush with 1 to 3 ml of heparin (10 to 100 U/ml).	
b. For *saline lock* flush with 1 to 3 ml of sterile normal saline.	Maintains patency of IV catheter.
25. Write date and time, gauge size and size of catheter, and placement of IV line on dressing.	Provides immediate access to data as to when IV was inserted and when subsequent dressing changes are needed.
26. Dispose of used needles in appropriate sharps container. Discard supplies. Remove gloves and wash hands.	Reduces transmission of microorganisms and protects staff from injury.

EVALUATION

STEPS	RATIONALE
1. Observe client every hour to determine if fluid is infusing correctly.	
a. Check if correct amount of solution infused as prescribed by looking at time tape.	
b. Count flow rate.	
c. Check patency of IV catheter or needle: briefly compress cannulated vein proximal to site. Observe for slowing or momentary cessation of IV rate.	Compression results in mechanical obstruction of vein. When IV catheter is patent, compression results in slowing or cessation of flow rate. No change in flow rate may indicate infiltration.

CRITICAL DECISION POINT If IV is positional, fluid will run less slowly depending on position of client's arm. Instruct client to position arm to maintain flow; if this continues, IV may have to be restarted.

STEPS	RATIONALE
d. Also observe client during compression of vessel for signs of discomfort.	
e. Inspect insertion site for absence of infiltration, phlebitis, or inflammation.	Provides continuous evaluation of type and amount of fluid delivered to client. Hourly inspection prevents accidental fluid overload or inadequate infusion rate and identifies early incidence of vein inflammation or tissue damage.

STEPS	RATIONALE
2. Observe client every hour to determine response to therapy (i.e., measure vital signs, conduct postprocedure assessments).	IV fluids and additives are given to maintain or restore fluid and electrolyte balance. They can also cause unexpected effects, which can be serious.
3. **Unexpected outcomes** that may occur include uncorrected fluid and electrolyte imbalances or inaccurate administration of IV fluids, which can result in:	
➤ **Fluid volume deficit (FVD)** as manifested by decreased urine output, dry mucous membranes, hypotension, tachycardia.	Prolonged fluid volume deficits increase risk for severe dehydration, shock, coma, death. Ordered 24-hour infusion may require readjustment by physician.
➤ Fluid volume excess as manifested by crackles in the lungs, shortness of breath, edema. Reduce IV flow rate if symptoms appear and notify physician.	Results when cardiovascular or renal systems cannot adapt to excess fluids and overload occurs.
➤ Electrolyte imbalances as manifested by abnormal serum electrolyte levels, changes in mental status, alterations in neuromuscular function, changes in vital signs, and other manifestations.	Can result from disease, trauma, prescribed therapies. Severity of symptoms relates directly to degree of electrolyte imbalance.
➤ **Infiltration** as indicated by swelling and possible pitting edema, pallor, coolness, pain at insertion site, possible decrease in flow rate. IV must be discontinued then reinserted if still needed.	Swelling results from increased fluid in interstitial tissue. If enough fluid accumulates, pitting edema forms. Pallor is caused by decreased circulation to region. In addition, fluid may be flowing through IV line at decreased rate or may have stopped because of increased tissue pressure. Pain may also occur with infiltration.
➤ Phlebitis is indicated by pain, increased skin temperature, erythema along path of vein. IV must be discontinued, then restarted if still needed.	**Phlebitis** is inflammation of a vein caused by an IV catheter or by chemical irritation of additives and medications given intravenously, or bacterial contamination.
➤ Bleeding occurs at venipuncture site.	Common in clients who have received heparin or who have a bleeding disorder or if site is at a bend. If bleeding occurs around venipuncture site and catheter is within vein, gauze dressing may be applied over site. Be aware that if gauze dressing is used, it must be removed in order to accurately assess insertion site. Bleeding from vein is usually slow, continuous seepage. Blood on the dressing can result when the administration set becomes disconnected from the catheter's hub. When blood appears on the dressing, verify that the system is intact and change the dressing.

RECORDING AND REPORTING

1. Record in nurse's notes number of attempts for insertion, type of fluid, insertion site by vessel, flow rate, size and type catheter or needle, and when infusion was begun. A special parenteral therapy flow sheet may be used (Fig. 20-3, p. 668).	Documents initiation of therapy as ordered by physician. A special form provides a record of total IV therapy.
2. Record client's response to IV fluid, amount infused, and integrity and patency of system every 4 hours or according to agency policy.	Documents ongoing IV therapy and client's tolerance and response to therapy.
3. Report to oncoming nursing staff: type of fluid, flow rate, status of venipuncture site, amount of fluid remaining in present solution, expected time to hang next IV bag or bottle, and any side effects.	Provides next nursing personnel with status of IV fluid. Allows new nursing staff to plan when new solution should be hung. Also provides information for accurate calculation of IV fluid intake.

STEPS	RATIONALE
4. Report to physician adverse reactions such as pulmonary congestion, shock, thrombophlebitis.	Prompt reporting of adverse reactions permits initiation of appropriate medical therapies.

Follow-up Activities

1. Monitor and chart resolution of unexpected outcomes (e.g., infiltration, phlebitis) every 4 hours.
2. Observe entire IV setup and correct flow rate (Skill 20-3), change solution (Skill 20-4), change infusion tubing (Skill 20-5), and change dressing (Skill 20-7) according to agency policy.
3. If intake and output are not being measured, this should be initiated.
4. When infiltration occurs, IV must be discontinued and, if necessary, new line reinserted into vein of other extremity if possible.
5. Peripheral IV access should be changed every 48 to 72 hours (CDC, 1996) or per physician orders if venous access is limited and more frequently if complications occur (i.e., phlebitis, infiltration, infection).

• • • • •

Special Considerations

- Obese clients present problems for venipuncture because of difficulty in locating superficial veins.
- Avoid using circulatory or neurologically impaired extremities.
- Use large-gauge (16-, 18-, or 20-gauge) catheter if it is anticipated that blood or blood components are going to be administered.
- Critically ill clients at all stages of life require more frequent assessment to monitor status of therapy.
- When solution has less than 100 ml remaining, present nursing shift should have new solution at client's bedside and slow flow rate. This reduces risk of solution emptying during change-of-shift report.
- Institutions that do not have IV safety devices may have policies for using a "one-handed" technique to recap IV stylets (OSHA, 1991). The care giver will lay the cap on a flat surface and *with one hand only,* will slide the needle into the cap.

Teaching Considerations

- Instruct client about signs and symptoms of infiltration, phlebitis, and inflammation. Client can report early onset to nurse.
- Instruct client to inform nurse if flow slows or stops or blood is seen in the tubing.
- Instruct client how to ambulate with IV pole or stand.
- Instruct client to ask for assistance when bathing or when changing gown.

Pediatric Considerations

- Pediatric veins are very fragile. Avoid sites that are easily moved or bumped. Use commercial protective device to cover area.
- In addition to the usual venipuncture sites, the veins in the scalp or the foot are used in infants.
- If clients are older children, allowing them to select IV site may increase cooperation because they have some control over their treatment.
- Most IV infusions in pediatric clients require a 22- to 24-gauge ONC (LaRocca and Otto, 1993).
- When child is critically ill or long-term IV access is anticipated, PICC catheter, Broviac atrial, or implanted port may be used to access larger vein.
- Choosing age-appropriate activities compatible with the maintenance of the IV infusion is important to maintain normal growth and development.

Gerontologic Considerations

- Gerontologic veins are very fragile. Avoid sites that are easily moved or bumped. (Use commercial protective device to protect site.)
- In older clients, use the smallest gauge possible, for example, 22-, 24-, or 26-gauge. This is less traumatizing to the vein and allows better blood flow to provide increased hemodilution of the IV fluids or medications (Coulter, 1992).
- If possible, avoid the back of the older adult's hand or the dominant arm for venipuncture because these sites greatly interfere with the older adult's independence.
- If the older adult has fragile skin and veins, use minimal tourniquet pressure or no tourniquet at all.
- When the older adult has lost subcutaneous tissue, the veins lose stability and roll away from the needle. To stabilize the vein, apply traction to the skin below the projected insertion point (Coulter, 1992).
- Using an angle of 5 to 15 degrees on insertion is helpful because the older adult's veins are more superficial (Coulter, 1992).

Home Care Considerations

- Ensure that the client is able and willing to self-administer IV therapy or that there is a reliable

ST. JOHN'S HOSPITAL
Springfield, Illinois

I.V. MAINTENANCE RECORD

I.V. FLUID & I.V. MEDICATION

Site Code

R.J. or L.J. – Right or Left Jugular
R.S.V. or L.S.V. – Right or Left Subclavian Vein
R.L.L. or L.L.L. – Right or Left Lower Leg
R.H. or L.H. – Right or Left Hand
R.F.A. or L.F.A. – Right or Left Forearm
R.U.A. or L.U.A. – Right or Left Upperarm
R.F. or L.F. – Right or Left Foot
R.S., L.S. or M.S. – Right, Left or Mid Scalp
R.F.V. or L.F.V. – Right or Left Femoral Vein
R.A.C. or L.A.C. – Right or Left Antecubital
R.W. or L.W. – Right or Left Wrist

K.V.O. – Keep Vein Open
H.L. – Heparin Lock
P.B. – Piggyback
P. – Push

Triple Lumen Catheter

Proximal - 18 gauge (White)	Middle - 18 gauge (Blue)	Distal - 16 gauge (Brown)
Draw blood Blood Adm Medications	TPN Medications	Blood Adm. Colloids Viscous Fluids CVP Monitoring Medications

Allergy:

No. of last I.V. __________ Letter of last expander __________

No. of last Blood/Component __________

Signature:

DATE		
Night Nurse		
Day Nurse		
Evening Nurse		

Order Date		Amount, Solution, Infusing Time or Rate, Medication, Dose, Time	Site(s)	Pump	Time	Time
		One Time I.V. Meds.				
	No.	I.V. Fluids				
		I.V. TUBING CHANGE. (Indicate I.V. No. & Time)				
	Stop Date	Intermittent & PRN I.V. Meds.				
		I.V.P.B. TUBING CHANGE (Indicate Drug & Time)				

Fig. 20-3 IV maintenance record. (Courtesy St. John's Hospital, Springfield, Ill.)

I.V. SITE ASSESSMENT

SITE CODE				TYPE CODE			
R.J. or L.J.	Right or Left Jugular			M.C.	Medicut	H.C.	Hickman Catheter
R.S.V. or L.S.V.	Right or Left Subclavian Vein	K.V.O.	Keep Vein Open	A.C.	Angiocath	B.C.	Broviac Catheter
R.L.L. or L.L.L.	Right or Left Lower Leg	H.L.	Heparin Lock	S.V.	Scalpvein	M.L.C.	Multi-lumen Catheter
R.H. or L.H.	Right or Left Hand	P.B.	Piggyback	A.S.	Angio-set	M.L.P.	Multi-lumen Proximal
R.F.A. or L.F.A.	Right or Left Forearm	P.	Push	C.D.	Cutdown	M.L.M.	Multi-lumen Middle
R.U.A. or L.U.A.	Right or Left Upperarm	Cath	Catheter	I.C.	Intracath	M.L.D.	Multi-lumen Distal
R.F. or L.F.	Right or Left Foot			I.P.	Infuse A Port	I.	Introducer
R.S., L.S. or M.S.	Right, Left or Mid Scalp						
R.F.V. or L.F.V.	Right or Left Femoral Vein						
R.A.C. or L.A.C.	Right or Left Antecubital						
R.W. or L.W.	Right or Left Wrist	NA	Not Applicable				

Document on each site once each shift & P.R.N. No space is to be left blank. Place "NA" in spaces which do not apply.

Date	Time	I.V. Site Start	I.V. Site d/c	Site Code	Cath Size	Type Code	Site Day	Cap Change	Dressing Change	I.V. Site: s̄ tenderness redness, edema, drainage	Signature

#1005
(2 of 2)

(Courtesy St. John's Hospital, Springfield, Ill.)

Fig. 20-3, cont'd IV maintenance record.

care giver or nursing support person at home to provide this IV therapy care.

- Determine the client's ability to obtain help, for example, availability of care giver, presence of and ability to use telephone.
- Ensure that all needles and equipment contaminated by blood are disposed of in puncture-resistant containers with lids, for example, plastic milk cartons, or coffee cans. Some suppliers will provide sharps containers for needle disposal (see Chapter 41).
- Instruct client and primary care giver about procedures of IV therapy, including hand washing, sterile technique while manipulating syringes and other supplies.
- Teach client and primary care giver to recognize potential problems with infusion and appropriate reaction to problems.
- Teach primary care giver to apply pressure with sterile gauze if catheter falls out and, if client is on anticoagulant therapy, to tape several pieces of sterile gauze in place for at least 20 minutes or until bleeding stops.
- Teach client and primary care giver to take tub bath but not to let IV tubing touch water and to unplug pump first if one is used. If showering is mandatory, the client must insert hand and forearm into a plastic bag. Tape bag in place to ensure that IV site is completely covered.
- Instruct client to wear clothes with wide sleeves.
- Teach client about activity restrictions, for example, avoiding strenuous exercise of the arm with the IV.
- In addition, for home care clients, teach client and family to monitor intake and output using household measuring devices.

SKILL 20-2 Inserting a Peripherally Inserted Central Catheter

Peripherally inserted central catheters (PICCs) provide alternate access when the client requires intermediate-length venous access (greater than 7 days to 3 months). In many states the PICC can be inserted by a registered nurse that has received special training. In some cases only IV therapy team members will insert PICC lines. The staff nurse must still understand what a PICC line is and be aware of its appropriate care and maintenance. In comparison to centrally placed venous catheters, the PICC has less risk of pneumothorax, hemothorax, or air embolism and is more cost effective. Compared with peripheral IV catheters, the PICC can be kept in place longer (more than 48 to 72 hours). In fact, PICC lines may remain in place as long as there are no signs of problems (infiltration, migration, infection, etc.). In addition, PICC lines are associated with less risk of infiltration and phlebitis because the IV fluids and medications are diluted in the greater volume of blood flow present in the larger veins (subclavian or superior vena cava) where the tip of the catheter is placed. For the catheter to be successfully placed, the client must have a palpable cephalic or basilic vein in the antecubital fossa. In addition to phlebitis, other complications associated with PICC use include clotting and leaking or breaking of the catheter.

PICCs vary in size from 16- to 24-gauge and in length from 40 to 60 cm (16 to 24 in). The length is chosen based on the distance from the client's antecubital fossa to the point desired for placement of the tip. They can have a single or double lumen. A guide wire or stylet can be used when inserting a PICC to make the catheter stiffer and easier to advance. The catheter is made of soft materials, which cause minimal irritation to the vein.

PICCs can be used to infuse IV fluids, parenteral nutrition, blood and blood products, and medications such as antibiotics. The smaller-gauge catheters cannot be used for some types of infusions, especially those of blood and blood products and parenteral nutrition. Not all PICCs can be used to draw blood. The nurse should be aware of product advantages and limitations of each device used.

EQUIPMENT

(Many manufacturers of PICCs provide an insertion kit that provides most of the required equipment; check how equipment is supplied in each agency. Not every kit contains same supplies.)

- 2 pairs of sterile gloves
- 2 sterile drapes (1 fenestrated, 1 nonfenestrated)
- Sterile forceps (nontoothed)
- Sterile scissors
- 2 sterile 4 × 4 gauze pads
- Tourniquet
- 3 povidone-iodine swab sticks
- 3 alcohol swab sticks
- 2 sterile 2 × 2 gauze pads
- Transparent dressing
- Steri-strips
- 6 10-ml syringes with 1-inch, 21-gauge needles
- Short extension tubing (one for each lumen)
- Injection cap (one for each lumen) (Luer lock)

- 2 10-ml vials of sterile normal saline for injection
- 10-ml vial of heparin (10 to 100 U/ml)
- PICC (size depends on size of client's vein and type of infusion ordered)
- Lidocaine (1% or 2% with or without epinephrine) or Enteric mixture of local anesthetics lidocaine and Prilocaine (EMLA) (topical lidocaine) for topical anesthesia
- 2 tape measures (one sterile and one unsterile)
- Face mask, gown, goggles

STEPS	RATIONALE
ASSESSMENT	
1. Review physician's order for type of catheter, type of infusion, and desired placement of the catheter. An order requesting the insertion of a PICC line and administration of an IV solution must be made by a licensed physician prior to the implementation of this procedure.	Ensures safe and correct initiation of the PICC. The catheter tip can be placed in either the subclavian vein or in the superior vena cava. (The superior vena cava is the most desired position.)
2. Know agency's policy concerning personnel who may start PICCs.	Most agencies require special training for RNs who insert PICCs.
3. Review manufacturer's directions concerning the catheter and insertion technique. Each manufacturer publishes guidelines for a particular catheter; adherence to the guidelines facilitates safe insertion. Several techniques exist for PICC insertion: a. Breakaway needle introducer (used for this procedure description) b. ONC c. Over a guide wire	
4. Assess client's understanding of length and type of therapy and management of PICC.	Client or significant other should be assessed to assume management of PICC once discharged home. Dressing changes are often done by home care agency, in a clinic, or in a doctor's office.
5. Assess client's fluid, **electrolyte,** and nutritional status.	Provides data to verify reason for IV therapy and to serve as a basis for evaluation.
6. Assess client's comfort, oxygenation, and elimination needs.	Anticipation of these needs prevents interruption of sterile procedure.
7. Assess for drug allergies.	Local lidocaine will be applied to skin for anesthetic purposes.

NURSING DIAGNOSIS

Clustering of defining characteristics from the assessment data may reveal the following nursing diagnoses for clients requiring this skill:

- Altered nutrition: less than body requirements
- Fluid volume deficit
- Risk for fluid volume deficit
- Risk for infection
- Knowledge deficit regarding use of PICC

Related factors are individualized based on a client's condition or needs.

PLANNING

1. **Expected outcomes** following completion of procedure:	
➤ Client tolerates positional changes during insertion of PICC line. ➤ The client will have no complaint of pain or erythema at the insertion site; PICC remains patent; catheter should be intact without visible breakage.	Catheter insertion performed correctly with good sterile technique. In one study, phlebitis occurred in 7% of the clients after an average time of 19 days, clotting occurred in 5.6% of the clients, and broken catheters ocurred 6.4% of the time (Loughran, Edwards, and McClure, 1992).
➤ Site is free of bleeding or hematoma.	Catheter inserted into vein without trauma to tissues or vein wall.
➤ Client is free of respiratory distress.	No introduction of air embolus occurs.

STEPS	RATIONALE
➤ Client's chest x-ray film shows proper placement of catheter tip.	
➤ Fluid and electrolyte balance will be normal as measured by normal vital signs, serum electrolyte levels, intake and output.	Reflects the correction or maintenance of normal fluid and electrolyte balance.
➤ Client will have normal body weight and other indicators of nutritional balance.	Body weight can be maintained or gained when the client receives parenteral nutrition.
➤ Client remains afebrile with normal white blood cell count (WBC).	Elevated body temperature is associated with catheter sepsis.
➤ Client explains purpose and type of PICC and discusses proper management skills for home care.	
➤ Client lists three signs and symptoms of infection, thrombosis, and air embolism and interventions for each. Enables client to initiate corrective measures at home.	
2. Explain the procedure to the client, including position that will be used and possible complications.	Decreases anxiety and promotes cooperation.
3. Verify that a consent form has been signed.	Many agencies require a consent form.
4. Measure circumference of client's upper arm and document.	Provides a baseline for subsequent comparison to determine swelling, which can be associated with the advent of complications (i.e., venous thrombosis).

IMPLEMENTATION

1. Wash hands.	Reduces transmission of microorganisms.
2. Organize equipment on a clean clutter-free bedside stand or clean over-bed table.	Reduces risk of contamination and accidents.
3. Instruct client to wash arms thoroughly from fingertips to midbiceps using antibacterial soap and warm water. (Assist client as needed.)	Decreases bacteria prior to insertion.
4. Clip hair around insertion site if necessary.	Helps dressing and tape adhere to skin. Makes dressing removal less painful. Clipping prevents microabrasions thus decreasing risk for infection.

➤ ***CRITICAL DECISION POINT*** **Do not shave area. Shaving causes microabrasions.**

5. Identify an appropriate vein in the antecubital fossa by placing a tourniquet around the right upper arm close to the axilla and examining the veins in the antecubital fossa; release tourniquet, leaving it in place beneath the arm.	Either the basilic or the cephalic vein may be used; the basilic vein is preferred because it is less tortuous. Releasing the tourniquet prevents venous engorgement.

➤ ***CRITICAL DECISION POINT*** **Veins that are sclerosed (often from frequent blood drawing) should be avoided because the catheter will, most likely, be difficult to advance.**

6. Position the client in a supine position in bed with the arm at a 45- to 90-degree angle (see agency policy) to the client's trunk.	This provides a straighter course for advancing the catheter to the large veins in the chest.
7. Measure the distance from the insertion site to the proposed site for the catheter tip using the unsterile tape measure. For subclavian placement, measure from the proposed insertion site up the arm to the shoulder and across to the midclavicular line. For superior vena cava placement, continue to the sternal notch and down to the third intercostal space on the right of the sternum.	Desired position of the catheter may be indicated in the physician's order or by the type of therapy to be given. These landmarks correspond to the venous structures underneath (see illustration).

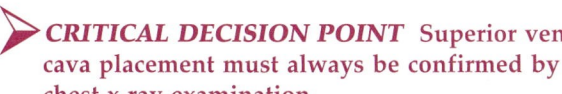

STEPS	RATIONALE
CRITICAL DECISION POINT Superior vena cava placement must always be confirmed by a chest x-ray examination.	
8. Put on mask, gown, and goggles. Client may also wear mask.	Reduces transmission of microorganisms.
9. Open the sterile supplies or kit. Using the kit's wrap as a sterile field, arrange supplies for efficient use; drop the 4 × 4 gauze, the extension tubings, and the injection cap(s) onto the field using sterile technique (see illustration). Cleanse the top of the normal saline, heparin, and lidocaine vials with alcohol and set aside.	Provides a sterile working surface. Facilitates efficient technique by having all supplies ready and accessible.
10. Put on sterile gloves.	Reduces transmission of microorganisms.
11. With another nurse or technician asisting, draw up lidocaine (optional), normal saline, and heparin for flushing.	
12. If using EMLA for anesthetic, prepare by applying to insertion site ½ to 1 hour before venipuncture and cover with a layer of Tegaderm dressing (see illustration).	Ensures skin is properly anesthetized.

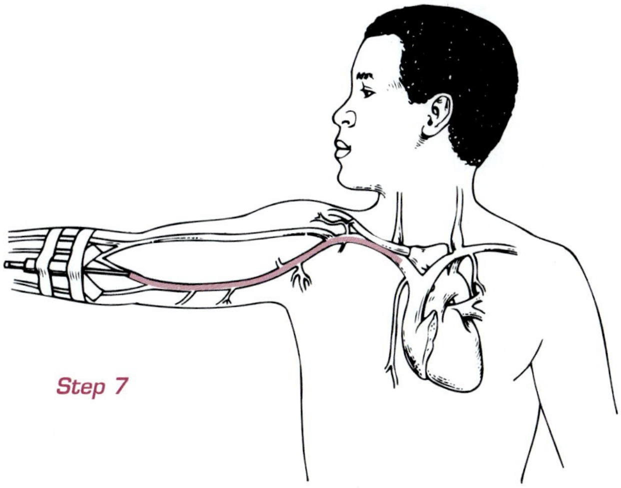

Step 7

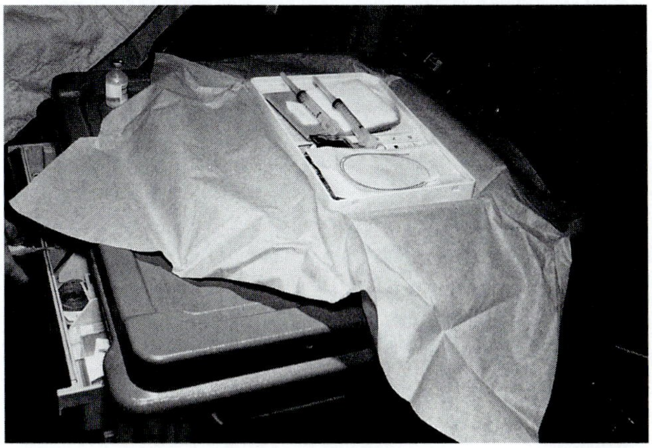

Step 9 Equipment for PICC insertion.

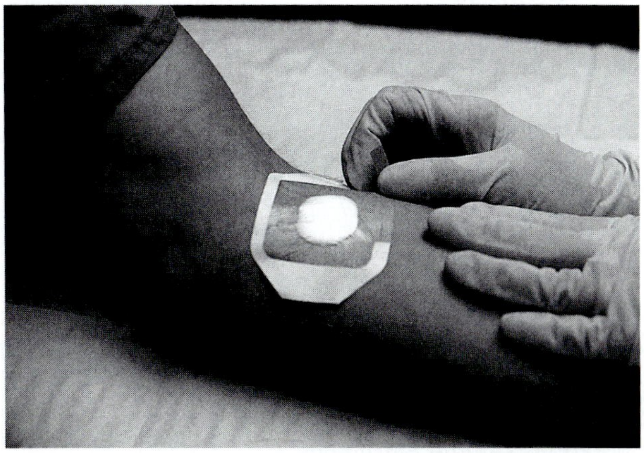

Step 12 Application of topical lidocaine to site chosen for PICC insertion.

STEPS	RATIONALE
13. Prepare catheter and tubing:	
a. Using the sterile tape measure, measure the catheter to the length previously determined plus 1 inch.	Ensures that distal tip of catheter will be properly positioned. The extra length will extend out from the venipuncture site.
b. Using the sterile scissors, cut the catheter at the appropriate length.	A straight cut may prevent the catheter end from lying on the intima and obstructing blood flow. A 45-degree bevel cut clearly identifies the tip of the catheter.
CRITICAL DECISION POINT **Check agency policy about whether a straight cut or a 45-degree bevel cut should be used. Not all catheters can be cut. Check product brochure.**	
c. Attach the injection cap to the extension tubing (one set for each lumen). Using a 4 × 4 gauze to hold the vial, draw up 5 ml of normal saline into a syringe for each lumen of the catheter and flush each cap and tubing with 2 ml. Remove the needle from the syringe and flush the catheter, leaving the syringe in place.	Removes air from tubing and catheter; ensures patency of catheter, detects any leaks.
d. Inspect the equipment for defects such as cracks or kinks. Verify patency of introducer.	Ensures proper function during and after insertion.
14. Prepare the insertion site:	
a. Place a sterile drape under the access arm.	Reduces transmission of microorganisms.
b. Vigorously scrub the insertion site using three alcohol swab sticks and allow to dry for 60 seconds. Follow by three povidone-iodine swab sticks (see illustration). A circular area from the middle of the forearm to the middle of the upper arm should be cleaned with each swab stick, starting at the venipuncture site and cleansing outward in a circular motion middle to outer edge. Cleansed area should be an approximate 6-inch concentric circular area from venipuncture site. Let the povidone-iodine dry completely (at least 2 minutes).	Alcohol defats the skin; povidone-iodine is a topical antiinfective that reduces skin surface bacteria. The circular motion moves bacteria on the skin away from the insertion site. Use of separate swab sticks prevents bacteria from being reintroduced to the venipuncture site. Povidone-iodine must dry to be effective in reducing microbial counts (Baranowski, 1993).

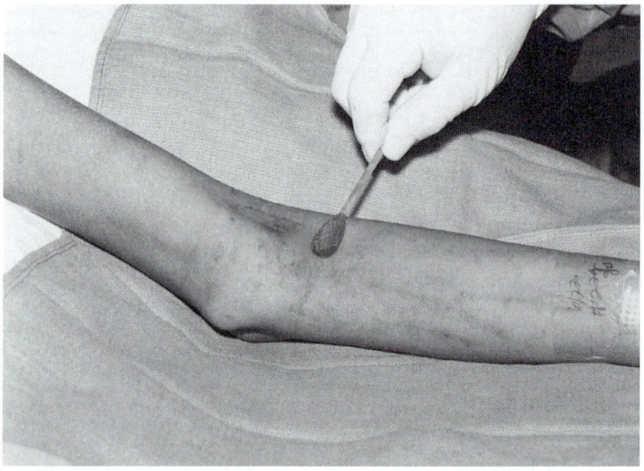

Step 14b PICC site prepping.

STEPS	RATIONALE
15. Remove gloves; reapply tourniquet if a single nonsterile tourniquet is used.	Tourniquet is not sterile; application of tourniquet impedes venous blood flow, resulting in an engorged vein to foster ease of venipuncture.
16. Put on a new pair of sterile gloves; use talc-free gloves or rinse gloves with sterile water.	Reduces the transmission of microorganisms; rinsing gloves prevents talc adherence to the catheter.
17. Place a sterile 4 × 4 gauze over the tourniquet or apply a sterile tourniquet.	Allows removal of tourniquet without contaminating glove.
18. Place fenestrated drape over the insertion site, being careful to avoid contamination of the site.	Provides a sterile field around the venipuncture site.

STEPS	RATIONALE
19. Administer 0.1 to 0.2 ml of 1% lidocaine at the insertion site. Check your agency's policy and the physician's order.	Local anesthetic reduces discomfort.
➤ ***CRITICAL DECISION POINT*** **Note lidocaine is used if EMLA has not been used. Do not use both.**	
20. Insert the introducer needle at a 20- to 30-degree angle, bevel up. Look for a brisk blood return through the introducer (see illustration).	Angle lessens risk of puncture of posterior wall of vein. The introducer is large bore.
➤ ***CRITICAL DECISION POINT*** **Verify that blood return is venous not arterial (arterial blood is pulsatile and bright red). The brachial vein is close to the brachial artery and the artery may be inadvertently cannulated.**	
21. Lower the introducer parallel to the skin and advance (½ to 1 cm) further into the vein.	Ensures that vein is securely cannulated.
22. Insert the catheter through the introducer needle and advance it slowly approximately 2 to 3 inches (5 to 7.5 cm) using the nontoothed forceps. Agency policy differs concerning the use of a guide wire or stylet. If a guide wire is used, ensure that it remains well within the lumen of the PICC during insertion. Take care that the catheter remains on the sterile field during insertion.	Allows the catheter to travel through the introducer into the vein. Slow advancement prevents trauma to the intima of the vein (Loughran, Edwards, and McClure, 1992). The guide wire provides more rigidity to the catheter to aid insertion. Otherwise, no significant difference was found between clients whose PICCs were begun with guide wires and those for whom guide wires were not used (Loughran, Edwards, and McClure, 1992).
➤ ***CRITICAL DECISION POINT*** **If the catheter leaves the sterile field, it is considered contaminated and cannot be inserted. A new sterile catheter must be used.**	
23. Release the tourniquet, while stabilizing the catheter, using the sterile 4 × 4 gauze if a nonsterile tourniquet is used.	Allows further catheter advancement. Prevents contamination of glove.
24. Advance the catheter an additional 6 inches (or more depending on client size) until tip of catheter is at the shoulder (see illustration). The catheter is marked at 10 cm intervals to facilitate identification of location of tip.	The client's position needs to change to facilitate entry into the subclavian vein.

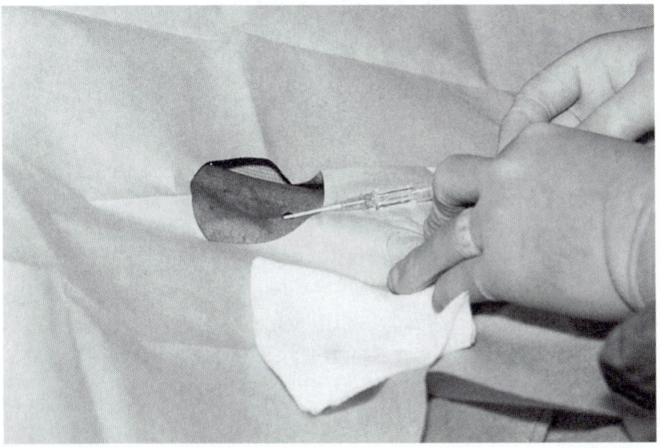

Step 20 Introduction of PICC introducer needle into antecubital fossa.

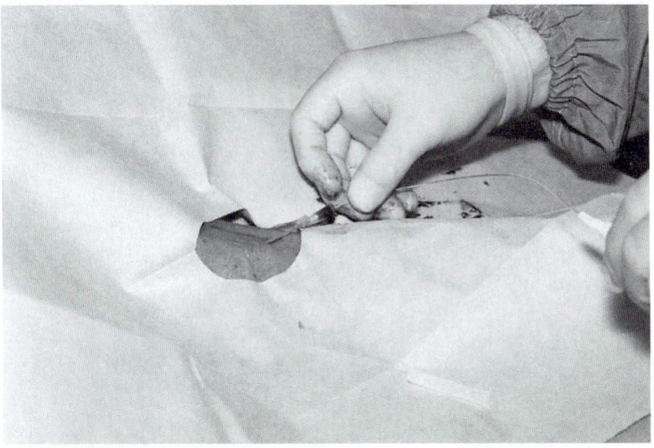

Step 24 Advancing PICC line through vein.

STEPS	RATIONALE
25. Instruct the client to turn the head toward the side of the venous access and drop the chin to the chest.	This position closes the internal jugular vein, preventing accidental cannulation.
26. Continue to slowly advance the catheter until the predetermined length is reached.	Aids proper placement of the tip of the catheter.
27. Fully withdraw the introducer needle. Either use the forceps to maintain the position of the catheter or apply light pressure 2 inches above the insertion site while the introducer is withdrawn.	The introducer is removed to prevent accidental puncture of the vein. Helps to ensure that the catheter will not be withdrawn with the introducer. Pressure any closer to the introducer may cause the introducer to nick the catheter.

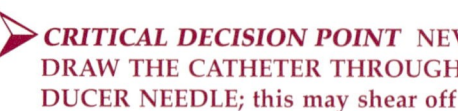

CRITICAL DECISION POINT NEVER WITHDRAW THE CATHETER THROUGH THE INTRODUCER NEEDLE; this may shear off the catheter, causing a catheter embolism.

STEPS	RATIONALE
28. When the introducer is out, press the wings together until they snap, then peel the needle from around the catheter.	Removes the needle so that the catheter cannot be inadvertently punctured.
a. Tell the client that a snapping sound will be heard.	Prevents anxiety.
29. Remove the guide wire using a gentle twisting motion.	Allows use of the lumen, prevents damage to the catheter and vein.
30. Attach a syringe filled with 3 ml of normal saline to the lumen where the guide wire had been, aspirate for a blood return, and flush the catheter.	Verifies patency of distal lumen, prevents clotting.
31. Remove the syringe from each lumen and attach the extension tubing and cap to the lumen.	Prevents blood loss, maintains closed system.
32. Cleanse the insertion site with antiseptic swab if there has been oozing of blood. Allow to dry (see illustration).	
33. Anchor the hub of the catheter to the skin with Steri-strips placed over the catheter's hub (see illustration). Some agencies suggest that the PICC should be sutured in place. Some state boards do not allow RNs to suture.	Helps to maintain the catheter's position for long-term use.
34. Place 2 × 2 gauze pads over the insertion site. Cover this with a transparent dressing (see illustration).	Provides pressure on the insertion site for 24 hours to control oozing caused by large-gauge introducer.

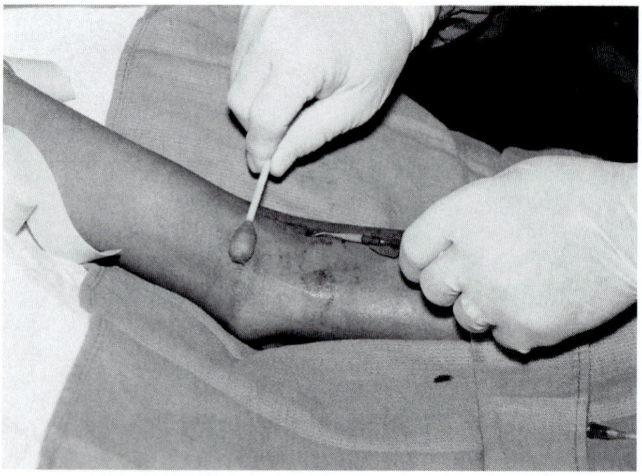

Step 32 Cleanse site if there has been oozing of blood.

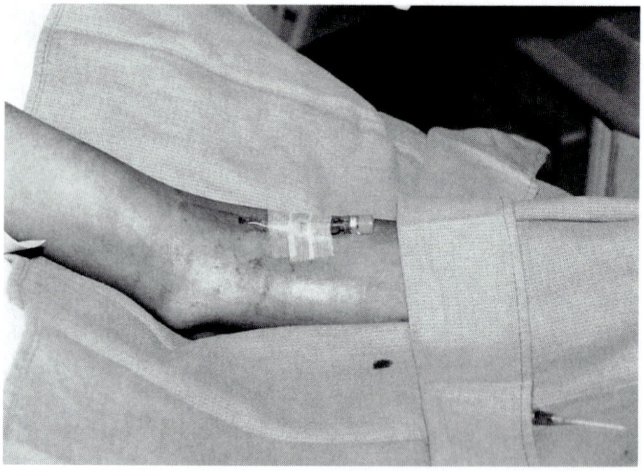

Step 33 Anchor PICC catheter hub with Steri-strips.

STEPS	RATIONALE
35. Coil the extension tubing and tape securely to the client's arm. Do not pull or apply undue pressure to the catheter when manipulating it. Label dressing with date and time of insertion and gauge of catheter.	Prevents inadvertent dislodgement. Prevents catheter breakage.
36. Flush each lumen with 3 ml of heparin solution.	Maintains patency of each lumen.
37. Dispose of equipment appropriately. Wash hands.	Reduces transmission of microorganisms.
38. Follow agency policy for x-ray verification of placement.	X-ray examination is usually done to verify placement in the superior vena cava before start of infusion therapy.
39. Document date, time of PICC placement, length and size of PICC catheter, vein accessed, and arm circumference.	Provides immediate access to data as to when PICC was inserted, length and size of PICC line, vein accessed, and when subsequent dressing changes are needed.

EVALUATION

1. Observe client and inquire about comfort level during insertion.	
2. Inspect and palpate PICC site immediately after insertion for bleeding or hematoma.	
3. Note respiratory status.	PICC line insertion can result in air embolism.
4. Once PICC has been inserted, call for chest x-ray examination.	Determines that catheter is positioned in superior vena cava.

CRITICAL DECISION POINT Chest x-ray examination is required for PICC lines placed in the superior vena cava.

5. Observe integrity of the PICC according to agency policy. a. Assess insertion site for phlebitis, exudate, leaking, clotting, catheter breakage. b. Verify that correct therapy is being delivered as ordered. c. Observe client for systemic complications such as air embolism, infection.	Provides information concerning the most frequent complications associated with PICCs.
6. Observe client to determine response to fluid and electrolyte therapy.	PICCs provide a reliable method for delivering IV fluids and electrolytes.
7. Weigh client daily.	PICCs can provide parenteral nutrition.
8. Measure client's body temperature every 4 hours.	Elevated body temperature provides evidence of infection, which may be related to the presence of the PICC.

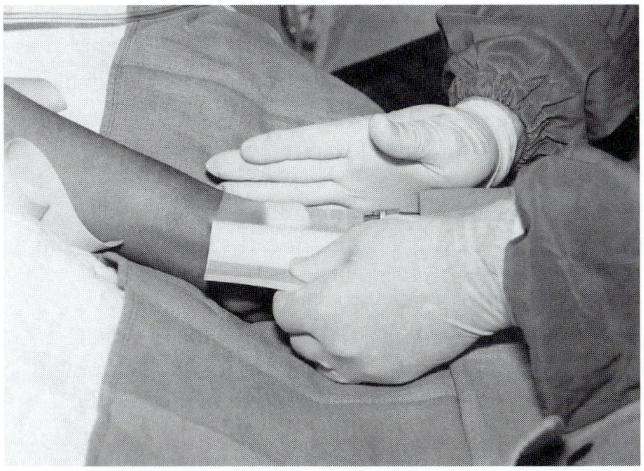

Step 34 Apply transparent dressing over PICC catheter.

STEPS	RATIONALE
9. Review with client and ask to describe signs and symptoms of complications and daily catheter maintenance.	
10. **Unexpected outcomes** that may occur include:	
➤ Client experiences pain and erythema at the insertion site; blood or fluids leak from PICC insertion site; PICC cannot be flushed; catheter is not intact.	These are the most frequent catheter-related complications associated with PICCs.
➤ Client develops a fever, elevated WBC; culture of PICC tip is positive.	These are signs and symptoms of catheter sepsis.
➤ Client develops fluid volume deficit, fluid volume excess, electrolyte imbalances.	If IV infusions are not administered accurately, the expected outcomes are not achieved.
➤ Client's body weight is less than ideal body weight.	If parenteral nutrition is not administered accurately, client receives insufficient nutrients to support normal body weight.
➤ Client develops sudden respiratory distress.	Indicates air embolism.
➤ Client develops irregular pulse.	May indicate catheter is in the right atrium. May need to be withdrawn several centimeters.

Recording and Reporting

1. Record PICC's gauge and length, insertion site, date and time of insertion, location of catheter tip, radiographic confirmation of location of catheter tip (if x-ray examination has been completed), presence or absence of signs and symptoms of complications.	Documents correct initiation of therapy, client's response.
2. Report status of PICC, the therapy being administered, and the development of complications and their treatment.	PICCs provide long-term venous access; information concerning the catheter and IV therapy should be kept up-to-date. Complications can occur at any time.

Follow-up Activities

1. Once catheter has been inserted verify radiographic confirmation of placement for all catheters intended to be placed in the superior vena cava before initiating IV infusions.
2. After the first 24 hours, replace the 2 × 2 gauze dressing with a sterile, transparent, occlusive dressing. This dressing can be left in place for 3 to 7 days, depending on agency policy.
3. Measure the amount of catheter that remains external with each dressing change to detect catheter migration.
4. Regularly aspirate for blood return and flush the catheter with normal saline followed by heparin solution (10 to 100 U/ml) (according to agency policy). Prevents clotting after any infusion.

• • • • •

Special Considerations

➤ When the PICC is to be placed in the superior vena cava, try to use the dominant arm because movement accelerates blood flow and reduces the risk of dependent edema. However, the placement of some catheters and their dressings may restrict flexion of the elbow on the side of insertion.

➤ Urokinase per physician order may be used to declot a PICC if necessary. See your agency's policy regarding this procedure.

Teaching Considerations

➤ Since PICC insertion and care may be unfamiliar to the client, careful and repeated verbal explanations with written follow-up are important.

➤ Instruct client and care giver about signs and symptoms of the most common complications: phlebitis, clotting, leaking at catheter insertion site, or breaking of the catheter. Instruct client on how to respond to each of these.

➤ Because the dressing is the anchor for the PICC, the client and care giver need to notify the nurse if the dressing becomes loose. The nurse does the dressing change.

- If the PICC becomes clotted, the client should promptly seek care so that declotting measures can be instituted.
- Instruct clients about allowed activities:
  - The PICC dressing should not become wet, so bathing must be adapted to keep the cannulated arm dry.
  - The client should avoid vigorous activities, e.g., weight lifting because the catheter may be damaged.
  - The client can move the arm freely because there is less chance of infiltration and dislodgement than with a peripheral venipuncture using a short catheter. However, elbow flexion may be hampered by the placement of the dressing.

Pediatric Considerations

- An advantage of the use of PICCs for neonates is the longer duration of use as compared with traditional peripheral catheters.
- In neonates the antecubital veins, long saphenous vein, superficial temporal vein, external jugular vein, popliteal vein, veins in the ankle, and axillary veins may be used.

Home Care Considerations

- Ensure that the client is able and willing to care for the PICC line and administer IV therapy or that there is a reliable care giver or nursing support personnel at home to provide IV therapy care prior to insertion.
- The catheter can be inserted in the home or the client may have it inserted prior to discharge from the hospital.
- Common uses for PICCs in the home are long-term antibiotic/antiviral administration, pain control, parenteral nutrition, and hydration.
- Since the client in the home setting may be more active, a secure dressing is required.
- Superior vena cava insertion is not practiced in the home setting since this requires an x-ray postinsertion.

SKILL 20-3 Regulating Intravenous Flow Rate

After the infusion is initiated and the line is patent, the nurse is responsible for regulating the rate of infusion according to the physician's orders. An infusion rate that is too slow can lead to further cardiovascular and circulatory collapse in a client who is dehydrated, in shock, or critically ill. In addition, if an infusion runs too slowly, the chances of the vein clotting off are greater. An infusion rate that is too rapid can result in fluid overload, which is particularly dangerous in certain cardiovascular, kidney, and neurological disorders and in the very young and very old. The nurse calculates the infusion rate to prevent too-slow or too-rapid administration.

Children, older adults, clients with severe head trauma, and clients susceptible to **fluid volume excess (FVE)** must be protected from sudden increases in infusion volumes. Sudden increases can occur accidentally. For example, a restless client may loosen the roller clamp with a sudden movement and thus increase the flow rate, or the flow rate may be accidentally increased if the client ambulates. A sudden increase in volume can make the client critically ill or even cause death in some cases. Two types of **electronic infusion devices (EIDs)** can assist the nurse to maintain correct flow rates, maintain catheter patency, prevent runaway bolus IV infusions, and alert the nurse when an IV bag or bottle is empty or when there is an IV occlusion. These are the infusion pump and the IV controller device. Many EIDs also record the volume of fluid infused.

An **infusion pump** is designed to deliver a measured amount of fluid over a period of time, that is, milliliters per hour. If the pump has a drop sensor, an alarm sounds if drops are not detected at the appropriate rate. This can occur if the IV bag or bottle is empty. An alarm also sounds if the pressure in the system increases, for example, when an infiltration of IV fluids into the subcutaneous tissue has occurred or the client's arm position is obstructing the flow

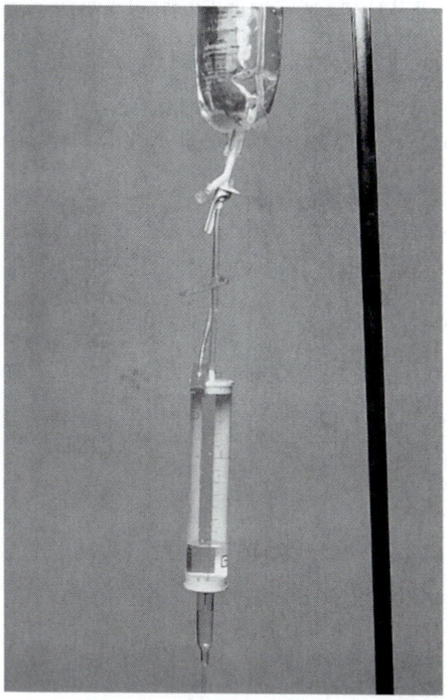

Fig. 20-4 Volume control device.

of fluid. Since the pump uses positive pressure, an infiltration may be extensive before the pump's alarm sounds. The nurse must use frequent inspection and palpation of the IV site to ensure timely detection of an infiltration. IV pumps have a high degree of accuracy and precision to ensure that IV fluid therapy is given correctly.

An IV controller delivers fluid with the aid of gravity. The IV container must be placed approximately 36 inches above the IV site to overcome venous resistance and operate properly (Elkin, Perry, and Potter, 1996). IV controllers deliver fluids based on a determination of drops per minute, which is in turn based on milliliters per hour. The nurse must monitor the volume delivered each hour to ensure that the calculated drops per minute deliver the actual volume desired. The actual volume delivered depends on the rate of infusion, the IV tubing size, and fluid viscosity. Because IV controllers cannot overcome increased resistance in the IV system, infiltrations can be more quickly detected by an IV controller than by a pump. This sensitivity also increases the number of nuisance alarms that occur when client movement is misinterpreted as increased resistance to flow. A volume control device is a calibrated chamber placed between the IV bag or bottle and the insertion spike and drip chamber of the administration set (Fig. 20-4). A small volume of IV fluid is placed in the chamber from the IV fluid container. This smaller volume is then delivered to the client. The advantage of this system is that only the smaller volume of fluid infuses if the rate of the IV is inadvertently increased.

EQUIPMENT

- **Watch with second hand**
- **Paper and pencil**
- **IV infusion pump (optional)**
- **Volume control device (optional)**

STEPS	RATIONALE
ASSESSMENT	
1. Observe for patency of IV line and catheter:	For fluid to infuse at proper rate, IV line and needle must be free of kinks, knots, clots.
a. Open drip regulator and observe for rapid flow of fluid from solution into drip chamber, then close drip regulator to prescribed rate (see Implementation section).	Rapid flow of fluid into drip chamber indicates patency of IV line. Closing drip chamber to prescribed rate prevents fluid overload.
b. Compress cannulated vein slightly proximal to the end of the catheter and observe the drip chamber.	Cessation of drops from drip chamber indicates catheter or needle is in vein. If fluid continues to drip, infiltration may be present and further assessment is needed.
2. Check client's medical record for correct solution and additives. Usual order includes solution for 24 hours, usually divided into 2 or 3 L. Occasionally, IV order contains only 1 L to keep vein open (KVO). Record also shows time over which each liter is to infuse.	
➤ ***CRITICAL DECISION POINT*** **IV fluids are medications. "Five rights" decrease chance of medication error (see Chapter 17).**	
3. Check client's knowledge of how positioning of the IV site affects flow rate.	Fosters client participation in maintaining most effective position of arm with IV equipment. Position or setting of control clamp or EID should be done only by health care provider.
4. Verify with client how venipuncture site feels, for example, determine if there is pain or burning.	Pain or burning may be early indication of phlebitis. Includes client in decision making.

NURSING DIAGNOSIS

Clustering of defining characteristics from the assessment data may reveal the following nursing diagnoses for clients requiring this skill:

➤ Fluid volume deficit

➤ Risk for fluid volume deficit

Related factors are individualized based on a client's condition or needs.

STEPS | **RATIONALE**

PLANNING

1. **Expected outcomes** following completion of procedure:
   - ➤ Serum electrolytes remain within normal limits.
   - ➤ Client receives prescribed volume of fluid over desired time interval.

   When infusion rate remains within prescribed range, the therapeutic aim is achieved.

2. Have paper and pencil to calculate flow rate.

   The beginning student is unfamiliar with IV fluid rates and should use mathematical calculations to obtain correct rate.

3. Know calibration **(drop factor)** in drops per milliliter (gtt/ml) of infusion set:
   Microdrip: 60 gtt/ml
   Macrodrip (Metheny, 1992):
   Abbott: 15 gtt/ml
   Travenol: 10 gtt/ml
   McGaw: 15 gtt/ml

   Microdrip tubing, also called pediatric tubing, universally delivers 60 gtt/ml and is used when small or very precise volumes are to be infused. However, there are different commercial parenteral administration sets for macrodrip tubing. Macrodrip tubing should be used when large quantities or fast rates are necessary.

➤ **CRITICAL DECISION POINT Nurses should know which company's infusion set an agency uses.**

4. Select one of the following formulas to calculate flow rate after determining ml/hr.

   ml/hr = total infusion (ml)/hours of infusion
   (a) ml/hr/60 minutes = ml/minute
   (b) Drop factor × ml/minute = drops/minute

   OR

   ml/hr × drop factor/60 minutes = drops/minute

   Once hourly rate has been determined, these formulas give correct flow rate.

IMPLEMENTATION

1. Read physician's orders and follow "five rights" for correct solution and proper additives.

   IV fluids are medications; following "five rights" decreases chance of medication error.

   a. IV fluids are usually ordered for 24-hour period, indicating how long each liter of fluid should run; for example, IV order for client is:
      Bottle 1: 1000 ml D_5W with 20 mEq KCl to run 8 hours
      Bottle 2: 1000 ml D_5W with 20 mEq KCl to run 8 hours
      Bottle 3: 1000 ml D_5W with 20 mEq KCl to run 8 hours
      Total 24-hour IV intake: 3000 ml

      Determines volume of fluid that should infuse hourly.

➤ **CRITICAL DECISION POINT It is common for physicians to write an abbreviated IV order such as: "D5W with 20 mEq KCl @ 125cc/hr continuous." This order implies that the IV should be maintained at this rate until discontinued.**

2. Determine hourly rate by dividing volume by hours, for example,
   1000 ml/8 = 125 ml/hr
   or if 3 L is ordered for 24 hours
   3000/24 = 125 ml = 125 ml/hour

   Provides even infusion of fluid over prescribed hourly rate.

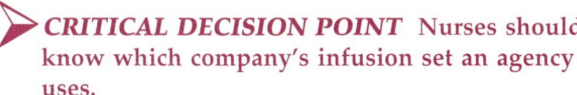

STEPS	RATIONALE
3. Place adhesive or fluid indicator tape on IV bottle or bag next to volume markings (see illustration based on 125 ml in 8-hour period beginning at 0800).	Time taping IV bag gives nurse visual cue as to whether fluids are being administered over correct period of time. Time tapes should be used for all IV infusions, including those on therapies infused via EIDs.

➤ *CRITICAL DECISION POINT* Avoid use of felt-tip pens or permanent markers on IV bags because the ink could contaminate the solution (Millam, 1992).

STEPS	RATIONALE
4. After hourly rate has been determined, calculate minute rate based on drop factor of infusion set. Microdrip infusion set has a drop factor of 60 gtt/ml. Regular drip or macrodrip infusion set used in this example has drop factor of 15 gtt/ml. Using formula, calculate minute flow rates: Bottle 1:1000 ml with 20 mEq KCl	Allows nurse to calculate minute flow rate based on this formula: total volume × drop factor/infusion time in minutes
Microdrip: 125 ml × 60 gtt/ml/60 minutes = 7500 gtt/60 minutes = 125 gtt/minute	When using microdrip, ml/hour always equals gtt/minute.
Macrodrip: 125 ml × 15 gtt/ml/60 minutes = 31 to 32 gtt/minute. Volume is multiplied by drop factor and the product is divided by time (in minutes).	
5. Time flow rate by counting drops in drip chamber for 1 minute by watch, then adjust roller clamp to increase or decrease rate of infusion (see illustration).	Determines if fluids are administered too slowly or too fast.

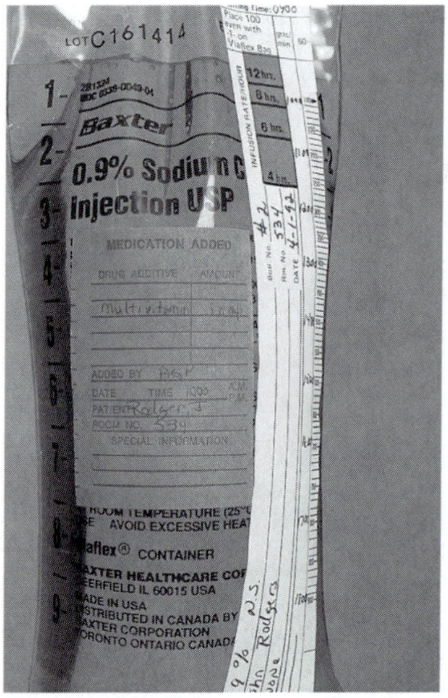

Step 3 IV fluid bag with time tape.

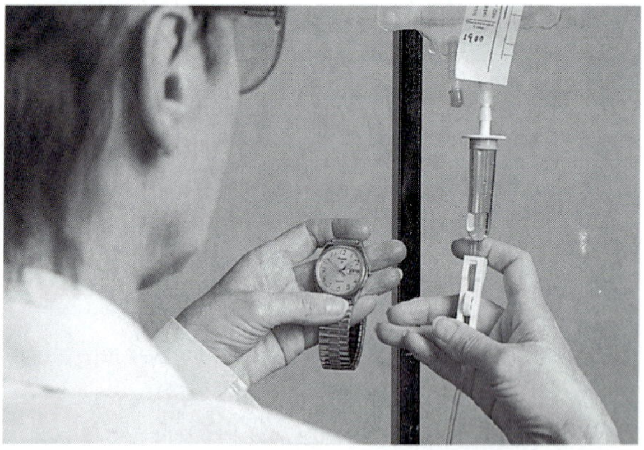

Step 5 Counting IV drip rate.

STEPS	RATIONALE
6. Follow this procedure for infusion controller or pump:	
a. Place electronic eye on drip chamber below origin of drop and above fluid level in chamber or consult manufacturer's directions for setup of the infusion (see illustration). If a controller is used, ensure that IV bag is 36 inches above the IV site.	The electronic eye counts the number of drops flowing from administration set to ensure that proper rate infuses. IV controller works by gravity.
b. IV infusion tubing is placed within ridges of control box in direction of flow (i.e., portion of tubing nearest IV bag at top and portion of tubing nearest client at bottom) or consult manufacturer's directions for use of pump (see illustration). Required drops per minute or volume per hour are selected, door to control chamber is closed, power button is turned on, and start button is pressed (see illustration).	Infusion pumps move fluid by compressing and milking IV tubing, thus propelling fluid through tubing.

CRITICAL DECISION POINT **Special infusion tubing is required for some pumps. Check agency equipment and associated policies.**

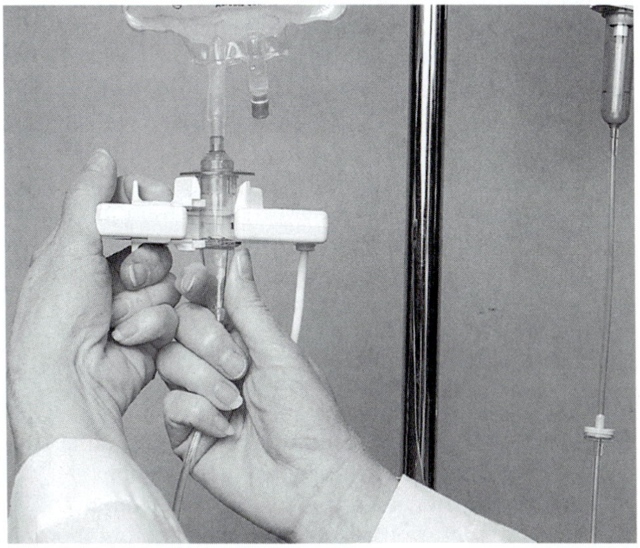

Step 6a Place electronic eye above fluid level in drip chamber.

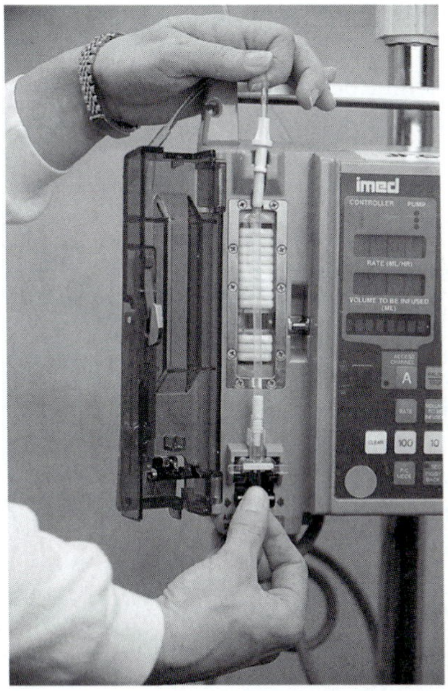

Step 6b (1) Insert IV tubing into pump chamber.

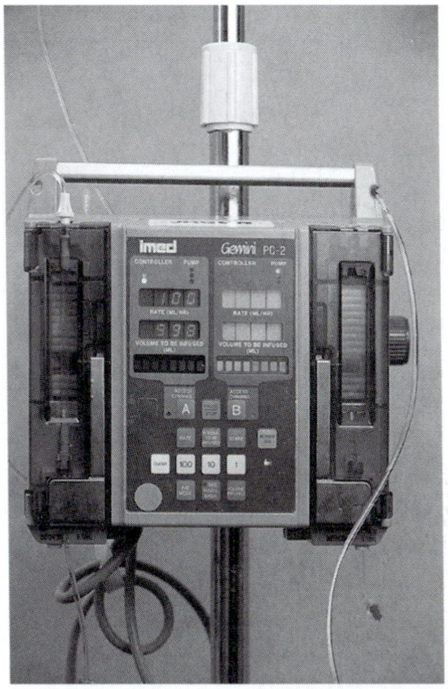

Step 6b (2) Press start button on IV pump.

STEPS	RATIONALE
c. Drip regulator must be open while infusion controller or pump is in use.	
d. Monitor infusion rates and IV site for infiltration according to agency policy.	Infusion controllers or pumps are not infallible and do not replace frequent, accurate nursing assessments. Infusion pumps may continue to infuse IV fluids after an infiltration has begun.
e. Assess patency of system when alarm sounds.	Alarm indicates that electronic eye has not noted precise number of drops from drip chamber. Alarm on infusion pump can be triggered by empty solution bag or bottle, kink in tubing, closed drip regulator, infiltrated or clotted needle, and/or air in the tubing.
7. Follow this procedure for volume control device:	
a. Place volume control device between IV bag and insertion spike of infusion set (see Fig. 20-4 p. 679).	Reduces risk of sudden increases in fluid volume.
b. Place 2 hours' allotment of fluid into device.	Prevents IV line from running dry if nurse does not return in exactly 60 minutes. In addition, if there is accidental increase in flow rate, client receives at most only a 2-hour allotment of fluid.
c. Assess system at least hourly; add fluid to volume control device. Regulate flow rate.	Maintains patency of system.

EVALUATION

1. Observe client for signs of overhydration or dehydration to determine response to therapy and restoration of fluid and electrolyte balance.	Signs and symptoms of dehydration or overhydration warrant changing rate of fluid infused.
2. Evaluate for signs of infiltration: inflammation at site, clot in catheter, kink or knot in infusion tubing.	Prevents decrease or cessation of flow rate.
3. Unexpected outcomes that may occur include:	
➤ Sudden infusion of large volume of solution occurs, causing fluid overload.	Result of rapid administration of large amount of fluid into circulating blood volume. Signs and symptoms indicate client's cardiovascular and/or renal status cannot adapt to large volume and include dyspnea and crackles in the lung.
➤ There is an empty IV solution container with subsequent loss of IV line patency.	Absence of IV fluid allows clot to form at tip of catheter and occlude line.
➤ The IV infusion is slower than ordered.	This can occur when the client changes position, decreasing the height between the IV bag or bottle and the IV site, or bends the extremity with the IV.

RECORDING AND REPORTING

1. Record rate of infusion, drops/min, and ml/hr in nurses' notes every 4 hours or according to agency policy.	Documents that the prescribed flow is delivered to client.
2. Immediately record in nurse's notes any new IV fluid rates.	Specifically documents at what point fluid rate was changed.
3. Document use of any EID or controlling device and number on that device.	Provides valuable risk management information if complications were to develop.
4. At change of shift or when leaving on break, report rate of infusion to nurse in charge or next nurse assigned to care for client.	Assists in maintaining continuity of therapy.

FOLLOW-UP ACTIVITIES

1. Monitor IV setup at least every hour, noting the volume of IV fluid infused and the rate of infusion.

STEPS **RATIONALE**

a. If the IV has infused at an incorrect rate, the drip should be reestablished to the ordered rate. If the volume of fluids infused is severely deficient, consult the physician for a new order to provide the ordered volume of fluids over a shorter period.

CRITICAL DECISION POINT The rate of the IV fluids should NOT be automatically increased, because the rapid increase in vascular volume might result in fluid volume excess and pulmonary edema.

b. If the volume of fluids is severely excessive, consult the physician immediately. and closely monitor the client for problems related to potential fluid overload. In addition, monitor IV setup at least every hour, noting client's response and the presence of any IV site complications. Ensure that the setup is intact.

Special Considerations

- If rapid flow of fluid is not observed and no kinks are visible, nurse may need to remove dressing to fully observe needle or catheter (Skill 20-6).
- Some agencies have conversion charts posted in medication area that specify desired flow rates in drops/min for a variety of IV fluid prescriptions.
- Many institutions use EIDs on all clients receiving IV fluids. Pediatric clients or clients with fluctuating fluid and electrolyte status should have volume control devices or EIDs to regulate IV fluid solution.
- Nurses should not depend entirely on visual cue provided by time taping. Nurse routinely monitors IV infusion rate and regulates flow accordingly.
- Rate of infusion should be checked by watch, even when infusion pump is used.

Teaching Considerations

- Client should know the prescribed hourly flow of IV fluids.
- If an infusion pump is used, the client should know its preset rate and the significance of alarms.

Home Care Considerations

- Ensure that client is able and willing to operate the EID (if applicable) and administer IV therapy or that there is a reliable care giver or nursing support personnel at home to provide this IV therapy care.
- Make sure nurse is in the home when IV pump is delivered. This enables nurse to determine that equipment works properly.
- Teach client and primary care giver to time drops per minute using watch with second hand.
- Ensure that client's electrical outlets are properly grounded.

SKILL 20-4 Changing Intravenous Solutions

Clients receiving IV therapy may require frequent changing of IV solutions. The nurse must allow adequate time for this procedure and follow proper technique in order to prevent infection. Occasionally clients have an infusion only to deliver IV medication every 4, 6, or 8 hours (see Chapter 19). In this case an hourly infusion flow of about 10 to 25 ml/hr is used to KVO in between doses, and usually a microdrip infusion set is used. Generally these clients do not use an entire IV solution bag. A new solution bag or bottle should be changed according to agency policy. The CDC (1996) does not have a recommendation for hang time of IV fluids.

on test

EQUIPMENT

- **Bottle/bag of IV solution as ordered by physician**
- **Time tape**

STEPS	RATIONALE
ASSESSMENT	
1. Check physician's orders.	Ensures that correct solution will be used.
2. If order is written for KVO or to keep open (TKO), note date and time when solution was last changed.	A hang time is no longer recommended by the Centers for Disease Control and Prevention (1996) to ensure sterility of solutions in bag or bottle. Refer to agency policy.
3. Determine the compatibility of all IV fluids and additives by consulting appropriate literature or the pharmacy.	Incompatibilities can cause physical, chemical, and therapeutic client changes.
4. Determine client's understanding of need for continued IV therapy.	Reveals need for client instruction.
5. Assess patency of current IV access site.	If patency is not verified, a new IV access site may be needed. Notify physician.

NURSING DIAGNOSIS

Clustering of defining characteristics from the assessment data may reveal the following nursing diagnoses for clients requiring this skill:

- Fluid volume deficit
- Risk for fluid volume deficit
- Risk for infection

Related factors are individualized based on a client's condition or needs.

STEPS	RATIONALE
PLANNING	
1. **Expected outcomes** following completion of procedure:	
➤ Fluid infusion is correct.	Client receives correct fluid volume.
➤ IV line remains patent.	Ensures infusion of fluid into intravascular space.
➤ Client's serum electrolyte level returns to normal.	When the correct fluids are infused, the therapeutic goal is achieved.
2. Have next solution prepared at least 1 hour before needed. If prepared in pharmacy, be sure it has been delivered to the client's hospital unit. Check that solution is correct and properly labeled. Check solution expiration date.	Adequate planning reduces risk of clot formation in vein caused by empty IV bag. Checking prevents medication error.
3. Prepare to change solution when fluid remains only in neck of bottle or bag.	Prevents air from entering tubing and vein from clotting from lack of flow.
4. Prepare client and family by explaining the procedure, its purpose, and what is expected of client.	Decreases anxiety and promotes cooperation.
5. Be sure drip chamber is at least half full.	Provides fluid to vein while bag is changed.
IMPLEMENTATION	
1. Wash hands.	Reduces transmission of microorganisms.
2. Prepare new solution for changing. If using plastic bag, remove protective cover from IV tubing port. If using glass bottle, remove metal cap and metal rubber disks.	Permits quick, smooth, and organized change from old to new solution.
3. Move roller clamp to stop flow rate.	Prevents solution remaining in drip chamber from emptying while changing solutions.
4. Remove old IV fluid container from IV pole.	Brings work to nurse's eye level.
5. Quickly remove spike from old solution bag or bottle and, without touching tip, insert spike into new bag or bottle.	Reduces risk of solution in drip chamber running dry and maintains sterility.
➤ **CRITICAL DECISION POINT** If spike is contaminated, a new IV tubing set is required.	
6. Hang new bag or bottle of solution.	Allows gravity to assist with delivery of fluid into drip chamber.

STEPS	RATIONALE
7. Check for air in tubing. If bubbles form they can be removed by closing the roller clamp, stretching the tubing downward, and tapping the tubing with the finger (the bubbles rise in the fluid to the drip chamber) (see illustration). For a larger amount of air, insert a needle and syringe into a port below the air and aspirate the air into the syringe. Swab port with alcohol and allow to dry prior to inserting needle into port. Reduce air in tubing by priming slowly instead of allowing a wide open flow.	Reduces risk of air embolus. Use of an air-eliminating filter also reduces this risk.
8. Make sure drip chamber is one-third to one-half full. If the drip chamber is too full, pinch off tubing below the drip chamber, invert the container, squeeze the drip chamber (see illustration), hang up the bottle, and release the tubing.	Reduces risk of air entering tubing.
9. Regulate flow to prescribed rate.	Maintains measures to restore fluid balance and deliver IV fluid as ordered.

EVALUATION

STEPS	RATIONALE
1. Observe client for signs of overhydration or dehydration to determine response to IV fluid therapy.	Provides ongoing evaluation of client's fluid and electrolyte status.
2. Monitor IV infusion for correct solution and additives.	Verifies that physician's order is being carried out.
3. An **unexpected outcome** that may occur is: ➤ Flow rate is incorrect; client receives too little or too much fluid.	Incorrect infusion of volume is a medication error and must be documented.

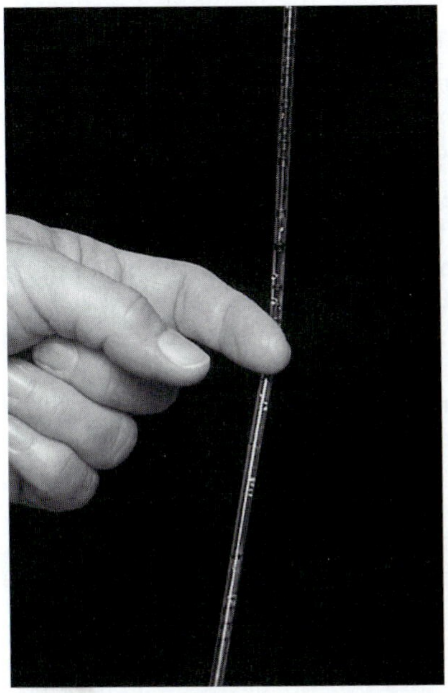

Step 7 Tap tubing to cause air bubbles to rise up to drip chamber.

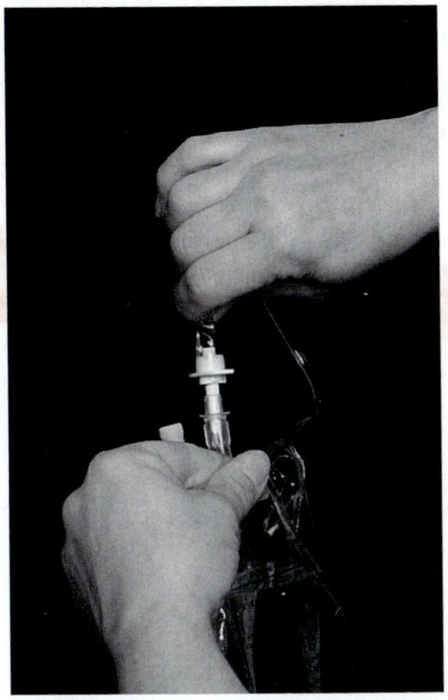

Step 8 Squeeze drip chamber to remove a portion of fluid. Be sure to leave chamber ⅓ to ½ full.

STEPS | **RATIONALE**

Recording and Reporting

1. Record amount and type of fluid infused and amount and type of new fluid according to agency policy. A special flow sheet may be used for parenteral fluids.

   Documents that solution has infused and new solution has been started.

Follow-up Activities

1. When incorrect infusion is delivered to client, change the solution to the correct one, assess the client for adverse effects, and document and report to physician as directed by agency policy.

• • • • •

Special Considerations

- IV fluid orders are usually written at least daily by physician.
- Contamination of infusion set increases risk of infection.
- If client is critically ill, nurse should plan to review client's medical orders at least every 2 hours.
- Some agencies require that changes of IV solution be noted in nurse's notes and on parenteral fluid flow sheet.

Teaching Considerations

- Inform client of new solution, additives, flow rate, and potential side effects.

Home Care Considerations

- Ensure that client is able and willing to self-administer IV therapy (including changing IV solutions) and care for IV access site or that there is a reliable care giver or nursing support person at home to provide this IV therapy care.
- If client or family must pick up antibiotics or other parenteral fluids from the hospital pharmacy, be sure the physician's orders have been completed to avoid needless waiting by the client or family at the hospital.
- Instruct client and primary care giver how to perform an IV solution change.
- If medications are delivered to client's home, be sure to instruct client/care giver on proper storage of these IV medications.

SKILL 20-5 Changing Infusion Tubing

Changing infusion tubing is much simpler and more efficient if the nurse changes the tubing when preparing to hang a new bag or bottle. However, the CDC (1996) recommends replacing tubing, including piggyback tubing and stopcocks, no more frequently than 72-hour intervals. This is assuming the system has not been contaminated. Situations arise when the nurse needs to change tubing without hanging a new bag. Such situations include accidental puncture of the tubing or after infusion of blood or a blood product (Chapter 21).

EQUIPMENT

IV infusion
- Infusion tubing
- 0.22 μmm filter and extension tubing (if necessary)

Heparin flush
- Injection cap, loop, or short extension tubing (if necessary)

Normal saline flush
- Syringes
- 2 sterile 2 × 2 gauze pads
- Tape
- Disposable nonsterile gloves

If a new IV dressing must be applied, assemble additional equipment (Skill 20-6).

STEPS	RATIONALE
ASSESSMENT	
1. Determine when new infusion set is needed:	
a. Agency policy will indicate frequency of routine change for IV administration sets and heparin flushes.	The CDC (1996) recommends tubing change no more often than 72-hr intervals.
b. Puncture of infusion tubing.	Punctured tubing results in fluid leakage and bacterial contamination.
c. Contamination of tubing.	Contamination of tubing allows entry of bacteria into client's bloodstream.
2. Observe for occlusions in tubing. Such occlusions can occur after infusion of packed red cells, whole blood, albumin, or other blood components.	Whole blood or blood component products can occlude or partially occlude tubing because viscous solutions adhere to walls of tubing and decrease the size of the lumen.
3. Determine client's understanding of the need for continued IV infusions.	Reveals need for client instruction.

NURSING DIAGNOSIS

Clustering of defining characteristics from the assessment data may reveal the following nursing diagnosis for clients requiring this skill:

➤ Risk for infection

Related factors are individualized based on a client's condition or needs.

PLANNING

STEPS	RATIONALE
1. **Expected outcomes** following completion of procedure:	
➤ Client's IV site will be free from signs of phlebitis.	Sterile IV tubing prevents bacterial growth.
➤ Client will experience no leakage of solution from tubing.	Intact system decreases risk of bacterial contamination.
➤ Client's IV tubing will be patent.	Brief interruption of IV infusion will not result in clotting of catheter.
➤ Client's IV site will be free from redness, swelling, pain or exudate.	Proper technique prevents infection.
2. Prepare client and family by explaining the procedure, its purpose, and what is expected of client.	Decreases anxiety, promotes cooperation and prevents sudden movement of extremity, which could dislodge IV needle or catheter.

IMPLEMENTATION

STEPS	RATIONALE
1. Wash hands.	Reduces transmission of microorganisms.
2. Open new infusion set, keeping protective coverings over infusion spike and connector and connector site for butterfly needle or IV catheter.	Provides nurse with ready access to new infusion set and maintains sterility of infusion set.
3. Apply nonsterile, disposable gloves.	Reduces risk of exposure to HIV, hepatitis, and other blood-borne bacteria (CDC, 1987; Garner, 1996).
4. If needle or catheter hub is not visible, remove IV dressing as directed in Skill 20-6. Do not remove tape securing needle or catheter to skin.	Needle hub must be accessible to provide smooth transition when removing old and inserting new tubing.
5. For IV Infusion:	
a. Move roller clamp on new IV tubing to "off" position.	Prevents spillage of solution after bag or bottle is spiked.
b. Slow rate of infusion by regulating drip rate on old tubing. Be sure rate is at KVO rate.	Prevents complete infusion of solution remaining in tubing. Complete infusion of solution remaining in tubing increases risk of occlusion of IV catheter or needle.

STEPS	RATIONALE
c. With old tubing in place, compress drip chamber and fill chamber.	Provides surplus of fluid in drip chamber so there is enough fluid to maintain IV patency while changing tubing.
d. Remove old tubing from solution and hang or tape drip chamber on IV pole 36 inches above IV site.	Allows fluid to continue to flow through IV catheter while nurse is preparing new tubing.
e. Place insertion spike of new tubing into old solution bag opening and hang solution bag on IV pole.	Permits flow of fluid from solution into new infusion tubing.
CRITICAL DECISION POINT **If spike becomes contaminated, a new IV tubing set is required.**	
f. Compress and release drip chamber on new tubing; slowly fill drip chamber one-third to one-half full.	Allows drip chamber to fill and promotes rapid, smooth flow of solution through new tubing.
g. Slowly open roller clamp, remove protective cap from needle adapter (if necessary), and flush tubing with solution. Replace cap.	Removes air from tubing and replaces it with fluid.
h. Turn roller clamp on old tubing to "off" position.	Prevents spillage of fluid as tubing is removed from needle hub.
6. For Heparin Lock:	
a. If a loop or short extension tubing is needed because of an awkward IV site placement, use sterile technique to connect the new **injection cap** to the loop or tubing.	
b. Swab injectin cap with alcohol. Insert syringe with 1 to 3 ml saline and inject through the injection cap into the loop or short extension tubing.	Removes air to prevent introduction into the vein.
7. Stabilize hub of catheter or needle and apply pressure over vein just above insertion site. Gently pull out old tubing (see illustration *A*). Maintain stability of hub and quickly insert needle adapter of new tubing or heparin lock into hub (see illustration *B*).	Prevents accidental displacement of catheter or needle. Prevents clot formation in catheter or needle and back flow of blood.
8. Open roller clamp on new tubing. Allow solution to run rapidly for 30 to 60 seconds.	Permits IV solution to enter catheter to prevent catheter occlusion.
9. Regulate IV drip according to physician's orders and monitor rate hourly.	Maintains infusion flow at prescribed rate.
10. If necessary, apply new dressing (Skill 20-6).	Reduces risk of bacterial infection from skin.

A

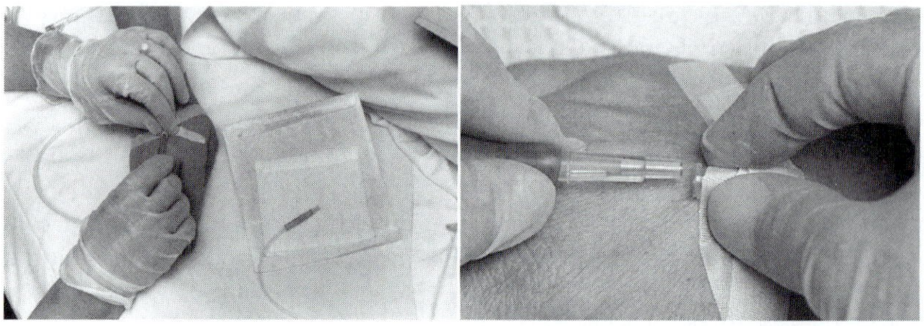

B

Step 7 **A,** Maintain stability of catheter hub. **B,** Connect new tubing to IV catheter hub.

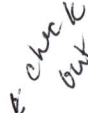

STEPS	RATIONALE
11. Discard old tubing in proper container.	Reduces accidental transmission of microorganisms.
12. Remove and dispose of gloves. Wash hands.	Reduces transmission of microorganisms.
E VALUATION	
1. Evaluate flow rate and observe connection site for leakage.	Maintains prescribed rate of flow of IV fluid and determines if fit is secure.
2. An **unexpected outcome** that may occur is: ➤ Decreased or absent flow of IV fluid is indicated by decreased rate.	Can occur if nurse fails to open drip regulator and recalibrate drip rate on new tubing. Infiltration or occlusion of catheter can also be the cause.
RECORDING AND REPORTING	
1. Record changing of tubing and solution on client's record. A special parenteral therapy flow sheet may be used.	Ensures regular change of equipment is performed.
2. Place a piece of tape or preprinted label with the date and time of tubing change and attach to tubing below the level of drip chamber.	Provides a visual cue to all care providers of when IV tubing was changed.

FOLLOW-UP ACTIVITIES

1. If solution flow rate is slowed or increased, assess for infiltration and recalibrate IV flow to prescribed rate.

• • • • •

Special Considerations

- ➤ Flushing with normal saline after administration of whole blood or blood components can reduce risk of occlusion of IV tubing.
- ➤ If disconnection of tubing from catheter is required to irrigate the catheter, IV should be turned off and distal end of IV tubing should be connected to a sterile needle with cap.
- ➤ If infusion pump is used, remove old tubing from pump and replace with new tubing.

Teaching Considerations

- ➤ Instruct client to notify nurse if fluid leaks around IV site or from the tubing itself or if tubing separates from catheter.

Home Care Considerations

- ➤ Instruct client or primary care giver in procedure for performing a sterile IV tubing change.
- ➤ Ensure that client is able and willing to change infusion tubing and maintain IV access site or that there is a reliable person at home to provide this IV therapy care.

SKILL 20-6 Changing a Peripheral Intravenous Dressing

Dressing applications are done for both IV infusion sites and heparin lock insertion sites at the time when the IV is inserted or when the IV site is changed. The IV site is usually changed every 72 hours and the peripheral IV dressing is applied then. Otherwise, the peripheral IV dressing is not changed unless it becomes, wet, soiled, or loosened/removed (CDC, 1996). There is no difference in technique for the two; however, dressing change of a PICC site requires rigorous sterile technique.

The type of material used for the IV dressing depends on agency policy. The advantage of the transparent dressing is that the IV site can be inspected constantly without removal of the dressing. However, if there is significant drainage at the insertion site, a gauze dressing should be utilized. The dressings provide some protection and stability for the insertion site.

Using sterile technique during dressing changes reduces the risk of phlebitis and infection at the venipuncture site. Phlebitis is an inflammation of the vein and is associated with pain, redness, swelling, and a palpable venous cord (Intravenous Nurses Society, 1990). The occurrence of phlebitis increases the risk for developing a catheter-related infection.

A secure IV dressing is essential. Applying tape and a

dressing that are not secure allows for IV catheter movement, which can result in infection or puncture of the vein by the catheter and flow of IV solution into the surrounding interstitial tissue. An infiltration is associated with slowed IV flow rate, tissue swelling around the IV site (especially proximal), and coolness. Changing a gauze dressing at routine intervals allows the visualization of the insertion site.

EQUIPMENT

- **Povidone-iodine swab stick (three are needed for PICC dressing change)**
- **Alcohol swab stick (three are needed for PICC dressing change)**
- **Adhesive remover (if needed)**
- **Strips of sterile, precut tape**
- **Steri-Strips (for PICC dressing)**
- **Disposable gloves (sterile gloves for PICC dressing change)**

For gauze dressing:

- **Sterile 2 × 2 gauze pad**

or

- **Sterile 4 × 4 gauze pad**

For transparent dressing:

- **Sterile transparent dressing**

STEPS	RATIONALE
ASSESSMENT	
1. Determine when dressing was last changed. Many institutions require nurse to write date and time on dressing and date the device was first placed.	Provides information regarding length of time that present dressing has been in place. In addition, nurse is able to plan for dressing change.
2. Observe present dressing for moisture and intactness.	Moisture is medium for bacterial growth. Moisture on sterile dressing renders dressing contaminated. Nonadhering dressing increases risk of bacterial contamination to venipuncture site or displacement of IV catheter.
3. Observe IV system for proper functioning or complications: kinks in infusion tubing or IV catheter. Palpate the catheter site through the intact dressing for inflammation or subjective complaints of pain or burning.	Unexplained decrease in flow rate requires the nurse to investigate placement and patency of the IV catheter. Pain can be associated with both phlebitis and infiltration.
4. Inspect exposed catheter site for swelling, infiltration.	Indicates fluid infusing into surrounding tissues. Will require removal of IV catheter.
5. Monitor body temperature.	Elevated temperature may be related to infection at the IV site.
6. Determine client's understanding for the need for continued IV infusion.	Reveals need for client instruction.

NURSING DIAGNOSIS

Clustering of defining characteristics from the assessment data may reveal the following nursing diagnosis for clients requiring this skill:

➤ Risk for infection
➤ Pain

Related factors are individualized based on a client's condition or needs.

PLANNING

1. **Expected outcomes** following completion of procedure:	
➤ Client will have patent IV as evidenced by absence of infiltration, phlebitis, or clot.	Maintains IV infusion as prescribed.
➤ Client's temperature remains normal.	
➤ IV insertion site is without pain, redness, swelling, or exudate.	Site remains uninfected.
2. Explain procedure and purpose to client and family. Explain that affected extremity must be held still and how long procedure will take.	Decreases anxiety, promotes cooperation, and gives client time frame around which personal activities can be planned.

STEPS	RATIONALE
IMPLEMENTATION	
1. Wash hands. Apply disposable gloves.	Reduces transmission of microorganisms. Infections related to IV therapy are most often caused by catheter hub contamination, so careful technique must be used throughout the dressing change. Gloves reduce nurse's risk of exposure to HIV, hepatitis, and other blood-borne viruses or bacteria.
2. Remove tape and gauze from old dressing one layer at a time, leaving tape that secures IV needle or catheter in place. Be cautious if catheter tubing becomes tangled between two layers of dressing.	Prevents accidental displacement of catheter or needle.
3. Observe insertion site for signs and/or symptoms of infection, namely redness, swelling, and exudate.	
4. If infiltration, phlebitis, or clot occur or if ordered by physician, discontinue infusion (Skill 20-8).	
5. If IV is infusing properly, gently remove tape securing needle or catheter (put on sterile gloves first for PICC dressing change). Stabilize needle or catheter with one finger. Use adhesive remover to cleanse skin and remove adhesive residue, if needed.	Exposes venipuncture site. Stabilization prevents accidental displacement of catheter or needle. Adhesive residue decreases ability of new tape to adhere tightly to skin.
CRITICAL DECISION POINT Keep one finger over catheter at all times until tape is replaced for security.	
6. Using circular motion, cleanse peripheral IV insertion site with alcohol, then povidone-iodine solution (see illustration) starting at insertion site and working outwards creating concentric circles. Allow each solution to dry for 2 minutes. For a PICC, cleanse with three alcohol swab sticks and allow to dry for 60 seconds (see illustration). Follow by three povidone-iodine sticks. Allow to dry for 2 minutes.	Circular motion prevents cross-contamination from skin bacteria near venipuncture site. Povidone-iodine is a topical antiinfective that reduces skin surface bacteria; the solution must be dry to be effective in reducing microbial counts (Baranowski, 1993).

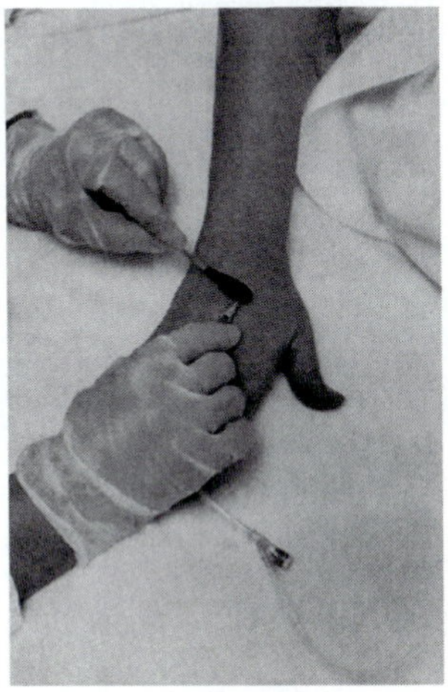

Step 6a Cleanse IV site with antiseptic swab.

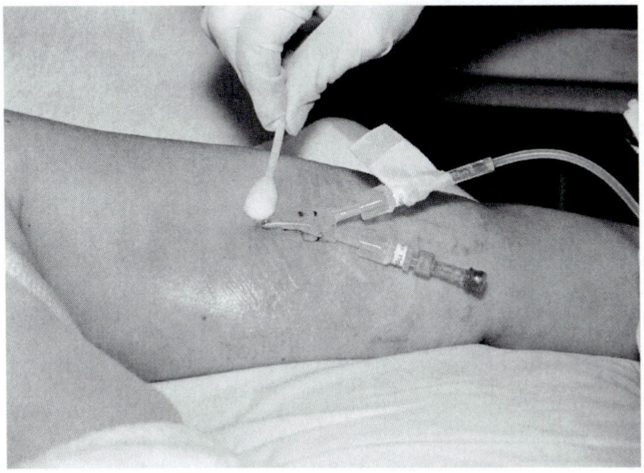

Step 6b Cleanse PICC site with alcohol.

STEPS	RATIONALE
CRITICAL DECISION POINT **Do not tape over connection of access tubing or port to IV catheter.**	
7. Gauze dressing:	
a. Place single strip of ½-inch nonallergenic tape under peripheral IV catheter with sticky side up to anchor IV catheter or needle. For PICC catheter place several Steri-strips over catheter (see illustration).	Prevents accidental displacement of catheter or needle.
b. Place a second piece of sterile tape directly across catheter at hub.	Further prevents accidental displacement of catheter.
c. Place 2 × 2 or 4 × 4 gauze over venipuncture site.	Provides barrier against bacteria.
8. Transparent dressing:	
a. Place a piece of sterile tape directly across catheter hub.	Further prevents accidental displacement of catheter.
b. Place transparent dressing over venipuncture site. Apply in the direction of hair growth (see illustration).	Provides barrier against bacteria. Reduces discomfort when dressing is removed.
9. Remove and discard gloves.	
10. Anchor IV tubing with additional pieces of tape. When using polyurethane dressing minimize the tape placed over dressing.	Prevents accidental displacement of IV needle or catheter or separation of IV tubing from needle adapter.
11. Place date and time of dressing change, and size and gauge of catheter directly on dressing.	Documents dressing change.
12. Discard equipment and wash hands.	Reduces transmission of microorganisms.

EVALUATION

1. Observe functioning and patency of IV system in response to changing dressing.	Validates that IV is patent and functioning correctly.
2. Monitor client's body temperature.	Elevated temperature indicates an infection that may be associated with bacterial contamination of the venipuncture site.

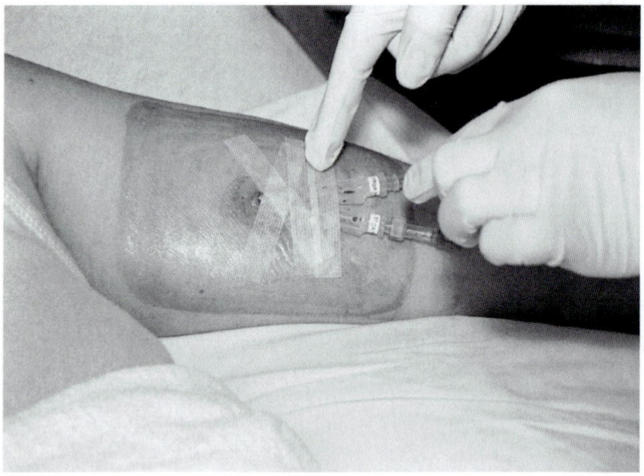

Step 7a Taping PICC.

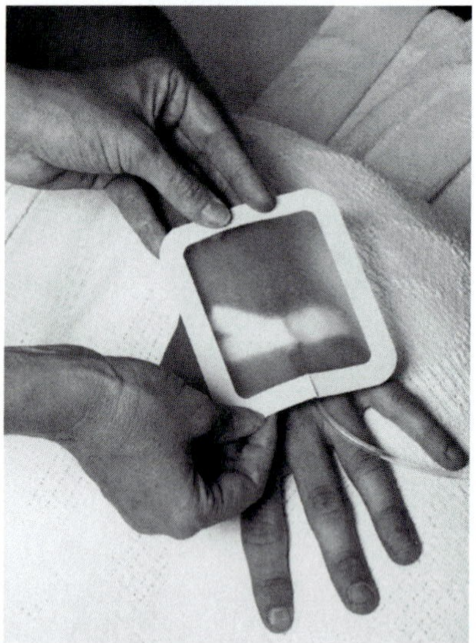

Step 8b Applying transparent dressing to peripheral IV.

STEPS	RATIONALE
3. **Unexpected outcomes** that may occur include:	
➤ IV catheter or needle is infiltrated, as evidenced by decreased flow rate or edema, pallor, or decreased temperature around insertion site.	Indicates fluid in interstitial space, which interferes with circulation and causes edema and coolness in the tissue.
➤ Phlebitis is present, as evidenced by erythema and tenderness along vein pathway.	Results from inflammation of vein.
➤ IV catheter or needle is accidently removed.	Can occur during incorrect removal of dressing or after application of a dressing that does not support the weight of the IV tubing.
➤ Client has an elevated temperature.	May indicate evidence that venipuncture site has become infected.
➤ Insertion site is red and/or edematous and/or painful and/or has presence of exudate.	Provides evidence that venipuncture site has become infected.
REPORTING AND RECORDING	
1. Record in nurse's notes time IV dressing was changed and type of dressing used. Include patency of system and observation of venipuncture site.	Documents that dressing was changed, description of functioning of IV system, and that venipuncture site is free of signs and symptoms of infection.
2. Report to nurse in charge or oncoming nursing shift that dressing was changed and any significant information about integrity of system.	Assists in verification of care delivered and planning of future nursing care.

FOLLOW-UP ACTIVITIES

1. When infiltration or phlebitis is present:
   a. Discontinue IV catheter or needle (Skill 20-8) and apply warm, moist heat to affected area.
   b. If needed, initiate another IV using another extremity.

• • • • •

Special Considerations

- ➤ If there is no date or time on gauze IV dressing, assume that present dressing is at least 48 hours old and plan to change it.
- ➤ Clients who have received heparin or have low platelet counts require longer pressure (5 to 10 minutes or more) on site because of action of heparin on blood-clotting mechanisms.

Teaching Considerations

- ➤ Client should be instructed to notify nurse if skin under dressing or tape becomes reddened, itches, or burns or if dressing becomes loosened.

Pediatric Considerations

- ➤ Pediatric clients may not be able to fully understand nurse's explanation. Presence of parent or security toy during procedure can help to decrease fear and increase cooperation.

Gerontologic Considerations

- ➤ In the older adult with fragile skin, prevent skin tears by minimizing the use of tape directly on the skin.

Home Care Considerations

- ➤ Ensure that the client is able and willing to perform this procedure and care for IV access site or that there is a reliable care giver or nursing support person at home to provide this IV therapy care.

SKILL 20-7 Caring for Vascular Access Devices

Clients with chronic disease often need long-term IV therapy, which requires safe, repeated access to the venous system for administration of drugs, fluids, nutrition, and blood products. Frequent venipuncture and multiple IV lines pose problems and risks, including infection, pain, and bruising. Clients with chronic disease are generally more susceptible to infection and bleeding. Clients receiving multiple doses of chemotherapeutic drugs experience vein sclerosis or hardening. Eventually, no suitable peripheral veins remain for drug administration.

The need for safe and convenient long-term IV therapy has led to the development of **venous access devices (VADs),** which are catheters, **cannulas,** or infusion ports designed for long-term, repeated access to the venous or arterial systems. The nurse must be able to maintain the integrity of central venous catheters (CVCs) and implanted infusion ports and educate clients about the care of catheters for eventual home use.

To manage long-term IV therapy effectively the nurse must be familiar with the various types of VADs. This can be confusing since catheters are often referred to by brand name instead of type and placement (e.g., Hickman, Groshong, Raaf, Port-a-Cath). Also, in the literature there is not universal acceptance of one term to describe a particular catheter. For this skill VADs will be divided into two types: CVCs (tunneled and percutaneous) and implanted infusion ports. **Central venous catheters** are inserted into a large vein, typically the superior vena cava that leads to the right atrium of the heart (Fig. 20-5). The large vessel lumen minimizes the risks of vessel irritation, inflammation, or sclerosis that commonly occur when smaller peripheral veins are used. These catheters are used to administer IV fluids, antibiotics, chemotherapy, and parenteral nutrition, to infuse medications and blood products, and to obtain blood samples.

-not venous

Tunneled CVCs are surgically inserted with the client in the operating room under general or local anesthesia. First a tunnel is made through subcutaneous tissue, usually between the clavicle and nipple. The **subcutaneous tunnel** allows the catheter to remain in place longer because it creates space between the end of the catheter and the actual vein. The risk of infection is lower. Next, the catheter tip is inserted through the cephalic, internal or external jugular vein, or a similar large vein, and is threaded into the right atrium (Fig. 20-6). The catheter is held in place with a Dacron cuff that surrounds the catheter located on the chest wall. These catheters have single, double, or triple lumens, which are hollow tubes inside the catheter that allow simultaneous administration of several infusions.

The second type of CVC is the percutaneously placed catheter. This **percutaneous** catheter is inserted directly through the skin and into a large vein of the neck (Fig. 20-7), usually the subclavian. It also may be inserted through the large veins of the antecubital fossa and threaded into the tip of the right atrium. This catheter is usually called a PICC line (see Skill 20-2). There are various types of percutaneously placed central catheters. The length of time they are left in place depends on the type and the manufacturer's recommendations, the length of therapy, and the condition/functionality of the catheter.

The third type of VAD is the **implanted infusion port,** which consists of a self-sealing injection port housed in a plastic or metal case (Fig. 20-8) and is connected most often to a silicone venous catheter. The port is also available with a double lumen catheter. The physician implants the

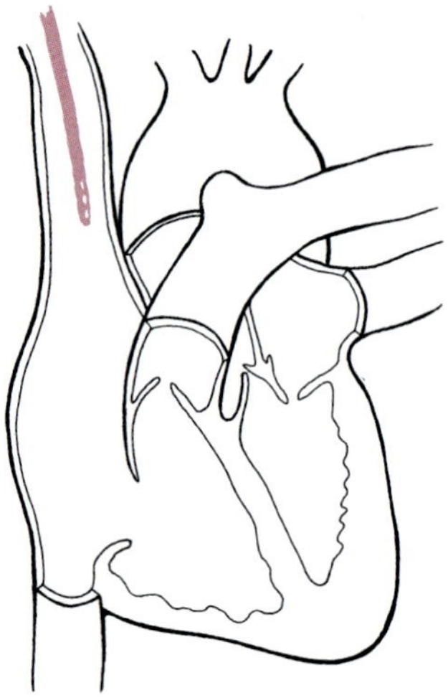

Fig. 20-5 Catheter tip lies in right atrium.

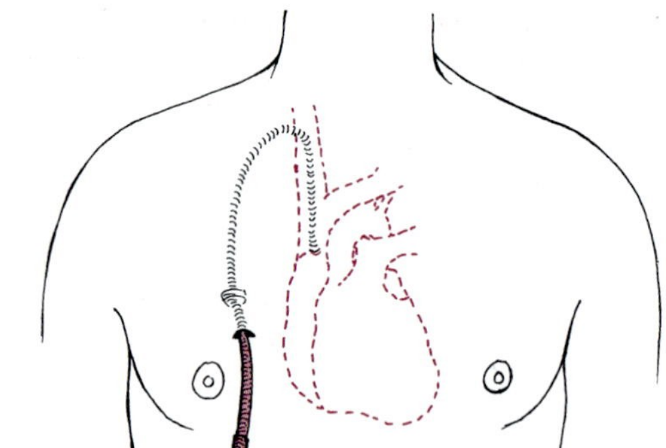

Fig. 20-6 Small gauge tunneled catheter is in place, threaded into right atrium.

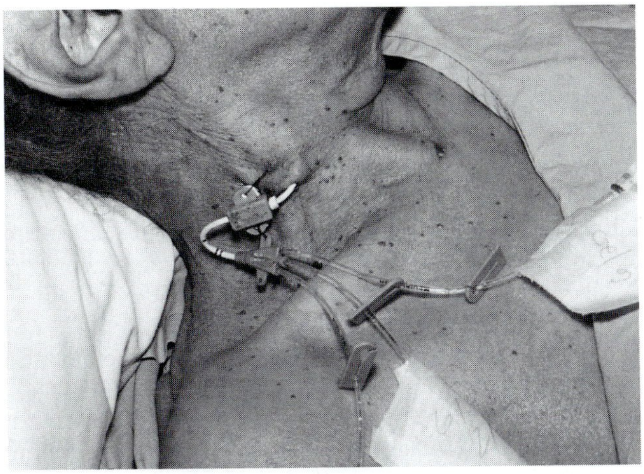

Fig. 20-7 CVC placed in jugular vein.

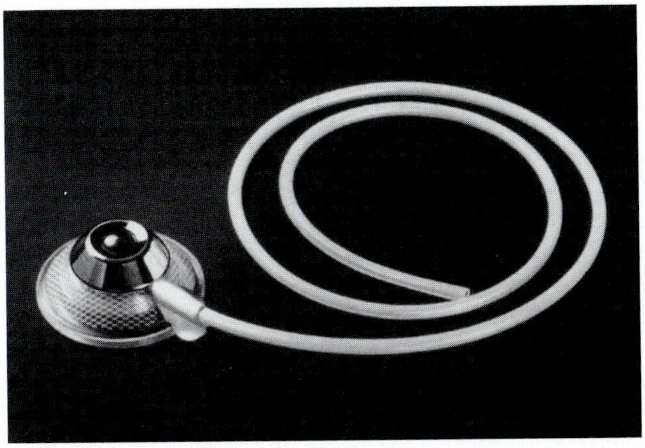

Fig. 20-8 Implantable infusion port.

infusion port under sterile conditions in an operating room with the client under local anesthesia. The infusion port usually rests in a subcutaneous pocket in the infraclavicular fossa, and the catheter is inserted into a large vein and threaded into the right atrium. The port can be easily palpated to determine placement. Specially designed **noncoring Huber needles** (straight or with 90-degree angles) are inserted through the skin to enter the port (Fig. 20-9). Implanted infusion ports are used for administration of injections and for continuous infusions of all types: medications, chemotherapy, parenteral nutrition, and blood products. When not in use no external catheter is present, and the port manufacturers recommend the port be heparinized every 4 weeks to maintain its patency. No other care is required for a port that is not being used.

Care of VADs is simple as long as nurses and clients are aware of the purpose and function of the devices and the two most common complications, infection and clotting. In the home, most clients learn to use clean technique for dressing changes and catheter care. Within 2 to 3 weeks a transparent dressing is sufficient to cover catheter insertion sites. Clients can learn to initiate infusions, heparinize devices, and discontinue infusions.

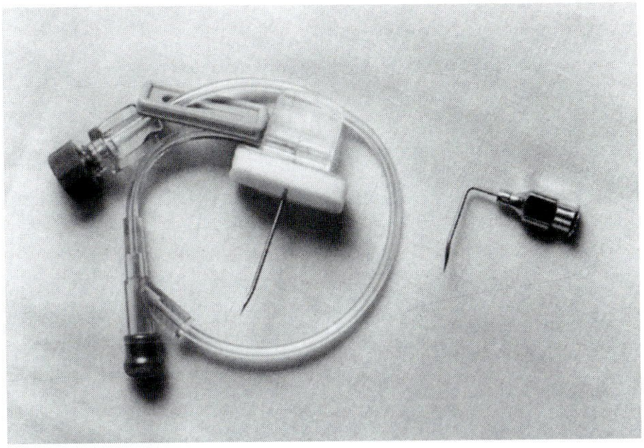

Fig. 20-9 Assortment of Huber needles.

EQUIPMENT

Blood drawing

- Povidone-iodine and alcohol preparation swabs
- 4 to 5 syringes (10 and 20 ml)
- Sterile drape
- Saline flush
- Heparin flush (10 U/ml or 100 U/ml)
- Plastic clamp
- Sterile Huber needle (20- to 22-gauge)
- Sterile needle (20- to 22-gauge)
- Blood tubes, labels, requisitions
- Gloves, gowns, masks

Administration of drugs, fluids, blood products

- Povidone-iodine and alcohol swabs
- Drug, fluid, blood product to be infused
- Sterile IV tubing
- IV pole, infusion pump, or blood pump
- Sterile drape
- Saline flush
- Sterile Huber needle (20- to 22-gauge)
- Sterile needle (20- to 22-gauge)
- Dressing supplies as indicated below
- Gloves, gown, masks

Dressing change

- Povidone-iodine and alcohol swabs
- Gloves
- Tape
- Sterile gauze 4 × 4 or 2 × 2 sponges (gauze dressing)
- Transparent occlusive dressing (transparent dressing)

Heparinization

- Povidone-iodine and alcohol preparation swabs
- Syringe (5 ml or 10 ml—see agency policy)
- Saline flush
- Heparin flush (10 U/ml or 100 U/ml)
- Plastic clamp
- Sterile needle (22-gauge)

STEPS	RATIONALE
ASSESSMENT	
1. Assess diagnosis of client's stage of disease and plan of therapy by review of medical record.	Allows nurse to understand need for vascular access in treatment of disease and in evaluation of response to therapy and to determine need to educate client about disease process and plan of therapy using VAD.
2. Assess treatment schedule: times for administration of fluids, drugs, blood products, nutrition.	Allows nurse to schedule use of VAD for simultaneous administration of products, to educate client about schedule of administration, and to provide for comfort and reduction of anxiety about therapy.
3. Assess type of VAD in place.	Care and management depend on type and size of catheter, number of lumens, type of infusion port.
4. Assess need to use VAD for blood sampling.	Scheduling sampling needs allows nurse to minimize entering VAD system and allows for timely collection of specimens to evaluate therapy. Risk of infection increases with multiple entries into vascular system, especially in immunocompromised clients.

CRITICAL DECISION POINT In some situations, several tests can be run from one blood tube sample. For example, potassium, calcium, and magnesium test results can all be obtained from one full tube of blood versus three separate tubes. Always anticipate the need for a blood test (i.e., blood cultures if a client has developed an elevated temperature). If your next task was to draw blood for electrolyte results, you could eliminate reaccessing the VAD at a later time by asking the physician if blood cultures are to be drawn.

STEPS	RATIONALE
5. Assess VAD placement site for skin integrity and signs of infection: redness, swelling, tenderness, exudate, bleeding.	Clients requiring long-term IV therapy often have conditions placing them at risk for alterations in skin integrity and immune function.
6. Assess for proper function of VAD before therapy: integrity of port or catheter, ability to irrigate or infuse fluid, ability to aspirate blood.	Ensures proper function of VAD with minimal complications.
7. Assess need for irrigation and dressing change by referring to medical record, nurses' notes, manufacturer's recommended guidelines for use.	Provides guidelines for catheter patency and prevention of infection.
8. Assess client's reaction to VAD and knowledge of purpose, care, maintenance. Ask client to discuss steps in care and to perform procedure (i.e., catheter site cleansing or dressing change).	Determines client's level of understanding. Allows nurse to educate client for home care of VAD.
9. Assess physician's order for medication, fluids, blood products, blood sampling.	

NURSING DIAGNOSIS

Clustering of defining characteristics from the assessment data may reveal the following nursing diagnoses for clients requiring this skill:

- Risk for infection
- Impaired skin integrity
- Knowledge deficit regarding use of VAD

Related factors are individualized based on a client's condition or needs.

PLANNING

STEPS	RATIONALE
1. **Expected outcomes** following completion of procedure:	
➤ Site is intact, has normal color, and has no swelling.	Local signs of infection are absent.

STEPS	RATIONALE
➤ Systemic signs of infection (fever, malaise, increased WBC) are absent.	Catheter system remains sterile.
➤ Fluids, medications, blood products infuse without difficulty.	Patency of catheter is maintained.
➤ Blood can be aspirated from catheter.	Indicates patency.
➤ Catheter and connecting tube are intact.	Integrity of system is maintained.
➤ Catheter tip is correctly placed, as confirmed by x-ray examination.	Correct placement minimizes chances of displacement or occlusion.
➤ Client and family are able to explain the purpose of VAD therapy and perform dressing changes and skin care.	Demonstrates that client and family are learning.
2. Position client in supine position with head slightly elevated.	Stabilizes client and prevents accidental pulling or tugging at catheter. Location of infusion port requires palpation and examination in supine position.
3. Explain procedure and purpose to client and family. Instruct client to lie still.	Decreases anxiety and promotes cooperation.

IMPLEMENTATION

ADMINISTRATION OF INFUSIONS OR SAMPLING OF BLOOD FROM IMPLANTED INFUSION PORT

1. Wash hands thoroughly. Mask self and client. Not all institutions require masking of the client. The client may, instead, be asked to turn head away from the port site. Refer to agency policy.	Reduces transfer of microorganisms, prevents spread of airborne microorganisms while needle insertion site is exposed.
2. Prepare sterile field and open sterile supplies.	Provides work space for use of sterile items.
3. Using alcohol, prepare client's skin overlying port septum, moving outward in concentric circles from insertion site out. Allow to dry for 60 seconds.	Rigorous skin preparation is necessary to prevent introducing bacteria into system.
4. In the same manner, use povidone-iodine swabs to cleanse skin overlying port septum.	Provides additional skin cleansing. Allow to dry for 2 minutes.
5. Apply sterile gloves.	Prevents transmission of microorganisms by nurse's hands.
6. As another nurse holds vial of saline, fill sterile syringe with saline solution.	Allows nurse filling syringe to not contaminate supplies.
7. Attach one end of sterile extension tubing to syringe and attach appropriate size Huber needle to other end. Fill tubing with saline solution.	Removes all air from tubing, reducing risk of air embolus.
8. Apply sterile drape to port site (may be optional in some agencies).	Provides sterile work area.
9. Palpate port septum, observing strict aseptic technique (see illustration).	Entry site for needle insertion must be located to ensure proper needle entry.
10. While holding wings or needle hub, insert Huber needle through skin at a 90-degree angle and push firmly down until needle penetrates silicone septum and hits the bottom of the portal chamber.	Do not push too hard. If tip of the needle bends, the septum can be damaged upon removal of needle.

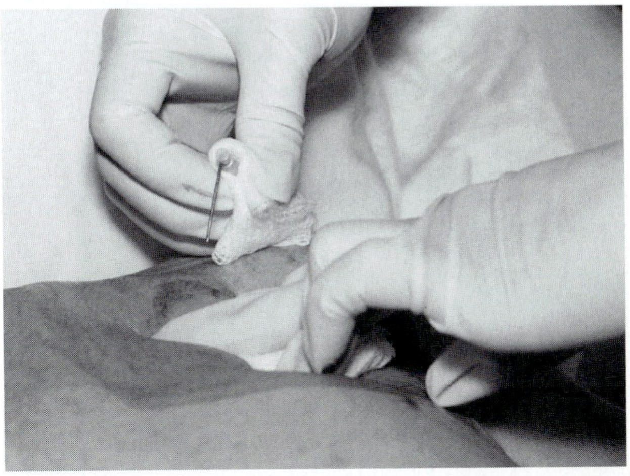

Step 9 Inserting Huber needle into vascular access port.

STEPS	RATIONALE
11. Check for proper placement by attempting to withdraw blood by aspirating with the attached syringe (see illustration).	
12. If a good blood return is present, flush the tubing with the remaining saline in the syringe. If a blood return is not obtained, fill another syringe, as in Step 6, and attempt to flush port with 10 ml normal saline.	Forceful irrigation against resistance may propel clotted blood into the client's muscular system.
➤ ***CRITICAL DECISION POINT*** **Do not irrigate forcefully if resistance is felt. If unable to flush, reposition the needle without completely withdrawing it from the skin or reprepping will be necessary. Never use a syringe less than 10 ml; exerts too high a pressure.**	
13. Observe for swelling. If swelling occurs around the needle insertion site, stop the procedure and notify physician.	This may indicate that needle is not in the port, but in the surrounding subcutaneous tissue or that there is a tear in the catheter.
14. To draw blood samples, first aspirate and discard 5 ml of fluid.	Avoids dilution of sample.
15. Withdraw necessary blood for each sample, using two 10 ml syringes equal to total volume withdrawn.	Eliminates repeated need to puncture infusion port for sampling.
16. Flush with 2 ml heparin (10 u/ml).	First clears fibrin after blood draw.
17. Refill saline syringe and flush port with 20 ml normal saline.	Any fluid other than normal saline has potential for clotting blood or precipitating in catheter.
18. If continuous infusion is not indicated, heparinize port by flushing with 5 ml heparin flush solution using positive pressure.	Prevents clot formation.
19. If IV fluid will be continuously administered, secure Huber needle with steri-strips. (see illustration). Cover the Huber needle and insertion site with a transparent dressing. If Huber needle does not sit flush on skin, place folded 2 × 2 gauze under hub and then cover with dressing.	Prevents accidental dislodging of needle at insertion site.
20. Connect IV infusion tubing with sterile tubing connected to Huber needle.	IV infusion system should be closed to maintain sterility.

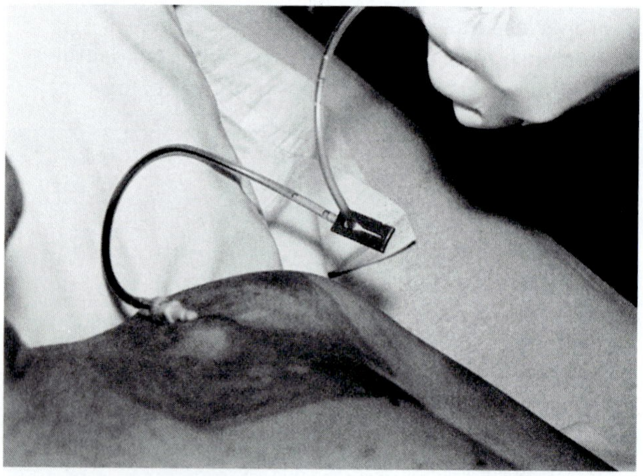

Step 11 Aspirating blood return from port.

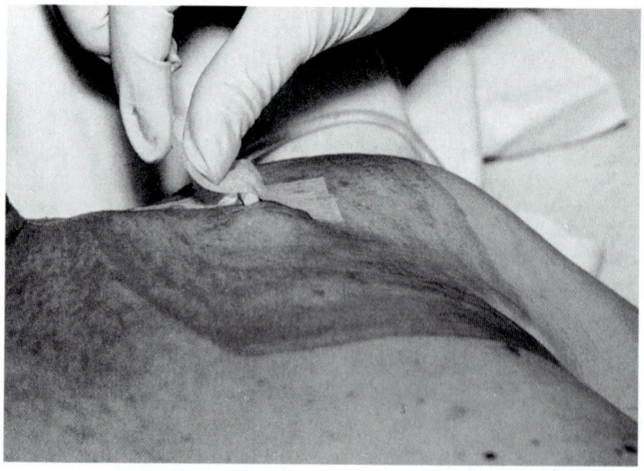

Step 19 Securing Huber needle.

STEPS	RATIONALE
21. Regulate IV infusion as ordered.	Maintains desired fluid intake and patency of catheter.
22. Dispose of all soiled supplies and used equipment. Send labeled specimens to laboratory. Wash hands.	Reduces spread of microorganisms.

ADMINISTRATION OF INFUSIONS OR SAMPLING OF BLOOD FROM CENTRAL VENOUS CATHETER

STEPS	RATIONALE
1. Wash hands thoroughly.	Reduces transmission of microorganisms.
2. Apply gloves. Apply gown and goggles (check agency policy) if blood sampling.	Prevents transfer of body fluids.
3. Use povidone-iodine and/or alcohol preparation swabs to cleanse injection cap or catheter hub according to your agency's policy.	Prevents introduction of microorganisms into catheter.
4. Prepare two syringes: one with 10 ml normal saline, the other with 20 ml saline.	Used to flush catheter.
5. If injection cap will be removed, clamp catheter.	Catheter must be clamped if injection cap is removed to prevent entrance of air.
6. If injection cap is in place, insert needle of syringe containing 10 ml normal saline and flush. If injection cap is removed, connect syringe tip to catheter hub, release clamp, flush with positive pressure, and reclamp.	Flushing ensures patency of catheter. Catheter must always be clamped during change of syringe or tubing to prevent exposure to air.
7. Connect syringe for blood sampling and release clamp. Aspirate 5 ml fluid, reclamp, and discard aspirate.	Avoids diluting sample.
8. Attach or insert syringe of size equal to volume of blood sample to withdraw to catheter. Release clamp. Withdraw necessary blood for samples and reclamp.	Samples should be collected at one time to minimize time needed to open catheter system.
9. Attach syringe filled with 2 ml heparin (10 u/ml) and flush. Clears fibrin left after blood draw.	
10. Attach or insert syringe filled with 20 ml normal saline to catheter. If clamp is present, release, flush vigorously, and reclamp.	Catheter should be cleared of all blood or medications that may clog catheter lumen or precipitate with additives in IV fluids.
11. If no continuous infusion is indicated, flush catheter with heparin or normal saline as appropriate. Connect syringe containing 5 ml heparin or normal saline flush solution. If clamp is present, release, flush with positive pressure, and reclamp.	A catheter not in use must be flushed to prevent clot formation. This is commonly done with heparin; however, Groshong catheters are flushed with normal saline only.
12. Replace new cap to end of catheter and remove clamp.	Maintains sterile seal to catheter.
13. If IV fluids will be administered, connect IV tubing to end of catheter, being sure both ends are sterile.	IV system should be closed to maintain sterility.
14. Regulate IV infusion as ordered.	Maintains ordered fluid intake and keeps catheter patent.
15. Tape all tubing connections and pin tubing to client's gown.	Prevents accidental tubing disconnection and catheter displacement.
16. Dispose of soiled equipment and used supplies. Wash hands.	Reduces transmission of microorganisms.

DRESSING CHANGE

STEPS	RATIONALE
1. Wash hands and apply clean gloves.	Reduces transmission of microorganisms.
2. Mask self and client, if indicated (check agency policy).	Prevents exposure of catheter exit or placement site to airborne microorganisms.
3. Carefully remove old dressing in the direction the catheter was inserted, noting drainage and appearance of catheter or needle insertion site.	Remove tape carefully because clients frequently have alterations in skin integrity.

STEPS	RATIONALE
4. Inspect placement or exit site for signs of redness, swelling, inflammation, tenderness, exudate.	This is a potential site of infection.
5. If catheter is tunneled, palpate Dacron cuff in subcutaneous tunnel.	Documenting position of cuff verifies proper placement.
6. Inspect catheter and hub for intactness and remove clean gloves.	Catheter may become torn, cut, displaced, cracked, split.
7. Wash hands thoroughly and open dressing kit in a sterile manner. Most agencies have dressing kits that contain all needed dressing change supplies.	
8. Apply sterile gloves.	Prevents direct transmission of microorganisms to skin **exit site.**
9. Clean placement or exit site with alcohol swabs by starting from inside moving out in circular fashion creating concentric circles. Maintain strict asepsis. Clean about a 3 cm area. Allow alcohol to remain on the skin for at least 60 seconds (see illustration).	It is impossible to sterilize skin. Organisms that accumulate must be eliminated by mechanical and chemical means.

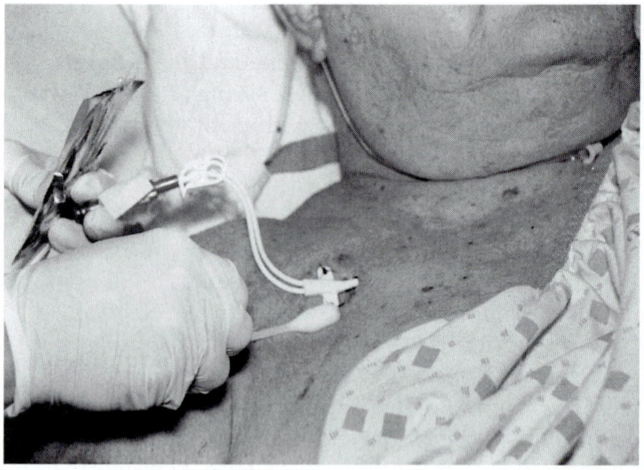

Step 9 Cleanse central venous catheter site.

10. Repeat Step 9 using the povidone-iodine swabs. Allow to dry for 2 minutes.	Povidone-iodine must be dry to be effective in reducing microbial count (Baranowski, 1993).
11. Redress site using sterile gauze and tape or transparent dressing as indicated.	Prevents entrance of bacteria into exit or placement site.
12. Secure tubing or needle to client's gown. If catheter is not in use, loop catheter and tape to client's skin.	Prevents accidental pulling and displacement.
13. Label date, time of dressing change, size of needle in place.	Documents dressing change. Provides guideline for time of next change.
14. Dispose of soiled supplies; remove gloves and wash hands.	Reduces transmission of microorganisms.

EVALUATION

1. When continuous infusions are administered, observe and calculate drip rate hourly. Note ease with which fluid rate can be increased.	To maintain proper fluid infusion, desired drip rate should be regulated continuously. A gradual slowing in rate or inability to increase rate may indicate catheter occlusion.
2. Routinely assess vital signs of client, noting changes symptomatic of infection.	Catheter-related sepsis can cause fever, chills, flushed skin, tachycardia.
3. Observe catheter or port exit or placement site when sites are exposed (Table 20-2).	Continual monitoring for signs of inflammation or infection is essential.
4. Observe all catheter connection points periodically.	An intact system prevents accidental blood loss or entrance of air.
5. Inspect condition of catheter and connecting tubing daily for leaks, holes, tears, splits, or cracked hubs.	Break in integrity of system predisposes client to hemorrhage or air embolus.

Table 20-2 Complications of VADs

Complication	Assessment	Prevention	Intervention
Catheter damage, breakage	Observe for pinholes, leaks, tears, every shift Assess for drainage after flushing	Follow proper clamping procedure Avoid sharp objects near the catheter Avoid using needles longer than 1 inch through the injection cap Avoid inserting larger than 21-gauge needles through the injection cap	Use a catheter stylet for temporary repair Use permanent repair kit Remove catheter
Occlusion: thrombus, precipitation, malposition	Assess for blood return Assess for inability to infuse Assess equipment If port, reaccess and verify needle placement Assess with syringe directly on catheter Assess for discomfort or pain in shoulder, neck, or arm at insertion site Assess for neck or shoulder edema Assess sutures to ensure no restriction	Follow routine flushing with positive pressure Avoid tugging on VAD Administer low-dose oral anticoagulant therapy Avoid using excessive force Flush between drugs Flush vigorously after viscous solutions Avoid mixing incompatible drugs Avoid kinking catheter	Reposition client Have client cough and deep breathe Raise client's arm Venogram Administer thrombolytics Remove catheter Use gentle push-pull technique with normal saline Obtain x-ray If precipitate, try hydrochloric acid or ethanol solution
Infection: exit site, tunnel, thrombus, port pocket	Assess exit site for redness, drainage, edema, or tenderness Assess vital signs Monitor laboratory findings	Use strict hand washing Use aseptic technique Adhere to dressing change technique Apply dressing over exit site Apply antibiotic or antimicrobial ointment at exit site	Administer antibiotic therapy Remove catheter Administer thrombolytic agent Replace catheter Obtain blood cultures peripheral and from VAD Do not use VAD if it has not been accessed
Dislodgement, Twiddler's syndrome	Assess length of catheter daily Inform client of possible catheter dislodgment Identify edema at exit site or drainage Palpate exit site and tunnel for coiling Assess distended neck veins	Loop and tape the catheter securely Use occlusive dressing Use athletic sock for PICC Avoid pulling on VAD Handle with care Avoid manipulating catheter (port) by hand	Reinsert catheter Secure catheter with sutures Teach client not to manipulate catheter
Catheter migration, pinch-off syndrome, port separation	Assess for client complaints of gurgling sounds Assess for change in patency of catheter Obtain x-ray Assess edema of arm and hand on side of insertion Assess distended neck veins Assess for inability to infuse fluids Assess length of catheter daily	Avoid trauma Avoid placement near site of local disease	Reposition under fluoroscopy Remove catheter Stop all fluid administration
Skin erosion, hematomas, cuff extrusion, scar tissue formation over port	Assess for loss of viable tissue over implantation Assess for separation of exit site edges Assess for drainage at exit site Assess for redness Assess for edema, contusions Note if tunneled catheter is exposed	Maintain nutritional status Minimize edema with cold packs Avoid pressure or trauma Rotate site with each port access	Remove VAD Improve nutrition Provide appropriate skin care

Continued.

Table 20-2 Complications of VADs—cont'd

Complication	Assessment	Prevention	Intervention
Infiltration, extravasation	Assess for erythema Assess for edema Assess for spongy feeling Assess for labored breathing Assess for no blood return Assess for complaints of pain Assess for no free-flow IV drip	Do not administer vesicants Use own judgment to use without a blood return Use astute assessment skills Administer medications according to drug literature	Apply warm compress Provide emotional support Obtain x-ray Use antidotes Discontinue IV fluids
Pneumothorax, hemothorax, air emboli, hydrothorax	Use astute assessment skills Assess for subcutaneous emphysema Assess for chest pain Assess for dyspnea, apnea, hypoxia, tachycardia, hypotension, nausea, confusion	Use cap on distal end when not in use Do not leave catheter open to air	Insert chest tubes Elevate feet Administer oxygen Aspirate air, fluid Remove catheter If air emboli suspected, place client on left side with head elevated slightly
Incorrect placement	Cardiac dysrhythmias Assess for hypotension Assess for neck distention Assess for narrow pulse pressure Assess for inadequate blood withdrawal Assess for retrograde of blood	Obtain x-ray after placement Reposition catheter as warranted Use astute assessment skills	Obtain x-ray and ECG Stop all fluid administration Discontinue catheter Administer support medications

Modified from Carter P et al: Access device guidelines: modules I and II, 1989, Oncology Nursing Society.
NOTE: Use clinical judgment in continuing to use VADs. Advanced skills must be taught and checked off in a clinical setting.

STEPS	RATIONALE
6. Consult x-ray reports for catheter placement.	A routine chest x-ray examination can locate position of catheter tip.
7. Evaluate ability of client and family to provide care and maintain catheter or infusion port through discussion and return demonstrations of dressing changes and skin care. Determine need for restrictions on daily activities.	Measures client's ability to care for self and any additional learning needs.
8. Unexpected outcomes that may occur include:	
➤ Client has redness, swelling, exudate, inflammation, tenderness at exit or placement sites.	Infection is present at sites.
➤ Client has fever, chills, positive blood cultures.	Signs and symptoms of systemic infection are caused by catheter-related sepsis.
➤ Client has a VAD from which no blood can be obtained.	
a. Assist client in positional changes (i.e., turning side to side, sitting up, lying flat), ask client to perform Valsalva maneuver, cough, take a deep breath, after which nurse repeats attempt to withdraw blood.	Moves catheter away from vessel wall.
b. Administer a bolus of IV fluids.	Sometimes moves catheter away from vessel wall.
c. Obtain physician's order for fibrinolytic therapy (urokinase); administer according to institutional policy and procedure.	Dissolves fiber sheath at catheter tip, which may be cause of inability to withdraw blood.
➤ There is damage to catheter: displacement, cut or tear, hole; loss of cap, crack in hub or cap. Clamp catheter immediately proximal to damaged site. Notify physician.	Requires immediate catheter repair (if repair kit is available) or discontinuation to prevent hemorrhage or air embolus.
➤ Air **embolus** forms. Symptoms depend on area of body affected.	Air bubbles enter and travel through circulatory system, blocking blood flow after lodged in vessel lumen.

STEPS	RATIONALE
➤ Client or family member is unable to explain or perform VAD care.	May indicate need for home health care referral or additional instruction.

Recording and Reporting

1. Chart date and time of medications, blood products, parenteral nutrition given, samples obtained, in nurses' notes or on medication administration record.	Timely documentation prevents administration errors and repetition of blood sampling.
2. Chart condition of exit site or port implantation site, including skin integrity, signs of infection, placement, integrity and functionality of catheter.	Documents ongoing condition and response to catheter site care.
3. Chart dressing change procedure, label date, time, type and size of needle in port.	Documents nursing care.
4. Chart patency of catheter, ability to draw blood, difficulty with infusions.	If complications arise, it is important to have documentation that preventive measures were performed.
5. Chart measures taken to educate client in self-care, response to education.	Provides continuity of care so that other staff members may contribute to education.
6. In emergency situations (damage to catheter, loss of patency, blood loss, air embolus, septic episode, local signs of infection), notify nursing or medical personnel immediately. Instruct client and family when to contact medical personnel.	Allows immediate attention by appropriate personnel.

Follow-up Activities

1. If redness, swelling, exudate, inflammation, tenderness at exit site is noted, obtain order for a culture and sensitivity of any exudate and reassess cleansing regimen and dressing techniques. Identifies infecting organism. Poor cleansing technique leads to infection.
2. After client's discharge, contact client to determine condition of VAD and client's ability to care for VAD. Allow opportunity for client to ask questions regarding care of VAD.

• • • • •

Special Considerations

- ➤ Most common complications are infection, bleeding, leakage at insertion site, occlusion, displacement of catheter or needle in port.
- ➤ Clients who have undergone radiation therapy or chemotherapy have compromised immune functions that increase risk of infection.
- ➤ Ready access to manufacturer's recommendations and familiarity with institutional policies and procedures are essential.
- ➤ Have a catheter repair kit available or know where to obtain one immediately.

Teaching Considerations

- ➤ Discuss and provide written emergency measures and telephone numbers of health care personnel to be used in case of catheter damage; needle displacement; swelling, redness, or leakage at insertion site; occlusion of port or catheter; temperature above 100° F; shaking chills.
- ➤ Provide written instruction for dressing changes, inspection of insertion site, irrigations, tubing changes.
- ➤ Arrange for instruction and return demonstration of skills by client or care giver.
- ➤ Have client or care giver maintain a list of care givers and telephone numbers (i.e., physician, nurse, social worker, pharmacist, dietitian).

Home Care Considerations

- ➤ Initiate early referral for discharge planning to social service, counselor, or home care coordinator for assessment of resources.
- ➤ Determine client and care giver's acceptance of client's altered body image.
- ➤ Provide client with written list of providers for supplies and equipment.
- ➤ Assess willingness and ability of primary care giver to assist in home management of device. Acceptance of altered body image influences primary care giver's readiness to assist with care.
- ➤ Instruct client and care giver in adaptations of hospital procedures that can be made at home (i.e., good hand washing instead of sterile gloves).
- ➤ Discuss troubleshooting and emergency care routines with care giver in home.
- ➤ Assess home environment and determine suitable area for dressing changes, avoiding areas where contaminants are potential hazards.
- ➤ Determine ability of client to meet expenses of equipment involved in caring for VAD.

SKILL 20-8 Discontinuing Peripheral Intravenous Access

EQUIPMENT

- Disposable gloves
- Sterile 2 × 2 or 4 × 4 gauze sponge
- Tape

STEPS	RATIONALE
ASSESSMENT	
1. Observe IV site for signs and symptoms of infection, infiltration, phlebitis.	Provides preassessment data that can be used for comparison when performing postassessments.
2. Review physician order for discontinuation of IV.	Order required for procedure
3. Determine client's understanding for the need for discontinued peripheral IV access.	Reveals need for client instruction.

NURSING DIAGNOSIS

Clustering of defining characteristics from the assessment data may reveal the following nursing diagnosis for clients requiring this skill:

➤ Risk for infection

Related factors are individualized based on a client's condition or needs.

PLANNING

1. **Expected outcomes** following completion of procedure:
   - ➤ IV will be removed with minimal trauma to client.
   - ➤ IV site will remain free of infection.
2. Explain procedure to client. Explain that affected extremity must be held still and how long procedure will take.

IMPLEMENTATION

STEPS	RATIONALE
1. Wash hands. Apply disposable gloves.	Reduces transmission of microorganisms. Gloves reduce the nurse's risk of exposure to HIV, hepatitis, and other blood-borne viruses or bacteria.
2. Turn IV tubing roller clamp to "off" position.	Prevents spillage of IV fluid.
3. Remove IV site dressing and tape securing needle or catheter.	Exposes the IV needle or catheter.
4. Hold needle or catheter and clean site with alcohol, then povidone-iodine solution.	Removes secretions around skin puncture site.
5. Place sterile gauze over venipuncture site and remove catheter or needle by pulling straight away from insertion site in a slow, steady motion. Inspect catheter for intactness after removal.	Prevents damage to client's vein; determines if catheter tip is intact.
➤ **CRITICAL DECISION POINT** **Do not elevate or lift catheter before it is completely out of the vein to avoid trauma or formation of a hematoma.**	
6. Apply pressure to site for 2 to 3 minutes.	Controls bleeding or hematoma formation.
➤ **CRITICAL DECISION POINT** **If client has received anticoagulants or has a low platelet count, apply steady pressure for 5 minutes and assess bleeding.**	
7. Apply folded gauze dressing over insertion site and secure with tape.	Maintains pressure to prevent bleeding and bacterial entry into puncture site.
8. Discard used supplies and wash hands.	Reduces transmission of microorganisms.

STEPS	RATIONALE
EVALUATION	
1. Observe site for evidence of bleeding.	Additional pressure may be needed.
2. Observe site for redness, pain, drainage, swelling.	May indicate infection at old IV site.
RECORDING AND REPORTING	
1. Record in nurses' notes time peripheral IV was discontinued. Include site assessment information.	Documents that peripheral IV was discontinued and indicates preassessment of IV insertion site.
2. Report to nurse in charge or oncoming nursing shift that peripheral IV was discontinued and any significant information related to the procedure.	Assists in verification of care delivered and planning of future nursing care.

• • • • •

Teaching Considerations

- Client should be instructed to notify nurse if bleeding is noted at insertion site.
- Client should be instructed to notify nurse if insertion site becomes reddened, painful, swollen, or if drainage is present.

CRITICAL THINKING EXERCISES

1. Mr. J. is visiting his daughter in the United States from Italy. He speaks no English. He is right-handed. While visiting, he develops pneumonia and requires IV antibiotics. He is found to have a rash on his left hand and wrist. What is the best place for his IV insertion site?
2. Mrs. C.'s IV order is 1000 ml normal saline (0.9 NS) with 20 mEq of KCl to run at 125 ml/hour.
   a. Which type of IV tubing should be used for this order (macrodrip = 10 gtt/ml or minidrip = 60 gtt/ml)?
   b. Calculate the drops per minute for this order.
   c. How long will a 1000 ml bag last?
3. Mr. K. has an IV infusion of 1000 ml D5 0.45% NaCl at 150 ml/hour. There was 700 ml left in the bag at the beginning of the shift. An hour later, you check the bag and note that there is 650 ml left in the bag. What are the possible causes for this? Describe how you should investigate to determine the actual cause.
4. Mrs. B. has chronic renal failure. She is to receive 1000 ml 0.45% NS to run at 50 ml/hour. When you check the IV, you discover that 1000 ml 0.9% NS is infusing at 150 ml/hour.
   a. What is the highest priority action in this situation?
   b. For what complication is Mrs. B. at risk because of the IV fluids that were infusing?
   c. What assessments would indicate this complication?
5. During a dressing change of a tunneled CVC, you discover that the exit site is red and tender and has puslike drainage. What actions would you take?
6. During the infusion of IV fluid through an implanted infusion port, the site surrounding the port becomes swollen and painful. The IV fluids will not infuse. What is the most likely cause?

REFERENCES

Association for Practitioners in Infection Control: Position paper: prevention of device-mediated blood-borne infections to health care workers, *American Journal of Infection Control* 21(2):76, 1973.

Baranowski L: Central venous access device: current technologies, users, and management strategies, *J Intraven Nurs* 16(3):167, 1993.

Centers for Disease Control: Guideline for prevention of intravascular device-related infections, *Infection Control and Hospital Epidemiology* 17(7):438-472, 1996.

Centers for Disease Control: Recommendations for prevention of HIV transmission in health care settings, *MMWR* 36(suppl 25):35, 1987.

Coulter K: Intravenous therapy for the elder client: implications for the intravenous nurse, *Journal of Intravenous Nursing* 15(suppl):S18, 1992.

Elkin M, Perry A, and Potter P: *Nursing interventions and clinical skills,* St Louis, 1996, Mosby.

Garner J: Guideline for isolation precautions in hospitals, *Infection Control and Hospital Epidemiology* 17(1):53, 1996.

Horne MM, Heitz UE, Swearingen PL: *Fluid, electrolyte, and acid-base balance: a case study approach,* St Louis, 1991, Mosby.

Horne MM, Swearingen PL: *Pocket guide to fluid, electrolyte, and acid-base balance,* ed 3, St Louis, 1997, Mosby.

Intravenous Nurses Society: Intravenous nursing standards of practice, *J Intraven Nurs* 13(suppl):S5, 1990.

LaRocca JC, Otto, SE: *Pocket guide to intravenous therapy,* St Louis, 1993, Mosby.

Loughran SC, Edwards S, McClure S: Peripherally inserted central catheters—guidewire versus non guide wire use: a comparative study, *J Intraven Nurs* 15(3):152, 1992.

Millam DA: Starting IVs: how to develop your venipuncture expertise, *Nurs '92* 22(9):33, 1992.

Occupational Safety and Health Act: Bloodborne pathogens, *Federal Register* 56(235):64, 175, Dec 6, 1991.

Tully JL et al: Complications of intravenous therapy with steel needles and Teflon catheters. A comparative study. *Am J Med* 70:702-706, 1981.

ADDITIONAL READING

Anderson KM, Holland JS: Maintaining the patency of peripherally inserted central catheters with 10 units/cc heparin, *J Intraven Nurs* 15(2):84, 1992.

Baldwin DR: Management of intravenous hazardous materials and hazardous wastes in the work environment, *J Intraven Nurs* 15(2):90, 1992.

Fabian B: Peripherally inserted central catheter exchange using a breakaway sheath, *J Intraven Nurs,* 18(2):92, 1995.

Hermey C: *Quick reference for IV therapy,* St Louis, 1995, Mosby.

Hoffmann K, et al: Transparent polyurethane film as an intravenous catheter dressing, *Journal of the American Medical Association* 267(15):2072, 1992.

Intravenous Nurses Society: Intravenous nursing standards of practice, *J Intraven Nurs* 14(suppl):546, 1990.

Journal of Intravenous Nursing: *Revised standards of practice,* Belmont, Mass, 1991,

Kelly C, et al: A change in flushing protocols of central venous catheters, *Oncol Nurs Forum* 19(4):599, 1992.

LaRocca J: *Handbook of homecare IV therapy,* St Louis, 1994, Mosby.

LaRue GD: Improving central placement rates of peripherally inserted catheters, *J of IV Nurs,* 18(1):24, 1995.

Williams EB, Kelman GB, Jacox M: A regional study of intravenous therapy practices, *J Intraven Nurs,* 17(4):195, 1994.

CHAPTER 21

Blood Therapy

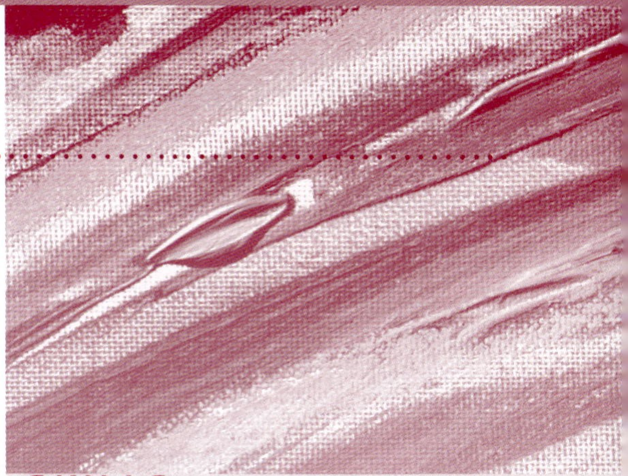

OBJECTIVES

Mastery of content in this chapter will enable the nurse to:

- Define key terms.
- Discuss indications for blood therapy.
- Describe various transfusion reactions.
- Demonstrate the following skills on selected clients: initiating blood therapy, assisting with autotransfusion, and monitoring for transfusion reactions.

SKILLS

21-1 Initiating Blood Therapy

21-2 Assisting with Autologous Blood Transfusion

21-3 Monitoring for Transfusion Reactions

KEY TERMS

Agglutinate
Autologous blood transfusion
Autotransfusion
Blood group
Blood transfusion
Blood type
Hemolysis
Reinfusion devices
Transfusion reaction

Transfusion therapy is the intravenous (IV) administration of whole blood or blood components for therapeutic purposes. It may be used to restore intravascular volume with whole blood or albumin, to restore the oxygen-carrying capacity of blood by replacing red blood cells, to replace clotting factors and/or platelets to reverse coagulopathy, or to replace white blood cells in neutropenic clients.

Despite precautions, blood component therapy is not without risk. Clerical errors, either in the collection or distribution of blood, may lead to the administration of incompatible units of blood. In addition, unforeseeable incompatibility and/or disease transmission remain a small possibility.

While the decision to transfuse is made by a physician, it is the nurse who must assess the client before, during and after a transfusion. It is important that the nurse understand the rationale for transfusion of any component to be given, the expected outcomes, and the possible unanticipated outcomes so that the nurse may immediately identify any adverse effects of the therapy.

ABO SYSTEM

Blood type in the ABO system is determined by the presence or absence of certain antigens on the surface of red blood cells. When the type A antigen is present, the blood group is called type A, and when the type B antigen is present, the blood group is type B. When both A and B antigens are present, the blood group is type AB, and when neither A nor B antigens are present, the blood group is type O.

Antibodies that react against the A and B antigens occur naturally in the plasma of people whose red blood cells do not carry them. Therefore, people with type A blood have anti-B antibodies, and people with type B blood have anti-A antibodies. People with type AB blood have neither antibody, and people with type O blood have both. These antibodies (agglutinins) react against the antigens (agglutinogens) causing the red blood cells to **agglutinate** (clump together), resulting in a life-threatening transfusion reaction.

Rh SYSTEM

Although six common types of Rh antigen may be present on the surface of red blood cells, the type D antigen is widely prevalent and is most likely to incite an immune response. It is the presence or absence of the D antigen that determines a person's Rh type. A person with the D antigen is considered Rh positive, and a person without the D antigen is considered Rh negative.

Unlike the ABO antigens, there are no naturally occurring antibodies to the Rh antigen. A person with Rh-negative blood must first be exposed to Rh-positive blood before any Rh antibodies are formed. A person with Rh-negative blood who is exposed to a large amount (≥200 ml) of Rh-positive blood will develop enough antibodies

Table 21-1 Adverse Reactions to Blood Transfusions

Reaction	Mechanism	Onset	Signs and Symptoms	Prevention	Management
Acute hemolytic	ABO, Rh incompatibility; causes intravascular destruction of RBCs as antibodies in recipient's plasma attach to antigens on donor RBCs	Within 5-15 min of initiation of transfusion	Sensation of heat and pain along vein in which blood is being infused; Chills, low back pain, headache, nausea, chest tightness, fever, dyspnea, hypotension, hemoglobinemia, hemoglobinuria, (Hgb molecules from donor blood released into recipient's bloodstream and excreted by kidneys), disseminated intravascular coagulation, renal failure, possibly death	Careful identification of client when blood sample is obtained for blood typing and compatibility screening, and when blood is released from blood bank; careful verification procedure at bedside prior to transfusion	This is potentially life-threatening. **1.** Stop transfusion **2.** Maintain IV access. **3.** Notify physician. **4.** Monitor vital signs at least every 15 min. **5.** Monitor intake and output hourly. (Attempts may be made to alkalinize the urine and initiate diuresis as this may prevent precipitation of hemoglobin within the renal tubules). Dialysis may be required. **6.** Obtain blood and urine samples and send to laboratory with unused portion of unit of blood. **7.** Document reaction according to agency policy.
Delayed hemolytic	Immune response mounted by recipient against non-ABO donor antigens	Several days to 2 weeks	Anemia, positive Coombs' test	Careful cross-matching of donor and recipient blood	Potential to be missed since it may occur several days posttransfusion. **1.** Monitor laboratory values for anemia. (Recognition is important because subsequent transfusions may cause an acute hemolytic reaction). **2.** If detected, notify physician and blood bank.
Febrile (nonhemolytic)	Most common reaction; possible sensitivity of recipient to the leukocytes or platelets in the donor's blood	30 min after initiation to 6 hr after completion of transfusion	Fever greater than 1° C above baseline, flushing, chills, headache, muscle pain	Utilizing leukocyte-reduced blood products	**1.** Stop transfusion **2.** Administer antipyretics as ordered. **3.** Monitor temperature every 4 hr.
Urticaria	Caused by recipient allergy to a plasma protein in the donor's blood	During transfusion to 1 hr post-transfusion	Local erythema, hives, and itching	May administer antihistamines pretransfusion if ordered	**1.** Stop transfusion. **2.** Notify physician and blood bank. **3.** Administer antihistamines as ordered. **4.** Monitor and document vital signs every 15 min. **5.** Transfusion may be restarted if fever, dyspnea, and wheezing are not present.

Modified from LaRocca J, Otto S: *Mosby's Pocket guide to intravenous therapy,* ed 3, St Louis, 1997, Mosby; National Blood Resource Education Program Nursing Education Working Group: Transfusion nursing: trends and practices for the '90s, *Am J Nurs* 91(6):42, 1991.

Table 21-1 Adverse Reactions to Blood Transfusions—cont'd

Reaction	Mechanism	Onset	Signs and Symptoms	Prevention	Management
Anaphylaxis	Caused by recipient allergy to a donor antigen (usually IgA)	Within 5-15 min of initiation of transfusion	Coughing, nausea, vomiting, respiratory distress, hypotension, loss of consciousness, possible cardiac arrest	Transfusion of saline-washed or leukocyte-depleted RBCs	This is a life-threatening reaction. **1.** Stop transfusion. **2.** Maintain IV access. **3.** Notify physician and blood bank. **4.** Administer antihistamines and antipyretics as ordered. **5.** Measure and document vital signs every 5-15 min. **6.** Initiate cardiopulmonary resuscitation if necessary.
Graft-versus-host disease	Reproduction of donor lymphocytes in an immunocompromised recipient, which attack the recipient's RBCs as if they were foreign proteins	Days to weeks	Skin rash, fever, jaundice due to liver dysfunction, bone marrow suppression	Administration of irradiated or saline-washed blood products as ordered	**1.** Administer methotrexate, corticosteroids as ordered.
Circulatory overload (adverse effect rather than allergic reaction)	Occurs with infusion of blood or components too rapidly for the client to tolerate	Any time during or within 1-2 hr after completion of the transfusion	Dyspnea, cough, crackles at lung bases, tachypnea, tachycardia, increased central venous pressure	Administering blood or component at rate prescribed by physician, based on client's size and health status; administering PRBCs instead of whole blood; minimizing amount of saline infused with a transfusion	**1.** Slow or stop transfusion as ordered. **2.** Elevate client's head. **3.** Notify physician. **4.** Administer diuretics, oxygen, and morphine as ordered.
Bacterial sepsis (adverse effect rather than allergic reaction)	Bacterial contamination of infused product	During the transfusion to 2 hr posttransfusion	Fever, chills, abdominal cramping, vomiting, diarrhea, profound hypotension	Proper care of blood or blood product from the time of procurement through the end of administration	**1.** Stop transfusion. **2.** Maintain IV access. **3.** Notify physician. **4.** Monitor and document vital signs. **5.** Obtain blood culture from recipient. **6.** Administer IV fluids, antibiotics, vasopressors, and steroids as ordered.

to mount a severe transfusion reaction with repeat exposure. These antibodies take up to 2 weeks to form. Therefore, in the case of massive transfusion as used in trauma situations, Rh-positive blood may be used for a person with Rh-negative blood without adverse effect, provided that the person has not been exposed to Rh-positive blood in the past.

An Rh-negative mother previously exposed to Rh antigen can transfer Rh antibodies across the placenta to an Rh-positive fetus. This can result in severe **hemolysis** (breakdown of red blood cells [RBCs]) with resultant anemia and jaundice, and can be fatal to the infant.

GUIDELINES

1. Review hospital or agency policy and procedure regarding administration of blood or blood products, because it is designed to ensure safe administration of blood products.
2. Know the client's normal range of vital signs. Administration of blood products increases intravascular volume and may elevate a client's blood pressure. This may be one of the desired effects of therapy. However, some clients cannot tolerate the volume load of a blood transfusion and may develop fluid volume excess, leading to markedly elevated blood pressure, tachycardia, pulmonary edema, or cardiac failure.
3. Monitor and document the client's vital signs immediately prior to initiation of therapy and closely during blood therapy as well. (Policies will differ between institutions regarding timing of vital sign monitoring throughout blood transfusions.) An elevation in temperature or heart rate may be one of the first signs that a person is having an adverse reaction to a transfusion. A client may also experience marked hypotension if a severe reaction occurs (Table 21-1).
4. Understand the indications for and the goal of the transfusion therapy. This will allow the nurse to assist the physician in evaluating the outcome and assessing the need for any further therapy.
5. Assess the client's most recent serum electrolyte values. When blood is stored, there is continual destruction of RBCs, which releases potassium from the cells into the plasma. If blood is transfused rapidly, there may be transient hyperkalemia before the potassium is reabsorbed. Blood that is preserved with citrate-phosphate-dextrose (CPD) contains a high concentration of citrate ions. The excess citrate may combine with the ionized calcium in the recipient's blood, resulting in transient low ionized calcium levels. While ionized calcium deficiency resulting from blood transfusions is rare, it is more likely to occur in young children, older adults, or osteoporotic clients.
6. Verify the client's understanding of the procedure and its rationale. This may help to alleviate any anxiety the client may have regarding receiving blood products.

DELEGATION CONSIDERATIONS

Unlicensed assistive personnel may obtain blood components from the blood bank in most institutions. Depending on the agency's policy, they may also assist the nurse in the verification procedure prior to the initiation of blood therapy. However, the skills of initiating blood therapy, assisting with blood transfusions, and monitoring for transfusion reactions require knowledge application unique to a professional nurse. For these skills, delegation is inappropriate.

SKILL 21-1 Initiating Blood Therapy

A variety of blood components are available for clients requiring blood therapy (Table 21-2). The indications for use differ from one product to another. It is the responsibility of the physician to determine which blood component should be administered to the client.

Prior to requesting a blood component for a client, the nurse must first ensure that a sample of the client's blood has been sent to the laboratory within the past 72 hours for blood typing and general compatibility screening.

EQUIPMENT

- Blood administration set
- 0.9% NaCl (normal saline) IV solution
- Alcohol wipes
- Disposable, clean gloves
- Tape
- Blood pressure cuff and stethoscope
- Thermometer
- Signed transfusion consent form

If needed:

- Infusion pump
- Leukocyte depleting filter
- Blood warmer
- Pressure bag

Table 21-2 Blood and Blood Component Products*

Blood Product and Source	Volume and Infusion Time	Able to Transmit HIV/HBV	ABO/Rh Testing Needed	Actions/Uses
Red blood cell products				
Whole blood (single donor: homologous, directed or autologous)	550 ml 2-3 hours	Yes	Yes/Yes	Replaces red cell mass and plasma volume. Expected to raise Hgb 1.0 gm/dl and Hct by 3% in non-hemorrhaging adult. (Rarely used.)
Packed red blood cells (PRBCs) (single donor: homologous or directed)	250-350 ml 2-3 hours	Yes	Yes/Yes	Preferred method of replacing red blood cell mass. Expected to raise Hgb and Hct same as whole blood.
Modified blood products				
Leukopoor red blood cells (single donor: homologous or directed)	200-250 ml 2-3 hours	Yes	Yes/Yes	Replaces red blood cells while preventing febrile non-hemolytic transfusion reactions. Reduces risk of CMV transmission.
Irradiated red blood cells (single donor: homologous or directed)	250-350 ml 2-3 hours	Yes	Yes/Yes	Replaces red blood cells while preventing transfusion-associated graft-versus-host disease. Used in immunodeficient clients.
Coagulation components				
Fresh frozen plasma (FFP) (single donor)	200-250 ml 1 hour	Yes	Yes/No	Replaces plasma without red blood cells or platelets. Contains most coagulation factors and complement. Used in the control of bleeding where replacement of coagulation factors is needed (disseminated intravascular coagulation, liver disease).
Cryoprecipitate (multiple donors: pooled)	5-20 ml/bag 1 bag/10 kg body weight 1-2 ml/minute	Yes	No/No	Replaces factors VIII, XIII, von Willebrand's factor and fibrinogen.
Factors VIII and IX concentrates (multiple: pooled)	10-30 ml 6 ml/minute	No	No/No	Replaces coagulation factors VIII and IX in clients with hemophilia A and B.
Platelets				
Multiple/random donor: pooled	40-70 ml/unit Give 1 unit/10 kg body weight 30 minutes-3 hours	Yes	Yes/Yes	Replaces platelets in patients with thrombocytopenia. Single donor platelets are most useful in immunologically refractory clients when given as HLA matched with recipient. 1 unit of platelets can raise the platelet count 5,000-10,000/ml in an average 70 kg adult.
Single donor, obtained by automated pheresis	200-500 ml 30 minutes-3 hours	Yes	Yes/Yes	
Colloid components				
Albumin (pooled) 5%	250-500 ml (1-10 ml/minute) Infuse within 1 hour	No	No/No	5% solution is oncotically equivalent to plasma—used to treat hypoproteinemia in burns, and hypoalbuminemia in shock and ARDS. Used to support blood pressure in dialysis and acute liver failure.
(pooled) 25%	50-100 ml (0.2-0.4 ml/minute) Infuse within 1 hour			Increases circulating blood volume by increasing intravascular oncotic pressure.

*Other rarely used blood components include granulocytes, immunoglobulin (IgG) and saline washed red blood cells.

Modified from McKenry L and Salerno E: *Mosby's pharmacology in nursing*, ed 19, St Louis, 1995, Mosby; American Red Cross: Transfusion medicine update, *Blood Component Therapy* 3(1), 1995.

STEPS	RATIONALE
ASSESSMENT	
1. Verify that the IV catheter to be used is an 18-gauge or larger and that it is patent (see Chapter 20).	A patent IV ensures that the transfusion will be initiated and infused within the time guidelines set forth. Large catheters promote optimal flow of blood components and guard against hemolysis. (Smaller bore catheters may damage red blood cells.) Infiltration or signs of infection at the IV site contraindicate the use of that line for blood therapy.
2. Obtain client's transfusion history.	Identifies client's prior response(s) to transfusion of blood components. If a client has experienced a reaction in the past, anticipate a similar reaction and be prepared to rapidly intervene.
3. Review the physician's order for the blood component transfusion. Check that transfusion consent has been properly completed.	A physician's order must be present before transfusing a blood product. Verifying the order helps to ensure that the appropriate blood component will be administered. Client consent must be obtained.
4. Know the indication for the blood product to be transfused (e.g., packed red blood cells [PRBCs] for a client with a low hematocrit from gastrointestinal bleeding).	Knowing the rationale for the product to be transfused facilitates evaluation of the outcome of therapy.
5. Obtain and record vital signs immediately prior to initiation of the transfusion.	Change from baseline vital signs will alert the nurse to a potential transfusion reaction or adverse effect of therapy.

NURSING DIAGNOSIS

Clustering of defining characteristics from the assessment data may reveal the following nursing diagnoses for clients requiring this skill:

- Activity intolerance
- Altered tissue perfusion
- Decreased cardiac output
- Fluid volume deficit
- Knowledge deficit regarding purpose and risks of blood transfusions

Related factors are individualized based on a client's condition or needs.

PLANNING

STEPS	RATIONALE
1. **Expected outcomes** following completion of the procedure:	
➤ Client's cardiac output returns to baseline.	Intravascular volume is restored.
➤ Mucous membranes are pink with brisk capillary refill.	Tissue perfusion is improved
➤ Client experiences improved activity tolerance.	Oxygenation status is improved.
➤ Client's systolic blood pressure > 100 mm Hg, urine output ½ to 1 cc/kg/hr.	Parameters reflect optimal fluid status.
➤ Laboratory values will reflect improvement in targeted areas (clotting factors, hematocrit).	
➤ Client will verbalize understanding of rationale for therapy.	
2. Explain procedure to client and family. Have client sign any necessary consent forms.	Some agencies require clients to sign consent forms prior to receiving blood component therapy.

IMPLEMENTATION

PREADMINISTRATION

1. Obtain blood component from blood bank following agency protocol.
2. Correctly verify the product and identify the client with a person considered qualified by your agency.

STEPS	RATIONALE

CRITICAL DECISION POINT Strict adherence to verification procedures before administration of blood or blood components reduces the risk of administering the wrong blood to the client. Most hemolytic transfusion reactions are caused by clerical errors (Boone et al., 1995). When a discrepancy is noted during the verification procedure, *do not administer the product.* Notify the blood bank and appropriate personnel as indicated by agency policy.

a. Check client's first and last names by having the client state name, if able. Also check client's identification number and date of birth on arm band and client record.
b. Record the verification process as directed by agency policy.
c. Verify that the component received from the blood bank is the component ordered by the physician.
d. Check that the client's blood type and Rh type are compatible with the donor blood type and Rh type.
e. Check that the unit number on the unit of blood and on the form from the blood bank match.
f. Check the expiration date and time on the unit of blood.
g. Check the appearance of the blood product.
   Air bubbles, clots or discoloration may indicate bacterial contamination or inadequate anticoagulation of the stored component and would be contraindications for transfusion of that product.

3. Empty urine drainage collection container or have client void.
   If a transfusion reaction occurs, a urine specimen containing urine produced after initiation of the transfusion will be sent to the lab.

ADMINISTRATION

1. Wash hands and apply clean, disposable gloves.
   Utilizing standard precautions reduces risk for transmission of microorganisms.

2. Open blood administration set.
   a. For single tubing administration, set roller clamp to "off" position.
   Moving roller clamps to off position prevents accidental spilling and wasting of product.
   b. For Y tubing set all three roller clamps to off position.

3. Prepare blood component for administration.

a. For Single-Tubing Administration

(1) Invert blood component bag gently, 2 to 3 times.
   Equally distributes cells throughout preservative solution.
(2) Spike blood component unit.
(3) Squeeze drip chamber, allowing filter to fill with blood.
(4) Open roller clamp slowly, and allow infusion tubing to fill with blood.
(5) Close roller clamp when tubing is filled with blood.
   Priming the tubing removes air from the system.
(6) Piggyback infusion of 0.9% saline IV solution to the single tubing blood administration set using a stopcock or needleless valve.
   Needle use should be minimized when infusing blood products since fragile blood cells can be damaged if forced through a needle. Also avoids risk of needlestick.

CRITICAL DECISION POINT Normal saline is used to prevent coagulation of the product. Solutions that contain dextrose will cause coagulation of donor blood.

STEPS | **RATIONALE**

b. For Y Tubing (see illustration)

Y tubing is used to facilitate maintenance of IV access in case a client will need more than 1 unit of blood. When utilizing Y tubing, normal saline can be easily infused following each transfusion (follow manufacturer's guidelines regarding the number of units that can be given before tubing must be changed).

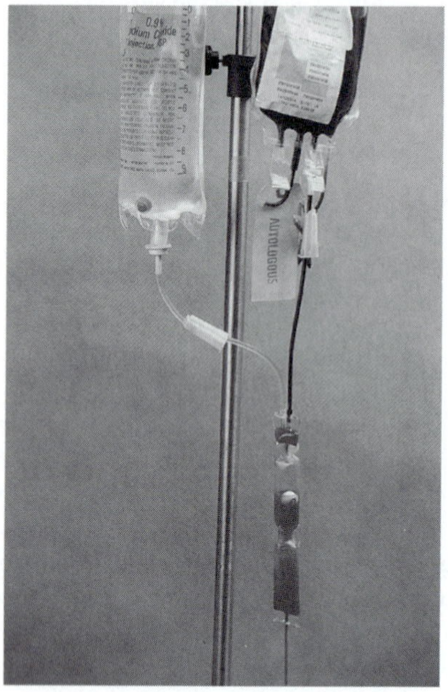

Step 3b Blood administration setup with Y tubing.

(1) Spike 0.9% normal saline IV bag.

(2) Open roller clamp on tubing attached to saline bag.

Having both roller clamps open will prime the tubing with saline. Priming the tubing removes air from the system.

(3) Squeeze drip chamber, allowing saline to cover the filter.

(4) Open roller clamp on common tubing.

(5) Close the lower roller clamp (the clamp on the common tubing) after the tubing is filled with saline.

This will prevent spilling or wasting of saline.

(6) Gently invert the blood component bag 2 to 3 times.

This will equally distribute the cells throughout the preservative solution.

(7) Spike and hang the blood component bag.

(8) Close the roller clamp leading from the saline bag to the drip chamber.

This will prevent blood from backing up into the saline bag.

(9) Open the roller clamp leading from the blood component bag to the drip chamber.

(10) Squeeze drip chamber, allowing blood to enter.

4. Maintaining asepsis, attach the primed tubing to the IV catheter. Open lower clamp.

This initiates the infusion of blood product into the client's vein.

5. Remain with client during the first 5 to 15 minutes of a transfusion. Initial flow rate during this time should be 2 ml/min.

CRITICAL DECISION POINT **Most transfusion reactions occur within the first 5 to 15 minutes of a transfusion. Infusing a small amount of blood component initially minimizes the volume of blood to which the client is exposed, thereby minimizing the severity of a reaction.**

STEPS	RATIONALE
6. Monitor client's vital signs 5 minutes after the blood product has begun infusing and per agency policy after that.	Frequent monitoring of vital signs will help to quickly alert the nurse to a transfusion reaction.
7. Regulate the rate of transfusion according to physician's orders. (The drop factor for blood tubing is 10 drops/ml.)	Maintaining the prescribed rate of flow decreases the risk of fluid volume excess while restoring vascular volume.
➤ ***CRITICAL DECISION POINT*** **A unit of blood should not hang for more than 4 hours because of the danger of bacterial growth.**	
8. After blood has infused, clear IV tubing with 0.9% normal saline and discard blood bag according to agency policy.	Infusing IV saline solution infuses the remainder of the blood in the IV tubing.
9. Appropriately dispose of all supplies. Remove gloves and wash hands.	Standard precautions during a transfusion reduce transmission of microorganisms.

EVALUATION

1. Monitor IV site and status of infusion each time vital signs are taken.	Detects the presence of infiltration or phlebitis, and verifies continuous and safe infusion of blood product.
2. Observe for any changes in vital signs, and for chills, flushing, itching, dyspnea, rash, or other signs of transfusion reaction.	These may be early signs of a transfusion reaction (see Table 21-1).
3. Observe client and assess laboratory values to determine response to administration of blood component.	This aids in determining whether the goals of therapy have been reached or if further blood component therapy will be required.
4. **Unexpected outcomes** that may occur include:	
➤ Client displays signs and symptoms of a transfusion reaction (see Table 21-1).	Occurs when donor blood is incompatible with recipient's blood or when the recipient has a sensitivity to a plasma protein in the transfused (donor's) blood.
➤ Client develops infiltration or phlebitis at venipuncture site.	Requires removal of IV line and insertion of new IV catheter in a different site.
➤ Rate of infusion slows in the absence of infiltration.	The blood component may be too viscous. The line may need to be gently flushed with normal saline, or a pressure bag may be used to increase the rate of flow of the product.

RECORDING AND REPORTING

1. Record type of blood component and amount administered, along with client's response to the therapy. This may be documented on the transfusion record itself or in your nurse's notes, depending on policy.	Documents component given and client's response.
2. Report signs and symptoms of a transfusion reaction immediately.	This will ensure prompt treatment of the reaction.

FOLLOW-UP ACTIVITIES

1. In the event of a transfusion reaction follow Table 21-1.
2. In the event of fluid overload:
   a. Slow or stop transfusion, elevate head of bed and inform physician of physical findings.
   b. Administer diuretics, morphine, oxygen as ordered by physician.
   c. Continue to closely monitor vital signs, intake and output.

STEPS | **RATIONALE**

3. In the event of infiltration or phlebitis at venipuncture site:
   a. Stop transfusion and discontinue infiltrated IV line.
   b. Obtain IV access at new venipuncture site.
   c. Restart transfusion if remainder of product can be infused within 4 hours of initiation of transfusion.
   d. Institute nursing measures to reduce discomfort at infiltrated or infected site.
4. Continue to monitor client's laboratory values to evaluate whether further blood component therapy may be necessary.

• • • • •

Special Considerations

- Saline solution should remain until transfusion is completed to flush line of blood or to keep IV line patent for supportive measures in case of a transfusion reaction.
- Never inject any medication into an IV line with a blood component infusing because of possible incompatibility with or bacterial contamination of the blood product.
- When clients require rapid transfusion of multiple units of blood products, the infusion tubing may be hung through a special blood warmer. Heating of the unit of blood itself (e.g., in a microwave or under hot water) is strongly discouraged because these methods can cause destruction of the cells.
- Rapid transfusion of cold blood through a central line is discouraged because it may cause ventricular dysrhythmias.
- If a client is bleeding severely, a pump with special blood tubing may be used to increase the flow rate of a blood product during transfusion.

Teaching Considerations

- Instruct client regarding the rationale for the transfusion and the anticipated amount of time for completion of transfusion.
- Discuss with client and family the rationale for frequent vital sign monitoring throughout transfusion.
- Inform client and family to notify nurse in case of itching, swelling, dizziness, dyspnea, low back pain, or chest pain.
- Instruct client to inform nurse if signs or symptoms of infiltration are present.
- Client and care giver should be instructed regarding signs and symptoms of long-term transfusion reactions (e.g., delayed hemolytic reaction) so that they can report them and receive treatment if necessary.

Pediatric Considerations

- The first 50 ml of a blood transfusion should be run very slowly in a pediatric client, and the nurse should stay with the child for that time (Wong, 1995).

Gerontologic Considerations

- Elderly clients may have decreased cardiac function, thus requiring a slower infusion time. Half-units may be obtained if a client is unable to tolerate the volume in a whole unit of blood or blood component.

Home Care Considerations

- Clients who have had prior transfusion reactions, acute angina, or congestive heart failure are not considered good candidates for home transfusion.
- If blood is given in the home setting, the nurse must follow meticulous cross-check procedures to ensure proper administration of the correct product.
- The transfusion must be initiated as soon as possible after the component is obtained from the blood bank. It should be transported in an insulated container with ice. The blood bank will determine the appropriate temperature.
- The nurse must plan for the client to have nursing personnel present during the entire transfusion process and for 30 to 60 minutes posttransfusion.
- When the blood sample is obtained for blood typing and cross-matching, an identity band should be attached to the client, with full name and identification number used by the laboratory. This provides clear identification of the client when the blood component transfusion is initiated.
- Home health agency policies and procedures should address legal implications, educational preparation of the nurse, client assessment, blood storage and transport, disposal of biohazardous material, and emergency procedures.

SKILL 21-2 Assisting with Autologous Blood Transfusion

Autologous blood transfusion is the collection and reinfusion of a client's own blood. The blood for an autologous blood transfusion can be obtained by preoperative donation when the surgery can be planned in advance (for example, open heart, orthopedic, plastic, or gynecologic procedures). The client may donate 1 to 5 units of blood, depending on the type of surgery and the client's ability to maintain an acceptable hematocrit. Acute infection is a contraindication to blood donation for autologous transfusion, just as it is for homologous transfusion. The autologous blood is tested for human immunodeficiency virus (HIV) and hepatitis B virus (HBV), just as homologous blood is tested. A person may donate blood on a schedule agreed upon by the client and physician. Typically a client will donate once a week, provided that his or her hematocrit remains above 33% and/or the hemoglobin is 11 g/dl. It is also recommended that donations be discontinued more than 72 hours prior to surgery (American Association of Blood Banks, 1995). A unit of RBCs can be stored for 35 to 42 days and can be stored frozen for several years, depending upon the rationale and the storage space available in the institution's blood bank.

An autologous transfusion can also be obtained through perioperative blood salvage. In this case a client undergoes a procedure (e.g., an orthopedic or vascular procedure) where there is significant blood loss into a space that can be drained for the purpose of reinfusion. (Arlington, Costigan, and Aievoli, 1992).

During intraoperative salvage, collection systems can reinfuse the blood directly or wash and spin the blood to increase the hematocrit and remove clotting factors, which eliminates the need for anticoagulation before reinfusion.

Postoperative salvage and infusion can be either continuous or intermittent, depending on the equipment used (Fig. 21-1). The client's blood is removed through tubes from the site of bleeding and filtered before reinfusion, and an anticoagulant such as heparin, acid citrate dextrose, or CPD may be used to prevent blood clots. The blood must be reinfused within 6 hours of the beginning of collection when an intermittent system is used, and if more than 50% of the client's total blood volume is reinfused, replacement of clotting factors is necessary.

There are several advantages to autologous transfusions. Autologous transfusions are safer for the client because they eliminate the risk of incompatibility reactions (except those due to clerical errors) and exposure to bloodborne infectious agents (except for bacterial contamination). When preoperative donation is used, the need to carefully identify the blood unit and the client is as important as it is for a homologous (donated by another person) transfusion. Otherwise the advantages are negated. When perioperative blood salvage is used, the same advantages are present. Additionally, the transfusion contains more viable red blood cells than does stored blood, its pH is normal, and there is a higher level of 2,3-diphosphoglycerate (2,3-DPG; a chemical that increases the oxygen-carrying capacity of hemoglobin) (Peterson, 1992). Another advantage of autologous transfusions is the conservation of the blood supply, especially if the client has a rare blood type.

A

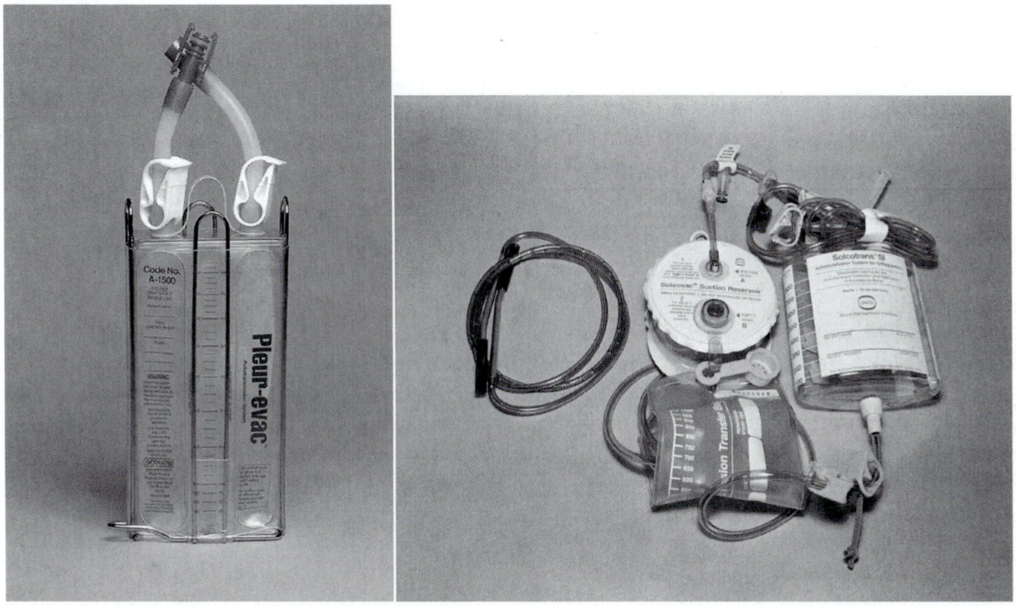

B

Fig. 21-1 **A,** Pleur-evac thoracic autotransfusion device. **B,** *Solcotrans* orthopedic autotransfusion device.

EQUIPMENT

- Cell saver or continuous or intermittent collection container and tubing
- 0.9% normal saline IV solution
- Anticoagulant, if needed
- Transfer bag and tubing
- Label
- Disposable gloves

STEPS	RATIONALE
ASSESSMENT	
1. Verify that the IV catheter to be used is 18-gauge or larger and that it is patent.	Larger catheters promote optimal flow of blood components and guard against hemolysis. Infiltration or signs of infection at the site contraindicates the use of that line for blood therapy. Another IV access would need to be initiated, and the infected or infiltrated line discontinued.
2. Verify blood product and client identification once blood is obtained (Skill 21-1).	
3. Obtain and record vital signs immediately prior to initiation of the transfusion.	Clients requiring **autotransfusion** are experiencing excessive blood loss, and hemodynamic status may be labile. It is important to be aware of baseline vital signs so that any deterioration in status may be quickly treated.
4. Assess client's level of comfort prior to initiating autotransfusion.	Pain increases oxygen demand. When RBCs are depleted, the body's ability to meet that demand is reduced. The client may need to be medicated for comfort to decrease the metabolic demand.
5. Assess client's understanding of the procedure and the rationale.	Clarifying the client's need for and the associated benefits of the therapy may alleviate some of the anxiety the client may have regarding this procedure.

NURSING DIAGNOSIS

Clustering of defining characteristics from the assessment data may reveal the following nursing diagnoses for clients requiring this skill:

- Altered tissue perfusion
- Decreased cardiac output
- Fluid volume deficit
- Knowledge deficit regarding benefits and risks of autotransfusion

Related factors are individualized based on a client's condition or needs.

STEPS	RATIONALE
PLANNING	
1. **Expected outcomes** following completion of procedure	
➤ Cardiac output returns to baseline.	
➤ Mucous membranes are pink and moist.	
➤ Capillary refill is brisk.	
➤ Urine output is ½ to 1 ml/kg/hr.	
➤ Client's systolic blood pressure is greater than 100 mm Hg.	Parameters reflect improved intravascular volume.
➤ Client will verbalize understanding of rationale for therapy.	Instruction is focused on purpose, benefits, and risks.
2. Explain procedure to client and family. Have client sign necessary consent forms.	Informed consent is necessary prior to a transfusion.
IMPLEMENTATION	
1. Wash hands and put on appropriate attire:	Reduces transmission of microorganisms and prevents exposure from splashes of blood.
a. Intraoperative: surgical garb as appropriate (see Chapter 36).	

STEPS	RATIONALE
b. Postoperative: disposable gloves; gown and goggles if necessary.	
2. Connect drainage tubes to collection container or cell processing system. Minimize air bubbles by establishing secure connections. Follow agency and manufacturer's procedure for setup and maintenance of system.	Allows collection of client's blood for reinfusion, storage (no longer than 6 hours), or washing and spinning.
3. Follow procedure outlined in Skill 21-1 for implementation of administration of autologous transfusion.	

EVALUATION

1. Observe client and laboratory values to determine response to administration of autologous blood transfusion.	Improvement in client's vital signs, cardiac output, tissue perfusion, fluid balance, and hemoglobin and hematocrit levels are expected.
2. Monitor IV site and status of infusion each time vital signs are measured.	Detects infiltration or phlebitis, verifies maintenance of constant infusion of autologous blood.
3. **Unexpected outcomes** that may occur include:	
➤ Client displays signs and symptoms associated with decreased cardiac output: hypotension, tachycardia, cold skin, decreased urine output.	If blood loss is too rapid, client may require homologous blood transfusions.
➤ Infiltration or phlebitis at venipuncture site is present.	Requires removal of intravenous line and insertion of new IV catheter.
➤ Rate of infusion slows in the absence of infiltration.	The blood may be too viscous, and the line may need gentle flushing with normal saline.

RECORDING AND REPORTING

1. Record amount of blood received by autotransfusion and client's response to blood therapy.	Documents amount of blood lost, administration of blood, and client's response.
2. Report number of units infused at change-of-shift report.	Provides oncoming nursing personnel with an exact number of units transfused.
3. Report to physician any deterioration in cardiac status.	May require emergent therapy to control bleeding.

FOLLOW-UP ACTIVITIES

1. Decreased cardiac output:
   a. Ensure that transfusion is infusing at ordered rate so that rate of volume replacement is sufficient.
2. Infiltration at venipuncture site:
   a. Stop transfusion.
   b. Restart IV at new venipuncture site.
   c. Institute nursing measures to reduce discomfort at previous site.

• • • • •

Special Considerations

- ➤ Although threat of adverse reactions is reduced during autologous transfusion, client's baseline and serial vital signs should be recorded in nurse's notes or on appropriate form.
- ➤ Hemolytic reactions occur because blood sample, blood unit, or client was improperly identified. Proper identification is mandatory, and agency procedure should be followed.
- ➤ Autologous donors do not always have to meet all of the criteria required for homologous blood donation. The autologous donation is tested for evidence of viral infection (hepatitis, HIV) and may be found to be positive. There is not a universal recommendation concerning whether this blood should be discarded. One reason to discard the blood is to prevent its inadvertent release to an uninfected client.

- Another method used by clients as an alternative to anonymous homologous transfusion is the directed donation: a friend or relative donates blood specifically for a particular client's use. These donations must meet the same standards as any homologous blood donation. Disadvantages include overt and covert pressure to donate that can be placed on the potential donor. Also, potential donors may engage in behaviors that place them at high risk of hepatitis or HIV infections that they may be reluctant to admit. Directed donations are no safer than other homologous donations.
- Some states require that clients be informed about autologous donation prior to a procedure being initiated that may require a blood transfusion (e.g., total knee replacement).

SKILL 21-3 Monitoring for Transfusion Reactions

During the transfusion of blood products, a client is at risk for adverse reactions, particularly during the first 15 minutes. The nurse should remain with the client for that period, to assess vital signs and the client's physiological response. Selected transfusion reactions are described in Table 21-1.

A **transfusion reaction** is a systemic response to the administration of a blood product incompatible with that of the recipient, containing allergens to which the recipient is sensitive or allergic, or contaminated with bacteria.

Several types of adverse reactions may result from a blood transfusion. General adverse reactions (see Table 21-1) may have symptoms ranging from fever, chills, and skin rash to hypotension and cardiac arrest. A client may also experience a delayed reaction, which will not manifest itself for days or weeks.

Other possible adverse outcomes that may result from transfusion therapy include circulatory overload and transmission of diseases such as malaria, hepatitis, cytomegalovirus, or HIV. Currently all units of blood undergo extensive serological testing, thereby minimizing the risk of acquiring a blood-borne disease.

STEPS	RATIONALE
ASSESSMENT	
1. Observe for fever with or without chills.	Fever may be indicative of the onset of an acute hemolytic reaction, febrile nonhemolytic reaction, graft-versus-host disease, or bacterial sepsis.
2. Observe client for tachycardia and/or tachypnea and dyspnea.	May indicate an acute hemolytic reaction or circulatory overload. These symptoms may be accompanied by a cough in the case of circulatory overload.
3. Observe client for hives or a skin rash.	These may be early indications of an urticarial reaction, anaphylaxis, or graft-versus-host disease. Itching would also be present with an urticarial reaction.
4. Observe client for flushing.	Flushing may be present in an acute hemolytic reaction or a febrile nonhemolytic reaction. Localized flushing may be present with an urticarial reaction.
5. Observe the client for gastrointestinal symptoms.	Nausea and vomiting may be present in acute hemolytic transfusion reactions, anaphylactic reactions, or sepsis. Diarrhea may be present in graft-versus-host disease or sepsis.
6. Observe the client for a fall in blood pressure.	Hypotension may be indicative of an acute hemolytic reaction, anaphylaxis, or sepsis.
7. Observe the client for wheezing, chest pain, and (ultimately) cardiac arrest.	These are all indications of an anaphylactic reaction.
8. Be alert to client complaints of headache or muscle pain in the presence of a fever.	Both may be indicative of a febrile nonhemolytic reaction.
9. Observe client for disseminated intravascular coagulation, renal failure, and hemoglobinemia/hemoglobinuria.	All are late signs of an acute hemolytic reaction.

STEPS	RATIONALE
10. Auscultate client's lungs, and monitor central venous pressure, if possible.	Crackles in the bases of the lungs and a rising central venous pressure (CVP) are indications of circulatory overload.
11. Observe client for jaundice and signs and symptoms of liver failure and bone marrow suppression.	These are indicative of graft-versus-host disease.
12. Observe client's laboratory values for anemia refractory to transfusion therapy.	This could signify a delayed hemolytic reaction.
13. Observe the client receiving massive transfusions. Client may be at risk for mild hypothermia, cardiac dysrhythmias, hypotension, and hypocalcemia.	Cold blood products can affect the cardiac conduction system, resulting in ventricular dysrhythmia. Other cardiac dysrhythmias, hypotension, and tingling may indicate hypocalcemia, which occurs when citrate (used as a preservative for some blood products) combines with the client's calcium.

NURSING DIAGNOSIS

Clustering of defining characteristics from the assessment data may reveal the following nursing diagnoses for clients requiring this skill:

- Anxiety
- Decreased cardiac output
- Fluid volume excess
- Hyperthermia
- Hypothermia
- Impaired gas exchange
- Pain

Related factors are individualized based on a client's condition or needs.

PLANNING

1. Expected outcomes following completion of procedure:	
➤ Client will have pink mucous membranes and brisk capillary refill. ➤ Client's cardiac output will return to baseline. ➤ Client will maintain core body temperature of 97° to 99° F. ➤ Client will have urine output of 0.5 to 1 ml/kg/hr. ➤ Client will maintain systolic blood pressure of 100 mm Hg or greater. ➤ Client will maintain oxygen saturation of greater than 95%. ➤ Client will be comfortable and calm.	Clinical signs indicate restored vascular volume and no transfusion reaction.
2. Explain treatment of a reaction to client and family.	

IMPLEMENTATION

In the Event of Transfusion Reaction:

1. Stop the transfusion.	Severity of reaction is related to the amount of component infused. (In the event of an urticarial reaction, the transfusion should be stopped and an antihistamine administered per the physician's order. The transfusion may then be restarted per physician's order. See Table 21-1.)
2. Remove tubing containing blood product and replace it with new tubing (see Chapter 20), except as noted above, in the case of urticaria.	Prevents the blood in the tubing from being infused.
3. Maintain patent IV line using 0.9% normal saline.	Medications and fluids will need to be administered for certain reactions.
4. Notify the physician and the blood bank.	Transfusion reactions require immediate medical intervention. The blood bank will have a procedure to follow when notified of a transfusion reaction.

STEPS	RATIONALE
5. Obtain blood samples (if needed) from the arm opposite the transfusion. Check agency policy regarding the number and type of tubes to be used.	Typically, one tube of blood will be crossmatched to the pretransfusion sample to ensure that correct blood was given to the recipient, and the blood will be checked for antibodies to determine the type of reaction. A second blood sample will be checked for free hemoglobin in the serum, indicating hemolysis, and a bilirubin level should be obtained.
6. Return remainder of blood component and attached blood tubing to the blood bank.	A sample of this blood will be crossmatched to the client's pretransfusion and posttransfusion samples to determine if an error in crossmatching occurred.
7. Monitor and document client's vital signs every 15 minutes or more frequently if needed.	Maintain ongoing assessment of client's cardiopulmonary status.
8. Administer prescribed medications according to type and severity of transfusion reaction.	
a. Epinephrine	Stimulates sympathetic nervous system to relieve respiratory distress and combat vasodilation in anaphylaxis.
b. Antihistamine (e.g., diphenhydramine)	Parenteral antihistamine diminishes some aspects of allergic response. May also be ordered pretransfusion in some cases.
c. Antibiotics	Administered when bacterial contamination/sepsis is suspected.
d. Antipyretics/analgesics	Administered to relieve fever and discomfort in acute hemolytic reactions, febrile nonhemolytic reactions, graft-versus-host disease, and bacterial sepsis.
e. Diuretics/morphine	May be administered in circulatory overload to reduce intravascular volume and decrease vascular tone.
f. IV fluids	Rapid administration of IV fluids may help to counteract some of the symptoms of anaphylactic shock.
9. Initiate cardiopulmonary resuscitation if necessary (see Chapter 16).	Anaphylaxis can quickly lead to cardiopulmonary arrest. Prompt resuscitation may prevent complications.
10. Obtain first voided urine sample and send to laboratory. A catheter may need to be inserted to obtain the urine (see Chapter 43).	Hemoglobinuria occurs with acute hemolytic reactions. The degree of damage to the kidneys is influenced by the pH of the urine and the rate of urinary excretion. Attempts will be made to initiate diuresis and alkalinize the urine. If kidney damage is severe, dialysis may be required.

EVALUATION

1. Observe client to determine response to discontinuing transfusion or instituting measures to reduce transfusion reaction.	Provides continued monitoring of client's cardiopulmonary status and physiological response.
2. **Unexpected outcome** that may occur is: ➤ Client's physiological status worsens.	Client's physiological status may worsen with severe transfusion reactions and can progress to cardiac arrest.

RECORDING AND REPORTING

1. Immediately report presence of transfusion reaction and client's physical assessment findings to nurse in charge and physician.	The assistance of an additional nurse will aid in administering prompt nursing care. Quickly alerting the physician ensures prompt medical attention.
2. Record exact time of transfusion reaction, assessment findings, nursing and medical actions taken.	Documents presence of transfusion reaction and treatment administered.

FOLLOW-UP ACTIVITIES

1. Maintain patent IV access.
2. Continue to monitor client's vital signs and assess physiological status.

Special Considerations

- Some physicians may order antihistamines and antipyretics to be given prior to initiation of transfusion to reduce the incidence or severity of febrile nonhemolytic reactions.
- Fatalities from transfusion reactions must be reported to the Food and Drug Administration by the agency.
- Sepsis and other infections due to blood transfusion should be reported to your agency's infection control department, which will then communicate that information to the state health department and the Centers for Disease Control and Prevention.

Teaching Considerations

- Clients and care givers should be taught the signs and symptoms of transfusion reactions, and the steps to be taken should they occur.

Pediatric Considerations

- A premature infant who receives blood transfusions is at high risk for graft-versus-host disease, because the immature immune system cannot adequately recognize and respond to foreign lymphocytes. RBCs with leukocytes removed are preferable in this case (Wong, 1995).

Gerontologic Considerations

- Elderly clients may have decreased cardiac function and are therefore more likely to develop circulatory overload than younger clients.

Home Care Considerations

- Certain adverse outcomes (development of hepatitis) or transfusion reactions (delayed hemolysis) occur days to weeks after a client has received the transfusion and may become evident in the home setting. It is important that client, family, and home health care workers are aware of the signs and symptoms of these adverse occurrences.

CRITICAL THINKING EXERCISES

1. A 45-year-old client, Mr. Canseco, is bleeding significantly from an abdominal wound. His blood pressure is 86/46 and his skin is cool and clammy. You and another nurse check the information on the bag of blood obtained from the blood bank with the information on the client's record and find the information below. What should you do?
   Name: John Smyth
   Room number: 352-1
   ID number: 123-45-67a
   Blood type: A-Pos.
2. You check a transfusion after it has been hanging for 45 minutes and find that the rate of infusion of PRBCs is slower than ordered. Which actions should you perform first?
3. Ten minutes after a transfusion of PRBCs was begun, your 26-year-old female client states she has a headache and feels tightness in her chest. What is the first thing you should do?

REFERENCES

American Association of Blood Banks: *Tech Man*, ed 11, 1995.

American Red Cross: Transfusion medicine update, *Blood Compon Ther* 3(1):, 1995.

Arlington R, Costigan K, and Aievoli C: Postoperative orthopaedic blood salvage and reinfusion, *Orthoped Nurs* 11(3):30, 1992.

Boone DJ et al: Transfusion medicine monitoring practices, *Arch Pathol and Lab Medicine* 119:999, 1995.

Kim MJ, McFarland GK, McLane AM: *Pocket guide to nursing diagnoses*, ed 7, St Louis, 1997, Mosby.

McKenry L, Salerno E: *Mosby's pharmacology in nursing*, ed 19, St Louis, 1995, Mosby.

Peterson K: Nursing management of autologous blood transfusion, *J Intraven Nurs* 15(3):128, 1992.

Wong DL: *Nursing care of infants and children*, ed 5, St Louis, 1995, Mosby.

ADDITIONAL READING

Baranowski L: Current trends in blood component therapy: the evolution of a safer, more effective product, *J Intraven Nurs* 15(3):136, 1992.

Carstens VL, Earnshaw MB: Postoperative orthopedic autotransfusion: successful management for the total knee arthroplasty patient, *AORN Journal* 56(2):272, 1992.

Gerber L: Autologous blood transfusion: why and how, *J Intraven Nurs*, 17(2):65, 1994.

Johnson GM, Bowman RJ: Autologous blood transfusion: current trends, nursing implications, *AORN Journal*, 56(2):282, 1992.

Murdock MA, Roberson ML: Reported use of autotransfusion systems in initial resuscitation areas by one hundred thirty-six United States hospitals, *J Emerg Nurs* 19(6):486, 1993.

Potter P, Perry A: *Fundamentals of nursing: concepts, process, and practice*, ed 4, St Louis, 1997, Mosby.

UNIT VIII

Nutrition

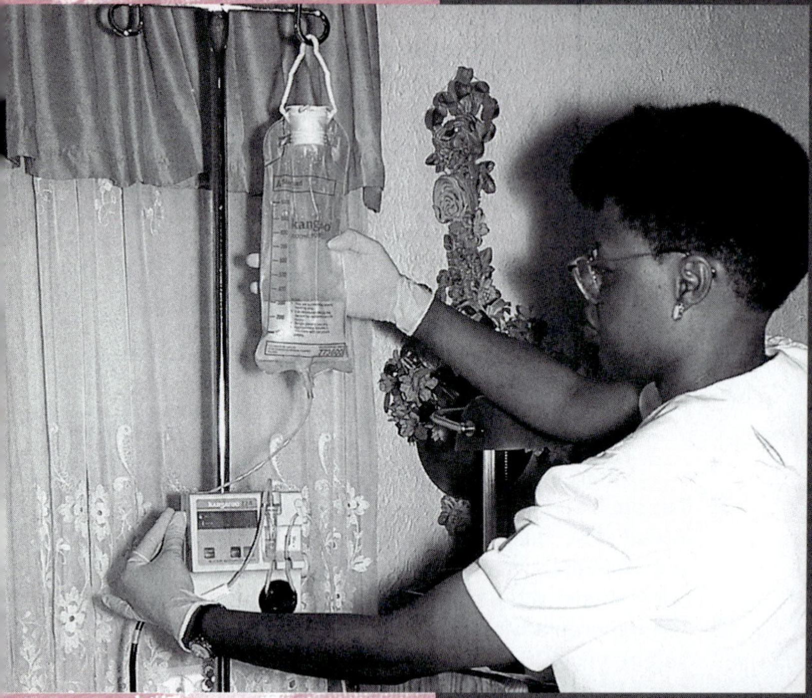

CHAPTER 22

Oral Nutrition

OBJECTIVES

Mastery of content in this chapter will enable the nurse to:

- Define key terms.
- Perform accurate nutritional assessment.
- Identify clients appropriate for nutritional assessment.
- Assess clients' ability to swallow and proper positioning before feeding.
- Provide mouth care after feeding a client.
- Demonstrate how to properly feed the client who cannot self-feed.
- Prepare the client to receive appropriate meals.
- Evaluate the client's tolerance of oral nutrition.
- Identify the client at risk for aspiration related to dysphagia.

KEY TERMS

Anthropometrics	Gag reflex
Aspiration	Kilograms
Basal energy expenditure (BEE)	Malnutrition
Bolus	Midarm circumference
Dysphagia	Prealbumin
Full liquid diet	Triceps skinfold

SKILLS

Nutritional status for clients of any age reflects general health and can affect rate of recovery from procedures, surgery, or illness. When a client with a functional GI tract is unable to obtain adequate oral nutrition, nutritional status can be compromised. A nurse's role may include performing nutritional assessment to determine if the client is already malnourished or at risk of becoming malnourished, feeding an adult client who cannot self-feed, and identifying a client who is at risk of aspiration during oral feeding.

Nutritional assessment includes collection of objective and subjective data that relate to nutritional status (see box on p. 728). No single biochemical test, such as serum albumin, can accurately indicate poor nutrition, but collectively biochemical tests, measurements of height and weight, and dietary histories can accurately reflect the client's nutritional status. Nurses can work with the registered dietitian to complete a nutritional assessment. Because nursing care involves frequent client contact, nurses who understand nutritional assessment can readily assess nutritional problems and evaluate the adequacy of the nutritional plan of care.

Adults usually eat independently, but they may need to be fed in the presence of physical or cognitive limitations. For example, neurological, neuromuscular, or orthopedic problems can impair a client's ability to manipulate feeding utensils. Clients' loss of independence and control when fed by another person can lead to psychological problems and depression. It is important for the nurse to understand the psychological and social impact of altered ability to self-feed and to give the client as much choice and independence as possible.

Dysphagia (difficulty swallowing) is the most common cause of aspiration in adults during oral feeding. Dysphagia can be caused by neurological and neuromuscular diseases and by trauma to or surgical procedures of the oral cavity or throat. The nurse should suspect the presence of dysphagia when the client coughs or gags during eating,

COMPONENTS OF A NUTRITIONAL ASSESSMENT

History
- Swallowing, gastrointestinal, and elimination symptoms
- Functional status
- Social support
- Psychological status
- Ability to purchase food

Physical Assessment
- Height
- Weight
- Usual weight
- Ideal body weight
- Frame size
- Anthropometrics, such as triceps skinfold, midarm circumference, and midarm muscle circumference

Biochemical Parameters
- Serum proteins, such as albumin, **prealbumin,** transferrin, retinol binding protein
- Nitrogen balance
- Delayed cutaneous hypersensitivity (skin tests)
- Resting energy expenditure

Dietary History
- 24-hour food recall
- Food frequency questionnaire

exhibits multiple attempts at swallowing, complains of food "getting stuck" in the throat, or has poor lip and tongue control. **Aspiration** of food can lead to pneumonia. Nursing interventions for the dysphagic client can help to avoid aspiration.

GUIDELINES

1. Be aware of clients who are at risk for malnutrition. The nurse can provide preventive care and seek appropriate resources for intervention.
2. Be aware of the signs and symptoms of malnutrition (see Table 22-2, p. 731). Clients who are not thin and visibly malnourished may still have nutritional problems (e.g., the obese client with adequate fat reserves but depleted circulating protein reserves). Nutritional care should be provided for all clients.
3. Use a systematical and organized approach to nutritional assessment. This allows the nurse to obtain complete, essential information without being redundant.
4. Be aware of the client's social history. Clients may be interested in healthy nutritional practices but may be unable to implement them (e.g., no refrigeration at home, lack of money to buy food or infant formula). The nurse needs to be aware of limitations and work with the client toward realistic goals.
5. Review the client's medical history. Certain diseases, medications, and medical problems can influence nutritional status. Clients with some medical problems or nonfunctioning GI tracts cannot be treated with oral nutrition. Parenteral therapies may be necessary (American Society for Parenteral and Enteral Nutrition, 1995).
6. Verify that the type of feeding ordered is what has been provided to the client. Knowledge of the different types of oral diets helps the nurse properly plan and recommend changes to meet client needs.
7. Promote factors that improve client's appetite such as pleasant and comfortable surroundings and an attractive meal presentation.
8. An organized approach when feeding a client of any age helps the client feel more at ease, and appetite may increase in an unhurried atmosphere.
9. Be aware of the psychological impact on the adult client who cannot self-feed. Feeding in an unhurried, understanding manner that allows maximal client independence can lessen the negative aspects of being fed by someone else. Instruct family members to provide an unhurried, social atmosphere when feeding the client and to allow the client to be as independent in feeding as possible. Assistive devices may enable the client to perform self-care.
10. Recognize symptoms such as coughing, gagging, multiple swallow attempts, or complaints of difficulty swallowing that may indicate dysphagia with aspiration.

SKILL 22-1 Performing Nutritional Assessment

Nutritional assessment is a specific, measurable means of identifying clients who may be malnourished. Clients may be assessed for a variety of reasons, including having diagnoses associated with nutrition problems (such as gastrointestinal problems, trauma, burns, sepsis, or malabsorption), recent rapid weight loss, or history of poor dietary intake. The Joint Commission for Accreditation of Healthcare Organizations (JCAHO) standards now require the identification of clients who are nutritionally at risk by means of an initial screening mechanism (JCAHO, 1996). Clients who are identified to be at risk should have a nutritional assessment.

Four components of nutritional assessment are evaluated: (1) client history (medical, psychological, and social);

(2) physical examination, which may include anthropometrics; (3) biochemical parameters; and (4) dietary history. Elements of the client history give background to factors influencing current nutritional status. The medical history indicates medications, surgery, and coexisting medical conditions compromising nutrition. Depression or abnormal psychiatric behavior leading to decreased food intake can be identified in the psychological history. A social history can give important insight into beliefs, the financial ability to obtain food, and food customs influencing nutrition. Assessment of dietary intake by sample menus, eating habits, or 24-hour recall can indicate food practices or avoidance of food groups that may impair nutritional status. A physical examination can also indicate impaired nutrition. Evaluation of body size, weight, and muscle wasting is accomplished through the use of **anthropometrics.** These can include measurements such as wrist circumference for body frame size, **midarm circumference** (MAC), and **triceps skinfold** (TSF) to measure muscle and fat reserves. Finally, biochemical parameters are evaluated that reflect the status of circulating proteins.

Nutritional assessment goals as outlined by the American Society of Parenteral and Enteral Nutrition (ASPEN, 1995) include the following:

1. Establish baseline subjective nutritional parameters.
2. Identify specific nutritional deficits.
3. Determine nutrition risk factors for individual clients.
4. Establish nutritional needs for individual clients.
5. Identify medical and psychosocial factors that may influence the prescription and administration of nutritional support.

EQUIPMENT

- **Assessment sheet and pen**
- **Tongue blade, stethoscope, penlight**
- **Scale**
- **Tape measure**
- **Lange Harpenden or Holtain skin calipers (optional—if anthropometric measurements are obtained)**

DELEGATION CONSIDERATIONS

The interpretation of data collected during a nutritional assessment is a skill that requires problem solving and knowledge application unique to a professional nurse, and delegation is inappropriate.

- Delegation of steps in data collection, such as obtaining height and weight or assisting the client to complete a 24-hour recall, may be appropriate.

STEPS	RATIONALE
ASSESSMENT	
1. Determine need to perform nutritional assessment based on diagnosis and history.	Certain conditions place the adult client at risk for malnutrition (see box below).
2. Assess client for usual body weight, noting changes (see Chapter 11).	
3. Review results of relevant laboratory tests (Table 22-1).	These biochemical parameters (tests ordered by physician) measure visceral and circulating protein status. Albumin and transferrin indicate visceral protein status. Total lymphocyte count (TLC) can reflect immunocompetence.

ADULTS AT NUTRITIONAL RISK

Actual or potential for developing malnutrition:

- Involuntary weight loss or gain of >10% of usual body weight within 6 months or >5% of usual body weight within 1 month
- >20% over or under ideal body weight
- Presence of chronic disease
- Increased metabolic requirements

Altered diets or diet schedules:

- Receiving parenteral or enteral nutrition
- Recent illness, surgery, or trauma

Inadequate nutrition intake including not receiving food or nutrition products for >7 days

From American Society for Parenteral and Enteral Nutrition (ASPEN): The 1995 ASPEN standards for nutrition support: hospitalized patients, *Nurs Care Pract* 10(6):208, 1995.

Table 22-1 Laboratory Tests for Nutritional Assessment

Laboratory Test	Normal Range	Implication of Abnormal Value
Serum albumin	3.5-4.5 mg/dl	Reflects liver's ability to synthesize plasma proteins; changes slowly
Transferrin	200-250 mg/dl	Main iron-storage protein; changes more rapidly than albumin
Prealbumin	15.7-29.6 mg/dl	Sensitive measure of visceral body protein
Urinary urea nitrogen	Positive balance when compared to nitrogen intake	$\text{Nitrogen balance} = \frac{\text{Protein intake}}{6.25} - 4$ A positive nitrogen intake indicates that nitrogen can be stored instead of broken down for energy
Hemoglobin	12-15 mg/dl	Anemia may be associated with **malnutrition**

STEPS	RATIONALE
4. Determine what medications client is taking (over-the-counter and prescribed).	Certain medications can inhibit or potentiate action of other medications. Also, medications and nutrients may interact to either decrease medication function (e.g., foods rich in vitamin K such as dark green vegetables and coumarin anticoagulants) or impair nutrient utilization (mineral oil laxatives). Nurses are expected to be aware of drug-drug and drug-nutrient interactions that may impair client care.

NURSING DIAGNOSIS

Clustering of defining characteristics from the assessment data may reveal the following nursing diagnoses for clients requiring this skill:

- Risk for aspiration
- Risk for fluid volume deficit
- Altered nutrition: more than body requirements
- Altered nutrition: less than body requirements
- Altered nutrition: risk for more than body requirements
- Feeding self-care deficit
- Knowledge deficit regarding nutritionally balanced diet
- Sensory/perceptual alterations (gustatory)
- Impaired swallowing

Related factors are individualized based on a client's condition or needs.

PLANNING

STEPS	RATIONALE
1. **Expected outcomes** following completion of procedure:	
➤ Client denies any gastric, swallowing, or chewing problems or food intolerances.	Indicates absence of gastric disturbance or food intolerance.
➤ Physical assessment and laboratory data are consistent with adequate nutritional status.	Indicates that client's nutritional intake is adequate to produce normal nutritional status.
2. Prepare equipment and supplies.	
3. Explain to client purpose for nutritional assessment.	Ensures client's participation in care.
4. Perform nutritional assessment in quiet, undistracting environment.	Helps nurse to better obtain needed information.

IMPLEMENTATION

STEPS	RATIONALE
1. Obtain complete and thorough nursing history, including social, economic, and psychological information (Chapter 11).	Allows nurse to determine client's nutritional baseline, potential problem areas, and current problems.
2. Either initiate diet diary or perform 24-hour recall interview. The use of food models may assist the client to recall portions more accurately.	Evaluates food consumption and eating habits.
3. Document findings on nutritional assessment sheet.	Prompt documentation prevents nurse from omitting essential information from late entry.
4. Assist client into bed.	Having client in bed facilitates physical assessment.

Table 22-2 Clinical Signs of Nutritional Status

Body Area	Signs of Good Nutrition	Signs of Poor Nutrition
General appearance	Alert, responsive	Listless, apathetic, cachectic
Weight	Normal for height, age, body build	Overweight or underweight (special concern for underweight)
Posture	Erect, arms and legs straight	Sagging shoulders, sunken chest, humped back
Muscles	Well-developed, firm, good tone, some fat under skin	Flaccid, poor tone, underdeveloped, tender, edematous, wasted appearance, cannot walk properly
Nervous control	Good attention span, not irritable or restless, normal reflexes, psychological stability	Inattentive, irritable, confused, burning and tingling of hands and feet (paresthesia), loss of position and vibratory sense, weakness and tenderness of muscles (may result in inability to walk), decrease or loss of ankle and knee reflexes, absent vibratory sense
Gastrointestinal function	Good appetite and digestion, normal regular elimination, no palpable organs or masses	Anorexia, indigestion, constipation or diarrhea, liver or spleen enlargement
Cardiovascular function	Normal heart rate and rhythm, no murmurs, normal blood pressure for age	Rapid heart rate (above 100 beats per minute) enlarged heart, abnormal rhythm, elevated blood pressure
General vitality	Endurance, energetic, sleeps well, vigorous	Easily fatigued, no energy, falls asleep easily, looks tired, apathetic
Hair	Shiny, lustrous, firm, not easily plucked, healthy scalp	Stringy, dull, brittle, dry, thin, and sparse, depigmented, can be easily plucked
Skin (general)	Smooth, slightly moist, good color	Rough, dry, scaly, pale, pigmented, irritated, bruises, petechiae, subcutaneous fat loss
Face and neck	Skin color uniform, smooth, healthy appearance, not swollen	Greasy, discolored, scaly, swollen, skin dark over cheeks and under eyes, lumpiness or flakiness of skin around nose and mouth
Lips	Smooth, good color, moist, not chapped or swollen	Dry, scaly, swollen, redness and swelling (cheilosis), or angular lesions at corners of the mouth, fissures or scars (stomatitis)
Mouth, oral membranes	Reddish pink mucous membranes in oral cavity	Swollen, boggy oral mucous membranes
Gums	Good pink color, healthy, red, no swelling or bleeding	Spongy, bleed easily, marginal redness, inflamed, gums receding
Tongue	Good pink color or deep reddish in appearance, not swollen or smooth, surface papillae present, no lesions	Swelling, scarlet and raw, magenta color, beefy (glossitis), hyperemic and hypertrophic papillae, atrophic papillae
Teeth	No cavities, no pain, bright, straight, no crowding, well-shaped jaw, clean, no discoloration	Unfilled caries, absent teeth, worn surfaces, mottled (fluorosis), malpositioned
Eyes	Bright, clear, shiny, no sores at corner of eyelids, membranes moist and healthy pink color, no prominent blood vessels or mound of tissue or sclera, no fatigue circles beneath	Eye membranes pale (pale conjunctivae), redness of membrane (conjunctival infection), dryness, signs of infection, Bitot's spots, redness and fissuring of eyelid corners (angular palpebritis), dryness of eye membrane (conjunctival xerosis), dull appearance of cornea (corneal xerosis), soft cornea (keratomalacia)
Neck (glands)	No enlargement	Thyroid enlargement
Nails	Firm, pink	Spoon shape (koilonychia), brittle, ridged
Legs, feet	No tenderness, weakness, or swelling; good color	Edema, tender calf, tingling, weakness
Skeleton	No malformations	Bowlegs, knock-knees, chest deformity at diaphragm, beaded ribs, prominent scapulas

Modified from Williams SR: Nutritional assessment and guidance in prenatal care. In Worthington-Roberts BS, Williams SR, editors: *Nutrition in pregnancy and lactation*, ed 5, St Louis, 1993, Mosby.

STEPS	RATIONALE
5. Perform physical assessment as described in Chapter 11.	Through use of physical assessment, nurse will be able to detect signs and symptoms of malnutrition (Table 22-2).
6. Assist client to standing position, and be sure client is free of restrictive clothing.	Clients must be standing for anthropometric measurements.
7. Have client stand on scale, or if client is unable to stand use chair, bed, or sling-type scales. Record weight; convert to **kilograms** (weight ÷ 2.2 = kg).	Weight is a useful index of client's state of nutrition. Ideally, client should be weighed with same scale at same time of day with same amount of clothing for comparison of weight changes over time.
8. Measure client's height. If client is unable to stand, measure from heel to top of head while lying flat on bed and record.	Correct height measurement assists in calculating ideal body weight.
9. Calculate, or determine via standard height and weight chart, ideal body weight (IBW) with a range for normal of 10% above and 10% below IBW. Calculation of IBW can be accomplished using the following formula: Male: 106 pounds (47.7 kg) for the first 5 feet, then add 6 pounds per additional inch (2.25 kg per 2.5 cm). Female: 100 pounds (45 kg) for the first 5 feet, then add 5 pounds per additional inch (2.25 kg per 2.5 cm).	Determination of IBW using a standard chart may require the calculation of frame size.
10. Using measuring tape, measure the smallest portion of wrist distal to styloid process (bony prominence at wrist) (see illustration).	Wrist circumference and height are used to calculate body frame size (Table 22-3).

➤ ***CRITICAL DECISION POINT*** **Additional anthropometric measurements are used in some settings. These measurements require some practice for accuracy and consistency. The measurements are most helpful for clients who will have a long-term episode of care. Single measurements on clients in acute care settings are of limited value.**

Table 22-3 **Calculation of Body Frame Size**

$$\text{Ratio} = \frac{\text{Height (cm)}}{\text{Wrist circumference (cm)}}$$

Frame Size	Values for Men	Values for Women
Small	10.4	11.0
Medium	9.6-10.4	10.1-11.0
Large	9.6	10.3

STEPS	RATIONALE
11. With client's nondominant arm relaxed, measure circumference at midpoint of arm in centimeters (between tip of acromial process of scapula and olecranon process of ulna) and record (see illustration). If client is bedridden, measurements may be taken with arm bent and placed across chest.	Mid–upper-arm circumference (MAC) estimates muscle wasting.
12. With thumb and forefinger, pinch a double fold of fat lengthwise about 1 cm above midpoint of MAC. With other hand, place teeth of calipers on either side of fat fold. Calipers are placed below fingers so pressure is exerted from calipers rather than fingers. Record three separate readings in mm and document (see illustration).	Skinfold measurements are used to estimate fat content of subcutaneous tissue (e.g., biceps, scapula, abdominal muscles). Triceps skinfold (TSF) is most common and easiest to measure. Average the three readings of TSF.
13. Assist client to comfortable position.	Remainder of assessment is composed of calculations and review of laboratory work.
14. Calculate midarm muscle circumference (MAMC) **(MAMC = MAC (cm) − [TSF (cm) × 3.14])** and record.	MAMC is estimation of skeletal muscle mass.

STEPS	RATIONALE
15. Wash hands.	Reduces transmission of microorganisms.
16. Explain to client that nutritional assessment is complete.	Allows time for client to ask questions about assessment.

EVALUATION

STEPS	RATIONALE
1. Review history and physical findings. Note abnormalities or areas of concern.	Completeness of data obtained from history and physical findings permits prompt interventions for nutritional alterations.
2. Discuss findings of diet history and 24-hour recall with client.	Determines status of dietary habits and client's knowledge.
3. Compare client's weight for height with ideal and usual weight.	Significant weight fluctuations or weight outside of normal range may indicate nutritional risk.
4. Review anthropometric data against normal measurements.	
5. Compare biochemical test levels with client's levels.	Abnormal values, when considered with other nutritional parameters, may indicate malnutrition.
6. Consult a dietitian to calculate client's caloric needs. A variety of formulas are available. Most commonly used formula is the Harris-Benedict equation for **basal energy expenditure (BEE).**	Provides timely identification of inadequate caloric intake in clients at risk for inadequate dietary intake.
7. Determine amount of protein client requires.	Protein based on ideal body weight in kg × 0.8 to 2.0 (normal to severe stress).
8. Determine route of nutrition (enteral [oral or tube] or parenteral).	If gastrointestinal tract functions, it should be used.
9. For parenteral nutrition (PN): the physician and dietitian will choose either peripheral or central PN, and determine whether fat is needed (see Chapter 24).	Parenteral nutrition and fat emulsion are necessary to promote and maintain nutritional balance during illness if GI tract is unavailable.

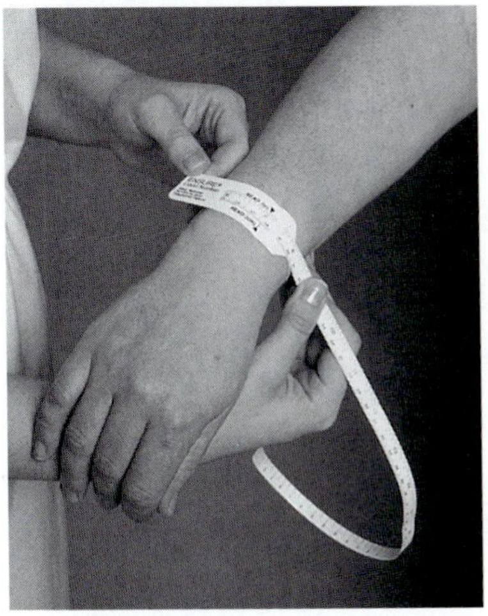

Step 10 Wrist circumference.

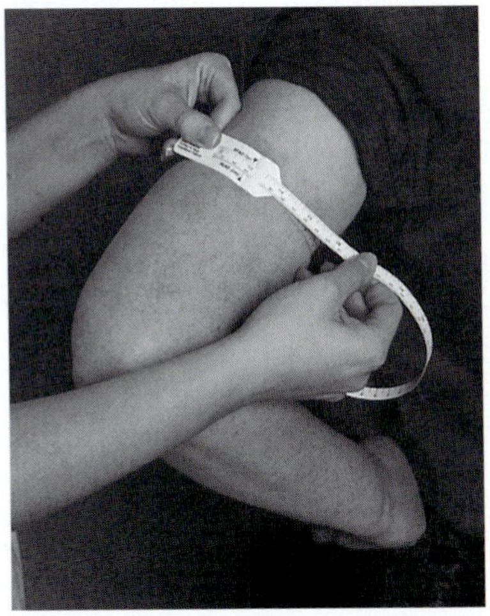

Step 11 Measurement of mid-upper arm circumference.

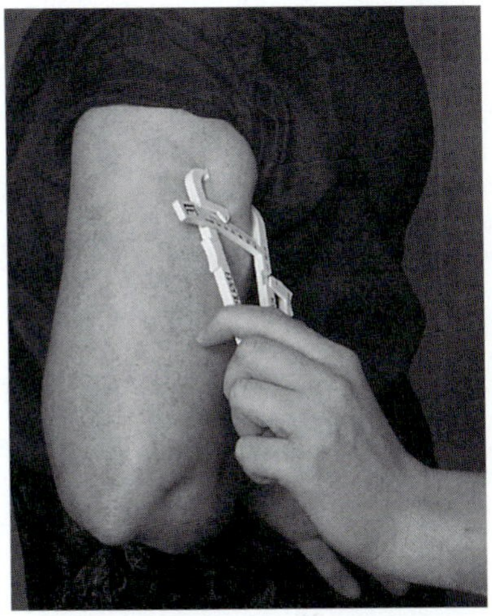

Step 12 Triceps skinfold.

Nutritional Assessment

Date 12/11 Admit Date 12/7

Unit No.

Name
Address

DOB

Client History:

Medical RADIATION ENTERITIS - CA
12/9 EXPLORATORY SURGERY
Social/Psych MILD DEPRESSION 2° DISEASE STATE
Diagnosis SMALL BOWEL OBSTRUCTION
Ht 183 cm Wt 71 Kg Usual Wt 82 Kg
%Change 13 IBW 80.9 (72.7 - 89)
Age 48 Sex (M) F

Drug Therapy ______ Insulin ______ Steriods
______ Narcotics ______ (Other:) ______
PROCHLORPERAZINE, FENTANYL

Contributing Factors:

✓ Fever ___ Infection/Sepsis
___ Dysphagia ✓ Emesis
___ Chewing Probs.
___ Polytrauma ___ Diarrhea
✓ Chemo/(Radiation)
✓ Surgery
___ Other ______

Anthropometrics:

Wrist Circum. 6 1/2"
MAC 28.5
TSF
1 11.8
2 11.4
3 11.6
Ave. 11.6

Estimation of Intake:

Less than requirements ✓
Meeting requirements ______
More than requirements ______
Gastointestinal Tract functional?
Yes ______ No ✓

Clinical/Lab Data:

	Normal		Mild		Moderate		Severe	
Albumin	>3.5		3.4-2.8		2.7-2.1	2.3	<2.1	
Total Lymph Count (TLC)	>1500		1499-1200		1199-800	1100	<800	
Transferrin	>200		199-150		149-100	138	<100	
% Usual Body Wt.	>95%		94-85%	86.5	84-75%		<74%	
% Ideal Body Wt.	>90%		89-80%	87.7	79-70%		<70%	
Skin Tests (#react./#placed)	4/4				1-2/4 (weak)	1/4	0/4 (anergic)	
Other ______								

Recomendations:

______ Calories/day ______ gm protein/day

Route: ______ enteral-oral ______ enteral-tube feeding ______ parenteral

______

Signature

Fig. 22-1

STEPS	RATIONAL
10. **Unexpected outcomes** that may occur include:	
➤ Body weight is below or above ideal body weight.	Indicates actual or potential malnourished status.
➤ Laboratory tests are not within normal limits.	

Recording and Reporting

1. Record results on nutritional assessment form, making recommendations to the dietician and documenting any significant differences from the norm (Fig. 22-1).	Timely documentation ensures accurate information.
2. Report unusual findings to nurse in charge or physician.	Enables early interventions to begin to correct nutritional alterations.

Follow-up Activities

1. Check weight weekly and assess for change. Report significant changes to physician.
2. Document significant changes in intake, especially if client is at risk of malnutrition.

• • • • •

Special Considerations

- Client or significant other should be reliable source of information for a dietary history.
- Both diet diary and 24-hour recall are effective methods for taking diet history. Diet diary is obtained over longer period and helps to determine food likes and dislikes, as well as allergies. The 24-hour recall is an account of everything the client has consumed over that period of time; it is less time consuming but not as accurate.
- To determine ideal body weight or percentage of change:

$$\% \text{ IBW} = \text{Actual weight} \times 100/\text{IBW}$$

or

$$\frac{\% \text{ Weight}}{\text{change}} = \frac{\text{Actual}}{\text{weight}} \times \frac{100/}{\text{Usual weight}}$$

- If client has lost more than 10% of body weight in a short time, weight-gain program is begun. 500 kcal daily increase in calories provides 1-lb weight gain over 1 week.
- Albumin is major protein produced by liver. It is a useful indicator for chronically malnourished clients. In an acute client, greater number of factors influence albumin (e.g., stress, hydration, surgery). Transferrin is more specific indicator of protein and calorie malnutrition than albumin.

Pediatric Considerations

- Anthropometric data for the infant, birth to 36 months, includes measurement of length, weight, and head circumference. These measurements are compared to standard growth charts to determine percentiles (see Chapter 11). The height and weight of children age 2 to 18 years is compared to standard growth charts for interpretation. Triceps skinfold measurements are performed for children in the same manner as for adults. Standards for triceps skinfold for children age 1 to 18 have been published (Wong, 1995).

Gerontologic Considerations

- Anthropometric standards were developed based on healthy middle-age men and may not accurately reflect muscle wasting in the older adult. Tools available in the Nutrition Screening Initiative (NSI, 1995) have been designed specifically for nutrition screening of older adults (Fig. 22-2).

The Warning Signs of poor nutritional health are often overlooked. Use this checklist to find out if you or someone you know is at nutritional risk.

DETERMINE YOUR NUTRITIONAL HEALTH

Read the statements below. Circle the number in the yes column for those that apply to you or someone you know. For each yes answer, score the number in the box. Total your nutritional score.

	YES
I have an illness or condition that made me change the kind and/or amount of food I eat.	2
I eat fewer than 2 meals per day.	3
I eat few fruits or vegetables, or milk products.	2
I have 3 or more drinks of beer, liquor or wine almost every day.	2
I have tooth or mouth problems that make it hard for me to eat.	2
I don't always have enough money to buy the food I need.	4
I eat alone most of the time.	1
I take 3 or more different prescribed or over-the-counter drugs a day.	1
Without wanting to, I have lost or gained 10 pounds in the last 6 months.	2
I am not always physically able to shop, cook and/or feed myself.	2
TOTAL	

Total Your Nutritional Score. If it's ---

0-2 **Good!** Recheck your nutritional score in 6 months.

3-5 **You are at moderate nutritional risk.** See what can be done to improve your eating habits and lifestyle. Your office on aging, senior nutrition program, senior citizens center or health department can help. Recheck your nutritional score in 3 months.

6 or more **You are at high nutritional risk.** Bring this checklist the next time you see your doctor, dietitian or other qualified health or social service professional. Talk with them about any problems you may have. Ask for help to improve your nutritional health.

These materials developed and distributed by the Nutrition Screening Initiative, a project of:

AMERICAN ACADEMY OF FAMILY PHYSICIANS

THE AMERICAN DIETETIC ASSOCIATION

NATIONAL COUNCIL ON THE AGING

Remember that warning signs suggest risk, but do not represent diagnosis of any condition. Turn the page to learn more about the Warning Signs of poor nutritional health.

Fig. 22-2 Tool for nutrition screening of older adults. (Courtesy, The Nutrition Screening Initiative, Washington, DC.)

The Nutrition Checklist is based on the Warning Signs described below. Use the word DETERMINE to remind you of the Warning Signs.

DISEASE

Any disease, illness or chronic condition which causes you to change the way you eat, or makes it hard for you to eat, puts your nutritional health at risk. Four out of five adults have chronic diseases that are affected by diet. Confusion or memory loss that keeps getting worse is estimated to affect one out of five or more of older adults. This can make it hard to remember what, when or if you've eaten. Feeling sad or depressed, which happens to about one in eight older adults, can cause big changes in appetite, digestion, energy level, weight and well-being.

EATING POORLY

Eating too little and eating too much both lead to poor health. Eating the same foods day after day or not eating fruit, vegetables, and milk products daily will also cause poor nutritional health. One in five adults skip meals daily. Only 13% of adults eat the minimum amount of fruit and vegetables needed. One in four older adults drink too much alcohol. Many health problems become worse if you drink more than one or two alcoholic beverages per day.

TOOTH LOSS/ MOUTH PAIN

A healthy mouth, teeth and gums are needed to eat. Missing, loose or rotten teeth or dentures which don't fit well or cause mouth sores make it hard to eat.

ECONOMIC HARDSHIP

As many as 40% of older Americans have incomes of less than $6,000 per year. Having less--or choosing to spend less--than $25-30 per week for food makes it very hard to get the foods you need to stay healthy.

REDUCED SOCIAL CONTACT

One-third of all older people live alone. Being with people daily has a positive effect on morale, well-being and eating.

MULTIPLE MEDICINES

Many older Americans must take medicines for health problems. Almost half of older Americans take multiple medicines daily. Growing old may change the way we respond to drugs. The more medicines you take, the greater the chance for side effects such as increased or decreased appetite, change in taste, constipation, weakness, drowsiness, diarrhea, nausea, and others. Vitamins or minerals when taken in large doses act like drugs and can cause harm. Alert your doctor to everything you take.

INVOLUNTARY WEIGHT LOSS/GAIN

Losing or gaining a lot of weight when you are not trying to do so is an important warning sign that must not be ignored. Being overweight or underweight also increases your chance of poor health.

NEEDS ASSISTANCE IN SELF CARE

Although most older people are able to eat, one of every five have trouble walking, shopping, buying and cooking food, especially as they get older.

ELDER YEARS ABOVE AGE 80

Most older people lead full and productive lives. But as age increases, risk of frailty and health problems increase. Checking your nutritional health regularly makes good sense.

The Nutrition Screening Initiative, 2626 Pennsylvania Avenue, NW, Suite 301, Washington, DC 20037

A5944(1.00)/DECEMBER 1995

Fig. 22-2, cont'd. For legend see opposite page.

SKILL 22-2 Assisting the Adult Client with Oral Nutrition

Assisting the adult with oral nutrition requires time, patience, knowledge, and understanding. Most people eat without assistance. However, with illness or trauma, the client may be physically unable to eat without assistance. Physical impairments that limit self-feeding include hemiplegia, fractured arm, quadriplegia, debilitating illness, or generalized weakness. The presence of intravenous catheters or tubings, dressings, and bandages can also limit self-feeding. In addition, some older adults tire quickly and may need to be assisted even though they can eat independently. Although adult feeding needs and techniques differ from those for infants, the adult who needs help to eat still needs compassion and understanding. Merely feeding the adult can be accomplished with common sense, but providing a socially meaningful mealtime requires education and experience on the part of the nurse.

DELEGATION CONSIDERATIONS

The skill of assisting the client with oral nutrition can be delegated to unlicensed assistive personnel.

- Instruct care provider to assist the client to a comfortable position in a chair or with the head of the bed elevated.
- Offer a washcloth and towel to the client before the meal tray is provided.
- Instruct care provider to assist the client with preparation of the tray or food, such as opening containers, cutting up meat, or pouring liquids. The tray should be at a comfortable height and distance from the client.
- Instruct care provider to observe for any swallowing problems and to notify nurse immediately. Clients with swallowing problems require the assistance of licensed personnel.

STEPS	RATIONALE
ASSESSMENT	
1. Assess that GI tract is functional, and determine what type of diet the client can tolerate (Table 22-4).	Nurse's awareness of specific diet order provides appropriate nutrition.
2. Assess client's ability to swallow. In clients with neurological condition, assess **gag reflex** (see Chapter 11).	Some clients (those who have neurological diseases or are handicapped) may be at risk for dysphagia and aspiration and may not be able to tolerate a regular diet. Change in consistency of diet (thickened liquids, pureed, soft), swallow training, or alternative means of nutrition may be needed.
3. Determine to what extent the client is able to self-feed.	Clients with any level of independence should not be totally fed by hospital staff.
Assess physical motor skills, level of consciousness, visual acuity and peripheral vision, and mood.	Thorough understanding of client's physical and cognitive limitations alerts the nurse to client's needs.
4. Assess client's appetite, tolerance of foods, cultural and religious preferences, and food likes and dislikes.	Awareness of client's needs before meals prevents misunderstanding and frustration for both nurse and client.
5. Assess whether client has food allergies.	Prevents allergic reaction to food groups.

NURSING DIAGNOSIS

Clustering of defining characteristics from the assessment data may reveal the following nursing diagnoses for clients requiring this skill:

- ➤ Risk for aspiration
- ➤ Risk for fluid volume deficit
- ➤ Feeding self-care deficit
- ➤ Sensory/perceptual alterations (gustatory)
- ➤ Impaired swallowing

Related factors are individualized based on a client's condition or needs.

Table 22-4 Routine Diets*

Diet Type	Description	Foods Allowed
Clear liquid	Nutritionally inadequate, low-residue diet to provide fluids and minimally stimulate GI tract after surgery or procedures	Clear soups, broth, clear fruit juices, and flavored gelatin; long-term use should be supplemented with clear liquid nutritional supplements
Full liquid	Transitional liquid diet for clients with chewing, swallowing, or digestive difficulties	Clear liquids, milk-based liquids or foods that melt, and thin cereals
Soft	Diet for clients with problems chewing or swallowing tough foods; also used for some GI disturbances	Soft foods low in fiber prepared without strong seasonings; meat may be ground if needed
Regular or house	Regular consistency for clients without nutritional problems	All foods that may be high fat, sodium, and sugar; approximately 2000 kcal per day

*Specific foods allowed and diet types vary from agency to agency. Refer to the diet manual at each facility.

STEPS	RATIONALE
PLANNING	
1. Expected outcomes following completion of procedure:	
➤ Client denies any gastric, swallowing, or chewing problems or food intolerances.	Indicates absence of gastric disturbance or food intolerance.
➤ Client's weight increases or remains the same over the time diet therapy is provided.	Nutritional intake exceeds or meets daily requirements.
➤ Client completes meal.	Prescribed dietary intake has been eaten; decreases risk of nutritional imbalances.
➤ Client is able to participate in independent feeding.	Enables client to be as independent as possible. Provide assistive devices as needed to promote independence. Involve family in mealtime if possible.
2. Prepare client's room for mealtime:	
a. Remove any unpleasant odors and sights (e.g., remove bedpans, bedside urinals, used dressings, trash).	Unsightly, odor-filled room can decrease client's appetite.
b. Clear overbed table.	
c. Set up chair for client and for nurse. Place bed in upright back position if the client is unable to be up in the chair.	
3. Prepare client for meal:	
a. Help client urinate or defecate.	
b. Help client wash hands.	Reduces spread of microorganisms.
c. Assist client with mouth care. Clients with dysphagia or dry mouth may benefit from clear water rinsing or swabbing.	Oral hygiene improves taste and increases appetite.
d. Clients with stomatitis (irritation of oral mucosa) may benefit from rinsing with a solution containing ½ to 1 teaspoon of salt to 1 pint of water.	
➤ ***CRITICAL DECISION POINT*** **Clients may avoid foods because of pain from mouth sores or esophagitis.**	
e. Assist client to put in dentures and put on eyeglasses or insert contact lenses if used. Check that dentures are not too loose.	Enhances client's ability to chew and see food. Loose dentures inhibit normal chewing and pose a safety risk.
f. Assist client to comfortable sitting position. If client is unable to sit, turn client on side with the head of the bed elevated.	Position minimizes risk of aspiration.

STEPS	RATIONALE
g. Obtain special devices and needed supplies to facilitate feeding (hand splints, built-up silverware, straw, large spoon, modified cup, towels) before meal.	Ensures organized, unhurried atmosphere.

IMPLEMENTATION

STEPS	RATIONALE
1. Wash hands before preparing client's tray.	Reduces spread of microorganisms.
2. Assess tray for completeness and correct diet.	Prevents ingestion of incorrect or incomplete meal.
3. Prepare tray to meet client's needs: open cartons, remove lids, cut food, season food after asking client's preferences.	Clients with cognitive or physical impairments may not have the fine motor coordination needed to prepare tray for eating.
4. If client is able to eat independently, stop here. Return after 10 to 20 minutes.	Determines how well client is tolerating diet.
5. For the client who cannot eat independently, begin feeding by assisting. Ask client about any religious or cultural preferences before beginning feeding.	Sitting or standing close to client during feeding promotes psychologically comforting and caring environment, which may increase appetite.
6. Ask in what order client would like to eat, and cut food into bite-size pieces (see illustration).	Allows client more independence and control. Small pieces are easier to chew and minimize risk of aspiration.
7. Feed client in a manner that facilitates chewing and swallowing.	
a. Older adult: feed small amounts at a time, assessing chewing, swallowing, and fatigue.	Decreased saliva production in the older adult can impair swallowing. Sauces, gravies, and frequent liquids with meals enhance swallowing. Chewing and sitting up for feeding may accelerate onset of fatigue. Frequent rests may be helpful (White, 1991; Whitehouse, 1992).
b. Neurologically impaired client: feed small amounts at a time and assess for ability to chew, manipulate tongue to form a **bolus,** and swallow. Give small amounts of thin liquids (soup, beverages) and assess for swallowing.	

CRITICAL DECISION POINT Clients with limited tongue strength and control may be unable to move bolus to back of mouth for swallowing. Checking for "pocketed" food in mouth prevents aspiration. Clients with dysphagia who aspirate thin liquids may benefit from liquids thickened with commercial thickening products or from change in consistency of diet.

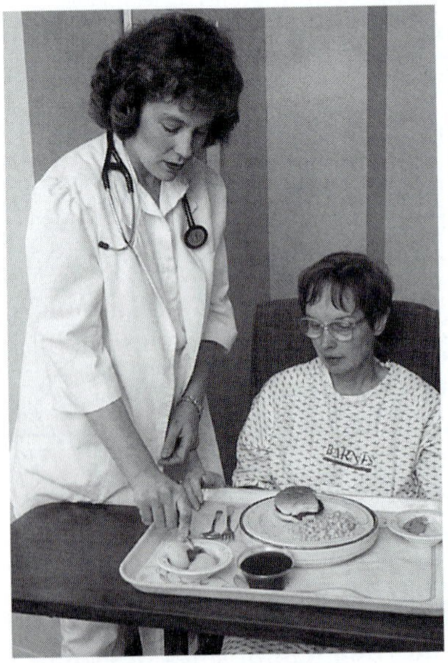

Step 6 Nurse assisting client at mealtime.

STEPS	RATIONALE
c. Cancer client: check for food aversions before and during the meal.	May have strong abnormal sense of taste and smell because of medications.
8. Provide fluids as requested. Do not allow client to drink all liquids at beginning of meal.	Assists swallowing. Prevents client from filling up on liquids.
9. Talk to client during meal.	Meal should be a pleasant event. Conversation promotes socialization. Involve family if possible.

STEPS	RATIONALE
10. Use meal as an opportunity to educate client (e.g., topics related to nutrition, postoperative exercises, discharge plans).	Education can occur whenever nurse and client are together.
11. Assist client to wash hands and perform mouth care.	Mouth care after meals helps prevent dental caries.
12. Assist client to resting position.	Client may feel tired after full meal. If client is prone to aspiration, leave head elevated 45 degrees for 30 minutes after meal.
13. Return client's tray to appropriate place and wash hands.	Reduces spread of microorganisms.

EVALUATION

1. During meal observe client's ability to swallow.	Determines if client develops dysphagia and becomes prone to aspiration.
2. Weigh client daily (if nutrition has been inadequate).	Gradual weight gain reflects improved nutritional status.
3. Assess client's tolerance to diet.	Overfeeding may cause nausea and vomiting. Underfeeding may leave client feeling hungry.
4. Assess client's fluid and food intake.	Helps to determine whether client's nutritional and fluid needs are being met.
5. Assess client's ability to feed self.	Determines if client is gaining independence in feeding.
6. **Unexpected outcomes** that may occur include:	
➤ Client is unable to complete meal.	Client may have taste abnormalities, early satiety (fullness), or decreased interest in eating because of hospital atmosphere.
➤ Client complains of nausea, vomiting, diarrhea, or food intolerances.	Gastrointestinal symptoms may indicate food intolerances, allergies, or presence of bacteria. Presence of such symptoms impairs absorption of nutrients.
➤ Client experiences weight loss.	Nutritional intake is inadequate.

RECORDING AND REPORTING

1. Document in client's chart: client's tolerance of diet, amount eaten, and intake and output.	Documentation facilitates communication among health care professionals.
2. Report any swallowing difficulties, food dislikes, refusal to eat to nurse in charge.	Enables nurse to further assess client's swallowing ability and change diet to foods more easily tolerated or the client's food preferences.

FOLLOW-UP ACTIVITIES

1. Determine why client is unable to finish meal (e.g., inadequate personnel for feeding assistance, ingestion of large volume of liquids immediately before meal, improper diet).
2. Notify physician of any unexpected outcomes.

• • • • •

Special Considerations

- ➤ If client is on calorie counts, record caloric intake on appropriate form; if intake and output are being evaluated, record fluid intake on appropriate form.
- ➤ Clients may be receiving oral nutritional supplements (special foods or medical nutritionals such as Ensure, Isocal, and Resource) to increase calories and protein between or during meals. Record the amount taken and communicate client tolerance (likes or dislikes, supplements to fill or replace meals) to the health care team to evaluate supplement effectiveness.
- ➤ Certain conditions, such as pressure ulcer, traction, or spinal surgery, may prevent positioning with head elevated.

Teaching Considerations

- ➤ Instruct client and primary care giver in required diet, including elimination of certain foods. Provide written instructions.
- ➤ Instruct client and primary care giver to maintain a nutritional balance of foods.
- ➤ Instruct client and primary care giver to monitor intake of fluids, calories, fats, and salt.
- ➤ Instruct client and primary care giver on importance of providing frequent mouth care.

Pediatric Considerations

- Infant feeding includes bottle or breast feeding and the introduction of semisolid foods such as cereals at around 6 months; strained vegetables, meats, and fruits at around 8 months; and bite-size table foods at around 1 year. Cup feeding and finger foods are introduced as the child's fine motor skills develop.

Gerontologic Considerations

- Older adult clients may have diminished appetite because of loss of taste and smell and decreased number of taste buds.

Home Care Considerations

- Assess familiarity of client and primary care giver with proper nutritional standards.
- Assess financial resources of client and family to determine if they are able to purchase proper foods for the client.
- Assess priority given by client and family to provision of a balanced nutritional plan.
- Verify physician's diet order for the client.
- Verify accuracy of food with physician's diet order.
- Teach family members to assist client to feed self. Help client do as much as possible in feeding self.
- Assist client, family, and primary care giver to make eating an enjoyable experience.

SKILL 22-3 Aspiration Precautions

Aspiration in the adult client usually occurs as a result of difficulties in swallowing (dysphagia). Dysphagia can result from neurological or neuromuscular diseases (stroke, amyotrophic lateral sclerosis, myasthenia gravis) and from trauma to or surgical procedures of the oral cavity or throat (cancer therapy, ingestion of caustic substances).

Symptoms that suggest dysphagia include coughing and gagging while eating, multiple swallow attempts, drooling, pockets of food in the mouth, a gargly sounding voice, and a sensation of food "getting stuck" in one's throat (Perspectives on Dysphagia, 1990). Clients who exhibit these symptoms should be evaluated for dysphagia. For clients with altered consciousness who ingest food orally, episodes of pneumonia may indicate aspiration of food or oral secretions.

Swallowing evaluations may be conducted by a speech therapist or radiologist. The speech therapist evaluates the client's ability to swallow foods of various thickness. Thin liquids are typically the most difficult substances for a client with dysphagia. Radiological studies using radiopaque dyes that are swallowed are also used to diagnose dysphagia with aspiration.

EQUIPMENT

- **Chair or electric bed (to allow client to sit upright)**
- **Thickening agents as needed (rice, cereal, yogurt, gelatin, commercial thickening agent)**
- **Tongue blade**
- **Penlight**

DELEGATION CONSIDERATIONS

This skill requires problem solving and knowledge application unique to a professional nurse. For this skill, delegation is inappropriate.

Instruct staff how to recognize signs associated with aspiration and to position client in an upright, sidelong position to protect airway.

STEPS	RATIONALE
ASSESSMENT	
1. Perform nutritional assessment (see Skill 22-1).	Clients with aspiration from dysphagia may alter their eating patterns or choose foods that do not provide adequate nutrition.
2. Assess clients who are at increased risk of aspiration for signs and symptoms of dysphagia.	Client may exhibit symptoms or demonstrate poor lip and tongue control. Clients at risk include those who have neurological or neuromuscular diseases and those who have had trauma to or surgical procedures of the oral cavity or throat.
3. Report signs and symptoms of dysphagia to the physician.	The client may need to have an evaluation performed by a radiologist or speech therapist.

STEPS | **RATIONALE**

NURSING DIAGNOSIS

Clustering of defining characteristics from the assessment data may reveal the following nursing diagnoses for clients requiring this skill:

- Risk for aspiration
- Sensory/perceptual alterations (gustatory)
- Impaired swallowing

Related factors are individualized based on a client's condition or needs.

PLANNING

1. **Expected outcomes** following completion of procedure:
   - Client will not exhibit signs or symptoms that suggest aspiration is occurring.
     - *Rationale:* Signs or symptoms associated with aspiration may indicate the need for further evaluation of swallowing, such as a fluoroscopic swallow study.

IMPLEMENTATION

1. Ask client about any difficulties with swallowing or chewing various textures of food.
   - *Rationale:* Be alert for symptoms such as coughing, dyspnea, or drooling that suggest difficulty handling food, especially thin liquids.
2. Using penlight and tongue blade, gently inspect mouth for pockets of food.
   - *Rationale:* Pockets of food in the mouth can indicate difficulty swallowing.
3. Elevate head of client's bed so that hips are flexed at a 90-degree angle and head is flexed slightly forward, or assist client to same position in a chair.
   - *Rationale:* Reduces risk of aspiration.
4. Offer client thicker foods, such as blenderized foods, yogurt, creamed soups, gelatin, custard, or mashed potatoes, and assess client for signs or symptoms of difficulty swallowing.
   - *Rationale:* Thicker foods are less likely to cause difficulty with swallowing.
5. If client manages thicker foods without difficulty, proceed gradually with foods of thinner consistency. Observe client closely for signs of dysphagia.

CRITICAL DECISION POINT **Thin liquids, such as coffee, tea, or sodas, are the most difficult foods for a client with dysphagia to swallow.**

6. If no signs or symptoms of dysphagia are evident, assist the client to complete the meal or place the meal within reach of the client for self-feeding.
   - *Rationale:* The client may not require adaptation of meal consistency but may still require appropriate positioning to reduce the risk of aspiration.
7. Ask client to remain sitting upright for at least 30 minutes after the meal.
   - *Rationale:* Reduces the risk of gastroesophageal reflux that can cause aspiration.
8. Assist client to wash hands and perform mouth care.
   - *Rationale:* Mouth care after meals helps prevent dental caries.
9. Return client's tray to appropriate place and wash hands.
   - *Rationale:* Reduces spread of microorganisms.

EVALUATION

1. Assess client's ability to ingest foods of various textures and thickness.
   - *Rationale:* Indicates whether aspiration risk is increased with thin liquids.
2. Assess client's food and fluid intake.
   - *Rationale:* Client may avoid certain types and textures of food that are difficult to swallow.
3. Weigh client weekly.
   - *Rationale:* Determines if weight is stable and reflects adequate calorie level.
4. Assess client's oral cavity after meal to detect pockets of food.
   - *Rationale:* Determines presence of pockets of food when meal has included foods of various textures.
5. **Unexpected outcomes** that may occur include:
   - Client coughs, gags, complains of food "stuck in throat," or has pockets of food in mouth.
     - *Rationale:* Client may require a swallowing evaluation.

STEPS	RATIONALE
➤ Client avoids certain textures of food.	Avoidance of certain food textures or thickness may occur if client is fearful of swallowing difficulty.
➤ Client experiences weight loss.	Nutritional intake is inadequate.

Recording and Reporting

1. Document the following in client's chart: client's tolerance of various food textures, amount of assistance required, position during meal, absence or presence of any symptoms of dysphagia, and amount eaten.	Documents client's nutritional intake as well as abiity to manage oral nutrition.
2. Report any coughing, gagging, choking, or swallowing difficulties to nurse in charge or physician.	Findings may indicate need for further diagnostic tests to evaluate client's swallowing before further oral intake is given.

Follow-up Activities

1. Notify physician of any symptoms that occurred during meal and which foods caused the symptoms.

• • • • •

Special Considerations

➤ Thickening agents or other food substances that thicken foods can be added to increase viscosity of food for a client with dysphagia.

Gerontologic Considerations

➤ Older adults who have had a stroke or have Parkinson disease are at risk for aspiration.

➤ Consider consultation with a speech therapist for swallowing exercises and techniques to improve swallowing and reduce risk of aspiration.

Critical Thinking Exercises

1. A client is 130% of normal body weight for height. What nutritional assessment parameters would assist the nurse to determine if the client is malnourished?
2. A client with cancer complains that the smell of food causes her to lose her appetite. What modifications in feeding can the nurse make to assist this client?
3. The nurse has performed a nutritional assessment for a client with myasthenia gravis. The client has lost 20 pounds over the last 6 months and has a serum albumin of 2.9 mg/dl. What are possible nursing interventions to determine the cause of this client's weight loss?

References

American Society for Parenteral and Enteral Nutrition (ASPEN): The 1995 ASPEN standards for nutrition support: hospitalized patients, *Nurs Care Pract* 10(6):206, 1995.

JCAHO Board of Directors: *1996 comprehensive accreditation manual for hospitals,* Oakbrook, Ill, 1996, JCAHO.

Nutrition Screening Initiative, 2626 Pennsylvania Avenue NW, Suite 301, Washington, DC, 20037, 1995.

Perspectives on Dysphagia: The Bristol-Myers Squibb Company, Evansville, Indiana, 1990.

White JV et al: Consensus of the nutrition screening initiative: risk factors and indications of poor nutritional status in older Americans, *J Am Diet Assoc* 91(7):783, 1991.

Whitehouse MJ: Nursing assessment of the elderly patient, *J Intr Nurs* 15:S14, 1992.

Williams SR: *Nutrition and diet therapy,* ed 7, St Louis, 1993, Mosby.

Williams SR: Nutritional assessment and guidance in prenatal care. In Worthington-Roberts BS, Williams SR, editors: *Nutrition in pregnancy and lactation,* ed 5, St Louis, 1993, Mosby.

Wong DL: *Whaley & Wong's nursing care of infants and children,* ed 5, St Louis, 1995, Mosby.

Additional Reading

Baker DM: Assessment and management of impairments in swallowing, *Nurs Clin North Am* 28(4):793, 1993.

Bradford KL: Dysphagia and the cancer patient. In Bloch A, editor: *Nutrition management of the cancer patient,* Rockville, Md, 1990, Aspen Publishers.

Diloro C, Price ME: Swallowing: an assessment guide, *Am J Nurs* 90(7):42, 1990.

Donahue PA: When it's hard to swallow: feeding techniques for dysphagia management, *J Gerontol Nurs* 16(4):6, 1990.

Emmick-Herring B, Wood P: A team approach to neurologically based swallowing disorders, *Rehab Nurs* 15(3):132, 1990.

Price ME, Diloro C: Swallowing: a practice guide, *Am J Nurs* 90(7):39, 1990.

CHAPTER 23

Enteral Nutrition

OBJECTIVES

Mastery of content in this chapter will enable the nurse to:

- Define key terms.
- Assess the client who is to receive enteral tube feedings.
- Determine the appropriate route of intubation for the client.
- Demonstrate ability to intubate the client.
- Demonstrate the appropriate technique for administering bolus tube feedings.
- Demonstrate the appropriate technique for administering continuous tube feedings.
- Demonstrate the appropriate technique for administering jejunal feedings.
- Demonstrate appropriate care of exit site for gastrostomy and jejunostomy tube.
- Evaluate the client's tolerance of enteral feeding.

KEY TERMS

Enteral nutrition
Gastrostomy feeding tube
Jejunal feeding tube
Nasogastric feeding tube
Nasointestinal feeding tube

SKILLS

23-1 Intubating the Client with a Small-Bore Nasogastric or Nasointestinal Feeding Tube

23-2 Verifying Tube Placement for a Large-Bore or Small-Bore Feeding Tube

23-3 Administering Enteral Feedings via Nasogastric Tube (Large or Small Bore)

23-4 Administering Enteral Feedings via Gastrostomy Tube

23-5 Administering Enteral Feedings via Nasointestinal Tube or Jejunostomy Tube

Enteral nutrition is the administration of nutrients directly into the gastrointestinal (GI) tract. The most desirable and appropriate method of providing nutrition is the oral route; unfortunately, this is not always possible. For clients with a functional GI tract who are unable or unwilling to ingest oral nutrients, enteral tube feedings are an alternative. A variety of enteral feeding formulas are available in whole protein or partially digested form. Special enteral formulas for renal disease, hepatic disease, pulmonary disease, or diabetes are also available. Adult and pediatric formulas can be chosen.

The skills presented in this chapter focus on the administration of nutritional feedings directly into the gastrointestinal tract and the goal of restoring the client's nutritional status. The nurse bases care on specific assessment findings.

GUIDELINES

1. Be aware of the purpose for the feeding and which clients are appropriate candidates. A feeding tube may not be appropriate for the client, and harm could occur at the time of insertion (e.g., upper GI bleeding or inadvertent placement of nasoenteral tube in the respiratory tract) or during the feeding (e.g., aspiration, electrolyte imbalance, or fluid imbalance).
2. Be aware of the psychological implications associated with the insertion of a feeding tube. The client may become frightened and will need reassurance and encouragement throughout the insertion procedure.
3. Be aware of safety measures to prevent dislodgment of the feeding tube and aspiration of gastric contents by the client. Clients who are disoriented or comatose are

at greater risk for aspiration than those who are alert and oriented.

4. Consider the client's medications and their route of delivery. Mixing medications with tube feeding formula should be avoided when possible. Some medications, particularly antibiotics and syrups, may lose their therapeutic effectiveness and disrupt emulsion of the feeding formula, resulting in a formula that resembles undigested milk. Tablets and pills, even when finely crushed, can clog a small-bore feeding tube. Certain medications should not be crushed because they have an enteric coating that protects the stomach mucosa from irritation; some medications should not be delivered directly into the intestine (see Chapter 18).
5. Know the client's exercise pattern. Clients requiring physical or occupational therapy should have their tube feedings completed at least 1 hour before activity to decrease the risk of vomiting or abdominal discomfort.

SKILL 23-1 Intubating the Client with a Small-Bore Nasogastric or Nasointestinal Feeding Tube

Large-bore nasogastric tubes are contraindicated when used primarily for enteral feedings, because they carry an increased risk of aspiration and are more irritating to the nasopharyngeal and esophageal mucosa (Lehmann, 1992). Occasionally, large-bore gastrointestinal tubes that were inserted for gastric decompression will be used to initiate enteral feeding because they are already in place. If the feeding continues for more than a few days, the nurse should consult with the physician about placement of a small-bore enteral feeding tube (Fig. 23-1). Small-bore feeding tubes are available in weighted (tungsten) or unweighted designs. Weighted tubes were thought to pass more easily into the duodenum or jejunum via peristalsis; however, research has not demonstrated an advantage of the weight in promoting intestinal passage (Lord et al., 1993). Because the tubes are flexible, a guidewire or stylet is used to provide rigidity and to facilitate positioning and then removed once correct placement is verified. Small-bore tubes can be left in place for an extended period with less irritation to the nasopharyngeal, esophageal, and gastric mucosa.

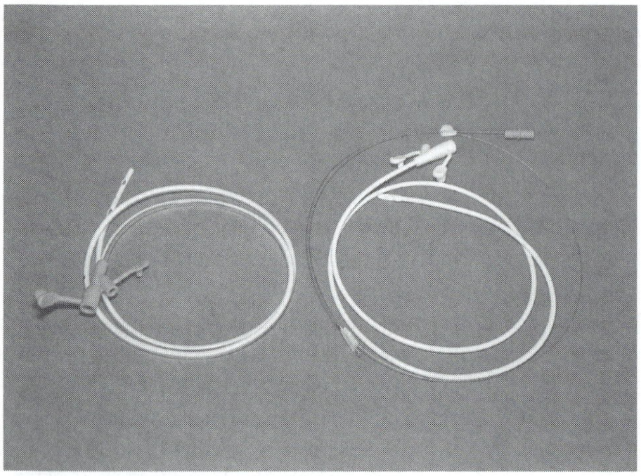

Fig. 23-1 Small bore feeding tube.

Placing a **nasogastric** (NG) or **nasointestinal** (NI) **feeding tube** requires a physician's order. Placement needs to be verified by radiograph to determine that the tube is in the stomach or intestine rather than in the airways (Chang et al., 1982; Metheny et al., 1990a; Metheny et al., 1990b). Complications of prolonged intubation may include nasal erosion, sinusitis, esophagitis, gastric ulceration, and pulmonary aspiration.

EQUIPMENT

- Nasogastric or nasointestinal tube (8 to 12 Fr) with guidewire or stylet
- 60-ml or larger Luer-Lok or catheter-tip syringe
- Stethoscope
- Hypoallergenic tape and tincture of benzoin
- pH Indicator strip
- Glass of water and straw
- Emesis basin
- Safety pin
- Rubber band
- Towel
- Facial tissues
- Clean gloves
- Suction equipment in case of aspiration
- Penlight to check placement in nasopharynx
- Tongue blade

DELEGATION CONSIDERATIONS

This skill requires problem solving and knowledge application unique to a professional nurse. For this reason, this skill is usually not delegated.

STEPS	RATIONALE
ASSESSMENT	
1. Assess client for need for enteral tube feedings and intubation: impaired swallowing, head or neck surgery, decreased level of consciousness, surgeries involving upper alimentary tract, or facial trauma; also assess weight for client's height, hydration status, electrolyte balance, and organ function.	Identifying clients who need tube feedings before they become nutritionally depleted facilitates preparation of nursing care plan and promotes client education. Enteral feeding preserves the function and mass of the gut, promotes wound healing, diminishes hypermetabolism in burn injuries, and may decrease the incidence of infection in critically ill clients (Zaloga, 1994).
2. Assess patency of nares. Have client close each nostril alternately and breathe. Examine each naris for patency and skin breakdown.	Nares may be obstructed or irritated, or septal defect or facial fractures may be present. Assessment determines most patent naris.
3. Assess client's medical history: nosebleeds; nasal surgery; deviated septum; anticoagulant therapy, coagulopathy.	If client has history of any of the problems listed, nurse may need to seek physician's order to change route of nutritional support.
4. Assess client for gag reflex. Place tongue blade in client's mouth, touching uvula.	Assists nurse in identifying client's ability to swallow and determines reduced risk of aspiration.
5. Assess client's mental status.	Alert client is better able to cooperate with procedure. If vomiting should occur, an alert client can usually expectorate vomitus, which can help to reduce the risk of aspiration.
6. Assess for bowel sounds. Consult the physician if bowel sounds are absent.	Absence of bowel sounds may indicate decreased or absent peristalsis and increased risk of aspiration or abdominal distention.

NURSING DIAGNOSIS

Clustering of defining characteristics from the assessment data may reveal the following nursing diagnoses for clients requiring this skill:

- Altered nutrition: less than body requirements
- Impaired swallowing
- Risk for aspiration

Related factors are individualized based on a client's condition or needs.

PLANNING

STEPS	RATIONALE
1. **Expected outcomes** following completion of procedure:	
➤ Tube is in stomach or intestine.	Correct placement.
➤ Feeding tube will remain patent.	Feeding tubes can become occluded with formula or medications; occlusion of feeding tube can result in need to insert new feeding tube.
➤ Client has no complaints or signs of discomfort or nasal trauma.	Tube correctly secured minimizes irritation to nares.
2. Explain procedure to client.	Increases client's cooperation with intubation procedure.
3. Explain to client how to communicate during intubation by raising index finger to indicate gagging or discomfort.	It is important for client to have a way of communicating to alleviate stress.
4. Position client in sitting or high Fowler's position. If client is comatose, place in semi-Fowler's position.	Reduces risk of pulmonary aspiration in event client should vomit.
5. Examine feeding tube for flaws: rough or sharp edges on distal end and closed or clogged outlet holes.	Flaws in feeding tube hamper tube intubation and can injure client.
6. Determine length of tube to be inserted and mark with tape or indelible ink.	Being aware of proper length to intubate determines approximate depth of insertion.

STEPS	RATIONALE

CRITICAL DECISION POINT **Tip of tube must reach stomach. Measure distance from tip of nose to earlobe to xyphoid process of sternum (see illustration). Add additional 20 to 30 cm (8 to 12 in) for nasointestinal tube (Welch, 1996; Lord et al., 1993; Hanson, 1979).**

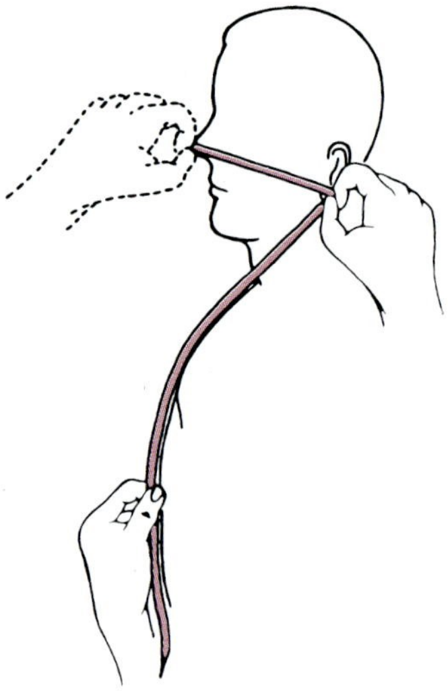

7. Prepare NG or NI tube for intubation:
   a. Plastic tubes should not be iced. — Tubes will become stiff and inflexible, causing trauma to mucous membranes.
   b. Wash hands. — Reduces spread of microorganisms.
   c. Inject 10 ml of water from 30-ml or larger Luer-Lok or catheter-tip syringe into the tube. — Aids in guidewire or stylet insertion.
   d. Make certain that guidewire is securely positioned against weighted tip and that both Luer-Lok connections are snugly fitted together. — Promotes smooth passage of tube into GI tract. Improperly positioned stylet can induce serious trauma.
8. Cut tape 10 cm (4 in) long.

IMPLEMENTATION

1. Put on clean gloves. — Reduces transmission of microorganisms.
2. Inspect nares for any irritation or obstruction.
3. Dip tube with surface lubricant into glass of water. — Activates lubricant to facilitate passage of tube into naris to GI tract.
4. Insert tube through nostril to back of throat (posterior nasopharynx). May cause client to gag. Aim back and down toward ear. — Natural contours facilitate passage of tube into GI tract.
5. Flex client's head toward chest after tube has passed through nasopharynx. — Closes off glottis and reduces risk of tube entering trachea.

CRITICAL DECISION POINT **Encourage client to swallow by giving small sips of water or ice chips when possible. Advance tube as client swallows. Rotate tube 180 degrees while inserting.** — Swallowing facilitates passage of tube past oropharynx. Rotating tube decreases friction.

6. Emphasize need to mouth breathe and swallow during the procedure. — Helps facilitate passage of tube and alleviates client's fears during the procedure.
7. Advance tube each time client swallows until desired length has been passed. — Reduces discomfort and trauma to client.

CRITICAL DECISION POINT **Do not force tube. If resistance is met or client starts to cough, choke, or become cyanotic, stop advancing the tube and pull tube back.**

8. Check for position of tube in back of throat with penlight and tongue blade. — Tube may be coiled, kinked, or entering trachea.

STEPS	RATIONALE
9. Check placement of tube (see Skill 23-2).	Proper position is essential before initiating feedings.
10. Apply tincture of benzoin or other skin adhesive on tip of client's nose and tube. Allow to dry.	Helps tape adhere better. Protects skin.
11. Remove gloves and secure tube with tape, avoiding pressure on naris.	A properly secured tube allows the client more mobility and prevents trauma to nasal mucosa.
a. Split one end of tape lengthwise 5 cm (2 in). Place the intact end of tape over bridge of client's nose. Wrap each of the 5-cm strips around tube as it exits nose (see illustrations).	Securing tape to nares prevents tissue necrosis.
b. Fasten end of nasogastric tube to client's gown by looping rubber band around tube in slip knot. Pin rubber band to gown.	Reduces traction on the naris if tube moves.
12. For intestinal placement, position client on right side when possible until radiological confirmation of correct placement has been verified. Otherwise, assist client to a comfortable position.	Promotes passage of the tube into the small intestine (duodenum or jejunum).
CRITICAL DECISION POINT **Leave guidewire or stylet in place until correct position is ensured by x-ray film. Never attempt to reinsert partially or fully removed guidewire or stylet while feeding tube is in place.**	Guidewire or stylet may perforate GI tract, especially esophagus or nearby tissue, and seriously injure the client.
13. Obtain x-ray film of abdomen.	Placement of tube is verified by x-ray examination (Metheny, 1988).
14. Apply gloves and administer oral hygiene (see Chapter 6). Cleanse tubing at nostril.	Promotes client comfort and integrity of oral mucous membranes.
15. Remove gloves, dispose of equipment, and wash hands.	Reduces transmission of microorganisms.

EVALUATION

1. Observe client to determine response to NG or NI tube intubation:	
a. Persistent gagging	Indicates prolonged irritation and stimulation of client's gag reflex. Can result in vomiting and increased risk of aspiration.
b. Paroxysms of coughing	May indicate presence of NG or NI tube in client's airway.

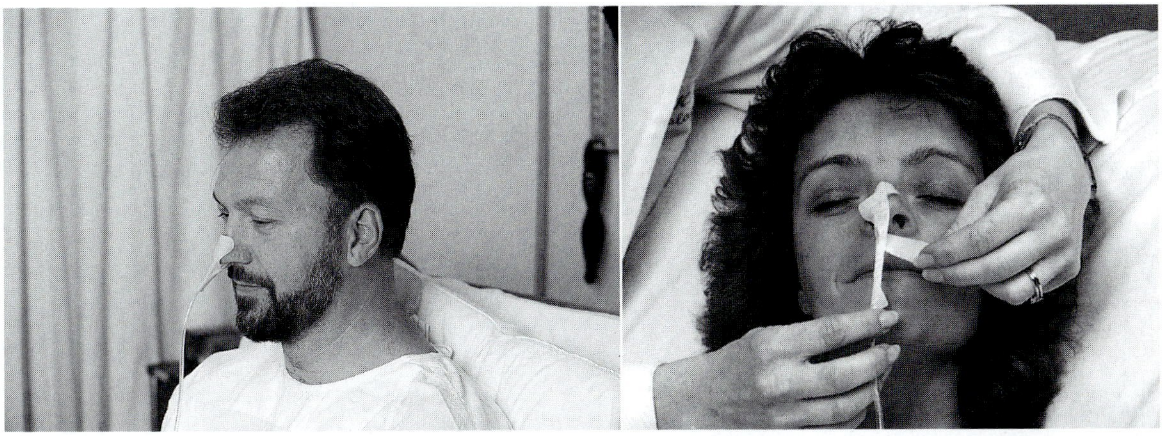

Step 11a

STEPS	RATIONALE
2. Confirm x-ray results.	Verifies tube position.
3. **Unexpected outcomes** that may occur include:	
➤ Aspiration of stomach contents into respiratory tract as evidenced by coughing, dyspnea, cyanosis, ascultation of crackles or wheezes, and fever.	An x-ray will confirm whether aspiration has occurred.
➤ Displacement of feeding tube to another site (i.e., from stomach to esophagus or duodenum to stomach).	May occur when client coughs or vomits or if frequent nasotracheal suctioning is done (Metheny et al., 1990a).

Recording and Reporting

1. Record and report type and size of tube placed, location of distal tip of tube, client's tolerance of procedure, and confirmation of tube position by x-ray.	Provides new nursing personnel with status of GI feeding. Allows new nursing staff to plan for next feeding.

Follow-Up Activities

1. Pulmonary aspiration of vomitus: notify physician; suction client; obtain chest x-ray film.
2. Aspirate GI contents and measure pH (Metheny et al., 1993). Correlate measured pH with x-ray results.
3. Displaced feeding tube: remove old tube and insert new tube.

• • • • •

Special Considerations

- NG or NI feeding tubes may be inserted in clients with decreased level of consciousness, but risk of pulmonary aspiration is increased if there is impaired gag reflex.
- Refer to agency policy for insertion of NI feeding tubes. Some agencies require a physician to insert tubes with a guidewire.
- Flushing with 30 ml of tap water every 4 hours during continuous feeding, before and after residual checks, and before and after medication administration will help to increase absorption of medication (Metheny, 1996) and ensure patency and continued smooth infusion of feeding formula into client's GI tract. Clients with fluid restriction should have a 10- to 30-ml flush.

Teaching Considerations

- Instruct primary care giver to offer oral hygiene frequently and to keep client's lips moistened.
- Teach primary care giver correct method for securing feeding tube to nares to eliminate pressure on nares and face and to allow enough tubing for movement.

Pediatric Considerations

- Premature infant and neonate: measure from bridge of nose to just beyond tip of sternum. Older child: measure from tip of nose to earlobe to tip of sternum.
- In infant, observe for vagal stimulation during insertion of feeding tube resulting in decreased heart rate.

Gerontologic Considerations

- Ensure adequate lubrication of tube to decrease discomfort for the older adult, who may have decreased oral or nasopharyngeal secretions.

Home Care Considerations

- Assess client or primary care giver's ability to maintain tube and feeding program.
- Assess environmental safety and sanitation of client's home to determine potential for infection or injury.
- Teach client or primary care giver method of GI fluid pH measurement and expected range (see Skill 23-2).

SKILL 23-2 Verifying Tube Placement for a Large-Bore or Small-Bore Feeding Tube

Testing placement of a large-bore or a small-bore feeding tube is a responsibility of the nurse. Tube position should be verified before each intermittent feeding and at least once every 4 hours before flushing the tube when continuous feedings are given. In addition, nurses assess for gastric versus respiratory placement when tubes are initially inserted.

Inadvertent respiratory placement or dislocation of feeding tubes must be detected to maintain client safety. Displacement of soft small-bore tubes is less easily detected than is displacement of firm large-bore tubes. However, failure to detect pulmonary placement in large- or small-bore tubes can lead to complications, especially if feedings are instilled. Therefore, the most accurate method for verifying tube placement is x-ray confirmation (Metheny et al., 1990b).

EQUIPMENT

- 30-ml or larger Luer-Lok or catheter-tip syringe
- Stethoscope
- Clean gloves
- pH Indicator strip

DELEGATION CONSIDERATIONS

The verification of tube placement is a skill that requires problem solving and knowledge application unique to a professional nurse. For this skill, delegation is inappropriate.

STEPS	RATIONALE
ASSESSMENT	
1. Identify signs and symptoms of inadvertent respiratory placement: coughing, choking, or cyanosis.	These signs and symptoms may indicate inadvertent respiratory placement.
2. Identify signs and symptoms that increase risk of tube dislocation: a. Coughing b. Retching or gagging c. Nasotracheal suctioning	Feeding tubes may become dislocated (e.g., stomach to esophagus or stomach to lungs).
3. Review client's record for history of prior tube displacement.	Clients who have a history of tube displacement are at increased risk.
4. Observe the external portion of the tube for a change in length related to displacement.	Increased external length of the tube may indicate that the distal tip is no longer in the correct location.

NURSING DIAGNOSIS

Clustering of defining characteristics from the assessment data may reveal the following nursing diagnoses for clients requiring this skill:

- ➤ Risk for aspiration
- ➤ Impaired gas exchange

Related factors are individualized based on a client's condition or needs.

PLANNING

STEPS	RATIONALE
1. **Expected outcomes** following completion of procedure:	
➤ Tube feeding formula infuses smoothly into client's GI tract.	Feeding tube is patent and properly positioned.
➤ Client does not experience respiratory distress (e.g., increased respiratory rate, coughing, poor color).	If feeding tube is displaced in respiratory tract, client can develop respiratory distress, but symptoms are more likely with displacement of a large-bore tube.
2. Explain procedure to client.	Increases client's cooperation. Well-informed client is more cooperative and relaxed.

STEPS	RATIONALE

IMPLEMENTATION

1. Wash hands and put on gloves. — Reduces transmission of microorganisms.
2. Perform measures to verify placement of tube:
   a. Inject 30 ml of air into the tube and aspirate GI contents with a syringe. — Obtain GI contents to determine proper placement (Metheny et al., 1993).
   b. Measure pH of aspirated GI contents (see illustration) (Metheny et al., 1993) (see box below). — Gastric sites usually have a pH range of 1 to 4. Intestinal sites have a pH of >6.

CRITICAL DECISION POINT Auscultation is no longer considered a reliable method for verification of tube placement because a tube inadvertently placed in the lungs, pharynx, or esophagus can transmit a sound similar to that of air entering the stomach (Metheny et al., 1990a; Chang et al., 1982).

3. Remove and dispose of gloves. Wash hands. — Reduces transmission of microorganisms.

OBTAINING GI FLUID FOR pH MEASUREMENT, LARGE- AND SMALL-BORE FEEDING TUBES: BOLUS AND CONTINUOUS FEEDING

- Flush tube with 30 ml warm water after medications or completed feedings.
- Wait 1 hour after feeding or medications.
- Plan pH testing at times when continuous feedings may be withheld, such as for chest physical therapy or avoidance of medication interaction.
- Flush tube with 30 ml of air.
- Aspirate GI contents.
- If unable to aspirate GI contents, reposition client to allow tip of tube to rest in GI fluid. Flush tube with 30 ml of air and attempt to aspirate.

Modified from Metheny N et al: Effectiveness of pH measurements in predicting feeding tube placement, *Nurs Res* 38(5):285, 1989.

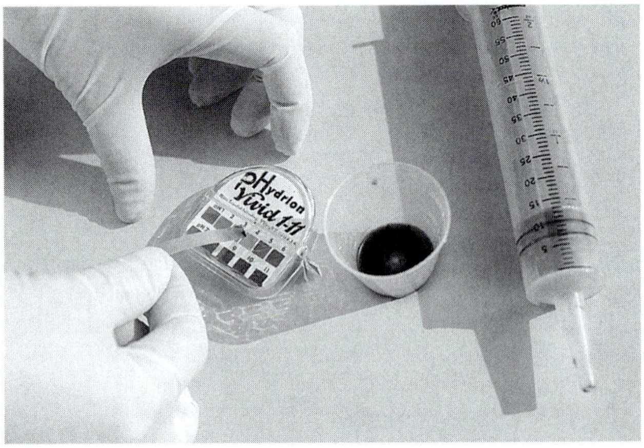

Step 2b

EVALUATION

1. Observe client for respiratory distress:
   a. Persistent gagging — May indicate prolonged irritation; stimulation of client's gag reflex can result in vomiting and increased risk of aspiration.
   b. Paroxysms of coughing — May indicate presence of nasogastric tube in client's airway.
   c. Respiratory patterns (e.g., rate) are not consistent with baseline parameters
2. Observe flow rate of enteral formula:
   a. A slower rate may indicate kink or clog within the feeding tube, inaccurate setting on feeding pump, or malfunction of the pump itself.
   b. Excessive flow may indicate inaccurate setting on the feeding pump or malfunction of the pump itself.

STEPS	RATIONALE
3. **Unexpected outcomes** that may occur include: ➤ Feeding tube is displaced (i.e., stomach to pulmonary system or intestine to stomach) because of severe coughing, nasotracheal suctioning, or vomiting.	Severe respiratory distress or abdominal distention may indicate displacement of feeding tube into the respiratory system or into the stomach when intestinal feedings are indicated.

Recording and Reporting

1. Record and report type of tube, length of tube inserted, pH, auscultation results, and client's tolerance to verifying tube placement.	Provides nursing personnel with status of GI feeding. Allows nursing staff to plan for next feeding.

Follow-up Activities

1. Displaced or occluded feeding tube: remove old tube and insert new tube.

• • • • •

Special Considerations

- If muffled or faint sound is present after injected air, tube may be in lungs.
- For obese clients, sound produced by injected air may be very faint, requiring air injection two or three times.
- In clients with gastric resections, do not withdraw or advance tube, because suture line could be interrupted, causing hemorrhage.
- If unable to aspirate GI contents, turn client on side. Tube opening may be against gastric or intestinal mucosa.

Pediatric Considerations

- In infant only, inject 0.5 to 1.0 ml of air during auscultation and before aspiration of gastric secretions for pH measurement.

Gerontologic Considerations

- Assess client for use of medications that may affect the pH of gastric secretions, such as histamine-receptor antagonists or antacids.

Teaching and Home Care Considerations

- Instruct client or primary care giver to check that tube is in correct position before administering formula or medications.
- Instruct client or primary care giver not to proceed with feedings if there is any doubt as to proper placement of tube.
- Teach client or primary care giver method of GI fluid pH measurement and expected range.

SKILL 23-3 Administering Enteral Feedings via Nasogastric Tube (Large or Small Bore)

Enteral feeding is preferred over parenteral nutrition because it improves utilization of nutrients, is generally safer for clients, maintains structure and function of the gut, and is less expensive. Not all clients are able to be fed enterally, but if the bowel can handle nutrients, this method should be used. The indications for enteral feeding include the following:

1. Clients who cannot eat (comatose clients with a functional gastrointestinal system, clients receiving mechanical ventilation, or clients recovering from oral, head, and neck surgeries)
2. Clients who will not eat (older adults or confused clients)
3. Clients who cannot maintain adequate oral nutrition (clients with cancer, sepsis, infection, trauma, or head injury)

EQUIPMENT

- Disposable feeding bag and tubing or ready-to-hang system
- 30-ml or larger Luer-Lok or catheter-tip syringe
- Stethoscope
- pH Indicator strip
- Infusion pump (required for intestinal feedings): use pump designed for tube feedings
- Prescribed enteral feedings
- Gloves

DELEGATION CONSIDERATIONS

Administration of enteral tube feeding via syringe is a procedure that can be delegated to unlicensed assistive personnel.

- The professional nurse should verify tube placement before the feeding and establish patency of the tube by flushing it with water.
- The nurse should also ensure that the client is sitting upright in a chair or in bed and instruct the assistive personnel to infuse the feeding slowly.
- Unlicensed personnel should be instructed to report any difficuly infusing the feeding or any discomfort voiced by the client.

STEPS	RATIONALE
ASSESSMENT	
1. Identify signs and symptoms of malnutrition (see Chapter 22).	Certain conditions, such as gastrointestinal diseases, cancer, severe infections, head injury, trauma, and metabolic diseases, place clients at risk for malnutrition.
2. Assess client for food allergies.	Prevents client from developing localized or systemic allergic responses.
3. Assess client's need for enteral tube feedings: impaired swallowing, decreased level of consciousness, head or neck surgery, facial trauma, surgeries of upper alimentary canal.	Identify clients who need tube feedings before they become nutritionally depleted.
4. Auscultate for bowel sounds before feeding.	Absent bowel sounds may indicate decreased ability of GI tract to digest or absorb nutrients.
5. Obtain baseline weight and laboratory values. Assess client for fluid volume excess or deficit, electrolyte abnormalities, and metabolic abnormalities such as hyperglycemia.	Enteral feedings are to restore or maintain a client's nutritional status. Provides objective data to measure effectiveness of feedings.
6. Verify physician's order for formula, rate, route, and frequency. Laboratory data and bedside assessments, such as finger-stick blood-glucose measurement, are also ordered by the physician.	Tube feedings, laboratory tests, and bedside tests must be ordered by physician.

NURSING DIAGNOSIS

Clustering of defining characteristics from the assessment data may reveal the following nursing diagnoses for clients requiring this skill:

- ➤ Altered nutrition: less than body requirements
- ➤ Impaired swallowing

Related factors are individualized based on a client's condition or needs.

STEPS	RATIONALE
PLANNING	
1. **Expected outcomes** following completion of procedure:	
➤ Nutritional status is improved, as evidenced by increasing weight, improving laboratory values, and improved intake and output.	Indicates that client's nutritional needs are being met.
➤ Client has no signs of respiratory distress (e.g., increased respiratory rate, coughing, poor color) or discomfort.	Entry of feeding tube into airways causes respiratory distress.
2. Explain procedure to client.	Well-informed client is more cooperative and at ease.
3. Wash hands.	Reduces transmission of microorganisms.

STEPS	RATIONALE
4. Prepare feeding container to administer formula:	
a. Have tubing feeding at room temperature.	Cold formula may cause gastric cramping and discomfort because the liquid is not warmed by mouth and esophagus.
b. Connect tubing to container as needed or prepare ready-to-hang container.	Tubing must be free of contamination to prevent bacterial growth.
c. Shake formula container well, and fill container and tubing with formula (see illustration).	Filling the tubing with formula prevents excess air from entering gastrointestinal tract.
5. Place client in high Fowler's position or elevate head of bed 30 degrees.	Elevated head helps prevent aspiration.

IMPLEMENTATION

CRITICAL DECISION POINT Check placement of gastric tube.

STEPS	RATIONALE
1. Apply gloves.	Reduces transmission of microorganisms.
a. Aspirate gastric contents to check for gastric residual (see illustration). Return aspirated contents to stomach unless the volume exceeds 150 ml.	Presence of gastric secretions indicates that the distal end of the tube is in the stomach. Residual volume indicates if gastric emptying is delayed. Delayed gastric emptying may be reflected by 150 ml or more remaining in the client's stomach.
b. Measure pH of aspirated GI contents.	Gastric contents usually have a pH range of 1 to 4. Intestinal sites have a pH of >6 (Metheny et al., 1993).
c. Auscultate over left upper quadrant with stethoscope.	Determines presence of peristalsis. Auscultation is no longer considered a reliable method for verification of placement of tube, because air in tube inadvertently placed in lungs, pharynx, or esophagus can transmit sound similar to that of air entering stomach (Metheny et al., 1990a, 1990b; Chang et al., 1982).

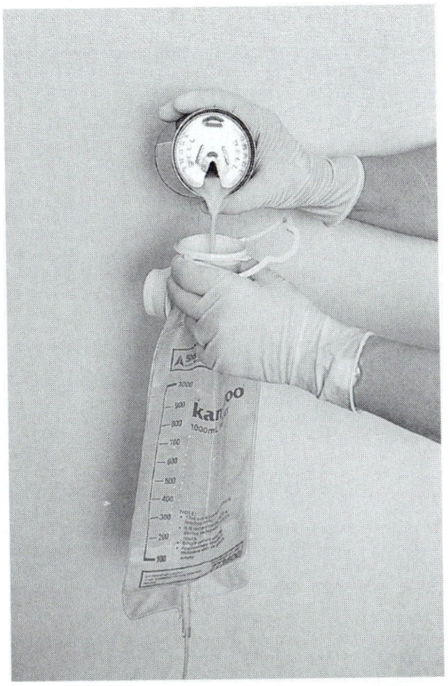

Step 4c

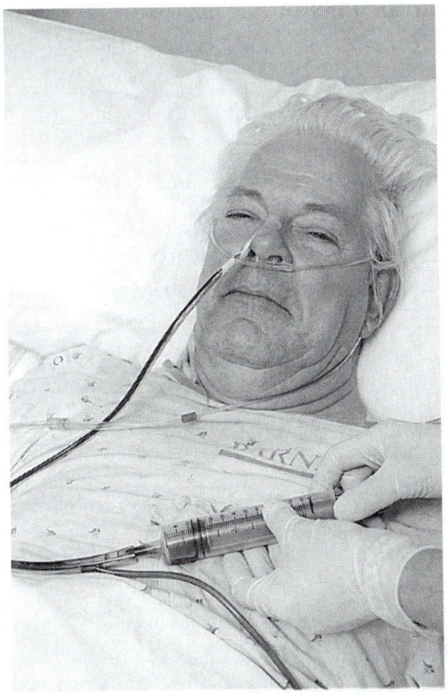

Step 1a

STEPS	RATIONALE
2. Initiate feeding:	
a. Bolus or intermittent feeding:	
➤ Pinch proximal end of the feeding tube.	Prevents air from entering client's stomach.
➤ Attach barrel of syringe to end of tube.	
➤ Fill syringe with measured amount of formula. Release tube and allow syringe to empty gradually by gravity, refilling until prescribed amount has been delivered to the client.	
➤ If feeding bag is used, hang feeding bag on an IV pole. Fill bag with prescribed amount of formula and allow bag to empty gradually over at least 30 minutes.	Gradual emptying of tube feeding by gravity from syringe or feeding bag reduces risk of abdominal discomfort, vomiting, or diarrhea induced by bolus or too-rapid infusion of tube feedings.
b. Continuous-drip method (see illustration):	
➤ Hang feeding bag and tubing on IV pole.	Continuous feeding method is designed to deliver prescribed hourly rate of feeding. This method reduces risk of abdominal discomfort. Clients who receive continuous drip feedings should have residuals checked every 4 hours and tube placement verified.
➤ Connect distal end of tubing to the proximal end of the feeding tube.	
➤ Connect tubing through infusion pump and set rate.	
3. When tube feedings are not being administered, cap or clamp the proximal end of the feeding tube.	Prevents air from entering stomach between feedings.
4. Administer water via feeding tube as ordered with diluted formula.	Provides client with source of water to help maintain fluid and electrolyte balance.
5. Rinse bag and tubing with warm water whenever feedings are interrupted.	Rinsing bag and tubing with warm water clears old tube feedings and reduces bacterial growth.

➤ ***CRITICAL DECISION POINT*** **Advance tube feeding rate gradually (see box below). Tube feedings should be advanced gradually to prevent diarrhea and gastric intolerance of formula.**

ADVANCING THE RATE OF TUBE FEEDING

Intermittent

1. Start formula at full strength for isotonic formulas (300 to 400 mOsm) or diluted to isotonicity.
2. Infuse formula over at least 20 to 30 minutes via syringe or feeding container.
3. Begin feedings with no more than 150 to 250 ml at one time. Increase by 50 ml per feeding per day to achieve needed volume and calories in six to eight feedings.

Continuous

1. Start formula at full strength for isotonic formulas (300 to 400 mOsm) or diluted to isotonicity.
2. Begin infusion rate at 30 to 50 ml per hour.
3. Advance rate by 10 to 20 ml per hour per day to target rate if tolerated.

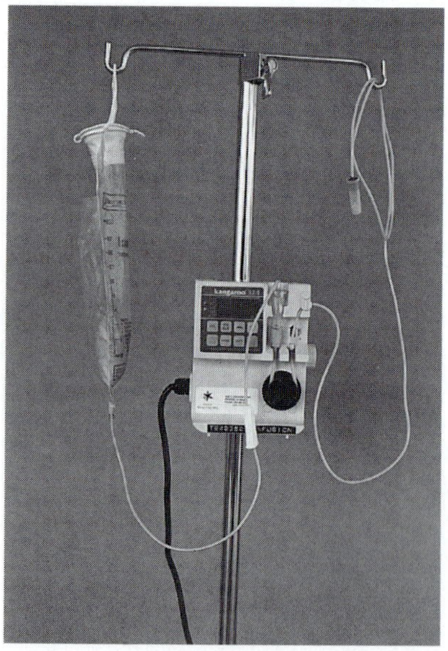

Step 2b

STEPS	RATIONALE
E VALUATION	
1. Evaluate amount of aspirate (residual) every 4 hours.	Evaluates tolerance of tube feeding.
2. Monitor finger-stick blood glucose every 6 hours until maximum administration rate is reached and maintained for 24 hours.	Alerts nurse to client's tolerance of glucose.
3. Monitor intake and output every 24 hours.	Intake and output are indications of fluid balance or fluid volume excess or deficit.
4. Weigh client daily until maximum administration rate is reached and maintained for 24 hours, then weigh client three times per week.	Weight gain is indicator of improved nutritional status; however, sudden gain of >2 pounds in 24 hours usually indicates fluid retention.
5. Observe return of normal laboratory values.	Improving laboratory values (i.e., albumin, transferrin, and prealbumin) indicate an improved nutritional status.
6. Observe client's respiratory status.	
7. Observe client's level of comfort.	
8. **Unexpected outcomes** that may occur include:	
➤ Client aspirates formula.	Aspiration can occur when tube is inappropriately placed or client coughs and displaces tube.
➤ Client develops diarrhea.	Clients receiving tube feedings may have loose stools, but diarrhea or liquid stools (three times or more in 24 hours) indicate intolerance. Antibiotics and medications containing sorbitol may induce diarrhea (Guenther et al., 1991; Benya, Layden, and Movarhan, 1991; Edes, Walk, and Austin, 1990).
➤ Client develops nausea and vomiting.	Vomiting is usually not caused by feeding but may indicate gastric ileus.

RECORDING AND REPORTING

1. Record amount of feeding.	Documents amount of feeding administered to client.
2. Record client's response to tube feeding, patency of tube, and any side effects.	Documents client's reaction to therapy and identifies presence of any adverse reactions (e.g., aspiration).
3. Record and report type of feeding, status of feeding tube, client's tolerance, and adverse effects.	Provides new nursing personnel with status of gastric feeding. Allows new nursing staff to plan for next feeding.

FOLLOW-UP ACTIVITIES

1. Aspiration: suction client, notify physician, obtain chest x-ray film.
2. Diarrhea: decrease feeding, review medications, notify physician.
3. Nausea and vomiting: withhold tube feeding, notify physician.

• • • • •

Special Considerations

- ➤ Some tube feedings are ordered as continuous drip over 24 hours.
- ➤ Change disposable bag and tubing every 24 hours.
- ➤ Formula can be hung 6 to 8 hours at room temperature in a standard feeding container or longer if given in a ready-to-hang system.
- ➤ If bowel sounds are absent or if the client's abdomen is distended, notify physician before initiating feeding.
- ➤ Review medications that should be given in liquid form and not crushed because they lose efficacy when crushed.
- ➤ Aspiration may be lessened if head of bed is elevated 30 to 45 degrees during feeding and for 1 hour after feeding.
- ➤ Client may need antidiarrheal agents or stool cultures if diarrhea occurs.

Teaching Considerations

- ➤ Instruct client or primary care giver to keep formula refrigerated between feedings.
- ➤ Instruct client or primary care giver to administer feedings at room temperature.

- Teach client and primary care giver to keep feeding tube capped or clamped between feedings and to give feedings with client in sitting position. If tolerated, client should remain upright for 1 hour after feedings.
- Instruct client or primary care giver to keep air from entering tubing via irrigating syringe and to irrigate with 30 to 60 ml of water before and after feedings, before and after medications, and before and after residual checks.
- Instruct client or primary care giver that client may complain of feelings of fullness, increased gas, belching, or diarrhea.
- Teach client or primary care giver method of GI fluid pH measurement and expected range.

Pediatric Considerations

- Intermittent feeding is preferred in infants because of possible perforation of the stomach, nasal airway obstruction, ulceration, and irritation to mucous membranes with continuous feedings.

Gerontologic Considerations

- Older adult clients may be more susceptible to hyperglycemia related to the glucose concentration in enteral formulas.

Home Care Considerations

- Instruct primary care giver and client to monitor intake and output using household measuring devices.

SKILL 23-4 Administering Enteral Feedings via Gastrostomy Tube

Gastric feeding takes advantage of the stomach's capacity as a natural reservoir, permitting delivery of partially digested nutrients to the bowel at a slow rate. Gastric feedings may be given through a nasogastric or a **gastrostomy feeding tube.** The nasogastric tube can be inserted by the nurse (see Skill 23-1).

A gastrostomy tube is an alternative route for gastric feedings. The tube is inserted in the operating room or endoscopy suite by a surgeon or gastroenterologist. A large tube is surgically placed in the stomach and exits through an incision in the upper left quadrant of the abdomen. An alternative is a percutaneous endoscopic gastrostomy (PEG) tube, which is inserted with endoscopic visualization of the stomach (Fig. 23-2). This tube exits through a puncture wound in the upper left quadrant of the abdomen. These tubes are used for clients unable to tolerate nasogastric tubes or who are expected to be receiving enteral feedings for a long time.

EQUIPMENT

- **Disposable feeding container and tubing**
- **30-ml or larger Luer-Lok or catheter-tip syringe**
- **Stethoscope**
- **Formula**
- **Infusion pump: use pump designed for tube feedings**
- **pH indicator strip**
- **Gloves**

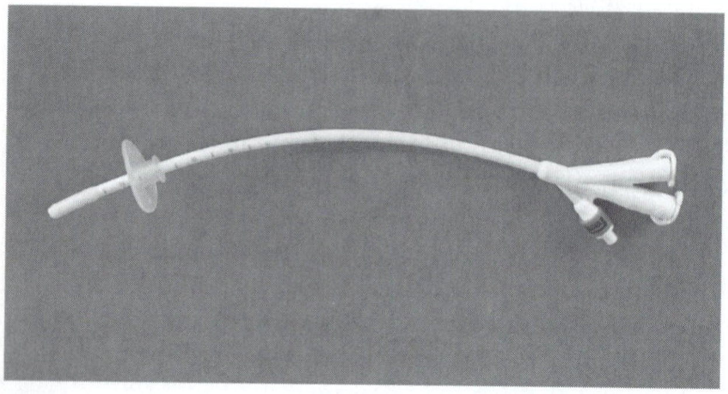

Fig. 23-2 Percutaneous endoscopic gastrostomy tube (PEG).

DELEGATION CONSIDERATIONS

Administration of enteral tube feeding via syringe is a procedure that can be delegated to unlicensed assistive personnel.

- The professional nurse should verify tube placement before the feeding and establish patency of the tube by flushing it with water.
- The nurse should also ensure that the client is sitting upright in a chair or in bed and instruct the assistive personnel to infuse the feeding slowly.
- Unlicensed personnel should be instructed to report any difficuly infusing the feeding or any discomfort voiced by the client.

STEPS	RATIONALE
ASSESSMENT	
1. Identify signs and symptoms of malnutrition (see Chapter 22).	Certain conditions place the client at risk for malnutrition.
2. Assess client for food allergies.	Prevents client from developing localized or systemic allergic responses.
3. Assess client's need for enteral tube feedings (see Skill 23-1): impaired swallowing, decreased level of consciousness, surgeries of upper alimentary canal, long-term need for enteral nutrition.	Identifies clients who need tube feedings before they become nutritionally depleted.
4. Auscultate for bowel sounds before feeding.	Bowel sounds indicate presence of peristalsis and ability of gastrointestinal tract to digest nutrients.
5. Verify physician's order for formula, rate, route, and frequency.	Tube feedings must be ordered by physician.
6. Assess gastrostomy site for breakdown, irritation, or drainage.	Infection, pressure from gastrostomy tube, or drainage of gastric secretions can cause skin breakdown.
7. Obtain baseline weight and laboratory values.	Enteral feedings are to restore or maintain a client's nutritional status. Provides objective data to measure effectiveness of feedings.

NURSING DIAGNOSIS

Clustering of defining characteristics from the assessment data may reveal the following nursing diagnosis for clients requiring this skill:

- Altered nutrition: less than body requirements

Related factors are individualized based on a client's condition or needs.

STEPS	RATIONALE
PLANNING	
1. **Expected outcomes** following completion of procedure:	
➤ Nutritional status is improved, as evidenced by increasing weight, improving laboratory values, and improving intake and output.	Indicates that client's nutritional needs are being met.
➤ There are no signs of respiratory distress (e.g., increased respiratory rate, coughing, poor color).	Signs occur if vomitus or regurgitated feeding enters the respiratory tract.
➤ Skin surrounding stoma site is dry and intact.	Skin breakdown around gastrostomy site occurs from pressure of feeding tube or seepage of gastric contents around tube.
2. Explain procedure to client.	Well-informed client is more cooperative and feels more at ease.
3. Wash hands.	Reduces transmission of microorganisms.
4. Prepare feeding container to administer formula:	
a. Connect tubing to container as needed or prepare ready-to-hang container.	Tubing must be free of contamination to prevent bacterial growth.
b. Fill container and tubing with formula.	Filling tubing with formula prevents excess air from entering gastrointestinal tract.
5. Elevate head of bed 30 to 45 degrees.	Elevating client's head helps prevent chance of aspiration.
IMPLEMENTATION	
1. Apply gloves and check placement of gastric tube:	
a. Aspirate gastric secretions and check gastric residual. Return gastric contents to stomach unless the volume exceeds 150 ml. If the volume is >150 ml, hold feeding and notify the physician.	Presence of gastric contents indicates that end of tube is in stomach. Gastric residual determines if gastric emptying is delayed. Delayed gastric emptying may be indicated by 150 ml or more remaining in client's stomach from previous feeding.
b. Measure pH of aspirated GI contents.	Gastric contents usually have a pH range of 1 to 4. Intestinal sites have a pH of >6 (Metheny et al., 1993).

STEPS	RATIONALE
2. Initiate feeding:	
a. **Bolus or Intermittent Feeding:**	
(1) Pinch proximal end of the gastrostomy tube.	Prevents air from entering the client's stomach.
(2) Attach barrel of syringe to end of tube.	
(3) Fill syringe with formula. Allow syringe to empty gradually, refilling until prescribed amount has been delivered to the client.	Gradual emptying of tube feeding by gravity from a syringe or gavage bag reduces the risk of diarrhea induced by bolus tube feedings.
(4) If feeding container is used, hang feeding container on an IV pole. Fill container with prescribed amount of formula and allow container to empty gradually over at least 30 minutes. Flush tube at end of feeding.	
b. **Continuous-Drip Method:**	
(1) Hang feeding container on IV pole.	
(2) Connect end of feeding tube container to the proximal end of the gastrostomy tube.	
(3) Connect tubing through infusion pump and set rate.	Continuous feeding method is designed to deliver a prescribed hourly rate of feeding. This method reduces the risk of diarrhea. Clients who receive continuous-drip feedings should have residuals checked every 4 hours.
3. When tube feedings are not being administered, cap or clamp the proximal end of the gastrostomy tube.	Prevents air from entering the stomach between feedings.
4. Administer water via feeding tube as ordered with or between feedings.	Provides client with source of water to help maintain fluid and electrolyte balance.
5. Rinse container and tubing with warm water after all intermittent feedings.	Rinsing container and tube with warm water clears old tube feedings and prevents bacterial growth.

CRITICAL DECISION POINT Advance tube feeding rate gradually (see the box on p. 756). Tube feedings should be advanced gradually to prevent diarrhea and gastric intolerance of formula.

STEPS	RATIONALE
6. The gastrostomy exit site is usually left open to air. However, if a dressing is needed because of drainage, change dressing daily or PRN and report the drainage to the physician; inspect exit site every shift.	Leakage of gastric drainage may cause irritation and excoriation. Skin around feeding tube should be cleansed daily with warm water and mild soap; a small precut gauze dressing may be applied to exit site.
7. Dispose of supplies and wash hands.	Reduces transmission of microorganisms.

EVALUATION

STEPS	RATIONALE
1. Evaluate client's tolerance of tube feeding. Check amount of aspirate (residual) every 4 hours.	Tolerance of tube feeding is evaluated by checking.
2. Monitor finger-stick blood glucose every 6 hours until maximum rate of administration is reached and maintained for 24 hours.	Alerts nurse to client's tolerance of glucose or fluid volume excess.
3. Monitor intake and output every 24 hours.	Intake and output are indications of fluid balance.
4. Weigh client daily until maximum administration rate is reached and maintained for 24 hours, then weigh client three times per week.	Weight gain is indicator of improved nutritional status; however, a sudden gain of >2 pounds in 24 hours usually indicates fluid retention.
5. Observe return of normal laboratory values.	Improving laboratory values (i.e., albumin, transferrin, and prealbumin) indicate return to normal nutritional status.

STEPS	RATIONALE
6. Observe stoma site for skin integrity.	Gastric secretions can cause injury and necrosis at stoma site.
7. **Unexpected outcomes** that may occur include:	
➤ Client aspirates formula.	Aspiration can occur when gastric emptying is delayed or formula is administered too rapidly and produces vomiting. Suction equipment should be available for the client who is receiving enteral nutrition.
➤ Client develops diarrhea.	Clients receiving tube feedings may have loose stools, but diarrhea or liquid stools (three times or more in 24 hours) indicate intolerance. Antibiotics and medications containing sorbitol may induce diarrhea (Edes, Walk, and Austin, 1990; Benya, Layden, and Movarhan, 1991; Guenther et al., 1991).
➤ Client develops nausea and vomiting.	Vomiting is usually not caused by feeding but may indicate gastric ileus.
➤ Skin surrounding gastrostomy site breaks down.	Pressure from tube or presence of gastric contents irritates skin.

Recording and Reporting

1. Record amount and type of feeding.	Documents amount and type of feeding administered to client.
2. Record client's response to tube feeding, patency of tube, and any untoward effects.	Documents client's reaction to therapy and identifies presence of any adverse reactions (e.g., aspiration).
3. Report to oncoming nursing staff: type of feeding, status of gastrostomy tube, client's tolerance, adverse effects.	Provides new nursing personnel with status of gastric feeding. Allows new nursing staff to plan for next feeding.

Follow-up Activities

1. Aspiration: suction client, notify physician, obtain chest x-ray film.
2. Diarrhea: decrease feeding, review medications, notify physician.
3. Nausea and vomiting: withhold tube feeding and notify physician.

• • • • •

Special Considerations

- ➤ If bowel sounds are absent, notify physician before initiating feeding.
- ➤ Formula can be hung 6 to 8 hours at room temperature in a standard feeding container or longer if given in a ready-to-hang system.
- ➤ Gastrostomy tube is easier and safer for client because of location and is more appropriate for long-term use.
- ➤ Risk of aspiration may be lessened if head of bed is elevated 30 to 45 degrees during feeding and for 1 hour after feeding.
- ➤ Client may need antidiarrheal agents or stool culture if diarrhea occurs.
- ➤ Some tube feedings are ordered as continuous drip over 24 hours; others are ordered for a specified amount given at intermittent intervals (e.g., 230 ml every 4 hours).

Teaching Considerations

- ➤ Teach client or primary care giver to clean around tube with warm water and mild soap. Hydrogen peroxide diluted with water can be used for the first few days after insertion of the tube to remove any crusting around the exit site. A dressing is usually not necessary or recommended.
- ➤ If client has a large-bore tube, instruct client or primary care giver to crush all pills and mix with water before administration through the tube. If client has a small-bore tube, medications in liquid form are less likely to clog the tube.
- ➤ Instruct client or primary care giver to keep air from entering tubing via irrigating syringe and to irrigate with 30 to 60 ml of water before and after feedings, before and after residual checks, and before and after medications.

Pediatric Considerations

- ➤ A low-profile gastrostomy tube (gastrostomy button) may be used for pediatric clients to decrease the chance of the child pulling out or dislodging the tube and for increased comfort. The low-profile tube has an adapter to allow syringe feeding or connection to a feeding container.

➤ Intermittent feeding is preferred in infants because of possible perforation of stomach and irritation to mucous membranes with continuous feedings.

Gerontologic Considerations

➤ Older adults may have decreased gastric transit time so that formula remains in the stomach longer than for younger clients. Gastric residual checks are of special importance to decrease the risk of vomiting and aspiration during gastric feeding.

Home Care Considerations

➤ Instruct primary care giver to maintain records of intake and output using household measuring devices.

SKILL 23-5 Administering Enteral Feedings via Nasointestinal Tube or Jejunostomy Tube

Nasointestinal (NI), that is, duodenal or jejunal feedings, are given to clients who have gastric ileus (decreased or absent peristalsis that affects the stomach but not the intestines), delayed gastric emptying, gastric resections precluding delivery of nutrients into the stomach, or neurological impairments that place them at greater risk of aspiration. Clients who do not require long-term support can benefit from use of the NI route. The advantage of these feedings is decreased gastric reflux, which reduces the risk of aspiration.

The **jejunal feeding tube** is inserted during surgery or in the endoscopy suite. Endoscopic insertion of a jejunostomy tube may be done in the same procedure with a percutaneous endoscopic gastrostomy (PEG) tube. The jejunostomy tube is inserted into the gastrostomy tube and passes through it into the small bowel (Fig. 23-3).

After insertion of a large-bore PEG tube, the percutaneous endoscopic jejunostomy (PEJ) tube is passed through the PEG tube and advanced into the jejunum. A Y-shaped connector attached to the jejunostomy tube caps the PEG tube and closes the system. This Y-shaped connector labels the gastrostomy tube and designates the jejunostomy tube for feeding. The nurse should be aware of which tube is gastric and which is jejunal.

EQUIPMENT

- Disposable feeding container or ready-to-hang bag
- 30-ml or larger Luer-Lok or catheter-tip syringe
- Formula
- Infusion pump: use pump designed for tube feedings
- pH indicator strips
- Stethoscope
- Gloves

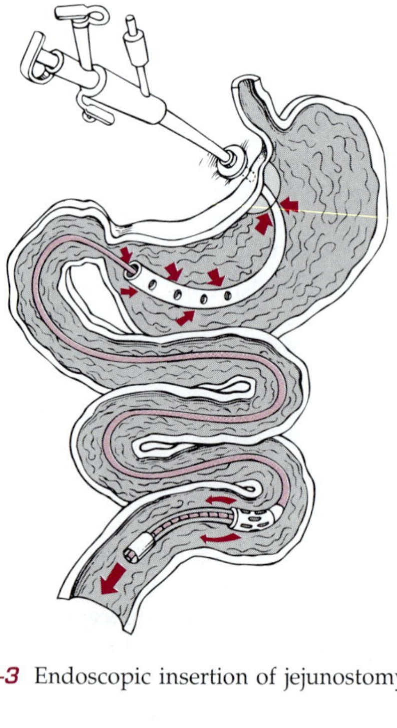

Fig. 23-3 Endoscopic insertion of jejunostomy tube.

DELEGATION CONSIDERATIONS

Administration of enteral tube feeding via a nasointestinal tube or a jejunal tube is a procedure that can be delegated to unlicensed assistive personnel.

- The professional nurse should verify tube placement before the feeding and establish patency of the tube by flushing it with water.
- The nurse should also ensure that the client is sitting upright in a chair or in bed and instruct the assistive personnel to infuse the feeding slowly.
- Unlicensed personnel should be instructed to report any difficulty infusing the feeding or any discomfort voiced by the client.

STEPS	RATIONALE
ASSESSMENT	
1. Identify signs and symptoms of malnutrition (see Chapter 22).	Certain conditions place the client at risk for malnutrition.
2. Assess client for food allergies.	Prevents client from developing localized or systemic allergic responses.
3. Assess client's need for enteral tube feedings (see Skill 23-1): impaired swallowing, decreased level of consciousness, surgeries of upper alimentary tract, need for long-term enteral nutrition.	Identifies clients who need tube feedings before they become nutritionally depleted. Enteral feeding preserves the function and mass of the gut, promotes wound healing, diminishes hypermetabolism in burn injuries, and may decrease infection in critically ill clients (Zaloga, 1994).
4. Auscultate for bowel sounds before feeding. Consult physician if bowel sounds are absent.	Absence of bowel sounds may indicate decreased or absent peristalsis and increased risk of aspiration or abdominal distention.
5. Obtain baseline weight and laboratory values.	Enteral feedings are to restore or maintain nutritional status. Provides objective data to measure effectiveness of feedings.
6. Verify physician's order for formula, rate, route, and frequency.	Tube feedings must be ordered by physician.

NURSING DIAGNOSIS

Clustering of defining characteristics from the assessment data may reveal the following nursing diagnosis for clients requiring this skill:

- Altered nutrition: less than body requirements

Related factors are individualized based on a client's condition or needs.

STEPS	RATIONALE
PLANNING	
1. **Expected outcomes** following completion of procedure:	
➤ Nutritional status is improved, as evidenced by increasing weight and improving laboratory values.	Indicates that client's nutritional needs are being met.
➤ Client verbalizes or demonstrates comfort.	
➤ There are no signs of respiratory distress.	
➤ There are no signs of pressure around nares.	
➤ Skin surrounding jejunostomy site is dry and intact.	
2. Explain procedure to client.	Well-informed client is more cooperative and feels more at ease.
3. Prepare feeding container to administer formula:	
a. Have tube feeding at room temperature.	Cold formula may cause gastric cramping and discomfort because the liquid is not warmed by mouth and esophagus.
b. Connect tubing to container as needed or prepare ready-to-hang bag.	Tubing must be free of contamination to prevent bacterial growth.
c. Fill container and tubing with formula.	Placement of formula through tubing prevents excess air from entering gastrointestinal tract.
4. Elevate head of bed 30 to 45 degrees.	Elevating client's head helps prevent chance of aspiration.
IMPLEMENTATION	
1. Wash hands and put on clean gloves.	Reduces transmission of microorganisms.
2. Measure pH of aspirated GI contents.	Gastric contents usually have a pH range of 1 to 4. Intestinal sites have a pH of >6 (Metheny et al., 1993).

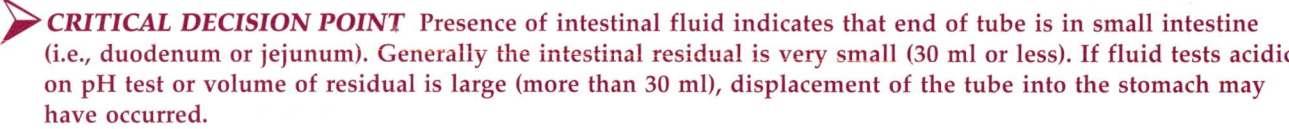

STEPS	RATIONALE
CRITICAL DECISION POINT **Presence of intestinal fluid indicates that end of tube is in small intestine (i.e., duodenum or jejunum). Generally the intestinal residual is very small (30 ml or less). If fluid tests acidic on pH test or volume of residual is large (more than 30 ml), displacement of the tube into the stomach may have occurred.**	
3. Flush with 30 ml of water.	
CRITICAL DECISION POINT **Initiate continuous tube feeding (see Skill 23-3, Implementation, "Continuous-drip method," Step 1b, p. 760).**	NI feedings are given continuously to ensure proper absorption.
4. Flush tube with 30 to 60 ml of water at the end of the feeding or before refilling the feeding container.	Maintains patency of tube and provides client with some free water (without concentrated formula fluid).
5. Advance tube feeding administration rate gradually (see p. 724).	To provide maximal nutrition, formula needs to be increased to meet client's nutritional requirements.
EVALUATION	
1. Evaluate amount of aspirate (residual) every 4 hours.	Evaluates tolerance of tube feeding.
2. Monitor finger-stick blood glucose every 6 hours until maximum administration rate is reached and maintained for 24 hours.	Alerts nurse to client's tolerance of glucose.
3. Monitor intake and output every 24 hours.	Intake and output are indications of fluid balance or fluid volume excess.
4. Weigh client daily until maximum administration rate is reached and maintained for 24 hours, then weigh client three times per week.	Weight gain is indicator of improved nutritional status; however, a sudden gain of >2 pounds in 24 hours usually indicates fluid retention.
5. Observe return of normal laboratory values.	Improving laboratory values (albumin, transferrin, prealbumin) indicate an improved nutritional status.
6. Inspect nares or jejunostomy site for signs of pressure.	Nasointestinal tubes can cause uncomfortable pressure areas on client's nares.
7. **Unexpected outcomes** that may occur include:	
➤ Client develops diarrhea.	Antibiotics and medications containing sorbitol may induce diarrhea (Edes, Walk, and Austin, 1990; Benya, Layden, and Movarhan, 1991; Guenther et al., 1991).
➤ Client develops nausea and vomiting.	Vomiting is usually not caused by feeding but may indicate displacement of the nasointestinal tube into the stomach or the need for gastric decompression (if the vomitus does not appear to be tube feeding).
➤ Client develops respiratory distress.	Results from vomitus or regurgitated feeding tube formula in respiratory tract.
➤ Skin surrounding nares breaks down.	Results from prolonged pressure from feeding tube on nares.
RECORDING AND REPORTING	
1. Record amount and type of feeding.	Documents amount and type of feeding administered to client.
2. Record client's response to tube feeding, patency of tube, and any side effects.	Documents client's reaction to therapy and identifies presence of any adverse reactions (e.g., aspiration).
3. Report to oncoming nursing staff: type of feeding, status of feeding tube, client's tolerance, adverse effects.	Provides new nursing personnel with status of intestinal feeding. Allows new nursing staff to plan for next feeding.

FOLLOW-UP ACTIVITIES

1. Diarrhea: decrease feeding, review medications, notify physician.
2. Nausea and vomiting: withhold tube feeding and notify physician.

• • • • •

Special Considerations

- Formula can be hung 6 to 8 hours at room temperature in a standard feeding container or longer if given in a ready-to-hang system.
- Aspiration may be lessened if head of bed is elevated 30 to 45 degrees during feeding.
- If bowel sounds are absent, notify physician before initiating feeding.
- Client may need antidiarrheal agents or stool cultures if diarrhea occurs.

Teaching Considerations

- Teach client or primary care giver to clean around tube with warm water and mild soap. Hydrogen peroxide diluted with water can be used for the first few days after insertion of the tube to remove any crusting around the exit site. A dressing is usually not necessary or recommended.
- Instruct client or primary care giver to keep air from entering tubing via irrigating syringe and to irrigate with 30 to 60 ml of water before and after feedings, before and after residual checks, and before and after medications.

Pediatric Considerations

- Infant enteral formulas are specially designed to mimic breast milk. Very small bore tubes (5 to 7 Fr) are used for enteral feeding in infants and young children.

Gerontologic Considerations

- The use of an intestinal feeding tube may reduce the risk of aspiration of tube feeding for the older adult.

Home Care Considerations

- Instruct primary care giver to maintain records of intake and output using household measuring devices.

CRITICAL THINKING EXERCISES

1. **Your client has a nasointestinal (NI) feeding tube for continuous tube feeding. He has just vomited 200 ml of fluid that resembles the tube feeding formula. What steps would you take to assess his airway and make decisions about the tube placement and feeding schedule?**
2. **Your client had a nasogastric feeding tube inserted 3 days ago. While checking for placement you obtain a pH of 7. What are the possible explantions for this value, and what actions would you take?**
3. **Your client has gained 5 pounds after 2 days of continuous enteral feeding. What would you do?**

REFERENCES

Benya R, Layden T, Movarhan S: Diarrhea associated with tube feeding: the importance of objective criteria, *J Clin Gastroenterol* 13(2):167, 1991.

Chang J et al: Inadvertent endobronchial intubation with nasogastric tube, *Arch Otolaryngol* 108:528, 1982.

Edes TE, Walk BE, Austin JL: Diarrhea in tube-fed patients: feeding formula not necessarily the cause, *Am J Med* 88:91, 1990.

Guenther P et al: Tube feeding–related diarrhea in acutely ill patients, *JPEN* 15(3):277, 1991.

Hanson RL: Predictive criteria for length of nasogastric tube insertion for tube feeding, *JPEN* 3:160, 1979.

Lehmann S: Parenteral and enteral access devices. In Teasley-Strausberg KM, editor: *Nutrition support handbook,* Cincinnati, 1992, Harvey Whitney Books.

Lord L et al: Comparison of weighted vs unweighted enteral feeding tubes for efficacy of transpyloric intubation, *JPEN* 17(3):271, 1993.

Metheny N: Measures to test placement of nasogastric and nasoenteral feeding tubes: a review, *Nurs Res* 37(6):323, 1988.

Metheny NM: *Fluid and electrolyte balance: nursing considerations,* ed 3, Philadelphia, 1996, Lippincott.

Metheny N et al: Detection of inadvertent respiratory placement of small-bore feeding tubes: a report of 10 cases, *Heart Lung* 19(6):631, 1990a.

Metheny N et al: Effectiveness of pH measurements in predicting feeding tube placement, *Nurs Res* 38(5):285, 1989.

Metheny N et al: Effectiveness of pH measurements in predicting feeding tube placement: an update, *Nurs Res* 42(6):323, 1993.

Metheny N et al: Effectiveness of the auscultatory method in predicting feeding tube location, *Nurs Res* 39(5):262, 1990b.

Welch SK: Certification of staff nurses to insert enteral feeding tubes using a research-based procedure, *NCP* 11(1):21, 1996.

Zaloga G: Timing and route of nutritional support. In Zaloga G, editor: *Nutrition in critical care,* St Louis, 1994, Mosby.

ADDITIONAL READING

Clochesy J: Evaluation of a system for intragastric pH monitoring of intensive care unit patients: preliminary report, *Am J Crit Care* 1(1):81, 1992.

Heather D et al: Effect of a bulk-forming cathartic on diarrhea in tube-fed patients, *Heart Lung* 1(20):409, 1991.

Hickey MS: *Handbook of enteral, parenteral, and ARC/AIDS nutritional therapy,* St Louis, 1992, Mosby.

Jacobs S et al: Continuous enteral feeding: a major cause of pneumonia among ventilated intensive care unit patients, *JPEN* 14(4):353, 1990.

Kohn C: The relationship between enteral formula contamination and length of enteral delivery set usage, *JPEN* 15(5):567, 1991.

CHAPTER 24

Parenteral Nutrition

OBJECTIVES

Mastery of content in this chapter will enable the nurse to:

- Define key terms.
- Identify clients who are candidates for parenteral nutrition.
- Identify appropriate sites to administer parenteral nutrition.
- Demonstrate appropriate nursing care of the client receiving all types of nutritional support.
- Assist the physician with placement of a central vein catheter.
- Demonstrate a central line dressing change application.

KEY TERMS

Amino acid	Malabsorption
Dextrose	Osmolality
Enteral nutrition	Parenteral nutrition
Hydrothorax	Trendelenburg position
Infusate	Valsalva maneuver
Iso-osmotic solutions	Visceral protein status
Lipid emulsion	

SKILLS

24-1 Caring for the Client Receiving Central Venous Placement for Central Parenteral Nutrition

24-2 Caring for the Client Receiving Central Parenteral Nutrition (CPN)

24-3 Caring for the Client Receiving Peripheral Parenteral Nutrition with Lipid (Fat) Emulsion

Parenteral nutrition (PN) is the intravenous (IV) infusion of nutrients, including amino acids (protein/nitrogen), glucose (hypertonic, isotonic solutions), fat emulsions (fatty acids), vitamins, electrolytes, minerals, and trace elements. Nutrition through the gastrointestinal tract **(enteral nutrition)** is best and should be used when the client's gastrointestinal tract is functional before initiating parenteral nutrition. However, certain disease states limit the ability to use enteral nutrition, and PN is indicated.

To provide comprehensive care, the nurse must be able to detect clients at risk for malnutrition and assess malnourished clients. Detection and assessment of these clients is discussed in Skill 22-1. Performing a nutritional assessment enables the nurse to determine a therapeutic approach that addresses the client's nutritional needs, as well as the appropriate route of administration. Parenteral nutrition can be administered as peripheral parenteral nutrition (PPN) or central parenteral nutrition (CPN). **Iso-osmotic solutions** (of similar **osmolality** as blood) can be given via peripheral veins; however, hypertonic (highly concentrated) solutions must be given via central veins. The final concentration of **dextrose** in the nutrition solution is the main factor that determines the osmolarity of PN.

Lipid emulsions were previously most often given as a separate infusion that was piggybacked into the PN solution. Today, total nutrient admixture or three-in-one emulsions are used to provide nutritionally complete PN. Fats provide significant calories in the American diet and supply essential and nonessential fatty acids that are used as energy. The essential fatty acid present in **lipid emulsion** is linoleic acid; this acid cannot be made from other fats in humans and must be supplied. Linoleic acid is an omega-6 fatty acid and a deficiency of linoleic acid is immunosuppressive. Current research is focused on structured lipid emulsions that are composed of a mixture of omega-6 and omega-3 (fish oil–based) fatty acids (Babineau et al., 1994).

A nutritional regimen that does not provide adequate

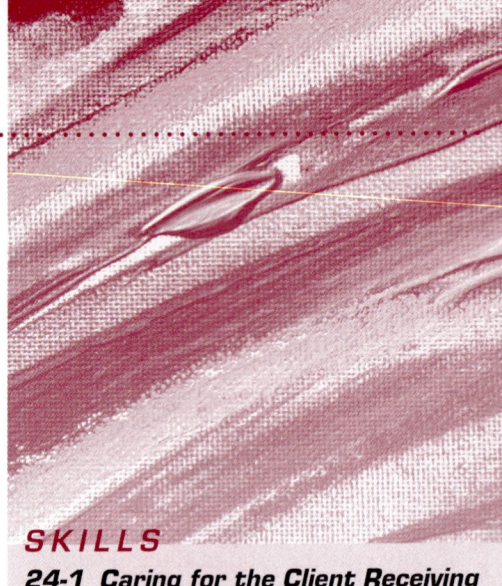

fatty acids can lead to essential fatty acid deficiency (EFAD). Signs and symptoms of EFAD include dry scaly skin, sparse hair growth, impaired wound healing, decreased resistance to stress, increased susceptibility to respiratory tract infections, anemia, thrombocytopenia, and liver function abnormalities.

Fat emulsion is a soybean or safflower oil base that is isotonic and may be infused with an amino acid and dextrose solution through a central or peripheral vein. Fats may be administered through a separate IV; given piggyback through a Y connector near the port of entry; or given through admixing the amino acid, dextrose, and fat emulsion solution in one container (three-in-one system) to infuse over 24 hours. When administering fat (lipid) emulsions via piggyback infusion, the solution must be added below the infusion filter and inserted in the port nearest to the venipuncture site.

Rapid infusion (6 to 8 hours) of lipids may produce symptoms of nausea, vomiting, and fever, which may be relieved by slowing the infusion rate.

Emulsified fats provide a high-calorie intake. For example, 500 ml of a 10% solution supplies 550 kcal, and 500 ml of a 20% solution supplies 1000 kcal.

Not all clients should receive fat emulsion. Individuals for whom fat emulsions are contraindicated include those who have a disturbance of normal fat metabolism, such as pathological hyperlipemia.

PN has physiological and psychological implications. Clients who are unable to eat may become socially isolated, suffer hunger pangs, have food cravings, or even hallucinate about food. A majority of social events focus around food, thereby excluding the client from complete participation. The nurse promotes the client's psychological well-being by discussing possible feelings and sensations with the client; describing possible alternatives to satisfy oral cravings, such as chewing gum or sucking on hard candies (if allowed); and describing ways in which the client may continue to participate in social interactions. Many clients who receive parenteral nutrition are capable of some oral intake. Client and family education helps to alleviate many of the client's and family's fears and concerns.

The nursing committee of the American Society of Parenteral and Enteral Nutrition (ASPEN) has defined nutritional support nursing practice, the scope of nutritional support nursing, and the goals of nutritional support (ASPEN, 1996):

> Nutritional support nursing practice is the care of individuals with potential or known nutrition alterations. The goal of nutrition support nursing is to assist individuals to restore and maintain optimal nutritional health.

GUIDELINES

1. Identify clients who are candidates for PN. Clients unable to take nutrition orally or enterally and who are at risk of malnutrition because of actual or anticipated prolonged inability to ingest, digest, or absorb nutrients should be considered for PN. In addition, clients who are severely injured may receive PN and enteral nutrition.
2. Know when peripheral vein access can be used instead of central vein access. Clients who require short-term nutrition support, for whom central access placement is contraindicated or not feasible, who have adequate peripheral access, and who can tolerate larger volumes of fluid are candidates for peripheral parenteral nutrition.
3. Know the limits of solutions used for peripheral vein versus central vein access. Solutions with a final dextrose concentration of >10% must be given via central vein.
4. Be aware of complications associated with PN. Major side effects include metabolic, fluid imbalance, technical, and infections.
5. Establish the client's normal range of vital signs, electrolyte balance, triglyceride levels, and fluid status. Clients who receive PN may have rapid changes in these values.
6. Know the client's recent temperature range. Clients with peripheral or central IV lines are susceptible to septicemia; an elevated temperature can be an early indicator of a bacterial process.

DELEGATION CONSIDERATIONS

The skills in this chapter require problem solving and knowledge application unique to a professional nurse. For these skills, delegation is inappropriate.

SKILL 24-1 Caring for the Client Receiving Central Venous Placement for Central Parenteral Nutrition

Central parenteral nutrition (CPN) is a form of nutritional support administered through central vein cannulation (Fig. 24-1). A catheter is usually placed in the subclavian vein through infraclavicular venipuncture. This site is preferred because it provides a flat, relatively immobile area on the chest and blood flows at a high rate, decreasing the risk of phlebitis or displacement.

The nurse has an important role when assisting the physician to place a CPN line. Attention to asepsis and positioning, being available to reassure the client during the procedure, and ensuring that the right equipment is available are critical to the success of the procedure. Because CPN is associated with numerous complications (Table 24-1), it is also vital that the nurse carefully monitor the CPN site and notify the physician of any symptoms or complications (Flowers, Ryan, and Gough, 1991; Hickey, 1992; Davis, 1991).

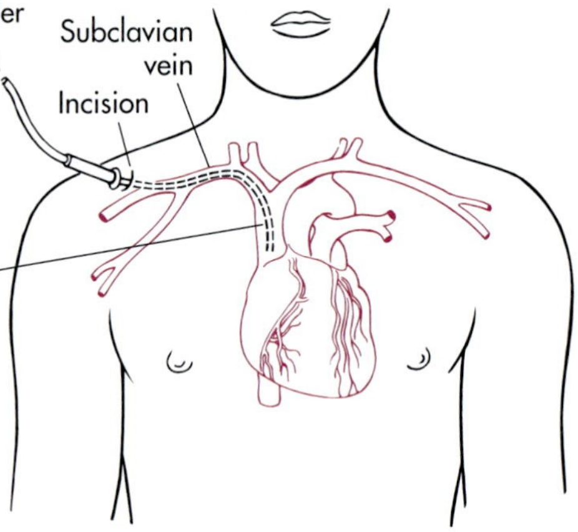

Fig. 24-1

Table 24-1 Complications of Central Parenteral Nutrition

Problem	Cause	Symptoms	Immediate Action	Prevention
Air embolism	IV tubing disconnected; part of catheter system open or removed without clamp on	Sudden respiratory distress; shortness of breath, coughing, chest pain	Clamp catheter; position client in Trendelenburg position; call physician	Make sure all catheter connections are secure; clamp catheter
Infection	Poor aseptic technique. Contaminated tubing or infusate; secondary contamination from septicemia	Unexplained hyperglycemia, redness at infection site, fever, chills	Call physician	Use proper aseptic technique
Hyperglycemia	Client receiving solution too quickly; too little insulin in solution; infection	Excessive thirst, urination, blood sugar >160 mg/ml	Call physician; may need to slow infusion rate (physician order)	Review medical history for glucose intolerance or diabetes; keep rate as ordered, never increase to "catch up." Use aseptic technique and routine blood glucose monitoring
Hypoglycemia	CPN abruptly discontinued; too much insulin	Client is shaky, dizzy, nervous, anxious	Call physician; if CPN discontinued abruptly, may need to restart D_{10}NS at previous CPN rate. If client has oral intake, give ½ cup fruit juice. Perform blood glucose monitoring; retest in 15 to 30 minutes	Decrease CPN, "tapering" gradually until discontinued; blood glucose monitoring is used to ensure adequate insulin

Modified from Davis CL: Nursing care of total parenteral and enteral nutrition. In Fischer JE, editor: *Total parenteral nutrition,* ed 2, Boston, 1991, Little, Brown; Hickey MS: *Handbook of enteral, parenteral, and ARC/AIDS nutritional therapy,* St Louis, 1992, Mosby; Pennington CR: Toward safer parenteral nutrition, *Aliment Pharmacol Ther* 4(5):427, 1990 (review article).

EQUIPMENT

- **Subclavian insertion tray** *or* the following:
- **Caps**
- **Sterile gowns**
- **Masks and protective eyewear (if there is a risk of "splash")**
- **Nonsterile gloves**
- **Sterile gloves**
- **Gauze pads**
- **Bottle of alcohol**
- **Alcohol swabs**
- **Surgical towels**
- **Povidone-iodine scrub**
- **Povidone-iodine swabsticks**
- **1% lidocaine (Xylocaine)**
- **Central line catheter kit**
- **Sterile drapes**
- **500-ml bottle D_5W**
- **Transparent dressing or gauze dressing for catheter insertion site**
- **Tape**
- **Intravenous infusion pump**
- **Tincture of benzoin (optional)**

STEPS	RATIONALE
ASSESSMENT	
1. Assess need for CPN and define client's current nutritional status.	Provides baseline to compare changes after CPN is started.
2. Check physician's order for insertion of central vein catheter and for size and type of catheter.	Invasive procedure requires a consent. Physician may request a certain type or size of catheter.
3. Assess client's hydration status.	Dehydration depletes fluid volume and may make insertion of a central vein catheter more difficult.
4. Assess client for any surgical procedures of the upper chest or anatomical irregularities.	Previous surgical procedures or central vein catheterizations may indicate that a particular site should not be used. Scoliosis or other spine deformities may make positioning difficult.

NURSING DIAGNOSIS

Clustering of defining characteristics from the assessment data may reveal the following nursing diagnoses for clients requiring this skill:

➤ Altered nutrition: less than body requirements
➤ Risk for infection

Related factors are individualized based on a client's condition or needs.

STEPS	RATIONALE
PLANNING	
1. **Expected outcomes** following completion of procedure:	
➤ Insertion occurs without complication.	Placement of a central vein catheter carries risks.
➤ Insertion site is free of inflammation.	Denotes absence of infection at central venous site.
2. Explain to client steps for central line placement, the **Valsalva maneuver,** the need for CPN, and follow-up care.	
3. Verify that consent was signed.	Consent document is required, because central line placement is considered an invasive procedure.
IMPLEMENTATION	
1. Nurse and physician wash hands.	Reduces transmission of microorganisms.
2. Physician, with the assistance of nurse, positions client flat in bed lying supine. Place rolled towel between client's scapulae and place protective pad under shoulder area.	Opens angle between clavicle and first rib; dilates veins.
3. Nurse puts on cap, mask, eyewear, and clean gloves. Physician should put on cap, gown, mask, and sterile gloves.	
4. Nurse opens central vein kit and adds any sterile equipment to the kit for use during the insertion.	Maintains sterile field.

STEPS	RATIONALE
5. Nurse saturates 4 × 4 gauze pads with alcohol, and physician scrubs area using circular motion from shoulder to ear to chin to nipple for approximately 1 minute.	Alcohol cleans and defats skin.
6. With povidone-iodine scrub, physician cleans same area for 1 minute.	Removes surface skin bacteria.
7. Physician wipes away excess scrub solution with sterile 4 × 4 gauze pad.	
8. Physician changes sterile gloves.	
9. Physician uses drapes and towels to create a sterile field. Physician finds anatomical landmarks and places fenestrated drape appropriately.	Provides sterile work space.
10. Physician prepares equipment in kit.	
11. Nurse sets up IV bag, fills tubing, and covers end of tubing with a sterile cap.	IV tubing is ready to be connected to IV catheter.
12. Nurse places client in **Trendelenburg position** and turns client's head away from site of insertion.	Promotes maximal filling and distention of subclavicular vein.
CRITICAL DECISION POINT **Trendelenburg position is contraindicated in clients with head injuries, increased intracranial pressure, and spinal cord injuries.**	
13. Nurse wipes off top of 1% lidocaine bottle with alcohol swabs and turns upside down.	Removes surface bacteria; allows physician to withdraw lidocaine while maintaining asepsis.
14. Physician injects needle into bottle and withdraws approximately 3 to 4 ml lidocaine. Physician injects needle into site for subclavian puncture and anesthetizes venipuncture site.	Minimizes discomfort client feels during venipuncture.
15. Physician inserts subclavian IV catheter into subclavian vein. Usually this is done by locating the vein with a large-bore cannula, removing the needle from the cannula, threading a wire into the cannula and vein, removing the cannula over the wire, and threading the central vein catheter over the wire to the appropriate location (Seldinger technique) (Nussbaum and Fischer, 1994).	Large vein is less irritated by CPN solution.
CRITICAL DECISION POINT **Nurse checks on client throughout to assess tolerance of procedure and asks client to perform Valsalva maneuver whenever the inserted catheter will be open to air.**	Valsalva maneuver increases intrathoracic pressure and prevents entry of air into the catheter.
16. When blood return is evident and catheter placement is appropriate, physician connects IV tubing to client's subclavian catheter.	Prevents air from entering venous system.
17. Nurse runs the IV fluid in at a rapid rate (macro drip 20-30 gtts/min, micro drip 60 gtts/min) for 5-10 minutes.	Assesses whether fluid is infusing easily.
18. Nurse lowers IV bag below heart level.	Provides blood return to determine presence of IV in venous system.
19. Nurse raises IV bag and slows rate to 30 to 40 ml per hour via infusion pump until chest x-ray study is obtained.	Central line cannulations increase risk of pneumothorax. Chest x-ray verifies absence of pneumothorax and confirms location before fluids are administered at a rapid flow.
20. Physician sutures central venous catheter in place.	Suturing catheter to skin at insertion site prevents accidental dislodgement.

STEPS	RATIONALE
21. Physician removes sterile drapes and completes procedure.	Occurs only if physician is not applying occlusive dressing to IV site.
Applying Occlusive Dressing	
1. Put on sterile gloves.	Maintains surgical asepsis.
2. With alcohol swab, start at catheter exit site and work in circular motion outward approximately 2 to 3 inches. (Do three times.)	Removes blood and defats skin.
3. With povidone-iodine swabs, repeat above step. Allow area to dry.	Disinfects skin. (Do not blow or fan dry.)
➤ ***CRITICAL DECISION POINT*** **It is no longer recommended to routinely apply** antimicrobial ointment **to catheter insertion site at time of insertion or during routine dressing changes (see Chapter 20).**	Studies of the efficacy of antimicrobial ointments are contradictory and, unless ointment contains a fungicide, it may contribute to colonization of *Candida* (Pearson, 1996).
4. Apply transparent or occlusive gauze dressing over site (see Chapter 37).	Reduces transmission of microorganisms to venipuncture site and allows observation of site.
5. Assist with chest x-ray examination.	Documents line position or presence of pneumothorax or other complications.
6. Reposition client.	Maintains comfort.
7. When position of central vein catheter is confirmed, prepare parenteral nutrition solution for infusion via infusion pump.	
8. Dispose of supplies and wash hands.	Reduces transmission of microorganisms.
EVALUATION	
1. Observe client for shortness of breath, pain, bleeding or swelling at the insertion site, and occlusiveness of the dressing.	Symptoms may indicate complications of insertion.
2. Observe insertion site for erythema, warmth, tenderness, edema, or drainage.	Symptoms may indicate infection at line insertion site.
3. **Unexpected outcomes** that may occur include (Table 24-1):	
➤ Displacement of the central vein catheter into veins of the neck or chest.	
➤ Pneumothorax.	
➤ Bleeding at the insertion site or into the pleural cavity.	
➤ Inability to place central vein catheter despite attempts.	Increases risk of pneumothorax.
RECORDING AND REPORTING	
1. Record condition of client before, during, and after the procedure.	Documents client's response to the procedure.
2. Document presence or absence of blood return after placement of the central vein catheter.	Establishes patency of line.
3. Document confirmation of appropriate position of the central vein catheter.	Establishes that catheter is in appropriate position before hypertonic dextrose is administered.

FOLLOW-UP ACTIVITIES

1. Shortness of breath or pain in the chest or shoulder within 24 to 48 hours after the insertion of a central venous catheter can be a sign of a delayed complication, such as a pneumothorax.

• • • • •

Special Considerations

- The site of insertion of the central venous catheter may affect the risk of contamination of the site or the ability to maintain an occlusive dressing. Femoral sites are more prone to contamination from urine or feces. Insertions via the internal jugular vein of the neck may be more prone to loss of occlusion from the client's movements.

Teaching Considerations

- Instruct client to report discomfort around the site; in either arm, shoulder, or side of the neck; or any shortness of breath.

Pediatric Considerations

- Central vein catheters that are of a smaller diameter and shorter length are available for children and infants.

Gerontologic Considerations

- Older adults may have difficulty with lying flat in bed, and a modification of the totally supine position may be necessary.

Home Care Considerations

- Clients or family members may need to learn to perform catheter site care for long-term implanted or tunneled central venous catheters.

SKILL 24-2 Caring for the Client Receiving Central Parenteral Nutrition (CPN)

Central parenteral nutrition (CPN) is a form of nutritional support indicated for correction or maintenance therapy for clients who are malnourished or at risk for malnutrition (Fig. 24-2). CPN involves the use of solutions infused through central veins (e.g., superior vena cava, femoral vein).

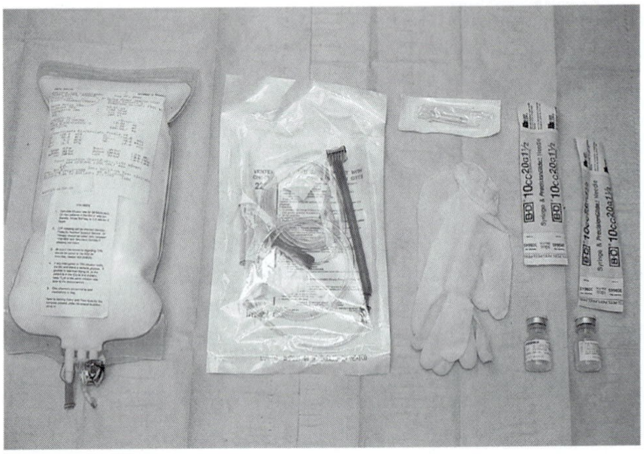

Fig. 24-2

EQUIPMENT

- IV infusion tubing
- CPN solution (IV)
- IV filter (optional—0.22 micron for dextrose/amino acids, 1.2 micron for three-in-one solutions)
- Intravenous infusion pump

STEPS	RATIONALE
ASSESSMENT	
1. Assess client's nutritional status (see Skill 22-1), caloric intake, laboratory values, and weight.	Nurse needs to be aware of client's nutritional needs to judge response to therapy.
2. Determine if client is candidate to receive CPN: client is NPO more than 6 days or there are symptoms of malnutrition (Table 24-2).	CPN should be used only for clients who are unable to be fed via the enteral route.
3. Assess factors influencing CPN administration.	Clients who have electrolyte disturbances, elevated blood glucose, renal dysfunction, or hepatic dysfunction may require their CPN therapy to be adapted.
4. Verify physician's order for nutrients, minerals, vitamins, trace elements, and electrolytes, as well as flow rate.	CPN must be ordered by physician and is often ordered daily in the hospital setting after review of laboratory values.

NURSING DIAGNOSIS

Clustering of defining characteristics from the assessment data may reveal the following nursing diagnoses for clients requiring this skill:

- Altered nutrition: less than body requirements
- Risk for infection

Related factors are individualized based on a client's condition or needs.

STEPS	RATIONALE

PLANNING

1. **Expected outcomes** following completion of procedure:
   - Client's ideal weight gain is usually between 1 and 2 lb per week.
     Weight is an indicator of how well the client is doing nutritionally and determines fluid volume. Weight gain greater than 1 lb per day indicates fluid retention.
   - Serum glucose levels are less than 200 mg/dl.
     Serum glucose levels are used to determine client's tolerance of the glucose solution.
   - Central access catheter or device is patent and site is free of pain, swelling, redness, inflammation, or phlebitis if a peripherally inserted central catheter is used.
     Ensures that CPN is infusing into the vein rather than into surrounding tissues and that there are no signs of an access device infection.
2. Explain purposes of CPN.
   Promotes understanding and reduces anxiety.

IMPLEMENTATION

1. Wash hands and put on gloves.
   Reduces transmission of microorganisms.
2. Inspect PN solution for particulate matter or, if it is a three-in-one solution, inspect emulsion for a cream layer or separation of the fat into a layer.

CRITICAL DECISION POINT Do not use the PN solution if it has particulate matter or if the lipids have separated. Notify the pharmacy and request a new solution.

3. Connect PN solution to appropriate intravenous tubing, prime tubing, and connect to central catheter line.
   PN solutions need to be connected to new, sterile intravenous tubing every 24 hours.
4. Place IV tubing into an intravenous infusion pump and regulate flow rate as ordered (see Chapter 20) (see illustration).
   CPN flow rates are ordered to meet client's metabolic and electrolyte needs. Rate must be maintained to prevent electrolyte imbalances. Typically, the initial administration rate is 40 to 60 ml per hour. The rate is advanced each day toward the target rate to provide adequate calories and protein.

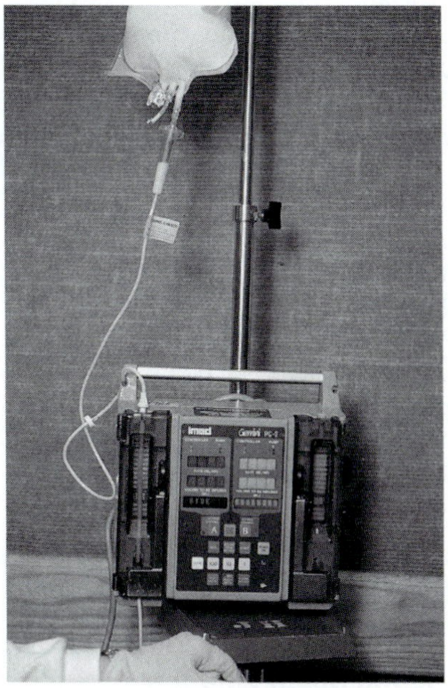

Step 4 TPN solution infusing via pump.

Table 24-2 Comparison of CPN and PPN

	CPN	PPN
Osmolality	1800 to 2000 mOsm	600 to 700 mOsm
Route of administration	Central venous catheter	Small peripheral vein
Usual daily caloric intake	2000 to 4000	700 to 2000
Fat emulsion	Minor caloric source; provides essential fatty acid	Major caloric source; provides essential fatty acid
Objectives	Weight maintenance; weight gain	Weight maintenance
Duration of therapy	6 days or longer	3 to 7 days

STEPS	RATIONALE
EVALUATION	
1. Obtain daily weights.	
2. Assess for fluid retention.	Weight gain in excess of 1 lb per day, dependent edema, lung crackles, and intake greater than output per each 24-hour period indicate fluid retention.
3. Monitor client's glucose and laboratory parameters to determine response to CPN.	Adequate tolerance is demonstrated by maintenance of normal electrolyte levels, satisfactory fluid balance, acceptable serum glucose levels, gradual increase in weight, and improvement in serum proteins.
4. Inspect central venous access site.	Determines presence of patency and absence of infection, infiltration, or phlebitis.
5. **Unexpected outcomes** that may occur include:	
➤ There is redness and swelling around the central vein access site.	Indicates possible central venous catheter infection. Assess the client for fever and consult with the physician about the need for cultures of the site or blood.
➤ The central venous access device is not patent.	The access device may have become occluded with fibrin or particulate matter. Report the occlusion to the physician. If the device is a surgically placed device or peripheral intravenous central catheter (PICC) (see Chapter 20), a thrombolytic agent such as urokinase may be ordered.
➤ Weight gain greater than 1 lb per day.	Indicates fluid retention rather than restoration of body proteins.
➤ Crackles auscultated over lung fields.	When fluid overload is present, excess fluid accumulates in lung fields.
➤ Taut skin turgor.	Indicates peripheral edema.
➤ Serum glucose is greater than 200 mg/dl.	Indicates client's intolerance to glucose load in the CPN solution. May document need for addition of insulin to the CPN, modification of CPN solution, or sliding scale insulin coverage.
➤ Serum electrolytes are out of normal range.	May indicate movement of electrolytes in response to infusion of fluids and glucose. The electrolyte levels in the solution may need to be adjusted.

RECORDING AND REPORTING

1. Record condition of central venous access device, rate of infusion, intake and output each shift, vital signs, and weights.	Documents infusion flow rate, client's response to therapy, electrolyte levels, and fluid status.
2. If signs of infection, occlusion, or infiltration occur, notify the physician.	Provides for timely intervention for complication.

FOLLOW-UP ACTIVITIES

1. Place warm, moist pack on extremity with infiltration or phlebitis (PICC line only). Warm, moist heat promotes circulation and reduces swelling and redness. Mild phlebitis that does not respond to heat or more severe phlebitis may require removal of the PICC.
2. If client shows signs of fluid retention, notify physician. Anticipate a change in CPN order, or physician may order restriction of oral fluids or administration of a diuretic.

• • • • •

Special Considerations

➤ Rate of CPN does need to be gradually increased to prevent metabolic and electrolyte abnormalities. CPN is hyperosmolar and is tolerated well by most clients if initiated in stepwise fashion.

➤ CPN is usually not abruptly discontinued, because it may lead to the occurrence of hypoglycemia. If the infusion of CPN must be stopped suddenly, an infusion of D_5W at the same infusion rate is sufficient to avoid hypoglycemia (ASPEN, 1995).

Teaching Considerations

➤ Instruct client and family about the purpose and goals of CPN.

- Teach client and primary care giver to monitor client's weight, calorie count, intake and output, and serum glucose.
- Teach client and primary care giver about actions to take in case of emergency or unexpected outcomes.

Pediatric Considerations

- Indications for parenteral nutrition for infants include gastroschisis, congenital anomalies of the gastrointestinal system, and short bowel syndrome.
- CPN can cause hepatobiliary dysfunction in infants.
- Catheter-related sepsis and thrombosis of central veins is more prevalent in the pediatric population (Chwals, 1994).

Gerontologic Considerations

- Older adults may have impaired ability to manage higher fluid volumes, lipid intolerance, or an increased incidence of hyperglycemia.

Home Care Considerations

- Observe client and primary care giver perform procedure in hospital before discharge (see Chapter 43).

SKILL 24-3 Caring for the Client Receiving Peripheral Parenteral Nutrition with Lipid (Fat) Emulsion

Peripheral access requires the use of lower concentrations of dextrose and amino acids to lower tonicity and lessen the risk of vein damage (see Table 24-2). For example, PPN consists of 5% to 10% dextrose and amino acids supplemented by IV fat emulsion to provide 2000 kcal/day. PPN is usually administered in conjunction with fat emulsion. Unfortunately, PPN is often difficult to maintain because of frequent episodes of phlebitis in superficial arm veins and infiltrations of solutions into subcutaneous tissue. Therefore the final dextrose concentration must be no greater than 10%, because the peripheral vein will sclerose at higher concentrations. However, solutions of lower concentration make it difficult to supply adequate calories and amino acids through a peripheral vein. This problem, with the scarcity of adequate access sites, is the reason many experts recommend PPN for only short periods of time. Nutrients given through central veins may be very concentrated (e.g., 1800 mOsm). However, concentrations this great are not tolerated in peripheral veins because of their relatively low blood flow. Indications for PPN include the following:

1. Short-term need for parenteral nutrition. NPO for more than 5 days but anticipation that the client will tolerate enteral or oral nutrition within 7 to 10 days.
2. History of problems with central vein access or inability to establish central vein access. Clients with a history of multiple central venous catheter infections or occlusions have increased risks associated with catheter placement. Multiple catheter placements may deplete access sites.
3. Adequate peripheral access. Despite its lower osmolality, PPN tends to cause phlebitis and may require frequent changes in the access location.
4. Ability to tolerate larger volumes of fluid. Because of the lower concentration of dextrose in PPN, a larger volume of fluid is required to attain adequate calories. Clients with impaired renal or cardiac function may not tolerate PPN.
5. Ability to tolerate lipid emulsions. Lipid is the most calorically dense nutrient, and PPN without lipid would not provide adequate calories unless very large volumes of fluid were provided. One liter of 10% dextrose provides only 340 kcal. Five hundred milliliters of 10% lipid provides 550 kcal.

EQUIPMENT

- PPN solution
- Lipid emulsion
- Two sets of IV tubing (filter optional—0.22 micron for amino acid/dextrose solution)
- Needle (19 gauge), Y connector, or stopcock
- Alcohol swab
- Infusion pump

STEPS	RATIONALE
ASSESSMENT	
1. Assess client for potential lipid intolerance. Assess serum triglyceride level. Serum triglyceride should be drawn before initiation of fat therapy (baseline) and 6 hours after fat has infused.	Determines client's ability to metabolize lipid.

STEPS	RATIONALE
2. Find appropriate functional IV site to administer PPN and lipid emulsion.	Fat emulsions may be given through separate IV, piggybacked through peripheral line, or admixed in solution bag.
3. Check administration time for fat emulsion.	Fat emulsions may cause adverse symptoms if infused too rapidly as a separate infusion. The infusion time should be at least 4 hours. Fat emulsions should hang no longer than 10 hours as a separate infusion. When admixed with the PPN, fats are administered over 24 hours.
4. Check physician's order for volume of fat emulsion and PPN solution.	Fat emulsions and PPN must be ordered by physician.
5. Assess for patency and function of intravenous system (see Chapter 20).	Patent and functioning intravenous system is needed for the delivery of peripheral parenteral nutrition.

NURSING DIAGNOSIS

Clustering of defining characteristics from the assessment data may reveal the following nursing diagnoses for clients requiring this skill:

- Altered nutrition: less than body requirements
- Risk for infection

Related factors are individualized based on a client's condition or needs.

PLANNING

STEPS	RATIONALE
1. **Expected outcomes** following completion of procedure:	
➤ Triglyceride level is stable.	Increased level indicates poor tolerance to fat.
➤ Venipuncture site is free of phlebitis, pain, swelling, redness, and inflammation.	Ensures proper administration of PPN with lipids.
➤ Client does not show signs of systemic infection (e.g., elevated temperature).	Temperature is an indication of possible systemic infection related to parenteral nutrition.
2. Explain purposes of PPN.	Promotes understanding and reduces anxiety.
3. Place client in a comfortable position.	When clients are comfortable, they tolerate procedures more readily.

IMPLEMENTATION

STEPS	RATIONALE
1. Wash hands and put on gloves.	Reduces transmission of microorganisms.
2. Connect tubing to solution and run fat emulsion into IV tubing.	To prevent air from entering vascular system, all tubing must be purged.
3. Clean peripheral line tubing injection port with alcohol swab (optional: use Y connector).	Removes surface organisms at injection site and prevents organisms from entering blood system.
4. Insert fat emulsion infusion into injection port proximal to the venipuncture site using needle or needleless system, below the infusion filter on the main parenteral nutrition line.	Fat emulsions cannot infuse through a 0.22 micron IV filter—the emulsion would separate.
5. Set flow rate on infusion pump.	Up to 2.5 g fat/kg/day may be infused, but fat emulsion should not exceed 60% of total kcal.
6. Begin PPN at ordered rate.	The rate of PPN administration does not need to be gradually increased. The lower concentration of dextrose allows most clients to tolerate the full administration rate without difficulty.
7. Discard supplies and wash hands.	Prevents transmission of infection.

EVALUATION

STEPS	RATIONALE
1. Assess client's response to therapy: proper weight gain, improved laboratory values.	Provides objective data to measure the response to therapy.
2. Monitor temperature every 4 hours and regularly inspect venipuncture site for signs of phlebitis or infiltration.	Determines onset of fever, a complication of intolerance to fat emulsion or sepsis. Determines integrity of IV system.

STEPS	RATIONALE
3. Assess client's response to fluid volume: weight changes, intake and output balance, absence of edema, absence of shortness of breath.	
4. **Unexpected outcomes** that may occur include:	
➤ There is intolerance to fat emulsion as evidenced by increased triglyceride levels, increased temperature (3° to 4° F), chills, headache, nausea and vomiting, muscle ache, backache, chest pain.	Lipoprotein lipase, which is responsible for clearance of fat from circulation, may not be activated; excess fat accumulation occurs.
➤ See unexpected outcomes in Skill 24-2.	

Recording and Reporting

1. Record intake and output every shift.	Indicates fluid status.
2. Record temperature every 4 hours.	Gradual elevation of temperature may indicate catheter sepsis.
3. Record condition of IV site and status of infusion.	Documents status of IV site.

Follow-up Activities

1. If fat emulsion is not tolerated, therapy must be discontinued per physician's order.

• • • • •

Special Considerations

- Do not shake fat emulsion bottle; this disrupts physical stability of microscopic fat globules. Inspect bottle for opacity and consistency in texture and color.
- 10% fat emulsions are infused over at least 4 hours, and 20% fats are infused over at least 6 hours. All fats can hang for 10 hours; admixing fats can hang for 24 hours. Initial rate is 1 ml/min for 15 to 30 minutes.

Teaching Considerations

- Teach client and primary care giver to monitor client's weight, calorie count, intake and output, and IV site.

Pediatric Considerations

- Indications for parenteral nutrition for infants include gastroschisis, congenital anomalies of the gastrointestinal system, and short bowel syndrome.
- CPN can cause hepatobiliary dysfunction in infants.
- Catheter-related sepsis and thrombosis of central veins is more prevalent in the pediatric population (Chwals, 1994).

Gerontologic Considerations

- Older adults may have impaired ability to manage higher fluid volumes, lipid intolerance, or an increased incidence of hyperglycemia.

Home Care Considerations

- See Home Care Considerations given for Skill 24-2, p. 775.

Critical Thinking Exercises

1. The nurse observes that the client who has had a bowel resection is still without bowel sounds and bowel movements on postoperative day 5. The client had been having difficulty eating before the operation and had lost about 10 pounds in 2 weeks. What further assessments and planning would be appropriate at this point?
2. The nurse assists the physician to place a central vein catheter. About 1 hour after the procedure, the client complains of pain and shortness of breath. The results of the chest x-ray are not yet available. What complication of central catheter placement might these symptoms indicate?
3. After 24 hours of receiving CPN, the client begins to complain about thirst, frequent urination, and hunger. What metabolic complication of CPN might these symptoms indicate?
4. The client is receiving PPN with a separate lipid infusion. What assessments should the nurse make to determine the client's tolerance of this therapy?

REFERENCES

American Society for Parenteral and Enteral Nutrition (ASPEN): Standards for nutrition support: hospitalized patients, *Nutr Clin Pract* 10(6):208, 1995.

American Society for Parenteral and Enteral Nutrition (ASPEN): Guidelines for the use of parenteral and enteral nutrition in adult and pediatric patients, *JPEN* 17(4)(suppl):1SA, 1993.

American Society for Parenteral and Enteral Nutrition (ASPEN): Standards of practice: nutrition support nurses, *Nutr Clin Pract* 11(3):127, 1996.

Babineau T et al: Lipids. In Zaloga GP, editor: *Nutrition in critical care,* St Louis, 1994, Mosby.

Chwals WJ: Infant and pediatric nutrition. In Zaloga GP, editor: *Nutrition in critical care,* St Louis, 1994, Mosby.

Davis CL: Nursing care of total parenteral and enteral nutrition. In Fischer JE, editor: *Total parenteral nutrition,* ed 2, Boston, 1991, Little, Brown.

Flowers JF, Ryan JA, Gough JA: Catheter-related complications of total parenteral nutrition. In Fischer JE, editor: *Total parenteral nutrition,* ed 2, Boston, 1991, Little, Brown.

Hickey MS: *Handbook of enteral, parenteral, and ARC/AIDS nutritional therapy,* St Louis, 1992, Mosby.

Nussbaum MS, Fischer JE: Parenteral nutrition. In Zaloga GP, editor: *Nutrition in critical care,* St Louis, 1994, Mosby.

Pearson ML (Hospital Infection Control Practices Advisory Committee): Guidelines for prevention of intravascular-devise–related infections, *Infection Control and Hospital Epidemiology* 17(7):438, 1996.

Pennington CR: Toward safer parenteral nutrition, *Aliment Pharmacol Ther* 4(5):427, 1990 (review article).

ADDITIONAL READING

ASPEN: Standards of practice: standards for home nutrition support, *Nutr Clin Pract* 7:65, 1992.

Orr M: Hyperglycemia during nutrition support, *Crit Care Nurs* 12(1):64, 1992.

Williams SR: *Basic nutrition and diet therapy,* ed 10, St Louis, 1995, Mosby.

UNIT IX

Elimination

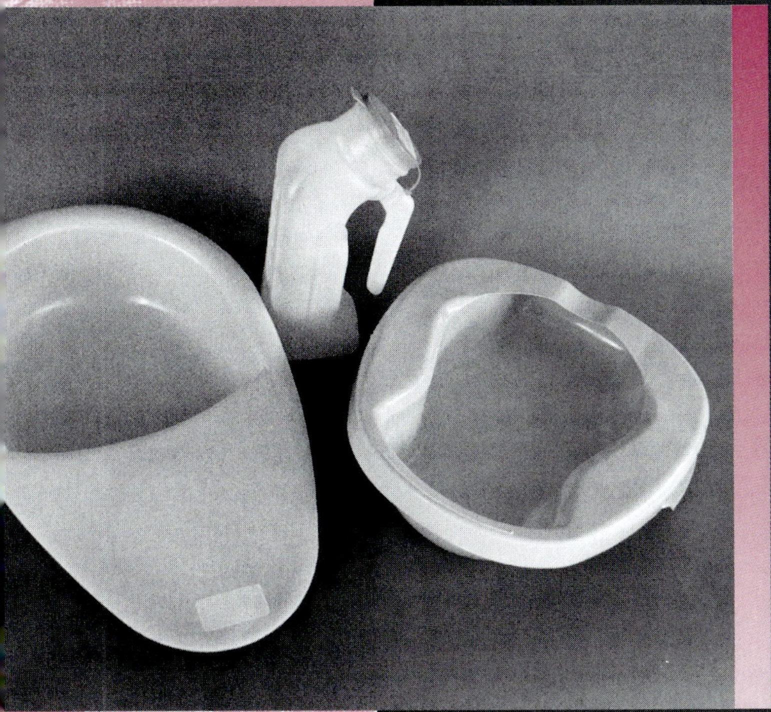

CHAPTER 25

Urinary Elimination

OBJECTIVES

Mastery of content in this chapter will enable the nurse to:

- Define key terms.
- Identify factors that alter normal voiding.
- Describe devices used to promote urinary drainage.
- Select appropriate clients for measurement of intake and output.
- Evaluate a client's hydration status.
- Perform the following skills: measure and record intake and output, place and remove urinal, insert urinary catheter, care for an indwelling urinary catheter, obtain residual urine, irrigate a catheter, remove a retention catheter, apply a condom catheter, and administer intermittent peritoneal and continuous ambulatory peritoneal dialysis.

KEY TERMS

Catheterization
Dialysis
External urethral sphincter
Incontinence
Intake
Micturition
Nosocomial (hospital-acquired) infections
Output
Residual urine
Urinary retention
Urinary tract infections
Urine
Urine-specific gravity

SKILLS

25-1 Measuring and Recording Intake and Output
25-2 Assisting a Client to use a Urinal
25-3 Inserting a Straight or Indwelling Catheter
25-4 Care of the Indwelling Catheter
25-5 Obtaining Catheterized Specimens for Residual Urine
25-6 Performing Catheter Irrigation
25-7 Removing a Retention Catheter
25-8 Applying a Condom Catheter
25-9 Care of Suprapubic Catheter
25-10 Peritoneal Dialysis and Continuous Ambulatory Peritoneal Dialysis

Urinary elimination is a natural and often private process individuals take for granted until it is altered by some uncontrollable physiological factor. Clients needing assistance with urinary elimination may require physiological and psychological assistance from the nurse. Physiological support may require use of an invasive procedure like the insertion of a catheter into the bladder. Psychological assistance may be needed to help the client adjust to an alteration in urinary elimination like a urine collection bag. Therefore the nurse must be competent in performing technical skills and sensitive to a client's psychological needs.

The urinary tract is susceptible to infections, particularly when invaded, as is the case when a sterile catheter is inserted. Therefore the nurse must be able to apply the principles of sterile asepsis.

When clients have altered or impaired urinary elimination, their **intake** and **output** (I&O) is measured to help monitor fluid and electrolyte balance. Monitoring I&O measurements requires cooperation and assistance from the client and the family. Intake measurements must include all liquids and semiliquids, such as gelatin and ice cream, and liquid medications taken orally. Fluids administered as enteral feedings through nasogastric, gastrostomy, or jejunostomy tubes are considered oral intake and should be recorded as such (see Chapter 23). Intravenous (IV) solutions (see Chapter 20), blood components (see Chapter 21), and parenteral nutrition (see Chapter 24) are recorded as fluid intake.

Output includes the measurement and recording of all liquid excreted or drained from the client. Thus all **urine,** vomitus, and liquid stool are recorded as output. Drainage from wounds, fistulas, and nasogastric and wound suction equipment is also considered output (see Chapter 40). The recording of all types of I&O is a procedure used to monitor fluid and electrolyte balance.

Certain disease processes, medications, and stages of growth and development influence fluid and electrolyte status. Physical assessment findings can indicate that a fluid or electrolyte imbalance exists. The nurse must know the factors influencing fluid and electrolyte balance and the signs and symptoms of fluid imbalances. When there is a potential or actual fluid and electrolyte imbalance, the nurse should institute I&O measurement.

GUIDELINES

1. Know the client's usual fluid intake pattern, including the types and amounts of fluids and when they are ingested.
2. Know the client's normal range of vital signs. Abnormal fluid and electrolyte balances can affect the amount of circulating blood volume. During dehydration, the blood pressure is decreased and the pulse and body temperature are elevated. Overhydration usually produces a bounding pulse; the rate may be either increased or decreased. Blood pressure may rise slightly, but body temperature remains unchanged.
3. Know the client's medical history including diseases and any therapies the client is receiving that may affect bladder function. Clients with injuries from burns or trauma or cardiopulmonary or renal disease frequently have fluid imbalances. Medications may affect fluid and electrolyte balance. Diuretics are successfully used to regulate fluid balance; however, side effects can further potentiate fluid and electrolyte imbalances.
4. Be aware of environmental conditions that can affect fluid balance. Prolonged exposure to extreme environmental temperatures can cause increased loss of body fluids through perspiration.
5. Institute measurement of I&O when there is an anticipated or suspicious change in fluid balance. The nurse is responsible for the maintenance of accurate records. Measurements are kept throughout the day and totaled every 8 hours, but the nurse may determine that more frequent measurements are required.
6. Know the client's most recent serum electrolyte measurements. Abnormal electrolyte values can affect fluid balance and, if uncorrected, can lead to deterioration of the client's health status or even death.
7. Practice asepsis conscientiously. Because **urinary tract infections** are the most prevalent **nosocomial (hospital-acquired) infections,** it is imperative that the nurse adhere to Standard Precaution guidelines. Glove changes and hand washing between care of different clients is critically important (Garner, 1996). The nurse should teach clients, particularly girls and women, proper perineal hygiene habits (see Chapter 6).
8. Know the client's level of comfort. A client uncomfortable physically or psychologically may be unable to relax the **external urethral sphincter** to void or completely empty the bladder. The nurse can promote comfort measures by providing privacy, offering the client a warm bedpan, assisting the client into a normal voiding position (standing for a man, squatting for a woman), or reducing pain by administering a prescribed analgesic before helping the client walk to the bathroom. Distraction measures, such as turning on a sink faucet so the client can hear water running, may help the client to void.
9. Identify conditions that weaken abdominal or pelvic muscles such as multiple abdominal or gynecological surgeries or pregnancies. Clients with weak abdominal or pelvic floor muscles can be taught exercises to strengthen these muscles and increase the ability of the bladder to contract and promote better control of the external urethral sphincter.
10. Know the client's normal patterns of **micturition.** The client should be taught never to ignore the urge to void. The nurse can assist by responding readily to the client's request to use a bedpan, urinal, bathroom, or commode. The nurse can also offer the client the opportunity to void after meals and before bedtime. Clients taking diuretic medications should receive them early in the morning so they do not need to void during the night.
11. Consider the client's age when assessing micturition habits. Toilet training and enuresis are concerns that arise in the toddler and preschooler. In the adult, increasing age may bring disease and physiological changes that predispose to **incontinence.**
12. Consider the client's mobility status as it influences access to toileting facilities. Assessments that should be made include use of walking aids, distance to the toilet, ability to remove clothing or to get in and out of the bathroom, and lighting (McCormick et al., 1992).

SKILL 25-1 Measuring and Recording Intake and Output

Measuring and recording all I&O during a 24-hour period helps to complete the assessment data base for fluid and electrolyte balance. The nurse is responsible for collecting and recording these data. Intake includes all liquids taken orally, by feeding tube, and parenterally. Liquid output includes urine, diarrhea, vomitus, gastric suction, and drainage from postsurgical tubes such as chest tubes or Penrose drains. Frequently, the recording of such data is referred to as the client's I&O.

EQUIPMENT

- Daily I&O record
- Graduated measuring container
- Pencil or pen
- Bedpan, urinal, bedside commode, or urine hat (a receptacle that fits inside the commode)
- Disposable gloves
- Sign alerting all personnel that I&O measurement is needed

DELEGATION CONSIDERATIONS

The skill of recording I&O can be delegated to unlicensed assistive personnel.

- Provide the care provider with the metric conversions for common liquid holding containers such as coffee cup and milk cartons.
- Ensure that the care provider knows Standard Precaution guidelines relating to body fluids.
- Caution the care provider to be sensitive to the privacy needs of the client.
- Clarify information that should be reported to the nurse about I&O such as changes in color, amount, or odor of stool or urine or presence of incontinence.

STEPS	RATIONALE
ASSESSMENT	
1. Identify clients who are susceptible to insufficient fluid intake, e.g., clients with impaired swallowing, unconscious clients, clients with impaired motility.	
2. Identify conditions that can increase fluid loss:	
a. Review client's graphic record for elevations in body temperature (see Chapter 10).	Prolonged fever diminishes body fluids by increasing insensible water losses from lungs through increased respiratory rate and from skin through diaphoresis.
b. Large amounts of fluids can be lost when clients have diarrhea and/or vomiting secondary to gastroenteritis.	Untreated diarrhea may lead to fluid and electrolyte imbalances especially in the very young and in the frail older adult. Gastroenteritis can lead to an excretion of potassium and chloride ions that affects fluid and electrolyte balance. Excretion of hydrogen ion from vomiting alters acid-base status.
c. Assess for surgical wound drainage. Wound drains are frequently present in clients suffering trauma and in those who have had chest or abdominal surgery.	Wound drainage represents plasma or whole blood loss. If drainage is significant or prolonged, fluid and electrolyte imbalance result. Wound suction removes plasma and whole blood. Excessive fluid loss from a wound must be replaced. Accurate recording of output assists in fluid replacement.
d. Identify presence of any wound (see Chapter 40) or gastric suction equipment. Clients who have undergone abdominal surgery or who have chest tube drainage, gastrointestinal hemorrhage, pancreatitis, or cholecystitis may have nasogastric suction (see Chapter 35).	Gastric suction removes hydrochloric acid, potassium, and other fluids from the stomach. Gastric suction decompresses the stomach and keeps the stomach empty.
e. Major burns may cause life-threatening changes in fluid and electrolyte status.	Fluid volume loss is directly proportional to amount and depth of injury. Major fluid shifts can occur with burns.
f. Severe trauma, especially crush injuries.	Hyperkalemia results from release of intracellular potassium from injured cells.

STEPS	RATIONALE
g. Endocrine imbalances:	
(1) Cushing's disease or Cushing's syndrome	Excessive amounts of corticosteroids cause sodium and water retention with potassium excretion.
(2) Addison's disease	Insufficient amounts of corticosteroids cause sodium and water excretion.
(3) Diabetic ketoacidosis	Osmotic diuresis resulting from increased blood sugar causes severe fluid volume deficit.
3. Assess patency and flow rate of IV and parenteral nutrition solutions (see Chapters 20 and 24).	Incorrect solutions and inaccurate flow rates can result in fluid and electrolyte imbalances.
4. Identify clients who are taking medications that can influence fluid balance status:	
a. Diuretics	Diuretics are generally used to reduce edema and lower blood pressure. There are many subgroups of diuretics, and each group achieves its desired effect by different actions, but fluid and electrolyte imbalances are possible with any diuretic. Therefore the I&O of clients receiving diuretics are often monitored and daily weights are obtained (Skidmore-Roth, 1994).
b. Steroids	Steroids (e.g., prednisone, cortisone) cause sodium and water retention and excretion of potassium.
5. Weigh clients daily and observe for weight changes that occur within 24 to 48 hours: 2% to 5% loss—Mild dehydration 6% to 9% loss—Moderate dehydration 10% to 14% loss—Severe dehydration 20% loss—Death 2% to 4% gain—Mild volume overload 5% to 7% gain—Moderate overload	Allows nurse to identify early assessment findings for dehydration or volume overload.
6. Assess client for signs of fluid overload or dehydration:	Kidneys attempt to excrete excess fluid during periods of overhydration and conserve body water during periods of dehydration.
a. Eyes—*Dehydration:* sunken eyes, dry conjunctivae, decrease or absence of tearing. *Fluid overload:* periorbital edema, blurred vision, papilledema.	
b. Mouth—*Dehydration:* sticky, dry mucous membrane; dry, cracked lips; decreased saliva; increased viscosity of saliva. *Fluid overload:* longitudinal furrows on tongue, swollen tongue, excessive salivation.	
c. Skin—*Dehydration:* increased skin temperature; dry, scaly skin; poor turgor. *Fluid overload:* edema.	Signs of dehydration result from reduction of fluid within tissues and circulatory system. Body compensates for overhydration by maintaining excess volume in extracellular fluid spaces and transferring fluid into tissues, causing edema.
d. Cardiovascular—*Dehydration:* increased pulse rate, weak pulse, hypotension, decreased capillary filling. *Fluid overload:* bounding pulse rate, blood pressure normal with or without orthostatic changes, third heart sound (S_3), distended neck veins.	
e. Gastrointestinal—*Dehydration:* sunken abdomen. *Dehydration* or *fluid overload:* vomiting, diarrhea, abdominal cramps.	
f. Renal—*Dehydration:* oliguria or anuria, **urine-specific gravity** increased. *Fluid overload:* decreased specific gravity, diuresis (if kidneys are normal).	
7. Inspect urine color and urine-specific gravity (normal is 1.010 to 1.030).	

STEPS	RATIONALE
8. Monitor hematocrit (Hct).	An increased Hct value may indicate dehydration.
9. Assess client's knowledge of the purpose for I&O measurement.	

NURSING DIAGNOSIS

Clustering of defining characteristics from the assessment data may reveal the following nursing diagnoses for clients requiring this skill:

- Altered urinary elimination
- Fluid volume deficit
- Risk for fluid volume deficit
- Fluid volume excess
- Impaired physical mobility
- Knowledge deficit regarding intake and output measures
- Total incontinence
- **Urinary retention**

Related factors are individualized based on a client's condition or needs.

PLANNING

STEPS	RATIONALE
1. **Expected outcomes** following completion of procedure:	
➤ Oral intake is 600 to 900 ml greater than output and at least 1500 ml per 24 hours.	Difference allows for insensible water loss from lungs, intestine, and skin.
➤ Weight remains within 2% of baseline.	
➤ Ambulatory clients will save urine for monitoring.	Monitors improving fluid status.
2. Select appropriate clients whose I&O should be measured.	Nurse can institute I&O measurement with any client. Clients whose conditions are unstable or potentially unstable require I&O measurement at least every 4 hours.
3. Explain procedure to client.	Reduces anxiety and improves cooperation.
4. Mark containers that measure output with client's name, room number, and container contents.	Clients who have numerous drainage sites like a urinary catheter and a colostomy should have each container labeled to decrease the chance of cross-contamination.
5. Post sign alerting personnel that I&O measurement has been instituted for client. Often the I&O record itself is posted on the door.	

IMPLEMENTATION

STEPS	RATIONALE
1. Explain to client and family why I&O measurements are important.	Family and alert active clients need to be active participants so that I&O measurements are not inadvertently omitted as they participate in care.
2. Provide client with copy of hospital's metric conversion chart.	Provides easy and accurate conversion method for recording intake.
3. Measure and record all intake of fluid:	
a. Liquids with meals, gelatin, custards, ice cream, popsicles, sherbets, ice chips	Liquids frozen into solid substances (e.g., ice cream, ice chips) or semisolid foods (e.g., custards, gelatin) are counted as liquid intake.
b. Liquid taken with medications	Many medications should be taken with a full glass of water. This liquid can add considerably to intake and must be included in I&O monitoring.
c. Parenteral fluids: IV (see Chapters 19 and 20), blood components (see Chapter 21), total parenteral fluid (see Chapter 24)	Parenteral fluids are instilled directly into intravascular space and distributed to interstitial and extracellular fluid and should be recorded as intake.
d. Enteral tube feedings (see Chapter 23)	High-calorie liquid meals are instilled directly into the gastrointestinal system through nasogastric, gastrostomy, or jejunostomy tubes.

➤ ***CRITICAL DECISION POINT*** **Intake should be recorded as soon as it is measured.**

STEPS	RATIONALE
4. Instruct client not to empty urinal, Foley catheter, drainage bag, bedpan, urine hat, or commode but to ask nurse to empty and record amount.	Maintains accurate record of output.
5. Apply disposable gloves before handling Foley catheter, nasogastric tube, and other equipment.	Prevents nurse's exposure to potentially infectious body fluids per Standard Precaution guidelines.
CRITICAL DECISION POINT **If emptying drainage and splashing is anticipated, wear mask, eye protection, and gown to protect skin, mucous membranes, and clothing.**	
6. Measure and record all drainage from Foley catheter, nasogastric suction, and wound suction at least every 8 hours.	Allows nurse to tabulate total output for each nursing shift.
CRITICAL DECISION POINT **The registered nurse in many agencies is responsible for evaluating the shift and 24-hour totals. Tabulating the 24-hour I&O totals may be delegated to a licensed practical nurse in some agencies.**	
7. Remove gloves and other protective gear after measuring and disposing of output fluids. Wash hands before recording information on the I&O record.	Reduces transmission of microorganisms.

EVALUATION

1. Evaluate condition of skin and mucous membranes.	Reflects hydration status.
2. Observe color, characteristics, and amount of urine.	Continual monitoring of client's fluid I&O provides opportunity to identify and correct actual or potential fluid imbalances. Check specific gravity if urine appears concentrated.
3. Note I&O balance.	
4. **Unexpected outcomes** that may occur include:	
➤ Fluid volume deficit is present.	Result of prolonged loss without replacement of circulating and interstitial fluid volume as evidenced by intake greater than output, weight gain greater than 2% over 24 to 48 hours, and an increased Hct value.
➤ Fluid volume overload is present.	Result of chemical or physiological imbalance within body that causes abnormal retention of fluid.

RECORDING AND REPORTING

1. At end of each nursing shift, calculate total I&O for each client for whom I&O measurement has been instituted (Fig. 25-1).	Provides assessment data on fluid balance for next nursing shift.
2. Calculate and record total 24-hour I&O on 24-hour fluid record sheet located in client's medical record (Fig. 25-1).	Allows entire health care team to review client's 24-hour I&O records over specific period.
3. Report immediately to physician any client whose urine output is less than 30 ml/hr.	

FOLLOW-UP ACTIVITIES

1. It may be necessary to weigh the client to help assess fluid status. Remember to obtain weights with the same scale, same time of day, and with comparable articles of clothing, including bed linen if bed weights are necessary.
2. Encouraging fluids is a nursing responsibility, therefore any client not restricted in total fluid intake should be assessed if oral intake is not minimally 1500 ml/day.

• • • • •

ROBINSON MEMORIAL HOSPITAL

DATE ______________ ***IV SOLUTION / FLUID BALANCE FLOW SHEET***

STOOL: 7-3
3-11
11-7

SPECIMENS:

OBSERVATIONS / INTERVENTIONS CODES:
1. Redness at Site
2. Swelling at Site
3. c/o Pain
4. Drainage at Site
5. Intact s̄ 1, 2, 3, 4,
6. IV Restart

SOLUTIONS / BLOOD / BLOOD PRODUCTS:
A. ______
B. ______
C. ______
D. ______
E. ______
F. ______

DIET: %
Feed ☐ Assist ☐ Self ☐
Breakfast ______
Lunch ______
Supper ______
Snacks ______
Tube Feeding ______
type ______
rate ______

Sol. Code	Time	Rate	Site	Observ	Catheter Size	Initials

Sol. Code	Time	Rate	Site	Observ	Catheter Size	Initials

INTAKE	7 A	8 A	9 A	10 A	11 A	12 P	1 P	2 P	TOTAL
Oral / NG									
IV									
IV									
IV									
IV									
IVPB									
Blood									

7 - 3 8 HOUR TOTALS ⇒

	3 P	4 P	5 P	6 P	7 P	8 P	9 P	10 P	TOTAL
Oral / NG									
IV									
IV									
IV									
IV									
IVPB									
Blood									

3 - 11 8 HOUR TOTALS ⇒

	11 P	12 A	1 A	2 A	3 A	4 A	5 A	6 A	TOTAL
Oral / NG									
IV									
IV									
IV									
IV									
IVPB									
Blood									

11 - 7 8 HOUR TOTALS ⇒

OUTPUT	7 A	8 A	9 A	10 A	11 A	12 P	1 P	2 P	TOTAL
Urine / Foley									
Gastric									
Drains									

7 - 3 8 HOUR TOTALS ⇒

	3 P	4 P	5 P	6 P	7 P	8 P	9 P	10 P	TOTAL
Urine / Foley									
Gastric									
Drains									

3 - 11 8 HOUR TOTALS ⇒

	11 P	12 A	1 A	2 A	3 A	4 A	5 A	6 A	TOTAL
Urine / Foley									
Gastric									
Drains									

11 - 7 8 HOUR TOTALS ⇒

24 HOUR TOTALS

INTAKE		OUTPUT	
Oral / NG		Urine	
IV		Gastric	
Blood		Drains	
TOTAL		TOTAL	
24 HOUR BALANCE			
CUMULATIVE BALANCE			

FORM #099951

Fig. 25-1 Daily intake and output and twenty-four hour intake and output record. (Courtesy, Robinson Memorial Hospital, Ravenna, Ohio.)

Special Considerations

- Symptoms of endocrine imbalances may also be present in clients receiving synthetic steroid preparations such as prednisone.
- Postoperative clients are frequently prescribed clear liquid diets and their diets are advanced to solid foods as the nurse determines that tolerance increases.
- Actual time for calculation of 24-hour I&O totals can vary. In some institutions totals are calculated at 12 midnight, in others at 6 AM.
- Monitoring and evaluating I&O is an ongoing process. I&O should be recorded immediately to prevent errors in reporting.
- If two clients in the same room require I&O measurement, clearly label the urine hats for each client.
- When two clients in the same room have Foley catheters, each client must have a graduated with each clearly marked with name and room number; that graduated must be used only for the client indicated.

Teaching Considerations

- Ambulatory client may require frequent reminders of need to measure and record all liquid I&O.
- Severely ill or disoriented client may be unable to understand reason for I&O measurement or to actively participate in any measuring or recording. However, family members may be able to help maintain accurate output records.
- Clients who have severe fluid restriction (e.g., renal failure, congestive heart failure) are at risk for fluid imbalances.
- Clients with visual impairments may not be able to use standard metric conversion I&O guide.
- Instruct client and primary care giver on use of household measuring devices to measure I&O.

Gerontologic Considerations

- Older adults are more susceptible to fluid and electrolyte imbalances secondary to prolonged fever. Clients with chronic illnesses or acute trauma, such as burns and abdominal injuries, have potential for further fluid and electrolyte imbalances with fever.
- Clients older than age 60 are at greater risk of fluid and electrolyte imbalances secondary to gastroenteritis.
- Incontinence may be discovered when I&O is monitored. It is a myth that incontinence is a function of age. The process of aging is not the sole cause of incontinence (Pearson and Larson, 1992).

Home Care Considerations

- Assess client and primary care giver to determine ability and motivation to maintain accurate records of client's I&O.
- Provide client and primary care giver with appropriate measuring containers and I&O chart. I&O measurements require conversion chart for household measures to metric measures. Demonstrate proper manner for measuring I&O.
- Provide opportunity for client and primary care giver to demonstrate measuring I&O.
- Instruct client and care giver that recording daily weight is an important adjunct to monitoring I&O.

SKILL 25-2 Assisting a Client to use a Urinal

The client's ability to void depends on feeling the urge to urinate and on being able to control the urethral sphincter. One factor that can interfere with micturition is bed rest or immobility, which does not allow the client to assume the normal position for emptying the bladder. The female client is accustomed to squatting, which promotes contraction of the pelvis and abdominal muscles that assist in sphincter control and bladder contraction. The nurse assists the bedridden woman to use a bedpan for voiding (see Chapter 26). A man voids more easily in the standing position. If a man cannot walk to the toilet facilities, he may stand at the bedside and void into a urinal (a plastic or metal receptacle for urine). If he is unable to stand at the bedside, the nurse needs to assist him to use the urinal in bed.

EQUIPMENT

- **Urinal (Fig. 25-2)**
- **Disposable gloves**
- **Graduated cylinder (used for measuring volume if urinal is not marked)**
- **Supplies for diagnostic urine tests specimen collection**

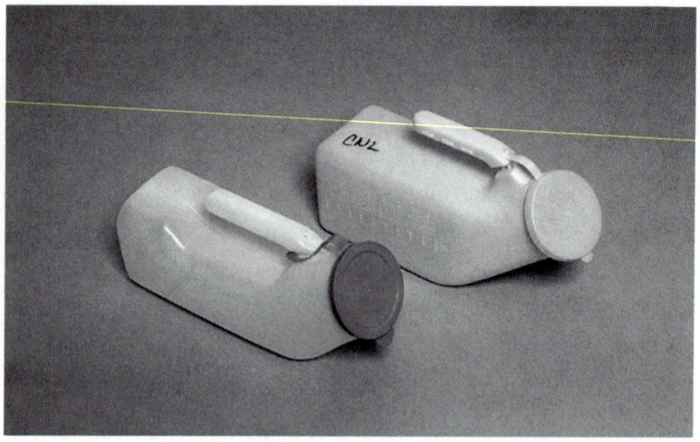

Fig. 25-2 Types of male urinals.

D ELEGATION CONSIDERATIONS

The skill of assisting a client to use a urinal can be delegated to unlicensed assistive personnel.

- Verify that the care provider knows how to place a urinal correctly.
- Ensure that care provider knows Standard Precaution guidelines relating to body fluids.
- Caution the care provider to be sensitive to the privacy needs of the client.
- Clarify information that should be reported to the nurse about urine such as changes in color, amount, or odor and the presence of incontinence.
- Inform care provider about the amount of assistance the client requires to use the urinal and if standing is permitted.

STEPS	RATIONALE

A SSESSMENT

STEPS	RATIONALE
1. Assess client's normal urinary elimination habits.	Identifies normal pattern of urination; helps nurse to recognize when client may require use of urinal.
2. Assess for periods of incontinence.	
3. Palpate for distended bladder.	Indicates if bladder is full and client needs to void.
4. Assess client's cognitive and physical status.	Provides nurse with information about how much assistance is required to use urinal.
5. Assess client's knowledge regarding urinal use.	Reveals need for client instruction.

N URSING DIAGNOSIS

Clustering of defining characteristics from the assessment data may reveal the following nursing diagnoses for clients requiring this skill:

- Altered urinary elimination
- Functional incontinence
- Impaired physical mobility
- Knowledge deficit regarding use of urinal
- Reflex incontinence
- Stress incontinence
- Toileting self-care deficit
- Urge incontinence
- Urinary retention

Related factors are individualized based on client's condition or needs.

P LANNING

STEPS	RATIONALE
1. **Expected outcomes** following completion of procedure:	
➤ Client is able to assist self with urinal.	Promotes self-care for toileting needs.
➤ Client remains continent.	
2. Obtain assistance from other nurses to position client if necessary.	Men find it easier to void when standing. Unless contraindicated, one or more nurses may help client to stand at bedside.
3. Explain procedure to client.	Promotes maximal cooperation.
4. Set up voiding routine.	Nurse offers urinal when client feels urge to void. A urinal should be provided and the client asked to void on a regular schedule so that habits can be reestablished in the incontinent adult (McCormick et al., 1992).

I MPLEMENTATION

STEPS	RATIONALE
1. Wash hands and apply gloves.	Reduces transmission of microorganisms.
2. Provide privacy by closing bedside curtain or room door.	Promotes relaxation.

STEPS	RATIONALE
3. Assist client into appropriate position: position on side, back, or sitting with head of bed elevated or assist to standing position.	Men find it easier to void and empty bladder while standing.
➤ ***CRITICAL DECISION POINT*** **Always determine mobility status before having a client stand to void.**	
4. If possible, client should hold urinal and position penis in urinal. If client needs assistance, position penis completely within urinal and hold urinal in place or assist client to hold urinal.	Penis is placed completely within urinal to avoid urine spills.
5. Once client has finished voiding, remove urinal and wash and dry penis.	Prevents growth of microorganisms. Prevents skin breakdown.
6. Assess urine, empty and cleanse urinal, and return it to client for future use.	Avoids spilling and reduces odors.
7. Allow client to wash hands after voiding.	Reduces spread of microorganisms.
8. Remove and dispose of gloves; wash hands.	Reduces spread of microorganisms.
EVALUATION	
1. Reassess client to determine ability to use urinal.	Promotes modification of nursing care plan to include more assistance or increased frequency to assist client to use urinal.
2. Note amount, appearance, and odor of urine.	Indicates abnormalities.
3. **Unexpected outcomes** that may occur include:	
➤ Client is unable to use urinal.	Increases risk of incontinence or urinary retention.
➤ Client is incontinent.	Increases anxiety and contributes to body image disturbance. Increases risk of skin breakdown.
RECORDING AND REPORTING	
1. Record and report client's ability to use urinal and characteristics of urinary output.	Communicates pertinent information to all health care personnel.
2. If I&O measurement is being monitored in client, include output data on flow sheet (see Skill 25-1).	Monitors fluid balance.
3. Report frequency of client's voiding patterns.	Promotes normal urinary elimination and prevents incontinence.

FOLLOW-UP ACTIVITIES

1. Incontinence:
   a. Offer urinal more frequently.
   b. Place urinal near client.
   c. Provide frequent skin care.
   d. Assess type of incontinence (e.g., overflow, stress, urge)
2. Inability to void using a urinal:
   a. Attempt to place client in standing position.
   b. Provide privacy.
   c. Provide relaxing environment.
3. Persistent urge, stress, or overflow incontinence may indicate a serious medical problem; referral for urological evaluation may be appropriate.

• • • • •

Special Considerations

- Nurse must consider possibility of orthostatic hypotension occurring in clients who are immobilized or who have been recumbent for prolonged period.
- If client is allowed privacy while voiding, ensure that call bell is within easy access so nurse can be summoned to empty and if necessary remove urinal.

- Urinals should not routinely be left sitting with urine. Stagnant urine is an excellent medium for bacteria growth.

Teaching Considerations

- Instruct client and primary care giver on appropriate urinal positioning technique.
- Instruct client and primary care giver on appropriate skin cleaning practices after urinal use.
- Instruct client and primary care giver to inspect the skin for breakdown.
- Instruct client and primary care giver on appropriate urinal cleansing techniques.

Gerontologic Considerations

- Aging process may impair micturition; elderly men may require urinal more frequently to avoid urinary incontinence.
- The older man who is accustomed to standing to void may empty his bladder more readily if allowed to stand when using the urinal.

Home Care Considerations

- Assess client and primary care giver to determine ability and willingness to use urinal.
- Assess level of assistance required by client to determine if additional medical equipment is necessary (e.g., overbed trapeze, bedside commode).
- Consider referral to home care agency to follow up and reinforce teaching concepts.

SKILL 25-3 Inserting a Straight or Indwelling Catheter

Catheterization of the bladder involves introducing a rubber or plastic tube through the urethra and into the bladder. The catheter provides for a continuous flow of urine in clients unable to control micturition or in those with obstruction to urine outflow. Because bladder catheterization carries the risk of the development of urinary tract infection (UTI), it is preferable to rely on other measures to promote bladder emptying.

Intermittent catheterization, in which a straight catheter is used, can be repeated as necessary. An indwelling or Foley catheter remains in place for an extended period. It may be necessary to change indwelling catheters periodically. The nurse uses sterile asepsis to reduce the risk of bladder infections.

EQUIPMENT (Fig. 25-3)

- Catheterization kit containing the following sterile items:
  - Gloves (extra pair optional)
  - Drapes, one fenestrated
  - Lubricant
  - Antiseptic cleansing solution
  - Cotton balls
  - Forceps
  - Prefilled syringe with sterile water to inflate balloon of indwelling catheter
  - Catheter of correct size and type for procedure (i.e., intermittent or indwelling)
  - Sterile drainage tubing with collection bag and multipurpose tube holder or tape, safety pin, and elastic band for securing tubing to bed if client is bedridden (for indwelling catheter)
  - Receptacle or basin (usually bottom of catheterization tray)
  - Specimen container
- Blanket
- Waterproof absorbent pad
- Disposable gloves, basin with warm water, soap, face cloth, towel
- Flashlight or other appropriate additional light as needed

DELEGATION CONSIDERATIONS

The skill of urinary catheterization is not usually delegated to unlicensed assistive personnel. The use of unlicensed assistive personnel for inserting urinary catheters may occur in some settings, but it has not become routine practice.

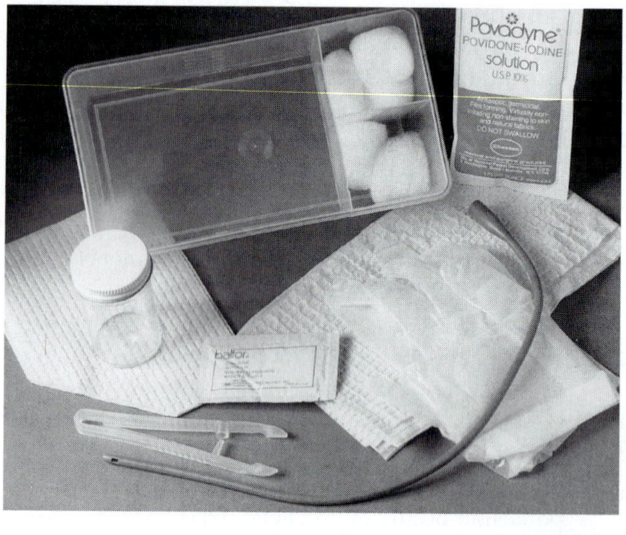

Fig. 25-3

STEPS	RATIONALE
ASSESSMENT	
1. Assess status of client:	
a. Time of last urination by asking client, checking I&O flow sheet, or palpating the bladder.	Bladder fullness may be detected with deep palpation above the symphysis pubis.
b. Level of awareness or developmental stage.	Reveals client's ability to cooperate and level of explanation needed.
c. Mobility and physical limitations of client.	Affect way that nurse positions client. Nurse can request additional nursing personnel to assist with this procedure if necessary.
d. Client's gender and age.	Determines catheter size: 8 to 10 Fr is generally used for children, 14 to 16 Fr is indicated for women, 12 Fr may be considered for young girls, and 16 to 18 Fr is used for male clients unless larger size is ordered by physician.
e. Distended bladder.	Causes pain. Can indicate need to insert catheter if client is unable to void independently.
f. Assess for anatomical landmarks, erythema, drainage, and odor.	Determines condition of perineum.
g. Any pathological condition that may impair passage of catheter (i.e., enlarged prostate gland in men).	Obstruction prevents passage of catheter through urethra into bladder.
h. Allergies.	Determines allergy to antiseptic, tape, latex, and lubricant. Betadine allergies are common; if the client is unaware of allergy, ask if allergic to shellfish.
2. Review client's medical record, including physician's order and nurses' notes.	Determine purpose of inserting catheter: preparation for surgery, urinary irrigations, collection of sterile urine specimen, or measurement of residual urine. Assess for previous catheterization including catheter size, response of client, and time of last catheterization.
3. Assess client's knowledge of the purpose for catheterization.	Reveals need for client instruction.

NURSING DIAGNOSIS

Clustering of defining characteristics may reveal the following nursing diagnoses for clients requiring this skill:

- Pain
- Urinary retention

Related factors are individulaized based on a client's condition or needs.

PLANNING

STEPS	RATIONALE
1. Expected outcomes following completion of procedure:	
➤ Bladder distention relieved.	Removal of urine from bladder relieves sensation of fullness.
➤ Client will verbalize relief of discomfort in bladder within 24 hours of catheter insertion.	Patent catheter system keeps bladder empty and client comfortable.
➤ Minimum of 30 ml of urine is present in urinary collection bag every hour.	Verifies presence of catheter in bladder, catheter patency, and adequate perfusion to kidneys.
➤ Client verbalizes minimal pain during procedure.	Localized trauma may result from catheterization.
2. Explain procedure to client.	Promotes cooperation.
3. Arrange for extra nursing personnel to assist as necessary.	Client may be unable to assume positioning for procedure.
4. Begin monitoring I&O.	Catheterized clients are at risk for urinary complications.

STEPS	RATIONALE
IMPLEMENTATION	
1. Wash hands.	Reduces transmission of microorganisms.
2. Close curtain or door.	Offers privacy, reduces embarrassment, and aids in relaxation during procedure.
3. Raise bed to appropriate working height.	Promotes use of proper body mechanics.
4. Facing client, stand on left side of bed if right-handed (on right side if left-handed). Clear bedside table and arrange equipment.	Successful catheter insertion requires nurse to assume comfortable position with all equipment easily accessible.
5. Raise side rail on opposite side of bed and put side rail down on working side.	Promotes client safety.
6. Place waterproof pad under client.	Prevents soiling of bed linen.
7. Position client:	Provides good visualization of perineal structures.
a. **Female client:**	
(1) Assist to dorsal recumbent position (supine with knees flexed). Ask client to relax thighs so the hip joints can be externally rotated.	Legs may be supported with pillows to reduce muscle tension and promote comfort.
(2) Position female client in side-lying (Sims') position with upper leg flexed at knee and hip if unable to be supine. If this position is used, nurse must take extra precautions to cover rectal area with drape during procedure to reduce chance of cross-contamination.	This alternate position is used if client cannot abduct leg at hip joint (e.g., if client has arthritic joints). Also, this position may be more comfortable for client. Support client with pillows if necessary to maintain position.
➤ ***CRITICAL DECISION POINT*** **Get assistance to position and to support weak or frail clients.**	
b. **Male client:**	
(1) Assist to supine position with thighs slightly abducted.	Comfortable position for client that aids in visualization.
8. Drape client:	
a. **Female client:**	
(1) Drape with bath blanket. Place blanket diamond fashion over client, with one corner at client's neck, side corners over each arm and side, and last corner over perineum.	
b. **Male client:**	
(1) Drape upper trunk with bath blanket and cover lower extremities with bed sheets, exposing only genitalia.	Avoids unnecessary exposure of body parts and maintains client's comfort.
9. Wearing disposable gloves, wash perineal area with soap and water as needed; dry (see Skill 6-2).	Reduces microorganisms near urethral meatus and allows further opportunity to visualize perineum and landmarks.
10. Position lamp to illuminate perineal area. (When using flashlight, have assistant hold it.)	Permits accurate identification and good visualization of urethral meatus.
11. Open package containing drainage system; place drainage bag over edge of bottom bed frame and bring drainage tube up between side rail and mattress.	
➤ ***CRITICAL DECISION POINT*** **This step is necessary only if indwelling catheter is to be inserted and drainage system is not part of the catheterization kit.**	

STEPS	RATIONALE
12. Open catheterization kit according to directions, keeping bottom of container sterile.	Prevents transmission of microorganisms from table or work area to sterile supplies. The materials in the kit are ordered in sequence of use.
CRITICAL DECISION POINT Place plastic bag that contains kit within reach of work area to use as waterproof bag to dispose of used supplies.	
13. Apply sterile gloves (see Chapter 34).	Allows nurse to handle sterile supplies without contamination.
CRITICAL DECISION POINT If underpad is first item in kit, place the pad plastic side down under the patient.	
14. Organize supplies on sterile field. Open inner sterile package containing catheter. Pour sterile antiseptic solution into correct compartment containing sterile cotton balls. Open packet containing lubricant. Remove specimen container (lid should be loosely placed on top) and prefilled syringe from collection compartment of tray and set them aside on sterile field.	Maintains principles of surgical asepsis and organizes work area.
15. Before inserting indwelling catheter, test balloon by injecting fluid from prefilled syringe into balloon port (see illustration).	Checks integrity of balloon. Do not use the catheter if the balloon does not inflate or leaks.
16. Lubricate 2.5 to 5 cm (1 to 2 inches) for women and 12.5 to 17.5 cm (5 to 7 inches) for men.	

A

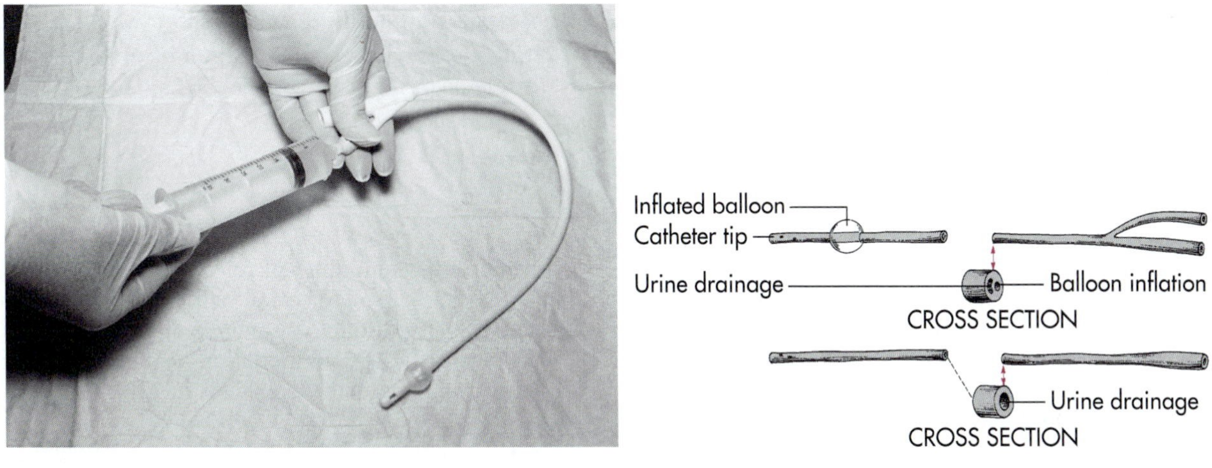

B

Step 15 Types of urinary catheters: **A,** indwelling (Foley) catheter; **B,** straight catheter.

STEPS	RATIONALE
17. Apply sterile drape:	
a. Female client:	
(1) Allow top edge of drape to form cuff over both hands. Place drape down on bed between client's thighs. Slip cuffed edge just under buttocks, taking care not to touch contaminated surface with gloves.	Outer surface of drape covering hands remains sterile. Sterile drape against sterile gloves is sterile.
(2) Pick up fenestrated sterile drape and allow it to unfold without touching an unsterile object. Apply drape over perineum, exposing labia and being sure not to touch contaminated surface.	Maintains sterility of work surface.
b. Male client:	
(1) Two methods are used for draping depending on preference. *First method:* Apply drape over thighs and under penis without completing opening fenestrated drape. *Second method:* Apply drape over thighs just below penis. Pick up fenestrated sterile drape, allow it to unfold, and drape it over penis with fenestrated slit resting over penis.	Maintains sterility of work surface.
18. Place sterile tray and contents on sterile drape between thighs. Open specimen container.	Provides easy access to supplies during catheter insertion. Maintains aseptic technique during procedure.
19. Cleanse urethral meatus.	
a. Female client:	
(1) With nondominant hand, carefully retract labia to fully expose urethral meatus. Maintain position of nondominant hand throughout procedure.	Full visualization of urethral meatus is provided. Full retraction prevents contamination of urethral meatus during cleansing.
CRITICAL DECISION POINT **Closure of labia during cleansing requires that the procedure be repeated because area has become contaminated.**	
(2) Using forceps in sterile dominant hand, pick up cotton ball saturated with antiseptic solution and clean perineal area, wiping front to back from clitoris toward anus. Using a new cotton ball for each area, wipe along the far labial fold, near labial fold, and directly over center of urethral meatus.	Cleansing reduces number of microorganisms at urethral meatus. Use of single cotton ball for each wipe prevents transfer of microorganisms. Preparation moves from area of least contamination to that of most contamination. Dominant hand remains sterile.
b. Male client:	
(1) If client is not circumcised, retract foreskin with nondominant hand. Grasp penis at shaft just below glans. Retract urethral meatus between thumb and forefinger. Maintain nondominant hand in this position throughout procedure.	Accidental release of foreskin or dropping of penis during cleansing requires process to be repeated because area has become contaminated.
(2) With dominant hand, pick up cotton ball with forceps and clean penis. Move it in circular motion from urethral meatus down to base of glans. Repeat cleansing three more times, using clean cotton ball each time.	Reduces number of microorganisms at urethral meatus and moves from areas of least to most contamination. Dominant hand remains sterile.

STEPS | **RATIONALE**

20. Pick up catheter with gloved dominant hand 7.5 to 10 cm (3 to 4 inches) from catheter tip. Hold end of catheter loosely coiled in palm of dominant hand (optional: may grasp catheter with forceps). Place distal end of catheter in urine tray receptacle if non-retention catheterization being done.

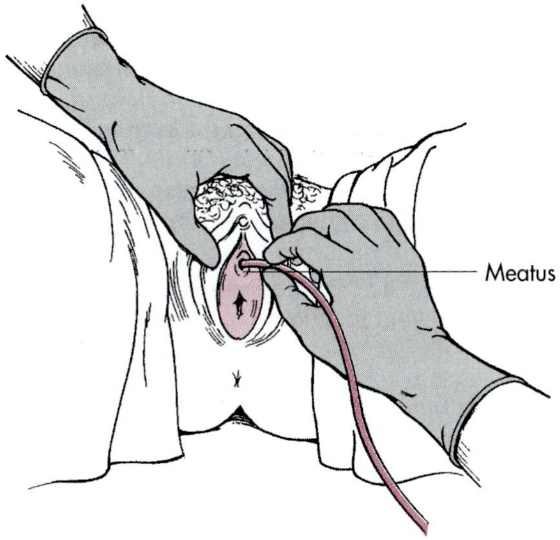

Step 21a(1)

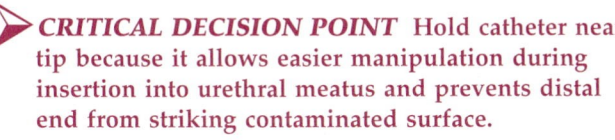

INFLATION OF BALLOON FOR INDWELLING CATHETER

Inflate balloon of indwelling catheter with amount of fluid recommended by the manufacturer.

a. While holding catheter with thumb and little finger of nondominant hand at urethral meatus, take end of catheter and place it between first two fingers of nondominant hand.
b. With free dominant hand, attach syringe to injection port at end of catheter.
c. Slowly inject total amount of solution. If client complains of sudden pain, aspirate solution and advance catheter farther.
d. Release catheter and pull gently to feel resistance. Then move catheter slightly back into bladder.

CRITICAL DECISION POINT Hold catheter near tip because it allows easier manipulation during insertion into urethral meatus and prevents distal end from striking contaminated surface.

21. Insert catheter:

a. Female client:

(1) Ask client to bear down gently as if to void and slowly insert catheter through urethral meatus (see illustration).

Relaxation of external sphincter aids in insertion of catheter.

(2) Advance catheter a total of 5 to 7.5 cm (2 to 3 inches) in adult or until urine flows out catheter's end. When urine appears, advance catheter another 2.5 to 5 cm (1 to 2 inches). Do not force against resistance. Place end of catheter in urine tray receptacle.

Female urethra is short. Appearance of urine indicates that catheter tip is in bladder or lower urethra. Advancement of catheter ensures bladder placement.

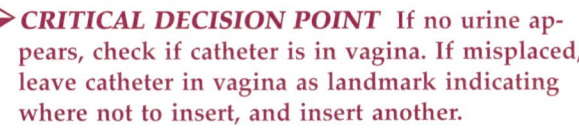

CRITICAL DECISION POINT If no urine appears, check if catheter is in vagina. If misplaced, leave catheter in vagina as landmark indicating where not to insert, and insert another.

(3) Release labia and hold catheter securely with nondominant hand. Inflate balloon if retention catheter is used (see box above).

Bladder or sphincter contraction may cause accidental expulsion of catheter.

STEPS	RATIONALE
b. Male client:	
(1) Lift penis to position perpendicular to client's body and apply light traction (see illustration).	Straightens urethral canal to ease catheter insertion.
(2) Ask client to bear down as if to void and slowly insert catheter through urethral meatus.	Relaxation of external sphincter aids in insertion of catheter.
(3) Advance catheter 17 to 22.5 cm (7 to 9 inches) in adult or until urine flows out catheter's end. If resistance is felt, withdraw catheter; do not force it through urethra. When urine appears, advance catheter another 2.5 to 5 cm (1 to 2 inches).	The adult male urethra is long. It is normal to meet resistance at the prostatic sphincter. When resistance is met, nurse should hold catheter firmly against sphincter without forcing catheter. After few seconds, sphincter relaxes and catheter is advanced. Appearance of urine indicates catheter tip is in bladder or urethra. Further advancement of catheter ensures proper placement.
(4) Lower penis and hold catheter securely in nondominant hand. Place end of catheter in urine tray receptacle. Inflate balloon if retention catheter is used (see box on p. 795).	Catheter may be accidentally expelled by bladder or urethral contraction. Collection of urine prevents soiling and provides output measurement.

CRITICAL DECISION POINT **Do not use force to insert a catheter.**

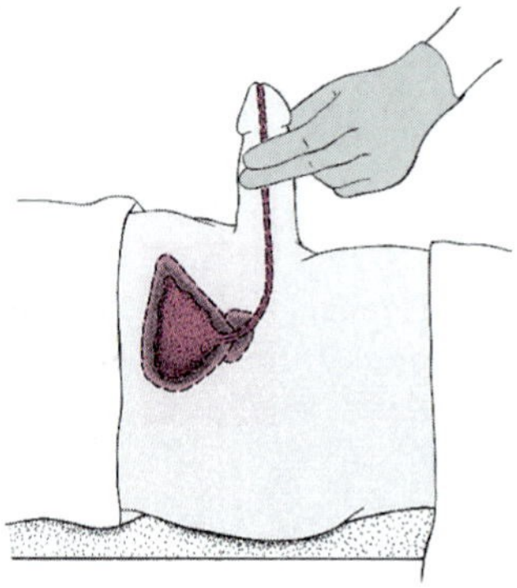

Step 21b(1) Structures of the male genitourinary system.

STEPS	RATIONALE
22. Collect urine specimen as needed. Fill specimen cup or jar to desired level (20 to 30 ml) by holding end of catheter in dominant hand over cup.	Allows sterile specimen to be obtained for culture analysis.
23. Allow bladder to empty fully unless institution policy restricts maximal volume of urine drained with each catheterization (about 800 to 1000 ml).	Retained urine may serve as reservoir for growth of microorganisms.
24. Remove straight, single-use catheter:	
a. Withdraw catheter slowly but smoothly until removed.	Minimizes discomfort to client.
25. After inflating balloon fully, release catheter with nondominant hand and pull gently to feel resistance.	Inflation of balloon anchors catheter tip in place above bladder outlet to prevent removal of catheter (see illustration).

STEPS	RATIONALE
26. Attach end of catheter to collecting tube of drainage system (see illustration). Drainage bag must be below level of bladder, do not place bag on side rails of bed.	Establishes closed system for urine drainage.
27. Anchor catheter:	
a. Female client:	
(1) Secure catheter tubing to inner thigh with strip of nonallergenic tape (commercial multipurpose tube holders with a Velcro strap are available). Allow for slack so movement of thigh does not create tension on catheter (see illustration).	Anchoring catheter to inner thigh reduces pressure on urethra, thus reducing possibility of tissue injury in this area.
b. Male client:	
(1) Secure catheter tubing to top of thigh or lower abdomen (with penis directed toward chest). Allow slack in catheter so movement does not create tension on catheter (see illustration).	Anchoring catheter to lower abdomen reduces pressure on urethra at junction of penis and scrotum, thus reducing possibility of tissue injury in this area.

CRITICAL DECISION POINT **Be sure there are no obstructions in tubing. Coil excess tubing on bed and fasten it to bottom sheet with clip from kit or with rubber band and safety pin.**

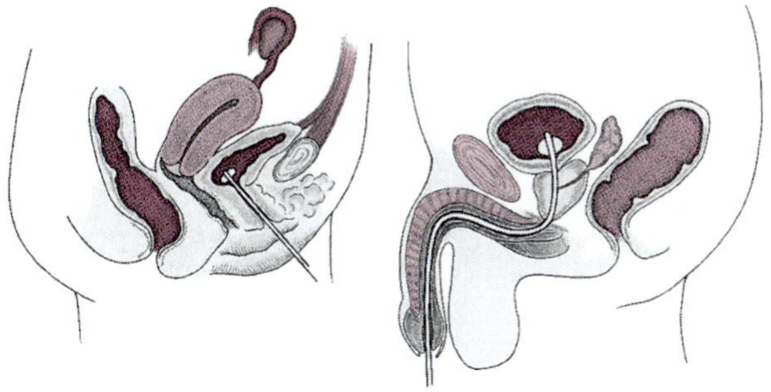

Step 25

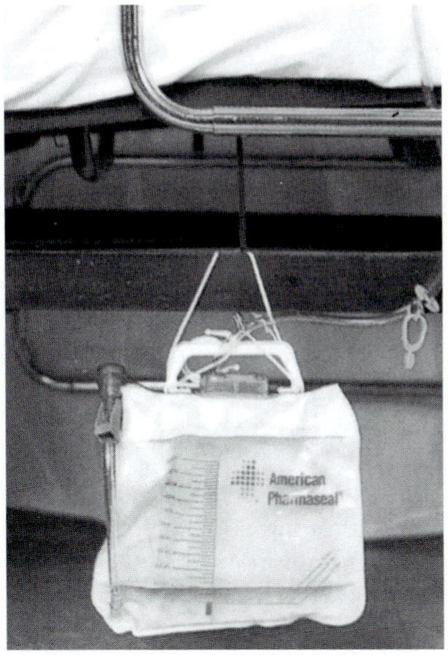

Step 26

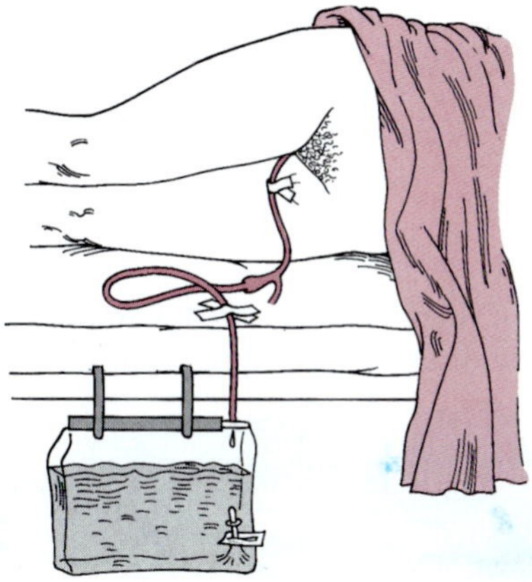

Step 27a Securing the female indwelling catheter.

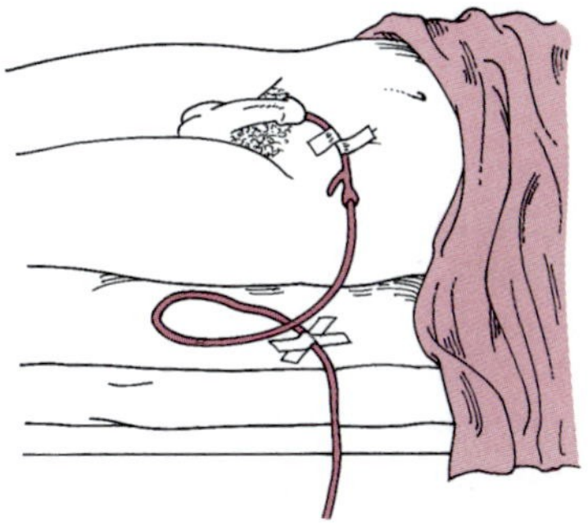

Step 27b Securing the male indwelling catheter.

STEPS	RATIONALE
28. Assist client to comfortable position. Wash and dry perineal area as needed.	Maintains comfort and security.
29. Remove gloves and dispose of equipment, drapes, and urine in proper receptacles.	Reduces transmission of microorganisms.
30. Wash hands.	Reduces spread of microorganisms.
EVALUATION	
1. Palpate bladder.	Determines if distention is relieved.
2. Ask about client's comfort.	Determine if client's sensation of discomfort or fullness has been relieved.
3. Observe character and amount of urine in drainage system.	Determines if urine is flowing adequately.
4. Determine that there is no urine leaking from catheter or tubing connections.	Prevents injury to client's skin.
5. **Unexpected outcomes** that may occur include:	
➤ No urine is present. *Female:* Catheter may be in vaginal opening. *Male:* Catheter may not be advanced far enough through prostatic urethra.	Urine should drain freely. If not, nurse must further assess catheter placement.
➤ Catheter in male client cannot be advanced.	Nurse must assess; if catheter cannot be advanced, physician is notified.
➤ Bladder discomfort despite catheter patency.	Indicates urethral spasm or infection.
➤ Leakage of urine from catheter.	Indicates improper catheter placement, possible balloon deflation, or too small a catheter.
➤ Inability to insert catheter resulting from urethral stricture.	Stricture causes resistance to procedure; physician may be required to insert catheter.

Recording and Reporting

1. Report and record type and size of catheter inserted, amount of fluid used to inflate balloon, characteristics of urine, amount of urine, reasons for catheterization, specimen collection, and, if appropriate, client's response to procedure and teaching concepts.	Identifies for other care providers pertinent information about the catheter and client's response to catheterization.
2. Initiate I&O records.	

Follow-up Activities

1. If urine is not draining once the catheter has been inflated, manipulate or roll the catheter. Assess the client for discomfort and check intake record. Do not advance catheter once the balloon has been inflated.
2. If at the time of insertion you are unable to advance the catheter, seek assistance from physician.
3. Monitor tubing and bag placement to prevent pooling of urine and reflux of urine into the bladder.
4. Avoid raising the drainage bag above the level of the client's bladder.
5. Empty the drainage bag at least every 8 hours.
6. Initiate routine catheter care minimally every 8 hours.

• • • • •

Special Considerations

- When client is incontinent, nurse should try alternate measures such as decreasing nighttime fluids or offering urinal or bedpan more frequently. Inserting catheter carries risk for UTI.
- Check institution policy before beginning catheterization; some agencies restrict maximal amount of urine that can be drained at one time. This amount may vary from 800 to 1000 ml. Research has not shown that there is a limit to the amount of urine that can be drained. (Williams, Wallhagen, and Dowling, 1993).
- Women who are newly postpartum or who have had gynecological surgery and immediately postoperative clients after bladder surgery are at risk for bladder distention.
- If catheter is definitely in bladder and no urine is

produced within an hour, absence of urine should immediately be reported to physician.

- Spinal cord–injured (SCI) clients run the risk of autonomic dysreflexia (hyperreflexia) when exposed to a noxious stimulus such as a full bladder. Hyperreflexia is an autonomic response of the sympathetic system that results in dangerously high blood pressure. SCI clients who require intermittent catheterization are especially susceptible to dysreflexia (Latham, 1994).

Teaching Considerations

- Instruct client on ways to lie in bed with catheter. In the side-lying position facing the catheter, the tubing should drape over the thigh. In the side-lying position facing away from the catheter, the tubing should extend between the legs.
- Explain to client that a burning and/or pressure sensation may be experienced during catheter insertion.
- Caution client against lying on tubing and against raising catheter bag and tubing above hips.
- Explain how the client can cooperate during the procedure.
- Explain what is involved in the care of the catheter and drainage system.

Pediatric Considerations

- Children require smaller catheters than adults; an 8 to 10 Fr catheter is generally used for children.
- For infant or child, nurse must explain procedures to parent.

Gerontologic Considerations

- A client with a catheter is especially vulnerable to UTI. The frail older adult client who is physically compromised runs the additional risk of developing septicemia, an infection that has spread to the blood. Septicemia is a potentially life-threatening complication. Therefore the client who is incontinent should not be routinely catheterized.
- An adequate oral fluid intake of 2000 ml/day and assisting the older adult to toilet on a regular timed basis will help bladder retraining and minimize the need for excessive catheterization.
- Attached equipment such as a catheter may make it more likely that the older adult will not be fully ambulatory, thereby increasing the risks associated with decreased mobility. When catheters are required, they should be removed as soon as the client's condition allows.

Home Care Considerations

- Clients who are at home may use a leg bag during the day and switch to a large-volume bag at night so that sleep can remain uninterrupted.
- Clients may catheterize themselves at home on an intermittent basis using clean technique. Self-catheterization has been shown to be successful in maintaining continence and results in less infections than the use of indwelling catheters.

SKILL 25-4 Care of the Indwelling Catheter

Clients with indwelling catheters require specific perineal hygiene care to reduce the risk of UTI. Any secretions or encrustation at the catheter insertion site must be completely removed. Perineal care and the cleansing of the first 2 inches of the catheter every 8 hours is minimally expected. This is often referred to as catheter care. The use of powders or lotions on the perineum is contraindicated because of the risk of growth of microorganisms, which may ascend the urinary tract.

EQUIPMENT

- Disposable gloves
- Bed protector
- Bath blanket
- Soap, washcloth, basin and water (to cleanse perineum before catheter care)
- Graduated cylinder (used if urine collection bag will be emptied)

DELEGATION CONSIDERATIONS

The skill of performing routine catheter care can be delegated to unlicensed assistive personnel.

- Ensure that care provider knows Standard Precaution guidelines relating to body fluids.
- Caution care provider to be sensitive to the privacy needs of the client.
- Clarify information that should be reported to the nurse about the catheter drainage (color, odor, amount), catheter tubing (leaks, discharge, encrustations), and perineum (color, discharge, contamination from fecal incontinence).
- Inform care provider about the amount of assistance the client requires with positioning and understanding.

STEPS	RATIONALE
ASSESSMENT	
1. Determine how long catheter has been in place. Check agency policy to determine how often indwelling catheter must be changed.	Catheters in place for 3 or more days are more likely to cause urethral irritation and buildup of encrustation.
2. Observe any discharge or encrustation around urethral meatus.	May indicate inflammatory process and may harbor bacteria.
3. Assess for complaints of pain or discomfort; determine location and type of pain client is experiencing; assess for presence of allergies (e.g., to antiseptic solution).	Indicates potential UTI.
4. Monitor client's temperature.	Possible symptom of UTI.
5. Determine client's fluid intake.	Lack of fluid intake reduces natural flushing of urinary system and increases chance of bacterial growth.
6. Assess urine color, clarity, odor, and amount.	Possible symptom of UTI, possible indicator of client's volume status.
7. Assess client's knowledge of catheter care procedure.	Reveals need for client instruction.

NURSING DIAGNOSIS

Clustering of defining characteristics from the assessment data may reveal the following nursing diagnoses for clients requiring this skill:

- Altered urinary elimination
- Knowledge deficit regarding perineal care
- Pain
- Risk for infection
- Toileting self-care deficit

Related factors are individualized based on client's condition or needs.

STEPS	RATIONALE
PLANNING	
1. **Expected outcomes** following completion of procedure:	
➤ Urethral meatus is free of secretions and encrustation.	Indicates absence of irritation.
➤ Urine is clear and volume is sufficient.	Indicates absence of UTI and adequate output.
➤ Client is afebrile.	Indicates absence of infection.
➤ Client will verbalize feeling of comfort after procedure is completed.	Cleansing relieves local discomfort.
2. Explain procedure to client.	Reduces anxiety and promotes cooperation throughout procedure.
3. Identify clients who need catheter care more often than every 8 hours.	Clients who are incontinent of stool or have wound drainage in the perineal area must have catheter care performed more frequently.
IMPLEMENTATION	
1. Wash hands and apply gloves.	Reduces transmission of microorganisms.
2. Close curtain or close door.	Provides privacy and reduces embarrassment to client, thus promoting relaxation.
3. Raise bed to appropriate working height. Raise side rails on opposite side of bed and lower side rail on working side.	Promotes use of proper body mechanics and client safety.
4. Organize equipment for perineal care.	Increases efficiency of procedure.
5. Position client correctly and cover with bath blanket, exposing only perineal area:	Reduces client's embarrassment.
a. Female in dorsal recumbent position.	
b. Male in supine position.	Ensures easy access to perineal tissues.
CRITICAL DECISION POINT Get assistance for positioning the weak or frail client as necessary.	
6. Place waterproof pad under client.	Protects bed from soiling.

STEPS	RATIONALE
7. Drape bath blanket on bedclothes so that only perineal area is exposed.	Prevents unnecessary exposure of body parts.
8. Provide routine perineal care as outlined in Skill 6-2.	
9. Assess urethral meatus and surrounding tissues for inflammation, swelling, and discharge.	Determines local infection and status of hygiene.
➤ ***CRITICAL DECISION POINT*** **Ask client if burning or discomfort is felt.**	
10. Use a clean washcloth and wipe in circular motion along length of catheter for about 10 cm (4 inches).	Reduces presence of secretions or drainage on outside catheter surface.
➤ ***CRITICAL DECISION POINT*** **Note the presence of any encrustation and clean thoroughly.**	
11. Replace as necessary the adhesive tape or multipurpose tube holder that anchors catheter to client's leg or abdomen. Remove adhesive residue from skin.	Secures catheter, thus reducing risk of catheter being pulled and exposing portion of catheter that was in urethra. Also prevents drag on catheter and avoids creating pressure from balloon on bladder floor.
➤ ***CRITICAL DECISION POINT*** **Avoid placing tension on the catheter.**	
12. Replace tubing and collection bag as necessary and/or according to agency policy, adhering to principles of surgical asepsis.	Urinary tubing and collection bag should be changed if there are signs of leakage, odor, or sediment buildup. The catheterization system including the catheter may need to be replaced if leaking or blockage occurs.
➤ ***CRITICAL DECISION POINT*** **Avoid routine changing of collection bags.**	
13. Check drainage tubing and bag to ensure that:	
a. No tubing loops hang below level of bladder or the entry into the collection bag.	Prevents pooling of urine and reflux of urine into bladder.
b. Tube is coiled and secured onto bed linen.	Prevents looping of tubing and subsequent pooling of urine.
c. Tube is not kinked or clamped.	Prevents stasis of urine in bladder. Also ensures that client is not lying on tubing, causing pressure on skin and increasing risk of pressure ulcer.
d. Collection bag is positioned appropriately on the bed frame.	Ensures appropriate drainage of urine.
14. Collection bag should be emptied as necessary but at least every 8 hours.	Urine in collection bag is excellent medium for growth of microorganisms.
15. Assist client to safe, comfortable position.	Promotes safety and comfort.
16. Lower the bed to its lowest position and position side rails accordingly.	Promotes safety.
17. Dispose of contaminated gloves and supplies and wash hands.	Reduces transmission of microorganisms.

EVALUATION

1. Inspect condition of urethra and surrounding tissue.	Determines if area is cleansed properly and if client has any tissue breakdown or irritation.
2. Note character and amount of urine.	Helps to indicate if infection is present and output is adequate.
3. Assess client's temperature.	Helps to indicate if infection is present.
4. Ask if client senses urethral discomfort.	Determines if cleansing reduced irritation.
5. **Unexpected outcomes** that may occur include:	
➤ Odor is present.	Indicates bacterial process.

STEPS	RATIONALE
➤ Urethral meatus is reddened and swollen.	Indicates irritation from catheter or tension from collection bag.
➤ Client has fever.	Source of fever can be UTI.
➤ Urine is leaking.	Indicates disruption of closed drainage system.
➤ Bleeding is present.	Indicates tension has been placed on tubing and caused irritation.
➤ Perineum is reddened and/or skin is broken.	Indicates irritation from urine or stool.

RECORDING AND REPORTING

1. Record in nurses' notes when catheter care was given, assessment of urethral meatus, and character of urine.	Documents care delivered and assessment factors to support presence or absence of inflammatory process or external irritation.
2. Report the presence of an odor, fever, reddened and swollen urethral meatus, or improper draining of urine.	May require further therapy.

FOLLOW-UP ACTIVITIES

1. Notify physician if urethral irritation is present.
2. Ensure that times for catheter care are set in the care plan. Clients with indwelling catheters should receive perineal and catheter care every 8 hours and after bowel movements.

• • • • •

Special Considerations

- Avoid disconnecting the catheter from the collection tubing and bag.
- Keep the collection bag off the floor where microorganisms are abundant.
- If the urine collection bag contains 1500 ml or more and the client is ambulatory, the bag may need to be emptied before the 8-hour interval.

Teaching Considerations

- Unless contraindicated, clients with a catheter should drink at least 2000 ml of fluid per day to promote continuous flushing of the bladder, preventing sediment from collecting in the catheter tubing.
- Instruct client to hold collection bag below the level of the bladder when ambulating.

Gerontologic Considerations

- The older adult client may exhibit atypical signs and symptoms of UTI. Although the usual symptoms of dysuria, urgency, frequency, odor, and hematuria should be assessed, they may not be present. The assessment must also include assessing for less specific signs such as fever and/or mental status changes including agitation, lethargy, and confusion.

Home Care Considerations

- Assess client and primary care giver for ability and motivation to participate in routine catheter care.
- Silicone catheters may be a better choice for the client in the home, where catheterization for longer periods of time may be done, because the silicone is less likely to become encrusted. Encrustations harbor microorganisms.

SKILL 25-5 Obtaining Catheterized Specimens for Residual Urine

Residual urine is the volume of urine in the bladder after a normal voiding. Clients suspected of retaining urine are assessed for residual urine. Urinary retention is the inability of the bladder to fully empty.

Clients at risk for large residual volumes include those receiving bladder training exercises, such as those with spinal cord injuries, those who have suffered a cerebrovascular accident, and those who have had bladder surgery.

DELEGATION CONSIDERATIONS

The skill of obtaining catheterized specimens for residual urine requires the knowledge and decision making skills unique to a professional nurse and is not routinely delegated to unlicensed assistive personnel.

EQUIPMENT

Assemble equipment (see Skill 25-3)

- Straight catheter

STEPS	RATIONALE
ASSESSMENT	
1. Review prior I&O record.	Identifies usual amount of urine voided during each voiding.
2. Determine if client experiences pain or discomfort when voiding.	Pain may be associated with bladder spasms.
3. Review physician's order to determine how often residual urine must be checked.	Order must be obtained from physician before nurse can catheterize client. Physician's order indicates when this procedure is no longer necessary (e.g., check residual urine twice a day until amount obtained is less than 100 ml).
4. Check time of last voiding before catheterization.	Residual urine determinations should be performed immediately after voiding to obtain accurate information about amount of urine remaining in bladder.
5. Assess client's knowledge regarding residual urine.	Reveals need for client education.

NURSING DIAGNOSES

Clustering of defining characteristics from the assessment data may reveal the following nursing diagnoses for clients requiring this skill:

- Altered urinary elimination
- Fluid volume deficit
- Risk for fluid volume deficit
- Fluid volume excess
- Functional incontinence
- Knowledge deficit regarding residual urine
- Pain
- Reflex incontinence
- Risk for infection
- Stress incontinence
- Total incontinence
- Urge incontinence
- Urinary retention

Related factors are individualized based on a client's condition or needs.

STEPS	RATIONALE
PLANNING	
1. **Expected outcomes** following completion of procedure:	
➤ Successive catheterizations result in decreasing amount of residual urine.	Client gains improved bladder control.
➤ Urine remains clear and dilute, without foul odor.	Removal of retained urine reduces medium for bacterial growth.
➤ Client will verbalize decrease in pain or discomfort with voiding.	Voiding at regularly scheduled times decreases residual volumes.
2. Explain procedure to client.	Helps to minimize anxiety.
IMPLEMENTATION	
1. Ask client to void completely and measure volume of urine.	Determines how much client is able to void compared to how much urine remains in bladder after catheterization.
CRITICAL DECISION POINT Remind ambulatory clients not to dispose of urine and that it must be measured.	
2. Wash hands.	Reduces transmission of infection.
3. Proceed as for inserting straight catheter (see Skill 25-3, Implementation).	Insertion of straight catheter drains residual urine.
4. Accurately measure urine obtained.	Allows amount retained to be compared to amount voided.
EVALUATION	
1. Compare amount of urine voided and amount obtained on catheterization.	Difference indicates whether procedure should be repeated. Volume should be less than 100 ml (Aridge, 1993).

STEPS	RATIONALE
2. **Unexpected outcomes** that may occur include:	
➤ Catheterization results in large and increasing volume of urine.	Indicates inadequate bladder emptying. Client who retains 25% of total bladder capacity is experiencing urinary retention. Total bladder capacity is calculated as sum of voiding and residual volume (Gray, 1992).
➤ Urinary incontinence of small amount of urine occurs.	Results from overflow incontinence from bladder distention.
➤ Client has signs and symptoms associated with bladder infection.	Retained urine contains bacterial growth.

RECORDING AND REPORTING

1. Report and record amount of urine voided, amount obtained from catheterization, and client's response.	Communicates information to all members of health care team, indicating progress of therapy.
2. Report presence of unexpected outcomes.	May require further therapy.

FOLLOW-UP ACTIVITIES

1. Notify physician about signs and symptoms of UTI.
2. Assist client in scheduling fluid intake at regular intervals. A voiding schedule will help prevent bladder distention, which contributes to detrusor muscle weakness (Gray, 1992).
3. Notify physician if residual urine volume is greater than 200 ml. Physician may request that indwelling catheter be placed.

• • • • •

Special Considerations

➤ Straight catheters are used to drain residual urine; however, physician may order indwelling Foley catheter insertion if residual urine volumes exceed a certain volume. If physician's order is written in such a manner, nurse may elect to perform residual catheterization with Foley catheter.

➤ Urine retention predisposes the client to UTI and urinary calculi. Signs and symptoms of UTI are a change in urinary elimination such as frequency or nocturia; pain in back or on urination (dysuria); changes in urine including odor, blood, or sediment in urine and color changes to dark yellow or pink; and systemic symptoms as fever and chills. The major symptom of urinary calculi is pain that is described as dull and aching to intense, and the pain can be localized in the flank, back, lower abdomen, or groin. In addition, the client may present with fever, chills, nausea, and vomiting.

Teaching Considerations

➤ Teach client to obtain I&O measurements (see Skill 25-1).

➤ Clients need to be informed about symptoms of UTI. Infections can increase bladder spasms and lead to worsening of urine retention.

Gerontologic Considerations

➤ Urine retention is not considered a normal part of aging and therefore should not be dismissed.

➤ UTI that occurs as a result of residual urine can be devastating to the frail older adult. Septicemia, an infection that spreads into the circulation, may be life threatening in the compromised older client.

Home Care Considerations

➤ Clients may need to be taught how to perform self-catheterization at home.

➤ Clients at home may use a double-voiding technique to help decrease the amount of residual urine. The client is instructed to void, wait about 5 minutes, and then void again. The relaxation between voidings may be helpful in cases of bladder outlet obstruction or weak contractility of the detrusor muscle (Gray, 1992).

SKILL 25-6 Performing Catheter Irrigation

Catheter irrigations are performed on an intermittent or continuous basis to maintain catheter patency. There are two types of irrigation systems: closed bladder irrigation systems and open irrigation systems using disposable trays. A closed bladder irrigation system provides intermittent or continuous irrigation of the system without disrupting the sterile alignment of the catheter and drainage system (Fig. 25-4). The closed system is used most frequently in clients who have had genitourinary surgery. These clients are at risk for occlusion of the Foley catheter by small blood clots and mucous fragments; they are also at risk for UTI. The closed bladder irrigation system allows bladder irrigation to maintain catheter patency without disrupting the system and increasing the risk of entry of bacteria into the urinary tract.

The open irrigation system is also used to maintain catheter patency. However, this system is used when bladder irrigations are required less frequently (e.g., every 8 hours) and there are no blood clots or large mucous shreds in the urinary drainage. This type of irrigation requires the nurse to aseptically break the closed drainage system and maintain surgical asepsis throughout the procedure.

Both systems can be used to irrigate the bladder with a medication to treat an infection or local bladder irritation.

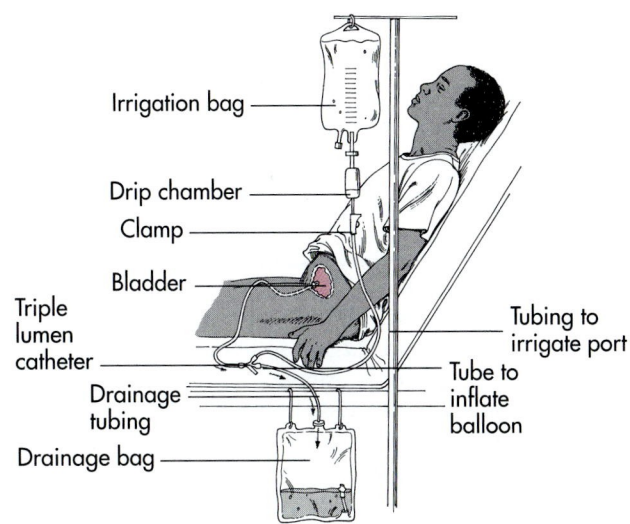

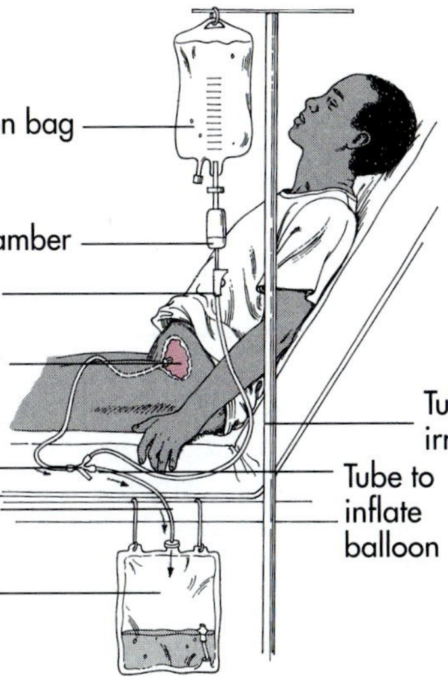

Fig. 25-4

EQUIPMENT

Closed continuous method
- Sterile irrigating solution
- Irrigation tubing with clamp (with or without Y connector) (clamp regulates irrigation flow rate; Y connector allows IV bags to be connected to tubing)
- IV pole
- Y connector (optional) (used to connect irrigation tubing to double-lumen catheter)

Closed intermittent method
- Sterile irrigating solution
- Sterile graduate
- Sterile 30 to 50 ml syringe (used to instill irrigant into catheter)
- Sterile 19- to 22-gauge 1-inch needle
- Antiseptic swab
- Screw clamp (used to temporarily occlude catheter as irrigant is instilled)

Open intermittent method
- Sterile irrigating solution
- Disposable sterile irrigation tray and set
  - Bulb syringe or 60 ml piston-type syringe
  - Sterile collection basin
  - Waterproof drape
  - Sterile solution container
  - Antiseptic swabs
- Gloves
- Tape

DELEGATION CONSIDERATIONS

The skill of catheter irrigations requires the knowledge and decision making skills unique to a professional nurse and is not routinely delegated to unlicensed assistive personnel.

STEPS	RATIONALE
ASSESSMENT	
1. Check client's record to determine:	
a. Purpose of closed bladder irrigation	Allows nurse to anticipate observations to make (e.g., blood or mucus in urine).
b. Physician's order for type and amount of irrigant	Order required to initiate therapy. Ensures that correct medication or solution and amount will be administered.

STEPS	RATIONALE
c. Type of irrigation: continuous or intermittent	Allows nurse to select proper equipment. In continuous irrigation, clamp regulates slow, steady flow into bladder. Because outflow should correspond to regulated irrigation drip, patency of catheter must be checked frequently to prevent distention of bladder. For intermittent irrigation, flow from irrigating solution is clamped for specified time and then opened, and designated amount of irrigating solution is allowed to flush into bladder. Intermittent irrigation requires close observation of catheter patency between irrigations.
d. Type of catheter used:	
(1) Triple lumen (one lumen to inflate balloon, one to instill irrigate solution, and one to allow outflow of urine)	Indicates if it is necessary to break system for irrigation.
(2) Double lumen (one lumen to inflate balloon, one to allow outflow of urine) (see Fig. 25-3)	
2. Assess the following:	
a. Color of urine and presence of mucus, clots, or sediment	Indicates if client is bleeding or sloughing tissue and determines necessity for increasing irrigation rates with continuous irrigations or increasing irrigation frequency with intermittent irrigations.
b. Patency of drainage tubing:	
(1) Note if fluid entering bladder and fluid draining from bladder are in appropriate proportions.	
c. Closed system:	
(1) Determine that drainage tubing is not kinked, clamped off incorrectly, or looped below bladder level.	Determines if system is obstructed. One would expect more output than fluid instilled because of urine production.
(2) Note amount of fluid remaining in existing irrigating solution container.	
3. Review I&O record.	Determines baseline for prior output measures. All clients with continuous bladder irrigations should have I&O measurements (see Skill 25-1).
4. Assess client for presence of bladder spasms and discomfort.	Reveals need for bladder irrigation.
5. Assess client's knowledge regarding purpose of performing catheter irrigation.	Reveals need for client instruction.

NURSING DIAGNOSIS

Clustering of defining characteristics from the assessment data may reveal the following nursing diagnoses for clients requiring this skill:

- Altered urinary elimination
- Fluid volume excess
- Impaired physical mobility
- Knowledge deficit regarding the need for bladder irrigation
- Pain
- Risk for infection

Related factors are individualized based on a client's condition or needs.

PLANNING

STEPS	RATIONALE
1. Expected outcomes following completion of procedure:	
➤ Output is greater than volume of irrigating solution used.	Indicates patency of drainage system.
➤ Absence of pain or discomfort.	Surgery involving bladder and urethral structures results in discomfort.

STEPS	RATIONALE
➤ Absence of fever; urine is not concentrated or foul smelling.	Patency of system promotes drainage of clots and mucus, which if trapped cause bladder spasms.
2. Explain procedure to client.	Helps client relax and promotes cooperation.
3. Have irrigant at room temperature.	Cold irrigant may cause discomfort and bladder spasm.
4. Normal saline is the most common solution used for irrigation.	If another solution is ordered, it may not be found on the unit. Order special solutions from pharmacy in a timely fashion.

IMPLEMENTATION

STEPS	RATIONALE
1. Wash hands.	Reduces transmission of microorganisms.
2. Provide privacy: pull curtains around bed and fold back covers so catheter is exposed at junction where it connects to drainage tubing. Cover client's chest with bath blanket.	Promotes client's self-esteem; shows respect for client while exposing only area nurse must see.
3. Position client in supine position and remove tape or Velcro tube holder that is anchoring catheter to client. Be careful not to pull on catheter.	Allows for client comfort. Removing tape enables nurse to manipulate catheter.
4. Assess lower abdomen for signs of bladder distention.	Detects if catheter or closed irrigation system is malfunctioning, blocking urinary drainage.
5. Closed intermittent irrigation:	
a. Pour prescribed room-temperature sterile irrigating solution in sterile container.	
b. Draw room-temperature sterile solution into syringe using aseptic technique.	Ensures sterility of irrigating fluid.

CRITICAL DECISION POINT **Avoid cold solution because it may cause bladder spasm.**

STEPS	RATIONALE
c. Clamp indwelling retention catheter below soft injection port.	Occlusion of catheter provides resistance against which irrigant can be forcefully instilled into catheter.
d. Apply gloves.	Reduces risk of exposure to body fluids.
e. Cleanse catheter injection port with antiseptic swab (this same port is used for specimen collections).	Reduces transmission of infection.
f. Insert needle of syringe through port at 30-degree angle.	Ensures needle tip enters lumen of catheter and that needle does not puncture tubing.
g. Inject fluid into catheter and bladder.	The injection dislodges clots and sediment. Too much pressure may traumatize the bladder wall.

CRITICAL DECISION POINT **Use slow even pressure when injecting fluid.**

STEPS	RATIONALE
h. Withdraw syringe and remove clamp; allow solution to drain into urinary drainage bag. (It is optional to keep tubing clamped temporarily to allow instilled fluid to remain in bladder.)	Allows drainage to flow via gravity.
6. Closed continuous irrigation:	
a. Apply gloves and using aseptic technique, insert (spike) tip of sterile irrigation tubing into bag containing irrigation solution.	Reduces transmission of microorganisms.
b. Close clamp on tubing and hang bag of solution on IV pole.	Prevents loss of irrigating solution.
c. Open clamp and allow solution to flow through tubing, keeping end of tubing sterile; close clamp.	Removes air from tubing.
d. Wipe off irrigation port of triple-lumen catheter or attach sterile Y connector to double-lumen catheter and then connect to irrigation tubing.	The third catheter lumen or Y connector provides means for irrigating solution to enter bladder. System must remain sterile. When attaching sterile connector, put on gloves to maintain Standard Precautions.

STEPS	RATIONALE
CRITICAL DECISION POINT Be sure drainage bag and tubing are securely connected to drainage port of Y connector when using double-lumen catheter.	
e. For continuous irrigation, calculate drip rate and adjust clamp on irrigation tubing accordingly; be sure clamp on drainage tubing is open and check volume of drainage in drainage bag.	Ensures continuous, even irrigation of catheter system. Prevents accumulation of solution in bladder, which may cause bladder distention and possible injury.
f. For intermittent flow, clamp tubing on drainage system, open clamp on irrigation tubing, and allow prescribed amount of fluid to enter bladder (100 ml is normal for adult); close irrigation tubing clamp and then open drainage tubing clamp.	Fluid is instilled through catheter into bladder, flushing system. Fluid drains out after irrigation is complete.
CRITICAL DECISION POINT Do not leave a clamped drainage bag unattended.	
7. Open irrigation:	
a. Apply gloves.	Reduces transmission of infection. Irrigation is a sterile procedure, but only parts of the system coming in contact with the inside of the catheter must remain sterile. The tip of the syringe, end of the catheter, end of the catheter tubing, and irrigant must remain sterile. Therefore the use of sterile gloves is optional.
b. Open sterile irrigation tray; establish sterile field and pour required amount of sterile solution into sterile solution container. Replace cap on large container of solution.	Adheres to principles of surgical asepsis.
c. Position waterproof drape under catheter.	Prevents soiling of bed linen.
d. Aspirate 30 ml of solution into irrigating syringe.	Prepares irrigant for instillation into catheter.
e. Move sterile collection basin close to client's thigh.	Prevents soiling of bed linen and prohibits reaching over sterile area.
CRITICAL DECISION POINT Wipe connection point between catheter and tubing with antiseptic wipe before disconnecting.	
f. Disconnect catheter from drainage tubing, allowing urine to flow into sterile collection basin; cover open end of drainage tubing with sterile protective cap and position tubing so it stays coiled on top of bed.	Maintains sterility of inner aspect of catheter lumen and drainage tubing; reduces potential of introducing pathogens into bladder.
g. Insert tip of syringe into lumen of catheter and gently instill solution.	Reduces incidence of bladder spasm but clears catheter of obstruction.
CRITICAL DECISION POINT If strong resistance is noted, do not force the irrigation.	
h. Withdraw syringe, lower catheter, and allow solution to drain into basin. Repeat, instilling solution and draining several times until drainage is clear of clots and sediment.	Allows drainage to flow by gravity. Provides for adequate flushing of catheter.
i. If solution does not return, have client turn onto side facing nurse; if changing position does not help, reinsert syringe and gently aspirate solution.	Change in position may move tip of catheter in bladder, increasing likelihood that fluid instilled will flow out.

STEPS	RATIONALE
CRITICAL DECISION POINT Watch client for indications of pain or discomfort.	
j. After irrigation is complete, remove protector cap from drainage tubing adapter, cleanse adapter with alcohol swab, and reinsert adapter into lumen of catheter to reestablish closed drainage system.	
8. Anchor catheter to client's leg or thigh with tape or Velcro multipurpose tube holder (see Step 26 in Skill 25-3).	Prevents trauma to urethral tissue.
9. Assist client into comfortable position.	Promotes relaxation and rest.
10. Lower bed to lowest position and position side rails accordingly.	Promotes client safety.
11. Dispose of contaminated supplies, remove gloves, and wash hands.	Reduces spread of microorganisms.

EVALUATION

STEPS	RATIONALE
1. Calculate fluid used to irrigate bladder and catheter and subtract from volume drained.	Determines accurate urinary output.
2. Assess characteristics of output: viscosity, color, and presence of clots.	Data serve as baseline to judge response to therapy.
3. Observe for catheter patency.	
4. Observe client for signs of pain and fever.	
5. Observe urine to determine clarity, concentration, and odor.	Determines presence of bacteria in urine.
6. **Unexpected outcomes** that may occur include:	
➤ Irrigating solution is not returned.	Indicates possible occlusion of Foley catheter, which can lead to urinary retention.
➤ Client complains of pain.	May indicate urinary retention.
➤ Signs of fever or cloudy, foul urine.	May indicate infection.
➤ Increase in bladder spasms.	May indicate occlusion of catheter with foreign object (e.g., blood clot).

RECORDING AND REPORTING

STEPS	RATIONALE
1. Record amount of solution used as irrigant, amount returned as drainage, characteristics of output, and urine output of drainage in nurses' notes and I&O sheet.	Documents procedure and client's tolerance of it.
2. Report catheter occlusion, sudden bleeding, infection, or increased pain to physician.	May require more aggressive therapy. Reduces risk of urinary retention.

FOLLOW-UP ACTIVITIES

1. Notify physician if irrigant is retained and bladder is distended.
2. Notify physician if large clots or sediment is returned. May need to change from intermittent to continuous irrigation.
3. Notify physician if bladder spasms increase or are unrelieved.

• • • • •

Special Considerations

- Triple-lumen catheter system does not have to be broken when irrigating bladder and is therefore often used after bladder surgery when frequent irrigations to prevent clotting are required.
- Double-lumen catheter system requires nurse to break system to irrigate bladder.
- Bleeding is common after transurethral prostatectomy. Nurse should expect bright red–tinged urine during first 48 hours postoperatively followed by

pink-tinged to clear urine by fifth postoperative day.

- Supplies for closed irrigation system may be kept at bedside. Irrigating solution should be at room temperature. This practice is similar to that when bag of IV fluid is added to IV infusion. Check that solution, volume, client, route, and time are correct. Discard any sterile solution not used within 24 hours of opening. Check institutional policy; some agencies call for new irrigant every shift when an open irrigation is performed. When irrigant is opened, it should be marked with the date and time.
- Room-temperature sterile normal saline is usually used; cold solution can cause bladder spasms.
- If blood is present, flow rate may need to be increased to keep system patent. Rate of infusion may be determined by independent nursing judgment.
- Amount of solution used to flush system may be a nurse judgment or indicated by physician or institutional policy. Frequency of irrigation is based on need of client (e.g., client who has just had prostate gland surgery may require irrigations every 5 to 10 minutes in first hour, which are then tapered to every 4 hours).

Teaching Considerations

- Instruct client and primary care giver to observe urine daily for changes in color, presence of mucus or blood, and changes in consistency and odor.
- Instruct client to maintain adequate oral intake of 2 L/day (unless contraindicated).

Gerontologic Considerations

- Benign prostatic hypertrophy is common as men age, and surgical intervention on the prostate gland may be required. After surgery, continuous and rapid irrigation of the bladder with a three-way Foley catheter is often necessary to prevent clotting and obstruction of the catheter.

Home Care Considerations

- Assess the client and primary care giver for ability and motivation to perform catheter irrigation.
- Assess client's environment for appropriate storage space for materials needed for procedure.
- Observe client and primary care giver while they perform procedure.
- Refer client to home care agency for in-home follow-up.

SKILL 25-7 Removing a Retention Catheter

Removal of a retention catheter is a skill requiring clean technique. When removing a retention catheter, the nurse must prevent trauma to the urethra. If the retention catheter balloon is not fully deflated, its removal can result in trauma and subsequent swelling of urethral meatus, and urinary retention can occur.

If the catheter was in place for more than several days, the client may experience dysuria resulting from inflammation of the urethral canal. Because of decreased bladder muscle tone, the client may urinate frequently.

EQUIPMENT

- **Syringe (same size as volume of solution used to inflate balloon) (Check balloon and inflate valve, which has this information printed on it.)**
- **Waterproof pad**
- **Alcohol swab**
- **Nonsterile disposable gloves**
- **Correctly labeled sterile specimen container and 25-gauge 1/2-inch needle (if culture and sensitivity are to be obtained before catheter removal)**

DELEGATION CONSIDERATIONS

The skill of removing a retention catheter can be delegated to unlicensed assistive personnel.

- Inform care provider to check the size of balloon and the size of syringe needed to deflate the balloon.
- Ensure that care provider knows Standard Precaution guidelines relating to body fluids.
- Caution the care provider to be sensitive to the privacy needs of the client.
- Clarify information that should be reported to the nurse about the deflation such as excessive burning or bleeding.
- Inform care provider not to use force when removing catheter.
- Instruct care provider to notify nurse if balloon does not deflate.
- Instruct care provider to assist client with perineal care (see Skill 6-2).
- Clarify whether client will need assistance to ambulate to bathroom for voiding.
- Instruct care provider to place measuring device (urine hat) labeled with client's name in bathroom if I&O is to be monitored (see Skill 25-1).
- Instruct care provider to teach client how to use measuring device.

STEPS	RATIONALE

ASSESSMENT

1. Review client's medical record for physician's order and the reason for removing catheter. — Physician may have ordered catheter to be removed, enabling client to void after removal. It may be removed to be replaced with another indwelling catheter.
2. Note period of time catheter was in place. — Assesses risk for loss of bladder tone.
3. Assess client's knowledge of procedure. — Reveals need for client instruction.

NURSING DIAGNOSIS

Clustering of defining characteristics from the assessment data may reveal the following nursing diagnoses for clients requiring this skill:

- Functional incontinence
- Reflex incontinence
- Risk for infection
- Stress incontinence
- Total incontinence
- Urge incontinence
- Urinary retention

Related factors are individualized based on a client's condition or needs.

PLANNING

1. **Expected outcomes** following completion of procedure:
   - Client voids a minimum of 250 ml of urine with each voiding within 6 to 8 hours of catheter removal. — Indicates return of voluntary bladder function.
   - Client voids without discomfort. — Indicates absence of urethral trauma.
   - Skin under tape site is intact and not abraded, open, or reddened.
2. Explain procedure to client. — Reduces anxiety and promotes cooperation.
3. If client is ambulatory, obtain a urine hat that fits into toilet so that the ambulatory client's output can be measured after catheter removal.

Step 8

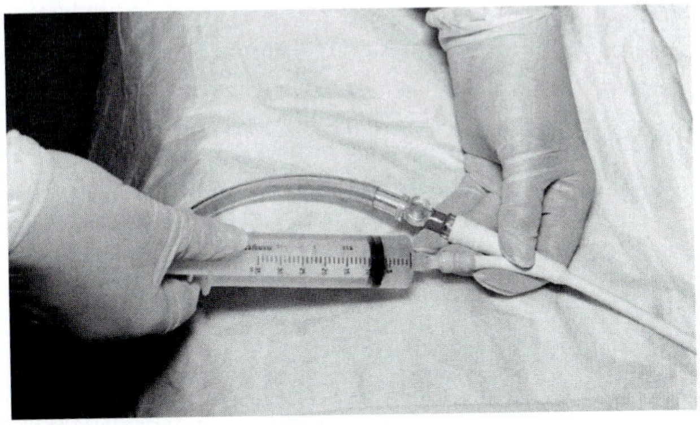

IMPLEMENTATION

1. Wash hands and apply gloves. — Reduces transmission of microorganisms.
2. Provide privacy by closing curtain and door. — Provides privacy, reduces embarrassment, and relaxes client.
3. Raise bed to appropriate working height. Raise side rail on opposite side of bed and lower side rail on working side. — Promotes use of good body mechanics and client safety.
4. Position client in supine position. — Provides easy access to visualize urethral meatus.
5. Place waterproof pad between female's thighs (if in supine position) or over male's thighs. — Prevents soiling of bed linen. Provides wrapper to cover contaminated catheter after removal, thus eliminating possibility of urine contaminating nurse's hand.
6. Obtain sterile urine specimen if required (see Skill 44-4). — Determines if bacteria are present in urine.
7. Remove adhesive tape or Velcro tube used to secure and anchor catheter. Cleanse any residue from skin. — Removes source of irritant on skin. Allows for positioning of catheter for removal.
8. Insert hub of syringe into inflation valve (balloon port). Aspirate entire amount of fluid used to inflate balloon (see illustration). — Deflates balloon to allow for removal. If solution is not completely aspirated, partially inflated balloon causes trauma to urethral wall as catheter is removed.

STEPS	RATIONALE
➤ ***CRITICAL DECISION POINT*** **Do not use force to make the syringe fit into the valve.**	
9. Pull catheter out smoothly and slowly.	Prevents trauma to urethral mucosa.
➤ ***CRITICAL DECISION POINT*** **Stop pulling catheter if resistance is met; balloon is probably still inflated.**	
10. Wrap contaminated catheter in waterproof pad. Unhook collection bag and drainage tubing from bed.	Prevents contamination of nurse's hands.
11. Reposition client as necessary. Lower level of bed and position side rails accordingly.	Promotes client comfort and safety.
12. Measure and empty contents of collection bag.	Provides accurate recording of urinary output.
13. Dispose of all contaminated supplies correctly, remove gloves, and wash hands.	Reduces spread of microorganisms.
➤ ***CRITICAL DECISION POINT*** **Handle catheter and drainage bag as biohazards.**	
14. If another catheter is to be inserted, proceed according to procedure for insertion of retention catheter (Skill 25-3).	
EVALUATION	
1. Observe time and amount of first voided specimen.	Indicates return of bladder function and ability of bladder to empty fully. If volume is small, residual urine must be measured.
2. Note any discomfort experienced by client when voiding.	It is normal for client to experience dysuria, especially if catheter had been in place for several days or weeks.
3. Note condition of skin at site where device was used to anchor catheter tubing to leg.	Determines presence of skin irritation.
4. **Unexpected outcomes** that may occur include:	
➤ Client is unable to void in 6 to 8 hours.	Indicates urinary retention.
➤ Bladder is distended; client voids small amounts frequently and complains of burning or pain.	Indicates urinary retention with overflow incontinence. UTI may be present.
➤ Skin under tape site is reddened and weeping fluid.	Indicates tape burn or allergic response.

Recording and Reporting

1. Record and report time catheter was removed and time and amount of next voiding.	Communicates pertinent information to all members of health care team.
2. Record presence of unexpected outcomes.	
3. Continue to monitor I&O as necessary.	

Follow-up Activities

1. Notify physician if bladder distends, client has not voided for 6 to 8 hours, or client complains of increasing urge to void.
2. Provide perineal care after catheter removal.
3. Monitor the client's first voiding for color, odor, and amount to evaluate return of bladder function.
4. I&O is often monitored for at least 24 hours after removal of catheter.

• • • • •

Special Considerations

- If client has not voided within 6 to 8 hours after catheter removal, the catheter (intermittent or indwelling, depending on order of physician) may have to be reinserted. Assess for signs of urinary retention.
- The practice of bladder training before removal of a catheter is not advised. Its effectiveness is not well documented and it may increase the risk of infection.

Teaching Considerations

- Explain to client that burning sensation may be felt as catheter is withdrawn.
- Instruct client regarding the use of over-the-counter medicines that may cause urinary retention (e.g., nasal decongestants, anticholinergic medications).
- Instruct client to maintain fluid intake of at least 2 L/day (unless contraindicated) to reduce risk of infection.
- Instruct client to ask for assistance when getting up to walk to toilet if client has not been ambulatory.
- Instruct client how to use urine hat if I&O is monitored.

SKILL 25-8 Applying a Condom Catheter

The external application of a urinary drainage device is a convenient, safe method of draining urine in male clients. The condom catheter is suitable for incontinent or comatose clients who still have complete and spontaneous bladder emptying. The condom is a soft, pliable rubber sheath that slips over the penis and is kept in place with the use of an elastic adhesive strip (Fig. 25-5). The catheter may be attached to a leg drainage bag or a standard urinary drainage bag.

A condom catheter may remain in place 24 hours, but it should be monitored every 4 hours to detect potential problems. With each catheter change, the nurse cleanses the urethral meatus and penis thoroughly and looks for signs of skin irritation.

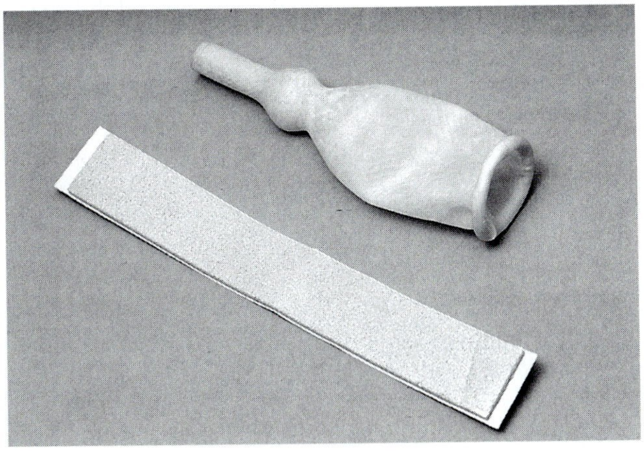

Fig. 25-5

EQUIPMENT

- **Condom catheter kit**
  - **Rubber condom sheath (appropriate size)**
  - **Strip of elastic adhesive**
  - **Skin preparation**
- **Urinary collection bag with drainage tubing or leg bag and straps**
- **Basin with warm water and soap**
- **Towels and washcloths**
- **Bath blanket**
- **Nonsterile disposable gloves**
- **Scissors and/or safety razor**

DELEGATION CONSIDERATIONS

The skill of applying a condom catheter can be delegated to unlicensed assistive personnel.

- Ensure that care provider knows Standard Precaution guidelines relating to body fluids.
- Caution care provider to be sensitive to the privacy needs of the client.
- Arrange for extra personnel to assist with moving dependent clients.
- Consult agency policy regarding condom catheter care; delegation may vary with agencies.
- Clarify that skin of penile shaft is intact and free from swelling, redness, or open lesions before condom catheter is applied.
- Clarify the care provider's understanding of how to apply the adhesive strip that secures the condom catheter.

STEPS	RATIONALE

ASSESSMENT

STEPS	RATIONALE
1. Assess urinary elimination patterns, client's ability to voluntarily urinate, and continence.	Clients who are incontinent are at risk for skin breakdown.
2. Assess mental status of client so appropriate teaching related to condom catheter can be implemented.	Some male clients may be incontinent only at night. Teaching can be implemented to instruct client on self-application.
3. Assess condition of penis.	Provides baseline to compare changes in condition of skin after condom catheter application.
4. Assess client's knowledge of the purpose of a condom catheter.	Reveals need for client instruction.

NURSING DIAGNOSIS

Clustering of defining characteristics from the assessment data may reveal the following nursing diagnoses for clients requiring this skill:

- Risk for impaired skin integrity
- Knowledge deficit regarding application of condom catheter
- Toileting self-care deficit
- Total incontinence

Related factors are individualized based on a client's condition or needs.

PLANNING

STEPS	RATIONALE
1. **Expected outcomes** following completion of procedure:	
➤ Client is continent with condom catheter intact.	Catheter is secure; normal voiding occurs.
➤ Penile shaft is free of skin irritation or breakdown.	Indicates absence of irritation.
2. Explain procedure to client.	Reduces anxiety and promotes cooperation.
3. Arrange for extra nursing personnel to assist with moving dependent client.	Promotes client safety and proper use of body mechanics by nurse.
4. Read the instructions on the package if a condom catheter kit is used.	Application of the adhesive strip before or after the condom is applied varies with brand.

IMPLEMENTATION

STEPS	RATIONALE
1. Wash hands.	Reduces transmission of microorganisms.
2. Provide privacy by closing room door or bedside curtain.	Maintains client's self-esteem.
3. Raise bed to appropriate working height. Raise side rail on opposite side of bed and lower side rail on working side.	Promotes use of good body mechanics and client safety.
4. Assist client into supine position. Place bath blanket over upper torso. Fold sheets so lower extremities are covered; only genitalia should be exposed.	Promotes comfort; draping prevents unnecessary exposure of body parts.
5. Prepare urinary drainage collection bag and tubing. Clamp off drainage bag port. Secure collection bag to bed frame; bring drainage tubing up through side rails onto bed. Prepare leg bag for connection to condom if necessary.	Provides easy access to drainage equipment after condom catheter is in place.
6. Apply disposable gloves. Provide perineal care (see Skill 6-2) and dry thoroughly.	Removes irritating secretions. Rubber sheath of condom rolls onto dry skin more easily.
7. Clip hair at base of penis. In some cases shaving the hair at the base of the penis may be necessary.	Hair adheres to condom and is pulled during condom removal or may get caught in rubber as condom catheter is applied.
8. Apply skin preparation to penis and allow to dry. If client is uncircumcised, return foreskin to normal position.	Skin preparation has an alcohol base. Evaporation is necessary to prevent irritation.
9. With nondominant hand, grasp penis along shaft. With dominant hand, hold condom sheath at tip of penis and smoothly roll sheath onto penis.	Prepares penis for easy condom placement.

STEPS	RATIONALE
CRITICAL DECISION POINT Allow 2.5 to 5 cm (1 to 2 inches) of space between tip of glans penis and end of condom catheter (see illustration).	
10. Spiral wrap penile shaft with strip of elastic adhesive. With some brands of catheters the adhesive strip is applied before the condom is applied. Condom must be secured firmly so it is snug and stays on but not tight enough to cause constriction of blood flow. Strip should be spiral wrapped and not overlap itself. Do not use any tape except that provided by the manufacturer. Other tapes will not provide the flexibility needed for spiral wrap and may impair circulation to the penis. Never use adhesive tape in the application of the condom catheter because it may impede circulation.	
11. Connect drainage tubing to end of condom catheter. Be sure condom is not twisted. Catheter can be connected to large-volume bag or leg bag (see illustration).	Allows urine to be collected and measured. Keeps client dry. Twisted condom obstructs urine flow.
12. Place excess coiling of tubing on bed and secure to bottom sheet.	Prevents looping of tubing and promotes free drainage of urine.
13. Place client in safe, comfortable position. Lower bed and place side rails accordingly.	Promotes safety and comfort.
14. Dispose of contaminated supplies and wash hands.	Reduces spread of microorganisms.

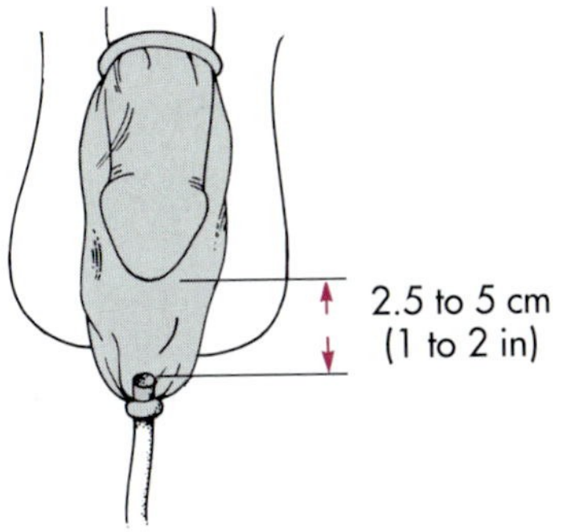

Step 9

EVALUATION

STEPS	RATIONALE
1. Observe urinary drainage.	Determines if normal voiding is occurring.
2. Inspect penis with condom catheter in place within 30 minutes after application. Look for swelling and discoloration and ask client if there is any discomfort.	Determines if catheter has been applied incorrectly.
3. Remove and change condom and inspect skin on penile shaft for signs of breakdown or irritation at least daily when hygiene is performed and when condom is reapplied.	Indicates if condom or urine is causing irritation or if adhesive is too restrictive. Frequent assessment of circulation of glans penis is important to determine if condom has been applied too tightly.
4. **Unexpected outcomes** that may occur include:	
➤ Skin around penis is reddened and excoriated.	Results from pressure of adhesive or contact with urine.
➤ Urination is reduced in amount and frequency.	Indicates urinary retention.
➤ Urine leaks from tubing.	Catheter is improperly secured to drainage, catheter has been improperly applied, or adhesive has been applied too snugly, which may result in impaired circulation.
➤ Penile swelling or discoloration.	

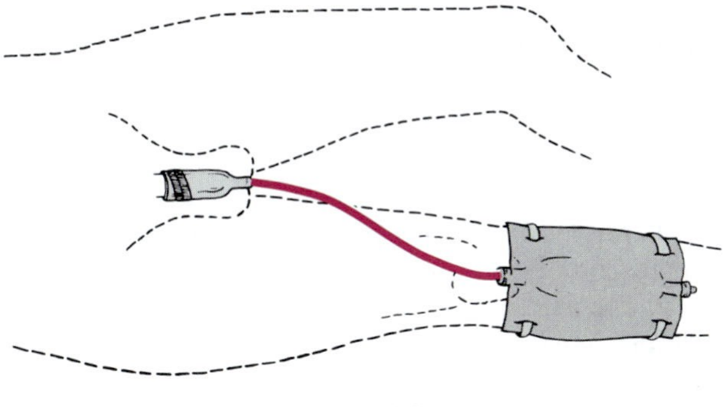

Step 11

STEPS	RATIONALE

Recording and Reporting

1. Report and record pertinent information: condom application, condition of penis skin and scrotum, and voiding pattern.	Communicates information to all members of health care team.
2. Monitor I&O as indicated.	

Follow-Up Activities

1. Increase frequency of perineal skin care to every shift and whenever necessary (see Chapter 6).
2. Assess condom application 30 minutes after applying and inspect every 4 hours to determine if the penis circulation is adequate.
3. Change condom catheter every 24 hours to allow appropriate perineal skin care.
4. Observe urinary drainage to make sure that urine drains from the condom device and does not pool, bathing the penis in urine.

• • • • •

Special Considerations

- Condom catheter is suitable for incontinent or comatose male clients with complete and spontaneous bladder emptying.
- Check institutional policy to determine if physician's order is required to apply condom catheter.
- Procedure should be explained, even if client is comatose, because he may be able to hear.
- Some institutions apply a thin layer of plasticized skin spray to skin of penile shaft to protect skin from ulceration and irritation caused by rubber condom and adhesive holding it in place.
- If leg bag is used, assess leg every 8 hours for circulatory impairment.

Teaching Considerations

- Teach client to keep condom and catheter kink free and positioned below the level of the bladder.
- Teach client with leg bag to periodically assess leg straps for tightness and to report pain in leg.
- Teach client a collection bag that fills completely may put unnecessary tension on the catheter and contribute to problems keeping the catheter intact (Smith, 1994).

Gerontologic Considerations

- Condom catheters are not recommended in clients with chronic obstruction such as benign prostatic hypertrophy (Urinary Incontinence Guideline Panel, 1992).
- Clients with neuropathy should be carefully evaluated before application of the condom catheter.

Home Care Considerations

- Care givers should be taught assessments to be made and what to report.
- Condom catheters are not meant for long-term use (Urinary Incontinence Guideline Panel, 1992).
- The use of condom catheters is associated with increased risk of UTI, and therefore the care giver should be alert to indicators of infection.
- Teach client to switch from leg bag to drainage bag at night.
- Modifications may need to be made in clothing to promote optimal drainage.

Skill 25-9 Care of a Suprapubic Catheter

Suprapubic catheters are inserted surgically into the bladder through the lower abdomen above the symphysis pubis (Fig. 25-6). Although most successfully used for short periods with clients who have had gynecological and bladder surgery, the suprapubic catheter may be used in older adult men who require a long-term alternative to urinary catheterization (McCormick et al., 1992).

As with the indwelling urinary catheter, the suprapubic catheter predisposes the client to UTI, but the incidence may be lower than that with the indwelling catheter. The advantages of the suprapubic catheter for the client are that the client may void naturally when the catheter is clamped and it is more comfortable than the indwelling catheter. The procedure can be performed at the bedside with the client under local anesthesia or it may be performed in surgery.

The nurse is responsible for maintaining the catheter while the client is in the nursing home or hospital and for teaching the client or care giver about routine care. Daily care will depend on the institution's policy, but the cleaning and dressing of the catheter site is similar to that for any surgical drain.

EQUIPMENT

- Gloves, sterile and clean
- Cleansing agent
- Sterile gauze for cleaning
- Sterile drain sponge (split gauze)
- Tape
- Dressing bag

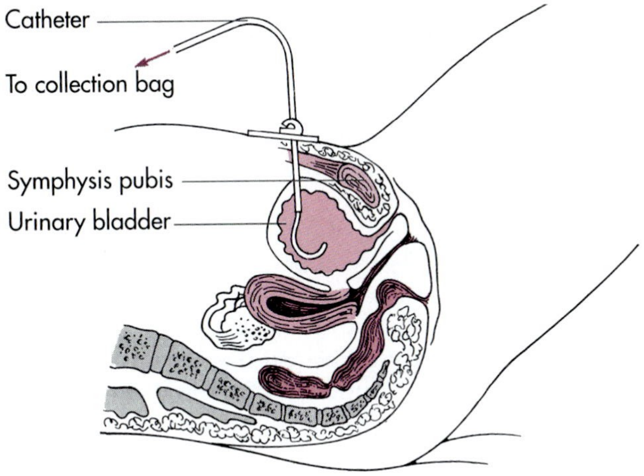

Fig. 25-6

DELEGATION CONSIDERATIONS

The skill of caring for a suprapubic catheter requires the knowledge and decision making skills unique to the professional nurse and is not usually delegated to unlicensed assistive personnel.

STEPS	RATIONALE
ASSESSMENT	
1. Assess urine in bag for amount, clarity, color, odor, and sediment.	Abnormal findings may indicate potential complications like UTI, decreased urinary output, and blockage.
2. Assess dressing for drainage and intactness.	Drainage indicates potential complication like infection. Dressing coming off may be caused by tape choice or client picking at dressing.
3. Assess catheter insertion site for signs of inflammation such as redness, swelling, and discharge. Ask client if there is any pain at site.	If insertion is new, slight inflammation may be expected as part of wound healing. May indicate potential infection.
4. Assess how catheter is held in place.	The catheter may be sutured or be retained by a commercial body seal.
5. Assess tape site for signs of irritation.	Taping over the same area over a prolonged period may lead to skin irritation and breakdown.
6. Assess for fever.	An increased temperature may indicate infection.
7. Check for allergies.	Client may be sensitive to tape or to antiseptic solution.

NURSING DIAGNOSIS

Clustering of defining characteristics from the assessment data may reveal the following nursing diagnoses for clients requiring this skill:

- Altered urinary elimination
- Fluid volume deficit
- Risk for fluid volume deficit
- Fluid volume excess
- Functional incontinence
- Impaired physical mobility
- Risk for knowledge deficit regarding care of suprapubic catheter
- Pain
- Reflex incontinence
- Risk for infection
- Total incontinence
- Urge incontinence
- Urinary retention

Related factors are individualized based on a client's condition or needs.

STEPS	RATIONALE
PLANNING	
1. **Expected outcomes** following completion of procedure:	
➤ Client will verbalize no pain or discomfort at insertion site.	Patent catheter system keeps bladder empty and client comfortable and without signs of infection.
➤ Minimum of 30 ml of urine is present in urinary collection bag every hour.	Verifies that there is adequate perfusion to kidneys and that catheter is not blocked.
➤ Urine remains clear and dilute without foul odor.	Removal of retained urine reduces medium for bacterial growth.
➤ Site remains dry, clean, and intact.	No indication of infection develops.
➤ Client remains afebrile.	Indicates that no infection is developing.
2. Explain procedure to client.	Helps to minimize anxiety.
IMPLEMENTATION	
1. Wash hands.	Reduces transmission of infection.
2. Close curtain or door.	Provides privacy, reduces embarrassment, and relaxes client.
3. Proceed as for applying a dry dressing (see Steps 2 to 11, Skill 37-1).	The catheter site is surgically made and therefore is similarly treated as other dressings.
4. Clean site by swabbing in circular motion starting closest to the drain and continuing in outward widening circles for approximately 2 inches (5 cm) (see illustration).	Follows principle of sterile technique to move from area of least contamination to most. Cleanses microorganisms that could migrate to site.
➤ ***CRITICAL DECISION POINT*** **Use nondominant sterile gloved hand to hold catheter erect while cleaning.**	
5. With dominant sterile gloved hand, apply split gauze around catheter and tape in place.	

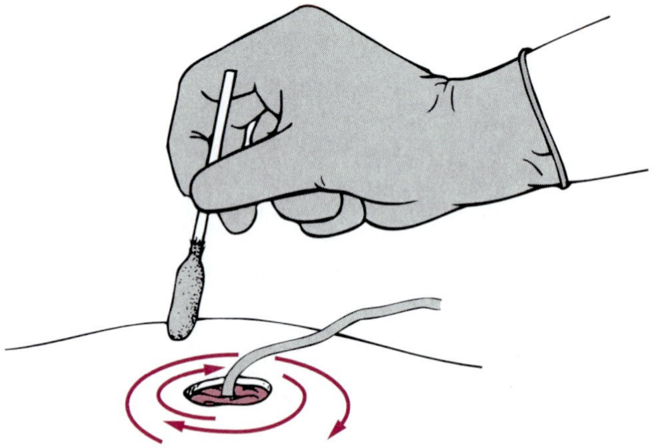

Step 4

STEPS	RATIONALE
6. Secure catheter to abdomen with tape or Velcro multipurpose tube holder to reduce tension on insertion site.	This technique is similar to that used for the indwelling urinary catheter. Secures catheter and reduces risk of excessive tension on suture and/or body seal.
7. Check bag and tubing placement.	
➤ ***CRITICAL DECISION POINT*** **Be sure there are no obstructions in tubing. Coil excess tubing on bed and fasten it to bottom sheet with clip from kit or with rubber band and safety pin.**	
EVALUATION	
1. Ask client whether there is any pain or discomfort from suprapubic catheter.	
2. Observe client's urine for sediment, odor, or discoloration.	Possible signs of infection when present.
3. Inspect dressing at least every shift.	

STEPS	RATIONALE
4. Monitor for signs of infection: elevated WBC, positive urine culture, or elevated temperature.	
5. **Unexpected outcomes** that may occur include:	
➤ Catheter becomes dislodged.	
➤ Catheter is blocked by clots, accumulation of sediment, or position of catheter in bladder.	The suprapubic catheter is often small bore and is easily blocked.
➤ Site bleeds after removal of old dressing.	May indicate disruption of incision or infection.
➤ Client develops a UTI.	Although associated with lower rates of infection than the indwelling urinary catheter, the suprapubic catheter is surgically introduced and can become infected, especially in the compromised client and or if there are breaks in the closed system.
➤ Leakage of urine at site and skin breakdown.	Inspection and dressing changes are important in monitoring for these problems.

Recording and Reporting

1. Report and record dressing replacement including assessments of wound and tolerance of client to dressing.	Communicates information to all members of health care team, indicating progress of therapy.
2. Report presence of unexpected outcomes.	May require further therapy.

Follow-up Activities

1. Notify physician about signs and symptoms of UTI.
2. Encourage client to drink at least 1500 ml of fluids per day if no restrictions.
3. Notify physician if signs of infection at catheter site are present.

Special Considerations

- Clients may have both an indwelling and a suprapubic catheter after gynecological or bladder surgery. Urine must be assessed in both drainage systems. (Most urine will be found in the suprapubic drainage system.)
- Clients with both suprapubic and indwelling catheters will have the indwelling urinary catheter removed first, usually between the second and fourth postoperative day.
- Bladder spasms may occur in clients with suprapubic catheters. The diameter of the suprapubic catheter is small and is easily occluded with clots, mucus, or sediment. Occlusion can lead to bladder irritation and spasms.
- Residual urine can be assessed by having client void while suprapubic drainage tubing is clamped; the residual urine is then measured by releasing the clamp. Residual urine amounts of less than 50 ml may indicate that bladder function has returned postoperatively.

Teaching Considerations

- Encourage clients to consume a minimum of 1500 ml of fluids daily.
- Clients should be taught to keep the drainage bag lower than the bladder and to keep tubing free of kinks.

Home Care Considerations

- With shortened hospital stays it is common for the postsurgery client to go home with a suprapubic catheter.
- Client or care giver needs to be taught how to clean and dress the suprapubic site.
- Client or care giver needs to be taught how to empty a catheter bag and assess urine for color, odor, clarity, and amount.

SKILL 25-10 Peritoneal Dialysis and Continuous Ambulatory Peritoneal Dialysis

The kidneys are organs that filter and excrete excess fluid and solute wastes. When the kidneys fail, little to no urine is produced, electrolyte imbalances occur, and toxins accumulate in the blood. If excess fluid and toxins are not removed, death results.

Dialysis is a process that removes fluid and solute wastes from the blood or lymph. There are two major types of dialysis: hemodialysis and peritoneal dialysis. Hemodialysis nursing is a specialty practice that involves the shunting of the client's blood through a machine. Peritoneal dialysis is a procedure that infuses a hypertonic solution into the peritoneal cavity. The solution is left for a specified period of time and then drained. The semipermeable peritoneum membrane serves as a filter to remove excess water, electrolytes, and toxins from the blood. Peritoneal dialysis has three steps, each of which varies in length: (1) infusing the dialysate into the cavity, (2) allowing the fluid to dwell in the cavity, and (3) draining the dialysate from the cavity. These are sometimes referred to as "fill, dwell, and drain times".

Peritoneal dialysis can be performed for the acutely ill client or for the client with chronic renal failure. Acute intermittent peritoneal dialysis (IPD) is used within the hospital setting and involves the surgical insertion of a temporary catheter into the peritoneal cavity (Fig. 25-7). An exchange or dialysis cycle in acute peritoneal dialysis ranges from ½ hour to 2 hours (Lancaster, 1995).

A second form of peritoneal dialysis is used with clients who need ongoing dialysis. Clients who require dialysis because of a chronic condition have long-term peritoneal catheters inserted and, based on need, may receive their dialysis in a variety of settings including their homes. Therapy can be intermittent or continuous depending on the need.

Continuous ambulatory peritoneal dialysis (CAPD) is a type of therapy that has made home peritoneal dialysis feasible for the client with end-stage renal disease. With this type of dialysis, a permanent catheter is surgically implanted into the peritoneal cavity, and the processes of osmosis and diffusion remove fluid, excess electrolytes, and toxins from the blood. CAPD has the same three phases as acute peritoneal dialysis; however, the time cycle differs. Exchanges during the day are 3 to 6 hours long, and nighttime exchanges last 8 to 12 hours. During the "dwell time" an empty bag and drainage tubing are folded and concealed under the client's clothes (unless a bagless system is used). Afterward, the client drains the abdominal cavity, which is followed by reinstillation of fresh dialysate into the peritoneal cavity. The dialysate must be changed three to five times a day. One major advantage of CAPD is that it allows the client to be out of the hospital, maintain the system at home, and continue with daily activities.

A variation of the CAPD is continuous cyclic peritoneal dialysis (CCPD), which uses a cycler that automates the infusion of the dialysate. CCPD is often used to automate nighttime exchanges for clients in the home or may be used by hospital staff to automate the cycling process. When used for the client at night in the home, this process is referred to as nightly intermittent peritoneal dialysis.

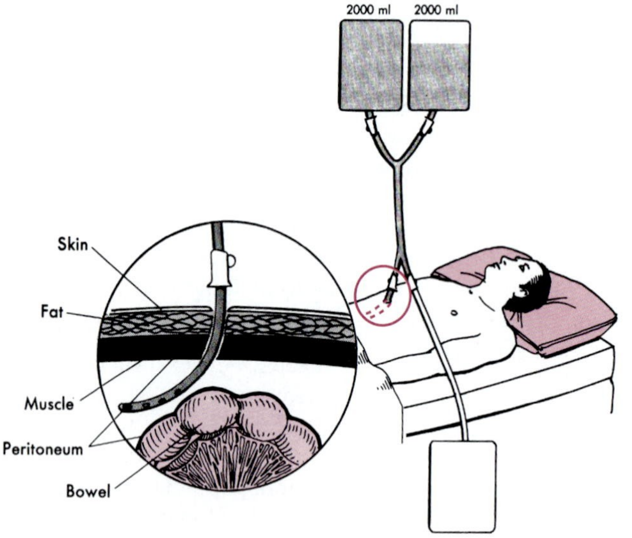

Fig. 25-7 Client receiving peritoneal dialysis. Dialysis fluid is being inserted into peritoneal cavity. (From Phipps WJ, Long BC, Woods NF, Cassmeyer VL: *Medical-surgical nursing,* ed 4, St Louis, 1995, Mosby.)

EQUIPMENT

- Ordered dialysate at 37° C (98° F)
- Sterile on-off pack containing titanium or plastic adapter and catheter cap
- Hydrogen peroxide
- Povidone-iodine solution
- Povidone-iodine ointment
- Mask, sterile gloves, goggles
- IV pole
- Connector tubing (CAPD clients may not need)
- Sterile drainage bag
- IV bag label (IPD only)
- Peritoneal dialysis flow sheet (Fig. 25-8)

DELEGATION CONSIDERATIONS

The skills of peritoneal and continuous ambulatory dialysis require the knowledge and decision making skills unique to a professional nurse and are not delegated to unlicensed assistive personnel.

St. Louis University Medical Center

PERITONEAL DIALYSIS FLOW SHEET

+ = fluid retained by the patient

– = fluid removed from patient in excess of amount instilled

Pre-Dialysis Weight 69.7 Kg

Post-Dialysis Weight 67.5 Kg

DATE	DINEAL 1.5%	DINEAL 2.5%	DINEAL 4.25%	MEDICATION ADDED	SIGNATURE	SOLUTION IN: FILL Start	SOLUTION IN: TIME Finish	SOLUTION IN: 10 MIN Vol	SOLUTION OUT: DRAIN Start	SOLUTION OUT: TIME Finish	SOLUTION OUT: 20 MIN Vol	DIFF (+) OR (–)	CUMULATIVE DIFFERENCE
4/12		✓		HEPAIN 1000 u TOBRA 8mg	Sl	08	0810	2 l	09	0920	2100	–	–100
"		✓		"	Sl	0920	0930	2 l	1030	1050	2200	–	–300
"		✓		"	Sl	1050	1100	2 l	12 N	1220	2300	–	–600
												TOTAL	–1000

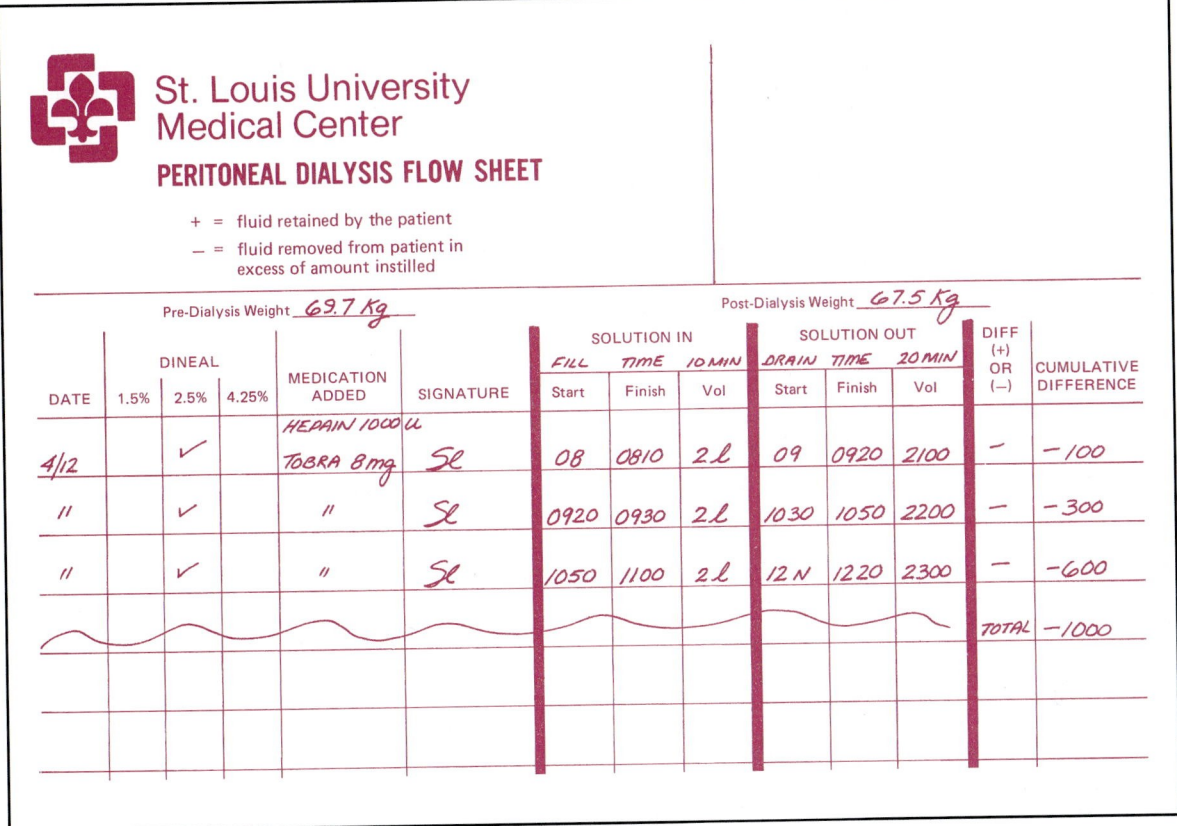

Fig. 25-8 Peritoneal dialysis flow sheet. (Courtesy St Louis University Medical Center, St Louis.)

STEPS	RATIONALE
ASSESSMENT	
1. Obtain client's weight.	Provides baseline information about weight attributed to fluid retention. A daily weight gain of 1 kg is equivalent to 1 L of fluid.
2. Obtain vital signs.	Fluid volume changes associated with dialysis increase risk for hemodynamic blood pressure changes. In clients undergoing IPD, increased abdominal pressure may lead to bradycardia subsequent to vagal nerve stimulation (Lancaster, 1995).
3. Assess respiratory rate and auscultate lungs.	Pressure from fluid that is cycled into the peritoneal cavity may cause difficulty with breathing. Fluid volume changes may lead to fluid volume overload.
4. Measure abdominal girth.	Mark midpoint of client's abdomen. Keep mark as reference for future measurements. Provides baseline data regarding amount of fluid in peritoneal cavity.
5. Monitor for fluid and electrolyte balance.	Clients may experience hypervolemia or hypovolemia. Signs of hypervolemia include increased blood pressure, difficulty breathing, edema, and neck vein distention. Signs of hypovolemia include tachycardia, hypotension, poor skin turgor, dry mucous membranes, and cramping in hands and feet (Smith, 1992). With potassium imbalance, either hypokalemia or hyperkalemia may occur. Laboratory work must be performed to monitor for a potassium alteration.
6. Inspect catheter site for erythema, tenderness, drainage, and swelling.	Indicates infection at catheter entry site, which increases risk for peritonitis.

STEPS	RATIONALE
7. Measure body temperature.	Provides baseline data about client's febrile status.
8. Review hospital or dialysis unit's procedure for IPD or CAPD.	There may be institutional variations regarding ordering of supplies; fill, dwell, and drain times; catheter care; and discharge teaching plan.
9. Review physician's orders: a. Verify dialysis solution and any medications added to solution. b. Verify number of exchanges and infusion and dwell and drain times.	IPD and CAPD require specific orders individualized to client's fluid needs and disease process.
10. Obtain laboratory data as ordered: a. IPD: every 12 to 24 hours. b. CAPD: can vary depending on individual needs.	Documents fluid and electrolyte status and changes that occur from IPD or CAPD.
11. Assess client's knowledge regarding the purpose of dialysis.	Reveals need for client instruction.

NURSING DIAGNOSIS

Clustering of defining characteristics from the assessment data may reveal the following nursing diagnoses for clients requiring this skill:

- Altered urinary elimination
- Fluid volume deficit
- Risk for fluid volume deficit
- Fluid volume excess
- Impaired home maintenance management
- Impaired physical mobility
- Knowledge deficit regarding peritoneal dialysis
- Pain
- Risk for infection
- Social isolation
- Urinary retention

Related factors are individualized based on the client's condition or needs.

PLANNING

STEPS	RATIONALE
1. **Expected outcomes** following completion of procedure:	
➤ Decreased weight.	Indicates that excess fluid was removed. Indicates that more dialysate was removed than was instilled.
➤ Stable vital signs.	Indicates that there are no adverse hemodynamic responses.
➤ Decreased abdominal girth.	Indicates that no fluid was retained in peritoneal cavity.
➤ No erythema, tenderness, or drainage at catheter site.	Indicates absence of local inflammation at catheter site.
➤ No fever.	Indicates that no systemic infection is present.
➤ Dialysate return is clear or slightly light yellow.	Expected color of returned fluid; indicates absence of blood or bacteria in peritoneal cavity.
➤ Client is able to discuss principles of asepsis and peritoneal dialysis.	Discussing principles allows nurse to document cognitive learning.
➤ Client or caregiver will perform CAPD.	Demonstration is an effective measure to evaluate psychomotor learning.
2. Explain procedure to client.	Assists in reducing anxiety and promoting cooperation.

IMPLEMENTATION

STEPS	RATIONALE
1. Wash hands and put on mask.	Reduces transmission of microorganisms.
CRITICAL DECISION POINT **Client and nurse must wear masks.**	
2. Place client in semi-Fowler's or high Fowler's position.	Instilling fluid into peritoneal cavity decreases diaphragmatic excursion. The semi-Fowler's or high Fowler's position promotes optimal lung expansion.

STEPS	RATIONALE
3. Add medications aseptically immediately before beginning instillation of dialysate. Disinfect multiple dose vials and injection ports of plastic bags. Label and record all medications added (Lancaster, 1995).	
CRITICAL DECISION POINT **Maintain strict asepsis when adding medications to dialysate.**	
a. Heparin	Reduces accumulation of fibrin around catheter tip.
b. Prophylactic antibiotics	Reduces risk of peritonitis.
c. Insulin	Regular insulin is added to control serum glucose (Lancaster, 1995).
4. Attach two warmed dialysate bags to inflow tubing and attach to IV pole. Bags are punctured exactly as IV solution bags (see Chapter 20) or with special spiking devices.	Dialysate is warmed by dry heat through the use of warming pad, incubator, or microwave warming device. Hanging two bags promotes timely, organized follow-up exchanges. Standard IPD usually includes 24 exchanges in 24 hours. CAPD clients are instructed to hang only one bag because these clients have three to five exchanges daily.
CRITICAL DECISION POINT **Immersing dialysate in warm water is not recommended because of the chance of contamination (Lancaster, 1995; Armstrong and Zalatan, 1992). Dialysate that is too cold results in intolerance, cramps, and hypothermia.**	
5. Apply sterile gloves.	
6. Disinfect catheter cap and end of catheter; remove cap and disinfect adapter. Connect tubing, maintaining asepsis.	
a. With the CAPD system a Y connector that attaches on one side to the dialysate and the other side to the drainage bag may be used. The Y connector is attached aseptically.	This connection allows for flushing about 100 ml of dialysate into the drainage bag and then draining dialysate from the peritoneum. Research has shown this procedure, called the "flush before fill," to be effective in reducing the incidence of peritonitis (Lancaster, 1995).
7. Open clamp on first dialysate bag and clamp on client line. Infuse solution over prescribed time (usually 2 L/10-15 minutes).	Permits instillation of dialysate into peritoneal cavity.
8. Clamp inflow tubing for prescribed dwell time:	
a. IPD: usually 30 minutes.	
b. CAPD: 3 to 5 hours (CAPD client folds tubing and infusion bag on abdomen, which is concealed by clothing, and uses same bag and tubing for drain cycle).	Prevents air from entering peritoneal cavity. Dwell time permits peritoneal membrane to exchange fluid, electrolytes, toxins from blood.
CRITICAL DECISION POINT **CAPD clients have increased abdominal girth during dwell time of exchange process.**	
CRITICAL DECISION POINT **Monitor infusion and dwell time carefully. A timer may be used to remind the nurse of the scheduled interval for each phase.**	
9. Remove first dialysate bag from IV pole. Place third warmed bag on pole.	Promotes organized procedure. When multiple exchanges are ordered, nurse should have two dialysate bags on IV pole.

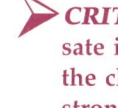

STEPS	RATIONALE
10. Unclamp outflow tubing and drain (usually for 20 minutes).	Permits drainage of dialysate and wastes from peritoneal cavity. During first two or three exchanges, it is common for dialysate to remain in cavity; excess should drain with later exchanges.
➤ ***CRITICAL DECISION POINT*** **Evaluate drainage for clarity and color.**	
11. Clamp outflow tubing.	Prevents untimed drain during subsequent exchange.
12. Empty and measure fluid in drainage bag.	Provides assessment of fluid balance of dialysate solution. If volume of fluid infused is more than amount drained, balance is positive (e.g., if 2000 ml of dialysate was infused and 1800 ml was drained, balance is positive 200 ml [+200 ml], meaning the client is retaining the fluid.)
➤ ***CRITICAL DECISION POINT*** **Wear gloves, mask, eye protection (or face shield), and gown when emptying because splashes may occur. Remove contaminated items. Wash hands.**	
13. Repeat steps until all exchanges are complete.	
14. During first exchanges, monitor client's vital signs every 15 minutes.	Promotes timely documentation of hemodynamic effects of IPD.
15. When all exchanges are complete:	
a. Acute use catheter (short-term use) Disinfect, disconnect connections, and discard tubing. Disinfect catheter rim and securely place sterile cap on end.	
b. Chronic use catheter (long-term use) See guidelines made specifically for catheter.	Maintains patency of catheter insertion site.
16. Inspect catheter site; if dressing is reapplied, apply a clear transparent occlusive dressing (see Skill 37-4).	Intact, dry dressing reduces risk of infection.
17. Wash hands and dispose of contaminated supplies according to agency policy.	Reduces transmission of microorganisms and blood-borne pathogens.

EVALUATION

1. Obtain weight.	Decrease indicates removal of excess fluid; increase indicates retention of fluid.
2. Obtain dialysis fluid balance measurements.	Determines adequacy of fluid removal.
3. Obtain vital signs.	Documents tolerance to IPD.
4. Obtain body temperature.	Denotes presence or absence of infection.
5. Measure abdominal girth.	Provides an indirect measurement of fluid retention in peritoneal cavity.
6. Inspect catheter site for erythema, tenderness, drainage, and swelling.	Documents symptoms of infection.
7. Auscultate lungs for crackles.	Provides a measurement of fluid overload. As intravascular fluid increases, crackles are auscultated in bases of lungs.
8. Inspect returned dialysate solution.	Notes blood, fecal contents, and urine.
9. Observe client performing CAPD.	Documents learning of skill.
10. Assess client's comfort level.	Clients may have incisional pain after access insertion. Clients undergoing peritoneal dialysis may also describe a feeling of fullness following instillation of a large volume of dialysate in the abdominal cavity.
11. Monitor laboratory work.	Imbalances in potassium may occur. A relative increase or decrease in hematocrit may indicate hypovolemia or hypervolemia, respectively.

STEPS	RATIONALE
12. **Unexpected outcomes** that may occur include:	
➤ Increased weight or no weight change.	Indicates fluid retained in peritoneal cavity.
➤ Positive fluid balance.	Indicates excess fluid retained (e.g., total of twelve 2 L [24,000 ml] exchanges instilled; total output: 20 L; 4 L [+4000 ml] remains in peritoneal cavity).
➤ Decreased blood pressure and tachycardia.	Client unable to tolerate fluid volume, or catheter may have perforated bowel.
➤ Increased abdominal girth.	Indicates retained fluid.
➤ Erythema, tenderness, and drainage at catheter site.	Indicates local inflammatory response.
➤ Fever.	Indicates systemic infection.
➤ Dialysate drainage is abnormal:	
• Cloudy.	Indicates possible infection.
• Bright red blood.	Indicates perforation of organ or major vessel.
• Brown color or presence of stool.	Indicates perforation of bowel.
➤ Cramps.	Indicates that dialysate is too cold, infusion is too rapid, volume is too much for client to tolerate, or electrolyte imbalances have occurred.
➤ Sudden respiratory distress.	Indicates that volume is too excessive for client to tolerate.
➤ Poor instillation flow.	Indicates kink in inflow tubing or catheter.
➤ Poor drainage.	Indicates kink or fibrin clot in outflow tubing or catheter.
➤ Leaking of dialysate from peritoneum.	Look for edema in abdominal wall, perineum, or penis (Lancaster, 1995).
➤ Leak at catheter site.	Indicates catheter displacement toward abdominal surface.

Recording and Reporting

1. Document client's weight, abdominal girth, and dialysis fluid balance before and after IPD.	Notes presence or absence of retained fluid in peritoneal cavity.
2. Document client's vital signs and respiratory status before, during, and after dialysis.	Notes hemodynamic response.
3. Document client's temperature and status of catheter site.	Notes presence or absence of local or systemic infection.
4. Record presence of pain or discomfort.	Identify location, quality, and duration of pain. Report pain that is severe or unexpected.
5. Record color of dialysate drainage.	Notes abnormalities in drainage color.
6. Record condition of catheter dressing or if new dressing is applied.	Records status of dressing's condition and most recent dressing change.
7. Note any unexpected outcomes and actions taken by nurse and physician.	Records continuing care of client and possible future complications.

Follow-up Activities

1. Report to physician if the following occur (physician may remove catheter):
   a. Signs of local infection
   b. Catheter displacement (verified by abdominal x-ray film)
2. Stop dialysis and/or notify physician for:
   a. Change in vital signs
   b. Respiratory distress
   c. Bright red blood in dialysate drainage
   d. Fecal contents in dialysate drainage
   e. Scrotal swelling
   f. Complaints of cramps not related to instillation of cold fluid
   g. Leak of dialysate fluid
   h. Inability to drain dialysate fluid from catheter

STEPS **RATIONALE**

3. Follow-up appointment for renal clinic for CAPD client.
4. Renal dietitian consultation.
5. Laboratory data as ordered by physician to determine the efficacy of treatment.

• • • • •

Special Considerations

- Catheter insertion is a physician responsibility. Insertion of acute-use catheters may be performed at the bedside. The chronic CAPD catheter is surgically placed in the operating room. The nurse may assist in the insertion of an acute catheter by obtaining supplies, positioning the client, starting dialysis after insertion, maintaining surgical asepsis, and observing Standard Precautions.
- Centers for Disease Control and Prevention (CDC) recommendations require proper disposal of IPD fluid.
- Changes in blood pressure and increased respiratory rate may signal intolerance to the amount of fluid instilled into the peritoneal cavity.
- Client receiving IPD should be encouraged to move around in bed. However, movements should avoid stressing catheter or tubing.
- Individual hospitals have individual flow sheets to record IPD fluids (Fig. 25-9, p. 821).
- Peritoneal dialysis solutions are available in four dextrose concentrations (1.5%, 2.5%, 3.5%, and 4.25%), each with increasing osmolality to enhance fluid removal by osmosis.
- If the client is losing fluid weight, a negative balance is achieved. A positive balance means the client is *retaining* instilled fluid.

Teaching Considerations

- Teach scrub and exchange procedures to CAPD clients according to policy.
- Instruct client about the common symptoms of fluid excess and deficit.
- Review teaching plan with client before discharge and during each clinic visit.
- Ask client to correctly demonstrate scrub and exchange procedure.
- Periodically review potential complications and signs and symptoms.
- Review medications and dietary and fluid restrictions.
- Instruct client when and whom to contact in emergency.
- Instruct client to take blood pressure correctly.
- Instruct client to weigh self correctly.
- Instruct client about common symptoms associated with peritonitis.

Gerontologic Considerations

- A major risk factor for death with CAPD is age greater than 65 years (Lancaster, 1995).
- The older adult client may be at risk for malnutrition related to loss of protein during dialysis, dietary restrictions, and loss of appetite.
- Clients on dialysis often suffer many complications; older adults are no exception. However, the older adult client may be taking medications for other chronic health problems. Monitoring and assessment of medication therapy are ongoing.

Home Care Considerations

- CAPD clients must do the following correctly to complete CAPD exchanges:
  - Achieve expected outcomes under Planning.
  - Demonstrate CAPD scrub and aseptic exchange procedure.
  - State signs of infection.
  - Adhere to fluid, dietary, and medication therapies.
  - Perform activities of daily living. CAPD is designed so client can maintain normal daily activities.
- The training interval for client undergoing CAPD is individualized to the client and family.

CRITICAL THINKING EXERCISES

1. Four hours after the removal of an indwelling catheter (at 2 PM), a client states that her bladder feels full. She says she has only minimal incisional discomfort (1 on a pain scale of 1 to 5). Two days earlier, she had undergone open cholecystectomy. The I&O was balanced in the first 24 hours postoperatively. She is not receiving IV fluids and has had 1000 ml of oral intake today. At 10 AM when the Foley catheter was removed, there was 400 ml in the bag. She has a dressing on the upper right abdomen and no drainage tubes. What assessments would you make to determine bladder status? What interventions would you implement to enhance urination?
2. You are making an initial shift assessment of a client who is undergoing continuous bladder irrigation after prostate surgery. What assessments tell you that the drip rate is adequate? What assessments tell you that the drip rate needs to be increased?
3. You are making a home visit to a client who has a condom catheter in place. His wife, who is the care giver, tells you that he was complaining of pain and discomfort around the penis after she reapplied the catheter this morning. What problems might cause this pain and discomfort? What assessments of the client do you need to make to determine the cause? If the catheter was applied incorrectly by the wife, what steps can be taken to ensure that she understands how to perform the procedure?

REFERENCES

Armstrong S, Zalatan S: Microwave warming of peritoneal dialysis fluid, *ANNA J* 19(6):535, 1992.

Beare P, Myers J: *Adult health nursing,* ed 2, St Louis, 1994, Mosby.

Garner J: Guidelines for isolation precautions in hospitals, *Infect Control Hosp Epidemiol* 17(1):51, 1996.

Gray M: *Genitourinary disorders,* St Louis, 1992, Mosby.

Lancaster L: *ANNA: curriculum for nephrology nursing,* ed 3, Pitman, N.J., 1995, Anthony J. Janetti.

Latham L: When spinal cord injury complicates med/surg care, *RN* 57(8):26, 1994.

McCormick K, et al: Urinary incontinence in adults, *Am J Nurs* 92(10):75, 1992.

Pearson B, Larson J: Urine control by elders: noninvasive strategies. In Funk E, et al, editors: *Key aspects of elder care: managing falls, incontinence, and cognitive impairment,* New York, 1992, Springer, pp 154-168.

Potter P, Perry A: *Fundamentals of nursing:* ed 4, St Louis, 1997, Mosby.

Skidmore-Roth L: *Mosby's 1994 nursing drug reference,* St Louis, 1994, Mosby.

Smith D: Devices for continence, *Nurse Pract Forum* 5(3):186, 1994.

Smith L: Peritoneal dialysis the critically ill patient, *AACN Clin Issues Crit Care Nurs* 3(3):558, 1992.

Williams M, Wallhagen M, Dowling G: Urinary retention in hospitalized elderly women, *J Gerontol Women* 19(2):7, 1993.

Urinary Incontinence Guideline Panel: *Urinary incontinence in adults: clinical practice guidelines,* AHCPR Pub. No. 92-0038. Rockville, Md., March 1992, Agency for Health Care Policy and Research, Public Health Services, U.S. Department of Health and Human Services.

ADDITIONAL READING

Brunier G, McKeever P: The impact of home dialysis on the family: literature review, *ANNA J* 20(6):653, 1993.

Doughty B: *Urinary and fecal incontinence: nursing management,* St Louis, 1991, Mosby.

Horne M, Swearingen P: *Fluids, electrolytes and acid-base balance,* St Louis, 1993, Mosby.

McDowell J: Care of urinary incontinence in the home, *Nurse Pract Forum* 5(3):138, 1994.

Penn C, et al: Assessment of urinary incontinence, *J Gerontol Nurs* 22(1):8, 1996.

Stokes R: Teaching during dialysis, *ANNA J* 4:407, 1991.

Urinary Incontinence Guideline Panel: *Urinary incontinence in adults: Quick reference guide for clinicians,* AHCPR Pub. No. 92-0041. Rockville, Md., March 1992, Agency for Health Care Policy and Research, Public Health Services, U.S. Department of Health and Human Services.

CHAPTER 26

Bowel Elimination

OBJECTIVES

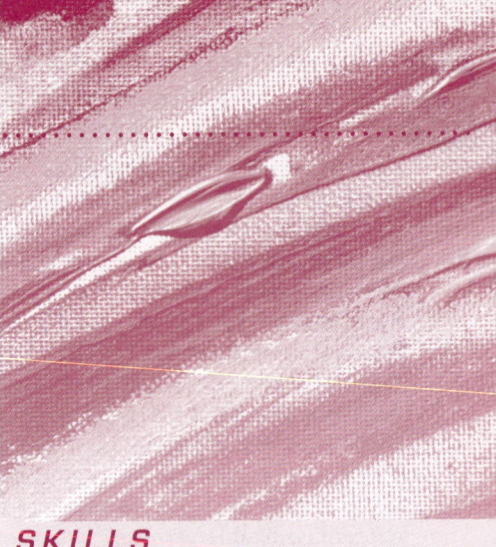

Mastery of content in this chapter will enable the nurse to:

- Define key terms.
- Describe factors that impede normal bowel elimination.
- Discuss methods to relieve constipation or impaction.
- Implement the following skills: assist client to use a bedpan, insert a rectal tube, digitally remove stool, administer an enema.

KEY TERMS

Carminative
Cathartic
Cleansing enema
Colon
Constipation
Defecation
Enema
Flatulence
Hemorrhoids
Impaction
Medicated enema
Occult blood
Oil-retention enema
Rectal tube
Rectum

SKILLS

26-1 Assisting the Client to Use a Bedpan
26-2 Inserting a Rectal Tube
26-3 Removing Fecal Impaction Digitally
26-4 Administering an Enema

The act of defecating is a normal body process essential to eliminate wastes from the body. People develop their own normal elimination patterns. However, these patterns might be disturbed by physiological and psychological factors. When ill at home or in a health care setting, people may not be able to maintain normal elimination habits and therefore might require a nurse's assistance to help with this body process.

To assist clients with bowel elimination, the nurse must have a clear understanding of normal elimination and factors that contribute to alterations. The nurse must be able to assist immobilized clients with the elimination process by helping them on and off bedpans. Often a nurse may be responsible for collecting stool specimens and ensuring that they are properly handled. If a client is constipated, the nurse may be expected to competently administer enemas or to digitally remove impacted stool. While completing any of these skills, the nurse must always show respect for a client's privacy and emotional needs.

GUIDELINES

1. Determine a client's normal pattern of bowel elimination and try to accommodate that pattern while the client is in a health care setting. Determine the time the client normally has a bowel movement and the amount of assistance needed.
2. Provide privacy and try to reduce the client's embarrassment. If possible, the client should be encouraged to use the bathroom. However, if the nature of the illness limits physical activity, ensure as much privacy as possible during use of the bedpan or bedside commode. Pull the curtains around the bed or close the door to the room.
3. Be aware of foods that promote normal peristaltic movement, including high-fiber foods such as raw fruit, whole grains, and green leafy vegetables, which are consistent with the client's prescribed diet. Immobilized clients should receive foods that promote peristalsis but not those that adversely affect bowel routine.

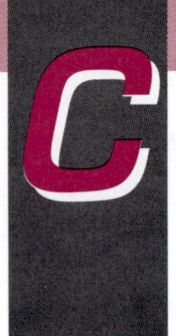

4. Unless contraindicated, encourage adequate hydration. Normally, a person should drink 6 to 8 glasses of water per day. Warm fluids are especially effective in increasing peristalsis.
5. Encourage clients to be as active as physically possible. Physical activity promotes peristalsis, whereas immobilization decreases it.
6. Promote client comfort. The client must be in a comfortable position to defecate.
7. Be aware of the side effects of medications the client is receiving. Some drugs may impair the normal elimination pattern by causing diarrhea or constipation (Tedesco, 1985). Also, general anesthetic agents used during surgery cause temporary cessation of peristalsis, which can affect the normal elimination pattern after surgery.
8. Consider the developmental changes that affect bowel functioning throughout the life span. For example, an elderly person might become less active, muscle tone might be decreased, and eating patterns might change. These factors could result in constipation.

SKILL 26-1 Assisting the Client to use a Bedpan

A client restricted to bed must use a bedpan for defecation. Women use bedpans to pass urine and feces, whereas men use bedpans only for defecation. Sitting on a bedpan can be extremely uncomfortable. The nurse should help the client assume a position similar to the natural squatting position.

Two types of bedpans are available (Fig. 26-1). The regular bedpan, made of metal or hard plastic, has a curved, smooth upper end and a tapered lower end. The pan is approximately 5 cm (2 inches) deep. A fracture pan, designed for clients with body or leg casts, has a shallow upper end approximately 1.3 cm (½ inch) deep that slips easily under a client. The upper end of either pan fits under the client's buttocks toward the sacrum, with the lower end just under the upper thighs.

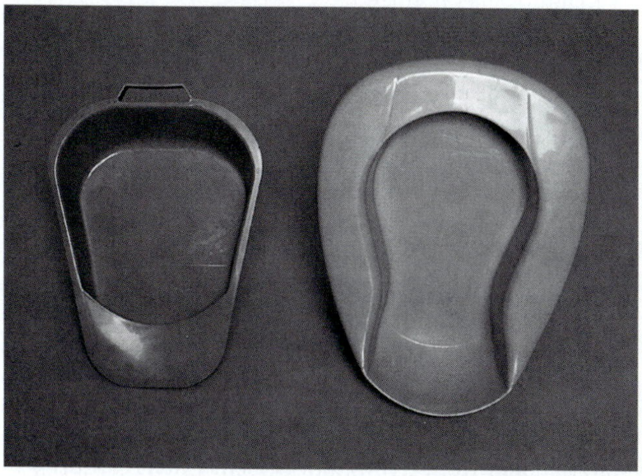

Fig. 26-1 Types of bedpans. *Left,* Fracture bedpan. *Right,* Regular bedpan.

EQUIPMENT

- **Disposable gloves**
- **Appropriate type of clean bedpan**
- **Bedpan cover**
- **Toilet tissue**
- **Specimen container (if necessary), plastic bag, clearly labeled with date, client's name, and identification number**
- **Washbasin, washcloths, towels, soap**
- **Waterproof, absorbent pads**
- **Clean draw sheet (optional)**

DELEGATION CONSIDERATIONS

The skill of assisting a client to use a bedpan can be delegated to unlicensed assistive personnel.

- Inform and assist care provider in proper way to position clients who have mobility restrictions.
- Caution care provider about transmission of pathogens.
- Inform care provider about how to position clients who also have therapeutic equipment present, such as drains, intravenous catheters, or traction.

STEPS	RATIONALE

ASSESSMENT

Steps	Rationale
1. Assess client's normal bowel elimination habits: routine pattern, effect of certain foods and eating habits on bowel elimination, effect of stress on normal bowel elimination patterns, current medications, normal fluid intake.	Nurse's competence in managing client's elimination problems depends on thorough understanding of normal elimination and factors that may create alterations. Mass peristalsis is strongest during the hour after first meal of the day.
2. Auscultate abdomen for bowel sounds and palpate for abdominal distention.	Normal bowel sounds occur irregularly at the rate of 5 to 35 per minute (Doughty and Jackson, 1993). A fecal-filled colon is palpated as a firm rounded mass. A distended bladder can be palpated as a smooth, round mass above the symphysis pubis (Barkauskas et al., 1994).
3. Assess client to determine level of mobility and amount of assistance required.	Nurse should know how much activity client is allowed. Elderly, obese, debilitated clients may require assistance of two or more nurses to help them onto or off of the bedpan. Assistance from additional personnel promotes safety for client and nurses.
4. Assess if client is allowed to sit up or must lie flat when using bedpan.	Determines most appropriate type of bedpan.
5. Assess for rectal or abdominal pain and hemorrhoids or irritation of skin surrounding anus.	Rectal or abdominal pain can reduce client's ability to bear down during defecation. Unexplained abdominal pain should be assessed by a physician before enema administration.
6. Determine if a stool specimen is needed.	Provides ample opportunity to obtain specimen container before placing the client on the bedpan.

NURSING DIAGNOSIS

Clustering of defining characteristics from the assessment data may reveal the following nursing diagnoses for clients requiring this skill:

- Bowel incontinence
- Constipation
- Diarrhea
- Impaired physical mobility

Related factors are individualized based on a client's condition or needs.

PLANNING

Steps	Rationale
1. **Expected outcomes** following completion of procedure:	
➤ Client is able to successfully defecate in bedpan.	Indicates normal elimination.
➤ Stool is soft and formed.	These are normal characteristics.
➤ Perianal skin is clear and intact.	No irritation has occurred.
➤ Client eliminates without pain.	
2. Explain procedure to client, including self-help tips.	Information promotes client's independence and reduces anxiety.
3. Obtain assistance from additional nursing personnel as warranted.	Adequate personnel resources minimize muscle strain for client and nurse.

IMPLEMENTATION

Steps	Rationale
1. Wash hands and apply gloves.	Reduces transmission of microorganisms.
2. Provide privacy by closing curtains around bed or door of room.	Reduces embarrassment and promotes bowel elimination.
3. Place bedpan under warm, running water for few seconds, then dry. Be careful that pan is not too hot.	Metal bedpans are very cold. Warm pan helps client to relax anal sphincter. Although plastic bedpans may not be as cold to touch as metal, warming them before use is still wise.
4. Put side rail up on opposite side of bed.	Protects client from falling out of bed. Client can use side rail to grasp onto and assist self to move about in bed.
5. Position bed in high level according to nurse's height.	Promotes use of good body mechanics and prevents muscle strain for nurse and client.

STEPS	RATIONALE
6. Ensure that client is positioned properly.	

CRITICAL DECISION POINT **Observe for the presence of drains, dressings, intravenous fluids, traction. These devices may impede a client from assisting with the procedure and may also necessitate more personnel to assist in placing the client on a bedpan.**

STEPS	RATIONALE
a. For client who is mobile in bed and can assist with procedure: Client and bed should bend at corresponding places.	
(1) Raise client's head 60 degrees.	Prevents hyperextension of back and provides support to upper torso when client raises hips. Sitting position promotes defecation.
(2) Remove upper bed linens just enough so they are out of the way, but do not unduly expose client.	Prevents embarrassment to client; demonstrates respect for client's sense of dignity.
(3) Remove bedpan cover and place in accessible location.	
(4) Instruct client to flex knees and lift hips upward.	Little effort should be required of client, whose body weight is supported by lower legs and feet and upper torso and arms.
(5) Place hand closest to the client under client's sacrum to assist lifting. At the same time, use other hand to slip bedpan under client. Be sure open rim of bedpan is facing toward foot of bed. (Or have the client use overhead trapeze frame.)	Nurse must ensure that bedpan is placed high enough under buttocks so feces enters pan. Incorrect placement of bedpan can cause discomfort for client and spillage of contents.
b. For immobile client:	
(1) Position bed in flat or level position.	Assists client for whom it is unsafe to exert effort when lifting hips, who must remain flat, or who is unable to lift hips to roll onto bedpan.
(2) Remove top linens as necessary to turn client while minimizing exposure.	Prevents embarrassment to client; demonstrates respect for client's sense of dignity.
(3) Ask client to roll into side-lying position or turn client into side-lying position. Simultaneously, place bedpan firmly against client's buttocks and down into mattress. Be sure that open rim of bedpan is facing toward foot of bed (see illustration). Client then rolls onto back with bedpan securely positioned under buttocks. The use of a fracture pan requires less maneuvering by the client (see illustration).	Incorrect placement can cause discomfort to client and spillage of contents.

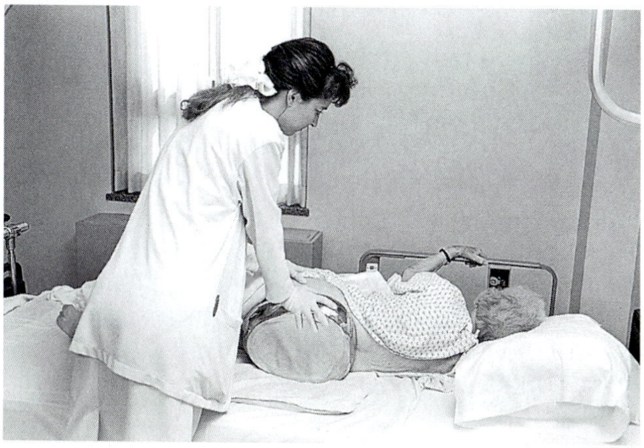

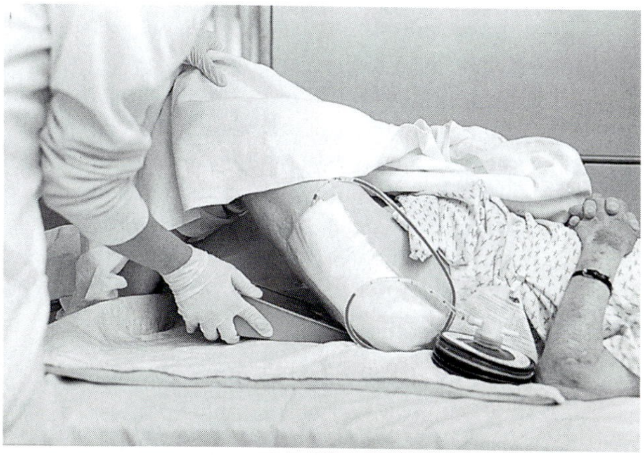

Step 6b(3)

STEPS	RATIONALE
(4) Client's head can then be raised to a comfortable level, unless contraindicated.	Client can assume sitting position unless the condition necessitates maintaining flat position. Sitting position promotes defecation.
7. Ensure that client is comfortable; cover client for warmth. Small pillow or rolled towel placed under lumbar curve of back provides added comfort.	Pain reduces or eliminates urge to defecate, which can result in bowel elimination problems.
8. Ensure that call bell and toilet tissue are within easy reach for client.	Promotes safety by preventing client from reaching over edge of bed for objects out of reach.
9. Ensure that bed is in lowest position and side rails are up.	Promotes client safety.
10. Allow client to be alone, but monitor status and respond promptly to call signal.	Reassures client that nurse has not forgotten. Client may not be able to call nurse; the nurse is responsible for assessing client's status while on bedpan.
11. Remove gloves and wash hands.	Reduces transmission of microorganisms.
12. Position client's bedside chair close to working side of bed. Place bedpan and contents on chair after removal from client.	Adheres to principles of medical asepsis. Prevents spillage that could occur if full bedpan was placed on bed.
13. Collect basin of warm water.	Allows client to wash hands after wiping perineal area (if appropriate); also allows nurse, wearing gloves, to use water to wash client's perineal area if client is unable to wipe thoroughly.
14. Reapply gloves and remove upper linens, minimally exposing client.	Prevents undue embarrassment; maintains privacy.
15. Determine if client is able to wipe own perineal area. If not, using several layers of toilet tissue, wipe from mons pubis toward rectal area (for female client only); dispose of contaminated tissue in bedpan.	Cleansing from area of lesser contamination to greater contamination reduces spread of microorganisms.
16. Remove bedpan.	
a. For mobile, independent client:	
(1) Ask client to flex knees, placing body weight on lower legs, feet, and upper torso; lift buttocks up from bedpan. At same time, place hand farthest from client on side of bedpan to support it (prevent spillage) and place other hand (closest to client) under sacrum to assist in lifting. After client is completely lifted off bedpan, remove pan and place it on bedside chair.	Nurse should avoid pulling or shoving pan from under hips because this action can pull skin and cause tissue injury.
(2) Offer client opportunity to wash hands after having wiped perineal area (if appropriate).	Reduces spread of microorganisms.
b. For immobile client:	
(1) Lower head of bed.	Facilitates turning of client.
(2) Assist client to roll onto side and off bedpan. Hold bedpan steady while client is rolling off it; otherwise spillage will occur. Place bedpan and contents on bedside chair.	
(3) Wipe client's anal area with tissue, depositing contaminated tissue in bedpan. If necessary, wash perineal area with warm, soapy water, drying area thoroughly.	Cleansing from area of lesser contamination to greater contamination reduces spread of microorganisms. Prevents excoriation and skin breakdown. Promotes personal hygiene. This is an excellent time to perform perineal hygiene (Chapter 6).
17. Cover bedpan and contents with bedpan cover as soon as possible.	Reduces spread of offensive odors.

STEPS	RATIONALE
18. Return client to comfortable position, ensuring that bottom linens are clean and as wrinkle-free as possible. Soiled linens must be changed.	Reduces chance of skin breakdown when bedridden client lies on dry, wrinkle-free linens.
19. Position bed in its lowest position. Ensure that call bell, drinking water, and desired personal items (e.g., books) are within easy access.	Promotes comfort and prevents injury to client.
20. If stool specimen is to be obtained, this is appropriate time to collect it. Wearing gloves, empty contents of bedpan into toilet or in special receptacle in appropriate utility room. Spray faucet attached to most institution toilets allows bedpan to be rinsed thoroughly.	This should be done as soon as possible to prevent spread of offensive odor. Client uses same bedpan each time. (If it becomes very soiled, it could be replaced with clean one and soiled one sent for resterilization).
21. Replace all used equipment in appropriate location for subsequent use when required.	
22. Dispose of soiled linens correctly.	Reduces spread of microorganisms.
23. Remove gloves and wash hands.	Reduces spread of microorganisms.

EVALUATION

1. Assess characteristics of stool. Note color, odor, consistency, frequency, amount, shape, and constituents. Also assess characteristics of urine, if client voided in bedpan.	Identifies significant changes or findings, which must be reported to correct member of health care team and recorded on appropriate sheet in client's record.
2. Evaluate client's ability to use bedpan.	Provides continual assessment of ability to use bedpan.
3. Inspect client's perianal area and surrounding skin while removing bedpan.	Liquid stool predisposes client to skin breakdown.
4. Evaluate client's overall activity tolerance and comfort.	Defecation and use of the bedpan can be energy consuming.
5. Unexpected outcomes that may occur include:	
➤ Incontinence.	Frequently caused by client's embarrassment in using bedpan or nursing staff delay in offering bedpan.
➤ Constipation.	Results from pain, dietary habits, immobility, and unnatural position for defecation.
➤ Skin breakdown.	Results from irritation of skin caused by urine or fecal materials.
➤ Blood in stool or black stool.	Important diagnostic finding that requires further testing (see Chapter 43).

RECORDING AND REPORTING

1. Record and report character and amount of stool in nurses' notes. Record urine output if client also voids.	Communicates pertinent information to all members of health care team.
2. Complete laboratory requisition if stool or urine specimen was collected, and send to laboratory.	Proper labeling ensures proper identification of test results.

FOLLOW-UP ACTIVITIES

1. Incontinence:
   a. Offer client bedpan every 2 hours and after meals.
   b. Reassess client's elimination pattern.
   c. Answer call light promptly.
2. Constipation:
   a. Increase fluids unless contraindicated.
   b. Provide fruits, vegetables, grains, if consistent with prescribed diet.
   c. Provide maximum activity.
3. Skin breakdown:
   a. Increase perineal care to every 4 hours and after each bedpan use (Chapter 6).
4. Blood in stool:
   a. Test specimen for occult blood in stool (Chapter 43).
   b. Bright red blood need not be tested but should be reported to appropriate personnel.

• • • • •

Special Considerations

- Barium, used as contrast medium when x-raying bowel, can cause constipation if not evacuated after procedure.
- If client is sharing room, roommates may wish to leave room to provide privacy. Request that visitors leave. Refresh air as needed, provide maximal amount of ventilation.
- Extra assistance may be required to turn totally or partially dependent client.
- Nurse must use correct body mechanics while positioning client to prevent muscle strain on client or self.
- If client has urinated in bedpan, amount of urine may need to be measured.

Teaching Considerations

- Some bedridden clients have overhead trapeze frame connected to bed to help lift themselves on and off bedpan. Teaching this activity can help to maintain strength of client's arms.
- Teach female clients to cleanse from area of lesser contamination to greater contamination (i.e., wiping from front to back). This reduces transmission of anal bacteria to urinary meatus and reduces risk of urinary tract infections.

Gerontologic Considerations

- Incidence of constipation is greater because of changes in the nerves impulses. With aging these impulses may be dulled and as a result the older adult does not perceive the need to defecate.
- Reinforce with older adult clients that as long as the consistency of the stool remains normal and that the bowel movements occur with regularity, they have no reason for concern (Lueckenotte, 1996).
- With increased age transit time through the bowel increases, causing a normal lengthening of the time between bowel movements (Lueckenotte, 1996).

Home Care Considerations

- Assess client and primary care giver to determine ability and motivation to carry out care of client.
- Assess client's environment to determine availability of privacy and adequate time to use bedpan.

SKILL 26-2 Inserting a Rectal Tube

A rectal tube may be used to aid in the relief of abdominal distention secondary to unexpelled flatus. Such distention frequently occurs after abdominal surgery. The tube may remain in place for several minutes to allow flatus to escape.

DELEGATION CONSIDERATIONS

The skill of inserting a rectal tube can be delegated to unlicensed assistive personnel.

- Inform and assist care provider in proper way to position clients who have mobility restrictions.
- Caution care provider about transmission of pathogens.
- Inform care provider regarding when a rectal tube is used and when it is contraindicated, as with rectal surgery.
- Inform care provider about how to correctly place rectal tube and what to expect regarding flatus, drainage from the tube.

EQUIPMENT

- Disposable gloves
- Rectal tube of correct size:
  - Adult: 22 to 26 Fr
  - Infant/child: 10 to 12 Fr
- Collection device for any drainage
- Water-soluble lubricant
- Waterproof, absorbent pad
- Tape (Use the appropriate type on client with a history of allergy to tape.)

STEPS	RATIONALE
ASSESSMENT	
1. Assess client for abdominal distention, amount of flatus client is passing, existing pathological condition related to intestinal disorders, bowel sounds.	Indicate extent of distention and/or status of peristalsis.
2. Check physician's order regarding specific instructions for use of rectal tube.	Depending on institutional policy, might or might not be independent nursing function.

STEPS	RATIONALE

NURSING DIAGNOSIS

Clustering of defining characteristics from the assessment data may reveal the following nursing diagnosis for clients requiring this skill:

➤ Pain

Related factors are individualized based on a client's condition or needs.

PLANNING

STEPS	RATIONALE
1. **Expected outcomes** following completion of procedure:	
➤ Abdomen is flat and soft.	Indicates procedure was effective.
➤ Client states that distention and cramping are relieved.	Indicates relief.
2. Explain procedure to client.	Information promotes client's cooperation with tube's insertion and retention and reduces anxiety.

IMPLEMENTATION

STEPS	RATIONALE
1. Wash hands and apply gloves.	Reduces transmission of microorganisms.
2. Provide privacy by pulling curtains.	Reduces client's embarrassment; helps client to maintain sense of dignity.
3. Raise bed to appropriate working height. Put side rail up on opposite side of bed.	Promotes good use of body mechanics by nurse and client safety.
4. Ask client to turn onto left side and assume side-lying or Sims' position. Assist client as necessary. Keep client draped except for rectal area.	Allows rectal tube to follow natural curve of rectum and sigmoid colon, thus reducing incidence of irritation or injury to rectal mucosa.
5. Place waterproof pad along buttocks.	Prevents soiling bed linens if fecal material leaks from tube.
6. Lubricate tip of rectal tube generously.	Prevents trauma to rectal mucosa and facilitates easier entry into rectum.
7. Take care to expose client minimally. Gently separate buttocks, locate anus, and ask client to take deep breath and slowly exhale through mouth.	Promotes relaxation and maintains client's sense of self-esteem. Slow exhalation helps to relax external rectal sphincter, thereby decreasing discomfort caused by insertion of rectal tube.

➤ ***CRITICAL DECISION POINT*** **Observe anal region for swelling, hemorrhoids, redness, irritation, or drainage. Presence of such findings may contraindicate placement of the rectal tube or indicate the need for other interventions to the perianal skin.**

STEPS	RATIONALE
8. Insert tip of rectal tube slowly, pointing it in direction of umbilicus, ensuring that a pad is in place to collect any drainage. Distance tube can be inserted: *Adult:* 15 cm (6 inches) *Child:* 5 to 10 cm (2 to 4 inches)	Careful insertion prevents trauma to rectal mucosa. Insertion beyond proper limit or forcing tube can result in bowel perforation.

➤ ***CRITICAL DECISION POINT*** **If obstruction or resistance is encountered, *do not continue.* Report finding to appropriate member of health care team.**

STEPS	RATIONALE
9. After inserting tube, tape it to lower buttock.	Prevents dislodging.
10. Allow rectal tube to remain in place for no longer than 30 minutes. Ensure bed is in lowest position. Leave call bell within easy access.	Can cause irritation to rectal mucosa. Call bell promotes client's safety.
11. Remove gloves and wash hands.	Reduces spread of microorganisms.
12. Don gloves and remove rectal tube. Clean client's rectal area. Note characteristics of drainage from rectal tube.	Removes excess lubricant and tape residue.
13. Return client to comfortable position.	Promotes sense of well-being.

STEPS	RATIONALE
14. Dispose of used supplies appropriately, and remove gloves and wash hands.	Reduces spread of microorganisms.

EVALUATION

1. Palpate client's abdomen for firmness and distention. Auscultate bowel sounds.	Determines effectiveness in removing flatus and determines if procedure must be repeated.
2. Ask client if relief was obtained from rectal tube.	Reveals effect of therapy.
3. **Unexpected outcomes** that may occur include:	
➤ Abdomen remains distended with bowel sounds.	Flatus is unrelieved.
➤ Client continues to complain of discomfort.	
➤ Nurse is unable to pass rectal tube.	Possible obstruction because of feces in rectum or unknown pathological condition (Saltzstein et al., 1988).

RECORDING AND REPORTING

1. Record and report physical assessment findings before and after rectal tube insertion.	Communicates data to all members of health care team.

FOLLOW-UP ACTIVITIES

1. Notify physician if rectal tube cannot be placed because of resistance.
2. Assess client for continued passage of flatus after tube removal.
3. Encourage ambulation as allowed.

Special Considerations

- ➤ If this is an independent nursing function, nurse should check institution's procedural manual for guidelines.
- ➤ Because fluid is not being instilled, rectal tube can be advanced farther than when administering enema to reach areas where flatus has accumulated.
- ➤ If flatulence persists, time between insertions should be determined by physician.
- ➤ Do not leave rectal tube in for longer than 30 minutes.

Teaching Considerations

- ➤ The client should be instructed to notify the nurse if pain intensifies before next nursing assessment.

Gerontologic Considerations

- ➤ The presence of excessive abdominal distention related to flatus in the older adult must be taken seriously. The nurse must conduct further assessment to determine if the presence of gas occurs with changes in bowel habits, abdominal pain, or other gastrointestinal tract symptoms (Lueckenotte, 1996).

SKILL 26-3 Removing Fecal Impaction Digitally

When an impaction is present, the fecal mass may be too large or hard to be passed voluntarily. Suppositories and enemas may be ordered to promote evacuation of stool. However, if the enema fails to promote defecation, the nurse must use a finger to break up and remove the fecal mass. This procedure can be very uncomfortable and embarrassing for the client. Excessive rectal manipulation may cause irritation to the mucosa, bleeding, and stimulation of the vagus nerve, which can cause a reflex slowing of the heart rate. Either constipation or diarrhea can suggest the presence of an impaction (Wright and Staats, 1986).

EQUIPMENT

- Disposable gloves
- Water-soluble lubricant
- Waterproof, absorbent pads
- Bedpan
- Bedpan cover
- Bath blanket
- Washbasin, washcloths, towels, and soap

DELEGATION CONSIDERATIONS

This skill requires problem solving and knowledge unique to a professional nurse. Delegation of this skill is inappropriate.

STEPS	RATIONALE

ASSESSMENT

STEPS	RATIONALE
1. Assess client to determine:	
a. Last bowel movement.	Infrequent defecation increases chances of hard stool forming in rectum.
b. Consistency of stool, seepage of liquid stool. This situation may occur particularly in immobilized client. Client seems to continually or frequently be incontinent of liquid stool.	Symptomatic of an impaction high in colon. Client may be able to pass small pieces of hard stool or have episodes of passing small amounts of liquid stool (Mager-O'Connor, 1984).
c. Expression of desire to defecate but inability to do so.	Large fecal mass causes rectal distention.
d. Complaints of pain when trying to defecate.	Pain often suppresses urge to defecate and compounds problem.
e. Normal bowel patterns, eating habits, exercise pattern or level of mobility, medications, especially narcotic analgesics.	Nurse must determine if these are contributing factors and attempt to include nursing actions in care plan that may help to prevent situation from recurring.
f. Client's normal vital signs.	Vagus nerve stimulation during digital stimulation may result in reflex slowing of heart rate.

➤ **CRITICAL DECISION POINT** **Clients with a history of dysrhythmia or heart disease have a greater risk of changes in heart rhythm. Be sure to monitor client's pulse before and during procedure. This procedure may be contraindicated in cardiac clients; if in doubt verify with physician.**

STEPS	RATIONALE
g. Bowel sounds and abdominal distention.	Indicates presence of peristalsis but does not conclusively confirm gastrointestinal patency. Distention can contribute to constipation.
2. Check client's record to determine if physician's order exists to remove stool manually.	Because this procedure may involve excessive stimulation of vagus nerve, physician's order must be written in client's record before nurse can perform procedure.

NURSING DIAGNOSIS

Clustering of defining characteristics from the assessment data may reveal the following nursing diagnoses for clients requiring this skill:

- ➤ Constipation
- ➤ Diarrhea
- ➤ Pain

Related factors are individualized based on a client's condition or needs.

PLANNING

STEPS	RATIONALE
1. Expected outcomes following completion of procedure:	
➤ Impacted stool is successfully removed.	Indicates rectum is clear of stool.
➤ Client is able to subsequently defecate voluntarily.	Removal of impacted stool should result in normal defecation.
➤ Client is free of abdominal or rectal discomfort.	Fecal impaction causes direct pain to rectum and indirect abdominal discomfort through abdominal distention.
➤ Vital signs remain normal.	Indicates absence of vagal stimulation.
2. Explain procedure to client.	Information reduces anxiety and encourages client participation in a therapeutic elimination protocol.

IMPLEMENTATION

STEPS	RATIONALE
1. Wash hands and apply gloves.	Prevents transmission of microorganisms.
2. Obtain assistance to help change client's position, if necessary:	Promotes client safety and use of good body mechanics by nurse.
a. Assist client to left side-lying position with knees flexed.	Provides access to rectum.

STEPS	RATIONALE
3. Provide for privacy: pull curtains around bed or close door to room, drape bath blanket over client so client is minimally exposed.	Maintains client's dignity.
4. Raise bed to comfortable working height. Put side rail up on opposite side of bed.	Incorporates good body mechanics; promotes client's safety.
5. Drape client's trunk and lower extremities with bath blanket.	Prevents unnecessary exposure of body parts.
6. Place waterproof pad under buttocks.	Prevents soiling of bed linen.
7. Place bedpan next to client.	Bedpan is receptacle for stool.
8. Lubricate gloved index finger with lubricating jelly.	Permits smooth insertion of finger into anus and rectum.
CRITICAL DECISION POINT **Observe for the presence of perianal skin irritation. Presence of such indicates the need for postprocedure skin care to the perianal region to reduce pain during subsequent bowel elimination.**	
9. Insert index finger into rectum and advance finger slowly along rectal wall toward umbilicus.	Allows nurse to reach impacted stool high in rectum.
10. Gently loosen fecal mass by massaging around it. Work finger into hardened mass.	Loosening and penetrating mass allows nurse to remove it in small pieces, resulting in less discomfort to client.
11. Work stool downward toward end of rectum. Remove small sections of feces.	Prevents need to force finger up into rectum and minimizes trauma to mucosa.
12. Periodically assess heart rate and look for signs of fatigue.	Vagal stimulation slows heart rate and may cause dysrhythmia. Procedure may exhaust client.
CRITICAL DECISION POINT **Stop procedure if heart rate drops or rhythm changes.**	
13. Continue to clear rectum of feces and allow client to rest at intervals.	Rest improves client's tolerance of procedure.
14. After removal of impaction, provide washcloth and towel to wash buttocks and anal area.	Promotes client's sense of comfort and cleanliness.
15. Remove bedpan and dispose of feces. Remove gloves by turning inside out and discarding in proper receptacle.	Reduces transmission of microorganisms.
16. Assist client to toilet or clean bedpan. (Procedure may be followed by enema or cathartic.)	Disimpaction may stimulate defecation reflex.
17. Wash hands.	Reduces transmission of microorganisms.

EVALUATION

1. Perform rectal examination for stool.	Determines if rectum is clear.
2. Reassess vital signs and compare to baseline values.	Determines extent of vagal stimulation.
3. Assess bowel sounds.	Determines peristaltic activity.
4. Palpate abdomen to determine if it is soft and nontender.	Discomfort is relieved.
5. **Unexpected outcomes** that may occur include:	
➤ Seepage of liquid fecal material occurs.	Indicates continued presence of hard fecal material high in rectum.
➤ Client experiences bradycardia, decreased blood pressure, decreased level of consciousness.	Vagal stimulation can decrease heart rate, which lowers blood pressure and cardiac output, resulting in decreased level of consciousness.
➤ Presence of blood on gloved finger or in stool.	May result from trauma to rectal mucosa.

RECORDING AND REPORTING

1. Record and report client's tolerance to procedure, amount and consistency of stool removed, and adverse effects.	Communicates relevant data to all members of health care team.

Follow-up Activities

1. In case of seepage of liquid stool:
   a. Contact physician before proceeding to cleansing enema and cathartics.
   b. Increase intake of oral and, if needed, parenteral fluids; increase bulk in diet; increase activity.
2. Monitor the client for 1 hour, assessing for decreased blood pressure or level of consciousness. If client experiences either of these, immediately notify the physician and institute appropriate actions.

• • • • •

Special Considerations

- Some institutions allow only the physician to perform this procedure. Check policy manuals.
- Physician may order oil-retention enema several hours before this procedure to soften stool for easier extraction (Skill 26-4).
- Physician may order analgesic to be administered before procedure.
- Physician may order procedure to be followed by administration of cleansing enema or cathartics.

Teaching Considerations

- If constipation and subsequent impaction are diet related, teach client about high-fiber nutritional products to increase bulk and the need for adequate fluid intake.
- If necessary, teach ancillary care givers about the effects of immobility, hydration, and nutrition on normal bowel elimination.

Gerontologic Considerations

- Many older adult clients are especially prone to dysrhythmia and other problems related to vagal stimulation; monitor heart rate and rhythm closely.
- At least 28% of elderly clients are constipated as a result of insufficient dietary bulk, inadequate fluid intake, laxative abuse, diminished muscle tone and motor function, decreased defecation reflex, mental or physical illness, and presence of tumors or structures (Ebersole and Hess, 1994).
- For the elderly, instituting a diet adequate in dietary fiber (6 to 10 grams per day) adds bulk, weight, and form to stool and improves defecation (Ebersole and Hess, 1994).
- Consider development of a regular toileting routine that includes responding to the urge to defecate (Lueckenotte, 1996).

SKILL 26-4 Administering an Enema

An enema is the instillation of a solution into the rectum and sigmoid colon. Cleansing enemas promote complete evacuation of feces from the colon. They act by stimulating peristalsis through infusion of large volumes of solution. Oil-retention enemas act by lubricating the rectum and colon. Feces absorb oil and become softer and easier to pass. Medicated enemas contain pharmacological therapeutic agents and may be prescribed to reduce dangerously high serum potassium levels, as with use of a sodium polystyrene sulfonate *(Kayexalate)* enema, or to reduce bacteria in the colon before bowel surgery, as with use of a neomycin enema.

The primary reason for an enema is promotion of defecation. The fluid, depending on volume and type, breaks up the fecal mass, stretches the rectal wall, and initiates the defecation reflex. Clients should not rely on enemas to maintain bowel regularity because enemas do not treat the cause of irregularity or constipation. Frequent enemas disrupt normal defecation reflexes, resulting in dependence on enemas for elimination (Clarke, 1989). Types of enemas:

- *Tap water (hypotonic)* enema should not be repeated after first installation because water toxicity or circulatory overload can develop.
- *Physiologic normal saline* is safest. Infants and children can tolerate only this type because of their predisposition to fluid imbalance. If solution is prepared at home, mix 500 ml (1 pint) of tap water with 1 teaspoon table salt.
- *Hypertonic solution* is useful for clients who cannot tolerate large volumes of fluid. Only 120 to 180 ml (4 to 6 ounces) is usually effective (e.g., commercially prepared *Fleets* enema).
- *Soapsuds solution* is pure soap added to either tap water or normal saline, depending on client's condition and frequency of administration. Use only Castile pure soap. Recommended ratio of pure soap to solution is 5 ml (1 teaspoon) to 1000 ml (1 quart) warm water or saline. Soap should be added to enema bag after water is in place.
- *Oil retention* enema uses an oil-based solution. Permits administration of a small volume, which is absorbed by the stool. The absorption of the oil softens stool for easier evacuation.
- *Carminative* solution provides relief from gaseous distention. An example is MGW solution, which contains 30 ml of magnesium, 60 ml of glycerin, and 90 ml of water.

EQUIPMENT

Enema bag administration

- Disposable gloves
- Enema container (Fig. 26-2)
- Tubing and clamp (if not already attached to container)
- Appropriate size rectal tube:
  Adult: 22 to 30 Fr
  Child: 12 to 18 Fr
- Correct volume of warmed solution:
  Adult: 750 to 1000 ml
  Child:
  150 to 250 ml, infant
  250 to 350 ml, toddler
  300 to 500 ml, school-age child
  500 to 700 ml, adolescent
- Water-soluble lubricant
- Waterproof, absorbent pads
- Bath blanket
- Toilet tissue
- Bedpan, bedside commode, or access to toilet
- Wash basin, washcloths, towel, and soap
- IV pole

Prepackaged enema

- Disposable gloves
- Prepackaged enema container with rectal tip (Fig. 26-3)
- Water-soluble lubricant
- Waterproof, absorbent pads
- Bath blanket
- Toilet paper
- Bedpan, bedside commode, or access to toilet
- Washbasin, washcloths, towel, and soap

DELEGATION CONSIDERATIONS

The skill of administering an enema can be delegated to unlicensed assistive personnel.

- Inform and assist care provider in proper way to position clients who have mobility restrictions.
- Caution care provider about transmission of pathogens.
- Inform care provider about how to position clients who also have therapeutic equipment present, such as drains, intravenous catheters, or traction.
- Inform care provider regarding signs and symptoms of client not tolerating the procedure, and when it must be stopped.

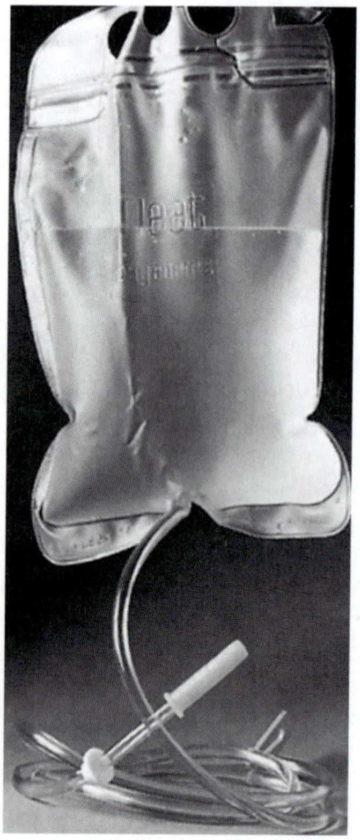

Fig. 26-2 High-volume enema bag with tubing.

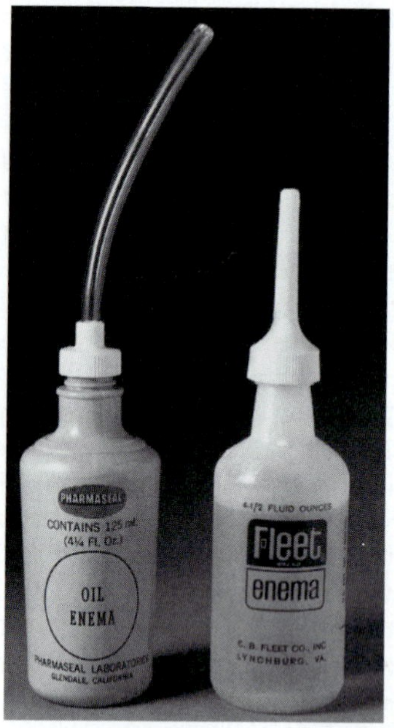

Fig. 26-3 Prepackaged enema container with rectal tip(s).

STEPS	RATIONALE

ASSESSMENT

STEPS	RATIONALE
1. Assess status of client: last bowel movement, level of awareness/developmental stage (so nurse can incorporate appropriate teaching instructions), normal bowel patterns, hemorrhoids, mobility, external sphincter control, abdominal pain (Davis, 1986).	Determines factors indicating need for enema and influencing the type of enema used. Particular care must be taken when inserting rectal tube to reduce irritation of hemorrhoidal tissues; use generous amount of lubricating jelly to reduce friction when passing rectal tube.
2. Determine client's level of understanding of purpose of enema.	Allows nurse to plan for appropriate teaching measures.
3. Check client's medical record to clarify the rationale for the enema.	Determines purpose of enema administration: preparation for special procedure or relief of constipation.
4. Review physician's order for enema.	Order by physician is usually required for hospitalized client. Used to determine how many enemas client will require, type of enema to be given (e.g., oil retention, carminative, medicated).

NURSING DIAGNOSIS

Clustering of defining characteristics from the assessment data may reveal the following nursing diagnoses for clients requiring this skill:

- Constipation
- Pain

Related factors are individualized based on a client's condition or needs.

PLANNING

STEPS	RATIONALE
1. **Expected outcomes** following completion of procedure:	
➤ Stool is evacuated.	Solution clears rectum and lower colon of stool.
➤ Enema return is clear.	All feces in colon have passed.
➤ Abdominal distention is absent.	Gas and feces have been expelled.
➤ Client's discomfort is relieved.	
2. Explain procedure to client.	Information promotes client cooperation and reduces anxiety.

IMPLEMENTATION

STEPS	RATIONALE
1. Wash hands and apply gloves.	Reduces transmission of microorganisms.
2. Provide privacy by closing curtains around bed or closing door.	Reduces embarrassment for client.
3. Raise bed to appropriate working height for nurse; raise side rail on opposite side.	Promotes good body mechanics and client safety.
4. Assist client into left side-lying (Sims') position with right knee flexed. Children may also be placed in dorsal recumbent position.	Allows enema solution to flow downward by gravity along natural curve of sigmoid colon and rectum, thus improving retention of solution.

➤ ***CRITICAL DECISION POINT*** **If client is suspected of having poor sphincter control, position the client on the bedpan in comfortable dorsal recumbent position. Clients with poor sphincter control cannot retain all of enema solution.**

STEPS	RATIONALE
5. Place waterproof pad under hips and buttocks.	Prevents soiling of linen.
6. Cover client with bath blanket, exposing only rectal area, clearly visualizing anus.	Provides warmth, reduces exposure of body parts, allows client to feel more relaxed and comfortable.
7. Place bedpan or commode in easily accessible position. If client will be expelling contents in toilet, ensure that toilet is free. (If client will be getting up to bathroom to expel enema, place client's slippers and bathrobe in easily accessible position.)	Used in case client is unable to retain enema solution.

STEPS	RATIONALE
8. Administer enema using prepackaged disposable container.	
a. Remove plastic cap from rectal tip. Tip is already lubricated, but more jelly can be applied as needed.	Lubrication provides for smooth insertion of rectal tube without causing rectal irritation or trauma (Saltzstein, 1988).
b. Gently separate buttocks and locate rectum. Instruct client to relax by breathing out slowly through mouth.	Breathing out promotes relaxation of external rectal sphincter.
c. Insert tip of bottle gently into rectum. *Adult:* 7.5 to 10 cm (3 to 4 inches) *Child:* 5 to 7.5 cm (2 to 3 inches) *Infant:* 2.5 to 3.75 cm (1 to 1½ inches)	Gentle insertion prevents trauma to rectal mucosa (Saltzstein, 1988).
d. Squeeze bottle until all of solution has entered rectum and colon. (Most bottles contain approximately 250 ml of solution.) Hypertonic solutions require only small volumes to stimulate defecation. Instruct client to retain solution until the urge to defecate occurs, usually 2 to 5 minutes.	
9. Administer enema using enema bag:	
a. Add warmed solution to enema bag: warm tap water as it flows from faucet, place saline container in basin of hot water before adding saline to enema bag, check temperature of solution with bath thermometer or by pouring small amount of solution over inner wrist.	Hot water can burn intestinal mucosa. Cold water can cause abdominal cramping and is difficult to retain.
b. Raise container, release clamp, and allow solution to flow long enough to fill tubing.	Removes air from tubing.
c. Reclamp tubing.	Prevents further loss of solution.
d. Lubricate 6 to 8 cm (3 to 4 inches) of tip of rectal tube with lubricating jelly.	Allows smooth insertion of rectal tube without risk of irritation or trauma to mucosa.
e. Gently separate buttocks and locate anus. Instruct client to relax by breathing out slowly through mouth.	Breathing out promotes relaxation of external anal sphincter.
f. Insert tip of rectal tube slowly by pointing tip in direction of client's umbilicus. Length of insertion varies: Adult: 7.5 to 10 cm (3 to 4 inches) Child: 5 to 7.5 cm (2 to 3 inches) Infant: 2.5 to 3.75 cm (1 to 1½ inches)	Careful insertion prevents trauma to rectal mucosa from accidental lodging of tube against rectal wall. Insertion beyond proper limit can cause bowel perforation.
g. Hold tubing in rectum constantly until end of fluid instillation.	Bowel contraction can cause expulsion of rectal tube.
h. Open regulating clamp and allow solution to enter slowly with container at client's hip level.	Rapid instillation can stimulate evacuation of rectal tube.
i. Raise height of enema container slowly to appropriate level above anus: 30 to 45 cm (12 to 18 inches) for high enema, 30 cm (12 inches) for low enema, 7.5 cm (3 inches) for infant. Instillation time varies with volume of solution administered (e.g., 1 L/10 min).	Allows for continuous, slow instillation of solution. Raising container too high causes rapid instillation and possible painful distention of colon. High pressure can cause rupture of bowel in infant.
j. Lower container or clamp tubing if client complains of cramping or if fluid escapes around rectal tube.	Temporary cessation of instillation prevents cramping, which may prevent client from retaining all fluid, altering effectiveness of enema.
k. Clamp tubing after all solution is instilled.	Prevents entrance of air into rectum.
10. Place layers of toilet tissue around tube at anus and gently withdraw rectal tube.	Provides for client's comfort and cleanliness.

STEPS	RATIONALE
11. Explain to client that feeling of distention is normal. Ask client to retain solution as long as possible while lying quietly in bed. (For infant or young child, gently hold buttocks together for few minutes.)	Solution distends bowel. Length of retention varies with type of enema and client's ability to contract rectal sphincter. Longer retention promotes more effective stimulation of peristalsis and defecation.
12. Discard enema container and tubing in proper receptacle or rinse out thoroughly with warm soap and water if container is to be reused.	Reduces transmission and growth of microorganisms.
13. Assist client to bathroom or help to position client on bedpan.	Normal squatting position promotes defecation.
14. Observe character of feces and solution (caution client against flushing toilet before inspection).	
➤ ***CRITICAL DECISION POINT*** **When enemas are ordered "until clear," it is essential to observe contents of solution passed. The enema return is considered "clear" when no solid fecal material exists, but the solution may be colored.**	
15. Assist client as needed to wash anal area with warm soap and water (if nurse administers perineal care, use gloves).	Fecal contents can irritate skin. Hygiene promotes client's comfort.
16. Remove and discard gloves and wash hands.	Reduces transmission of microorganisms.
EVALUATION	
1. Inspect color, consistency, amount of stool and fluid passed.	Determines if stool is evacuated or fluid is retained. Note abnormalities such as presence of blood or mucus.
2. Assess condition of abdomen.	Determines if distention is relieved.
3. **Unexpected outcomes** that may occur include:	
➤ Abdomen is rigid and distended.	Results from perforation of bowel. Enemas should never be given when appendicitis or bowel obstruction is suspected.
➤ Abdominal cramping occurs.	Results from excessive volume or incorrect temperature of instilled solution.
RECORDING AND REPORTING	
1. Record pertinent information: a. Type and volume of enema given. b. Characteristics of results.	Communicates pertinent information to all members of health care team. Improves documentation of treatment results.
2. Report failure of client to defecate to physician.	May indicate need for further therapies.

FOLLOW-UP ACTIVITIES

1. Stop enema if severe cramping, bleeding, or sudden abdominal pain occurs. Physician should be notified of any adverse effect.

• • • • •

Special Considerations

- ➤ If client cannot control external sphincter, such as a client with paralysis, then client must be placed on bedpan because enema solution cannot be retained.
- ➤ Administering enema with client sitting on toilet is unsafe because curved rectal tubing can abrade rectal wall.
- ➤ "Enemas until clear" order means that enemas are repeated until client passes fluid that is clear and contains no fecal matter. Check agency policy, but usually client should receive only three consecutive enemas to avoid disruption of fluid and electrolyte balance.
- ➤ Some commercial enema kits come with a rectal tube, so ensure that size is appropriate.

➤ Some disposable kits come with prelubricated tip. Add additional lubricant as needed.

Teaching Considerations

➤ Client should be instructed that enemas should not be given to treat cause of constipation.

➤ For self-administration, client should be instructed to lie in dorsal recumbent position with knees and hips flexed toward chest.

➤ Caution client against flushing toilet before nurse has inspected contents.

Pediatric Considerations

➤ For infant or child, nurse may wish to involve parent in procedure.

➤ Children and infants usually do not receive prepackaged hypertonic enemas.

Gerontologic Considerations

➤ Caution is needed when enemas are ordered "until clear" in the older adult population. Older adults may become fatigued, are at risk for fluid and electrolyte imbalances, and may experience changes in vital signs.

➤ Instruct older adults and their care givers on how to modify diet to avoid constipation. (See Skill 26-2).

Home Care Considerations

➤ Assess client's and primary care giver's ability and motivation to administer enema and provide instruction as needed.

➤ Assess client's ability to administer enema if enema ordered is self-administrative type.

➤ Assess client's environment to identify location where enema may be administered with privacy.

➤ Teach skill; observe to determine level of understanding. Review possible complications and what action to take.

CRITICAL THINKING EXERCISES

1. You have just manually removed a fecal impaction from an older adult, immobilized client. What measures could you institute to prevent further impaction?
2. Your client has watery diarrhea. What other assessments are necessary to determine if this watery diarrhea is a symptom of a fecal impaction?
3. You are providing perineal care to a patient after return of a high-volume saline enema and notice a small amount of bright red blood on the washcloth. How would you proceed, and what are your rationales?
4. Identify and explain four important strategies that can help prevent constipation.

REFERENCES

Barkauskas VH, et al.: *Health and physical assessment*, St Louis, 1994, Mosby.

Davis A, et al.: Bowel management: A quality assurance approach to upgrading programs, *J Gerontol Nurs* 12(5):13, 1986.

Doughty DB, Jackson DB: *Gastrointestinal disorders, Mosby's clinical nursing series*, St Louis, 1993, Mosby.

Ebersol P, Hess P: *Toward healthy aging: Human needs and nursing response*, ed 3, St Louis, 1994, Mosby.

Lueckenotte AG: *Gerontologic Nursing*, St Louis, 1996, Mosby.

Mager-O'Connor E: How to identify and remove fecal impaction, *Geriatr Nurs* 5(3):158, 1984.

Saltzstein R, Quebbeman L, Melvin JL: Anorectal injuries incident to enema administration: A recurring avoidable problem, *Am J Phys Med Rehabil* 67:186, 1988.

Tedesco FJ: Laxative use in constipation, *Am J Gastroenterol* 80:303, 1985.

Wright BA, Staats DO: The geriatric implications of fecal impaction, *Nurs Pract* 11(10):53, 1986.

ADDITIONAL READING

Alterescu V: Theoretical foundations for an approach to fecal incontinence, *J Enterost Ther* 13:44, 1986.

Briterman RA: Getting the bowels under control, *Emerg Med Clin North Am* 19:69, 1987.

Burggraf V, Donlin B: Assessing the elderly, *Am J Nurs* 85:872, 1985.

Erickson EP: Bowel management plan for homebound elderly, *J Gerontol Nurs* 14(1):16, 1988.

Lewis N: Nursing mangement of altered patterns of elimination, *J Home Health Care Pract* 1(1):35, 1988.

Lind CD: Diagnosis: GI complaints in the geriatric patient, *Hosp Med* 23(10):183, 1987.

Potter PA, Perry AG: *Fundamentals of nursing: concepts, process, and practice*, ed 4, St Louis, 1997, Mosby.

Whaley LF, Wong DL: *Nursing care of infants and children*, ed 5, St Louis, 1996, Mosby.

CHAPTER 27

Ostomy Care

OBJECTIVES

Mastery of content in this chapter will enable the nurse to:

- Define key terms.
- Identify types of bowel and bladder diversions.
- Explain differences in color and consistency of drainage based on the location of an ostomy.
- Discuss factors influencing enterostomy drainage.
- Describe methods used to maintain skin integrity during pouching of ostomies.
- Pouch an incontinent urinary diversion.
- Irrigate a colostomy.
- Catheterize a urinary diversion.

SKILLS

KEY TERMS

Allergen
Anastomosis
Colon conduit
Colostomy
Conduit
Continent ostomy or diversion
Cystectomy
Effluent
Enterostomy
Fascia
Ileal conduit
Ileostomy
Intubation
Maceration
Maculopapular
Noncontinent (incontinent) ostomy/diversion
Nosocomial infection
Ostomy
Peristalsis
Peristomal
Peritonitis
Skin barrier
Stent
Stoma
Ureterostomy
Urinary diversion

Certain diseases or conditions require surgical intervention to create an opening into the abdominal wall for fecal or urinary elimination. A portion of intestinal mucosa or segment of ureter is brought out to the abdominal wall, and a stoma, or opening, is formed to allow feces or urine to drain.

An **ostomy** is an opening made to allow passage of urine or feces. The piece of intestine that is brought out onto the client's abdomen is called a **stoma.** An **enterostomy** is any surgical procedure that produces an artificial stoma in a portion of intestine through the abdominal wall. The drainage from the stoma is often called **effluent.** The forms of enterostomy are ileostomy, which involves the ileum of the small intestine, and colostomy, which can involve various segments of the colon. Ostomies can be temporary or permanent (Fig. 27-1) and continent or noncontinent. The surgical procedures (see Fig. 27-2) involved in creating a stoma for urinary drainage are called **urinary diversions,** for which two categories of urinary diversions exist, continent and noncontinent (incontinent). Clients who have a noncontinent urinary diversion cannot control when the urine exits from their stoma and therefore must wear an external urinary ostomy pouch at all times. Examples of noncontinent urinary diversions are an ileal conduit and other forms of ureterostomies (Fig. 27-2). Continent urinary diversion surgery creates an internal pouch where urine is stored. Clients who have continent urinary diversions, such as the Kock or Indiana pouch, do not need to wear an external ostomy pouch over their urinary stoma. Instead, these clients are taught to insert a catheter periodically throughout the day into their stoma to drain out the urine (see Skill 27-5).

For diseases or conditions of the bowel, the location of the ostomy determines the consistency of stool passed. An ileostomy bypasses the entire large intestine; thus stools are liquid and frequent, and contain digestive enzymes.

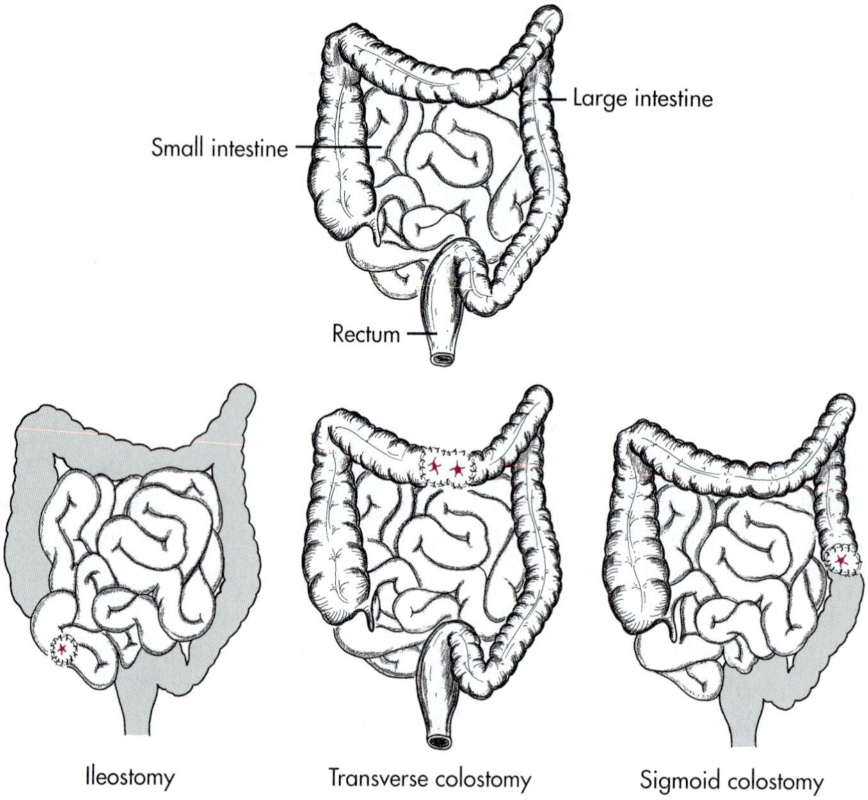

Fig. 27-1 Types of enterostomies: ileostomy, transverse colostomy, sigmoid colostomy.

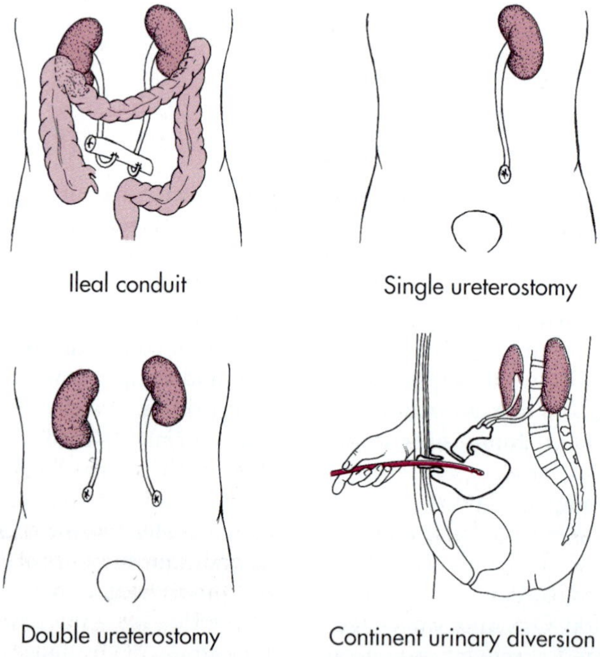

Fig. 27-2 Types of ureterostomies: ileal loop, single ureterostomy, double ureterostomy, continent urinary diversion (Indiana pouch).

The same fecal characteristics hold true for a colostomy of the ascending colon. A colostomy of the transverse colon generally results in a thicker, formed stool. The sigmoid colostomy emits stool almost identical to that normally passed through the rectum. A person with any of the above incontinent ostomies must cover the stoma with a disposable or reusable pouch to collect the effluent.

Ostomies that emit frequent liquid stools must be pouched at all times. The pouch must be emptied throughout the day. Skin care is vital to prevent irritation from fecal irritants.

A colostomy in the transverse colon has to be pouched at all times. The regularity of bowel movements is unpredictable. The transverse colostomy cannot be managed by daily irrigation.

Because of its anatomical location, a sigmoid colostomy can be managed (no fecal output between irrigations) by irrigation. Scheduled irrigations of the descending or sigmoid colostomy allow the person to empty the bowel and may eliminate the need for a pouch (see Skill 27-2). Some clients continue to wear pouches for a feeling of security and in case of fecal spillage between irrigations. Irrigation is optional since many clients prefer natural bowel evacuation.

Over the past years, many developments have occurred in the field of pediatric gastrointestinal surgery that have improved survival rates for neonates having gastrointestinal ostomy surgery. Because pediatric clients have unique needs, refer to the articles that give a more in depth explanation of these surgical procedures and the associated care (Bastawrous et al., 1995; Boarini, 1989; Brown and Ricketts, 1994; Foster, 1995; Hull and Erwin-Toth, 1996). In *Pediatric Considerations* at the end of the skills in this chapter, some of the major points that are pertinent for these clients and their care givers are highlighted.

Figure 27-2 illustrates urinary diversions. The ileal loop may be called an ileal conduit. The surgical procedure may or may not involve cystectomy (removal of the bladder). For an ileal conduit, usually 6 to 8 inches of ileum are separated from the bowel. One end is used to create an external stoma, usually in the lower right quadrant, and the other end is sutured closed. The ureters are internally implanted into this piece of bowel. The client must wear an external ostomy pouch or appliance at all times to collect the urine. The rest of the bowel is sutured together so the client has normal bowel movements as before surgery.

A ureterostomy involves bringing the end of one or both ureters directly to the abdominal surface. A ureterostomy is difficult to pouch, may become occluded in certain body positions, or may become obstructed, with no urine flow. Irritation of the skin from leakage of urine is a common problem. The ureterostomy is the type of urinary diversion usually done in neonates (Boarini, 1989).

Regardless of the type of ostomy, a threat to body image may be perceived (Kluka and Kristijanson, 1996; Piper and Mikols, 1996; Piper, Mikols, Grant, 1996; Quayle, 1994; Walsh et al., 1995). Researchers have shown that clients with ostomies have concerns about stool leakage and odor, body image changes, self-care, and surgical complication management. Some other concerns the client may have are fears of mutilation, rejection by friends or family, and even a loss of normal sexual function (Golis, 1996). Foul-smelling odors, spillage or leakage of liquid stools or urine, and the inability to regulate bowel movements give the client a sense of powerlessness and loss of self-esteem.

Education and counseling of clients with ostomies is a major intervention for the nurse (Piper and Mikols, 1996). Instruction for clients should begin upon admission during the preoperative period and resume early postoperatively as the client's physical condition permits. The nurse must help the client to understand that a normal lifestyle is possible with an ostomy.

GUIDELINES

1. Know what type of effluent is expected from the ostomy. Some ostomies, such as an ileostomy, normally have liquid drainage. Ileostomy drainage is most damaging to skin. Copious output may result in dehydration and electrolyte imbalance. An ileal conduit, though draining urine, normally has mucus because the bowel still produces mucus.
2. Know if the ostomy is continent or noncontinent (incontinent). This information indicates to the nurse whether the lack of spontaneous drainage signals a problem (i.e., noncontinent ostomy) or whether it requires insertion of a catheter to drain the effluent (i.e., continent ostomy). Just because a client has a stoma does not mean that the drainage will spontaneously flow from it. Clients who have continent ostomies (Kock or Indiana pouches) need to have the stoma intubated with a catheter periodically during the day to drain the fecal or urine contents (Hull and Erwin-Toth, 1996) (see Skill 27-5).
3. Know the client's usual elimination pattern so the client can return to or maintain a usual schedule while receiving nursing care.
4. Know the client's routine for self-care of the ostomy. A client who has independently cared for an ostomy should be encouraged to resume self-care as soon as possible.
5. Know the equipment options available. Various types of equipment are used for different types of stomas, ostomy drainage, and skin irritations.

DELEGATION CONSIDERATIONS

This skills in this chapter require problem solving and knowledge application unique to a professional nurse. Delegation of skills in this chapter is inappropriate. The one exception, in some agencies, is pouching of established colostomies.

SKILL 27-1 Pouching an Enterostomy

Immediately after surgical diversion or removal of a portion of bowel, it is necessary to place a pouch over the newly created stoma because in noncontinent ostomies effluent may begin immediately. The pouch collects all effluent and protects the skin from irritating drainage. A pouch with its skin barrier should fit comfortably, cover the skin surface around the stoma, and create a good seal. The postoperative pouch should allow visibility of the stoma.

The technique of pouching a newly formed stoma differs from techniques used to pouch a stoma several days or weeks old. The new stoma is edematous during the postoperative healing process. An incision line from the bowel resection may lie close to the stoma (Fig. 27-3). The stoma itself often has a series of small stitches around its perimeter. A pouch and its skin barrier must be applied so that they do not constrict the stoma or traumatize healing tissues. Initially, the pouch over a postoperative colostomy may not need to be emptied frequently because drainage is diminished or lacking. Several days may pass before a client's normal elimination pattern returns. In the case of an ileostomy, the client will have frequent stools when peristalsis returns.

Many types of pouches and skin barriers are available. Some pouches have skin barriers directly preattached and are called one-piece pouching systems. Some of these one-piece pouches already are precut to size by the manufacturer while others must be custom cut to size for the client's stoma measurement. Other systems are two separate pieces. The pouch can be applied to the skin barrier by attaching it to the flange (a plastic ring) on the barrier. Often the skin barrier needs to be custom cut to the client's specific stoma size. For two-piece systems, the skin barrier with flange must be used with the corresponding size pouch that fits that flange *from the same manufacturer* to use the system correctly without leakage. Nurses should understand how to use each of these different pouching systems (Fig. 27-4).

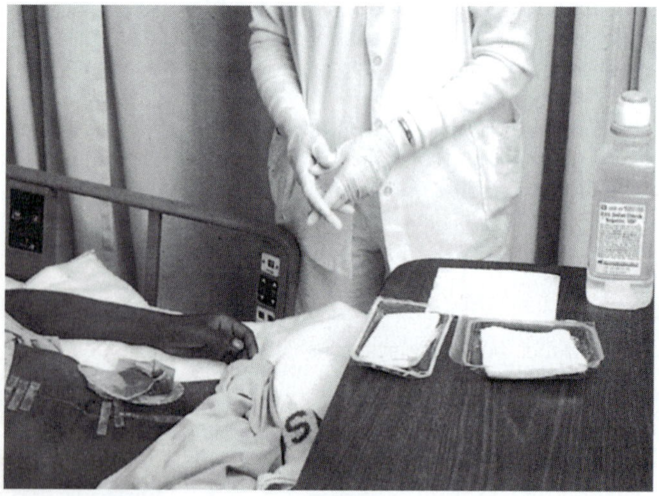

Fig. 27-3 Ostomy pouch near suture line.

EQUIPMENT

- **Pouch, clear drainable colostomy/ileostomy in correct size for two-piece system (see Fig. 27-4, *A*) or custom cut-to-fit one-piece type with attached skin barrier (see Fig. 27-4, *B*).**
- **Pouch closure device, such as a clamp**
- **Adhesive remover (optional)**
- **Clean disposable gloves**
- **Deodorant**
- **Gauze pads or wash cloth**
- **Towel or disposable waterproof barrier**
- **Basin with warm tap water**
- **Scissors**
- **Skin barrier such as sealant wipes or wafer**
- **Tape or ostomy belt**

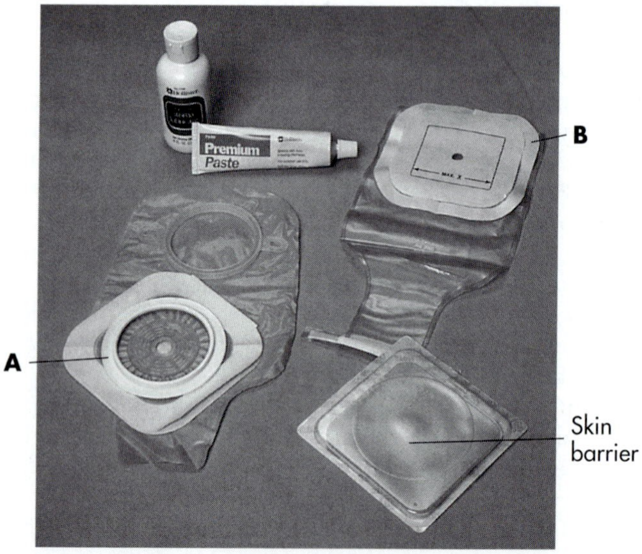

Fig. 27-4 Examples of some pouching systems. **A**, Two-piece detachable system (NOTE: the skin barrier would need to be custom cut by the client according to self-stoma size obtained by measurement). The pouch opening is already precut by the manufacturer to fit the size of the flange on the skin barrier. **B**, One-piece pouch with skin barrier attached.

STEPS	RATIONALE

ASSESSMENT

1. Auscultate for bowel sounds. — Documents presence of peristalsis.
2. Observe skin barrier and pouch for leakage and length of time in place. Depending upon type of pouching system used (such as with an opaque pouch), the nurse may have to remove the pouch in order to fully observe the stoma. Clear pouches permit the viewing of the stoma without their removal.
3. Observe stoma for color, swelling, trauma, and healing; stoma should be moist and reddish-pink. Assess type of stoma. Stomas can be flush with the skin or be a budlike protrusion on the abdomen. An example of a normal bud stoma can be found in the illustration.

   Rationale: Stoma characteristics should be one of the factors to consider when selecting an appropriate pouching system.

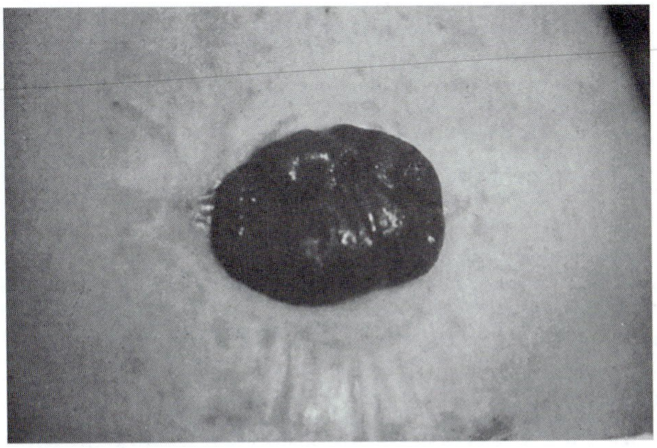

Step 3 Viable, matured transverse loop colostomy and normal peristomal skin. (Courtesy Hollister, Inc, Libertyville, Ill.)

CRITICAL DECISION POINT **The stoma should be measured each pouching system change to determine the correct size of equipment needed. Follow each ostomy pouch manufacturer's directions and measuring guide as to which size ostomy pouch to use based on the client's actual stoma measurement size.**

4. Observe abdominal incision (if present).

   Rationale: Relationship to stoma determines proper placement of pouch.

5. Observe effluent from stoma and keep a record of intake and output. Ask client about skin tenderness.
6. When assessing skin for irritation, check that the pouching system is not leaking.

   Rationale: May indicate need for different type of pouch or sealant.

CRITICAL DECISION POINT **Some clients because of stomal and abdominal characteristics may need convexity in their ostomy pouching system to avoid leakage (Rolstad and Boarini, 1996).**

7. To minimize skin irritation, avoid unnecessary changing of the entire pouching system. A one-piece pouch with attached skin barriers or the skin barrier of a two-piece pouching system should be changed every 3 to 7 days, *not* daily.

   Rationale: Pouches should be emptied when one third to half full because the weight of contents may dislodge the skin seal, and ostomy drainage is irritating to the skin. Also, pouches collect flatus (gas), which needs to be expelled since it can disrupt the skin seal.

CRITICAL DECISION POINT **Do not put holes in the pouch for flatus to escape.**

8. Assess abdomen for best type of pouching system to use. Consider:
   a. Contour and peristomal plane
   b. Presence of scars, incisions
   c. Location and type of stoma

   Rationale: Determines pouching system selection and need for other equipment.

9. Assess the client's condition as to the best type of pouching system to use.

STEPS	RATIONALE
CRITICAL DECISION POINT **Pouching system options include the following: one-piece pouch with skin barrier already attached, precut pouch and skin barrier, or two-piece pouch system, which consists of a pouch that can detach from the skin barrier, which remains around the client's stoma for several days. The bottom of ostomy pouches are either open ended, closed only with a clip, or have a rubber band or some other type of closure device between emptying; or closed ended, where the end of the pouch is sealed closed. One-piece pouches should be open-ended pouches that can be opened periodically to empty the effluent *without* removing the pouch from around the stoma. Two-piece pouches give the client the choice of using either an open-ended or closed-ended pouch. This is because the client can remove the pouch from the skin barrier to empty the effluent.**	Clients who have difficulty using their hands or who have limited vision may find a one-piece system or a precut pouch and skin barrier more desirable to use, others prefer being able to keep the skin barrier in place for several days, changing just the pouch, and therefore prefer the two-piece system. Even clients who are blind can be taught to change their own ostomy equipment (Ramos and Glosson, 1996).
10. After skin barrier and pouch removal, assess skin around stoma, noting scars, folds, skin breakdown, and peristomal suture line if present.	Determines need for barrier paste to increase adherence of pouch to skin or to fill in irregularities.
11. Determine client's emotional response and knowledge and understanding of an ostomy and its care.	Assists in determining extent to which client is able to participate in care and need for teaching and information clarification.

NURSING DIAGNOSIS

Clustering of defining characteristics from the assessment data may reveal the following nursing diagnoses for clients requiring this skill:

- Constipation
- Diarrhea
- Risk for impaired skin integrity
- Ineffective individual coping
- Knowledge deficit regarding ostomy self-care
- Pain

Related factors are individualized based on a client's condition or needs.

PLANNING

STEPS	RATIONALE
1. **Expected outcomes** following completion of procedure:	
➤ Client denies discomfort.	
➤ Stoma is moist and reddish-pink. Skin is intact and free of irritation; sutures are intact.	Normal findings in client with postoperative enterostomy that is healing. Stoma initially is edematous and shrinks over next 6 to 8 weeks.
➤ Stoma is functioning with moderate amount of liquid or soft stool and flatus in pouch. (Flatus is noted by bulging of pouch in absence of drainage; flatus initially indicates return of peristalsis after surgery.)	Snug seal around stoma has been attained. Skin is free of irritation.
➤ Client observes stoma and steps of procedure carefully.	Reveals acknowledgment of body alteration and interest in self-care.
➤ Client asks questions about procedure and may attempt to assist with pouch change.	Asking to assist indicates readiness to learn and to begin self-care.
2. Explain procedure to client; encourage client's interaction and questions.	Lessens anxiety and promotes client's participation.
3. Assemble equipment and close room curtains or door.	Optimizes use of time; conserves client's and nurse's energy. Provides privacy.

STEPS	RATIONALE
IMPLEMENTATION	
1. Position client either standing or supine and drape. If seated position either on or in front of the toilet.	When client is supine fewer wrinkles allow for ease of application of pouching system; maintains client's dignity.
2. Wash hands and don disposable gloves.	Reduces transmission of microorganisms.
3. Place towel or disposable waterproof barrier under the client.	Protects bed linen.
4. Remove used pouch and skin barrier gently by pushing the skin away from the barrier. An adhesive remover may be used to facilitate removal of the skin barrier.	Reduces trauma; jerking irritates the skin and can cause tears.
5. Cleanse peristomal skin gently with warm tap water using gauze pads or clean washcloth; do not scrub the skin; dry completely by patting the skin with gauze or towel.	Avoid use of soap since it leaves a residue on the skin that interferes with pouch adhesion to the skin. Skin must be dry as skin barrier; pouch does not adhere to wet skin. If blood appears on the gauze pad, do not be alarmed; the stoma, if rubbed, may ooze some blood from the cleaning process. Bleeding into the pouch is abnormal. The stoma's surface is highly vascular mucous membrane.
6. Measure the stoma for correct size of pouching system needed using the manufacturer's measuring guide (see illustration below and on p. 852).	Ensures accuracy in determining correct pouch size needed. Stoma shrinks and does not reach usual size for 6 to 8 weeks.
7. Select appropriate pouch for client based on client assessment. With a custom cut-to-fit pouch, use an ostomy guide to cut opening on the pouch 1/16 to 1/8 inch larger than stoma before removing backing. Prepare pouch by removing backing from barrier and adhesive (see illustration). With ileostomy, apply thin circle of barrier paste around opening in pouch; allow to dry.	The paste facilitates seal and protects skin. Size of pouch opening keeps drainage off skin and lessens risk of damage to stoma during peristalsis or activity. Pouch and skin barrier are changed whenever leaking. Change when client is comfortable; before a meal is better since this avoids increased peristalsis and chance of evacuation during the pouch change. Can also be changed before or after tub bath or shower. Stool is alkaline and this irritates the skin; fecal bacteria can colonize on the skin and increase risk of infection.
8. Apply the skin barrier and pouch. If creases next to stoma occur, use barrier paste to fill in; let dry 1 to 2 minutes.	

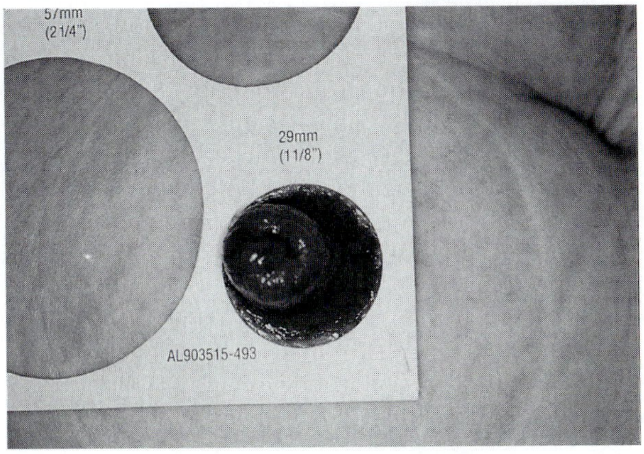

Step 6 Measuring an ostomy.

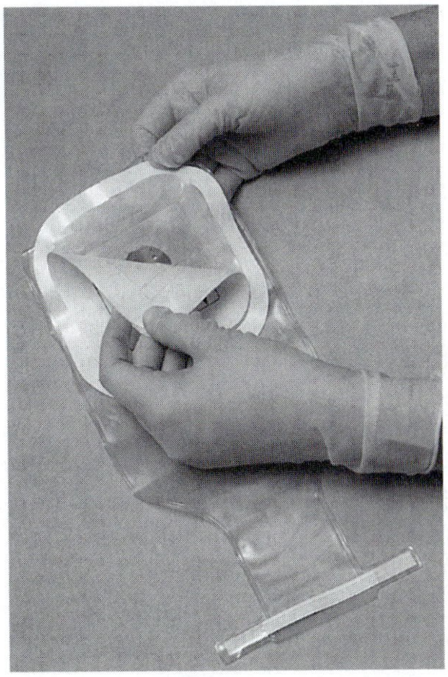

Step 7

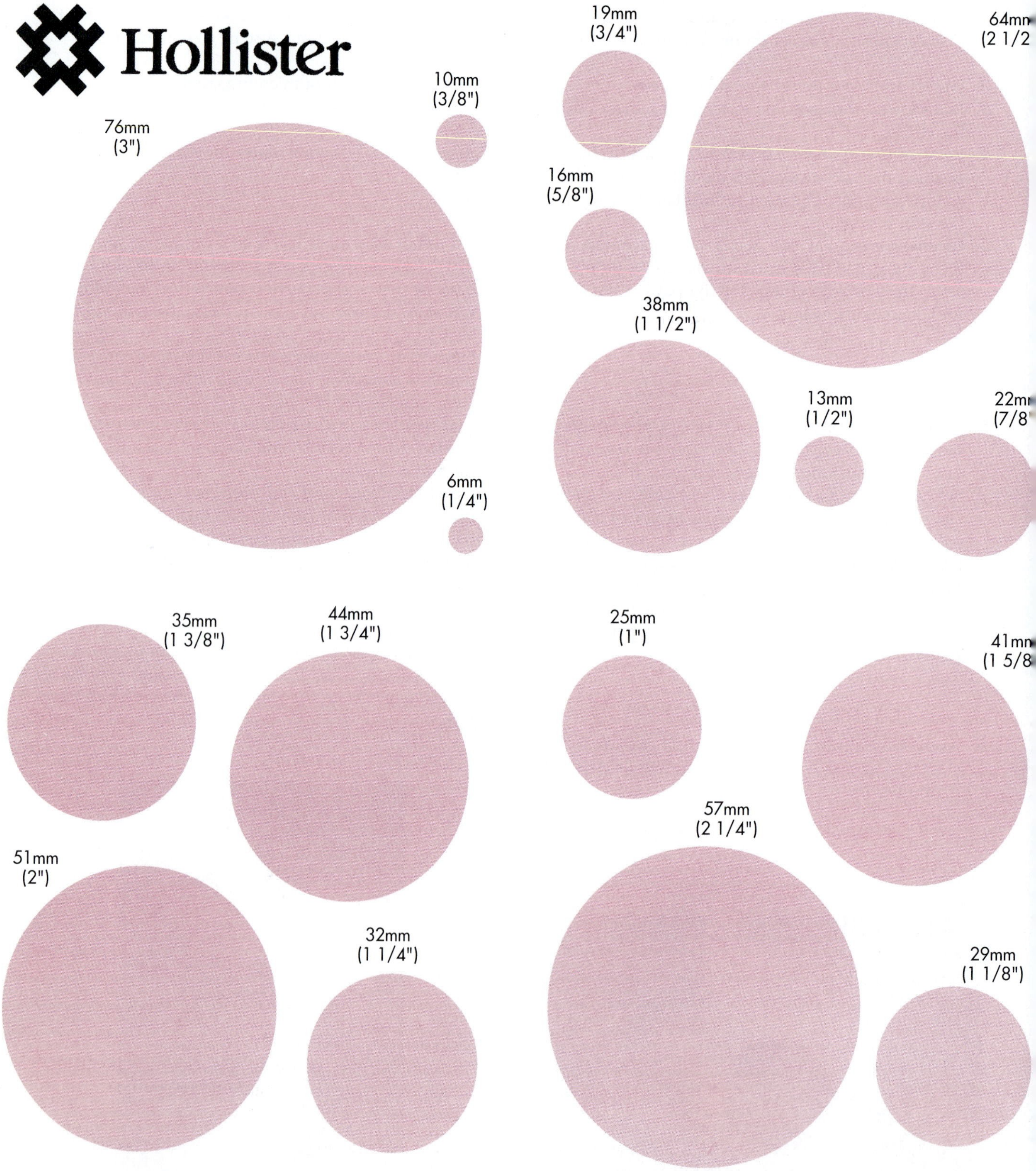

Step 6 Measuring card. (Courtesy, Hollister Inc. Libertyville, Ill.)

STEPS	RATIONALE

CRITICAL DECISION POINT **When applying a skin barrier to a stoma that is close to a client's abdominal incision, the skin barrier may have to be trimmed in order for it to fit.**

a. For one-piece pouching system:
(1) Use skin sealant wipes on skin directly under adhesive skin barrier or pouch; allow to dry. Press the adhesive backing of the pouch and/or skin barrier smoothly against the skin, starting from the bottom and working up and around the sides.
(2) Hold pouch by barrier, center over stoma, and press down gently on barrier; bottom of pouch should point toward client's knees.
(3) Maintain gentle finger pressure around the barrier for 1 to 2 minutes.

b. If using a two-piece pouching system:
(1) Apply flange (barrier with adhesive) as in steps above for one-piece system. Then snap on pouch and maintain finger pressure. — Creates wrinkle-free, secure seal; decreases irritation from the adhesive on skin.

9. Apply nonallergeric paper tape around the pectin skin barrier in a "picture frame" method. Half of the tape should be on the skin barrier and half on the client's skin. Some clients may prefer a belt attached to the pouch for extra security rather than tape. — "Picture framing" the pectin skin barrier adds to the security of keeping the pouch system attached securely.

CRITICAL DECISION POINT **Make sure a client who chooses to wear an ostomy belt does not have the belt too tight. To check for appropriate tightness, two fingers should be able to be placed between belt and skin.**

10. Although many ostomy pouches are odor-proof, some nurses and clients like to add a small amount of ostomy deodorant into the pouch. Do not use "home remedies," which can harm the stoma, to control ostomy odor.

CRITICAL DECISION POINT **Aspirin should never be added to the ostomy pouch. It can cause stomal bleeding.**

11. Fold bottom of drainable open-ended pouches up once and close using a closure device such as a clamp (or follow manufacturers' instructions for closure). — Maintains secure seal to prevent leaking.
12. Properly dispose of old pouch and soiled equipment. Consider spraying deodorant in room if needed. — Lessens odors in room.
13. Remove gloves and wash hands. — Reduces transmission of microorganisms.
14. Change pouch every 3 to 7 days unless leaking; pouch can remain in place for tub bath or shower; after bath, pat adhesive dry. — Avoids unnecessary trauma to skin from too frequent changes. Drying ensures adhesion of pouch.

CRITICAL DECISION POINT **Sometimes the nonallergic paper tape needs to be reapplied after showering or bathing.**

EVALUATION

1. Ask if client feels discomfort around stoma. — Determines presence of skin irritation.

STEPS	RATIONALE
2. Note appearance of stoma around skin and existing incision (if present) while pouch is removed and skin is cleansed. Reinspect condition of skin barrier and adhesive.	Determines condition of tissues and progress of healing. Determines presence of leaks.
3. Auscultate bowel sounds and observe characteristics of stool.	Determines return of peristalsis and bowel elimination.
4. Observe client's nonverbal behaviors as pouch is applied. Ask if client has any questions about pouching.	May indicate emotional response to stoma and readiness for teaching. Determines level of understanding of procedure.
5. **Unexpected outcomes** that may occur include:	
➤ Skin around stoma is irritated, has burning sensation. Mucosal layer of stoma separates from skin.	May be caused by undermining of pouch seal by fecal contents. An allergic reaction can be manifested by erythema and blistering, usually confined to one area immediately under allergen. (Stop use of suspected allergen.) Rapid removal of pouch can cause redness or irritation of skin. Yeast infection around stoma causes redness and burning with maculopapular rash. May indicate breakdown of sutures or poor healing. Some skin barrier pastes and sealants contain alcohol that may burn irritated skin. To enhance client comfort, *avoid* using them in these situations.
➤ Necrotic stoma is manifested by purple or black color, dry instead of moist texture, failure to bleed when washed gently, tissue sloughs.	Can reveal inadequate circulation to stoma caused by excessive edema or excessive tension on bowel suture line.
➤ Client complains of irritation and burning around stoma.	Symptoms of skin inflammation, maceration, breakdown.
➤ Client refuses to view stoma or participate in care.	Each person moves through grieving phase at different rate. Knowledge and acceptance by staff facilitate understanding and adjustment. Acceptance and understanding of significant others should be encouraged by staff because this is an integral part of adjustment by client.

RECORDING AND REPORTING

1. Chart type of pouch and skin barrier applied.	Documents care provided. Indicates specific pouch and appropriateness for client.
2. Record amount and appearance of stool or drainage in pouch, size of stoma, color of stool, texture, condition of peristomal skin, and sutures.	Documents postoperative return of bowel function, and ongoing condition of skin.
3. Report any of the following to the charge nurse and/or physician:	
a. Abnormal appearance of stoma, suture line, peristomal skin, character of output, absence of bowel sounds.	May indicate need for closer nursing and medical observation or intervention to correct problems.
b. No flatus in 24 to 36 hours and no stool by third day.	
4. Document abdominal distention and excessive tenderness, nature of bowel sounds.	May indicate postoperative ileus.
5. Record client's level of participation and need for teaching.	Aids in developing teaching goals and evaluation of progress.

FOLLOW-UP ACTIVITIES

1. Obtain referral for enterostomal therapy (ET) nurse.
2. Advise client of ostomy support groups in community.
3. Consult with dietitian for list of gas-forming foods and foods that increase odor or cause constipation and diarrhea (Hampton and Bryant, 1992).
4. Consider referral to social service.

• • • • •

Special Considerations

- Use only pectin skin barriers with urinary stoma. Karaya skin barriers are destroyed by urine.
- Use barrier paste around the base of an ileostomy stoma so that no skin is visible when the pouch is applied. The paste also can be placed around the opening in the pouch; allow to dry before applying the pouch (or flange in two-piece system).
- Remember that ileostomy drainage is very irritating to the skin since the feces are highly alkaline and contain digestive enzymes. If output exceeds 2400 ml/day the client is at risk for fluid and electrolyte imbalance; notify the physician.
- Before disposing of old pouch, remove the clamp, wash it, and save it; measure output.
- The stoma has no nerve endings and touching it will not hurt the client.
- Clients with wide perineal resections may experience sexual dysfunction and need intervention in coping with this (Cohen, 1991).
- Initially, ileostomy output is copious, dark greenish-brown liquid. This gradually thickens to a more brownish color; monitor output carefully. A colostomy may not function for 3 to 5 days after surgery regarding evacuation of stool.
- Notify physician of signs of necrosis of stoma. First 24 to 72 hours present greatest risk for compromise of blood flow. A normal stoma oozes blood if rubbed. Bleeding into the pouch from the inside of the stoma is abnormal and should be reported immediately to the physician.
- Return of peristalsis causes an increase in flatus. Advise clients that this is indicative of bowel functioning and that this is "good news" to lessen their possible embarrassment. Also tell them that they cannot voluntarily control passing flatus since the stoma does not have a sphincter. Wearing a pouch cover may decrease the sound.
- Some clients can avoid permanent stoma placement by undergoing ileal-anal anastomosis as an alternative as determined by their physician (Hull and Erwin-Toth, 1996).

Teaching Considerations

- Include family members or significant other in teaching since this may facilitate client's readiness to learn.
- Client's readiness to learn may be judged, for example, by willingness to look at stoma and asking questions. If client is apprehensive about touching or looking at stoma, have client hold gauze pad over stoma and clean around stoma.
- Some clients acknowledge stoma with minimal emotional difficulty; some may never completely adjust to it. Individualize care according to client's situation and circumstances (Cohen, 1991).
- Teach client to avoid constipation by eating a balanced diet and having adequate fluids.
- If client has limitations affecting dexterity, select a pouching system that can easily be managed by client.
- Client should be given a teaching manual with steps clearly stated, or audiotaped instructions. With client who has learning disability, a "picture book" of the steps may be more appropriate.
- Client should be given a list of equipment and the name, address, and phone number of a supplier in client's community. Some insurance companies pay some of the cost of ostomy supplies (Halvorson and Kertz, 1996). Utilization limits exist for amount of ostomy supplies that insurance reimburses the client (Halvorson and Kertz, 1996).
- Adult clients may wear usual clothes since peristalsis pushes stool out of stoma, and snug clothes do not interfere with the effluent emptying into the external pouch. Tight girdles and undergarments, however, should not be worn without the consent of the surgeon. For babies, one-piece garments are preferred as they can deter the baby from pulling off the ostomy pouch.
- Clients should avoid placing pouches in extremely hot or cold locations since temperature may affect the barrier and adhesive materials.
- Clients may find that wearing a pouch cover increases their comfort especially when it is hot and sticky. Another advantage to a pouch cover is that it hides the effluent from the client's view.

Pediatric Considerations

- Because most ostomy surgery done on neonates is for emergency situations, often no time is available for preoperative selection of the stoma site. Most stomas, however, are temporary with the stoma being "taken down" (removed or closed) when the baby is about 1 year old. Colostomies are the most frequent type of stomas in neonates. They are usually done because the baby has necrotizing enterocolitis (NEC), Hirschsprung's disease, or imperforate anus (Boarini, 1989; Brown and Ricketts, 1994).
- Use equipment that is designed by manufacturers for use with pediatric clients (Brown and Ricketts, 1994). The preterm baby's skin is immature and thus has a weaker cohesion between the dermis and epidermis layers of the skin. Therefore it is more permeable, leading to a greater risk of toxicity from absorption of products and an increased risk for damage from stripping of the skin (Boarini, 1989).
- Usually, a baby triples its birth weight in the first year. The stoma does not delay the baby's growth. As the baby grows in size, so too does the stoma. Therefore, the stoma should be measured frequently and appropriate adjustments in pouching and skin barrier size be made accordingly (Boarini, 1989).

- Changes in the baby's sleeping, teething, and eating patterns require changes in the management of the ostomy (Boarini, 1989).
- Neonates often have multiple stomas on their tiny abdomens. Select a cut-to-fit pouch that allows multiple stoma openings in the skin barrier, yet still fits on the neonate's tiny abdomen (Brown and Ricketts, 1994).
- Because babies swallow large amounts of air while sucking, it is normal to expect considerable amounts of flatus. Make sure the pouch can accommodate the increased amount of flatus or be prepared to release the flatus frequently (Brown and Ricketts, 1994).
- Consider using a one-piece pouching system for better adherence with premature infants and neonates. Older babies and children may like the advantage of the two-piece ostomy system for ostomy pouch emptying (Brown and Ricketts, 1994).
- Parents of pediatric clients need support to express their feelings about their loss of a perfect baby (Boarini, 1989).
- Baby's skin can be easily mechanically damaged. Remove the old ostomy pouch slowly and gently to avoid mechanical trauma to the skin. Use only warm water to wash the peristomal skin. Avoid using harsh soaps and cleansers (Brown and Ricketts, 1994).
- Normally, an ostomy pouching system should be used to contain the effluent. Diapering does not provide adequate peristomal skin protection from the digestive enzymes in the stool for most ileostomies. Parents of a child with sigmoid colostomy caused by an imperforate anus may opt not to use an ostomy pouch, but rather use diapers and skin protection products (Brown and Ricketts, 1994).
- Brown and Ricketts (1994) have described characteristics of pouch skin barriers for pediatric clients:
  - Flexible to cover an infant's rounded abdominal contour.
  - Thin enough to avoid undermining of stool beneath the skin barrier.
  - Large enough to accommodate multiple stomas in one skin barrier.
- Stoma prolapse occurs more frequently in pediatric clients because of the increase in intraabdominal pressure that occurs with crying (Brown and Ricketts, 1994).
- Encourage the older child to do ostomy self-care independently (Brown and Ricketts, 1994).
- One-piece outfits help prevent the normally curious exploring baby from dislodging the ostomy pouch (Boarini, 1989).
- While the normal stoma color is red, a temporary change in stoma color to white or purple may occur when the baby is crying (Boarini, 1989).

Gerontologic Considerations

- Evaluate the older adult's cognitive status for understanding ostomy self-care instructions.
- Evaluate the older adult's motor and visual ability to prepare ostomy equipment. For clients who are unable to custom cut the size of their skin barriers, consider having barriers precut by the ostomy equipment supplier or using a precut two-piece system.
- Avoid hot water and harsh soaps when washing the peristomal skin.
- Older clients need teaching about the change in the number of eliminations (from an incontinent ostomy) that would be normal on a daily status.
- Financial concerns about the cost of ostomy supplies and reimbursement may be an important issue for clients on Medicare (Halvorson and Kertz, 1996).

Home Care Considerations

- Evaluate the client's home toileting facilities. This includes:
  - The presence of adequate toileting facilities in the client's home.
  - Flushable toilet facilities.
  - Number and location of toileting facilities.
  - Number of other people living with the client who must share the toileting facilities.
  - Identification of the toileting facilities pattern of use as to time of day and amount of time spent in bathroom by the other people living with the client.
- Evaluate the client's ostomy routine in relationship to usual lifestyle after discharge.
- Caution the client that most ostomy pouches and barriers cannot be flushed down the toilet; they clog the system. Dispose of used ostomy pouch according to local sanitation regulations.
- Client should understand that while the nurse may have used sterile gauze to clean the stoma, it is *not* necessary to use sterile gauze. In fact, gauze is not needed at all; a washcloth or any soft material can be used.

SKILL 27-2 Irrigating a Colostomy

The purpose of a colostomy irrigation is to cleanse the bowel of feces before tests or surgical procedures, to relieve constipation, or to establish a pattern of regular bowel elimination after ostomy surgery. Irrigation of a colostomy is a simple procedure that clients can learn. The muscular quality of the colon allows it to be safely irrigated with a relatively large amount of fluid. Clients who perform irrigations at home learn to establish an irrigation routine so that regular evacuation of the bowel occurs without stomal discharge between irrigations. Irrigations for achieving regular bowel evacuation can be achieved only with descending and sigmoid end colostomies.

Irrigating an ileostomy is rarely necessary, except in cases of food blockage near the stomal outlet. Then, a gentle lavage may be performed, but only by a qualified person such as an ET nurse. An ileostomy produces a liquid drainage containing a high concentration of electrolytes such as sodium, chloride, potassium, magnesium, and bicarbonate. Because excessive lavage could lead to a serious fluid and electrolyte imbalance, normal saline is used.

EQUIPMENT

- Ostomy irrigation set that consists of an irrigation solution bag and tubing with a fluid control clamp and cone tip
- Irrigation sleeve (with belt tabs or stick-on ring and end-closure device)
- Water-soluble lubricant
- Ostomy pouch and skin barrier or stoma cap cover
- Clean disposable gloves

Toilet facilities that include:

- A flushable toilet
- A hook or some device to hold the irrigation container
- Toilet tissue
- Running water (that is suitable for use)

For clients who are bedridden:

- Bedpan
- Towels
- Waterproof pad

STEPS	RATIONALE
ASSESSMENT	
1. Assess frequency of defecation, character of stool, and placement of stoma, as well as nutritional pattern.	May indicate need to irrigate to stimulate elimination function; consistency of stool varies along length of GI tract.
2. Assess time when client normally irrigates colostomy. In the case of a new ostomy, confer with physician about when irrigations can begin. Obtain written order. Confer with client for best time to irrigate.	Maintains established routine for bowel emptying. Irrigation initiates attempt to establish regular bowel emptying. Bowel must be totally healed so irrigation fluid will not cause perforation. This usually occurs 3 to 7 days after surgery.
3. Review orders for diagnostic or surgical procedures involving the bowel.	Procedures may indicate need to cleanse bowel of fecal contents or delay starting irrigation procedure.
4. Assess client's understanding of procedure and ability to perform techniques.	Determines level of participation to expect from client and level of explanations nurse should provide and if irrigation is appropriate for client.

NURSING DIAGNOSIS

Clustering of defining characteristics from the assessment data may reveal the following nursing diagnoses for clients requiring this skill:

- Anxiety
- Constipation
- Knowledge deficit regarding irrigation management

Related factors are individualized based on a client's condition or needs.

PLANNING

STEPS	RATIONALE
1. **Expected outcomes** following completion of procedure:	
➤ Large amount of flatus, formed stool, and fluid returns. Client denies abdominal pain or cramping. Spillage of stool does not occur between irrigations.	Normal defecation with full return of water occurs. Absence of abdominal discomfort indicates that irrigant was instilled at proper rate.

STEPS	RATIONALE
➤ Client performs the irrigation procedure with minimal emotional distress.	Ability to perform irrigation strengthens client's sense of control.
➤ Client understands and can perform procedure with minimal assistance.	Client is ready to perform self-care.
2. Explain procedure and anticipated responses (e.g., some abdominal cramping) to client, encourage client's participation and questions.	Lessens anxiety and promotes client's participation.
3. Assemble equipment and close room curtains or door.	Optimizes use of time; conserves client's and nurse's energy. Provides privacy.

IMPLEMENTATION

STEPS	RATIONALE
1. Position client:	
a. On toilet or in chair in front of toilet, if ambulatory.	
b. On side, with head slightly elevated, if unable to be out of bed.	Allows for placement of irrigation sleeve into toilet or bedpan.
2. Apply disposable gloves.	Reduces transmission of microorganisms.
3. For adult clients, fill irrigation bag with 500 to 1000 ml warm irrigation solution (either tap water or normal saline); clear tubing of air (see illustration). 500 to 1000 ml is sufficient to distend the colon and effect evacuation. Start with 500 ml.	Allows solution to slowly enter colon and avoids cramping. Cold irrigation solution could trigger syncope; hot water could damage stoma and intestinal mucosa. Air entering the colon may trigger cramping.
4. Hang the irrigation solution container on a hook so that the end of the bag is no higher than client's shoulder height when sitting or 18 to 20 inches (45 to 50 cm) above stoma. (See illustration.)	This position prevents too high a pressure and reduces possibility of bowel damage.

➤ ***CRITICAL DECISION POINT*** **Assess if client is capable of sitting on the toilet. Make sure the end of the irrigation sleeve is sufficiently into the toilet to prevent stool from getting on the floor or the client.**

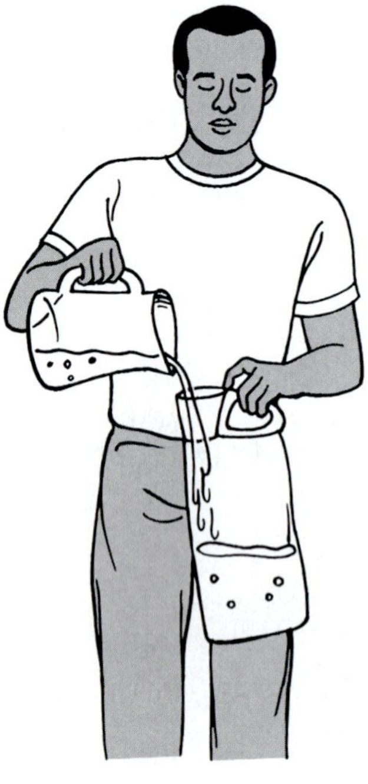

Step 3

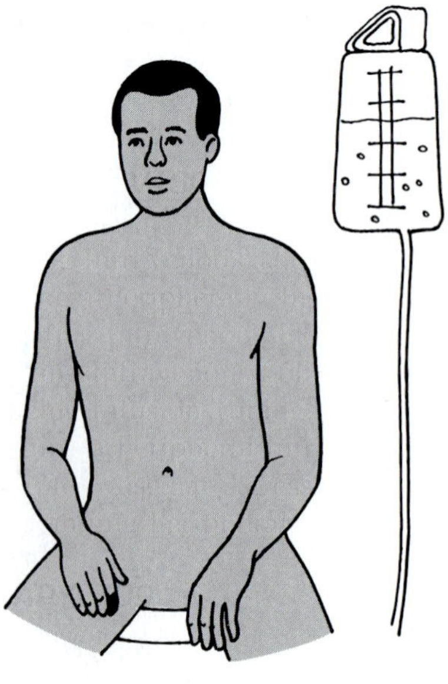

Step 4

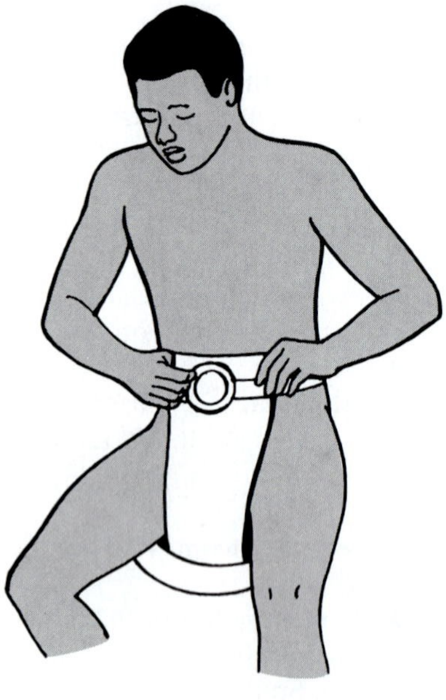

Step 6

STEPS	RATIONALE
5. Remove used pouch by gently pushing skin from adhesive and barrier; properly dispose of used pouch (save clamp, if attached to pouch) and remove gloves and wash hands.	Prevents skin irritation; controls odor in room.
6. Apply irrigation sleeve over stoma; tip of sleeve should rest in water in toilet or in bedpan (see illustration).	Directs flow of stool into toilet or bedpan; if in toilet, also controls odor and splashing.
7. Apply gloves, lubricate cone tip, reach through the top of the irrigation sleeve and hold cone tip snugly against stomal opening (see illustration A). *Do not* force the cone into the stoma. Start inflow of solution. Adjust direction of cone to facilitate inflow of solution. Illustration B shows client performing self-irrigation; gloves are not required for client.	Prevents trauma to stoma; cone tip avoids perforation of bowel. Cone aids in retaining solution during inflow. Aiming flow of solution toward direction of bowel aids inflow.

CRITICAL DECISION POINT **Only use a cone tip to do irrigations. Do *not* use a tube without a cone tip. It carries a higher risk for perforation of colon.**

STEPS	RATIONALE
8. Allow solution to flow in over 5- to 10-minute period.	Avoids rapid distention of bowel; if cramping or nausea occurs, stop the inflow of solution until either subsides; have client take a few slow, deep breaths.
9. After the desired amount of solution has entered the colon, clamp the tubing and wait 15 seconds before removing the cone. Discard gloves. Close the top of the irrigation sleeve.	Avoids sudden backflow of solution from the stoma.
10. Allow 15 to 20 minutes for initial evacuation; don gloves. Dry tip of irrigation sleeve and close bottom (use ostomy pouch clamp or rubber band). Fold the sleeve up and over the top as per manufacturer's specific directions for each brand of irrigation sleeve, leave in place for 30 to 45 minutes. Discard gloves. Client may walk around.	Prevents leakage; optimizes evacuation of stool. Entire procedure should take approximately 1 hour. Assists in evacuation of stool.
11. Don gloves; unclamp sleeve, empty any fecal contents; remove sleeve. Rinse with liquid cleanser and cool water. Hang sleeve to dry.	Maintains sleeve in clean condition for future use.

CRITICAL DECISION POINT **Most irrigation sleeves are meant to be reused. Do not throw out reusable irrigation sleeves after each use. This is very costly.**

A

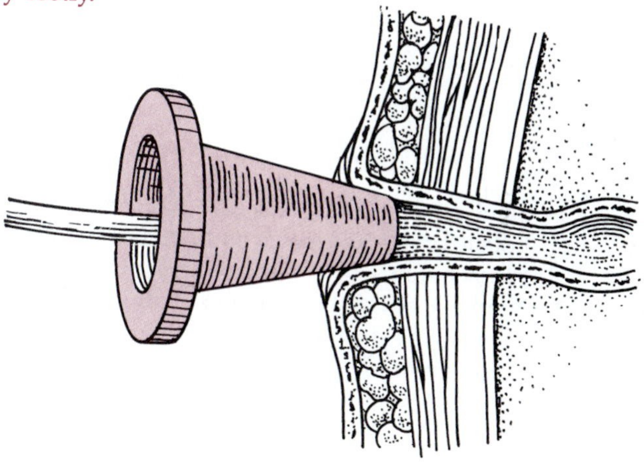

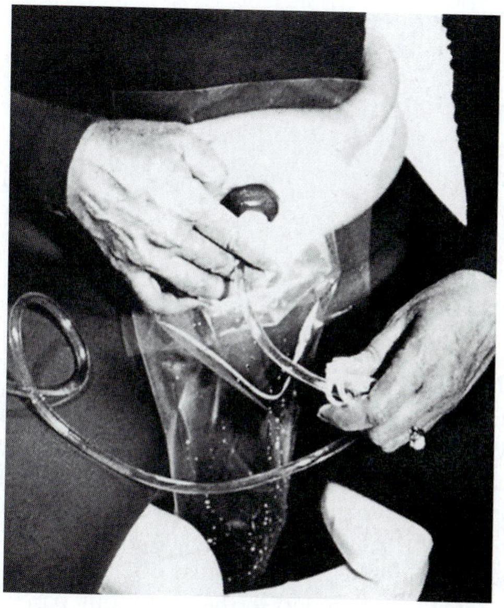

B

Step 7

STEPS	RATIONALE
12. Apply new colostomy pouch or stoma cap covering per procedure (see Skill 27-1).	Avoids soiling of clothes or skin irritation from accidental leakage.
13. Remove gloves and wash hands.	Reduces transmission of microorganisms.

EVALUATION

STEPS	RATIONALE
1. Inspect volume and character of fecal material and fluid that returns after irrigation.	Determines if solution is retained. If client is dehydrated, bowel may absorb irrigation solution and fecal output will be limited or nil. Character and amount of stool reveal success in evacuation.
2. Note client's response during irrigation. Assess client's radial pulse. Ask if cramping or abdominal pain is felt.	Reveals tolerance of irrigation.
3. Ask client to describe steps of procedure.	Evaluates client's learning.
4. **Unexpected outcomes** that may occur include:	
➤ Client is unable to retain sufficient solution to result in desired effect. Client retained all of solution with no return.	May be caused by nausea, instillation that is too rapid, solution that is too cold, or improper technique with the irrigation cone. Frequently seen when client is dehydrated or tense.
➤ Client experiences pain during insertion and during or after administration. Abdomen is hard and painful with no bowel sounds. No output through ostomy occurs except for small amount of blood. Pulse may be weak and rate may change from normal baseline.	Symptoms of perforation.
➤ Client experiences diarrhea or spillage between irrigation.	May be caused by medication, infection, or diet. If colon is obstructed, may put out some liquid stool, but irrigation does not return properly.
➤ Client is unable to explain or perform procedure.	Indicates additional instruction is needed.

RECORDING AND REPORTING

STEPS	RATIONALE
1. Record procedure, time of irrigation, volume, and type of solution, amount and type of return, client's tolerance.	Documents procedure and results. Data used for comparison for future irrigations.
2. Record reapplication of skin barrier and pouch and condition of stoma and skin.	Documents procedure. Data used to compare change in condition of skin or stoma.
3. Report symptoms of extreme discomfort, onset of severe diarrhea, poor results, or excessive bleeding to nurse in charge or physician.	Indicates need for additional therapy.

FOLLOW-UP ACTIVITIES

1. Consult with dietitian.
2. Obtain referral for ET nurse.

• • • • •

Special Considerations

- Debilitated, confused, or unconscious clients are at risk for constipation or impaction. Irrigate only with physician's order if obstruction is suspected.
- *Only* clients with stomas in the lower descending or sigmoid colon are candidates for colostomy irrigation for routine bowel evacuation.
- Many clients who had regular bowel movements before surgery revert to their previous pattern without needing irrigation.
- Some clients feel more secure with a small, closed pouch; others use gauze pads, colostomy dressings, or stoma cover caps with charcoal gas filters.
- Normally irrigation is done in bathroom.
- Clients who develop diarrhea should discontinue irrigation until stool thickens. Diarrhea can be caused by diet, medication, radiation, chemotherapy, bacterial infection, and other factors.

Teaching Considerations

- Client should be instructed in community resources such as ostomy groups, home health agencies, suppliers.
- Clients should be given a teaching manual with steps clearly stated, or audiotaped instructions.

Pediatric Considerations (See also Skill 27-1)

- Irrigations to regulate bowel movements are not usually done for pediatric clients.
- Sometimes irrigations of the distal ostomy limb are done for clean out purposes for pediatric clients with Hirschsprung's disease.
- Amount of irrigation solution used differs from amount used for adults. Physician orders the amount of irrigation solution to use, usually based on pediatric client's weight and size.

Gerontologic Considerations (See also Skill 27-1)

- Assess client's willingness to do ostomy self-irrigations. This takes a time commitment to be able to perform the skill correctly.
- Assess client's physical ability to do ostomy self-irrigations. Motor and/or visual limitations may make it difficult but not impossible for client to do the procedure. Some adaptions in the irrigation technique may need to be made to enable older clients with motor and/or visual limitations to successfully do self-irrigation.
- Some older adults become upset if they do not have a daily bowel movement. With some irrigation routines, irrigation is not done daily, therefore the client will not have a daily bowel movement. Client needs to understand and accept this.

Home Care Considerations

- Assess home environment for bathroom privacy for ostomy care.
- Establish scheduled time (approximately 1 hour) for uninterrupted ostomy care.
- Assess bathroom for towel rack, hook, or other device from which irrigation device may be hung; end of irrigation solution bag should hang at shoulder level when client is sitting on the toilet.
- Irrigation sleeve may be attached by a belt, stick on, or by snapping directly onto the flange of the skin barrier. For home care, two-piece system is easier to use and more cost effective; it allows client to remove pouch from flange and then attach irrigation sleeve, then snap on a clean pouch or stoma cap when evacuation is completed.
- Tell clients if they travel in a foreign country that if they cannot drink the water, they should not irrigate with it.

SKILL 27-3 Pouching a Noncontinent Urinary Diversion

Because urine flows continuously from a noncontinent urinary diversion, a urinary pouch is usually placed over the opening immediately after surgery. Placement of the pouch may be more challenging than the enterostomy because urine flow keeps the skin moist and in the immediate postoperative period urinary stents may be in place in the stoma.

The stoma of a urinary diversion is normally red or pink. It is made from a portion of the gastrointestinal tract, either the ileum or the colon, and has the same mucosal surface. Ideally the stoma should protrude ½ to ¾ inch above the skin. An ileal conduit is usually located in the right lower quadrant; a colon conduit is usually located in the left lower quadrant. Ureterostomies are usually performed in infants, and a conduit is performed when the child approaches school age (see Fig. 27-2, p. 846).

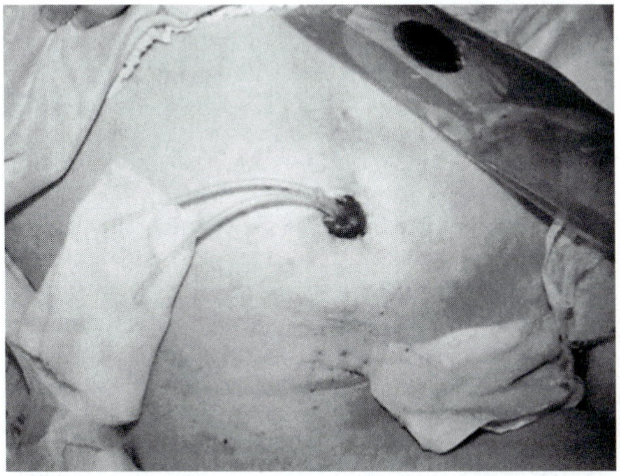

Fig. 27-5 Urinary stoma with stents. (From Broadwell DC, Jackson BS: *Prinicples of ostomy care*, St Louis, 1982, Mosby.)

EQUIPMENT

- **Pouch, urinary (with antireflex flap) and skin barrier NOTE: use two-piece system (pouch and flange) if stents are present (Fig. 27-5); use measuring guide to measure the stoma to determine the correct size of pouch and skin barrier.**

- Bedside urinary drainage bag
- Clean nonsterile disposable gloves
- Hand-held hair dryer
- Sterile gauze pads
- Towel or disposable waterproof barrier
- Basin with warm tap water
- Scissors
- Skin-sealant wipes
- Sterile forceps (if stents present)
- Vinegar

STEPS	RATIONALE
ASSESSMENT	
1. Check pouch for leakage; length of time in place; ask client about skin tenderness or discomfort. Check stoma for color, healing. Check abdominal incision (if present) for relationship to stoma for proper placement of pouch. To prevent skin irritation, pouch should be changed, if not leaking, every 3 to 7 days, or when checking for skin irritation. Stoma should be moist and reddish-pink; immediately after surgery it is edematous and usually has urinary stents in place.	Pouches should be emptied when one third to one half full since weight of urine in pouch may weaken or dislodge skin seal.
2. Observe output from stoma. Immediately after surgery, ureteral stents are in place and remain for 10 to 14 days. The physician then removes the stents.	Urinary output must be monitored on all postoperative clients with urinary diversions to monitor renal status and patency of stents; output should never be less than 30 ml/hr. Stents are used to maintain patency of ureters at anastomotic sites. These stents are sutured in place with dissolvable sutures.
3. Assess abdomen for best type of pouch to use. After pouch is off, assess skin around stoma, observing scars, folds, skin breakdown; also check peristomal suture line if present.	Maximizes secure fit and minimizes chance of leakage. Pouch and skin barrier are changed with any leakage. Determines need for barrier paste and additional intervention.
4. Determine client's emotional response, knowledge, and understanding of ostomy. Determine client's family and other significant support.	Helps determine extent client is able to participate in care, and need for teaching. Helps anticipate discharge needs.

NURSING DIAGNOSIS

Clustering of defining characteristics from the assessment data may reveal the following nursing diagnoses for clients requiring this skill:

- ➤ Body-image disturbance
- ➤ Risk for impaired skin integrity
- ➤ Knowledge deficit regarding ostomy self-care

Related factors are individualized based on a client's condition or needs.

STEPS	RATIONALE
PLANNING	
1. **Expected outcomes** following completion of procedure:	
➤ Stoma is moist, reddish-pink, oozes blood only slightly if rubbed. Peristomal skin is free of irritation and is intact. Sutures are intact, and incision is well approximated.	
➤ Urine drains freely from stents or stoma. Urine is yellowish with mucous shreds and is without foul odor. Volume of output is within acceptable limits (30 ml/hr).	These are normal findings in postoperative phase. The mucosal surface of the stoma is easily traumatized. Mucous shreds are normal when bowel is used as urinary diversion. Urine should flow freely if unobstructed.
➤ Client denies discomfort.	Reflects ongoing healing without complications.
➤ Client, family member, or significant other is willing to view stoma and asks questions about procedural steps.	Shows adjustment to body image change and willingness to learn self-care.
2. Assemble equipment.	Optimizes use of time; conserves client's and nurse's energy.

STEPS	RATIONALE
3. Close room curtains or door.	Provides privacy.
4. Explain procedure to client; encourage client's participation and questions.	Lessens anxiety and promotes client's participation.

IMPLEMENTATION

STEPS	RATIONALE
1. Position client standing or supine and drape. Some clients may prefer to do the pouch change while sitting as this may make it easier for them to see the stoma. However, when a skin barrier and pouch are applied in the sitting position, the skin may have folds and wrinkles. Because of this, skin barriers and pouches applied with the client in the sitting position may leak.	When client is supine fewer wrinkles occur, allowing for ease of pouch application; maintains client's dignity.
2. Prepare pouch by removing backing from barrier and adhesive; if using cut-to-fit, cut opening 1/16 to 1/8 inch larger than stoma before removing backing. Some urinary pouches have special skin barrier that melts and forms secure seal around base of stoma.	Barrier facilitates seal and protects skin; size of opening keeps urine off skin and lessens risk of maceration with skin irritation; avoids risk of damage to stoma. Stoma shrinks and does not reach optimal size for 6 to 8 weeks. Pouch and skin barrier is changed whenever leaking. Change when client is comfortable; better time is in morning on arising since urinary output is reduced.
3. Wash hands and apply gloves.	Reduces transmission of microorganisms.
4. Place towel or disposable waterproof barrier under client. Tightly roll several gauze pads separately (should resemble tampon). If gauze pads (called "wicks") come in contact with stents, roll with sterile gloves on. Place wicks on sterile barrier (can use inside of gauze wrapper).	Protects bed linen. Rolled gauze pads used to absorb urine during pouch change.
5. Remove used pouch carefully and gently by pushing the skin away from the barrier. If stents are present, *do not pull.* Immediately place a wick or sterile gauze pad over stomal opening. If stents are present, place sterile gauze pad underneath tips.	Reduces risk of trauma to skin and risk of injury to ureters if stents are present; jerking irritates skin and can cause skin tears. Keeps urine from leaking onto skin. Immediately after surgery copious mucus exists over stoma since bowel has not adjusted to presence of urine.
6. Cleanse peristomal skin gently with warm tap water using gauze pads; do not scrub the skin.	Avoid soap. It leaves residue on skin, which interferes with pouch adhesion. Pouch does not adhere to wet skin. Stents are sutured in place to decrease risk of damage. If blood appears on gauze pad used to cleanse skin, do not be alarmed since stomal surface may ooze blood if rubbed. Bleeding into the pouch is abnormal. Doing a vinegar soak removes the uric acid crystals that may be deposited on the peristomal skin.

➤ *CRITICAL DECISION POINT* If uric acid crystals are present on skin, apply a washcloth with a vinegar soak (1/3 vinegar and 2/3 warm water) to the peristomal skin. Rinse with warm tap water, dry completely by patting the skin with dry gauze or towel. Can use hand-held dryer set on cool. If copious mucus is on surface of stoma, carefully remove while stabilizing stents with sterile forceps.

STEPS	RATIONALE
7. Wick stoma continuously during pouch measurement and change. Place tip of gauze at the stomal opening. Measure the stoma.	Using a wick at the stoma tip prevents the peristomal skin from becoming wet with urine during the pouching change procedure.
a. If creases form next to stoma, use barrier paste to fill in; let dry 1 to 2 minutes.	

STEPS	RATIONALE
CRITICAL DECISION POINT **Barrier paste fills in the irregularities in the abdominal contour and helps with better adherence. For some clients, a pouch system with convexity may be needed.**	
b. Apply skin sealant in circular area around base of stoma to any skin not protected by barrier; let dry. Hold pouch by barrier, center over stoma and stents, and press down gently on barrier. Bottom of pouch should be angled slightly to attach to bedside urinary drainage bag. Use another skin sealant on skin coming in contact with adhesive; allow to dry. Press adhesive backing smoothly against the skin starting from the bottom and working up and around the sides. Never use a Karaya skin barrier with a urinary diversion.	Urine renders karaya ineffective and results in leakage.
c. Maintain gentle finger pressure around barrier for 1 to 2 minutes.	Helps to ensure molding and adherence of the skin barrier.
d. If using two-piece pouch, apply flange (barrier with adhesive) as above, then snap on pouch.	Urine drains almost continuously. Waterproofs any skin that may contact urine. Creates wrinkle-free secure seal. Angling pouch avoids uneven twisting, which can disrupt seal (if client is mostly out of bed, apply pouch vertically). Prevents trauma to skin.
8. During the night, open the drain spout, attach the specific manufacturer adaptor piece to the end of the pouch and then attach this to bedside urinary bag. Place the bag at a point close to the foot of the bed.	Constant flow of urine results in frequent emptying; overfilling of pouch may break skin seal. Placing bag at foot of bed maximizes straight drainage that avoids urine accumulation in the pouch.
CRITICAL DECISION POINT **Know the specific urinary equipment that is being used. Many urinary pouches need an adaptor piece that is specific to their brand to attach the urinary pouch to a bedside urinary drainage bag. Even within some manufacturers, the adaptor piece varies with the different types of urinary pouches available.**	Failure to use the correct adaptor piece causes leakage of urine.
9. Properly dispose of used pouch and soiled equipment.	Avoids odor in room.
CRITICAL DECISION POINT **Do *NOT* throw used pouch and skin barrier into the toilet. Most pouching equipment clogs the toilet.**	
10. Remove gloves; wash hands.	Reduces transmission of microorganisms.
11. Change skin barrier and pouch every 3 to 7 days unless leaking; pouch can remain in place for tub bath or shower; after bath pat adhesive dry or use hand-held dryer on cool.	Avoids unnecessary trauma to skin from too-frequent changes. Drying ensures adhesion of pouch.
EVALUATION	
1. Observe appearance of stoma, peristomal skin, suture line during pouch change.	Determines condition of stoma and peristomal skin and progress of wound healing.
2. Evaluate character and volume of urinary drainage.	Determines if stoma or stents are patent. Character of urine can reveal degree of concentration and alterations in renal function.
3. Ask if client notes discomfort around stoma.	Evaluates presence of skin irritation.

STEPS	RATIONALE
4. Observe client's, family member's, or significant other's willingness to view stoma and ask questions about procedure.	Determines level of adjustment and understanding of stoma care and pouch application.
5. **Unexpected outcomes** that may occur include:	
➤ Peristomal skin is irritated, reddened, tender, or has overgrowth. Maceration may be present. Stoma is necrosed (blackened and dry). Mucosal separation of stoma from skin (mucocutaneous suture line).	Can be caused by allergy to barrier and adhesive, mechanical trauma, infection. Opening of pouch may be too small or too large. Too small a skin barrier and pouch pressing into the stoma can cause cuts and bruises of the stoma. Peristomal necrosis can result from inadequate blood supply from excessively edematous stoma, suture line tension on bowel. Separation may be caused by infection, delayed wound healing, poor nutritional status, and other factors.
➤ No urinary output for several hours or output is less than 30 ml/hr. Urine has foul odor.	Obstruction of stents or stoma; compromised renal function. Alkaline urine has foul smell and predisposes client to infection, crystalization, stomal stenosis.
➤ Client reports burning sensation around base of stoma.	Peristomal skin irritation. Yeast infection around stoma causes itching, burning; appears as reddened area with maculopapular rash.
➤ Client, family member, or significant other is unable to observe stoma, ask questions, or participate in care.	Adjustment takes time, and process of grieving is individualized.

Recording and Reporting

1. Record type of pouch, time of change, condition and appearance of stoma and peristomal skin, character of urine.	Documents procedure. Provides data on condition of stoma and skin for future comparisons.
2. Record urinary output.	Provides ongoing record of fluid balance and functioning of urinary diversion.
3. Document client's, family's, or significant other's reaction to stoma, and level of participation. Some clients may have sexual dysfunction as a result of surgical exploration in the perineal area.	Allows staff to provide continuity of care while supporting client and family through grieving.
4. Report abnormalities in stoma or peristomal structures and absence of urinary output to nurse in charge or physician.	The sooner proper treatment is initiated, the less chance for the client to experience complications.

Follow-up Activities

1. Obtain referral for ET nurse.
2. Advise client of ostomy support groups.

• • • • •

Special Considerations

- Observe stoma for necrosis or separation during immediate postoperative phase.
- During hospitalization pouch may be connected to leg bag when client is out of bed.
- Some mucus is always present in the urine.
- Clients with cystectomy may experience sexual dysfunction and need intervention.

Teaching Considerations

- Give instruction according to client's level of understanding.
- Use opportunity to teach whenever doing pouch change even if client does not appear interested. *Do not* force client to look at stoma; allow time for adjustment.
- Teach clients significance and importance of drinking at least 2 quarts of water daily and of keeping urine acidic through intake of acid ash foods such as cranberry juice, cereals, poultry. Clients need to check this with physician (Walsh, 1992).
- Teach clients that some mucus in urine is expected; they should report any blood in their urine, excessively cloudy urine, chills, fever, and back pain to their physician.

- Client should be given a teaching manual with steps clearly stated, or audiotaped instructions.
- Clients should be given a list of equipment and the name, address, and phone number of a supplier in their community.

Pediatric Considerations

- In neonates, urinary diversions are less common than fecal ostomies (Boarini, 1989).
- The type of urostomy done in neonates is usually a ureterostomy. Because these stomas are very tiny, are flush to the skin and often in skin creases in the flank area, they are VERY difficult to pouch and maintain a good intact seal with the skin barrier and pouch. Sometimes the parents may decide not to use an ostomy pouching system. Because urine is less erosive to the skin than fecal effluent, some parents can opt to use diapers with good skin care to manage their baby's urostomy (Boarini, 1989).

Gerontologic Considerations

- Some older clients feel that they can cope with the continuous flow of urine from the stoma by decreasing the amount of fluid they drink so they will have less output. This can be very dangerous to client's health. Client needs appropriate teaching to change this misconception.
- Limitations in physical and visual ability may require adjustments in self-ostomy routine.

Home Care Considerations

- Assess home environment to assist client in arranging for privacy, adequacy of lighting, obtaining and storing equipment, and emergency assistance.
- At home, pouch spout should be opened and connected to straight drainage at night. Make sure client understands that using the wrong adaptor piece causes leakage.
- Many different types of pouching systems are available. Some are one piece and others two piece. All disposable pouches are odor proof and most have an antireflux valve. Clients should be encouraged to find a pouch that they can apply easily and that satisfies them.
- Clients should avoid placing pouches in extremely hot or cold locations since temperature may affect the barrier and adhesive materials.
- Pouch covers are available or can be easily made. Special underwear and sleep garments are also available.
- Clients may prefer to wear a leg bag during the day versus attaching to a bedside urinary drainage bag.
- Advise clients when they travel to always keep spare ostomy supplies with them in case luggage gets lost.
- While swimming, clients may find that applying waterproof tape to the skin barrier and/or wearing an ostomy belt prevents the pouch and skin barrier from becoming dislodged.
- Clients may wear usual clothes since urine is "pushed" through by peristaltic waves.

SKILL 27-4 Catheterizing a Noncontinent Urinary Diversion

Catheterization is performed to screen for infection and is the only way to obtain an accurate culture and sensitivity specimen (Chapter 43). When necessary to obtain a specimen from a urinary diversion, the best method is to insert a sterile double-tip catheter into the stoma. Obtaining a specimen from the pouch does not provide an accurate finding.

With the use of strict aseptic technique, catheterization is relatively safe and easy. To prevent trauma of tissues, the nurse should understand how the stoma and ureteral tract are constructed.

Reflux of urine can cause infection. Incorrect pouch placement, the use of a urinary pouch without an antireflux valve, stagnant urine, or large volumes of urine promote reflux. The risk for reflux of urine into the ureter can be reduced by attaching straight drainage to the urinary pouch during sleep or when high urinary output is expected. A client must understand the importance of draining the pouch frequently and using clean technique during stomal and skin care.

EQUIPMENT

Urinary catheterization supplies (may be contained in prepackaged sterile catheter kit or may need to be gathered separately). *All items must be sterile.*

- 14 to 16 Fr red rubber catheter (most use a double-tip catheter)
- Water-soluble lubricant
- Povidone-iodine swabs
- Sterile disposable gloves
- Sterile specimen container
- Gauze pads
- Bed protection barrier
- Towels
- Urinary diversion pouch (if client is using one-piece system; if using two-piece system, pouch can be snapped off for the procedure)
- Nonsterile disposable gloves

STEPS	RATIONALE
ASSESSMENT	
1. Determine need to perform catheterization to obtain a sterile specimen from urinary diversion; note signs and symptoms of urinary tract infection (UTI) such as elevated temperature, chills, foul-smelling urine, elevated WBC count.	Urinary diversion may pose risk for reflux of urine back to kidneys, resulting in infection.
2. Obtain physician's order for catheterization.	Invasive procedure requires physician's order.
3. Assess client's understanding of need for procedure and how procedure is done.	Determines willingness to cooperate and indicates extent of explanation nurse should provide.

NURSING DIAGNOSIS

Clustering of defining characteristics from the assessment data may reveal the following nursing diagnoses for clients requiring this skill:

- Risk for infection
- Knowledge deficit regarding urinary diversion catheterization

Related factors are individualized based on a client's condition or needs.

STEPS	RATIONALE
PLANNING	
1. **Expected outcomes** following completion of procedure:	
➤ No bacteria are present in urine.	No infection is present.
➤ Skin and stoma are intact, without signs of irritation.	Urinary pouch is intact.
➤ Client describes risks of infection and techniques to prevent infection.	Demonstrates client's learning.
2. Assemble equipment.	Optimizes use of time; conserves client's and nurse's energy.
3. Close room curtains or door.	Provides privacy.
4. Explain procedure to client; if possible attempt to obtain specimen when client is due to change pouch if using one-piece system.	Lessens anxiety and promotes client's cooperation. Changing pouch too frequently can result in skin breakdown.
IMPLEMENTATION	
1. Position client sitting, if possible, and drape towel across pelvic area.	Gravity facilitates flow of urine. Maintains client's dignity. Towel absorbs urine.
2. Wash hands and open barrier. Prepare several gauze wicks and place on edge of barrier. Apply nonsterile gloves.	Reduces transmission of microorganisms; wicks absorb urine from stomal opening.
3. Remove used pouch according to Skill 27-3, *Implementation, Steps 5 through 9.*	Protects skin from trauma.
4. Remove and discard gloves. Open sterile catheterization set according to instructions or open needed equipment and place on sterile barrier. If not using kit, place gauze pad on sterile field and squeeze small amount of lubricant onto gauze. If possible, have client wick stoma while waiting.	Avoids contamination.
5. Don sterile gloves. Cleanse "face" of stoma with povidone-iodine swabs using circular motion from center outward. Using new swab each time, repeat twice.	Removes surface bacteria.
6. Allow some urine to flow out of stoma.	Flushes povidone-iodine off face of stoma. Iodine in specimen alters results.
7. Lubricate catheter with water-soluble lubricant.	Lubricant facilitates passage of catheter through stoma.
8. Remove lid from specimen container. Place distal end of catheter into specimen container. Hold catheter in container with nondominant hand.	Only a few drops of urine are obtained; care should be used to direct all into container.

STEPS	RATIONALE
9. With dominant hand, gently insert catheter 2 to 2½ inches (5 to 6.5 cm) into stoma. If using a double-tip catheter, insert the catheter into the stoma first, then gently advance the inner catheter. Redirect course as needed. Use gentle but firm pressure similar to regular catheterization of urethra. Have client cough or turn slightly to facilitate passage of catheter.	Care must be taken to avoid perforation. Some resistance is common at muscle level in conduit. Allow catheter to enter slowly. May relax abdominal muscles.
10. Maintain container below level of stoma. Have client cough as needed. Urine may flow around and through catheter. This is acceptable, but only urine from catheter is desired. Normally, wait 5 minutes; if no urine is in container, pinch catheter and remove; direct urine "trapped" in catheter into cup.	Facilitates drainage of urine. Only 3 to 5 ml of urine is needed for culture and sensitivity studies.
11. After withdrawing catheter, place gauze pad over stoma.	Keeps skin dry.
12. Apply lid to specimen container. Remove gloves and label specimen with required information.	Prevents accidental spillage. Labeling ensures acceptance of specimen by laboratory and processing.
13. Reapply new pouch.	Pouch is necessary to contain urine; proper technique is important to avoid skin and stoma irritation.
14. Remove used pouch and equipment and dispose of properly.	Avoids unpleasant odor in room and eliminates source of bacterial colonization.
15. Wash hands and send specimen to laboratory at once.	Avoids transmission of infection. Allowing urine to sit for long periods at room temperature affects laboratory results.

EVALUATION

1. Refer to laboratory report and compare results of culture and sensitivity with normal expected findings. Remember that mucus is a normal finding in the urine of a client with an ileal or colon conduit.	Determines presence of infection. If contamination appears likely, second specimen will need to be sent.
2. Observe stoma and peristomal area for skin breakdown.	Exposure of skin to urine increases the risk of skin breakdown.
3. Check that urinary pouch and skin barrier are intact with no leakage.	A properly applied pouch and skin barrier that are the correct size minimize chance of leakage.
4. Ask client about signs and symptoms of UTI.	
5. **Unexpected outcomes** that may occur include:	
➤ Culture reveals evidence of bacteria in urine.	Infection is present.
➤ Skin or stoma reveals complications.	Indicates infection, allergy, urine leakage, mechanical trauma.
➤ Client is unable to describe risks of infection.	Indicates need for further instruction.

RECORDING AND REPORTING

1. Record time specimen collected, client's tolerance of procedure, appearance of urine, skin, stoma.	Documents procedure. Provides data for future comparison.
2. Report results of laboratory test to nurse in charge or physician.	Infection will require supportive therapies.

FOLLOW-UP ACTIVITIES

1. Monitor temperature, WBC count, urine characteristics.

Special Considerations

- Before beginning this procedure, become familiar with how to pouch a noncontinent urinary diversion (Skill 27-3).
- Only a small amount of urine will be obtained when inserting catheter if urinary diversion is functioning correctly.
- Unless contraindicated, give fluids to client 1 hour before procedure to increase urinary flow.
- Client may want to remove and apply appliance while nurse does actual catheterization. Client who is unable to cooperate may require some restraint to avoid contamination of specimen.
- Allow a 30-minute wait for specimen, especially if client has been NPO for intravenous pyelogram or other test, if possible. If client complains of severe pain or if urine flow is diminished, perforation of conduit or severe infection may be indicated.
- Avoid forcing catheter because conduit has no sensory fibers.
- Some pouches are reusable. Always check with client regarding what to do with the pouch, and assist as needed.
- Be patient and do not expect to obtain specimens as quickly as when catheterizing a urinary bladder.

Teaching Considerations

- Explain common symptoms of UTI: flank pain, dark or bloody urine, foul-smelling urine, fever, nausea.
- Encourage client to maintain fluid intake, and notify physician if symptoms of infection develop.
- Instruct client or primary care giver about clean technique during pouch application.
- Reinforce importance of fluid intake (2 liters/day).

SKILL 27-5 Maintaining a Continent Diversion

Continent diversions can be done to contain either urine or stool. These newer surgical procedures provide clients with the option of having an ostomy that does not spontaneously drain effluent, but rather must be drained from the internal pouch by the client. Figure 27-6 shows an example of an internal pouch created for a continent stool diversion. A more detailed description of the surgical procedure done to create an internal pouch for stool diversions can be found in the article by Hull and Erwin-Toth (1996). The pouch is emptied when the client inserts a catheter or tube into the external stoma to drain the stool. Because the ostomy is continent, the client does not have to wear an external ostomy pouch over the external stoma.

A continent urinary diversion is a reservoir or pouch that collects urine. Urine is evacuated only when a catheter is inserted into the stoma to empty the urine. This is unlike a conventional urinary diversion such as an ileal conduit, which serves only as a passageway for urine to flow to the outside of the abdomen. Many techniques are available for its construction using various portions of the small and/or large bowel (see Fig. 27-2, p. 846). Depending on the surgical technique used, the continent urinary diversion may be a Kock pouch, an Indiana continent urinary diversion, or some other type (Atta, 1991).

Because this reservoir is continent, the client does not have to wear an external pouch. The reservoir is intubated (or catheterized) at scheduled times to drain urine, and it must be irrigated. The opening (called a stoma) into the reservoir generally is placed in the right lower quadrant of the abdomen below where an ileal conduit would be. The stoma is flush with the skin or slightly budded and is reddish-pink. Skinfolds and creases do not present the same type problem as they would with an ileal conduit (Cavas and Makay, 1991).

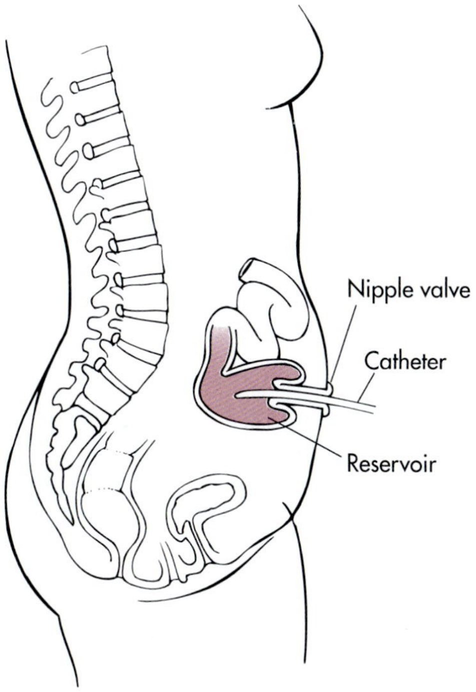

Fig. 27-6 A catheter is inserted and secured in the pouch before conclusion of the operation. (Modified from Hull, Erwin-Toth, *Journal of WOCN*, 1996, Mosby.)

EQUIPMENT

Varies with recovery phase. Postoperative care to 3 weeks:

- Sterile normal saline (NS)
- Sterile catheter tip irrigating syringe
- Sterile gauze pads
- Sterile gloves
- Povidone-iodine swabs
- Sterile specimen cup
- Sterile water
- Towels

Postoperative care 4 to 6 weeks:

- Sterile NS
- Sterile catheter tip irrigating syringe
- Sterile gauze pads
- Sterile gloves
- Povidone-iodine swabs
- Sterile basin
- Sterile 14 to 16 Fr red rubber catheter
- Water-soluble lubricant
- Stoma cover (commercial or Band-Aid or nonstick dressing)
- Liquid antimicrobial soap
- Towels

STEPS	RATIONALE
ASSESSMENT	
1. Observe all tubes for intactness and patency, nature of drainage, and connection to appropriate collection system. Label all collecting bags with origin of urine or drainage contained in them. Keep intake and output record.	Clients return immediately after surgery with a catheter in the stoma. Avoids errors in input and output record. Minimal acceptable urine output is 30 ml/hr from all sources.
➤ ***CRITICAL DECISION POINT*** **If client had a continent urinary diversion, then ureteral stents that exit through the stoma or another site on the abdomen will also be present; the stents are connected to a separate drainage system. Usually another large tube (e.g., a cecostomy) is placed into the pouch for extra drainage.**	
2. Observe stoma for color, peristomal skin for maceration, and all external suture lines.	Determines potential problems and reflects healing progress.
3. Assess bowel sounds and lung sounds. Assess serum values of chloride and creatinine.	Manipulation of large portions of bowel may lead to an ileus. Underventilation by client after surgery may lead to respiratory complications. Immediately after surgery, intestinal segment used for reservoir may absorb chloride and hydrogen ions. Creatinine measures effectiveness of kidney function (Golomb, Klutke, and Raz, 1989).
4. Palpate lightly around the stoma, noting any localized tenderness or guarding.	May be sign of infection along the internal suture lines.
5. Determine client's emotional response, knowledge, and understanding of continent reservoir or pouch, family and other significant support.	Helps determine extent client is able to participate in care, and need for teaching. Assists in anticipating discharge needs.

NURSING DIAGNOSIS

Clustering of defining characteristics from the assessment data may reveal the following nursing diagnoses for clients requiring this skill:

- ➤ Altered patterns of elimination (either urinary or bowel)
- ➤ Body-image disturbance
- ➤ Risk for impaired skin integrity
- ➤ Knowledge deficit regarding ostomy self-care

Related factors are individualized based on a client's condition or needs.

STEPS	RATIONALE
PLANNING	
1. **Expected outcomes** following completion of procedure:	
➤ Stoma is moist, reddish-pink, oozes blood only slightly if rubbed. Peristomal skin is free of irritation and intact. Sutures are intact, and incision is well approximated. Client denies discomfort.	These are normal findings in postoperative phase. Reflects ongoing healing without complications.
➤ Effluent is normal depending on type of continent diversion:	
• Urine drains freely from stents, stomal catheter, or intubation catheter. Urine is yellowish with mucous shreds and is without foul odor. Volume of output is within acceptable limits.	Mucous shreds are normal when bowel is used as reservoir. Urine should flow freely if unobstructed.
• Stool is brown, semiformed.	
➤ Client has no pain at the stoma or the peristomal skin.	Pain might be an indicator of infection.
➤ Client, family member, or significant other is willing to view stoma and asks questions about procedural steps.	Shows adjustment to body image change and willingness to learn self-care.
➤ Client is able to intubate and irrigate pouch before discharge.	Reflects comprehensive teaching. Continent diversion requires a knowledgeable client to maintain optimal functioning. If unable to care for self, client is at risk for complications.
2. Assemble equipment.	Optimizes use of time; conserves client's and nurse's energy.
3. Close room curtains or door.	Provides privacy.
4. Explain procedure to client; encourage client's interaction and questions.	Lessens anxiety and promotes client's participation.
IMPLEMENTATION	
POSTOPERATIVE CARE TO 3 WEEKS	
1. Position client supine or sitting and drape with towels.	Facilitates instilling NS into reservoir; sitting is a better position for drainage. Maintains client's dignity.
2. Wash hands and open sterile equipment. Remove lid from sterile specimen cup and place lid with open side up. Pour 20 to 30 ml sterile NS into sterile specimen cup. Open sterile syringe and povidone-iodine swabs and position them for use.	Reduces transmission of microorganisms.
3. Put on sterile gloves and draw 20 to 30 ml sterile NS into syringe. Cleanse connection point of indwelling stomal catheter and drainage tubing with povidone-iodine swabs using a circular motion; use each swab once; wait 30 seconds.	Reduces risk of nosocomial infection.
4. Disconnect and gently irrigate stomal catheter; do not contaminate tip of drainage tubing.	Large numbers of internal anastomotic sites require strict asepsis during postoperative phase.
➤ ***CRITICAL DECISION POINT*** **Do not aspirate since this increases risk of damage to internal suture lines. Irrigation maintains patency of stomal catheter since large amount of mucus is secreted initially by reservoir (Davidson, 1990).**	
5. Reconnect drainage system. Record volume used for irrigation. For urinary diversions, subtract this from total urine output at end of each shift. Follow hospital protocol for changing bedside urinary drainage bags.	Keeps accurate urinary output record. Reduces risk of colonization of microorganisms.

STEPS	RATIONALE
6. Using remaining povidone-iodine swabs, cleanse the "face" of the stoma around the catheter. Use another swab and cleanse the skin around the base of the stoma; allow to dry 30 seconds and gently remove iodine with a gauze pad moistened with sterile water.	Mucus accumulates on the face of the stoma and seeps onto the skin. Maintains skin integrity and reduces risk of infection. Some clients are allergic to iodine.
7. Discard soiled equipment; remove gloves. Maintain sterile specimen cup and sterile NS, water containers for next irrigation. Label these with date, time, nurse's initials. NOTE: Hospital protocols vary; generally, immediately after surgery continent diversions are irrigated every 2 to 4 hours to maintain patency of the stomal catheter, allowing urine to drain freely.	Reduces transmission of microorganisms. Maintains sterility of cup so it can be used for 8 hours; helps reduce costs. Some supplies can stay at bedside for 8 hours if strict aseptic technique is followed; this helps contain costs.

POSTOPERATIVE CARE OF 4 TO 6 WEEKS

STEPS	RATIONALE
1. Follow steps 1 and 2 in preceding section. Omit setting up sterile specimen cup.	Generally stomal catheter is removed the third postoperative week.
2. Open sterile basin and maintain inside of wrapper as sterile field. Pour 30 to 60 ml of sterile N/S into basin. Open gauze pads onto sterile wrapper; squeeze small amount of water-soluble lubricant onto gauze pad. Open wrapper of sterile red catheter for use or place catheter onto sterile basin wrapper.	Maintains strict aseptic technique to reduce risk of nosocomial infection during the recovery phase.
3. Apply sterile gloves and draw 30 to 60 ml of sterile NS into syringe. Cleanse "face" of stoma with povidone-iodine swab starting from center and using circular movements to outer edge; wait 30 seconds.	Reduces risk of nosocomial infection; removes any accumulation of mucus.
4. Lubricate catheter well. Insert into stoma by gently rotating during insertion; insert until urine starts to drain.	Reduces trauma to continence mechanism (valve) during insertion; some resistance to insertion is normal as the catheter passes through the layer of abdominal fascia. The client may need to change position to facilitate insertion. Taking slow, deep breaths also helps (Davidson, 1990).
5. If no effluent starts to drain, problem solving is needed. The illustration can be used to help solve the problem of inadequate effluent from the pouch. For example, try moving catheter in and out slightly. If this is unsuccessful, irrigate the pouch as in Skill 27-2, Step 7 under *Implementation*. If this is a scheduled time for irrigation, proceed after effluent has drained and irrigate with 30 to 60 ml of sterile NS; allow to drain.	Mucus may plug the catheter. Continent diversions must be irrigated at scheduled times.
6. Before withdrawing the catheter, have the client cough three or four times, then slowly remove.	Positive pressure inside the abdomen clears residual urine from the pouch and continence valve; clears mucus from catheter.
7. Gently cleanse the peristomal skin with gauze pads and liquid antimicrobial soap; rinse; pat dry.	Reduces bacterial colonization and removes any dried mucus to maintain skin integrity.
8. Cover stoma with stomal covering.	Some leakage of effluent occurs until full recovery from the surgery; mucus will always be produced.
9. Discard soiled equipment; remove gloves. Maintain sterile NS, label with date, time, nurse's initials.	Reduces transmission of microorganisms. Some equipment can stay at bedside for 8 hours if strict aseptic technique is followed; this helps reduce costs.

STEPS	RATIONALE
10. Record output and amount used for irrigation. NOTE: Postoperative week 3: stoma is intubated every 2 to 3 hours and once at night to drain urine; it is irrigated every 4 hours. A schedule should be known to the client and to all care givers. A time card at the bedside facilitates this. Week 4 through 5: intubate every 4 hours and PRN at night; irrigate bid and PRN. Fully recovered client with continent urinary diversion must intubate (or be intubated if unable to do) every 4 hours and PRN at night; irrigate bid and PRN. Physician's protocols may vary somewhat.	Keeps accurate output record. The scheduled intubation times allow for gradual expansion of the pouch. Pouches or reservoirs vary as to maximum amount of urine they can hold after complete recovery; may range from 150 to 600 ml. Reservoirs constructed from bowel always secrete mucus and must be routinely irrigated.

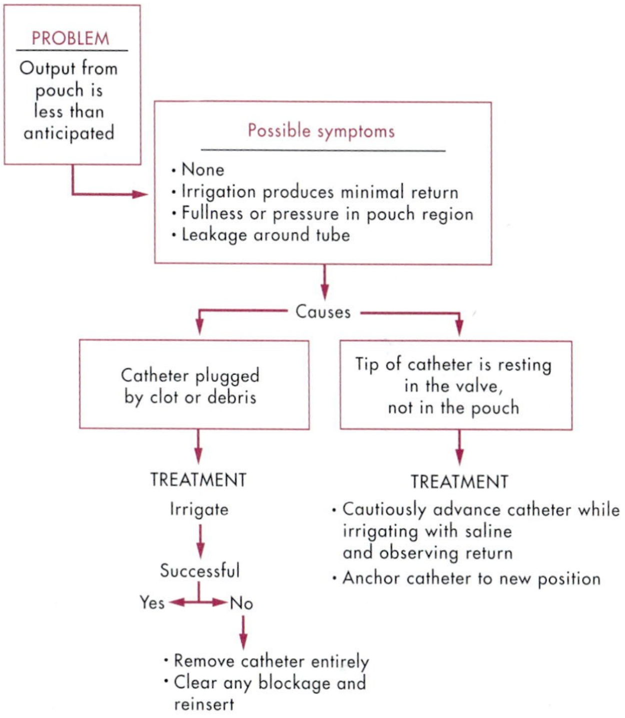

Step 5 Problem solving when output from the pouch is lower than anticipated. (Modified from Hull, Erwin-Toth, *Journal of WOCN,* 1996, Mosby.)

EVALUATION

STEPS	RATIONALE
1. Note appearance of stoma, peristomal skin, abdominal suture lines.	Determines condition of stoma and peristomal skin and progress of wound healing.
2. Evaluate character and volume of output.	Determines if stomal catheter, stents, and residual catheter (e.g., cecostomy tube) are patent. Alerts nurse for need to irrigate stomal catheter. Minimal urinary output is 30 ml/hr.
3. Palpate for discomfort over pouch site and over peristomal skin.	May indicate large amount of residual urine or infection. Determines if any skin irritation is present.
4. Observe client's, family member's, or significant other's willingness to participate in care.	Determines level of adjustment, need for teaching, and risk for complications.
5. **Unexpected outcomes** that may occur include:	
➤ Continence valve leaks excessively and continuously after stomal catheter is removed.	Dysfunction of valve is major complication that may result from stricture of stoma, incomplete healing, anastomotic leaks, failure to empty reservoir at scheduled times (overdistention), damage from improper catheter insertion (perforation).
➤ Intubation cannot be performed.	Catheter enters area of valve's interior wall; overdistention of pouch causes pressure against valve.
➤ Stool is especially thick.	Encourage client not to take a laxative but rather to increase daily fluid intake including intake of prune juice (Hull and Erwin-Toth, 1996).
➤ Client's renal function is compromised with abnormal creatinine values; electrolyte status may be affected.	Failure of antirefluxing anastomoses between ureters and reservoir occurs. Intestinal reservoirs absorb chloride and hydrogen ions.

STEPS	RATIONALE
➤ Bacterial contamination of urine or alkaline pH of urine may occur.	Frequent intubation and irrigation increase risk for bacterial invasion. Alkaline urine has strong, foul odor, and it predisposes client to infection, crystalization of urine, stomal stenosis, pouchitis.
➤ Client reports heavy, full, aching sensation over pouch.	May be internal leakage of effluent from anastomotic sites with leakage into peritoneal cavity; infected anastomotic sites; possible peritonitis, pouchitis.
➤ Skin is irritated in peristomal area and macerated. Stoma is necrosed (blackened and dry).	Moisture from mucus on skin predisposes to irritation and infection. Inadequate blood supply may result from excessive edema of structures or suture line tension.
➤ No urinary output occurs for several hours, or output is less than 30 ml/hr.	Obstruction of catheter or valve or reduced renal function occurred. Client also may be dehydrated.
➤ Client, family member, or significant other is unable to observe stoma, ask questions, or participate in care.	Adjustment takes time, and process of grieving is individualized.

Recording and Reporting

1. Record time of irrigation and/or intubation, size of catheter used, ease of intubation, amount of NS used, amount and character of output, and client's tolerance.	Documents procedure; provides data on condition of valve, urinary output, and potential complications.
2. Document client's, family's, and significant other's responses and their level of participation in care.	Allows staff to provide continuity of care while supporting client through adjustment phase.
3. Report abnormalities of stoma and peristomal skin.	Allows for prompt intervention.

Follow-up Activities

1. Obtain referral for ET nurse.
2. Advise client of ostomy support groups.
3. Before discharge obtain a Medic-Alert bracelet or necklace with the following message: "Continent urinary or stool diversion; must insert catheter to drain every 4 hours" (Heneghan et al., 1990).

• • • • •

Special Considerations

- ➤ Observe stoma in immediate postoperative period for necrosis or separation.
- ➤ During immediate postoperative period catheters are connected to bedside urinary drainage bags.
- ➤ Some mucus will always be present in the urine when a portion of bowel is used.
- ➤ Clients with cystectomy may experience sexual dysfunction and need intervention and follow-up in this area (Salter, 1992).
- ➤ In addition to scheduled irrigations, scheduled emptying times *must* be followed to avoid risk of complications.

Teaching Considerations

- ➤ Give instruction according to client's level of understanding and ability and readiness.
- ➤ Use the opportunity to teach whenever doing pouch irrigation or intubation even if client does not appear interested. Do not force the client to look at stoma; allow time for adjustment.
- ➤ Include family member or significant other in teaching if possible.
- ➤ Client should be given a teaching manual with steps clearly stated, or audiotaped instructions. For someone with a learning disability, a "picture book" of steps may be more appropriate.
- ➤ Client should be given a list of equipment and the name, address, and phone number of a supplier in the community.
- ➤ Teach clients that some mucus in the urine is expected; they should report any blood in urine, excessively cloudy urine, chills, fever, and back pain to physician immediately.
- ➤ Teach clients to do Kegel exercises (Hull and Erwin-Toth, 1996).

Gerontologic Considerations

- ➤ Clients should be carefully assessed preoperatively for their suitability for having a continent diversion. Clients must have the physical, visual, and mental ability to intubate the stoma and drain the internal pouch on prescribed schedule.

Home Care Considerations

- Teach clients proper care of intubation catheters: After use, rinse inside to clear any mucus and wash with warm, soapy water; rinse well inside and out; suspend catheter so that it hangs to dry. Dry completely and keep in a clean plastic bag or toothbrush holder container.
- Clients must always carry their catheter with them.
- Teach clients to *not* use petroleum-based products for lubricating the catheter since this increases the risk of infection; client may use plain warm tap water or water-soluble lubricant (preferred). May use plain warm tap water to irrigate after week 6 (this may vary with physician's protocol).
- Discard catheter after 1 month's use.
- Taking deep breaths facilitates intubation since it helps to relax abdominal muscles; massaging the lower abdomen aids emptying; coughing periodically while draining effluent helps clear mucus from catheter because of increasing positive pressure.
- Client must always wear Medic-Alert bracelet or necklace.
- Keeping a small card in pocket or purse with time schedule for intubation and irrigation is a helpful reminder.
- Client may use moist towel or nonalcohol towelette to cleanse face of stoma before intubation; may use catheter-tip syringe or bulb syringe for irrigation.
- Client can sit on stool or stand next to a sink to perform irrigation and intubation. Teach client to not let end of catheter come in contact with fixtures or water in toilet or sink.

CRITICAL THINKING EXERCISES

1. The parents of a pediatric client with an incontinent ileostomy state, "We don't understand why we just can't diaper our baby." What would be an appropriate answer by the nurse? Explain the rationale behind the nurse's response.
2. During a colostomy irrigation, a client complains of cramping in the abdomen. What should be done at this time and why?
3. State the physiological reasons for use of a wick when changing a pouch on a client with a noncontinent urinary diversion.
4. A client who needs to have a urinary diversion asks the nurse about the differences between a continent and noncontinent urinary diversion. How should the nurse respond?
5. An older client with a transverse colostomy is having leakage from the skin barrier. What nursing assessments are important to make at this time? Explain why.

REFERENCES

Atta MA: A new technique for continent urinary reservoir reconstruction, *J Urol* 145:960, 1991.

Bastawrous AAL, et al: Trends in pediatric ostomy surgery: Intestinal diversion for necrotizing enterocolitis and biliary diversion for biliary hypoplasia syndromes, *JWOCN,* 22(6):280, 1995.

Boarini JH: Principles of stoma care for infants, *J Enterostom Ther* 16(1):21, 1989.

Brown KC, Ricketts RR: Current management of the neonatal patient with an ostomy. *Progressions,* 6(3):3, 1994.

Cavas M, Makay S: The Indiana pouch, *AORN* 54:494, 1991.

Cohen A: Body image in the person with a stoma, *J Enterostom Ther* 18:68, 1991.

Davidson MW, et al: Continent Indiana reservoir: nursing management, *Ostomy/Wound Manag* 31:50, 1990.

Foster ME: Surgical options for managing chronic fecal incontinence in children, *Progressions,* 7(1):13, 1995.

Golis AM: Sexual issues for the person with an ostomy, *JWOCN* 23:1, 1996.

Golomb J, Klutke CG, Raz S: Complications of bladder substitution and continent urinary diversion, *Urol* 34:329, 1989.

Halvorson ML, Kertz JM: Changes in Medicare reimbursement for ostomy supplies: An overview, *JWOCN,* 23:26, 1996.

Heneghan GM, et al.: The Indiana pouch: A continent urinary diversion, *J Enterostom Ther* 17:231, 1990.

Hull TL, Erwin-Toth P: The pelvic pouch procedure and continent ostomies: Overview and controversies, *JWOCN,* 23(3):156, 1996.

Kulka S, Kristijanson LJ: Development and testing of the ostomy concerns scale: Measuring ostomy-related concerns of cancer patients and their partners, *JWOCN,* 23(3):166, 1996.

McConnell EA: How to irrigate a colostomy, *Nursing '90* 20:78, 1990.

Piper B, Mikols C: Predischarge and postdischarge concerns of persons with an ostomy, *JWOCN* 23(2):105, 1996.

Piper B, Mikols C, Grant TRD: Comparing adjustment to an ostomy for three groups, *JWOCN,* 23(4):197, 1996.

Quayle BK: Making positive choices: Body image and the new ostomy patient, *Ostomy/Wound Manag* 40:4, 1994.

Ramos L, Glosson A: Teaching ostomy care to a patient who is blind, *JWOCN,* 23(4):235, 1996.

Rolstad BS, Boarini J: Principles and techniques in the use of convexity, *Ostomy/Wound Manag* 42:1, 1996.

Salter MJ: Aspects of sexuality for patients with stomas and continent pouches, *J Enterostom Ther* 19:126, 1992.

Walsh BA: Urostomy and urinary pH, *J Enterostom Ther* 19:110, 1992.

Walsh BA, et al.: Multidisciplinary management of altered body image in the patient with an ostomy. *JWOCN,* 22(5):227, 1995.

UNIT X

Posture, Mobility, and Ambulation

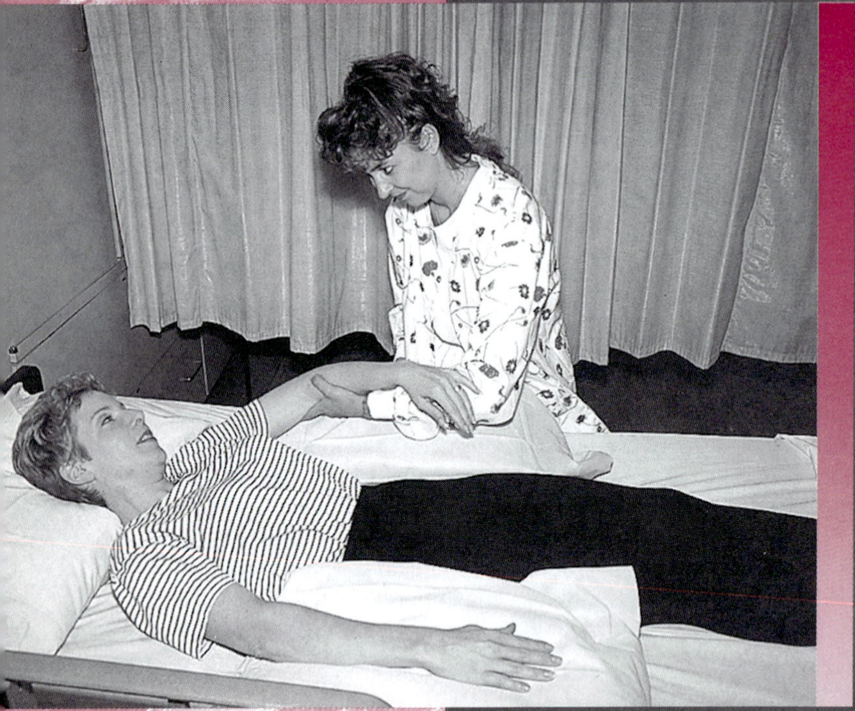

CHAPTER 28

Body Alignment and Mechanics

OBJECTIVES

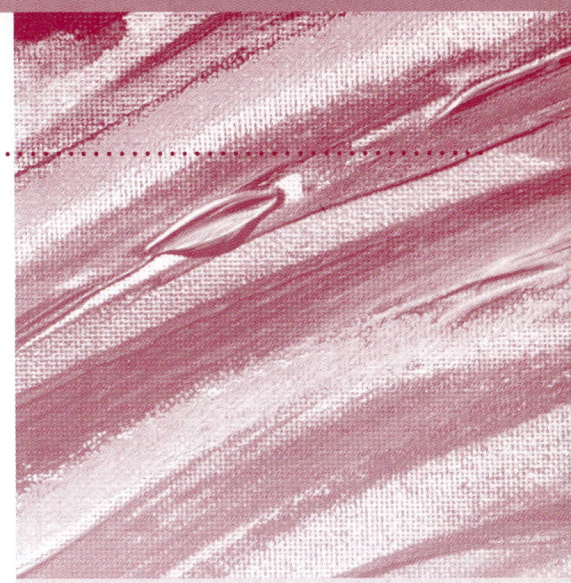

Mastery of content in this chapter will enable the nurse to:

- Define key terms.
- Describe body mechanics and its importance in caring for clients.
- Describe normal body alignment for standing, sitting, and lying down.
- Assess for alterations in body alignment.
- Describe procedures for lifting.

KEY TERMS

Balance
Base of support
Body alignment
Body mechanics
Center of gravity
Gravity
Leverage
Line of gravity
Posture
Turning sheet
Weight

SKILLS

28-1 Maintaining Body Alignment

28-2 Performing Safe and Efficient Lifting Techniques

Coordinated body movement involves the integrated function of the skeletal system, skeletal muscles, and nervous system. Because these systems cooperate so closely in the mechanical support of the body, they can almost be considered a single functional unit. The skeleton and skeletal muscles contribute in part to the body's shape.

The skeleton is the supporting framework of the body and consists of 206 bones. The four types of bones in the skeleton are long, short, flat, and irregular. Long bones contribute to height (e.g., femur, fibula, tibia in the leg) and length (e.g., phalanges of the fingers and toes). Short bones (e.g., carpal bones in the foot) occur in clusters and, when combined with ligaments and cartilage, usually permit movement of the extremities. Flat bones (e.g., bones in the skull, ribs in the thorax) provide structural contour. Irregular bones make up the vertebral column and some bones of the skull, such as the mandible.

The muscles associated primarily with movement are located near the skeletal region, where leverage results in movement. **Leverage** is an inducing or compelling force. Leverage occurs when specific bones, such as the humerus, ulna, and radius, and the associated joints, such as the elbow joint, act together as a lever. Thus force is applied to one end of the bone to lift a **weight** as another point tends to rotate the bone in the direction opposite that of the applied force. The skeletal muscles that attach to the bones of leverage provide the necessary strength to move the object.

Muscles associated primarily with maintaining posture are short and shaped like a feather because they converge obliquely at a common tendon. Muscles of the lower extremities, trunk, neck, and back are associated primarily with posture. These muscle groups work together to stabilize and support body weight when a person is standing or sitting.

Movement and posture are regulated by the nervous system. The major area of the nervous system that controls voluntary motor function is the precentral gyrus or motor strip, which is located in the cerebral cortex. Thus the motor fibers from the right motor strip initiate voluntary movement for the left side of the body and vice versa for the right side.

Body mechanics is the coordinated effort of the musculoskeletal and nervous systems to maintain **balance, posture,** and **body alignment** during lifting, bending, moving, and performing activities of daily living. Body mechanics also facilitates body movement so that a person can carry out a physical activity without using excessive muscle energy.

The knowledge and application of body mechanics enable the nurse to care safely for clients with varying levels of independent mobility throughout the life span. Knowledge and practice of body mechanics protect the client and nurse from injury to their musculoskeletal systems.

Application of body mechanics enables the nurse to use correct muscle groups when completing nursing care. Thus the nurse is able to position, transfer, and help clients ambulate safely and efficiently. In addition, this knowledge provides the nurse with a basis for assessing a client's body alignment and position and further reduces the risks related to immobility.

GUIDELINES

1. Know the physiological influences on body alignment and mobility that affect clients throughout the life span. The greatest impact of the physiological changes on the musculoskeletal system is observed in the early and later years of life. In the child, the major consequences of decreased muscle activity are loss of muscle strength, endurance, muscle mass, and joint mobility; bone demineralization; and contracture. Inactive older adults are at risk for muscle atrophy, loss of bony mass, contractures of joints, and pressure ulcers.
2. Know the pathological conditions that affect a client's body alignment and mobility. Postural abnormalities can affect body mechanics. For example, a client with severe kyphosis may not be able to lift an object safely because the **center of gravity** is not aligned. Diseases affecting bone formation (e.g., osteoporosis) alter body alignment and mobility. Degenerative joint diseases (e.g., osteoarthritis), impaired muscle development (e.g., muscular dystrophy), and central nervous system damage (e.g., paralysis) can interfere with normal body alignment and mobility. Therefore the client's risk of musculoskeletal injury is increased.
3. Know the client's medical history and determine if the client is taking medications that can affect body alignment. For example, tranquilizers can affect coordination and steroids can affect bone formation.
4. Control factors that can indirectly affect body mechanics by altering the safety of the environment. Cluttered hallways and bedside areas increase the client's risk of falling (see Chapters 4 and 41).
5. Use an organized, systematic approach to assess and improve body mechanics. Continued nursing assessment promptly identifies risks to normal body alignment and promotes immediate nursing interventions.
6. Safe and knowledgeable use of equipment, ambulatory aids, and accessible supplies for client positioning and comfort indirectly contributes to the mechanical protection of the client and nurse.

DELEGATION CONSIDERATIONS

The skills of maintaining body alignment and mechanics and proper lifting can be delegated to unlicensed, assistive personnel.

- Caution care provider to elevate bed to waist level.
- Inform care provider in proper body mechanics.
- Inform care provider in proper body alignment.
- Instruct care provider to seek assistance when moving or lifting heavy objects.

SKILL 28-1 Maintaining Body Alignment

The term *body alignment* refers to the conditions of the joints, tendons, ligaments, and muscles in various body positions. When the body is aligned, whether standing, sitting, or lying, no excessive strain is placed on these structures. Body alignment means the body is in line with the pull of **gravity** and contributes to body balance. Without this balance, the center of gravity is displaced, which increases the force of gravity and predisposes the person to falls and injuries.

Body balance is achieved when a wide **base of support** exists, the center of gravity falls within the base of support, and a vertical line can be drawn from the center of gravity through the base of support. Body balance also is enhanced by posture. The more aligned the posture, the greater the balance. Clinical nursing activities require the nurse to maintain body alignment. It is essential for the nurse to provide an opportunity for the client to observe correct posture and to identify the client's learning needs for maintaining body alignment. In addition, the nurse needs to identify trauma, muscle damage, or nerve dysfunction in the client.

STEPS	RATIONALE
ASSESSMENT	
1. Observe alignment of client in standing, sitting, or lying position.	
2. **STANDING** (see illustration):	Determines if client assumes body alignment.
a. Head is erect and at midline.	Maintains body alignment in relation to body's normal center of gravity.
b. Shoulders and hips are straight and parallel.	
c. Vertebral column appears straight when viewed posteriorly.	
d. Lateral observation indicates head is erect and spinal curves are aligned in reverse-S pattern.	In reverse-S pattern, cervical vertebrae are anteriorly convex, thoracic vertebrae are posteriorly convex, and lumbar vertebrae are anteriorly convex.
e. Lateral observation indicates that abdomen is comfortably tucked in and knees and ankles are slightly flexed.	Maintains abdomen and trunk directly over body's center of gravity.
f. Arms are comfortably positioned at each side.	
g. Feet are placed slightly apart, with toes pointed forward.	Produces broad base of support and improves balance.
h. Center of gravity is located midline and forms vertical line from middle of forehead to midpoint between feet. A pregnant woman's center of gravity is more anterior to adapt to normal weight gain and growing fetus. Thus she leans slightly backward, and spinal column is slightly sway-backed (see illustration).	Laterally, **line of gravity** runs vertically from middle of skull to posterior one third of foot.
3. **SITTING** (see illustration):	
a. Head is erect, and vertebrae are in straight alignment.	Prevents stress on intravertebral joints.
b. Body weight is evenly distributed on buttocks and thighs.	Prevents increased pressure over bony prominences and reduces damage to underlying musculoskeletal system.

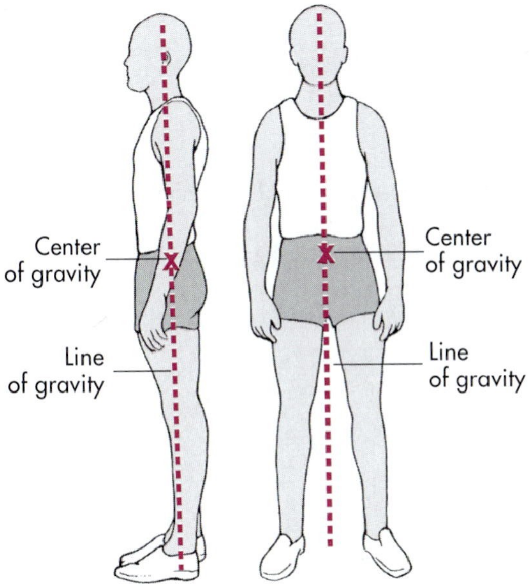

Step 2 Body alignment when standing.

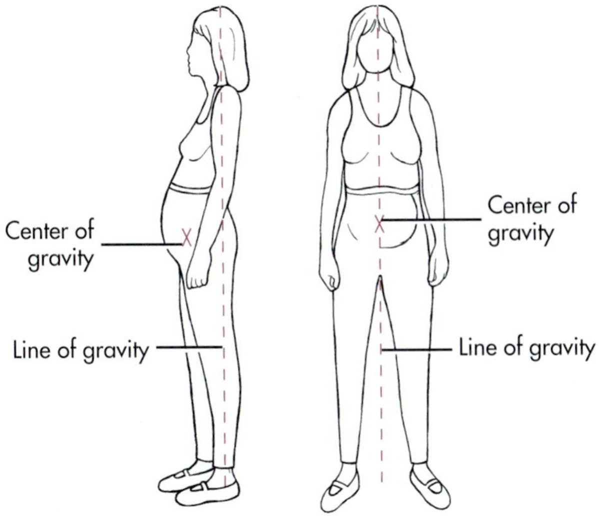

Step 2h Center of gravity in pregnant woman.

STEPS	RATIONALE
c. Thighs are parallel and in horizontal plane.	Maintains flexion of hips and provides broad base of support.
d. Both feet are supported on floor and ankles are comfortably flexed.	Maintains plantar flexion and reduces risk of footdrop.

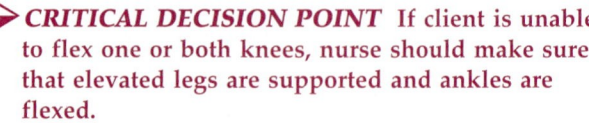

CRITICAL DECISION POINT **If client is unable to flex one or both knees, nurse should make sure that elevated legs are supported and ankles are flexed.**

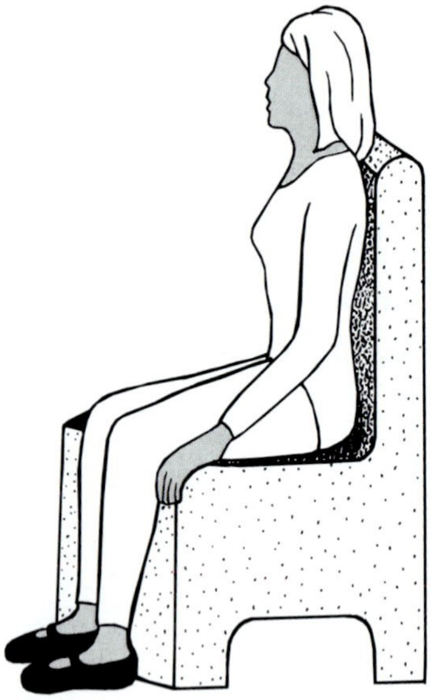

Step 3 Center of gravity when sitting.

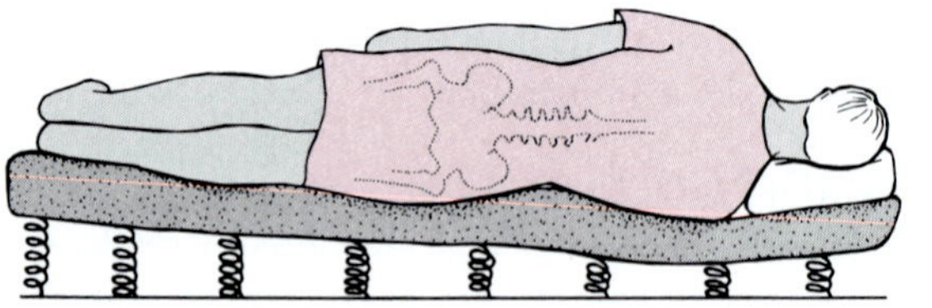

Step 4 Body alignment in lateral position.

STEPS	RATIONALE
e. A 2.5 to 5 cm (1 to 2 inch) space is maintained between edge of seat and popliteal space on posterior surface of knee.	Ensures that no excessive pressure is placed on popliteal artery or nerve, which could decrease circulation or impair nerve function.
f. Client's forearms should be supported on armrest, in lap, or on table in front of chair.	Reduces force of gravity on shoulder joint and chance of accidental shoulder dislocation.
4. LYING (see illustration):	
a. Client is in lateral position, with positioning supports removed.	Allows nurse to observe spinal alignment and any pressure points.
b. Client's body should be supported by adequate mattress.	Reduces strain on joints and ligaments.
c. Vertebral column should be in alignment without observable curves.	Allows for even distribution of body weight.

NURSING DIAGNOSIS

Clustering of defining characteristics from the assessment data may reveal the following nursing diagnoses for clients requiring this skill:

- Impaired physical mobility
- Knowledge deficit concerning body mechanics
- Knowledge deficit concerning proper positioning
- Risk for activity intolerance
- Risk for disuse syndrome
- Risk for impaired skin integrity
- Risk for injury

Related factors are individualized based on a client's condition or needs.

STEPS	RATIONALE
PLANNING	
1. **Expected outcomes** following completion of procedure:	
➤ Body is positioned without skin surfaces being exposed to undue pressure.	Extremities are not crossed or aligned to cause pressure.
➤ While sitting, lying, or standing, client aligns body straight and in correct position.	Avoids strain on musculoskeletal structures.
➤ Client is able to explain benefits of body alignment.	Increases likelihood of good postural habits being followed.
2. Instruct client or care giver on proper body alignment for standing, sitting, or lying.	Provides client or care giver with necessary knowledge to identify potential altered body alignment.
IMPLEMENTATION	
1. Demonstrate to client and caregiver correct body alignment for standing, sitting, and lying.	Demonstration is reliable technique for teaching psychomotor skills and enables client and caregiver to ask questions.
2. Provide opportunity for return demonstration.	Allows evaluation of client or family learning.
3. Discuss with client and care giver the hazards of prolonged immobility on body alignment and mobility (see Chapter 8).	Alerts client and caregiver to early assessment factors associated with incorrect body alignment and impaired mobility.
4. Provide client and care giver with resources (e.g., community health agency, physician) to contact when mobility or body alignment is impaired.	Alerts resource persons to assist with minor problems of body alignment before severe, irreversible problems occur.
EVALUATION	
1. Inspect skin surfaces.	Reveals pressure sites.
2. Have client demonstrate body alignment for standing, sitting, and lying.	Return demonstration reveals if learning occurred.
3. Ask client to describe benefits of body alignment.	Evaluates cognitive learning.
4. **Unexpected outcomes** that may occur include:	
➤ Incorrect body alignment is indicated by poor posture or decreased joint mobility.	Indicates need for follow-up learning activities.
➤ Damage to skin and musculoskeletal system (e.g., pressure sore, contracture) occurs.	
RECORDING AND REPORTING	
1. Record information presented to client and client's progress toward learning selected knowledge.	Documents client teaching with plan of care.
2. Report information taught to client at change of shift.	Alerts oncoming nursing personnel to information already presented.

FOLLOW-UP ACTIVITIES

1. Review care plan with client and care giver and modify as needed.

• • • • •

Special Considerations

- Clients with lower extremity weakness, paralysis, or immobilization are at risk for musculoskeletal trauma because of uneven or prolonged distribution of body weight.
- Clients with upper extremity weakness or paralysis are at risk for shoulder dislocation if the forearms are unsupported.
- Clients with impaired mobility, decreased sensation, or lack of voluntary muscle control are at risk for musculoskeletal damage and must have their positions changed frequently.

Teaching Considerations

- Shorter clients should be taught to use a footstool when sitting.
- Clients at risk for thrombophlebitis, such as postoperative or postpartum clients or clients taking

anticoagulants or medication that can increase platelet production, should be taught to maintain space between edge of chair and popliteal space and not cross their legs.

- If client has cognitive or sensory impairment, is a young child, or is severely debilitated, family is primary focus of instruction.
- When client is immobilized or confined to bed, family must be taught proper positioning and transfer techniques (see Chapter 29).

Pediatric Considerations

- The use of play is an integral part of relationships with children. Play can be used as a teaching mode, for expression of feeling, or as a method to achieve a therapeutic goal.
- Play activities such as painting or drawing on large sheet of paper placed on bed or wall can encourage movement. Play activities to encourage ambulation include push/pull toy (toddler) and wagon (school age).

Gerontologic Considerations

- Older adult client may take smaller steps with feet closer together and may be at risk for falling.
- During aging process, cervical vertebrae may become more flexed, and kyphotic posture may result.

Home Care Considerations

- Teach family members or friends of clients who are permanently disabled proper body mechanics and proper body alignment.
- Bed must be at care giver's waist level.
- Teach family members or friends to place clients in positions that maintain musculoskeletal alignment and reduce pressure on bony prominences.
- Provide family members and care givers a turning schedule for the client.

SKILL 28-2 Performing Safe and Efficient Lifting Techniques

The rate of injuries in occupational settings has increased during recent years. More than half of these injuries are back injuries and the direct result of unsafe lifting and bending techniques. The most common back injury is strain of the lumbar muscle group, which includes the muscles surrounding the lumbar vertebrae (Owen and Garg, 1993). Muscle injury to this area affects the person's ability to bend forward, backward, and side to side. In addition, the ability to rotate the hips and lower back from left to right and right to left is decreased.

By becoming knowledgeable about safe, efficient lifting techniques, nurses can promote safe transferring of clients without causing injury to the client or their own musculoskeletal systems.

STEPS	RATIONALE
ASSESSMENT	
1. Assess position of weight to be lifted.	Position of weight to be lifted should be as close to the lifter's center of gravity as possible.
CRITICAL DECISION POINT Client whose position is restricted because of traction, trauma, or body cast requires two or more persons to lift regardless of weight or height.	
2. Assess height of object to be lifted.	Best height for lifting vertically is slightly above level of middle finger when arm is hanging at person's side.
3. Assess lifter's body position.	Body should be positioned so multiple muscle groups are able to work together. Use arms and legs (not back). Tighten abdominal and gluteal muscles in preparation for moving.
4. Know maximal weight that can be safely carried.	Maximal weight that can be safely carried is approximately no more than 30% of the person's body weight. The lifter must always get assistance if in doubt about own ability to safely lift or transfer.

STEPS	RATIONALE

NURSING DIAGNOSIS

Clustering of defining characteristics from the assessment data may reveal the following nursing diagnoses for clients requiring this skill:

- Impaired physical mobility
- Knowledge deficit concerning proper positioning
- Risk for activity intolerance
- Risk for disuse syndrome
- Risk for impaired skin integrity
- Risk for injury

Related factors are individualized based on a client's condition or needs.

PLANNING

STEPS	RATIONALE
1. **Expected outcomes** following completion of procedure:	
➤ Nurse and client safely use lifting techniques.	Provides feedback that safe lifting techniques are used.
➤ No injuries result from lifting procedure.	Avoids strain on musculoskeletal system.
2. When lifting involves transferring client, prepare client by removing excess linen from bed or chair and explaining procedure.	Reduces risk of injury from tripping. Explanation increases understanding and cooperation.
3. When lifting object, remove excess clutter from environment.	Provides clear path to lift and transfer object.

IMPLEMENTATION

STEPS	RATIONALE
1. Lift object from below center of gravity (see illustration):	
a. Come close to object to be moved.	Increases body balance during lifting procedure.
b. Enlarge base of support.	Maintains body balance and reduces risk of falling.
c. Lower center of gravity to object.	Increases body balance and enables muscle groups to work together.
d. Maintain alignment of head and neck with vertebrae.	Reduces risk of injury to lumbar vertebrae and associated muscle groups.
e. Use a **turning sheet** to move client.	Prevents shearing force on client's skin.

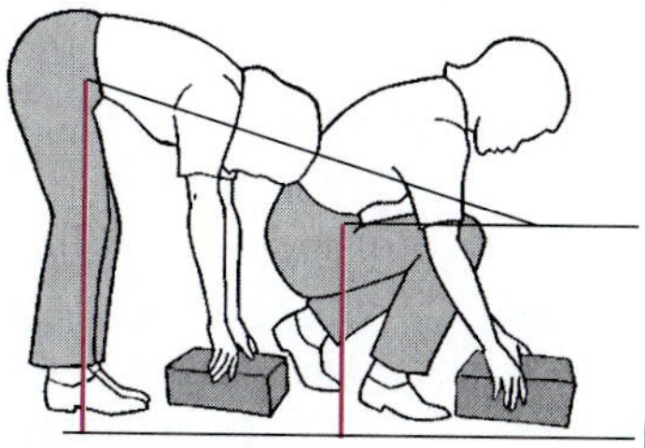

Step 1 Comparison of lifting techniques by lowering center of gravity of object to be lifted.

STEPS	RATIONALE
2. Lift object from shelf above center of gravity:	
a. Use safe, stable stepstool.	Raises center of gravity closer to object.
b. Stand as close to shelf as possible.	Moves center of gravity closer to object.
c. Quickly transfer weight of object from shelf to arms and over base of support.	Reduces danger of falling by moving lifted object close to center of gravity over base of support.

EVALUATION

STEPS	RATIONALE
1. Observe nurse and client to determine ability to safely use lifting techniques.	Determines effective use of lifting techniques.
2. Observe environment to ensure it is free of clutter.	
3. **Unexpected outcomes** that may occur include:	
➤ Lifter suffers injury to musculoskeletal system or client experiences injury during transfer technique.	Indicates need for follow-up learning activities.

STEPS	RATIONALE
RECORDING AND REPORTING	
1. Record type of lifting techniques taught to client or care giver.	Provides documentation of information given to client or care giver regarding lifting techniques.
2. Immediately report any lifting injury to nurse or client.	Necessary for risk management to prevent future injuries. Nurse is eligible for worker's compensation.

FOLLOW-UP ACTIVITIES

1. Review care plan with client and care giver and modify as needed.

• • • • •

Special Considerations

- If lifting injury is sustained, some institutions also require incident report to be completed and filed in nursing office.

Teaching Considerations

- Lifting load that is too heavy can result in muscle tears. Sudden twisting or bending also can tear muscles and ligaments.
- Teach primary care giver to use correct body mechanics in moving, lifting, transferring, and positioning client.
- Teach primary care giver to use turning sheet to reduce possibility of skin damage caused by shearing force.

Pediatric Considerations

- Place child on pressure-reducing surface. Change position frequently. Protect pressure points. Inspect skin surfaces frequently for signs of irritation, redness, and evidence of pressure. Keep side rails up at all times (Wong, 1995).
- Children can be transported in a stroller or wagon.

Gerontologic Considerations

- Shearing force against the sacrum causes tissue damage.
- In the older adult client who is thin, has fragile skin, or is nutritionally compromised, lubricants or protective films or padding can reduce friction injuries.
- Use a turning sheet to avoid shearing force on client's skin.

Home Care Considerations

- Teach care givers safe, efficient lifting techniques.
- Teach care givers safe transferring techniques.

CRITICAL THINKING EXERCISES

1. You are caring for two clients: a 71-year-old man who suffered a stroke resulting in left hemiparesis and a 65-year-old man who has had back surgery. What aspects of their care will be similar? Different?
2. An 80-year-old woman is recovering from a musculoskeletal injury that requires limited mobility and bed rest. How will she be affected during this period of decreased mobility?
3. The employee health nurse at your hospital would like your assistance in developing a teaching manual for nurses directed toward preventing back-related injuries. What items would you include in this manual?

REFERENCES

Owen B, Garg A: Back stress isn't part of the job, *Am J Nurs* 93(2):48, 1993.

Wong DL: *Whaley & Wong's nursing care of infants and children*, ed 5, St Louis, 1995, Mosby.

ADDITIONAL READING

Butler D, et al: The influence of load knowledge on lifting techniques, *Ergonomics* 36(12):1489, 1993.

Elkins M, Perry A, Potter P: *Nursing interventions and clinical skills*, St Louis, 1996, Mosby.

Potter PA, Perry AG: *Fundamentals of nursing: Concepts, process, and practice*, ed 4, St Louis, 1997, Mosby.

Snell J: Raising awareness . . . new guidance that spells out the message to nurses: "Avoid all manual lifting," *Nurs Times* 91(31):20, 1995.

Stacey N: Moving people, *Nurs Times* 90(19):47, 1994.

Winklemolen GHM, Landerweerd JA, Drost MR: An evaluation of patient lifting techniques, *Ergonomics* 37(5):921, 1994.

Witt PL: Preventing back pain: a guide for your patients, *Consultant* 34(4):515, 1994.

Wong DL: *Clinical manual of pediatric nursing*, ed 4, St Louis, 1996, Mosby.

CHAPTER 29

Transfer and Positioning

OBJECTIVES

Mastery of content in this chapter will enable the nurse to:

- Define key terms.
- Describe body alignment for standing, sitting, and lying.
- Describe positioning techniques for the supported Fowler's, supine, prone, side-lying, and Sims' positions.
- Describe the procedures for helping a client to move up in bed, helping a client to a sitting position, and transferring a client from a bed to a chair.
- Describe the procedure for a three-person carry.

KEY TERMS

Foot board
Footdrop
Friction
Hand rolls
Hemiparesis
Hemiplegia
Hoyer lift (mechanical/hydraulic lift)
Orthostatic hypotension
Paralysis
Paresis
Proprioceptive function

SKILLS

29-1 Using Safe and Effective Transfer Techniques

29-2 Moving and Positioning Clients in Bed

Transfer and positioning are basic skills learned early in the education of the professional nurse. Knowledge of these skills and the nurse's ability to implement them properly help maintain the client's mobility and independence and protect the nurse from injury.

The principles of body mechanics and alignment are important in transferring and positioning the physically dependent client (see Chapter 28). Practical application of these principles reduces the risk of injury to clients and health care personnel. Back injuries are a significant problem for nursing personnel; many of these injuries are sustained each year as a result of improper lifting and bending techniques.

Too often the client develops complications independent of illness because the principles of alignment and body mechanics are not followed. Improper alignment of the dependent client can result in joint contractures or injuries that may take months to correct or that may even result in permanent disability.

Positioning to maintain correct body alignment is essential in the prevention of complications. Improper positioning has many implications. Incorrect positioning, especially of the client with circulatory system impairment, may result in a decubitus ulcer, which can develop in 24 hours and require months of time and thousands of dollars to correct (Lueckenotte, 1996). Contractures and **footdrop** occur within a few days when muscles, tendons, and joints become less flexible because of lack of mobility and incorrect alignment (Elkin, Perry, and Potter, 1996). The force of gravity pulls an unsupported, weakened foot into a footdrop position, and calf muscles and heel cords shorten, complicating future attempts at walking. Pillows placed under the knees or an elevated knee gatch can produce knee and hip contractures. A sagging mattress increases the risk of hip contractures. These knee and hip contractures can cause future gait and posture problems, making mobility more difficult.

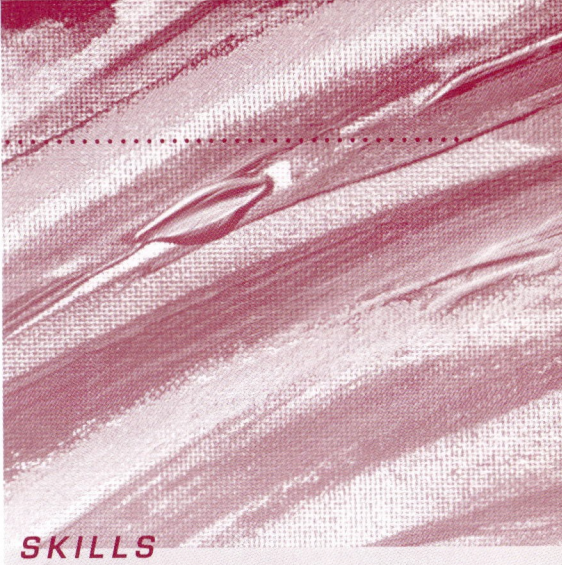

Some clients are at especially high risk for complications of improper positioning and have increased risk of injury during transfer. A number of pathological factors and congenital or acquired postural abnormalities alter alignment, mobility, or both. Pathophysiological mechanisms altering bone formation or joint mobility present special risks, as does impaired muscle development, which results in muscle wasting and weakness. Central nervous system (CNS) damage may result in motor impairment, proprioceptive loss, or cognitive dysfunction, all of which affect mobility. Direct trauma also affects body mechanics.

Use of proper transfer and positioning techniques ensures the outcome of the client achieving an optimal level of independence. The loss of independence can result in the client's needing assistance in the home or even being required to live in a nursing home. The ability to maintain independence is also important in preventing social isolation and maintaining body alignment essential to well-being.

GUIDELINES

1. Know the client's fluid balance status. Dehydration or edema may require more frequent position changes because clients with alterations in fluid balance are prone to skin breakdown.
2. Know the client's range of joint motion (ROJM). Contractures or spasticity limit joint and muscle mobility; the nurse must take care not to position the limb in an unnatural way. This could result in injury to or dysfunction of the affected limb.
3. Identify circulatory alterations such as venous ulcers, which may prevent the client from having the extremity in a dependent position. A history of deep-vein thrombosis may restrict the length of time a client can remain in a sitting position.
4. Determine the client's level of sensory perception. Loss of sensation increases vulnerability to the hazards of immobility. Clients with decreased sensation must have their positions evaluated and changed frequently to avoid damage to the integumentary and musculoskeletal systems.
5. Identify the client with incontinence or profuse sweating. Moisture from incontinence or sweating can decrease tensile strength and alter skin resiliency to external forces.
6. Know the client's baseline vital signs. The client with low blood pressure may not be able to tolerate sudden position changes and is at risk of fainting while transferring from bed to chair. The febrile client who becomes diaphoretic may require more frequent position changes to avoid skin breakdown.
7. Know underlying conditions such as chronic disease (e.g., diabetes, chronic obstructive pulmonary disease) or malnutrition. Clients with underlying chronic conditions are at risk for skin breakdown and other hazards of immobility and as a result require more frequent position changes.
8. Know the client's cognitive status and stage of psychological adaptation to illness. Both factors affect the ability to learn and participate in transfer and positioning.

DELEGATION CONSIDERATIONS

The skills of safe and effective transfer techniques and moving and positioning clients in bed can be delegated to unlicensed assistive personnel. Clients who have spinal cord trauma usually require transfer and moving by professional nurses.

- Caution care giver about level of the bed for selected skills.
- Caution care giver to maintain proper body mechanics.
- Instruct care giver on safe transfer techniques.
- Instruct care giver on moving and positioning in bed.
- Evaluate care giver's transfer and positioning skills.

SKILL 29-1 Using Safe and Effective Transfer Techniques

Transferring is a nursing skill that helps the dependent client attain positions to regain optimal independence as quickly as possible. Physical activity maintains and improves joint motion, increases strength, promotes circulation, relieves pressure on skin, and improves urinary and respiratory functions. It also benefits the client psychologically by increasing social activity and mental stimulation and providing a change in environment. Thus mobilization plays a crucial role in the client's rehabilitation.

One of the major concerns during transfer is the safety of the client and the nurse. The nurse prevents self-injury by using correct posture, minimal muscle strength, and effective body mechanics and lifting techniques.

The nurse must be aware of the client's motor deficits, ability to aid in transfer, and body weight. As a rule of thumb, nurses should always get assistance if in doubt about their ability to transfer a client.

Many special problems must be considered in transfer. A client who has been immobile for several days or longer may be weak or dizzy or may develop **orthostatic hypotension** (a drop in blood pressure) when transferred. A client with neurological deficits may have **paresis** (muscle weakness) or paralysis unilaterally or bilaterally, which complicates safe transfer. A flaccid arm may sustain injury during transfer if unsupported. As a general rule, a nurse should use a transfer belt and obtain assistance for mobilization of such clients.

EQUIPMENT

- **Transfer belt (if needed), sling or lap board (as needed), nonskid shoes, bath blankets, pillows**
- **Wheelchair: position chair at 45-degree angle to bed, lock brakes, remove footrests, lock bed brakes.**
- **Stretcher: position at right angle (90 degrees) to bed, lock brakes on stretcher, lock brakes on bed**
- **Mechanical/hydraulic lift: use frame, canvas strips or chains, and hammock or canvas strips**

STEPS	RATIONALE
ASSESSMENT	
1. Assess physiological capacity to transfer and cognitive ability to understand.	Determines neuromuscular integrity for transfer and special adaptive techniques that are necessary. Clients with impaired cognition may require more assistance to transfer.
a. Muscle strength (legs and upper arms)	Immobile clients have decreased muscle strength, tone, and mass. Affects ability to bear weight or raise body.
b. Joint mobility and contracture formation	Immobility or inflammatory processes (i.e., arthritis) may lead to contracture formation and impaired joint mobility.
c. Paralysis or paresis (spastic or flaccid)	Client with CNS damage may have bilateral **paralysis** (requiring transfer by swivel bar, sliding bar, **Hoyer lift**) or unilateral paralysis, which requires belt transfer to "best" side. Weakness (paresis) requires stabilization of knee while transferring. Flaccid arm must be supported with sling during transfer.
d. Bone continuity (trauma, amputation)	Clients with trauma to one leg or hip may be non-weight-bearing when transferred. Amputees may use sliding board to transfer.
2. Assess presence of weakness, dizziness, postural hypotension.	Determines risk of fainting or falling during transfer. Immobile clients may have decreased ability for autonomic nervous system to equalize blood supply, resulting in drop of 15 mm Hg or more in blood pressure when rising from sitting position.
3. Assess level of endurance:	
a. Assess ability to use arms and legs for moving up and down in bed and repositioning.	Estimates ability to participate in transfer.
b. Assess level of fatigue during activity.	Ability to transfer may be limited by fatigue. Strength may be evaluated by participation in activities of daily living (ADLs). Planned rest periods before transfer may enhance function.
c. Assess vital signs.	Vital sign changes such as increased pulse and respiration may indicate activity intolerance (see Chapter 10).
4. Assess client's **proprioceptive function** (awareness of posture and changes in equilibrium):	Determines stability of balance for transfer.
a. Ability to maintain balance while sitting in bed or on side of bed	Determines risk of fainting or falling during transfer.
b. Tendency to sway to or position self to one side	Clients with brain dysfunction may have proprioceptive losses. This may cause them to lean to one side or lose balance during transfer.
5. Assess client's sensory status: a. Adequacy of central and peripheral vision b. Adequacy of hearing	Determines influence of sensory loss on ability to make transfer. Visual field loss decreases client's ability to see in direction of transfer. Peripheral sensation loss

STEPS	RATIONALE
c. Loss of peripheral sensation	decreases proprioception. Clients with visual and hearing losses need transfer techniques adapted to deficits. Clients with cerebrovascular accident (CVA) may lose area of visual field, which profoundly affects vision and perception. Clients with **hemiplegia** also may "neglect" one side of the body (deny its existence), which distorts perception of the visual field.
6. Assess client's level of comfort: a. Pain b. Muscle spasm	Pain may reduce client's motivation and ability to be mobile. Pain relief before transfer enhances client participation.
7. Assess client's cognitive status: a. Ability to follow verbal instructions b. Short-term memory c. Appropriateness of response d. Recognition of physical deficits and limitations to movement	Determines client's ability to follow directions and learn transfer techniques. May indicate clients at risk for injury. Clients with short-term memory deficits may have difficulty with transfer, initial learning, or consistent performance. Clients with head trauma or CVA may have perceptual cognitive deficits that create safety risks. If client has difficulty in comprehension, simplify instructions and maintain consistency.
8. Assess client's level of motivation: a. Client's eagerness versus unwillingness to be mobile b. Whether client avoids activity and offers excuses	Altered psychological states reduce client's desire to engage in activity.
9. Assess previous mode of transfer (if applicable).	Determines mode of transfer and assistance required to provide continuity. Transfer belts should be used with hemiplegic clients being transferred for the first time and all other high-risk clients.
10. Assess client's specific risk of falling when transferred, sustaining injury in fall.	Certain conditions increase client's risk of falling or potential for injury. Neuromuscular deficits, motor weakness, calcium loss from long bones, cognitive and visual dysfunction, and altered balance increase risk of injury.

NURSING DIAGNOSIS

Clustering of defining characteristics from the assessment data may reveal the following nursing diagnoses for clients requiring this skill:

- Activity intolerance
- Impaired physical mobility
- Impaired skin integrity
- Risk for injury
- Pain

Related factors are individualized based on a client's condition or needs.

PLANNING

STEPS	RATIONALE
1. Expected outcomes following completion of procedure:	
➤ Client dangles legs or sits without dizziness, weakness, or orthostatic hypotension.	Precautions during transferring prevent vascular compromise.
➤ Client tolerates increased activity.	
➤ Client can bear more weight.	Repeated transfers usually result in improved endurance and greater independence of client.
➤ Client transfers without injury.	Proper techniques avoid injury.
➤ Client is more motivated to be mobile.	
➤ Client transfers with minimal or no assistance.	
➤ Client increases independence in ADLs.	
➤ Client's skin remains clear and intact, without redness.	Absence of pressure ulcer formation.

STEPS	RATIONALE
2. Explain procedure to client. Repeat instructions simply and with continuity to client with cognitive dysfunction.	Promotes cooperation and reduces anxiety.

IMPLEMENTATION

STEPS	RATIONALE
1. Wash hands.	Reduces transfer of microorganisms.
2. Assist client to sitting position (bed at waist level):	
a. Place client in supine position.	Enables nurse to assess client's body alignment continually and to administer additional care, such as suctioning or hygiene needs.
b. Face head of bed and remove pillows.	Proper positioning reduces twisting of the nurse's body when moving the client. Pillows may cause interference when the client is sitting up in bed.
c. Place feet apart with foot nearer bed behind other foot.	Improves nurse's balance and allows transfer of body weight as client is moved to sitting position.
d. Place hand farther from client under shoulders, supporting client's head and cervical vertebrae.	Maintains alignment of head and cervical vertebrae and allows for even lifting of client's upper trunk.
e. Place other hand on bed surface.	Provides support and balance.
f. Raise client to sitting position by shifting weight from front to back leg.	Improves nurse's balance, overcomes inertia, and transfers weight in direction in which client is moved.
g. Push against bed using arm that is placed on bed surface.	Divides activity between nurse's arms and legs and protects back from strain. By bracing one hand against mattress and pushing against it as client is lifted, part of weight that would be lifted by nurse's back muscles is transferred through nurse's arms onto mattress.
3. Assist client to sitting position on side of bed with bed in low position:	
a. With client in supine position, raise head of bed 30 degrees.	Decreases amount of work needed by client and nurse to raise client to sitting position.
b. Turn client to side, facing nurse on side of bed on which client will be sitting (see illustration).	Prepares client to move to side of bed and protects from falling.
c. Stand opposite client's hips. Turn diagonally so nurse faces client and far corner of foot of bed.	Places nurse's center of gravity nearer client. Reduces twisting of nurse's body because nurse is facing direction of movement.
d. Place feet apart with foot closer to head of bed in front of other foot.	Increases balance and allows nurse to transfer weight as client is brought to sitting position on side of bed.
e. Place arm nearer head of bed under client's shoulders, supporting head and neck.	Maintains alignment of head and neck as nurse brings client to sitting position.
f. Place other arm over client's thighs (see illustration).	Supports hip and prevents client from falling backward during procedure.

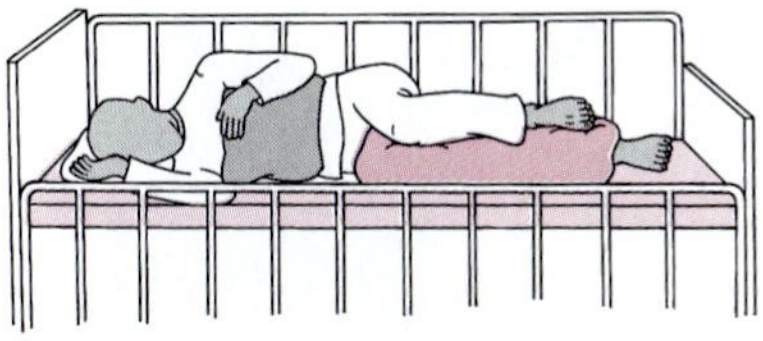

Step 3b Side-lying position.

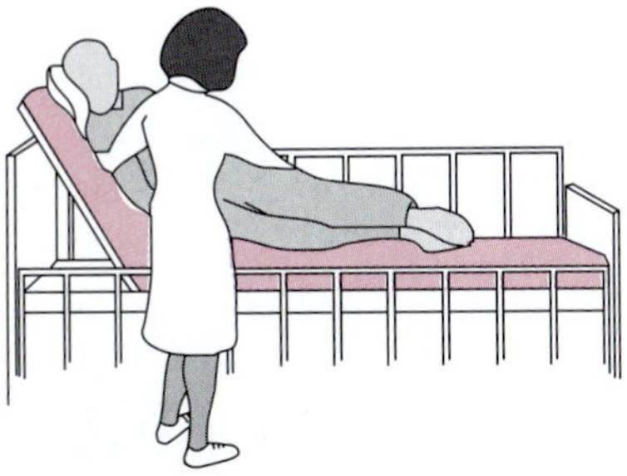

Step 3f Nurse places arm over client's thigh.

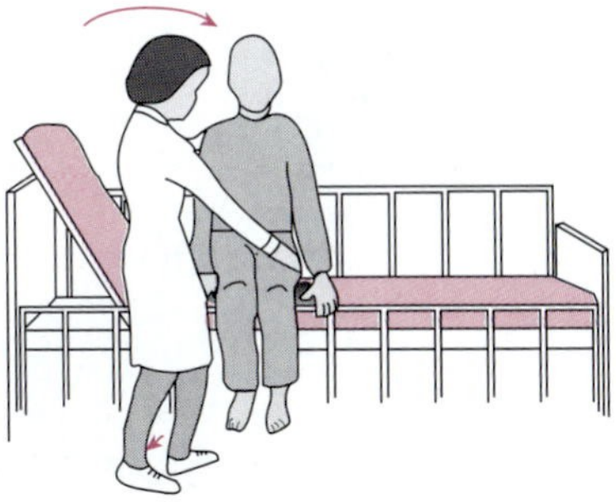

Step 3h Nurse shifts weight to rear leg and elevates client.

STEPS	RATIONALE
g. Move client's lower legs and feet over side of bed. Pivot toward rear leg, allowing client's upper legs to swing downward.	Decreases friction and resistance. Weight of client's legs when off bed allows gravity to lower legs, and weight of legs assists in pulling upper body in sitting position.
h. At same time, shift weight to rear leg and elevate client (see illustration on p. 889).	Allows nurse to transfer weight in direction of motion.
CRITICAL DECISION POINT **Remain in front until client regains balance.**	Reduces risk of falling.
CRITICAL DECISION POINT **Continue to provide physical support to weak or cognitively impaired client.**	These clients are at high risk for falling.
4. Transferring client from bed to chair with bed in low position:	
a. Assist client to sitting position on side of bed. Have chair in position at 45-degree angle to bed.	Positions chair within easy access for transfer.
b. Apply transfer belt or other transfer aids, if needed.	Transfer belt allows nurse to maintain stability of client during transfer and reduces risk of falling. Client's arm should be in sling if flaccid paralysis is present.
c. Ensure that client has stable nonskid shoes. Weight-bearing or strong leg is placed forward, with weak foot back.	Nonskid soles decrease risk of slipping during transfer. Always have clients wear shoes during transfer; bare feet increase risk of falls. Client will stand on stronger, or weight-bearing, leg.
d. Spread feet apart.	Ensures balance with wide base of support.
e. Flex hips and knees, aligning knees with client's knees (see illustration).	Flexion of knees and hips lowers nurse's center of gravity to object to be raised; aligning knees with client's allows for stabilization of knees when client stands.
f. Grasp transfer belt from underneath, if used, or reach through client's axillas and place hands on client's scapulas.	Lifting client with hands on scapulas reduces pressure on axillas and maintains client stability. Clients with upper extremity paralysis or paresis should never be lifted by or under arms. Transfer belt is grasped at each side to provide movement of client at center of gravity.

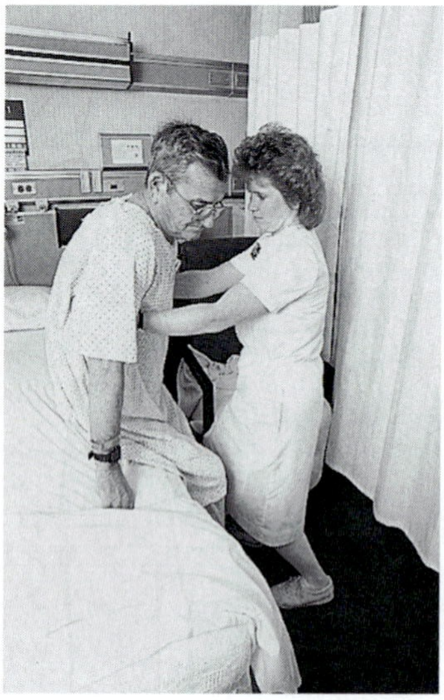

Step 4e Nurse flexes hips and knees, aligning knees with client's knees.

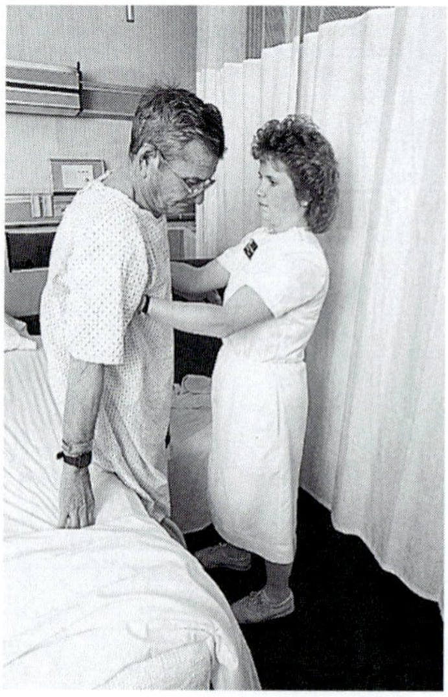

Step 4g Nurse rocks client to standing position.

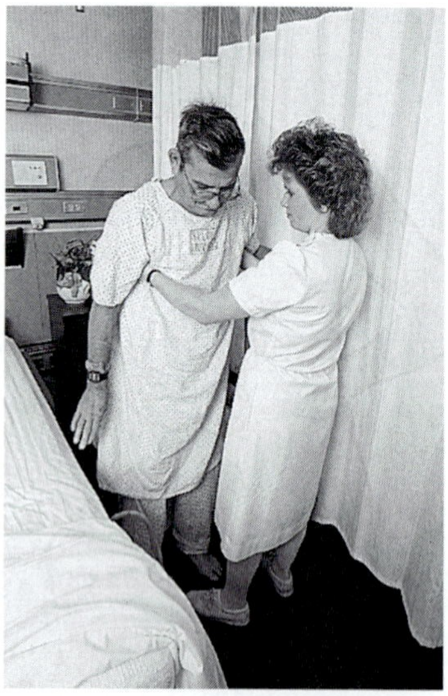

Step 4j Client uses armrests for support.

STEPS	RATIONALE
g. Rock client up to standing position on count of three while straightening hips and legs and keeping knees slightly flexed (see illustration). Client may be instructed to use hands to push up if applicable.	Rocking motion gives client's body momentum and requires less muscular effort to lift client.
h. Maintain stability of client's weak or paralyzed leg with knee.	Ability to stand can often be maintained in paralyzed or weak limb with support of knee to stabilize.
i. Pivot on foot farther from chair.	Maintains support of client while allowing adequate space for client to move.
j. Instruct client to use armrests on chair for support and ease into chair (see illustration).	Increases client stability.
k. Flex hips and knees while lowering client into chair (see illustration).	Prevents injury to nurse from poor body mechanics.
l. Assess client for proper alignment for sitting position. Provide support for paralyzed extremities. Lap board or sling will support flaccid arm. Stabilize leg with bath blanket or pillow.	Prevents injury to client from poor body alignment.
m. Praise client's progress, effort, performance.	Continued support and encouragement provide incentive for client perserverance.
5. Perform three-person carry from bed to stretcher (bed at stretcher level):	
a. Three nurses stand side by side facing side of client's bed. Individuals performing the procedure should be of equal height.	Prevents twisting of nurses' bodies. Client's alignment is maintained.
b. Each person assumes responsibility for one of three areas: head and shoulders, hips, and thighs and ankles.	Distributes client's body weight evenly.
c. Each person assumes wide base of support with foot closer to stretcher in front and knees slightly flexed.	Increases balance and lowers center of gravity of person lifting.
d. Arms of lifters are placed under client's head and shoulders, hips, and thighs and ankles, with fingers securely around other side of client's body (see illustration).	Distributes client's weight over forearms of lifters.

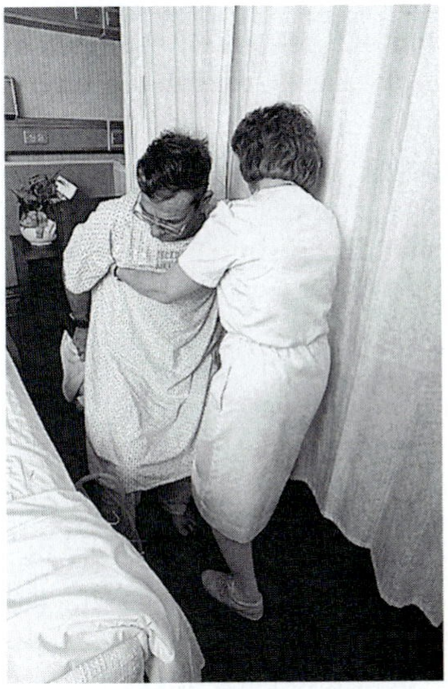

Step 4k Nurse eases client into chair.

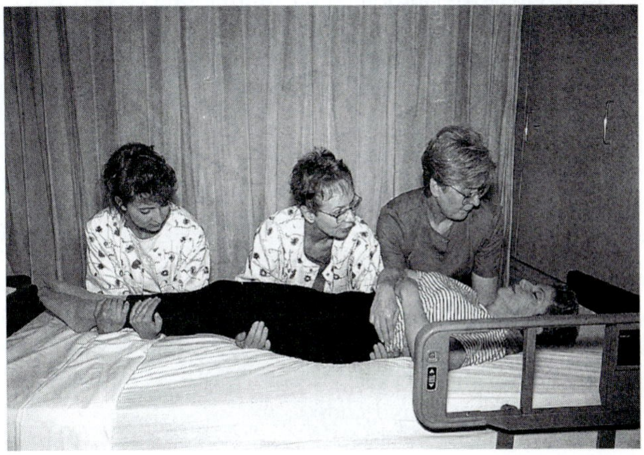

Step 5d Proper positioning of lifters during three-person transfer.

STEPS	RATIONALE
CRITICAL DECISION POINT Spinal cord injuries must be stabilized before transfer.	
e. Lifters roll client toward their chests. On count of three, client is lifted and held against nurses' chests.	Moves workload over lifters' base of support. Enables lifters to work together and safely lift client.
f. On second count of three, nurses step back and pivot toward stretcher, moving forward if needed.	Transfers weight toward stretcher.
g. Nurses gently lower client onto center of stretcher by flexing knees and hips until elbows are level with edge of stretcher.	Maintains nurses' alignment during transfer.
h. Nurses assess client's body alignment, place safety straps across body, and raise side rails.	Reduces risk of injury from poor alignment or falling.
6. Use mechanical/hydraulic lift to transfer client from bed to chair:	
a. Bring lift to bedside.	Ensures safe elevation of client off bed. (Before using lift, be thoroughly familiar with its operation.)
b. Position chair near bed, and allow adequate space to maneuver lift.	Prepares environment for safe use of lift and subsequent transfer.
c. Raise bed to high position with mattress flat. Lower side rail.	Allows nurse to use proper body mechanics.
d. Keep bed side rail up on side opposite nurse.	Maintains client safety.
e. Roll client away from nurse.	Positions client for use of lift sling.
f. Place hammock or canvas strips under client to form sling (see illustration). With two canvas pieces, lower edge fits under client's knees (wide piece), and upper edge fits under client's shoulders (narrow piece).	Two types of seat are supplied with mechanical/hydraulic lift: hammock style is better for clients who are flaccid, weak, and need support; canvas strips can be used for clients with normal muscle tone. Hooks should face away from client's skin. Place sling under client's center of gravity and greatest portion of body weight.
g. Raise bed rail.	Maintains client safety.
h. Go to opposite side of bed and lower side rail.	
i. Roll client to opposite side and pull hammock (strips) through.	Completes positioning of client on mechanical/hydraulic sling.
j. Roll client supine onto canvas seat.	Sling should extend from shoulders to knees (hammock) to support client's body weight equally.
k. Remove client's glasses, if appropriate.	Swivel bar is close to client's head and could break eyeglasses.
l. Place lift's horseshoe bar under side of bed (on side with chair).	Positions lift efficiently and promotes smooth transfer.
m. Lower horizontal bar to sling level by releasing hydraulic valve. Lock valve.	Positions hydraulic lift close to client. Locking valve prevents injury to client.
n. Attach hooks on strap (chain) to holes in sling. Short chains or straps hook to top holes of sling; longer chains hook to bottom of sling.	Secures hydraulic lift to sling.
o. Elevate head of bed.	Positions client in sitting position.
p. Fold client's arms over chest.	Prevents injury to paralyzed arms.
q. Pump hydraulic handle using long, slow, even strokes until client is raised off bed.	Ensures safe support of client during elevation (see illustration).
r. Use steering handle to pull lift from bed and maneuver to chair.	Moves client from bed to chair.
s. Roll base around chair.	Positions lift in front of the chair in which client is to be transferred.
t. Release check valve slowly (turn to left) and lower client into chair.	Safely guides client into back of chair as seat descends.

STEPS	RATIONALE
u. Close check valve as soon as client is down and straps can be released.	If valve is left open, boom may continue to lower and injure client.
v. Remove straps and mechanical/hydraulic lift (see illustration).	Prevents damage to skin and underlying tissues from canvas or hooks.
w. Check client's sitting alignment.	Prevents injury from poor posture.
7. Wash hands.	Reduces transmission of microorganisms.

E VALUATION

STEPS	RATIONALE
1. Monitor vital signs. Ask if client feels fatigued.	Evaluates client's response to postural changes and activity.
2. Observe for correct body alignment and presence of pressure points on skin.	Minimizes risk of immobility complications.
3. Note client's behavioral response to transfer.	Reveals level of motivation and self-care potential.
4. Ask if client experienced pain during transfer.	Determines need for additional pain control.
5. **Unexpected outcomes** that may occur include:	
➤ Client is unable to comprehend and follow directions for transfer.	Cognitive impairment affects learning and retention. Reassess continuity and simplicity of instruction.
➤ Client sustains injury on transfer.	Indicates improper transfer technique was used. Evaluate incident that caused injury (e.g., assessment inadequate, change in client status, or improper use of equipment).
➤ Client's level of weakness does not permit active transfer.	Physical impairments require increased assistance from nursing personnel. Increase bed activity and exercise to heighten tolerance.
➤ Client continues to bear weight on non–weight-bearing limb.	Certain conditions (e.g., hip fractures) need to be non–weight-bearing through healing process. Reassess client's understanding of weight-bearing status.
➤ Client transfers well on some occasions, poorly on others.	Transfers may be difficult when client is fatigued; periodic confusion may alter performance.
➤ Client is unable to stand for time required in transfer.	Results from increased fatigue, orthostatic hypotension, or pain.

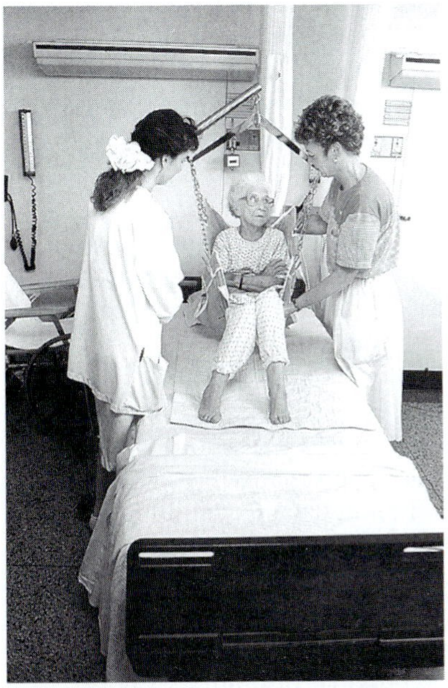

Step 6f Proper placment of sling under client.

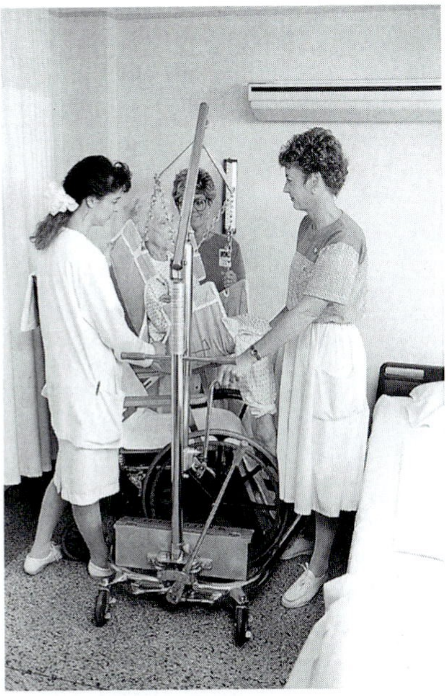

Step 6q Use of hydraulic lift to lower client into chair.

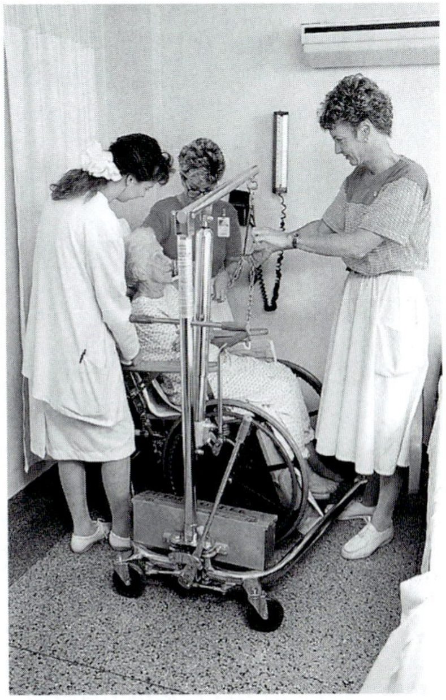

Step 6v Removal of hydraulic lift.

STEPS	RATIONALE
➤ Localized areas of erythema develop that do not disappear quickly.	Early signs of pressure sores.

RECORDING AND REPORTING

1. Record procedure, including pertinent observations: weakness, ability to follow directions, weight-bearing ability, balance, ability to pivot, number of personnel needed to assist, amount of assistance (muscle strength) required.	Documents transfer procedure and client's response to transfer.
2. Report any unusual occurrence to nurse in charge. Report transfer ability and assistance needed to next shift or other care givers. Report progress or remission to rehabilitation staff (physical therapist, occupational therapist).	Transfer techniques and adaptive aids used for client, as well as client's response, must be conveyed to other health care personnel to provide continuity of care.

FOLLOW-UP ACTIVITIES

1. Schedule transfer after periods of rest.
2. Gradually increase number of transfers and period of time out of bed.
3. Assess special transfer equipment needed for home setting.
4. Assess home environment for hazards.

• • • • •

Special Considerations

- ➤ Older adult client with short-term memory loss or client with cognitive dysfunction related to disease or trauma may be unable to follow directions regarding positioning and transfer or may attempt to climb out of bed or get up from chair.
- ➤ Alterations in neuromuscular function, alterations in physiology of bone formation related to disease or aging process, loss of joint mobility, CNS damage, and hazards of immobility increase risk of injury during transfer.
- ➤ Profound weakness, cardiac dysfunction, and hypotension are also risk factors. Many facilities have developed "fall risk" assessments to aid in identifying such high-risk persons.
- ➤ Psychological support and encouragement are very important considerations for immobile clients.

Teaching Considerations

- ➤ For many clients the return to home is coupled with enhanced psychological well-being and increased levels of motivation and ability for self-care function. Appropriate teaching of self-care skills and use of aids to maximize ability enhance outcome.
- ➤ Teach family and client transfer skills. Information should include principles of body mechanics and hazards of immobility. Incorporate return demonstration into discharge planning.

Pediatric Considerations

- ➤ Whenever possible, transporting the child by stretcher, stroller, or wheelchair outside the confines of the room will increase environmental stimuli and provide social contact with others. The child will benefit from frequent visitors, clocks and calendars, and a program of diversonal therapy.

Gerontologic Considerations

- ➤ Immobilized older adult clients are at risk of developing complications that affect all body systems. These complications include muscle atrophy, contractures, pressure ulcers, cardiovascular and respiratory problems, constipation, urinary stasis, and mental confusion.
- ➤ Use a turning sheet to avoid shearing force on the older adult client who has fragile skin.

Home Care Considerations

- ➤ Transfer ability at home is greatly enhanced by prior teaching of family and support persons, assessment of home for safety risks and functionality, and provision of applicable aids.
- ➤ Family or support person should practice transfer in hospital to achieve success before taking client home. Alternatively, client (if living alone) should practice transfer skills in bed that will be used at home, commode, and bath. Clients should be taught to transfer to chairs with arms for ease of rising and sitting.
- ➤ Home should be free of risks (i.e., throw rugs, electric cords, slippery floors). If wheelchair is used, access must be possible through all doors, and space for transfer must be available in bedroom and bathroom.

➤ Aids that enhance transfer ability are shower stools, commode elevators, handrails on tub, and nonskid shower surface. Many self-care devices are available for wheelchair-bound clients or clients with weak or poor muscle function. These are best prescribed by occupational or physical therapist; however, many medical supply stores can provide excellent information and catalogs of such supplies.

SKILL 29-2 Moving and Positioning Clients in Bed

Correct positioning of clients is crucial for maintaining body alignment and comfort, preventing injury to the musculoskeletal system, and providing sensory, motor, and cognitive stimulation. A client with impaired mobility, decreased sensation, impaired circulation, or lack of voluntary muscle control can develop damage to the musculoskeletal system while lying down. The nurse must minimize this risk by maintaining unrestricted circulation and correct body alignment while moving, turning, or positioning the client.

EQUIPMENT

- Pillows
- Foot board (optional)
- High-top sneakers
- Trochanter roll
- Sandbag
- Hand rolls
- Side rails

STEPS	RATIONALE
ASSESSMENT	
1. Assess client's body alignment and comfort level while client is lying down.	Provides baseline data for later comparisons. Determines ways to improve position and alignment.
2. Assess for risk factors that may contribute to complications of immobility:	Increased risk factors require client to be repositioned more frequently.
a. Paralysis: **hemiparesis** resulting from CVA; decreased sensation.	Paralysis impairs movement; muscle tone changes; sensation is affected. Because of difficulty in moving and poor awareness of involved body part, client is unable to protect and position body part for self.
b. Impaired mobility: traction or arthritis or other contributing disease processes.	Traction or arthritic changes of affected extremity result in decreased ROJM.
c. Impaired circulation	Decreased circulation predisposes client to pressure sores.
d. Age: very young, aged	Premature and young infants require frequent turning because their skin is fragile. Normal physiological changes associated with aging predispose older adults to greater risks for developing complications of immobility.
3. Assess client's level of consciousness.	Determines need for special aids or devices. Clients with altered levels of consciousness may not understand instructions and may be unable to help.
4. Assess client's physical ability to help with moving and positioning: a. Age b. Level of consciousness c. Disease process d. Strength e. ROJM f. Coordination	Enables nurse to use client's mobility and strength. Determines need for additional help. Ensures client and nurse safety.
5. Assess for tubes, incisions, and equipment (e.g., traction).	Will alter positioning procedure.

STEPS	RATIONALE

NURSING DIAGNOSIS

Clustering of defining characteristics from the assessment data may reveal the following nursing diagnoses for clients requiring this skill:

- Activity intolerance
- Impaired physical mobility
- Impaired skin integrity
- Risk for impaired skin integrity

Related factors are individualized based on a client's condition or needs.

PLANNING

STEPS	RATIONALE
1. Expected outcomes following completion of procedure:	
➤ Client retains ROJM.	Correct positioning allows client to achieve optimal joint mobility and alignment.
➤ Client's skin shows no evidence of breakdown.	Frequent position changes decrease risk of skin breakdown.
➤ Client's comfort is increased.	Proper positioning reduces stress on joints.
➤ Client's level of independence in completing ADLs is increased.	Maintaining good body alignment and joint mobility increases client's level of independence and overall mobility. Client with inadequate joint mobility may need assistance to carry out ADLs.
2. Raise level of bed to comfortable working height.	Raises level of work toward nurse's center of gravity.
3. Remove all pillows and devices used in previous position.	Reduces interference from bedding during positioning procedure.
4. Get extra help as needed.	Provides for client and nurse safety.
5. Explain procedure to client.	Helps to decrease anxiety and increase cooperation.

IMPLEMENTATION

STEPS	RATIONALE
1. Wash hands.	Reduces transmission of infection.
2. Close door to room or close bedside curtains.	Provides for client privacy.
3. Put bed in flat position.	Provides easy access to client and allows nurses to reposition client without working against gravity.
4. Move immobile client up in bed (one nurse):	
a. Place client on back with head of bed flat. Stand on one side of bed.	Enables nurse to assess body alignment. Reduces gravity's pull on client's upper body.
b. Remove pillow from under head and shoulders and place pillow at head of bed.	Prevents striking client's head against head of bed.
c. Begin at client's feet. Face foot of bed at 45-degree angle. Place feet apart with foot nearest head of bed behind other foot (forward-backward stance). Flex knees and hips as needed to bring arms level with client's legs. Shift weight from front to back leg, and slide client's legs diagonally toward head of bed.	Positioning is begun at client's legs because they are lighter and easier to move. Facing direction of movement ensures proper balance. Shifting nurse's weight reduces force needed to move load. Diagonal motion permits pull in direction of force. Flexing knees lowers nurse's center of gravity and uses thigh muscles rather than back muscles.
d. Move parallel to client's hips. Flex knees and hips as needed to bring arms level with client's hips.	Maintains nurse's correct body alignment. Brings nurse closest to object to be moved and lowers center of gravity. Uses thigh muscles rather than back muscles.
e. Slide client's hips diagonally toward head of bed.	Aligns client's hips and feet.
f. Move parallel to client's head and shoulders. Flex knees and hips as needed to bring arms level with client's body.	Maintains nurse's proper body alignment. Brings nurse closer to object to be moved. Lowers nurse's center of gravity. Uses thigh muscles rather than back muscles.
g. Slide arm closest to head of bed under client's neck, with hand reaching under and supporting client's shoulder.	Supports client's head and neck, maintaining alignment and preventing injury during movement.
h. Place other arm under client's upper back.	Supports client's body weight and reduces friction during movement.

STEPS	RATIONALE
i. Slide client's trunk, shoulders, head, and neck diagonally toward head of bed.	Realigns client's body on one side of bed.
j. Elevate side rail. Move to other side of bed and lower side rail.	Protects client from falling out of bed.
k. Repeat procedure, switching sides until client reaches desired position in bed.	
l. Center client in middle of bed, moving body in same three sections.	Maintains proper body alignment. Provides ample room for turning, positioning, and other nursing activities.
5. Assist client to move up in bed (one or two nurses):	
a. Place client on back with head of bed flat.	Enables nurse to assess body alignment. Reduces gravity's pull on client's upper body.
b. Remove pillow from under head and shoulders and place pillow at head of bed.	Prevents striking client's head against head of bed.
c. Face head of bed.	Facing direction of movement prevents twisting of nurse's body while moving client.
(1) Each nurse should have one arm under client's shoulders and one arm under client's thighs.	
(2) Alternative position: position one nurse at client's upper body. Nurse's arm nearest head of bed should be under client's head and opposite shoulder; other arm should be under client's closest arm and shoulder. Position other nurse at client's lower torso. This nurse's arms should be under client's lower back and torso.	Prevents trauma to client's musculoskeletal system by supporting shoulder and hip joints and evenly distributing weight.
d. Place feet apart, with foot nearest head of bed behind other foot (forward-backward stance).	Wide base of support increases nurse's balance. Stance enables nurse to shift body weight as client is moved up in bed, thereby reducing force needed to move load.
e. When possible, ask client to flex knees with feet flat on bed.	Enables client to use femoral muscles during movement.
f. Instruct client to flex neck, tilting chin toward chest.	Prevents hyperextension of neck when moving client up in bed.
g. Instruct client to assist moving by pushing with feet on bed surface.	Reduces **friction.** Increases client mobility. Decreases nurse's workload.
h. Flex knees and hips, bringing forearms closer to level of bed.	Increases balance and strength by bringing nurse's center of gravity closer to client. Uses thighs instead of back muscles.
i. Instruct client to push with heels and elevate trunk while breathing out, thus moving toward head of bed on count of three.	Prepares client for move. Reinforces assistance in moving up in bed. Increases client cooperation. Breathing out avoids Valsalva maneuver.
j. On count of three, rock and shift weight from front to back leg. At the same time client pushes with heels and elevates trunk.	Rocking enables nurse to improve balance and overcome inertia. Shifting nurse's weight counteracts client's weight and reduces force needed to move load. Client's assistance reduces friction and nurse's workload.
6. Move immobile client up in bed with drawsheet or pullsheet (two nurses):	
a. Place drawsheet or pullsheet under client, extending from shoulders to thighs.	Supports client's body weight and reduces friction during movement.
b. Place client on back with head of bed flat.	
c. Position one nurse at each side of client.	Distributes weight equally between nurses.
d. Grasp drawsheet or pullsheet firmly near the client.	

STEPS	RATIONALE
e. Place feet apart with forward-backward stance. Flex knees and hips. Shift weight from front to back leg, and move client and drawsheet or pullsheet to desired position in bed.	Facing direction of movement ensures proper balance. Shifting weight reduces force needed to move load. Flexing knees lowers nurses' center of gravity and uses thighs instead of back muscles.
7. Realign client in correct body alignment.	Prevents injury to musculoskeletal system. Nurses may assist client to one of the positions listed here.
a. Position client in supported Fowler's position (see illustration):	
(1) Elevate head of bed 45 to 60 degrees.	Increases comfort, improves ventilation, and increases client's opportunity to socialize or relax.
(2) Rest head against mattress or on small pillow.	Prevents flexion contractures of cervical vertebrae.
(3) Use pillows to support arms and hand if client does not have voluntary control or use of hands and arms.	Prevents shoulder dislocation from effect of downward pull of unsupported arms, promotes circulation by preventing venous pooling, and prevents flexion contractures of arms and wrists.
(4) Position pillow at lower back.	Supports lumbar vertebrae and decreases flexion of vertebrae.
(5) Place small pillow or roll under thigh.	Prevents hyperextension of knee and occlusion of popliteal artery from pressure from body weight.
(6) Place small pillow or roll under ankles.	Prevents prolonged pressure of mattress on heels.
CRITICAL DECISION POINT **To keep feet in proper alignment, place** foot board **at bottom of client's feet or apply high-top sneakers on client's feet.**	Maintains dorsiflexion and prevents footdrop.

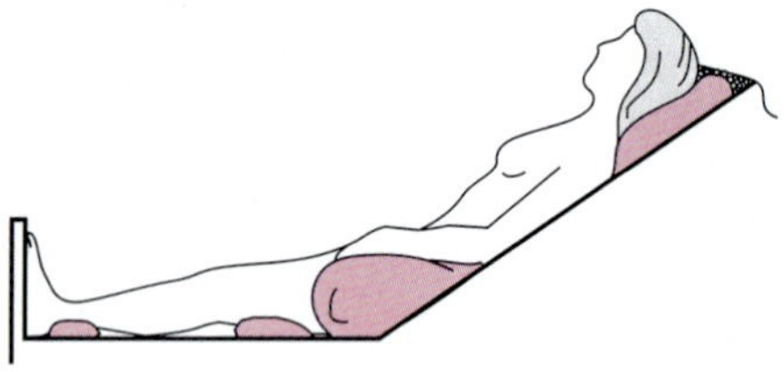

Step 7a Foot board in place (Fowler's position).

STEPS	RATIONALE
b. Position hemiplegic client in supported Fowler's position:	
(1) Elevate head of bed 45 to 60 degrees.	Increases comfort, improves ventilation, and increases client's opportunity to relax.
(2) Position client in sitting position as straight as possible.	Counteracts tendency to slump toward affected side. Improves ventilation and cardiac output; decreases intracranial pressure. Improves client's ability to swallow and helps to prevent aspiration of food, liquids, and gastric secretions.
(3) Position head on small pillow with chin slightly forward. If client is totally unable to control head movement, hyperextension of the neck must be avoided.	Prevents hyperextension of neck. Too many pillows under head may cause or worsen neck flexion contracture.
CRITICAL DECISION POINT **Provide support for involved arm and hand on overbed table in front of client. Place arm away from client's side and support elbow with pillow.**	Paralyzed muscles do not automatically resist pull of gravity as they do normally. As a result, shoulder subluxation, pain, and edema may occur.
CRITICAL DECISION POINT **Position** ***flaccid*** **hand in normal resting position with wrist slightly extended, arches of hand maintained, and fingers partially flexed; may use section of rubber ball cut in half; clasp client's hands together.**	Maintains hand in functional position. Prevents contractures.

STEPS	RATIONALE
CRITICAL DECISION POINT Position *spastic* hand with wrist in neutral position or slightly extended; fingers should be extended with palm down or may be left in relaxed position with palm up.	Maintains hand in functional position. Inhibits flexor spasticity.
(4) Flex knees and hips by using pillow or folded blanket under knees.	Ensures proper alignment. Flexion prevents prolonged hyperextension, which could impair joint mobility.
(5) Support feet in dorsiflexion with firm pillow, foot board, or high-top sneakers.	Prevents footdrop. Stimulation of ball of foot by hard surface has tendency to increase muscle tone in client with extensor spasticity of lower extremity.
c. Position client in supine position:	
(1) Place client on back with head of bed flat.	Necessary for placing client in supine position.
(2) Place small rolled towel under lumbar area of back.	Provides support for lumbar spine.
(3) Place pillow under upper shoulders, neck, or head.	Maintains correct alignment and prevents flexion contractures of cervical vertebrae.
(4) Place trochanter rolls or sandbags parallel to lateral surface of client's thighs.	Reduces external rotation of hip.
(5) Place small pillow or roll under ankle to elevate heels (see illustration in Step 7a).	Reduces pressure on heels, helping to prevent pressure sores.
(6) Place foot board or firm pillows against bottom of client's feet.	
(7) Place high-top sneakers on client's feet.	Maintains feet in dorsiflexion. Prevents footdrop.
(8) Place pillows under pronated forearms, keeping upper arms parallel to client's body (see illustrations).	Reduces internal rotation of shoulder and prevents extension of elbows. Maintains correct body alignment.
(9) Place **hand rolls** in client's hands. Consider physical therapy referral for use of hand splints.	Reduces extension of fingers and abduction of thumb. Maintains thumb slightly adducted and in opposition to fingers.
d. Position hemiplegic client in supine position:	
(1) Place head of bed flat.	Necessary for positioning in supine position.
(2) Place folded towel or small pillow under shoulder or affected side.	Decreases possibility of pain, joint contracture, and subluxation. Maintains mobility in muscles around shoulder to permit normal movement patterns.

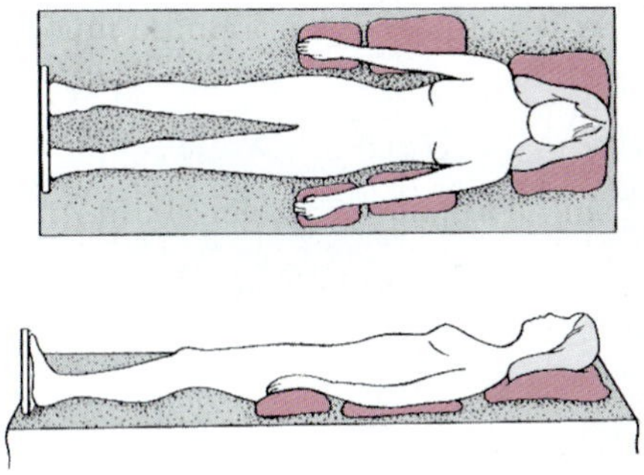

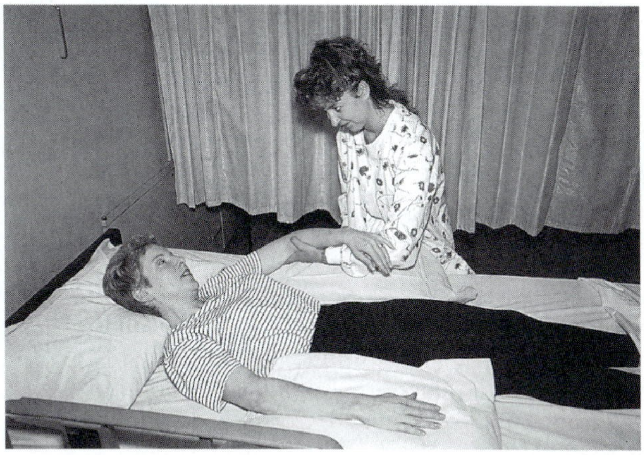

Step 7c(8) Supine position with pillows in place.

STEPS	RATIONALE
(3) Keep affected arm away from body with elbow extended and palm up. (Alternative is to place arm out to side, with elbow bent and hand toward head of bed.)	Maintains mobility in arm, joints, and shoulder to permit normal movement patterns. (Alternative position counteracts limitation of ability of arm to rotate outward at shoulder [external rotation]. External rotation must be present to raise arm overhead without pain.)
CRITICAL DECISION POINT **Position affected hand in one of recommended positions for flaccid or spastic hand.**	Maintains hand in functional position.
(4) Place folded towel under hip of involved side.	Diminishes effect of spasticity in entire leg by controlling hip position.
(5) Flex affected knee 30 degrees by supporting it on pillow or folded blanket.	Slight flexion breaks up abnormal extension pattern of leg. Extensor spasticity is most severe when client is supine.
(6) Support feet with soft pillows at right angle to leg.	Maintains foot in dorsiflexion and prevents footdrop. Pillows prevent stimulation to ball of foot by hard surface, which has tendency to increase muscle tone in client with extensor spasticity of lower extremity.
e. Position client in prone position:	
(1) Roll client over arm positioned close to body, with elbow straight and hand under hip. Position on abdomen in center of bed.	Positions client correctly so alignment can be maintained.
(2) Turn client's head to one side and support head with small pillow (see illustration).	Reduces flexion or hyperextension of cervical vertebrae.
(3) Place small pillow under client's abdomen below level of diaphragm (see illustration).	Reduces pressure on breasts of some female clients and decreases hyperextension of lumbar vertebrae and strain on lower back. Improves breathing by reducing mattress pressure on diaphragm.
(4) Support arms in flexed position level at shoulders.	Maintains proper body alignment. Support reduces risk of joint dislocation.
(5) Support lower legs with pillow to elevate toes (see illustration).	Prevents footdrop. Reduces external rotation of legs. Reduces mattress pressure on toes.
f. Position hemiplegic client in prone position:	
(1) Move client toward unaffected side.	Ensures proper client alignment in center of bed when client is rolled onto abdomen.

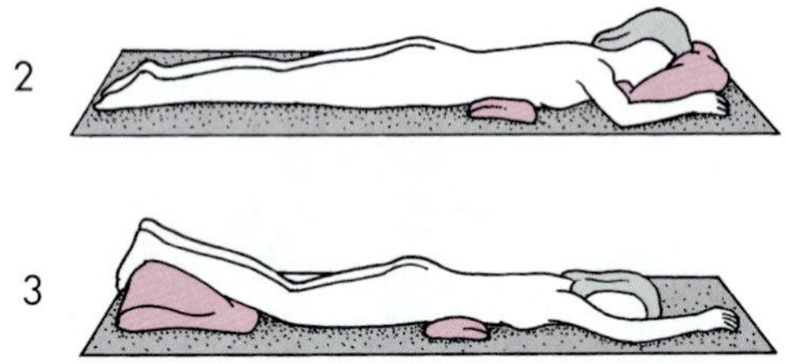

Step 7e(2-3) Prone position with pillows in place.

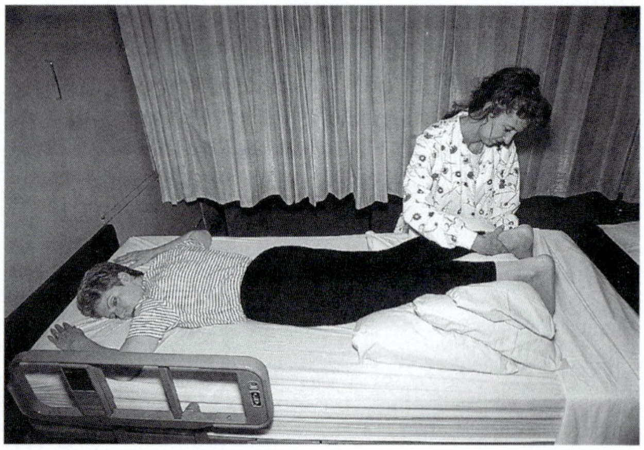

Step 7e(5)

STEPS	RATIONALE
(2) Roll client onto side.	
(3) Place pillow on client's abdomen.	Prevents sagging of abdomen when client is rolled over; decreases hyperextension of lumbar vertebrae and strain on lower back.
(4) Roll client onto abdomen by positioning involved arm close to client's body, with elbow straight and hand under hip. Roll client carefully over arm.	Prevents injury to affected side.
(5) Turn head toward involved side.	Promotes development of neck and trunk extension, which is necessary for standing and walking.
(6) Position involved arm out to side, with elbow bent, hand toward head of bed, and fingers extended (if possible).	Counteracts limitation of arm's ability to rotate outward at shoulder (external rotation). External rotation must be present to raise arm over head without pain.
(7) Flex knees slightly by placing pillow under legs from knees to ankles.	Flexion prevents prolonged hyperextension, which could impair joint mobility.
(8) Keep feet at right angle to legs by using pillow high enough to keep toes off mattress and use high-top sneakers.	Maintains feet in dorsiflexion.

g. Position client in lateral (side-lying) position:

STEPS	RATIONALE
(1) Lower head of bed completely or as low as client can tolerate.	Provides position of comfort for client and removes pressure from bony prominences on back.
(2) Position client to side of bed.	Provides room for client to turn to side.
(3) Turn client onto side.	To turn helpless client onto side, flex client's knee that will not be next to mattress. Place one hand on client's hip and one hand on client's shoulder.

CRITICAL DECISION POINT **Clients at risk for pressure ulcer development require the 30° lateral position (see Chapter 8).**

STEPS	RATIONALE
(4) Roll client onto side toward nurse.	Client is positioned so leverage on hip makes turning easy.
(5) Rolling client toward nurse lessens trauma to tissues.	
(6) Place pillow under client's head and neck.	Maintains alignment. Reduces lateral neck flexion. Decreases strain on sternocleidomastoid muscle.
(7) Bring shoulder blade forward.	Prevents client's weight from resting directly on shoulder joint.
(8) Position both arms in slightly flexed position. Upper arm is supported by pillow level with shoulder; other arm, by mattress.	Decreases internal rotation and adduction of shoulder. Supporting both arms in slightly flexed position protects joint. Ventilation is improved because chest is able to expand more easily.
(9) Place tuck-back pillow behind client's back. (Make by folding pillow lengthwise. Smooth area is slightly tucked under client's back.)	Provides support to maintain client on side.
(10) Place pillow under semiflexed upper leg level at hip from groin to foot (see illustrations on p. 902).	Flexion prevents hyperextension of leg. Maintains leg in correct alignment. Prevents pressure on bony prominence.
(11) Place sandbag parallel to plantar surface of dependent foot. Place high-top sneakers on client's feet.	Maintains dorsiflexion of foot. Prevents footdrop.

h. Position client in Sims' (semiprone) position:

STEPS	RATIONALE
(1) Lower head of bed completely.	Provides for proper body alignment while client is lying down.
(2) Place client in supine position.	Prepares client for position.

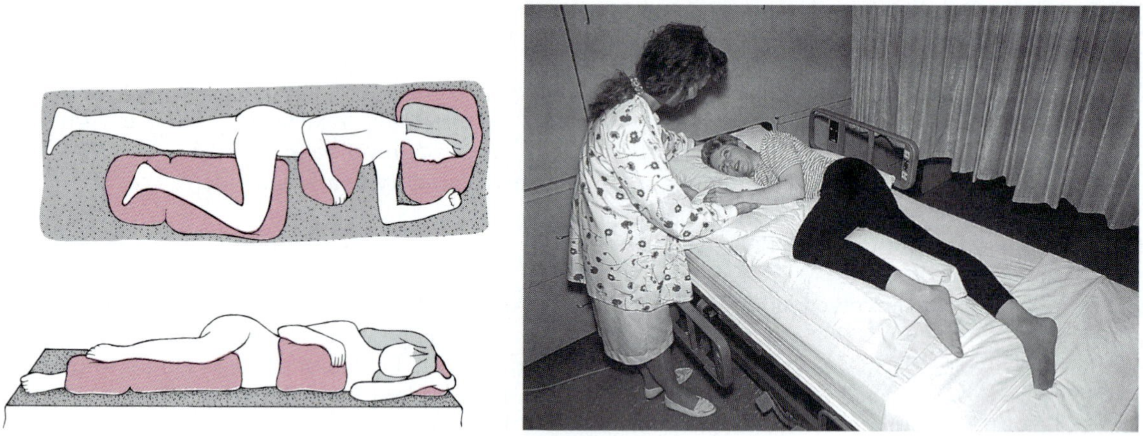

Step 7g(10) Lateral position with pillows in place.

STEPS	RATIONALE
(3) Position client in lateral position, lying partially on abdomen.	Client is rolled only partially on abdomen.
(4) Place small pillow under client's head.	Maintains proper alignment and prevents lateral neck flexion.
(5) Place pillow under flexed upper arm, supporting arm level with shoulder.	Prevents internal rotation of shoulder. Maintains alignment.
(6) Place pillow under flexed upper legs, supporting leg level with hip.	Prevents internal rotation of hip and adduction of leg. Flexion prevents hyperextension of leg. Reduces mattress pressure on knees and ankles.
(7) Place sandbags parallel to plantar surface of foot (see illustration).	

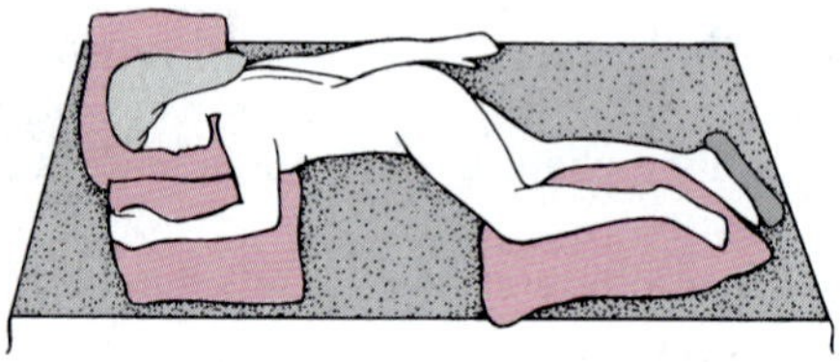

Step 7h(7) Sandbag supporting foot in dorsiflexion.

(8) Place high-top sneakers on client's feet.	Maintains foot in dorsiflexion. Prevents footdrop.
8. Wash hands.	Reduces transmission of infection.

EVALUATION

1. Assess client's body alignment, position, and level of comfort.	Determines effectiveness of positioning. Additional supports (e.g., pillows, bath blankets), may be added or removed to promote comfort and correct body alignment.
2. Measure ROJM.	Determines if joint contracture is developing.
3. Assess for areas of erythema or breakdown involving skin.	Provides ongoing observation regarding client's skin and musculoskeletal systems. Indicates complications of immobility or improper positioning of body part.
4. **Unexpected outcomes** that may occur include:	
➤ Joint contractures develop or worsen.	Improper positioning results in shortening of muscles.
➤ Skin shows areas of erythema and breakdown.	Frequency of repositioning is inadequate.
➤ Client avoids moving.	Indicates fear of pain.

RECORDING AND REPORTING

1. Record procedure and observations (e.g., condition of skin, joint movement, client's ability to assist with positioning).	Documents procedure, client's response, and effectiveness of nursing care.
2. Report observations at change of shift and document in nurses' notes.	Individualizes nursing care given to client.

FOLLOW-UP ACTIVITIES

1. Increase frequency of positioning if pressure areas begin to appear, joint mobility becomes impaired or worsened, or client complains of discomfort.
2. Consult with physical and occupational therapists as needed.

• • • • •

Special Considerations

- The Occupational Safety and Health Administration (OSHA) has identified standards on back safety. Health care providers are required to provide employees with safety information and training to use when transferring and positioning clients.
- Client experiencing severe pain may require analgesia before moving or positioning.
- Some positions may be contraindicated in certain situations (e.g., respiratory difficulties, certain neurological conditions, and presence of incisions, drains, or tubings).
- Use aids such as pillows to relieve concentrated areas of pressure under client's body.
- Reposition clients, especially debilitated, unconscious, or paralyzed clients, at least every 2 hours.

Teaching Considerations

- Include family in explanations, especially when caring for infant, young child, or confused or unconscious client.
- Teach client ways to assist with positioning.
- Provide opportunity for return demonstration.
- Teach client and family signs and symptoms of pressure sores and contractures.

Pediatric Considerations

- Children should be encouraged to be as active as their condition and restrictive devices allow. Opportunity, materials, or objects to stimulate activity and encouragement and participation of others must be available.
- Children who are unable to move will need passive exercise and movement.

Gerontologic Considerations

- Position older adult client to avoid strain on joints, tendons, ligaments, and muscles.
- Older adult clients must be repositioned every 2 hours and a regular program of ROJM exercises must be maintained.

Home Care Considerations

- Assess ability and motivation of client, family members, and primary care giver to participate in moving and positioning client in bed.
- Assess home to determine compatibility of environment with assistive devices (e.g., overbed trapeze, Hoyer lift, hospital bed).
- Assess skin for pressure areas and friction burns.

CRITICAL THINKING EXERCISES

1. Develop a discharge teaching plan for a client who has right hemiparesis.
2. In what ways could you involve the family of a client who has been prescribed bed rest?
3. While resting in bed some evening, imagine yourself being unable to reposition yourself without help. How would this make you feel?
4. Some clients have alterations in their proprioceptive function and may not be sensitive to touch, pressure, heat, cold, or pain. Can you identify special needs of these clients and specific ways you can intervene during ambulation or transfer?
5. If no pillows are available, what other devices could you use to position a client in alignment?

REFERENCES

Elkin MK, Perry AG, Potter PA: *Nursing interventions and clinical skills,* St Louis, 1996, Mosby.

Leuckenotte AG: *Gerontologic nursing,* St Louis, 1996, Mosby.

CHAPTER 30

Exercise and Ambulation

OBJECTIVES

Mastery of content in this chapter will enable the nurse to:

- Define key terms.
- Discuss indications for assisting with ambulation or using devices to assist ambulation.
- Discuss indications for performing range-of-motion and isometric exercises.
- Describe measures to minimize orthostatic hypotension.
- Identify significant assessment data to be noted before assisting with ambulation, range-of-motion, and isometric exercises.
- Demonstrate the following skills on selected clients: assisting with ambulation, assisting ambulation with the use of an ambulation aid, assisting with range-of-motion exercises, assisting with isometric exercises, applying elastic stockings, and instituting measures to minimize orthostatic hypotension.
- Develop teaching plans for selected clients for safety precautions to use at home while using an ambulation aid, applying and monitoring effects of elastic stockings, and performing range-of-motion and isometric exercises.

SKILLS

30-1 Performing Range-of-Motion Exercises

30-2 Performing Isometric Exercises

30-3 Applying Elastic Stockings

30-4 Changing Client's Position to Minimize Occurrence of Orthostatic Hypotension

30-5 Assisting with Ambulation

KEY TERMS

Abduction
Active range-of-motion exercises
Active-assisted range-of-motion exercises
Activity tolerance
Adduction
Atrophy
Bed rest
Circumduction
Contractures
Crutch gait
Crutch palsy
Dangling
Dorsal
Dorsiflexion
Eversion
Exercises
Extension
External rotation
Flexion
Footboard
Gait
Hazards of immobility
Hyperextension
Immobility
Internal rotation
Inversion
Isometric contractions
Isometric exercise
Isotonic exercises
Joint
Mobility
Orthostatic hypotension
Passive range-of-motion exercises
Plantar flexion
Posture
Pronation
Resistive isometric exercise
Supination
Thrombus
Walking belt

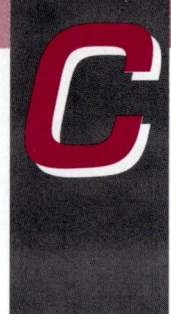

Mobility refers to a person's *ability* to move about freely, and **immobility** refers to a person's *inability* to move about freely. Mobility and immobility are best understood as the end points of a continuum, with many degrees of partial mobility in between. Some clients move back and forth on the mobility–immobility continuum, but for other clients, immobility is absolute and continues for an indefinite period.

The ability to move body parts independently is a function most people take for granted. The level of mobility has a significant impact on an individual's physiological, psychosocial, and developmental well-being (Hamilton and Lyon, 1995). When there is an alteration in mobility, many body systems are at risk for impairment. Impaired mobility may result in "decreased joint range of motion, loss of muscular strength and endurance, loss of bone mass and strength, cardiovascular deterioration, respiratory problems, metabolic imbalances, pressure ulcers, and decreased urinary function" (Hamilton and Lyon, 1995).

Research has demonstrated that there is a measurable decrease in the range of motion and as much as a 15% loss of muscle strength after only 1 week of immobility (Dittmer and Teasell, 1993). The severity of the impairment depends on the client's age, overall health status, and the degree of immobility experienced. For example, pronounced effects of immobility develop more quickly in older adult clients with chronic illnesses than they do in younger clients. Older adults may experience **orthostatic hypotension,** syncope, confusion, increased risk of fractures, and functional incontinence as a result of decreased mobility from **bed rest** (Creditor, 1993; Hamilton and Lyon, 1995; Wanich et al., 1992). Alterations in mobility can have profound psychosocial and developmental effects. For adults, immobility may alter employment, family role functions, and social interactions. Such changes can lead to altered self-concept and lowered self-esteem. Children also are affected by immobility. Activity for them is a way of releasing energy and expressing themselves. When deprived of physical activity, children become restless and may even show signs of anger and aggression.

Changes in a client's mobility can result from various health problems. Examples of medical conditions that can alter mobility are musculoskeletal conditions such as fractured extremities or muscle sprains, neurological conditions such as spinal cord trauma, degenerative neurological conditions such as myasthenia gravis, and head injuries. Some clients may not actually be immobilized for therapeutic reasons (e.g., prescribed bed rest, reduced activity). Some examples are a cardiovascular condition or infectious problems. Nursing measures attempt to maintain and/or restore optimal mobility as well as to decrease the hazards associated with immobility (Hamilton and Lyon, 1995; Wanich et al., 1992). Frequent repositioning, deep breathing and coughing exercises, muscle and joint exercises, increased fluid intake, and dietary intake of fiber foods are measures that help to reduce the hazards of immobility.

GUIDELINES

1. Check the physician's orders to determine the client's activity level and type of **exercises** or assistive device to be used. This action must be done to protect the physician and nurse legally and to determine the frequency of intervention and type of ambulation or exercise to be used.
2. Know the client's past medical history. The nurse should know why the client needs assistance with ambulation and any contraindication or limits to exercise.
3. Know the client's normal ranges for vital signs. Vital signs vary. Exercise and mobility can be fatiguing and stressful, so a set of baseline vital signs is necessary.
4. Assess baseline muscle strength. The client may need muscle-strengthening exercises before ambulation.
5. Assess baseline **joint** function. This knowledge helps the nurse to determine whether range-of-motion exercises are needed and provides a baseline for comparison of joint function after range-of-motion exercises are performed.
6. Obtain and become familiar with the type of assistive device to be used. There are various assistive devices available. Nurses need to know proper preparation and use of devices to be able to teach clients to use them safely and correctly.
7. Prepare the client. The client may be afraid of falling. Schedule other activities so that the client is not fatigued. Obtain extra personnel, safety devices, and flat, nonskid shoes for the client.
8. Determine the type and frequency of intervention. The intervention is based on assessment findings and the physician's order. Activity that is appropriate for 1 day or one shift can change, resulting in an increased or decreased need for assistance with ambulation or change in the type of intervention.
9. Know the client's home care plan. The client may need to continue the exercise regimen or use an assistive device at home.

SKILL 30-1 Performing Range-of-Motion Exercises

Regardless of whether the cause of immobility is permanent or temporary, the immobilized client must receive some type of exercise to prevent excessive muscle **atrophy** and joint **contractures.** The total amount of activity required to prevent disuse syndrome is about 2 hours for every 24-hour period, but this activity must be scheduled throughout the day to prevent the client from remaining inactive for long periods.

Exercises performed in bed can help to promote joint mobility, muscle strength, and muscle endurance (Recker, 1992). Exercise prevents some of the complications of immobility and helps to prepare a client for ambulation. Three types of exercises the nurse may use to help the client maintain muscle and joint function are range-of-motion (ROM) exercise, **isometric exercise** (see Skill 30-2), and **resistive isometric exercises.**

ROM exercises put each joint through as full a range of motion as possible without causing discomfort. ROM exercises may be *active, passive,* or *active-assisted* (Ruda, 1996). **Active range-of-motion exercises** are defined as exercises the client is able to perform independently, and **passive range-of-motion exercises** are performed for the client by someone else. **Active-assisted range-of-motion** exercises are performed by a client with some assistance (Dawe and Curran-Smith, 1994). A client who is weak or partially paralyzed may be able to move a limb partially through its range of motion. In this case the nurse can help the client perform active-assisted ROM exercises by helping the client finish the full ROM. Another form of active-assisted ROM exercise is when a client uses the strong arm to exercise the weaker or paralyzed arm.

DELEGATION CONSIDERATIONS

The skill of performing range of motion exercises can be delegated to unlicensed assistive personnel. Clients with spinal cord or orthopedic trauma usually require exercise by professional nurses or physical therapists. The following information is needed when delegating this skill to nursing staff or family members:

- Perform exercises slowly.
- Provide adequate support to joint being exercised.
- Do not exercise joints beyond the point of resistance or to the point of fatigue or pain.

Table 30-1 Incorporating Active Range-of-Joint-Motion Exercises into Activities of Daily Living

Joint Exercised	Activity of Daily Living	Movement
Neck	Nodding head yes	Flexion
	Shaking head no	Rotation
	Moving right ear to right shoulder	Lateral flexion
	Moving left ear to left shoulder	Lateral flexion
Shoulder	Reaching to turn on overhead light	Extension
	Reaching to bedside stand for book	Extension
	Scratching back	Hyperextension
	Rotating shoulders toward chest	Abduction
	Rotating shoulders toward back	Adduction
Elbow	Eating, bathing, shaving, grooming	Flexion, extension
Wrist	Eating, bathing, shaving, grooming	Flexion, extension, hyperextension, abduction, adduction
Fingers and thumb	All activities requiring fine motor coordination (e.g., writing, eating, hobbies)	Flexion, extension, abduction, adduction, opposition
Hip	Walking	Flexion, extension, hyperextension
	Moving to side-lying position	Flexion, extension, abduction
	Moving from side-lying position	Extension, adduction
	Rolling feet inward	Internal rotation
	Rolling feet outward	External rotation
Knee	Walking	Flexion, extension
	Moving to and from side-lying position	Flexion, extension
Ankle	Walking	Dorsiflexion, plantar flexion
	Moving toe toward head of bed	Dorsiflexion
	Moving toe toward foot of bed	Plantar flexion
Toes	Walking	Extension, hyperextension
	Wiggling toes	Abduction, adduction

ROM exercises remain the same regardless of whether the client can do the exercises independently or some degree of assistance is required by the client. Active ROM exercises should be encouraged if the client's health status allows because they involve the client in self-care and increase independence, self-control, and self-esteem (Dawe and Curran-Smith, 1994). Active and active-assisted ROM exercises help to prevent muscular atrophy and joint contracture. Passive ROM exercises help to maintain joint function but do not result in sufficient muscle tension to maintain muscle tone. Active ROM exercises can be incorporated into activities of daily living (Table 30-1) as well as into children's play activities. Examples of exercise through play include having the child act like a butterfly or throw a bean bag or wadded piece of paper into a trash can or at a target.

STEPS	RATIONALE
ASSESSMENT	
1. Review client's chart to determine client's medical history and obtain physician's order if needed.	Any type of joint problem, cardiac problem, or other conditions that may be aggravated by energy expenditure or joint movement indicate need to discuss ROM exercises with client's physician. Therefore the nurse must use some judgment in deciding whether to institute exercises independently or to consult the physician before beginning exercises.
2. Assess baseline joint function:	
a. Observe client's ability to perform ROM exercises during normal activities of daily living.	Assessment of baseline ROM capabilities is important for evaluating later ROM capabilities.
b. During ROM exercises assess for the following:	
(1) Any limitation in normal ROM or any unusual increase in mobility of joint	Decreased ROM may indicate arthritis, inflammatory process, or contracture.
(2) Any signs of redness or increased heat in skin overlying joint	May indicate joint problem that contraindicates ROM exercises or may indicate septic arthritis.
(3) Tenderness in or around joint	
(4) Crepitation produced by motion of joint	Crepitation suggests roughening of articular cartilages and is also felt in stenosis and tenosynovitis.
(5) Deformities	Deformities suggest bony enlargement (e.g., degenerative joint disease) or contracture.
3. Assess client's or care giver's understanding of ROM exercises to be used.	Allows client to verbalize concerns and identifies educational needs of client or care giver.

NURSING DIAGNOSIS

Clustering of defining characteristics from the assessment data may reveal the following nursing diagnoses for clients requiring this skill:

- Activity intolerance
- Anxiety
- Decreased cardiac output
- Fatigue
- Fear
- Impaired physical mobility
- Knowledge deficit regarding ROM exercise techniques
- Pain
- Risk for impaired skin integrity

Related factors are individualized based on a client's condition or needs.

STEPS	RATIONALE
PLANNING	
1. **Expected outcomes** following completion of procedure:	
➤ Range of joint motion is within normal limits or client's baseline range for each joint.	Indicates full joint mobility and decreases risk of contracture formation.
➤ Client denies discomfort during exercises.	Joints are exercised safely.
➤ Client demonstrates ROM during activities of daily living.	Incorporation of teaching into routine care makes skill relevant to client's needs.
2. Explain procedure and reason for performing ROM exercises.	Relieves client's anxiety and encourages cooperation and participation.
3. Assist client to comfortable position.	Positioning allows easy access to joints for complete ROM.

STEPS	RATIONALE
IMPLEMENTATION	
1. Wash hands.	Reduces transmission of microorganisms.
2. Expose only limb to be exercised.	Provides privacy and avoids embarrassing client.
3. Raise bed to comfortable position and stand on side of bed of joints to be exercised.	Maintains proper body mechanics to prevent back strain as exercises are carried out.
4. Be sure ROM exercises are performed slowly and gently.	Rapid, jerky movements may cause muscle spasms with resulting discomfort.
5. When performing ROM exercises, support joint by holding distal and proximal areas adjacent to joint (see illustration [1]), by cradling distal portion of extremity (see illustration [2]), or by using cupped hand to support joint (see illustration [3]).	Support is provided to joint while ROM exercises are performed.
6. Begin following exercises in sequence outlined. Each movement should be repeated five times during exercise period. NOTE: Discontinue exercise if client complains of discomfort or if there is resistance or muscle spasm.	It is easiest to perform exercises in head-to-toe format.

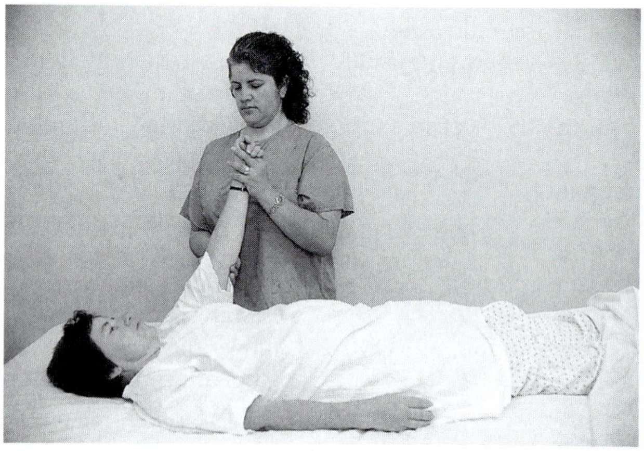

Step 5(1)

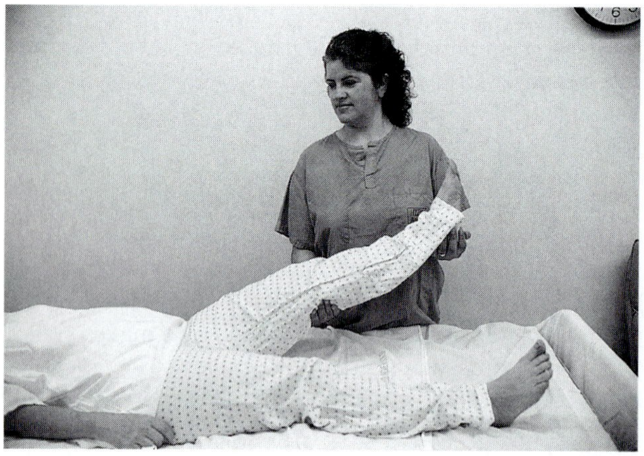

Step 5(2)

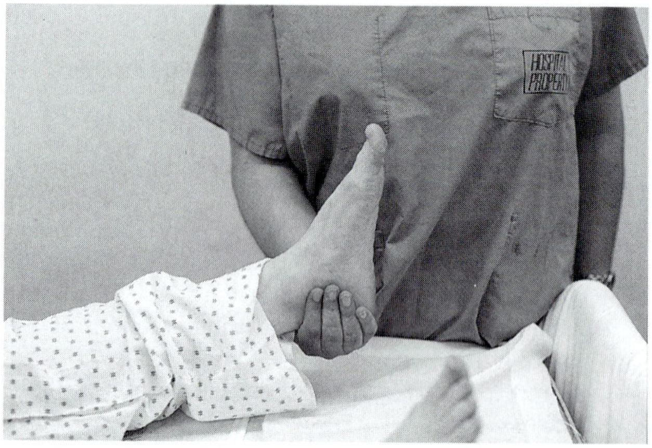

Step 5(3)

STEPS	RATIONALE
a. Neck	
(1) ***Flexion:*** Bring chin to rest on chest (ROM: 45 degrees) (see illustration 6a [1]). (2) ***Extension:*** Return head to erect position (ROM: 45 degrees) (see illustration 6a [1]). (3) ***Hyperextension:*** Bend head as far back as possible (ROM: 10 degrees) (see illustration 6a [1]). (4) *Lateral flexion:* Tilt head as far as possible toward each shoulder (ROM: 40 to 45 degrees) (see illustration 6a [2]). (5) *Rotation:* Rotate head in circular motion (ROM: 360 degrees) (see illustrations 6a[3] and 6a[4]).	If flexion contracture of neck occurs, client's neck is permanently flexed with chin to or actually touching chest. Ultimately, client's total body alignment is altered, visual field is changed, and overall level of independent functioning is decreased.

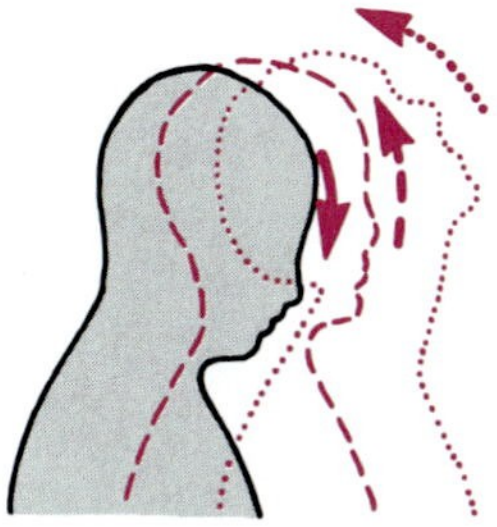

Step 6a(1)

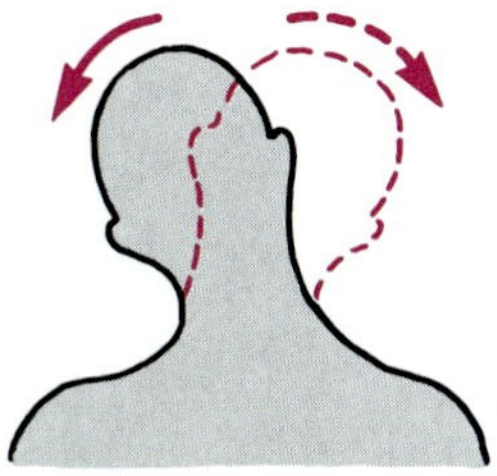

Step 6a(2)

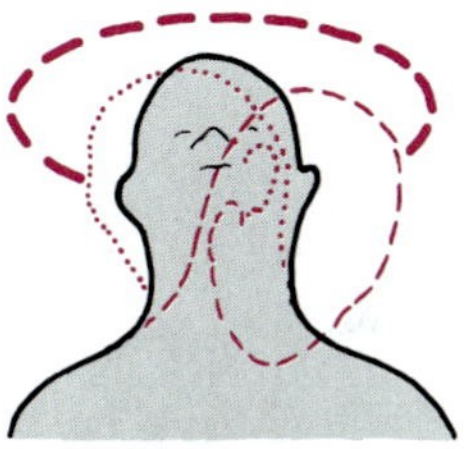

Step 6a(3)

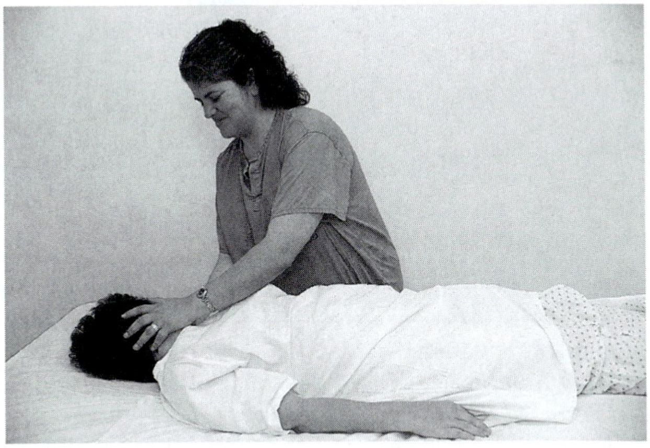

Step 6a(4)

b. Shoulder	
(1) *Flexion:* Raise arm from side position forward to above head (ROM: 180 degrees) (see illustration). (2) *Extension:* Return arm to position at side of body (ROM: 180 degrees). (3) *Hyperextension:* Move arm behind body, keeping elbow straight (ROM: 45 to 60 degrees) (see illustration).	Exercising shoulder effectively increases power of deltoid muscle. This strength will help if client needs to use an ambulation device, such as crutches, later.

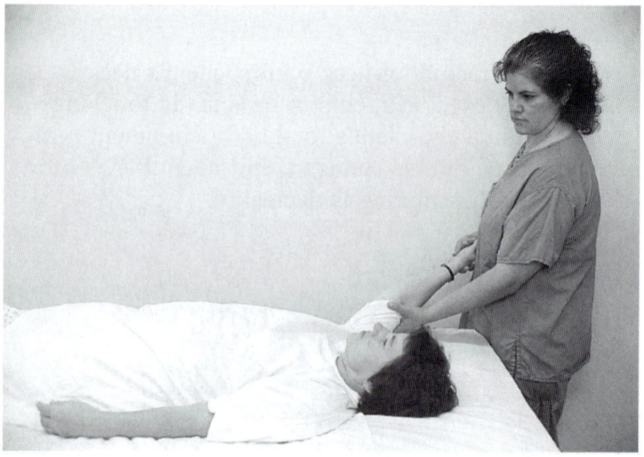

Step 6b(1)

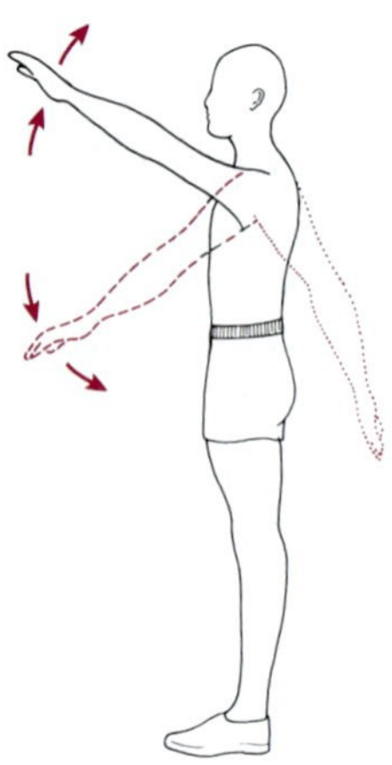

Step 6b(3)

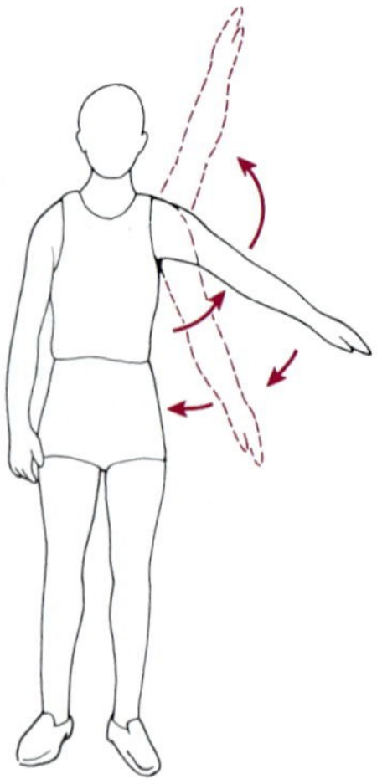

Step 6b(4)

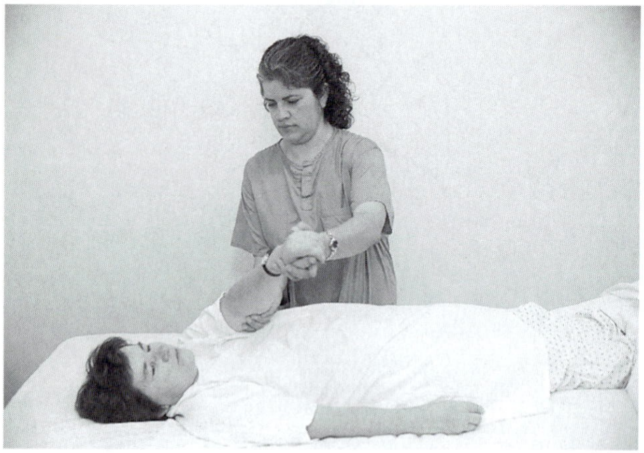

Step 6b(5)

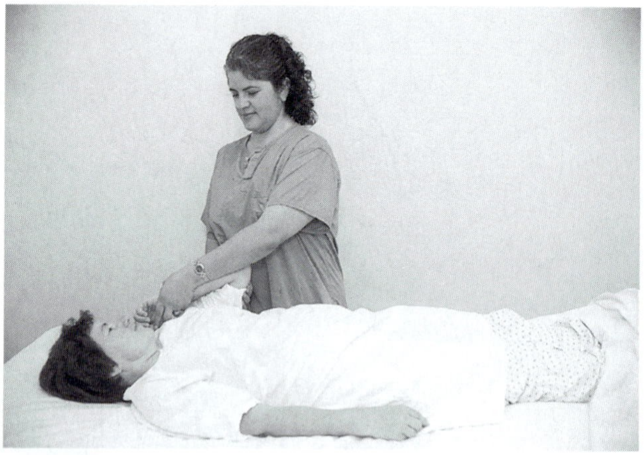

Step 6b(6)

STEPS	RATIONALE
(4) **Abduction:** Raise arm to side to position above head with palm away from head (ROM: 180 degrees) (see illustration).	
(5) **Adduction:** Lower arm sideways and across body as far as possible (ROM: 320 degrees) (see illustration).	A frozen shoulder makes it impossible to reach overhead.
(6) *Internal rotation:* With elbow flexed, rotate shoulder by moving arm until thumb is turned inward and toward back (ROM: 90 degrees) (see illustration).	
(7) **External rotation:** With elbow flexed, move arm until thumb is upward and lateral to head (ROM: 90 degrees) (see illustration).	
(8) **Circumduction:** Move arm in full circle. Circumduction is a combination of all movements of ball-and-socket joint (ROM: 360 degrees) (see illustration).	

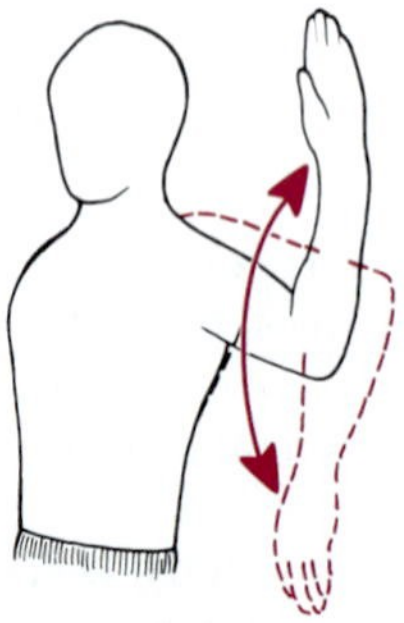

Step 6b(7)

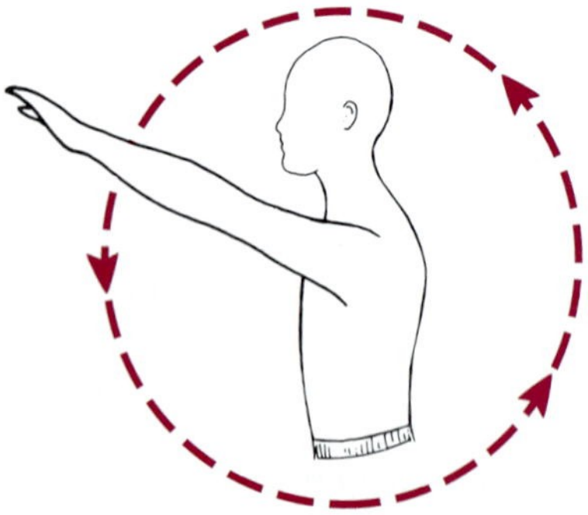

Step 6b(8)

STEPS	RATIONALE

c. Elbow

(1) *Flexion:* Bend elbow so that lower arm moves toward its shoulder joint and hand is level with shoulder (ROM: 150 degrees) (see illustration).

(2) *Extension:* Straighten elbow by lowering hand (ROM: 150 degrees) (see illustration 6c(1)).

(3) *Hyperextension:* Bend lower arm back as far as possible (ROM: 10 to 20 degrees).

Elbow fixed in full extension is very disabling and limits client's independence.

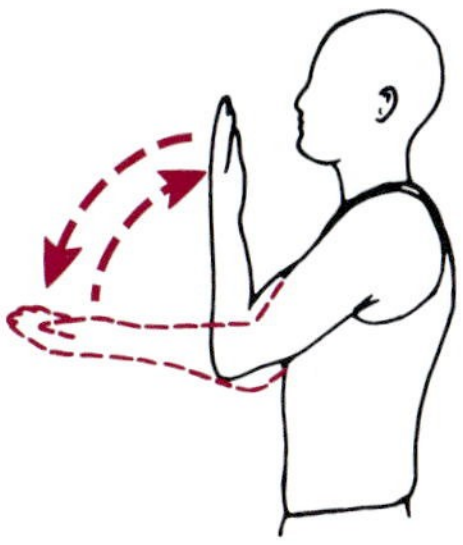

Step 6c(1)

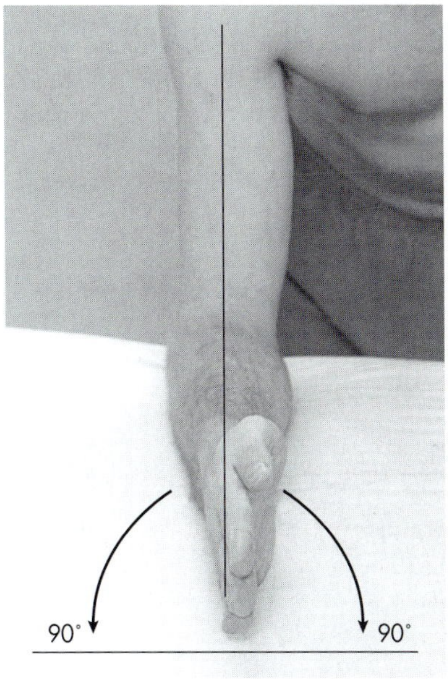

Step 6d(1) From Mourad LA: *Orthopedic disorders,* Mosby's Clinical Nursing Series, St Louis, 1991, Mosby.

d. Forearm

(1) **Supination:** Turn lower arm and hand so that palm is up (ROM: 70 to 90 degrees) (see illustration).

(2) **Pronation:** Turn lower arm so that palm is down (ROM 70 to 90 degrees) (see illustration 6d(1)).

For optimal functioning, forearm must be able to rotate from supination to pronation.

e. Wrist

(1) *Flexion:* Move palm toward inner aspect of forearm (ROM: 80 to 90 degrees) (see illustration).

(2) *Extension:* Move fingers so fingers, hands, and forearm are in same plane (ROM: 80 to 90 degrees).

If wrist becomes fixed in even slightly flexed position, person's grasp is weakened. Wrist strength is necessary to be able to use crutches.

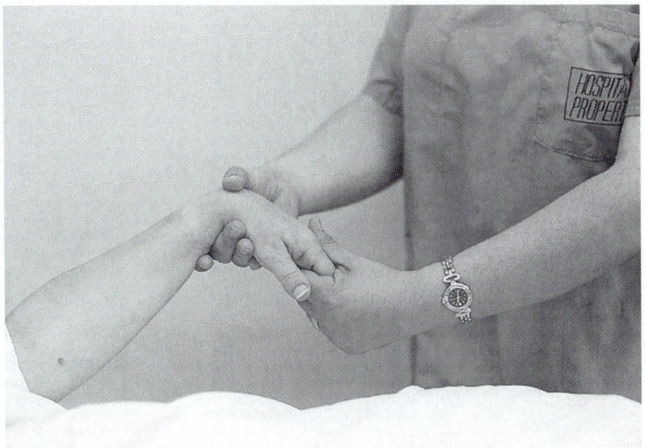

Step 6e(1)

STEPS | **RATIONALE**

(3) *Hyperextension:* Bring **dorsal** surface of hand back as far as possible (ROM: 80 to 90 degrees) (see illustration).
(4) *Abduction (radial flexion):* Bend wrist medially toward thumb (ROM: up to 30 degrees) (see illustration).
(5) *Adduction (ulnar flexion):* Bend wrist laterally toward fifth finger (ROM: 30 to 50 degrees) (see illustration).

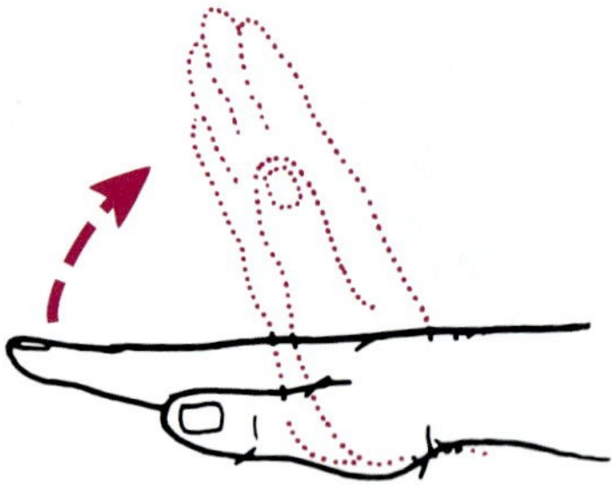

Step 6e(3)

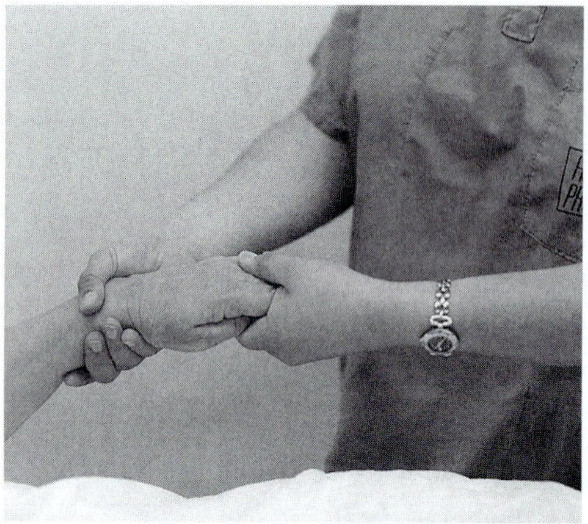

Step 6e(4)

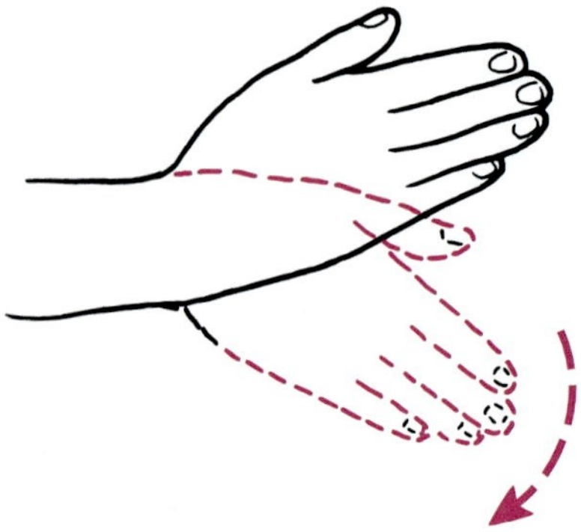

Step 6e(5)

f. Fingers

(1) *Flexion:* Make fist (ROM: 90 degrees) (see illustration).
(2) *Extension:* Straighten fingers (ROM: 90 degrees).
(3) *Hyperextension:* Bend fingers back as far as possible (ROM: 30 to 60 degrees) (see illustration).
(4) *Abduction:* Spread fingers apart (ROM: 30 degrees) (see illustration).
(5) *Adduction:* Bring fingers together (ROM: 30 degrees) (see illustration 6f(4)).

Flexibility of fingers and thumb is necessary to grasp items (e.g., holding onto crutch).

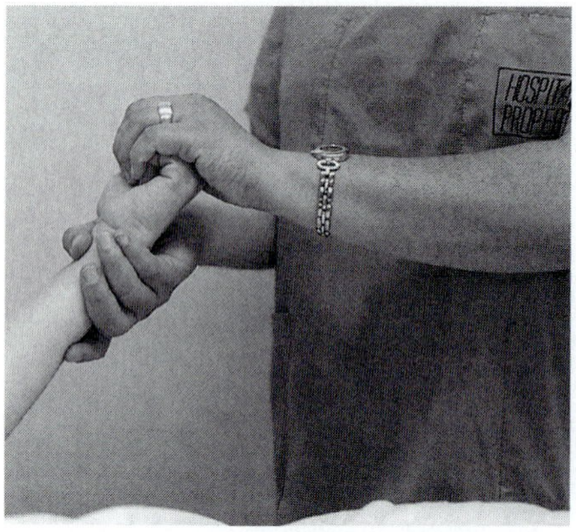

Step 6f(1)

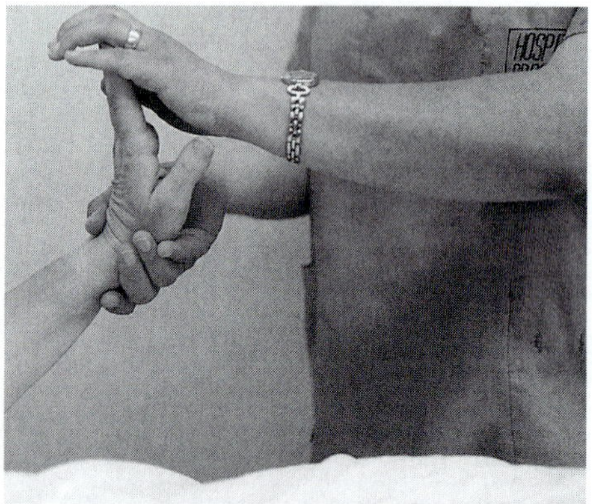

Step 6f(3)

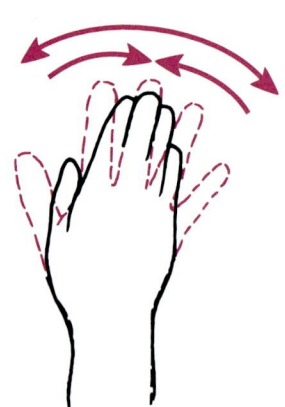

Step 6f(4)

STEPS | **RATIONALE**

g. Thumb

(1) *Flexion:* Move thumb across palmar surface of hand (ROM: 90 degrees) (see illustration).
(2) *Extension:* Move thumb straight away from hand (ROM: 90 degrees).
(3) *Abduction:* Extend thumb laterally (usually done when placing fingers in abduction and adduction) (ROM: 30 degrees).
(4) *Adduction:* Move thumb back toward hand (ROM: 30 degrees).
(5) *Opposition:* Touch thumb to each finger of same hand (see illustration).

Flexibility of thumb maintains coordination for fine motor activities.

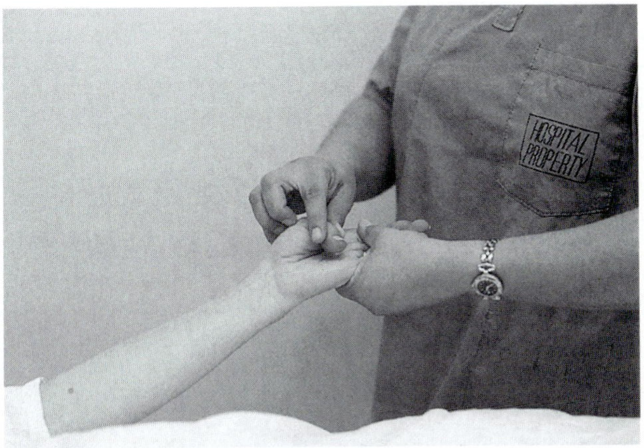

Step 6g(1)

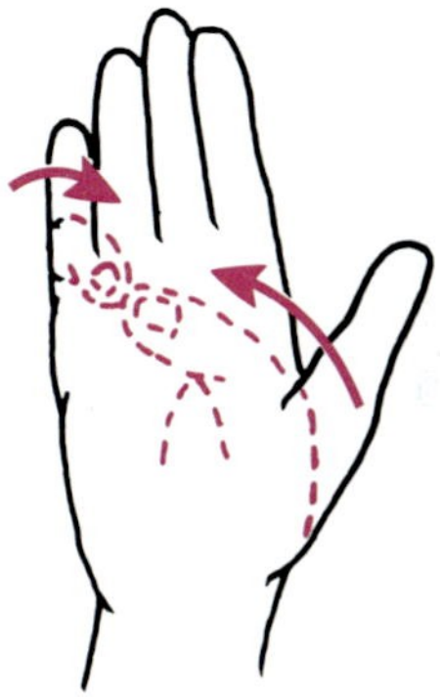

Step 6g(5)

h. Hip

(1) *Flexion:* Move leg forward and up (ROM: 90 to 120 degrees) (see illustration).
(2) *Extension:* Move leg back beside other leg (ROM: 90 to 120 degrees) (see illustration 6h(1)).
(3) *Hyperextension:* Move leg behind body (ROM: 30 to 50 degrees) (see illustration).

Contracture of hip can cause unsteady gait or difficulty ambulating.

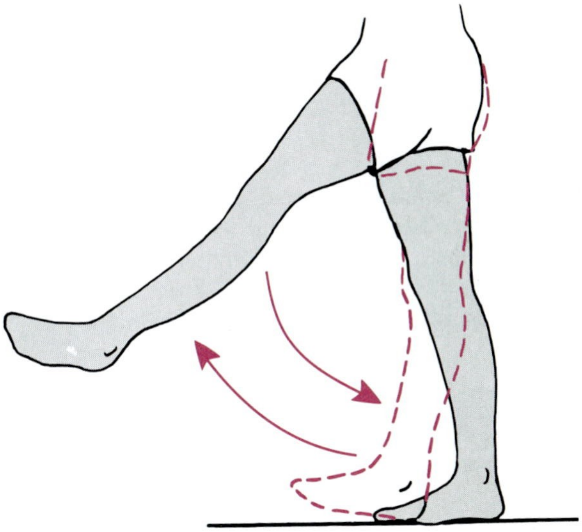

Step 6h(1)

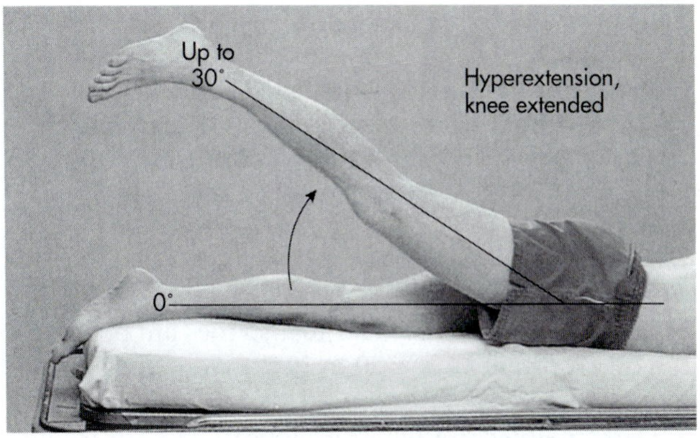

Step 6h(3) From Mourad LA: *Orthopedic disorders,* Mosby's Clinical Nursing Series, St Louis, 1991, Mosby.

STEPS	RATIONALE

(4) *Abduction:* Move leg laterally away from body (ROM: 30 to 50 degrees) (see illustration).

(5) *Adduction:* Move leg back toward medial position and beyond if possible (ROM: 30 to 50 degrees) (see illustration 6h(4)).

(6) *Internal rotation:* Turn foot and leg toward other leg (ROM: 90 degrees) (see illustration).

(7) *External rotation:* Turn foot and leg away from other leg (ROM: 90 degrees) (see illustration 6h(6)).

(8) *Circumduction:* Move leg in circle (ROM: 360 degrees) (see illustration).

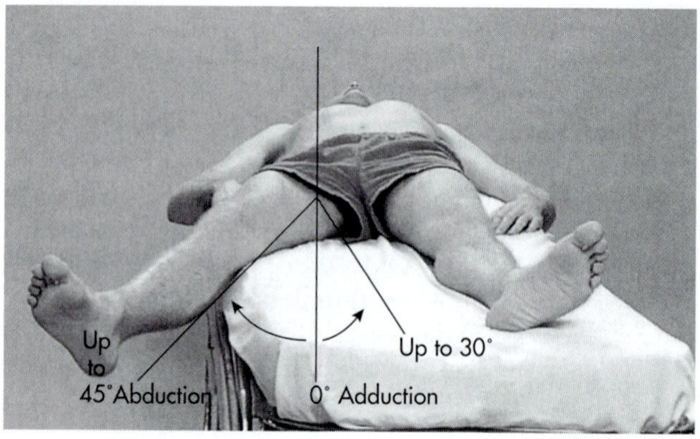

Step 6h(5) From Mourad LA: *Orthopedic disorders,* Mosby's Clinical Nursing Series, St Louis, 1991, Mosby.

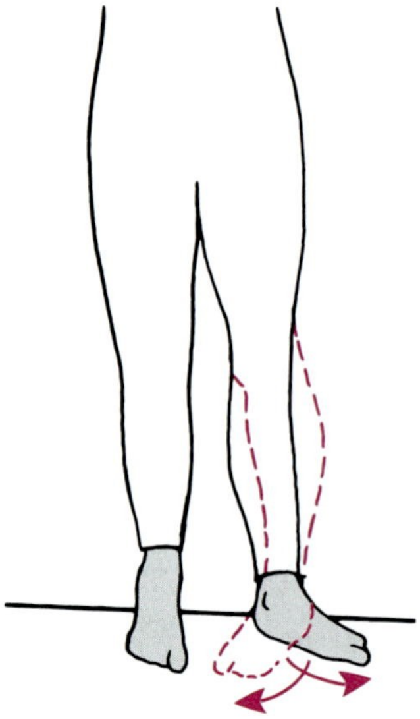

Step 6h(6)

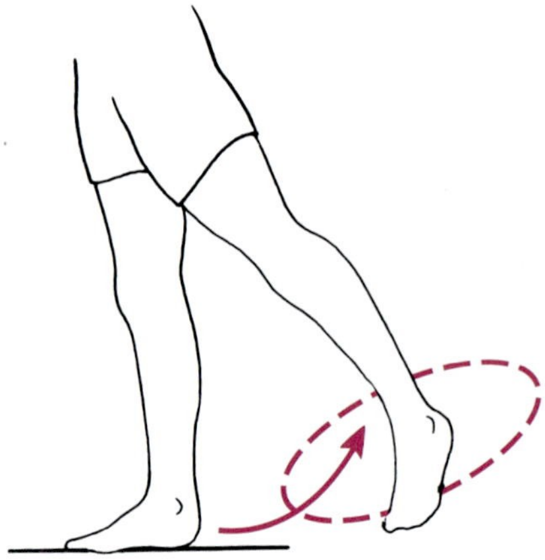

Step 6h(8)

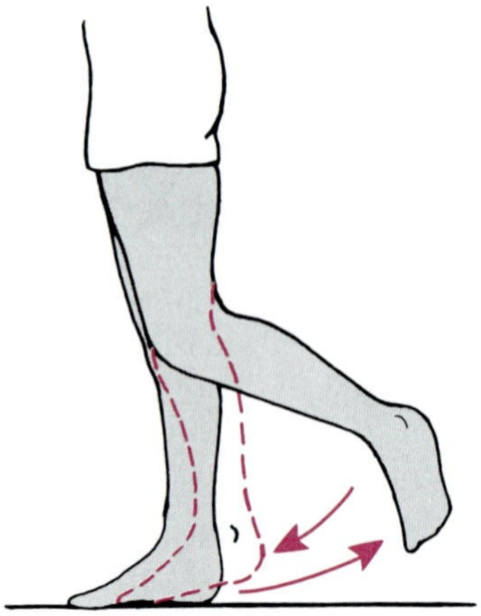

Step 6i(1)

i. Knee

(1) *Flexion:* Bring heel toward back of thigh (ROM: 120 to 130 degrees) (see illustration).

(2) *Extension:* Return leg to floor (ROM: 120 to 130 degrees) (see illustration 6i(1)).

Stiff knee can result in severe disability, the degree of which depends on position in which knee is stiffened. If knee is fixed in full extension, person must sit with leg thrust straight out in front. If knee is fixed in flexed position, person limps when walking.

j. Ankle

(1) **Dorsiflexion:** Move foot so toes are pointed upward (ROM: 20 to 30 degrees) (see illustration 6j(1)).

(2) **Plantar flexion:** Move foot so toes are pointed downward (ROM: 45 to 50 degrees) (see illustration 6j(1)).

Deformity of ankle can impair client's ability to walk.

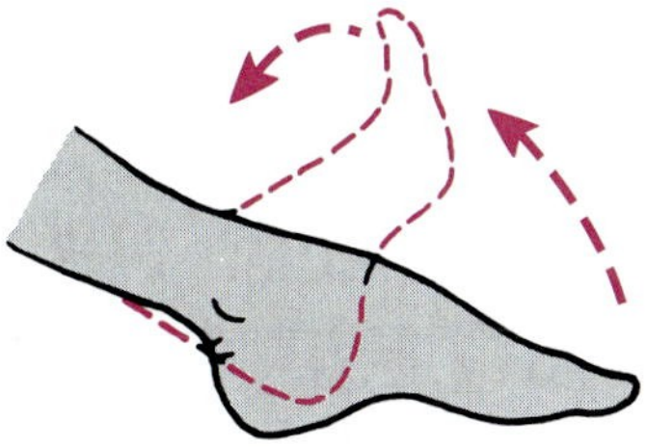

Step 6j(1)

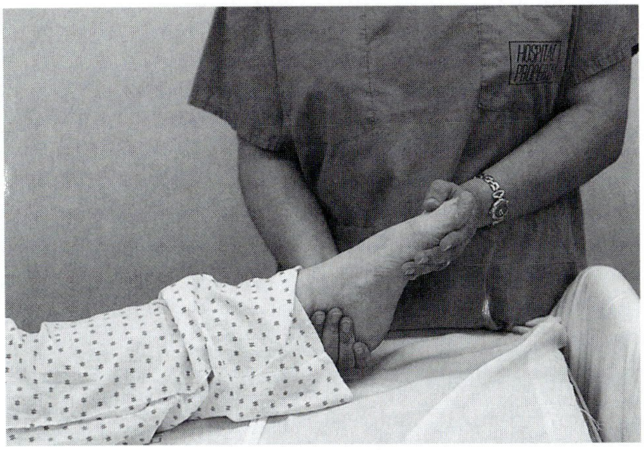

Step 6k(1)

STEPS	RATIONALE
k. Foot	
(1) **Inversion:** Turn sole of foot medially (ROM: 10 degrees or less) (see illustration).	Adequate ROM in lower extremities allows client to walk.
(2) **Eversion:** Turn sole of foot laterally (ROM: 10 degrees or less) (see illustration 6k(1)).	
(3) *Flexion:* Curl toes downward (ROM: 30 to 60 degrees) (see illustration).	
(4) *Extension:* Straighten toes (ROM: 30 to 60 degrees 6k(3)).	
(5) *Abduction:* Spread toes apart (ROM: 15 degrees or less) (see illustration).	
(6) *Adduction:* Bring toes together (ROM: 15 degrees or less) (see illustration 6k(4)).	
7. Reposition client to position of comfort and wash hands.	

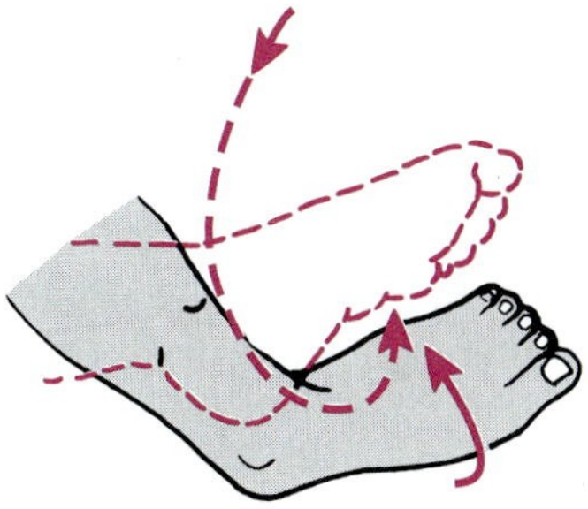

Step 6k(2)

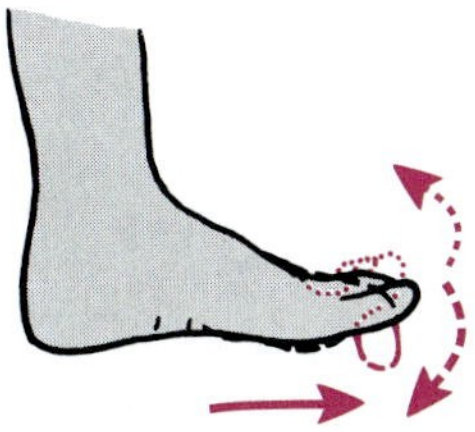

Step 6k(3)

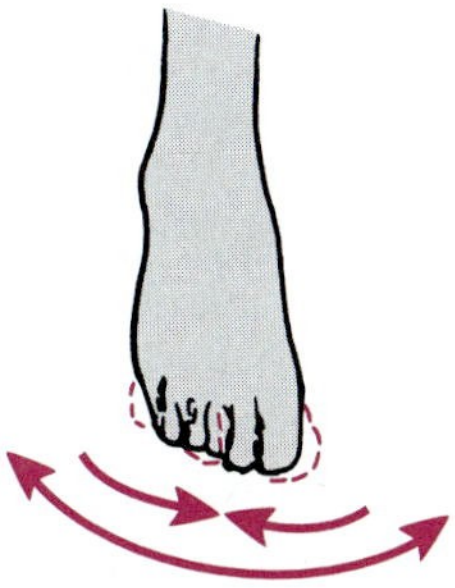

Step 6k(4)

EVALUATION

1. Observe range of various joints as compared to baseline range of those joints.	Determines whether exercises have had desired effect of increasing or maintaining joint mobility.
2. Ask for client's subjective statements regarding experience (e.g., complaints of discomfort, level of fatigue).	Evaluates client's tolerance of exercise.
3. Determine degree of assistance required to perform exercises.	Establishes guidelines to maximize self-care ability.
4. Ask client to independently perform exercises.	Determines that client performs exercises correctly.

STEPS	RATIONALE
5. **Unexpected outcomes** that may occur include:	
➤ Client experiences discomfort on ROM exercise.	Could indicate inflammation, infection, or joint contracture.
➤ Resistance is encountered when performing ROM exercise.	Could indicate beginning of joint contracture or joint disease.
➤ Spastic muscle contraction develops during ROM exercises.	Could indicate muscle fatigue. Movement of affected part is stopped, and continuous gentle pressure is placed on muscle group until it relaxes. Exercises are then restarted, using slower steady movement.

Recording and Reporting

1. Record in nurses' notes the joints exercised, type of exercise, extent to which joints can be moved, any joint abnormalities, client's subjective statements regarding tolerance of activity, and nurse's objective observation of tolerance.	Documents performance and subsequent effect of ROM exercises.
2. Report immediately to nurse in charge or physician if there is resistance on performance of ROM exercises, if client complains of pain on movement of joint, or if there are signs of swelling, redness, or heat in joint.	Notifies physician of alteration so necessary treatment can be started.

Follow-up Activities

1. Notify physician if there was resistance on performance of ROM exercises, if the client complained of pain on movement of a joint, or if there are signs of swelling, redness, or heat in joint.

• • • • •

Special Considerations

- It is essential to maintain joint flexibility. Contracted or immobile joints make protective positioning of a client difficult or impossible. It is hard to relieve pressure over bony prominences and to protect the client from pressure sores. Adequate skin care is difficult because it is hard to separate the skin folds adequately. If the client is in a curled or fetal position, chest expansion is restricted, and changes in abdominal pressure make elimination difficult.
- Contractures can begin shortly after onset of immobility. ROM exercises should be started as soon as possible. However, not all clients require ROM exercises. Assess to determine which joints obtain full ROM during client's normal activities.
- Performing ROM exercises during a warm bath helps decrease muscle tension and establishes ROM exercises as a part of the daily routine (Dawe and Curran-Smith, 1994).

Teaching Considerations

- Instruct client to exercise only to point of resistance and to stop if client expresses pain.
- Provide opportunity for return demonstration.

Pediatric Considerations

- Children should have ROM exercises incorporated into play activities to encourage participation and increase self-esteem.

Gerontologic Considerations

- Older adults may need ROM exercises in two or more sessions to control fatigue.

Home Care Considerations

- Assess family or primary care giver's ability, availability, and motivation to assist client with exercises client is unable to perform independently.
- Assist family or primary care giver to arrange home environment to promote exercise program (e.g., space allocation, lighting, temperature, safety precautions).
- Consult physical therapist for additional assistance or exercises and client's response to exercise program.
- Develop schedule for implementing the performance of the exercise program.

SKILL 30-2 Performing Isometric Exercises

In addition to ROM exercises, some immobilized clients may be able to perform some muscle-strengthening exercises. These include isotonic (dynamic), isometric (static), and resistive exercises. **Isotonic exercises** cause muscle contraction and change in muscle length. Examples of isotonic exercises are walking, performing aerobics, and moving arms and legs against light resistance. Isotonic exercises increase circulation and respiratory rate and have beneficial effects on the entire body (Topp, Mikesky, and Bawel, 1994). Some individuals, however, are unable to tolerate such increases in activity. For these individuals, isometric exercises are more appropriate. Isometric exercises involve tightening or tensing of muscles without moving body parts **(isometric contractions).** They increase muscle tension but do not change the length of muscle fibers. Therefore improvements in muscle strength apply only at the joint angle where isometric exercises are performed (Topp, Mikesky, and Bawel, 1994). Isometric exercises are easily accomplished by an immobilized client in bed. Both isotonic and isometric exercises help to prevent muscular atrophy and combat osteoporosis.

Isometric exercises may also be resistive. Resistive isometric exercises are those in which the individual contracts the muscle while pushing against a stationary object or resisting the movement of an object (Borgman-Gainer, 1996). A gradual increase in the amount of resistance and length of time that the muscle contraction is held will increase muscle strength and endurance (Topp, Mikesky, and Bawel, 1994). Examples of resistive isometric exercises are performing push-ups, pushing against a **footboard** to move up in bed, and hip lifting. In hip lifting, the individual, who is in a sitting position, pushes with the hands against a sitting surface such as a chair to raise the hips. Resistive isometric exercises help to promote muscular strength and provide the necessary stress for bone maintenance and growth. Without sufficient stress against bone, osteoclastic activity (activity by cells responsible for bone tissue absorption) increases over osteoblastic activity (activity by bone-forming cells). The result is demineralization of the bone and eventual osteoporosis.

DELEGATION CONSIDERATIONS

The skill of performing isometric exercises can be delegated to unlicensed assistive personnel. Clients with cardiovascular disease require evaluation by a professional nurse when initially performing these exercises. The following information is needed when delegating skills to nursing staff or family members:

- Gradually increase amount of time and frequency of isometric exercises.

STEPS	RATIONALE
ASSESSMENT	
1. Review client's chart for contraindications to isometric exercises.	Isometric exercises raise blood pressure and pulse and temporarily obstruct flow around tensed muscle (Topp, Mikesky, and Bawel, 1994). Client's medical condition, especially if history of cardiac problems is present, may be a contraindication.
2. Assess client's baseline vital signs.	Isometric exercises may raise blood pressure. Documentation of baseline vital signs is necessary to determine whether exercises cause a deterioration in vital signs.
3. Assess baseline muscle strength: a. Ask client to perform task against resistance (e.g., push one foot against palm of hand). b. Assess grasp strength by having client grasp nurse's hands. Note whether hand grasps are equal. c. Have client grasp two fingers of nurse's right hand with client's left hand and two fingers of nurse's left hand with client's right hand. d. Observe client's abilities to do daily activities (e.g., whether client has adequate strength to bathe self, pull self up in bed, move from bed to chair). e. Obtain client's subjective statements related to muscle strengths. Does client feel weaker?	Enables nurse to compare muscle strength before and after exercise.

STEPS	RATIONALE
4. Assess client's or care giver's understanding of isometric exercises to be used.	Allows client to verbalize concerns and identifies educational needs of client or care giver.

N URSING DIAGNOSIS

Clustering of defining characteristics from the assessment data may reveal the following nursing diagnoses for clients requiring this skill:

- Activity intolerance
- Fatigue
- Impaired physical mobility
- Knowledge deficit regarding exercises
- Pain

Related factors are individualized based on a client's condition or needs.

P LANNING

1. **Expected outcomes** following completion of procedure:
   - Client will gradually increase number of exercise repetitions. — Client will gradually become stronger and be able to increase number of repetitions. Isometric exercises increase muscle tone.
   - Vital signs will remain stable. — Documents client's **activity tolerance.**
2. Explain procedure and demonstrate exercises. — Relieves anxiety and encourages client's cooperation.
3. Assist client to comfortable position. — Reduces stress and promotes client participation.

I MPLEMENTATION

1. Provide privacy. — Prevents client embarrassment.
2. Instruct client to perform following exercises as prescribed and gradually increase repetitions. Muscle groups used for walking should be exercised isometrically four times per day until client is ambulatory. Muscle group is tightened (contracted) for 8 seconds then completely relaxed for several seconds (Borgman-Gainer, 1996). Repeat 8 to 10 times for each muscle group during each exercise session several times a day. Exercises are as follows:

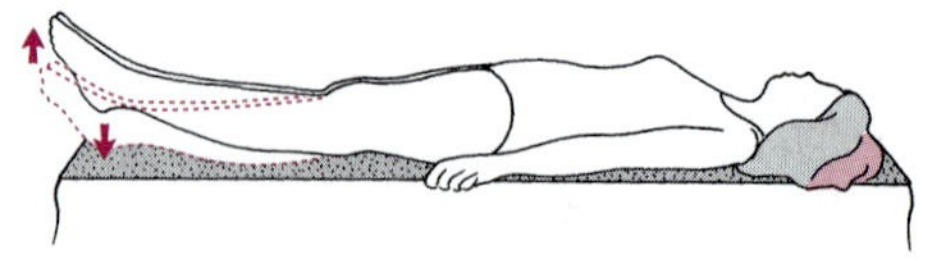

Step 2a(2)

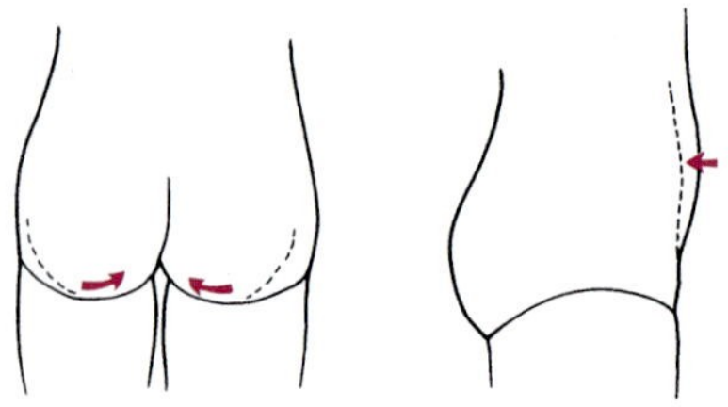

Step 2b(2) Step 2c

CRITICAL DECISION POINT Clients doing isometric exercises should be taught to exhale while exerting effort. Many persons hold their breath when exerting effort (Valsalva maneuver). This increases intrathoracic pressure, causing decrease in venous return to heart. When breath is released, intrathoracic pressure decreases, causing large surge of blood to return to the heart and increase cardiac work load (Borgman-Gainer, 1996; Griego and House-Fancher, 1996).

a. Quadriceps isometric exercises:

(1) Assist to supine recumbent position.
(2) Instruct client to press back of the knee against mattress while trying to lift heel from bed (see illustration).
(3) Hold muscles tightly contracted for 8 seconds and then relax completely for several seconds.
(4) Repeat.

For person to ambulate and get out of chair, large muscles of thigh (quadriceps) must be strong enough for client to extend knees and stabilize them.
Nurse can assist client in learning this exercise by placing hand between client's knee and mattress and asking client to press hand against mattress with the knee.

b. Gluteal muscle isometric exercises:

(1) Assist client to recumbent position. — Improves client's balance when sitting.
(2) Instruct client to pinch buttocks muscles together and hold for 8 seconds and then relax

STEPS	RATIONALE
completely for several seconds (see illustration 2b(2)).	
(3) Repeat.	
c. Abdominal muscle isometric exercises (see illustration):	
(1) Pull abdominal muscles in as tightly as possible.	Improves trunk stability.
(2) Hold for 8 seconds.	
(3) Release muscles gradually.	
(4) Repeat.	
d. Foot muscle isometric exercises:	
(1) Instruct client to move foot in a circle in all directions and flex foot toward and away from knee.	Increases muscle activity in leg and thereby promotes venous return to heart.
e. Hand muscle isometric exercises:	
(1) Obtain sponge rubber ball. (Size of ball depends on size of client's hand.)	Strengthens grip to hold onto crutch or walker more effectively.
(2) Grip ball with entire hand five to ten times.	
(3) Dig each fingertip, one at a time, into ball five to ten times each.	
(4) Gradually increase frequency of exercise until client can grip ball and exercise once or twice a day.	
f. Biceps isometric exercises:	
(1) Raise arms to shoulder height and interlock fingertips of both hands.	Strengthens biceps and thereby helps with ambulation if ambulatory assistive device is used.
(2) Try to pull hands apart using arm muscles.	
(3) Hold for 8 seconds.	
(4) Relax muscles.	
(5) Repeat.	
g. Triceps muscle isometric exercises (see illustration):	
(1) Raise arms to shoulder height.	Strengthens triceps to assist with transfer techniques and use of crutches or walker.
(2) Make fist with one hand and place against palm of other hand.	
(3) Push hands together as hard as possible for 8 seconds.	
(4) Relax and repeat after 2 minutes.	

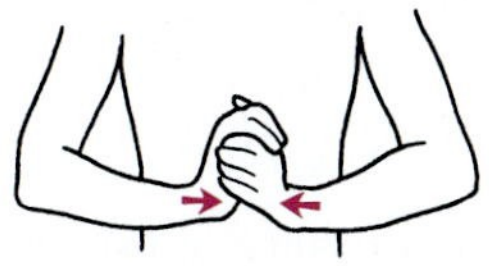

Step 2g

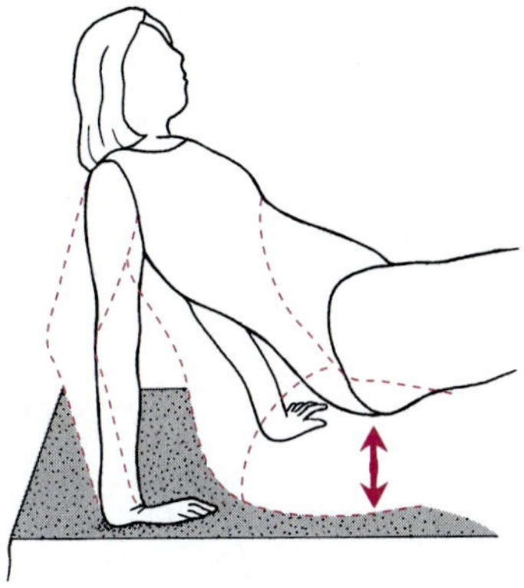

Step 3a

STEPS	RATIONALE
3. Instruct client in the following resistive isometric exercises:	
a. Triceps muscle resistive isometric exercises (see illustration):	
(1) Assist client to sitting position on edge of bed or in chair. If mattress is soft, blocks or books are placed on bed under client's hands.	To use crutches or walker effectively, client must have enough strength in the triceps to extend and stabilize the elbows while lifting or shifting body weight.

STEPS	RATIONALE
(2) Instruct client to try to lift buttocks off bed or seat of chair by pressing down on mattress or chair seat with hands.	
(3) Hold muscle tight for 8 seconds, then relax.	
(4) Repeat.	
b. Quadriceps muscle resistive isometric exercises:	
(1) Push feet against footboard. Hold muscles tight for 8 seconds, then relax.	Builds strength, size, and shape of leg muscles and provides stress against bone that is needed to maintain a balance between osteoblasts and osteoclasts. Without sufficient stress, the osteoclastic activity increases over the osteoblastic activity and bone demineralization occurs.
(2) Repeat.	

EVALUATION

1. Observe client's ability to perform exercises.	
2. Determine client's level of energy, muscular strength, and comfort following exercises.	Assesses whether client is performing exercises accurately and whether the exercises are increasing muscle strength.
3. Obtain vital signs.	Assesses tolerance to activity.
4. **Unexpected outcomes** that may occur include:	
➤ Client is unable to perform exercises.	Client may be too weak. Continue ROM exercises and reposition client to try to increase strength. Make sure nutrition and rest are adequate.
➤ Client is unwilling to perform exercises.	Lack of understanding of significance of exercises may be the problem. Stress importance of the exercises.
➤ Muscular strength is not increasing.	Client may not be performing exercises as described or as often as instructed. Stress importance of following routine.
➤ Client's blood pressure and heart rate increase significantly during exercises.	Client may not be able to tolerate procedure. Discontinue exercises and consult physician.

RECORDING AND REPORTING

1. Record in nurses' notes the type of isometric exercises used, length of time contractions held, number of repetitions of each exercise, assessment of client's muscular strength after exercises, and client's subjective statements regarding muscular strength.	Provides documentation of client's progress in using isometric exercises.
2. Report client's tolerance or untoward effect to nurse in charge or physician.	Notifies appropriate personnel of untoward effects and possible need for modification of exercise plan.

FOLLOW-UP ACTIVITIES

1. Assess client's understanding of significance of exercises.
2. Notify physician if having difficulty performing exercises or if muscle strength is not improving.

• • • • •

Special Considerations

- ➤ It may be more effective to instruct client to perform exercises before each meal and at bedtime instead of four times per day.
- ➤ Proper nutrition is essential if client is to be able to perform exercises. The promotion of protein anabolism involves conservation and replenishment of energy stores.

Teaching Considerations

- ➤ Instruct client to gradually increase exercises each day and to exhale on exertion to avoid Valsalva maneuver (Riegel and Thomason, 1995).

SKILL 30-3 Applying Elastic Stockings

Thrombophlebitis is one of the most common venous disorders. Thrombophlebitis is the development of a **thrombus** or clot along with the inflammation of the vein and may be classified as superficial or deep. Superficial thrombophlebitis may be caused by varicose veins or intravenous (IV) medications. It has been reported that "65% of all patients receiving IV therapy develop superficial thrombophlebitis" (Rudolphi and Doyle, 1996). After injury or surgery, clients are at risk for deep vein thrombosis (DVT). It has been called the greatest single threat to postoperative recovery (Rudolphi and Doyle, 1996; von Rueden and Harris, 1995). Complications of DVT are pulmonary embolism and increased susceptibility to recurrent DVT. Since DVT usually occurs during a client's recovery phase, nurses need to incorporate various interventions to try to prevent this potentially fatal complication (Campbell, 1992).

Three elements contribute to the development of a DVT; they are commonly referred to as Virchow's triad. These elements are hypercoagulability of the blood, venous wall damage, and stasis of blood flow (Carroll, 1993; Rudolphi and Doyle, 1996). Elastic stockings help reduce two of the elements of Virchow's triad: blood stasis and venous wall injury. First, they promote venous return by maintaining pressure on superficial veins to prevent venous pooling, thereby reducing the risk of clot formation in the lower extremities. Second, an increased incidence of DVT has been found in clients in whom the venous diameter had increased. In these cases, the endothelial layer can tear. It has been suggested that elastic stockings prevent passive dilation of the veins, thereby decreasing the risk of endothelial tears.

EQUIPMENT

- Tape measure
- Talcum powder
- Elastic support stockings

DELEGATION CONSIDERATIONS

The following information is needed when delegating the application of elastic stockings to nursing staff or family members:

- Avoid activities that promote venous stasis (e.g., crossing legs, wearing garters, or elevating legs on pillows).
- When possible, elevate legs to improve venous return.
- Do not massage legs.
- Elevate legs before applying stockings.
- Avoid wrinkles in the stockings.
- Observe for allergic reactions, skin irritation, and thrombophlebitis.

STEPS	RATIONALE
ASSESSMENT	
1. Assess client for risk factors in Virchow's triad to determine need for elastic stockings: a. *Hypercoagulability:* all clients with clotting disorders, fever, dehydration, pregnancy and first 6 weeks postpartum if the woman was confined to bed, and oral contraceptive use (especially if client smokes) b. *Venous wall abnormalities:* local trauma, orthopedic surgeries, major abdominal surgery, varicose veins, atherosclerosis c. *Blood stasis:* immobility, obesity, pregnancy	Potential candidates for elastic stockings are clients who have an alteration in one of the elements of Virchow's triad (Bright and Georgi, 1992; Rudolphi and Doyle, 1996; von Rueden and Harris, 1995).
2. Observe for signs, symptoms, and conditions that might contraindicate use of elastic stockings. Signs and symptoms include:	
a. Dermatitis or open skin lesion	Elastic stockings may aggravate skin condition or cause it to spread. Also, physician may want medication and dressing applied to lesion.
b. Recent skin graft	Continuous pressure is necessary to keep graft adherent to recipient bed, but pressure should not be so firm as to cause death of graft (Long and Phipps, 1992; Solotkin and Knipe, 1996).

STEPS	RATIONALE
c. Disproportionately large thighs	Elastic stockings may not fit correctly, causing excessive pressure and constriction around thighs, thereby reducing venous return (Bright and Georgi, 1992; Galindo-Ciocon, 1995).
d. Severe atherosclerosis	Persons with atherosclerosis should not wear clothing that constricts and further impedes circulation and so should avoid rolled garters and socks with tight bands.
e. Pulmonary edema	Elastic stockings promote venous return. Treatments for pulmonary edema are to decrease venous return and circulating blood volume to decrease workload on heart (Bright and Georgi, 1992).
f. Decreased circulation in lower extremities as evidenced by cyanotic, cool extremities	Elastic stockings may further impede circulation.
3. Obtain physician's order.	Protects nurse, physician, and client. May be needed for legal or reimbursement reasons.
4. Assess client's or care giver's understanding of application of elastic stockings.	Identifies potential educational needs of client or care giver.
5. Assess and document the condition of client's skin and circulation to the legs (i.e., presence of pedal pulses, edema, discoloration of the skin, temperature, lesions, or cuts).	Identifies a baseline for skin integrity and quality of peripheral pulses in lower extremities.

NURSING DIAGNOSIS

Clustering of defining characteristics from the assessment data may reveal the following nursing diagnoses for clients requiring this skill:

- Activity intolerance
- Altered peripheral tissue perfusion
- Decreased cardiac output
- Impaired physical mobility
- Knowledge deficit regarding application of elastic stockings
- Risk for impaired skin integrity

Related factors are individualized based on a client's condition or needs.

PLANNING

STEPS	RATIONALE
1. **Expected outcomes** following completion of procedure:	
➤ Client shows no evidence of skin irritation or thrombophlebitis.	Ensures that there are no side effects to the circulatory system or client's skin.
➤ Client is able to demonstrate application of elastic stockings.	Verifies correct psychomotor learning.
➤ Client has reduction of edema in lower extremities.	Elastic stockings decrease venous pooling in lower extremities.
2. Explain procedure and reasons for applying stockings.	Reduces anxiety and encourages client cooperation.
3. Use tape measure to measure client's legs to determine proper stocking size.	Stockings must be measured according to manufacturer's directions. Elastic stockings come in two lengths: knee length and thigh length. The choice of length depends on physician's order.

CRITICAL DECISION POINT Compare client's measurements with the manufacturer's sizing chart. If too large, stockings will not adequately support extremities. If too small, stockings may impede circulation. The optimum stocking pressure is 20 to 30 mm Hg at the ankle, decreasing to 8 mm Hg at the middle to upper thigh. This change in pressure produces the greatest increase in venous flow velocity that is both safe and practical (Bright and Georgi, 1992).

STEPS	RATIONALE
IMPLEMENTATION	
1. Wash hands.	Reduces transmission of microorganisms.
2. Position client in supine position. Elevate head of bed to comfortable level.	Promotes good body mechanics for nurse. Client position eases application. Also, the stockings should be applied before standing to prevent stagnation of blood in lower extremities. If client has been standing, client should sit in chair or lie in bed for 15 minutes with legs elevated before applying elastic stockings (Bright and Georgi, 1992).
3. After legs are cleansed, apply small amount of talcum powder to legs and feet, provided client does not have sensitivity to talcum powder.	Talcum powder reduces friction and allows for easier application of stockings.
4. Apply stockings:	
a. Turn elastic stocking inside out by placing one hand into sock, holding toe of sock with other hand, and pulling (see illustration).	Allows easier application of stocking.
b. Place client's toes into foot of elastic stocking, making sure that sock is smooth (see illustration).	Wrinkles in sock can impede circulation to lower region of extremity (Bright and Georgi, 1992).
c. Slide remaining portion of sock over client's foot, being sure that the toes are covered. Make sure the foot fits into the toe and heel position of the sock. Sock will now be right side out (see illustration).	If toes remain uncovered, they will become constricted by elastic and their circulation can be reduced.

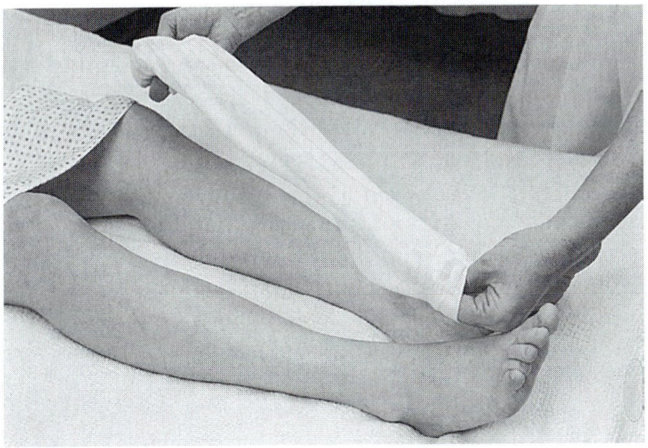

Step 4a

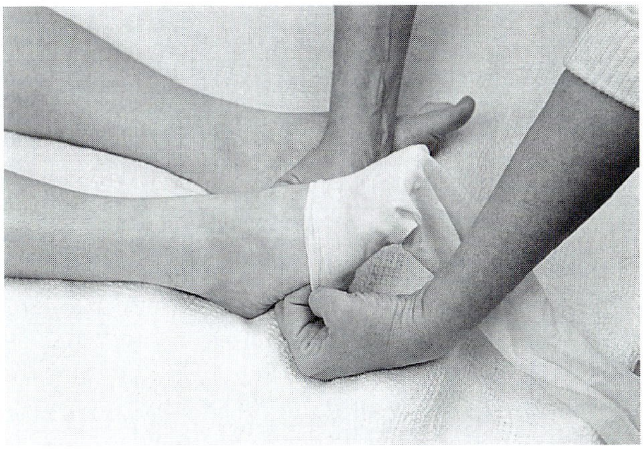

Step 4b

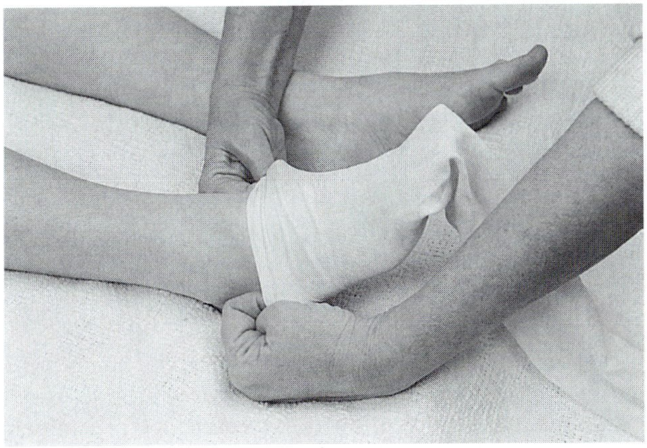

Step 4c

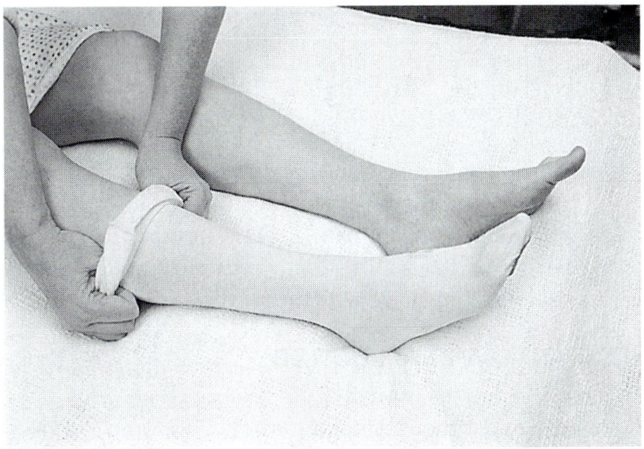

Step 4d

STEPS	RATIONALE
d. Slide sock up over client's calf until sock is completely extended. Be sure sock is smooth and no ridges are present (see illustration).	Ridges impede venous return and can counteract overall purpose of elastic stocking (Bright and Georgi, 1992).
e. Instruct client not to roll socks partially down.	Rolling sock partially down has a constricting effect and can impede venous return.
5. Reposition client to position of comfort and wash hands.	Maintains proper body alignment and promotes comfort. Reduces transmission of microorganisms.

EVALUATION

1. Inspect stocking to make sure there are no wrinkles or binding at top of stocking.	Wrinkles lead to increased pressure and alter circulation.
2. Observe circulatory status of lower extremities. Observe color, temperature, and condition of skin.	Ensures circulatory status in lower extremities has not been compromised.
3. Observe client's reaction to stockings.	Ensures client is adapting to stockings and is not experiencing any discomfort from stockings.
4. Observe client or care giver apply stockings.	Determines ability to perform skill accurately.
5. **Unexpected outcomes** that may occur include:	
➤ Skin reaction to elastic stockings develops. Observe for evidence of redness, skin lesions, and client's subjective complaint of itching or burning.	Some clients may have skin reaction to material used in elastic socks. May indicate allergic reaction.
➤ Decrease in circulation in lower extremities develops. Assess for coolness in lower extremities, cyanosis, decrease in pedal pulses, decrease in blanching, and numbness or tingling sensation.	Elastic stockings may be too small or have wrinkles or folds that impede circulation. Signs and symptoms may indicate obstruction of arterial blood flow.

➤ *CRITICAL DECISION POINT* Thrombophlebitis can develop in lower extremity. Clinical manifestations of thrombophlebitis vary according to size and location of thrombus. Signs and symptoms of superficial thrombosis include palpable vein and the surrounding area being tender to touch, reddened, and warm. There may be slight temperature elevation. Edema of extremity may or may not occur. Signs and symptoms of DVT include swollen extremity; pain; warm, cyanotic skin; and temperature elevation (Galindo-Ciocon, 1995; Rudolphi and Doyle, 1996). If calf is involved, positive Homans' sign may be present (pain in calf on dorsiflexion of foot) (Fig. 30-1). Venous stasis with resultant clot formation may have occurred even though stockings were in place. Other causes could be injury to vein or hypercoagulability. Extremity with phlebitis will be larger than opposite limb. Area over inflamed vein may be reddened and skin may be warm in area of phlebitis.

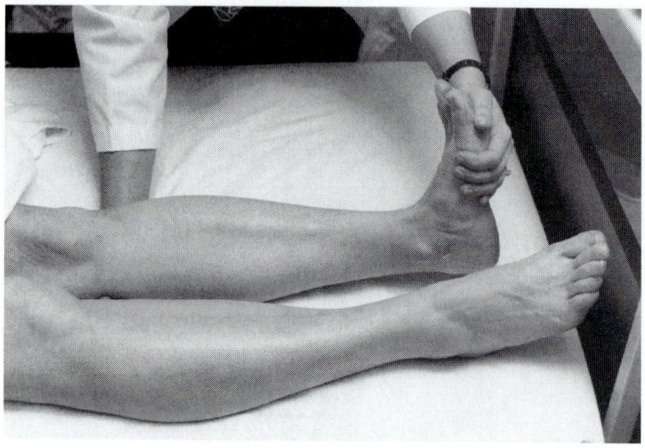

Fig. 30-1 Assessing Homans' sign.

➤ Pulmonary embolism develops. Signs and symptoms include tachypnea, shortness of breath, anxiety, pleuritic chest pain, cough, hemoptysis, tachycardia, and signs of right ventricular failure (i.e., distended neck veins) (Rudolphi and Doyle, 1996).	At least 90% of pulmonary emboli originate from thrombi in the lower extremities (Coffman, 1992). The risk is decreased if elastic stockings are used, but it is still a potential complication if the client has an alteration in one of the elements of Virchow's triad.

RECORDING AND REPORTING

1. Record in nurses' notes:	
a. Date and time of stocking application and condition of skin before application.	Documents condition of lower extremities before and after application of elastic stockings.

STEPS	RATIONALE
b. Circulatory status of lower extremities before stocking application.	
c. Stocking length and size.	
d. Date and time stockings are removed.	
e. Condition of skin and circulatory status after removal.	
f. Calf or thigh circumferences (daily if client is at risk for thrombophlebitis).	Unexplained increase in circumferences of the calf or thigh could indicate thrombophlebitis.
2. Immediately report signs of thrombophlebitis or impeded circulation in lower extremities to charge nurse or physician. (See signs and symptoms in Evaluation, Step 5.)	Institutes prompt therapy to restore circulation. Remove stockings and elevate leg until given further orders.
3. Report any signs of skin irritation to physician.	

FOLLOW-UP ACTIVITIES

1. Remove stockings at least once each shift.
2. Demonstrate application of elastic stockings.
3. If any signs of thrombophlebitis or skin irritation are noted, remove stockings and contact physician.

Special Considerations

- Lower extremities should not be massaged.
- Clients may require two pairs of elastic stockings: one for wear while the other is laundered.
- Replace stocking every 6 months to maintain proper compression (Bright and Georgi, 1992).
- Another measure to reduce DVT is the use of sequential pneumatic compression stockings. These devices consist of an air pump, connecting tubing, and extremity sleeves that sequentially inflate and deflate chambers within the stocking (Fig. 30-2). The intermittent pumping action drives superficial blood into deep veins, where it is evacuated proximally by the venous valves, thus removing pooled blood and preventing both venous stasis and the accumulation of clotting factors (Bright and Georgi, 1992; Ciocon, Fernandez, and Ciocon, 1993).

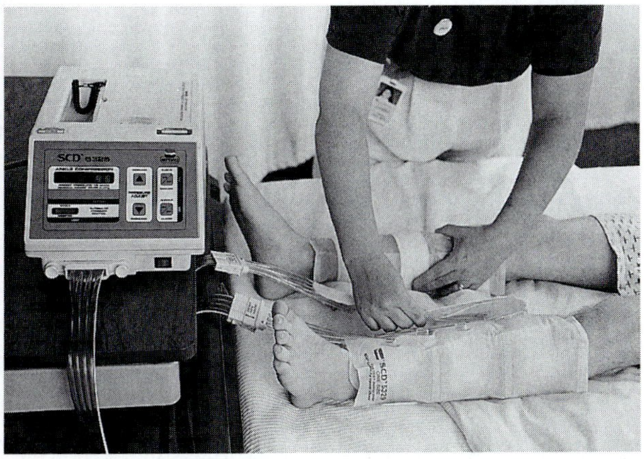

Fig. 30-2 Sequential pneumatic compression stockings.

Teaching Considerations

- Have client demonstrate stocking application.
- Instruct client to launder stockings as follows:
  - Every 2 days with mild detergent.
  - Lay flat to dry (dryer heat weakens elastic, and hanging stockings causes elastic to stretch out of shape).
- Discourage clients from activities that promote venous stasis (e.g., crossing legs, wearing garters, elevating legs on pillows).
- When possible, elevate legs to improve venous return (Bright and Georgi, 1992; Ciocon, Galindo-Ciocon, and Galindo, 1995; Galindo-Ciocon, 1995; Rudolphi and Doyle, 1996).

Pediatric Considerations

- Assess for wrinkles in stockings. Encourage children not to roll or fold stockings on lower legs.
- Assess for proper fit. Stockings that are too tight will impede circulation. Stockings that are too loose will be inefficient.

Gerontologic Considerations

- Assess for early signs of venous insufficiency. Venous insufficiency is the most common cause of leg edema in older adults (Ciocon, Galindo-Ciocon, and Galindo, 1995).
- Perform comprehensive assessments of older adults. Normal physiological aging can mask the signs and symptoms of venous insufficiency (Galindo-Ciocon, 1995).

Home Care Considerations

- Assess and evaluate proper fit and application of stockings at regularly scheduled intervals.
- Assess if client is adhering to prescribed use of stockings. Potential reasons for discontinuing use are socioeconomic causes, cosmetic concerns, discomfort, lack of knowledge regarding reasons for use, and difficulty with application (Bright and Georgi, 1992).

SKILL 30-4 Changing Client's Position to Minimize Occurrence of Orthostatic Hypotension

One of the most common complications of immobility is orthostatic hypotension (Hamilton and Lyon, 1995). Orthostatic or postural hypotension is a drop in blood pressure that occurs when the client changes from a horizontal to vertical position (e.g., when the client rises from a lying to a sitting position or from a sitting to a standing position). Although research findings indicate that there is a wide range of normal orthostatic responses to position changes, it is agreed that a 15 mm Hg decrease in systolic pressure or a 10 mm Hg decrease in diastolic pressure with symptoms of dizziness, pallor, or fainting indicates postural hypotension. Immobilized clients and those undergoing prolonged bed rest are at risk for orthostatic hypotension. Orthostatic hypotension is thought to be caused by two factors.

Although orthostatic hypotension cannot be prevented, its effects can be minimized. Interventions are directed toward maintaining muscle tone to increase venous return to the heart and to decrease stasis of blood in the lower extremities. Two interventions to help clients maintain muscle tone are the previously mentioned ROM and isometric exercises (see Skills 30-1 and 30-2) and the application of elastic stockings (see Skill 30-3) (Doering, 1993; Borgman-Gainer, 1996). Another intervention to reduce the effects of orthostatic hypotension is helping the client become progressively mobile as soon as possible (i.e., sitting in an upright [90-degree] position in bed, sitting on the side of the bed with legs in a dependent position and wiggling the feet **[dangling]**, transferring from bed to chair, or walking) (Doering, 1993; Winslow, Lane, and Woods, 1995). Before a client is helped out of bed, certain client assessments must be made and necessary safety precautions taken.

EQUIPMENT

- Elastic stockings (if ordered)
- Robe
- Safety belt
- Nonskid shoes or slippers

DELEGATION CONSIDERATIONS

The following information is needed when delegating the skill of position changes to minimize orthostatic hypotension to nursing staff or family members:

- Have client wear shoes with a nonslip surface during transfer or ambulation.
- Make slow, gradual position changes.
- Observe for nausea, pallor, and dizziness.
- Have client sit in chair or return to bed if client has symptoms of orthostatic hypotension.

When assisting with ambulation:

- Do not try to hold clients if they become dizzy or faint. Ease them into a sitting position in a chair or on the floor.
- Be sure the area is free of clutter, wet areas, and rugs that may slide.

STEPS	RATIONALE
ASSESSMENT	
1. Review client's chart to assess previous activity level, vital signs, and current activity order.	Determines how long client has been assigned bed rest and current activity order. The longer a client has been immobile, the greater the risk for orthostatic hypotension.
2. Obtain client's vital signs in supine position.	Provides baseline for comparison when client changes from supine to upright position; dizziness and/or a decrease of 15 mm Hg in systolic blood pressure and 10 mm Hg in diastolic blood pressure when upright is indicative of postural hypotension (Winslow, Lane, and Woods, 1995).
3. Assess client's environment for potential safety hazards before ambulation or transfer (e.g., wet floor, clutter).	Protects client from falls and other injuries.

STEPS	RATIONALE
PLANNING	
1. **Expected outcomes** following completion of procedure:	
➤ Client will have no symptoms of orthostatic hypotension: dizziness, decrease in blood pressure greater than 15 mm Hg (systolic) to 10 mg (diastolic).	Client is able to maintain a stable blood pressure during transfer.
2. Explain procedure and reasons for getting client out of bed.	Reduces anxiety and encourages client cooperation.
3. Assess whether another staff member is needed before transferring or ambulating client.	Prevents accidental lifting injuries to client and nurse.
IMPLEMENTATION	
1. Wash hands.	Reduces transfer of microorganisms.
2. Place bed in low position.	Have bed as close to floor as possible in case client becomes dizzy and falls.
3. Slowly raise head of bed to high Fowler's position and obtain blood pressure.	Raising slowly allows body to adjust to change in position. Note whether blood pressure decreases or client complains of dizziness when changing from supine to upright position.
4. Observe client for signs of orthostatic hypotension: nausea, pallor, dizziness, seeing spots, or lightheadedness.	Indicates orthostatic hypotension. Procedure may need to be postponed until client is able to tolerate high Fowler's position without signs and symptoms of orthostatic hypotension (Winslow, Lane, and Woods, 1995).
5. Assist client to sit with legs dangling over side of bed for 1 to 3 minutes. "Have client wiggle feet and move their legs intermittently while they are dangling their legs. Avoid pressure on the backs of the knees" (Winslow, Lane, and Woods, 1995).	Allows autonomic nervous system to adapt to postural change. Decreases pooling of blood into the legs while dangling. Prevents decrease of venous return (Winslow, Lane, and Woods, 1995).
6. Continue to talk with client and assess for orthostatic hypotension.	Decreases in blood pressure and increases in heart rate may occur as long as 2 minutes after position changes (Winslow, Lane, and Woods, 1995).
7. If there are no signs of dizziness or lightheadedness, assist client to stand, transfer to a chair, or ambulate.	Absence of dizziness or lightheadedness indicates that it is safe to attempt to transfer client to chair or ambulate.
8. Wash hands.	
EVALUATION	
1. Observe client for signs of orthostatic hypotension.	Dizziness can indicate reduced blood pressure, and the nurse must safely guide client into chair or back to bed.
2. Recheck client's blood pressure while client is sitting the first few times client is mobile.	Indicates how well the client is tolerating the activity.
3. **Unexpected outcomes** that may occur include:	
➤ Client becomes lightheaded and begins to fall.	Results from orthostatic hypotension.
RECORDING AND REPORTING	
1. Record in nurses' notes:	
a. Supine and upright blood pressures.	Documents client's tolerance of increased activity level.
b. Any changes in respiratory rate, skin color, or temperature noted when client is placed in upright position.	
c. Client's subjective statements regarding upright position.	Documents any symptom the client perceived during transfer.

STEPS	RATIONALE
d. If client sat in chair, note length of time client was able to sit and how well activity was tolerated. Recheck and document blood pressure while client is sitting up.	Documents client's activity tolerance when transferring to a chair or ambulating.
e. If client ambulates, note distance walked, stability of gait, any assistance needed, and how procedure was tolerated.	Documents client's activity tolerance.
2. Report immediately if client sustains injury or is unable to tolerate activity.	Provides prompt follow-up care of any injuries.

FOLLOW-UP ACTIVITIES

1. If client experiences dizziness, instruct client to sit down and lower the head or lie down.
2. If client starts to fall while walking with nurse, nurse should put both arms around client's waist and stand with feet apart to provide broad base of support. Extend leg and let client slide against it to floor. As client slides, nurse bends knees to lower body.

• • • • •

Special Considerations

- Before attempting to get a client out of bed, be sure adequate assistance is available.
- Use caution when attempting to transfer or ambulate a client who has recently been given an antihypertensive or narcotic medication because these drugs may predispose the client to hypotension, dizziness, or instability (Burden, 1995).

Teaching Considerations

- Instruct client or care giver on the importance of having the client wear shoes with a nonslip surface during transfer or ambulation.
- Instruct client or care giver on the importance of slow, gradual position change (Radwanski and Hoeman, 1996).
- Instruct client to report any symptoms of dizziness, lightheadedness, or seeing spots.

Pediatric Considerations

- Children who have volume losses resulting in dehydration have an increased potential for orthostatic hypotension.
- Maintain hydration and provide safety precautions to prevent falls.
- When assisting a child, be sure to assess weight correctly—looks can be deceiving.

Gerontologic Considerations

- Older adults who have volume losses or have undergone prolonged bed rest have greater risk for hypotension with postural change.
- Provide 1500 to 2000 ml of fluid every 24 hours unless contraindicated to ensure hydration (Radwanski and Hoeman, 1996).
- Clients using medications to reduce blood pressure are at greater risk for orthostatic hypotension.

Home Care Considerations

- Safety belt can be made from cotton webbing by wrapping it around client's waist over clothing and tying it into square knot. Belt can be made at home or purchased commercially and is used by primary care giver to provide secure grip on client while changing client's position.

SKILL 30-5 Assisting with Ambulation

Clients who have been immobile for even a short time may require assistance with ambulation. Assistance may mean walking alongside the client while providing support (Fig. 30-3) or the client may require the use of an assistive device to aid in ambulation. An assistive device may be ordered to increase stability, to support a weak extremity, or to reduce the load on weight-bearing structures such as hips, knees, or ankles. These devices range from standard canes, which provide minimal support, to crutches and walkers, which can be used by clients who are unable to bear complete weight on the lower extremities or who bear weight on one lower extremity. Selection of the appropriate device depends on the client's age, diagnosis, muscular coordination, and ease of maneuverability (Borgman-Gainer, 1996). Use of assistive devices may be temporary, such as during recuperation from a fractured extremity or orthopedic surgery, or permanent, such as in the case of a client with paralysis or permanent weakness of the lower extremities.

Canes are lightweight, easily movable devices that extend about waist high and are made of wood or metal. Canes help to maintain balance by widening the base of support. They are indicated for clients with hemiparesis and are used to ease the strain on weight-bearing joints. Canes are not recommended for clients with bilateral leg weakness; for such clients, crutches or a walker is more appropriate (Borgman-Gainer, 1996). There are three types of commonly used canes. The *standard crook cane* provides the least support and is used by clients requiring only minimal assistance to walk. It has a half-circle handle, which allows it to be hooked over chairs (Fig. 30-4). The *T-handle cane* has a bent shaft and a straight-shaped handle with grips, which makes it easier to hold. It provides greater stability than the standard cane and is especially useful for clients with hand weakness (Fig. 30-5). The *tripod cane* (pyramid cane) has three legs and the *quad cane* has four legs; the additional legs provide a wide base of support. This type of cane is useful for clients with unilateral, partial, or complete leg paralysis. It also has the advantage in that it stands alone, freeing the arms to help the client rise from a chair (Borgman-Gainer, 1996) (Fig. 30-6).

A crutch is a wooden or metal staff that reaches from the ground almost to the axilla. Crutches are used to remove weight from one or both legs. They are used by clients who must transfer more weight to their arms than is possible with canes. There are three types of crutches: axillary, Lofstrand or Canadian, and platform. The axillary crutch is frequently used by clients of all ages on a short-term basis (Fig. 30-7).

The Lofstrand crutch has a hand grip and a metal band that fits around the client's forearm. Both the metal band and the hand grip are adjusted to fit the client's height. This type of crutch is useful for clients with a permanent disability, such as paraplegic clients. The metal arm band stabilizes and assists in guiding the crutch. The metal arm band offers other advantages as well. First, the encircling arm band allows clients to use their hands for other activities, such as opening doors, without dropping the

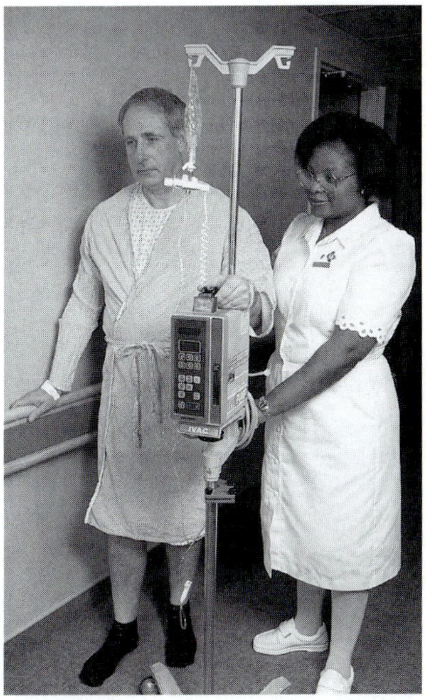

Fig. 30-3 Assisting a client with ambulation.

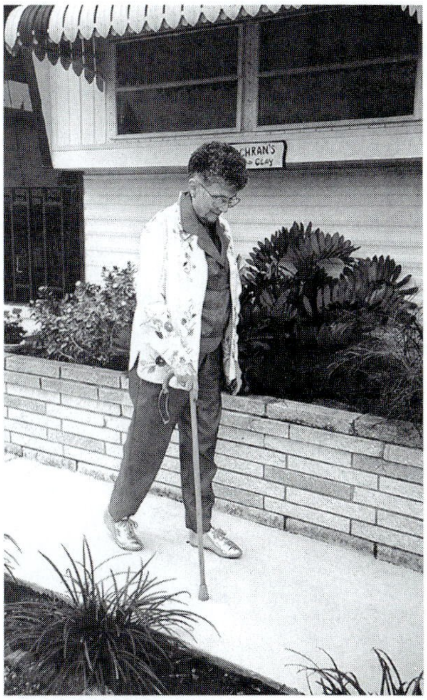

Fig. 30-4 Standard crook cane.

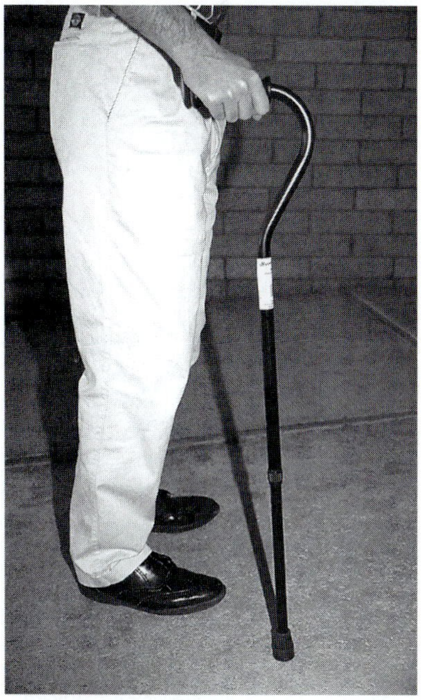

Fig. 30-5 T-handled cane.

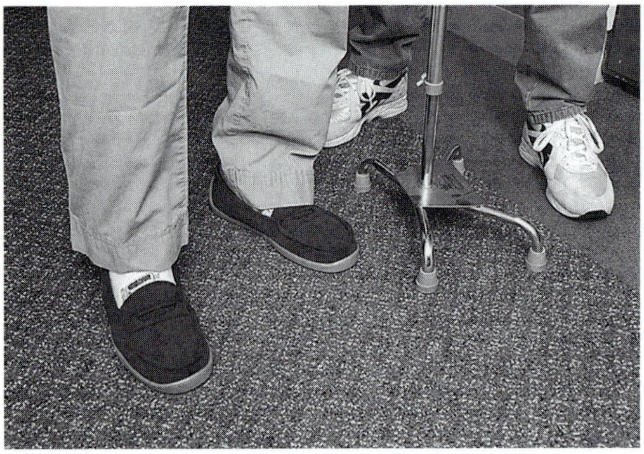

Fig. 30-6 Quad cane.

crutches. Second, the anterior opening of the band allows clients to free themselves of the crutches if a fall occurs.

The Canadian crutch is like the Lofstrand only it has an additional cuff for the upper arm to give added support. The platform crutch is used by clients who are unable to bear weight on their wrists. It has a horizontal trough on which the clients can rest their forearms and wrists and a vertical handle for the client to grip.

A walker is an extremely light, movable device, about waist high, consisting of a metal frame with handgrips, four widely placed, sturdy legs, and one open side. Because it has a wide base of support, the walker provides great stability and security. A walker can be used by a client who is weak or who has problems with balance (Borgman-Gainer, 1996) (Fig. 30-8). In addition to the standard walker, there are several other models available: a foldable version that is easy to transport, one with a fold-down seat, and one with wheels on the front legs. Walkers with wheels are useful for clients who have difficulty lifting the walker as they walk because of limited balance or endurance. The disadvantage, however, is that the walker can roll forward when weight is applied (Borgman-Gainer, 1996).

EQUIPMENT

- **Ambulation device (crutch, walker, cane)**
- **Safety device (walking belt;** Fig. 30-9)
- **Well-fitting, flat shoes for client**
- **Robe or sweatpants**

DELEGATION CONSIDERATIONS

The skill of assisting the client with ambulation may be delegated to unlicensed personnel. The following information is needed when delegating this skill to nursing staff or family members:

- Have client wear shoes with a nonskid surface during ambulation.
- Do not try to hold clients if they become dizzy or faint. Ease them into a sitting position in a chair or on the floor.
- Be sure the area is free of clutter, wet areas, and rugs that may slide or buckle.

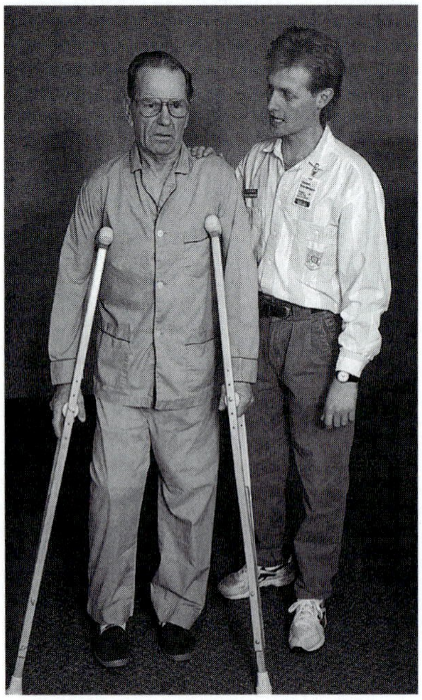

Fig. 30-7 Axillary crutch.

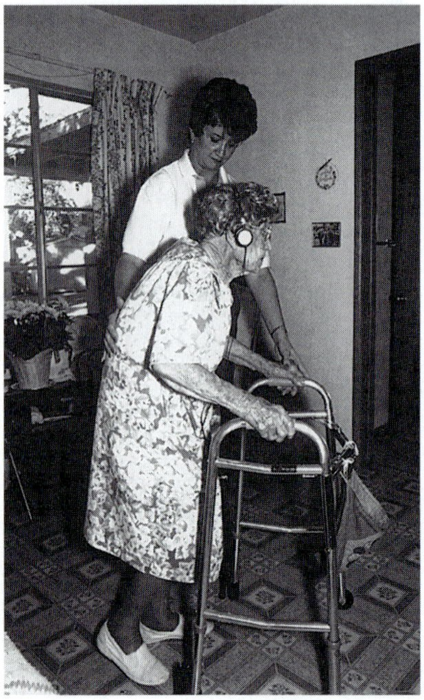

Fig. 30-8 Walker.

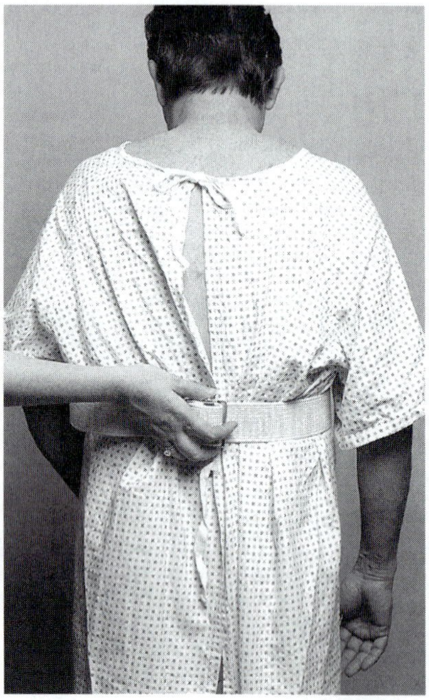

Fig. 30-9 Walking belt.

STEPS	RATIONALE
ASSESSMENT	
1. Review client's chart including:	
a. Client's medical history	Certain medications, chronic illness, history of falling may influence the client's ability to ambulate independently.
b. Client's previous activity level	Identifies client's previous activity level. Client may tire easily or be prone to orthostatic hypotension if rest has been prolonged.
c. Current activity order	Verifies if an ambulation aid is needed and specifies amount of activity permitted.
2. Assess client's physical readiness:	
a. Assess client's vital signs and orientation to time, place, and person.	Ambulation following immobility can be fatiguing and stressful. Baseline vital signs offer means for comparison after exercise. The oriented client is able to understand instructions.
b. Evaluate ROM and muscle strength and assess for the presence of foot deformities.	Determines if client has enough flexibility and muscle strength to ambulate safely and if client needs muscle-strengthening exercises. Determines if any foot deformities are present to affect ambulation.
c. Assess client for any visual, perceptual, or sensory deficits.	Determines if client can use assistive device safely. Ambulation after immobility can be fatiguing and stressful.
d. Assess environment for potential threats to client safety.	Protects client from potential injury.
e. Assess client for discomfort.	Client may be in pain or may fear pain resulting from exercise. If necessary, administer analgesic before exercise.
3. Assess client's or care giver's understanding of technique of ambulation to be used.	Allows client to verbalize concerns. Clients who have been immobile for a long time may be hesitant to ambulate. Care giver may be hesitant to learn how to assist with ambulation.
4. Determine optimal time for ambulation.	Client's personal habits must be considered when planning activities.
5. Assess degree of assistance client needs.	For safety, another person may be needed initially to assist with client ambulation. Allow the client as much independence as possible.

NURSING DIAGNOSIS

Clustering of defining characteristics from the assessment data may reveal the following nursing diagnoses for clients requiring this skill:

- Activity intolerance
- Altered peripheral tissue perfusion
- Decreased cardiac output
- Fatigue
- Impaired physical mobility
- Risk for impaired skin integrity
- Risk for injury

Related factors are individualized based on a client's condition or needs.

PLANNING

STEPS	RATIONALE
1. Expected outcomes following completion of procedure:	
➤ Client will ambulate without episode of injury. ➤ Client is able to ambulate without excessive fatigue or dizziness. ➤ Client will state correct assigned ambulation **gait.** ➤ Client will demonstrate assigned gait. ➤ Client will resume social and self-care activities.	Progressive ambulating activities increase client's endurance and independence.

STEPS	RATIONALE
2. Prepare client for procedure:	
a. Explain reasons for exercise and demonstrate specific gait technique to client or care giver.	Teaching and demonstration enhance learning, reduce anxiety, and encourage cooperation.
b. Decide with client how far to ambulate.	Determines mutual goal.
c. Schedule ambulation around client's other activities.	Schedule rest periods between activities so client does not become too fatigued.
d. Place bed in low position and slowly assist client to upright position. Let client sit or stand for a few minutes until balance is gained.	Prevents orthostatic hypotension and potential injuries. If client becomes dizzy when position is changed from supine to upright, refer to Skill 30-4 for measures to minimize orthostatic hypotension.
e. If ambulation device is used, make sure it is appropriate height:	Promotes optimal support and stability.
(1) Crutch measurement includes three areas: client's height, distance between crutch pad and axilla, and angle of elbow flexion. Use one of two methods:	
• *Standing*—Position crutches with crutch tips at point 4 to 6 inches (10 to 15 cm) to side and 4 to 6 inches in front of client's feet and crutch pads 1½ to 2 inches (4 to 5 cm) below axilla. • *Supine*—Crutch pad should be 3 to 4 finger widths under axilla with crutch tips positioned 6 inches (15 cm) lateral to client's heel (Borgman-Gainer, 1996) (see illustration 2e(1)).	Radial nerve passes under axillary area superficially. If crutch is too long, it can cause pressure on axilla and radial nerve. Injury to radial nerve causes paralysis of elbow and wrist extensors, commonly called **crutch palsy.** Also, if crutch is too long, shoulders are forced upward and client cannot push body off the ground. If ambulation device is too short, client will be bent over and uncomfortable (Borgman-Gainer, 1996; Deathe, Hayes, and Winter, 1993; McConnell, 1992).

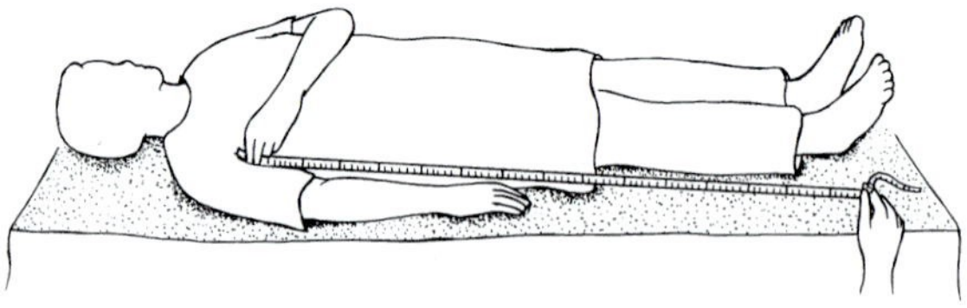

Step 2e(1) Supine method.

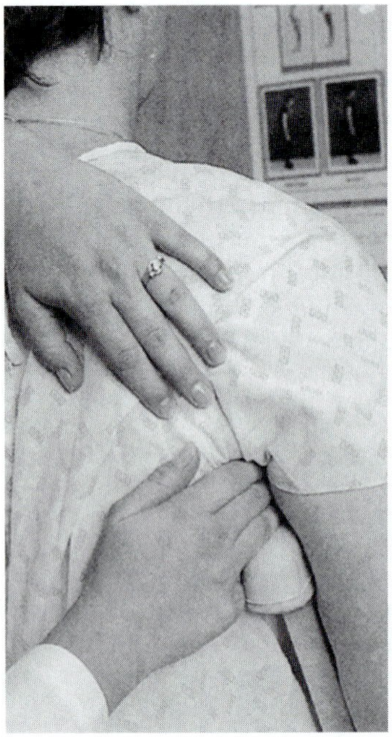

Step 2e(1)a Top of crutch.

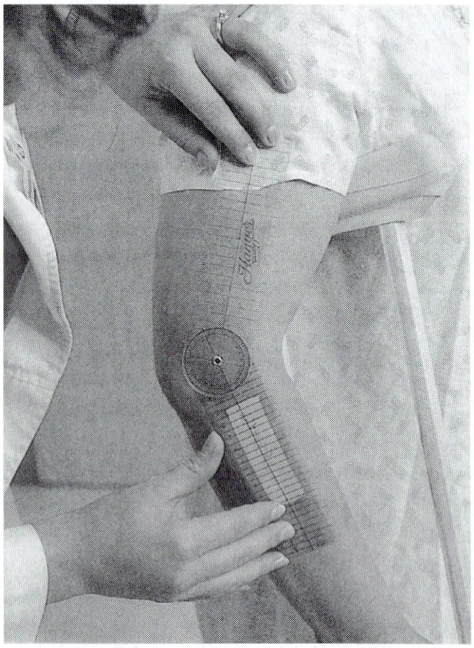

Step 2e(1)b Elbows flexed.

STEPS	RATIONALE
• Instruct client to report any tingling or numbness in the upper torso.	May mean crutches are being used incorrectly or that they are wrong size.
• Following correct crutch adjustment, two or three fingers should fit between top of crutch and axilla (see illustration 2e(1)a).	
• With either measurement method, elbows should be flexed 15 to 30 degrees. Elbow flexion is verified with goniometer (see illustration 2e(1)b).	
• In addition to overall *length* of axillary crutch, *height* of handgrip is important. Both dimensions are adjustable on well-made crutch, and this ability to adjust these dimensions is an important feature for a growing child. Handgrip should be adjusted so that client's elbow is *slightly flexed.*	If handgrip is too low, radial nerve can be damaged even if overall crutch length is correct because extra length between handgrip and axillary bar can force bar up into axilla as client stretches down to reach handgrip. If handgrip is too high, client's elbow is sharply flexed, and strength and stability of arms are decreased.
(2) Cane measurement: Client should hold cane on uninvolved side 4 to 6 (10 to 15 cm) inches to side of foot. Cane should extend from greater trochanter to floor. Allow approximately 15 to 30 degrees of elbow flexion.	Offers most support when on stronger side of body. Cane and weaker leg work together with each step. If cane is too short, client will have difficulty supporting weight and be bent over and uncomfortable. As weight is taken on by hands and affected leg is lifted off floor, complete extension of elbow is necessary (Borgman-Gainer, 1996; Deathe, Hayes, and Winter, 1993).
(3) Walker measurement: Upper bar of walker should be slightly below client's waist. Elbows should be flexed at approximately 15 to 30 degrees when standing within walker with hands on handgrips.	As weight is taken on by hands and client's legs are lifted off floor, complete extension of elbows is necessary. Walker of the wrong height causes the client to expend more energy, experience greater discomfort, and feel unable to achieve adequate weight transmission through the arms (McConnell, 1992).
(4) Make sure the ambulation device has rubber tips.	Rubber tips increase surface tension and prevent the device from slipping (McConnell, 1992).
(5) Make sure surface client will walk on is clean, dry, and well-lighted. Remove any objects that might obstruct the pathway.	Prevents injuries.

IMPLEMENTATION

ASSISTED AMBULATION WITH ONE NURSE

STEPS	RATIONALE
1. Review how to minimize effects of orthostatic hypotension (see Skill 30-4).	Helps client gain balance before attempting ambulation and ensures that client will not become faint while walking.
2. Apply walking belt if unsure of client's stability and assist client to standing position; observe balance.	Prevents injury. Walking belt encircles client's waist and has space for nurse to hold while client walks. If client appears weak or unsteady, return client to bed.
3. Have client take a few steps while nurse is positioned on client's stronger side. If an assistive device (e.g., cane, walker) is used, then nurse stands on client's weak side.	If client has hemiplegia (one-sided paralysis) or hemiparesis (one-sided weakness), stand next to client's unaffected side and support client by placing arm closest to client on the walking belt or around client's waist and other arm around inferior aspect of client's upper arm.
4. Grasp walking belt in middle of client's back or place hands at client's waist if no walking belt is used.	Provides support at waist so client's center of gravity remains midline.
5. Take a few steps forward with client. Then assess for strength and balance.	Ensures client has satisfactory strength and balance to continue.
6. If client becomes weak or dizzy, return to bed or chair, whichever is closer.	Allows client to rest.

STEPS	RATIONALE
7. If client begins to fall, use procedure Follow-up Activity 2, Skill 30-4, for lowering client to floor.	Nurse can cause more damage to self and client by trying to catch client.

ASSISTED AMBULATION WITH TWO NURSES

STEPS	RATIONALE
1. Follow Steps 1 and 2, Assisted Ambulation with One Nurse.	
2. Stand on either side of client.	
3. Place arms nearest client around client's waist and other arms so that both nurses' hands support client's axillae.	Provides secure grip for each nurse.
4. Step forward in unison with client, keeping speed and step size same as client's.	Ensures stability of client.
5. Gradually increase distance walked.	Strengthens muscles, increases endurance, and prevents client from becoming too fatigued.
6. Follow Steps 6 and 7, Assisted Ambulation With One Nurse.	

AMBULATION WITH ASSISTIVE DEVICES

STEPS	RATIONALE
1. Assist client in crutch-walking by choosing appropriate **crutch gait.**	To use crutches, client supports self with hands and arms; therefore strength in arm and shoulder muscles, ability to balance body in upright position, and stamina are necessary. Exercises such as squeezing a rubber ball, raising and lowering both arms in a slow, rhythmic manner while holding weights, push-ups, and pull-ups will assist in strengthening the upper extremities. The type of gait the client uses in crutch-walking depends on amount of weight client is able to support with one or both legs.

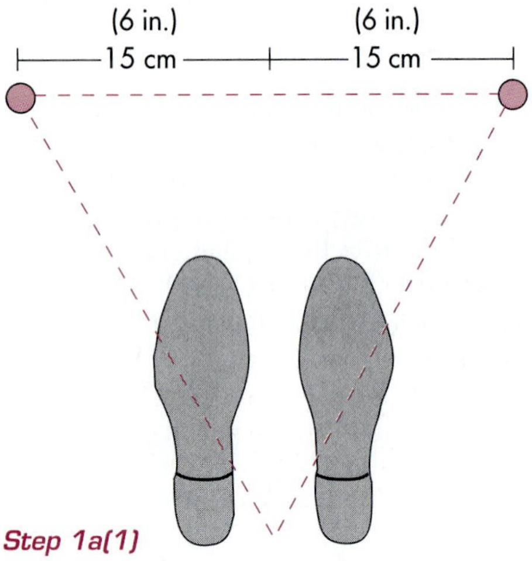

Step 1a(1)

STEPS	RATIONALE
a. Four-point gait:	This is the most stable of crutch gaits because it provides at least three points of support at all times. Requires bearing weight on both legs. Often used when client has some form of paralysis, such as for spastic children with cerebral palsy (Wong, 1995). May also be used for arthritic clients.
(1) Begin in tripod position (see illustration). Crutches are placed 6 inches (15 cm) in front and 6 inches to side of each foot. The client's weight should be placed on the handgrips, not under the arms.	Improves client's balance by providing wide base of support. Client should have a posture of erect head and neck, straight vertebrae, and extended hips and knees.
(2) Move right crutch forward 4 to 6 inches (10 to 15 cm) (see illustration).	Crutch and foot position is similar to arm and foot position during normal walking.
(3) Move left foot forward to level of left crutch.	
(4) Move left crutch forward 4 to 6 inches (10 to 15 cm).	
(5) Move right foot forward to level of right crutch.	
(6) Repeat above sequence.	

STEPS	RATIONALE
b. Three-point gait:	Requires client to bear all weight on one foot. Weight is borne on uninvolved leg and then on both crutches. Affected leg does not touch ground during early phase of three-point gait. May be useful for client with broken leg or sprained ankle.
(1) Begin in tripod position (see illustration 1a(1)).	Improves client's balance by providing wide base of support.
(2) Advance both crutches and affected leg (see illustration).	
(3) Move stronger leg forward.	
(4) Repeat sequence.	

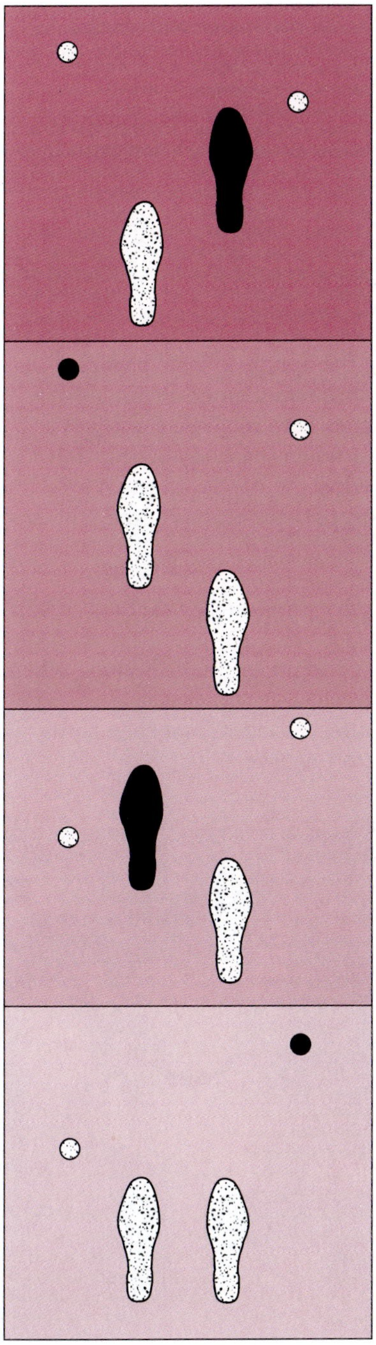

Step 1a(2)

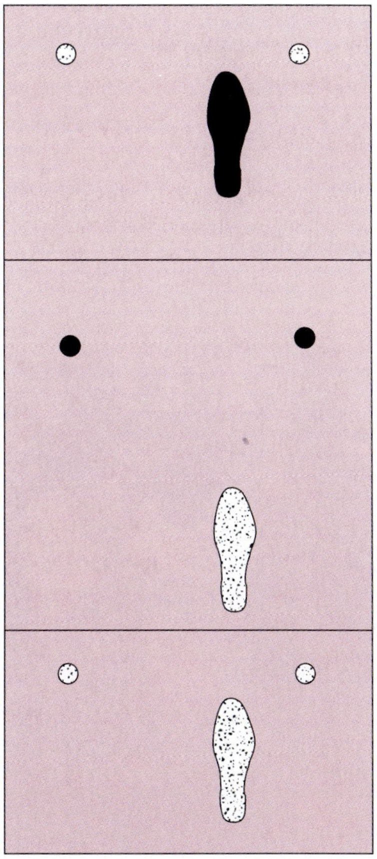

Step 1b(2)

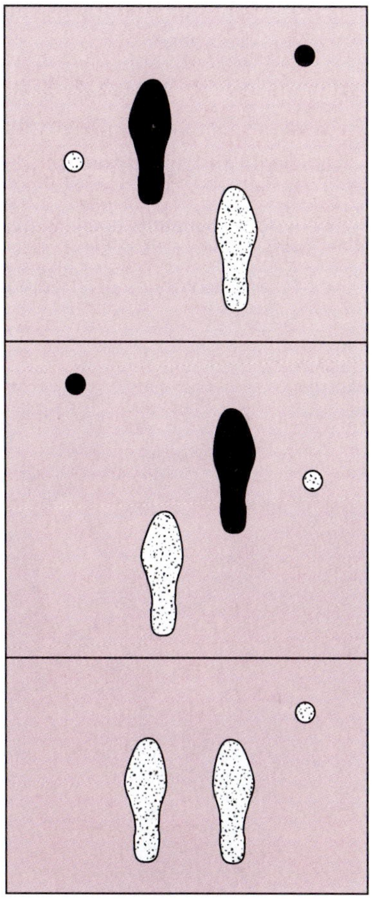

Step 1c(2)

STEPS	RATIONALE
c. Two-point gait:	Requires at least partial weight-bearing on each foot. Is faster than the four-point gait. Requires more balance because only two points support body at one time (Borgman-Gainer, 1996).
(1) Begin in tripod position (see illustration 1a[1]).	Improves client's balance by providing wide base of support.
(2) Move left crutch and right foot forward (see illustration 1c[2] on p. 935).	Crutch movements are similar to arm movement during normal walking.
(3) Move right crutch and left foot forward.	
(4) Repeat sequence.	
d. Swing-to gait:	
(1) Begin in tripod position (see illustration 1a[1]).	Frequently used by clients whose lower extremities are paralyzed or who wear weight-supporting braces on their legs.
(2) Move both crutches forward.	This is the easier of the two swinging gaits. It requires the ability to partially bear body weight on both legs (Borgman-Gainer, 1996).
(3) Lift and swing legs to crutches, letting crutches support body weight.	
(4) Repeat two previous steps.	
e. Swing-through gait:	
(1) Begin in tripod position (see illustration 1a[1]).	Requires that client have the ability to bear partial weight on both feet (Borgman-Gainer, 1996).
(2) Move both crutches forward.	Initial placement of crutches is to increase the client's base of support so that when the body swings forward, the client is moving the center of gravity toward the additional support provided by the crutches.
(3) Lift and swing legs through and beyond crutches.	
2. Assist client in climbing stairs with crutches:	
a. Begin in tripod position.	Improves client's balance by providing wide base of support.
b. Client transfers body weight to crutches (see illustration).	Prepares client to transfer weight to unaffected leg when ascending first stair.
c. Client advances unaffected leg to stair (see illustration).	Crutch adds support to affected leg. Client then shifts weight from crutches to unaffected leg.

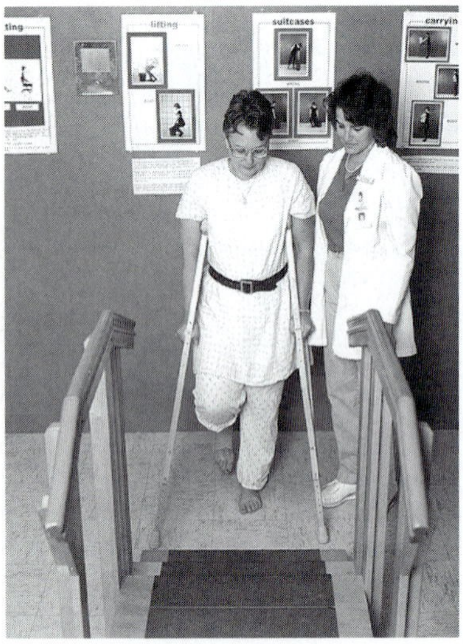

Step 2b

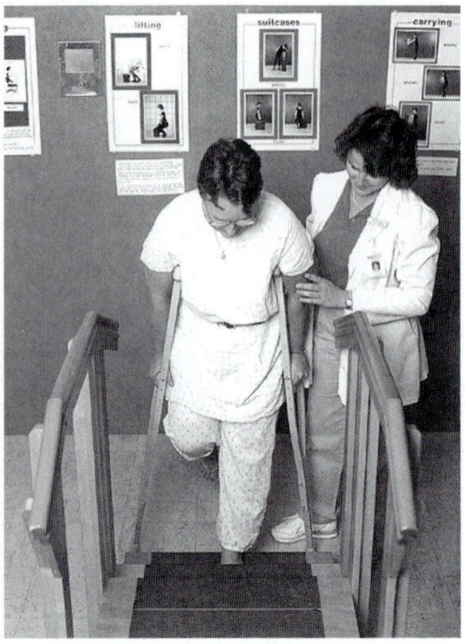

Step 2c

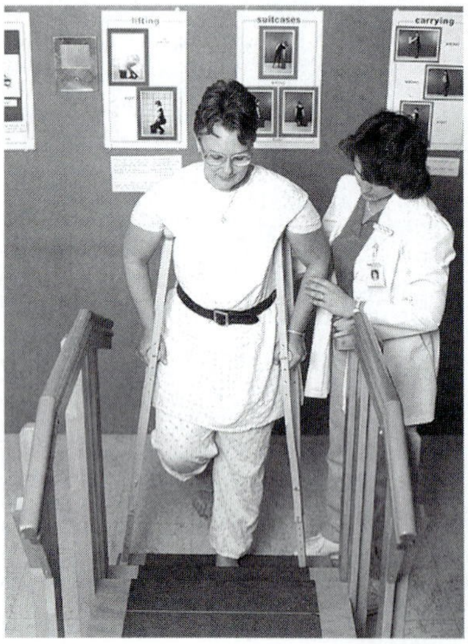

Step 2d

STEPS	RATIONALE
d. Both crutches are aligned with unaffected leg on stairs (see illustration p. 936).	Maintains balance and provides wide base of support.
e. Repeat sequence until client reaches top of stairs.	
3. Assist client in descending stairs with crutches:	
a. Begin in tripod position.	Improves client's balance by providing wide base of support.
b. Client transfers body weight to unaffected leg (see illustration).	Prepares client to release support of body weight maintained by crutches.
c. Move crutches to stair and instruct client to begin to transfer body weight to crutches (see illustration) and move affected leg forward.	Maintains client's balance and base of support.
d. Client moves unaffected leg to stair and aligns with crutches (see illustration).	Maintains balance and provides base of support.
e. Repeat sequence until stairs are descended.	
4. Assist client in ambulating with walker:	Walker is used by clients who are able to bear partial weight. Walkers do need to be picked up, so client does need sufficient strength to be able to pick up walker. Four-wheeled model, which does not need to be picked up, is not as stable.
a. Have client stand in center of walker and grasp handgrips on upper bars.	Client balances self before attempting to walk (McConnell, 1992).
b. Lift walker, move it 6 to 8 inches (15 to 20 cm) forward, and then set it down, making sure all four feet of the walker stay on the floor. Take a step forward with either foot. Then follow through with the other leg.	Provides broad base of support between walker and client. Client then moves center of gravity toward the walker. Keeping all four feet of the walker on the floor is necessary to prevent tipping of the walker.
c. If there is unilateral weakness, after the walker is advanced, instruct the client to step forward with the weaker leg, support self with the arms, and follow through with the uninvolved leg. If client is unable to bear weight on one leg, after advancing walker have the client swing onto it, supporting weight on hands.	

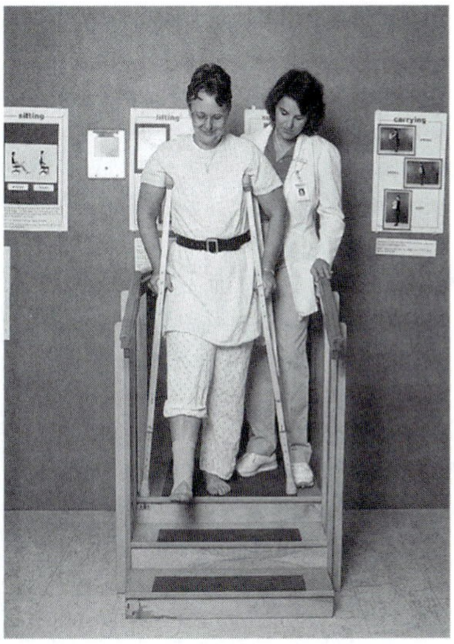

Step 3b

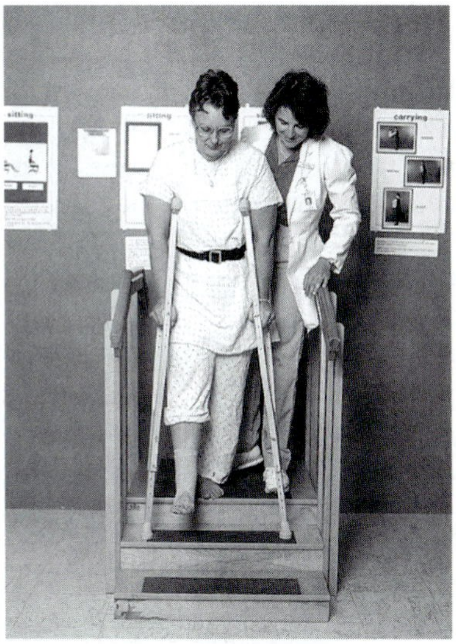

Step 3c

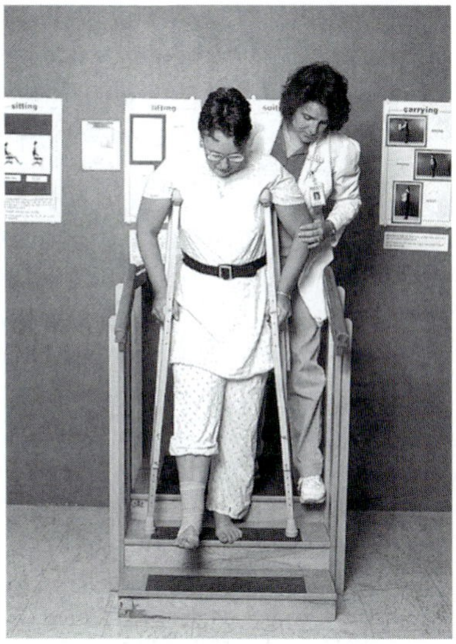

Step 3d

STEPS	RATIONALE
5. Assist client in ambulating with cane (same steps are taught whether standard or quad canes are used):	
a. Begin by placing cane on the side opposite the involved leg.	Provides added support for the weak or impaired side.
b. Place cane forward 6 to 10 inches (15 to 25 cm), keeping body weight on both legs.	Distributes body weight equally.
c. Move involved leg forward, even with the cane.	Body weight is supported by cane and uninvolved leg.
d. Advance uninvolved leg past cane.	Body weight is supported by cane and involved leg.
e. Move involved leg forward, even with uninvolved leg.	Aligns client's center of gravity. Returns client body weight to equal distribution.
f. Repeat these steps.	

EVALUATION

1. After ambulation, obtain client's vital signs, heart rate, respiratory rate, and temperature; observe skin color, and ask about the client's energy level.	Assesses how client tolerated procedure and evaluates whether there was progress in ambulation. Assesses stage of client's illness and degree of convalescence when evaluating the process.
2. Assess client's subjective statements regarding experience.	
3. Assess gait of client, observing body alignment in standing position and balance.	Determines if client is correctly using supportive aids for ambulation. Keep in mind the client's previous manner of ambulating when assessing gait.
4. Observe client's ability to perform self-care activities.	
5. **Unexpected outcomes** that may occur include:	
➤ Client will be unable to ambulate.	Possible reasons include fear of falling, physical discomfort, upper body muscles that are too weak to use ambulation device, and lower extremities that are too weak to support body.
➤ Client sustains injury.	Obstacles were in client's path, incorrect technique was used, or proper safety precautions were not taken.

RECORDING AND REPORTING

1. Record in nurses' notes type of gait the client used, amount of assistance required, distance walked, and client's tolerance of activity.	Documents technique used and client's progress using technique.
2. Immediately report any injury sustained during attempts to ambulate, alteration in vital signs, or inability to ambulate to nurse in charge or physician.	

FOLLOW-UP ACTIVITIES

1. Inspect rubber tips on bottom of ambulation device frequently.
2. If wooden crutch is used, examine it for cracks.
3. Remove obstacles from pathways, including throw rugs, and wipe up any spills immediately.
4. Avoid large crowds. Crowds increase the risk of the crutch, cane, or walker being kicked or jarred and client losing balance.
5. Notify medical personnel if there are symptoms of tingling or numbness when client uses crutches.
6. Instruct client to continue muscle-strengthening exercises at home.

• • • • •

Special Considerations

- Use caution when attempting to ambulate a client who has recently been given an antihypertensive or analgesic medication because the medication may cause dizziness or instability.
- When client is ambulating with or without assistive device, emphasize need to always look ahead, to prevent injuries, and to use good **posture.** Slouching and looking down will cause the client to tire more easily and increases risk of injury.
- Care must be taken if the client has IV tubings or a Foley catheter. Obtain an IV pole with wheels that can be pushed as the client walks. Urinary catheter drainage bags must stay at or below the level of the bladder, so a second person may be needed to assist.
- Caution should be used if the client uses a walker or other assistive devices on uneven terrain or on inclines.
- Walkers have the disadvantage of being difficult to maneuver in small spaces and on stairs. A walker specifically designed for stairs is available, but its extra weight has limited its use.
- Clients should be taught more than one gait so they may change from one gait to another. Shifting crutch gaits relieves fatigue.

Teaching Considerations

- If a walker is used, the client is taught to examine the frame daily. When inspecting a walker, the client should observe for signs of bending or deformation of the frame, protruding screws that can scratch, and loose or missing screws that weaken the joints of the frame. Handgrips should be assessed for any cracks or signs of being loose (McConnell, 1992).
- Clients should be instructed to use the arms of a chair rather than the walker to give them leverage when getting up from a chair; the walker is likely to tip if used for this purpose (McConnell, 1992).
- Instruct clients to always wear shoes that are approximately the same heel height as the shoes worn when the measurements for the ambulation device were taken. This will ensure that the assistive device fits accurately.
- Blistering or soreness of the hands can result from continual pressure between the hand and the handle of a crutch. Advise client to release pressure intermittently and wear gloves or pad the handle to reduce friction.

Pediatric Considerations

- It is important to remember that children and adolescents are also subject to potential problems of immobility—for example, a child with cerebral palsy, a teenager with a sprained ankle.
- Children who are immobilized may exhibit sluggish intellectual or motor responses and decreased communication skills (Wong, 1995).
- Aids that are adjustable in length are useful when a client is first fitted and for children who require that their aids grow with them.
- For rehabilitation of a small child who has not yet learned to walk or who is unsteady, special crutches with three or four legs provide needed stability to allow the child to maintain an upright posture and learn to walk (Wong, 1995).

Gerontologic Considerations

- The older adult with arthritis may require additional time in the morning before resuming activities.

Home Care Considerations

- Client should be instructed on how to use the ambulation aid on various terrains (e.g., carpet, stairs, rough ground, inclines). Client should also be instructed on how to maneuver around obstacles such as doors and how to use the aid when transferring such as to and from a chair, toilet, tub, and car (Borgman-Gainer, 1996).
- Assess whether client is using the ordered ambulation aid correctly. If client is noncompliant, try to determine cause. Potential reasons for noncompliance are:
  - Lack of perception of reason and benefits of the aid
  - Time lapse between onset of disability and training with equipment
  - Lack of proper training
  - Decreased ability to attend to tasks

CRITICAL THINKING EXERCISES

1. An elderly client is admitted to the hospital for a fractured left hip resulting from a fall at home. The client is scheduled for a total hip replacement tomorrow. What are the client's primary immobility risks at this time?
2. What interventions could the nurse implement to prevent or reduce the identified hazards of immobility?
3. After removing a client's elastic support hose, the nurse notes an area on the right leg that is reddened and warm to the touch. What could these signs signify, and what steps should the nurse take?
4. Use of the knee gatch or placing pillows under the knees could lead to what potential problems in an immobilized client?
5. To assist a client who is going to ambulate with crutches after recent knee surgery, what interventions could be implemented to improve the chances of success?

REFERENCES

Borgman-Gainer M: Independent function: movement and mobility. In Hoeman S, editor: *Rehabilitation nursing: process and application,* ed 2, St Louis, 1996, Mosby.

Bright L, Georgi A: How to protect your patient from DVT, *Am J Nurs* 94(12):28, 1992.

Burden N: A case study: identification and treatment of narcotic depression in the ambulatory surgical patient, *J Post Anesth Nurs* 10(2):94, 1995.

Campbell A: How to use pneumatic compression stockings, *Nursing* 22(9):32BB, 1992.

Carroll P: Deep venous thrombosis: implications for orthopaedic nursing, *Orthop Nurs* 12(3):33, 1993.

Ciocon J, Fernandez B, Ciocon D: Leg edema: clinical clues to the differential diagnosis, *Geriatrics* 48(5):34, 1993.

Ciocon J, Galindo-Ciocon D, Galindo D: Raised leg exercises for leg edema in the elderly, *Angiology* 46(1):19, 1995.

Coffman J: Venous thrombosis and the diagnosis of pulmonary emboli, *Hosp Pract* 27(4A):99, 1992.

Creditor M: Hazards of hospitalization of the elderly, *Ann Int Med* 118(3):219, 1993.

Dawe D, Curran-Smith J: Going through the motions, *Can Nurse* 90(1):31, 1994.

Deathe A, Hayes K, Winter D: The biomechanics of canes, crutches, and walkers, *Crit Rev Phys Rehabil Med* 5:15, 1993.

Dittmer D, Teasell R: Complications of immobilization and bedrest. Part I: musculoskeletal and cardiovascular complications, *Can Fam Phys Med Fam Can* 39:1428, 1993.

Doering L: The effects of positioning on hemodynamics and gas exchange in the critically ill: a review, *Am J Crit Care* 2(3):208, 1993.

Galindo-Ciocon D: Nursing care of elders with leg edema, *J Gerontol Nurs* 21(2):7, 1995.

Griego L, House-Fancher M: Coronary artery disease. In Lewis S, Collier I, Heitkemper M, editors: *Medical surgical nursing: assessment and management of clinical problems,* ed 4, St Louis, 1996, Mosby.

Grubb B, Kosinski D, Samoil D: Recurrent unexplained syncope: the role of head-upright table testing, *Heart Lung* 22(6):502, 1993.

Hambleton N: Dealing with complications of epidural analgesia, *Nursing* 24(1):55, 1994.

Hamilton L, Lyon P: A nursing-driven program to preserve and restore functional ability in hospitalized elderly patients, *J Orthop Nurs Assoc* 25(4):30, 1995.

Long B, Phipps W: *Medical-surgical nursing: A nursing process approach,* ed 3, St Louis, 1992, Mosby.

McConnell E: Using a stationary walker, *Nursing* 22(1):75, 1992.

McConnell E: What's wrong with this patient? Investigating orthostatic hypotension, *Nursing* 25(9):76, 1995.

Radwanski M, Hoeman S: Geriatric rehabilitation nursing. In Hoeman S, editor: *Rehabilitation nursing: process and application,* ed 2, St Louis, 1996, Mosby.

Recker D: Overcoming the obstacles to caring for the long-term critical care patient, *Crit Care Nurse* 12(5):40, 1992.

Riegel B, Thomason A: NTI research abstracts. Are nurses still practicing "coronary precautions" with acute myocardial infarction patients? *Am J Crit Care* 4(3):246, 1995.

Ruda S: Nursing assessment: Musculoskeletal system. In Lewis S, Collier I, Heitkemper M, editors: *Medical surgical nursing: assessment and management of clinical problems,* ed 4, St Louis, 1996, Mosby.

Rudolphi D, Doyle J: Nursing role in management: Vascular disorders. In Lewis S, Collier I, Heitkemper M, editors: *Medical surgical nursing: assessment and management of clinical problems,* ed 4, St Louis, 1996, Mosby.

Solotkin K, Knipe C: Nursing role in management: Burn patient. In Lewis S, Collier I, Heitkemper M, editors: *Medical surgical nursing: assessment and management of clinical problems,* ed 4, St Louis, 1996, Mosby.

Topp R, Mikesky A, Bawel K: Developing a strength training program for older adults: planning, programming, and potential outcomes, *Rehabil Nurs* 19(5):266, 1994.

von Rueden K, Harris J: Pulmonary dysfunction related to immobility in the trauma patient, *AACN Clin Iss Adv Pract Acute Crit Care* 6(2):212, 1995.

Wanich C, et al: Functional status outcomes of a nursing intervention in hospitalized elderly, *Image* 24(3):201, 1992.

Wild L, Coyne C: The basics and beyond: epidural analgesia, *Am J Nurs* 92:26, 1992.

Winslow E, Lane L, Woods R: Dangling: a review of relevant physiology, research, and practice, *Heart Lung* 24(4):263, 1995.

Wong D: *Whaley & Wong's nursing care of infants and children,* ed 5, St Louis, 1995, Mosby.

ADDITIONAL READING

Herzog J: Deep vein thrombosis in the rehabilitation client: diagnostic tools, prevention, and treatment modalities, *Rehabil Nurs* 18(1):8, 1993.

Manson D, Redeker N: Measurement of activity, *Nurs Res* 42:87, 1993.

Neuberger G, et al: Determinants of exercise and aerobic fitness in outpatients with arthritis, *Nurs Res* 43(1):11, 1994.

Phipps W, et al: *Medical-surgical nursing: concepts and clinical practice,* ed 5, St Louis, 1995, Mosby.

Seeley J: A comprehensive method of management for patients with chronic venous insufficiency and venous ulcers, *Ostomy Wound Manag* 38(8):45, 1992.

Verderber A, Gallagher K: Effects of bathing, passive range-of-motion exercises, and turning on oxygen consumption in healthy men and women, *Am J Crit Care* 3(5):374, 1994.

Verderber A, Gallagher K, Severino R: The effect of nursing interventions on transcutaneous oxygen and carbon dioxide tensions, *West J Nurs Res* 17(1):76, 1995.

CHAPTER 31

Orthopedic Measures

OBJECTIVES

Mastery of content in this chapter will enable the nurse to:

- Define key terms.
- Explain benefits of the use of casts for clients with musculoskeletal injuries.
- Describe how to assist in application of casts.
- Describe neurovascular assessments of a client in specific casts.
- Describe techniques for drying casts.
- Describe toileting techniques for clients in casts.
- Describe turning and positioning techniques for clients in casts.
- Describe elements of client education for the client with a cast and after removal of cast.
- Explain the purposes of placing clients in skin or skeletal traction.
- Explain the rationale for the use of skin versus skeletal traction.
- Describe client conditions requiring the use of each form of skin or skeletal traction.
- Describe steps for applying each form of skin or skeletal traction.

SKILLS

31-1 Assisting with Cast Application

31-2 Assisting with Cast Removal

31-3 Assisting with Application of Skin Traction

31-4 Assisting with Insertion of Pins, Wires, or Nails for Skeletal Traction

KEY TERMS

Cast
Cast brace
Cast saw
Cast shoe
Cast stabilization
Cast syndrome
Casting tape
Cervical halter
Countertraction
Crepitation
External fixation
Four-poster cast
Harris splint
Knee exercise
Knee sling
Minerva jacket
Neurovascular assessment
Pearson attachment
Pelvic belt
Pelvic sling
Petaling
Pulleys
Reduction
Sheet wadding
Spica cast
Spreader bar
Stockinette
Thomas splint
Traction
Traction boot
Walking heel
Webril
Weight holder

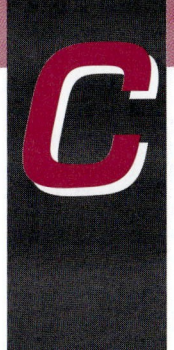

Clients in a cast or traction are susceptible to problems that can affect all body systems. Depending on the extent of a client's injury or illness, an orthopedic device may affect a single body part or the entire body. Changes in the client's immobility require extensive nursing care.

The adequacy of central and peripheral circulation to the injured area must be carefully assessed, because delivery of oxygen and removal of wastes are vital for bone healing, muscle growth and strength, and regaining mobility. Color, temperature, and capillary refill assessments provide data about the adequacy of circulation to the injured extremity. Inflammation, cellulitis, or edema may indicate venous stasis or infection.

Integumentary tissues inside and outside the cast must remain healthy and well nourished. Assessment of the tissues detects pressure, inflammation, or lesions that could lead to infection or pressure sores. Gentle and thorough cleansing of skin, careful drying, and lubrication with lotions provide moisture and stimulation to the integumentary tissues to maintain a healthy state.

Turning and positioning help to maintain the health of integumentary and musculoskeletal tissues of individuals in casts. After application of a cast, especially a **spica cast** or body cast (Fig. 31-1) or **Minerva jacket,** the client must be turned from side to side and prone to facilitate thorough drying of the cast. Turning the client every 2 to 3 hours while keeping the damp cast uncovered facilitates drying. Turning also aids circulation throughout the body and helps to maintain muscle strength and tone. Placement of pillows, rolls, or blankets helps the client to maintain the side-lying or prone position. In addition, musculoskeletal tissues maintain strength through regularly performed active range of joint motion (ROJM) exercises with or without resistance or weight. Quadriceps-, gluteus-, triceps-, biceps-, and hamstring-setting exercises, performed routinely and steadily, help to maintain muscle mass and tone (see Chapter 30).

A major challenge for nurses caring for clients in body, spica, or Minerva jacket casts is to maintain respiratory function. Turning facilitates moving air and fluids in the airways, but it is also vital that clients be encouraged to breathe deeply and cough. Bed rest over time affects the respiration, resulting in decreased functioning. Clients who develop respiratory complications may require respiratory therapy and at times administration of antibiotics. Preventive measures should be sufficient to avoid such necessities.

Additional challenges center around intake and maintenance of functions of the gastrointestinal and genitourinary systems. Clients in casts who are confined to bed frequently develop anorexia, constipation, and at times fecal impaction. Maintaining a high (3000 ml or more) fluid intake plus a high-bulk or high-residue diet fosters proper bowel elimination. Fluid intake also facilitates renal circulation and urinary output to lessen the possibility of a urinary tract infection or renal calculi.

Clients immobilized in casts or traction may lose

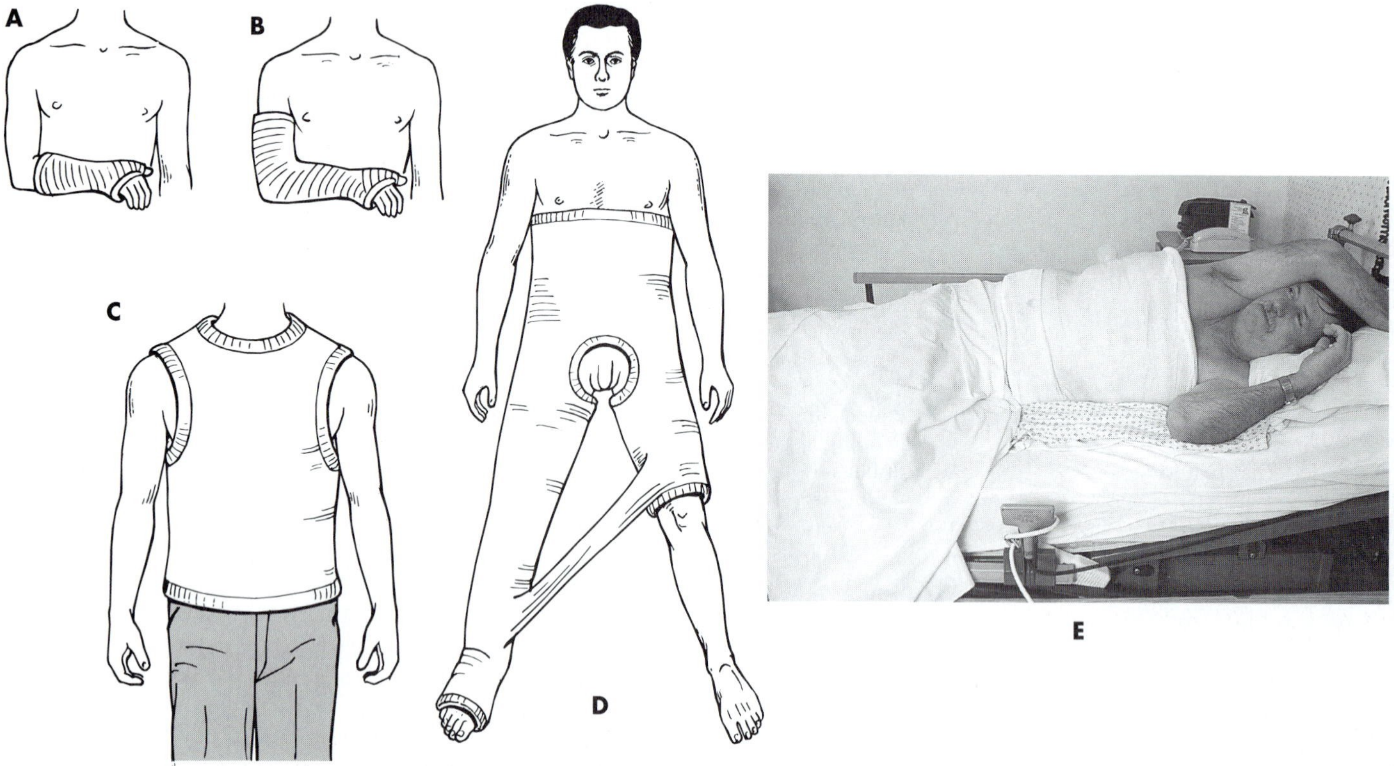

Fig. 31-1 Types of casts. **A,** Short arm cast. **B,** Long arm cast. **C,** Plaster body jacket cast. **D,** One-and-a-half hip spica cast. **E,** Body cast.

weight. Diets should be high in protein, carbohydrates, vitamins, bulk, and fluids and should contain a moderate amount of fat, unless contraindicated. Because of individual metabolic and endocrine stress responses, the client will experience catabolism with muscle mass loss for a period of 10 to 20 or more days. Remodeling of bone, a process by which bone resorption and bone deposit occurs, is governed by hormones and stress placed on the bone. When serum calcium levels decrease, parathyroid hormone (PTH) is released. This stimulates osteoclast activity (bone resorption), calcium is released from the bone, and the serum calcium level rises. With an elevated serum calcium level, calcitonin from the thyroid gland is released, bone resorption is suppressed, and calcium salts are deposited in the bone matrix.

Motor and sensory functions are greatly affected when a client is placed in a cast. Motor changes may lead to muscle and joint weakness from disuse or pressure. Sensory changes, also from pressure or trauma, may lead to complaints of pain, numbness, and tingling. When such sensory signs are present, they may be relieved by changing the client's position. It is essential to monitor for the five P's (pain, pallor, pulselessness, paresthesia, and paralysis) of neurovascular status, because permanent damage may result if the circulation is not restored or pressure is not removed (Dykes, 1993). Bivalving, or cutting the cast, removes the pressure or tightness and increases circulation. Motor weakness may be restored to normal ranges through ROJM exercises and physical therapy. Full muscle function returns slowly and consistent performance of exercises is required.

Psychologically, clients in casts may experience alterations in self-concept and body image. They may lose some independence, mobility, and work income during their "cast days"; however, if clients perceive these changes as temporary, they usually regain full independence and mobility and return to work sooner than those in casts who do not experience regression periods.

Clients in traction or those with casts who are confined to bed may become easily tired during the day and may take short, frequent naps. Thus they may be less sleepy at night and may lie awake past their usual bedtime. To offset this syndrome, clients should remain active, engage in stimulating activities, and avoid napping.

Traction is a force or pull applied to the bones directly or indirectly to overcome deformity and to help restore alignment. When bones are fractured, muscle spasms pull the distal fragments out of their normal positions. Sufficient pull must be applied to the injured tissues to overcome muscle spasms and thus permit the bones to realign themselves in the usual anatomical positions. In situations of severe muscle spasms, marked deformity, or displacement, traction must be applied directly to the distal fragments by means of a strong nail or pin to which traction is applied through a bar, ropes, pulleys, and weights. Such skeletal traction may be applied to one or more bones, including the bones of the skull, upper and lower extremities, and pelvic bones.

Traction to the skin, also known as "skin traction," is applied indirectly to the bones. It is typically between 5 and 7 pounds and is commonly used for minor trauma. Because of the lower tolerance of skin tissues, traction is applied for shorter periods, with less weight, and at times can be interrupted. **Neurovascular assessment** is essential to ensure that circumferential dressings (dressings that encircle an extremity) do not impede circulation or place pressure on neurological tissue.

Skeletal traction, if used for severe trauma, is applied for longer periods, requires much heavier weights, and is never interrupted.

Knowledge of normal mobility and the findings from the nursing assessment enable the nurse to provide care to the client with a cast or traction. The following guidelines can help the nurse individualize the client's care plan.

GUIDELINES

1. Identify the client's dietary preferences. Wound healing and repair of bone and tissues require additional nutritional intake. Providing foods the client can enjoy meets these additional nutritional needs.
2. Determine the limits of range of joint motion (ROJM) to the casted extremity or extremity in traction. Although it is important to maintain joint mobility, the nurse must not move the affected extremity beyond the limits imposed by the cast or traction. Excessive movement can impair wound healing, extremity alignment, and new bone growth.
3. Determine the client's level of independent functioning. Knowing what the client is capable of doing enables the nurse to properly plan for assisting the client with activities of daily living (ADLs) such as bathing, eating, dressing, and grooming.
4. Identify the client's normal elimination patterns. Restrictions on mobility imposed by the cast or traction can result in altered elimination patterns.
5. Determine the client's understanding of the normal bone-healing process. This knowledge assists the nurse in developing a teaching plan for the client to care for the casted extremity at home.
6. Identify the results of recent laboratory tests. Serum calcium and phosphorus are two minerals that compose callus, the precursor to bone ossification. Hemoglobin, hematocrit, and red blood cell levels will decrease in blood loss anemia.
7. Determine the frequency and type of analgesics ordered for the client by the physician. The client may experience acute, continuous pain and/or muscle spasms during the first 4 to 7 days (the acute inflammatory stage) and thus require 24-hour administration of analgesics and/or muscle relaxants during this time.
8. Identify the materials used in cast application and traction setup. Various materials affect drying time, resistance to pressure, and weight bearing.
9. With traction, maintain the established line of pull, maintain countertraction, maintain continuous traction unless otherwise ordered, maintain correct body alignment, and prevent friction.

SKILL 31-1 Assisting with Cast Application

A **cast** is an externally applied structure used to hold musculoskeletal tissues in a specific position to permit healing of injuries or fractures or to align malpositioned tissues, such as in clubfoot or congenital hip dislocation. The rigidity of the cast overcomes the tension, tone, or rotational forces of the muscles or bones for the time required to heal or align the diseased or injured tissues. Because a cast holds tissue in the position in which it is applied, it must be applied carefully and properly to achieve the goals for its use.

Casts are made from plaster of Paris or synthetic materials (Fig. 31-2). A plaster of Paris cast has multiple rolls of open-weave cotton saturated with calcium sulfate crystals. These casts are heavier than synthetic casts and take up to 48 hours with no weight bearing or application of pressure to dry. Plaster of Paris is easy to mold and shape around unstable fractures. Synthetic casts are composed of polyester and cotton, which is impregnated with a water-activated polyurethane resin. Synthetic casts are also made of fiberglass or plastic. Although the newer synthetic casts are more expensive than plaster, they can withstand contact with water without crumbling. These casts are lightweight, set in 15 minutes, and can sustain weight bearing or pressure in 15 to 30 minutes.

Client safety is important as the nurse helps apply the cast. The nurse provides optimal skin care to the client before, during, and after cast application. The nurse cleans the extremity, removing dirt, glass, or debris beneath the cast that would irritate the skin. After application of the cast, the nurse ensures that plaster crumbs are removed and rough edges are petaled to prevent skin breakdown.

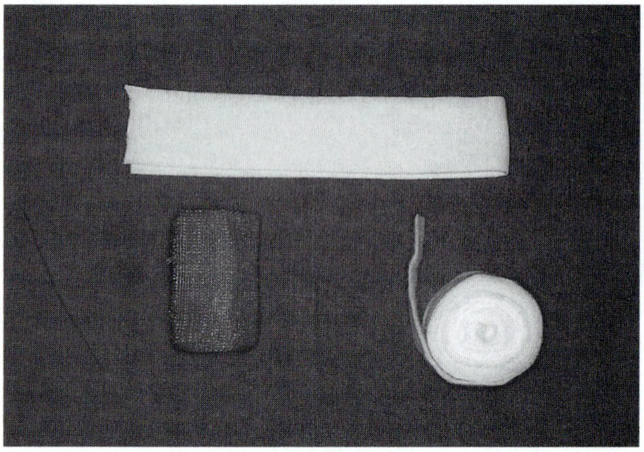

Fig. 31-2 Plaster roll and padding material.

EQUIPMENT

NOTE: **Equipment may be preassembled on "cast cart"**

- **Plaster rolls (sizes include 2-, 3-, 4-, and 6-in rolls); depending on purpose of cast or specific client condition, other cast materials such as glass fiber,** casting tape, **or plastic may be used instead of plaster**
- **Padding material (felt,** stockinette, sheet wadding, Webril, **or other material; various thicknesses and lengths are available)**
- **Plastic-lined bucket or basin filled three-fourths full with warm water**
- **Disposable gloves and aprons**
- **Scissors**
- **Paper or plastic sheets**
- Cast saw **(if old cast is to be removed)**
- **Cart, chair, fracture table**

DELEGATION CONSIDERATIONS

The skills of assisting with cast application may be delegated to unlicensed assistive personnel.

- Inform and assist care provider in proper method of cast application.

STEPS	RATIONALE
ASSESSMENT	
1. Assess client's previous health status, including conditions affecting wound healing (e.g., diabetes, peripheral vascular disease, malnutrition, age).	Client's health status is pertinent to potential healing of tissues enclosed by cast.
2. Assess client's understanding of upcoming cast application.	Relieves client's anxiety and helps nurse determine whether additional information is needed.
3. Assess condition of tissues to be in the cast, including circulation and temperature to extremities. Note presence of skin breakdown, bruising, rash, and irritation. Skin of babies, children, and older adults may contain less subcutaneous fat.	Determines need for additional skin care before cast application. Determines need for close observation.

CRITICAL DECISION POINT Clients with skin breakdown may not be candidates for casting.

STEPS	RATIONALE
4. Determine client's pain status.	Fractures are painful; client responses vary, as does need for an analgesic.
CRITICAL DECISION POINT Muscle spasms may be more effectively treated with skeletal muscle relaxants than with narcotics.	
5. Determine extent to which client will be able to use casted extremity.	Predicts degree of assistance needed for self-care and/or ambulation.

NURSING DIAGNOSIS

Clustering of defining characteristics from the assessment data may reveal the following nursing diagnoses for clients requiring this skill:

- Bathing/hygiene and dressing/grooming self-care deficit
- Risk for impaired skin integrity
- Risk for peripheral neurovascular dysfunction
- Altered peripheral tissue perfusion
- Impaired home maintenance management
- Impaired physical mobility
- Knowledge deficit regarding casting procedure
- Pain
- Risk for injury

Related factors are individualized based on a client's condition or needs.

PLANNING

STEPS	RATIONALE
1. **Expected outcomes** following completion of procedure:	
➤ Client experiences only slight edema, soreness, mild pain, and some limitation of active ROJM from being in cast.	Cast limits normal function of affected tissues.
➤ Skin of tissues below cast is warm and of normal color with capillary refill of 3 seconds or less. Client verbalizes no abnormal or unusual sensations and is able to move fingers or toes below casted part.	Neurovascular function to body part is maintained.
➤ Client is able to perform limited ROJM actively.	Other joints should move without impairment.
➤ Client has some impaired function in mobility initially.	Cast may be heavy, or it may impair mobility because of size or area of body in cast.
➤ Client uses assistance with usual ADLs if head, neck, or upper extremity is in cast.	Cast can interfere with ability to dress, feed, or bathe oneself.
➤ Client verbalizes increase in comfort after cast application.	Injured tissues and bone are stabilized.
➤ Client demonstrates cast-care techniques.	Demonstrates learning.
2. Instruct client, parent, and other assistants how they can facilitate application of cast by maintaining affected part in desired position.	Cast will hold tissues in the position in which they are held during cast application. Client teaching reduces anxiety and increases cooperation.

IMPLEMENTATION

STEPS	RATIONALE
1. Administer analgesic before cast application: PO 30 to 40 minutes prior; IM 20 to 30 minutes prior; IV 2 to 5 minutes prior.	Reduces pain during cast application. Provides optimal analgesic effect.
2. Wash hands and put on gloves.	Reduces transmission of microorganisms. Synthetic cast can leave gluelike resin on hands.
3. Position client as needed; client may be lying, sitting, or standing, depending on type of cast and tissues to be casted.	Parts to be put in cast must be supported and in optimal position for cast application.
4. Prepare skin for cast if necessary; may involve cleansing with soap and water, changing dressing, and trimming long hair. Use gentle strokes to maintain skin integrity.	Reduces complications to underlying tissues after casting. Gentle manipulation prevents pain or additional injury.

STEPS	RATIONALE
5. Explain that client may experience warmth during the cast application process.	Plaster gives off heat from a chemical reaction when drying.
6. Depending on type of cast material being applied, do *one* of the following:	
a. Hold plaster roll under water in a casting bucket or plastic basin until bubbles stop, then squeeze slightly and give roll to person applying cast.	Dampened plaster rolls are unrolled and molded to fit part being casted. Some have resin for easy moldability.
b. Submerge synthetic cast roll in lukewarm water for 10 to 15 seconds. Squeeze to remove excess water.	Initiates chemical reaction that produces heat and hardens tape.
c. Hold body part or parts to be put in cast in position requested by person applying cast.	Support of body part may involve applying slight manual traction, if desired, to maintain optimal position.
d. Hold parts while casting tape is applied and molded (see illustration, p. 947). Synthetic tape is applied with slight tension. When wrapping is completed, gently compress with hands.	Casting tape is impregnated with synthetic adhesive or glass fiber materials, which dry quickly and are lightweight. Compression promotes bonding of cast layers.
7. Continue to supply dampened rolls of plaster, synthetic cast roll, or cast tape or to hold parts as necessary until cast is finished.	Plaster must be of sufficient thickness to give strength to cast.
8. Supply **walking heel** cast, **cast brace,** bar, or other **cast stabilization** material as requested by physician or practitioner.	Ambulation (after cast dries) may be permitted with partial weight bearing, which is facilitated by walking **cast shoe,** heel or sole. Bars stabilize spica cast, or "posts" (metal poles) stabilize **"four-poster" cast.** Brace can be incorporated into cast to aid in maintaining joint motion and mobility.
9. Assist with "finishing" by folding stockinette or other padding down over outer edge of cast to provide smooth edge. Damp plaster is then unrolled over padding to hold it securely outside cast.	Smooth edges lessen possible skin irritation. By finishing cast with stockinette, later **"petaling"** is not required when cast is dry.
10. Supply scissors to trim plaster rolls around thumb, fingers, and toes as necessary.	Cast should be snug but should not constrict joint movement or circulation.
11. Depending on tissues casted:	
a. Place damp cast on cloth-covered pillows (two to three) to prevent deformation or pressure points as it sets. Maintain elevation above heart level as long as neurovascular assessments are normal (see Evaluation section).	Pillows prevent cast from hardening in undesirable position. Elevation enhances venous return and decreases edema. If there is evidence of neurovascular deficit, then lower to the heart level to negate the effects of gravity.
CRITICAL DECISION POINT **Handle casted extremity with palms only. Fingers can cause indentations that can lead to pressure areas.**	
b. Place casted tissues in sling, making sure sling just holds, and does not encase, cast.	Covering (encasing) impedes air movements and delays drying.
c. Remove and dispose of gloves.	Reduces transmission of microorganisms.
d. Cover client or reclothe as needed, leaving damp, casted areas uncovered.	Covering blocks air movement, delays drying, and retains heat, which can lead to skin damage with plaster.
12. Assist with transfer of client to stretcher or wheelchair for return to nursing unit, to prepare client for discharge. May accompany client to room and assist with transfer to bed if necessary. Client may have cast applied in room.	Safety in transfer requires use of pillows to support cast, side rails, restraints, and sufficient personnel to support client and cast. Safety in transfer requires more than one person to accompany client in body, spica, long arm, long leg, and Minerva jacket cast to prevent falls.
13. Clean equipment (pail, scissors, cast saw, and so on), and return to usual places; discard used materials. Wash hands.	Facilitates use of equipment and area for next client. Reduces transmission of infection.

STEPS	RATIONALE
14. Explain purposes of exposure for faster drying, use of fans or lights to facilitate drying, use of elevation if pertinent, or application of ice bags if ordered.	Casts must dry from inside out for thorough drying. Fans should not be used in open areas or under cast; organisms may be blown in to cause infection. Hot blow dryers or heat lamps can burn tissues. Elevation and use of ice decreases edema formation.

CRITICAL DECISION POINT **Synthetic casts are dry or set by time of transfer, because they set in 7 to 15 minutes. Soft tissues around affected area may swell from processes of "reducing" or manipulating before cast was applied.**

CRITICAL DECISION POINT **Ice is placed to the side rather than the top of the cast to prevent indentations.**

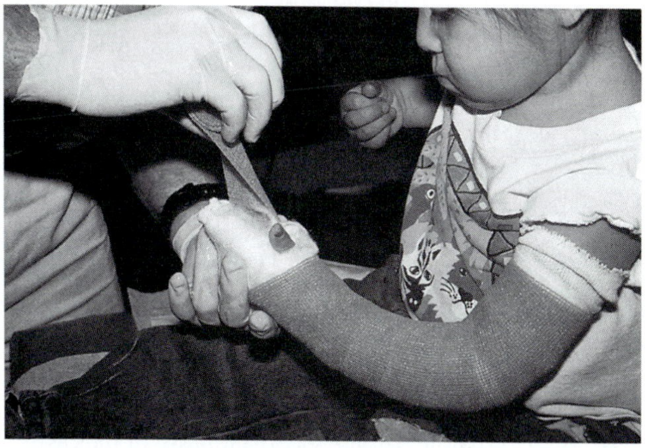

Step 6d Applying long arm cast.

STEPS	RATIONALE
15. Reposition client every 2 to 3 hours.	Prevents any one area of the cast from receiving continuous pressure. Avoids indentation of cast.
16. Inform client to notify personnel of any alteration in sensation, abnormal sensation, or inability to move fingers or toes.	Pressure within a casted extremity may increase with edema and lead to compartment syndrome. Compartment syndrome occurs when pressure within the muscle compartment increases as a result of edema, bleeding, or decreased venous return. The fascia covering the muscle group acts as a tourniquet directing the pressure to structures within the compartment: nerves, blood vessels, and muscle tissue. Neurovascular assessments are used to determine development of compartment syndrome.

EVALUATION

STEPS	RATIONALE
1. Observe client for signs of pain or anxiety: severe edema, uncontrollable pain, inability to move body parts distal to cast, hyperventilation, swallowing air (aerophagia), tachycardia, and blood pressure increases.	These are signs of development of "compartment syndrome," **"cast syndrome,"** or severe claustrophobia from snugness of cast (common for clients in spica or body cast).
2. Evaluate neurovascular status by performing neurovascular assessment every 1 to 2 hours for the first 24 hours.	Neurovascular status determines circulation and oxygenation of tissues and functioning of neurological tissues.

CRITICAL DECISION POINT **A deterioration in neurovascular status requires immediate action, because irreversible tissue death occurs within 4 to 12 hours without adequate oxygenation.**

STEPS	RATIONALE
a. Observe color of tissues distal to cast (may be pink, whitish, or bluish). Older adult clients may have bluish color normally; however, no other signs of circulatory compromise should be present.	Pink indicates arterial pressure is normal, whitish signifies decreased arterial supply, and bluish color signifies venous stasis.
b. Observe for edema distal to cast. Older adults may have concurrent dependent edema because of health state.	Edema results from trauma or venous stasis. Rarely, heat of plaster drying contributes to development of edema.

STEPS	RATIONALE
c. Compare neurovascular status with preapplication neurovascular assessment. Assess temperature of tissues above and below or around cast. Older adult clients frequently have cooler-than-usual extremities because of decreased peripheral circulation.	Warmth of tissues distal or proximal to cast usually indicates adequate perfusion.

CRITICAL DECISION POINT If tissues are cold or cool, compare with similar unaffected tissues, such as opposite fingers, toes, or foot, to determine if coolness is excessive, which would indicate decreased arterial perfusion.

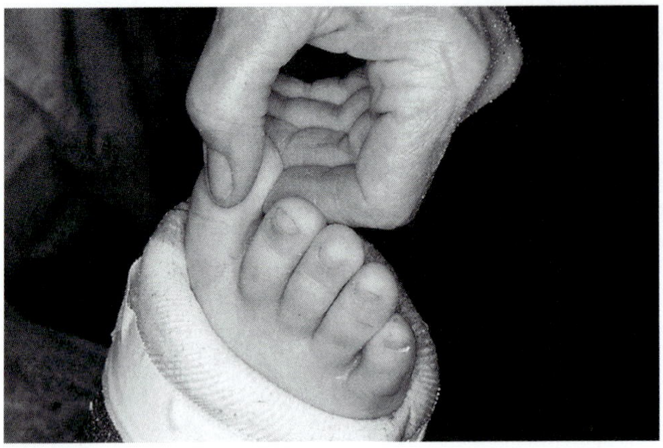

Step 2e Assessing capillary refill. The nailbed is compressed. When released it should "pink up" in 3 seconds or less.

STEPS	RATIONALE
d. When possible palpate the distal pulse of the casted extremity; note presence and strength of pulse.	Weak or absent pulse may indicate decreased circulation to casted area.
e. Assess capillary refill by pressing on toe or fingernail (if cast is on extremity), releasing, and noting "pinking" of nail; nail should "pink up" in 3 seconds or less (see illustration).	"Blanching" on pressure with subsequent capillary refill is indicative of arterial perfusion. Capillary refill is too sluggish if refill takes more than 3 seconds. It takes 2 seconds to say "capillary refill" slowly and 4 seconds to repeat it once.

CRITICAL DECISION POINT Older adult clients may have slow or even poor capillary refill because of peripheral vascular conditions; use more than one neurovascular assessment to determine circulatory adequacy.

STEPS	RATIONALE
f. Determine amount and severity of pain if present. Ask client for descriptions; avoid coaching client with words to describe pain.	Manipulation and reduction may produce dull, aching pain as a result of pressure on nerve endings. Clients vary in perception and tolerance of pain. Sudden increase in pain, unrelenting pain, or pain out of proportion should be investigated further because it may signify thrombus formation or compartment syndrome.
g. Compare tissues in cast with contralateral tissues to determine current condition.	Comparison with normal tissues assists in forming judgment of neurovascular status.
h. Inspect condition of skin around edges of cast.	This area is susceptible to pressure and friction.
i. Ask client to move parts in ROJM if possible; note if client is unable to do active ROJM of uncasted areas. Older adult clients may have stiffness of joints or edema from other health conditions.	Range of motion should be performed within limitations imposed by cast. Only tissues out of cast can, or should, be moved.
j. If client cannot do *active* ROJM to contiguous tissues, perform *passive* ROJM on these joints, noting responses or complaints of increased pain.	Passive movements decrease edema and demonstrate ability of part to be moved. However, inability to perform active ROJM and increased pain during passive movement may signify development of compartment syndrome and should be reported.
k. Ask client to describe sensations or feelings of tissues in cast. Listen for descriptions such as pins and needles, asleep, numb, burning, or throbbing; do not prompt client by using those words.	May signify pressure or anoxia affecting normal transmission of nerve impulses.
3. Smell the cast edges; a sour smell is normal.	Detects early sign of infection (foul odor).

STEPS	RATIONALE
4. Observe the client performing cast care.	Return demonstration objectively measures the client's learning.
5. **Unexpected outcomes** that may occur include:	
➤ Client experiences malunion or malposition of affected parts.	May be caused by insufficient **reduction** (placement) in cast.
➤ Client experiences nonunion.	May result from local or systemic factors, such as infection, foreign objects in area, diabetes, or malnutrition.
➤ Client develops osteomyelitis if open wound was present at time of casting.	Causes of osteomyelitis may be bacterial, fungal, tubercular, or other and may not develop for years after injury and cast.
➤ Client develops pressure ulcer over bony prominence.	May result from inward pressure of cast on tissues.
➤ Client experiences muscle weakness.	May result from prolonged immobility
➤ There is decreased circulation or sensation distal to cast, as indicated by cold extremity, decreased capillary refill, numbness, tingling, or diminished pulse.	Indicates cast is constricting circulation to extremity. If constriction remains, bivalving and splitting underlying soft dressing or removal may be necessary to prevent permanent damage.
➤ Client experiences increased pain with swelling, pallor, and reduced movement of distal parts.	Signs of compartment syndrome and muscle ischemia.
➤ Client experiences altered sensations such as tingling, numbness, and/or alteration in motion.	Signs of compartment syndrome and muscle ischemia.
➤ Client is unable to demonstrate cast care.	Reinstruction is necessary. Adaptation of teaching interventions is made to fit client situation.

Recording and Reporting

1. Record application of cast and condition of skin and circulation. Report abnormal or untoward findings from neurovascular checks; report the following *immediately:* bluish color to distal parts, marked increase in edema or pain, delayed capillary refill (longer than 3 seconds), inability to palpate distal peripheral pulses if originally palpable, increased numbness or tingling, cold tissues, and inability to move tissues actively.	All are signs of circulatory compromise, stasis, and, possibly, development of compartment syndrome.

Follow-up Activities

1. If edges of cast begin to fray, apply "petals" to further protect cast. Small pieces of adhesive tape 2.5 to 5.0 cm (1 to 2 in) are cut and taped over edge of cast (optional).
2. If odor and drainage from cast are noted:
   a. Contact physician.
   b. Draw circle on cast around drainage site. Record time and date on circle (optional).
3. If circulation to extremity is compromised:
   a. Call physician.
   b. Anticipate bivalving or removing cast.

• • • • •

Special Considerations

- ➤ If cast is applied for clubfoot, person applying cast can usually mold cast in desired position.
- ➤ Clients in casts may be more comfortable than when not in cast if deformity or **crepitation** (fractured ends rubbing against each other) is present.
- ➤ Client with wet large-limb or wet spica cast requires three people to assist in turning. Proper assistance prevents undue pressure on cast.
- ➤ Realign pillows to promote cast drying when client is repositioned.

Teaching Considerations

- ➤ Client must be taught to care for cast in home to protect it from moisture and unnecessary wear.
- ➤ Teach client about effects of pressure from cast on underlying skin and tissue.
- ➤ Prepare client for itching sensations under cast. Client should avoid sticking objects down or in cast to scratch, because these objects can cause breaks in underlying skin and subsequent infections. May require medication to control the itching.

- If client must use crutches, instruct in crutch-walking techniques (see Skill 30-5).
- Teach client proper ROM and isometric exercises for affected extremity.
- Caution client against drying wet cast with a hair dryer; this can cause plaster to crack or skin underneath to be damaged.

Pediatric Considerations

- Parents or other care givers must be taught to protect the cast from moisture or unnecessary wear. Plastic wrap placed around the perineal area during defecation prevents soiling.
- If child has clubfoot, parents and child should be taught that frequent cast changes are necessary. Cast changes accommodate normal bone and tissue growth and correction of abnormality.
- Babies in casts for treatment of clubfoot have limited maneuverability.
- Children are particularly prone to placing objects into a cast to scratch. They must be monitored closely. Medication can be used to control itching.
- Babies or children may signify pain through crying or restlessness.
- Casts are removed earlier in babies and children because of speedy healing and to facilitate muscle and joint function.
- Plaster of Paris casts on babies and children may have less plaster, to aid in moving or lifting.

Gerontologic Considerations

- Older nonverbal clients may signify pain through crying or restlessness.
- Lightweight, synthetic casts are better for older adult clients. Cast is less restrictive, and light weight helps clients maintain better balance.
- Plaster of Paris casts on older adults may have less plaster, to aid in moving or lifting.
- Older adult clients may have reduced sensation and be less able to detect compression (Lewis and Knortz, 1993).
- Older adult clients may take longer for bone healing than younger clients.

Home Care Considerations

- Client must inspect cast and petal rough edges to reduce risk of trauma to underlying skin and need for cast changes.
- Client must inspect cast daily for foul odor, which indicates skin excoriation or infection under cast.
- Client must inspect skin daily for pressure or friction areas.
- Client must inspect cast daily for cracks or changes in alignment.
- Client must keep plaster of Paris cast dry. When bathing, casted extremity must not be submerged because cast absorbs water, loses structural integrity, and crumbles. If cast becomes wet, dry immediately.
- Synthetic casts may be cleaned with warm water and mild soap.

SKILL 31-2 Assisting with Cast Removal

Cast removal consists of removing the cast and padding with a mechanical device such as a cast saw (Fig. 31-3). The nurse must prepare for this procedure so the client remains still and cooperates during cast removal. The removal of a cast is painless but can be noisy. A child or confused client may need to be gently restrained during the procedure to prevent injury by the equipment. After the cast is removed, the nurse provides appropriate skin care.

EQUIPMENT

- Cast saw
- Plastic sheets or papers
- Cold water enzyme wash
- Skin lotion
- Basin, water, washcloths, towels
- Scissors
- Clean gloves

DELEGATION CONSIDERATIONS

The skill of cast removal may be delegated to unlicensed assistive personnel.

- Inform and assist care provider in proper method of cast removal.

A B

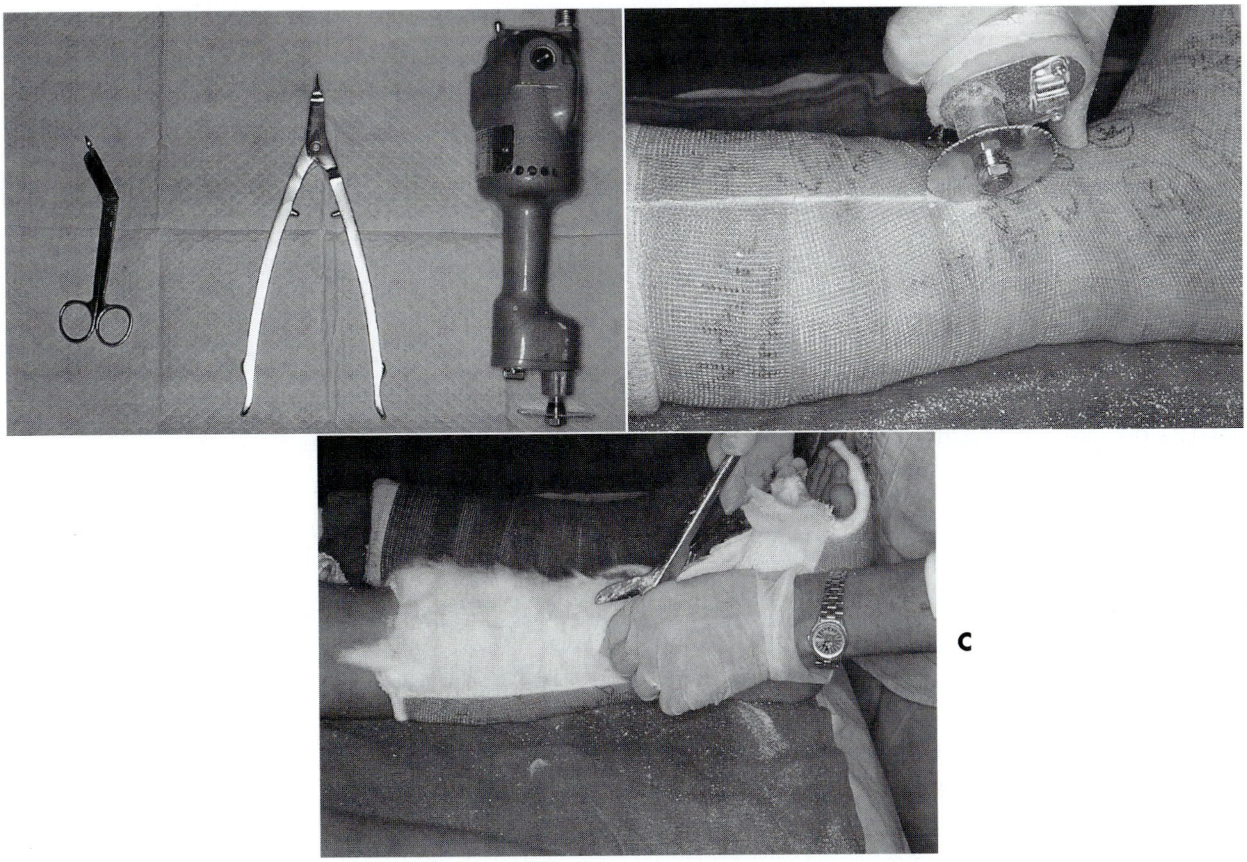

C

Fig. 31-3 **A,** Equipment for removing a cast. From *left to right:* scissors, cast spreader, cast saw. **B,** Cast saw is used to remove cast. To bivalve a cast, it is cut longitudinally on either side and the wadding is cut with scissors. The two halves may be secured together with an elastic wrap, or the top is removed and the bottom shell of the cast becomes a posterior splint. **C,** Cutting through wadding under cast with scissors.

STEPS	RATIONALE
ASSESSMENT	
1. Assess client's understanding of and response to upcoming cast removal.	Helps develop a teaching plan that aids in reducing anxiety.
2. Assess client's readiness for cast removal (client's physical findings, physician's orders, x-ray results).	Determines level of healing and readiness to remove cast.
3. Ask client if any itching or irritation under cast is felt.	Indicates healing and accumulation of dried skin layers.

NURSING DIAGNOSIS

Clustering of defining characteristics from the assessment data may reveal the following nursing diagnoses for clients requiring this skill:

- ➤ Risk for impaired skin integrity
- ➤ Knowledge deficit regarding cast removal
- ➤ Anxiety
- ➤ Risk for injury

Related factors are individualized based on a client's condition or needs.

STEPS	RATIONALE
PLANNING	
1. **Expected outcomes** following completion of procedure:	
➤ Client incurs no underlying tissue or skin injury; there is buildup of dry, dead skin. Client skin remains intact.	Cast is removed safely. Layers of dead skin cells that accumulate are removed over time without scrubbing.
➤ Client verbalizes understanding of normal physical sensations and the procedural steps of cast removal.	Understanding lessens anticipatory anxiety.
➤ Client is able to describe and demonstrate the level of activity and weight bearing allowed.	Allows client to safely assume activity at home.
➤ Client is able to explain skin care measures.	Allows client to assume self-care.
2. Explain the physical sensations to expect during cast removal. Cast saw vibrates cast loose; client will feel heat and vibration.	Explanation minimizes fear of possible injury.
3. Describe the procedural steps for cast removal: appearance of saw, removal of outer cast, appearance of padding, cleansing of skin.	Client is prepared to witness and participate in procedure.
IMPLEMENTATION	
1. Apply gloves if drainage is anticipated, and assist person removing cast by positioning, turning, and holding cast and tissues in cast.	Prevents injury from saw.
➤ ***CRITICAL DECISION POINT*** **Client must remain still during cast removal.**	
2. After removal of cast and padding, inspect tissues for general condition, redness, warmth, and drainage.	May signify inflammation or infection of tissues.
3. If skin is intact, gently apply cold water enzyme wash to skin; let stay on skin 15 to 20 minutes.	Helps dissolve or emulsify dead cells and fatty deposits on tissues. Prevents injury to delicate tissue.
➤ ***CRITICAL DECISION POINT*** **Do not scrub skin, because this may lead to skin breakdown. It may take several days before all residue is removed from skin.**	
4. After elapsed time, gently wash off enzyme wash; if possible, immerse tissues in basin or tub to aid in removal of tissue debris without undue rubbing or pressure.	Removes as much debris as possible.
5. After patting tissues dry (avoid rubbing), apply generous coating of skin lotion, gently massaging into skin.	Rubbing could traumatize tender tissues. Lotion lubricates skin.
6. Obtain a physician's order to gently put joints through active and passive ROJM. Clarify level of activity allowed.	Joints and muscles will be stiff and weak. Activity is resumed slowly to avoid reinjury.
7. Assist in transfer of client for return to room or for discharge if anticipated.	
8. All equipment and casts should be cleaned or discarded according to standard precautions. Remove gloves. If cast is soiled with blood, discard as biohazard waste.	Reduces transmission of microorganisms.
EVALUATION	
1. Observe underlying skin.	Reveals condition of skin.
2. Assess client's verbal and nonverbal responses.	Expressions, tone of voice, and movement reveal level of anxiety or fear.

STEPS	RATIONALE
3. Ask client to explain ordered exercise plan and demonstrate exercises.	Demonstrates learning.
4. Have client explain and perform skin care.	Demonstrates learning of self-care.
5. **Unexpected outcomes** that may occur include:	
➤ Client becomes tense and restless and withdraws from cast saw.	Anxiety requires further explanation and support.
➤ Client experiences extensive edema, pain, or limited use of affected tissues.	Patterns may be related to malunion, nonunion, or extreme muscle weakness.
➤ Client is unable to perform ADLs and exercises.	May be related to nonunion or pain. Physician will assess the nonunion by x-ray film.
➤ Underlying skin may be scratched.	Result of friction from saw.
➤ Client is unable to explain self-care measures.	Reinstruction or clarification is needed.

RECORDING AND REPORTING

1. Record cast removal, condition of tissues formerly in cast, and person removing cast in nurse's notes.	Provides for completeness of care and documentation for legal concerns. Provides baseline data to ensure continuity of care.

FOLLOW-UP ACTIVITIES

1. Client may have transient symptoms after cast removal. Physician or nurse should instruct client to:
   a. Elevate body part if edema returns.
   b. Use nonnarcotic analgesics every 4 hours for up to 24 hours if needed.
   c. Slowly perform ROJM exercises every 4 hours. (If marked weakness exists, physician may order client to receive physical therapy or to use sling or immobilizer for 1 to 2 days for continued rest.)
2. Report changes in movement, severe swelling, and increased pain to physician.

• • • • •

Special Considerations

➤ Amount of cellular debris under client's cast depends on length of time tissues are in cast and overall skin integrity.
➤ Use caution with tender skin areas or joints.

Teaching Considerations

➤ Instruct client to call physician if unable to perform ADLs, if excessive edema occurs, if client experiences limited use of joints or muscles, or if mobility is affected. If client is treated for congenital deformity with repeated cast changes, instruct when next cast change is due; give client written appointment.
➤ Provide client with scheduled exercises to increase mobility and muscle strength.

Pediatric Considerations

➤ Babies and children may be frightened of the cast saw. Demonstration of the saw before removal of the cast may alleviate anxiety.

Gerontologic Considerations

➤ Older adult clients may experience marked stiffness or weakened muscles, depending on length of time in cast.
➤ Older adult client's skin is drier, thinner, and more fragile than that of a baby, child, or younger adult.

Home Care Considerations

➤ Client should have chair or bed with pillows to elevate extremity for intermittent edema.
➤ Suggest regular use of moisturizers for dry, scaly skin of casted extremity.
➤ Assess client's environment for potential safety risks.

SKILL 31-3 Assisting with Application of Skin Traction

Skin traction is one of the two basic types of traction used for the treatment of fractured bones and correction of orthopedic abnormalities. Skin traction applies pull to an affected body structure by straps attached to the skin around the structure. For traction to be effective, there must be a pull in the opposite direction **(countertraction)** by using the weight of the client's body or by elevating part of the bed toward the traction. Recovery is facilitated through immobilization and alignment of body parts. The nurse provides safe care through skillful application of traction. The following are the major forms of skin traction, with some variation within some of the types.

1. Bryant's traction—vertically held type of bilateral traction to the legs (Fig. 31-4, *A*). This type of traction can be used for children weighing less than 40 lb. Adhesive strips are applied to the lateral surfaces of each leg and wrapped with elastic bandages to secure them in place. A **spreader bar** is attached to the strips and then to ropes, pulleys, and weights. Bryant's traction, called Gallow's traction in England, is used for children with fractures of the femur. After the muscle spasms are overcome and the fragments are aligned with some evidence of union, the child is removed from traction and placed in a spica cast to continue recovery and for callus formation to progress. Children may remain in Bryant's traction for only 7 to 10 days.
2. Buck's extension—horizontally applied unilateral or bilateral traction (Fig. 31-4, *B*). Buck's traction is applied in one of two ways: adhesive strips are applied to the lateral surfaces of the limb or limbs (usually one leg or forearm) and wrapped with elastic bandages, or a commercially prepared foam boot with Velcro straps is applied. A spreader bar is attached to the adhesive strips as in Bryant's traction or to the foam boot and then to ropes, pulleys, and weights. Buck's extension is used before repair of hip fractures to reduce muscles spasms, contractures, and dislocations and occasionally as an interim treatment for lumbosacral muscle spasms causing low back pain.
3. Cotrel's traction—skin traction consisting of two separate forms: head halter and pelvic belt (Fig. 31-4, *C*). Cotrel's traction is used occasionally as a preoperative treatment to help straighten spinal curvatures before insertion of skeletal rods for correction of scoliosis. The pull in opposite directions on the head and pelvis helps to overcome the deforming muscle pull causing the curvature. **Cervical halter** traction and **pelvic belt** traction are explained later in this section.
4. Dunlop's traction—simultaneous horizontal form of Buck's extension to the humerus with an accompanying vertical Buck's extension to the forearm (Fig. 31-4, *D*). The horizontal Buck's extension is the "treating"

A

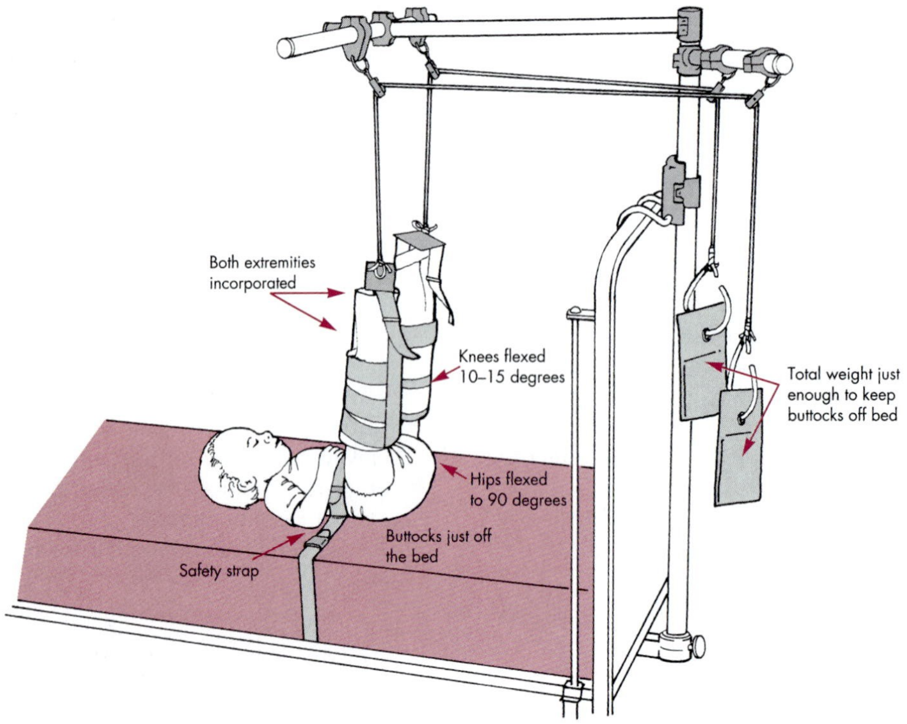

Fig. 31-4 **A,** Bryant's traction. (**A, B,** and **D** From Folcik M, Carini-Garcia G, Birmingham J: *Traction: assessment and management,* St Louis, 1994, Mosby.)

traction for fractures of the humerus, whereas the vertical Buck's extension is primarily used to maintain the forearm in the desired position relative to the humerus.

5. Cervical (head halter)—traction involving a specially shaped halter with cutout areas for the ears, face, and top of the head (Fig. 31-5, *A*). The halter cups the chin and has straps leading from the occipital skull area that attach to the chin portion and then connect to one or two spreader bars on either side of the head; the bar or bars are then attached to ropes, pulleys, and weights. Cervical traction should be used only for degenerative or arthritic conditions of the cervical vertebrae, not for fractures of the vertebrae. Because cervical traction must be removed occasionally for client safety and care and because this traction does not result in total spinal immobilization, it is unsafe and potentially dangerous for a client with a fracture of cervical vertebrae. Release of the weights in such a situation could lead to paralysis.
6. Pelvic belt—traction consisting of a girdlelike belt that fits around the lumbosacral and abdominal areas, fastening in the middle of the abdomen with pressure-sensitive straps or buckles (Fig. 31-5, *B*). The belt has long straps that attach to a wide spreader bar beyond the feet; the bar is then connected to ropes, pulleys, and weights. The client is placed in Williams' position (supine with the head of the bed slightly elevated and the knees bent) to decrease the stress on the lumbosacral spine. This pelvic belt, or lumbosacral traction, is used for clients with low back pain, muscle spasms, and a ruptured nucleus pulposus (herniated or ruptured disk). This traction basically serves to keep the client in bed, thus relieving inflammation and irritation of the injured nerves or muscles. It does not overcome the her-

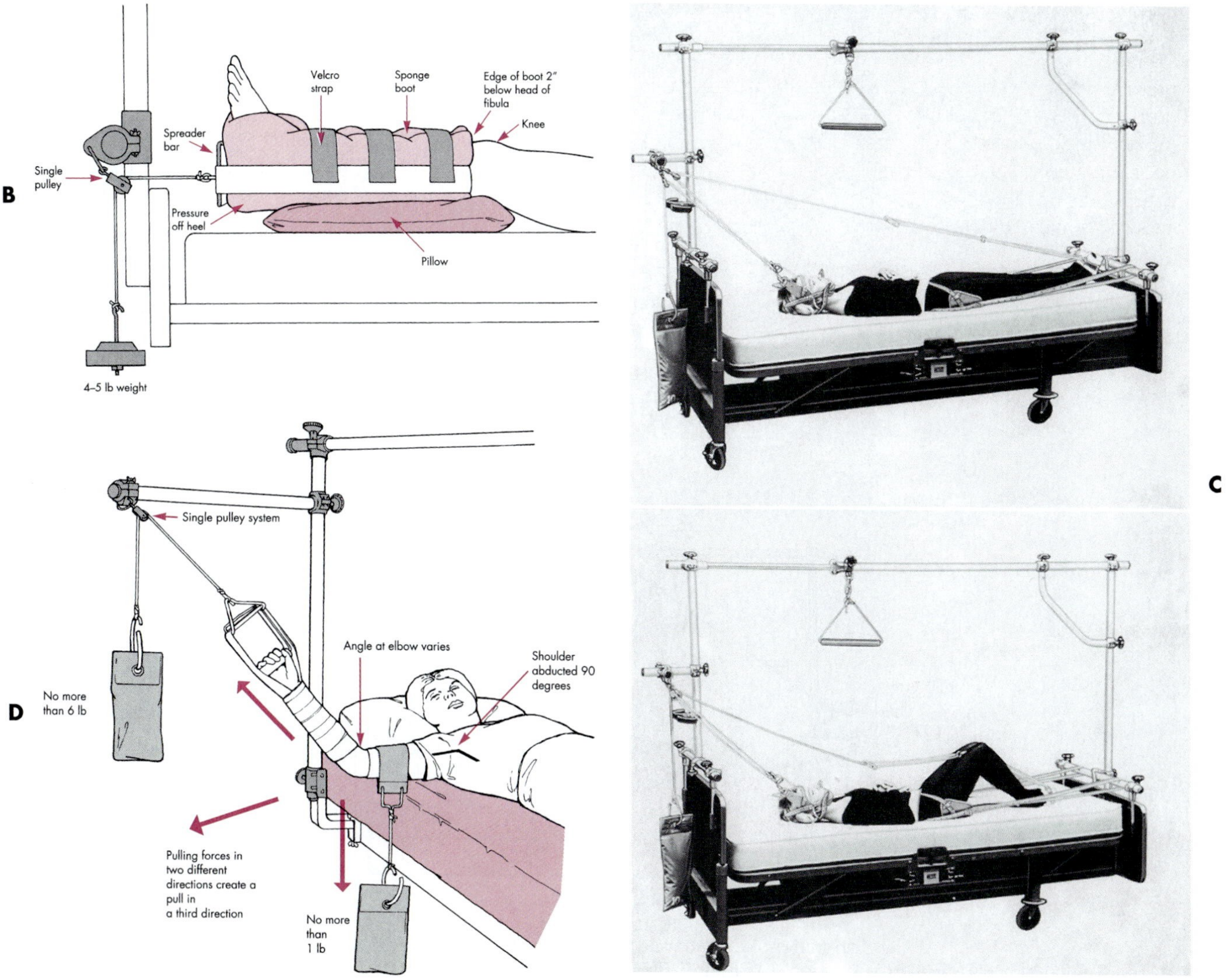

Fig. 31-4, cont'd **B,** Buck's extension. **C,** Cotrel's traction. **D,** Dunlop's traction.

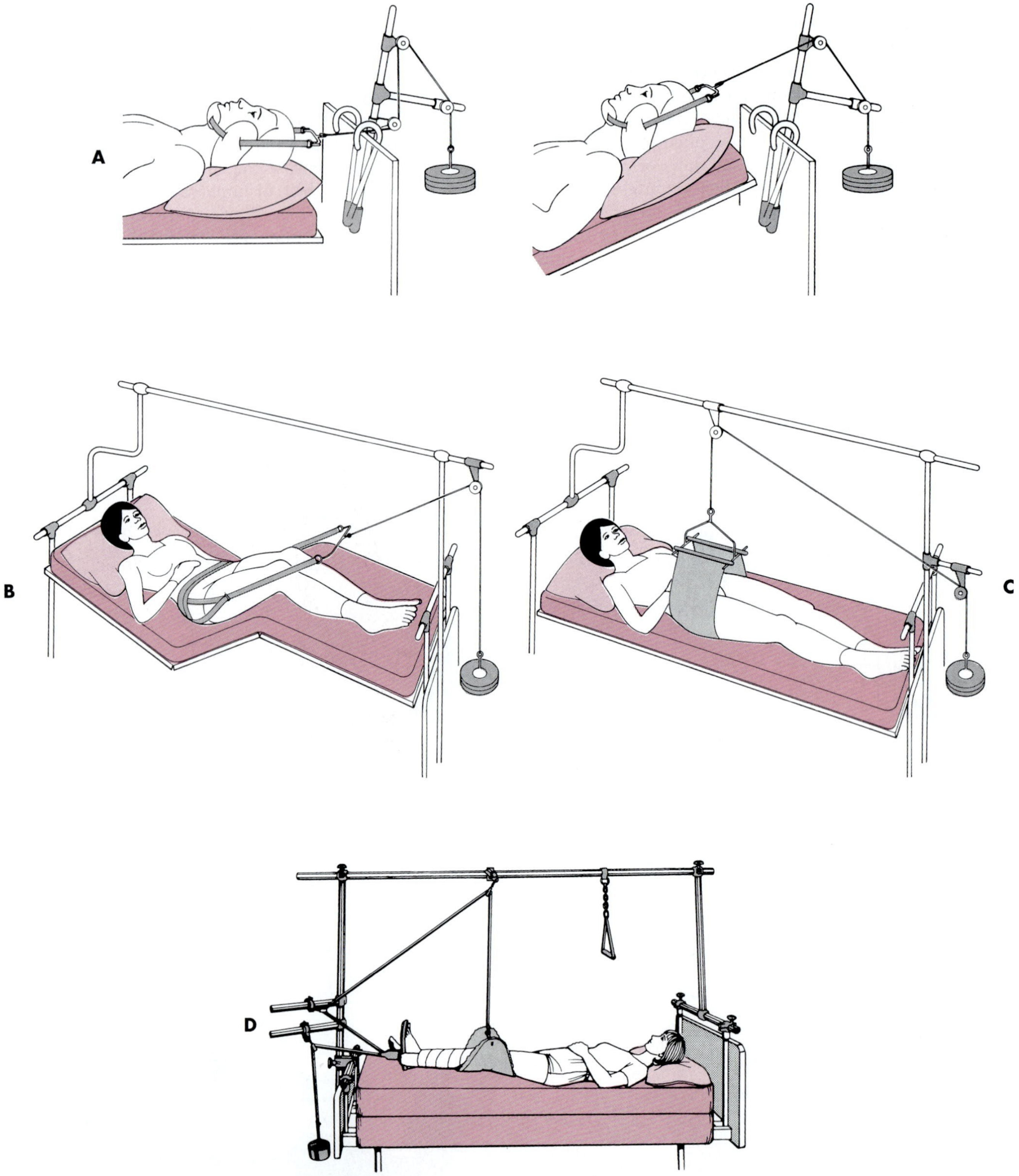

Fig. 31-5 **A,** Cervical halter skin traction. **B,** Pelvic belt traction (skin). **C,** Pelvic sling (skin). **D,** Russell's traction. (**A, B,** and **C** From Beare PG, Myers JL: *Principles and practice of adult health nursing,* ed 2, St Louis, 1994, Mosby. **D** From Phipps W et al.: *Medical-surgical nursing: concepts and clinical practice,* ed 15, St Louis, 1995, Mosby.)

nation of the nucleus pulposus. Additional treatments, including diathermy, use of muscle relaxant drugs, and physical therapy, are used in conjunction with this traction.

7. **Pelvic sling** (Weil sling)—"traction" consisting of a hammocklike belt wherein the sling cradles the pelvis in its boundaries for treatment of one or more fractures of the pelvic bones. The sling is attached on each side to a pin threaded through a sewn tunnel; each pin is then placed in a grooved spreader bar attached to ropes, pulleys, and weights. The sling applies gentle inward pressure to the injured tissues, thereby providing comfort and security to the client (Fig. 31-5, *C*).
8. Russell's traction—modification of Buck's extension using Newton's second law of thermodynamics (for each force in one direction there is an equal force in the opposite direction) to double the amount of pull through the arrangement of ropes, pulleys, and weights (Fig. 31-5, *D*).

Because skin tissues and subcutaneous attachments cannot tolerate great amounts of weight without losing strength and continuity, skin traction uses weights varying from 1 to 2 lb for children in Bryant's traction to 7 to 10 lb for cervical skin traction. Average weights are 5 to 7 lb for Buck's extension, 7 to 10 lb for Dunlop's traction, 10 to 15 lb for pelvic belt traction (weight is distributed over the entire pelvis and lower back), and 10 to 20 lb for a pelvic sling (the sling is really a form of hammock suspension rather than traction).

Each form of skin traction mentioned above has a usual or "classic" position used for the majority of clients in that traction. Variations may be needed to treat a specific injury or condition. If pertinent, these variations are noted in the discussion of each type of traction.

EQUIPMENT

- **Ropes,** pulleys, **weights,** weight holder **(ropes are nylon for strength; weights vary from 1 to 5 lb—have several of each weight) (Babies, children, and older adults require less weight than do young adults)**
- **Bed frame for attachment of traction or portable frames that attach to bed**
- **One or more spreader bars**
- **Adhesive-backed moleskin**
- **Elastic bandages**
- **Heel or elbow protectors (optional)**
- **Knee sling for** Russell's traction
- **Wastebasket with plastic bag liner**

DELEGATION CONSIDERATIONS

The skill of assisting with application of skin traction may be delegated to unlicensed assistive personnel.

- Inform and assist care provider in proper method of aiding in application of skin traction.

STEPS	RATIONALE
ASSESSMENT	
1. Assess condition of client's overall health, including degree of mobility and current medical conditions such as diabetes or peripheral vascular disease.	Determines client's health state and ability to tolerate traction.
2. Assess condition of specific tissues to be placed in traction; note skin condition, excessive hair, bruises, rash, or other lesions.	Determines ability of local tissues to tolerate traction.
CRITICAL DECISION POINT **Irritated or broken skin should not have skin traction placed over the damaged tissues.**	
a. Cervical halter: assess occipital area of head, ears, chin, and neck.	
b. Bryant's traction: assess one or both legs.	
c. Buck's extension: assess one or both legs.	
d. Dunlop's traction: assess arm and forearm.	
e. Pelvic belt: assess lower back and abdomen.	Pain and spasms should be relieved by traction.
f. Pelvic sling: assess back and abdomen.	
g. Russell's traction: assess lower limbs.	Bruises may indicate trauma that would be relieved by traction.
CRITICAL DECISION POINT **Cotrel's traction includes head halter and pelvic belt and is not considered separately.**	
3. Assess client's understanding of reason for traction.	Determines concerns, acceptance, and need for instruction.

STEPS	RATIONALE
4. Assess client's level of pain.	Serves as baseline for later comparison.
5. Assess client's neurovascular status.	Serves as baseline for later comparison.

NURSING DIAGNOSIS

Clustering of defining characteristics from the assessment data may reveal the following nursing diagnoses for clients requiring this skill:

- Bathing/hygiene and dressing/grooming self-care deficit
- Risk for impaired skin integrity
- Risk for peripheral neurovascular dysfunction
- Altered peripheral tissue perfusion
- Impaired home maintenance management
- Impaired physical mobility
- Knowledge deficit regarding the type and use of traction
- Pain

Related factors are individualized based on a client's condition or needs.

PLANNING

STEPS	RATIONALE
1. **Expected outcomes** following completion of procedure:	
➤ Client participates in bathing and feeding.	Activities are performed safely and without injury.
➤ Skin around straps and moleskin remains intact, without irritation.	Skin is free of pressure and/or pulling.
➤ X-ray studies confirm satisfactory alignment of fracture fragments with or without evidence of beginning callus formation (evidence of callus may not become apparent for 7 to 10 days or longer) if client is in traction for fracture.	Objective evidence is required for comparison with subjective relief of symptoms.
➤ Client describes purpose for traction and follows activity restrictions.	Client learns and accepts need for restrictions.
➤ As result of being in one specific type of skin traction, one of the following occurs:	
• Cervical halter: client notes relief of spasms and pain in neck and back of neck and head (may require administration of muscle relaxant and narcotic medications while in traction).	Each type of traction is designed to relieve muscle spasms; restore alignment or lessen shortening, overriding, or rotation; relieve pain; and increase comfort.
• Bryant's traction: child is able to maintain positioning with distraction by parents or care givers.	
• Buck's extension: client is able to maintain leg in alignment. Older adult clients with severe hip pain noticeably relax.	Narcotic use may be required for 1 to 3 days for acute pain.
• Dunlop's traction: same result occurs as for Buck's extension (used for upper extremity).	Clients may require narcotics for 1 to 3 days for acute pain of fractured humerus.
• Pelvic belt: client notes lessening of spasms of lumbosacral muscles, possibly slight lessening of sensory signs of pressure on sciatic nerve (numbness, tingling, or "pins and needles" radiating down back of leg to toes), and possibly less pressure in vertebral area at site of injury. Client is usually ordered to be in traction for 2 hours, out of traction for 2 hours, and out of traction at night, plus have orders for muscle relaxant medications, narcotic analgesics, and physical therapy.	Pull may lessen pressure on spinal or peripheral nerves, thereby alleviating symptoms.
• Pelvic sling: client experiences almost immediate comfort and relief from pelvic and abdominal discomfort, pain, and feeling of "coming apart."	Sling compresses tissues together. Clients are very comfortable in sling and develop sense of security while in it.
• Russell's traction: client notes lessening of pain in hip area (if traction is for hip trauma), relief	Russell's traction exerts double pull with less weight than Buck's extension because of pulley arrangement.

STEPS	RATIONALE
of muscle spasms, and ease in ability to maintain more normal anatomical position of leg and thigh.	
➤ Cotrel's traction: client experiences some straightening of curvature of spine.	Surgical correction may be required for marked curvature.
➤ Sufficient time in traction (varying from 1 to 10 or more days) elicits symptom relief.	Time is required for inflammation to abate and tissues to regain more normal functions.
➤ Neurovascular status remains stable.	There is no evidence of increased pressure within the muscle compartment and no neurovascular deficit.
2. Explain procedure to client, including traction setup and mobility restrictions.	Promotes cooperation and reduces anxiety.

IMPLEMENTATION

STEPS	RATIONALE
1. Prepare client and area of body to be in traction:	
a. Cervical halter: cleanse face and neck; shave man unless he has beard.	Lessens irritation under cervical halter.
b. Bryant's traction: cleanse both legs gently if necessary (change diaper if necessary for baby).	
c. Buck's extension: wash affected leg (or legs) very gently and dry carefully. Do not shave legs.	Shaving may create micronicks that could become inflamed under traction strips.
d. Dunlop's traction: cleanse arm and forearm gently if needed.	
e. Pelvic belt: check back and iliac crests for lesions.	
f. Pelvic sling: ask female client to void before being placed in sling if no catheter is in place.	Sling must be removed for placement of fracture bed pan. Male client can use urinal with no change in position of sling.
g. Russell's traction: cleanse lower extremity to knee as needed.	
2. Position client as requested by physician: a. Cervical halter: client flat on back. b. Bryant's traction: child flat on back. c. Buck's extension: client on back; head of bed flat or elevated no more than 30 degrees. d. Dunlop's traction: client flat on back. e. Pelvic belt: client flat on back. f. Pelvic sling: client flat on side or back. g. Russell's traction: client on back; head of bed slightly elevated.	Position varies with part of body to be placed on traction, plus effects of weight and gravity.
3. Assist with application of specific cervical halter, adhesive strips and elastic bandages, and pelvic belt or sling as needed. Nurse may be asked to hold client in desired position or apply halter, strips, or elastic bandages while physician and other assistants hold client's tissues in desired positions.	For lower extremity, adhesive strips are applied beginning below head of fibula on lateral surface of leg to avoid pressure over peroneal nerve. Ensures proper alignment of body parts under traction. Elastic bandages are applied from distal to proximal to promote venous return.
4. Assist with attachment of spreader bars, ropes, and pulleys. Ropes are tied securely in knots, passed in grooves of pulleys to weights, and are not frayed.	Provides proper weighted traction for extremity alignment.
5. When all traction materials and spreader bars are in place, weights are placed on weight holder and attached to loop in rope. The weights are then *lowered slowly and gently* until rope is taut. Physician determines exact amount of weight to be applied and position to be maintained for majority of time by client (clients should have written orders for specific traction weights, bed position, and turning regimen when pertinent).	Traction is slowly established to avoid involuntary muscle spasms or pain for client. Weight should be sufficient to create enough pull to overcome muscle spasms but not to cause distraction or marked increase in pain.

STEPS	RATIONALE
6. Before physician leaves, check client's position and ask about additional permissible positions for client and bed.	Ensures safety of care and position for effective traction.
a. Cervical halter: client stays flat on back, or head of bed may be elevated 15 to 20 degrees if ordered.	Angle of pull may allow head to be up to use body weight as countertraction.
b. Bryant's traction: baby or child must stay on back at all times; buttocks are held slightly off bed if traction weight is correct amount.	Child cannot turn to side or abdomen, because traction would be ineffective and reinjury could occur.
c. Buck's extension: client is primarily on back; may be allowed to turn to unaffected side for brief periods (10 to 15 minutes). Pillow placed under leg in traction may be used only when client is on side.	Positioning on side permits back care and rest to tissues. Pillows under leg or legs in traction should not be used, because they lessen traction's effectiveness.
d. Dunlop's traction: client must lie on back. Bed may be tilted on low-shock blocks toward side opposite traction. Head of bed is kept flat.	Tilting uses body for some countertraction.
e. Pelvic belt: client lies on back; knee portion of Gatch bed and head of bed may be raised so hips and knees are flexed at 45-degree angles (Williams' position).	Flexion of hips and knees relaxes lumbosacral muscles to lessen spasms.
f. Pelvic sling: client lies on back when in sling; sling should have enough weight attached to raise buttocks slightly off bed. If sling is off, it can be used carefully as turning sheet if client's fractures permit side lying.	Hammock effect of sling is most effective with client on back. Sling must be removed for placement of bedpan.
g. Russell's traction: client lies on back; head of bed may be elevated 30 to 45 degrees, depending on injury.	Low Fowler's position creates most effective traction pull.
h. Cotrel's traction: client must lie flat on back.	
7. Ask client how traction is affecting injured tissues if client is able to respond (ask parents of baby or child how client has been responding since traction has been on). Babies or young children may cry when weights are initially applied but soon cease crying and appear more comfortable.	Initial reaction may be slight increase in soreness or pain until client is able to relax and allow traction to perform as designed.
8. For safety, raise side rails as appropriate. Client's in Bryant's traction should always have someone in attendance.	Promotes client safety.
9. Assess neurovascular status 15 minutes after application of skin traction and every 1 to 2 hours for 24 hours (see Skill 31-1, Evaluation, Step 2).	If skin traction is applied too tightly then pressure is applied to nerves and vascular structures, resulting in a potentially irreversible deficit.
10. Gather unused materials and return to storage areas.	Promotes safety and cleanliness.
11. Wash hands.	Reduces transmission of microorganisms.
EVALUATION	
1. Observe client's participation in self-care.	Client may refrain from activity unnecessarily or may try to do too much.
2. Assess condition of skin around traction straps or bandages.	Ensures early identification of irritation or breakdown.
3. Observe entire traction setup and functioning: check all knots, ropes in pulleys, weights on weight holder; whether apparatus is hanging freely; position of halter, sling, belt, and other material for specific traction.	Reassessment is necessary to determine if traction is functioning as designed or desired or to make needed adjustments. Malfunctioning traction interferes with healing.

STEPS	RATIONALE
4. Ask if client understands mobility restrictions.	Feedback demonstrates learning.
5. Ask if client is experiencing pain, spasms, or muscle burning.	Indicates misalignment of bones or presence of muscle spasms.
6. Conduct neurovascular assessments every 1 to 2 hours for first 24 hours, then extend to every 4 hours if client is stabilizing.	Provides objective data concerning peripheral perfusion to tissues.
7. **Unexpected outcomes** that may occur include:	
➤ Child in Bryant's traction continues to turn to abdomen and disrupts traction.	
➤ Client experiences increased pain, soreness, or stiffness.	Pull on injured tissues may cause pressure on injured nerve endings, increasing pain.
➤ Client suffers frequent or severe muscle spasms.	Muscle irritation may lead to muscle spasms.
➤ Client experiences displaced alignment (evident on x-ray film) if fracture is present.	Too much weight, improper alignment, or improper positioning may keep fragments apart, altering healing.
➤ Client experiences sense of claustrophobia or being "held down" in one or another type of traction.	Restraint and position required may cause client to experience such feelings.
➤ Specific unexpected outcomes:	
• Cervical halter: client has pain in temporomandibular joint and chin or may develop headaches.	Pull of cervical halter is incorrect; straps need to be shortened between chin and occipital part of halter to direct pull from occipital area and away from chin and jawline.
• Bryant's traction: baby or child develops edema of feet. Peripheral pulses are not palpable.	Elastic bandages may be too snugly applied. Bandages can be removed and reapplied with two persons performing rewrapping; one person holds limb in vertical position as other rewraps bandage.
• Buck's extension: client develops pressure area on heel, or client is unable to dorsiflex or evert foot in traction if **traction boot,** adhesive straps, or elastic bandages exert pressure over head of fibula.	Pressure area is related to lack of circulation and insufficient position changes. Peroneal nerve courses over head of fibula down anterolateral surfaces of leg. Pressure on peroneal nerve results in inability to dorsiflex or evert foot.
• Dunlop's traction: client experiences pressure on elbow, or client is unable to approximate thumb to rest of fingers and may complain of numbness of thumb or tingling along sides of thumb and index finger.	Pressure ulcers may develop because of bony prominence of olecranon (use of elbow pad relieves pressure). Elastic bandage is too tight over radial nerve at wrist. Elastic bandage should be removed from forearm *only* and rewrapped more loosely; symptoms should then be rechecked for alleviation or continuance.
• Pelvic belt: client experiences marked increase in pain or numbness or other sensory pressure signs when in belt.	Pull of belt may increase pressure on edematous or injured nerves. Removal of traction should ease complaints.
• Pelvic sling: client becomes very dependent on sling and refuses to allow its discontinuance or becomes anxious when out of sling.	Security felt in sling leads to anxiety and concern for comfort when sling is removed. Weaning may be required and involves releasing sling for short to longer periods of time to permit adjustment to being out of sling.
• Russell's traction: client has pain behind knee or nonpalpable popliteal pulse.	**Knee sling** may cause knee to be flexed in too-acute angle, causing pressure signs. Knee sling can be adjusted for proper size and rope pulled down at knee to permit proper position and pull to relieve symptoms.
8. Client experiences burning, weeping, or drainage under adhesive strips or moleskin.	Reactions may be caused by allergic reactions, skin hypersensitivity, or too much weight causing loss of skin attachments to subcutaneous tissues. Loss of skin continuity necessitates removal of traction.

STEPS	RATIONALE
RECORDING AND REPORTING	
1. Record assessment of skin underneath traction apparatus and nursing interventions to maintain skin integrity.	Ensures continuity of care and provides documentation for legal considerations.
2. Record neurovascular assessment of bilateral body parts (see Skill 31-1, Evaluation, Step 2).	Bilateral comparison provides objective evidence for assessments.
3. Record length of time client is in or out of specific traction. NOTE: Clients in cervical halter and pelvic belt traction are usually in 1 to 2 hours, out 1 to 2 hours, and out to sleep.	Skin traction can be removed for care (with specific orders or based on institutional policies) for brief periods unless orders give specific directions.

FOLLOW-UP ACTIVITIES

1. After final discontinuance of specific traction, one of the following may occur:
   a. Cervical halter: client may be taught to apply traction for home care.
   b. Bryant's traction: client may be placed in spica cast.
   c. Buck's extension: client may have hip nailing, prosthesis, or muscle-lengthening procedures.
   d. Dunlop's traction: client may be placed in hanging cast to humerus.
   e. Pelvic belt: client may be discharged or may undergo outpatient physical therapy. Surgical repair may involve laminectomy, spinal fusion, or chemonucleolysis.
   f. Pelvic sling: client is ambulatory with walker, crutches, or cane. Occasionally, client with multiple fractures may have external fixation with Hoffman or other apparatus.
   g. Russell's traction: client may have surgical correction of hip fracture or release of muscle contractures.
   h. Cotrel's traction: client may be placed in brace or undergo surgery.

• • • • •

Special Considerations

- If institutional policies or physician's orders specify, clients are removed from traction for skin care or as ordered. If removed for skin care, client is out of traction only for 10 to 15 minutes before it is reapplied.
- Muscles and joints may be weakened from bed rest or traction and need time to regain strength.

Teaching Considerations

- Explain procedure to client. If client is a child, then explain to parents, who can clarify for child.
- Disoriented clients may need repeated explanations.
- Explain that traction may increase muscle weakness, spasms, and pain in older adult clients.
- Client is taught to ambulate slowly within medical guidelines, gradually increasing length of time out of bed and distance walked.
- Client should be taught to notify physician of undesirable signs, such as marked increase in pain, muscle spasms, and increased numbness. Symptoms may signify reinjury or insufficient healing.

Pediatric Considerations

- Babies and children have immature musculoskeletal tissues and are almost constant "movers."
- Babies and children in Bryant's traction must sleep in traction; it is rarely removed once established, except to loosen elastic bandages for marked edema of feet.

Gerontologic Considerations

- Older adults may have keratoses, rashes, or other lesions that could become irritated in skin traction.
- Older adults may have long-standing conditions of musculoskeletal tissues such as arthritis or gout that could lead to inflamed tissues and skin breakdown.
- Older and chronically ill clients may have increased need for position changes resulting from limitations from osteoporosis, osteomalacia, weakened muscles, or increased risk of skin breakdown.

Home Care Considerations

- If client is to be discharged to home, relatives or care givers should be instructed on care needs (including home traction) and mode of ambulation.
- Home environment must be assessed and adapted to accommodate hospital bed and traction.
- Integrity of traction should be inspected daily—weights hang freely, traction ropes rest in groove of pulley, and client's body is not allowed to interfere with countertraction. In many cases the client's body is the countertraction.

SKILL 31-4 Assisting with Insertion of Pins, Wires, or Nails for Skeletal Traction

Skeletal traction is the second kind of traction used for the treatment of fractures or correction of orthopedic abnormalities. As with skin traction, skeletal traction may be applied to one or several bones. Skeletal traction begins externally but continues internally directly through the bones. Weights are then attached to the skeletal pin, wire, or nail via ropes and pulleys. Amounts of weights for skeletal traction vary from 10 lb for Dunlop's skeletal traction to 20 to 25 lb for cervical traction, to 30 to 40 lb for balanced suspension to the femur. Amounts of weights used are also dictated by age, overall condition of the client in traction, and the purpose of the traction.

The procedure can also involve **external fixation,** which consists of a metal frame that secures pins inserted through the bone above and below a fracture site. The external fixation stabilizes a fracture with hardware visible outside the body. It fosters the healing of complex fractured bones, usually in the lower extremities.

Skeletal traction is often used when continuous traction is desired to properly immobilize, position, and align a fractured bone during the healing process. The nurse provides safe care after skillful application of traction. Common forms of skeletal traction include the following:

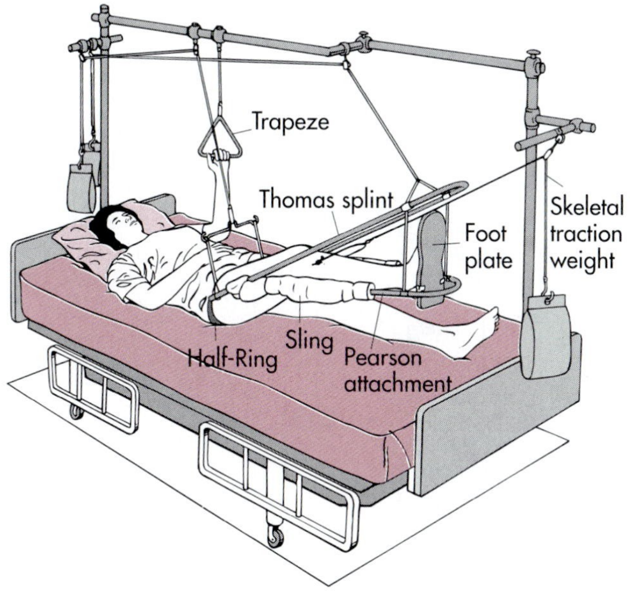

Fig. 31-6 Balanced-suspension skeletal traction. Traction in long axis of right thigh is applied by means of Kirschner wire through proximal portion of tibia. Limb is supported by Thomas splint beneath thigh and Pearson attachment beneath leg. Footplate attachment prevents foot-drop. Weights apply countertraction to upper end of Thomas splint and suspend its lower end. By using the left arm and leg as shown, client can shift position of the hips without change in amount of traction.

1. Balanced-suspension skeletal traction (BSST) to the femur—traction used for displaced or overriding fractures of the femur. Balanced suspension brings about relief of muscle spasms, realignment of the fracture fragments, and callus formation (Fig. 31-6). This form of traction is used less frequently because of the length of time required for hospitalization when it is used as the major form of treatment. It is now used primarily before surgical implantation of an internal fixation pin, plate, or nail until the client's condition or other injuries stabilize to permit

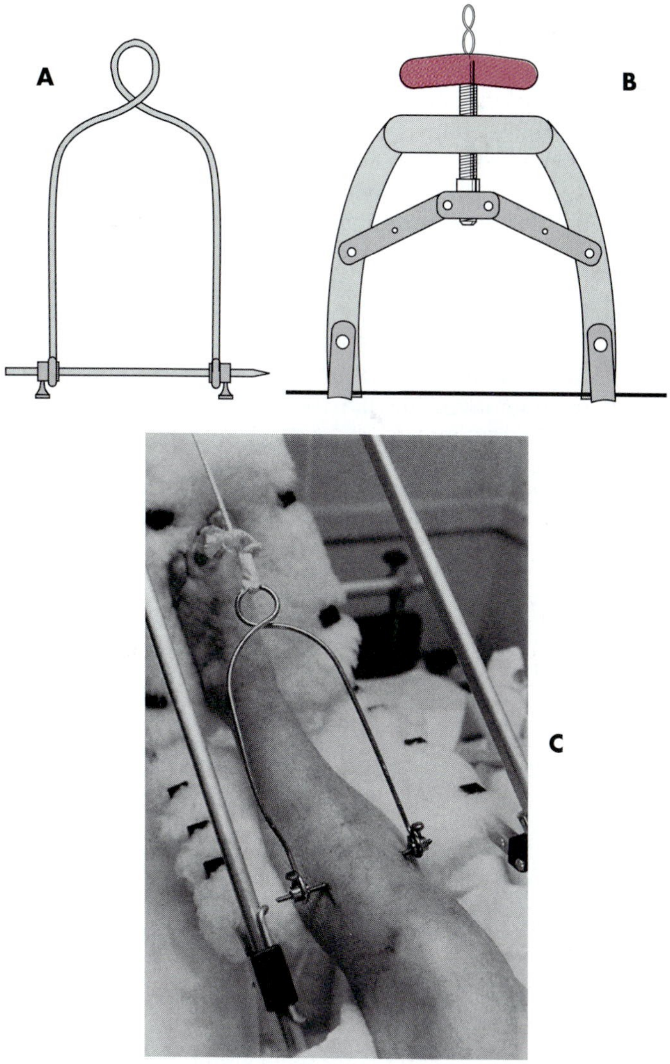

Fig. 31-7 **A,** Kirshner wire and tractor. **B,** Steinmann pin and holder. **C,** Steinmann pin placed in tibial plateau for treatment of distal femoral fracture. (**C** From Phipps W et al.: *Medical-surgical nursing: concepts and clinical practice,* ed 15, St Louis, 1995, Mosby.)

surgery. Balanced suspension involves the use of splints under the thigh and leg to suspend them off the bed, with a Steinmann pin or Kirschner wire supplying the traction (Fig. 31-7, *A* and *B*). The pin or wire is drilled through the upper tibia and attached to a spreader, which is then attached to ropes, pulleys, and weights (Fig. 31-7, *C*). Sufficient weights are hung to overcome the quadriceps and hamstring muscle spasms; sometimes weights of 30 to 40 lb or more may be required initially. Suspension weights may be 7 to 8 lb, and they are balanced by 7 to 8 lb of countertraction.

2. Upper extremity traction:
   a. Side-arm traction—skeletal form of Dunlop's traction (Fig. 31-8, *A*). The difference consists mainly of a pin drilled through the lower humerus (instead of the horizontal Buck's extension mentioned previously) and attached to a spreader, ropes, pulleys, and weights. The forearm is held in vertical Buck's extension, as it would be in Dunlop's skin traction. Side-arm skeletal traction is used for severe fractures, in which the greater pull permitted with the skeletal pin is required to overcome muscle spasms, resulting in effective alignment and union.
   b. 90-90 Overhead traction—humerus is placed at 90 degrees to the trunk, and elbow is flexed at 90 degrees. A sling supports the forearm. A Kirschner wire is placed through the olecranon process of the ulna (Fig. 31-8, *B*).
3. External fixation—commonly used form of skeletal traction involving the use of one of a variety of frames to hold pins drilled into or through bones (Fig. 31-9). External fixation is frequently used with comminuted fractures having soft-tissue injury. External fixation frames are used for skull and facial fractures, ribs, all bones of the upper and lower extremities, and pelvic bones. Frames may fit on one side of a bone or bones or may be attached to pins on either side of an injured limb.
4. Skull tong traction—traction involving the use of one of a variety of tongs (Crutchfield, Vinke, Gardner-Wells, or Barton) drilled into the skull or placed below the scalp and attached to ropes, pulleys, and weights. This type of traction is used for fractures of cervical vertebrae and involves the use of special beds or turning frames to facilitate nursing care.

EQUIPMENT

- **Sterile gloves for physician**
- **Wastebasket with plastic liner**

For balanced-suspension skeletal traction (BSST):

- **Sterile tray for insertion of Kirschner wire or Steinmann pin (secure from operating suite)**
- **Skin preparation solutions as desired**
- **Local anesthetic of physician's choice, usually 1% to 2% lidocaine**
- **Thomas splint or Harris splint**
- **Pearson attachment**
- **Foot support**
- **Ropes, pulleys, weights, weight holders**
- **Towels, felt, stockinette**

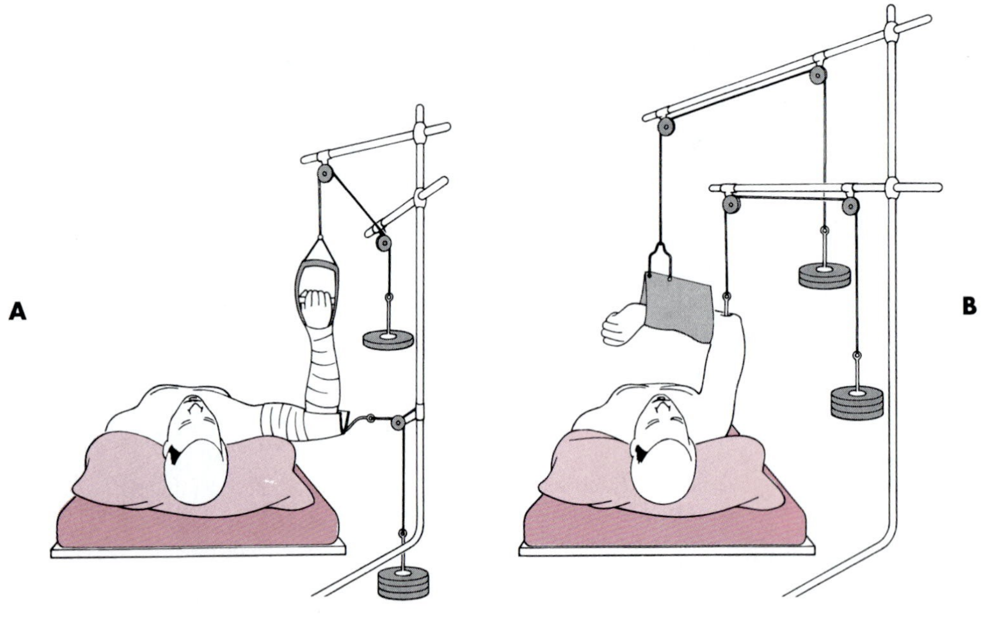

Fig. 31-8 **A,** Side-arm traction (skin/skeletal). **B,** Overhead 90-90 traction (skeletal). (From Beare PG, Myers JL: *Principles and practice of adult health nursing,* ed 2, St Louis, 1994, Mosby.)

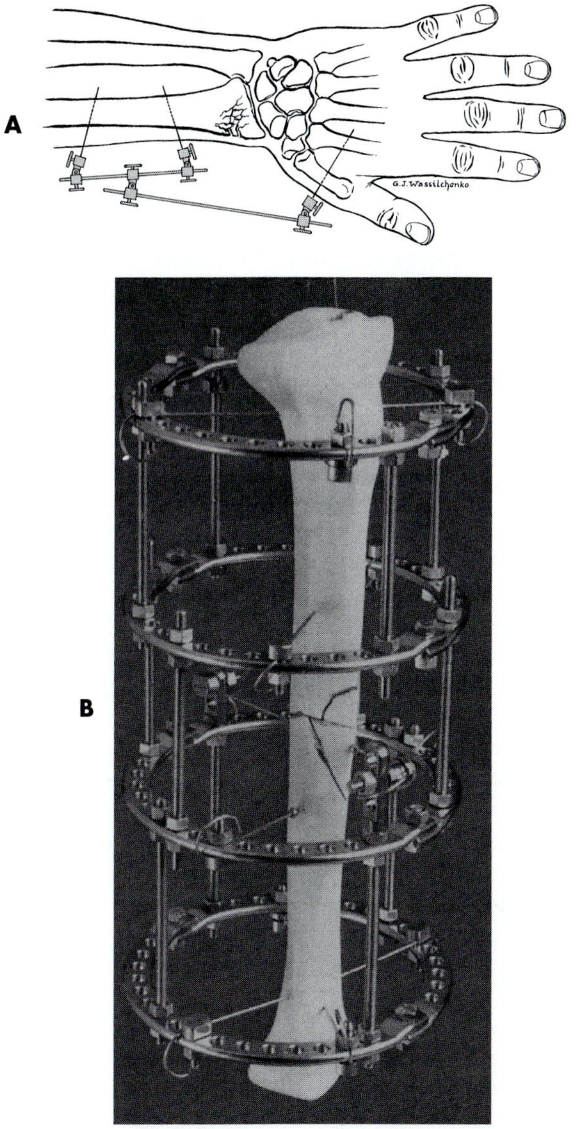

Fig. 31-9 External fixators. **A,** Roger Anderson fixator. **B,** Ilizarhov fixator for treatment of comminuted fractures. (**B** From Phipps W et al.: *Medical-surgical nursing: concepts and clinical practice,* ed 15, St Louis, 1995, Mosby.)

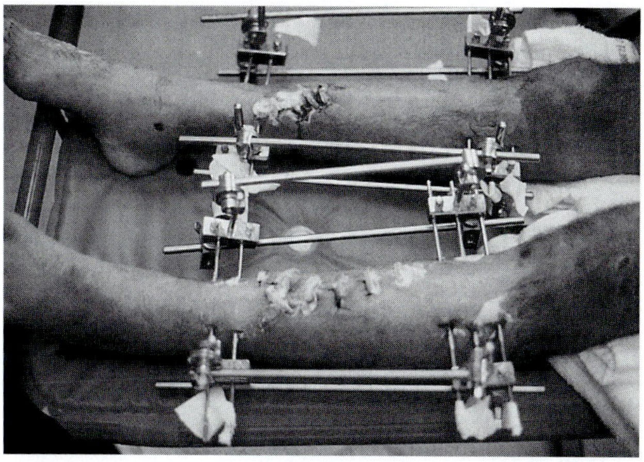

Fig. 31-10 Bilateral Hoffman devices for treatment of comminuted fractures of tibia/fibula.

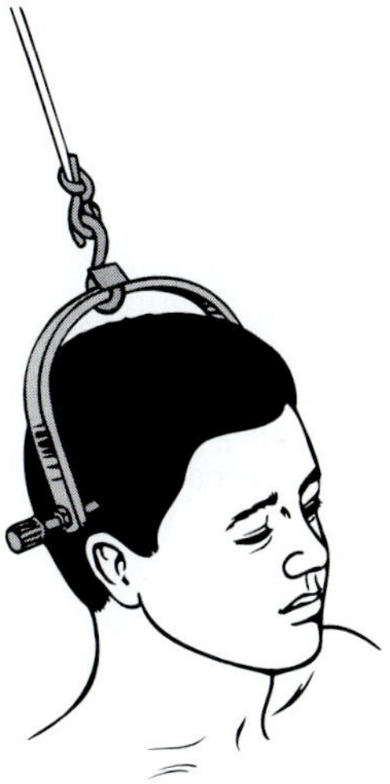

Fig. 31-11 Gardner-Wells tongs for stabilization of cervical vertebral fractures.

- Drill and extension cord if needed
- Antiseptic ointment
- Adhesive tape

For upper extremity skeletal traction:

- Sterile tray with Kirschner wire or Steinmann pin (secure from operating suite)
- Adhesive strips or moleskin
- Elastic bandages
- Handgrip bar
- Ropes, pulley, weights, weight holders
- Low-shock blocks (optional)
- Local anesthetic of physician's choice, usually 1% to 2% lidocaine
- Antiseptic ointment
- Skin preparation materials as desired

For external fixation:

- External fixator, usually Hoffman or Roger Anderson apparatus, Vital fixator, AO fixator, or other fixator (Fig. 31-9, A; 31-10)
- Sterile tray with pins for insertion (secure from operating room)
- Antiseptic ointment
- Skin preparation materials

Skull tong traction:

- Tongs: Crutchfield, Vinke, Gardner-Wells, or Barton (Fig. 31-11)

- Sterile tray: usually traction is applied in operating room
- Antiseptic ointment
- Skin preparation materials

Pin care:
- Sterile applicators
- Normal saline solution *or* hydrogen peroxide/normal saline solution in 1 : 1 solution or plain hydrogen peroxide
- Sterile containers
- Sterile gauze barrier (optional)
- Povidone-iodine solution (optional)
- Topical antibiotic ointment (optional)
- Clean gloves

DELEGATION CONSIDERATIONS

The skills of assisting with insertion of skeletal pins and pin site care may be delegated to unlicensed assistive personnel.
- Instruct personnel of signs and symptoms associated with infection or inflammation at pin insertion site.

STEPS	RATIONALE
ASSESSMENT	
1. Assess overall health condition of client, including mobility status.	Determines client's health state and ability to tolerate bed rest and skeletal traction.
2. Carefully assess specific tissues to be placed in skeletal traction. Note marked edema, rash, or other open lesions.	Determines ability of tissues to tolerate traction. Skeletal pin goes through skin to bone and out through skin.
3. Assess client's knowledge of upcoming traction, application, and purposes.	Determines willingness and ability to participate in care.
4. Assess client's level of pain.	Used as baseline for later comparisons.
5. Observe client's nonverbal behaviors and questions.	May reveal anxiety about impending procedure.

NURSING DIAGNOSIS

Clustering of defining characteristics from the assessment data may reveal the following nursing diagnoses for clients requiring this skill:
- ➤ Bathing/hygiene and dressing/grooming self-care deficit
- ➤ Risk for impaired skin integrity
- ➤ Risk for peripheral neurovascular dysfunction
- ➤ Risk for infection
- ➤ Impaired physical mobility
- ➤ Knowledge deficit regarding traction
- ➤ Pain
- ➤ Anxiety
- ➤ Risk for injury

Related factors are individualized based on a client's condition or needs.

PLANNING

STEPS	RATIONALE
1. **Expected outcomes** following completion of procedure:	
➤ Client participates in bathing and feeding.	Activities are performed safely, without injury. Client reduces risks of complications of immobility.
➤ Client's skin remains intact without redness, especially over pressure points.	Indicates no development of pressure sores.
➤ Client demonstrates adequate neurovascular functioning in extremity.	Adequate neurovascular functioning is essential to the health and well-being of the extremity.
➤ Skin around pin site shows no inflammation or drainage.	Regular cleansing prevents infection.
➤ Client retains ROJM in unaffected extremities and verbalizes understanding of activity restrictions. Demonstrates use of trapeze.	Routine exercise prevents contractures and muscle wasting.
➤ Client describes purpose of skeletal traction and follows activity restrictions.	Demonstrates learning and acceptance of restrictions.

STEPS	RATIONALE
➤ Client experiences reduced pain and muscle spasm.	Alignment of fracture reduces stress on bone fragments and adjoining muscle groups.
➤ Client does not become tense or withdrawn.	Demonstrates absence of anxiety.
➤ Client complies with restrictions imposed by traction apparatus.	No injury is sustained.

IMPLEMENTATION

TRACTION SETUP

STEPS	RATIONALE
1. Position client according to physician's request. Nurse or other assistant may be asked to support tissues to be placed in traction. Client will most often be on back with head of bed slightly elevated. Client will be flat in bed for Dunlop's skeletal traction.	Ensures proper alignment during and after traction application.
2. Physician performs skin preparation and discards materials in wastebasket.	Reduces possibility of wound and bone infection.
3. Physician injects local anesthetic into sites as desired. Nurse and other assistants support client, limb, or other tissues to be placed in traction.	Anesthetic acts quickly to create painless area. Client will feel pressure of pin being drilled through or into bones and will hear drill but should feel no pain.
4. Assist (usually by holding spreader bar, splint, or Pearson attachment) while physician continues to use drill to insert number of pins or nails desired for traction. Support area of joints not at injury site. Do not move distal portion unnecessarily.	Movement can cause severe pain or additional trauma.
5. Complete traction setup (Skill 31-3):	
a. BSST:	
(1) Assist with placement of Thomas or Harris splint, Pearson attachment, foot support, ropes, pulleys, and weights. Gently lower weights to establish traction. Apply antiseptic ointment to pin exit sites.	Splint and attachment are usually previously prepared for quick use. Ointment is applied to cover open wounds to prevent infection.
(2) Assist with application of Buck's extension to forearm, place handgrip, and establish skin traction by *slowly* lowering weights until rope is taut.	Skin traction allows forearm to remain in vertical position without undue effort from client.
(3) Assist with preparing sling for forearm in 90-90 traction (Fig. 31-8, *B* p. 964).	
(4) Assist with application of spreader to hold skeletal pin; tie rope to spreader and thread through pulleys to weight holder and weights. Slowly lower weights until rope is taut. Place shock blocks if requested. Apply antiseptic ointment to pin exit sites.	Amount of weight depends on severity of client's injury. Amounts vary from 5 to 10 or more lb. Shock blocks allow one side of bed to be raised to help client maintain desired position. Ointment is applied to prevent infection.
b. External fixation:	
(1) Hold affected tissues or limb while physician attaches and tightens fixator screws or clamps. Apply antiseptic ointment to pin exit sites.	Proper tension or tightness to pins is vital to prevent twist or "torque," which would delay healing. Ointment is applied to prevent infection.
c. Skull tong traction:	
(1) Client's cervical vertebrae are maintained in proper alignment with a Thomas cervical collar. Collar remains in place until skull tong traction is surgically placed. Traction is applied by weights ordered by physician.	Maintains proper cervical vertebrae alignment, thus reducing further injury and/or paralysis to the cervical segment of the spinal cord.

STEPS	RATIONALE
6. Assess client's initial reaction or response to traction before physician leaves.	Adjustments may be required immediately.
7. Raise side rails if appropriate.	Provides for client's safety.
8. Gather equipment and supplies and return to proper storage places.	Provides for safety and cleanliness.
9. Wash hands.	Prevents transmission of infection.

PIN CARE

Although there are commonalities in care, there are currently no accepted clinical standards for pin site care. Some institutions have policies outlining pin site care, and others permit pin site care only with a physician's orders. There is no research to support the effectiveness of pin site care in preventing infections (Jones-Walton, 1991).

STEPS	RATIONALE
1. Wash hands and apply clean gloves.	Reduces transmission of infection.
2. Remove old gauze dressing around pins and discard in receptacle.	
3. Prepare supplies and apply new gloves.	Aseptic technique reduces infection transmission.
4. Begin by cleaning pins on one side of extremity, then do same on other side.	
CRITICAL DECISION POINT **Never touch one pin site with material used on another.**	Prevents cross-contamination.
5. Dip sterile applicator into sterile container of hydrogen peroxide and saline. Place applicator by the pin and roll it along the skin, away from insertion site. Dispose of applicator.	Removes crusts from pin site. Crusts can obstruct drainage, which leads to bacterial buildup. (Some institutions use only hydrogen peroxide.)
6. Dip a new sterile applicator in normal saline; roll applicator across skin away from pin.	Removes peroxide solution to reduce skin irritation.
7. Using a sterile applicator, apply a small amount of povidone-iodine ointment or topical antibiotic ointment to pin site and cover with a sterile 2×2 split gauze dressing. (NOTE: some physicians leave site uncovered.)	Antiinfective reduces bacterial growth.
8. Repeat procedure for other pin site.	
9. Discard supplies. Remove and dispose of gloves. Wash hands.	Reduces transmission of infection.

EVALUATION

STEPS	RATIONALE
1. Observe entire traction setup and functioning: check all knots, ropes, pulleys, and weights. a. Knots are not caught in pulleys. b. Ropes are running straight through pulleys. c. Ropes are not frayed. d. Correct weight is hanging (do not add or remove weight without physician order). e. Weight is hanging freely (not caught on bed or resting on the floor). f. Bedclothes are not interfering with traction apparatus. g. Body is in proper alignment.	Determines if traction is functioning as desired.
2. Determine client's response to traction; client should begin to note relief of pain, sense of comfort, and lessening of muscle spasms.	Skeletal traction takes longer for client to note relief of symptoms because of more involvement of tissue trauma.
3. Evaluate for presence of pain and muscle spasms.	Determines need for analgesics, muscle relaxants, and success of traction in stabilizing fracture.
4. Inspect pin sites for drainage or inflammation.	Early signs of infection.
5. Assess for other indicators of infection, such as fever; elevated white blood count; continuous, dull aching pain; redness; or warmth in extremity.	Early signs of osteomyelitis.

STEPS	RATIONALE
6. Perform neurovascular assessment (see Skill 31-1).	Determines peripheral perfusion to tissues, as well as client's voluntary motor activity.
7. Perform motor assessment.	Checks for status of client's voluntary motor activity.
8. **Unexpected outcomes** that may occur include:	
➤ Client experiences delayed union, malunion, or nonunion.	Too much weight may cause distraction or pulling of fragments. Too little weight may allow misalignment.
➤ Client has severe edema, marked increase in pain, inability to actively move joints, or increased pain on passive movement.	Indicates compartment syndrome, which leads to increased venous stasis and decreased arterial perfusion; tissue anoxia may be developing.
➤ Client develops infection at pin site or at fracture site with development of osteomyelitis.	Interruption in skin continuity may lead to infection being carried into fracture site.
➤ Client experiences prolonged bleeding or frank hemorrhage. Chronically ill or older clients may have preexistent iron-deficiency anemia made worse by bleeding or hemorrhage.	Bleeding into joints, soft tissues, or cavities is common with bone fractures; as much as 2 to 3 units of blood loss is common in fractures of hip, femur, humerus, and pelvis. Replacement of blood loss may be required. (Autologous transfusion is frequently the treatment of choice.)
➤ Client experiences nerve damage:	
• Peroneal nerve: foot-drop with inability to evert and dorsiflex foot.	There may be excessive pressure or pin trauma to nerve at head of fibula.
• Radial or median nerve at wrist with inability to approximate thumb and fingers (radial) and numbness and tingling of thumb, index, middle fingers (median) with wrist-drop.	Elastic bandage in side-arm traction may be too tight at wrist. Sling for overhead 90-90 traction may exert pressure at the wrist. Median nerve pressure can result in carpal tunnel syndrome. Supracondylar fractures of the elbow may result in Volkmann's contracture from compartment syndrome, causing claw hand and wrist-drop.
➤ Client experiences fat embolism (more common in fractures of long bones) with symptoms of anoxia: restlessness, mental changes, tachycardia, tachypnea, dyspnea, low blood pressure, and petechial rash over upper chest and neck.	Fat molecules are released. They travel in the bloodstream to the lungs. It is also thought that release of fat molecules results in a chemical reaction in the blood stream that activates fatty acids. Fifty percent of persons with fat emboli die. Emboli occur most frequently in the first 24 to 72 hours after long bone fractures.
➤ Client experiences deep vein thrombosis.	Venous stasis from immobility can lead to deep vein thrombosis.
➤ Client experiences declining voluntary motor responses.	There may be some edema or further injury to the spinal cord (skull tong traction only).

Recording and Reporting

1. Record in nurse's notes type of traction applied, persons applying traction, site to which traction was applied, time of application, amount of weights, and client's initial response.	Provides for continuity of care and documentation for legal concerns.
2. Record all findings of neurovascular assessment (see Skill 31-1) every 1 to 2 hours or as ordered.	Enables nurse or physician to note beginning changes in patterns as soon as they develop.

Follow-up Activities

1. After discontinuance of specific form of skeletal traction, client may be treated with:
   a. Open reduction and internal fixation of fracture
   b. Application of cast
2. Client should be assisted in dangling legs at bedside and in ambulating (see Chapter 30, Skill 30-4). Older adult clients adjust more slowly to upright positions and may experience postural hypotension. A tilt-table is often used in assisting these clients to acclimate to an upright position.

Special Considerations

- Clients need frequent encouragement and praise during drilling periods.
- After traction procedure, nurse needs to discuss with physician whether pin care will be performed. The type and frequency of pin site care varies according to physician preference.
- Client may complain of heaviness of entire apparatus, depending on number of pins used and whether bilateral fixators are applied.
- The skin in the groin area and the proximal outer thigh should be inspected for pressure from the half-ring of the splint.

Teaching Considerations

- Client should be taught use of ambulatory aid (cane, walker, or crutches); instructions in writing should be given to client and significant others.
- Client should have written instructions for home cast maintenance.
- Clients should have dietary instructions if necessary.
- Client should be taught to notify physician of undesirable signs, including increase in pain, muscle spasms, increased numbness or tingling, appearance of drainage, redness, or soreness at operative or traction pin sites.

Pediatric Considerations

- Parents are taught that babies may cry when traction is established.
- Children may experience boredom, regression, and interference with school work. Parents and other care givers must look for ways to divert the child's attention and support the child. School work should be obtained from school and the child assisted when able to perform tasks. Parents are counseled regarding regression to decrease their anxiety.

Gerontologic Considerations

- Older adult clients may suffer from diabetes or peripheral vascular disease, adding risks to use of traction.

CRITICAL THINKING EXERCISES

1. You are preparing to autotransfuse your client after orthopedic surgery, and she expresses fear about getting blood. How would you respond?
2. What suggestions could you offer a 10-year-old child who has a cast on her right arm and wishes to take a tub bath?
3. The doctor is preparing to use the cast saw to remove your client's leg cast. The client expresses fear, and states, "I am on Coumadin. My heart doctor told me not to use anything sharp that might cut me!" How would you respond?
4. The nursing assistant asks the staff nurse if she can remove the skeletal traction while she bathes the client and changes the linens. How would you respond?
5. On the fifth postoperative day your client complains of a "pins and needles" feeling in his casted arm. After further inspection, you assess cyanotic and cool fingertips. These assessments are reported to the charge nurse, who states, "Elevate the arm, apply an ice bag, and leave a note on the front of the chart for the doctor to see in the morning." How would you respond?

REFERENCES

Beare PG, Myers JL: *Principles and practice of adult health nursing,* ed 2, St Louis, 1994, Mosby.

Dykes P: Minding the five p's of neurovascular assessment, *Am J Nurs* 93(6):38, 1993.

Folcik M, Carini-Garcia G, Birmingham J: *Traction: assessment and management,* St Louis, 1994, Mosby.

Jones-Walton P: Clinical standards in skeletal traction pin site care, *Orthop Nurs* 10(2):12, 1991.

Lewis C, Knortz K: *Orthopedic assessment and treatment of the geriatric client,* St Louis, 1993, Mosby.

Phipps W et al: *Medical-surgical nursing: concepts and clinical practice,* ed 15, St Louis, 1995, Mosby.

ADDITIONAL READING

Elkin MA, Perry AG, Potter PA: *Nursing interventions and clinical skills,* St Louis, 1996, Mosby.

Instructions for Gish Orthofuser, Irvin, Calif, 1994, Gish Biomedical.

Karpowicz J: *Using the Boehringer Autovac autotransfusion system,* Norristown, Pa, 1994, Boehringer Laboratories.

Mourad L: *Orthopedic disorders,* St Louis, 1991, Mosby.

Salmond S, Mooney N, Verdisco L, editors: *Core curriculum for orthopaedic nursing,* ed 2, New Jersey, 1991, Anthony J Jannetti.

Webber-Jones J et al: Managing traction: do you know Carol P Smith? *Nurs '94,* 94(7):66, 1994.

Zimmer: *The traction handbook,* Warsaw, Ind, 1990, Zimmer Manufacturing.

Chapter 32

Support Surfaces and Special Beds

OBJECTIVES

Mastery of content in this chapter will enable the nurse to:

- Define key terms.
- Identify the different types of support surfaces used to prevent pressure sore formation.
- Explain why preventive nursing care is still essential when using special mattresses and beds.
- Describe guidelines to follow when placing clients on special mattresses and beds.
- Describe mechanisms by which skin breakdown can occur on either an air-suspension or air-fluidized bed, a bariatric bed, or a support surface mattress.
- Describe correct placement of a client on an air-fluidized bed, an air-suspension bed, a bariatric bed, or a support surface mattress.

KEY TERMS

Air-fluidized bed
Air-suspension bed
Bariatric bed
Flotation pads
Friction
Immobility
Kinesthetic
Morbidly obese
Orthopedic
Pressure ulcers
Shearing

SKILLS

32-1 Placing a Client on a Support Surface Mattress
32-2 Placing a Client on an Air-Suspension Bed
32-3 Placing a Client on an Air-Fluidized Bed
32-4 Placing a Client on a Bariatric Bed

Approximately 1.7 million persons in the United States develop pressure ulcers yearly, which translates to billions of dollars in health care costs annually (Kuhn and Coulter, 1992). With the challenges of health care reform to improve quality while reducing costs, it is essential for the nurse to identify persons at risk for skin breakdown. Factors that contribute to pressure ulcer formation are both extrinsic (e.g., skin moisture, friction, shear) and intrinsic (e.g., protein malnutrition, loss of sensation, impaired mobility, advanced age, impaired mental status, infection, incontinence) (Ketts, 1995).

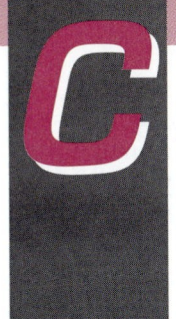

Current understanding is incomplete concerning soft tissue metabolism and the etiology of pressure ulcers. However, tissue damage occurs when the pressure exerted on the capillaries is high enough to close the capillaries. Capillary closing pressure is the pressure needed to close capillaries (e.g., when the pressure exceeds normal capillary pressure range of 16 to 32 mm Hg) (Maklebust, 1987). Pressure is the main factor in development of **pressure ulcers.** Because vessels collapse and thrombose when pressure is greater in tissues than in capillaries, tissue hypoxia and ischemia result from lack of transport of oxygen and nutrients to the tissues (Pontieri-Lewis, 1995). The standard hospital mattress should not be used for clients at risk for pressure ulcer formation, because it exerts high pressures on tissues overlying bony prominences (sacrum, heels, trochanters) (Wilson, 1994).

When a client is confined to bed, the tissues between the skeleton and supporting bed surface become compressed and the blood vessels within the tissues become occluded. A client lying supine on a hospital bed may exert as much as 150 mm Hg pressure (2.9 psi) on skin and soft tissue. Once pressure reaches more than 78 mm Hg for a period of time, a person usually feels discomfort and changes position. However, the client with altered sensation or one who cannot move independently is at risk for pressure ulcers of superficial and deep tissues unless pressure is significantly reduced. Pressures in excess of 20 to 40 mm Hg for prolonged periods can cause tissue injury (Koziak, 1961).

Special beds and mattresses have been designed to reduce the hazards of immobility to the skin and musculoskeletal system. It is important to understand the difference between a pressure reducing and pressure relieving support surface. The former reduces the interface pressure, between the body and support surface, below 32 mm Hg. Pressure reducing devices reduce the interface pressure, but not necessarily below capillary closing pressure (AHCPR, 1994). Many of the beds make it easier for nurses to lift, turn, or position clients with reduced strain on the nurses' back muscles. The three purposes of support surfaces include: comfort, postural control, and pressure management (Krouskop and van Rijswijk, 1995). Many mattresses or support devices can be applied over an ordinary bed mattress and frame to help reduce pressure on dependent body parts by dispersing the pressure over a larger area (Bryant et al., 1992).

No bed or mattress totally eliminates the need for meticulous nursing care. Turning devices can still injure soft tissues, requiring a nurse to be especially observant for signs of pressure sore formation (Bryant et al., 1992; Panel for the Prediction and Prevention of Pressure Ulcers in Adults, 1992).

With the use of technologically advanced special mattresses, the incidence of pressure ulcer formation should be reduced. However, these devices need to be used along with frequent repositioning, meticulous skin care, and nutrition that is high in vitamin C and protein, as well as hydration (Wilson, 1994).

GUIDELINES

1. Know the reason for the client's reduced mobility. A totally immobilized client benefits from support devices other than those used for a partially immobile client.
2. Perform client assessment to determine selection of appropriate special mattresses and beds.
3. Continue to provide basic preventive care measures against the hazards of **immobility,** for example, turning, correct positioning, skin assessment and care, or range-of-motion exercises (when allowed).
4. Use proper body mechanics when positioning or working with clients.
5. Follow all safety measures to prevent accidental falls or improper positioning when clients are placed on special beds or mattresses.
6. Encourage clients to remain as mobile as possible within the limits of their physical conditions and prescribed activity levels.
7. Educate family members/significant others about the advantages, disadvantages, and methods of operation of all support devices to ensure their proper use in the home care setting.
8. Perform baseline nutritional and fluid assessment.
9. Consult with health care professional (e.g., clinical nurse specialist) who has expertise in this area (if available).
10. Anticipate need to consult with social service or home health department regarding third-party reimbursement, as well as arrangements for delivery of special beds to the home.

DELEGATION CONSIDERATIONS

The skills of applying support surface mattresses or preparation of an alternative bed can be delegated to unlicensed assistive personnel.

- Inform and assist care provider in proper method of applying support surface to bed.
- Encourage care provider to obtain assistance when positioning client to reduce risk of friction and shear and to prevent self-injury.
- Explain to care provider the rationale for client to be routinely repositioned even though on support surfaces.
- Caution care provider to routinely inspect bony prominences and heels for signs of pressure and to notify RN to conduct assessment when abnormalities are noted.
- Caution care provider to wear gloves when inspecting mattress surfaces for wetness.
- Educate care provider on importance of maintaining adequate nutritional and fluid status in the client.
- Inform care providers to replace soiled bed linens or straighten wrinkled sheets.
- Explain to care provider how to clean and monitor special mattresses and beds.
- Explain to care provider how to determine if air mattress needs to be reinflated.

STEPS	RATIONALE
6. Verify physician's order for type of support surface.	In the United States, mattress may be placed before a physician's order is received, unless there is a question that it will be ordered. A physician's order is required to ensure third-party payment of the support surface. (NOTE: A physician's order is not required in Canada.)

NURSING DIAGNOSIS

Clustering of defining characteristics from the assessment data may reveal the following nursing diagnoses for clients requiring this skill:

- Altered peripheral tissue perfusion
- Anxiety
- Impaired home maintenance management
- Impaired physical mobility
- Impaired skin integrity
- Knowledge deficit regarding use of support surface mattress
- Pain
- Risk for impaired skin integrity
- Risk for infection

Related factors are individualized based on a client's condition or needs.

PLANNING

STEPS	RATIONALE
1. **Expected outcomes** following completion of procedure:	
➤ Skin is without erythema or mottling.	
➤ Existing pressure ulcer shows signs of healing.	Skin remains free of new pressure ulcers. Support surface does not interfere with circulation to dependent areas.
➤ Client expresses sense of comfort.	Localized areas of discomfort have been eliminated by equalized pressures.
➤ Client is removed from therapeutic surface when risk for pressure ulcers decreases.	Provides for efficient, cost-effective care while maintaining high-quality outcomes.
2. Explain purpose of mattress and method of application to client.	Relieves anxiety and promotes cooperation.
3. Apply gloves (should be worn if linens are soiled or wet). Obtain assistance as needed.	Gloves prevent contact with body fluids. Assistance reduces risk of friction and shear in transfer to new surface.

IMPLEMENTATION

➤ *CRITICAL DECISION POINT* Perform application of support surface mattress or transfer to bed in an organized, efficient manner. Clients whose medical conditions are unstable may not tolerate prolonged periods of position change (i.e., lying flat or turning from side to side).

STEPS	RATIONALE
1. Close room door or bedside curtain.	Provides client privacy during application of mattress to bed or transfer to alternate bed.
2. Apply support surface to bed or prepare alternate bed (bed may be occupied or unoccupied).	
a. Mattress replacement:	
(1) Apply mattress to bed frame after removing standard hospital mattress.	Hospital mattress needs to be stored. In some instances, mattress replacements may be standard procedure.
(2) Apply sheet over mattress.	Sheet reduces soiling.
b. Air mattress/overlay:	
(1) Apply deflated mattress flat over surface of bed mattress. (There may be directions on pad indicating which side to place up.)	Provides smooth, even surface.

STEPS	RATIONALE
(2) Bring any plastic strips or flaps around corners of bed mattress.	Secures air mattress in place.
(3) Attach connector on air mattress to inflation device. Inflate mattress to proper air pressure determined by air pump or blower.	Mattresses vary as to requiring one-time or continuous inflation cycle. Manufacturer's directions indicate desired air pressure designed to distribute client's body weight evenly. Directions are included with each mattress.
(4) Place sheet over air mattress, being sure to eliminate all wrinkles.	Prevents soiling of mattress and reduces direct contact of skin against plastic surface.
(5) Check air pumps to be sure pressure cycle alternates.	Alternating air-flow mattress produces intermittent cycling, inflating only parts of mattress at any one time. Intermittent cycle continually alternates pressure against skin and soft tissue.
c. Integrated air-surface bed:	
(1) Obtain and make bed.	In some instances bed may be available in all client rooms; if not, an ordering system exists to obtain one as needed (see agency policy).
(2) Place switch in the "Prevention" mode.	In the "Prevention" mode, surface pressures change automatically with client position to equalize pressure and eliminate points of pressure.
d. Water mattress (supplemental and self-contained):	
(1) Apply unfilled supplemental mattress flat over the surface of standard bed mattress. (Self-contained water mattress would replace bed mattress.)	Provides a smooth, even surface.
(2) Bring any plastic strips or flaps around corners of bed mattress.	Secures water mattress in place.
(3) Attach connector on water mattress to water source and fill mattress to level recommended by manufacturer. Follow manufacturer's directions regarding temperature of water. Mattress should be filled in close proximity to water source. Manufacturer's directions (enclosed with mattress) indicate desired water level designed to distribute client's body weight evenly (usually determined by client weight or height and weight).	
(4) Place sheet over water mattress, being sure to eliminate all wrinkles.	Reduces soiling of mattress and prevents direct contact of skin against plastic surface.
3. Position client comfortably as desired over support surface. Reposition routinely.	Location of existing pressure sore might influence type of positioning.

CRITICAL DECISION POINT **Support surfaces do not replace the need for regular turning.**

STEPS	RATIONALE
4. Remove gloves and wash hands.	Reduces transmission of microorganisms.

EVALUATION

STEPS	RATIONALE
1. Reinspect condition of client's skin at routine intervals.	Determines if pressure sores develop or if the condition of existing sores changes.
2. Reassess client's risk for pressure sore formation at routine intervals.	Documents change in status, which is critical for evaluating continued need for therapeutic surface.
3. Evaluate client's level of comfort.	If pressure-relief mattress is effective, client generally experiences less discomfort.
4. Evaluate inflation of mattress periodically.	Regular inspection of mechanical components of mattress ensures proper functioning.
5. **Unexpected outcomes** that may occur include:	

STEPS	RATIONALE
➤ Skin develops localized areas of erythema, mottling, swelling, and tenderness, with evidence of skin breakdown.	
➤ Existing pressure ulcers fail to heal or increase in size or depth.	Support surface fails to relieve pressure over dependent sites and bony prominences. Method and frequency of positioning, client's weight, and exposure of skin to moisture may cause pressure ulcer formation.
➤ Client expresses inability to achieve a sense of comfort and demonstrates restlessness, difficulty sleeping, or agitation.	Support surface fails to optimize level of comfort. May require change in air or water to appropriate level or the selection of a different surface.
➤ Bed or mattress develops a leak (air, water, or gel).	Leak or dysfunction of support surface decreases effectiveness of device in reducing pressure ulcer risk.

Recording and Reporting

1. Record type of support surface applied, extent to which client tolerated procedure, and condition of client's skin in nurse's notes or skin assessment flow sheet.	Documents therapy initiated; provides data for other nurses to compare in determining changes in condition of skin. For rental surfaces, provides documentation of use for reimbursement purposes.
2. Report evidence of pressure ulcer formation to nurse in charge or to physician.	Onset of pressure ulcer may require different type of therapy (see Chapter 8).

Follow-up Activities

1. Keep client's skin clean and dry.
2. Remove and replace any foam pad that becomes soiled with diaphoresis, feces, urine, or wound drainage. Dispose of soiled pad following institution's policy for standard precautions.
3. Evaluate for alternate surface and revise turning or positioning schedule.

• • • • •

Special Considerations

➤ Risk factors for pressure sore formation include reduced physical mobility, inadequate nutrition, anemia, moist skin, and reduced tactile sensation resulting in less independent turning (Panel for the Prediction and Prevention of Pressure Ulcers in Adults, 1992).

➤ Support surfaces are available to fit all types of beds.

➤ Keep linens between surface and client's skin to a minimum. Multiple layers decrease surface effectiveness.

➤ Foam pad or mattresses:
- Replace when wet or soiled.
- Washing removes fire-retardant chemicals.
- Replace at regular intervals (refer to hospital policy or manufacturer's recommendations), because foam compresses over time and no longer acts as a pressure-relieving device.
- Consider selecting alternate support surface if client becomes frequently soiled with diaphoresis, feces, urine, or wound drainage.

➤ Air mattresses:
- Keep sharp objects away from air mattresses. Tears can cause loss of air, making mattress ineffective.
- Assist client with transferring in and out of bed, because mattress surface may be slippery.
- Surface may be wiped clean with disinfectant solution.

➤ Integrated air-surface beds:
- Beds are equipped with a CPR switch to instantly lower head section from an elevated position and to deflate the mattress to provide a firm surface for chest compressions (Fig. 32-5).

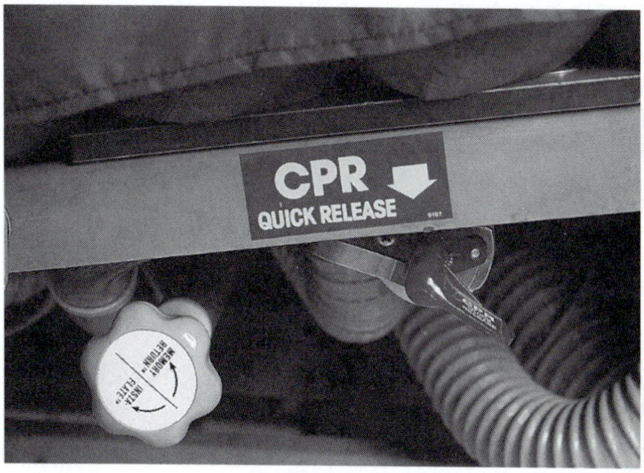

Fig. 32-5 CPR quick-release switch.

- Water mattresses:
  - Keep sharp objects away from water mattresses. Tears and punctures result in loss of water, making mattress ineffective.
  - Surface may be wiped clean with disinfectant solution.
  - Filled mattresses are heavy. Obtain assistance to move beds with water mattresses.

Teaching Considerations

- Explain risks of immobility to client and family members.
- Instruct in positioning and pressure relief.
- Explain risks for pressure ulcers.
- Explain purpose and function of the pressure-relief surface. Include reminder that the surface augments care and does not replace the need for turning and pressure-relief maneuvers.
- Explain precautions regarding sharp objects, fire hazard, and other concerns.
- Reeducate client as to need of support surface and discuss alternatives, including client's right to refuse a recommended surface.

Gerontologic Considerations

- Implement preventive measures for older adults, because the aging process causes their skin to become drier, thinner, and less pressure sensitive, increasing the risk of skin breakdown.

Home Care Considerations

- Most of the devices covered in this section may be adapted for home use on a standard twin bed or hospital bed.
- Selection should be based on client needs and environmental audit. For example:
  - The client on total bed rest who smokes would not be an ideal candidate for a foam mattress because of the potential for fire.
  - The client with pets who sleep in the bed may not be suited for a water- or air-filled mattress because of the risk of puncture.
- Reimbursement varies by surface type and payor source.

SKILL 32-2 Placing a Client on an Air-Suspension Bed

Air-suspension beds are indicated for clients who are immobile or otherwise confined to the bed. The **air-suspension bed** supports a client's weight on air-filled cushions. The bed minimizes pressure and reduces shear in a low–air-loss system (Fig. 32-6). If a client has large stage III or stage IV pressure ulcers on multiple turning surfaces, a low–air-loss bed or air-fluidized bed may be indicated (AHCPR, 1994).

For clients requiring high air loss under a given body part, for example, under the buttocks, high–air-loss cushions may be substituted. High air loss provides for selective drying while not having the effect of substantially increasing insensible fluid losses.

It is also possible to adapt the air-suspension beds to individual client needs with specialty cushions for positioning, foot support, and lateral arm supports. Another adaptation of the air-suspension bed is the kinetic low–air-loss bed. This bed is marketed widely to intensive care areas and has the ability to provide a pressure-relief surface while rotating approximately 30 to 35 degrees. This surface should not be used with a client who has an unstable spine or who is in traction.

EQUIPMENT

- Air-suspension bed (KinAir, Therapulse, Flexicare, Mediscus, Biodyne, RestCue)
- Gore-Tex sheet (supplied by rental company)
- Disposable bed pads, if indicated
- Disposable gloves (optional)

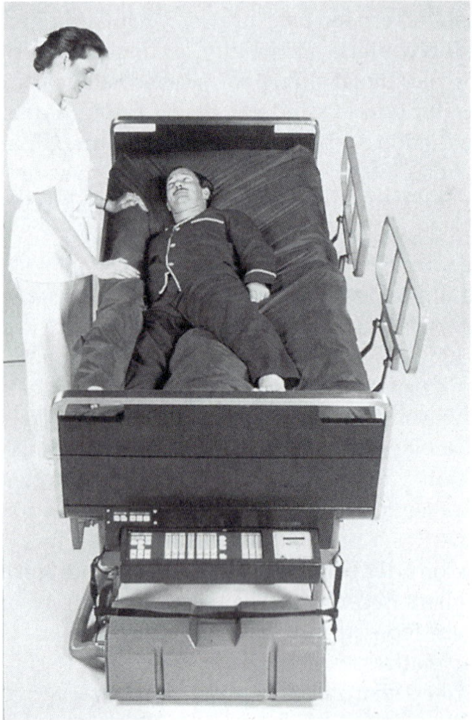

Fig. 32-6 Air-suspension bed. (Courtesy Kinetic Concepts, Inc, San Antonio, Tex.)

STEPS	RATIONALE
ASSESSMENT	
1. Identify clients who would benefit from air-suspension therapy, such as immobilized or burn clients.	Beds effectively minimize pressure on fragile tissues and dependent body parts. Selected for clients who require pressure relief for treatment of or prevention of pressure ulcers.
➤ ***CRITICAL DECISION POINT*** **This surface should not be used with a client who has an unstable spine or who is in traction.**	
2. Assess client for pain.	Helps to anticipate client's need for analgesic prior to transfer. Serves as baseline for change in condition.
3. Review client's medical orders.	In the United States a physician's order is needed to receive third-party reimbursement for the cost of the bed.
4. Wash hands and apply gloves. Assess condition of client's skin, paying particular attention to potential pressure sites and any existing skin lesions.	Prevents spread of microorganisms. Data provide baseline to determine any change in client's condition while on bed.
5. Assess client's level of consciousness.	Baseline used to detect change while client is on bed.
6. Assess client's and family members' understanding of purpose of bed.	Bed inflation is maintained by one or two blowers, which make a sound that may create anxiety for the client.
7. Review client's serum electrolyte levels in medical record, if available.	Baseline data used to compare with subsequent laboratory results to determine electrolyte imbalances.

NURSING DIAGNOSIS

Clustering of defining characteristics from the assessment data may reveal the following nursing diagnoses for clients requiring this skill:

- ➤ Altered peripheral tissue perfusion
- ➤ Anxiety
- ➤ Impaired home maintenance management
- ➤ Impaired physical mobility
- ➤ Impaired skin integrity
- ➤ Knowledge deficit regarding use of support surface mattress
- ➤ Pain
- ➤ Risk for fluid volume deficit
- ➤ Risk for impaired skin integrity
- ➤ Sensory/perceptual alterations, **kinesthetic**

Related factors are individualized based on a client's condition or needs.

PLANNING

STEPS	RATIONALE
1. **Expected outcomes** following completion of procedure:	
➤ Skin remains warm, clean, and intact, or existing lesions show evidence of healing.	Skin is free from pressure effects of immobility.
➤ Client rates comfort level as acceptable.	Bed's surface is soft, minimizing pain stimulation.
➤ Client remains alert and oriented or shows no change in level of orientation.	Client does not experience sensory perceptual changes from flotation.
2. Explain procedure and purpose of bed to client and family.	Reduces anxiety and promotes client's cooperation.
3. Wash hands and prepare the necessary equipment and supplies.	Reduces transmission of microorganisms.
4. Review instructions supplied by bed manufacturer.	Promotes safe and correct use of bed.
5. For clients with severe to moderate pain, premedicate approximately 30 minutes before transfer.	Promotes client's comfort and ability to cooperate during transfer to bed.
6. Obtain any additional personnel needed to transfer client to bed.	Ensures client's safety by having sufficient personnel to assist in transferring.

IMPLEMENTATION

STEPS	RATIONALE
1. Close client's room door or bedside curtain.	Maintains client's privacy during transfer.

STEPS	RATIONALE
2. Explain steps of transfer.	Reduces anxiety and helps client be a part of decision making during maneuvering.
3. Transfer client to bed using appropriate transfer techniques (see Chapter 29).	Appropriate transfer techniques maintain alignment and reduce risk of injury during procedure. Company representative will adjust bed to client's height and weight.
4. Turn bed on by depressing switch; regulate temperature.	Suspension minimizes pressure against skin's surface and reduces friction and shear force when client moves (Seila and Stahelin, 1992).
5. Position client and perform range-of-motion (ROM) exercises as appropriate.	Promotes comfort and reduces contracture formation. The bed reduces pressure on skin, but clients must still be turned and exercised to avoid joint deformity or contractures.
6. To turn clients, position bedpans, or perform other therapies, set instaflate. Once procedure is completed, release instaflate.	Instaflate firms the bed surface to facilitate turning and handling client. Client will not receive pressure relief while bed is in this mode.
7. In emergencies when resuscitation is required, press CPR switch to deflate bed immediately (see Fig. 32-5, p. 977).	Creates firm surface against which cardiopulmonary resuscitation can be performed.
8. Remove gloves. Wash hands.	

EVALUATION

1. Inspect condition of client's skin periodically while client is on bed.	Evaluates healing progress of any existing pressure sores. Determines if any new pressure areas are forming.
2. Ask client to rate level of comfort.	Flotation effects of bed minimize pain stimuli.
3. Assess client's orientation.	Determines onset of perceptual changes.
4. **Unexpected outcomes** that may occur include:	
➤ Areas of existing skin breakdown worsen.	Continued advancement of pressure ulcers can indicate deep tissue necrosis and need for surgical debridement of wound.
➤ Client is restless or agitated.	Low-pressure flotation devices may cause a sense of "lack of support," which some clients find unacceptable.
➤ Client becomes disoriented and complains of nausea.	Constant flotation may cause dizziness and sensory perceptual changes.
➤ Bed breaks.	

RECORDING AND REPORTING

1. Record transfer of client to bed, tolerance of procedure, and condition of skin in nurse's notes or skin assessment flow sheet.	Documents therapy initiated and records baseline data for other nurses to compare findings.
2. Report changes in condition of skin and electrolyte levels to physician.	Changes may indicate need for additional therapies.
3. Report restlessness or change in orientation.	May indicate client's inability to tolerate bed and need to discontinue therapy.

FOLLOW-UP ACTIVITIES

1. Repeat risk assessment for skin breakdown (see Chapter 8) at regular intervals to validate continued need for air-suspension bed or alternate surface.
2. Monitor pressure ulcers for further treatment needs.
3. Monitor client's skin hydration, because bed surface may be drying.

• • • • •

Special Considerations

- Scales are available in some air-suspension beds and available as under-bed units for clients who require frequent weights or for those who cannot be moved for weighing.
- Some beds are equipped with a seat deflate to assist with transferring clients in and out of bed.
- Gore-Tex sheet may cause pressure from hammocking if applied too tightly to bed. Check lateral client surfaces for reddening (e.g., lateral ankles, thighs, shoulders).
- Transport units are available to maintain inflation during interruption of primary power source.
- Experience has shown less analgesia is usually required by clients while on the bed.
- Specialty cushions are available to permit lying prone.
- Beds are usually rented; bed rental company is responsible for proper cleaning.
- Bed surface may be slippery, and transfers should not be attempted without assistance.
- The kinetic low–air-loss bed will provide approximately 30 degrees of turning continuously to the client while providing a pressure-relief surface.

Teaching Considerations

- Explain function and purpose of air-suspension therapy.
- Explain the need to continue to change position at intervals to diminish the effects of immobility.
- Explain the need for adequate fluid intake, because bed surface may be drying and may cause dehydration.

Gerontologic Considerations

- When hospitalized, older adult clients may experience significant misperceptions of their environment. This type of sensory perceptual change may be intensified by the constant flotation of the air-suspension bed.

Home Care Considerations

- A version of the bed is available for home use for rent or purchase.
- Instruct family on importance of maintaining client hydration.
- Instruct family regarding the need to provide client's skin care.

SKILL 32-3 Placing a Client on an Air-Fluidized Bed

An **air-fluidized bed** (Fig. 32-7) is designed to distribute a client's weight evenly over its support surface. The bed minimizes pressure and reduces shear force and friction through the principle of fluidization. Fluidization is created by forcing a gentle flow of temperature-controlled air upward through a mass of fine ceramic microspheres. The microspheres fluidize and take on the appearance of boiling milk and all the properties of a fluid. The client lies directly on a polyester filter sheet that allows air to pass through but does not allow the microspheres to escape. Clients feel as though they are floating on a surface like a warm waterbed. The contact pressure of the client's body against the filter sheet stays at 11 to 16 mm Hg.

Air-fluidized beds are useful in the care of clients who require minimal movement to prevent skin damage by shearing force and for clients who experience significant pain when being turned or positioned. Clients who can benefit from the bed include burn clients, those who have undergone extensive skin grafts or who have existing pressure ulcers, and victims of multiple trauma. Clients tend to perspire and lose body fluids while on the bed (Bryant et al., 1992; Fowler, 1987). The surface of the filter sheet warms; as clients perspire, moisture is quickly absorbed into the circulating microspheres. Diaphoresis can go undetected, and thus insensible fluid loss may not be noticed until a client develops fluid and electrolyte imbalances. This individual is often already compromised in relation to hydration, fluids, and electrolytes.

EQUIPMENT

- **Air-fluidized bed (Clinitron, Fluidair, Skytron)**
- **Foam positioning wedges**
- **Filter sheet (supplied by rental company)**
- **Disposable gloves (optional)**

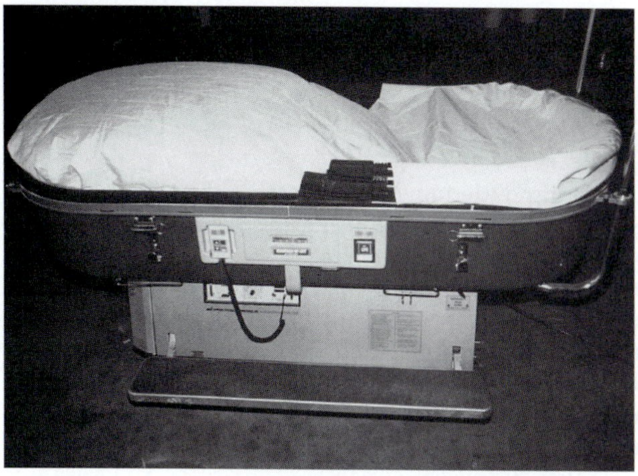

Fig. 32-7 Clinitron bed.

STEPS	RATIONALE
ASSESSMENT	
1. Wash hands.	Reduces transmission of organisms.
2. Perform pressure ulcer risk assessment to identify clients who would benefit from air-fluidized therapy.	Selected for clients who must not move because of risk of increased pain or trauma (see Chapter 8).
CRITICAL DECISION POINT The bed may not provide a stable surface for clients requiring skeletal traction.	
3. Assess condition of client's skin; pay particular attention to potential pressure sites and any existing pressure ulcers.	Data provide baseline to determine any change in client's condition while on bed.
4. Review client's medical orders.	Physician's order is needed to receive third-party reimbursement for cost of bed (not required in Canada).
5. Assess client's level of comfort.	Helps to anticipate client's need for analgesic prior to transfer. Serves as baseline for change in condition.
6. Assess client's level of orientation.	Baseline used to detect change while client is on bed. Flotation effect may cause altered sensory perceptions.
7. Assess client's and family members' understanding of purpose of bed.	Bed is large and makes sound when air blower is operating, which may create anxiety for client.
8. Review client's serum electrolyte levels in medical record (if available).	There is a tendency for clients to lose body fluids through diaphoresis. Baseline data are used to compare with subsequent laboratory results to determine electrolyte imbalances.
9. Identify clients at risk for complications of air-fluidized therapy: a. Older adult clients may become dehydrated from the airflow, which may increase insensible fluid losses. b. Clients receiving enteric tube feedings are at risk for aspiration due to the inability to elevate head of bed, which is limited to placing foam wedges under client's head and shoulders. c. Clients who have limited ability to change positions and who are susceptible to dehydration may have tenacious pulmonary secretions that are difficult to remove. d. Clients with specific positioning requirements such as elevating the head of bed are limited to use of foam wedges.	
CRITICAL DECISION POINT The prone position should *never* be attempted.	

NURSING DIAGNOSIS

Clustering of defining characteristics from the assessment data may reveal the following nursing diagnoses for clients requiring this skill:

- Altered health maintenance
- Altered peripheral tissue perfusion
- Anxiety
- Impaired home maintenance management
- Impaired physical mobility
- Impaired skin integrity
- Knowledge deficit regarding use of support surface mattress
- Pain
- Risk for altered body temperature
- Risk for fluid volume deficit
- Risk for impaired skin integrity
- Risk for infection
- Sensory/perceptual alterations, kinesthetic

Related factors are individualized based on a client's condition or needs.

STEPS	RATIONALE
PLANNING	
1. **Expected outcomes** following completion of procedure:	
➤ Skin remains warm, clean, and intact, or there is evidence of healing of pressure ulcers.	Skin is free from pressure effects of immobility.
➤ Client rates comfort level as acceptable.	Bed's surface effective in promoting comfort.
➤ Skin remains well hydrated, with good turgor; mucous membranes are moist; and electrolytes are in normal range.	Client's fluid and nutrient intake balance any insensible fluid loss from being on bed.
➤ Client remains alert and oriented or shows no change in level of consciousness.	Client does not experience sensory perceptual changes from flotation.
2. Explain procedure and purpose of bed to client and family.	Reduces anxiety and promotes client's cooperation.
3. Review instructions supplied by bed manufacturer.	Promotes safe and correct use of bed.
4. For clients with severe to moderate pain, premedicate approximately 30 minutes before transfer.	Promotes client's comfort and ability to cooperate during transfer to bed.
5. Obtain any additional personnel needed to transfer client to bed.	Ensures client's safety by having sufficient personnel to assist in transferring.
IMPLEMENTATION	
1. Close client's room door or bedside curtain.	Maintains client's privacy during transfer.
2. Explain steps of transfer.	Reduces anxiety and helps client be a part of decision making during maneuvering.
3. Wash hands and put on gloves (if bed linens or surface is soiled).	Reduces transmission of microorganisms.
4. Transfer client to bed using appropriate transfer techniques (see Chapter 29).	Appropriate transfer techniques maintain alignment and reduce risk of injury during procedure.
➤ ***CRITICAL DECISION POINT*** ***Never*** **attempt to place a client in a face-down position on an air-fluidized bed. Suffocation may occur.**	
5. Turn fluidization cycle on by depressing switch; regulate temperature.	Fluidization minimizes pressure against skin's surface and reduces friction and shear force when client moves.
6. Position client for comfort and perform range-of-motion (ROM) exercises as appropriate.	Promotes comfort and reduces contracture formation. The bed reduces pressure on skin, but clients must still be turned and exercised to avoid joint deformity or contractures.
7. To turn clients, position bedpans, or perform other therapies, stop fluidization. Once procedure is completed, set to continuous fluidization.	Stopping fluidization provides firm, molded support that facilitates turning and handling client. Continuous fluidization provides permanent fluid support.
8. In emergencies when resuscitation is required, press CPR switch and unplug unit to defluidize bed immediately (see Fig. 32-5).	Creates firm surface against which cardiopulmonary resuscitation can be performed. Unplugging bed prevents automatic start of fluidization, which occurs 30 minutes after cycle is stopped.
9. Remove gloves and wash hands.	Reduces transmission of infection.
EVALUATION	
1. Inspect condition of client's skin periodically while on bed, and monitor risk assessment.	Evaluates healing progress of any existing pressure ulcers. Determines if any new pressure areas are forming.
2. Ask client to rate ability to rest.	Bed surface is soft and conforming, minimizing pain stimulation.
3. Review client's serum electrolyte levels, monitor body temperature, and note hydration status of skin and mucous membranes.	Factors may reveal fluid and electrolyte losses.

STEPS	RATIONALE
4. Measure client's level of orientation.	Determines onset of perceptual changes.
5. **Unexpected outcomes** that may occur include:	
➤ Client becomes restless or agitated, with increased somatic complaints.	Sense of constant flotation may not be universally acceptable. Complaints of sinking or inability to adjust to bed may necessitate transfer to another surface.
➤ Areas of existing breakdown worsen.	Continued advancement of pressure ulcers can indicate deep tissue necrosis and need for surgical debridement of wound. Risk factors other than pressure may be underlying problem (e.g., nutrition, low perfusion pressures) (Bryant et al., 1992).
➤ Client's skin and mucous membranes are dehydrated, with abnormal electrolyte levels.	Temperature and evaporative effects of bed's surface cause fluid and electrolyte loss.
➤ Client becomes disoriented and complains of nausea.	Constant flotation can cause dizziness and sensory perceptual changes.
➤ Filter sheet tears.	Small microspheres will be released, potentially contaminating open wounds and causing hard surfaces to become slippery.

Recording and Reporting

1. Record transfer of client to bed, tolerance to procedure, and condition of skin in nurse's notes or skin assessment flow sheet.	Documents therapy initiated and records baseline data for other nurses to compare findings.
2. Report changes in condition of skin and electrolyte levels to nurse in charge or to physician.	Changes may indicate need for additional therapies.
3. Report change in orientation.	Change may require stopping therapy.

Follow-up Activities

1. Increase fluid intake and monitor intake and output.
2. Repeat risk assessment for skin breakdown (see Chapter 8) at regular intervals to validate continued need or plan for alternate surface.
3. Beds are equipped with special loose-fitting filter sheets that allow for optimal fluidization and pressure relief. Sheets should be inspected for tears, which allow the escape of microspheres contained in tank. Tears may be mended with adhesive tape as temporary measure until sheet can be replaced. Use of additional sheets or pads should be discouraged, because they interfere with optimal bed operation.

• • • • •

Special Considerations

- Use foam wedges as positioning aids.
- Beds weigh between 1700 and 2100 pounds and are not recommended for clients who require frequent transport in bed.
- Some beds allow nurse to adjust fluidization cycle.
- Experience has shown that less analgesia is usually required over time by clients during air-fluidized therapy.
- Sheets are available that control high air loss normally observed with air-fluidized therapy.
- When stopping fluidization, allow client to settle without disturbance onto surface of bed. Surface will mold to dependent surfaces of client and pressures will be equalized with no points of pressure.
- Company renting bed is responsible for cleaning tank of microspheres (usually by sieving) at regular intervals. Interval will vary from 1 to 4 weeks depending on need as body fluids (i.e., wound drainage, perspiration, urine) drain into the bed.
- Special cleaning is required between clients and occasionally during use to clean (sieve) the tank of microspheres. Cleaning is the responsibility of the bed rental company.

Teaching Considerations

- Explain function and purpose of air-fluidized therapy.
- Explain that client will require assistance to change positions.
- Explain the need to maintain adequate hydration of client.

Gerontologic Considerations

- Encourage client to be an effective participant in care.

- Older adult clients are at increased risk for dehydration.
- When hospitalized, older adult clients may experience significant misperceptions of their environment. This type of sensory perceptual change may be intensified by the flotation of the air-fluidized bed.

Home Care Considerations

- Beds weigh between 1700 and 2100 pounds; therefore the company leasing the bed needs to inspect the home for accessibility and structural support.
- Consult with social worker or case manager to determine third-party reimbursement.

SKILL 32-4 Placing a Client on a Bariatric Bed

A nursing adjunct in the care of the **morbidly obese** client (a person who weighs more than 100 pounds above ideal weight) is the bariatric bed that provides a safe, adaptable surface. The **bariatric bed** is capable of allowing upright or sitting positioning, client transport, and in-bed scales. The bed is equipped with hand controls that allow self-positioning and facilitate independence for the obese client. Since the bariatric bed is capable of supporting weights up to 850 pounds, it provides a stable, balanced surface that limits hospital liability should the standard bed frame collapse or the electric motor burns out.

The full-function hand controls allow the nurse caring for the obese client to change the bed position and thus facilitate care while reducing risk of staff injury in moving the client. The in-bed scale provides the nurse with a means of obtaining accurate weights, which is frequently a problem with the obese client, and thus improves health care and client dignity. The bed is slightly wider than a standard hospital bed, yet it is within the guidelines for standard door width, which allows movement into and out of a room without difficulty.

A limitation of this bed is the lack of pressure reduction or relief in the mattress. The at-risk obese client should have some type of pressure-relief mattress placed on the bariatric bed. Usual choices for pressure relief are the 4-inch foam, static air, or alternating air mattress overlays.

EQUIPMENT

- Bariatric bed
- Pressure-relief mattress overlay
- Sheets
- Overhead frame (optional)

STEPS	RATIONALE
ASSESSMENT	
1. Identify clients who would benefit from the bariatric bed system; assess their mobility status.	Selected for clients who are morbidly obese and who have the potential of being independent in positioning with assistance of a stable surface.
2. Assess condition of client's skin, paying particular attention to potential pressure sites and skinfolds. Determine the need for client to have pressure-relief mattress placed on the bariatric bed.	Data provide baseline to determine any change in client's condition while on the bed.
3. Assess client's and family members' understanding of purpose of bed.	Bed accommodates up to 850 pounds and adapts to a chair.
4. Review client's medical orders.	In the United States, a physician's order is needed to receive third-party reimbursement for the cost of the bed.

NURSING DIAGNOSIS

Clustering of defining characteristics from the assessment data may reveal the following nursing diagnoses for clients requiring this skill:

- Altered health maintenance
- Altered peripheral tissue perfusion
- Impaired home maintenance management
- Impaired physical mobility
- Impaired skin integrity
- Knowledge deficit regarding use of support surface mattress
- Risk for care giver role strain
- Risk for impaired skin integrity

Related factors are individualized based on a client's condition or needs.

STEPS	RATIONALE
PLANNING	
1. **Expected outcomes** following completion of procedure:	
➤ Client is independent for position changes.	Bed surface is adaptable by hand-operated controls.
➤ Skin remains intact, or existing lesions show evidence of healing.	Skin is free from pressure effects of immobility.
➤ Client remains free of injury.	Bed is stable to allow for positioning without tipping or bending.
2. Explain procedure and purpose of bed to client and family.	Reduces anxiety and promotes client's cooperation.
3. Review instructions supplied by bed manufacturer.	Promotes safe and correct use of bed.
CRITICAL DECISION POINT Do not exceed weight limits indicated by the manufacturer.	Client weight-limit accommodations vary according to various bariatric treatment systems.
4. For clients with severe to moderate pain, premedicate approximately 30 minutes before transfer.	Promotes client's comfort and ability to cooperate during transfer to bed.
5. Obtain any additional personnel needed to transfer client to bed.	Ensures safety of client and staff by having sufficient personnel to assist in transferring.
IMPLEMENTATION	
CRITICAL DECISION POINT Use of this bed is contraindicated in clients with spinal cord injuries.	
CRITICAL DECISION POINT Client weight-limit accommodations vary according to individual bariatric treatment systems.	
1. Close client's room door or bedside curtain.	Maintains client's privacy during transfer.
2. Explain steps of transfer.	Reduces anxiety and helps client be a part of decision making during maneuvering.
3. Wash hands and put on gloves (if needed) before assisting client to bed using appropriate transfer techniques (see Chapter 29). Depending on client's mobility status, it may be necessary to call for assistance.	Appropriate transfer techniques maintain alignment and reduce risk of injury to the client and health care workers during procedure.
4. Cover and position client, and place hand controls within reach. Be certain that the out-of-bed alarm is on, if needed. Attach overhead frame if needed.	Allows for maximal client independence. Alerts care giver that client has left the bed surface.
5. Remove gloves and wash hands.	Reduces transmission of microorganisms.
EVALUATION	
1. Inspect condition of client's skin periodically while client is on bed.	Evaluates healing of any existing pressure ulcers. Determines if any new pressure areas are forming.
2. Ask client to rate sense of comfort and safety.	Bed frame is stable for movement and position changes.
3. Evaluate client's risk for injury.	Surface is balanced and allows maximal client independence.
4. Evaluate client's ability to move in bed.	
5. **Unexpected outcomes** that may occur include:	
➤ Areas of existing skin breakdown worsen or new areas form.	Surface is not relieving pressure and may not be adequate for the at-risk client. Assess areas where the morbidly obese client is especially at risk for skin breakdown (e.g., between skinfolds of breasts and abdomen, areas exposed to moisture, and body surfaces in contact with bed frame).
➤ Client is unable to operate bed for position changes independently.	Surface is intended for the independent obese client to facilitate position change.

with aseptic techniques and barrier protection cannot be overemphasized. Today's nurse plays a vital role in the prevention and control of infections.

The presence of a pathogen does not mean that an infection will begin. Development of an infection occurs in a cyclical process that depends on the following six elements:

1. An infectious agent or **pathogen**
2. A reservoir or source for pathogen growth
3. A portal of exit from the reservoir
4. A mode of transmission
5. A portal of entry to the host
6. A susceptible host

An infection develops if this chain remains intact (Fig. 33-1). Nurses use infection control practices to break an element of the chain so that infection will not be transmitted (Table 33-1). The nurse's efforts to minimize the onset and spread of infection are based upon asepsis and the principles of aseptic technique. **Asepsis** is defined as the absence of disease-producing (pathogenic) organisms (Crow, Planchock, and Hendrick, 1995; DeCastro, Fauerback, and Masters, 1996). The two types of **aseptic technique** the nurse practices are medical and surgical asepsis.

Medical asepsis, or clean technique, includes procedures used to reduce the number of and prevent the spread of microorganisms. Hand washing, barrier techniques, and routine environmental cleaning are examples of medical asepsis. Principles of medical asepsis are commonly followed in the home, as in the case of washing hands before preparing food.

Surgical asepsis, or sterile technique, includes procedures used to eliminate microorganisms from an area. Sterilization destroys all microorganisms and their spores (Rutala, 1996). Sterile technique is practiced by nurses in the operating room (OR) and treatment areas, where sterile instruments and supplies are used. The techniques used in maintaining surgical asepsis are more rigid than those performed under medical asepsis (see Chapter 34).

GUIDELINES

1. Remember that hand washing with an appropriate soap or antiseptic is an essential part of client care and infection prevention. (Antiseptics are recommended for use in intensive care units, the OR, and special procedure areas.)
2. Always know a client's susceptibility to infection. Age, nutritional status, stress, disease processes, and forms of medical therapy can place clients at risk.
3. Recognize the elements of the infection chain and initiate measures to prevent the onset and spread of infection.
4. Incorporate consistently the basic principles of asepsis into client care.
5. Protect fellow health care workers from exposure to infectious agents through proper use and disposal of equipment. Nosocomial infections occur with greater frequency when clients are exposed to health care workers who are carriers of infection.
6. Be aware of body sites where nosocomial infections are most likely to develop. This enables the nurse to direct preventive measures.

DELEGATION CONSIDERATIONS

Hand washing is a basic procedure that should be performed correctly by all care givers. The skill involving care of a client under isolation precautions can be delegated to unlicensed assistance personnel.

- Instruct and observe hand-washing techniques by care provider.
- Review procedures for isolation precautions; stress steps necessary to prevent transmission of microorganisms.

SKILL 33-1 Hand Washing

The most important and most basic technique in preventing and controlling transmission of **infection** is hand washing. Hand washing is a vigorous, brief rubbing together of all surfaces of hands lathered in soap, followed by rinsing under a stream of water. The purpose is to remove soil and transient organisms from the hands and to reduce total microbial counts over time (Larson, 1995).

Contaminated hands are a prime cause of cross-infection. For example, a nurse caring for a client who has excessive pulmonary secretions assists the client in expectorating mucus and disposes of the tissues in a bedside container. The client's roommate asks the nurse to open containers of food on the meal tray. The nurse then leaves the client's room to pour a dose of medication due in 5 minutes. If the nurse fails to wash hands before each of these actions, organisms from the first client's mucus could easily be transmitted to the roommate's food and to the medication container.

The decision regarding when hand washing should occur depends on the following: the intensity of contact with clients or contaminated objects; the degree or amount of **contamination** that could occur with that contact; the susceptibility of the client or the health care worker to infection; and the procedure or activity to be performed (Larson, 1996). For example, if a nurse touches an object that is not visibly soiled, hand washing may not be required.

In contrast, prolonged and intense contact with a client's wound drainage would require thorough hand washing. Larson (1995) recommends that nurses wash hands in the following situations:

1. When visibly soiled
2. Before and after client contact
3. After contact with a source of **microorganisms** (blood or body fluids, mucous membrane, nonintact skin, or inanimate objects that might be contaminated)
4. Before the performance of **invasive procedures** such as placement of intravascular catheters or indwelling catheters (antimicrobial soap recommended)
5. After removing gloves (wearing gloves does not remove the need to wash hands)

The Centers for Disease Control and Prevention (CDC) and the U.S. Public Health Service note that washing times of at least 10 to 15 seconds (Garner, 1996) will remove most transient microorganisms from the skin. If hands are visibly soiled, more time may be needed. The frequency of washing also affects the type and number of bacteria on the hands. Larson (1996) stated that nurses who wash their hands 8 times a day are less likely to carry gram-negative bacteria on their hands. Routine hand washing may be performed with soap in any convenient form (bar, leaflets, liquid, or powder). However, bar soap that remains wet or in pooled water may harbor microorganisms. The use of antimicrobial soap (antiseptic) is encouraged when nurses need to reduce total microbial counts on their hands, such as situations where nurses are in contact with children or older adult clients who are **immunocompromised** or clients who have damage to their integumentary system (wounds or bruises). Additionally, an antimicrobial soap should be used prior to performing an invasive procedure such as care or insertion of an intravascular catheter. There are a number of effective antimicrobial soaps that contain chlorhexidine gluconate (CHG), alcohols, and iodophors. Certain antimicrobial soaps can irritate the skin, and the need for antimicrobial soap must be weighed against potential skin irritation.

EQUIPMENT

- **Easy-to-reach sink with warm running water**
- **Antimicrobial or regular soap**
- **Paper towels or air dryer**
- **Clean orangewood stick (optional)**

STEPS	RATIONALE
ASSESSMENT	
1. Inspect surface of hands for breaks or cuts in skin or cuticles. Report and cover lesions before providing client care.	Open cuts or wounds can harbor high concentrations of microorganisms. Agency policy may prevent nurse from caring for high-risk clients. If dermatitis occurs, additional interventions may be needed.
2. Inspect hands for heavy soiling.	Requires lengthier hand washing.
3. Assess client's risk for or extent of infection, for example, white blood cell count, extent of open wounds, or known medical diagnosis.	Use of antimicrobial soaps is encouraged for clients who are immunosuppressed (Larson, 1995).

NURSING DIAGNOSIS

Clustering of defining characteristics from the assessment data may reveal the following nursing diagnoses for clients requiring this skill:

➤ This skill is required for clients having a variety of nursing diagnoses.

Related factors are individualized based on a client's condition or needs.

PLANNING

1. **Expected outcome** following completion of procedure:	
➤ Hands and areas under fingernails are clean and free of debris.	Procedure is effective.

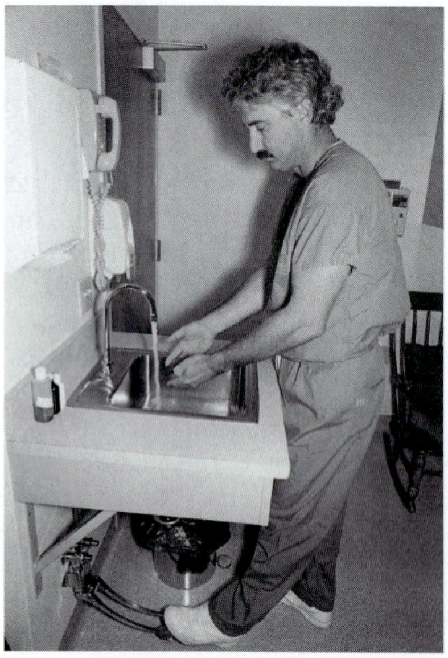

Step 4 Hand washing—turning on water.

STEPS	RATIONALE
IMPLEMENTATION	
1. Push wristwatch and long uniform sleeves above wrists. Avoid wearing rings. If worn, remove during washing.	Provides complete access to fingers, hands, wrists. Wearing of rings increases number of microorganisms on hands (Garner, 1995).
2. Be sure fingernails are short, filed, and smooth.	Most microbes on hands come from the subungual region (beneath the fingernails).
3. Stand in front of sink, keeping hands and uniform away from sink surface. (If hands touch sink during hand washing, repeat.)	Inside of sink is a contaminated area. Reaching over sink increases risk of touching edge, which is contaminated.
4. Turn on water. Turn faucet on or push knee pedals laterally or press pedals with foot to regulate flow and temperature (see illustration).	
5. Avoid splashing water against uniform.	Microorganisms travel and grow in moisture.
6. Regulate flow of water so that temperature is warm.	Warm water removes less of the protective oils than hot water.
7. Wet hands and wrists thoroughly under running water. Keep hands and forearms lower than elbows during washing.	Hands are the most contaminated parts to be washed. Water flows from least to most contaminated area, rinsing microorganisms into sink.
8. Apply a small amount of soap or antiseptic, lathering thoroughly (see illustration). Soap granules and leaflet preparations may be used.	The use of antiseptic exclusively can be drying to the hands and cause skin irritations.
CRITICAL DECISION POINT **The decision whether to use an antiseptic or not should be dependent on the procedure to be performed and the client's immune status.**	
9. Wash hands using plenty of lather and friction for at least 10-15 seconds. Interlace fingers and rub palms and back of hands with circular motion at least 5 times each. Keep fingertips down to facilitate removal of microorganisms.	Soap cleanses by emulsifying fat and oil and lowering surface tension. Friction and rubbing mechanically loosen and remove dirt and transient bacteria. Interlacing fingers and thumbs ensures that all surfaces are cleansed.
10. Areas underlying fingernails are often soiled. Clean them with fingernails of other hand and additional soap or clean orangewood stick.	Area under nails can be highly contaminated, which will increase the risk for infections for the nurse or the client.
CRITICAL DECISION POINT **Do not tear or cut skin under or around nail.**	
11. Rinse hands and wrists thoroughly, keeping hands down and elbows up (see illustration).	Rinsing mechanically washes away dirt and microorganisms.

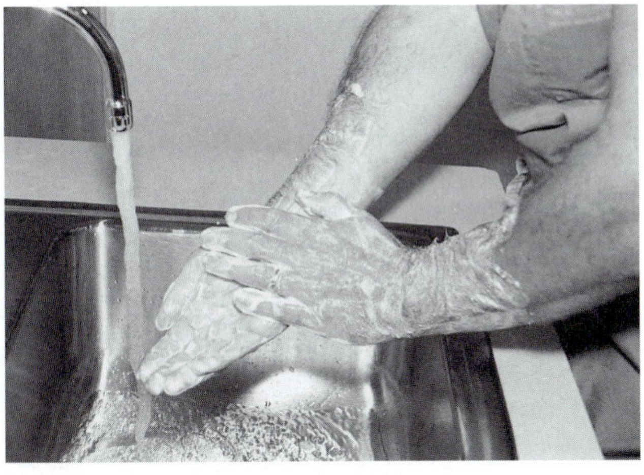

Step 8 Hand washing—lather hands thoroughly.

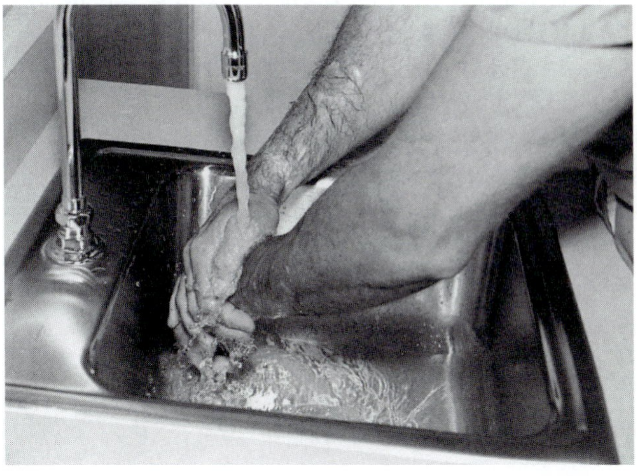

Step 11 Hand washing—rinsing hands.

STEPS	RATIONALE
12. Dry hands thoroughly from fingers to wrists and forearms with paper towel, single-use cloth, or warm air dryer.	Drying from cleanest (fingertips) to least clean (forearms) area avoids contamination. Drying hands prevents chapping and roughened skin.
13. If used, discard paper towel in proper receptacle.	Prevents transfer of microorganisms.
14. Turn off water with foot or knee pedals. To turn off hand faucet, use clean, dry paper towel, avoiding touching handles with hands.	Wet towel and hands allow transfer of pathogens by capillary action.

EVALUATION

1. Inspect surface of hands for obvious signs of dirt or other contaminants.	Determines if hand washing is adequate.
2. **Unexpected outcomes** that may occur include:	
➤ Hands or areas under fingernails remain soiled.	Requires nurse to repeat hand washing.
➤ Repeated use of soaps or antiseptic may cause dermatitis or cracked skin.	Requires methods to alleviate complications of hand washing. • Rinse and dry hands thoroughly. • Avoid excessive amounts of soap or antiseptic. • Try various products. • Use hand lotions or barrier creams. (Use small individual-use container because large containers have been associated with nosocomial infections.) • Wear gloves. (This should be on a temporary basis because glove wearing can increase bacterial growth and may increase latex allergies among clients and health care workers.)

RECORDING AND REPORTING

1. It is not necessary to record or report this procedure.
2. Report any dermatitis to employee health and/or infection control per your agency's policy.

FOLLOW-UP ACTIVITIES

1. Keep hands and cuticles well lubricated with hand lotion or moisturizer.

• • • • •

Special Considerations

- Clear nail polish that is well maintained may be worn with no increase in microbial count on nails (Larson, 1996). Colored polish makes dirt difficult to see under nails.
- When preparing for sterile procedure, use antiseptic hand wash rather than simple hand soap.
- Timing of hand wash varies, depending on purpose of wash.

Teaching Considerations

- Instruct the client and primary care giver in proper techniques and situations for hand washing.

Home Care Considerations

- Evaluate client and primary care giver to determine their understanding of the transmission of microorganisms and their ability and motivation to perform hand washing according to medical asepsis.
- Evaluate the hand-washing facilities in the home to determine the possibility of contamination, proximity of the facilities to the client, and the ability to maintain supplies and equipment.

SKILL 33-2 Caring for Clients Under Isolation Precautions

There is a risk of transmitting nosocomial infection or infectious disease among clients or health care workers. When a client has a known source of infection, health care workers follow specific infection control practices and preventions.

The majority of organisms causing nosocomial infections are found in the colonized body substances of clients, regardless of whether or not a culture has confirmed infection and a diagnosis has been made (Jackson and Lynch, 1992). Body substances such as feces, urine, mucus, and wound drainage can contain potentially infectious organisms.

Isolation or barrier precautions include the appropriate use of gowns, masks, eyewear, and other protective devices or clothing. Nurses should assess the need for barrier precautions for each task they plan and for all clients regardless of their diagnoses (Lynch, 1995). Because of increased attention to the prevention of blood-borne pathogens and tuberculosis (TB), the Centers for Disease Control and Prevention (CDC) (1988, 1994) and the Occupational Safety and Health Administration (OSHA) (1994, 1991) have stressed the importance of barrier protection.

In 1996, the Hospital Infection Control Practice Advisory Committee (HICPAC) of the CDC published revised guidelines for isolation precautions. These recommendations were based on current epidemiological information regarding disease transmission in hospitals. Although primarily intended for care of clients in acute care, the recommendations can be applied to clients in subacute care or long-term care facilities. HICPAC recommended that hospitals modify the recommendations according to their needs and as dictated by federal, state, or local regulations (Centers for Disease Control and Prevention, 1996; Garner, 1996).

The new guidelines contained two tiers of precautions. The first and most important tier (see the box at right) is called standard precautions and is designed for care of all clients regardless of risk or presumed infection status. **Standard precautions** are the primary strategies for prevention of infection transmission. The second tier (Table 33-2) is precautions designed for care of clients with specific infections or diagnoses. These precaution are used for clients known or suspected to be infected, or **colonized,** with microorganisms transmitted by droplets, by airborne route, or by contact with contaminated surfaces or dry skin (Table 33-3).

Standard precautions apply to contact with (1) blood, (2) body fluids, (3) nonintact skin, and (4) mucous membranes. These combined precautions are the major features of universal precautions and body substance isolation.

There are three types of **transmission-based precautions:** airborne, droplet, and contact. They may be combined together for diseases that have multiple routes of transmission, for example, chickenpox. When used either singularly or in combination, they are to be used in addition to standard precautions when required by the specific infection or colonization with a specific organism.

When a client requires isolation in a private room, the nurse must remember that loneliness can easily develop. Isolation disrupts normal social relationships with visitors and care givers. A client who suffers from an infectious disease may also experience self-concept or body image changes. Unless the nurse acts to minimize feelings of psychological and physical isolation, the client's emotional state can interfere with recovery.

EQUIPMENT

- **Disposable gloves, mask, eyewear or goggles, gown, and other equipment as appropriate**

STANDARD PRECAUTIONS (TIER ONE)* FOR USE WITH ALL CLIENTS

- Standard precautions apply to blood, all body fluids, secretions, excretions, nonintact skin, and mucous membranes.
- Hands are washed if contaminated with blood or body fluid, immediately after gloves are removed, between client contact, and when indicated to prevent transfer of microorganisms between clients or between clients and environment.
- Gloves are worn when touching blood, body fluid, secretions, excretions, nonintact skin, mucous membranes, or contaminated items. Gloves should be removed and hands washed between client care.
- Masks, eye protection, or face shields are worn if client care activities may generate splashes or sprays of blood or body fluid.
- Gowns are worn if soiling of clothing is likely from blood or body fluid. Wash hands after removing gown.
- Client care equipment is properly cleaned and reprocessed, and single-use items are discarded.
- Contaminated linen is placed in leakproof bag and is handled to prevent skin and mucous membrane exposure.
- All sharp instruments and needles are discarded in a puncture-resistant container. CDC recommends that needles be disposed of uncapped or a mechanical device be used for recapping.
- A private room is unnecessary unless the client's hygiene is unacceptable. Check with infection control professional.

Adapted from Centers for Disease Control and Prevention, Hospital Infection Control Practice Advisory Committee: Guidelines for isolation precautions in hospitals, *A J Infection Control* 24:24, 1996.
*Formally universal precautions and body substance isolation.

Table 33-2 Transmission Categories Tier Two (for Use with Clients Infected or Colonized with Specific Organisms)

Category	Disease	Barrier Protection
Airborne precautions	For diseases transmitted by small droplet nuclei (smaller than 5 microns), such as measles; chickenpox; disseminated varicella zoster; pulmonary or laryngeal TB*	Private room, negative airflow of at least six air exchanges per hour; respirator or mask*
Droplet precautions	For diseases transmitted by large droplets (larger than 5 microns), such as streptococcal pharyngitis, pneumonia, and scarlet fever in infants or small children, pertussis, mumps, meningococcal pneumonia or sepsis, pneumonic plague	Private room or cohort client; mask when at least 3 ft from client
Contact precautions	For diseases transmitted by direct client or environmental contact, such as colonization or infection with multidrug-resistant organisms, respiratory syncytial virus, major wound infections, herpes simplex, scabies	Private room or cohort clients; gloves, gowns

Adapted from Centers for Disease Control and Prevention, Hospital Infection Control Practice Advisory Committee: Guidelines for isolation precautions in hospitals, *A J Infection Control* 24:24, 1996.
*See CDC TB guidelines.

STEPS	RATIONALE
ASSESSMENT	
1. Assess the client and review medical history for possible indications for isolation, for example, risk factors for TB, major draining wound, or purulent productive cough. Review the precautions necessary for the specific isolation system.	Mode of transmission for infectious microorganism determines type and degree of precautions followed.
2. Review laboratory test results.	Informs nurse of the type of microorganism for which client is being isolated and body fluid in which it was identified.
3. Consider types of care measures to be performed while in client's room.	Enables nurse to organize procedures and time spent in client's room.
4. Review nurses' notes or confer with colleagues regarding client's emotional state and reaction/adjustment to isolation.	Determines need for emotional support, teaching, etc.
5. Prepare all equipment needed to be taken into client's room.	Prevents nurse from making more than one trip into room.
6. Determine from chart or significant other if client and family understand the purpose of isolation or procedures to anticipate.	Determines client's level of knowledge.
7. Before donning latex gloves, assess if the client has a known latex allergy.	Client with latex allergy can have a serious reaction even after brief exposure.

NURSING DIAGNOSIS

Clustering of defining characteristics from the assessment data may reveal the following nursing diagnoses for clients requiring this skill:

- Impaired social interaction
- Knowledge deficit regarding purpose of isolation
- Risk for infection

Related factors are individualized based on a client's condition or needs.

PLANNING

STEPS	RATIONALE
1. **Expected outcomes** following completion of procedure:	
➤ Client spontaneously engages in discussions with nurse and family.	Active interaction reveals client's willingness and/or ability to communicate and to be taught and to understand information.
➤ Client asks for information about disease transmission.	

Table 33-3 Synopsis of Types of Precautions and Patients Requiring the Precautions*

Standard Precautions

Use Standard Precautions for the care of all patients

Airborne Precautions

In addition to Standard Precautions, use Airborne Precautions for patients known or suspected to have serious illnesses transmitted by airborne droplet nuclei. Examples of such illnesses include:

(1) Measles
(2) Varicella (including disseminated zoster)*
(3) Tuberculosis†

Droplet Precautions

In addition to Standard Precautions, use Droplet Precautions for patients known or suspected to have serious illnesses transmitted by large particle droplets. Examples of such illnesses include:

(1) Invasive *Haemophilus influenzae* type b disease, including meningitis, pneumonia, epiglottitis, and sepsis
(2) Invasive *Neisseria meningitidis* disease, including meningitis, pneumonia, and sepsis
(3) Other serious bacterial respiratory infections spread by droplet transmission, including:
  (a) Diphtheria (pharyngeal)
  (b) Mycoplasma pneumonia
  (c) Pertussis
  (d) Pneumonic plague
  (e) Streptococcal pharyngitis, pneumonia, or scarlet fever in infants and young children
(4) Serious viral infections spread by droplet transmission, including:
  (a) Adenovirus*
  (b) Influenza
  (c) Mumps
  (d) Parvovirus B19
  (e) Rubella

Contact Precautions

In addition to Standard Precautions, use Contact Precautions for patients known or suspected to have serious illnesses easily transmitted by direct patient contact or by contact with items in the patient's environment. Examples of such illnesses include:

(1) Gastrointestinal, respiratory, skin, or wound infections or colonization with multidrug-resistant bacteria judged by the infection control program, based on current state, regional, or national recommendations, to be of special clinical and epidemiologic significance
(2) Enteric infections with a low infectious dose or prolonged environmental survival, including:
  (a) *Clostridium difficile*
  (b) For diapered or incontinent patients: enterohemorrhagic *Escherichia coli* 0157:H7, *Shigella,* hepatitis A, or rotavirus
(3) Respiratory syncytial virus, parainfluenza virus, or enteroviral infections in infants and young children
(4) Skin infections that are highly contagious or that may occur on dry skin, including:
  (a) Diphtheria (cutaneous)
  (b) Herpes simplex virus (neonatal or mucocutaneous)
  (c) Impetigo
  (d) Major (noncontained) abscesses, cellulitis, or decubiti
  (e) Pediculosis
  (f) Scabies
  (g) Staphylococcal furunculosis in infants and young children
  (h) Zoster (disseminated or in the immunocompromised host)*
(5) Viral/hemorrhagic conjunctivitis
(6) Viral hemorrhagic infections (Ebola, Lassa, or Marburg)

From: Centers for Disease Control and Prevention, Hospital Infection Control Practice Advisory Committee: Guidelines for isolation precautions in hospitals, *American Journal of Infection Control* 24:24, 1966.

*Certain infections require more than one type of precaution.

†See CDC *Guidelines for Preventing the Transmission of Tuberculosis in Health-Care Facilities.*

STEPS	RATIONALE

IMPLEMENTATION

1. Wash hands.
   Rationale: Reduces transmission of microorganisms.
2. Apply gown, mask, gloves, and goggles as appropriate:
   a. Apply gown, being sure it covers all outer garments. Pull sleeves down to wrist. Tie securely at neck and waist (see illustration).
   Rationale: Protective garments prevent transmission of organisms from nurse to client and protect nurse from contact with infectious pathogens.
   b. Apply disposable gloves. If worn with gown, bring cuffs over edge of gown sleeves.

CRITICAL DECISION POINT NOTE: **Unpowdered latex-free gloves should be worn if the client or the health care worker has a latex allergy.**

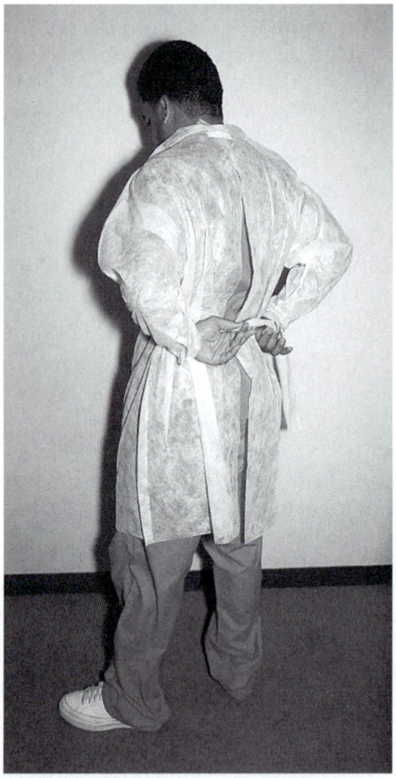

Step 2a Isolation—tying gown.

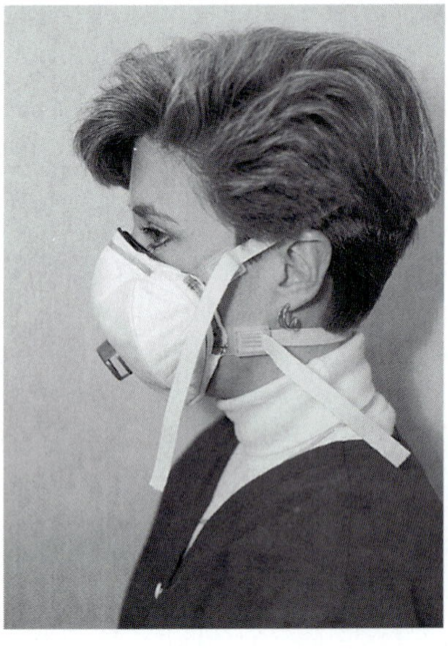

Step 2c(1) Isolation—nurse wearing HEPA respirator.

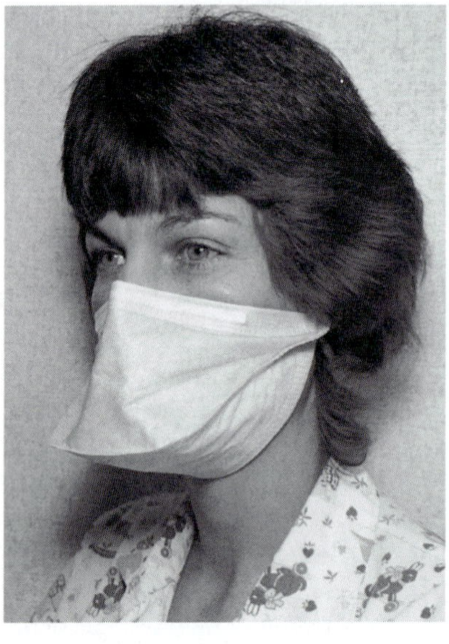

Step 2c(2) Isolation—nurse wearing N-95 respirator.

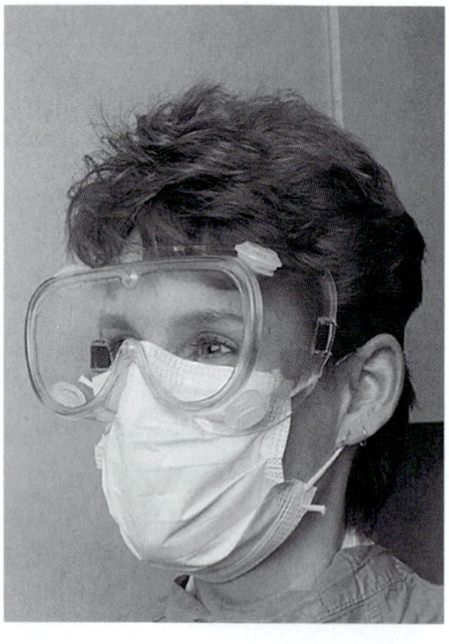

Step 2d Isolation—nurse wearing goggles.

STEPS	RATIONALE
c. Apply either surgical mask or respirator around mouth and nose (see illustration).	Type of mask or respirator will depend on type of isolation and facility policy (see illustrations).
d. Apply goggles to fit snugly around face and eyes (see illustration).	Goggles are worn when exposure to splashing body fluids is likely.
3. Enter client's room. Arrange supplies and equipment.	Prevents extra trips entering and leaving room.
4. Explain purpose of isolation and precautions necessary to client and family. Offer opportunity to ask questions. Assess for emotions that may be related to the isolation, such as loneliness or boredom, and for signs/symptoms of depression, for example, lack of appetite or difficulty sleeping.	Improves client's and family's ability to participate in care and minimizes anxiety.
5. Assess vital signs.	
a. Avoid contact of stethoscope or blood pressure cuff with infective material.	

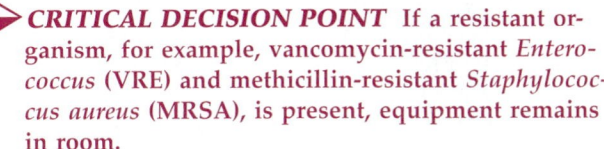

CRITICAL DECISION POINT If a resistant organism, for example, vancomycin-resistant *Enterococcus* (VRE) and methicillin-resistant *Staphylococcus aureus* (MRSA), is present, equipment remains in room.

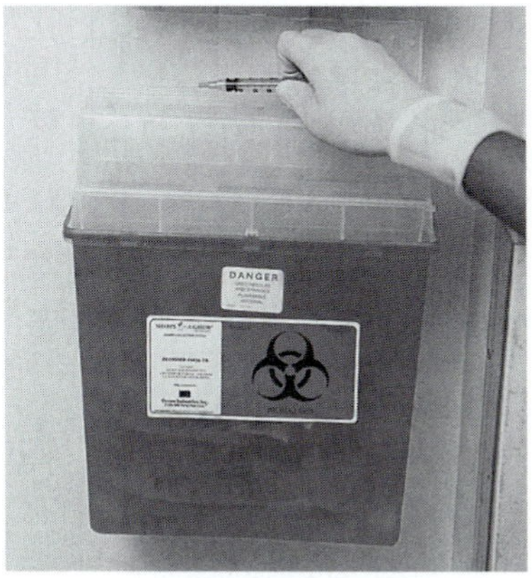

Step 6d Isolation—disposal of syringes and uncapped needle.

STEPS	RATIONALE
b. If stethoscope is to be reused, clean diaphragm or bell with alcohol. Set aside on clean surface.	Equipment is either cleaned between clients or used only for client in isolation.
c. Individual or disposable thermometers should be used.	
6. Administer medications (see Chapter 18):	
a. Give oral medication in wrapper or cup.	Supplies are handled and discarded to minimize transfer of microorganisms.
b. Dispose of wrapper or cup in plastic-lined receptacle.	
c. Administer injection, being sure gloves are worn.	
d. Discard syringe and uncapped needle or sheathed needle into special container (see illustration).	
e. Place reusable syringe on clean towel for eventual removal and disinfection.	Prevents added contamination of syringe.
7. Administer hygiene, encouraging the client to verbalize any questions or concerns regarding isolation.	

CRITICAL DECISION POINT During this time, informal teaching can be provided.

STEPS	RATIONALE
a. Avoid allowing isolation gown to become wet; carry washbasin outward away from gown; avoid leaning against wet tabletop.	Moisture allows organisms to travel through gown to uniform.
b. Assist client in removing own gown; discard in impervious linen bag.	
c. Remove linen from bed; if excessively soiled, avoid contact with isolation gown. Place in impervious linen bag.	Linen soiled by client's body fluids is handled so as to prevent contact with clean items.

STEPS	RATIONALE
CRITICAL DECISION POINT In case of excess soiling, a gown impervious to moisture should be worn.	
d. Provide clean bed linen and set of towels.	
e. Change gloves and wash hands if they become excessively soiled and further care is necessary.	
8. Collect specimens (see Chapter 43):	
a. Place specimen containers on clean paper towel in client's bathroom.	Specimens of blood and body fluids are placed in well-constructed containers with secure lids to prevent leaks during transport.
b. Follow procedure for collecting specimen of body fluids.	
c. Transfer specimen to container without soiling outside of container. Place container in a plastic bag.	
d. Check label on specimen for accuracy. Send to laboratory (warning labels may be used, depending on hospital policy).	

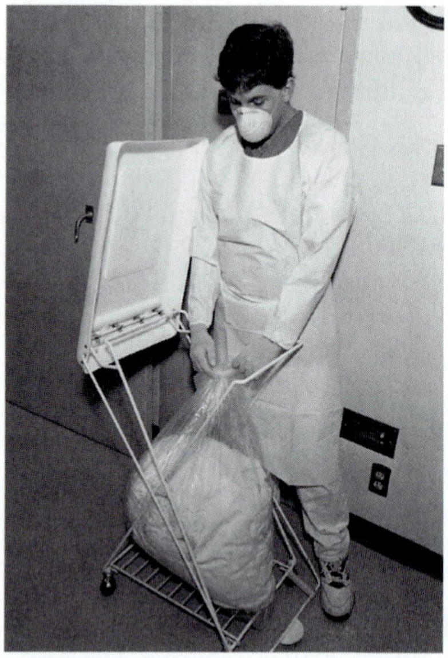

Step 9b Tie bags.

STEPS	RATIONALE
9. Dispose of linen, trash, and disposable items:	
a. Use single bags that are impervious to moisture and sturdy to contain soiled articles.	Linen or refuse should be totally contained to prevent exposure of personnel to infective material.
b. Tie bags securely at top in knot (see illustration).	
10. Remove all reusable pieces of equipment. (Refer to institution policy for method of removal.)	All items must be properly disinfected for reuse.
11. Resupply room as needed.	Limiting trips of personnel into and out of room reduces nurse's and client's exposure to microorganisms. Quality time should be spent with the client when in the room.
12. Leave isolation room.	
a. Remove eyewear or goggles.	Gloved hands are used to remove eyewear or goggles that may be splattered with body fluids.
b. Untie gown at waist. Remove one glove by grasping cuff and pulling glove inside out over hand (see illustration).	
c. Discard glove. With ungloved hand, tuck finger inside cuff of remaining glove and pull it off, inside out (see illustration).	
d. Untie mask strings; drop mask into trash receptacle.	
CRITICAL DECISION POINT Do not touch outer surface of mask.	

STEPS	RATIONALE
e. Untie neck strings of gown. Allow gown to fall from shoulders. Remove hands from sleeves without touching outside of gown. Hold gown inside at shoulder seams and fold inside out (see illustration). Discard in laundry bag.	Gloves and gown are removed by avoiding contamination of hands.
f. Wash hands for a minimum of 10 seconds.	
g. Retrieve wristwatch and stethoscope (unless it must remain in room) and note vital sign values on paper.	Clean hands can contact clean items.

➤ *CRITICAL DECISION POINT* Note stethoscope should be washed off with disinfectant before reuse.

STEPS	RATIONALE
h. Explain to client when you plan to return to room. Ask whether client requires any personal care items. Offer books, magazines, etc. that may assist the client from being bored or feeling restricted.	Include client in planning care.
i. Leave room and close door, if necessary.	Door should be closed if client is in negative airflow room.

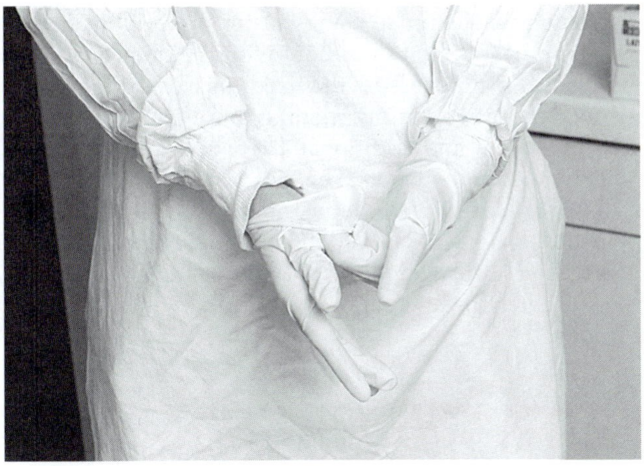

Step 12b Removal of gloves.

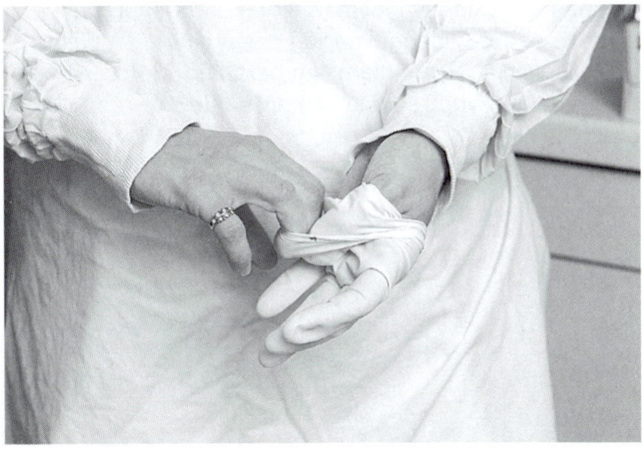

Step 12c Removal of gloves.

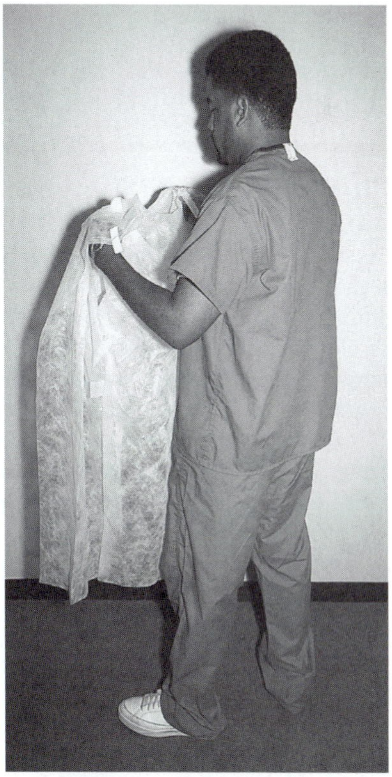

Step 12e Removal of gown.

STEPS	RATIONALE
EVALUATION	
1. While in room, ask if client has had sufficient opportunity to discuss health problems, course of treatment, or other topics important to client.	Measures client's perception of adequacy of discussions with care givers.
2. **Unexpected outcomes** that may occur include:	
➤ Client avoids social and therapeutic discussions.	Isolation may create loneliness and sense of depression.
➤ Client or health care worker may have an allergy to latex gloves.	

RECORDING AND REPORTING

1. Document client's response to social isolation in nurse's progress notes.	Directs other care givers to provide adequate support through communication.

• • • • •

Pediatric Considerations

➤ Isolation creates a sense of separation from family and a loss of control. The strange environment adds to the confusion a child feels during isolation. Preschoolers are unable to understand the cause-effect relationship for isolation. Older children may be able to understand the cause but still fantasize. Children require simple explanations, for example, "You need to be in this room to help you get better." All barriers to be used must be shown to the child. Parents must be actively involved in any explanations. The nurses let a child see their faces before applying masks so that the child does not become frightened.

Gerontologic Considerations

➤ Isolation also can be a particular concern for older adults, especially those who have signs and symptoms of confusion or depression. Many times clients become more confused when they are confronted with a nurse using barrier precautions or when they are left in a room with the door closed. The nurse must assess the need for closing the door (negative airflow room) along with the safety of the client and additional safety measures that may need to be taken. The older adults should be assessed for signs of depression such as loss of appetite or decrease in verbal communications. If necessary, this should be brought to the attention of the health care team for appropriate interventions.

CRITICAL THINKING EXERCISES

1. The nurse is assisting Mrs. Jones in bed and notices that her urinary catheter drainage bag has become disconnected from the catheter. The nurse cleanses the end of the catheter and connects a new drainage bag. In what way does this procedure break the chain of infection?
2. If you as a nurse are practicing standard precautions and you walk into a room to assist a physician with a wound irrigation, what type of protective barriers would you wear?
3. Based on the concepts of standard precautions, explain when a nurse would wear gloves while handling a sputum specimen.
4. The nurse has performed a phlebotomy procedure and has been wearing clean gloves. A client calls to the nurse from the next bed. Before responding, what should the nurse do?

REFERENCES

Bobo L: The microbiologic environment. In Soule B, Larson E, Preson G, editors: *Infection and nursing practice: prevention and control,* St Louis, 1995, Mosby.

Centers for Disease Control: Update: universal precautions for prevention of transmission of human immunodeficiency virus, hepatitis B virus, and other bloodborne pathogens in health care setting, *MMWR* 37(24):377, 1988.

Centers for Disease Control and Prevention: Guidelines for preventing the transmission of mycobacterium tuberculosis in health-care facilities, *Fed Regis* 59(208):54242, 1994.

Centers for Disease Control and Prevention, Hospital Infection Control Practice Advisory Committee: Guidelines for isolation precautions in hospitals, *AJ Infection Control* 24:24, 1996.

Crow S, Planchock N, Hendrick E: Antisepsis: disinfection and sterilization. In Soule B, Larson E, and Preston G, editors: *Infection and nursing practice: prevention and control,* St Louis, 1995, Mosby.

DeCastro M, Fauerback L, Masters L: Aseptic technique. In Olmsted R, editor: *APIC infection control and applied epidemiology,* St Louis, 1996, Mosby.

Garner B: Infection control. In Meeker MH, Rothrock JC, editors: *Alexander's care of the patient in surgery,* St Louis, 1995, Mosby.

Garner J: Isolation systems. In Olmsted R, editor: *APIC infection control and applied epidemiology,* St Louis, 1996, Mosby.

Goldrick B, Turner J: Education and behavior change in prevention and control of infection. In Soule B, Larson E, Preston G: *Infection and nursing practice: prevention and control,* St Louis, 1995, Mosby.

Jackson M, Lynch P: Body substance isolation, *Infect Contr and Hosp Epidem* 13(14):191, 1992.

Larson E: APIC guidelines for handwashing and hand antisepsis in health care settings, *AJIC,* 23(4):251, 1995.

Larson E: Antiseptic. In Olmsted R, editor: *APIC infection control and applied epidemiology,* St Louis, 1996, Mosby.

Lynch P: Barrier precautions and personal protection. In Soule B, Larson E, Preston G, editors: *Infections and nursing practices,* St Louis, 1995, Mosby.

Occupational Safety and Health Administration: Occupational exposure to bloodborne pathogens: final rule, 29 CFR 1919:1030, *Fed Regis* 56:64003, 1991.

Occupational Safety and Health Administration: Respiratory protection, *Fed Regis* 59(219):58884, 1994.

Rutala W: Disinfection and sterilization of patient-care items, *Infect Contr and Hosp Epidem* 17(6):377, 1996.

ADDITIONAL READING

Benenson A: *Control of communicable disease in man,* Washington, DC, 1995, APHA.

Grimes D, Grimes B: *Infectious disease,* St Louis, 1995, Mosby.

Kim MJ, et al: *Pocket guide to nursing diagnoses,* ed 7, St Louis, 1997, Mosby.

Maki DG et al: Double-bagging of items from isolation rooms is unnecessary as an infection control measure: a comparative study of surface contamination with single and double-bagging, *Infect Contr* 7(11):535, 1986.

Rutala W: *Chemical germicides in health care,* Washington, DC, 1995, APIC.

Schaffer S, et al: *Pocket guide to infection prevention and safe practice,* St Louis, 1996, Mosby.

Smith P, Rusnak P: APIC guideline for infection prevention and control in the long-term care facility, *Am J Infect Contr* 19(4):198, 1991.

Springer L, et al: Anticipated care for HIV-infected clients: nurses' reactions, *J Assoc Nurses in AIDS Care* 5(1):29, 1994.

CHAPTER 34

Sterile Technique

OBJECTIVES

Mastery of content in this chapter will enable the nurse to:

- Define key terms.
- Discuss settings where surgical aseptic techniques may be used.
- Describe conditions when surgical asepsis should be used.
- Identify principles of surgical asepsis.
- Explain the importance of organization and caution when using surgical aseptic techniques.
- Apply and remove a cap and mask correctly.
- Apply sterile gloves using open glove method.
- Prepare a sterile field.
- Apply a sterile drape correctly.

KEY TERMS

Asepsis
Microorganisms
Pathogenic microorganisms
Standard precautions
Sterile
Sterile field
Surgical asepsis

SKILLS

34-1 Donning and Removing Cap and Mask

34-2 Preparing a Sterile Field

34-3 Open Gloving

Surgical asepsis or aseptic techniques and practices are designed to render and maintain objects and areas free from **pathogenic microorganisms** (Crow, Planchock, and Hendrick, 1995). As in medical **asepsis,** hand washing with an appropriate soap or antiseptic is essential before the initiation of an aseptic procedure. Surgical asepsis does require more precautions than medical aseptic technique (see Chapter 33). Any break in technique could result in contamination, increasing the client's risk for an infection. Although surgical asepsis is commonly practiced in an operating room (OR), a labor and delivery area, and a major diagnostic area; the nurse may use surgical aseptic techniques at the client's bedside (see box on p. 1005) in three primary situations:

- During procedures that require intentional perforation of a client's skin (e.g., insertion of intravenous [IV] catheters and administration of injections [see Chapters 19 and 20])
- When the skin's integrity is broken due to a surgical incision or burns
- During procedures that involve insertion of devices or surgical instruments into normally sterile body cavities (e.g., insertion of a urinary catheter, [see Chapter 25])

The skills in this chapter can be used at the client's bedside; portions of Skills 34-1 and 34-2 also could be practiced in the OR and/or delivery room. Chapter 35 describes additional skills specific to the OR and labor and delivery areas. A nurse in an OR follows a series of steps towards **sterile** technique, such as applying a mask, protective eyewear, and a cap; performing a surgical hand scrub; and applying a sterile gown and gloves. In contrast, a nurse performing a sterile dressing change at a client's bedside may only wash the hands and apply sterile gloves. Regardless of the procedures followed in different settings, the use of surgical asepsis depends on the nurse developing a surgical aseptic awareness. The nurse must always recognize the importance of strict adherence to aseptic principles (Roth, 1996). Additionally, the nurse can play an active role in enforcing these same principles with other

PRINCIPLES OF SURGICAL ASEPSIS

1. All items used within a sterile field must be sterile.
2. A sterile barrier that has been permeated by punctures, tears, or moisture must be considered contaminated.
3. Once a sterile package is opened, the edges are considered unsterile.
4. Gowns, once put on, are considered sterile in front from chest to waist or table level; sleeves are considered sterile from 5 cm (2 inches) above elbows to fingertips of gloved hand. (NOTE: Cuffs are not considered sterile once glove has been removed.)
5. Tables draped as part of sterile field are considered sterile only at table level.
6. If there is any question or doubt of an item's sterility, the item is considered to be unsterile.
7. Sterile persons or items contact only sterile areas; unsterile persons or items contact only unsterile areas.
8. Movement around and in the sterile field must not compromise or contaminate the sterile field.

members of the health care team. The nurse can be an excellent role model and client advocate, reinforcing proper practice when another care giver breaks technique.

In the OR, control of aseptic practice is more easily enforced because of the controlled environment. In treatment areas and at the bedside, it is important to have a client's full cooperation. The nurse must prepare a client before any procedure. Certain clients may fear moving or touching objects during a sterile procedure; whereas others may even try to assist. The nurse explains how a procedure is to be performed and what a client can do to avoid contaminating sterile items, including avoiding sudden body movement, refraining from touching sterile supplies, and avoiding coughing or talking over a sterile area.

The Centers for Disease Control and Prevention (CDC) (1996) has established standard precautions as the minimum standard for infection control. Standard precautions should be used for potential contact with blood and certain body fluids (peritoneal, pericardial, pleural, cerebrospinal fluid [CSF], vaginal, seminal, and amniotic). These are considered infectious for human immunodeficiency virus (HIV), hepatitis B virus (HBV), hepatitis C virus (HCV), and other blood-borne pathogens. Standard precautions also apply to body fluids containing visible blood. The use of standard precautions calls for the wearing of masks in combination with eye protection devices such as goggles or glasses with solid side shields whenever splashes, spray, spatter, or droplets of blood or other potentially infectious fluids may be generated. These barriers keep the eye, nose, and mouth free from exposure. Similarly, gowns are to be worn when there is risk of being splattered with blood or other infectious materials. All health care institutions should ensure that personal protective equipment and instructions for their use are provided to all employees (Meeker and Rothrock, 1995; Soule, Larson, and Preston, 1995).

GUIDELINES

1. Incorporate the principles of surgical asepsis when conducting any sterile procedure.
2. Use barrier techniques to decrease the transmission of **microorganisms** from health care personnel to the client.
3. Always assess the client's potential for infection before choosing the barrier to be used, for example, masks, caps, etc.
4. Always review your facility's policies and procedures before conducting a sterile procedure.
5. Remember that hand washing is essential before initiating any sterile procedure.
6. Always follow standard precautions with all clients.

DELEGATION CONSIDERATIONS

The skills of surgical asepsis can be delegated to unlicensed assistive personnel. However, procedures performed under sterile technique may not be delegated. It is the nurse's responsibility to determine what can be delegated:

- Instruct and observe techniques by unlicensed assistive personnel.
- Review procedures for aseptic techniques, stressing adherence to essential steps.

SKILL 34-1 Donning and Removing Cap and Mask

Although masks and caps are usually worn in the OR or labor and delivery areas, there are certain surgical aseptic procedures performed at a client's bedside that might require these barriers. For example, it may be a facility's policy for a nurse to wear a mask during the changing of a central line dressing. Other polices might require that a nurse wear a mask and a cap to secure hair during dressing changes on a client with extensive burns. The nurse should assess the client's potential for acquiring an infection before applying a mask (e.g., does the client have a large open wound, does the nurse have a respiratory infection). If a mask is worn, it should be changed if it becomes moist or soiled (e.g., splattered with blood). Nurses may choose to wear a surgical cap to secure loose hair that might contaminate a sterile area (Meeker and Rothrock, 1995). As in all situations that require protection from splatters from blood or body fluid, the nurse should follow standard precautions and wear personal protective equipment such as eyewear, a mask, and a gown.

EQUIPMENT

- Mask (different types are available for people with different skin sensitivities)
- Paper surgical cap (NOTE: use only if hospital policy requires or use to secure hair if there is a possibility of contamination of a sterile field)
- Hairpins, rubber bands, or both

STEPS	RATIONALE
ASSESSMENT	
1. Consider type of sterile procedure to be performed and consult facility's policy for use of mask and/or caps.	Not all sterile procedures require mask or cap.
2. If you have symptoms of a cold or respiratory infection, either avoid participating in procedure or apply a mask.	A greater number of pathogenic microorganisms reside within respiratory tract when infection is present.
3. Assess the client's potential for infection when choosing barriers for surgical asepsis.	Some clients may be at a greater risk for acquiring an infection.

NURSING DIAGNOSIS

Clustering of defining characteristics from the assessment data may reveal the following nursing diagnosis for clients requiring this skill:

➤ Risk for infection

Related factors are individualized based on a client's condition or needs.

STEPS	RATIONALE
PLANNING	
1. **Expected outcomes** following completion of procedure:	
➤ Client will not develop signs of localized infection.	Indicates the lack of microorganism transfer to the client and sterile field.
2. Prepare equipment.	Ensures availability before the procedure.
IMPLEMENTATION	
1. DONNING CAP	
a. If hair is long, comb back behind shoulders and arrange on crown of head.	Cap must cover all hair entirely.
b. Secure hair in place with pins.	Long hair should not fall down or cause cap to slip and expose hair.
c. Apply cap over head as you would apply hairnet. Be sure all hair fits under cap's edges (see illustration).	Loose hair hanging over sterile field may result in contamination of objects on field.

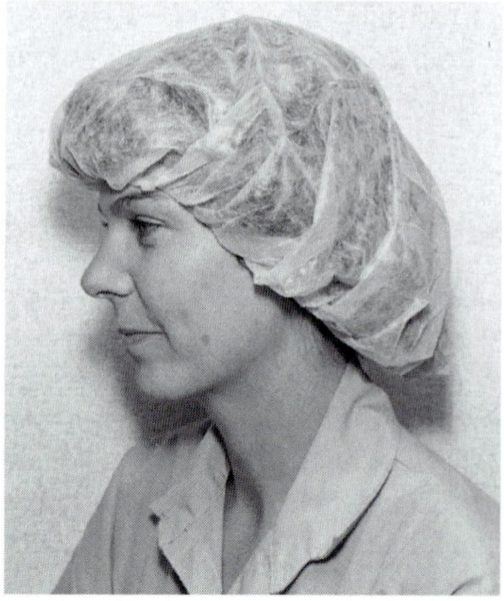

Step 1c

STEPS	RATIONALE
2. DONNING MASK	
a. Find top edge of mask (usually has a thin metal strip along edge).	Pliable metal fits snugly against bridge of nose.
b. Hold mask by top two strings or loops, keeping top edge above bridge of nose.	Prevents contact of hands with clean facial portion of mask. Mask will cover all of nose.
c. Tie two top strings at top of back of head, with strings above ears (see illustration).	Position of ties at top of head provides tight fit. Ties over ears may cause irritation.
d. Tie two lower ties snugly around neck with mask well under chin (see illustration).	Prevents escape of microorganisms through sides of mask as nurse talks and breathes.
e. Gently pinch upper metal band around bridge of nose.	Prevents microorganisms from escaping around nose.

Step 2c

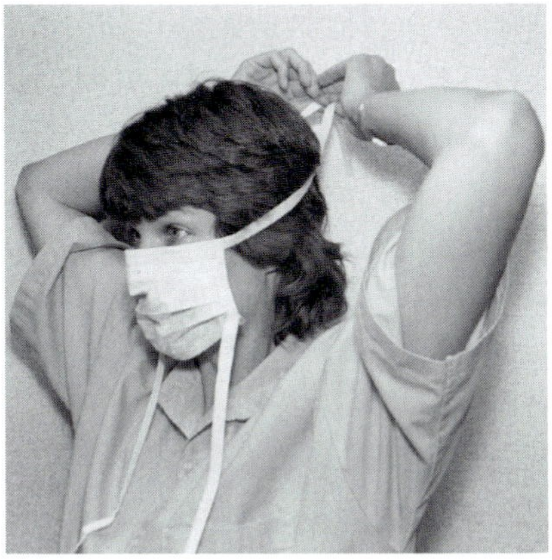

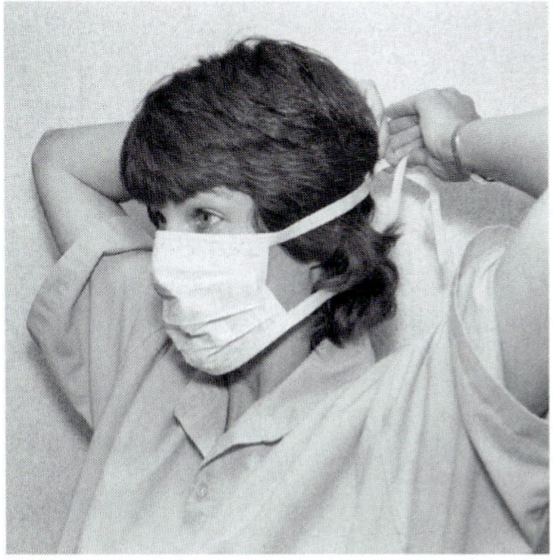

Step 2d

STEPS	RATIONALE
3. DISPOSING OF CAP AND MASK	
a. Untie bottom strings of mask first.	Prevents top part of mask from falling down over nurse's uniform. Contaminated surface of mask could then contaminate uniform.
b. Untie top strings and remove mask from face, holding ties securely (see illustrations).	Avoids contact of nurse's hands with contaminated mask.
c. Grasp outer surface of cap and lift from hair.	Minimizes contact of hands with hair.
d. Discard cap and mask in proper receptacle and wash hands (see illustration).	Reduces transmission of infection.

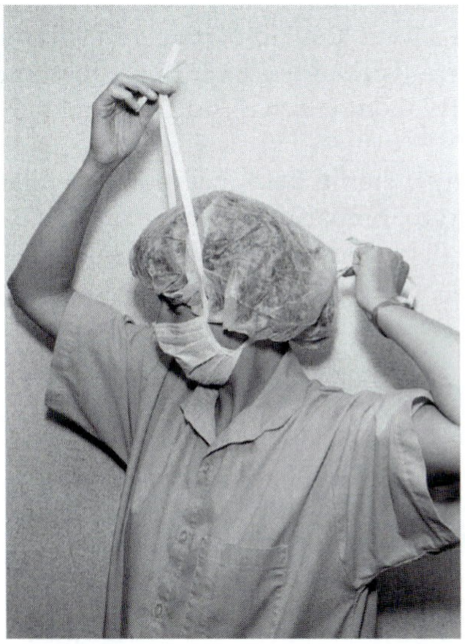

Step 3b(1)

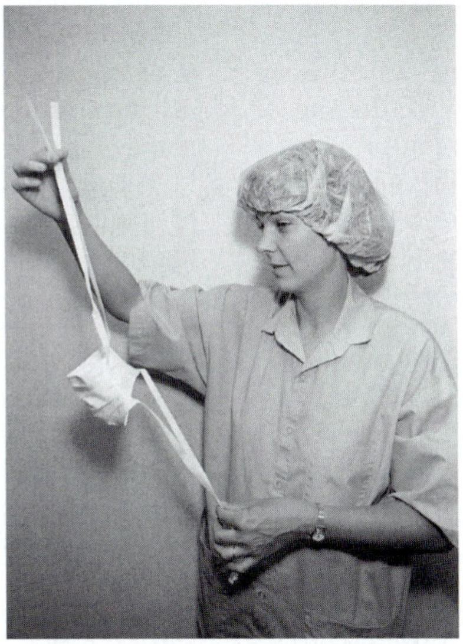

Step 3b(2)

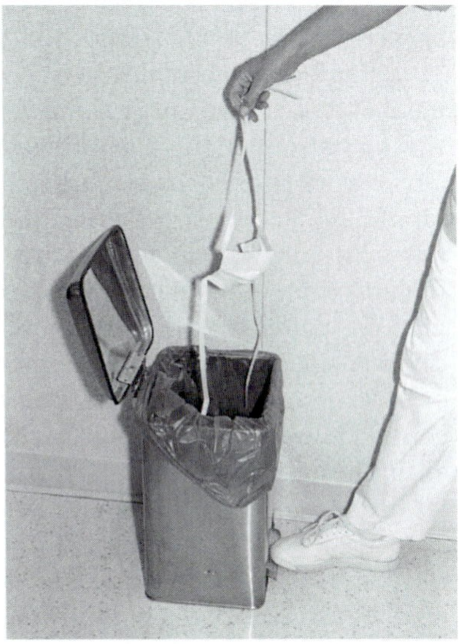

Step 3d

STEPS	RATIONALE
E VALUATION	
1. Following the procedure, assess the surgical site or area of the body treated for drainage, tenderness, edema, or change in temperature or color of skin.	Rules out presence of localized infection.
2. **Unexpected outcomes** that may occur include:	
➤ Redness, heat, edema, pain, or purulent drainage at wound or treatment site.	Indicates possible infection at site.

Recording and Reporting

1. Record procedure performed and client's status, for example, condition of surgical site.	Correct documentation allows nurses to continue to monitor the site for proper healing.

• • • • •

Special Considerations

- ➤ Procedures that usually require cap and mask include major dressing changes, wound debridement, assistance to physician when inserting central line IV catheters, major invasive diagnostic procedures, surgical procedures, and delivery of an infant.
- ➤ When cap is worn, ties fit over cap at top of head.

Teaching Considerations

- ➤ Instruct client and primary care giver to observe site for signs of infection.

SKILL 34-2 Preparing a Sterile Field

When performing sterile aseptic procedures, the nurse must have a work area in which objects can be handled with minimal risk of contamination. A **sterile field** serves such a purpose. It is an area considered free of microorganisms and may consist of a sterile tray or a surface draped with a sterile towel or wrapper (Crow, Planchock, and Hendrick, 1995).

A sterile drape establishes a sterile field around a treatment site, such as a surgical incision, venipuncture site, or site for introduction of a catheter. The drape provides a larger work surface for placing sterile supplies and for manipulating items with sterile gloves. It also allows the nurse to manipulate body parts underlying the drape without contaminating sterile gloves. Drapes are available in cloth, paper, and plastic. They may be wrapped in individual sterile packages or be included within sterile kits or trays. Many styles, shapes, and sizes are available to accommodate different areas or body parts to be covered. For example, a fenestrated drape has a slitlike hole in the center used to cover the perineal area during urinary catheter insertion.

Many sterile items come prepackaged within containers that serve as both sterile fields and work areas for the nurse. For example, bladder catheterization kits and tracheal suction kits contain sterile items that can be moved within the tray and containers into which sterile solutions can be poured. It is the responsibility of the nurse to monitor the field for contamination potential.

In surgery, there are additional precautions. Any unsterile member needs to stay at least 1 foot from the field. All sterile members should consider the field sterile at tabletop level only or inside a 5 cm (2 inch) border if the drape does not cover the entire working surface. Items that are of questionable sterility should be considered contaminated.

The skill of preparing a sterile field incorporates skills of opening sterile packages, preparing a sterile drape, adding sterile supplies to a field, and pouring sterile solutions.

EQUIPMENT

- Sterile gloves
- Sterile water-repellent drapes
- Sterile water-repellent gown (see facility's policy)
- Proper scrub attire (see facility's policy)
- Disposable cap and mask (see facility's policy)
- Sterile supplies and solutions specific to the procedure
- Waist-high table
- Protective eyewear

STEPS	RATIONALE
ASSESSMENT	
1. Verify that the procedure requires surgical aseptic technique.	Some procedures require medical rather than surgical aseptic technique.
2. Assess client's comfort, oxygen requirements, and elimination needs before preparing for procedure.	Certain procedures for which sterile field is prepared may last a long time. The nurse anticipates client's needs so that client can relax and avoid any unnecessary movement that might disrupt procedure.
➤ ***CRITICAL DECISION POINT*** **Position client for maximum comfort and ease of breathing.**	
3. Check sterile package integrity for punctures, tears, discoloration, moisture, or any other signs of contamination. If using commercially packaged supplies or if the facility's policy dictates, check for outdates. NOTE: Some facilities use event rather than time for outdates.	
4. Anticipate number and variety of supplies needed for procedure.	Not all sterile kits contain sufficient amounts or types of supplies. Failure to have necessary supplies causes nurse to leave sterile field, increasing risk of contamination.

NURSING DIAGNOSIS

Clustering of defining characteristics from the assessment data may reveal the following nursing diagnosis for clients requiring this skill:

➤ Risk for infection

Related factors are individualized based on a client's condition or needs.

STEPS	RATIONALE
PLANNING	
1. **Expected outcomes** following completion of procedure:	
➤ The client will not develop signs of infection.	Indicates the lack of microorganism transfer to the client and sterile field.
2. Prepare equipment at bedside.	Ensures availability before the procedure and prevents break in sterile technique. (Note that povidone-iodine and chlorhexidine are not considered sterile solutions and require separate work surfaces for prepping.)
3. Position client comfortably for specific procedure to be performed. If a body part is to be examined or treated, position client so part is accessible.	Client should be able to lie still in one position comfortably during procedure. Movement can cause contamination of sterile items.
4. Explain to client purpose of procedure and importance of sterile technique.	Ensures client's ability to cooperate. Teaching before procedure eliminates need to talk during procedure, which can cause air-droplet contamination of sterile area.
IMPLEMENTATION	
1. Apply cap, mask, and/or gown (may be optional; consult facility's policy, may need to include protective eyewear).	Controls spread of airborne microorganisms.
2. Select a clean, flat, dry work surface above waist level.	A sterile object below a person's waist is contaminated.
3. Wash hands thoroughly (the decision whether to use a soap or antiseptic depends on the procedure).	Reduces transmission of infection.

STEPS	RATIONALE
PREPARING STERILE WORK SURFACE	
1. Place sterile kit or package containing sterile items on clean, flat work surface above waist level.	Items placed below waist level are considered contaminated.
2. Open sterile kit or package containing sterile items.	
a. Sterile commercially packaged kit:	
(1) Remove kit from dust cover; place on surface.	
(2) Grasp outer surface of tip of outermost flap.	Outer surface of package is considered unsterile. There is a 2.5 cm (1 inch) border around any sterile drape or wrap that is considered contaminated.
(3) Open outermost flap away from body, keeping arm outstretched and away from sterile field (see illustration).	Reaching over sterile field contaminates it.
(4) Grasp outside surface of edge of first side flap.	Outer border is considered unsterile.
(5) Open side flap pulling to side, allowing it to lie flat on table surface. Keep your arm to side and not over sterile surface (see illustration).	Drape or wrapper should lie flat so it will not accidentally rise up and contaminate inner surface or sterile contents.
(6) Repeat steps for second side flap (see illustration).	
(7) Grasp outside border of last and innermost flap (see illustration).	Outer border is considered unsterile.
(8) Stand away from sterile package and pull flap back, allowing it to fall flat on table (see illustration).	Never reach over a sterile field.
b. Sterile linen-wrapped package: Remove tape seal and unwrap both layers as with the kit above (see illustration).	Linen-wrapped items have two layers. The first is a dust cover. The second layer must be opened to view the chemical indicator. If the item is dropped on the floor, it is considered contaminated.
(1) Use opened kit or package wrapper as sterile field.	Inner surface of kit and wrapper are considered sterile.

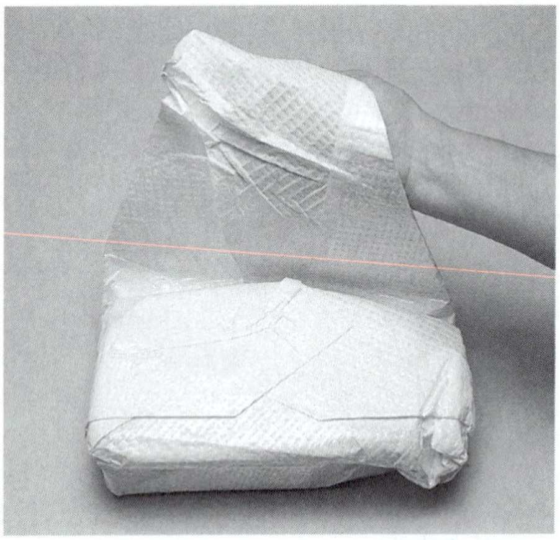

Step 2a(3)

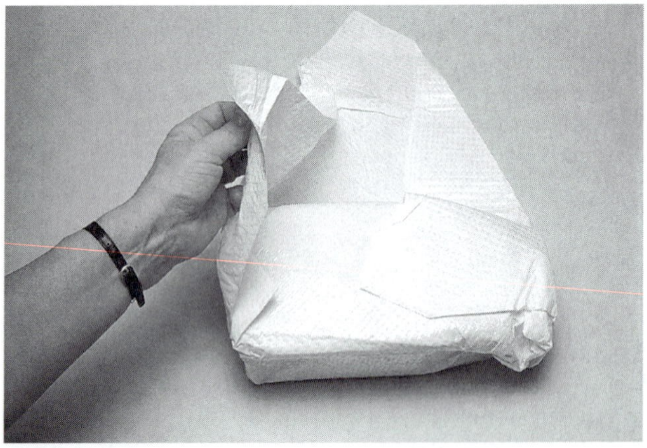

Step 2a(5)

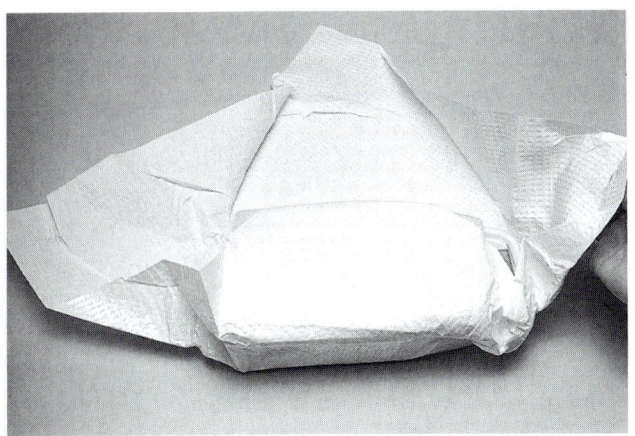

Step 2a(6)

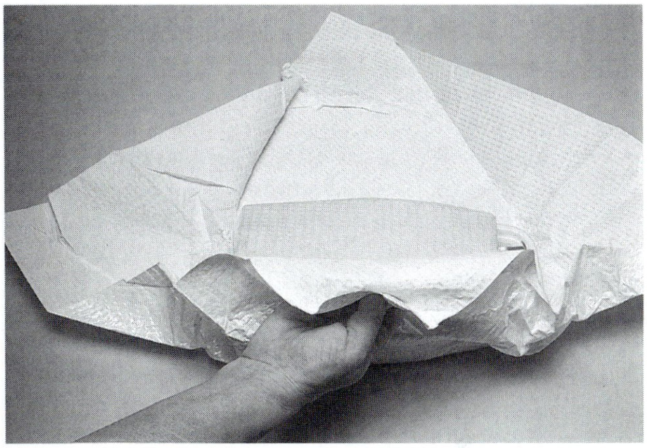

Step 2a(7)

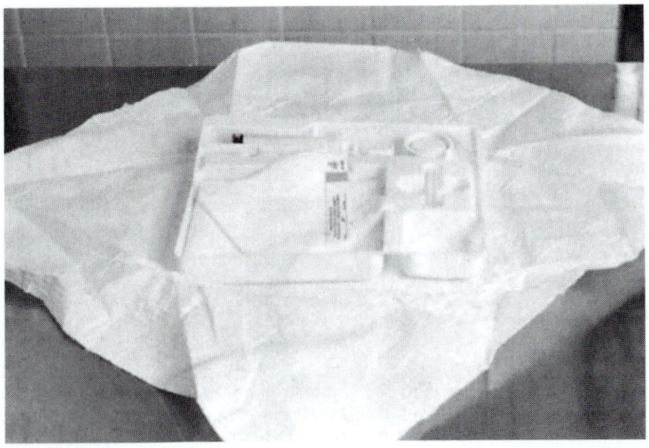

Step 2a(8)

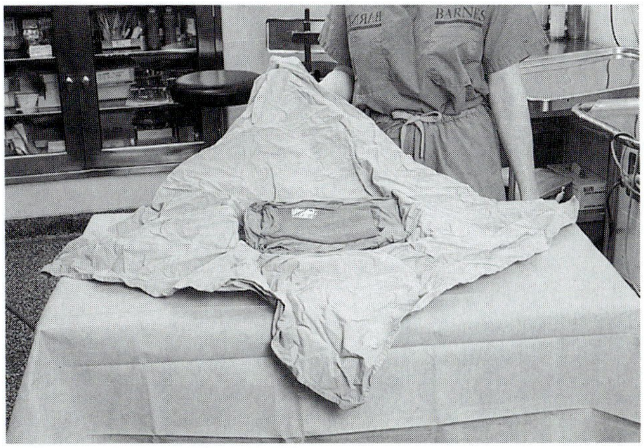

Step 2b

STEPS	RATIONALE
PREPARING A STERILE DRAPE *(This technique may be optional but is useful when a large work surface is desirable.)*	
1. Place pack containing sterile drape on flat surface and open as described (Step 2a, p. 1010) for package.	Ensures sterility of packaged drape.
2. Don sterile gloves and/or sterile gown (see Chapter 36).	Only sterile members may contact sterile items.
3. Grasp folded top edge of drape with the fingertips of one hand. Gently lift the drape up from its wrapper without touching any object (see illustration).	If a sterile object touches any nonsterile object, it becomes contaminated.
4. Allow drape to unfold, keeping it above the waist and away from the body. (Discard wrapper with the other hand.)	Drape can now be properly placed using two hands. Drape must be held away from unsterile surfaces.
5. With other hand, grasp adjacent corner of drape, holding it straight (see illustration).	Drape can now be properly placed with two hands.
6. Holding the drape, first position the bottom half over the top half of intended work surface (see illustration).	Prevents nurse from reaching over sterile field.
7. Then allow the top half of the drape to be placed over the bottom half of the work surface (see illustration).	Creates flat sterile work surface.
8. Option—gowned nurse should place top half of the drape over the work surface first.	Sterile objects may cross over sterile fields. The nurse is also shielded from an unsterile area.
ADDING STERILE ITEMS	
1. Open the sterile item (following package directions) while holding the outside wrapper in the nondominant hand.	Frees dominant hand for unwrapping outer wrapper.
2. Carefully peel the wrapper onto the nondominant hand.	Item remains sterile. Inner surface of wrapper covers hand, making it sterile.

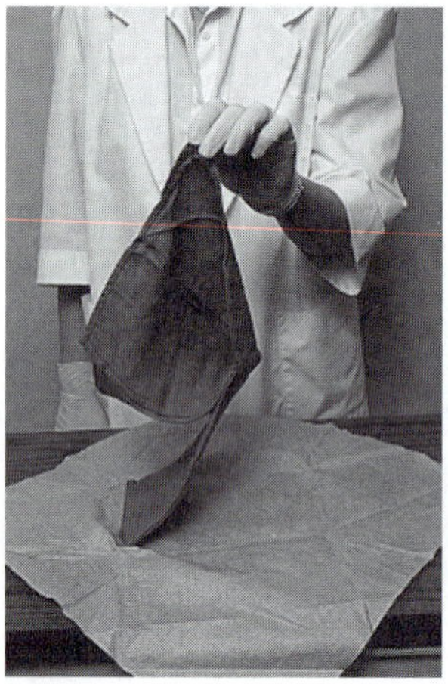

Step 3

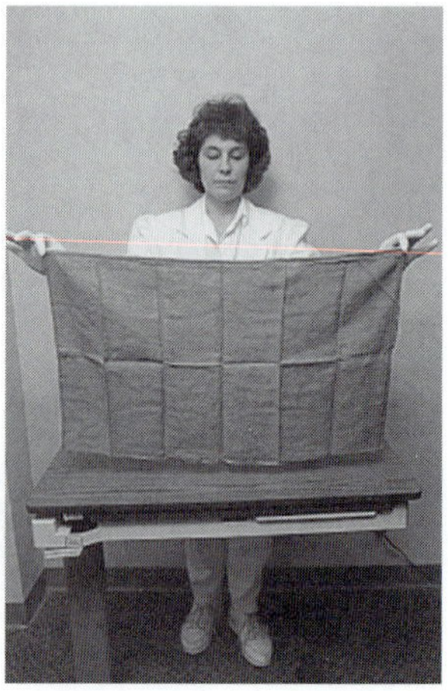

Step 5

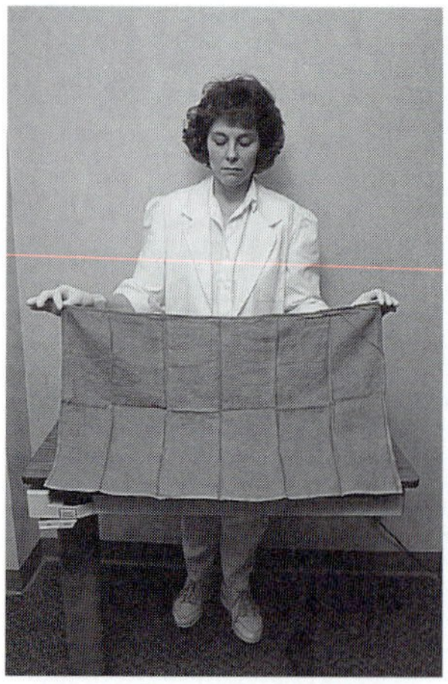

Step 6

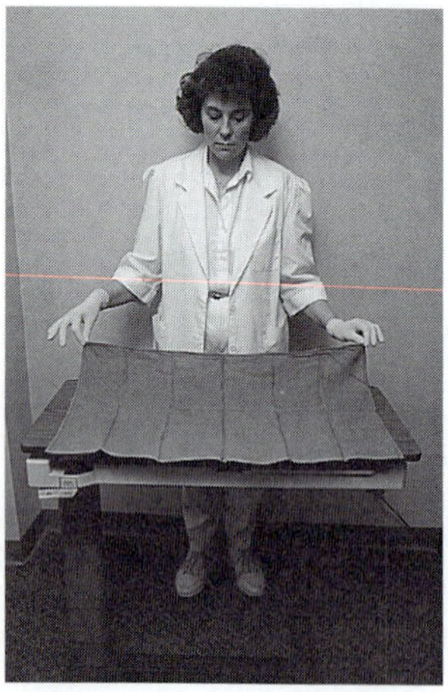

Step 7

STEPS	RATIONALE
3. Being sure the wrapper does not fall down on the sterile field, place the item onto the field at an angle (see illustration). Do not hold arm over the sterile field.	Prevents reaching over field and contaminating its surface.
CRITICAL DECISION POINT **Do not flip or throw objects onto a sterile field.**	
4. Dispose of outer wrapper.	Prevents accidental contamination of sterile field.

POURING STERILE SOLUTIONS

STEPS	RATIONALE
1. Verify contents and expiration date of the solution.	Ensures proper solution and sterility of contents.
2. Remove seal and cap from bottle in an upward motion.	Prevents contamination of the bottle lip.
3. With edge of bottle held away from edge and above inside of sterile receiving container, slowly pour solution (see illustration).	Edge of bottle is considered contaminated. Slow pouring prevents splashing that can contaminate underlying sterile field.
4. Discard any remaining fluid and bottle.	Surplus solution on the outer edge contaminates the lip of the bottle when it is brought upright.

EVALUATION

STEPS	RATIONALE
1. Assess the wound site or treated area for edema, drainage, change in temperature or color.	Rules out presence of localized infection.
2. **Unexpected outcomes** that may occur include:	
➤ Redness, heat, edema, pain, or purulent drainage at treatment site.	Indicates infection at site.

RECORDING AND REPORTING

STEPS	RATIONALE
1. Record area and description of treatment site.	Correct documentation allows nurses to continue to monitor the site for proper healing.

• • • • •

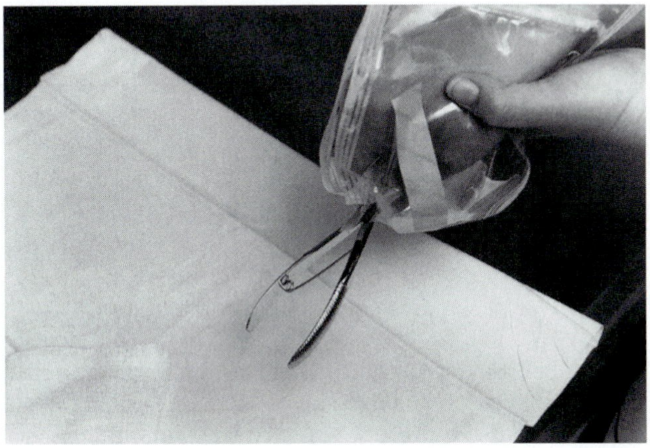

Step 3 Adding item to sterile field.

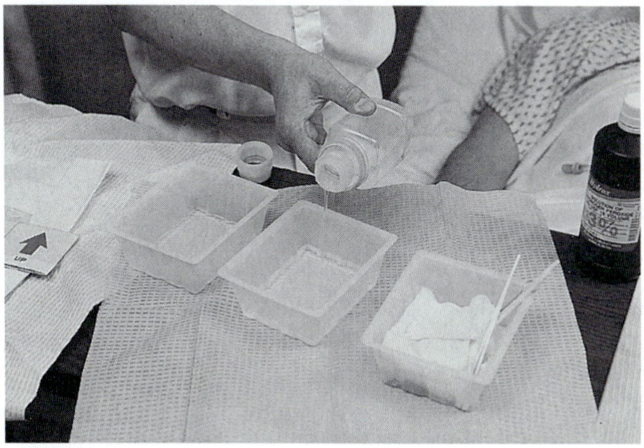

Step 3 Pouring sterile solution.

Special Considerations

- It is always helpful to have another nurse stand by to offer assistance and collect supplies should you overlook an item.
- Many sterile kits have cups or plastic molded sections into which fluids can be poured.
- The sealed edge of peel-packed items is considered contaminated.
- In the OR, sterile items that cannot be safely transferred to a sterile field should be handed to the sterile team member
- When liquids permeate the sterile field or barrier, it is called "strike through," resulting in contamination.
- The most common methods of sterilization are by steam and ethylene oxide. The chemical indicators should reflect the appropriate methods of sterilization.

Teaching Considerations

- Instruct client and primary care giver to observe site for signs of infection.
- Instruct client and primary care giver on further wound and dressing care.

Home Care Considerations

- In the home setting, most care will be performed in a clean environment. In the event that a sterile environment is ordered, the client and family need to be aware of the principles that apply to the sterile environment. For example, the family can be taught how to correctly use the package wrapper as a sterile drape/barrier when applying a sterile dressing, or the family can be taught the correct procedure for removing a sterile item from a package without contaminating the item.
- Assess the client's and family's understanding and ability to provide a sterile environment when needed to perform a specific procedure.

SKILL 34-3 Open Gloving

Gloves help prevent the transmission of pathogens by direct and indirect contact. Nurses apply sterile gloves before performing sterile procedures such as inserting urinary catheters, changing dressings on central IV catheters, or applying sterile dressings. It is important to select the proper-sized glove. The gloves should not stretch so tightly over the fingers that they can easily tear, yet they should be tight enough that objects can be picked up easily. Gloves are made in whole and half sizes, such as sizes 6, 6½, and 7. It is important to choose not only the right size of glove but also the correct material. For example, many clients and health care workers have known allergies to latex (*APIC infection control and applied epidemiology,* 1996). For those individuals, it is important to choose latex-free gloves. Studies have shown that for individuals who are highly sensitive to latex, local and/or systemic reactions occur when someone in close proximity removes a pair of latex gloves and the latex glove powder particles are suspended in the air (Beezhold et al., 1994).

Once gloves are applied, the nurse should always be conscious of the position of the hands during procedures. If a sterile glove touches a clean, a contaminated, or a questionably contaminated object, it becomes unsterile. It is helpful to interlock the fingers and hold the hands together in front of the body while waiting to handle sterile items. If a tear develops in a sterile glove, the nurse applies a new glove immediately.

EQUIPMENT

- **Package of proper-sized sterile gloves; latex or latex-free**

STEPS	RATIONALE
ASSESSMENT	
1. Consider the type of procedure to be performed and consult institutional policy on use of gloves.	Ensures proper use of gloves when needed.
2. Consider client's risk for infection—for example, preexisting condition, and size or extent of area being treated.	Directs nurse to follow added precautions if necessary.
3. Examine glove package to determine if it is dry and intact.	Torn or wet package is considered contaminated.
4. Inspect condition of hands for cuts, open lesions, or abrasions.	Lesions harbor microorganisms and should be covered with an impervious dressing. When strict surgical asepsis is used, presence of such lesions may prevent nurse from participating in procedure.
5. Assess if the client has a known latex allergy before donning latex gloves.	

STEPS | **RATIONALE**

NURSING DIAGNOSIS

Clustering of defining characteristics from the assessment data may reveal the following nursing diagnoses for clients requiring this skill:

➤ Risk for infection
➤ Risk for injury

Related factors are individualized based on a client's condition or needs.

PLANNING

1. **Expected outcomes** following completion of procedure:
   - ➤ Client will not develop signs or symptoms of infection after procedure.
     Rationale: Indicates microorganisms not introduced into sterile body cavities or sites (such as skin or urinary tract).
   - ➤ Client with history of allergy will not be exposed to latex.
2. Select correct size and type of gloves.
   Rationale: There is less chance of contamination if correct size of gloves is worn.

CRITICAL DECISION POINT Remember to assess if client has a latex allergy before donning latex gloves.

CRITICAL DECISION POINT Unpowdered latex-free gloves should be worn if client or health care worker has a latex allergy.

3. Place glove package near work area.
   Rationale: Ensures availability before procedure.

IMPLEMENTATION

GLOVE APPLICATION

1. Perform thorough hand washing.
   Rationale: Reduces the number of bacteria on skin surfaces and reduces transmission of infection.
2. Remove outer glove package wrapper by carefully separating and peeling apart sides (see illustration).
   Rationale: Prevents inner glove package from accidentally opening and touching contaminated objects.
3. Grasp inner package and lay it on clean, flat surface just above waist level. Open package, keeping gloves on wrapper's inside surface (see illustration).
   Rationale: Sterile object held below waist is contaminated. Inner surface of glove package is sterile.
4. If gloves are not prepowdered, take packet of powder and apply lightly to hands over sink or wastebasket.
   Rationale: Powder allows gloves to slip on easily. (Some staff members do not use powder for fear of promoting growth of microorganisms.)
5. Identify right and left glove. Each glove has cuff approximately 5 cm (2 inches) wide. Glove dominant hand first. (In illustrations left hand is dominant.)
   Rationale: Proper identification of gloves prevents contamination by improper fit. Gloving of dominant hand first improves dexterity.

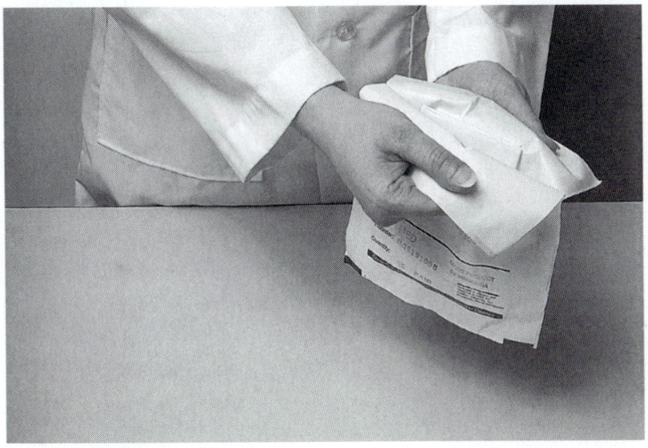

Step 2

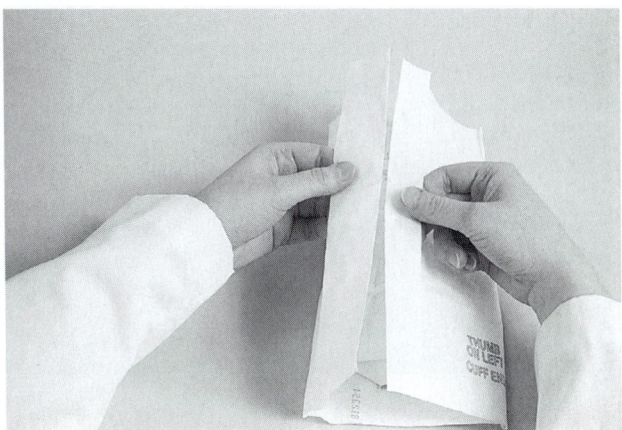

Step 3

STEPS	RATIONALE
6. With thumb and first two fingers of nondominant hand, grasp edge of cuff of glove for dominant hand. Touch only glove's inside surface (see illustration).	Inner edge of cuff will lie against skin and thus is not sterile.
7. Carefully pull glove over dominant hand, leaving cuff and being sure cuff does not roll up wrist. Be sure thumb and fingers are in proper spaces (see illustration).	If glove's outer surface touches hand or wrist, it is contaminated.
8. With gloved dominant hand, slip fingers underneath second glove's cuff (see illustration).	Cuff protects gloved fingers. Sterile touching sterile prevents glove contamination.
9. Carefully pull second glove over nondominant hand.	Contact of gloved hand with exposed hand results in contamination.

CRITICAL DECISION POINT **Do not allow fingers and thumb of gloved dominant hand to touch any part of exposed nondominant hand. Keep thumb of dominant hand abducted back.**

10. After second glove is on, interlock hands together. The cuffs usually fall down after application. Be sure to touch only sterile sides (see illustration).	Ensures smooth fit over fingers.

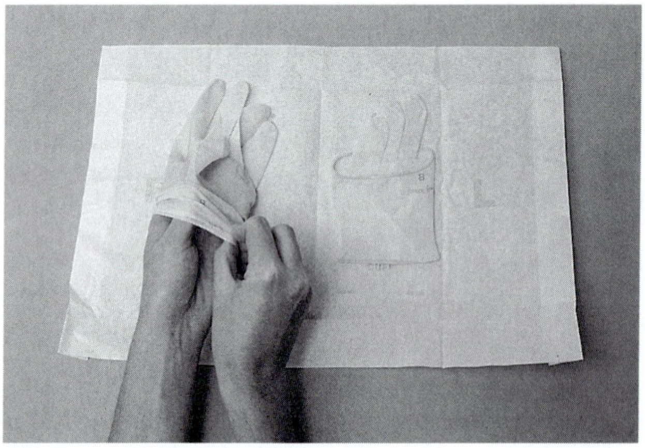

Step 6

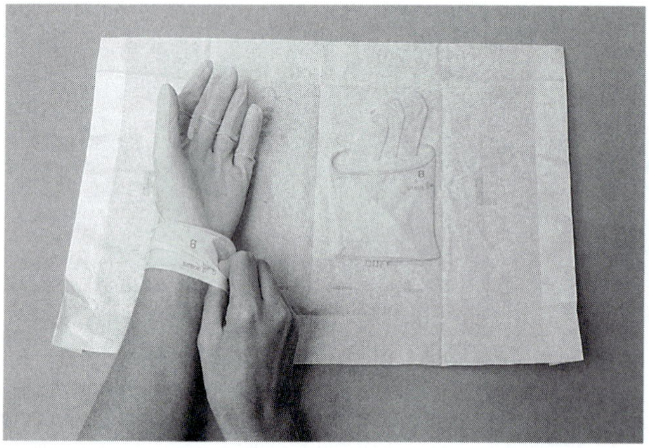

Step 7

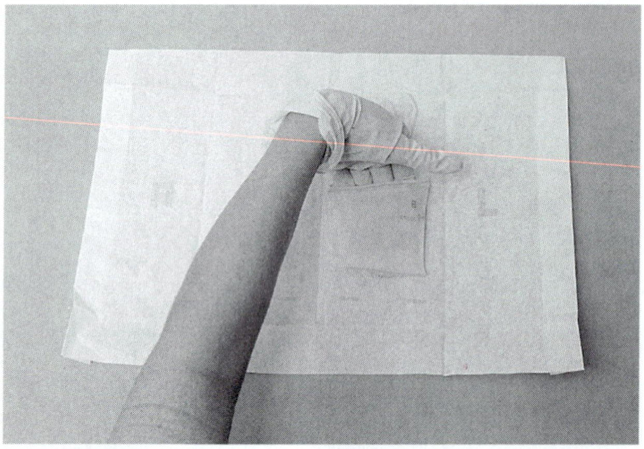

Step 8

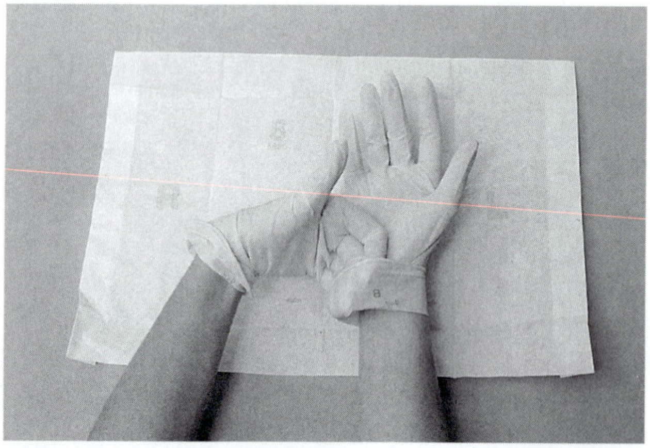

Step 10

STEPS	RATIONALE
GLOVE DISPOSAL	
1. Grasp outside of one cuff with other gloved hand; avoid touching wrist.	Minimizes contamination of underlying skin.
2. Pull glove off, turning it inside out. Discard in receptacle.	Outside of glove does not touch skin surface.
3. Take fingers of bare hand and tuck inside remaining glove cuff. Peel glove off inside out.	Discard in receptacle.
4. Wash hands thoroughly.	This protects the health care worker from any unseen tears or pinholes in the gloves, also removing the powder from the hands helps to prevent skin irritations.
EVALUATION	
1. Assess client for signs of infection, focusing on area treated.	Improper technique may contribute to the development of an infection.
2. **Unexpected outcomes** that may occur include:	
➤ Development of localized signs of infection—for example, urine becomes cloudy or odorous; wound becomes painful, edematous, reddened with purulent drainage.	Local infection, result of microorganism infecting normally sterile body sites.
➤ Development of systemic signs of infection—for example, fever, malaise, increased white blood cell count.	Infectious microorganism enters the bloodstream to cause systemic infection.
➤ Development of local latex allergy.	
RECORDING AND REPORTING	
1. Record procedure performed and client's response and status.	Documentation establishes a baseline for later comparison if client's condition changes.

CRITICAL THINKING EXERCISES

1. In the middle of a sterile procedure on the nursing division, you discover that a sterile item is missing. What are your options for obtaining the item?
2. A prepackaged item has a dry brown spot on the paper side. Is it sterile?
3. Why is it inappropriate to touch the mask when removing it from your face?
4. The nurse enters the client's room to begin a series of procedures: measurement of urine for intake and output, irrigation of a nasogastric tube, insertion of a urinary catheter, and measurement of the client's blood pressure. Which procedure requires use of sterile gloves?

REFERENCES

APIC infection control and applied epidemiology, St Louis, 1996, Mosby.

Beezold D, Kostyol D, and Wiseman J: The transfer of protein allergens from latex gloves, *AORN J,* 59(30), 1994:605-613.

Centers for Disease Control and Prevention, Hospital Infection Control Practice Advisory Committee: Guidelines for isolation precautions in hospitals, *AJIC* 24:24, 1996.

Crow S, Planchock N, Hendrick E: Antisepsis: disinfection and sterilization. In Soule B, Larson E, Preston G, editors: *Infections and nursing practices,* St Louis, 1995, Mosby.

Meeker MH, Rothrock JC: *Alexander's care of the patient in surgery,* ed 10, St Louis, 1995, Mosby.

Occupational Safety and Health Administration: Occupational exposure to blood-borne pathogens: final rule, 29 CFR 1919:1030, *Fed Regis* 56:64003, 1991.

Roth A: Infection prevention in the operating room, *Asepsis* 18(1):12, 1996.

Soule B, Larson E, and Preston G: *Infection and nursing practices,* St Louis, 1995, Mosby.

UNIT XII

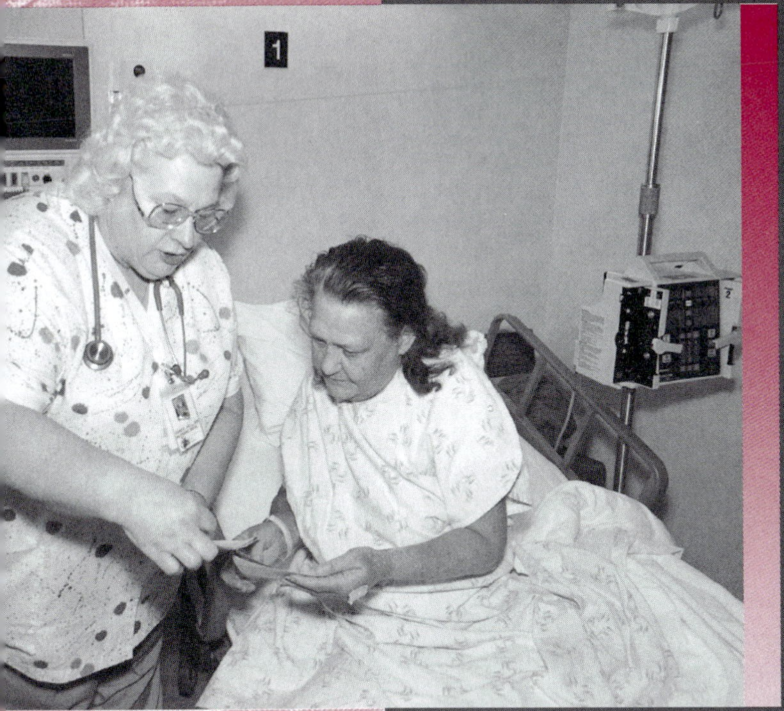

Care of the Surgical Client

CHAPTER 35

Preoperative and Postoperative Care

OBJECTIVES

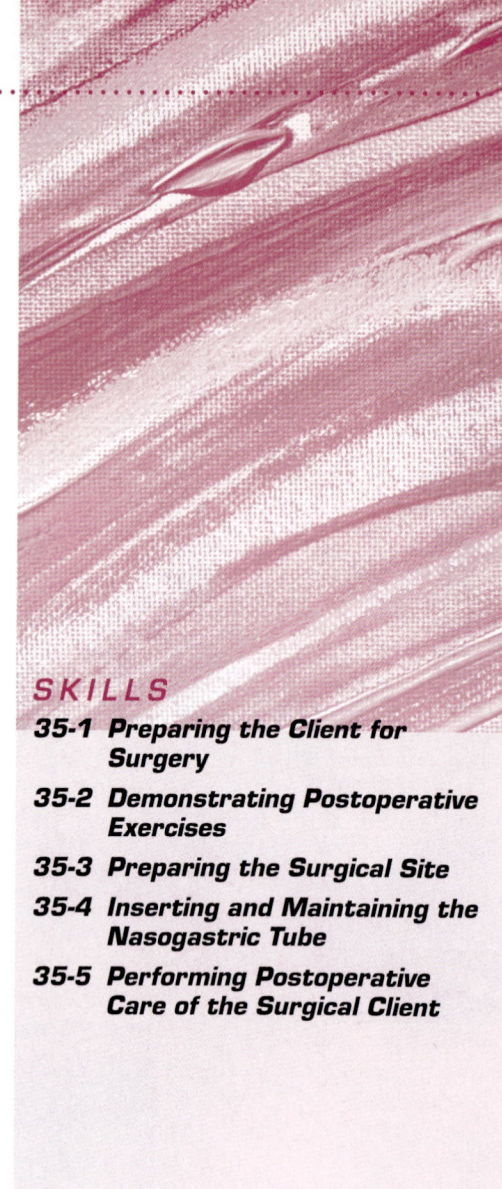

Mastery of content in this chapter will enable the nurse to:

- Define key terms.
- Describe the activities needed to prepare a client for surgery.
- Explain the rationale for preoperative procedures.
- Adequately prepare a client for surgery.
- Describe the benefits of structured preoperative teaching.
- Explain the rationale for each of the four postoperative exercises.
- Successfully instruct a client in performing postoperative exercises.
- Identify the benefits and risks associated with shaving a surgical site.
- Correctly prepare a surgical site.
- Describe purposes for nasogastric tube insertion.
- Correctly insert, check placement, irrigate, and discontinue a nasogastric tube.
- Discuss the differences in nursing assessment during the immediate postoperative period and the convalescent phase of recovery.
- Conduct an assessment of a postoperative client.

KEY TERMS

Anesthesia
Aspiration
Atelectasis
Decompression
Dehiscence
Hypovolemic shock
Paralytic ileus
Postoperative
Preoperative

SKILLS

35-1 Preparing the Client for Surgery
35-2 Demonstrating Postoperative Exercises
35-3 Preparing the Surgical Site
35-4 Inserting and Maintaining the Nasogastric Tube
35-5 Performing Postoperative Care of the Surgical Client

Any form of surgery is a stressful event, whether it is a major surgical procedure occurring in a large medical center or a minor procedure taking place in an outpatient center. The client must frequently make the decision to undergo a procedure that is associated with pain, possible disfigurement, dependence, or even the threat of death. Physiologically, the more complex the surgery, the more likely a client will undergo changes in most major body systems. The nurse uses a variety of skills to help the surgical client adequately prepare for the physiological and psychological stressors that surgery imposes.

During the **preoperative** phase the nurse performs a thorough assessment of the client's physical and emotional status. Coordination of a variety of diagnostic tests ensures that the surgeon has the information needed to determine the client's risks during surgery. In preparation for surgery, the nurse instructs the client in **postoperative** exercises so that the client can actively participate in the recovery process. Certain procedures, such as surgical skin preparation or the insertion of an indwelling catheter or nasogastric (NG) tube, may be performed to protect the client from risks associated with surgery. The nurse also communicates pertinent information to all members of the health care team so that the client receives the comprehensive, holistic care required.

During the postoperative phase, when the client returns from the operating room (OR), the nurse is initially responsible for assessing the client's physical status to monitor any changes during the recovery process. Once the client's condition stabilizes, the nurse focuses efforts on returning the client to a functional level of wellness as soon as possible within the limitations created by surgery. The speed of a client's recovery depends on how effectively the nurse can anticipate potential complications, initiate necessary supportive and preventive therapies, and actively involve the client and family in the recovery process. Each client's plan of care is individualized to provide an improved state of wellness and to maximize an ultimate level of independence.

GUIDELINES

1. Know the type and nature of any previous surgery. Anatomical and physiological alterations may affect the client's health care needs.
2. Identify the factors and conditions that may increase a client's risks during surgery. Preoperative preparation and postoperative care depend upon these risks.
3. Know the rationale for and extent of impending surgery. Each type of surgical procedure requires a different type of nursing care.
4. Administer pain relief therapies according to the client's needs postoperatively. Pain can slow the surgical client's recovery.
5. Encourage the client's independence as soon as possible during the postoperative period. This minimizes the occurrence of postoperative complications.
6. Anticipate how surgery will affect the client's ability to return home to a functional lifestyle. Early discharge planning, client education, referral to community resources, and rehabilitation measures are needed to prepare the client to return home.
7. Identify cultural and religious beliefs and practices that may impact clients' and family members' reactions to the surgical experience, such as transfusions and disposal of body parts.

SKILL 35-1 Preparing the Client for Surgery

Preparing the client for surgery involves activities and procedures that help to decrease anxiety, to ensure client safety, and to decrease the risks of complications. A thorough nursing assessment is needed to document baseline data for future comparisons, to determine teaching needs, and to identify clients at risk for complications during the perioperative experience.

Anxiety can interfere with the effectiveness of **anesthesia** and the ability of clients to actively participate in their care. Providing information to clients about what will occur during the perioperative experience, as well as what sensations the client can expect to feel, will help to decrease anxiety. Demonstration of a caring attitude to the client, family members, and significant others can increase feelings of trust and reduce anxiety (Fig. 35-1). Sedatives are frequently prescribed to inpatients to aid in sleep the night before surgery, and preoperative medications are administered the day of surgery to promote relaxation.

Client safety is ensured through a number of interventions and activities. Informed consent is required by law to help protect clients' rights, their autonomy, and their privacy. Failure to obtain informed consent may result in charges of "assault and battery or negligence" (Brick, 1996) being brought against the health care providers. The cli-

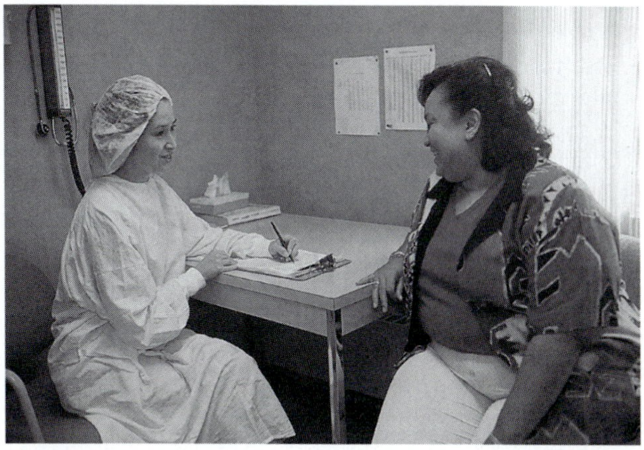

Fig. 35-1 Before beginning the assessment, the nurse establishes a trusting relationship with the client.

ent is provided information by the surgeon about the extent and type of surgery, alternative therapies, and usual risks and benefits. A consent form that includes this information must be signed by the client or the client's legal guardian and the surgeon. It must also be signed by a witness to verify that the client has been provided the required information. It is the nurse's responsibility, acting as the client's advocate, to ensure that the client understands the information and that the form has been signed and witnessed prior to the client receiving preoperative medication. Client safety is also promoted by restricting activity after administration of sedatives and by completion of a preoperative checklist to ensure that all procedures have been carried out.

The risks for postoperative complications are decreased in a number of ways, some of which are specific to the type of procedure. For example, any client with a surgical incision of the upper abdomen or thorax will be encouraged to use an incentive spirometer postoperatively to reduce the incidence of **atelectasis.** Skin preparation and coughing and deep breathing exercises are examples of other procedures used to reduce complications. Food and fluids are usually withheld for 4 to 8 hours prior to surgery requiring general anesthesia. Clients who are dehydrated or are at risk for hypovolemia will have parenteral fluids ordered. Medications may be given to decrease respiratory and gastrointestinal (GI) secretions, as an adjunct to anesthesia, and to decrease the risk of infection and development of stress ulcers. Low-residue and clear liquid diets, enemas, and cathartics are ordered for clients prior to undergoing bowel surgery. Povidone-iodine douches are used prior to many gynecological procedures. Eyedrops may need to be instilled prior to ophthalmic surgery.

Because many clients are admitted on the day of surgery, much of the preoperative preparation is the responsibility of the client or the primary care giver. It is important that the nurse provide adequate instructions both verbally and in writing and that the nurse assess adherence to the instructions on the client's admission to the surgical unit.

EQUIPMENT

- Stethoscope
- Informed consent form
- Preoperative checklist
- Enema set and prescribed solution (if ordered)
- Douche set and prescribed solution (if ordered)
- Intravenous (IV) solutions and equipment (if ordered)
- Indwelling catheter set (if ordered)
- Medications (if ordered)

DELEGATION CONSIDERATIONS

The skills of assessment and teaching that are part of preparing the client for surgery require problem solving and knowledge application unique to a professional nurse. For these skills delegation is inappropriate. Unlicensed assistive personnel may administer an enema or a douche, obtain vital signs, apply antiembolism stockings, and assist clients in removing clothing, jewelry, and prostheses.

- Instruct personnel on proper steps and precautions for delegated procedures.

Table 35-1 Assessment of the Surgical Client

Assessment Category	Key Criteria
Nursing history	Previous experience with surgery and anesthesia Client's and family's perceptions and understanding of surgery Medication history Physical or mental impairments Mobility limitations Prostheses (including hearing aids) Allergies (including latex) Smoking habits Alcohol ingestion Family support and coping mechanisms Occupation Emotional health
Physical examination	Temperature, blood pressure Pulse and respiratory rates Height and weight Oxygen saturation Electrocardiogram Laboratory values Radiology findings General system review: Head and neck Integument Thorax and lungs Heart and vascular Abdomen Neurological status
Risk factors	Age Nutrition Radiotherapy Fluid and electrolyte balance Preexisting infection Chronic respiratory disease (emphysema, bronchitis, asthma) Immunological disorders (leukemia, acquired immunodeficiency syndrome) Allergies (drugs, food, latex)

STEPS	RATIONALE
ASSESSMENT	
1. Determine ability of client to answer questions regarding health history and pending surgery.	Identifies reliability of client and need to supplement with information from family members or significant others. May indicate need for further information for informed consent.
2. Obtain nursing history (Table 35-1).	Provides information regarding risk factors and past patterns of behavior.
3. Perform physical examination (Table 35-1 and see Chapter 11).	Provides baseline data for future assessments and interventions.
CRITICAL DECISION POINT If client is having emergent surgery, assessment will focus on primary body systems affected.	
4. Identify risk factors (Table 35-1).	Allows for anticipation of possible complications and planning for interventions to reduce risks. Allergies, particularly to latex, can be life-threatening.
5. Ask client's and family members' expectations of surgery and the care to be provided.	Allows nurse to anticipate client's priorities and to adapt plan so that appropriate instruction and support can be given.
6. Assess client's preoperative orders.	Identifies specific procedures and diagnostic tests to be done and medications to be given.

NURSING DIAGNOSIS

Clustering of defining characteristics from the assessment data may reveal the following nursing diagnoses for clients requiring this skill:

- Anxiety
- Fear
- Body image disturbance
- Risk for infection
- Risk for ineffective airway clearance
- Risk for ineffective breathing pattern
- Risk for impaired gas exchange
- Pain
- Altered tissue perfusion
- Risk for aspiration
- Impaired physical mobility
- Knowledge deficit regarding the surgical experience
- Risk for impaired skin integrity
- Altered oral mucous membrane
- Risk for perioperative positioning injury

Related factors are individualized based on a client's condition or needs.

STEPS	RATIONALE
PLANNING	
1. **Expected outcomes** following completion of procedure:	
➤ Client can state what surgical procedure is being performed and the risks and benefits of the surgery.	Identifies readiness to sign informed consent.
➤ Client will participate in preoperative and postoperative care.	Preoperative preparations were effective.
➤ Client states anxiety is decreased.	Anxiety may interfere with effectiveness of anesthesia.
2. Prepare client chart with appropriate forms and assemble equipment as needed.	Ensures that all preoperative procedures will be completed.
3. Explain procedures and allow client, family members, and significant others to ask questions.	Decreases anxiety and increases cooperation.
IMPLEMENTATION	
1. Orient client to room or presurgical area.	Decreases anxiety and promotes feelings of control.
2. Check medical record and complete preoperative checklist (see illustration on p. 1024).	Ensures that pertinent laboratory and diagnostic test results are available and that all preoperative preparations are completed.
3. Assist with informed consent. Act as client advocate as needed. Witness form if allowed by agency.	Surgery cannot be legally performed without client receiving information about need and extent of the surgery, alternatives, risks, and benefits. Client may be afraid to ask questions.

A-1c PREOPERATIVE/PREPROCEDURAL CHECKLIST

● File with other A-1c's of same date. ●

PROCEDURE: ______________________________

DATE OF PROCEDURE: ______________________________

1. Place initials in appropriate box: YES, NO, N/A (not applicable, or was not ordered). Each item must have an entry.
2. Explain any "No." This can be done in the space after the item or in the "Comments" section. Use back of form, if needed.
3. To give more information on any item, use the space after the item. If more space needed, use the "Comments" section or back of form.

DATE

HOSP. NO.

NAME

BIRTHDATE

ADDRESS

IF NOT IMPRINTED, PLEASE PRINT DATE, HOSP. NO., NAME AND LOCATION

YES	NO	N/A	
			Special Information (e.g., blind, O_2, combative)
			Preoperative orders written.
			(If "NO", Dr. ______________ notified at ______________ date/time.)
			Consent complete and in medical record.
			Allergies (or NKA) labelled on cover of medical record.
			Specify Allergies:
			Isolation label on cover of medical record. Specify type:
			Ordered lab results in medical record.
			Urinalysis results in medical record.
			Chest x-ray completed. (Report in medical record: Yes ____ No ____)
			EKG in medical record.
			Type and cross/screen (circle) done. Date drawn:
			History and physical in medical record.
			Forms complete and in medical record:
			1. Nursing documentation with assessment, VS, and wt./ht.
			2. IV Solution Administration Cardex.
			3. Medication Administration Cardex.
			Addressograph plate on cover of medical record. All volumes to procedure, if required.

COMMENTS:

YES	NO	N/A	
			Blood band on patient and legible. Specify location ____________ and blood band # ____________
			Identification band on patient and legible. Specify location:
			Bathed and in proper attire.
			Nail polish, makeup, and hairpins removed.
			Jewelry removed. Specify item(s) removed and disposition:
			Prosthesis removed: hearing aid, dentures, eye glasses, contact lenses (circle).
			Other: Disposition:
			Anti-embolism stockings on.
			Sequential compression device sleeves on and controller to OR.
			NPO since:
			Teaching completed and documented.
			Preps/tests completed as ordered. Specify:
			Voided/catheterized (circle). Time:
			Medication(s) given.
			Medication(s)/article(s) sent with patient. Specify:

COMMENTS:

Date	Initials	Signature and Title of Individuals Filling Out Form

Date	Initials	Signature of RN Sending Patient to Procedure

41006/4-93/H7528 THE UNIVERSITY OF IOWA HOSPITALS AND CLINICS

A 1c | B CLIN. NOTES | C LABORATORY | D X-RAY EXAM | E CONSULTATION | F SPEC. EXAM | G THERAPY | H PATHOLOGY | I DIAGNOSIS

196EN18.9

Step 2 Preoperative/preprocedural checklist. (Courtesy University of Iowa Hospitals and Clinics.)

STEPS	RATIONALE
CRITICAL DECISION POINT Clients who are illiterate can sign with a mark with proper witness. Minors, unless married or declared emancipated, or individuals considered incompetent cannot sign consent form. Parent or legal guardian must provide consent.	
4. Provide preoperative teaching including postoperative exercises (Skill 35-2), skin preparation (Skill 35-3), pain control measures (see Chapter 5), and postoperative care in recovery room and nursing division (Skill 35-5).	Decreases anxiety and promotes cooperation in care.
5. Instruct client on the need and rationale for ingesting nothing by mouth (NPO) for 4 to 8 hours prior to surgery.	GI tract should be empty to decrease the risk of vomiting and **aspiration.**
CRITICAL DECISION POINT Client may brush teeth but should not swallow water. Client may take oral medications with a sip of water (30 ml) if specifically ordered to be taken preoperatively. All other oral medications are withheld.	
6. Provide for hygiene measures, ensuring client privacy. Instruct client to remove all clothing, including undergarments, and to don disposable cap and hospital gown with opening in back.	Provides easy access to client in OR.
7. Instruct client to remove hairpins, clips, wigs, hairpieces, jewelry, and makeup (including nail polish). Religious medals may be pinned to gown if agency policy permits. In some institutions, nail polish may need to be removed from only one finger if a pulse oximeter is used. Check institution's policy.	Hair appliances and jewelry may become dislodged and cause injury during positioning and intubation. Rings may decrease circulation in fingers. Assessment of skin and oxygenation is impeded by makeup and nail polish.
CRITICAL DECISION POINT Wedding rings may be taped in place. Be careful not to create tourniquet effect with tape around finger.	
8. Assist client in removing prostheses, including dentures and oral appliances, glasses and contact lenses, artificial limbs and eyes, artificial eyelashes, and hearing aids. Inventory items and give to family members or have security lock them up.	Prostheses can be lost or damaged during surgery and could cause injury. Oral appliances may occlude airway.
CRITICAL DECISION POINT If client will be required to follow instructions in the OR, hearing aid may be left in place. Check agency policy.	
9. Secure all valuables or give to family member or significant other. Have release form signed if required by agency.	Valuables may be lost or stolen.
10. Apply antiembolism stockings as ordered (see Skill 30-3).	Promotes venous return and reduces risk of thrombus formation.
11. Assess vital signs immediately before going to OR.	Abnormal vital signs may indicate conditions that increase risk for surgery.
CRITICAL DECISION POINT Vital signs not within normal range or client's baseline must be reported to physician and may require surgery to be postponed. Document in nurse's notes and/or preoperative checklist.	

~EPS	RATIONALE
12. Assist client to void prior to receiving preoperative medication.	Prevents incontinence and bladder distention during surgery. Preoperative medication may cause drowsiness and decreased voiding sensation.
13. Administer preoperative medications as ordered.	Reduces pain, anxiety, respiratory secretions, and amount of anesthesia required. Promotes relaxation.

➤ ***CRITICAL DECISION POINT*** **Check that informed consent is signed before giving medications. Preoperative medications may alter level of consciousness and make the consent invalid.**

14. Client is placed on bed rest with side rails up and call light within reach.	There is an increased chance of injury in attempting to ambulate to void when client is sedated and unattended.

EVALUATION

1. Compare all assessment data with client's baseline and expected normals.	Evaluates client's risk for complications and possible need to postpone surgery.
2. Have client repeat preoperative instructions and demonstrate postoperative exercises.	Client understands preoperative instructions and teaching.
3. Assess client for signs and symptoms of anxiety.	Increased heart rate and blood pressure, dilated pupils, dry mouth, increased sweating, and muscle rigidity or shaking are responses to stress and anxiety.
4. **Unexpected outcomes** that may occur include:	
➤ Vital signs are above or below client's baseline or expected range.	May indicate infection, anxiety, pain, or cardiovascular problem. Increases surgical risk.
➤ Informed consent not signed and witnessed.	Physician did not provide information and ensure consent form was signed. Client is not ready for surgery.
➤ Client did not remain NPO. Surgery may be cancelled.	Client did not understand instructions or forgot.
➤ Client unable to state instructions or demonstrate postoperative exercises.	Assessment of client's level of understanding or method of instruction was insufficient. Reinstruction necessary.
➤ Client did not void prior to receiving preoperative medication.	Client did not have need to void or was unable to void. Assess for bladder distention.

RECORDING AND REPORTING

1. Document all preoperative preparations in nurse's notes and/or checklist.	Documents care provided. Data provide baseline to compare changes in client's condition. Information ensures continuity of care.
2. Document client condition on transfer to OR.	Provides basis for comparison on admission to OR.
3. Report any abnormal assessment findings, lack of signed and witnessed consent form, failure of client to maintain NPO status.	May result in postponement of surgery.

FOLLOW-UP ACTIVITIES

1. Reinforce preoperative teaching as needed.
2. Perform additional assessment when findings are not within normal range.

• • • • •

Special Considerations

➤ In emergency situations where client is unable to give consent and family members are unavailable, telephone consent may be obtained. The oral consent must be witnessed by two persons. Documentation must include that oral consent was obtained and so witnessed. Later, a written consent signed by the person giving oral consent may be required. A signed telegram or a signed fax may also be considered an oral consent.

➤ Clients who are dehydrated or malnourished may require hydration with IV solutions (see Chapter 20) and parenteral nutrition (see Chapter 24).

Teaching Considerations

- Thorough preoperative teaching should prepare client for preoperative procedures and reduce the possibility of postponement of surgery and risk of complications.
- Teach client and primary care giver about surgical procedure, healing process, sutures, dressing, drains, feeding tubes, pain control, and diet. State rationale for each.

Pediatric Considerations

- Parents should be involved in preoperative preparation to decrease children's anxiety. Preadmission programs to prepare parents and children for same day surgery have been shown to decrease anxiety in both parents and children (Ellerton and Merriam, 1994).
- Preoperative preparation should take into consideration the developmental level of the child, for example, toys and games may be used to demonstrate preoperative procedures.

Gerontologic Considerations

- Physiological changes that occur with aging may require admission to hospital before surgery for additional diagnostic tests and stabilization of condition.
- Age-related changes such as decreased vision, hearing, and short-term memory may require the presence of family members or primary care giver during preoperative preparation.

Home Care Considerations

- Clients admitted on the day of surgery must be instructed about NPO status, skin preparation, and procedures such as enemas and douches before admission. Often the enemas or douches are done at home.
- Clients having surgery performed in ambulatory surgery centers must be accompanied by a family member or friend to allow for discharge after the procedure.

SKILL 35-2 Demonstrating Postoperative Exercises

Structured preoperative teaching has a positive influence on a surgical client's recovery. The nurse provides information and teaches skills that help clients understand the surgical experience and participate actively in the recovery process. Ideally a client should have adequate time to learn about the surgical experience. In the past, teaching occurred the evening before surgery when clients were most anxious. But due to cost reduction efforts, many clients are admitted to the hospital or ambulatory surgery center on the day of surgery. Preoperative teaching done at this time may not be highly effective because of the client's high anxiety level. Health care institutions are realizing the value of preparing clients well in advance so that clients gain the knowledge and skills needed to participate in their own care. Clients now frequently receive instruction before admission to a hospital or an outpatient surgical clinic. Teaching booklets and videotapes are available to supplement any instruction a nurse provides.

One study has found that clients prefer receiving preoperative information between admission to the hospital and the time of surgery, even if the time span is only a few hours or less (Schoessler, 1989). Therefore it seems ideal to attempt outpatient preoperative education just before admission and to reinforce the information before surgery. Ultimately a well-designed preoperative teaching program can improve a client's physical functioning and sense of well-being and shorten the length of hospital stay.

Postoperative exercises include diaphragmatic breathing and effective coughing, turning, and leg exercises. The use of incentive spirometry to encourage voluntary deep breathing through a machine that provides visual feedback may also be included. Incentive spirometry may be ordered by the physician for clients especially at risk for atelectasis or pneumonia (chronic smokers or clients on prolonged bed rest). During the discussion of these exercises, the nurse explains the relationship between the exercises and the physiological principles that make them important. Through specific explanations and guided practice the nurse helps develop client commitment to the recovery process. The nurse demonstrates the exercises and then continues to coach the client through several return practice sessions. Commitment to the exercise regimen is evidenced by the client's independent practice.

Whenever possible the nurse includes family members or other significant persons in the practice sessions. Frequently these individuals are with the client during the postoperative period and can thus serve as coaches. The nurse also provides clients with information about the sensations typically experienced after surgery, such as incisional pain and tightness of dressings. The information helps clients interpret realistically the events that occur in the postoperative period. As a result, clients are able to conserve their energies and attend to performing the exercises that assist in their recovery.

EQUIPMENT

- Pillow (optional; used to splint the incision when coughing to reduce discomfort)
- Incentive spirometer
- Elastic stockings or pneumatic compression cuffs

DELEGATION CONSIDERATIONS

The skill of teaching postoperative exercises requires problem solving and knowledge application unique to a professional nurse. Unlicensed assistive personnel can reinforce and assist clients in performing postoperative exercises.

- Review with unlicensed assistive personnel any precautions unique for a particular client.
- Be sure staff know when to inform the nurse if the client is unable to perform the exercises correctly.

STEPS	RATIONALE
ASSESSMENT	
1. Assess client's risk for postoperative respiratory complications: identify presence of chronic pulmonary condition (e.g., emphysema or asthma); any condition that affects chest wall movement, such as obesity or abdominal or thoracic surgery; history of smoking; and presence of reduced hemoglobin.	General anesthesia predisposes client to respiratory problems because lungs are not fully inflated during surgery; cough reflex is suppressed, and mucus collects within airway passages. Postoperatively, inadequate lung expansion can lead to atelectasis and pneumonia, creating greater risk for developing respiratory complications if chronic lung conditions are present. Smoking damages ciliary clearance and increases mucus secretion. A reduced hemoglobin level can lead to reduced oxygen delivery.
CRITICAL DECISION POINT Observe and report to physician if client has had a cold or upper respiratory infection within past week.	
2. Assess client's ability to cough and deep breathe by placing hand on client's abdomen, having client take a deep breath, and observing movement of shoulders, chest wall, and abdomen. Measure chest excursion during a deep breath. Ask client to cough after taking a deep breath.	Reveals maximum potential for chest expansion and ability to cough forcefully; serves as baseline to measure client's ability to perform exercises postoperatively. Diaphragmatic breathing allows for lung expansion and improved ventilation and increases blood oxygenation. Coughing loosens secretions and removes the secretions from the pulmonary alveoli.
3. Assess client's risk for postoperative thrombus formation (elderly, immobilized clients are most at risk). Observe for a positive Homans' sign (which may or may not be present) by monitoring calf pain when dorsiflexing the client's foot with the knee flexed. Observe for calf pain, redness, swelling, or vein distention.	Following general anesthesia, circulation is slowed, and when rate of blood flow is slowed there is a greater tendency for clot formation. Immobilization results in decreased muscular contraction in lower extremities, which promotes venous stasis.
CRITICAL DECISION POINT If present, notify the physician and do not manipulate the extremity any further. Antiembolism stockings or pneumatic compression cuffs may be ordered for clients at risk for thrombus formation (Skill 30-3).	
4. Assess client's ability to move independently while in bed.	Clients confined to bed rest, even for limited periods, will need to turn regularly. Determines existence of any mobility restrictions.
5. Assess client's willingness and capability to learn exercises; note factors such as attention span, anxiety, level of consciousness, and language level.	Ability to learn depends on readiness, ability, and learning environment.

STEPS	RATIONALE
CRITICAL DECISION POINT **Highly anxious clients or those in severe pain have difficulty learning and performing postoperative exercises.**	
6. Assess family members' or significant other's willingness to learn and to support client postoperatively.	Family's or significant other's presence postoperatively can be potential motivating factor for client's recovery; family member or significant other can coach clients on exercise performance.
7. Assess client's medical orders preoperatively and postoperatively.	May require adaptations in way exercises are performed.

NURSING DIAGNOSIS

Clustering of defining characteristics from the assessment data may reveal the following nursing diagnoses for clients requiring this skill:

- Risk for infection
- Risk for ineffective airway clearance
- Risk for ineffective breathing pattern
- Risk for impaired gas exchange
- Pain
- Altered tissue perfusion
- Impaired physical mobility
- Risk for impaired skin integrity

Related factors are individualized based on a client's condition or needs.

PLANNING

STEPS	RATIONALE
1. **Expected outcomes** following completion of procedure:	
➤ Client is able to correctly deep breathe, use incentive spirometer, cough, turn, and perform leg exercises throughout postoperative period.	Client's ability to perform exercises should be ensured by return demonstration.
➤ Postoperatively, chest excursion meets or exceeds preoperative level.	
➤ Lungs are clear to auscultation.	
➤ Negative Homans' sign, no redness in lower extremities, and client denies pain or tenderness in lower extremities.	Exercises help client maintain full lung expansion and clear airways and prevent circulatory and mobility problems postoperatively.
➤ Client initiates exercises spontaneously.	Client values importance of exercises to recovery.
2. Prepare equipment as needed.	
3. Prepare room for teaching.	

IMPLEMENTATION

Teaching Diaphragmatic Breathing

STEPS	RATIONALE
1. Assist client to a comfortable semi-Fowler's or high Fowler's position with knees flexed. If client chooses to sit, assist to side of bed or to upright position in chair.	Upright position facilitates diaphragmatic excursion.
CRITICAL DECISION POINT **Postoperatively, client can usually be positioned upright with head of bed elevated. If client must remain flat in bed, stress that exercises can still be performed.**	
2. Stand or sit facing client.	Client will be able to observe breathing exercises performed by nurse.
3. Instruct client to place palms of hands across from each other, down, and along lower borders of anterior rib cage; place tips of third finger lightly together (see illustration on p. 1030). Demonstrate for client.	Position of hands allows client to feel movement of chest and abdomen as diaphragm descends and lungs inside chest wall expand.

STEPS	RATIONALE
4. Have client take slow, deep breaths, inhaling through nose, and pushing abdomen against hands. Tell client to feel middle fingers separate as client inhales. Explain that client will feel normal downward movement of diaphragm during inspiration. Explain that abdominal organs descend and chest wall expands. Demonstrate for client.	Slow, deep breath prevents panting or hyperventilation. Inhaling through nose warms, humidifies, and filters air. Explanation and demonstration focus on normal ventilatory movement of chest wall. Client learns to understand how diaphragmatic breathing feels.
5. Avoid using chest and shoulders while inhaling and instruct client in same manner.	Using auxiliary chest and shoulder muscles during breathing increases useless energy expenditures and does not promote full lung expansion.
6. Take a slow, deep breath and hold for count of 3, and then slowly exhale through mouth as if blowing out a candle (pursed lips). Explain that client will feel middle finger tips touch as chest wall contracts.	Allows for gradual expulsion of air.
7. Repeat breathing exercise three to five times.	Allows client to observe slow, rhythmical breathing pattern.
8. Have client practice exercise. Client is instructed to take 10 slow, deep breaths every 2 hours while awake during postoperative period until mobile. Another option is to have client use incentive spirometry (see Chapter 12) (see illustration).	Repetition of exercise reinforces learning. Regular deep breathing will prevent postoperative complications.

Controlled Coughing

STEPS	RATIONALE
1. Explain importance of maintaining an upright position.	Position facilitates diaphragm excursion and enhances thorax expansion.
2. Demonstrate coughing. Take two slow, deep breaths, inhaling through nose and exhaling through mouth.	Deep breaths expand lungs fully so that air moves behind mucus and facilitates effects of coughing.
3. Inhale deeply a third time and hold breath to count of 3. Cough fully for two to three consecutive coughs without inhaling between coughs. (Tell client to push all air out of lungs.)	Consecutive coughs help remove mucus more effectively and completely than one forceful cough.

CRITICAL DECISION POINT **Coughing may be contraindicated after brain, spinal, or eye surgery.**

STEPS	RATIONALE
4. Caution client against just clearing throat instead of coughing.	Clearing throat does not remove mucus from deeper airways.

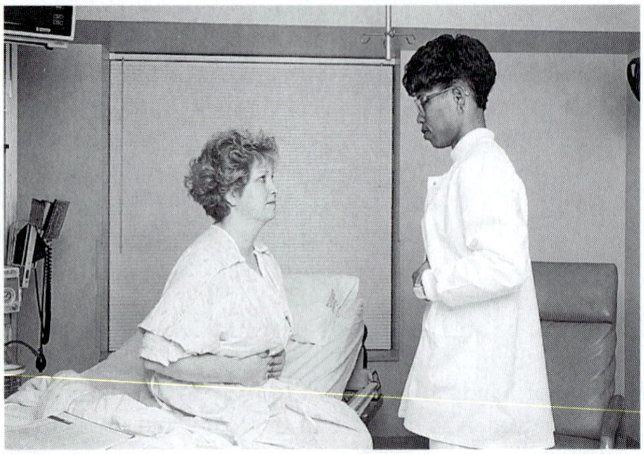

Step 3 Client and nurse practicing deep breathing.

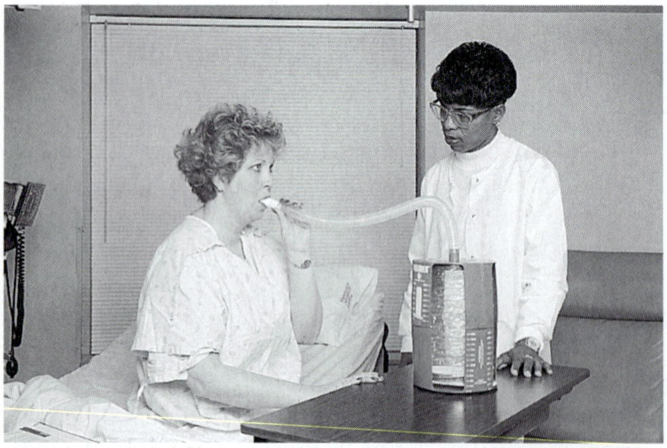

Step 8 Client demonstrates incentive spirometry.

STEPS	RATIONALE
CRITICAL DECISION POINT **Warn client that postoperative incisional pain will make it more difficult but that coughing will not cause injury to incision.**	
5. If surgical incision is to be either abdominal or thoracic, teach client to place pillow over incisional area and place hands over pillow to splint incision (see illustration). During breathing and coughing exercises, press gently against incisional area for splinting or support.	Surgical incision cuts through muscles, tissues, and nerve endings. Deep breathing and coughing exercises place additional stress on suture line and cause discomfort. Splinting incision with hands or pillow provides firm support and reduces incisional pulling.
6. Client continues to practice coughing exercises, splinting imaginary incision. The client is instructed to cough two to three times every 2 hours while awake.	Value of deep coughing with splinting is stressed to effectively expectorate mucus with minimal discomfort.
7. Instruct client to examine sputum for consistency, odor, amount, and color changes.	Sputum consistency, odor, amount, and color changes may indicate the presence of a pulmonary complication such as pneumonia.
CRITICAL DECISION POINT **For clients with preexisting pulmonary disease, know the character of sputum.**	

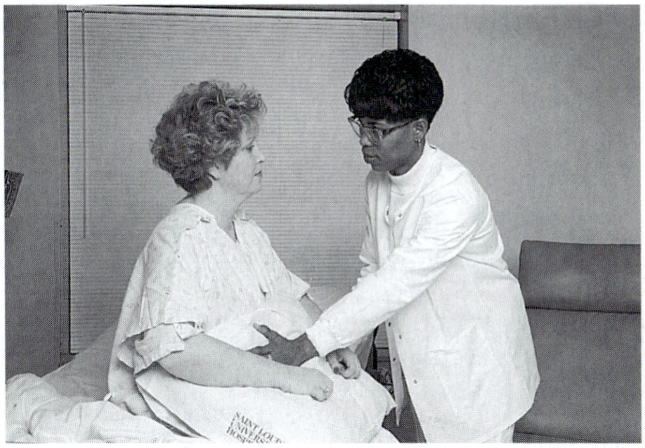

Step 5 Client splinting abdomen with pillow.

Turning

STEPS	RATIONALE
1. Instruct client to assume supine position toward right side of bed.	Positioning begins on right side of bed so that turning to left side will not cause client to roll toward bed's edge.
CRITICAL DECISION POINT **If client has decreased strength or mobility on the right side, have client assume position on left side of bed.**	
2. Have client place the left hand over incisional area to splint it.	Splinting incision supports and minimizes pulling on suture line during turning.
3. Instruct client to keep left leg straight and flex right knee up and over left leg.	Straight leg stabilizes the client's position. Flexed right leg shifts weight for easier turning.
CRITICAL DECISION POINT **Some clients may be restricted from flexing their legs postoperatively, such as those who have had back surgery or vascular repair. Client may be restricted from turning or may need assistance for positioning.**	
4. Have client grab left side rail with right hand, pull toward left, and roll onto left side.	Pulling toward side rail reduces effort needed for turning.

STEPS	RATIONALE
CRITICAL DECISION POINT If client is unable to perform the above maneuver, note in chart that turning must be done by staff or primary care giver every 2 hours. May need to place pillows behind client to help maintain side-lying position.	
5. Instruct client to turn every 2 hours while awake.	Reduces risk of vascular and pulmonary complications.

Leg Exercises

STEPS	RATIONALE
1. Have client assume supine position in bed. Demonstrate leg exercises by performing passive range of motion exercises and simultaneously explaining exercise.	Provides normal anatomical position of lower extremities.
CRITICAL DECISION POINT If client's surgery involves one or both extremities, surgeon must order leg exercises in postoperative period. Legs unaffected by surgery can be safely exercised unless client has preexisting phlebothrombosis (blood clot formation) or thrombophlebitis (inflammation of vein wall).	
2. Rotate each ankle in complete circle. Instruct client to draw imaginary circles with big toe. Repeat five times.	Leg exercises maintain joint mobility and promote venous return.
3. Alternate dorsiflexion and plantar flexion by moving both feet up and down. Direct client to feel calf muscles contract and relax alternately (see illustration).	Stretches and contracts gastrocnemius muscles.
4. Client continues leg exercises by alternately flexing and extending knees. Repeat five times (see illustration).	Contracts muscles of upper legs and maintains knee mobility.
5. Client alternately raises each leg straight up from bed surface, keeping legs straight. Repeat five times.	Promotes contraction and relaxation of quadriceps muscles.
CRITICAL DECISION POINT If client is unable to perform exercises, note in chart that passive range of motion must be done by staff or primary care giver.	

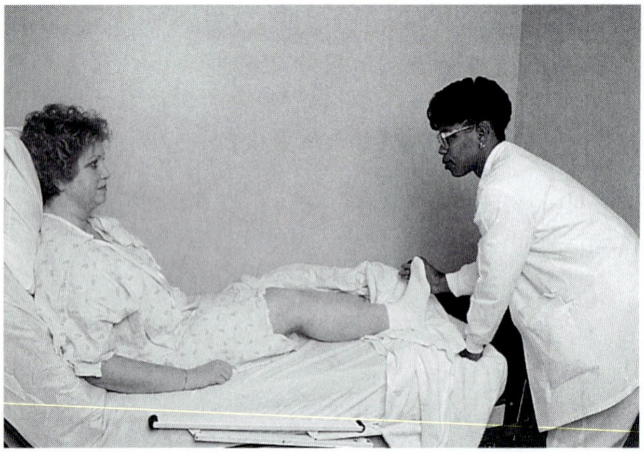

Step 3 Client and nurse demonstrate exercise, flexing feet.

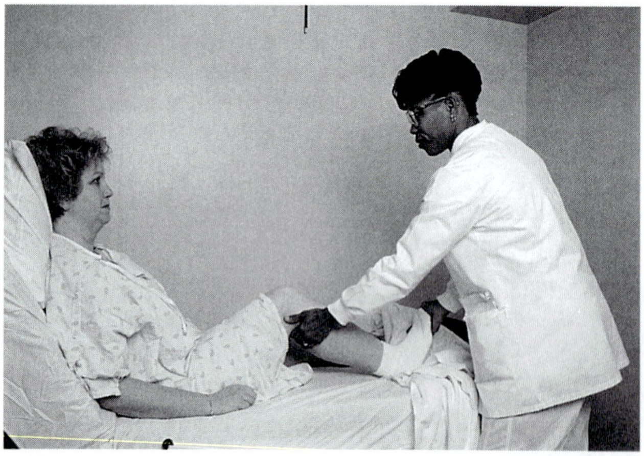

Step 4 Client and nurse demonstrate knee raising, flexion.

STEPS	RATIONALE
6. Have client continue to practice exercises at least every 2 hours while awake. Client is instructed to coordinate turning and leg exercises with diaphragmatic breathing, incentive spirometry, and coughing exercises.	Repetition of exercise sequence reinforces learning. Establishes routine for exercises that develops habit for performance. Sequence of exercises should be leg exercises, turning, breathing, and coughing.

EVALUATION

1. Observe client performing all four exercises independently.	Provide opportunity for practice and return demonstration of exercises. Ensures client has learned correct technique.
2. Observe family members' or significant other's ability to coach client.	Family member or significant other can assist positively or interfere with correct technique.
3. Evaluate client's chest excursion.	Determines degree of lung expansion.
4. Auscultate client's lungs.	Breath sounds reveal if airways are clear.
5. Assess for Homans' sign.	Negative sign indicates no venous thrombosis.
6. **Unexpected outcomes** that may occur include:	
➤ Client is unable to perform exercises correctly.	Additional instruction needed. Anxiety, pain, complications, or fatigue alter client's performance. Client may benefit from stress reduction techniques and pain management strategies.
➤ Client develops pulmonary and circulatory complications such as atelectasis, venous stasis, and thrombus postoperatively.	Deep breaths shallow, cough ineffective, and leg exercises inadequate.

RECORDING AND REPORTING

1. Record which exercises have been demonstrated to client and whether client can perform exercises independently or not.	Ensures continuity of instruction.
2. Record physical assessment findings in nurse's notes or flow sheet.	Documents baseline for later comparisons.
3. Report any problems client has in practicing exercises to nurse assigned to client on next shift.	Informs staff so that reinforcement can be provided.

FOLLOW-UP ACTIVITIES

1. Instead of diaphragmatic breathing, the client can benefit from the use of incentive spirometry.
2. Increase frequency of observation of exercises if client has difficulty practicing exercises.

• • • • •

Special Considerations

- ➤ Surgery involving thorax or upper abdomen impairs client's ability to effectively deep breathe or cough because of incisional pain.
- ➤ Encourage client to ask for pain medication ½ hour before performing cough and deep breathing or leg exercises postoperatively or use patient-controlled analgesia (PCA) immediately prior to exercising.

Teaching Considerations

- ➤ Explain postoperative exercises to the client and primary care giver, including their importance to recovery and physiological benefits.

Pediatric Considerations

- ➤ Parents should encourage and allow children to move within the limits posed by the surgery.
- ➤ Adolescents should receive the same preoperative instructions and teaching as adults to support their developmental stage.
- ➤ Children's normal responses of crying and moving extremities will maintain lung expansion and peripheral circulation. Therefore teaching coughing, deep breathing, and leg exercises is not necessary for young children.
- ➤ Children need family members and nursing staff to assume the coach's role.

Gerontologic Considerations

- Changes related to aging such as decreased vision, hearing, and short-term memory may affect teaching effectiveness. Shorter sessions with frequent reinforcement and the use of teaching aids with large print may be necessary. Including family members or primary care giver in teaching sessions is strongly encouraged. Take time to instruct client properly.
- The aging process decreases ventilatory capacity and increases risk for respiratory complications.

Home Care Considerations

- Review coughing, deep breathing, and relaxation exercises before admission to hospital or surgical clinic and after discharge.

SKILL 35-3 Preparing the Surgical Site

The body's first line of defense against infection is intact skin. A break in the integrity of the skin as a result of a surgical incision can become a potential source of infection. Before surgery, the skin overlying the proposed surgical site is thoroughly cleansed to minimize skin contamination and the risk of postoperative wound infection. Preparation of the incisional area sometimes begins the evening before surgery and involves washing the skin and removing hair around the incision site.

The skin is cleansed by scrubbing with an antimicrobial soap (e.g., chlorhexidine) two or more times. The client can perform the scrubbing during either a bath or shower. If an enema is given in preparation for surgery, the final shower or bath should be given after the enema. The client also may be required to shampoo hair if surgery involves the head, neck, or even the upper chest.

Hair removal should be performed only as necessary. The three methods of hair removal are clipping, use of a depilatory, and wet shaving. Shaving the surgical site removes hair that serves as a reservoir for infection. However, evidence shows that infections of small cuts made by a razor occur more often in clients who are shaved preoperatively than clients who are not shaved. Shaving is usually done immediately before the operation in the OR or holding area to reduce the time for potential bacterial growth. The procedure may be done by a nurse or surgical technician. The Centers for Disease Control and Prevention (CDC) (1985) recommends clippers or a depilatory to remove hair to minimize skin abrasions and cuts.

EQUIPMENT

- Portable lamp
- Bath blanket
- Towel or waterproof pad
- Disposable gloves
- Solvent solution to remove adhesives or nail polish

Depilatory
- Depilatory cream
- Basin with liquid antiseptic soap mixed with water

Clipping
- Electric clippers (used to remove short hair)
- Scissors (used to remove long hair)
- Towel
- Cotton balls, applicators, and antiseptic solution (optional)

Wet shave:
- Razor with extra blade or disposable razor
- Clean basin with warm water
- Gauze sponges
- Basin with liquid antiseptic soap mixed with water (avoid using povidone-iodine for clients with allergies to iodine or shellfish)
- Waterproof underpad or towels
- Washcloth, bath blanket
- Cotton balls, cotton applicators, and antiseptic solution (optional)

DELEGATION CONSIDERATIONS

The skill of preparing the surgical site can be delegated to unlicensed assistive personnel. Be sure to assess client's risk for bleeding tendencies before delegating skill.

- Inform personnel of appropriate antimicrobial soap and length of time for skin preparation.
- Review procedure for removal of hair.
- Review information to be reported to the nurse after completion of procedure.

STEPS	RATIONALE
ASSESSMENT	
1. Inspect general condition of skin.	Lesions, irritations, or infection increases chance for postoperative wound infections.
CRITICAL DECISION POINT If lesions, irritations, or signs of skin infection are present, shaving should not be done.	
2. Assess for allergy to iodine or shellfish.	Povidone-iodine solutions should not be used if client is allergic to iodine. Shellfish contain iodine.
3. Assess for bleeding tendency.	Presence of bleeding tendency would contraindicate use of a razor.
4. Review physician's order or the agency's procedure book for specific area to be shaved.	Extent of area for hair removal depends on site of incision, nature of surgery, and physician's preference. Area is always larger than actual incision to ensure wide perimeter with minimal bacteria.
5. Assess client's understanding and acceptance of purpose for hair removal.	Client may be anxious regarding removal of hair and implications regarding change in appearance.
CRITICAL DECISION POINT Certain cultures and religious groups have restrictions on removal and disposal of body hair.	

NURSING DIAGNOSIS

Clustering of defining characteristics from the assessment data may reveal the following nursing diagnoses for clients requiring this skill:

- Pain
- Risk for infection
- Risk for impaired skin integrity
- Risk for trauma
- Risk for body image disturbance

Related factors are individualized based on a client's condition or needs.

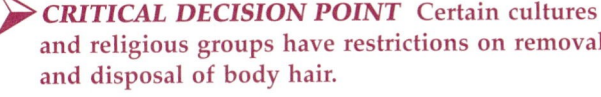

STEPS	RATIONALE
PLANNING	
1. **Expected outcomes** following completion of procedure:	
➤ Client's skin is free of all hair over shaved area.	Skin has received initial preparation for surgical incision to eventually be made.
➤ Skin is free of visible cuts, nicks, areas of inflammation.	Less likelihood of skin infections developing.
➤ Client denies burning or discomfort.	Skin intact without abrasions or cuts.
2. Prepare equipment at client's bedside.	
3. Explain procedure, extent of hair removal, and rationale for removal of hair over large surface area.	Promotes cooperation and minimizes anxiety because client may think incision will be as large as shaved site.
CRITICAL DECISION POINT Scissors may be used to trim especially long hair. Never dispose of client's scalp hair without permission, since this is considered personal property. Some clients use their hair for wig.	
IMPLEMENTATION	
1. Wash hands.	Reduces transmission of microorganisms.
2. Close room doors or bedside curtains and raise bed to high position.	Provides client privacy. Bed position prevents nurse from having to bend over for long periods. Promotes correct body mechanics and decreases back injury.
3. Position client comfortably with surgical site accessible. Rearrange drapes as necessary.	Hair removal and skin preparation can take several minutes. Nurse should have easy access to hard-to-reach areas. Prevents unnecessary exposure of body parts.

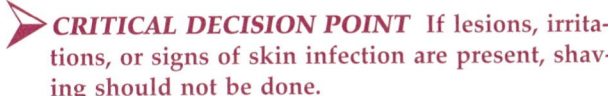

STEPS	RATIONALE
4. Don disposable gloves.	Use of disposable gloves safeguards the client and the nurse, minimizing nurse's exposure to blood-borne pathogens.
5. Depilatory hair removal:	
a. Apply depilatory cream to area; be sure entire area is adequately covered.	Hair removal by depilation leaves skin intact and free from cuts. If the client is not sensitive to the depilatory, it is a safer method of hair removal than shaving.
b. Wait the required number of minutes and then wipe off the cream.	Hair is removed simultaneously when wiping off the depilatory.
c. Wash skin with antiseptic soap and rinse thoroughly.	Removes microorganisms from the skin.
6. Hair clipping:	
a. Lightly dry area to be clipped with towel.	Removes moisture, which interferes with clean cut of clippers.
b. Hold clippers in dominant hand, about 1 cm (½ in) above skin, and cut hair in direction it grows. Clip small area at a time.	Prevents pulling on hair and abrasion of skin.
c. Lightly brush off cut hair with towel.	Removes contaminated hair and promotes comfort. Improves visibility of area being clipped.
d. When clipped area is over body crevices, for example, umbilicus or groin, clean crevices with cotton-tipped applicators or cotton ball dipped in antiseptic solution, then dry.	Removes secretions, dirt, and hair clippings, which harbor microorganisms.
7. Wet shave:	
a. Place towel or waterproof pads under body part to be shaved.	Prevents soiling of bed linen.
b. Drape client with bath blanket, leaving only area to be shaved at one time (10 to 20 cm [4 to 8 inches]) exposed.	Prevents unnecessary exposure of body parts and reduces client's anxiety.
c. Adjust lamp.	Provides maximum skin illumination.
d. Lather skin with gauze sponges dipped in antiseptic soap.	Softens hair and reduces friction from razor.
e. Shave small area at a time. With nondominant hand hold gauze sponge to stabilize skin. Hold razor at 45-degree angle in dominant hand and shave hair in direction it grows. Use short, gentle strokes (see illustration).	Shaving small areas minimizes cutting skin; shaving in direction hair grows prevents pulling.

CRITICAL DECISION POINT **Shaving too slowly can pull hair.**

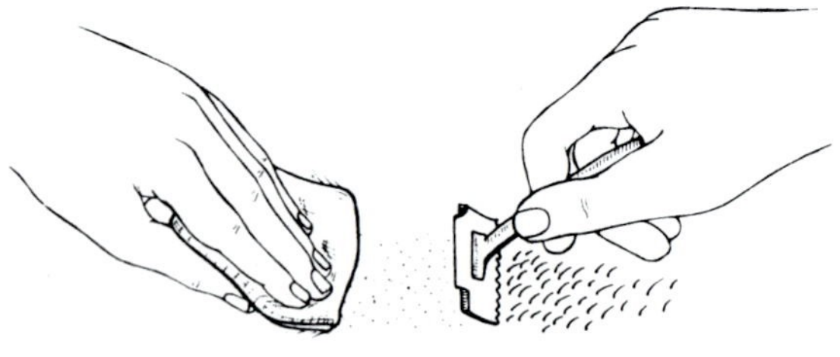

Step 7e Shaving.

STEPS	RATIONALE
f. Rinse razor in basin of water as soap and hair accumulate on the blade. Change and discard blades as they become dull.	Maintains clean, sharp razor edge to promote client's comfort and reduces the risk of abrasions.
g. Rearrange bath blanket as each portion of shave is completed.	Maintains client's comfort and privacy.
h. Use washcloth and warm water to rinse away remaining hair and soap solution. Change water as needed.	Reduces skin irritation and potential contamination; allows good visualization of skin.

STEPS	RATIONALE
i. If shaved area is over body crevices, for example, umbilicus or groin, cleanse with cotton-tipped applicators or cotton balls dipped in antiseptic solution.	Removes secretions, dirt, and remaining hair clippings, which harbor microorganisms.
j. Dry crevices with towel or applicators.	Reduces maceration of skin from retained moisture.
k. Discard waterproof towel or pad.	Reduces spread of microorganisms.
l. Observe skin closely for any nicks or cuts.	Any break in skin integrity increases risk of wound infection.
8. Tell client that procedure is completed.	Relieves client's anxiety.
9. Clean and dispose of equipment according to policy. Do not recover razor blade. Dispose of gloves.	Reduces spread of infection and reduces risk of injury from razor blades.
10. Wash hands.	Reduces spread of microorganisms.
EVALUATION	
1. Inspect condition of skin after completion of hair removal.	Determines if there is remaining hair or if skin was cut.
2. Question if client feels burning or discomfort.	Indicates presence of skin cut or irritation.
3. **Unexpected outcomes** that may occur include:	
➤ Client's skin is not totally clear of all hair.	Exceptionally thick hair is difficult to remove the first time. Additional depilatory or another shave is necessary.
➤ Client's skin becomes cut, nicked, or inflamed.	Blade may be dulled, angle of blade was not correct, or too much pressure was applied. Even minor skin wounds become infected.
➤ Client experiences burning over shaved site.	Local nicks or cuts cause burning.
RECORDING AND REPORTING	
1. Record procedure, area clipped or shaved, and condition of skin before and after in nurse's notes.	Documents status of surgical site for comparison over time.
2. Report any skin alterations or nicks or cuts in skin to surgeon.	Skin problems may require cancellation of surgery.

FOLLOW-UP ACTIVITIES

1. After shave, client should be checked to be sure that sheets are dry, bath blanket is removed, hospital clothing is being worn, and client is placed in comfortable position.

• • • • •

Special Considerations

➤ Most OR departments have a manual describing areas to be shaved for each type of surgery. (e.g., Eyebrows are not shaved unless ordered by the physician because hair does not grow back over scar tissue.)

➤ During emergencies, client may be shaved in OR to save critical time. If this is the case, heavy lather should be used to help control hair clippings removed by the razor. Following shave, carefully remove loose hair so that it does not remain on linen and possibly get into surgical wound.

➤ Most hospitals use disposable razors to prevent transmission of blood-borne infection from a contaminated razor. If disposable razor is not available, an autoclaved razor and new blade should be used for each client. Never share razors between clients.

➤ If client's skin becomes nicked or cut, some institutional policies and procedures may require an incident report to be completed.

➤ Occupational Safety and Health Administration (OSHA) guidelines require gloves to be worn, safe disposal of razor blades, and sterilization of reusable items. Razor blades are discarded into contaminated sharp holders.

Pediatric Considerations

➤ The face and neck of children are not usually shaved.

➤ Parents may want to save the hair if child's head is shaved.

Gerontologic Considerations

- Skin changes that occur with aging makes the skin more susceptible to irritation and injury, which increases the risk for infection.

Home Care Considerations

- Some surgeons may encourage clients to use a chlorhexidine skin cleanser or soap product containing hexachlorophene at home prior to an elective procedure.

SKILL 35-4 Inserting and Maintaining the Nasogastric Tube

An NG tube is a pliable plastic tube that is inserted through the client's nasopharynx and into the stomach. The tube is hollow and allows for removal of gastric contents and the introduction of liquids into the stomach. The primary use of the NG tube in the surgical client is for **decompression** or removal of air and fluids from the stomach. The NG tube helps prevent postoperative vomiting and distention caused by reduced peristalsis resulting from general anesthesia, manipulation of the viscera during surgery, or obstruction of the operative site by edema. When used for decompression, it is usually connected to an intermittent gastric suction device. The nurse routinely measures contents of the suction container to monitor intake and output.

The tubes most commonly used for decompression are the Levin and Salem sump tubes. The Levin tube is single lumen and has several holes near the tip. The Salem sump tube is a double-lumen tube: one provides an air vent and the other is for removal of gastric contents.

The client with an NG tube presents several nursing care problems. One of the greatest problems is maintaining the client's comfort. Some clients state that the discomfort from the tube exceeds the pain from the surgical incision. The tube is a source of constant irritation to the nasal mucosa and posterior pharynx. To lessen this discomfort, the tube should be secured with tape to the nose and then to the client's gown with a pin to prevent unnecessary movement. Other comfort measures include removing excess secretions from around the nares and lubricating the nostrils and tube with a water-soluble lubricant to avoid crusting of secretions. With one nostril occluded, the client tends to breathe through the mouth, and the lips and tongue may become dry and cracked. Mouth care should be provided at least every 2 hours to minimize dehydration. Frequent mouth rinses with cool water are helpful, although the nurse should caution the client not to swallow the water. The client may be allowed to chew gum to increase salivation or suck on small ice chips, which helps relieve the dryness in the throat. Sometimes an ice bag applied externally to the throat provides relief.

Another nursing care problem is maintaining patency of the tube. The tip of the tube may become occluded because the tube rests against the stomach wall or because it becomes blocked with thick secretions. The NG tube should be irrigated regularly with normal saline injected in an Asepto or catheter-tipped syringe. Turning the client facilitates draining the stomach. If necessary, the nurse should reposition the tube by advancing or withdrawing it slightly. However, some surgical procedures require that only a physician reposition the tube. For example, a nurse should not reposition an NG tube for a client who has had gastric or esophageal surgery.

EQUIPMENT

- No. 14 or no. 16 Fr NG tube (smaller lumen catheters are not used for decompression in adults because they must be able to remove thick secretions)
- Water-soluble lubricating jelly
- pH test strips (to measure gastric aspirate acidity)
- Tongue blade
- Flashlight
- Asepto bulb or catheter-tipped syringe
- 1 inch (2.5 cm) wide hypoallergenic tape
- Safety pin and rubber band
- Clamp, drainage bag, or suction machine or pressure gauge if wall suction is to be used
- Bath towel
- Glass of water with straw
- Facial tissues
- Normal saline
- Tincture of benzoin (optional)
- Disposable gloves

DELEGATION CONSIDERATIONS

The skill of inserting and maintaining the NG tube requires problem solving and knowledge application unique to a professional nurse. Unlicensed assistive personnel may measure and record the drainage from the NG tube and provide oral and nasal hygiene and comfort measures.

STEPS	RATIONALE
ASSESSMENT	
1. Inspect condition of client's nasal and oral cavity.	Baseline condition of nasal and oral cavity determines need for special nursing measures for oral hygiene after tube placement.
2. Ask if client has had history of nasal surgery and note if deviated nasal septum is present.	Nurse should insert tube into uninvolved nasal passage.
CRITICAL DECISION POINT Procedure my be contraindicated if surgery is recent.	
3. Palpate client's abdomen for distention, pain, and rigidity. Auscultate for bowel sounds.	Baseline determination of level of abdominal distention later serves as comparison once tube is inserted.
4. Assess client's level of consciousness and ability to follow instructions.	Determines client's ability to assist in procedure.
CRITICAL DECISION POINT If client is confused, disoriented, or unable to follow commands obtain assistance from another staff member to insert the tube.	

NURSING DIAGNOSIS

Clustering of defining characteristics from the assessment data may reveal the following nursing diagnoses for clients requiring this skill:

- Anxiety
- Risk for trauma
- Risk for aspiration
- Altered oral mucous membrane
- Impaired swallowing

Related factors are individualized based on a client's condition or needs.

STEPS	RATIONALE
PLANNING	
1. **Expected outcomes** following completion of procedure:	
➤ Client denies congestion of uninvolved naris.	Nares remain clear.
➤ NG tube drains light, green-colored gastric contents.	If tube is patent and in correct position, gastric contents drain easily.
➤ Abdomen remains soft and flat.	Indicative of abdominal decompression.
➤ Nares and surface of nose remain clear, without abrasions or excoriation, and nares remain moist.	Absence of mucosal and skin irritation.
➤ Client describes feeling of irritation in throat but not of severe nature.	Presence of tube causes some pharyngeal irritation.
2. Check medical record for surgeon's order, type of NG tube to be placed, and whether tube is to be attached to suction or drainage bag.	Procedure requires physician's order. Adequate decompression depends on NG suction.
3. Prepare equipment at the bedside.	
4. Identify client and explain procedure.	Identification prevents error of placing tube in wrong client. Explanation gains client's cooperation and lessens possibility that client will remove tube.
IMPLEMENTATION	
1. Wash hands and don disposable gloves.	Reduces transmission of microorganisms.
2. Position client in high Fowler's position with pillows behind head and shoulders. Raise bed to a horizontal level comfortable for the nurse.	Promotes client's ability to swallow during procedure. Good body mechanics prevent injury to nurse or client.
3. Pull curtain around the bed or close room door.	Provides privacy.
4. Stand on client's right side if right-handed, left side if left-handed.	Allows easiest manipulation of tubing.
5. Place bath towel over client's chest; give facial tissues to client.	Prevents soiling of client's gown. Tube insertion through nasal passages may cause tearing and coughing with increased salivation.

STEPS	RATIONALE
6. Instruct client to relax and breathe normally while occluding one naris. Then repeat this action for other naris. Select nostril with greater air flow.	Tube passes more easily through naris that is more patent.
7. Measure distance to insert tube:	
a. Traditional method: measure distance from tip of nose to earlobe to xiphoid process (see illustration).	
b. Hanson method: first mark 50 cm point on tube, then do traditional measurement. Tube insertion should be to midway point between 50 cm (20 inches) and traditional mark.	Tube should extend from nares to stomach; distance varies with each client.
8. Mark length of tube to be inserted with small piece of tape placed so it can easily be removed.	Marks amount of tube to be inserted from nares to stomach.
9. Cut a 10 cm (4 inch) piece of tape. Split one end down the middle lengthwise 5 cm (2 inches). Place on bed rail or bedside table.	Tape will be used after tube insertion to anchor the tube securely.
10. Curve 10 to 15 cm (4 to 6 inches) of end of tube tightly around index finger; then release.	Curving tube tip aids insertion and decreases stiffness of tube.
11. Lubricate 7.5 to 10 cm (3 to 4 inches) of end of tube with water-soluble lubricating jelly.	Minimizes friction against nasal mucosa and aids insertion of tube.
12. Alert client that procedure is to begin.	Decreases client anxiety and increases client cooperation.
13. Initially instruct client to extend neck back against pillow; insert tube slowly through naris with curved end pointing downward (see illustration). Gently lifting up tip of nose may aid insertion.	Facilitates initial passage of tube through naris and maintains clear airway for open naris.
14. Continue to pass tube along floor of nasal passage, aiming down toward ear. When resistance is felt, apply gentle downward pressure to advance tube (do not force past resistance).	Minimizes discomfort of tube rubbing against upper nasal turbinates. Resistance is caused by posterior nasopharynx. Downward pressure helps tube curl around corner of nasopharynx.
15. If resistance is met, try to rotate the tube and see if it advances. If still resistant, withdraw tube, allow client to rest, relubricate tube, and insert into other naris.	Forcing against resistance can cause trauma to mucosa. Helps relieve client's anxiety.

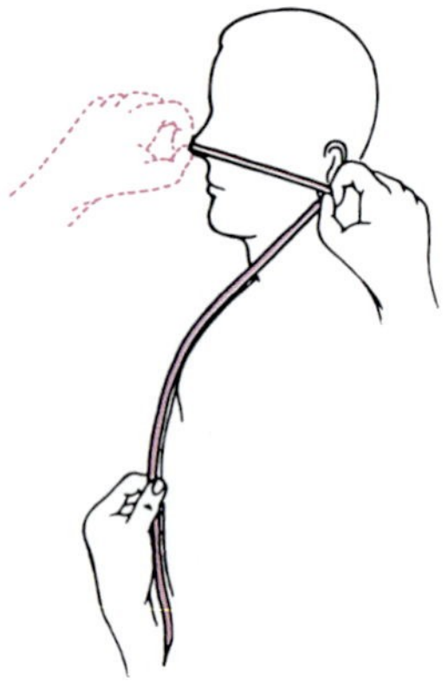

Step 7a Measuring length of NG tube.

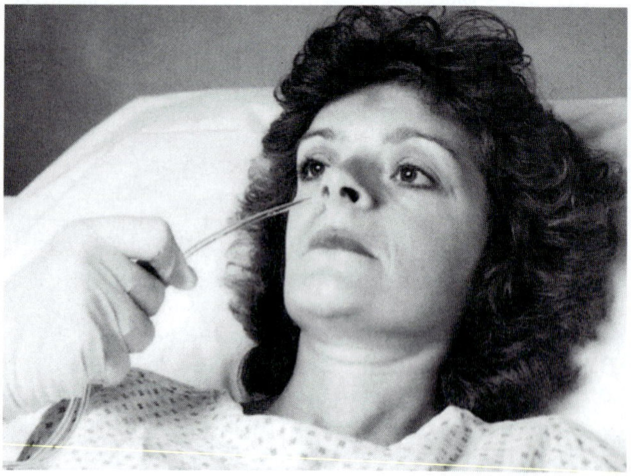

Step 13 Inserting NG tube.

STEPS	RATIONALE
CRITICAL DECISION POINT If unable to insert tube in either naris, stop procedure and notify physician.	
16. Continue insertion of tube until just past nasopharynx by gently rotating tube toward opposite naris.	
a. Stop tube advancement, allow client to relax, and provide tissues.	Relieves client's anxiety; tearing is natural response to mucosal irritation, and excessive salivation may occur due to oral stimulation.
b. Explain to client that next step requires that client swallow. Give client glass of water unless contraindicated.	Sipping of water aids passage of NG tube into esophagus.
17. With tube just above oropharynx, instruct client to flex head forward, take a small sip of water, and swallow. Advance tube 2.5 to 5 cm (1 to 2 inches) with each swallow of water. If client is not allowed fluids, instruct to dry swallow or suck air through straw. Advance tube with each swallow.	Flexed position closes off upper airway to trachea and opens esophagus. Swallowing closes epiglottis over trachea and helps move the tube into the esophagus. Swallowing water reduces gagging or choking. Water can be removed later from stomach by suction.
18. If client begins to cough, gag, or choke, withdraw slightly and stop tube advancement. Instruct client to breathe easily and take sips of water.	Tubing may accidentally enter larynx and initiate cough reflex. Gagging is eased by swallowing water. Risk for aspiration increases if vomiting occurs.
CRITICAL DECISION POINT If vomiting occurs, do not proceed until airway is cleared.	
19. If client continues to cough during insertion, pull tube back slightly.	Tube may enter larynx and obstruct airway.
20. If client continues to gag, check back of pharynx using flashlight and tongue blade.	Tube may coil around itself in back of throat and stimulate gag reflex.
21. After client relaxes, continue to advance tube desired distance.	Tip of tube should be within stomach to decompress properly.
22. Once tube is correctly advanced, remove tape used to mark length of tube and place the prepared split tape with nonsplit side on nose. Anchor with one of split ends while checking tube placement.	Tube should be partially anchored before placement is checked.
Checking Tube Placement	
1. Ask client to talk.	Client is unable to talk if NG tube has passed through vocal cords.
2. Inspect posterior pharynx for presence of coiled tube.	Tube is pliable and can coil up in back of pharynx instead of advancing into esophagus.
3. Draw up 10 to 20 ml of air into catheter-tipped syringe and attach to end of tube. Auscultate over left upper quadrant of abdomen while quickly injecting air into tube.	A whooshing or gurgling sound may indicate tube is correctly placed in stomach. Sounds transmitted by insufflation of air may also be transmitted from pleural space to upper abdomen, giving false impression of placement (Metheny, 1988; Metheny et al., 1990).
CRITICAL DECISION POINT This method used alone is not considered the most effective in determining placement of tube in stomach and should be used with other methods to accurately assess tube placement, such as x-ray examination. Check institutional policy for preferred methods for checking tube placement.	
4. Aspirate gently back on syringe to obtain gastric contents, observing color.	Gastric contents are usually cloudy and green, but may be off-white, tan, bloody, or brown in color. Aspiration of contents provides means to measure fluid pH and thus determine tube tip placement in GI tract.

STEPS	RATIONALE
5. Measure pH of aspirate with color-coded pH paper with range of whole numbers 1 to 11 (see illustration).	Gastric aspirates have decidedly acidic pH values, preferably 4 or less; compared with intestinal aspirates, which are usually greater than 4, or respiratory secretions, which are usually greater than 5.5 (Metheny et al., 1993; Metheny et al., 1994).
6. If tube is not in stomach, advance another 2.5 to 5.0 cm (1 to 2 inches) and repeat steps 3, 4, and 5 to check tube position.	Tube must be in stomach to provide decompression.

Anchoring Tube

STEPS	RATIONALE
1. After tube is properly inserted and positioned, either clamp end or connect it to drainage bag or suction machine.	Drainage bag is used for gravity drainage. Intermittent suction is most effective for decompression. Client going to OR often has tube clamped.
2. Tape tube to nose; avoid putting pressure on nares.	Prevents tissue necrosis. Tape anchors tube securely.
a. Before taping tube to nose, apply small amount of tincture of benzoin to lower end of nose and allow to dry (optional). Be sure top end of tape over nose is secure.	Benzoin prevents loosening of tape if client perspires.
b. Carefully wrap two split ends around tube (see illustration).	
3. Fasten end of NG tube to client's gown by looping rubber band around tube in slip knot. Pin rubber band to gown (provides slack for movement).	Reduces pressure on the nares if tube moves.
4. Unless physician orders otherwise, head of bed should be elevated 30 degrees.	Helps prevent esophageal reflux and minimizes irritation of tube against posterior pharynx.
5. Explain to client that sensation of tube should decrease somewhat with time.	Adaptation to continued sensory stimulus.
6. Remove gloves and wash hands.	Reduces transmission of microorganisms.

Tube Irrigation

STEPS	RATIONALE
1. Wash hands and don gloves.	Reduces transmission of microorganisms.
2. Check for tube placement in stomach (see Checking Tube Placement). Reconnect NG tube to connecting tube.	Prevents accidental entrance of irrigating solution into lungs.

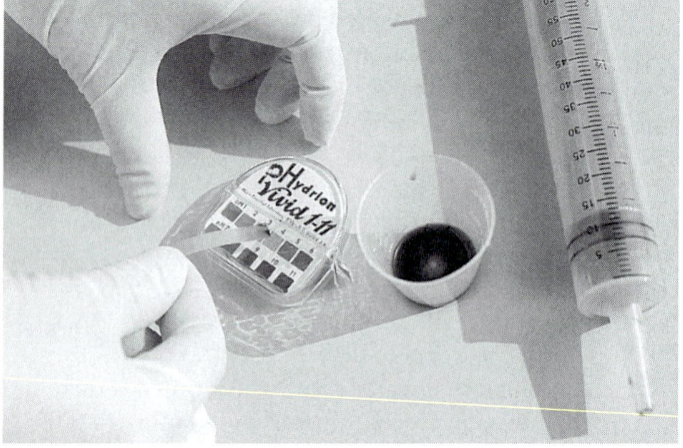

Step 5 Comparing pH tape to color chart.

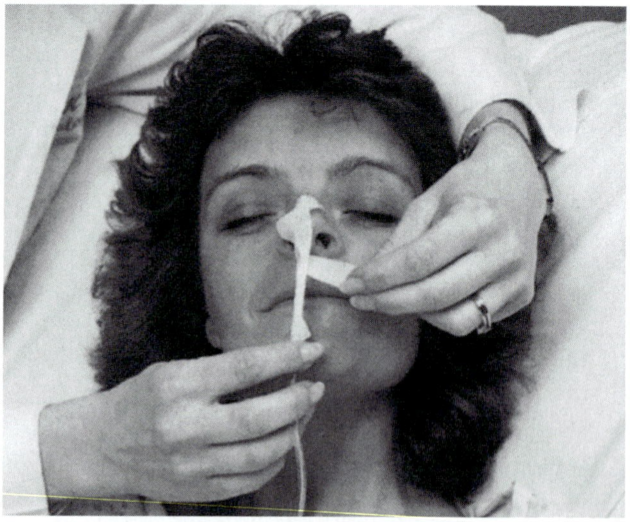

Step 2b Taping NG tube to client's nose.

STEPS	RATIONALE
3. Draw up 30 ml of normal saline into Asepto or catheter-tipped syringe.	Use of saline minimizes loss of electrolytes from stomach fluids.
4. Clamp NG tube. Disconnect from connection tubing and lay end of connection tubing on towel.	Reduces soiling of client's gown and bed linen.
5. Insert tip of irrigating syringe into end of NG tube. Remove clamp. Hold syringe with tip pointed at floor and inject saline slowly and evenly. Do not force solution.	Position of syringe prevents introduction of air into vent tubing, which could cause gastric distention. Solution introduced under pressure can cause gastric trauma.

➤ *CRITICAL DECISION POINT* Do not introduce saline through blue colored "pigtail" air vent of Salem sump tube.

STEPS	RATIONALE
6. If resistance occurs, check for kinks in tubing. Turn client onto left side. Repeated resistance should be reported to surgeon.	Tip of tube may lie against stomach lining. Repositioning on left side may dislodge tube away from the stomach lining. Buildup of secretions will cause distention.
7. After instilling saline, immediately aspirate or pull back slowly on syringe to withdraw fluid (see illustration). If amount aspirated is greater than amount instilled, record difference as output. If amount aspirated is less than amount instilled, record the difference as intake.	Irrigation clears tubing so stomach should remain empty. Fluid remaining in stomach is measured as intake.

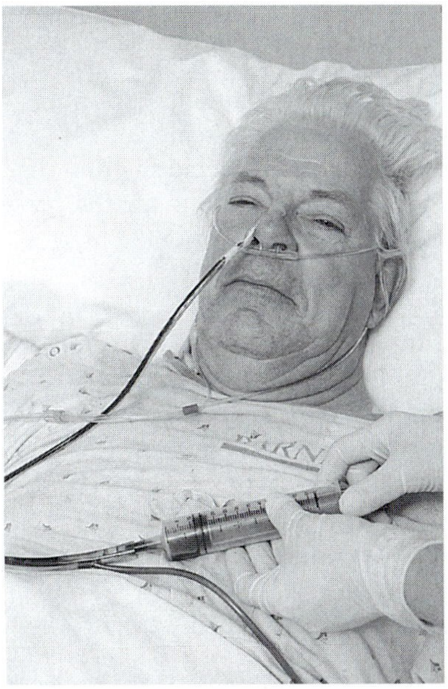

Step 7 Aspiration of NG tube.

STEPS	RATIONALE
8. Reconnect NG tube to drainage or suction. (If solution does not return, repeat irrigation.)	Reestablishes drainage collection; may repeat irrigation or repositioning of tube until NG tube drains properly.
9. Remove gloves and wash hands.	Reduces transmission of microorganisms.

Discontinuation of NG Tube

STEPS	RATIONALE
1. Verify order to discontinue NG tube.	Physician's order required for procedure.
2. Explain procedure to client and reassure that removal is less distressing than insertion.	Minimizes anxiety and increases cooperation. Tube passes out smoothly.
3. Wash hands and don disposable gloves.	Reduces transmission of microorganisms.
4. Turn off suction and disconnect NG tube from drainage bag or suction. Remove tape from bridge of nose and unpin tube from gown.	Have tube free of connections before removal.
5. Stand on client's right side if right-handed, left side if left-handed.	Allows easiest manipulation of tube.

EPS	RATIONALE
6. Hand the client facial tissue; place clean towel across chest. Instruct client to take and hold a deep breath.	Client may wish to blow nose after tube removed. Towel may keep gown from getting soiled. Airway will be temporarily obstructed during tube removal.
7. Clamp or kink tubing securely and then pull tube out steadily and smoothly into towel held in other hand while client holds breath.	Clamping prevents tube contents from draining into oropharynx. Reduces trauma to mucosa and minimizes client's discomfort. Towel covers tube, which can be an unpleasant sight. Holding breath helps to prevent aspiration.
8. Measure amount of drainage and note character of content. Dispose of tube and drainage equipment.	Provides accurate measure of fluid output. Reduces transfer of microorganisms.
9. Clean nares and provide mouth care.	Promotes comfort.
10. Position client comfortably and explain procedure for drinking fluids, if not contraindicated.	Depends on physician's order. Sometimes clients are NPO for up to 24 hours. When fluids are allowed the order usually begins with small amount of ice chips each hour and increases as client is able to tolerate more.
11. Clean equipment and return to proper place. Place soiled linen in utility room or proper receptacle.	Proper disposal of equipment prevents spread of microorganisms and ensures proper exchange procedures.
12. Remove gloves and wash hands.	Reduces transmission of microorganisms.

EVALUATION

1. Observe amount and character of contents draining from NG tube. Ask if client feels nauseated.	Determines if tube is decompressing stomach of contents.
2. Palpate client's abdomen periodically, noting any distention, pain, and rigidity and auscultate for the presence of bowel sounds. Turn off suction while auscultating.	Determines success of abdominal decompression and the return of peristalsis. The sound of the suction apparatus may be transmitted to abdomen and be misinterpreted as bowel sounds.
3. Inspect condition of nares and nose.	Evaluates onset of skin and tissue irritation.
4. Observe position of tubing.	Determines if tension is being applied to nasal structures.
5. Ask if client feels sore throat or irritation in pharynx.	Evaluates level of client's discomfort.
6. **Unexpected outcomes** that may occur include:	
➤ NG tube fails to drain fluid.	Tubing occluded, kinked, or malpositioned in upper stomach or esophagus.
➤ Client experiences vomiting.	Symptomatic of distention and/or reduced peristalsis. Tube not functioning properly.
➤ Abdomen becomes distended and tight, with reduced bowel sounds.	Symptomatic of distention and/or reduced peristalsis. Tube not functioning properly.
➤ Redness, tenderness, and excoriation of naris are present.	Result of tube rubbing against surface of naris and tape irritating skin on nose.
➤ Tube is pulling on naris.	Tube has inappropriate slack; retape.
➤ Client complains of severe sore throat, irritation in swallowing, nasal fullness.	Symptomatic of pharyngeal irritation.

RECORDING AND REPORTING

1. Record in nurse's notes time and type of NG tube inserted, client's tolerance of procedure, confirmation of placement, character of gastric contents, pH value, and whether tube is clamped or connected to drainage device.	Description of gastric contents provides baseline to determine any change.
2. Record in nurse's notes and/or flow sheet amount and character of contents draining from NG tube every shift, unless ordered more frequently by physician.	Maintains accurate record of intake and output.

STEPS	RATIONALE
3. Record each irrigation, type and amount of solution used, character and volume of aspirate, balance of fluid instilled and aspirated on intake and output sheet, nurse's notes, or flow sheet.	Balance reflects fluid gained or lost.
4. Record in nurse's notes presence or absence of bowel sounds.	NG tube cannot be removed until peristalsis is present.
5. Record time NG tube discontinued and client's tolerance of procedure.	
6. Report failure of tube to be inserted or drain, abdominal distention, and unusual character of drainage (e.g., blood) to physician.	Findings indicate need to reposition tube or administer additional therapies.

FOLLOW-UP ACTIVITIES

1. Increase frequency of NG tube irrigations or tube repositioning if client has nausea or is vomiting or if abdomen becomes hard or distended.
2. Continue to provide nursing measures for mouth care, care of nares, and client comfort. If naris is excoriated, apply lubrication or antiseptic ointment as ordered.

• • • • •

Special Considerations

- If client is confused or disoriented, obtain assistance from another nurse to insert tube.
- Comatose or semiconscious clients have reduced or absent gag reflex, making it difficult to determine if tube has passed correctly. If tube is in esophagus, client may often belch when air is instilled to check tube's placement.
- Periodically, check to be sure surface of tube is not taped against inside surface of nares. This will cause tissue erosion. Change tape at least daily or whenever soiled to minimize irritation.
- To provide additional comfort for client, apply petrolatum to nares to prevent crusting of secretions. When tube is in nostril, client tends to breathe through mouth, causing lips and tongue to become dry and crusted. Petrolatum applied to lips helps prevent dryness. Physician may allow sucking on small ice chips, gargling solution, throat lozenges, or chewing gum to increase saliva and decrease irritation. Sometimes frequently changing client's position helps relieve pressure from tube on one area in throat.
- Unless otherwise ordered, NG tube should be irrigated every 2 hours. Sometimes after instilling fluid, large amounts of air are aspirated. Continue to aspirate air and check client's abdomen to determine if hardness or distention is reduced.
- If gastric bleeding occurs, the physician may order an iced saline solution for irrigation.
- To prevent leakage of fluid from airway vent of Salem sump tubes, nurse should introduce 30 ml of air into airway lumen to clear tube, maintain patency of NG tube by checking drainage from main lumen, secure airway lumen above stomach level to avoid siphoning effect, and keep collection apparatus below client's midline to prevent reflux. Do not clamp airway vent.

Pediatric Considerations

- NG tubes may be of smaller size for children.

Gerontologic Considerations

- Severely debilitated or neurologically depressed elderly clients are at risk for inadvertent respiratory placement of an NG tube.

SKILL 35-5 Performing Postoperative Care of the Surgical Client

Nursing care of the postoperative surgical client is divided into two phases. During both phases the nurse must make comprehensive and detailed assessments of the client's condition. The effects of anesthesia and the physiological stressors imposed by surgery can place the client at risk for a variety of physiological alterations. It is also important for the nurse to facilitate communication among all members of the health care team, the client, and the client's family or significant other.

The first phase of postoperative care takes place during the immediate recovery period. For hospitalized clients this extends from the time the client leaves the OR to the time the client has stabilized in the recovery room (RR), postanesthesia room (PAR), or postanesthesia care unit (PACU) and has been transferred to the nursing division. For an ambulatory surgical client, the first phase of recovery normally lasts 1 to 2 hours before discharge home. The first phase is the most critical postoperative phase for assessing after effects of anesthesia, airway clearance, cardiovascular complications, temperature control, and neurological function. The client's condition can change rapidly. The nurse in the recovery area must make timely, intelligent, and accurate assessments to select the most appropriate measures of care for the client.

Each hospital has its own policies directing the process for recovering clients during the immediate postoperative period. Frequently, for example, clients transfer from the OR to an intensive care unit. In this situation the client is not sent to the RR area. The conditions of these clients are potentially so unstable as to require the monitoring available only in an intensive care unit.

The second phase of recovery is the postoperative convalescent period. This period extends from the time the client is discharged from the RR to the time the client is discharged from the hospital for inpatient clients. Outpatient surgical clients undergo convalescence at home. All clients who have undergone surgical procedures have similar postoperative needs. However, nursing care becomes very individualized depending on the nature of the client's surgery, preexisting medical conditions, the onset of complications, and the speed of recovery. Not all surgical clients recover at the same rate. During the convalescent period the nurse begins preparation for discharge and actively includes client, family, and significant others in the process. The nurse promotes the client's independence, educates the client about any limitations imposed by surgery, and provides resources needed for the client to assume an improved state of wellness.

EQUIPMENT

Recovery Room

- Stethoscope, sphygmomanometer, thermometer
- Pulse oximeter and monitor
- IV fluid poles
- Oxygen equipment such as mask, nasal cannula, tubing, oxygen regulator
- Continuous suction equipment (to suction airway)
- Dressing supplies
- Intermittent suction (for NG tube suction)
- Warmed blanket
- Additional equipment for physical assessment

Nursing Division

- Stethoscope, sphygmomanometer, thermometer
- IV fluid poles
- Intermittent external pneumatic compression equipment (if ordered)
- Emesis basin
- Washcloth and towel
- Waterproof pads
- Equipment for oral hygiene (see Chapter 6)
- Pillows
- Facial tissue
- Oxygen equipment
- Continuous suction equipment (for airway suction and wound drainage systems)
- Dressing supplies
- Intermittent suction (for NG suction)
- Orthopedic appliances (if traction needed)

DELEGATION CONSIDERATIONS

The skill of initiating and managing postoperative care of the client requires problem solving and knowledge application unique to a professional nurse. Unlicensed assistive personnel may obtain vital signs, apply nasal cannula or oxygen mask, and provide comfort and hygiene measures.

STEPS	RATIONALE

ASSESSMENT

Immediate Recovery Period

STEPS	RATIONALE
1. Receive report from circulating nurse, including procedure performed, range of vital signs, any complications, estimated blood loss (EBL), other fluid loss, fluid replacement, type of anesthesia, medications given, type of airway and size, extent of surgical wound, and any preoperative problems.	Determines client's general status and allows nurse to anticipate need for special equipment, nursing care, and activities in RR.
CRITICAL DECISION POINT Clients frequently first complain of pain. Know how much sedative and/or analgesic has been given.	
2. Upon client's arrival in RR, obtain report from surgeon and anesthesiologist.	Review provides detailed analysis of client's physiological status, allowing nurse to make appropriate observations and interventions. Provides baseline data to determine any change in condition.
3. Consider type of surgery client underwent, restrictions to movement, and anesthetic used.	Influences type of assessments nurse initiates, type of complications to observe for, and specific nursing interventions.
4. After receiving report, perform thorough client assessment including respiratory, cardiac, neurological, GI, GU, and fluid status; temperature; surgical site and drains; skin integrity; comfort and safety; and anxiety.	Provides baseline for further postoperative evaluations. Identifies priority nursing interventions.
CRITICAL DECISION POINT Be sure to turn client on side (when possible) to observe underlying skin.	

Convalescent Period

STEPS	RATIONALE
1. Obtain phone report from nurse in RR.	Preliminary report allows nurse to prepare hospital room with necessary supplies and equipment for client's special needs.
2. Upon client's arrival at division, collect more detailed report from nurse accompanying client.	Detailed report helps nurse plan appropriate assessment and nursing care measures. Data provide baseline to detect any change in client's condition.
3. Review client's chart for information pertaining to type of surgery, complications, medications administered, preoperative medical risks, and baseline vital signs.	Nature of surgery, intraoperative complications, and presence of medical risks dictate complications for which to observe. Vital signs provide means to measure postoperative changes.
4. Review surgeon's postoperative orders.	Offers additional guidelines for type of care to provide.

NURSING DIAGNOSIS

Clustering of defining characteristics from the assessment data may reveal the following nursing diagnoses for clients requiring this skill:

- Ineffective airway clearance
- Ineffective breathing pattern
- Impaired gas exchange
- Knowledge deficit regarding postoperative care
- Pain
- Altered tissue perfusion
- Risk for aspiration
- Impaired physical mobility
- Body image disturbance
- Impaired verbal communication
- Acute confusion
- Impaired skin integrity
- Fluid volume deficit
- Fluid volume excess
- Ineffective thermoregulation
- Inability to sustain spontaneous ventilation
- Altered protection
- Sensory perceptual alterations: visual, auditory
- Impaired swallowing
- Urinary retention

Related factors are individualized based on a client's condition or needs.

STEPS	RATIONALE
PLANNING	
1. Expected outcomes following completion of procedure:	
➤ Client's vital signs, including oxygen saturation, remain within previous baseline or normal expected range.	No cardiovascular, pulmonary, or thermoregulatory changes except those expected from effects of anesthetic or analgesic.
➤ Client reports relief of discomfort after analgesic or other pain relief measures.	Pain relief measures effectively alter client's reception or perception of pain.
➤ Breath sounds remain clear to auscultation; cough is clear.	Postoperative exercises and activity promote lung expansion and alveolar stability.
➤ Normal bowel sounds present within 48 to 72 hours after bowel surgery or general anesthetic. Normal bowel sounds are heard within 24 hours in cases of minor surgery.	Indicates return of intestinal peristalsis.
➤ Intake and output remain relatively in balance.	Adequate urinary elimination maintained. Fluid intake maintained.
➤ Client is able to discuss recovery and discharge plans. Verbalizes no specific physical complaints.	Client coping with stress of surgery.
2. Prepare the equipment as necessary at bedside.	
3. Explain to client all procedures you are to perform and rationale for each. On nursing division include family members and/or significant other in explanations.	Involves client in plan of care and minimizes anxiety. As recovery progresses, client is able to make more choices regarding how procedures should be performed.
➤ ***CRITICAL DECISION POINT*** **In ambulatory surgery centers, families are allowed at the bedside.**	
IMPLEMENTATION	
Immediate Recovery Period	
1. Wash hands.	Reduces transmission of microorganisms.
2. Check equipment setup in cubicle of RR.	All equipment must be operational and ready to use on client's arrival.
3. As client enters RR on stretcher, immediately attach oxygen tubing to regulator, hang IV fluids, check IV flow rates, and attach pulse oximeter (see Skill 10-6). Connect any drainage tubes to gravity drainage or intermittent suction as ordered. Attach cardiac monitor. Ensure indwelling catheter and bag are in drainage position.	Maintaining oxygenation and circulation are two priorities. Inhaled oxygen improves percentage delivered to alveoli. Pulse oximeter provides information on arterial oxygen saturation. IV fluids maintain circulatory volume and provide route for emergency drugs. Drainage tubes must remain patent and in proper position to allow fluid to drain from wound bed.
4. Conduct complete assessment of all vital signs. Compare findings with client's normal baseline. Continue assessing vital signs every 15 minutes or more often until client stabilizes.	Vital signs can reveal onset of postoperative complications, for example, respiratory depression, hypothermia or hyperthermia, pulse irregularity, or hypotension.
➤ ***CRITICAL DECISION POINT*** **If client underwent short procedure under IV sedation, check agency policy for sedation recovery guidelines.**	
5. Maintain patent airway:	
a. Position client on the side with head facing down and neck slightly extended.	Extension prevents occlusion of airway at pharynx. Downward position of head moves tongue forward, and mucus can drain out of mouth.
b. Place small folded towel under client's head. If client is restricted to supine position, elevate head of bed approximately 10 to 15 degrees, extend neck, and turn head to side.	Supports head in extended position. Prevents aspiration.

STEPS	RATIONALE
CRITICAL DECISION POINT If client is not able to hyperextend neck, turn head to side if possible, suction frequently.	
c. Encourage client to cough and deep breathe on awakening.	Promotes lung expansion and expectoration of mucous secretions.
d. Suction artificial airway and oral cavity as secretions accumulate.	Clears airway of secretions.
e. Once gag reflex returns, client spits out oral airway (see illustration). Do not tape oral airway.	Indicates client can clear airway independently. If airway is taped, client will gag and may obstruct airway.
6. Call client by name in moderate tone of voice. If there is no response, attempt to arouse the client by touching or gently moving a body part. Explain that the client is in the RR.	Determines client's level of consciousness and ability to follow commands.
7. Assess circulatory perfusion by inspecting color of nail beds and skin. Palpate for skin temperature.	Pink or normal skin color indicates adequate perfusion. Warm extremities reveal adequate circulation.
8. Observe condition of dressing and drains for any evidence of bright red blood. Also look underneath client for any pooling of bloody drainage.	Hemorrhage from a surgical wound usually occurs within first few hours, indicating that blood vessel was improperly tied or cauterized during surgery. When a dressing becomes saturated, blood oozes down client's side and collects under bedclothes.
9. Inspect surgical area for swelling or discoloration. Note condition of surgical dressing, including amount, color, odor, and consistency of drainage. Mark dressing with a circle around drainage using a black pen or marker. Place time of marking and check area every 10 to 15 minutes, marking any changes and noting vital signs.	A spread of an inch or more per three checks warrants a call to the surgeon because it could indicate hemorrhage. Determines extent of fluid loss and condition of underlying wound.
10. Refer to physician's order and reinforce or change dressing as indicated.	Dressing helps to maintain hemostasis and absorb drainage.
11. Inspect condition and contents of any drainage tubes and collecting devices. Note character and volume of drainage (see illustration).	Determines drainage tube patency and extent of wound drainage.

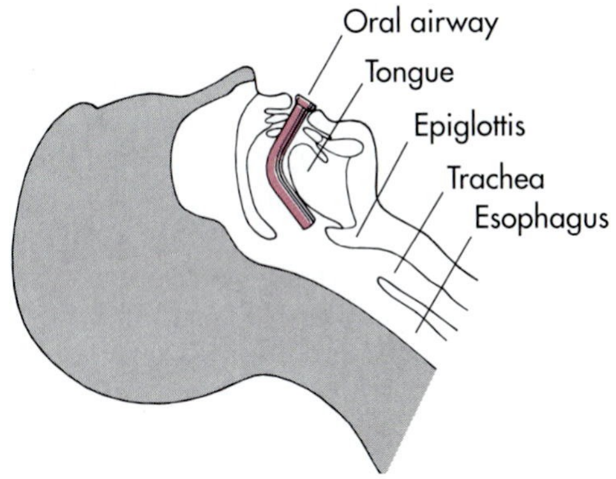

Step 5e Oral airway position before removal.

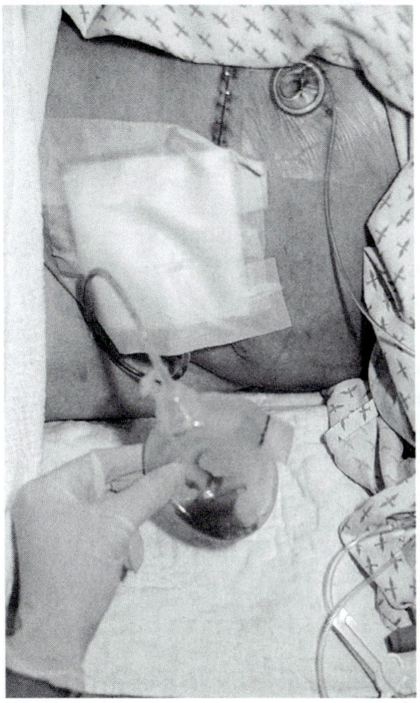

Step 11 Jackson-Pratt drain and client's wound.

STEPS	RATIONALE
12. Observe patency, intactness, volume, and character of urine from indwelling Foley catheter (if present).	Patent drainage system prevents bladder distention. Urine volume monitored to measure renal function.
13. If NG tube is present, irrigate periodically (Skill 35-4) with normal saline.	Maintains patency of tube to ensure gastric decompression.
14. Continue monitoring of IV fluid rates. Observe IV site for signs of infiltration, such as swelling, pitting edema, redness, warmth, discomfort, and leakage of IV fluid.	Continuous regular infusion of IV fluids maintains client's fluid intake to maintain adequate hydration and circulatory function.
15. As client awakens, provide mouth care by placing moistened washcloth to lips, swabbing oral mucosa with dampened swab, or applying petrolatum to lips.	Client still at risk for aspirating and should not be given fluids to rinse mouth. Moist cloth or swab can be soothing to dry mucosa.
16. Assess level of pain as client awakens. Provide pain medication as ordered and when vital signs have stabilized.	Pain can increase the stress response and interfere with postoperative exercises. Pain medication can further depress vital signs if anesthetic's effect still present.
17. Explain how client is progressing and that plans for transfer to a nursing division are being made.	Helps client remain oriented to surroundings and recovery activities.
18. Once all physiological signs have stabilized, contact physician for order to release client to floor.	Physician responsible for dictating level of observation and care required by client.

Convalescent Period

STEPS	RATIONALE
1. Make final check of equipment setup in client's room. Be sure bed is placed in high horizontal position and to side so that stretcher can easily be moved beside bed.	During transfer, client's status may change, necessitating quick interventions upon arrival. Availability of equipment ensures smooth transfer process.
2. Upon arrival at client's room assist RR staff and use three-person carry to transfer client to bed.	Technique avoids strain on nurses' back muscles and maintains client's safety.
3. Once client is transferred to bed, immediately attach any existing oxygen tubing, hang IV fluids, check IV flow rate, attach NG tube to suction, and place indwelling catheter in drainage position.	Maintains client's oxygenation and circulation.
4. Conduct complete assessment of all vital signs. Compare findings with vital signs in recovery area as well as client's baseline values. Continue monitoring as ordered.	Client should be stabilized once transferred to nursing division. Change in vital signs can reveal early onset of postoperative complications.

CRITICAL DECISION POINT **Report to the physician any findings deviating from previous assessment.**

STEPS	RATIONALE
5. Maintain client's airway:	
a. If artificial airway is still present, suction any secretions.	During transfer period, secretions can accumulate within airway.
b. Position client on side (if allowed); if client remains sleepy or lethargic, keep head extended.	Positioning minimizes chances of aspiration.
c. Encourage coughing and deep breathing.	Promotes lung expansion and expectoration of mucus.
6. Be sure any drainage tubes are connected to proper suction or drainage device. If NG tube is present, irrigate as ordered and connect to proper drainage device.	Maintains drainage tube patency so that wound beds remain dry for healing. Occlusion of NG tube can lead to abdominal distention.
7. Assess client's surgical dressing for intactness and presence and character of drainage. Reinforce as ordered. If no dressing present, inspect condition of wound.	Wound can hemorrhage quickly during early postoperative period. Observations of wound and dressings provides data to measure progress of wound healing.

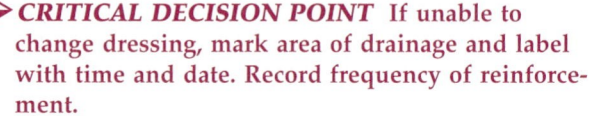

CRITICAL DECISION POINT **If unable to change dressing, mark area of drainage and label with time and date. Record frequency of reinforcement.**

STEPS	RATIONALE
8. Assess client for bladder distention. Offer bedpan if client senses urge to void.	Anesthetics and analgesics depress sensation of bladder fullness.
CRITICAL DECISION POINT Initiate measures to stimulate voiding within 4 hours of surgery.	
9. Measure all sources of fluid intake and output.	Assists in monitoring fluid and electrolyte balance.
10. Position client for comfort, maintaining airway and correct body alignment. Avoid positioning on surgical wound site or with pressure on popliteal space.	Good positioning reduces stress on suture line and decreases risks of aspiration and impaired circulation. Comfortable position helps client relax.
11. If ordered, apply elastic stockings or pneumatic compression cuffs to lower extremities and attach to compressor (see Skill 30-3). Explain to the client that the compression cuffs will inflate and deflate intermittently.	Increases venous return.
12. Explain to client that you have completed all observations and that you will ask family members or significant other to enter room. Place call light within reach and raise side rails.	Promotes client's orientation and sense of well-being. Call light and side rail positioning ensure client's safety as effects of anesthetic continue to diminish.
13. Explain client's general status to family and/or significant other, describe purpose of any equipment in room, and explain reason for frequent observations and procedures.	Family and significant others are normally anxious to learn about client's status. Unfamiliar sights (equipment and client's appearance) can be anxiety provoking. Family's and significant other's understanding can promote their participation in client's care.
CRITICAL DECISION POINT It can be helpful to give family simple tasks to perform, such as wiping client's face with washcloth and coaching postoperative exercises.	
14. Refer to recovery record to determine if pain medication administered. Administer analgesic if vital signs remain stable or initiate PCA, if ordered (see Skill 5-3).	Pain relief is essential for client to be able to begin postoperative exercises.
15. Provide oral hygiene and repeat as needed.	Maintenance of moist mucous membranes facilitates expectoration of secretions and promotes comfort.
16. As client stabilizes over the next hours or days, perform the following measures:	
a. Have client participate in postoperative exercises.	Promotes pulmonary and circulatory function to minimize onset of postoperative complications.
b. Encourage use of incentive spirometer as ordered. Watch client use spirometer first few times to judge efficacy of breathing.	Promotes lung expansion.
c. Begin activity orders. (Assess vital signs first time client sits or stands to judge tolerance.)	Promotes circulation, lung expansion, and peristalsis. (Sudden positional changes can cause postural hypotension.)
d. Begin dietary orders slowly according to client's tolerance.	Promotes normal fluid and electrolyte balance, restores nutritional intake, promotes normal GI function and wound healing.
e. Assist client in assuming normal urinary voiding pattern.	Promotes normal urinary elimination and prevents bladder distention.
CRITICAL DECISION POINT If client does not void within 8 hours after surgery, notify physician. Urinary catheter may have to be inserted.	
f. Closely monitor progress of wound healing and change dressings as ordered.	Wound infection occurs most often within 3 to 6 days postoperatively. Wound **dehiscence** occurs most often 3 to 11 days postoperatively.

STEPS	RATIONALE
CRITICAL DECISION POINT Delayed wound healing may result in wound dehiscence or evisceration. This occurs most frequently after coughing, sneezing, vomiting, or getting up from a sitting position. Caution should be observed when the client performs these activities.	
g. Monitor and maintain wound drainage devices, such as Jackson-Pratt, Hemovac, or Penrose drains.	Wound drainage devices promote healing from inside to outside.
CRITICAL DECISION POINT Be sure devices are draining properly.	
17. Gradually increase client's involvement in decision making and in any explanations about surgery and related implications.	Promotes client's sense of control and independence. Encourages feeling of self-esteem.
18. Discuss with client and family or significant other plans for discharge.	Discharge planning is continuous process, beginning with client's admission.

EVALUATION

STEPS	RATIONALE
1. Compare all vital sign assessment measurements with client's baseline and expected normals.	Evaluates client's respiratory, cardiovascular, and thermoregulatory status throughout recovery.
2. Evaluate effects of pain relief measures, such as positioning, and use of analgesics.	Determines level of comfort achieved and effectiveness of pain relief measures.
3. Monitor changes in surgical wound at least every shift.	Provides data to measure progress of wound healing.
4. Monitor lung sounds following postoperative exercises.	Determines status of airways.
5. Auscultate bowel sounds at least each shift.	Evaluates return of peristalsis and diet tolerance.
6. Monitor intake and output balance for each shift.	Can reveal onset of fluid imbalances.
7. Hold discussion with client regarding general level of comfort and progress toward recovery.	Gives client sense of participation in care. Client's perceptions can also be helpful in noting onset of complications. Reveals readiness to learn about discharge.
8. Conduct physical assessments according to client's unique type of surgery.	Monitors course of recovery.
9. **Unexpected outcomes** that may occur include:	
➤ Vital signs are above or below client's baseline or expected range.	Alterations may result from anesthetic effects, pain, or surgical complications such as **hypovolemic shock,** airway obstruction, fluid and electrolyte imbalances, or malignant hypothermia.
➤ Client continues to experience incisional pain.	Factors may heighten client's pain perception, such as anxiety, isolation, and fatigue. Analgesic ordered may be of insufficient dosage.
➤ Abnormal breath sounds are auscultated.	Result of atelectasis or mucous secretions in larger airways.
➤ Client complains of calf tenderness; exhibits positive Homans' sign and redness in lower extremity.	Signs of venous thrombosis or thrombophlebitis.
➤ Bowel sounds are absent or decreased.	**Paralytic ileus** can develop as common complication after bowel surgery. Intestinal motility may return slowly depending on anesthetic effects.
➤ Client develops fever, tenderness, and pain at wound site; increased white blood cell count or purulent drainage is present.	Signs of wound infection.
➤ Client reports feeling something in wound "give way." Increased serosanguinous drainage is noted.	Signs of wound dehiscence or evisceration.

STEPS	RATIONALE
CRITICAL DECISION POINT **Report immediately as could be life-threatening.**	
➤ Intake and output measurements reflect imbalance.	Indicates possible fluid volume excess or deficit. Client is at risk for electrolyte imbalance, pulmonary edema, and renal insufficiency.
➤ Client is unable to discuss discharge plans or has negative view of recovery.	May indicate client is coping poorly with stress of surgery.

Recording and Reporting

1. Document client's arrival at RR or nursing division; describe vital signs, assessment findings, and all nursing measures initiated in nurse's notes. Continue documentation at least every shift.	Documents care provided. Data provide baseline to compare changes in client's condition. Information ensures continuity of care among health team members.
2. Record vital signs and intake and output on appropriate flow sheet.	Provides means to record repetitive types of data over frequent time intervals. Provides graphic view of trends.
3. Report any abnormal assessment findings and signs of complications to nurse in charge or physician.	Certain physiological changes may require emergency measures.

Follow-up Activities

1. Increase frequency of monitoring should complications arise.
2. Increase frequency of supportive care, such as postoperative exercises and ambulation, if signs of complications develop.

• • • • •

Special Considerations

➤ Client under spinal anesthesia may benefit from being placed in quiet area of RR.

➤ Client with spinal anesthesia is unable to feel sensation below the level of the spinal cord.

➤ To prevent spinal headache, clients with spinal anesthesia must be positioned supine, without elevation of head, for 24 hours. Fluids should be encouraged.

➤ Report between surgeon and nurse should include level of anesthesia, vital signs, IV fluids or blood products used in surgery, presence of drains under surgical dressing, special concerns such as risk for hemorrhage or dysrhythmias, and incidence of complications during surgery.

➤ Postoperative orders usually include frequency of vital signs and special assessments, types of IV fluids and infusion rate, postoperative medications, fluids or foods allowed by mouth, level of activity or type of positioning, intake and output, laboratory tests or x-ray studies to be done, and special directions such as dressing changes, care of traction, and use of incentive spirometers.

➤ Client's level of consciousness is usually altered upon arrival in RR. Factors influencing consciousness include anesthetic, medications, electrolyte and metabolic changes, pain, and emotions.

➤ In early postoperative phase, clients tend to be lethargic and less responsive because of lingering effects of general anesthetic.

➤ Respiratory depression can result from anesthetic. Client may have endotracheal tube or airway in place when arriving in RR. Each requires special oxygen adaptor. Do not elicit gag reflex because client may vomit secretions that could be aspirated. Never position client with hands over the chest (reduces chest expansion).

➤ Hypotension may result from anesthetic or acute blood loss. Acute blood loss may lead to hypovolemic shock with signs of reduced blood pressure, elevated heart and respiratory rates, pale skin, and restlessness. Clients who suffer severe blood loss postoperatively may receive blood products.

➤ Lowered level of metabolism causes hypothermia. Rare complication of anesthetic is malignant hyperthermia and is an emergency.

➤ Size, location, and depth of wound influence amount of drainage (see Chapter 40). Changing dressings immediately postoperatively can disrupt wound edges and aggravate drainage. Most physicians prefer reinforcement with additional dressings only. First dressing changes most often occur 24 hours postoperatively and are usually done by the physician. Minor surgical wounds may not have dressings but simply skin closure.

➤ Male client may need assistance to stand to void.

If client is unable to void within 8 hours after surgery, it may be necessary to insert urinary catheter.

- Many nurses are hesitant to administer pain medications until client requests them. Nurse is best judge to provide pain control independently during time when client is at high risk for discomfort. Client with spinal anesthetic usually feels no pain. Remember that pain can sometimes lower blood pressure, thus analgesic may restore vital signs to normal. Use with judgment.
- Clients who had abdominal surgery usually resume their diet with clear liquids. If these are tolerated, diet is advanced to full liquids, soft, or regular diet. Some clients have surgeries that allow them to advance to regular diet once nausea subsides.
- Clients are usually ordered to sit in a chair the evening of surgery or the next day. Activity progresses to walking in room and then in hallways. Allow clients to use toilet facilities as soon as activity allows.

Teaching Considerations

- If client had spinal anesthetic, remind family or significant other that loss of extremity movement is normal for several hours.
- Instruct client and primary care giver to identify signs and symptoms and appropriate actions for infection; respiratory, circulatory, or GI difficulties; and wound disruptions.
- Reinforce preoperative teaching regarding coughing, deep breathing, and leg exercises; ambulation; and pain control.
- Provide important phone numbers to client and primary care giver to use in event of emergency and for follow-up care on discharge.
- Teach client about appropriate wound care and diet recommendations.
- Inform client of activity restrictions.

Pediatric Considerations

- Parent-child separation should be kept to the minimum time possible.
- Vomiting is more common among children postoperatively than adults (Zuckerberg, 1994).
- Mandatory fluid intake guidelines are not usually necessary because of aggressive fluid replacement in children.
- Voiding prior to discharge from ambulatory surgery is not usually required for children.

Gerontologic Considerations

- The ability of the elderly to tolerate surgery depends on the extent of physiological changes that have occurred with aging, the presence of any chronic diseases, and the duration of the surgical procedure.

Home Care Considerations

- Teach primary care giver about any postoperative exercises, home modifications, or activity limitations.
- If client is discharged with dressing changes, bedroom or bathroom is usually ideal for procedure. Have primary care giver perform return demonstration of dressing change.

CRITICAL THINKING EXERCISES

1. **Before the client's abdominal surgery, the nurse assesses that the client has a history of smoking one pack of cigarettes per day for 30 years. What is essential for the nurse to incorporate in preoperative teaching?**
2. **While shaving the surgical area, the unlicensed technician notices a small cut and break in the skin. What action would indicate that the nurse had provided appropriate instruction regarding this procedure?**
3. **While irrigating an NG tube, the nurse obtains aspirate with a pH of 3. The client is able to speak and appears to be breathing easily, but is complaining of a "sore throat." What does this indicate about the positioning of the NG tube?**
4. **What are the most important parameters for the nurse to assess during the immediate recovery period for the client who has undergone an abdominal hysterectomy?**

REFERENCES

Brick J: Informed consent and perioperative nursing, *JAORN* 63(1):258, 1996.

Centers for Disease Control: *Guidelines for prevention of surgical wound infections,* Atlanta, 1985, Hospital Infection Control Programs, US Department of Health and Human Services.

Ellerton M, Merriam C: Preparing children and families psychologically for surgery: an evaluation, *J Adv Nurs* 19(6):1057, 1994.

Joint Commission on Accreditation of Health Care Organizations: *Accreditation manual for hospitals,* Chicago, 1996, The Commission.

Metheny N: Measures to test placement of nasogastric and nasointestinal feeding tubes: a review, *Nurs Res* 37:324, 1988.

Metheny N, et al: Effectiveness of the auscultatory method in predicting feeding tube location, *Nurs Res* 39:262, 1990.

Metheny N, et al: Effectiveness of pH measurements in predicting feeding tube placement: an update, *Nurs Res* 42(6):324, 1993.

Metheny N, et al: Visual characteristics of aspirates from feeding tubes as a method for predicting tube location, *Nurs Res* 43(5):282, 1994.

Roach J, Tremblay L, Bowers D: A preoperative assessment and education program: implementation and outcomes, *Patient Ed Couns* 25:83, 1995.

Schoessler M: Perceptions of preoperative education in patients admitted the morning of surgery, *Patient Ed Couns* 14:127, 1989.

Zuckerberg A: Perioperative approach to children, *Pediat Clin N Am* 41(1):15, 1994.

ADDITIONAL READING

American Society of Post Anesthesia Nursing: *Standards of post anesthesia nursing practice,* Richmond, Va, 1991, The Association.

Association of Operating Room Nurses: *Standards and recommended practices for perioperative nursing,* Denver, 1995, The Association.

Chalfin D, Nasraway S: Preoperative evaluation and postoperative care of the elderly patient undergoing major surgery, *Crit Ill in Elder* 10(1):51, 1994.

Garner JS: *Guidelines for prevention of surgical wound infections,* Atlanta, 1985, Hospital Infections Program, CDC, PHS, and US Department of Health and Human Services.

Hallstrom R, Beck S: Implementation of the AORN skin shaving standard, *JAORN* 58(3):498, 1993.

Lunow K, Jung L: Comprehensive perioperative care: patient assessment, teaching, documentation, *JAORN* 57(5):1167, 1993.

Metheny N, et al: Detection of inadvertent respiratory placement of small-bore feeding tubes, *Heart Lung* 19:631, 1990.

Oetker-Black S: Preoperative preparation: Historical development, *JAORN* 57(6):1402, 1993.

Phipps W, et al: *Medical-surgical nursing concepts and clinical practice,* ed 5, St Louis, 1995, Mosby.

CHAPTER 36

Intraoperative Care

OBJECTIVES

Mastery of content in this chapter will enable the nurse to:

- Define key terms.
- Describe the roles of the circulating and scrub nurse.
- Identify guidelines for use of sterile technique in the operating room.
- Correctly don a sterile surgical gown.
- Correctly apply sterile gloves using the closed technique.

KEY TERMS

Asepsis
Aseptic technique
Circulating nurse
Contamination
Scrub nurse
Sponge
Sterile
Sterile conscience
Sterile field
Strike through
Surgical scrub

SKILLS

36-1 Surgical Hand Washing

36-2 Donning a Sterile Gown and Gloves (Closed Gloving)

The perioperative role of the operating room (OR) nurse encompasses the client's surgical experience from the preoperative throughout the intraoperative period and into the postoperative phase (see Chapter 35). The activities that the registered nurse performs as part of the perioperative role are carried out using the nursing process. Members of the surgical team include the surgeon and assistant(s), certified registered nurse anesthetist (CRNA) and/or physician anesthesiologist, circulating nurse, and scrub nurse or surgical technologist.

The intraoperative phase begins when the client enters the OR suite and ends with admission to the postanesthesia care unit or recovery area. The OR nurse provides support, safety, and comfort for the client during the intraoperative phase.

During the intraoperative phase the registered nurse assumes the role of either scrub nurse or circulating nurse. The *scrub nurse* (see box on p. 1057) provides the surgeon with instruments and supplies, disposes of soiled sponges, and accounts for sponges, needles, and instruments on the surgical field. Registered nurses, licensed practical nurses, or surgical technologists may assume the scrub nurse role. The *circulating nurse* (see box on p. 1057) is always a registered nurse and is considered to be the charge nurse in the room (Association of Operating Room Nurses, 1995a). The circulating nurse assumes responsibility and accountability for maintaining client safety and continuity of quality care. The conduct of the nonprofessional staff is supervised by the circulating nurse. In addition, the circulating nurse is an assistant to the scrub nurse and surgeon. When a client enters the OR, the **circulating nurse** helps position the client and applies necessary monitoring and/or safety equipment. During the procedure the circulating nurse works with the scrub nurse to be sure aseptic technique is followed and that the client receives necessary supportive care. A registered nurse may also function as first assistant to the surgeon. The registered nurse first assistant (RNFA) is an expanded role requiring advanced education.

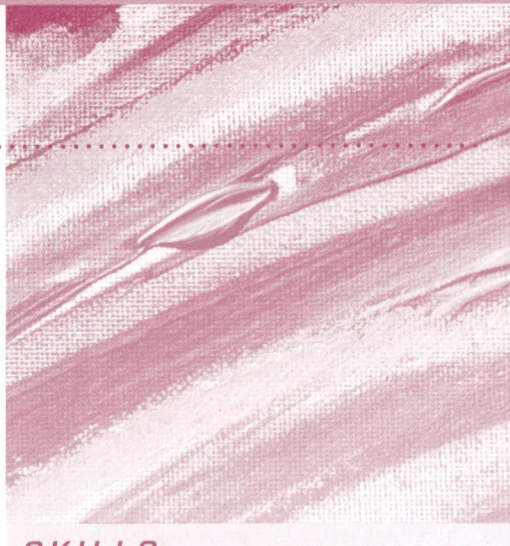

It is essential that perioperative nurses fully understand and follow the principles of **aseptic technique.** The over-

ROLE OF THE SCRUB NURSE

- Assists circulating nurse in preparing OR.
- Performs surgical hand scrub and dons sterile gown and gloves.
- Sets up sterile field with procedure-appropriate supplies and instruments, verifying all are in working order.
- Performs **sponge,** sharp, and instrument counts with circulating nurse prior to incision.
- Gowns and gloves surgeons and assistants as they enter the OR.
- Assists surgeons with sterile draping of client.
- Keeps sterile field orderly and monitors progress of procedure and any breaks in aseptic technique.
- Passes instruments and supplies to surgeons and assistants.
- Handles surgical specimens per institutional policy.
- Constantly monitors location of all sponges and sharps in the field and performs closing sponge, sharp, and instrument counts with circulating nurse.

all goal of **asepsis** is to minimize contamination of the surgical wound. Before the client reaches the OR, supplies, instruments, and equipment must be thoroughly sterilized to remove all microorganisms. Members of the surgical team follow specific guidelines for performing a **surgical scrub** and donning surgical attire before handling **sterile** items. The special preparation of the client's skin before application of sterile drapes helps reduce the numbers of microorganisms around the surgical incision. The **scrub nurse** and surgeons create a **sterile field** around the surgical wound and maintain it throughout the procedure in accordance with strict aseptic principles. The surgical procedure itself finally ends with sterile application of dressings.

All members of the health care team in the OR must develop a **sterile conscience,** or personal commitment to safe, quality client care. It requires discipline, integrity, honesty, and assertiveness concerning any shortcomings in aseptic practice. The scrub nurse, who accidentally touches the faucet with one hand, while rinsing rescrubs the hands; the circulating nurse, who accidentally touches a sterile item, has it removed from the field; the surgeon, who contaminates a sterile glove, has the affected glove changed. These are all examples of following one's sterile conscience.

During the postoperative phase the OR nurse assists in transferring the client to the recovery room or postanesthesia room (see Chapter 35). The OR nurse is an important resource in planning the client's postoperative care.

ROLE OF THE CIRCULATING NURSE

- Organizes and prepares OR prior to start of case; checks to see equipment works properly
- Gathers supplies for case and opens sterile supplies for scrub nurse
- Counts sponges, sharps, and instruments with scrub nurse prior to incision being made
- Sends for client at appropriate time
- Conducts preoperative client assessment, including the following:
  - Explains role and identifies client
  - Reviews medical record and verifies procedure and consents
  - Confirms client's allergies, nothing by mouth (NPO) status, laboratory values, electrocardiogram (ECG), x-ray films, skin condition
- Safely transfers client to operating table and positions client according to surgeon preference and procedure type
- Applies return electrode pad to client if electrocautery used; may prepare client's skin; may apply ECG electrodes for local case
- Explains briefly what the circulating nurse and the scrub nurse are doing
- Assists surgical team by tying gowns and arranging tables
- Assists anesthesiologist during induction and extubation
- Continuously monitors procedure for any breaks in aseptic technique or to anticipate needs of the team; opens additional sterile supplies for scrub nurse; ensures standard precautions maintained
- Handles surgical specimens per institutional policy
- Documents care on perioperative nurse's notes
- Performs sponge, sharp, and instrument counts with scrub nurse at beginning of wound closure

GUIDELINES

1. All items used within a sterile field must be sterile.
2. Gowns used by scrub persons must be sterile before donning. Once in place, gowns are considered sterile in front from the chest to table level and on the sleeves to 2 inches (5 cm) above the elbow.
3. Sterile persons must keep hands in sight, above waist level and below neckline to avoid **contamination.**
4. When wearing a sterile gown, arms should *not* be folded with hands tucked in the axillary region. This area is not considered sterile once the gown is donned. Perspiration can lead to **strike through,** or contamination that occurs when moisture permeates a sterile barrier.
5. Draped tables should be considered sterile only at table level. Sides of the drape extending below table level are unsterile.

6. All personnel moving around or within a sterile field must do so in a manner consistent with maintaining the sterility of that field. Scrubbed persons move from sterile areas to other sterile areas, contacting a sterile field only with sterile gowns and gloves. Unscrubbed persons should always stay at least 1 foot away from the sterile field while keeping it in constant view and should contact only unsterile areas.
7. All sterile supplies and equipment should be grouped around the sterile-draped client.
8. Unsterile persons must avoid reaching over the sterile field.
9. Scrubbed persons should remain close to the sterile field. When changing position, they should turn face to face or back to back.

DELEGATION CONSIDERATIONS

The circulating nurse must always be a registered nurse. The role of the scrub nurse can be delegated to a surgical technologist or licensed practical nurse. Nonlicensed personnel can assist the registered nurse in the circulating role by opening sterile supplies, setting up sterile fields, and running errands under the direction of the registered nurse.

SKILL 36-1 Surgical Hand Washing

The procedure for surgical hand washing requires greater effort than does medical aseptic practice (see Chapter 33). Since strict surgical procedures are to be carried out, the nurse must use extra precautions to rid hand surfaces of microorganisms. The skin can never be rendered sterile; however, it can be made surgically clean through scrubbing. Surgical hand washing is necessary for nurses working in ORs or delivery rooms and in special diagnostic test areas.

The Association of Operating Room Nurses (AORN) (1995b) recommends a 5 to 10 minute surgical scrub before each surgical procedure. Exceptions to the rule include procedures such as bronchoscopies, laryngoscopies, esophagoscopies and certain laser procedures. These procedures require only a thorough hand washing of 3 to 5 minutes.

For maximum elimination of bacteria, the nurse removes all jewelry and keeps fingernails short, clean, healthy, and free of artificial nails. Brushes are used during scrubbing. Some experts caution that too much brushing removes outer layers of the epidermis, thereby exposing bacterial flora in the deeper skin layers.

If harsh soaps are used, the nurse's skin can become irritated, providing an environment for additional microorganism growth. Antiseptic solutions such as chlorhexidine and Hibiclens improve removal of bacteria from the hands and arms.

EQUIPMENT

- **Deep sink with foot or knee controls for dispensing water and soap (faucets should be high enough for hands and forearms to fit comfortably)**
- **Antiseptic detergent (nonirritating, broad-spectrum, fast-acting, effective in reducing skin microorganisms, and having a residual effect) (Association of Operating Room Nurses, 1995)**
- **Surgical scrub brush with plastic nail pick**
- **Paper mask and cap or hood**
- **Sterile towel**
- **Proper scrub attire**
- **Protective eyewear (glasses or goggles)**

STEPS	RATIONALE
ASSESSMENT	
1. Consult institutional policy regarding required length of time for hand wash.	Guidelines vary regarding ideal time needed for surgical scrub.
2. Be sure fingernails are short, clean, and healthy. Artificial nails should be removed. **CRITICAL DECISION POINT** Nail polish should be removed if chipped or worn longer than 4 days because it may harbor greater numbers of bacteria (Association of Operating Room Nurses, 1995c).	Long nails and chipped or old polish increase number of bacteria residing on nails. Long fingernails can puncture gloves, causing contamination. Artificial nails are known to harbor gram-negative microorganisms and fungus.

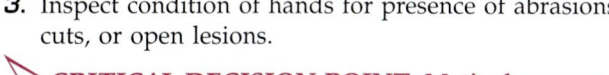

STEPS	RATIONALE
3. Inspect condition of hands for presence of abrasions, cuts, or open lesions.	These conditions increase likelihood of more microorganisms residing on skin surfaces.

CRITICAL DECISION POINT **Meticulous care of the hands may decrease potential for open areas.**

NURSING DIAGNOSIS

Clustering of defining characteristics from the assessment data may reveal the following nursing diagnoses for clients requiring this skill:

- Risk for infection

Related factors are individualized based on a client's condition or needs.

PLANNING

STEPS	RATIONALE
1. **Expected outcomes** following completion of procedure:	
➤ The client will not develop signs of surgical wound infection.	Indicates lack of microorganism transfer to the client and sterile field.
2. Prepare equipment.	Ensures availability prior to the procedure.
3. Remove all jewelry, including rings, watch, and bracelets.	Jewelry harbors microorganisms and interferes with access to all surfaces of skin to be cleaned.
4. Be sure sleeves are above elbows and uniform is fitted or tucked at waist.	Scrubbed hands and arms can become contaminated by brushing against loose garments.

IMPLEMENTATION

STEPS	RATIONALE
1. Apply surgical shoe covers, cap or hood, face mask, and protective eyewear (Skill 34-1).	Mask prevents escape into air of microorganisms that can contaminate hands. Other protective wear prevents exposure to blood and body fluid splashes during the procedure.
2. Turn on water using knee or foot controls and adjust to comfortable temperature.	
3. Wet hands and arms under running lukewarm water and lather with detergent to 2 inches above elbows (see illustration). (Hands need to be above elbows at all times.)	Water runs by gravity from fingertips to elbows. Hands become cleanest part of upper extremity. Keeping hands elevated allows water to flow from least to most contaminated areas. Washing a wide area reduces risk of contaminating overlying gown that the nurse later applies.

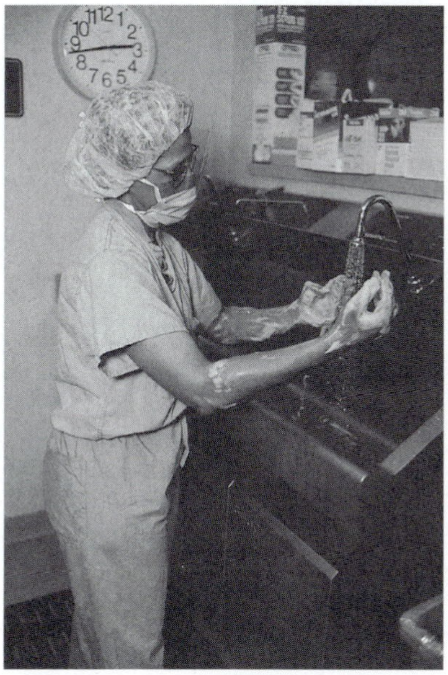

Step 3 Surgical scrub technique: prescrub wash/rinse.

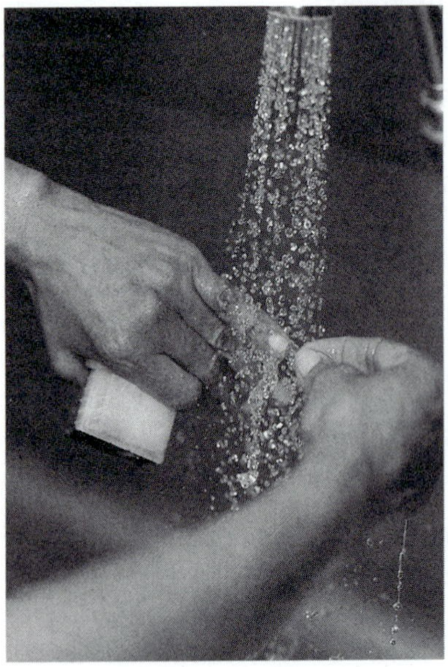

Step 5 Surgical scrub technique: cleaning under fingernails.

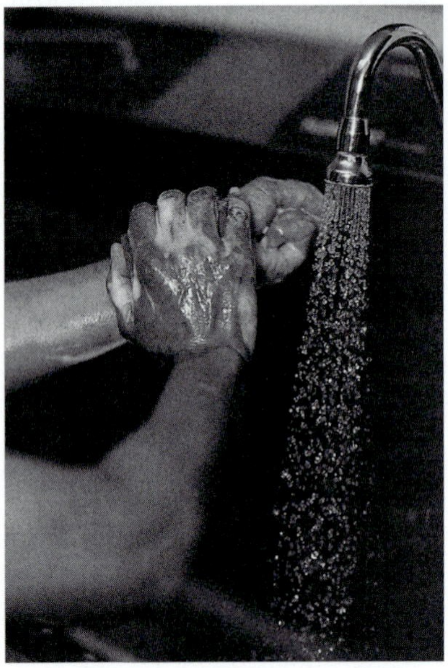

Step 6 Surgical scrub technique: scrubbing forearms.

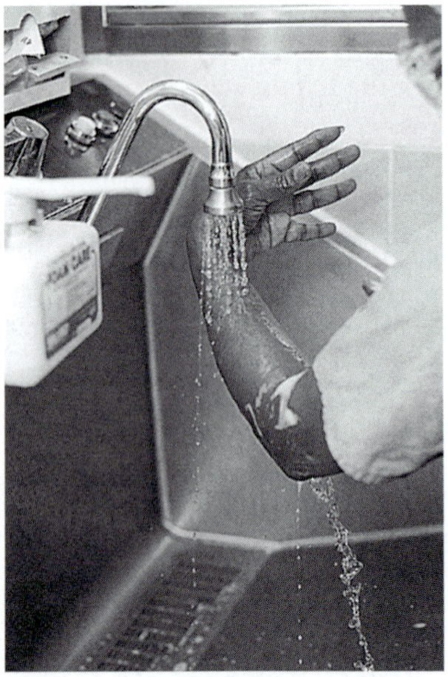

Step 7 Surgical scrub technique: rinsing arm.

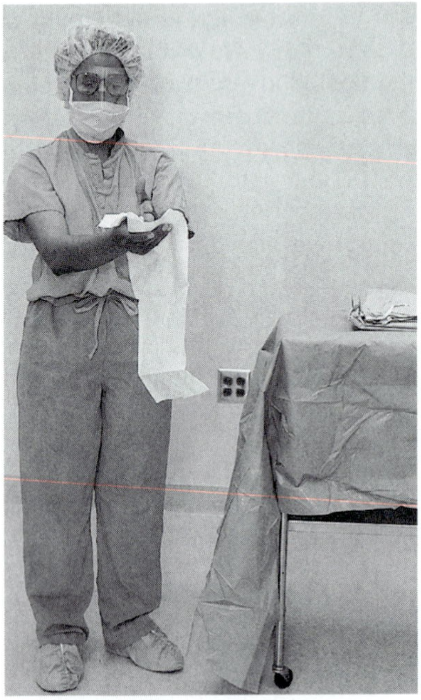

Step 8 Surgical scrub technique: drying sequence.

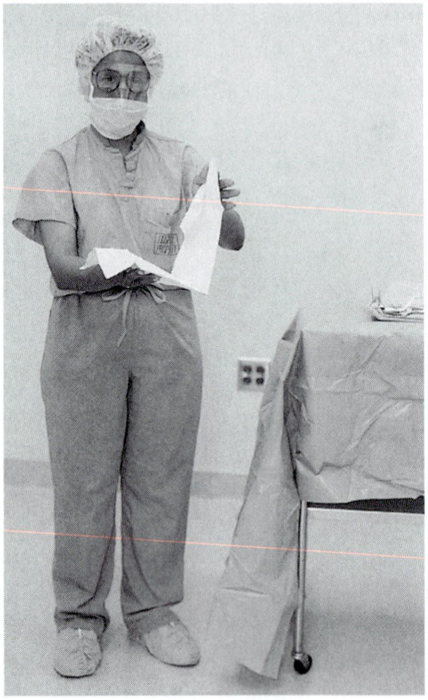

Step 9

STEPS	RATIONALE
4. Rinse hands and arms thoroughly under running water. **Remember to keep hands above elbows.**	Rinsing removes transient bacteria from fingers, hands, and forearms.
5. Under running water, clean under nails of both hands with file. Discard after use (see illustration).	Removes dirt and organic material that harbor large numbers of microorganisms.
6. Wet brush and apply antimicrobial detergent. Scrub the nails of one hand with 15 strokes. Holding brush perpendicular scrub the palm, each side of the thumb, and fingers, and the posterior side of the hand with 10 strokes each. The arm is mentally divided into thirds and each third is scrubbed 10 times (see illustration). Entire scrub should last 5 to 10 minutes. Rinse brush and repeat the sequence for the other arm. A two-brush method may be substituted. Check institution's policy.	Scrubbing loosens resident bacteria that adhere to skin surfaces. Ensures coverage of all surfaces. Scrubbing is performed from cleanest area (hands) to marginal area (upper arms).
7. Discard brush and rinse hands and arms thoroughly (see illustration). Turn off water with foot or knee control and back into room entrance with hands elevated in front of and away from the body.	After touching skin, brush is considered contaminated. Rinsing removes resident bacteria. Prevents accidental contamination.
8. Bending slightly forward at the waist, use a sterile towel to dry one hand thoroughly moving from fingers to elbow. Dry in a rotating motion (see illustration). Dry from cleanest to least clean area.	Drying prevents chapping and facilitates donning of gloves. Leaning forward prevents accidental contact of arms with scrub attire.
9. Repeat drying method for other hand, using a different area of the towel or a new sterile towel (see illustration).	Prevents accidental contamination.

EVALUATION

1. Observe the client for signs of localized wound infection.	Signs of infection include redness, heat, swelling, pain, and drainage.
2. **Unexpected outcomes** that may occur include:	
➤ Redness, heat, swelling, pain, or drainage at surgical site.	Indicates infection at site.

RECORDING AND REPORTING

1. Record area and description of surgical site postoperatively.	Correct documentation allows nurses to continue to monitor the site for proper healing.

• • • • •

Special Considerations

- Certain antiseptic detergents may cause skin irritations; therefore the nurse should not interchange different brands.
- Cuts or abrasions of the hands can contraindicate nurse's participation in procedure.
- Nurses often pin rings or watches to uniforms to prevent loss.
- Nurses in OR and labor and delivery areas wear special scrub suits.

SKILL 36-2 Donning a Sterile Gown and Gloves (Closed Gloving)

Attiring oneself correctly for the OR begins with personal hygiene. Potentially pathogenic bacteria are present on the skin, hair, and in the respiratory tract of all persons. Daily bathing and clean hair are necessary to minimize numbers of microorganisms. All persons entering a surgical suite must wear OR apparel (Association of Operating Room Nurses, 1995b). A clean scrub suit (pants and top) is worn to contain bacterial shedding. If scrub suits become visibly soiled or wet, they should be changed. Sleeves should be short enough to allow scrubbing to 2 inches above the elbow, and the top should be tucked in to prevent brushing against sterile areas and to decrease the amount of bacteria shed from the thoracic and abdominal skin.

OR apparel should be worn only within the surgical suite. If it is worn outside the OR, it should be covered or changed before the person reenters the area. Street clothes should never be worn in the restricted areas of the surgical suite.

All possible head and facial hair should be covered when one is in the surgical suite. The cap or hood should be the first piece of OR attire that is donned to prevent hair from collecting on the scrub clothes. A clean hat should be worn each day and should not be worn outside the surgical suite.

Shoe covers may be worn inside the OR for sanitation purposes. Knee high shoe covers may be worn as personal protective equipment for cases in which large amounts of fluid or blood may be lost. All shoe covers should be removed upon leaving the restricted areas of the suite, and new shoe covers may be put on when returning to the OR. Clean shoe covers should be worn each day and should be changed if they become soiled. Sandals are not recommended in the OR because they are not considered safe.

Masks must be worn in specified restricted areas of the surgical suite. Examples of restricted areas include rooms with open sterile supplies and areas designed to sterilize instruments. The surgical mask should completely cover the mouth and nose since its purpose is to filter organisms from exhaled air. The mask should be secured over the nose, along the sides of the face, and under the chin to keep air from escaping around it (see Chapter 34). As a mask becomes moist, its effectiveness decreases since bacteria can pass through it. Surgical masks should be changed between procedures and should not be allowed to hang around the neck, harboring bacteria from the nasopharyngeal airway. Only mask strings should be touched when removing a mask to reduce contamination of hands by bacteria from the airway.

Jewelry should not be worn in the surgical suite. Rings, watches, and necklaces serve as reservoirs for bacteria. Dangling earrings that hang outside the cap can fall onto the sterile field.

Before donning a sterile gown and gloves in the OR, a complete surgical scrub (Skill 36-1) must be performed.

EQUIPMENT

- **Package of proper-sized sterile gloves**
- **Sterile pack containing sterile gown (prepared by circulating nurse)**
- **Surgical cap, mask, and footwear**
- **Equipment needed for surgical hand washing (Skill 36-1)**
- **Protective eyewear**

STEPS	RATIONALE
ASSESSMENT	
1. Inspect condition of hands for cuts, open lesions, or abrasions.	Lesions harbor microorganisms and may prevent nurse from performing procedure.
2. Check fingernails as per procedure in Skill 36-1.	Fingernails harbor microorganisms.
3. Choose proper size and type of glove.	Ill-fitting gloves impede the ability to grasp objects and provide an opportunity for needle punctures. Skin sensitivities may occur with certain gloves.
4. Choose proper size and type of gown.	Ill-fitting gown may impede movement of nurse's extremities.

NURSING DIAGNOSIS

Clustering of defining characteristics from the assessment data may reveal the following nursing diagnoses for clients requiring this skill:

➤ Risk for infection

Related factors are individualized based on a client's condition or needs.

STEPS	RATIONALE
PLANNING	
1. **Expected outcomes** following completion of procedure:	
➤ Client will not develop signs of surgical wound infection.	Indicates microorganisms not introduced into sterile body cavity/site.
2. Prepare for surgical hand washing. Alert OR or treatment area that scrubbing is to begin. (OR staff will prepare gown and glove packs.)	OR assistant must be available to assist nurse with gowning once scrub is completed.
IMPLEMENTATION	
1. Perform surgical hand scrub (Skill 36-1).	
2. Enter operating suite keeping elbows bent and hands above waist.	Prevents hands from touching contaminated object.
3. Ask circulating nurse to assist by opening sterile gown (folded inside out) and glove package on a clean, dry, flat surface (see illustration).	Gown's outer surface remains sterile.
4. Reach down to sterile gown package; pick up the gown, grasping the inside surface of gown at the collar.	The hands are not completely sterile. The inside surface of the gown will contact the skin's surface and is thus considered contaminated.
5. Lift folded gown directly upward and step back away from table.	Provides wide margin of safety, avoiding contamination of gown.
6. Holding folded gown, locate neckband. With both hands, grasp inside front of gown just below neckband.	Clean hands may touch inside of gown without contaminating outer surface.
7. Hold gown at arm's length away from your body. Allow gown to unfold, keeping inside of gown toward body. Do not touch outside of gown with bare hands.	Outside of gown remains sterile.
8. With hands at shoulder level, slip both arms into armholes simultaneously (see illustration). Ask circulating nurse to bring gown over shoulders by reaching inside to arm seams. Gown is pulled on, leaving sleeves covering hands.	Careful application prevents contamination. Gown covers hands to prepare for closed gloving.

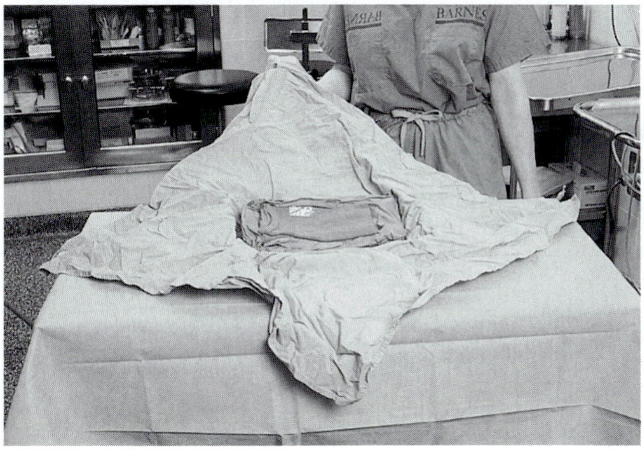

Step 3 Circulating nurse opening sterile gown.

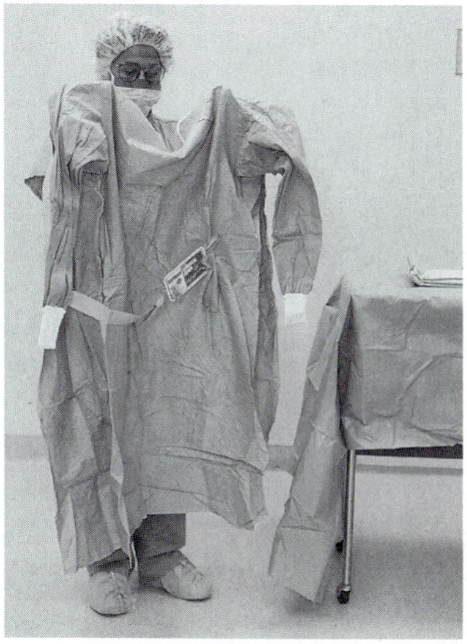

Step 8 Gowning technique: placing arms in sleeves.

STEPS	RATIONALE
9. Have circulating nurse securely tie back of gown at collar and waist (see illustration). (If gown is a wrap-around style, sterile flap to cover gown is not touched until the nurse has gloved.)	Gown must completely enclose underlying garments.

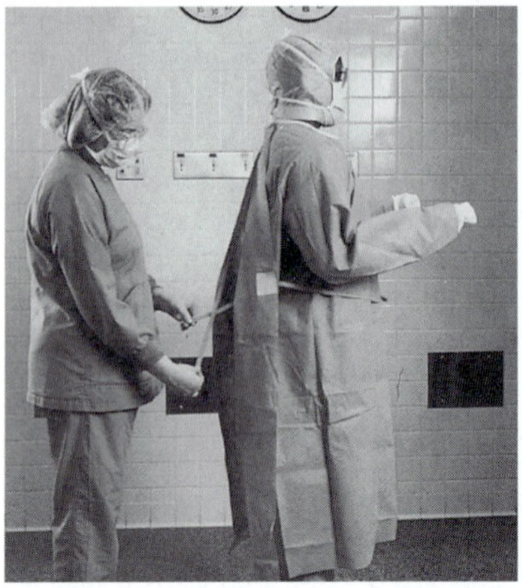

Step 9 Gowning technique: circulating nurse ties scrub gown.

A D F(1) F(2)

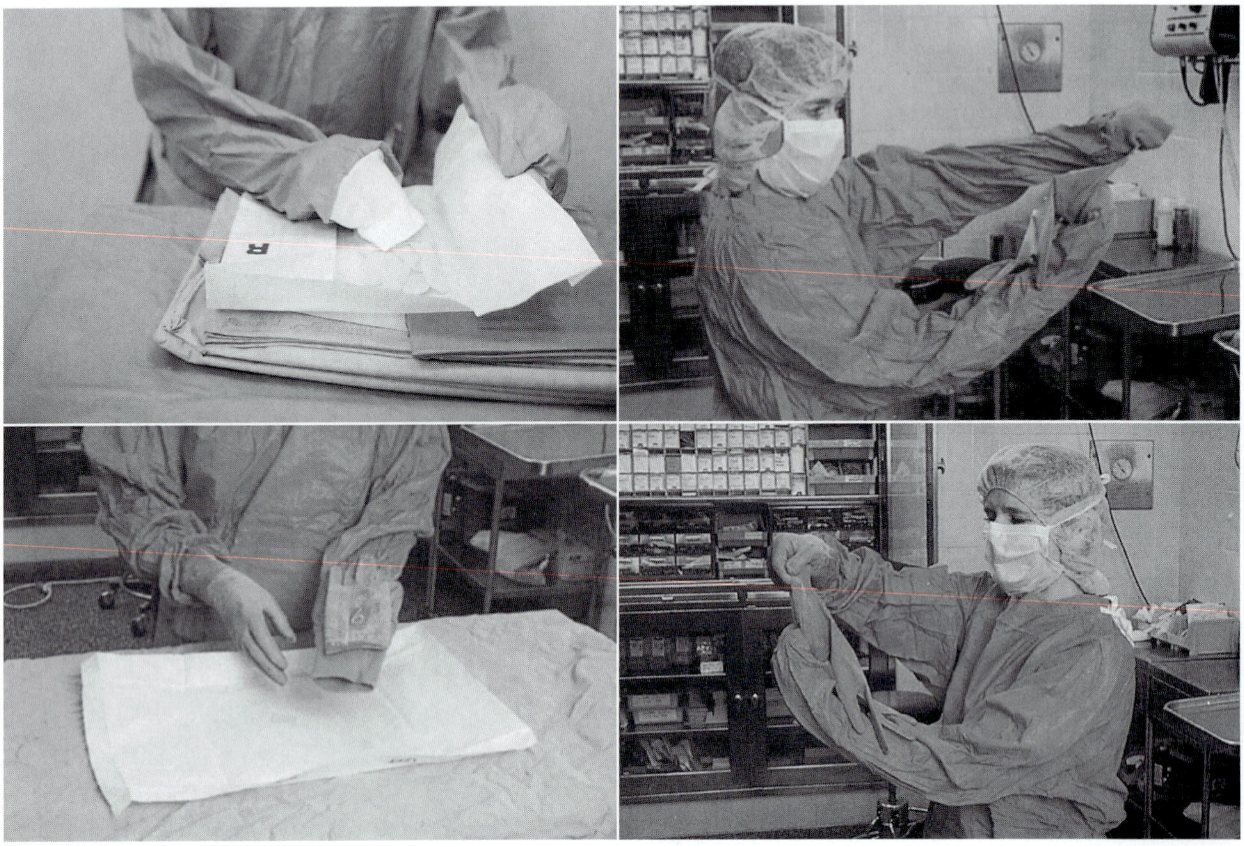

Step 10 Closed gloving sequence.

STEPS	RATIONALE
10. Apply gloves using the closed-glove method:	
a. With hands covered by gown sleeves, open inner sterile glove package (see illustration).	Hands remain clean. Sterile gown cuff will touch sterile glove surface.
b. With nondominant hand inside gown cuff, pick up glove for the dominant hand by grasping folded cuff.	Sterile gown touches sterile glove.
c. Extend dominant forearm with palm up and place palm of glove against palm of dominant hand. Glove fingers will point toward elbow.	Positions glove for application over cuffed hand, keeping glove sterile.
d. While holding glove cuff through gown with dominant hand on which it is placed, grasp back of glove cuff with nondominant hand and turn glove cuff over end of dominant hand and gown cuff (see illustration).	
e. Grasp top of glove and underlying gown sleeve with covered nondominant hand. Carefully extend fingers into glove, being sure glove's cuff covers gown's cuff.	Seal created by glove cuff over gown prevents exit of microorganisms over operative sterile field.
f. Glove nondominant hand in same manner, reversing hands (see illustration). Use gloved dominant hand to pull on glove (see illustration).	Sterile touches sterile.
CRITICAL DECISION POINT **Keep hand inside sleeve.**	
g. Be sure fingers are fully extended into both gloves.	Ensures that nurse has full dexterity while using gloved hand.
11. For wraparound sterile gowns: take gloved hand and release fastener or ties in front of gown.	Front of gown is sterile.
12. Enclose ties or snaps in a sterile towel and hand the towel to sterile team member who stands still (see illustration). Allowing margin of safety, turn around one-half turn to the left, covering back with extended gown flap. Take back tie from team member and secure tie to gown.	Contact with team member could contaminate gown and gloves. Gown must enclose undergarments.
CRITICAL DECISION POINT **On disposable sterile gowns, there is often a disposable tab attached to the tie that can be passed to a nonsterile team member for turning.**	

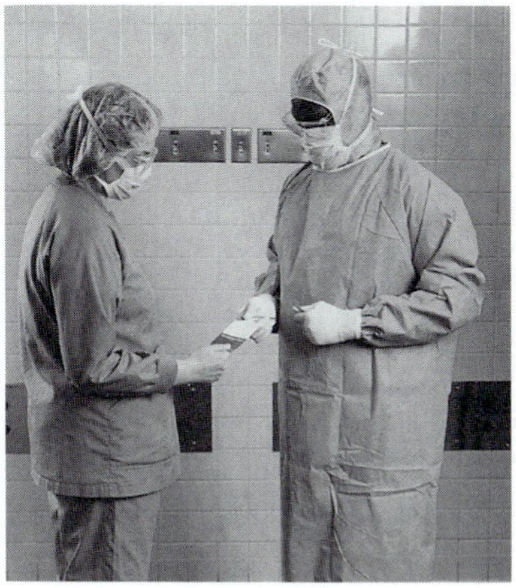

Step 12 Turning wrap-around gown.

EVALUATION

1. Unexpected outcomes that may occur include:	
➤ Client develops signs of infection—redness, heat, swelling, pain, and drainage at surgical site.	Symptomatic of wound infection.
➤ Client develops fever, malaise, and elevated white blood cell count.	Signs of systemic infection.

STEPS	RATIONALE

Recording and Reporting

1. Record the area and description of surgical site postoperatively. — Correct documentation allows nurses to continue to monitor site for proper healing.

• • • • •

Special Considerations

- When one glove becomes contaminated during a procedure, the open gloving method is used to reglove (see Skill 34-3).
- When both gloves are contaminated during a procedure, the nurse should regown and reglove or have a sterile member of the team do the regloving.
- Double gloving may be warranted in longer procedures, when handling heavier instruments, or when required by institutional policy.
- Nurse with cut or lesions on hands may not be allowed to assume role of scrub nurse.
- Upon completion of the procedure, the gown is always removed first, followed by the gloves, and all are disposed of in biohazardous receptacles according to institutional policies.

Teaching Considerations

- Instruct client and family or significant other to observe surgical site for signs of infection.

Critical Thinking Exercises

1. You are the circulating nurse for a thyroidectomy. As the surgical technologist sets up the sterile field you notice the technologist's gloved hand brushes against a nonsterile surface. How would you handle this situation?
2. A colleague tells you that your scrubbed arm hit the faucet, but you did not feel it. What would you do in this situation?
3. Karen, a medical student, is new in the OR. Upon presenting to be gowned and gloved you notice she has scrubbed without removing her ring. The surgeon is asking her to hurry because the case is a wonderful learning experience. What is the best response to this situation?
4. John, a nursing student, asks you the rationale for removing his soiled gown before his gloves. How would you respond?

References

Association of Operating Room Nurses: Position statement: resolution on the necessity for the registered nurse in the operating room, *AORN standards and recommended practices for perioperative nursing,* Denver, 1995a, The Association.

Association of Operating Room Nurses: Recommended practices for surgical attire, *AORN standards and recommended practices for perioperative nursing,* Denver, 1995b, The Association.

Association of Operating Room Nurses: Recommended practices for surgical hand scrubs, *AORN standards and recommended practices for perioperative nursing,* Denver, 1995c, The Association.

Additional Reading

Atkinson LJ: *Berry and Kohn's operating room technique,* ed 8, St Louis, 1996, Mosby.

Elkin MK, Perry AG, and Potter PA: *Nursing interventions and clinical skills,* St Louis, 1996, Mosby.

Meeker MH and Rothrock JC: *Alexander's care of the patient in surgery,* ed 10, St Louis, 1995, Mosby.

Potter PA and Perry AG: *Fundamentals of nursing: concepts, process, and practice,* ed 4, St Louis, 1997, Mosby.

UNIT XIII

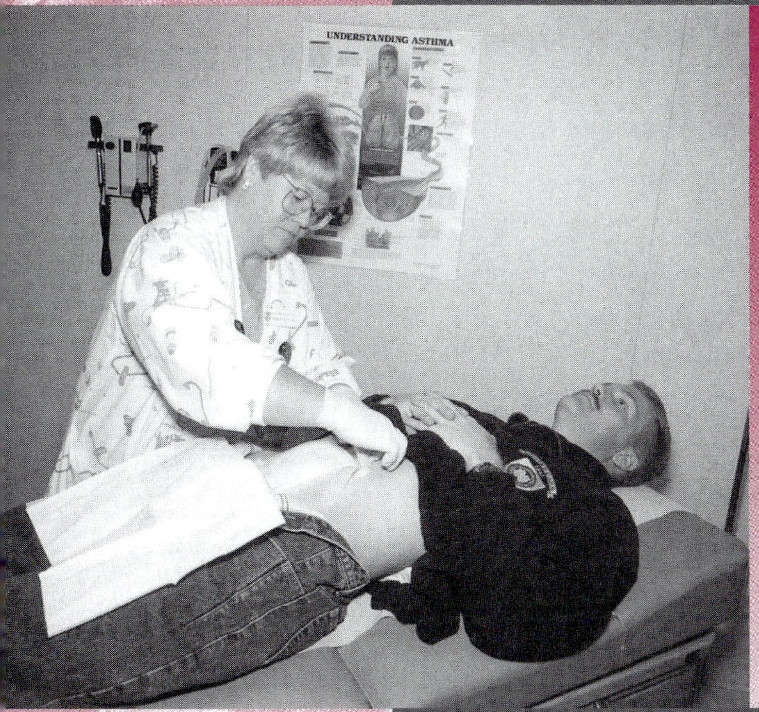

Dressings and Wound Care

CHAPTER 37

Dressings

OBJECTIVES

Mastery of content in this chapter will enable the nurse to:

- Define key terms.
- Properly assess a wound.
- Choose the correct dressing for a wound.
- Understand the technique of a dressing application.
- State advantages and disadvantages of the types of dressings used.
- Correctly apply dry, wet-to-dry, pressure, and synthetic dressings.

KEY TERMS

Dead space
Debridement
Dehiscence
Epithelialization
Erythema
Evisceration
Excoriated
Exudate
Granulation
Hydrocolloid
Hydrogel
Macerated
Neovascularization
Primary dressing
Pseudomonas aeruginosa
Secondary dressing

SKILLS

37-1 Applying a Dry Dressing
37-2 Applying a Wet-to-Dry Dressing
37-3 Applying a Pressure Bandage
37-4 Applying a Transparent Dressing
37-5 Applying a Hydrocolloid or Hydrogel Dressing
37-6 Applying a Foam Dressing
37-7 Applying Absorption and Alginate Dressings

Wound characteristics identified during assessment along with treatment goals determine the type of dressing needed (AHCPR, 1994) (see box at right). Health care professionals once thought that wounds healed best in a dry environment. Since the research of Winter in the 1960s and others, a moist rather than a dry environment is now believed to be better for wound healing. This concept of moist wound healing revolutionized wound management and served as a catalyst for the development of many moisture-retentive dressings (see Skills 37-4 through 37-7). Dressings that come in direct contact with the wound bed are called **primary dressings. Secondary dressings** are used to cover or hold primary dressings in place.

A properly applied dressing can decrease pain, enhance healing, and improve cosmetic results. Assessment of the exudate absorbed by the dressing provides valuable diagnostic information. Dressings serve several functions including maintenance of a moist environment (Field and Kerstein, 1994), protection from outside contaminants, protection from further injury, prevention of the spread of microorganisms, increased client comfort, and control of

AHCPR 1994 DRESSING RECOMMENDATIONS

- Use a dressing that keeps the ulcer bed continuously moist. Wet-to-dry dressings should be used only for debridement and are not considered continuously moist saline dressings.
- Use clinical judgment to select a type of moist wound dressing suitable for the ulcer. Studies of different types of moist wound dressings showed no differences in pressure ulcer healing outcomes.
- Choose a dressing that keeps the surrounding (periulcer) intact skin dry while keeping the ulcer bed moist.
- Choose a dressing that controls exudate but does not desiccate the ulcer bed.
- Consider care giver time when selecting a dressing.
- Eliminate wound **dead space** by loosely filling all cavities with dressing material. Avoid overpacking the wound.
- Monitor dressings applied near the anus, since they are difficult to keep intact.

bleeding. The ideal dressing should be easy to apply, able to conform to body contours, durable but flexible, cost effective, able to absorb or contain exudate, easily removed without damage to the healing surface, and acceptable in appearance (Bolton, Rijswijk, 1991).

When changing a dressing the nurse must be knowledgeable about wound healing in order to differentiate a normal or expected appearance from abnormal changes. Primary healing takes place when tissue is cleanly cut and the margins are reapproximated. Repair should occur without complication. New capillary circulation bridges the wound quickly in 3 to 4 days, and once normal tissue

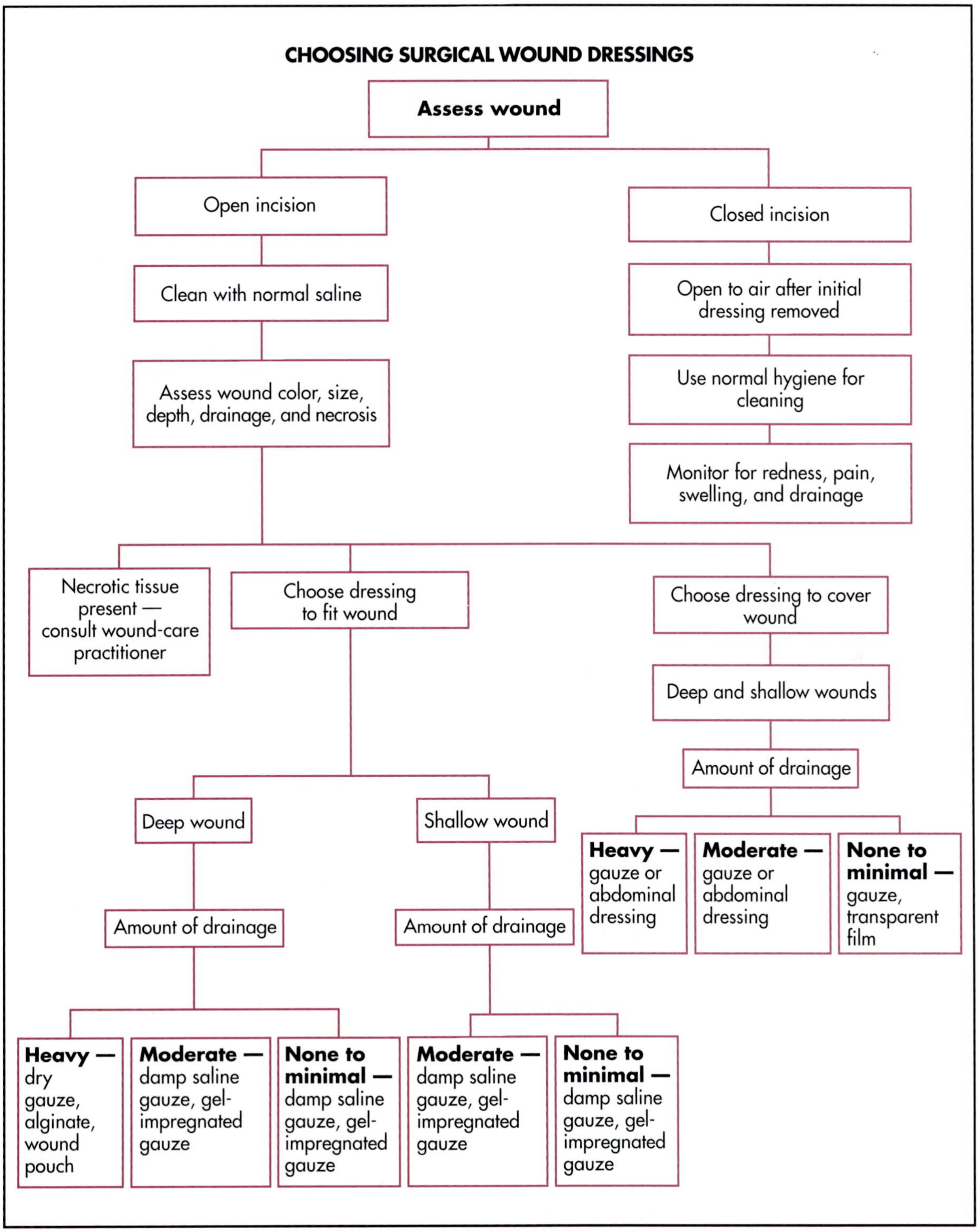

Fig. 37-1

oxygenation is achieved, the wound is considered to be healed. A wound closed for primary healing is most susceptible to infection during the first 4 days. Healing by secondary intention occurs when a wound is left open. Healing results in the formation of **granulation** tissue from the bottom of the wound and eventual **epithelialization** from the sides of the wound to close the defect made by the wound. Burns, infected wounds, and deep pressure ulcers heal in this manner (Wysocki, 1995; Wysocki and Bryant, 1992).

The type of dressing used depends upon the wound characteristics and the goal of wound management, which can be wound **debridement** or wound healing. Various types of dressings can be applied to wounds (Erwin-Toth and Hocevar, 1995; Krasner, 1992a, 1992b, 1995; Motta, 1995). Given the many types of dressings that are now available, the nurse may find it difficult to decide which dressing is best to use on a particular wound. Some nurses may find the decision tree in Fig. 37-1 helpful in selecting the appropriate dressing to care for a particular wound (Maklebust and Palleschi, 1996).

Woven gauze dressings, the oldest and most common type, do not interact with wound tissues and thus cause little wound irritation (Aronovitch, 1995). Gauze comes in a variety of sizes and shapes. The nurse applies gauze either wet or dry depending upon whether the wound needs debridement, a moist healing environment, or a covering to prevent trauma. Wet-to-dry dressings are used for wounds requiring debridement (see Skill 37-2). The nurse moistens the gauze layer that touches the wound surface (primary dressing). This dressing should not be so moist that it will never dry out. The moistened gauze increases the absorptive ability of the dressing to collect exudate and wound debris. This then is covered with a secondary dressing layer that is dry. When the inner moistened gauze dressing is dried, it is then removed from the wound. As the gauze is pulled from the wound, the wound tissue that has adhered to the wound bed is removed, thus effectively debriding the wound. Wet-to-dry dressings are an example of mechanical nonselective debridement, and are effective in cleansing infected and necrotic wounds (Johnson, 1992). To maintain the moist environment needed for wound healing, wet-to-wet (damp-to-damp or moist-to-moist) dressings rather than dry dressings should be used in a clean granulating wound.

Telfa gauze dressings contain a shiny, nonadherent surface on one side. When used as a contact layer the Telfa gauze does not stick to incisions or wound openings. Drainage passes through the nonadherent surface to the softened gauze above.

The **hydrocolloid** dressings (*DuoDERM, Comfeel, Restore, RepliCare,* and others) represent a category of hydroactive dressings (see Skill 37-5). These dressings provide a moist environment for wound healing while facilitating the softening and subsequent removal of wound debris. The dressing promotes wound healing by providing an occlusive protective barrier that absorbs drainage from the wound into the dressing. In addition, the dressing stays in place through an adhesive backing, reduces local pain, and may be used with wound **exudate** absorbers (e.g., *DuoDerm* granules) to increase time between dressing changes (Krasner, 1992a).

Hydrogel dressings (e.g., *Vigilon, Biolex, Nu-Gel, Intra-Site Gel, Saf-Gel,* etc.) have a high moisture content (95%) causing them to swell and retain fluid (see Skill 37-5). They are useful over clean, moist, or **macerated** tissues. The dressing provides a nonadherent, protective barrier with the ability to absorb wound drainage (Krasner, 1992b). These dressings are very soothing and cooling, thus making them especially useful for painful burn wounds. A secondary dressing is needed to hold these dressings in place.

Foam dressings (e.g., *Allevyn, LYOfoam, Reston, Epi-Lock, BIOPATCH, CURAFORM,* etc.) absorb light-to-heavy amounts of exudate, are conformable, and can easily be made to fit a wound. These properties make them especially useful for treating leg ulcers.

Dressings are also available as thin, self-adhesive elastic films (e.g., *Op-Site, Bioclusive, Blisterfilm, Acu-derm, Tegaderm, PRO-CLUDE, Polyskin,* etc.) (see Skill 37-4). The dressing is a synthetic permeable membrane that acts as a temporary second skin. This type of dressing has several advantages: (1) it adheres to undamaged skin to contain exudate and minimize wound contamination, (2) it serves as a barrier to external fluids and bacteria but allows the wound surface to "breathe," (3) it promotes a moist environment that speeds epithelial cell growth, and (4) it can be removed without damaging underlying tissues (Krasner, 1992a). Other advantages are that it allows the client to shower, and it permits direct observation of the wound. A disadvantage of such a dressing is that it cannot debride an infected wound. The film is ideal for small, superficial wounds. These dressings can be used to autolytically debride necrotic wounds. It is also useful as a dressing over an intravenous catheter site. The transparent film allows the nurse to assess the wound without removing the dressing.

GUIDELINES

1. Know the goal of management for the wound. For example, certain dressings can be used to debride wounds while others can be used to maintain a moist wound environment necessary for granulation tissue to fill in the wound defect in a clean wound.

TYPES OF WOUND EXUDATE

- *Serous,* which is a clear, watery plasma.
- *Sanguineous,* which indicates fresh bleeding.
- *Serosanguineous,* which is a pale, more watery drainage than sanguineous drainage.
- *Purulent,* which is a thick, yellow, green, or brown drainage.

2. Know the etiology or type of wound. Wounds caused by vascular insufficiency, diabetes, pressure, trauma, and surgery are all very different and must have an individualized treatment plan (Baranoski, 1995). Not knowing the etiology of the wound can have serious negative effects if the nurse uses treatments that are contraindicated for certain types of wounds.
3. Know the expected amount and type (see box on p. 1070) of wound exudate or drainage. Wounds that have large amounts of drainage require more frequent dressing changes or need dressings that are capable of absorbing large amounts of drainage. Such wounds include fresh postoperative sites, open wounds, and fistulae.
4. Know the type of dressing ordered by the physician. Wet-to-dry dressings require more equipment than do dry dressings. Pressure dressings require elastic bandages to maintain the pressure.
5. Determine if wound drainage tube(s) are present. This prevents their accidental dislocation when the old dressing is removed (see Skill 40-3).
6. Determine the presence of any further break in skin integrity adjacent to the wound. Breaks in skin integrity further increase the client's risk for infection, and further skin breakdown because of excoriation from wound drainage or pressure.
7. The location of the wound and the care setting that the client is in influence the decision of what dressing to use.

SKILL 37-1 Applying a Dry Dressing

A dry dressing may be chosen for management of a wound healing by primary intention with little drainage. The dressing protects the wound from injury, prevents introduction of bacteria, reduces discomfort, and speeds healing.

Dry dressings are most commonly used for abrasions and nondraining postoperative (primary intention healing) incisions. The dry dressing does not debride the wound and should not be selected for wounds requiring debridement. It is not appropriate for an open wound that is healing by secondary intention. If a dry dressing adheres to a wound, the nurse should moisten the dressing with sterile normal saline or water before removing the woven gauze. Moistening the dressing in this manner decreases the adherence of the dressing to the wound and reduces the risk of further trauma to the wound.

EQUIPMENT

- Gloves, clean or sterile (check institution policy)
- Dressing set (sterile), scissors, forceps
- Sterile drape (optional)
- Gauze dressings, sterile
- Sterile basin (optional)
- Antiseptic ointment (if ordered)
- Cleansing solution such as sterile saline or water
- Tape, ties, or bandage as needed
- Waterproof bag
- Extra gauze dressings
- ABD pads
- Adhesive remover (optional)
- Measurement device (optional): tape measure, camera
- Protective gown (optional)
- Mask (optional)
- Goggles (optional)

DELEGATION CONSIDERATIONS

Controversy about delegating wound care to other personnel exists. All nurses should check their specific state practice act as to what interventions are considered within the scope of nursing practice and which can be delegated to others including unlicensed assistant personnel. In some states, aspects of wound care such as dressing change can be delegated. This may include the changing of dressings using *clean* technique for chronic wounds. The care of acute new wounds and those that require sterile technique for dressing change generally remain within the domain of professional nursing practice. The *assessment* of the wound remains within the scope of the professional nurse even if the dressing change is delegated to others.

STEPS	RATIONALE
ASSESSMENT	
1. Assess size of wound to be dressed.	Assists nurse to plan for proper type and amount of supplies needed.
2. Assess location of wound.	Wound location alerts nurse as to dressing type needed and if assistance is needed to hold dressings in place.
3. Assess client's level of comfort.	Removal of dry dressing can be painful; client may require pain medication before dressing change to allow drug's peak effect during procedure.
4. Assess client's knowledge of purpose of dressing change.	Determines level of support and explanation required by client.
5. Assess need for client or family member to participate in dressing wound.	Prepares client or family member if dressing must be changed at home.
6. Review medical orders for dressing change procedure.	Indicates type of dressing or applications to use.
7. Identify clients at risk for wound healing problems, including:	
a. Older clients.	Physiological changes of aging alter the immune system, resulting in decreased resistance to pathogens.
b. Prematurely born infants.	The skin of premature babies is not mature and does not have the immune functions of normal skin.
c. Obesity.	Subcutaneous tissue has diminished vascularity.
d. Diabetes.	Vascular changes associated with diabetes reduce blood flow to peripheral tissues, also leukocyte malfunction occurs secondary to hyperglycemia.
e. Compromised circulation.	Results in inadequate supply of nutrients, blood cells, and oxygen to wound.
f. Poor nutritional state.	Impairs stages of inflammation and collagen formation states.
g. Immunosuppressive drugs.	Decreases inflammatory response and decreases collagen synthesis.
h. Irradiation in area of wound.	Decreases blood supply to tissues.
i. High levels of stress.	Increased cortisol levels reduce number of lymphocytes and decrease inflammatory response.
j. Steroids.	Slows rate of epithelialization and **neovascularization** and inhibits contraction.

NURSING DIAGNOSIS

Clustering of defining characteristics from the assessment data may reveal the following nursing diagnoses for clients requiring this skill:

- Risk for infection
- Impaired skin integrity
- Knowledge deficit regarding dressing application
- Pain

Related factors are individualized based on a client's condition or needs.

PLANNING

STEPS	RATIONALE
1. Expected outcomes following completion of procedure:	
➤ Client's wound is free of infection; drainage begins to diminish in amount.	Indicates wound is healing appropriately.
➤ Client reports minimal discomfort.	Indicates dressing procedure and choice are appropriate.
➤ Client explains method of dressing application.	Indicates learning has occurred.
2. Explain procedure to client.	Decreases client's anxiety.
3. Assess need for pain medication.	Dressing change is better tolerated by client if pain medication has been administered before dressing change.

STEPS	RATIONALE
IMPLEMENTATION	
1. Close room or cubicle curtains. Wash hands. Apply gown, goggles, and mask if risk of spray exists.	Provides for privacy and reduces transmission of microorganisms.
2. Position client comfortably and drape to expose only wound site. Instruct client not to touch wound or sterile supplies.	Draping provides access to the wound yet minimizes unnecessary exposure.
3. Place disposable bag within reach of work area. Fold top of bag to make cuff. Put on clean disposable gloves.	Ensures easy disposal of soiled dressings. Prevents contamination of bag's outer surface. Prevents transmission of infectious organisms.
4. Remove tape: pull parallel to skin, toward dressing. Remove remaining adhesive from skin.	Pulling tape toward dressing reduces stress on suture line or wound edges.
5. With gloved hand remove dressings. Keep soiled undersurface from client's sight.	Appearance of drainage may be upsetting to client.
6. Observe appearance of drainage on dressing. Assess for odor. Assess the wound.	Provides qualitative assessment of drainage and assessment of wound's condition.
CRITICAL DECISION POINT **Dressings that are heavily saturated with drainage indicate a need to change type of dressing to one that can adequately absorb amount of wound drainage.**	
7. Dispose of soiled dressings in disposable bag. Remove gloves by pulling them inside out. Dispose of in bag.	Reduces transmission of microorganisms to other persons.
8. Open sterile dressing tray or individually wrapped sterile supplies. Place on bedside table (see illustration).	Sterile dressings remain sterile while on or within sterile surface. Preparation of all supplies prevents break in technique during dressing change.
9. Open cleansing solution and pour over sterile gauze.	Keeps supplies sterile. Solution may be packaged to spray/pour directly on wound. Microorganisms move from unsterile environment through dressing package to dressing itself by capillary action (see Chapter 34).
CRITICAL DECISION POINT **If sterile drape or gauze packages become wet from solution, repeat preparation of supplies.**	
10. Put on gloves, clean or sterile depending on institution policy.	Sterile gloves allow handling of sterile supplies without contamination.
11. Inspect wound for appearance, drains, exudate, and integrity (see illustration). Measure wound size (length, width, and depth [if indicated]) (see Chapter 40). Avoid contact with contaminated material.	Indicates status of healing.

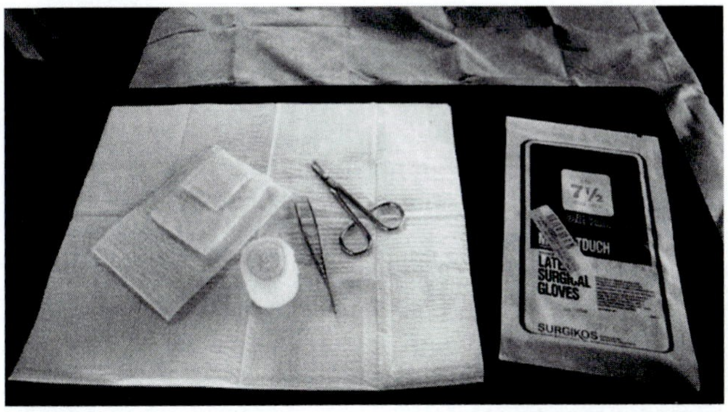

Step 8

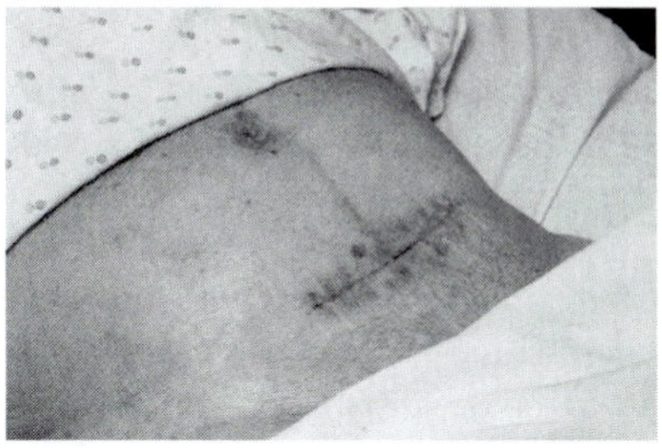

Step 11

STEPS	RATIONALE
12. Cleanse wound (see Chapter 40):	
a. Use separate swab for each cleansing stroke, or spray wound surface.	Prevents contaminating previously cleaned area.
b. Clean from least contaminated area to most contaminated.	Cleansing in this direction prevents introduction of organisms into wound.
13. Use dry gauze to blot in same manner as in Step 12 to dry wound.	Drying reduces excess moisture, which could eventually harbor microorganisms.
14. Apply antiseptic ointment if ordered, using same technique as for cleansing.	Helps reduce growth of microorganisms.
15. Apply dry sterile dressings to incision or wound site:	
a. Apply loose woven gauze as contact layer.	Promotes proper absorption of drainage.
b. Cut 4 × 4 gauze flat to fit around drain if present or use precut split drain flat.	Secures drain and promotes drainage absorption at site (see Chapter 40, Skill 40-3).
c. Apply second layer of gauze.	Layering ensures proper coverage and optimal absorption.
d. Apply thicker woven pad (surgi-pad).	Protects wound from external environment.
16. Secure dressing with tape, Montgomery ties or straps (which are applied perpendicular to the wound) (see illustration), or binder. Sometimes strips of a hydrocolloid dressing are placed on the skin under the Montgomery ties to further protect the skin.	Supports wound and ensures placement and stability of dressing.

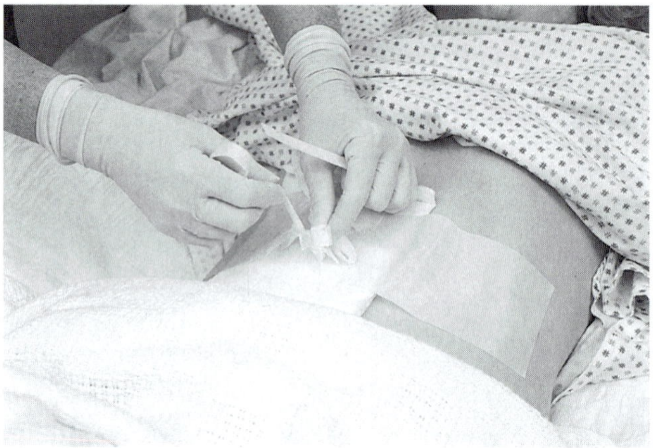

Step 16

STEPS	RATIONALE
17. Remove gloves, gown if worn, and dispose in bag. Dispose of all supplies. Remove goggles if worn.	Reduces transmission of microorganisms. Clean environment enhances client comfort.
18. Assist client to comfortable position.	Promotes client's sense of well-being.
19. Wash hands.	Reduces transmission of microorganisms.

EVALUATION

STEPS	RATIONALE
1. Inspect condition of wound and presence of any drainage.	Determines rate of healing.
2. Ask if client notes discomfort during procedure.	Pain may be early indication of wound complication or result of dressing pulling tissue.
3. Inspect condition of dressing at least every shift.	Determines status of wound drainage.
4. Ask client to describe steps and techniques of dressing change.	Evaluates client's learning.
5. **Unexpected outcomes** that may occur include:	
➤ Wound drainage increases, resulting in frequent dressing changes.	May indicate disruption of incision, dehiscence, hemorrhage, or onset of infection.
➤ Wound bleeds after removal of dry dressing.	Indicates disruption of epidermal surface.
➤ Client is unable to describe proper application of dressing.	Reinstruction is necessary.

STEPS	RATIONALE
RECORDING AND REPORTING	
1. Report and record:	
a. Appearance of wound and drainage.	
b. Change in wound characteristics, especially drainage amount, to physician.	Change may indicate need for different management plan.
c. Unexpected appearance of wound drainage or accidental removal of drain within an hour to physician.	Unless client shows evidence of wound **dehiscence** or **evisceration,** notification of physician of unexpected findings within an hour is adequate.
d. Type of dressing applied in client's medical record.	Documents progress of wound healing and promotes continuity in dressing change techniques.
e. Tolerance of client to dressing change during shift change.	Allows nurses to provide continuity in pain control.
2. Record frequency of dressing change and supplies needed on care plan.	Alerts staff members to dressing change times and supplies needed.
3. Write nurse's initials, date, and time of dressing change on the new dressing or tape in ink (not marker).	Maintains record of time dressing changed for reference should condition change.

FOLLOW-UP ACTIVITIES

1. Provide feedback to client and family regarding their ability to perform dressing change if teaching self-wound care or family participation.

• • • • •

Special Considerations

- Circumferential wounds may require assistance to cover.
- Tape located over hairy areas should be removed in direction of hair growth to reduce irritation and discomfort.
- If drains are present, slowly and carefully remove dressings one layer at a time to avoid accidental removal of drain.
- Wounds requiring a dressing change more often than every 4 hours may indicate need for drain placement or alternate dressing type.
- Personnel resources to assist in wound care include enterostomal therapist, clinical nurse specialist (surgery or oncology), and infection control nurse.
- Client may be allowed (and able) to shower for cleansing; this may eliminate *Implementation,* Steps 10 and 12.
- Another alternative to sterile technique is to have a clean glove on the nondominant hand and apply a sterile glove to the dominant hand in *Implementation,* step 10. One must be careful not to contaminate the sterile hand.

Teaching Considerations

- Wounds out of client's reach and vision require a family member's assistance.
- Explain expected wound appearance, what should be reported, and risks of improper wound care.
- After demonstrating wound care, allow client or family member to perform dressing change with and without supervision.

Pediatric Considerations

- Check that dressings products are safe to use on pediatric clients especially on premature infants.
- Pediatric clients may be fearful of dressing changes. Obtaining the client's cooperation and/or having another person available to keep the child from moving during the dressing change procedure may be needed.

Gerontologic Considerations

- The dressing change procedure may be a source of pain and misunderstanding by a confused or disoriented client.
- Prevent injury to older skin by avoiding skin tears from tape removal or products that can cause skin injury.

Home Care Considerations

- Assess extent of wound or incision in relation to client's level of activity to determine type of dressing that will achieve desired purpose.
- Assess area where procedure will be performed for adequate lighting. Determine if a table or cabinet is available on which sterile supplies may be placed with reasonable security.

SKILL 37-2 Applying a Wet-to-Dry Dressing

Wet-to-dry dressings are gauze moistened with an appropriate solution. For this reason, wet-to-dry dressings are sometimes called moist- or damp-to-dry dressings since this terminology more accurately describes what the dressing should be. In clinical practice, these terms (wet-to-dry, moist-to-dry, damp-to-dry) are considered synonymous.

The primary purpose of wet-to-dry dressings is to mechanically debride a wound. The moistened contact layer of the dressing (primary dressing) increases the absorptive ability of the dressing to collect exudate and wound debris (Provan and Phillips, 1991). As the dressing dries, it adheres to the wound and debrides the wound of the tissue when the dressing is removed. One must *take care not to apply a dressing so wet that it remains wet continuously* (Table 37-1). A dressing that is too wet may cause tissue maceration and bacterial growth. It also does not dry out and therefore does not remove the necrotic tissue when being removed from the wound. The moistened gauze must be covered with a secondary dressing layer that is dry.

Woven gauze should be used to pack wounds (Aronovitch, 1995). Principles for correctly packing a wound can be found in the box on p. 1077. Commonly used wetting agents include normal saline and lactated Ringer's solution, which are isotonic solutions that aid in mechanical debridement. Acetic acid is effective against **Pseudomonas aeruginosa,** but is toxic to fibroblasts in standard dilutions. Povidone-iodine, usually one-quarter to one-half strength, is a rapid-acting antimicrobial agent for cleansing *intact* skin. In open wounds, the solution is toxic to fibroblasts and has questionable efficacy in infected wounds and therefore should not be used. Other antibiotic solutions may be ordered, although their use is controversial. See Chapter 40, for a more detailed discussion of appropriate solutions to use to clean wounds. Because they can harbor microorganism growth, solutions should be discarded 24 to 48 hours after opening and replaced with fresh solutions.

EQUIPMENT

- Sterile gloves
- Dressing set (scissors and forceps)
- Sterile drape (optional)
- Thin, fine-mesh gauze or packing strip (Fig. 37-2)
- Gauze dressings and pads
- Sterile solution (as prescribed) to moisten dressing
- Waterproof pad
- Sterile solution such as saline
- Clean disposable gloves

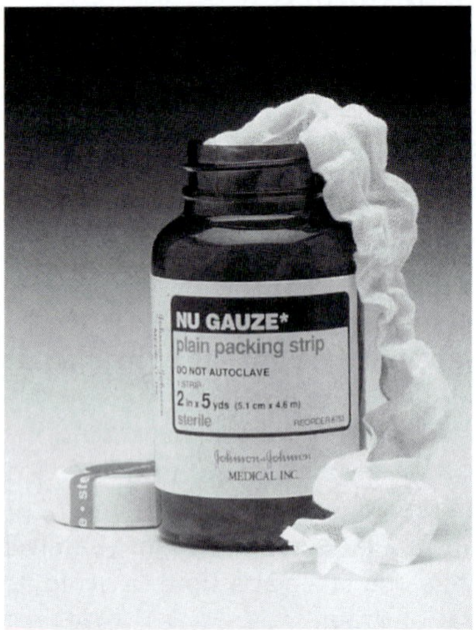

Fig. 37-2 Packing strip gauze.

Table 37-1 Problems Associated with Wounds Requiring Debridement

Problem	Nursing Activities
Solutions used may be irritating to healthy skin around wound.	Protect healthy skin with protective barrier, such as stomahesive, or apply topical ointments, such as zinc oxide. If zinc oxide is used, it should be removed with mineral oil.
Wound becomes excessively dry.	Continually moist dressing (with a physician's order) might be tried. Eliminate fine mesh gauze and lightly pack wound with fluffy gauze dampened with prescribed solution.
Wound is deep and retention of dressing in cavity is suspected.	Irrigate wound copiously with prescribed solution to remove. Use continuous "ribbon" or strip of gauze to dress deep wounds.
Wound drainage is damaging healthy tissue.	Protect healthy tissue with skin barrier, such as a hydrocolloid. Wounds with large amounts of drainage may benefit from occlusive drainage collection device.
Client's skin is irritated by tape.	Use hydrocolloid under tape, use Montgomery ties as needed, use fabric tape that has multidirection stretch, secure dressing with binder, or wrap with roll gauze if on extremity.

- Tape, ties, or bandage as needed
- Waterproof bag
- Adhesive remover
- Moisture proof gown (optional)
- Goggles (optional)
- Mask (optional)

PRINCIPLES FOR PACKING A WOUND

- Use the wound characteristics to decide what type of packing is appropriate.
- Make sure the packing material can be safely used to pack a wound.
- Moisten the packing material with a noncytotoxic solution such as normal saline. Never use cytotoxic solutions to pack a wound.
- If using woven gauze, fluff it before packing it into the wound.
- Loosely pack the wound.
- Do not let the packing material drag or touch the surrounding wound tissue before you put it into the wound.
- Fill all the wound dead space with the packing material.
- Pack the wound untill you reach the wound surface; never pack the wound higher than the wound surface.

STEPS	RATIONALE
ASSESSMENT	
1. Assess location and size of wound to be dressed, see Skill 37-1, Assessment (see Chapter 40).	Allows nurse to determine supplies needed and if assistance is required.

NURSING DIAGNOSIS

Clustering of defining characteristics from the assessment data may reveal the following nursing diagnoses for clients requiring this skill:

- Risk for infection
- Impaired skin integrity
- Knowledge deficit regarding wet-to-dry dressings
- Pain

Related factors are individualized based on a client's condition or needs.

STEPS	RATIONALE
PLANNING	
1. **Expected outcomes** following completion of procedure:	
➤ Exudate and necrotic debris are decreased; wound becomes clean with granulation tissue present.	Indicates progress in wound healing.
➤ Client describes minimal discomfort.	Pain medication and positioning are effective.
➤ Client explains procedure correctly.	Indicates learning has occurred.
2. Explain procedure to client. Instruct client not to touch sterile supplies.	Relieves anxiety and promotes understanding of dressing change. Prevents contamination of supplies.
3. Position client to allow access to area to be dressed.	Facilitates application of dressing.
IMPLEMENTATION	
1. Close room curtain or door and keep sheet or gown draped over body parts not requiring exposure.	Provides privacy.
2. Make cuff at top of disposable waterproof bag and place within reach of work area.	Cuff prevents accidental contamination of top of outer bag.
3. Place waterproof pad under client where dressing is to be changed.	Prevents soiling of bed linens.

STEPS	RATIONALE
4. Wash hands thoroughly. Put on mask, goggles, and moistureproof gown if spray potential. Put on clean disposable gloves and remove tape or bandage or untie Montgomery ties. Remove tape by loosening end and pulling gently parallel to skin and toward dressing.	Prevents transmission of infectious organisms. Reduces tension against wound edges.
5. With gloved hand or forceps, lift old outer secondary cover dressings off first, then remove the inner dressing (called the primary dressing) that is in direct contact with the wound bed. Keep soiled undersurface away from client's sight. Gently remove this inner dressing and inform client about possible discomfort. Because of this, premedication before this procedure may be necessary.	Purpose of dressing is to remove necrotic tissue and exudate. Appearance of drainage may be upsetting to client.

CRITICAL DECISION POINT **Inner primary dressing if applied properly will have dried and will adhere to underlying tissues, do *not* moisten it. This is a very critical point! It is incorrect technique and a common error by some clinicians to moisten the dried gauze prior to removing it so it does not stick to the wound and cause the client extreme discomfort. This defeats the purpose of using this type of dressing.**

Step 13

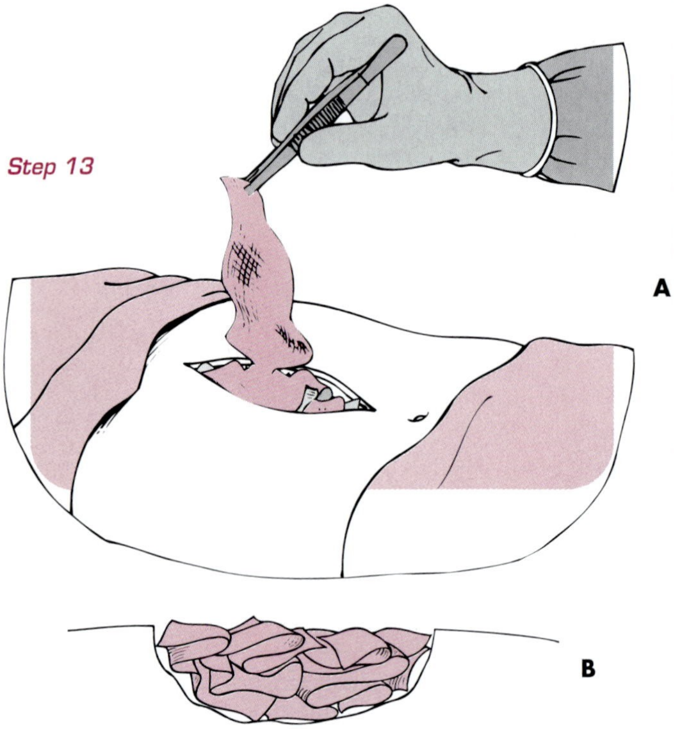

STEPS	RATIONALE
6. Observe character of drainage on dressings, and condition of the wound bed. Check for unexpected odor.	Provides assessment of wound's condition.
7. Dispose of soiled dressings in prepared waterproof bag.	Reduces transmission of microorganisms.
8. Remove disposable gloves by pulling them inside out and dispose of them properly.	Reduces transmission of microorganisms.
9. Prepare sterile dressing supplies.	Reduces risk of break in sterile technique resulting in contamination.

CRITICAL DECISION POINT **Open or "fluff" the woven gauze that will be placed directly against the wound bed. Sometimes "packing strip" may be used to pack the wound (see Fig. 37-2). When using packing strip, with a sterile scissor, cut the amount of dressing that is anticipated to be used to pack the wound. Do not let the packing strip touch the side of the bottle. Pour prescribed solution over the packing gauze or strip to moisten it. Contact layer must be totally moistened to increase dressing's absorptive abilities.**

STEPS	RATIONALE
10. Put on sterile gloves.	Allows handling of sterile supplies without contamination.
11. Inspect wound for type of tissue, color, characteristics of drainage, presence and type of sutures, presence of any drains.	Provides assessment of wound healing.
12. Cleanse wound with prescribed solution. Clean from least to most contaminated area.	Assists in debridement and cleanses wound of debris.
13. Wring out excess fluid and apply moist "fluffed" woven-mesh gauze or "packing strip" directly onto wound surface without having the gauze touch the surrounding skin (see illustration A, p. 1078).	Moist gauze absorbs drainage and adheres to debris.

➤ *CRITICAL DECISION POINT* If wound is deep, gently lay gauze over wound surface with forceps until all surfaces are in contact with moist gauze and the wound is loosely filled with the moistened woven gauze. Fill the wound but avoid packing the wound too tightly or having the gauze extend beyond the top of the wound (see illustration B, p. 1078).

➤ *CRITICAL DECISION POINT* The inner gauze should be moist but not dripping wet. The moist gauze must be able to dry in the wound. Having the inner gauze too wet so it does not dry is a common error in technique for this type of dressing.

14. Make sure any dead space from sinus tracts, undermining, or tunneling are loosely packed with gauze.

➤ *CRITICAL DECISION POINT* Do not overpack the wound too tightly; it can cause wound trauma.

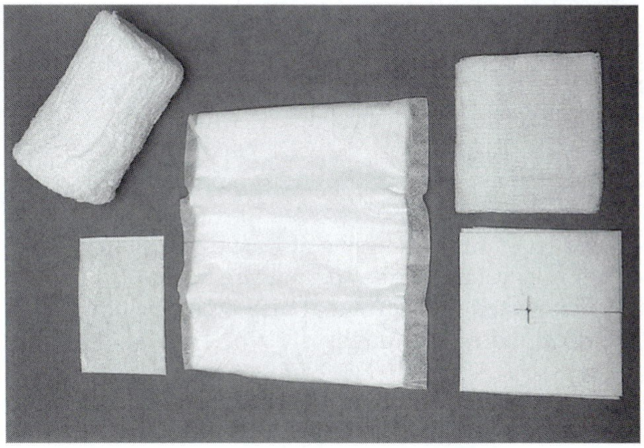

Step 16

STEPS	RATIONALE
15. Apply dry sterile gauze over wet gauze.	Dry layer pulls moisture from wound.
16. Cover the packed wound with a secondary dressing such as with ABD pad, surgi-pad, or gauze (see illustration).	Protects wound from the entrance of microorganisms.
17. Apply roll gauze (for circumferential dressings) (see illustrations), or Montgomery ties. For application of Montgomery ties or straps (see Skill 37-1):	Secures dressing in place.

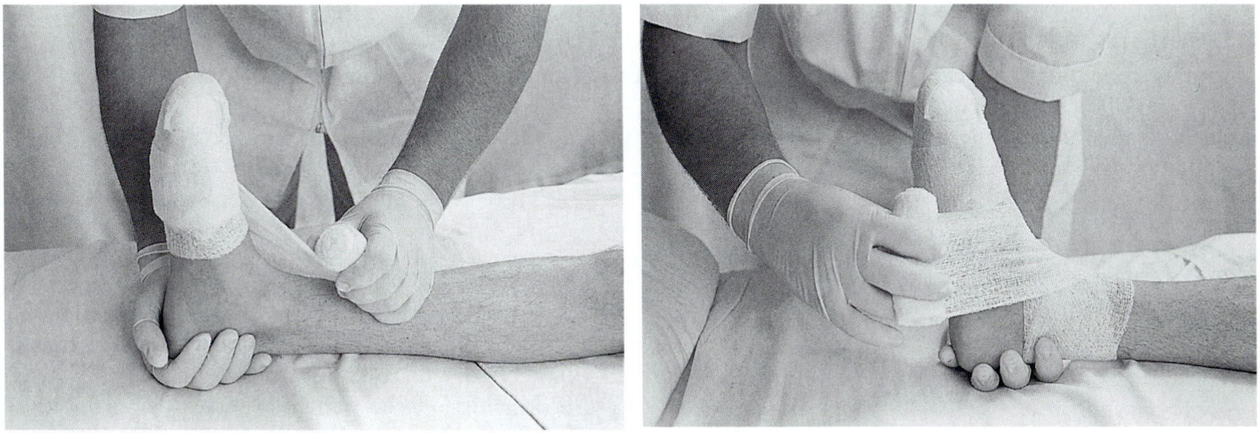

Step 17 Applying a roll gauze as a secondary circumferential dressing.

STEPS	RATIONALE
CRITICAL DECISION POINT Montgomery tie allows for frequent dressing changes without removal of adhesive tape.	
a. Expose adhesive surface of tape end.	
b. Place ties on opposite sides of dressing.	
c. Adhesive may be placed directly on client's skin or skin barrier may be used.	Skin barrier (strips of a hydrocolloid dressings) protects intact skin from stretch and tension of adhesive tape.
d. Secure dressing by lacing ties across dressing.	
18. Remove and dispose of gloves and cover gown (optional). Remove goggles.	
19. Assist client to comfortable position.	Restores client's sense of well-being.
20. Wash hands thoroughly.	Reduces transfer of microorganisms.

EVALUATION

1. Observe wound for healing.	Monitoring wound characteristics provides evidence of wound healing.
2. Ask if client has pain during procedure.	Determines client's comfort level and need for pain management.
3. Inspect status of dressing at least every shift.	Evaluates extent of drainage and integrity of dressing.
4. Ask client to describe wound care method.	Evaluates level of client's understanding of procedure.
5. **Unexpected outcomes** that may occur include:	
➤ Wound eschar toughens.	Eschar may require surgical debridement before resumption of wet-to-dry dressing changes.
➤ Character of wound drainage changes (increases, purulent).	May indicate dehiscence or infection.
➤ Skin around wound margins becomes red, mascerated, or **excoriated.**	May indicate solution in contact with skin or acidity of wound drainage.
➤ Client is unable to explain wound care.	Reinstruction is necessary.

Recording and Reporting

1. Report brisk bright red bleeding or evidence of wound dehiscence or evisceration to physician immediately.	Requires immediate intervention.
2. Report wound appearance and characteristics of drainage at shift change.	Ensures continuity of care by nursing staff.
3. Record wound appearance, color, presence and characteristics of exudate, type and amount of dressings used, and tolerance of client to procedure.	Documents client's progress and therapy provided.
4. Write date and time dressing applied on tape in ink (not marker).	Maintains record of time dressing changed for reference should condition change.

Follow-up Activities

1. Encourage client or significant other to participate in dressing changes (if it is anticipated that dressings will need changing after discharge).
2. Discuss change in dressing procedure with physician as wound surface becomes clean and granulation tissue is evident.

• • • • •

Special Considerations

- ➤ Saturated dressing will remain wet, and bacteria will grow.
- ➤ If drains are present, remove dressings one layer at a time (see Chapter 40).
- ➤ Rapid removal of adherent gauze layer may cause unnecessary discomfort and bleeding.
- ➤ If dressing is to be changed twice a day or more frequently, Montgomery ties reduce skin irritation from adhesives.

- Resources to assist in wound care include enterostomal therapist, clinical nurse specialist (surgery or oncology), infection control nurse, and home health nurse.

Teaching Considerations

- Explain risks of improper wound care.
- Explain expected appearance of wound and what should be reported.
- Wounds out of client's reach and vision require assistance for learning self-care.
- After demonstrating wound care, allow client or family member to perform dressing change with supervision.

Gerontologic Considerations

(see Skill 37-1)

Pediatric Considerations

(see Skill 37-1)

Home Care Considerations

- The ability of the care giver and the amount of time needed to change a particular dressing should be considered when selecting a dressing procedure in the home care setting. "In the home care setting, caregivers may choose more expensive dressing materials to reduce the frequency of dressing changes" (AHCPR, 1994).

SKILL 37-3 Applying a Pressure Bandage

A pressure bandage is a temporary treatment for the control of excessive bleeding. The bleeding is usually sudden and not anticipated. It may follow surgical intervention, or it may be a life-threatening occurrence related to accidental trauma, stabbing, suicide attempt, or other injury.

An adult weighing 154 lbs (70 kg) has a total volume of 5 L of circulating blood. All nursing actions must be rapidly and effectively executed when excessive blood loss occurs. Once pressure has been applied, it must continue until definitive actions can be executed by the health care team. Surgical repair is most often the option of choice.

EQUIPMENT

- **Sterile gauze**
- **Gauze roll bandage**
- **Adhesive tape**
- **Gloves**

STEPS	RATIONALE
ASSESSMENT	
1. Identify clients at risk for unexpected bleeding: a. Traumatic injury b. Donor graft site c. Arterial puncture sites d. Postoperative wounds e. Wounds after surgical debridement	Nurse should be familiar with conditions associated with unexpected bleeding to rapidly respond to bleeding.
PHASE I: IMMEDIATE ACTION—FIRST NURSE "ON THE SCENE"	
1. Identify client with sudden hemorrhage:	
a. Locate external bleeding site.	Maintaining asepsis and privacy are considered only if time and severity of blood loss permit inclusion of these activities.
b. Apply direct pressure immediately.	Hemostasis maintained as supplies are prepared.
2. Seek assistance.	Bandage must be quickly secured.
PHASE II: APPLYING PRESSURE BANDAGE—SECOND NURSE "ON THE SCENE"	
1. Quickly observe location of bleeding.	Bleeding source determines method and supplies needed for applying pressure bandage.
2. Quickly assess client's pulse, blood pressure, skin color, anxiety/restlessness, changes in level of consciousness.	Findings of tachycardia, hypotension, diaphoresis, restlessness, and diminished urinary output indicate impending hypovolemic shock.

STEPS	RATIONALE

NURSING DIAGNOSIS

Clustering of defining characteristics from the assessment data may reveal the following nursing diagnoses for clients requiring this skill:

- Altered peripheral tissue perfusion
- Decreased cardiac output
- Impaired skin integrity
- Fluid volume deficit

Related factors are individualized based on a client's condition or needs.

PLANNING

Steps	Rationale
1. **Expected outcomes** following completion of procedure:	
➤ Bleeding is temporarily controlled.	Source of bleeding controlled with pressure.
➤ Circulation to distal parts is adequate.	Blood flow to periphery maintained.
➤ Fluid loss is minimal.	
➤ Client's blood pressure and pulse remain within normal range.	Minimal volume of blood lost.

IMPLEMENTATION

Steps	Rationale
1. Apply clean gloves. *If client's condition permits,* wash hands, apply clean gloves, and provide privacy.	Maintaining asepsis and privacy are considered only if time and severity of blood loss permit inclusion of these activities.
2. First person presses on site of bleeding. Second person unwraps roller bandage and places within easy access.	Hemostasis maintained as supplies are prepared. Pressure dressing provides interim control of bleeding.
3. Second person quickly cuts 3 to 5 lengths of adhesive tape and places them within easy reach.	Bandage must be quickly secured.
4. In *simultaneous coordinated actions:*	
a. Rapidly cover bleeding area with many thicknesses of gauze compresses. First person slips fingers out as other nurse exerts adequate pressure to continue controlling bleeding.	Gauze is absorbent. Layers provide bulk against which local pressure can be applied to bleeding site.
b. Adhesive strips are placed 7 to 10 cm (3 to 4 inches) beyond width of dressing with even pressure on both sides of nurse's fingers as close as possible to central bleeding source. Secure tape on distal end, pull tape across dressing, and maintain firm pressure as proximate end of tape is secured.	Tape exerts downward pressure, promoting hemostasis.

➤ ***CRITICAL DECISION POINT*** **Do not tape around the circumference.**

Steps	Rationale
c. Remove fingers and quickly cover center of area with third strip of tape.	Provides pressure to source of bleeding.
d. Continue reinforcing area with tape as each successive strip is overlapped on alternating sides of center strip.	Prevents tape from loosening.
e. When pressure bandage is on extremity, apply roller gauze: apply two circular turns tautly on both sides of fingers that are pressing gauze. Compress over bleeding site. Simultaneously remove finger pressure and apply roller gauze pressure over center. Continue with figure-eight turns. Secure end with two circular turns and strip of adhesive.	Roller gauze acts as pressure bandage, exerting more even pressure over extremity. To ensure blood flow to distal tissues and prevent tourniquet effect, adhesive tape must not be continued around entire extremity.

➤ ***CRITICAL DECISION POINT*** **Start pressure bandage from *distal* to proximal.**

STEPS	RATIONALE
5. Remove gloves and wash hands.	Reduces the spread of microorganisms.

EVALUATION

1. Immediately evaluate client to determine response to pressure dressing. Observe for:	
a. Control of bleeding.	Effective pressure bandage controls bleeding without blocking distal circulation.
b. Adequacy of circulation (distal pulse, skin characteristics).	Determines level of perfusion to distal body parts.
c. Estimated volume of blood loss (e.g., count number of dressings used, weigh saturated dressing).	Determines blood and fluid replacement needs.
d. Vital signs.	Identifies early stages of hypovolemic shock.
2. Unexpected outcomes that may occur include:	
➤ Excessive pressure is exerted that results in pain; weak or absent pulses; edema of distal body part; tissue necrosis.	Impaired distal circulation.
➤ Uncontrolled hemorrhaging progresses to fluid and electrolyte imbalance, tissue hypoxia, confusion, hypovolemic shock, cardiac arrest, death.	Source of bleeding too large to control by local pressure, or bleeding was extensive before care giver arrived.

RECORDING AND REPORTING

1. Report immediately to physician present status of client's bleeding control, time bleeding was discovered, estimated blood loss, nursing interventions (including effectiveness of applied pressure bandage), apical and distal pulses, blood pressure, sensorium level, signs of restlessness, and need for physician to administer to client without delay.	Provides physician with data describing client's status and type of therapies indicated.
2. Record and implement physician's verbal orders in response to above reporting. (NOTE: Institutional policy on telephone/verbal orders varies.)	Nurse must act quickly on basis of client's status.
3. Shift-change report includes emergency situation, intervention and evaluation as reported to physician, and need for continuous bedside monitoring of bleeding control, distal pulse, vital signs, IV, consciousness level, oxygenation or hypoxia, and anxiety level.	Provides nurses with data regarding client's status and types of interventions needed to maintain continuity of care.
4. Record on progress note exact findings and care administered in relation to application of pressure bandage.	Documents therapy administered.

FOLLOW-UP ACTIVITIES (IMMEDIATE)

1. Initiate IV therapy (physician's order is required) for fluid replacement.
2. Initiate NPO order because surgical intervention may be needed.
3. Apply pressure to pressure point PRN; place client in Trendelenburg position; provide warmth.
4. Monitor vital signs every 15 minutes (apical, distal rate, BP).
5. Monitor dressing for signs of bleeding.
   a. Reinforce dressing with tape as needed to prevent seepage.
   b. If dressing is saturated, replace only top layers so as not to disturb any clot formation at the wound site.

FOLLOW-UP ACTIVITIES (AFTER DEFINITIVE INTERVENTION)

1. Determine client's emotional status.
2. Obtain client's hemoglobin and hemocrit levels. Changes in blood values will be delayed.

Special Considerations

- *Arterial bleeding* is bright red and gushes forth in waves, related to heart rhythm; if vessel is very deep, flow will be steady. *Venous bleeding* is dark red and flows smoothly. *Capillary bleeding* is oozing of dark red blood; self-sealing controls this bleeding. *Hemorrhage* is loss of a large amount of blood either externally or internally in short period of time.
- Establish IV line quickly if signs and symptoms of hypovolemic shock are present.
- Outside pressure does not exclude possibility of extended bleeding into tissues and body cavities.

Teaching Considerations

- Explain purpose of pressure bandage.
- Explain need to monitor vital signs.
- Explain need for client to remain quiet and stay in position to reduce bleeding.
- Teach primary care giver how to apply a pressure dressing if client is at risk of hemorrhage.

Pediatric Considerations

(see also Skill 37-1)

- Assess skin below pressure bandage and pulse points distal to pressure bandage to monitor for vascular compromise.

Gerontologic Considerations

(see also Skill 37-1)

- Assess skin below pressure bandage and pulse points distal to pressure bandage to monitor for vascular compromise.

Home Care Considerations

- At home client may apply pressure with clean towels or linen.
- Emergency system (911) should be activated.
- Client should be positioned to promote elevation of affected body part (if extremity) and promote relaxation.

SKILL 37-4 Applying a Transparent Dressing

A film dressing is a "clear, adherent, nonabsorptive, polymer-based dressing that is permeable to oxygen and water vapor but not to water" (AHCPR, 1994) (Fig. 37-3). Polyurethane moisture and vapor-permeable film dressings were developed to manage superficial wounds. They can also be used for autolytic debridement of small wounds. Pain and discomfort are diminished with the use of a transparent dressing, and the film conforms well to different body contours. Therefore, bodily movement is less restricted. Transparent dressings may be with or without adhesives.

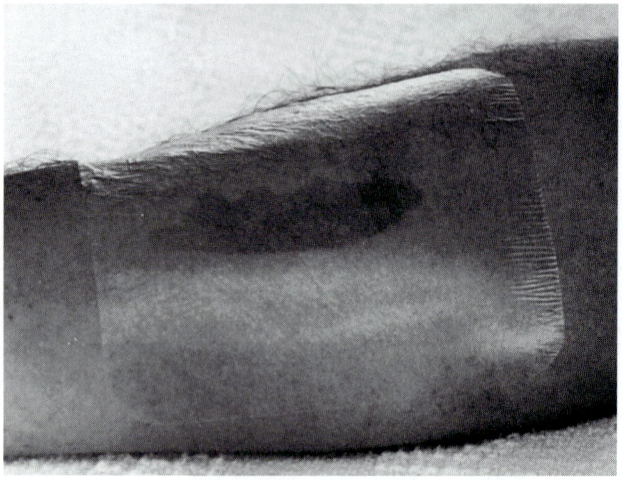

Fig. 37-3

With the use of a transparent dressing, a moist exudate forms over the wound surface, which prevents tissue dehydration and allows for rapid, effective healing by speeding epithelial cell growth. As these dressings are clear, the wound can be visualized without removing the dressing.

For best results these dressings should be used on clean, debrided wounds that are not actively bleeding. The film should be applied wrinkle free but not stretched over the skin. Should the fluid accumulation take on a white, opaque appearance with **erythema** of the surrounding tissue, one must assume an infectious process is underway, and the dressing should be removed and a wound culture obtained.

EQUIPMENT

- Sterile gloves (optional)
- Dressing set (optional)
- Sterile saline, or other agent (as ordered)
- Clean disposable gloves
- Cotton swabs
- Waterproof bag for disposal
- Mineral oil (optional)
- Transparent dressing (size as needed)
- Sterile gauze pads (4 × 4s)
- Skin preparation materials (optional)
- Moistureproof gown (optional)
- Goggles (optional)
- Mask (optional)

STEPS	RATIONALE
ASSESSMENT	
1. Assess location and size of wound to be dressed (see Chapter 40).	Allows nurse to determine supplies and assistance needed.
2. Review physician's orders for frequency and type of dressing change.	Physician orders frequency of dressing changes and special instructions.
3. Assess client's level of comfort.	Client who is comfortable during procedure is less likely to move suddenly, causing wound or supply contamination. Dressing change procedure can be painful and client may need pain management.
4. Assess client's knowledge of purpose of dressing.	Identifies client's learning needs.
5. Assess risk for wound healing (see Chapter 40).	

NURSING DIAGNOSIS

Clustering of defining characteristics from the assessment data may reveal the following nursing diagnoses for clients requiring this skill:

- Impaired skin integrity
- Pain
- Risk for infection

Related factors are individualized based on a client's condition or needs.

STEPS	RATIONALE
PLANNING	
1. **Expected outcome** following completion of procedure:	
➤ Wound heals rapidly with little pain and mobility restriction for client.	Dressing effective in preventing infection and promoting healing.
2. Explain procedure to client.	Relieves anxiety and promotes understanding of healing process.
3. Position client to allow access to dressing site.	Facilitates application of dressing.
IMPLEMENTATION	
1. Close door or cubicle curtains, keep sheet or gown draped over body parts not requiring exposure.	Provides privacy and decreases transfer of microorganisms.
2. Cuff top of disposable waterproof bag and place within reach of work area.	Cuff prevents accidental contamination of tip of outer bag.
3. Wash hands and put on clean disposable gloves. Moistureproof gown, mask, and eye goggles are worn when risk of spray exists.	Reduces transmission of infectious organisms from soiled dressings to nurse's hands.
4. Remove old dressing. For easier removal, ease off using cotton swab soaked in mineral oil, or secure piece of tape to corner of dressing and pull back slowly across dressing in direction of hair growth. Avoid letting client see old dressing because drainage can be upsetting to the client.	Reduces excoriation or irritation of skin following dressing removal.
5. Dispose of soiled dressings in waterproof bag and remove disposable gloves by pulling them inside out and dispose of them in waterproof bag.	Reduces transmission of microorganisms.
6. Prepare sterile dressing supplies.	Reduces risk of break in sterile technique.
7. Pour saline or prescribed solution over 4 × 4s.	Maintains sterility of dressing.
8. Put on gloves (sterile if institution policy).	Allows nurse to handle dressings.
9. Cleanse area gently with moist 4 × 4s, swabbing toward area of most exudate, or spray with wound cleanser.	Reduces introduction of organisms into wound.
10. Pat dry skin around wound thoroughly with dry 4 × 4s. Transparent dressing with adhesive backing does not adhere to damp surface. Nonadhesive transparent dressing clings to moist wound surface.	

STEPS	RATIONALE
CRITICAL DECISION POINT **Do not rub the skin to dry it.**	
11. Inspect wound for tissue type, color, odor, and drainage; measure if indicated.	Appearance indicates state of wound healing.
CRITICAL DECISION POINT **If wound has a large amount of drainage, choose another dressing that can absorb this amount of wound drainage rather than the transparent film dressing that can absorb light-to-moderate amounts of drainage.**	
12. Apply transparent dressing according to manufacturer's directions (Fig. 37-3, p. 1084). *Film should not be stretched during applications.* Avoid wrinkles in film.	Wrinkles would provide tunnel for exudate drainage.
CRITICAL DECISION POINT **Know the specific characteristics of the brand of film dressing you are applying. Some film dressings can be removed during the application process and reapplied to correct application errors such as being applied too tight or too loose with wrinkles.**	
13. Remove gown and goggles. Remove gloves by pulling inside out and discard in prepared bag.	Reduces risk of microorganism transfer.
14. Assist client to comfortable position.	Enhances client comfort and relaxation.
15. Discard soiled dressing change materials properly and wash hands.	Reduces transmission of microorganisms.
EVALUATION	
1. Inspect condition of wound on ongoing basis.	Determines status of wound healing. Wound can be easily viewed.
2. Evaluate client's level of comfort.	Determines if pain resulted from procedure.
3. **Unexpected outcomes** that may occur include:	
➤ Wound becomes infected.	Dressing changes may need to be done more frequently, or different type of dressing may be required.
➤ Dressing does not stay in place.	Evaluate size of dressing used for adequate wound margin (1 to 1½ inches [2.5 to 3.75 cm]) or dry skin more thoroughly before reapplication.
➤ Skin tears can occur with this type of dressing.	
RECORDING AND REPORTING	
1. Report unusual observations immediately, then chart what was reported and when.	Change in wound's condition may require different dressing or treatments.
2. Record characteristics of wound, color, odor, viscosity, and amount of drainage, and application of dressing in nurses' notes.	Documents status of wound and ensures continuity of care.
3. Write date and time on a sticker and place on peripheral aspect of dressing.	Documents by whom and when dressing was changed.

FOLLOW-UP ACTIVITIES

1. Observe wound, without disturbing dressing, every shift.

• • • • •

Special Considerations

- Transparent dressings may stay in place up to 7 days if complete occlusion is maintained.
- Measure wound after cleansing using greatest and smallest dimensions.
- Transparent dressings may be used over "island" dressing, such as Telfa, cut to fit area of wound.
- Appearance of wound may not be tolerated by client. Cover transparent dressing with dry gauze dressing taking care not to place tape directly on transparent dressing.
- If wound exudate builds up to cause bulge in dressing, either change dressing or aspirate fluid using small-gauge needle; patch hole with small piece of film.
- Topical medications may be applied over nonadhesive transparent dressings without disturbing dressing.
- Nonadhesive transparent dressings fall off as wound heals. If removal is needed, moisten with normal saline.

Teaching Considerations

- Explain wound healing process with film dressing.
- Explain need to change dressing should edges loosen.
  - Explain to client and family that collection of wound fluid under the dressing is not "pus," but the normal interaction of body fluids with the dressing.
- Allow client or care giver to demonstrate dressing change should self-care need be identified.

Pediatric Considerations

- Adhesive backing may cause skin tears on premature babies' immature skin.

Gerontologic Considerations

- Adhesive backing may be too strong for the skin of the elderly. Do not use a film dressing that has an adhesive backing that has a stronger bond to the epidermis than the epidermis has to the dermis.

Home Care Considerations

- Wound may be cleansed in shower, if approved by physician.
- Client may shower or bathe with dressing in place.
- Many types of transparent dressings exist. Explore types with client and recommend type client finds easy to work with and has access to.
- Make sure client has a source of dressing supplies for purchase after discharge.
- Cost of dressing supplies and lack of insurance coverage may be an issue for some clients.

SKILL 37-5 Applying a Hydrocolloid or Hydrogel Dressing

Hydrocolloid dressings can be used for a variety of reasons. These include: (1) maintaining a moist wound environment for healing of clean shallow to moderately deep wounds, (2) autolytic debridement of necrotic wounds, and (3) protection of intact skin. For example, by applying the dressing beneath Montgomery ties or on bony prominences to prevent shearing or friction injuries including pressure ulcers (see Chapter 8). Pain and discomfort are diminished with the use of a hydrocolloid dressing. Their "cushioning" effect provides protection to the wound and skin beneath bony prominences. These adhesive-backed dressings conform well to different body contours. Hydrocolloids come in the form of granules, paste, or wafer dressings.

With the use of a hydrocolloid dressing, wound exudate is absorbed into the dressing, forming a jellylike substance next to the wound surface. The dressing maintains a moist, insulated environment that promotes rapid, effective healing.

A hydrogel dressing is a "water-based nonadherent, polymer based dressing that has some absorptive properties" (AHCPR, 1994). These dressings are available in several forms including a "sheet" (see Fig. 37-4, *A* and *B*), amorphous gels (see illustration, Step 14b on p. 1090), and impregnated gauze that can be placed in the wound.

Hydrogel dressings facilitate wound debridement by rehydration; they absorb exudate and encourage healing by maintaining a moist wound healing environment. The gel dressings are nonadherent and must be covered with a secondary dressing to hold them in place.

The hydrogels may be used over leg ulcers, pressure ulcers, and burns. They can also be used to protect skin from radiation.

The hydrocolloid or hydrogel dressings are used frequently over venous stasis ulcers, arterial ulcers, and pressure ulcers. When used in combination with wound exudate absorbers, these dressings are useful over stage 3 pressure ulcers (see Chapter 8). Hydrogels do not stick to the wound and can be easily removed. Their "cooling" and soothing properties make them especially useful on painful wounds such as burns.

A B

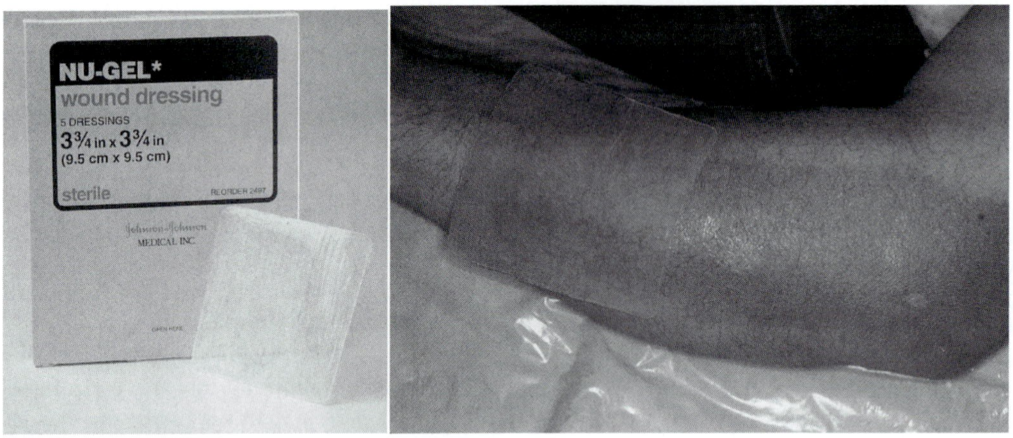

Fig. 37-4

EQUIPMENT

- Sterile gloves (optional)
- Dressing set (optional)
- Sterile saline, or other cleansing solution (as ordered)
- Clean disposable gloves
- Waterproof bag for disposal
- Hydrocolloid dressing (size as needed) or hydrogel dressing
- Sterile gauze pads (4 × 4s)
- Moistureproof gown (optional)
- Goggles (optional)
- Mask (optional)

STEPS	RATIONALE
ASSESSMENT	
1. Assess wound location and size of wound to be dressed see also Assessment, Skill 37-1. (See Chapter 40).	Allows nurse to determine supplies and assistance needed.
2. Determine the type of hydrocolloid dressing.	
CRITICAL DECISION POINT Some brands of hydrocolloid dressings are available in custom shapes and sizes to better fit certain difficult body parts such as the sacrum, heels, or elbows. The variety of shapes aids in flexibility of dressing selection and better dressing adherence.	
3. Review physician's orders for frequency and type of dressing change.	Physician orders mode of therapy.
4. Assess client's level of comfort.	Client who is comfortable during procedure is less likely to move suddenly, causing wound or supply contamination. Some dressing change procedures can cause client discomfort, and pain management may be necessary.
5. Assess client's knowledge of purpose of dressing.	Identifies client's learning needs.

NURSING DIAGNOSIS

Clustering of defining characteristics from the assessment data may reveal the following nursing diagnoses for clients requiring this skill:

- Impaired skin integrity
- Knowledge deficit regarding hydrocolloid dressing application
- Pain
- Risk for infection

Related factors are individualized based on a client's condition or needs.

STEPS	RATIONALE
PLANNING	
1. **Expected outcomes** following completion of procedure:	
➤ Wound heals rapidly with little pain and mobility restriction for client.	Dressing effective in preventing infection and promoting healing.
➤ Wound exudate is adequately absorbed.	
➤ Client explains procedure correctly.	Indicates learning has occurred.
2. Explain procedure to client.	Relieves anxiety and promotes understanding of healing process.
3. Position client to allow access to dressing site.	Facilitates application of dressing.
IMPLEMENTATION	
1. Close room door or cubicle curtains.	Provides for client privacy.
2. Expose wound site and cover client with bath blanket.	Draping provides access to wound while minimizing exposure.
3. Cuff top of disposable waterproof bag and place within reach of work area.	Cuff prevents accidental contamination of top of outer bag. Nurse should not reach across sterile field.
4. Wash hands and put on clean disposable gloves. Moistureproof gown, mask, and goggles are worn when risk of spray exists.	Reduces transmission of infectious organisms.
5. Remove old dressing. For easier removal, ease off with adhesive remover and pull back slowly across dressing in direction of hair growth.	Reduces irritation and possible injury to skin.
6. The hydrocolloid dressing interacts with wound fluids and forms a soft whitish-yellowish gel that may have a faint odor to it. This is a normal occurrence with hydrocolloid dressings and should not be confused with pus or purulent exudate or malodorous infected wounds.	
➤ **CRITICAL DECISION POINT** **Important to be able to distinguish the usual normal dressing interactions for accurate wound assessment.**	
7. Dispose of soiled dressings in waterproof bag. Remove disposable gloves by pulling them inside out and dispose of them in waterproof bag. Avoid having client see old dressing because the site of wound drainage may be upsetting to the client.	Reduces transmission of microorganisms.
8. Prepare sterile dressing supplies.	Reduces risk of break in sterile technique.
9. Pour saline or prescribed solution over 4 × 4s.	Maintains sterility of dressing.
10. Put on gloves, sterile if required by policy.	Allows nurse to handle dressings.
11. Cleanse area gently with moist 4 × 4s, swabbing exudate away from wound, or spray with wound cleanser (see also Chapter 40).	Reduces introduction of organisms into wound.
12. Thoroughly pat area dry with dry 4 × 4s.	Dressing will not adhere to damp surface. Hydrocolloid dressing has adhesive backing.
13. Inspect wound for tissue type, color, odor, and drainage. Measure wound size and depth (see also Chapter 40).	Appearance indicates state of wound healing.
➤ **CRITICAL DECISION POINT** **For some brands of hydrocolloid wafers, the size of the dressing used should be larger enough in comparison to the wound size to leave a 1- to 1½-inch margin of dressing beyond the wound end.**	Proper dressing size is necessary for the dressing to function properly.

STEPS | **RATIONALE**

14. Apply dressing.

a. Apply **hydrocolloid dressing** according to manufacturer's directions. Apply hydrocolloid granules or paste before wafer dressing in deeper wounds.

Dressing should not be stretched during applications. Avoid wrinkles that would provide tunnel for exudate drainage. Hydrocolloid granules assist in absorbing drainage to increase wearing time of dressing.

➤ **CRITICAL DECISION POINT** **Edges may be notched to help mold around wound. Consider using custom shapes to better conform to certain parts of the body such as heels, elbows, and sacrum.**

Tape applied around the edges of the hydrocolloid dressing may assist in keeping the dressing in place.

b. Apply amphorous gels approximately ¼- to ½-inch thick across wound surface (see illustration) or put hydrogel sheet over wound bed (see Fig. 37-4b). Cover with secondary dressing such as: gauze, hydrocolloid, foam.

Fluid gels take form of cavity-type wounds. A secondary dressing must be used with a hydrogel to hold it in place; it has no adhesive.

15. Remove sterile gloves by pulling them inside out and discard in prepared bag.

Reduces transfer of microorganisms.

16. Assist client to comfortable position.

Enhances client comfort and relaxation.

17. Discard soiled dressing change materials properly. Wash hands.

Reduces transmission of microorganisms.

EVALUATION

1. Inspect condition of wound on ongoing basis.

Determines status of wound healing.

2. Evaluate client's level of comfort.

Determines if pain resulted from procedure.

3. Ask client to describe wound care method.

Evaluates client's level of learning.

4. **Unexpected outcomes** that may occur include:

➤ Wound becomes infected.

Dressing changes may need to be done more frequently, or different type of dressing may be required.

➤ **CRITICAL DECISION POINT** **Client has a skin reaction from the product.**

Discontinue use of the dressing.

➤ Dressing does not stay in place.

Evaluates size of dressing used for adequate margin (1- to 1½-inch [2.5 to 3.75]), or dry skin more thoroughly before reapplication.

➤ **CRITICAL DECISION POINT** **Consider custom shapes for difficult body parts. "Picture-frame" the edges of the hydrocolloid dressing using tape.**

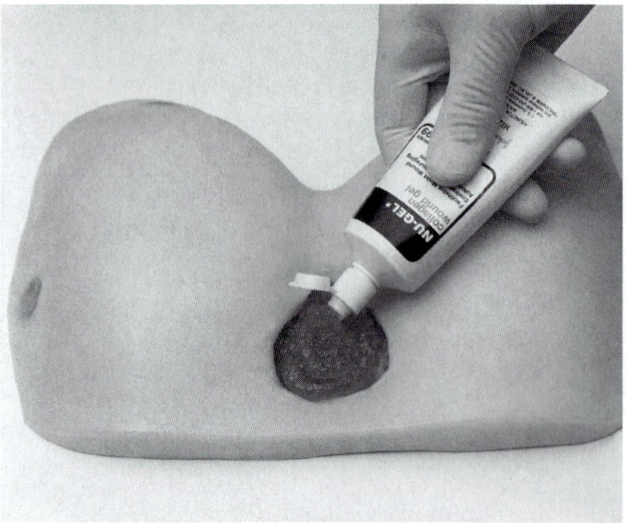

Step 14b Hydrogel amorphous gel being applied to a "wound".

STEPS | **RATIONALE**

- ➤ Wound develops more necrotic tissue and increases in size.

In rare instances, wounds do not tolerate hypoxia induced by hydrocolloid dressings. In these clients use should be discontinued.

➤ *CRITICAL DECISION POINT* Wound exudate is more than hydrogel can absorb. Consider switching to another more absorbent dressing; hydrogel dressings are not recommended for wounds with heavy exudate.

- ➤ Wound drainage is more than dressing can absorb.

Change type of dressing to one that can absorb amount of wound drainage.

- ➤ Client is unable to explain dressing technique.

Reinstruction is necessary.

Recording and Reporting

1. Report unusual observations immediately, then chart what was reported and when.

   Change in wound's condition may require different therapy.

2. Record characteristics of wound tissue type, color, odor, viscosity and amount of drainage, and application of dressing in client's medical record.

   Documents status of wound and ensures continuity of care.

3. Write date, time, and nurse's initials in ink (not marker) on the dressing.

Follow-up Activities

1. Observe dressing for adhesion every shift.

• • • • •

Special Considerations

- ➤ Some hydrocolloid dressings may be left in place for as long as 7 days if complete occlusion is maintained.
- ➤ Some hydrocolloid dressings swell as dressing absorbs wound exudate; change when dressing has changed or swollen to within ½ inch of dressing edge.
- ➤ Edge of dressing may be "picture framed" with hypoallergenic tape to prevent accidental pulling on edge of dressing.
- ➤ Excessive odor may indicate yeast. Topical miconazole gel if ordered may be used under hydrocolloid dressing.
- ➤ Hydrocolloid dressings should be left in place for at least 48 hours. If wound appearance must be evaluated more frequently, an alternative dressing should be used.

A

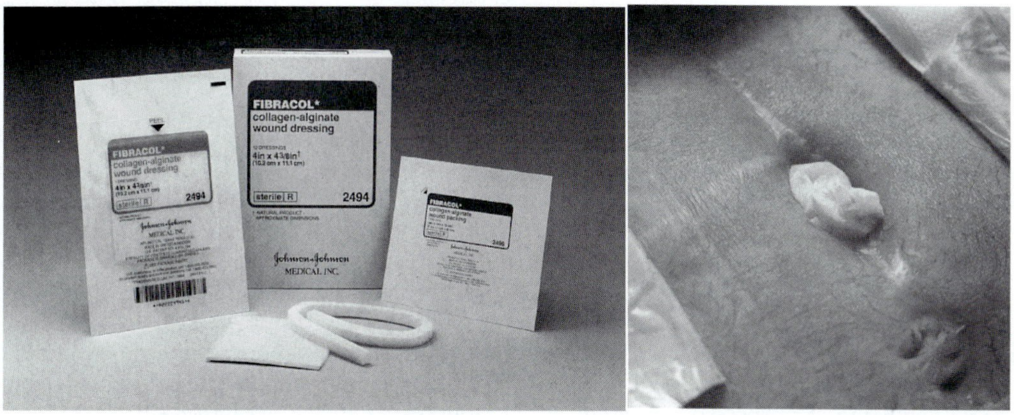

B

Fig. 37-5 **A,** Example of alginate dressing package. Alginate sheet *(left)* and alginate rope *(right)*. **B,** Alginate dressing placed in an abdominal wound.

- Hydrogel dressings may be used as carrier for topical medications.
- Frequency required for dressing changes depends on amount of exudate produced by wound. Fluid gels should not be left in place more than 3 days.

Teaching Considerations

- Instruct client and family regarding proper handling of hydrocolloid dressing to avoid contamination of the sterile adhesive surface.
- Advise client and family that fluid that may collect under dressing will have an odor and may appear purulent but is **not** an infection with purulent drainage but a normal occurrence as a result of the interaction of the hydrocolloid with wound fluid.
- Hydrogel dressings will feel cool when first applied.

Pediatric Considerations

(see Skills 37-1, 2, and 4)

Gerontologic Considerations

(see also Skills 37-1, 2, and 4)

- Avoid early and frequent removal of a hydrocolloid dressing to reduce injury to surrounding intact skin.

Home Care Considerations

- Dressing is easily applied and readily adaptable for home use.
- Dressing may not be available at every pharmacy. Client may need assistance locating dressing.
- Client may need to consider the cost of the dressing.

SKILL 37-6 Applying a Foam Dressing

A foam dressings is "a sponge like polymer dressing that may or may not be adherent; it may be impregnated or coated with other materials and has some absorptive properties" (AHCPR, 1994). These hydrophilic dressings are used in full-thickness wounds with minimal to moderate amounts of drainage. More heavily draining wounds may be covered with foam dressings when absorptive wound fillers are also used. These dressings require a secondary dressing to secure the foam in place, or they may be secured with tape or a sheet of flexible tape.

The foam dressings protect the wound surface while maintaining a moist, insulated environment. The result is a well-hydrated wound bed that can heal rapidly with little discomfort to the client. Application directions for the different brands of foam dressings vary. The nurse should read and follow the specific directions for the particular brand of foam dressings that is being used.

EQUIPMENT

- **Sterile gloves (optional)**
- **Dressing set (optional)**
- **Cleansing solution (as ordered) or sterile saline**
- **Waterproof bag**
- **Foam dressing**
- **Sterile gauze pads (4 × 4s)**
- **Moistureproof gown (optional)**
- **Goggles (optional)**
- **Mask (optional)**
- **Wound measurement devices (tape measure, tracing paper, camera)**

STEPS	RATIONALE
ASSESSMENT	
1. Assess wound location and size of wound to be dressed see Assessment, Skill 37-1. (See Chapter 40).	Allows nurse to determine supplies and assistance needed.
2. Assess client's level of comfort.	Client who is comfortable during procedure is less likely to move suddenly, causing wound or supply contamination. Dressing change procedure can be painful. Client may need pain management during this procedure.
3. Review physician's orders for frequency and type of dressing change.	Physician orders mode of therapy; the nurse frequently suggests dressings for local management of wound.
4. Assess client's knowledge of purpose of dressing.	Identifies client's learning needs.
5. Identify client's risk for poor wound healing (see Skill 37-1, *Assessment*, Step 7).	

STEPS	RATIONALE

NURSING DIAGNOSIS

Clustering of defining characteristics from the assessment data may reveal the following nursing diagnoses for clients requiring this skill:

- Impaired skin integrity
- Pain
- Knowledge deficit regarding wound care

Related factors are individualized based on a client's condition or needs.

PLANNING

STEPS	RATIONALE
1. **Expected outcomes** following completion of procedure:	
➤ Wound heals rapidly with little pain or mobility restriction for client.	Dressing effective in preventing infection and promoting healing.
➤ Wound exudate is adequately absorbed.	Dressing is effective in exudate management for draining wounds.
➤ Client explains procedure correctly.	Indicates learning has occurred.
2. Explain procedure to client.	Relieves anxiety and promotes understanding of healing process.
3. Position client to allow access to dressing site.	Facilitates application of dressing.

IMPLEMENTATION

STEPS	RATIONALE
1. Close room door or cubicle curtains.	Provides for client privacy and decreases transfer of microorganisms.
2. Expose wound site and drape client.	Draping provides access to wound while minimizing exposure.
3. Cuff top of disposable waterproof bag and place within reach of work area.	Cuff prevents accidental contamination of top of outer bag.
4. Wash hands and put on clean disposable gloves. If a risk of spray exists don protective gown, goggles, and mask.	Reduces transmission of infectious organisms.
5. Remove old dressing. For easier removal, ease off, pulling back slowly. Avoid having client see the old dressing as wound drainage can be upsetting to the client.	Reduces irritation and possible injury to intact skin. Foam dressing may fall off on its own as wound heals underneath.

➤ **CRITICAL DECISION POINT** **Check the removal directions for the specific brand of foam dressing that is being used. Some brands need to have the old dressing soaked or moistened to remove the dressing.**

STEPS	RATIONALE
6. Dispose of soiled dressings in waterproof bag. Remove disposable gloves by pulling them inside out and dispose of them in waterproof bag.	Reduces transmission of microorganisms.

➤ **CRITICAL DECISION POINT** **Do not confuse the normal discoloration that occurs with some brands of foam dressings as a sign of infection or deterioration of the wound.**

STEPS	RATIONALE
7. Prepare sterile dressing supplies.	Reduces risk of break in sterile technique.
8. Pour saline or prescribed solution over 4 × 4s, or open spray wound cleanser.	Maintains sterility of dressing.
9. Put on gloves (sterile if required by policy).	Allows nurse to handle dressings.
10. Cleanse area gently with moist 4 × 4s, swabbing exudate away from wound, or spray wound directly (see Chapter 40).	Reduces introduction of organisms into wound.

STEPS	RATIONALE
CRITICAL DECISION POINT With some brands of foam dressings, the wound must be *thoroughly* irrigated to remove all of the old dressing.	
11. Blot excess moisture from wound surface, dry intact skin around wound.	Periwound skin should be kept dry.
12. Inspect wound for tissue type, color, odor, and drainage, obtain wound measurements (see Chapter 40).	Appearance indicates state of wound healing. Measurements provide a basis for monitoring wound closure.
CRITICAL DECISION POINT Do not use foam dressings on nonexuding wounds. Most foam dressings are designed to absorb moderate amounts of wound drainage.	
13. *Apply foam dressing according to manufacturer's directions.* Application techniques differ for the different brands of foam dressings.	Most foam dressings should be applied smoothly; avoid wrinkles. May be used with absorptive dressings to accommodate more highly draining wounds.
a. Make sure you know which side of the foam dressing should be placed towards the wound bed and which side should be facing away from the wound bed.	Check with the manufacturer as to which types of secondary dressings to avoid when covering the foam dressing that could reduce the effectiveness of the foam dressing.
b. Choose the correct size dressing to use in the wound.	
CRITICAL DECISION POINT Some brands need a margin left around the wound edges. For some brands the dressing should extend beyond the wound edges; for others it is important to not overlap the dressing onto the skin surrounding the wound.	
c. With some brands, the dressings can be trimmed to fit the wound size while for other brands they cannot be cut.	
CRITICAL DECISION POINT Some brands of foam dressings need slight tension on the dressing while being applied. Some brands of foam dressings need to be covered with a secondary dressing.	
d. Know the removal and application characteristics of the specific brand of foam dressing you are using.	
14. Remove gloves by pulling inside out and discard in prepared bag.	Reduces risk of microorganism transfer.
15. Assist client to comfortable position.	Enhances client comfort and relaxation.
16. Discard soiled dressing change materials properly.	Reduces transmission of microorganisms.
17. Wash hands.	Reduces risk of microorganism transmission.
EVALUATION	
1. Inspect condition of wound, especially amount of exudate on ongoing basis.	Determines status of wound healing.
2. Evaluate client's level of comfort.	Determines if pain resulted from procedure.
3. Ask client to explain wound care method.	Evaluates client's level of learning.
4. Unexpected outcomes that may occur include:	
➤ Wound becomes infected.	Dressing changes may need to be done more frequently, or a different type of dressing regimen may be required.

STEPS	RATIONALE
➤ Dressing does not stay in place.	Evaluate size of dressing used for adequate margin.
➤ Wound increases in size.	Evaluate appropriateness of wound care protocol and look for other impediments to wound healing.
➤ ***CRITICAL DECISION POINT*** **Wound exudate is not adequately absorbed.**	Consider using a different type of dressing for more heavily draining wounds.

RECORDING AND REPORTING

STEPS	RATIONALE
1. Report unusual observations immediately, then chart what was reported and when.	Change in wound's condition may require new therapy.
2. Record characteristics of wound; color, odor, viscosity, and amount of drainage; and application of dressing in nurses' notes.	Documents status of wound and ensures continuity of care.
3. Graph wound surface area or volume if the wound is a chronic wound.	Graphing wound size facilitates monitoring of change over time. A plateau in size over several weeks may respond to a change in local care.
4. Write nurse's initials, date, and time of dressing change on the new dressing or tape in ink (not marker).	Maintains record of time dressing changed for reference should condition change.

FOLLOW-UP ACTIVITIES

1. Be sure client has access to dressing supplies if being followed as an outpatient.
2. If wound is the result of pressure necrosis, ensure client's pressure relief needs are evaluated and supported.
3. If wound is the result of venous insufficiency, ensure client has acceptable method of edema control (compression therapy).

• • • • •

Special Considerations

- For some brands, foam dressings may be left in place for as long as 7 days; if adherent may be allowed to fall off on its own.
- Foam dressings may be used over wound exudate absorbers.
- Dressing may be secured with roll gauze, tape, transparent dressing, or dressing sheet (*Mefix* or *Hypafix*).
- Foam dressings may be used in the presence of cellulitis.
- Since the application technique varies with the different brands of foam dressings, knowing which specific brand is being used and following the manufacturer's directions for removal and application is important.

Teaching Considerations

- Explain expected wound appearance with use of foam dressing.
- Explain frequency of dressing changes required.
- Instruct client and care giver to observe wound for signs and symptoms of infection.
- Since application technique can vary with different brands, tell client and care giver not to purchase a different brand other than the one they were given instructions for by the nurse. If a different brand must be used, the client and care giver should check with the nurse for any additional instructions or modification in foam dressing removal and application technique needed.

Pediatric Considerations

(see *Pediatric Considerations,* Skill 37-1)

Gerontologic Considerations

(see *Gerontologic Considerations,* Skill 37-1)

Home Care Considerations

(see *Home Care Considerations,* Skill 37-1)

SKILL 37-7 Applying Absorption and Alginate Dressings

Absorption dressings can contain large amounts of wound exudate. They may take the form of pastes, granules, sheeting, or rope. This group of dressings includes calcium alginate materials (see Fig. 37-5, *A*), which are manufactured from natural material (sea weed) and are known for their absorptive properties, forming a gel over the wound surface as exudate is contained. The exudate absorbers are nonadhesive, nonocclusive dressings that can be used in combination with other dressings. These dressings are appropriate for full thickness wounds with moderate-to-high amounts of drainage. Deep tracking wounds can safely be packed with calcium alginate rope, which allows easy removal with little risk of retained dressing deep in the wound cavity. Calcium alginate dressings may be further useful in control of wound odor, achieving hemostasis, and control of pain.

Generally, absorption and alginate dressings require a secondary dressing and that dressing can be changed as needed. The typical frequency of dressing changes is daily to once or twice a week.

EQUIPMENT

- **Sterile gloves (optional)**
- **Dressing set (optional)**
- **Sterile saline or other wound cleanser (as ordered)**
- **Clean disposable gloves**
- **Waterproof bag for disposal**
- **Absorption dressing**
- **Sterile gauze pads (4 × 4s)**
- **Secondary dressing of choice**
- **Moistureproof gown (optional)**
- **Goggles (optional)**
- **Mask (optional)**

STEPS	RATIONALE
ASSESSMENT	
1. Assess wound location and size of wound to be dressed (see Chapter 40).	Allows nurse to determine supplies and assistance needed.
2. Review physician's orders for frequency and type of dressing change.	Physician orders frequency of dressing changes and special instructions.
3. Assess client's level of comfort.	Client who is comfortable during procedure is less likely to move suddenly, causing wound or supply contamination.
4. Assess client's knowledge of purpose of dressing.	Identifies client's learning needs.

NURSING DIAGNOSIS

Clustering of defining characteristics from the assessment data may reveal the following nursing diagnoses for clients requiring this skill:

➤ Impaired skin integrity
➤ Pain

Related factors are individualized based on a client's condition or needs.

PLANNING

STEPS	RATIONALE
1. Develop individualized goals for the client based on nursing diagnoses:	
a. Client achieves wound healing.	Proper use of dressing promotes healing.
b. Client achieves pain control.	Proper application minimizes discomfort.
c. Client achieves control of wound exudate and odor.	Proper use of dressing controls drainage protecting skin around wound.
2. Expected outcomes following completion of procedure:	
➤ Wound heals rapidly with little pain or mobility restriction to client.	Dressing effective in preventing infection and promoting healing.
➤ Wound drainage is contained, and skin surrounding wound remains intact.	Dressing effective in controlling wound exudate.
3. Explain procedure to client.	Relieves anxiety and promotes understanding of healing process.
4. Position client to allow access to dressing site.	Facilitates application of dressing.

STEPS	RATIONALE
IMPLEMENTATION	
1. Close room door or cubicle curtains.	Provides for client privacy and reduces transmission of organisms.
2. Expose wound site and cover client.	Draping provides access to wound while minimizing exposure.
3. Cuff top of disposable waterproof bag and place within reach of work area.	Cuff prevents accidental contamination of top of outer bag.
4. Wash hands and put on clean disposable gloves. If risk of spray exists don protective gown, goggles, and mask.	Reduces transmission of infectious organisms from soiled dressings to nurse's hands.
5. Remove old dressing and dispose of in waterproof bag. Remove gloves.	Reduces transmission of microorganisms.

➤ *CRITICAL DECISION POINT* **Do not confuse the residual gel substance in the wound bed that occurs with some brands of alginate dressings with pus. The gel in the wound bed is not a sign of infection or deterioration of the wound.**

STEPS	RATIONALE
6. Prepare sterile dressing supplies.	Reduces risk of break in sterile technique.
7. Pour saline or cleansing solution over 4 × 4s.	Maintains sterility of dressing.

➤ *CRITICAL DECISION POINT* **With most brands of alginate dressings, the wound must be *thoroughly* irrigated to remove all of the old dressing.**

STEPS	RATIONALE
8. Put on gloves, sterile if required by policy, and cleanse area gently with 4 × 4s (see Chapter 40).	Allows nurse to handle sterile dressings and reduces introduction of organisms into wound.

➤ *CRITICAL DECISION POINT* **Irrigating the wound *gently* effectively removes any residual dressing gel without injuring the newly formed delicate granulation tissue that is forming in the healing wound bed.**

STEPS	RATIONALE
9. Inspect wound for tissue type, color, odor, and drainage, measure wound (see Chapter 40).	Appearance and measurements indicate state of wound healing.

➤ *CRITICAL DECISION POINT* **Do not use alginate or absorption dressings on nonexuding wounds. Most of these dressings are designed to absorb moderate-to-large amounts of wound drainage and therefore should not be used in wounds with minimal or no drainage. For some brands the dressing technique may need to be further modified if the wound is infected.**

STEPS	RATIONALE
10. Apply absorption or alginate dressing according to manufacturer's directions (see Fig. 37-5,*B*, p. 1091).	Application techniques differ for the different brands of dressings.

➤ *CRITICAL DECISION POINT* **For most brands of alginate dressings, the dressing can be cut or folded to fit the wound. For others, it is important not to completely fill the wound bed with the dressing, but rather to allow space for the alginate dressing to expand to fill the wound bed. Most exudate absorbers and alginates should not completely fill wound cavity, but fill ½ to ⅔ to allow for expansion with absorption. For some brands the alginate dressing should be applied moist and for others it should be dry. Some brands need a secondary dressing that extends at least 1¼ inch from the wound edges. Check with the manufacturer as to which types of secondary dressings to avoid when covering the dressing that could reduce the effectiveness of the alginate or absorption dressing.**

STEPS	RATIONALE
11. Remove gloves by pulling inside out and discard in prepared bag.	Reduces risk of microorganism transfer.
12. Assist client to comfortable position.	Enhances client comfort and relaxation.
13. Discard soiled dressing change materials properly. Wash hands.	Reduces transmission of microorganisms.

EVALUATION

1. Inspect condition of wound on ongoing basis, note drainage and odor.	Change in wound condition may require new therapy.
2. Note length of time before dressing needed to be changed.	Dressing is intended for moderate to highly draining wounds. If wound is dry, an alternative dressing should be chosen, for example, a hydrogel.
3. An **unexpected outcome** that may occur is: ➤ Wound dressing is dry and adherent when removed.	Wound drainage has diminished and an alternative dressing should be considered.

RECORDING AND REPORTING

1. Report unusual observations immediately.	Change in wound condition may require new therapy.
2. Record wound characteristics and measurements in client's medical record.	Documents status of wound and ensures continuity of care.
3. Graph wound surface area or volume if the wound is a chronic wound.	Graphing wound size facilitates monitoring of change over time. A plateau in size over several weeks may respond to a change in local care.
4. Write nurse's initials, date, and time of dressing change on the new dressing or tape in ink (not marker).	Maintains record of time dressing changed for reference should condition change.

FOLLOW-UP ACTIVITIES

1. Observe secondary dressing for strike through or leakage of exudate every shift.
2. Be sure client has access to dressing supplies if needed for home care.

• • • • •

Special Considerations

- ➤ Absorption dressings must be used with a secondary dressing.
- ➤ Frequency required for dressing changes depends on amount of exudate produced by the wound.
- ➤ Since the application technique varies with the different brands of alginate and absorption dressings, knowing which specific brand is being used and following the manufacturer's directions for removal and application is important.

Teaching Considerations

- ➤ Instruct client and care giver to observe wound for signs and symptoms of infection.
- ➤ Explain expected wound appearance with use of dressing. Instruct client and care giver in appearance of alginate dressings as dressing becomes a gelatinous mass when maximal absorption has occurred.
- ➤ Dressing may have a "low tide" or fishy odor when removed.
- ➤ Explain frequency of dressing changes required. Often the dressing is not changed daily.
- ➤ Since application technique can vary with different brands, tell client and care giver not to purchase a different brand other than the one they were given instructions for by the nurse. If a different brand must be used, the client and care giver should check with the nurse for any additional instructions or modification in alginate or absorption dressing removal and application technique needed.

Pediatric Considerations

(see *Pediatric Considerations,* Skill 37-1)

Gerontologic Considerations

(see *Gerontologic Considerations,* Skill 37-1)

Home Care Considerations

(see *Home Care Considerations,* Skill 37-1)

CRITICAL THINKING EXERCISES

1. Your client has ordered wet-to-dry dressings for debridement of a wound healing by secondary intention. In change of shift report, the nurse tells you that even though the dressing was dripping wet when it was applied, the dressing stuck to the wound so it should be moistened with saline prior to removing the dressing. What do you think about the nurse's statement? How do you plan to do this dressing change during your shift?
2. A client has a large, draining wound that is being cared for with an alginate dressing. When removing the old dressing, the nurse notices a "fishy" smell from the jellylike substance in the wound. Based on this assessment, what clinical decision should the nurse make?
3. A client's spouse is being taught how to change a burn dressing using a hydrogel sheet dressing. The spouse states "I don't understand why this dressing does not stick better to the wound, what am I doing wrong?" How should the nurse answer?

REFERENCES

Agency for Health Care Policy and Research (AHCPR): *Clinical practice guideline #15—Treatment of pressure ulcers,* US Department of Health and Human Services, Public Health Service, Rockville, MD, 1994.

Aronovitch S: Selecting the best dressing sponge, *Nursing 95* 25(7):52-54, 1995.

Baranoski S: Wound assessment and dressing selection, *Ostomy/Wound Manage* 41(7A Suppl):7S-13S, 1995.

Bolton L, Rijswijk L: Wound dressings: Meeting clinical and biological needs, *Derm Nursing* 3(3):146, 1991.

Erwin-Toth P, Hocevar BJ: Wound Care: Selecting the right dressing, *Am J Nurs* 95:46, 1995.

Field CK, Kerstein MD: Overview of wound healing in a moist environment, *Am J Surg* 167(1A suppl):2S, 1994.

Johnson A: A short history of wound dressings, *Ostomy/Wound Manage* 38(2):36, 1992.

Krasner D: Resolving the dressing dilemma: Selecting wound dressings by category, *Plast Surg Nurs* 12(1):22, 1992a.

Krasner D: Using a hydrogel, foam and dressing retention sheet, *Ostomy/Wound Manage* 38(3):28, 1992b.

Krasner D: Wound care: How to use the Red-Yellow-Black System, *Am J Nurs* 5:44, 1995.

Maklebust J, Palleschi M: Promoting surgical wound healing, *Nursing 96* 26(6):24c, 1996.

Motta GJ: Moistening up for good healing, *Nursing 95* 25:32H-32J, 1995.

Provan A, Phillips TJ: An overview of moist wound dressings: The under cover story, *Derm Nurs* 3(6):393, 1991.

Wysocki, AB: A review of the skin and its appendages, *Advances in Wound Care* 8:53, 1995.

Wysocki AB, Bryant, RA: Skin. In Bryant RA: *Acute and chronic wounds: nursing management,* (1-30), St Louis, 1992, Mosby.

ADDITIONAL READING

Foresman PA, et al.: A relative toxicity index for wound cleansers, *Wounds* 5(5):226-231, 1993.

Hebda PA, Lee CI: Occlusive dressings for surgical and other acute wounds, *Wounds* 4(3):84, 1992.

Willey T: A decision tree to choose wound dressings, *Am J Nurs* 43, 1992.

Wright RW, Orr R: Fibroblast cytotoxicity and blood cell integrity following exposure to dermal wound cleaners, *Ostomy/Wound Manage* 39(7):33-40, 1993.

CHAPTER 38

Binders and Bandages

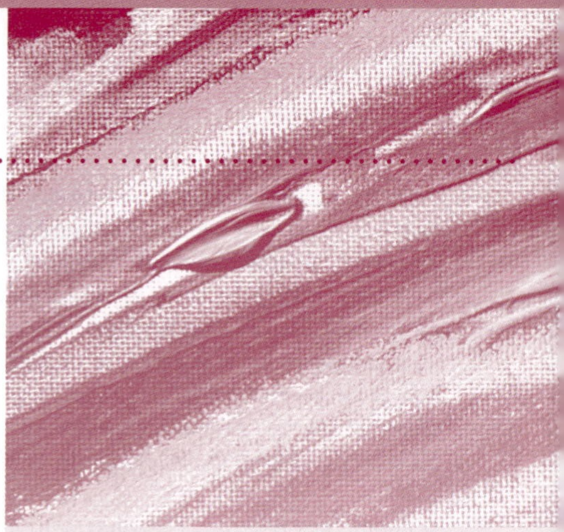

OBJECTIVES

Mastery of content in this chapter will enable the nurse to:

- Define key terms.
- Discuss the purposes of binders and bandages.
- Describe the precautions for use of binders and bandages.
- Demonstrate correct technique for applying turned bandages.
- Demonstrate correct application of binders.
- Document application of bandage and binder, including client's response, in the client's medical record.

KEY TERMS

Binder
Elastic bandage
T-binder

SKILLS

38-1 Applying an Elastic Bandage

38-2 Applying an Abdominal Binder, T-Binder, or Breast Binder

Binders and bandages applied over or around dressings can provide extra protection and therapeutic benefits by:

1. Creating pressure over a body part (e.g., an elastic pressure bandage applied over an arterial puncture site).
2. Immobilizing a body part (e.g., an elastic bandage applied around a sprained ankle).
3. Supporting a wound (e.g., an abdominal binder applied over a large abdominal incision and dressing).
4. Reducing or preventing edema (e.g., a breast binder used to minimize swelling between skin and tissue layers after a mastectomy).
5. Securing a splint (e.g., a bandage applied around hand splints for correction of deformities).
6. Securing dressings (e.g., elastic webbing applied around leg dressings after a vein stripping).
7. Maintaining the position of special equipment for applying traction (e.g., Buck's extension).
8. Enabling the client to participate in effective respiratory functions of deep breathing, coughing, and clearing of airway secretions; for example, a breast or abdominal binder supports local incisions, reducing the pain from respiratory maneuvers.

Bandages are available in rolls of various widths and materials, including gauze, elasticized knit, elastic webbing, flannel, and muslin. Gauze bandages are lightweight and inexpensive, mold easily around contours of the body, and permit air circulation to prevent skin maceration. **Elastic bandages** conform well to body parts but can also be used to exert pressure over a body part. Elastic bandages are used to secure dressings on extremities, stumps, and the hand (Table 38-1). Flannel and muslin bandages are thicker than gauze and thus stronger for supporting or applying pressure. A flannel bandage also insulates to provide warmth.

Binders are bandages made of large pieces of material specially designed to fit a specific body part. Most binders are made of elastic, cotton, muslin, or flannel. The most common types of binders are the breast binder, abdominal binder, and T-binder.

A breast binder looks like a tight-fitting sleeveless vest. It conforms to the shape of the chest wall and is available in different sizes. Breast binders can provide support after breast surgery or exert pressure to reduce lactation in a woman after childbirth.

An abdominal binder supports large abdominal incisions that are vulnerable to tension or stress as the client

Table 38-1 Types of Bandage Turns

Type	Description	Purpose or Use
Circular	Bandage turn overlapping previous turn completely 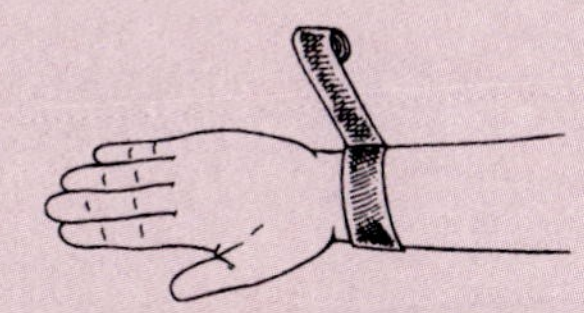	Anchors bandage at the first and final turn; covers small part (finger, toe)
Spiral	Bandage ascending body part with each turn overlapping previous one by one-half or two-thirds width of bandage 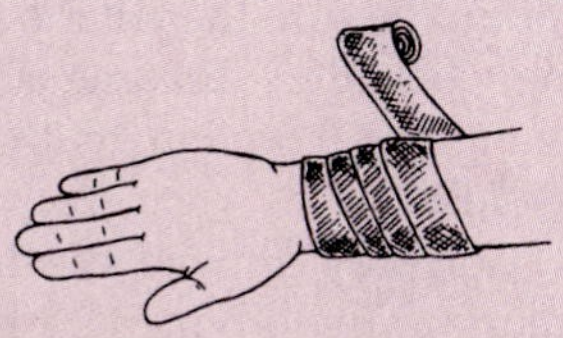	Covers cylindrical body parts such as wrist or upper arm
Spiral—reverse	Turn requiring twist (reversal) of bandage halfway through each turn 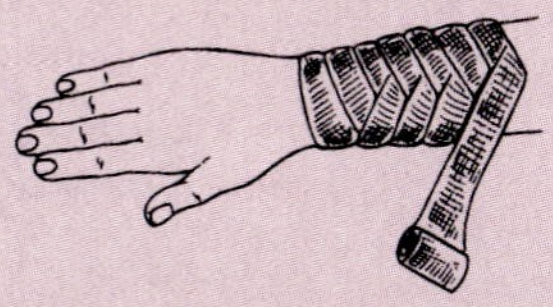	Covers cone-shaped body parts such as the forearm, thigh, or calf; useful with nonstretching bandages such as gauze or flannel
Figure eight	Oblique overlapping turns alternately ascending and descending over bandaged part; each turn crossing previous one to form figure eight 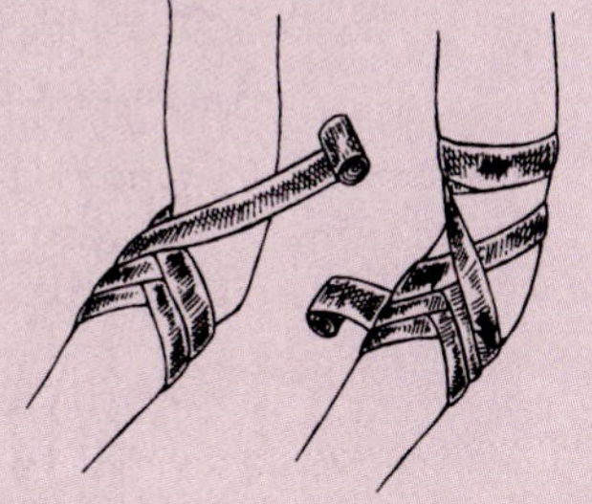	Covers joints; snug fit provides excellent immobilization

Continued.

Table 38-1 Types of Bandage Turns—cont'd

Type	Description	Purpose or Use
Recurrent	Bandage first secured with two circular turns around proximal end of body part; half turn made perpendicular up from bandage edge; body of bandage brought over distal end of body part to be covered with each turn folded back over on itself 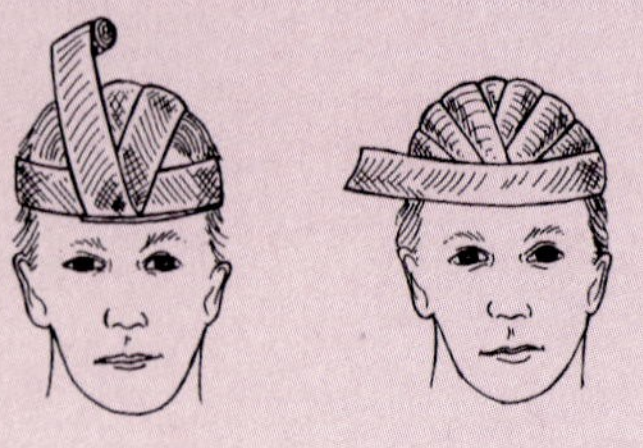	Covers uneven body parts such as head or stump

moves or coughs (Fig. 38-1). The nurse secures a binder with Velcro strips, metal fasteners, or safety pins.

As the name implies, the **T-binder** looks like the letter T (Fig. 38-2) and is used to secure rectal or perineal dressings. The single-T-binder fits female clients, and the double-T-binder fits male clients.

The belt of the T-binder fits securely around the client's waist, with the tail passing between the client's legs from back to front and attaching to the belt's front. The nurse should be sure the tail fits smoothly and against the dressing. T-binders become soiled easily and often require changing. Irritation to the urethra or scrotum must be avoided.

Correctly applied bandages and binders do not cause injury to underlying and nearby body parts or create discomfort for the client. For example, an abdominal binder must be applied correctly to allow for normal chest expansion.

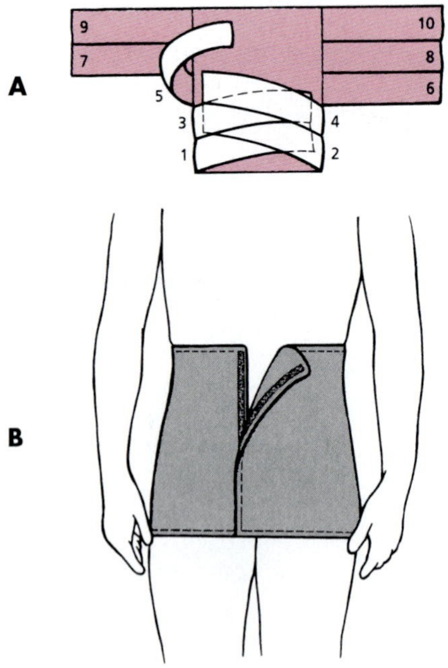

Fig. 38-1 Abdominal binders. **A,** Scultetus binder. **B,** Straight.

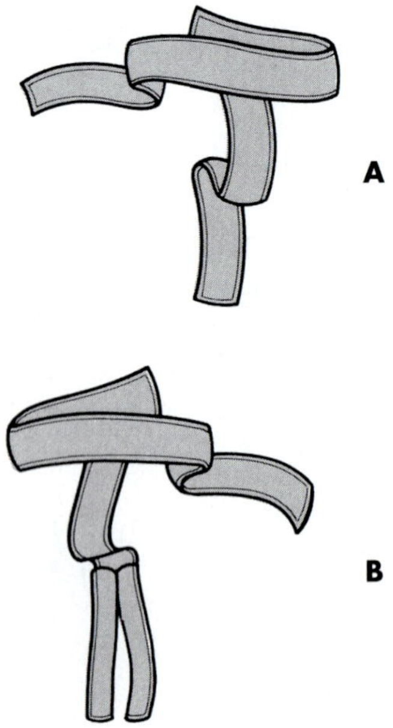

Fig. 38-2 **A,** T-binder (female). **B,** Double-T-binder (male).

GUIDELINES

1. The nurse who applies a bandage or binder can loosen or readjust it as necessary. The nurse should have a physician's order before loosening or removing a bandage or binder applied by a physician.
2. Before applying a bandage or binder, consider the client's cultural beliefs regarding exposure of the body.

DELEGATION CONSIDERATIONS

The skills of applying a bandage and binder (abdominal, T, or breast) can be delegated to unlicensed assistive personnel.

- Be sure personnel are trained on the appropriate procedures and have demonstrated competency.
- Nurse should complete an assessment of client's ability to breathe deeply, cough effectively, and move independently; of skin for irritation/abrasion; of incision/wound and dressing; and of comfort level before a binder or sling is applied for the first time. (See assessment criteria under individual skill.)
- Nurse should evaluate the client's response to bandage or binder application.
- Caution care giver that skin should not be wrinkled, and dressing should be clean and dry before bandage or binder is applied.

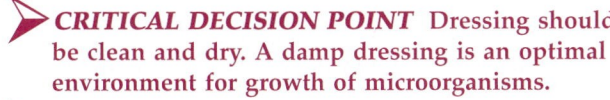

SKILL 38-1 Applying an Elastic Bandage

An elastic bandage is used to apply compression to an area. It is used most often on the lower extremities to prevent edema and support varicosities. Other uses include support of the knee, ankle, elbow, and wrist in conditions such as strains and sprains (Phipps, 1995). When fully stretched, the elastic bandage extends to 3 yards (270 cm). Shorter lengths of 1½ yards (135 cm) are available for bandaging the wrist or a child's foot or knee. Bandages are available in widths of 2 inches (5.0 cm), 3 inches (7.5 cm), 4 inches (10 cm), 6 inches (15 cm), and 8 inches (20 cm). The bandage is always rolled loosely, without any tension, in preparation for application. When fully rolled, the outside is placed next to the skin as a starting point. Even tension is applied, and the bandage is started at the site farthest from the heart (distal) and proceeds toward the heart (proximal). The type of bandage turn and selected width are determined by the size and shape of the body part to be bandaged. For example, 3- and 4-inch bandages are most commonly used for the adult leg.

EQUIPMENT

- **Correct width and number of bandages**
- **Safety pins, clips, or adhesive tape**
- **Disposable gloves, if wound drainage is present**

STEPS	RATIONALE
ASSESSMENT	
1. Inspect skin (especially skin over boney prominences) for alterations in integrity as indicated by presence of abrasion, discoloration, chafing, edema.	Altered skin integrity contraindicates the use of an elastic bandage.
2. Inspect any surgical dressing.	Surgical dressing replacement or reinforcement precedes application of any bandage.

➤ ***CRITICAL DECISION POINT*** **Dressing should be clean and dry. A damp dressing is an optimal environment for growth of microorganisms.**

➤ ***CRITICAL DECISION POINT*** **If incision/wound is to be covered by a bandage, it should be covered entirely to avoid soiling of bandage and irritation of wound.**

STEPS	RATIONALE
3. Observe adequacy of circulation by noting surface temperature, skin color, pulses (distal to area to be bandaged), presence of edema, and sensation and movement of body parts to be wrapped.	Comparison of area before and after application of bandage is necessary to ensure continued adequate circulation. Impairment of circulation may result in pain, coolness to touch when compared with opposite side of body, cyanosis or pallor of skin, diminished or absent pulses, edema or localized pooling, numbness and/or tingling of body part.
4. Review client's medical record and nursing prescriptions for specific orders related to application of elastic bandage. Note area to be covered, type of bandage required, frequency of change, previous response to treatment.	Specific prescription may direct procedure, including such factors as extent of application (i.e., toe to knee, toe to groin) or duration of treatment.
5. Identify client's and primary care giver's present knowledge level of skill if bandaging will be continued at home.	Ensures that planning and teaching are individualized.

NURSING DIAGNOSIS

Clustering of defining characteristics from the assessment data may reveal the following nursing diagnoses for clients requiring this skill:

- Impaired physical mobility
- Impaired tissue integrity
- Knowledge deficit regarding bandage application
- Pain

Related factors are individualized based on a client's condition or needs.

PLANNING

1. **Expected outcomes** following completion of procedure:
   - Client states pain or discomfort is decreased or absent. — All are indicators of proper application of the elastic bandage.
   - No tingling or numbness is noted by client.
   - Distal parts (toes, fingers) feel warm (symmetrically) to touch, no cyanosis or blanching is present, and motion is not unnecessarily impaired. — Indicates adequate circulation to distal regions.
   - Client applies bandage correctly. — Demonstrates learning and ensures continuity of care after discharge.
2. Explain procedure to client. — Increased knowledge promotes cooperation and reduces anxiety.

CRITICAL DECISION POINT Reinforce teaching that smooth, even, light pressure will be applied to improve venous circulation; prevent clot formation; reduce or prevent swelling; immobilize body part; secure surgical dressings; provide pressure.

3. Teach skill to client or significant other. — Reduces anxiety and ensures continuity of care after discharge.

IMPLEMENTATION

STEPS	RATIONALE
1. Wash hands and apply gloves if drainage is present.	Reduces transmission of microorganisms.
2. Close room door or curtains.	Maintains client's comfort and dignity.
3. Assist client to assume comfortable, anatomically correct position.	Maintains alignment. Prevents musculoskeletal deformity.

CRITICAL DECISION POINT Bandages applied to lower extremities are applied before client sits or stands.

STEPS	RATIONALE
CRITICAL DECISION POINT **Elevation of dependent extremities for 20 minutes before bandage application will enhance venous return.**	
4. Hold roll of elastic bandage in dominant hand and use other hand to lightly hold beginning of bandage at distal body part. Continue transferring roll to dominant hand as bandage is wrapped.	Maintains appropriate and consistent bandage tension.
CRITICAL DECISION POINT **Toes or finger tips should be visible for follow-up circulatory assessment (see illustration).**	

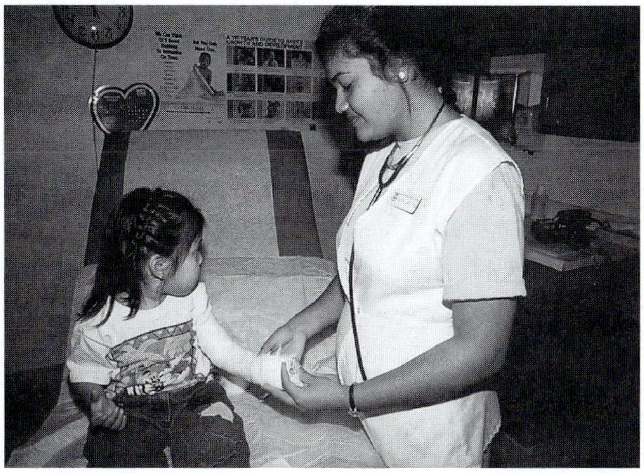

Step 4

STEPS	RATIONALE
5. Apply bandage from distal point toward proximal boundary using variety of turns to cover various shapes of body parts (see Table 38-1). (For bandaging of amputation stump, see illustration, p. 1106.)	Bandage is applied in manner that conforms evenly to body part and promotes venous return.
6. Unroll and very slightly stretch bandage.	Maintains uniform bandage tension.
CRITICAL DECISION POINT **Avoid wrapping bandage too tightly since this may cause numbness and tingling from impaired circulation.**	
7. Overlap turns by ½ to ⅔ width of bandage roll.	Prevents uneven bandage tension and circulatory impairment.
8. Secure first bandage with clip or tape before applying additional rolls.	
a. Apply additional rolls without leaving any uncovered skin surface. Secure last bandage applied.	Prevents wrinkling or loose ends.
9. Remove gloves if worn and wash hands.	Reduces transmission of microorganisms.

EVALUATION

STEPS	RATIONALE
1. Assess distal circulation when bandage application is complete and at least twice during 8-hour period.	Early detection and management of circulatory impairment ensures healthy neurovascular status.
a. Observe skin color for pallor or cyanosis.	
b. Palpate skin for warmth.	
c. Palpate pulses and compare bilaterally.	
d. Ask if client is aware of pain, numbness, tingling, or other discomfort.	Neurovascular changes indicate impaired venous return.
e. Observe mobility of extremity.	Determines if bandage is too tight, which restricts movement, or determines if joint immobility is attained.
2. Have client demonstrate bandage application.	Return demonstration documents learning.
3. **Unexpected outcomes** that may occur include:	
➤ Tingling or numbness is present in portions distal to wrap.	Neurovascular changes indicate impaired venous return because wrap was applied too tightly. Need to reapply.

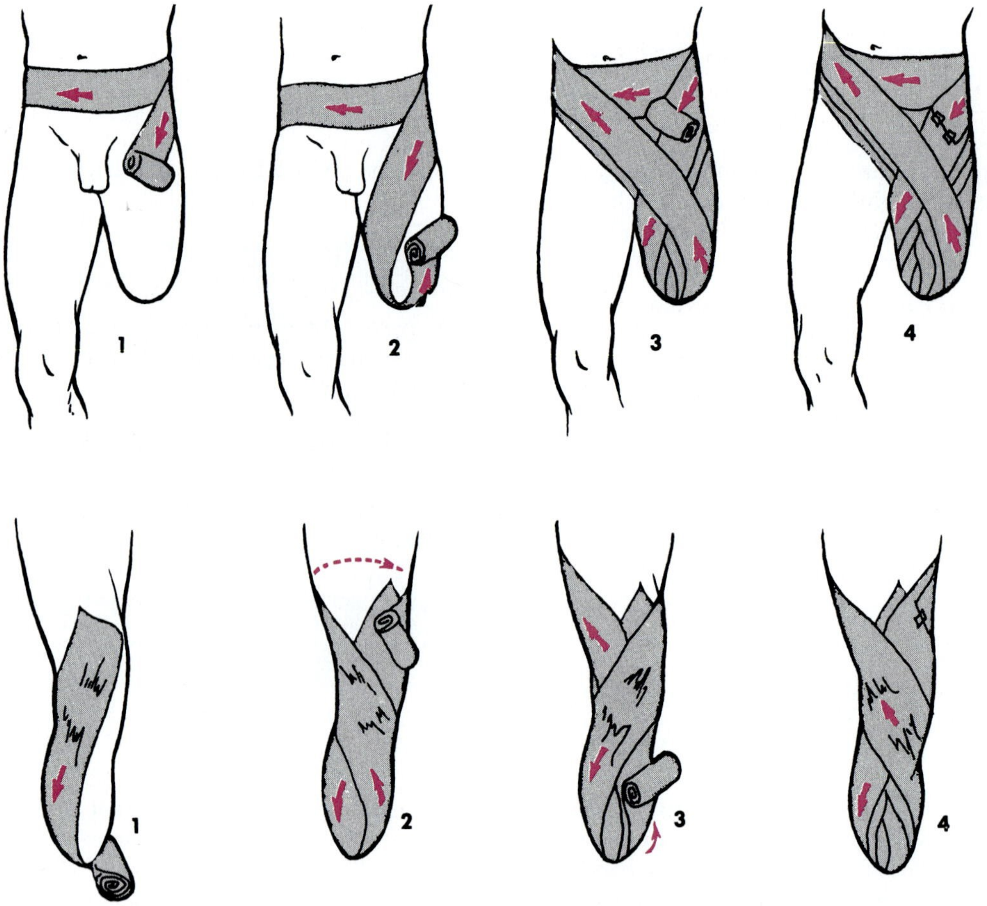

Step 5 *Top,* Correct method for bandaging midthigh amputation stump. Note that bandage must be anchored around patient's waist. *Bottom,* Correct method for bandaging midcalf amputation stump. Note that bandage need not be anchored around the waist.

STEPS	RATIONALE
➤ Extremity distal to wrap is cool, cyanotic, or blanched.	Indicates impaired circulation because wrap was applied too tightly. Need to reapply.
➤ Dressing is loose or improperly wrapped.	Improper support is provided to area.
➤ Extremity has decreased range of joint motion.	Wrap was applied too tightly or incorrectly.
Recording and Reporting	
1. Document condition of wound, integrity of dressing, application of bandage, circulation, and client's comfort level.	Promotes continuity of care and meets legal requirements regarding documentation of care given and client's response.
2. Report any changes in neurological or circulatory status to nurse in charge or physician.	May require change in type of dressing and/or bandage utilized.

Follow-up Activities

1. Remove and reapply elastic bandage:
   a. Once every 8 hours unless otherwise directed by physician.
   b. Assess PRN for wrinkles, looseness, or tightness; client discomfort or itchiness; changes including drainage; tingling or numbness; cool, cyanotic, or blanched extremity.

Special Considerations

- Avoid using safety pins to secure bandages.
- Heels, elbows, and ankles are subject to edema resulting from pooling if circulation is impaired or restricted.
- Preexisting vascular problems, copious wound drainage, client comfort level, and quality of pulses determines need for additional nursing interventions.
- Unless total immobilization is prescribed, range of motion exercises are continued.
- Use increasingly wider bandages as size of body part increases (e.g., 3-inch, 4-inch, and 6-inch bandages may be used to cover foot, calf, and thigh, respectively).

Teaching Considerations

- Applying elastic bandage to oneself is difficult. Teach significant other if treatment will continue after hospitalization.

Pediatric Considerations

- Use adhesive tape rather than loose clips to fasten bandage on small child or infant.

Gerontologic Considerations

- As clients age, skin becomes more fragile, which increases their susceptibility to skin breakdown. Once skin/tissue injury occurs, would healing is delayed. Assess these clients more frequently for evidence of skin breakdown or decrease in circulation over the areas covered by and distal to the bandage.

Home Care Considerations

- Assess client and primary care giver's ability, motivation, and availability to participate in bandaging procedure.
- Assess client's understanding of bandaging and willingness to leave bandage in place.
- Assess client's environment to determine potential for permitting bandaged area to remain free from contaminants.
- The elastic bandage is washable and is placed in large folds over a line to dry.

SKILL 38-2 Applying an Abdominal Binder, T-Binder, or Breast Binder

Binders are indicated for the support of underlying muscles and large incisions. The muscles and viscera surrounding an operative site may require support during the postoperative period. This promotes healing and permits a client to move more freely without additional discomfort. Assorted binders are available with the basic shape being a rectangle that is wide enough to extend from the groin to the waistline and long enough to encircle the area with an overlap for closure.

EQUIPMENT

- Gloves, if wound drainage present
- Abdominal binder:
  - Correct size cloth/elastic straight binder
  - Safety pins (unless Velcro closure or metal fasteners are attached): 6 to 8 safety pins are usually adequate for abdominal binders
- T- and double-T-binders:
  - Correct size binder
  - Safety pins: two pins for T-binder; three pins for double-T-binder
- Breast binder:
  - Correct size binder
  - Safety pins (approximately 12) unless Velcro closure is attached

STEPS	RATIONALE
ASSESSMENT	
1. For client who needs support of abdomen, observe ability to breathe deeply, cough effectively, and turn or move independently.	Baseline assessment determines client's ability to breathe and cough. Impaired ventilation of lung can lead to alveolar atelectasis and inadequate arterial oxygenation.
2. Determine if client has allergy to adhesive tape.	Contraindicates use of tape to secure binder.

STEPS	RATIONALE
3. Inspect skin for actual or potential alterations in integrity. Observe for irritation; abrasion; skin surfaces that rub against each other; allergic response to adhesive tape used to secure dressing.	Actual impairments in skin integrity can be worsened with application of a binder. Binder can cause pressure and excoriation.
4. Inspect any surgical dressing.	Dressing replacement or reinforcement precedes application of any binder.
➤ ***CRITICAL DECISION POINT*** **Dressing should be clean and dry and incision/wound should be entirely covered by dressing.**	Prevents nosocomial infection. Avoids soiling of bandage and irritation of wound.
5. Assess client's comfort level, using analog scale of 0 to 10 (see Chapter 5) and noting any objective signs and symptoms.	Data will determine effectiveness of binder placement.
➤ ***CRITICAL DECISION POINT*** **Expect client in moderate-to-severe pain to have diaphoresis, tachycardia, and elevated blood pressure.**	
6. Gather necessary data regarding size of client and appropriate binder.	Ensures proper fit of binder.

NURSING DIAGNOSIS

Clustering of defining characteristics from the assessment data may reveal the following nursing diagnoses for clients requiring this skill:

- ➤ Impaired physical mobility
- ➤ Impaired skin integrity
- ➤ Ineffective breathing pattern
- ➤ Knowledge deficit regarding binder application
- ➤ Pain

Related factors are individualized based on a client's condition or needs.

PLANNING

STEPS	RATIONALE
1. Expected outcomes following completion of procedure:	
➤ Client states pain is absent or reduced.	Support to incision area promotes comfort during postoperative exercises of coughing, deep breathing, turning, and ambulating.
➤ Client's suture line is intact, with no drainage or separation.	Decreases tension on suture line to promote healing. Snug support helps maintain intact suture line. Wrinkle-free application of binder encourages healthy skin response.
➤ Client's respirations are unrestricted. Coughing is effective, and secretions are expectorated.	The ability to fully expand the lungs and cough must continue after application of the binder to enhance oxygenation and avoid pulmonary complications.
2. Explain procedure to client.	Promotes client's understanding and cooperation.
3. Teach skill to client or significant other.	Reduces anxiety and ensures continuity of care after discharge.

IMPLEMENTATION

STEPS	RATIONALE
1. Wash hands and apply gloves (if likely to contact wound drainage).	Reduces transmission of microorganisms.
2. Close curtains or room door.	Maintains client's comfort and dignity.
3. Apply abdominal binder.	
a. Position client in supine position with head slightly elevated and knees slightly flexed.	Minimizes muscular tension on abdominal organs.
b. Fanfold far side of binder toward midline of binder.	Reduces time client remains in uncomfortable position.
c. Instruct and assist client to roll away from nurse toward raised side rail while firmly supporting abdominal incision and dressing with hands.	Reduces pain and discomfort.

STEPS	RATIONALE
d. Place fanfolded ends of binder under client.	Permits placement and centering of binder with minimal discomfort.
CRITICAL DECISION POINT Binders extend from just above symphysis pubis to just below costal margin.	
e. Instruct or assist client to roll over folded ends.	
f. Unfold and stretch ends out smoothly on far side of bed.	Maintains skin integrity and comfort.
g. Instruct client to roll back into supine position.	Facilitates chest expansion and adequate wound support when the binder is closed.
h. Adjust binder so that supine client is centered over binder using symphysis pubis and costal margins as lower and upper landmarks.	Centers support from binder over abdominal structures, which reduces incidence of decreased lung expansion.
CRITICAL DECISION POINT Cover any exposed areas of an incision or wound with sterile dressing.	
i. Close binder. Pull one end of binder over center of client's abdomen. While maintaining tension on that end of binder, pull opposite end of binder over center and secure with Velcro closure tabs, metal fasteners, or horizontally placed safety pins.	Provides continuous wound support and comfort.
CRITICAL DECISION POINT Recheck client's ability to breathe deeply and cough effectively.	Determines ventilation and clears the airways of pulmonary secretions.
CRITICAL DECISION POINT Shallow respirations, continuing after a tight binder has been loosened, may indicate beginning of serious respiratory problems, including alveolar atelectasis and pulmonary embolus, among others.	
j. Assess client's comfort level.	Helps determine effectiveness of binder placement.
k. Adjust binder as necessary.	Promotes comfort and chest expansion.
4. Apply single-T and double-T binders.	
a. Assist client to dorsal recumbent position, with lower extremities slightly flexed and hips rotated slightly outward.	Minimizes muscular tension on perineal organs.
b. Have client raise hips and place horizontal band around client's waist (or above iliac crests) with vertical tails extending past buttocks. Overlap waistband in front and secure with safety pins.	Permits placement of binder. Secures binder around client.
c. Complete binder application:	
(1) *T-binder:* Bring remaining vertical strip over perineal dressing and continue up and under center front of horizontal band. Bring ends over waistband and secure all thicknesses with safety pin.	Single-T and double-T-binders provide support to perineal muscles and organs and help maintain placement of perineal or suprapubic dressing.
(2) *Double-T-binder:* Bring remaining vertical strips over perineal or suprapubic dressing with each tail supporting one side of scrotum and proceeding upward on either side of penis. Continue drawing ends behind and then downward in front of horizontal band. Secure all thicknesses with one horizontally placed safety pin.	

STEPS	RATIONALE
d. Assess client's comfort level with client in lying, sitting, and standing positions. Readjust front pins and tails as necessary, ensuring that tails are not too tight. Increase padding if any area rubs against surrounding tissues.	Determines efficacy of binder to maintain dressings and support perineal structures.
➤ *CRITICAL DECISION POINT* Binder should hold perineal or suprapubic dressing in place as the client ambulates without applying pressure to urethra or scrotum.	
e. Instruct client regarding removal of binder before defecating or urinating and need to replace binder after performing these bodily functions.	Cleanliness of binder reduces infection risk.
5. Apply breast binder.	
a. Assist client in placing arms through binder's armholes.	Eases binder placement process.
b. Assist client to supine position in bed.	Supine positioning facilitates normal anatomical position of breasts; facilitates healing and comfort.
c. Pad area under breasts if necessary.	Prevents skin contact with undersurface.
d. Using Velcro closure tabs or horizontally placed safety pins, secure binder at nipple level first. Continue closure process above and then below nipple line until entire binder is closed.	Horizontal placement of pins may reduce risk of uneven pressure or localized irritation.
e. Make appropriate adjustments including individualizing fit of shoulder straps, pinning waistline darts to reduce binder size.	Maintains support to client's breasts.
f. Instruct and observe skill development in self-care related to reapplying breast binder.	Self-care is integral aspect of discharge planning. Skin integrity and comfort level goals are ensured.
6. Remove gloves and wash hands.	Prevents cross-infections.

EVALUATION

1. Observe site for skin integrity, circulation, and characteristics of the wound. (Periodically remove binder and surgical dressing to assess wound characteristics.)	Determines that binder has not resulted in complication to skin, wound, or underlying organs.
2. Assess comfort level of client, using analog scale of 0 to 10 and noting any objective signs and symptoms.	Binders should not increase discomfort.
3. Assess client's ability to ventilate properly including deep breathing and coughing.	Identifies any impaired ventilation and potential pulmonary complications.
4. Identify client's need for assistance with activities such as hair combing, dressing, ambulating.	Mobility of upper extremities may be limited depending on severity and location of incision.
5. **Unexpected outcomes** that may occur include:	
➤ Impaired breathing leads to ineffective oxygenation.	Restrictive application of binder with too much tension inhibits client's ability to fully expand lungs.
➤ Tight binder causes impaired circulation.	Postoperative risks of venous stasis, clot formation, and embolization can result from restrictive application of binder.
➤ Skin integrity is impaired.	Uneven pressure occurs in presence of wrinkles and leads to irritation. Rubbing together of skin surfaces causes excoriation of area.
➤ Pain and discomfort are increased.	Incorrect application of binder increases discomfort.

STEPS	RATIONALE
RECORDING AND REPORTING	
1. Report any skin irritation to nurse at between-shift report.	Promotes continuity of care and prevention of complications.
2. Record application of binder, condition of skin, circulation, integrity of dressing, and client's comfort level.	Promotes continuity of care and meets legal requirements regarding documentation of care given and client's response.
3. Report ineffective lung expansion to physician immediately.	Loosening of tight binder should permit client to fully expand lungs. Rapid reporting and appropriate intervention may prevent change from becoming serious emergency or irreversible complication.

FOLLOW-UP ACTIVITIES

1. Observe every 4 hours:
   a. Ability to deep breathe.
   b. Cough effectiveness.
   c. Objective and subjective symptoms of pain and discomfort.
2. Remove binder and inspect dressing and skin condition every 8 hours and PRN.
3. Bathe area daily and PRN.

• • • • •

Special Considerations

- Because of certain diagnostic procedures (e.g., x-ray, magnetic resonance imaging) as well as the potential for injury, using safety pins to secure binders is prohibited in some institutions.
- Thoroughly wash and dry under pendulous breasts before applying a breast binder to reduce risk of growth of microorganisms.
- Before applying breast binder for management of engorgement and suppression of lactation, note condition of nipples and physiological changes. Pad nipple areas with soft dressings to prevent seepage of fluid.
- If safety pins are used, place pins in cake of soap while applying or changing binder. Prevents loss or injury to client and eases gliding pin through thicknesses of cloth.
- In the extremely thin client, padding of boney prominences prevents excessive pressure and skin irritation.
- For postsurgical application of scultetus abdominal binder, precede upward from bottom to minimize pull on suture line.
- T-binders are easily soiled and require frequent replacement.
- Properly fitting brassiere that extends to lower rib cage and has front closure may be substituted for breast binders for postsurgical and postpartum clients.
- Elastic thoracic binders designed to provide support to area below breasts are commercially manufactured. This binder may be used for bruised and cracked ribs (in good alignment) on both male and female clients if medically indicated.
- When applying an abdominal binder on a very thin client, pad iliac prominences.

Teaching Considerations

- Consider client's dexterity in reapplying binder to self, opportunities to practice skill, and need to teach significant other.

Pediatric Considerations

- Use adhesive tape rather than loose clips or pins to fasten binder on small child or infant.

Gerontologic Considerations

- As clients age, skin becomes more fragile, which increases their susceptibility to skin breakdown. Once skin/tissue injury occurs, healing is delayed. Assess these clients more frequently for evidence of skin breakdown over the area covered by the binder.

Home Care Considerations

- Assess primary care giver's understanding, ability, and motivation to participate in application of binder.
- Assess client's understanding of purpose of binder and willingness to permit binder to remain in place.
- Abdominal, T, and breast binders are washable and are placed over a line to dry.

CRITICAL THINKING EXERCISES

1. An elastic bandage is to be applied to a client's ankle. What must the nurse take into consideration to safely apply the wrap?
2. An obese client recovering from abdominal surgery has an open abdominal wound that requires irrigation every 8 hours. How should the nurse support this client's abdominal tissues when ambulating?
3. A client underwent surgical repair of the right hand after sustaining an injury. The dressing of the hand is dry and intact with distal interphalangeal joints exposed. Describe nursing considerations when applying a sling to the affected arm.

REFERENCE

Phipps J, et al.: *Medical-surgical nursing: Concepts and clinical practice,* ed 5, St Louis, 1995, Mosby.

ADDITIONAL READING

Bobak I, Jensen M, Lowdermilk D: *Maternity & gynecologic care: The nurse and the family,* ed 6, St Louis, 1997, Mosby.

Ebersole P, Hess P: *Toward healthy aging: human needs and nursing response,* ed 4, St Louis, 1994, Mosby.

Harden J, Girard N: Breast reconstruction using an innovative flap procedure, *JAORN* 60(2):184-191, 1994.

Lewis S, Collier I, Heitkemper M: *Medical-surgical nursing: Assessment and management of clinical problems,* ed 4, St Louis, 1996, Mosby.

Seidel H, et al.: *Mosby's guide to physical examination,* ed 3, St Louis, 1995, Mosby.

Williamson V: Amputation of the lower extremity: An overview, *Orthop Nurs* 11(2):55-65, 1992.

CHAPTER 39

Hot and Cold Therapy

OBJECTIVES

Mastery of content in this chapter will enable the nurse to:

- Define key terms.
- Identify the effects of heat and cold on the client.
- Differentiate the types of injuries or conditions that benefit from hot and cold applications.
- Identify the risks to clients related to hot and cold applications.
- Explain common guidelines used to protect clients who receive hot and cold applications.
- Correctly apply hot and cold applications.

KEY TERMS

Compress
Conduction
Evaporation
Insulator
Neuropathy
Piloerection
Sitz bath
Vasoconstriction
Vasodilation

SKILLS

39-1 Applying a Moist Hot Compress to an Open Wound

39-2 Assisting with Warm Soaks and Sitz Baths

39-3 Applying Aquathermia and Heating Pads

39-4 Applying Cold Applications

39-5 Caring for Clients Requiring Hypothermia or Hyperthermia Blankets

The local application of heat and cold to body parts can have a beneficial effect. To use heat and cold therapies safely, the nurse must understand how the body normally responds to temperature variations and the risks connected with these applications.

Exposure to heat or cold causes both systemic and local responses. The hypothalamus acts as the thermostat of the body to maintain body temperature at approximately 37° C, or 98.6° F. Systemically, when the skin is exposed to warm or hot temperatures, **vasodilation** and perspiration occur to promote heat loss. As perspiration evaporates from the skin, cooling occurs. When the skin is exposed to cool or cold temperatures, the systemic response includes **vasoconstriction** and **piloerection** to conserve heat. Shivering also occurs in response to cooler temperatures. Shivering produces heat through muscular contraction.

The local response to heat and cold results from changes in blood vessel size, which affect blood flow to the exposed area. This physiological response explains the effectiveness of hot and cold therapies (see Table 39-1).

When receptors for heat or cold are stimulated, sensory impulses travel via somatic afferent fibers to the hypothalamus and cerebral cortex. The cerebral cortex makes a person aware of temperature sensations. The person can then adapt as necessary to maintain normal body temperature; if cold, the person can put on additional clothing. The hypothalamus simultaneously controls physiological reflexes needed to regulate normal body temperature. The body also has a protective reflex response for exposure to temperature extremes. Exposure to an extremely hot or cold stimulus sends impulses traveling to the spinal cord, synapsing at the spinal cord, and returning by way of motor nerves to cause withdrawal from the stimulus. The person becomes aware of the discomfort as withdrawal occurs.

Sensory adaptation to local temperature extremes can occur quickly within the body. Although a person may initially feel a temperature extreme, once the sensory receptors adapt, the person may become unaware of any temperature variation. Eventually excessive heat causes a burning sensation; excessive cold causes a numbing sensation before pain is sensed. Because of this physiological

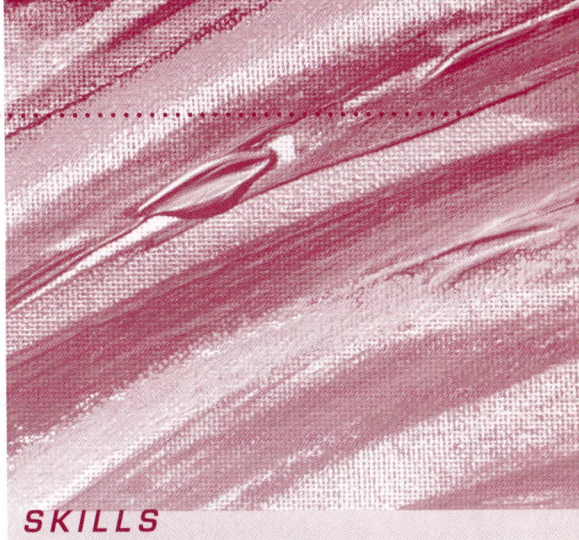

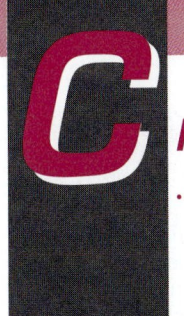

Table 39-1 Therapeutic Effects of Heat and Cold Applications

Therapy	Physiological Responses	Therapeutic Benefit	Examples of Conditions Treated
Heat	Vasodilation	Improves blood flow to injured body part, promotes delivery of nutrients and removal of wastes, lessens venous congestion in injured tissues	Inflamed or edematous body part; new surgical wound; infected wound; arthritis, degenerative joint disease; localized joint pain, muscle strains; low back pain, menstrual cramping; hemorrhoidal, perianal, and vaginal inflammation; local abscesses
	Reduced blood viscosity	Improves delivery of leukocytes and antibiotics to wound site	
	Reduced muscle tension	Promotes muscle relaxation and reduces pain from spasm or stiffness	
	Increased tissue metabolism	Increases blood flow; provides local warmth	
	Increased capillary permeability	Promotes movement of waste products and nutrients	
Cold	Vasoconstriction	Reduces blood flow to injured body part, prevents edema formation, reduces inflammation	Immediately after direct trauma such as sprains, strains, fractures, muscle spasms, after superficial laceration or puncture wound; after minor burn; when malignancy is suspected in area of injury or pain; after injections; for arthritis, joint trauma
	Local anesthesia	Reduces localized pain	
	Reduced cell metabolism	Reduces oxygen needs of tissues	
	Increased blood viscosity	Promotes blood coagulation at injury site	
	Decreased muscle tension	Relieves pain	

Table 39-2 Conditions That Increase Risk of Injury From Heat and Cold Application

Condition	Risk Factors
Very young; older adults	Thinner skin layers in children increase risk of burns; older adults have reduced sensitivity to pain
Open wounds, broken skin, stomas	Subcutaneous and visceral tissues more sensitive to temperature variations; also contain no temperature receptors and fewer pain receptors than normal skin
Areas of edema or scar formation	Reduced sensation to temperature stimuli because of thickening of skin layers from fluid buildup or scar formation
Peripheral vascular disease (e.g., diabetes, arteriosclerosis)	Body's extremities less sensitive to temperature and pain stimuli because of circulatory impairment and local tissue injury; cold application would further compromise blood flow
Confusion or unconsciousness	Reduced perception of sensory or painful stimuli
Spinal cord injury	Alterations in nerve pathways preventing reception of sensory or painful stimuli
Abscessed tooth or appendix	Infection highly localized; application of heat may cause rupture with systemic spread of microorganisms

phenomenon, the risk of tissue injury from hot and cold applications is great. Certain clients are more at risk than others for injury from hot and cold applications (Table 39-2). The nurse plays an important role in maintaining the client's safety in the application of heat and cold. The nurse must always have an order for a hot or cold application, and the order should include the desired temperature to be used when settings can be controlled (Table 39-3). Because many of these therapies can be used at home, the nurse must instruct clients and their families on the proper use of these therapies.

When using hot or cold therapies, the nurse can use either dry or moist applications. The selection of dry or moist application is determined by the nature of tempera-

Table 39-3 Temperature Ranges for Hot and Cold Applications

Temperature	Centigrade Range	Fahrenheit Range
Very hot	41° to 46° C	106° to 115° F
Hot	37° to 41° C	98° to 106° F
Warm	34° to 37° C	93° to 98° F
Tepid	26° to 34° C	80° to 93° F
Cool	18° to 26° C	65° to 80° F
Cold	10° to 18° C	50° to 65° F

ture **conduction** and the result desired from therapy. Temperature travels from an external source such as a compress or water pad to the skin's surface. A substance that conducts temperatures poorly is a good **insulator** and thus a protector for skin and tissues. For example, cloth placed over a heating pad insulates the skin from hot temperature extremes. Plastic, which is the external covering for most commercial heating pads, and the fluid in moist compresses both conduct heat well, thus placing the client at risk for injury during heat applications. However, there are distinct advantages to using both dry and moist applications (Table 39-4). The nurse should be familiar with the effects of each application type.

GUIDELINES

1. Protect damaged skin layers. Exposed layers of skin are more sensitive to temperature variations than intact skin layers.
2. Time all applications carefully. A person tolerates temperature extremes better when the duration of exposure is short (10 to 20 minutes). Prolonged exposure can injure tissues and eliminate the benefits of therapy (Bayles, 1991). Keep a timer or clock close by so that the client can help the nurse time applications.
3. Know the temperature of the application being used. Many devices, such as heating pads or water flow pads, have thermostats to regulate temperature. Always check the temperature of moist compresses applied directly to the skin.
4. Certain body parts are more sensitive than others to temperature extremes. The nurse can modify the intensity of heat and cold when sensitive skin areas are being treated.
5. Check the client frequently during a hot or cold application. The condition of the skin indicates whether tissue injury is occurring.
6. Know the client's risk for injury from heat or cold. Certain clients are more predisposed to injury than others (see Table 39-2).
7. Do not allow the client to adjust temperature settings. It is common for the client to adapt to a temperature extreme and then think that the temperature should be adjusted. Instruct all clients about adaptation.
8. Never position the client so that the client cannot move away from the temperature source. This avoids the risk of injuries from temperature exposure. The hospitalized client should always have a call light within reach.
9. Do not leave the client unattended, especially one who is unable to sense temperature changes or move away from the temperature source. The nurse is responsible for the client's safety.
10. Discourage the client from moving an application. This may cause injury to an unprotected area of the body and decrease the effectiveness of therapy.

Table 39-4 Choice of Dry or Moist Warm Applications

Type	Advantages	Disadvantages
Moist applications	Reduce drying of skin and soften wound exudate	Prolonged exposure can cause maceration of skin
	Conform well to body area being treated	Cool rapidly because of moisture evaporation
	Penetrate deeply into tissue layers	Create greater risk for burns to skin since moisture conducts heat
	Lessen sweating and insensible fluid loss	
Dry applications	Less likely to burn skin	Increase body fluid loss through sweating
	Do not cause skin maceration	Do not penetrate deep into tissues
	Retain temperature longer, since not influenced by evaporation	Cause increased drying of skin

DELEGATION CONSIDERATIONS

The skills outlined in this chapter can be delegated to unlicensed assistive personnel.

- Ensure care giver can perform skill competently.
- Caution care giver to maintain proper temperature of application during the duration of treatment.
- Caution care giver to keep application in place for only the length of time specified in the physician's orders.
- Have care giver notify the nurse when treatment is complete so that an evaluation of client's response can be made.

SKILL 39-1 Applying a Moist Hot Compress to an Open Wound

A hot compress is a section of sterile or clean gauze moistened with a prescribed heated solution and applied directly to an open wound or the skin's surface. A sterile compress is necessary only when there is a break in skin integrity. Commercially packaged sterile, premoistened compresses are available in some agencies. They require the use of a special infrared lamp to heat. Plain sterile or clean gauze can be heated by adding the gauze to a container of warmed solution. Often the nurse applies an aquathermia heating pad over a compress to deliver a continuous, controlled source of heat to improve the application's therapeutic effects (see Skill 39-3). Moist hot compresses are used to improve circulation, relieve edema, promote consolidation of exudate in a wound, and promote comfort.

EQUIPMENT

- Prescribed solution warmed to appropriate temperature
- Sterile gauze dressings or commercially prepared compresses
- Sterile container for solution
- Dry bath towel
- Disposable gloves
- Sterile gloves
- Waterproof pad
- Ties or tape
- Aquathermia or heating pad (optional)
- Bath blanket

STEPS	RATIONALE
ASSESSMENT	
1. Refer to physician's order for type of compress, location and duration of application, desired temperature, and institutional policies regarding temperature of compress.	Ensures safe and correct application.
2. Inspect condition of exposed skin and wound on which compress is to be applied.	Provides baseline to determine changes in skin during heat application.
CRITICAL DECISION POINT Very thin or damaged skin is more susceptible to injury from heat. Nonintact skin and drainage from wounds are indications to wear gloves.	
3. Assess client's extremities for sensitivity to temperature and pain by measuring light touch, pin-prick, and temperature sensation (see Chapter 11).	Clients insensitive to heat or cold sensations must be monitored closely during treatment.
CRITICAL DECISION POINT Diabetic clients, victims of stroke, and clients with peripheral neuropathy are particularly at risk for thermal injury.	
4. Refer to medical record to identify any systemic contraindications to heat application.	Heat causes vasodilation, which aggravates active bleeding. Heat applied to localized area of acute inflammation or tumor may cause rupture or activate cell growth.
CRITICAL DECISION POINT Use caution when there is an area of active bleeding or inflammation.	
5. Assess client's understanding of application and its purpose.	Determines need for health teaching.

NURSING DIAGNOSIS

Clustering of defining characteristics from the assessment data may reveal the following nursing diagnoses for clients requiring this skill:

STEPS	RATIONALE
➤ Altered peripheral tissue perfusion ➤ Impaired physical mobility ➤ Impaired skin integrity ➤ Knowledge deficit regarding moist heat applications	➤ Pain ➤ Risk for injury ➤ Sensory perceptual alterations (tactile)

Related factors are individualized based on a client's condition or needs.

PLANNING

1. **Expected outcomes** following completion of procedure:	
➤ Affected site is pink and warm to touch immediately after application.	Vasodilation increases blood flow to site.
➤ After multiple applications, wound shows signs of healing (e.g., granulation; reduced edema, inflammation, drainage).	Moist heat increases blood flow, enhances white blood cell infiltration, and removes waste products from the cells.
➤ Client denies burning sensation.	Indicates appropriate temperature.
➤ Client able to safely apply therapy.	Measures level of learning.
2. Assemble equipment and supplies.	Organization of supplies prevents unnecessary delays in the procedure.
3. Explain steps of procedure and purpose to client. Describe sensations to be felt, such as decreasing warmth and wetness. Explain precautions to prevent burning.	Minimizes client's anxiety and promotes cooperation during the procedure.

IMPLEMENTATION

1. Close door and bedside curtains.	Decreases drafts, thus decreasing the transmission of microorganisms. Provides for client privacy.
2. Assist client in assuming comfortable position in proper body alignment, and place waterproof pad under area to be treated.	Compress remains in place for several minutes. Limited mobility in uncomfortable position causes muscular stress. Pad prevents soiling of bed linen.
3. Expose body part to be covered with compress and drape client with bath blanket.	Prevents unnecessary cooling and exposure of body part.
4. Wash hands.	Reduces transmission of microorganisms.
5. Prepare compress:	Ensures orderly procedure.
a. Pour solution into sterile container.	
b. If using portable heating source, warm solution. Commercially prepared compresses may remain under infrared lamp until just before use. Open sterile packages and drop gauze into container to become immersed in solution.	Compresses must retain warmth for therapeutic benefit.

➤ ***CRITICAL DECISION POINT*** **Temperature must be tested by applying sterile solution to nurse's forearm (without contaminating solution).**

c. Adjust temperature of aquathermia pad (if needed) (see Skill 39-3).	
6. Apply disposable gloves. Remove any existing dressing covering wound. Dispose of gloves and dressings in proper receptacle.	Reduces transmission of microorganisms.
7. Assess condition of wound and surrounding skin. Inflamed wound appears reddened but surrounding skin is less red in color.	Provides baseline to determine skin changes following compress application.

➤ ***CRITICAL DECISION POINT*** **If skin surrounding wound is reddened, application may be contraindicated.**

STEPS	RATIONALE
8. Apply sterile gloves.	Allows nurse to manipulate sterile dressing and touch open wound.
9. Pick up one layer of immersed gauze, wring out any excess solution, and apply it lightly to open wound.	Excess moisture macerates skin and increases risk of burns and infection. Skin is sensitive to sudden change in temperature.
CRITICAL DECISION POINT **Watch client's response and ask if client feels discomfort.**	
10. In few seconds, lift edge of gauze to assess for redness.	Increased redness indicates burn.
11. If client tolerates compress, pack gauze snugly against wound. Be sure all wound surfaces are covered by hot compress.	Packing of compress prevents rapid cooling from underlying air currents.
12. Cover moist compress with dry sterile dressing and bath towel. If necessary, pin or tie in place. Remove sterile gloves.	Dry sterile dressing will prevent transfer of microorganisms to wound via capillary action caused by moist compress. Towel insulates compress to prevent heat loss.
13. Apply aquathermic or waterproof heating pad over towel (optional) (Skill 39-3). Keep it in place for desired duration of application.	Provides constant temperature to compress.
CRITICAL DECISION POINT **Removing hot compress after 20 minutes and then reapplying in 15 minutes if desired maintains vasodilation and positive therapeutic effects.**	Local application of heat for greater than 20 minutes often results in reflex vasoconstriction.
14. If an aquathermia pad is *not* used to maintain temperature of application, change hot compress using sterile technique every 5 minutes or as ordered during duration of therapy.	Prevents cooling and maintains therapeutic benefit of compress.
15. After prescribed time, apply disposable gloves and remove pad, towel, and compress. Reassess wound and condition of skin, and replace dry sterile dressing as ordered.	Continued exposure to moisture will macerate skin. Prevents entrance of microorganisms into wound site.
16. Assist client to preferred comfortable position.	Maintains client's comfort.
17. Dispose of equipment and soiled compress. Wash hands.	Reduces transmission of microorganisms.

EVALUATION

1. Inspect affected area covered by compress and heating pad every 5 to 10 minutes.	Assists in determining effects of application.
2. Ask every 5 to 10 minutes if client notices any unusual burning sensation not felt before application.	It may be difficult to assess burn merely by color changes if wound is inflamed or drainage is present.
3. Have client explain and demonstrate application.	Evaluates client's understanding of and ability to perform procedure.
4. **Unexpected outcomes** that may occur include:	
➤ Presence of redness and tenderness at affected site.	Temperature of compress is too extreme for condition of skin. Increased redness and tenderness are signs of first-degree burn.
➤ Client complains of burning and discomfort.	Extreme temperature for client to tolerate. Individuals vary in their tolerance to heat and pain.
➤ Client unable to explain or apply compress correctly.	Reinstruction needed.

RECORDING AND REPORTING

1. Record type, location, and duration of application. Note solution and temperature.	Documents therapy administered.

STEPS	RATIONALE
2. Describe condition of wound and skin before and after treatment as well as client's response to therapy.	Documents client's response to therapy.
3. Describe any instructions given and client's ability to explain and perform procedure.	Documents client's learning.
4. Report unusual findings to nurse in charge or physician.	Burn or other changes may require discontinuation of heat and initiation of different therapies.

Follow-up Activities

1. If heat applications are to be continued after discharge, have client or family member give a return demonstration before discharge.

• • • • •

Special Considerations

- Review agency's safety or infection control manual for disposal of soiled soaks and dressings in accordance with Occupational and Safety Health Administration's (OSHA) Blood-Borne Pathogens Act.

Teaching Considerations

- Teach client to gently pack wound to avoid discomfort.
- Care givers and clients need to be taught that careful assessment is needed for clients with reduced sensation to determine if temperature of compress is too hot.

Pediatric Considerations

- The skin of infants and children is thin and fragile and therefore easily damaged. Use special caution in this population.

Gerontologic Considerations

- The older adult and clients receiving long-term steroid therapy can develop thin, fragile skin, which is more easily damaged.

Home Care Considerations

- When necessary, assess availability of primary care giver to assist clients in application of compress, their understanding of purpose of procedure, their willingness to comply with procedure and not leave client with compress in place beyond prescribed time limit.
- Assess physical environment to determine existence of adequate facilities to prepare hot compress and provide for sterile technique.

SKILL 39-2 Assisting with Warm Soaks and Sitz Baths

Moist heat application also includes the use of warm baths, soaks, and sitz baths. A warm bath or soak usually involves immersion of a body part into a warmed solution. Warm soaks and sitz baths are used to promote circulation, reduce edema and inflammation, promote muscle relaxation, debride wounds, and apply medicated solutions. If a body part is too large to immerse, a soak can be accomplished by wrapping the affected body part in a dressing saturated with the prepared, warmed solution.

A **sitz bath** is given by use of a special tub or chair basin that allows a client to sit in water without immersing the legs, feet, and upper trunk (Fig. 39-1). Sitz basins are disposable and especially easy to use in the home. Clients who have undergone perineal or rectal surgery, who have had an episiotomy during childbirth, or who have painful hemorrhoids or perineal inflammation may benefit from a sitz bath.

When preparing a soak or bath, the nurse should remember that the heated solution is in direct contact with the client's skin. It is very important to check water temperature carefully to prevent burns. It is also desirable to keep the solution temperature constant to enhance the moist heat's therapeutic effects. Whenever heated solution is added to a soak basin or bath, the client's body part should be removed and then reimmersed once the solution has mixed.

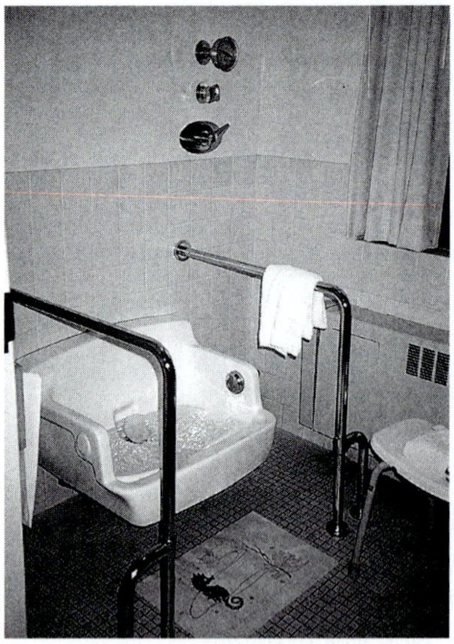

Fig. 39-1 Sitz bath.

EQUIPMENT

- Clean basin, tub, or sitz bath (basin may need to be sterile if body part to be soaked has open wound)
- Prescribed solution warmed to proper temperature (tap water is commonly used for sitz baths)
- Bath towel
- Bath blanket
- Absorbent gauze or cloth rolls (optional)
- Prescribed medication (if ordered)
- Waterproof pad for soak
- Gloves

STEPS	RATIONALE
ASSESSMENT	
1. Check physician's order for desired solution, body part to be soaked, and desired temperature as per institutional policy.	Ensures safe use of moist heat.
2. Refer to medical record to determine client's risk for reduced temperature sensation.	Certain conditions alter conduction of sensory impulses that transmit temperature and pain stimuli.
3. Refer to medical record to identify any systemic contraindications to immersion in warm baths.	Certain cardiovascular conditions and side effects of certain medications place clients at risk for sudden changes in blood pressure and blood flow caused by vasodilation.
CRITICAL DECISION POINT Clients with history of myocardial infarction, angina pectoris, and hypotension are at risk for sudden changes in blood pressure caused by vasodilation.	
4. Assess and document client's blood pressure and pulse.	Establishes a baseline for comparison.
5. Assess and document condition of skin of body part to be immersed.	Identifies thin or sensitive skin that is prone to injury from temperature extremes. Provides baseline to determine changes in skin during therapy. Identifies open wound, which necessitates use of sterile technique.
CRITICAL DECISION POINT Sitz baths are frequently used for episiotomy wounds in female clients. Inspect condition of suture line.	
6. Assess and document client's ability to position self in bath/soak.	Determines level of assistance needed to place client into sitz bath and to remove at the end of treatment.
7. Assess and document client's level of comfort using a visual analog scale.	Provides baseline for client's comfort level. Inflamed or injured body parts may be soothed by soak or bath.
8. Assess and document client's understanding of therapy and its purpose.	Determines need for health teaching.

NURSING DIAGNOSIS

Clustering of defining characteristics from the assessment data may reveal the following nursing diagnoses for clients requiring this skill:

- Altered peripheral tissue perfusion
- Impaired physical mobility
- Impaired skin integrity
- Knowledge deficit regarding sitz bath/warm soaks
- Pain
- Risk for injury
- Sensory perceptual alterations (tactile)

Related factors are individualized based on a client's condition or needs.

PLANNING

STEPS	RATIONALE
1. **Expected outcomes** following completion of procedure:	
➤ Client's skin is pink and warm to touch immediately after soak.	Vasodilation increases blood flow to area.
➤ Client will relate a measurable decrease in pain.	Moist heat reduces edema/inflammation and relaxes stiff and strained muscles. Heat applications lower pain perception by activating large-diameter sensory fibers that block painful stimuli.
➤ Blood pressure and pulse are within client's normal range.	No systemic vascular changes occurred. The goal of therapy is to achieve a localized vascular response.
➤ Client correctly uses heat application.	Demonstrates learning.
2. Prepare equipment and supplies.	Organization of supplies prevents unnecessary delays in the procedure.
3. Explain steps of procedure and purpose to client.	Minimizes client's anxiety and promotes cooperation during the procedure.

IMPLEMENTATION

STEPS	RATIONALE
1. Close door and bedside curtains.	Maintains privacy and reduces transmission of microorganisms.
2. Wash hands.	Reduces transmission of microorganisms.
3. Fill basin or tub with warmed solution. Check temperature.	Checking for correct temperature reduces risk of burns.

CRITICAL DECISION POINT Test temperature of solution by applying small amount to forearm.

STEPS	RATIONALE
4. For soaks, position client comfortably and place waterproof pad under area to be treated.	Prevents soiling of bed linen or clothing.
5. Assist client to immerse body part in tub or basin.	Prevents falls.
6. Cover client with bath blanket or towel as desired.	Prevents chilling and enhances client's ability to relax.
7. Maintain constant temperature throughout 15- to 20-minute soak:	
a. Keep large sheet or blanket over container or basin.	Prevents heat loss through **evaporation.** Therapeutic effects of soak can be obtained only from constant temperature.
b. After 10 minutes, remove body part from soak, check to see that skin is not burned, empty cooled solution, add newly heated solution, and reimmerse body part.	Maintains constant therapeutic temperature.

CRITICAL DECISION POINT Presence of burn contraindicates completing the soak. Adding warmed solution to basin with body part immersed can cause burn.

STEPS	RATIONALE
8. After 15 to 20 minutes, remove client from soak or bath; dry body parts thoroughly. (Clean gloves are required if drainage is present.)	Avoids chilling. Enhances client's comfort.

STEPS	RATIONALE
9. Assist client into comfortable position.	Maintains comfortable environment for client.
10. Drain solution from basin or tub. Clean tub and place in proper storage area. Dispose of soiled linen and gloves (if used); wash hands.	Reduces transmission of microorganisms.

EVALUATION

1. Inspect condition of body part immersed for redness, burns, and pain.	Evaluates effects of treatments.
2. Question client regarding presence of burning sensation, severity of pain, and general response to therapy.	Determines if client was exposed to temperature extreme resulting in burn. Evaluates client's subjective response to therapy.
3. Assess vital signs if client complains of dizziness or lightheadedness.	Determines if vascular response to vasodilation has occurred.
4. Ask client to demonstrate procedure and explain purpose of soak or sitz bath.	Measures level of learning.
5. **Unexpected outcomes** that may occur include:	
➤ Client's skin is reddened and sensitive to touch.	Extreme warmth caused burning of skin layer.
➤ Client experiences hypotension and complains of dizziness, nausea, and lightheadedness.	Result of systemic vasodilation.
➤ Client is unable to explain purpose of procedure or uses soak/bath incorrectly.	Reinstruction is required.

RECORDING AND REPORTING

1. Record procedure, including temperature and duration of soak, in nurses' notes.	Documents therapy delivered to client.
2. Describe condition of body part before and after therapy and client's response.	Documents response to therapy.
3. Record preprocedure and postprocedure vital signs.	Documents systemic response to treatment.
4. Describe any instruction given and client's success in demonstrating procedure.	Documents client's response to teaching efforts.
5. Report all client complaints and any unusual observations (e.g., change in vital signs) to nurse in charge or physician.	Provides guidelines for repeating therapy. Change in client's condition may mean different therapy is required.

FOLLOW-UP ACTIVITIES

1. Review agency's safety or infection control manual for disposal of soiled soaks and dressings.

• • • • •

Special Considerations

- ➤ Clients with thin skin include older adults, children, and those receiving long-term steroid therapy. Moist heat therapy by immersion may be contraindicated.

Teaching Considerations

- ➤ Client may resume therapy at home and should understand risks of burns. Explain risks of using warm baths and methods to ensure safety.
- ➤ If heat applications are to be continued after discharge, have client or family member give a return demonstration before discharge.

Pediatric Considerations

- ➤ The skin of infants and children is thin and fragile and therefore easily damaged. Use special caution in this population.

Gerontologic Considerations

- ➤ Older adult clients tolerate somewhat cooler temperature better because of less stable temperature regulation mechanisms.
- ➤ In some clients, such as frail, older clients with cardiac conditions, it may be necessary to monitor vital signs throughout procedure.

Home Care Considerations

- ➤ When necessary, assess availability of primary care giver to assist client. If care giver is not available, evaluate client as to ability, willingness, and understanding of preparing soaks or baths.
- ➤ Assess home environment to determine adequacy of facilities for use by client. Medical equipment companies may be contacted for assistance in determining best product for client.

SKILL 39-3 Applying Aquathermia and Heating Pads

Aquathermia and heating pads are common forms of dry heat therapy used in health care settings as well as in the home (Fig. 39-2). Both are covered and applied directly to the skin's surface, and for this reason extra precautions are needed to prevent burns. The aquathermia (water flow pad) consists of a waterproof rubber or plastic pad connected by two hoses to an electrical control unit that has a heating element and motor. Distilled water circulates through hollowed channels in the pad to the control unit where water is heated (or cooled). The temperature setting is adjusted by a plastic key that inserts into the control unit. In most health care institutions, the central supply department sets the temperature regulators to the recommended temperature, approximately 40.5° to 43° C (105° to 109.4° F). Because of the constant temperature control, aquathermia pads tend to be safer than heating pads. If distilled water in the unit runs low, the nurse simply adds more distilled water to the reservoir at the top of the control unit. Rubber and plastic conduct heat, so the pad should be encased in a towel or pillowcase to avoid direct exposure to the skin.

The conventional heating pad consists of an electric coil enclosed in a waterproof covering. A cotton or flannel cloth covers the outer pad. The pad connects to an electrical cord that has a temperature-regulating unit for high, medium, or low settings. Because it is so easy to readjust temperature settings on heating pads, clients should be instructed not to turn the setting higher once they have adapted to the temperature. It is wise to avoid ever using the highest setting.

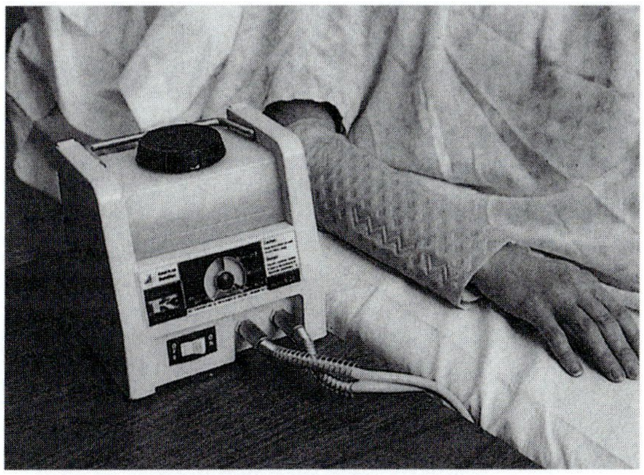

Fig. 39-2 Aquathermia pad.

EQUIPMENT

- **Aquathermia or heating pad**
- **Electrical control unit**
- **Distilled water (for aquathermia pad)**
- **Bath towel or pillowcase**
- **Tape, ties, or gauze roll**

STEPS	RATIONALE
ASSESSMENT	
1. Refer to physician's order for location of application and duration of therapy. Institutional policy usually sets recommended temperature.	Order required to help ensure client's safety.
2. Assess condition of skin over which pad is to be applied.	Provides baseline to determine change in skin condition after heat application.
3. Assess level of discomfort and range of motion if client is being treated for muscle sprain.	Provides baseline to determine if pain relief is achieved.
4. Assess area to be treated for sensitivity to temperature, light touch, and pain (see Chapter 11).	Determines if client is insensitive to heat extremes.
5. Check electrical plugs and cords for obvious fraying or cracking.	Prevents injury from accidental electrical shock.
6. Determine client's or family members' knowledge of procedure including steps for application and safety precautions.	Heating pads are frequently used in home. Assessment determines extent of health teaching required.

NURSING DIAGNOSIS

Clustering of defining characteristics from the assessment data may reveal the following nursing diagnoses for clients requiring this skill:

- Altered peripheral tissue perfusion
- Impaired physical mobility
- Impaired skin integrity
- Knowledge deficit regarding moist heat applications
- Pain
- Risk for injury
- Sensory perceptual alterations (tactile)

Related factors are individualized based on a client's condition or needs.

STEPS	RATIONALE
PLANNING	
1. **Expected outcomes** following completion of procedure:	
➤ Skin is pink and warm to touch after application.	Vasodilation from heat exposure increases blood flow to affected part.
➤ Client reports less discomfort of inflamed tissues or strained muscles.	Heat applications lower pain perception by stimulating large-diameter sensory nerve fibers and blocking pain impulses of smaller nerve fibers.
➤ Client may be able to move strained muscles more freely.	Reduced stiffness and improves range of motion.
➤ Client correctly applies pad.	Documents learning.
2. Prepare equipment and supplies.	Organization of supplies prevents unnecessary delays in procedure.
3. Explain procedure and precautions.	Improves likelihood of client's compliance with therapy.
IMPLEMENTATION	
1. Close room door and bedside curtain, wash hands, and position client comfortably so area to be treated may be exposed.	Provides for client's privacy. Reduces transfer of microorganisms. Client must be able to assume position for several minutes during application.
2. For aquathermia or uncovered heating pad, cover or wrap affected area with bath towel or enclose pad with pillowcase.	Prevents heated surface from touching client's skin.
➤ ***CRITICAL DECISION POINT*** **Do not pin the wrap to pad because this may cause a leak in device.**	
3. Place pad over affected area (see Fig. 39-2), and secure with tape, tie, or gauze as needed.	Pad delivers dry warm heat to injured tissues. Pad should not slip onto different body part.
➤ ***CRITICAL DECISION POINT*** **Never position client so that client is lying directly on pad. This position prevents dissipation of heat and increases risk of burns.**	
4. Turn heating pad on to low or medium setting and check temperature of aquathermia pad.	Prevents exposure of client to temperature extremes.
5. Monitor condition of skin every 5 minutes during application and question client regarding sensation of burning.	Determines if heat exposure is resulting in burn.
6. After 20 to 30 minutes (or time ordered by physician), remove pad and store.	Continued exposure will result in burns. Some clients should not have access to pad without supervision.
7. Assist client in returning to preferred comfortable position, dispose of soiled linen, and wash hands.	Promotes relaxing environment. Reduces spread of microorganisms.
EVALUATION	
1. Inspect condition of skin exposed to heat.	Evaluates response of skin to heat exposure.
2. Ask client if strained muscle or inflamed area continues to be painful.	Heat reduces edema and relieves pain from muscle stiffness and spasm.
3. Note if client is able to move strained muscle with less discomfort.	Heat relaxes strained muscle.
4. Observe client apply pad.	Measures level of learning.
5. **Unexpected outcomes** that may occur include:	
➤ Skin is reddened and sensitive to touch.	Symptoms indicate first-degree burn.
➤ Edema and inflammation are increased.	Applying heat too soon after an injury can increase edema through vasodilation.
➤ Body part is painful to move.	Movement stretches burn-sensitive nerve fibers in skin.

STEPS	RATIONALE
➤ Client applies heat incorrectly or is unable to relate precautions.	Reinstruction is necessary.

Recording and Reporting

1. Record site of application, duration of therapy, and client's response.	Documents therapy administered and results of care.
2. Describe any instruction given and client's success in demonstrating procedure.	Documents client's response to teaching efforts.
3. Report changes in skin integrity such as burns.	Further therapy may be needed to treat burn.

Follow-up Activities

1. If applications are to be done at home, have client apply pad and explain safety measures.

• • • • •

Special Considerations

- Review agency's safety or infection control manual for disposal of soiled soaks and dressings.
- Heating and aquathermia pads are rarely applied over open wounds.
- Do not actively exercise muscle to evaluate results of therapy. Active exercise can aggravate muscle strain.

Teaching Considerations

- Highlight safety precautions as they are followed during application.

Pediatric Considerations

- The skin of infants and children is thin and fragile, therefore easily damaged. Use special caution in this population.

Gerontologic Considerations

- Older adults are more at risk for burns because of loss of heat sensation. Check the site frequently during all treatments.

Home Care Considerations

- Assess client and primary care giver as to understanding, ability, and motivation to comply with procedure.
- Assess home environment for facilities to comply with implementation of procedure.

SKILL 39-4 Applying Cold Applications

Application of cold, which can be accomplished through the use of a moist cold compress, cool water flow pad and immersion of a body part into a cold soak, form of therapy used after the sudden onset of acute inflammation or swelling (see Table 39-1). Second, the application of an ice pack, bag, or collar is a simple way to apply cold to a small, localized area. The applications do not create moisture, so the client is spared the discomfort from cold solutions running down a body part. Vasoconstriction resulting from cold application reduces blood flow to the injured part and thus limits fluid accumulation and slows bleeding. The lower temperature also suppresses inflammation and produces a local anesthetic response. When used appropriately, cold applications can significantly lessen pain and immobility by reducing swelling of injured tissues (Sheehy, 1992; Murphy and Tkach, 1996). This is an important point for nurses to know when deciding on the choice of heat or cold for the treatment of acute injuries.

A cold compress usually consists of a gauze dressing or a washcloth that has been immersed in iced or chilled solution to achieve the desired temperature. The compress may be sterile or clean; however, a clean compress is most commonly used. Any open wounds require sterile applications. A variety of sizes or thicknesses of gauze can be used depending on the site of injury. For example, a cold compress to the eye requires a thicker gauze that fits a small area to maintain a cold temperature. Thin gauze works more effectively for larger areas such as the face.

There is now an electrically controlled cooling device that works much like an aquathermia pad (see Skill 39-3). The cooling pad has the advantage of delivering a constant cool temperature.

Ice bags and packs come in a variety of sizes to fit different body parts (Fig. 39-3). When a person is away from home or a health care setting, a plastic bag or glove can serve as an ice bag as long as a towel or cloth is also avail-

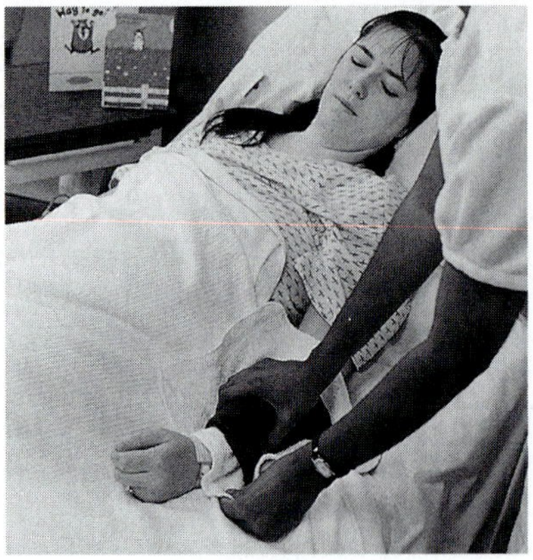

Fig. 39-3 Placement of ice pack (or bag) on extremity.

able to wrap around the bag to prevent direct exposure of the bag against the person's skin (Murphy and Tkach, 1996).

EQUIPMENT

Cold compress
- **Absorbent gauze (clean or sterile) folded to desired size**
- **Clean or sterile basin with ice and water at desired temperature**
- **Bath towel or absorbent pad**
- **Two pairs of disposable or sterile gloves (according to agency policy)**

Cool water flow pad
- **Cooling pad and electrical pump**
- **Tapes, ties, gauze roll, or Ace bandage**
- **Ice bag or collar with water**
- **Ice pack**
- **Towel or pillowcase**
- **Cloth ties or tape**
- **Gloves (if blood or body fluids are present)**

STEPS	RATIONALE
ASSESSMENT	
1. Refer to physician's order for location and duration of application.	Physician's order is required for all cold applications.
2. Inspect and document condition of injured or affected part. Gently palpate area.	Provides baseline for determining change in condition of injured tissues.
CRITICAL DECISION POINT **Keep injured part immobilized and in alignment. Movement can cause further injury to strains, sprains, or fractures.**	
3. Consider time in which injury occurred.	Cold should be applied quickly after an injury to prevent edema. Application of cold is most effective if started within 24 hours of injury.
4. Ask client to describe severity and character of pain using a visual analog scale.	Provides baseline for determining pain relief with therapy.
5. Assess area to be treated for sensitivity to temperature, light touch, and pain and for adequate circulation (see Chapter 11).	Determines if client is insensitive to cold extremes.
6. Assess client's understanding of procedure.	Determines need for health teaching.

NURSING DIAGNOSIS

Clustering of defining characteristics from the assessment data may reveal the following nursing diagnoses for clients requiring this skill:

- ➤ Altered peripheral tissue perfusion
- ➤ Impaired physical mobility
- ➤ Impaired skin integrity
- ➤ Knowledge deficit regarding moist cold applications
- ➤ Pain
- ➤ Risk for injury
- ➤ Sensory perceptual alterations (tactile)

Related factors are individualized based on a client's condition or needs.

STEPS	RATIONALE
PLANNING	
1. **Expected outcomes** following completion of procedure:	
➤ Affected area is slightly pale and cool to touch.	Result of vasoconstriction.
➤ Extent of edema is decreased.	Cold reduces blood flow to affected part, reducing edema formation.
➤ Client relates measurable decrease in pain.	Cold creates local anesthetic effect.
➤ Client correctly states how to apply cold compress and provides demonstration.	Documents learning.
2. Prepare equipment and supplies.	Organization prevents unnecessary delays.
3. Explain procedure and precautions.	Improves likelihood of client's compliance with therapy.
IMPLEMENTATION	
1. Close room door and bedside curtain.	Reduces spread of microorganisms via drafts. Provides privacy for client.
2. Wash hands.	Reduces spread of microorganisms.
3. Position client carefully, keeping body part in proper alignment and exposing only the area to be treated.	Prevents further injury to body part. Avoids unnecessary exposure of body parts, maintaining client's comfort and privacy.
➤ ***CRITICAL DECISION POINT*** **In cases of strains, sprains, or fractures, extremity or body part should remain aligned to prevent further injury.**	
4. Place towel or absorbent pad under area to be treated.	Prevents soiling of bed linen.
5. Apply disposable gloves.	Reduces spread of infection.
6. Cold compress:	
a. Check temperature of solution and submerge gauze into filled basin at bedside; wring out excess moisture.	Extreme temperature can cause tissue damage. Dripping gauze is uncomfortable to client.
b. Apply compress to affected area, molding it gently over site.	Ensures that cold is directed over site of injury.
7. Electrically controlled cooling device:	
a. Wrap cool water flow pad around body part (see illustration).	
b. Be sure correct temperature is set.	
c. Secure with Ace bandage, gauze roll, or ties.	

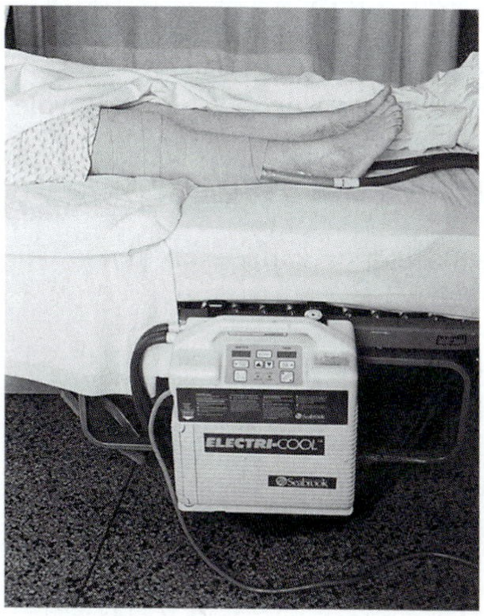

Step 7 Cooling device.

STEPS	RATIONALE
8. Prepare ice bag or collar:	
a. Fill bag with water, secure cap, and invert.	Checks for leaks.
b. Empty water, then fill bag two thirds full with small ice chips.	Bag can be more easily molded over body part.
c. Release excess air from bag by squeezing its sides before securing cap.	Excess air interferes with cold conduction.
d. Wipe bag dry.	Prevents skin maceration.
e. Apply snugly over area. Secure with tape as needed.	Cold should be directly over injury.
9. Prepare ice pack:	
a. Commercial packs are squeezed or kneaded.	Releases alcohol-based solution to create cold temperature.
b. Apply pack directly over area.	Cold should be applied directly over injury.

CRITICAL DECISION POINT **Cover prepared bag or pack with towel or pillowcase. Prevents direct exposure of cold against client's skin.**

CRITICAL DECISION POINT **Do not reapply ice pack to reddened or bluish areas; continual use of ice pack worsens ischemia.**

STEPS	RATIONALE
10. Remove gloves and dispose of in proper container.	Reduces transfer of microorganisms.
11. Check condition of skin every 5 minutes for duration of application.	Determines if there are adverse reactions to cold. These include mottling, redness, burning, blistering, and numbness.
12. After 15 to 20 minutes (or as ordered by the physician), apply clean gloves, remove compress or pad, and gently dry off any moisture.	Drying prevents maceration of skin. Prolonged application of cold can result in diminished blood flow and tissue ischemia or compensatory vasodilation to provide warmth to the area being treated.
13. Assist client to comfortable position.	Maintains relaxing environment.
14. Empty basin, dry, and store. Dispose of soiled linen and gloves; wash hands.	Reduces transfer of microorganisms.

EVALUATION

STEPS	RATIONALE
1. Inspect affected area for changes in condition of skin.	Determines reaction to cold compress application.
2. Palpate affected area gently.	Determines level of edema.
3. Question client about level of comfort.	Determines if pain has been relieved.
4. Ask client to apply cold application and explain risks of treatment.	Measures level of learning.
5. **Unexpected outcomes** that may occur include:	
➤ Skin takes on mottled, reddened, or bluish purple appearance.	Result of prolonged exposure, causing tissue ischemia.
➤ Client complains of burning-type pain and numbness.	Symptoms of ischemia.
➤ Client is unable to describe application or use compress correctly.	Reinstruction is necessary.

RECORDING AND REPORTING

STEPS	RATIONALE
1. Record procedure, including type, location, duration of application, and client's response in nurses' notes.	Documents therapy provided and client's response.
2. Describe any instruction given and client's success in demonstrating procedure.	Documents client's response to teaching efforts.
3. Report undesirable changes in condition of skin to nurse in charge or physician.	Injury from prolonged exposure requires different therapy.

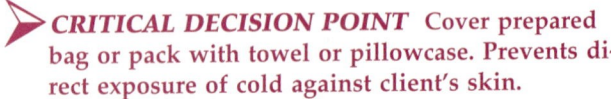

STEPS **RATIONALE**

Follow-up Activities

1. Cold compresses may be reapplied at intervals.
2. If compresses are to be applied at home, have client demonstrate procedure and explain precautions.

• • • • •

Special Considerations

- Review agency's safety or infection control manual for disposal of soiled soaks and dressings.
- If area is edematous, sensation may be reduced and extra caution must be used during cold therapy.
- Numbness and tingling are common sensations with cold applications and indicate adverse reactions only when severe and coupled with other symptoms.
- Moisture may form on outside of bag if room temperature is warm. This does not indicate a leak.
- Some commercial packs have soft insulated coverings so they can be applied directly to the skin.

Teaching Considerations

- Injuries requiring this type of therapy usually occur away from health care settings. Clients active in sports should know steps to take to minimize extent of injury.

Pediatric Considerations

- A greater metabolic rate and larger trunk in relation to the rest of the body make children more prone to hypothermia (Thomas, 1996). Exercise caution with young clients.
- Infants have an unstable temperature control mechanism, so mottling of the extremities is common and may not indicate an adverse reaction if this symptom is seen alone (Thomas, 1996).

Gerontologic Considerations

- Older adults are more at risk for tissue damage due to loss of cold sensation. Check the site frequently during all treatments

Home Care Considerations

- Clean cloth can be used in home setting as long as there is no open wound.
- Assess client and primary care giver as to understanding, ability, and motivation to comply with procedure.
- Assess client's home environment for adequacy of facilities with which to implement procedure.
- An ice pack can be improvised by placing ice cubes in a zip lock plastic bag.

SKILL 39-5 Caring for Clients Requiring Hypothermia or Hyperthermia Blankets

Clients can have high prolonged fevers from infectious and neurological diseases and as side effects from anesthesia. When there is difficulty controlling a fever in a client, one measure is the use of a hypothermia (cooling) blanket. Hypothermia blankets are fluid-filled rubberized blankets that circulate cooled solution (usually distilled water) through the blanket. When the client lies on the device, the cooling blanket helps to reduce the client's body temperature (Fig. 39-4).

Conversely, clients whose body temperature is abnormally low because of extreme exposure to cold or because of hypothermia induced for neurological or cardiac surgery require a hyperthermia (warming) blanket to assist the body to return to near-normal temperature. In the case of hyperthermia or rewarming therapy, a warmed solution is circulated through the blanket to help return the client's body temperature to normal.

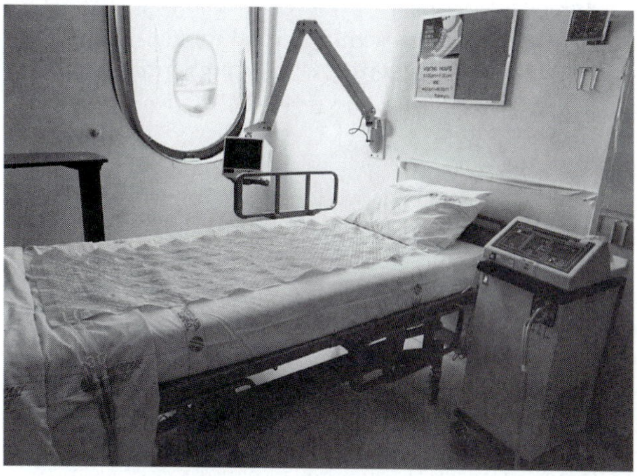

Fig. 39-4 Hypothermia cooling blanket before sheet applied to bed.

EQUIPMENT

- **Hypothermia or hyperthermia blanket with control panel and rectal probe**
- **Sheet or thin bath blanket**
- **Distilled water to fill the units if necessary**
- **Disposable gloves**
- **Rectal thermometer**

STEPS	RATIONALE
ASSESSMENT	
1. Refer to physician's order and double-check that client's current body temperature requires use of hypothermia or hyperthermia blanket.	Institution of therapy requires physician's order.
2. Assess vital signs, neurologic status, mental status, and peripheral circulation.	Establishes baseline data to use for comparison during therapy.
3. Verify that client's body temperature cannot be returned to normal by other, less intensive measures.	Use of hypothermia and hyperthermia blanket is not without risk and should be instituted only when other measures are not effective.
CRITICAL DECISION POINT Antipyretic therapy should be attempted for fever.	
4. Assess client's skin on ears, hands, fingers, heels, sacrum, and other bony prominences before therapy. Inspect scrotal surface of male client.	These areas are more exposed to blanket and consequently are at greater risk for injury. Baseline data enable the nurse to quickly determine if injury to skin is result of therapy.

NURSING DIAGNOSIS

Clustering of defining characteristics from the assessment data may reveal the following nursing diagnoses for clients requiring this skill:

- Altered peripheral tissue perfusion
- Impaired physical mobility
- Impaired skin integrity
- Knowledge deficit regarding implications of hypothermia or hyperthermia blanket
- Pain
- Risk for injury
- Sensory perceptual alterations (tactile)

Related factors are individualized based on a client's condition or needs.

PLANNING

STEPS	RATIONALE
1. **Expected outcomes** following completion of procedure:	
➤ Temperature is within normal range.	Indicates that therapy is effective.
➤ Absence of shivering with hypothermia blanket.	Shivering increases metabolic rate and heat production. This mechanism contributes to body temperature elevation and can cause client's body temperature to rise (Rakel, 1995). In addition, shivering causes vasoconstriction, which can injure the skin of distal body regions.
➤ Skin clear without signs of injury or burns.	Distal regions of client's skin are at greatest risk for injury from blanket.
2. Explain procedure to client.	Increases cooperation and reduces anxiety.
3. Prepare client:	
a. Prepare the blanket according to agency policy and manufacturer's instruction.	Agencies have specific policies as to who should maintain the equipment in functional order. Each type of blanket varies from one manufacturer to another. Manufacturer's instructions are located on the machine. Read before using.

STEPS	RATIONALE
IMPLEMENTATION	
1. Wash hands and apply gloves.	Reduces transmission of microorganisms.
2. Turn on blanket and observe that the cool or warm light is on. Precool or prewarm the blanket, setting the pad temperature to desired level.	Verifies that blanket is correctly set to assist in reducing (cool) or increasing (warm) client's body temperature. Prepares blanket for prescribed therapy.
3. Verify that pad temperature limits are set at desired safety ranges.	Safety ranges prevent excessive cooling or warming. The blanket automatically shuts off when preset body temperature is achieved.
4. Place sheet or thin bath blanket over hypothermia or hyperthermia blanket.	Protects client's skin from direct contact with blanket, thus reducing risk of injury to skin.
5. Position hypothermia or hyperthermia blanket under client.	
CRITICAL DECISION POINT **If using the blanket for hypothermia, wrap client's hands and feet in towels. Elevate scrotum off blanket surface with towels. This reduces the risk of thermal injury to the body's distal areas.**	Protects client's skin from direct contact with blanket, thus reducing risk of injury to skin.
6. Lubricate rectal probe and insert into client's rectum.	When using hypothermia or hyperthermia blanket, it is imperative that the nurse continuously monitor client's core internal (rectal) temperature.
7. Position client to protect from pressure ulcer development and impaired body alignment (see Chapter 8).	Client has an increased risk of pressure ulcer development because of the skin moisture created by the blanket and client's body temperature.
CRITICAL DECISION POINT **Turn client frequently (based on condition of skin) while on blanket.**	
8. Double-check the fluid thermometer on control panel of blanket before leaving room.	Verifies that pad temperature is maintained at desired level.
9. Remove gloves and wash hands.	Reduces transmission of microorganisms.
EVALUATION	
1. Monitor client's temperature and vital signs every 15 minutes during the first hour, every 30 minutes during the second hour, and every hour of therapy thereafter.	Provides continuous evaluation of response of client's body temperature to therapy during initial and continual therapy.
2. Evaluate the automatic temperature control every 30 minutes visually and every 4 hours by taking client's rectal temperature with glass thermometer.	Ensures removal of hypothermia or hyperthermia blanket when client's temperature returns to desired level. Verifies accuracy of rectal probe and automatic temperature control device.
3. Observe skin for indications of burns, change in color, and other signs of injury.	Hypothermia and hyperthermia blankets have the potential to cause skin injuries.
4. Determine client's level of comfort.	Therapy has the potential to cause discomfort. Prompt assessment reduces risk for severe injuries.
5. **Unexpected outcomes** that may occur include:	
➤ Client's core body temperature decreases or rises rapidly.	Indicates rapid response to therapy.
➤ Client's core temperature remains unchanged.	Client may need hypothermic or hyperthermic treatment of additional sites, such as axilla, groin, and neck, in addition to those covered by the blanket.
➤ Client begins to shiver.	Shivering increases metabolic rate and heat production, causing client's core body temperature to rise.
➤ Skin breaks down.	Indicates that the client's skin may have received thermal injury (frostbite or burn) from the blanket.

STEPS	RATIONALE
RECORDING AND REPORTING	
1. Record baseline data: vital signs, neurological and mental status, status of peripheral circulation and skin integrity when therapy was initiated, temperature control setting, and client response to therapy.	Documents client's status before instituting therapy, care provided, and client's response to therapy.
2. Chart on temperature graphic repeated VS measurements.	Documents response to therapy.
3. Report any unexpected outcome to physician.	Further treatment may be indicated.

FOLLOW-UP ACTIVITIES

1. *Rapid change in body temperature:* Turn off blanket. May need to adjust therapy.
2. *Client's core temperature remains unchanged:* Verify that equipment is set up and working correctly. Institute hypothermic or hyperthermic treatment of additional body sites such as groin, axilla, and neck.
3. *Client begins to shiver:* Turn off hypothermia (cooling) blanket. If ordered, warm the solution in the blanket a few degrees. Monitor temperature.
4. *Skin breakdown:* Assess condition of skin. Do not massage areas because massage can cause further injury. Pressure ulcer prevention measures may be needed (see Chapter 8).

• • • • •

Special Considerations

- Review agency's safety or infection control manual for disposal of soiled soaks and dressings in accordance with OSHA's Blood-Borne Pathogens Act.
- The material of the hypothermia or hyperthermia blanket itself can cause client's skin to become moist, thus increasing the risk of skin breakdown.
- Some clients may display early signs of shivering: ECG changes, facial muscle twitching, hyperventilation.

Teaching Considerations

- Clients and their families need to be instructed not to move the client off the blanket.

Pediatric Considerations

- A greater metabolic rate and larger trunk in relation to the rest of the body make children more prone to hypothermia (Thomas, 1996). Exercise caution with young clients.
- Infants have an unstable temperature control mechanism, so mottling of the extremities is common and may not indicate an adverse reaction.

Gerontologic Considerations

- Older adults are more at risk for tissue damage because of loss of cold sensation. Check the client frequently during all treatments.

CRITICAL THINKING EXERCISES

1. Your diabetic client requires a cold compress to the left ankle for 48 hours after suffering a fracture. What discharge instructions will you provide?
2. Explain the hazards associated with direct water contact as occurs with warm soaks.
3. How do cold or heat applications reduce pain?

REFERENCES

Bayles FH: Heat and cold injury guide, *Health You* 7(1):34, 1991.

Murphy PM, Tkach T: The heat is on: treating heat related emergencies, *J of Emer Medical Services* 1996.

Nanneman D: Thermal modalities: heat and cold. A review of physiologic effects with clinical applications, *Am Assoc Occupat Health Nurs* 39(2):70, 1991.

Occupational and Safety Health Administration: Occupational exposure to blood born pathogens: Final rule, 29CFR Part 1910:1030, *Federal Register,* 56:64003-64182, 1991.

Rakel RE: *Conn's current therapy,* Philadelphia, 1995, WB Saunders.

Sheehy SB: *Emergency nursing: principles and practice,* St Louis, 1992, Mosby.

Thomas DO: Assessing children: it's different, *RN* 59(4):38, 1996.

ADDITIONAL READING

McConnell EA: Clinical do's and dont's: how to apply an ice bag, ice collar, or ice glove, *Nurs 92* 22(7):18, 1992.

Wong DL: *Whaley and Wong's nursing care of infants and children,* ed 5, St Louis, 1995, Mosby.

CHAPTER 40

Wound Care and Irrigations

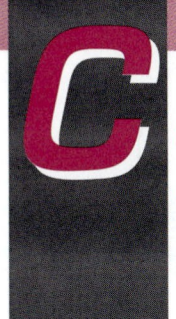

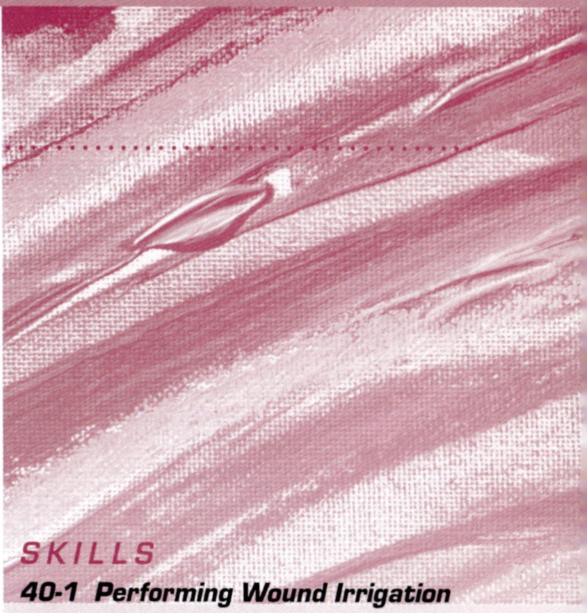

OBJECTIVES

Mastery of content in this chapter will enable the nurse to:

- Define key terms.
- Discuss the body's response during each stage of the wound-healing process.
- Differentiate between primary and secondary intention.
- Explain factors that impair or promote normal wound healing.
- Administer a wound irrigation.
- Remove sutures or staples.
- Demonstrate care of a wound-drainage system.

KEY TERMS

Dehiscence
Eschar
Evisceration
Granulation tissue
Healing ridge
Hemostasis
Hemovac drain
Irrigation
Jackson-Pratt (JP) drain
Keloid
Penrose drain
Primary intention
Secondary intention
Staples
Tertiary intention

SKILLS

40-1 Performing Wound Irrigation

40-2 Performing Suture and Staple Removal

40-3 Performing Drainage Evacuation

Proper wound care is necessary to promote an intact skin layer during healing. The integumentary system is the body's first line of defense against invasion by infectious microorganisms. The skin defends the body in other ways by serving as a sensory organ for pain, touch, and temperature. It has an acid pH, which is often called the "acid mantle."

The skin or integument, the largest external organ, has two layers: the epidermis and the dermis (Fig. 40-1). The outer layer, the epidermis, has five layers. The outermost layer, the stratum corneum, consists of flattened dead keratinized cells. The thin layer of the stratum corneum prevents dehydration of underlying cells and is a physical barrier to the entry of certain chemicals. The barrier is selective; it does allow absorption of topical medications in paste form. The next layers in the epidermis are the stratum lucidum, stratum granulosum, and stratum spinosum. The innermost layer of the epidermis, the stratum germinativum, is sometimes called the "basal layer." It is from this single layer of keratinocytes that cells migrate up toward the stratum corneum. An important feature of the stratum germinativum are the epidermal protrusions or "peaks and valleys" that point downward into the dermis. They provide resiliency and integrity to the skin structure. Also found in this layer are the melanocytes, which are the cells that give the skin its color. The area that separates the epidermis from the dermis is called the *dermoepidermal junction* or the *basement membrane zone*.

Beneath the epidermis is the dermis. The dermis contains no skin cells. Collagen (a tough fibrous protein layer), blood vessels, and nerves compose the dermal layer. Collagen composes about 70% of the dermis and is therefore extremely important in wound healing. The dermis restores the physical properties of the skin and its structural integrity. Restoration of both the epidermal and dermal layers is necessary to promote healing. Risk of local or systemic infection, impaired circulation, and breakdown of tissue is directly influenced by the ability of the dermal layer to heal (Bonier, 1985).

Physiologically, wound healing occurs in the same way for all clients, with skin cells and some tissues (including the vascular tissues) regenerating quickly and others regenerating slowly or not at all. The latter group includes cells of the liver, renal tubules, and central nervous system neurons (Potter and Perry, 1997).

Wound healing involves a series of physiological processes (see box below). These processes can be affected by the location, severity, and extent of the injury. The ability of cells and tissues to regenerate, return to normal structure, or resume normal functioning also affects heal-

STAGES OF WOUND HEALING

Defensive or Inflammatory Stage

Starts when skin integrity is impaired and continues from 4 to 6 days.

- **Hemostasis**—Blood vessels constrict, gathering of platelets stops bleeding. Clots form a fibrin matrix. Scab forms, preventing entry of infectious organisms.
- Inflammatory response—Increases blood flow to wound and vascular permeability to plasma resulting in localized redness and edema.
- White blood cells arrive at wound.
  Neutrophils ingest bacteria and small debris, then die in a few days and leave enzyme exudate, which either attacks bacteria *or* interferes with tissue repair.
  Monocytes become macrophages.
  Macrophages clean cell of debris by phagocytosis; aid in wound repair by recycling normal amino acids and sugars.
- Epithelial cells move from wound margins to base of clot or scab (for period of approximately 48 hours).

Reconstruction or Proliferative Stage

Closure begins on day 3 or 4 of defensive stage and continues for 2 to 3 weeks.

- Fibroblasts—Function with help of vitamins B and C; oxygen and amino acids synthesize collagen.
- Collagen—Provides strength and structural integrity to the wound.
- Epithelial cells—Differentiate to duplicate damaged cells (e.g., intestinal mucosal cells acquire their columnar appearance).

Maturation Stage

This final healing stage may continue for 1 year or more as collagen scar strengthens.

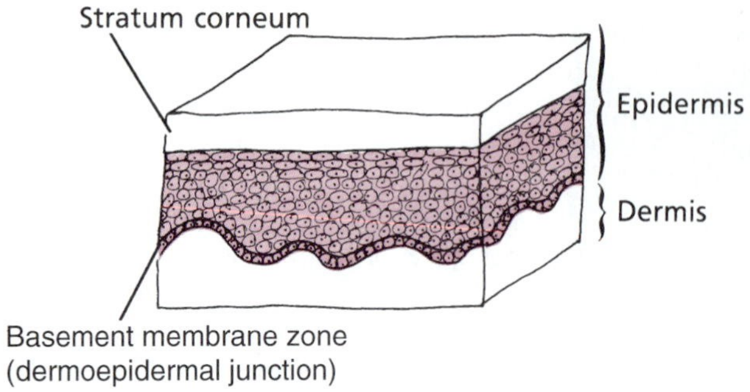

Fig. 40-1 Layers of the integument.

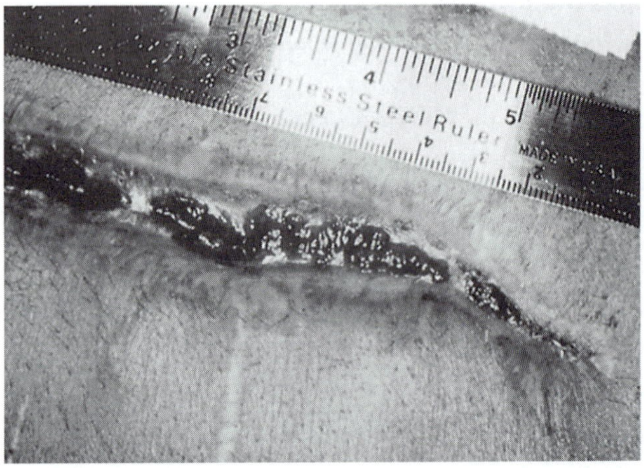

Fig. 40-2 Surgical wound with epithelialization occurring: epithelial healing ridge apparent. (Courtesy Dr. Diane Cooper, San Francisco. From Bryant RA, editor: *Acute and chronic wounds*, St Louis, 1992, Mosby.)

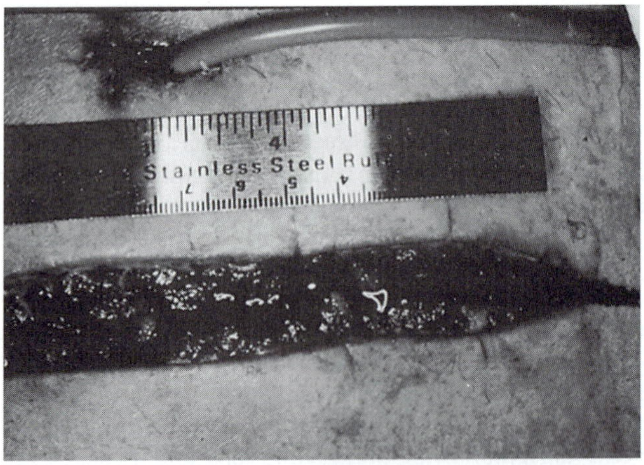

Fig. 40-3 Surgical wound lacking evidence of healing epithelial ridge. (Courtesy Dr. Diane Cooper, San Francisco. From Bryant RA, editor: *Acute and chronic wounds*, St Louis, 1992, Mosby.)

ing. Collagen deposition begins in the inflammatory phase and peaks during the proliferative phase (Cooper, 1992). It is important for nurses to assess for the accumulation of this new tissue (Cooper, 1992). This **"healing ridge"** is an "induration beneath the skin extending to about 1 cm (½ inch) on each side of the wound" (Hunt, 1979) (Fig. 40-2). It is usually present directly under the suture line between days 5 and 9 (Cooper, 1992). Absence of the healing ridge may indicate a wound at risk for dehiscence or infection (Hunt, 1979) (Fig. 40-3).

Types of healing are **primary intention, secondary intention, and tertiary intention.** Healing by primary intention is expected when the edges of a clean surgical incision remain close together. Tissue loss is minimal or absent. The skin cells quickly regenerate, and capillary walls stretch across under the suture line to form a smooth surface as they join.

Healing by secondary intention is quite the opposite and accompanies an open wound with tissue loss and jagged edges. **Granulation tissue** gradually fills in the area of the defect with scar tissue (Fig. 40-4). This process is typical of severe laceration or massive surgical intervention with skin loss. The risk of infection is directly related to the length of time it takes for the body surface to be covered with an intact skin layer. In secondary intention there is some gap between the edges. A thin fibrinous exudate covers the edges of the wound, prevents bacterial invasion, and coagulates surface bleeding. New capillaries are supported by connective tissue. This form of healing results in a thicker surface closure. The slowness of this process places the client at greater risk for infection and collection of body fluids that must be drained to permit healing. Some clients who heal by secondary-intention may develop an excessive amount of connective tissue in the scar surface. This tissue is known as a **keloid.** Other developments may include the formation of a fistula in response to the presence of bacteria in the wound.

Healing by tertiary intention is sometimes called delayed primary intention or closure. It occurs when surgical wounds are not closed immediately but left open for 3 to 5 days to allow edema or infection to diminish. Then the wound edges are sutured or stapled closed. Scarring is usually minimal (Maklebust and Palleschi, 1996). During the healing process a wound may have some type of dressing covering it. The initial dressing is not removed for direct wound inspection until a physician writes a medical order to remove it. Certain situations and some institutional policies govern who changes the dressing the first time. Special attention is paid to maintaining the position of drains during dressing changes (Doughty, 1992). An analgesic, as ordered, should be administered 30 to 45 minutes before changing the dressing. However, the nurse's assessment determines the best time for analgesic administration before wound care. Skin cleansing in the area of the suture line or drain site is indicated when an excessive amount of drainage occurs. The presence of wound exudate is an expected stage of epithelial cell growth.

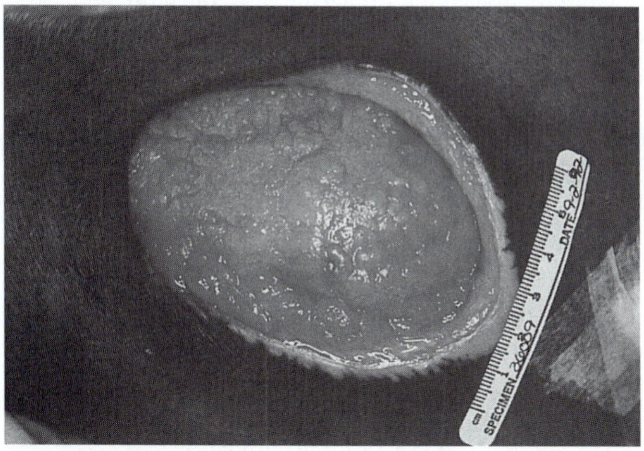

Fig. 40-4 Open wound with granulating base.

Meticulous hand washing and proper infection control procedures before and after removing soiled dressings, coupled with proper wound cleansing procedures, limit the risk of nosocomial infection. Using clean gloves prevents exposure from body fluids, exudate, or bloody drainage from wound. Wound cleansing "delivers a fluid or cleansing solution to the wound surface by means of a specific mechanical force and assists with the separation and removal of necrotic debris, particulate matter, bacteria, and residue of wound care products" (Barr, 1995). Effective wound cleansing can be accomplished by using an appropriate cleansing solution that does not harm the tissue and is delivered by adequate mechanical cleansing force action of either soaking, scrubbing, or irrigation (Barr, 1995). Irrigation is the method of wound cleansing most used by nurses.

Irrigation uses the mechanical force (either high or low) of a stream of solution to loosen particulate matter on the wound surface. The phase of wound healing and goal of wound cleansing determines whether high pressures (which are measured in psi or pounds per square inch) (4 to 25 psi) or low irrigation (<4 psi) is used (Barr, 1995) (Table 40-1). A commonly used high-pressure irrigation system is a 35-cc syringe with a 19-gauge needle or angiocath, which delivers a psi of 8 (AHCPR, 1994). This nursing intervention is used for wounds on any part of the torso or extremities. In addition to cleansing an area, prescribed medications may be introduced in solution form. Principles of basic wound irrigation include the following:

1. Cleanse in a direction from the least contaminated area to the most contaminated.
2. When irrigating, all the solution flows from the least contaminated to the most contaminated area.

When administering an irrigation be sure that the flow of irrigation moves from the area being cleansed to an area that is both distal to and lower than that area. In wound care, the area being cleansed is considered "clean" and the surrounding skin surfaces are considered "contaminated" without respect to whether the wound is infected. Within

Table 40-1 Wound Cleansing Protocol

Mechanical Force	High Pressure	Low Pressure
Phase of healing	Inflammatory	Proliferative
Wound base characteristics	• Presence of necrotic tissue (eschar, fibrin slough), debris, or other particulate matter • Significant bacterial burden • Moderate/large amount of exudate • Residue from wound care products	• Presence of granulation tissue or new epithelial cells • Non/minimum serous or sero-sanguinous exudate • Residue from wound care products
Clinical outcome(s)	• Loosen, soften, and remove devitalized tissue from wound • Separate eschar from fibrotic tissue/fibrotic tissue from granulating base • Remove wound care product residue	• Prevent trauma to viable wound tissue • Remove wound care product residue
Solutions	• Normal saline • Wound cleansers • Amount depends on size of wound	• Normal saline • Amount depends on size of wound
Delivery systems*	• 35 cc syringe/19 gauge angiocath • Irrijet® DS • Pleurovac	• Pouring saline directly from bottle • Bulb syringe • Piston syringe

From Barr JE: Principles of wound cleansing, *Ostomy/Wound Manag* 7A(suppl 41):155, 1995.
*This is not an all-inclusive list of delivery systems available. Inclusion does not imply endorsement.

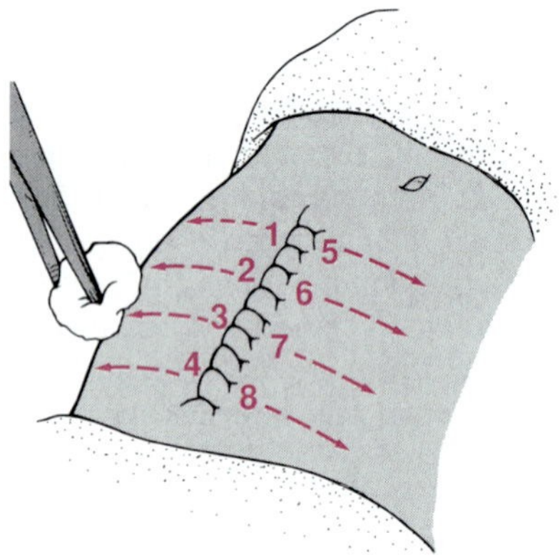

Fig. 40-5 Method of cleansing the suture line area.

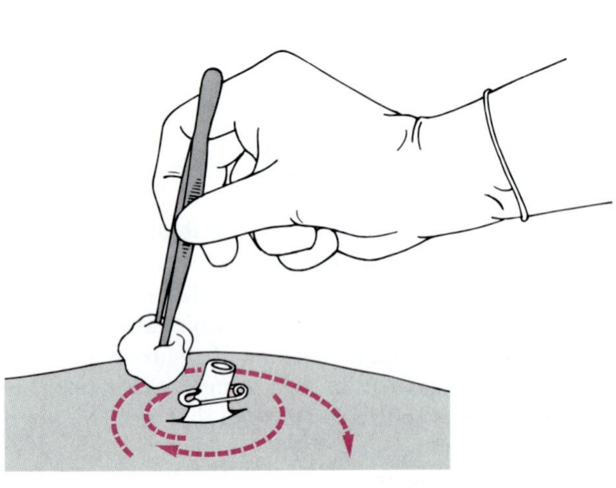

Fig. 40-6 Cleansing a drain site.

the wound, the flow is directed from healthy tissue toward infected tissue.

The suture line is the "least contaminated" area and is always cleansed first (Fig. 40-5). The center is the most important part of the suture line; therefore, clean the suture line itself by starting at the center of the suture line and working toward one end. With another sterile swab or gauze, start at the center of the incision and work toward the other end. All other cleaning involves moving from one end to the other on each side of the incision on the skin surrounding the incision. Work in straight lines, moving away from the suture line with each successive stroke. Use a sterile gauze 2 × 2 containing antiseptic or an antiseptic swab for each stroke.

Irrigating solutions are sterile. In the event that the irrigant has caustic or irritating properties, protect the skin with a skin protectant product and place the collection basin close to the area of the exiting fluid.

The drain site is cleansed using a circular stroke starting with the area immediately next to the drain (Fig. 40-6). With each new swab start immediately next to drain and attempt to cleanse a little further out from the drain.

GUIDELINES

1. Know the client's age. With age, there are vascular changes, collagen tissue is less pliable, and scar tissue is tighter. Because the epidermodermal junction becomes flatter in older adults, their skin tears more easily from mechanical trauma such as tape removal.
2. Know the client's nutritional status. Tissue repair and infection resistance are directly related to adequate nutrition, including proteins, carbohydrates, lipids, vitamins, and minerals (Brylinsky, 1995). Nutrition requirements can double in the presence of infection.

3. Observe for obesity. Inadequate vascularization decreases delivery of nutrients and cellular elements required for healing. The obese client is at greater risk for wound infection and dehiscence or evisceration.
4. Identify factors that decrease oxygenation, such as decreased hemoglobin and smoking. Small wounds heal more quickly when exposed to air. Tissue repair is negatively influenced by a hematocrit value below 33% and a hemoglobin value below 10 g/dl. Hemoglobin is reduced and oxygen release to tissues is reduced in smokers.
5. Know the types of medications prescribed. Steroids reduce inflammatory response and slow collagen synthesis. Cortisone depresses fibroblast activity and capillary growth. Chemotherapy depresses bone marrow.
6. Identify the presence of chronic diseases or chronic trauma, such as diabetes or radiation. Decreased tissue perfusion and failure to release oxygen to tissues result from diabetes. In radiation therapy, wound healing is most effective when surgery is performed within 4 to 6 weeks of irradiation before the anticipated vascular scarring and fibrosis.
7. Unwounded skin is always stronger than healed skin that has been wounded.

SKILL 40-1 Performing Wound Irrigation

Wound cleansing and irrigation is accomplished using sterile technique (surgical wounds) or clean technique (some chronic wounds). The cleansing solution is introduced directly into the wound with either a syringe, syringe and catheter, shower, or whirlpool. When a syringe is used, the tip should remain 2.5 cm (1 inch) above the wound. If the client has a deep wound with a narrow opening, a soft catheter is attached to the syringe to permit the fluid to enter the wound. Irrigation should not cause tissue injury or discomfort. Fluid retention is avoided by positioning the client on the side to encourage the flow of the irrigant away from the wound. With small wounds, it is often helpful to use a 35-ml syringe with a 19-gauge needle attached to facilitate optimal pressure for cleansing with minimal risk of tissue injury (Rodeheaver, 1990). Ambulatory clients may benefit from the use of a hand-held shower for wound cleansing, holding the shower spray approximately 12 inches (30 cm) from the wound. If the force applies too much pressure for the client's comfort, a clean washcloth may be tied around the shower head to disperse the force. An alternative is the shower table (Fig. 40-7), frequently utilized in burn and trauma wound care, which allows cleansing in the acute care area. For clients who require mechanical debridement and cleansing but cannot tolerate the above methods, the whirlpool is a useful method. The whirlpool procedure is frequently performed by or with the assistance of physical therapists, who then help apply dressings.

Wound irrigations promote wound healing through removing debris from a wound surface, decreasing bacterial counts, and loosening and removing eschar. **Eschar** is "thick, leatherly, necrotic, devitalized tissue" (AHCPR, 1994). Solutions used for irrigations include normal saline, warm water, or mild wound cleansers such as Cara Klenz, Saf Clens, and Biolex. Skin cleansers are not the same as wound cleansers and should not be indiscriminately substituted for them.

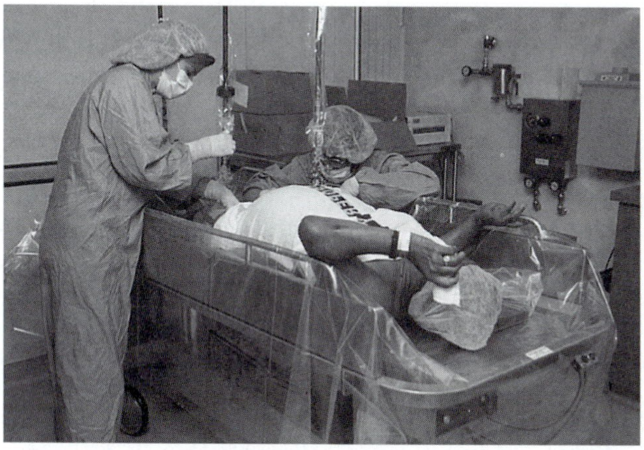

Fig. 40-7 Shower table.

EQUIPMENT

- Irrigant/cleansing solution (volume 1.2 to 2 times the estimated wound volume)
- Irrigation delivery system depending on amount of pressure desired:
  - Sterile irrigation 35-cc syringe with sterile soft angiocath or 19-gauge needle (AHCPR, 1994) *or*
  - Hand-held shower or whirlpool
- Clean gloves
- Sterile gloves
- Waterproof underpad, if needed
- Dressing supplies
- Disposable waterproof bag
- Gown, if risk of spray
- Goggles, if risk of spray

DELEGATION CONSIDERATIONS

Check institutional policy and the state's nurse practice act regarding which wound care interventions can be delegated to unlicensed assistive personnel. The skill of wound irrigation requires problem solving and knowledge application unique to a professional nurse, particularly regarding the assessment of any wounds and care of acute new wounds. However, cleansing of chronic wounds using *clean* technique can be delegated to assistive personnel. In this situation, instruct staff on what to report when a wound is cleansed. Assistive personnel must also know how to use clean technique so as to avoid cross-contamination from irrigation syringes and equipment.

STEPS	RATIONALE
ASSESSMENT	
1. Review physician's order for irrigation of open wound and type of solution to be used.	Open wound irrigation requires medical order including type of solution(s) to use.
2. Assess recent recording of signs and symptoms related to client's open wound:	
a. Extent of impairment of skin integrity, including size of wound (measure length, width, and depth). Wounds should be measured in cm and in the following order: length, width, and depth.	This assesses volume of irrigation solution needed. Data also used as baseline to indicate change in condition of wound.
b. Elevation of body temperature.	May indicate response to infection.
c. Drainage from wound (amount and color). Amount can be measured by part of dressing saturated or in terms of quantity (e.g., scant, moderate, copius).	Expect amount to decrease as healing takes place. Serous drainage is clear; sanguineous or bright red drainage indicates fresh bleeding; serosanguineous drainage is pink; purulent drainage is thick and yellow, pale green, or white.
d. Odor. Must state that there is no odor if none is present. More frequent cleansing is needed if the wound has a foul odor (AHCPR, 1994).	Strong odor indicates infectious process.
e. Consistency of drainage.	Leukocytes produce thick drainage.
f. Culture reports.	Remember that chronic wounds healing by secondary intention are often colonized.
g. Stage of healing of the client's wound.	Client's wound characteristics determine the type and amount of pressure to use during irrigation.
h. Dressing: dry and clean; evidence of bleeding, profuse drainage.	Provides an initial assessment of present wound drainage.
3. Assess comfort level or pain and identify symptoms of anxiety.	Discomfort may be related directly to wound or indirectly to muscle tension or immobility. Anxiety results from multiple factors e.g., surgery, diagnosis, awaiting pathology reports, and anticipation of unknown nursing interventions (e.g., first wound irrigation).
4. Identify client's history of allergies.	Known allergies suggest application of a sample of prescribed antiseptic as skin test before flushing wound with large volume of solution.

NURSING DIAGNOSIS

Clustering of defining characteristics from the assessment data may reveal the following nursing diagnoses for clients requiring this skill:

- Impaired skin integrity
- Impaired tissue integrity
- Pain
- Risk for injury

Related factors are individualized based on client's condition or needs.

STEPS	RATIONALE
PLANNING	
1. Expected outcomes following completion of procedure:	
➤ Client is comfortable after wound irrigation.	Premedication, gently administered irrigation, application of clean dressing, and repositioning client ensure comfort.
➤ Wound begins to heal; dressing is clean and dry; wound is free of drainage and inflammation, or drainage is decreased in amount or type (e.g., less bloody or serous as opposed to serosanguineous).	Healing progresses in absence of debris and presence of protective covering.
➤ Skin integrity is maintained; no redness, edema, or inflammation noted in surrounding tissue.	No further skin and tissue damage has resulted from wound irrigation.
2. Explain procedure of wound irrigation and cleansing.	Information will reduce client's anxiety.
3. Administer prescribed analgesic 30 to 45 minutes before starting wound irrigation procedure.	Increased comfort level permits client to move more easily and be positioned to facilitate wound irrigation.
4. Position client comfortably to permit gravitational flow of irrigating solution through wound and into collection receptacle (see illustration). Position client so that wound is vertical to collection basin.	Directing solution from top to bottom of wound and from clean to contaminated area prevents further infection. Positioning client during planning stage provides bed surfaces for later preparation of equipment.

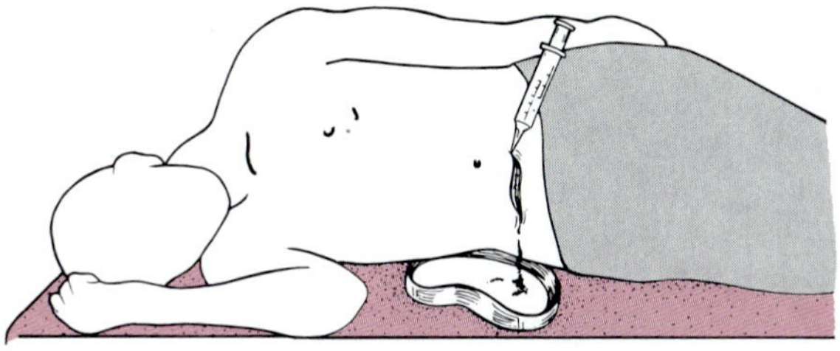

Step 4 Client position for wound irrigation.

STEPS	RATIONALE
IMPLEMENTATION	
1. Warm irrigation solution to approximate body temperature.	Warmed solution increases comfort and reduces vascular constriction response in tissues.
2. Wash hands.	Reduces transmission of microorganisms.
3. Form cuff on waterproof bag and place it near bed.	Cuffing helps to maintain large opening, thereby permitting placement of contaminated dressing without touching refuse bag itself.
4. Close room door or bed curtains.	Maintains privacy.
5. Apply gown and goggles if needed.	Protects nurse from splashes or sprays of blood and body fluids (CDC, 1995).
6. Put on clean gloves and remove soiled dressing and discard in waterproof bag. Discard gloves.	Reduces transmission of microorganisms.
7. Prepare equipment; open sterile supplies.	
8. Put on sterile gloves.	
9. To irrigate wound with wide opening:	
a. Fill 35-cc syringe with irrigation solution.	Flushing wound helps remove debris and facilitates healing by secondary intention.
b. Attach 19-gauge needle or angiocath.	Provides ideal pressure for cleansing and removal of debris.
c. Hold syringe tip 2.5 cm (1 inch) above upper end of wound and over area being cleansed.	Prevents syringe contamination. Careful placement of the syringe prevents unsafe pressure of the flowing solution.

STEPS	RATIONALE
d. Using continuous pressure, flush wound; repeat Steps 9a, b, and c until solution draining into basin is clear.	Clear solution indicates all debris has been removed.
10. To irrigate deep wound with very small opening:	
a. Attach soft angiocatheter to filled irrigating syringe.	Catheter permits direct flow of irrigant into wound. Expect wound to take longer to empty when opening is small.
b. Lubricate tip of catheter with irrigating solution; then gently insert tip of catheter and pull out about 1 cm (½ inch).	Removes tip from fragile inner wall of wound.
c. Using slow, continuous pressure, flush wound.	

CRITICAL DECISION POINT **CAUTION: Splashing may occur during this step.**

STEPS	RATIONALE
d. Pinch off catheter just below syringe while keeping catheter in place.	Avoids contamination of sterile solution.
e. Remove and refill syringe. Reconnect to catheter and repeat until solution draining into basin is clear.	
11. To cleanse wound with hand-held shower:	Useful for clients able to shower with assistance or independently. May be accomplished at home. A shower table (see Fig. 40-7, p. 1132) is helpful for bed-bound or acutely ill clients.
a. With client seated comfortably in shower chair, adjust spray to gentle flow; water temperature should be warm.	
b. Cover shower head with clean washcloth if needed.	
c. Shower for 5 to 10 minutes with shower head 12 inches (30 cm) from wound.	
12. To cleanse wound with whirlpool:	
a. Adjust water level and temperature; add prescribed cleansing agent.	
b. Assist client into whirlpool or place extremity into whirlpool.	
c. Allow client to remain in whirlpool for prescribed interval.	

CRITICAL DECISION POINT **Position client so that the water jets are not directly over the clean granulating wound tissue.**

STEPS	RATIONALE
13. Obtain cultures (see Chapter 43), if needed, after cleansing with nonbacteriostatic saline.	Routine culturing of open wounds is not recommended by AHCPR (1994). AHCPR (1994) recommends using quantitative bacterial cultures (tissue biopsy or wound fluid by needle aspiration) rather than swab cultures, which often detect only surface bacterial contaminants.

CRITICAL DECISION POINT **Consider culturing a wound if it has a foul, purulent odor; inflammation surrounds the wound; a nondraining wound begins to drain; or client is febrile.**

STEPS	RATIONALE
13. Dry wound edges with gauze; dry client if shower or whirlpool is used.	Prevents maceration of surrounding tissue from excess moisture.
14. Apply appropriate dressing (see Chapter 37).	Maintains protective barrier and healing environment for wound.
15. Remove gloves, and if worn, mask, goggles, and gown.	Prevents transfer of microorganisms.

STEPS	RATIONALE
16. Assist client to comfortable position.	
17. Dispose of equipment and soiled supplies. Wash hands.	Reduces transmission of microorganisms.

EVALUATION

1. Assess type of tissue in the wound bed.	Identifies wound healing progress and determines type of wound cleansing needed.
2. Inspect dressing periodically.	Determines client's response to wound irrigation and need to modify plan of care.
3. Evaluate skin integrity.	Determines if extension of wound has occurred.
4. Observe client for signs of discomfort.	Client's pain should not increase as a result of wound irrigation.
5. Observe for presence of retained irrigant.	Retained irrigant is a medium for bacterial growth and subsequent infection.
6. **Unexpected outcomes** that may occur include:	
➤ Bleeding or serosanguineous drainage appears.	Client has increased vulnerability to hemorrhage based on fragility of capillaries, inadequate cellular nutrition, and infectious process. May also indicate that wound irrigation pressure is too high for the wound. Reduce pressure during next irrigation.
➤ Retained fluid and debris appears.	Client is at risk for fistulization or infection.
➤ Increased pain or discomfort occurs.	May indicate further wound trauma or infection.
➤ Suture line opening extends. Notify physician and reevaluate amount of pressure to use for next wound irrigation.	Risk for dehiscence exists.

RECORDING AND REPORTING

1. Record wound irrigation and client response on progress notes.	Recording fulfills legal responsibility of nurse and provides information needed to ensure continuity of care.
2. Immediately report any evidence of fresh bleeding, sharp increase in pain, retention of irrigant, or signs of shock to attending physician.	These are presenting signs of tissue damage and fistula or sinus tract development. Shock phenomena may indicate internal bleeding or tissue damage.
3. At change of shift, report expected and unexpected outcomes that have actually occurred.	Continuity of care is facilitated by accurately reporting findings.

FOLLOW-UP ACTIVITIES

1. Shower or whirlpool should be cleansed with disinfectant solution after use.

• • • • •

Special Considerations

➤ Do not use cytotoxic solutions (e.g., Dakin's solution, acetic acid, hydrogen peroxide, povidone-iodine) to irrigate wounds. These cytotoxic solutions kill fibroblasts that lay down collagen, which is necessary for wound repair. Dakin's solution that has been improperly prepared can cause chemical burns to the tissue, because it is made with bleach. Hydrogen peroxide can cause air embolus. Client allergy and iodine toxicity have been reported with povidone-iodine use.

➤ Plan wound irrigation at time that permits physician and nurse to inspect wound simultaneously. This reduces number of dressing changes and possible client discomfort, limiting exposure to pathogens.

➤ Call light should be within reach of client in shower or whirlpool.

Teaching Considerations

➤ Instruct client and primary care giver to observe wound care, and provide time for return demonstrations.

➤ Explain the need for specialized supplies such as irrigating solutions and dressings and the need to maintain asepsis when performing care.

➤ Instruct client and care giver where and how additional supplies are obtained.

➤ Instruct client and primary care giver about signs of improper wound healing and wound infection.

Pediatric Considerations

- Pediatric clients may be very frightened. They might verbally and physically try to prevent the nurse from cleaning the wound. Having the child active in parts of the procedure or working out the child's feelings about wound irrigation using play therapy on a doll with a wound may help the child to be more cooperative with the procedure.
- Skin on neonates is immature and can easily be damaged from pressure and wound care products. Check that the products are approved for use with this population. Remember that in neonates the skin readily absorbs products.
- Assess need for pain management. Provide pain management before performing wound irrigation.

Gerontologic Considerations

- Wound irrigations can be traumatic, frightening, and painful to some older adult clients. The nurse should assess the client's cooperation before doing a wound irrigation. The nurse should be mindful of the client's cognitive level of understanding when performing a wound irrigation.
- Older skin loses many of its normal characteristics; therefore it is more easily damaged from trauma due to the cleaning process.
- Use one of the pain scales to assess if client has pain from the wound. Provide pain management before performing wound irrigation.

Home Care Considerations

- Assess client's and primary care giver's understanding of need for and methods of wound care.
- Assess client's home environment to determine adequacy of facilities for performing wound care; check especially for adequate lighting, running water, and storage of supplies.
- Teach client and care giver how to make normal saline, especially if cost is an issue. Normal saline can be made by using 2 teaspoons of salt in 1 liter (1 quart) of boiling water (Barr, 1995).
- Tell client and care giver that because normal saline has no preservatives, it should be thrown out 24 to 48 hours after it is first opened or made (Barr, 1995).

SKILL 40-2 Performing Suture and Staple Removal

Institutional policy determines whether *only* the physician or the physician *and* nurse may remove sutures and staples. The physician's written order is always obtained before implementing either skill. The time of removal is based on the stage of incisional healing and extent of surgery.

Sutures and staples are generally removed within 7 to 10 days after surgery if healing is adequate. Timing the removal of sutures and staples is important. They are left in long enough to ensure initial wound closure with enough strength to support internal tissues and organs. Leaving them in too long increases the risk of infection at the puncture sites. The physician determines and orders removal of all sutures or staples at one time or removal of every other suture or staple as the first phase, with the remainder removed in the second phase.

Sutures are threads of wire or other materials used to sew body tissues together. Sutures are placed within tissue layers in deep wounds and superficially as the final means for wound closure. The deeper sutures are usually an absorbable material that disappears in several days.

Staples are made of stainless steel wire. Their use is restricted by the location of the incision, because there must be adequate distance between the skin and structures that lie below the skin, including bone and vascular structures. The cosmetic result may not be as desirable as that obtained with finer suture material. Staples do provide ample strength. Removal requires a sterile staple extractor and maintenance of aseptic technique.

The client's history of wound healing, site of wound, tissues involved, and the purpose of the sutures determine the suture material selected. For example, a client with repeated abdominal surgeries might require wire sutures for greater strength to promote wound closure.

The physician and/or nurse judge whether to remove all sutures if any sign of suture line separation is evident during the process of suture or staple removal. It is not uncommon to remove every other suture initially, removing the balance several days to a week later.

EQUIPMENT

- Disposable waterproof bag
- Sterile suture removal set (forceps and scissors) or sterile staple extractor
- Sterile applicators or antiseptic swabs
- Steri-Strips or butterfly adhesive strips
- Clean gloves
- Sterile disposable gloves

DELEGATION CONSIDERATIONS

This skill requires problem solving and knowledge application unique to a professional nurse. For this skill, delegation is inappropriate.

STEPS	RATIONALE
ASSESSMENT	
1. Identify client with need for suture or staple removal: check physician's order.	Removal of sutures or staples is a dependent intervention. Adequate healing should have taken place within this time frame.
a. Review specific directions related to suture or staple removal.	Indicates specifically which sutures are to be removed (e.g., every other suture).
b. Determine history of conditions that may interfere with healing.	
(1) Conditions that place client at risk for impaired healing include advanced age, cardiovascular disease, diabetes, immunosuppression, radiation, obesity, smoking, poor cellular nutrition, very deep wounds, and infection.	Preexisting health disorders affect speed of healing and may result in dehiscence.
2. Assess client for history of allergies.	Determines if client is sensitive to antiseptic.
3. Inspect skin integrity of suture line for uniform closure of wound edges, normal color, and absence of drainage and inflammation.	Indicates adequate wound-healing for support of internal structures without continued need for sutures or staples.

NURSING DIAGNOSIS

Clustering of defining characteristics from the assessment data may reveal the following nursing diagnoses for clients requiring this skill:

- Impaired skin integrity
- Risk for impaired skin integrity
- Risk for infection

Related factors are individualized based on a client's condition or needs.

STEPS	RATIONALE
PLANNING	
1. **Expected outcomes** following completion of procedure:	
➤ All suture material or staples are removed.	Removes source of infection or irritation from retained sutures.
➤ Suture line is intact.	Wound is dry and intact and does not require protective dressings.
2. Explain to client that suture removal is usually not a painful procedure but that client may feel pulling or tugging of the skin.	Gains client cooperation and reduces anxiety.

CRITICAL DECISION POINT For client who is highly anxious or who has an extensive wound, consider need to administer analgesic 30 minutes before suture removal.

STEPS	RATIONALE
IMPLEMENTATION	
1. Close curtains or room door.	Provides privacy.
2. Position client comfortably, while exposing suture line.	Prepares area for staple or suture removal.
3. Ensure direct lighting is on suture line.	Aids visibility and correct placement of forceps or extractor during removal process, ultimately reducing soft tissue injury.
4. Wash hands.	Reduces risk of infection.
5. Place cuffed refuse disposal bag within easy reach.	Provides for easy disposal of contaminated dressings and prevents passing items over sterile work area.
6. Prepare sterile field with dressing change supplies:	Allows nurse to freely handle sterile supplies.
a. Open sterile suture removal tray or staple extract tray and slide contents onto prepared field, maintaining sterility of inside surface of wrapper or tray (see Chapter 34).	

STEPS	RATIONALE
b. Open sterile antiseptic swabs and place on inside surface of tray.	
c. Open sterile glove package, exposing cuffed ends.	
7. Apply clean gloves, remove dressing, and discard dressing and clean gloves in prepared refuse disposal bag.	Reduces transmission of infection.
8. Inspect wound (see illustration).	Determines adequacy of wound healing.
9. Apply sterile gloves, if required by policy.	Allows nurse to handle sterile supplies.
10. Cleanse sutures or staples and healed incision with antiseptic swabs.	Removes surface bacteria from incision and sutures or staples.
11. Remove staples:	
a. Place lower tips of staple extractor under first staple. As you close handles, upper tip of extractor depresses center of staple, causing both ends of staple to be bent upward and simultaneously exit their insertion sites in the dermal layer (see illustrations).	Avoids excess pressure to suture line and secures smooth removal of each staple.
b. Carefully control staple extractor.	Avoids suture-line pressure and pain.
c. As soon as both ends of staple are visible, move it away from skin surface and continue on until staple is over refuse bag (see illustration).	Prevents scratching tender skin surface with sharp pointed ends of staple for comfort and infection control.

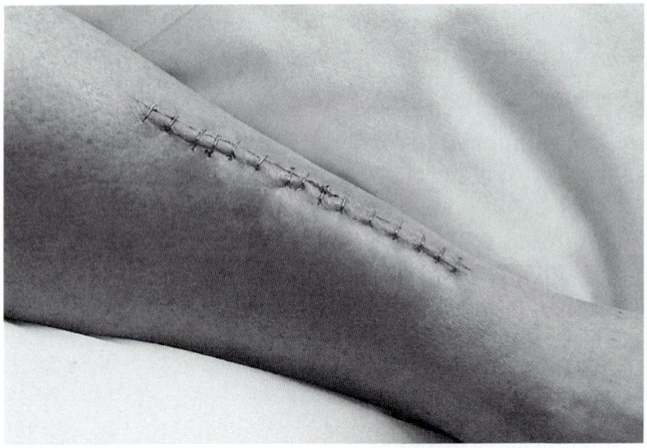

Step 8

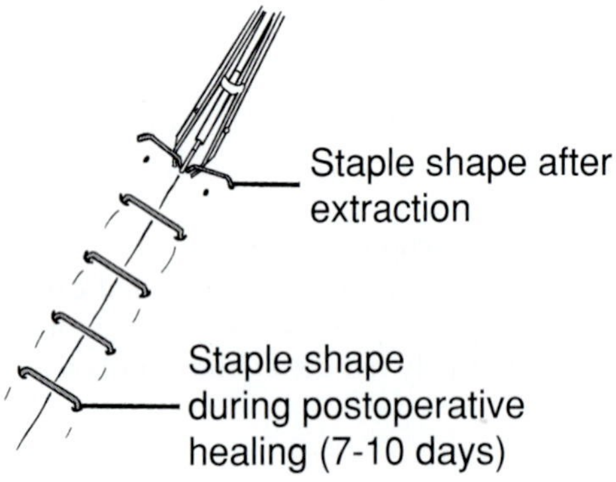

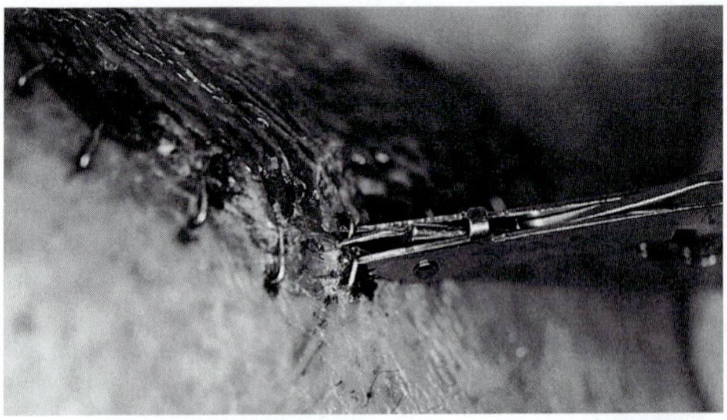

Step 11a

STEPS	RATIONALE
d. Release handles of staple extractor, allowing staple to drop into refuse bag.	Avoids contaminating sterile field with used staples.
e. Repeat Steps a through c until all staples are removed.	
12. Remove intermittent sutures* (see illustration):	
a. Place gauze a few inches from suture line. Grasp scissors in dominant hand and forceps in nondominant hand.	Gauze serves as receptacle for removed sutures. Placement of scissors and forceps allows for efficient suture removal.

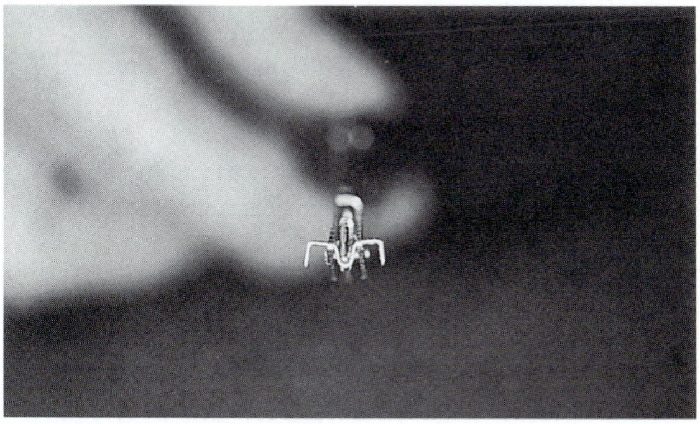

Step 11c

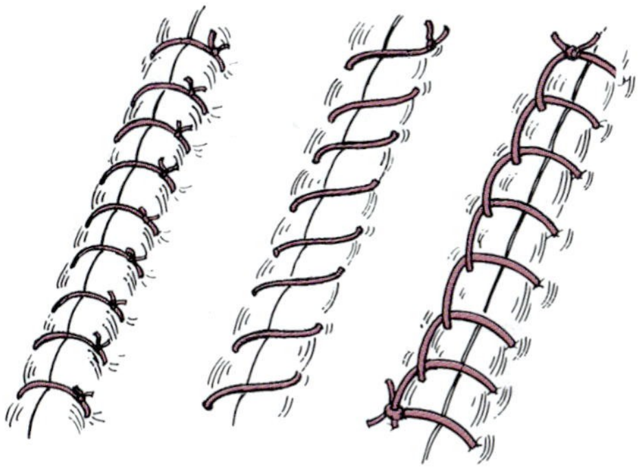

Step 12 *Left,* Intermittent; *middle,* continuous; *right,* blanket.

CRITICAL DECISION POINT **Placement of scissors and forceps is very important. Avoid pinching the skin around the wound when lifting up the suture. Likewise, avoid cutting the skin around the wound by accident when snipping the suture.**

b. Snip suture, close to skin surface, at end distal to knot (see illustration). Be sure ends are completely severed by gently lifting exposed end away from skin.	Releases suture.

*Each suture has a knot. Each interrupted suture is secured with its own knot. Knots are lined up on same side of incision.

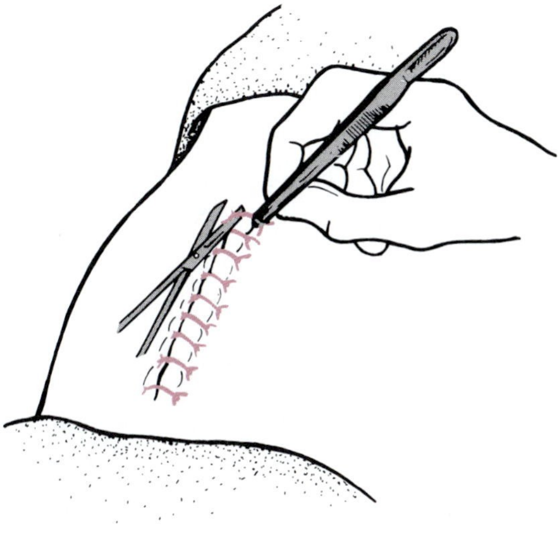

Step 12b Removal of intermittent suture. Nurse cuts suture as close to skin as possible, away from the knot.

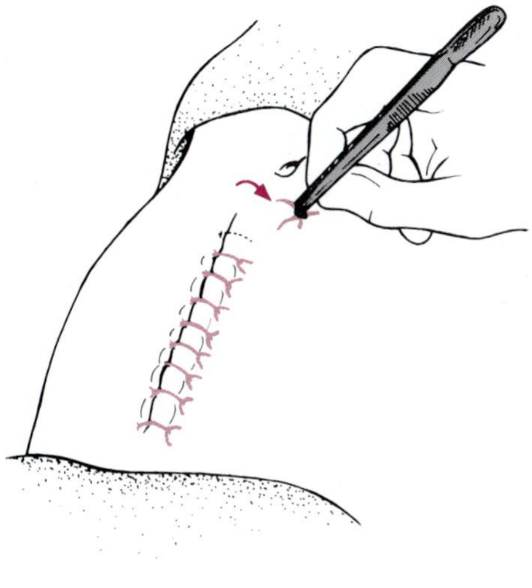

Step 12c Nurse removes suture and never pulls the contaminated stitch through tissues.

STEPS	RATIONALE
CRITICAL DECISION POINT Never snip both ends of suture; there will be no way to remove half of suture situated below the surface.	
c. Grasp knotted end with forceps and in one continuous smooth action remove entire suture (see illustration). Place suture on gauze.	Smoothly removes suture without additional tension to suture line.
CRITICAL DECISION POINT Never pull exposed surface of any suture into tissue below epidermis. The exposed surface of any suture is considered contaminated.	
d. Repeat Steps a through c until every other suture has been removed.	
e. Observe healing level. Based on observations of wound response to suture removal and physician's original order, determine whether remaining sutures will be removed at this time. If so, repeat Steps a through c until all sutures have been removed.	Determines status of wound healing and if suture line will remain closed after all sutures are removed.
f. If any doubt, stop and notify physician.	
13. Remove continuous sutures including blanket stitch sutures (see illustration Step 12):	
a. Place sterile gauze a few inches from suture line. Grasp scissors in dominant hand and forceps in nondominant hand.	Gauze serves as receptacle for removed sutures. Placement of scissors and forceps allows for efficient suture removal.
b. Snip first suture close to skin surface at end distal to knot.	
CRITICAL DECISION POINT Never snip both ends of suture; there will be no way to remove half of suture situated below surface.	
c. Snip second "suture" on same side.	Releases interrupted sutures from knot.
d. Grasp knotted end and remove first line of spiral in continuous smooth action, pulling away from severed end. Place "suture" on gauze compress.	Smoothly remove sutures without additional tension to suture line.
e. Repeat Steps a through d in consecutive order until the entire line has been removed.	
14. Inspect incision site and identify any trouble areas. Gently wipe suture line with antiseptic swab to remove debris and cleanse wound.	Reduces risk of further incision line separation.
CRITICAL DECISION POINT Make sure that all of the suture has been removed and that no part of it has been retained in the client's wound.	
15. If *any* separation is apparent, place supportive butterfly closures across area to maintain contact between wound edges.	Prevents further wound separation.
16. Apply light dressing or expose to air if no clothing will come in contact with suture line. Instruct client about applying own dressing if it will be needed at home.	Healing by primary intention eliminates need for dressing.

STEPS	RATIONALE
17. Discard all contaminated materials and remove and dispose of gloves.	Reduces transmission of infection.
18. Route reusable items such as staple extractor for resterilization, and wash hands.	Reduces transmission of infection.

EVALUATION

1. Assess site where sutures or staples were removed; inspect condition of soft tissues, including skin. Look for any pieces of removed suture that were left behind.	Sources of infection have been removed.
2. Determine if client has pain along incision.	Determines comfort level. Can indicate if suture material remains in skin.
3. **Unexpected outcomes** that may occur include:	
➤ Retained suture.	On rare occasions suture may become obscured or imbedded so deeply in clotted scab formation that it is not recognized. This multiplies risk of infection.
➤ Wound separation or drainage secondary to healing problems.	Predisposition to wound healing problems includes diabetes, immunosuppression, radiation, wound stress, age, inadequate cellular nutrition, obesity, smoking, inadequate tissue oxygenation, and depth of wound.

RECORDING AND REPORTING

1. Record on client's progress note *number* of sutures or staples removed and appearance of wound. Indicate that entire suture was removed.	Documents condition of suture line and status of wound healing.
2. Report time sutures were removed, level of healing of wound, and client's response to suture removal.	Notifies all personnel of procedure and status of wound healing.
3. Notify physician immediately of any of the following findings: suture line separation, **dehiscence, evisceration,** bleeding, or purulent drainage.	Facilitates rapid response and intervention.

FOLLOW-UP ACTIVITIES

1. Inspect incision site every shift and PRN if client identifies change in sensation.

• • • • •

Special Considerations

- ➤ Wire sutures are removed by the physician.
- ➤ When used, Steri-Strips or butterfly tape closures should be allowed to fall off.
- ➤ Skin testing may be advisable before use of antiseptic swabs at wound site.
- ➤ Limit amount of dressing supplies, because either a very light dressing or no dressing will be needed after suture or staple removal.
- ➤ Inadequate wound healing justifies discontinuing removal of all staples. Notify physician immediately.
- ➤ Continuous suture has one knot at each end of entire incision. One long "thread" spirals around entire line at evenly spaced intervals. Surface appearance will be very similar to line of interrupted sutures, except that each section crossing incision line does not have knot (see illustration p. 1145).
- ➤ Another type of continuous stitch is "blanket continuous suture." This spirals along incision with each turn pulled over to one side. Thread is looped around thread of previous stitch before making the next turn in spiral (see illustration, Step 12, p. 1145).

Teaching Considerations

- ➤ Crusting from around sutures can be removed with half-strength hydrogen peroxide as long as skin is intact.
- ➤ Teach client to observe for any sign of separation of wound edges before removing remaining sutures.
- ➤ Have client apply own dressing and inspect suture line for continued healing. Continue instruction on resumption of showering activities, prevention of abdominal strain during defecation, and provision of adequate nutrition and ambulation. Explain

gradual suture line skin color changes (e.g., in light-tone clients from red to natural color).
- Teach client not to put additional stress on the suture line from such activities as lifting or bending (Maklebust and Palleschi, 1996). Client with abdominal surgery or injury must avoid lifting heavy packages or equipment for several weeks.
- Determine whether client can bathe once sutures are removed.
- Instruct primary care giver and client to maintain clean technique when treating suture line and changing dressings.
- Instruct client that sometimes there may be a small amount of drainage from the wound immediately after suture removal.

Pediatric Considerations
- Assistance may be needed to keep babies from moving during the suture removal procedure.

Gerontologic Considerations
- Older adults may need reassurance about the suture removal procedure. Depending on their mental status, they may not understand the procedure.
- Older skin may be at higher risk for dehiscence after sutures are removed.

SKILL 40-3 Performing Drainage Evacuation

A wound heals only if drainage does not accumulate in the wound bed. Removal of even small amounts of drainage is accomplished by either a closed or open drain system. The drain may be inserted directly through the suture line into the wound or through a small stab wound near the suture line into the wound.

An open drain system (e.g., a **Penrose drain** [Fig. 40-8]) removes drainage from the wound and deposits it onto the skin surface. A safety pin is inserted through this drain, outside the skin, to prevent the tubing from moving into the wound.

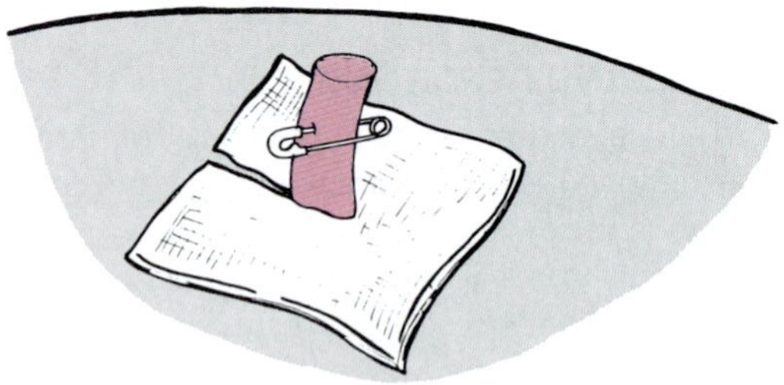

Fig. 40-8 Penrose drain with a drain-split gauze.

A

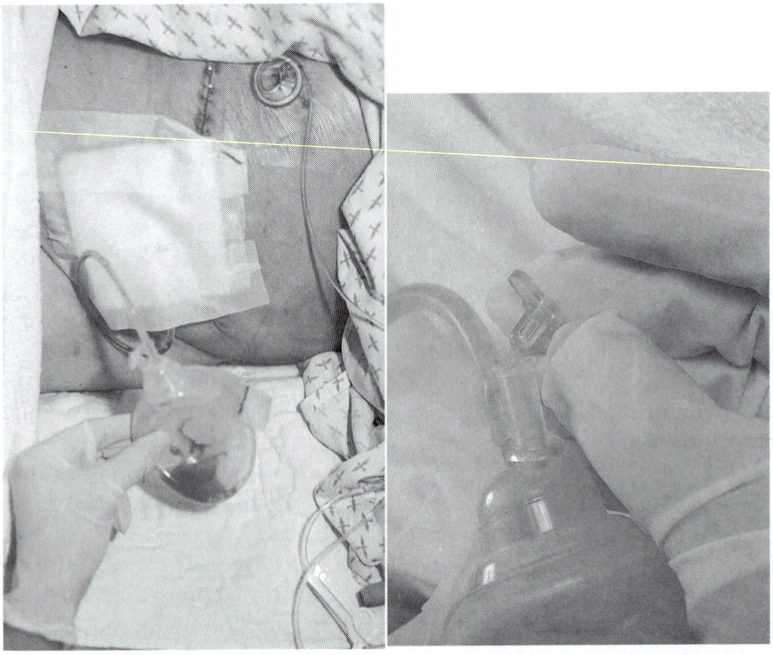

B

Fig. 40-9 **A,** Jackson-Pratt wound drainage system. **B,** Emptying Jackson-Pratt device.

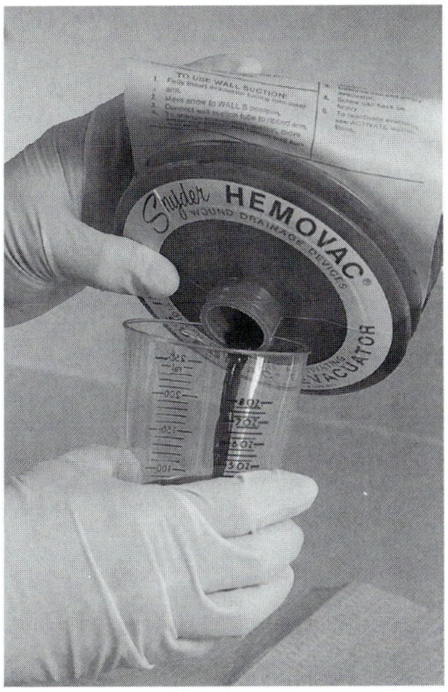

Fig. 40-10 Hemovac wound drainage system.

To remove the Penrose drain the physician advances the tubing in stages as the wound heals from the bottom up. Nursing interventions include caution to prevent accidental removal of the drain during dressing changes and to protect skin surfaces in direct contact with the irritating drainage. Because of the danger of accidental dislodgement and need to assess the drain placement accurately, Penrose drains that are covered with gauze pads are usually changed by the nurse and are not delegated to unlicensed assistive personnel. Some Penrose drains are contained within wound pouches. For these drains, the *emptying* of the wound pouch container can be safely delegated to unlicensed assistive personnel.

A closed drain system (e.g., the **Jackson-Pratt [JP] drain** [Fig. 40-9]), **Hemovac drain** (Fig. 40-10), VacuDrain, or Constavac relies on the presence of a vacuum to withdraw accumulated drainage through multiple perforations in clear plastic tubing into the closed reservoir, suction bladder, or bag. The closed system ensures dry skin but operates only if the tubing is patent and a vacuum exists. Drainage is emptied periodically from the reservoir, and the vacuum is reestablished.

EQUIPMENT

- **Graduated measuring cylinder**
- **Alcohol sponge**
- **Gauze sponges**
- **Goggles**
- **Sterile specimen container, if culture is needed**
- **Sterile dressings or pouch, if drain is needed**
- **Clean disposable gloves**
- **Safety pin(s)**

DELEGATION CONSIDERATIONS

Assessment of wound drainage and maintenance of drains and the drainage system requires problem solving and knowledge application unique to a professional nurse. However, an unlicensed assistive personnel may be delegated the skill of emptying a closed drainage container, measuring the amount of drainage, and reporting the amount on the client's I&O record. The nurse should assist the staff in reviewing I&O procedure.

STEPS	RATIONALE
ASSESSMENT	
1. Identify presence, location, and purpose of closed wound drain and drainage system as client returns from surgery.	Drainage tubing may be placed within wound or through small surgical incision near major wound.
2. Identify *number* of wound drain tubes and what drainage each one ought to be draining. Label each drain tube with a number or label.	Assigning a labeling system to each drain helps with consistent documentation when client has multiple drainage tubes.
3. Assess if the drain tube needs self-suction, wall suction, or no suction by checking the physician orders.	Some drain tubes such as Hemovacs can be used with self-suction or wall suction.
4. Inspect system to determine presence of one straight tube or Y tube arrangement with two tube insertion sites.	To plan skin care and identify quantity of sterile dressing supplies.
5. Inspect system to ensure proper functioning. A complete systematic inspection should include the insertion site, drainage moving through tubing in direction of reservoir (tubing patent), airtight connection sites, and presence of any leaks or kinks in the system.	Properly functioning system maintains suction until reservoir is filled; drainage is no longer being produced or accumulated. Tension on drainage tubing increases injury to skin and underlying muscle.

STEPS	RATIONALE
CRITICAL DECISION POINT **Attach the drainage tubing with tape and a safety pin to the client's gown so that it does not pull on the insertion site.**	
6. Be sure the Penrose drain has a sterile safety pin in place. Penrose drains may be covered with a gauze dressing or a closed wound container.	Pin prevents drain from being pulled below the skin's surface.
7. Identify type of drainage container client has.	Determines frequency for emptying drainage.

NURSING DIAGNOSIS

Clustering of defining characteristics from the assessment data may reveal the following nursing diagnoses for clients requiring this skill:

- Impaired skin integrity
- Risk for infection
- Risk for injury

Related factors are individualized based on a client's condition or needs.

PLANNING

1. **Expected outcomes** following completion of procedure:	
➤ Wound healing continues.	Client will be comfortable and epithelialization will continue in the absence of infectious pathogens or accumulated debris.
➤ Vacuum is reestablished.	Suction system is intact.
➤ Tubing is patent.	Fluid is draining away from wound.
2. Explain procedure to client.	Promotes client's cooperation.

IMPLEMENTATION

1. Close room door or bedside curtains.	Provides privacy.
2. Wash hands and apply gloves. Goggles should be worn only if the potential for splashing exists.	Reduces transmission of microorganisms.
3. Place open specimen container or measuring graduate on bed between you and client.	Permits measuring and discarding of wound drainage.
4. When emptying evacuator, maintain asepsis while opening port:	Avoids entry of pathogens.
a. Hemovac (see Fig. 40-10):	
(1) Open plug on port indicated for emptying drainage reservoir.	Vacuum will be broken and reservoir will pull air in until chamber is fully expanded.
(2) Tilt evacuator in direction of plug.	
(3) Slowly squeeze two flat surfaces together while draining into sterile laboratory specimen container if culture is ordered and remainder into graduated cylinder. Cover specimen container.	Prevents splashing of contaminated drainage.
(4) Hold uncovered alcohol sponge in dominant hand; place evacuator on flat surface with open outlet facing upward; continue pressing downward until bottom and top are in contact; hold surfaces together with one hand, quickly cleanse opening and plug with other hand, and immediately replace plug; secure evacuator on client's bed.	Compression of surface of Hemovac creates vacuum. Cleansing of plug reduces transmission of microorganisms into drainage evacuation.
(5) Check evacuator for reestablishment of vacuum, patency of drainage tubing, and absence of stress on tubing.	Facilitates wound drainage and prevents tension on drainage tubing.

STEPS	RATIONALE
b. Jackson-Pratt evacuator (see Fig. 40-9, *A*):	
(1) Open emptying port on opposite side of bulb-shaped reservoir (see Fig. 40-9, *B*).	
(2) Compress bulb over drainage container.	Empties drainage and reestablishes vacuum.
• Cleanse ends of emptying port with alcohol sponge. Replace cap immediately. Secure evacuator below wound site with safety pin through indicated perforation to client's gown.	Reduces transmission of microorganisms into drainage evacuator and prevents tension on drainage tubing.
5. Place and secure drainage reservoirs to prevent any pull on tubing insertion sites.	Pinning the drainage tubing to the client's gown will prevent tension or pulling on the tubing and insertion site.

CRITICAL DECISION POINT **Be sure there is slack in the tubing from the reservoir to wound.**

STEPS	RATIONALE
6. Route labeled specimen to laboratory if ordered by physician *or* if purulence is noted.	Allows for culture testing to reveal infection.
7. Discard soiled supplies, remove gloves, and wash hands.	Reduces transmission of microorganisms.
8. Apply new sterile gloves and proceed with dressing change (see Chapter 37) around drain site and inspection of skin if indicated or ordered. Split-drain sponge dressings are often used around drain tubes (see illustration A-B) and then covered with gauze. Penrose drains are either covered with gauze dressings or a wound pouch.	Prevents entrance of bacteria into surgical wound.
9. Discard contaminated materials and wash hands.	Reduces transmission of microorganisms.

EVALUATION

STEPS	RATIONALE
1. Observe for drainage in drainage evacuator.	Indicates presence of vacuum, patency of tubing, and functioning of drainage evacuator.
2. Inspect wound for drainage or collection of drainage fluid under the skin causing a seroma.	Drainage should not be significant under suture line. Indicates inadequate functioning of drainage evacuator.

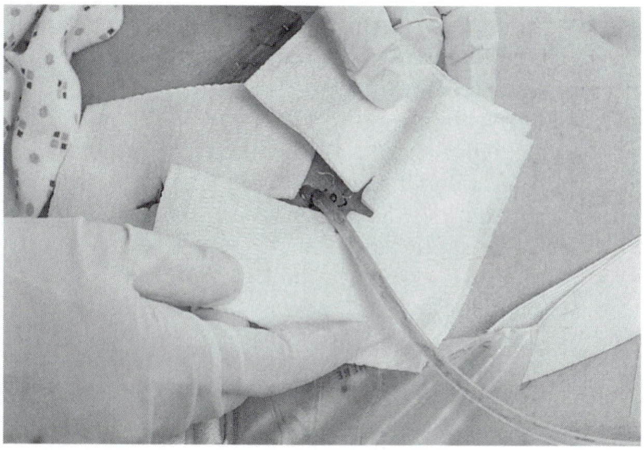

Step 8a Jackson-Pratt drain-split gauze dressing. Applying a split-drain dressing around a JP drain tube.

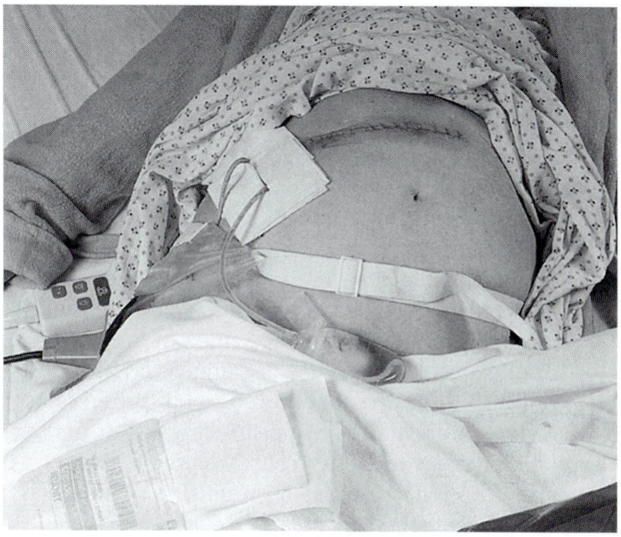

Step 8b Split-drain dressing in place around a JP drain tube.

STEPS	RATIONALE
3. Assess client's level of comfort.	Procedure should not increase client's pain.
4. Unexpected outcomes that may occur include:	
➤ There is nosocomial infection, indicated by purulent drainage, increased WBC count, and temperature elevation.	May indicate absence of scrupulous aseptic technique by care giver.
➤ There is soft-tissue injury indicated by bleeding and pain.	Tension on client's drainage tube insertion site.
➤ Drainage evacuator system is not accumulating drainage.	Air leaks at any connection site or in reservoir. Kinks in tubing or occluded tubing prohibits drainage flow.
CRITICAL DECISION POINT **Clots or large collections of debris may prohibit drainage flow. An area especially prone to clogging from drainage is the Y site in the drainage tubing.**	
➤ Pain.	Pain can result from infection, wound edema, increased drainage, and manipulation of drainage device.

Recording and Reporting

1. Record results of emptying wound drainage evacuator and dressing change (when performed) on progress notes and I&O record. Note characteristics of drainage; measure volume and discard.	Documents amount of drainage in client's record in appropriate place (e.g., I&O sheet). Documents progress of healing and continuity of care.
2. Quickly report to the physician:	
a. Sudden change in amount of drainage, either output or absence of drainage flow.	If vacuum drainage system is functioning, this may indicate occlusion of openings in tubing within wound.
b. Pungent odor of drainage or new evidence of purulence.	Infectious process requires intervention.
c. Severe pain.	
d. Dislodgement of the drainage tube.	Penrose drains often are not sutured in place and can become dislodged.
3. Report presence of functioning drainage evacuator and emptying frequency at change-of-shift report to nurse.	Ensures continuity of care and evaluation of wound-healing progress.

Follow-up Activities

1. Obtain suture removal set before removal of tubing by physician.

• • • • •

Special Considerations

- ➤ Placement of drainage tubing in major suture line is avoided to promote healing and decrease risk of infection. Drainage tubing has series of perforations to facilitate removal of accumulated debris and drainage.
- ➤ Drainage collection reservoir is emptied every 8 hours and PRN for large drainage volume. The nurse collects diagnostic specimen in the presence of unexpected purulence or pungent odor, reports findings to physician, and records in progress note.
- ➤ New wound drainage appears very red at first and later changes to lighter color. Volume decreases after 2 to 3 days and as it diminishes, whole system can be removed.
- ➤ Both Hemovac and Jackson-Pratt drainage evacuators have two openings. One is attached to tubing that carries drainage from client's wound to drainage chamber or reservoir. Second port is used to empty collected drainage.
- ➤ Attaching wall suction to Hemovac:
  - Connect graduated adaptor to emptying port and then to wall suction tubing.
  - Set suction level as prescribed, or on *low* if suction level not specified.
- ➤ Attaching wall suction to the Jackson-Pratt:
  - Attach connecting adaptor to suction tubing.
  - Set suction level as prescribed, or at *low* if not specified.
  - Attach tubing with graduated connector to open port and secure with tape.
- ➤ Drainage reservoirs fill slowly. If rapid expansion occurs after reestablishing drainage system, check

all connections, wound site, and reservoir for source of air leakage.
- To prevent cross-infections, maintain individualized equipment for drainage collection.

Teaching Considerations

- Instruct client about anticipated postoperative drainage, expected progress of wound healing and drainage volume, and estimated date of removal of drain as volume diminishes.
- Unexplained dark red drainage is major concern to any client. Being aware of what to expect reduces anxiety.
- Instruct primary care giver and client on how to change dressings located around drain site.
- Instruct client to wear loose-fitting clothes.
- Instruct client to keep drain lower than waist level when ambulating, sitting, or lying down.
- Instruct client not to pull or tug on tubing; secure drain with safety pin.

Pediatric Considerations

- Have parents help to prevent pediatric clients from dislodging drainage tubes.

Gerontologic Considerations

- Be aware that clients with large amounts of drainage will need additional fluid intake to prevent dehydration.
- Measures may need to be taken to prevent a confused client from pulling out the drain collector.

Home Care Considerations

- Dispose of drainage in commode.
- Wear clean gloves and wash hands after procedure.

CRITICAL THINKING EXERCISES

1. You are teaching a client's family how to irrigate the midabdominal wound that is healing by secondary intention. The spouse states, "I always thought it was best to paint the wound with povidone-iodine to prevent infection." How should the nurse respond to the spouse? What is the rationale behind the nurse's response? What does the spouse need to know about irrigating the wound?
2. You plan to irrigate a client's sacral pressure ulcer with a 35-ml syringe and a 19-gauge needle. How do you protect yourself from exposure to microorganisms?
3. It is your client's sixth postoperative day. When assessing the wound you note that several sutures remain. What actions do you take?
4. A client has two Jackson-Pratt drainage collectors on the left side of the abdomen. What nursing assessments should be made to ensure proper functioning of this system? Can any aspects of care for this type of drain collector be delegated? Explain the rationale for your answer.

REFERENCES

Agency for Health Care Policy and Research (AHCPR): Clinical practice guidelines No. 15: *Treatment of pressure ulcers,* AHCPR Pub No, 95-0653 U.S. Department of Health and Human Services, Public Health Service, Rockville, MD, 1994.

Barr JE: Principles of wound cleansing, *Ostomy/Wound Manag* 7A(suppl 41):15S, 1995.

Bonier P: Wound care forum, an unusual alternative, *Am J Nurs* 85:418, 1985.

Bryant RA, editor: *Acute and chronic wounds,* St Louis, 1992, Mosby.

Brylinsky CM: Nutrition and wound healing: an overview, *Ostomy/Wound Manag* 41(10):14, 1995.

CDC: Guideline for isolation precautions in hospitals, *Am J Infect Control* 24:24, 1996.

Cooper DM: Acute surgical wounds. In Bryant RA, editor: *Acute and chronic wounds,* St Louis, 1992, Mosby.

Doughty DB: Principles of wound healing and wound management. In Bryant R, editor: *Acute and chronic wounds,* St Louis, 1992, Mosby.

Hunt TK: Disorders of repair and their management. In Hunt TK, Dunphy JE, editors: *Fundamentals of wound management,* New York, 1979, Appleton-Century Crofts.

Maklebust J, Palleschi M: Promoting surgical wound healing, *Nurs '96* 26(6):24C, 1996.

Potter P, Perry A: *Fundamentals of nursing: concepts, process, and practice,* ed 4, St Louis, 1997, Mosby.

Rodeheaver GT: Controversies in topical wound management: wound cleansing and wound disinfection. In Krasner D, editor: *Chronic wound care,* King of Prussia, Pa, 1990, Health Management Publications.

Wong D, Baker C: Pain in children: comparison of assessment scales, *Pediatr Nurs* 14(1):9, 1988.

ADDITIONAL READING

Sussman C: Physical therapy modalities and the wound recovery cycle, *Ostomy/Wound Manag* 28(2):43, 1992.

VanDover D: Topical wound management, *Ostomy/Wound Manag* 32:40, 1991.

UNIT XIV

Home Care

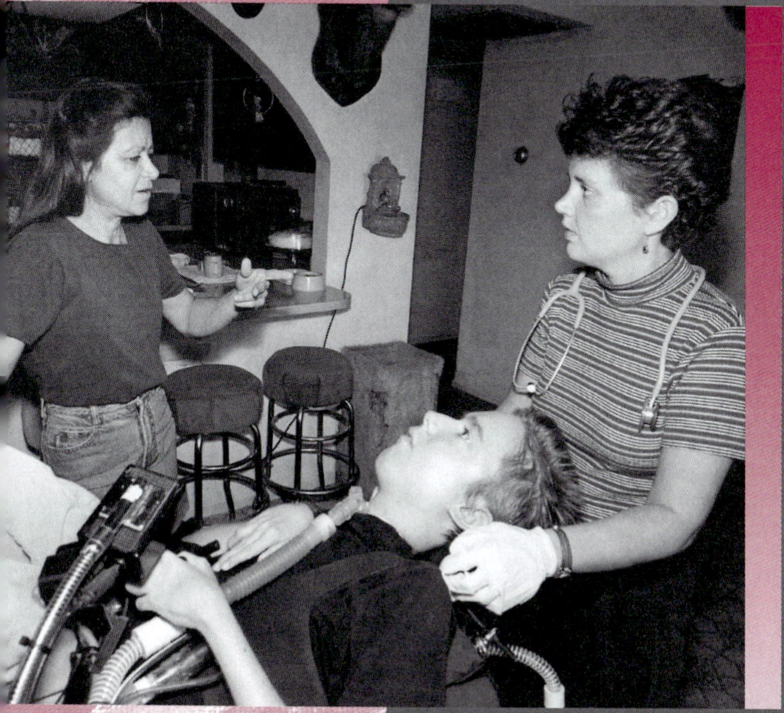

CHAPTER 41

Home Care Safety

OBJECTIVES

Mastery of content in this chapter will enable the nurse to:

- Define key terms.
- Identify clients at risk for accidents.
- Describe factors within a home environment that create risks for injury for clients.
- Perform a home safety risk assessment.
- Identify interventions that will modify the home environment for physical safety.
- Identify interventions to reduce safety risks for clients with sensory, cognitive, and mental status alterations.
- Recommend strategies to ensure safe drug administration within the home.

KEY TERMS

Alzheimer's disease
Amnesic syndromes
Dementia
Polypharmacy
Reminiscing
Respite care

SKILLS

41-1 Modifying Safety Risks in the Home Environment

41-2 Adapting the Home Setting for Clients with Cognitive Deficits

41-3 Medication and Medical Device Safety

Safety implies that people feel secure in their surroundings. In Maslow's hierarchy of needs, safety includes security, stability, protection, and freedom from fear and anxiety (Maslow, 1954). Thus safety has both a physical as well as an emotional component. The two often go hand-in-hand. For example, if a wheelchair-bound client has renovated a home with entry ramps and better bathroom access, the improved physical changes will make the client know there will be less risk in maneuvering within the home. In addition, the client will emotionally feel less anxious to interact within the environment.

Accidents are a common health problem within the United States, as well as in Canada and other nations. Billions of dollars are spent annually as a result of accidents occurring in the home. These accidents occur as a result of environmental threats and limitations and disabilities experienced by individuals. Of course, common sense is a variable as well. Many clients do not have the resources needed to ensure a safe home environment by keeping the home in good repair. Whatever resources a client brings to a situation, the nurse can play an important role in improving a client's safety conscience. The nurse collaborates with clients, family members, and other health care providers in the community in finding the best approaches for meeting a client's safety needs.

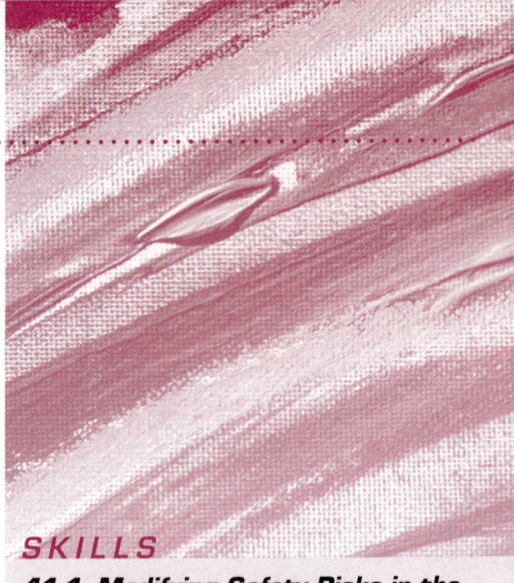

A nurse faces many situations when assisting clients in making the necessary adaptations to ensure a safe home environment. In acute care a nurse will care for clients who develop serious physical limitations and who are unable to fully recover before having to return home. Anticipation of the client's needs is essential so that modifications can be made by the family before the client's discharge. Sometimes the limitations are temporary, although often they may be permanent. Home health nurses must continually be alert for safety factors that place clients at risk for injury. The home health nurse becomes very adept at partnering closely with clients and family members so that modifications within the home do not disrupt normal lifestyles dramatically. Finally, nurses in any setting must assess for patterns of health care problems (e.g., falls, burns, medication errors) that may point to safety problems in the home. For example, recurrent burns may indicate a problem with a client's tactile sensation and inability to sense extremes in hot water temperature in the bathroom or kitchen.

Clients most at risk for experiencing threats to safety within the home are older adults because of the physiological changes that accompany aging, including a slower reaction time, muscular weakness, reduced pain perception, reduced depth perception and color discrimination, and reduced visual acuity. Despite the older adult's risks, Ebersole and Hess (1994) stress that older adults learn how to negotiate their environments relatively well and are usually more aware of potential dangers. Thus older adults may often be more cautious than younger persons.

In addition to physical changes, there is a percentage of the older adult population affected by cognitive and mental status alterations such as **dementia,** delirium, or **Alzheimer's disease.** The nature and implications of behavioral manifestations for each of these syndromes is beyond the scope of this textbook. However, it is important to recognize that if a client suffers memory loss, confusion, poor orientation, or reduced attention span, accidents can easily occur. Care providers are challenged with the choice of maintaining a person's autonomy versus taking steps to ensure their physical safety and protection (Lueckenotte, 1996).

Clients of any age will have safety risks when they experience alterations that impair their mobility, sensory function, or cognitive thought processes. If a loss or reduction in a person's ability to function within the environment occurs suddenly, the person may resist environmental changes, attempting to deny any limitations. In this case, the client may try to initiate self-care actions without necessary guidance or modification to the environment. For the client whose functional loss has been gradual, the accommodation may require only minimal revision. However, for the client whose alteration has been gradual and unnoticed by the client, more aggressive revisions may be needed from the client, family, and/or nurse.

Lueckenotte (1996) defines preventive safety as the interruption of a sequence of events that results in an accident. To successfully prevent or reduce the number of accidents in the home, it is necessary to consider what predisposes a person to an accident and how the environment can be modified to minimize the risk. The skills within this chapter are focused on helping clients retain their independence while implementing preventive safety measures within the home. Chapter 5 focuses more on safety interventions within a health care setting.

GUIDELINES

1. Any changes in a client's home environment should be made to retain as much of the client's independence as possible.
2. Before making any revisions to a client's home, know the client's financial resources.
3. Whenever possible let the client be the final decision maker in the types of alterations to be made.
4. Remember that some structural changes to a room or portion of the home can be expensive. Know the client's resources.
5. Family or friends who assume the role of care giver must learn the importance of preserving client autonomy as much as possible.
6. Any modifications to the home environment should be made considering the client's physical strengths and remaining functional abilities and not merely the client's disabilities.

SKILL 41-1 Modifying Safety Risks in the Home Environment

The home environment should be a place that is healthy, comfortable, and safe. People want to be able to move about freely within their homes, regardless of the home's size, and to have a sense of control over daily living routines. This requires maintenance of personal space and a sense of privacy. Ebersole and Hess (1994) point out that older adults in particular maintain a sense of personal space by clutter and placement of personal items. However, all persons create a personal space in their homes with which they can identify and maneuver about without having to think about every action or movement.

Sometimes illness or the progressive physical changes of aging require changes to be made in a person's home environment. The changes should compliment not only whatever deficit the client has but also any strengths remaining. For example, if a client has poor balance but good upper arm strength, modifications should be made so that the client can safely walk throughout the house, ascend and descend stairs, and enter and exit a bathtub or shower. Side rails along hallways and stairwells and grab bars in the bathroom are good solutions. A nurse who cares for a client who requires changes in the home environment must respect the concept of personal space. Making changes too rapidly without the client's consent may cause more problems than benefits. The nurse must appreciate the arrangement of the client's space within the home and not move things or suggest modifications without permission. Knowing the rooms the client most frequently uses can help in making the adjustments that will most likely create a safe environment.

An important part of making changes in the home environment is conducting a safety assessment. The home safety assessment covers all major living areas and helps to identify what changes are of greater priority over others. Well-planned environmental changes can reinforce the capabilities rather than the disabilities of a client. Independence can be enhanced to secure a better quality of life for clients and family members.

EQUIPMENT

- **Home safety checklist**

DELEGATION CONSIDERATIONS

Some of the principles that are involved in changing the home environment are both practical and common sense in approach. Unlicensed care providers such as home health aides often interact with clients and make suggestions for ways to make the home safer. However, an RN is best qualified to conduct a thorough home safety assessment and to determine what alterations or revisions are preferred on the basis of the client's physical and/or cognitive limitations. The RN should provide supervision to any unlicensed personnel who suggests changes to be sure they do not create any risks for the client.

STEPS	RATIONALE
ASSESSMENT	
1. Review previous physical findings or conduct an assessment of the client's vision, hearing, musculoskeletal, and neurological function (see Chapter 11).	May reveal sensory alterations or problems with strength, coordination, or balance that predispose client to injury.
2. Determine if client has had a history of falls or other injuries within the home.	Helps to focus on the type of accident client is most at risk of having.
3. Review any risk factors the client may have for being predisposed to accidents within the home:	
a. Known visual impairment	Reduced visual function may alter the client's balance, prevent clear perception of objects along the client's normal walkways, or interfere with adaptation to the dark or glaring light.
b. Hearing impairment	Prevents client from hearing normal environmental sounds clearly as a source of orientation. Also prevents clear perception of any home-installed alarms (e.g., smoke alarm).
c. Neuromuscular dysfunction	Unsteady gait or muscular weakness predisposes client to fall. Recurrent falls are associated with difficulty standing up from a chair (Corbett and Pennypacker, 1992).
d. Decreased energy or fatigue	Predisposes to falls.
e. Incontinence	Frequent trips to the bathroom often cause a client with other deficits to accidentally trip or fall over barriers.
f. History of stroke, diabetes, or spinal cord injury	Conditions cause changes in peripheral sensation of the extremities, preventing client from perceiving hot or cold extremes.
g. Postural hypotension	Dizziness or light-headedness predisposes to falls.
h. Amputation	Can cause client to be less steady or coordinated in maneuvering throughout home.
CRITICAL DECISION POINT Use the family as a resource in the assessment. Family may witness accident trends or patterns.	
4. With the client and family as active participants, conduct a home safety assessment:	Provides a comprehensive review of all areas within the home that may pose barriers and hazardous situations.
a. Front and back entrances	Entrances may pose barriers in the surfaces over which client must walk.
(1) Are walkways to the front/back door even and free from holes or cracks?	

STEPS	RATIONALE
(2) Are home entrances well lighted, including walkways?	
(3) Does the client have nonskid strips/safety treads or rough textured paint on outdoor steps?	Safety devices such as handrails and safety treads provide greater support and lessen chances of falls.
(4) Are doormats in good repair with a nonskid backing and a tapered edge?	
(5) Can the client open and close all doors easily?	
(6) Is there a sturdy handrail on both sides of the stairs leading to the entrance?	
(7) Are steps in good condition with even, flat surfaces?	
(8) Does the client have a shelf or bench by the front/back door to place grocery bags or other packages to make entry easy?	
(9) Can the client see who is outside without having to open the door?	
b. Kitchen	The kitchen is one of the most hazard-oriented rooms in the house and poses serious hazards for fire. Client learns the importance of staying attentive when cooking and minimizing risks.
(1) Does the client wear clothing with short or close-fitting sleeves when cooking?	
(2) Does the client always stay in the kitchen when cooking?	
(3) Does the client have a loud timer to signal when food is cooked?	
(4) Does the client keep the stove top and oven clean and grease free?	
(5) Are stove control dials easy to see and use?	
(6) Is an easy-to-use fire extinguisher close at hand?	
CRITICAL DECISION POINT **Have client walk through steps of how to use extinguisher.**	
(7) Are there emergency numbers for police, fire, and poison control posted on or near the telephone?	Emergency phone numbers and extinguisher ensure a quick response should a fire break out.
(8) Can items in the kitchen cabinets and shelves be reached without climbing on a stool or chair?	
(9) Is the step stool sturdy and in good repair?	Climbing on step stools or chairs poses risks for falls.
(10) Is there adequate lighting over the sink, stove, and work areas?	
(11) Does the client wipe up spills on the floor immediately?	
(12) Are kitchen throw rugs and mats slip-resistant?	
c. Bathrooms	The bathroom is also a hazard-oriented room. Wet floors and tub or shower bottoms can be very slippery, causing risk of falls.
(1) Can the bathroom door lock be unlocked from both sides of the door?	
(2) Is the tub or shower equipped with nonskid mats, abrasive strips, or surfaces that are not slippery?	
(3) Does the bathroom floor have a nonslip surface or a rug with a nonskid backing?	
(4) Does the client avoid using slippery bath oils when bathing?	

STEPS	RATIONALE
CRITICAL DECISION POINT **If client uses oils, recommend draining tub and placing towel in bottom of tub before attempting to get out.**	
(5) Do bathtub and shower have at least one grab bar?	Grab bars provide extra support while maneuvering into and out of tubs or showers.
(6) Is the grab bar a different color than that of the wall?	
(7) Is the client careful not to place towels on grab bars?	
(8) Does the shower have a stool and hand-held sprayer?	
(9) Are soap dishes recessed?	
(10) Are cold and hot water faucets clearly marked?	Accidental burns can occur from exposure to hot water.
(11) Is the water temperature on the water heater 120 degrees or lower?	
d. Bedroom	
(1) Is a night-light placed in the bedroom and/or bath?	Older adults have poor night vision.
(2) Is a working smoke detector just outside the bedroom door?	
(3) Can the client turn on a light without having to get out of bed in the dark?	Getting out of bed, without proper lighting or the ability to adjust to light changes, and reaching for necessary objects can predispose client to a fall.
(4) Is a flashlight kept near the bedside in case of a power outage?	
(5) Is furniture arranged to provide a clear path from bed to bathroom?	
(6) Is the client who smokes, careful to never smoke in bed?	
(7) Is a phone with emergency numbers within easy reach of the bed?	Clients may develop physical symptoms while in bed, requiring easy access to a phone.
e. Living room/family room	Clients can easily trip or fall over electrical cords, clutter, loose rugs, and furniture. The common walkway through the house should be clutter and barrier free.
(1) Are electrical cords removed from under furniture and carpeting?	
(2) Has the chimney been cleaned within the past year?	
(3) Can the client turn on a light without having to walk into a dark room?	
(4) Are lamp, extension, or phone cords kept out of the way of traffic?	
(5) Are hallways and walkways free from objects and clutter?	
(6) Are loose area rugs securely attached to the floor and not placed over carpeting? (For best safety, consider removal of throw rugs.)	
(7) Is furniture arranged in each room so that the client can walk around easily?	
(8) Is all furniture steady and without sharp edges?	
(9) Can the client sit and stand up easily from couches or chairs?	Some physical conditions make it difficult to bend at the knees and hips, making it hard to sit in low-lying chairs or couches.
f. Around the house	Assesses for hazards that may cause falls.
(1) Are all living areas well lighted?	

STEPS	RATIONALE
(2) Is flooring or carpeting throughout the house in good repair?	
(3) Are all thresholds level with the floor or no more than ½ inch in height?	
(4) Are stairways well lighted?	
(5) Is there a light switch at both the top and bottom of the stairs?	
(6) Does lighting produce glare or shadows on the stairs?	
(7) Do handrails run continuously from the top to the bottom of flights of stairs?	
(8) Are step coverings in good condition?	
(9) Are all stairs kept free of clutter?	
g. General fire safety	Smoke alarms properly located and well functioning can provide a timely alert for a fire.
(1) Does the client have properly working smoke detectors?	
(2) Does client routinely check detector alarms to be sure batteries are good?	
CRITICAL DECISION POINT Check to see when battery was last changed.	
(3) Does client have several emergency exit plans in case of fire?	
(4) Has family determined a meeting place in the event of an emergency, such as at the mailbox in front of home or parking area in front of house?	
(5) Does client use portable space heaters? Are they kept 3 feet away from flammable items?	Heaters, furnaces, and chimneys pose risks for fire.
(6) Is the furnace area free of things that can catch on fire?	
(7) During holidays does the client have a Christmas tree, and is it kept well watered?	
(8) Does a qualified professional check the furnace and chimney annually?	
h. General electrical safety	
(1) Are electrical cords in good condition, not frayed, spliced, or cracked?	
(2) Are electrical cords kept away from water?	
(3) Does the client use extension cord/outlet extenders with a built-in circuit breaker or fuse?	
(4) Do all wall outlets and switches have cover plates?	
(5) Does the client use light bulbs of the correct wattage for each fixture?	
(6) Is the fuse box easily accessible and clearly labeled?	
(7) Are lamp switches easy to turn so as to avoid burns from hot light bulbs?	
5. Assess the client's financial resources; determine monthly income used for ongoing expenses.	Determines potential for making repairs to the home. May reveal need for low-cost community service support.
6. Assess client's and family member's willingness to make changes. Has client accepted limitations that pose risk for injury? Determine how important functional independence is for the client.	Nurse's attempt to improve safety within the home can be perceived as intrusive. If it can be shown that necessary revisions to the home environment will preserve independence, client may participate more willingly.

STEPS | **RATIONALE**

NURSING DIAGNOSIS

Clustering of defining characteristics from the assessment data may reveal the following nursing diagnoses for clients requiring this skill:

- Altered health maintenance
- Health-seeking behaviors regarding home safety
- Impaired home maintenance management
- Impaired memory
- Impaired physical mobility
- Knowledge deficit regarding home safety risks
- Risk for injury
- Sensory/perceptual alterations (visual, auditory, and/or tactile)

Related factors are individualized based on a client's condition or needs.

PLANNING

1. **Expected outcomes** following completion of procedure:
   - Client will describe potential environmental risks within the home that may predispose to accidents.
     Rationale: During the home safety assessment the nurse instructs the client on those risks that are of greatest concern.
   - Client will initiate actions to correct environmental risks.
     Rationale: Client sees value in altering living environment.
   - Client will remain free of injury.
     Rationale: Environmental barriers are reduced or removed to minimize injuries.
2. Prioritize with client and family the environmental barriers that pose the greatest risk.
   Rationale: Client's own physical and/or cognitive deficits will make certain environmental risks more hazardous. Prioritization helps client make best choices.
3. Recommend calling in a reliable contractor if major home repairs are necessary.
   Rationale: Ensures repairs are made safely and correctly.

IMPLEMENTATION

1. Take steps to reduce physical hazards that can predispose to falls:
   a. Paint the edges of concrete stairs bright yellow or orange.
      Rationale: This highlights visual target for client to see edge of stairs more clearly.
   b. Rearrange furniture to open up space through hallway, living room, family room, and bedroom.
      Rationale: Creates unobstructed pathway for ambulation.
   c. Reduce clutter within living areas, including footstools, flower pots, extension cords, and children's toys.
   d. Remove all doormats and area rugs and replace with mat or carpet that has nonskid backing.
      Rationale: Reduces chance of client slipping when stepping on rug surface.
   e. Have enough electrical outlets installed to be able to plug a light or electronic device (TV, video) into a nearby outlet.
      Rationale: Prevents need to run extension cords across walkways.
   f. Have any rough edges on flooring or carpeting repaired.
      Rationale: Reduces risk of tripping over rough surface.
   g. Install nonskid strips on the surface of bathtub and/or shower stall.
      Rationale: Reduces chances of slipping on slippery surface.
   h. Have a grab bar installed in studs at the tub, toilet, and/or shower (see illustration). Have client select vertical or horizontal placement if choice available.
      Rationale: Bar provides stability for maneuvering in bathroom.

CRITICAL DECISION POINT **Be sure the bar is a different color than that of the wall for easy visibility.**

   i. Have handrails installed along the side of any stairway (see illustration). Be sure the stairways
      Rationale: Older adults have difficulty seeing edges of stairs.

STEPS	RATIONALE
are well lighted, with switches at the top and bottom of the steps.	
j. Install appropriate broad-beam lighting for outside walkways.	
k. Keep a lighted phone easily accessible, next to the client's bed.	Prevents client from having to get up out of bed, often in the dark.
2. Make modifications to promote safe practice of activities of daily living:	
a. Provide a direct light source in areas where the client reads, cooks, uses tools, or conducts hobby work. High-intensity light on the object or surface that is involved works best.	Older adults require three times as much light to see objects as they did when they were in their twenties (Ebersole and Hess, 1994).
CRITICAL DECISION POINT **Avoid fluorescent lighting, because it can create excessive glare.**	
b. Install satin and nongloss finishes for walls, cabinets, and counter tops in the kitchen. Have sheer curtains or adjustable shades in other living areas.	Reduces the glare to which older adults are very sensitive.
c. Apply colored tape or paint to the color-code controls of the stove, oven, dryer, toaster, and other appliances.	Clients with reduced visual acuity may adjust appliance to wrong setting, creating potential risk of fire or burning.
d. Install lazy Susans and pullout drawers with glide mechanisms in kitchen cabinets. Also install C-ring handles in lower cabinets.	Makes access to food and kitchen supplies easier.
3. Take steps to eliminate fire hazards:	
a. Have smoke detectors installed near each bedroom, the kitchen, and in the basement of the home. Be sure a detector is on each floor of the home.	Fires most frequently start in the basement near the furnace, dryer, or electrical wiring; kitchen; or in living areas where extensive wiring can be found. Alarm should be close by to alert client and family when sleeping.

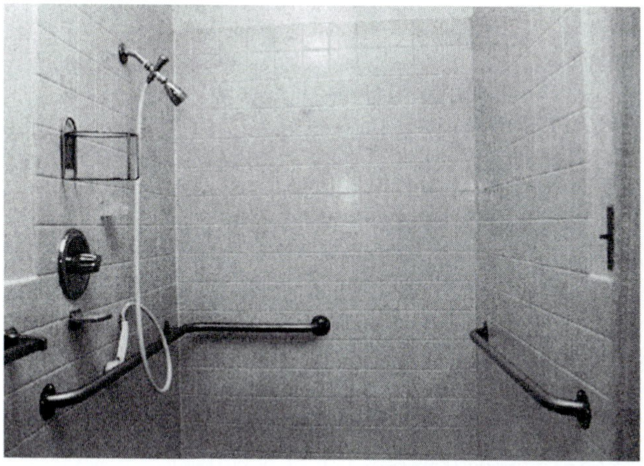

Step 1h Grab bars installed in a shower. (From Lueckenotte A: *Gerontologic nursing,* St Louis, 1996, Mosby.)

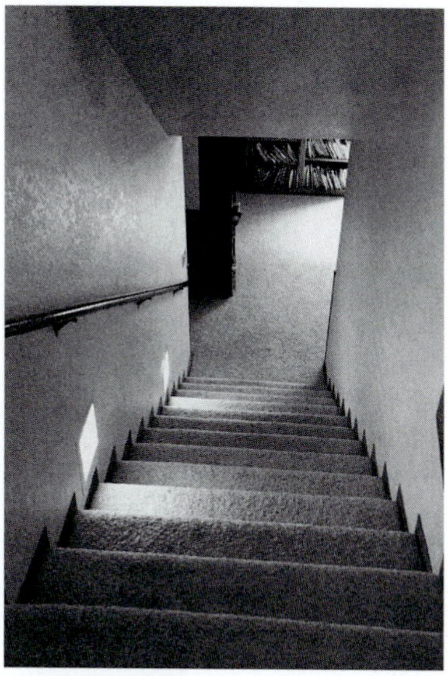

Step 1i Handrails installed along stairways provide security for clients with visual, balance, and coordination problems.

STEPS	RATIONALE
b. Have client select a fire extinguisher that is easy to handle and manipulate (see illustration). Ask client to read instructions and discuss its proper use.	Older adult or client with disability may have difficulty gripping mechanisms on certain extinguishers.
c. Have area around furnace cleared of any flammable items.	Reduces risk for fire.
d. Instruct client to never place a portable space heater within 3 feet of flammable items. Have client buy a model that turns off automatically if tipped over.	Intense heat can ignite flammable items easily.
e. Have client make appointments for maintenance of furnace and chimney cleaning.	
f. Have client check lightbulbs in all fixtures.	Ensures proper wattage being used.
g. Have client establish routine during cooking that keeps client in kitchen. Be sure cooking range is kept clean and items such as potholders and towels are kept away from burners.	Food cooking on stove can easily boil over or begin to burn when unattended.
h. If client is a smoker, review need to keep ashtrays clean and emptied as much as possible. Placing a small amount of water or sand in the bottom of an ashtray is useful if client is visually impaired.	Client with reduced vision may be unable to tell if cigarette, cigar, or match has extinguished.
4. Take steps to reduce chances of injury from burns:	
a. Have setting on hot water heater adjusted to 120 degrees or lower.	
b. Instruct client to always turn the cold water on first.	
c. Install touch pads to lamps.	Light can be easily turned on without risk of touching a hot lightbulb.
d. Use color codes of red for hot and blue for cold on water faucets. (If client cannot distinguish colors, choose two that are easily distinguished.)	Prevents accidental burning from turning on wrong faucet.

EVALUATION

1. Have client and family member(s) identify the safety risks that they perceive were revealed in the home safety assessment.	This will demonstrate what client recognizes as a risk and its relative importance for changing.

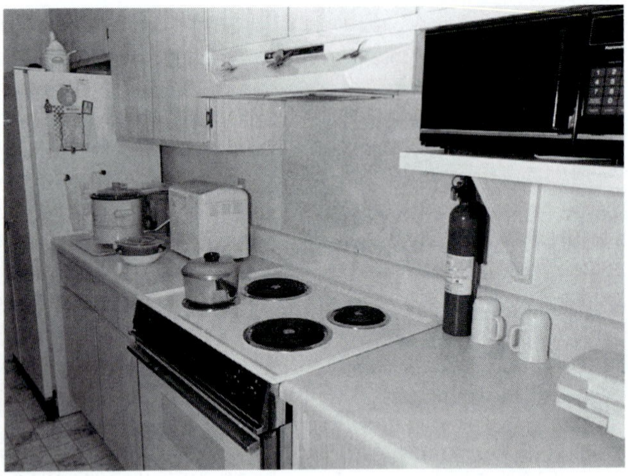

Step 3b Fire extinguisher.

STEPS	RATIONALE
2. During follow-up visits to the home ask client to discuss plans for making any modifications and observe what changes have been implemented.	Evaluates extent to which client sees risks as potentially harmful and complies with suggested changes.
3. During follow-up visit or call, ask if client has experienced any falls or other injuries within the home.	May reveal if risks have been eliminated, depending on client's previous history of injury.
4. **Unexpected outcomes** that may occur include:	
➤ Client and family do not acknowledge all of the risks revealed on the home safety assessment.	Client may perceive threat to personal space and environment, sensing a loss of control. Nurse should review those factors that pose the greatest risk for client first. Determine whether client's concern is over loss of independence or inadequate resources to make changes.
➤ Client fails to make changes agreed on in previous plan.	Reassess what factors are influencing client's willingness or unwillingness to make modifications.
➤ Client suffers fall or other injury within the home.	May reveal an environmental risk has not been corrected, that a new risk has developed, or that client's physical or cognitive condition has worsened. Reassess risks and determine if there are options for correction.

Recording and Reporting

1. Retain copy of home safety assessment in client's home health record.	Provides a baseline for future evaluation.
2. Record any instruction provided, client's response, and changes made within environment in progress notes.	Ensures continuity of care for next home visit.

Follow-up Activities

1. Encourage client to conduct a home safety check annually.

• • • • •

Special Considerations

- ➤ If client is wheelchair bound, there may be a need to lower light switches and other control devices within easy reach. Similarly, kitchen cabinets and other storage closets can be redesigned for access. A high-rise toilet with vertically hinged arm support allows the client to transfer sideways from wheelchair to toilet seat (Shamberg and Shamberg, 1994). Another option is placing a bedside commode (with bedpan removed) over a conventional toilet seat. The commode level is usually higher than the toilet. Then the toilet seat can also be placed near the bedside for nighttime use.
- ➤ For clients who have difficulty getting into and out of a tub, a bathtub transfer seat can be helpful.
- ➤ Wearing flat, nonskid, rubber-soled shoes reduces risk of trips and falls.

Teaching Considerations

- ➤ Care givers may benefit from learning how to safely assist a client to ambulate or transfer from bed to chair or wheelchair to chair, depending on client's mobility limitations.
- ➤ Instruct client and care giver on what to do in case client falls, including access to emergency assistance and how to prevent further injury. Many communities have a service available that is designed for persons who live alone. The service company provides a small device worn around a client's neck and a special monitor connected to the client's telephone. A client can summon help by pressing the button on the device if a phone is inaccessible. The alarm is received by the company, and the company then calls the client to assess the possibility of a false alarm. If there is no answer, the company will contact family members or friends or a rescue squad to check on the client. This service is a valuable option to frail older adults who are competent to live alone or be left at home while family members are away.

Pediatric Considerations

- ➤ Children with muscular dystrophies and spinal cord injuries will require use of a wheelchair. Modifications to the home are necessary if the child is to have any degree of freedom.

SKILL 41-2 Adapting the Home Setting for Clients with Cognitive Deficits

An important aspect of safety is a person's ability to perform routine activities of daily living and to make the correct decisions necessary to conduct home management activities. Home management includes use of the telephone, cleaning, shopping, money management, meal preparation, and taking medication. A person who is unable to perform these activities or who requires assistance from another may have physical disabilities and/or cognitive limitations. When the limitations are cognitive, a person's autonomy is clearly threatened. Family often misunderstand certain behaviors associated with cognitive and mental changes and become concerned as to whether the individual can function safely within the home. The nurse may enter into situations where decisions must be made as to whether a client is competent to perform self-care.

It is a myth that all older adults experience cognitive dysfunction. However, it is the older adult that the nurse most commonly cares for with cognitive dysfunction and who needs support within the home to remain functional. Making the right decisions about safety within the home and the care that will be required depends on an accurate assessment of mental health, physical health, social and economic status, functional status, and environmental characteristics (Solomon, 1988; Ebersole and Hess, 1994). The difficulty lies in distinguishing between normal and diverse characteristics of aging and pathological conditions (Ebersole and Hess, 1994).

Making accurate assessments of older adults' mental status and cognitive function takes considerable practice. First of all, the two processes are not the same (see Chapter 11). Mental status is an overlap between affective and cognitive function. A person may have certain mental processes intact (e.g., orientation to name, time, and place), while at the same time other processes are diminished or compromised (e.g., short-term memory of life events). Often nurses and other care providers make assumptions about a client's cognitive functioning from inadequate data. Assessment of a client's level of orientation alone is not an accurate indicator of cognitive functioning (Ebersole and Hess, 1994; Palmateer and McCartney, 1985).

To complicate the issue of differentiating mental status and cognitive changes, it must be remembered that older adults commonly suffer from depression. Depression is an emotional disorder that can result in cognitive impairment (Lueckenotte, 1996). It can occur alone or in combination with cognitive disorders such as dementia.

Clients may experience mental status and cognitive changes across a wide continuum from **amnesic syndromes** to Alzheimer's disease. A common complaint in an older adult is forgetting names, misplacing items, and poor recall of recent events or conversations (Lueckenotte, 1996). There are simple interventions that help the client adapt to these difficulties. In contrast, Alzheimer's disease is a progressive disorder that eventually makes a client unable to perform self-care due to loss of the ability to make decisions and judgments and to follow directions. Loss of verbal abilities, incontinence, and loss of the ability to walk occurs in the later stages.

This skill does not cover the complexity of assessing the full range of cognitive dysfunction in older adults. Instead it attempts to give the nurse guidelines for how to help clients who have varying degrees of cognitive dysfunction make adaptations to preserve their ability to function safely within the home. Similarly the skill addresses techniques for the family to use in assisting older adults.

EQUIPMENT

- Mini–Mental State Exam (see Chapter 11)
- Calendar
- Paper for making lists
- Bulletin board or poster board (optional)

DELEGATION CONSIDERATIONS

This skill requires problem solving and knowledge application unique to a professional nurse. For this skill delegation is inappropriate.

STEPS	RATIONALE
ASSESSMENT	
1. Conduct the assessment during a short session and be sensitive to the client's sensory needs or disabilities.	Improves likelihood of gathering relevant data (Ebersole and Hess, 1994).
2. Be sure the room in which you meet with the client and family is well lit with minimal outside noises or interruptions. Speak clearly and in a normal tone of voice.	An optimal environment for the assessment of the client's cognitive and mental status will provide a more valid assessment.

STEPS	RATIONALE
3. Ask client to describe own level of health and how it affects the ability to maintain self-care skills (e.g., bathing, dressing, eating, toileting).	Question will require client to attend to one topic. Allows nurse to assess attention and concentration. Also determines if client is fully perceptive of physical capabilities.
CRITICAL DECISION POINT **Family members may be used to confirm description. Do not create situation in which client feels you are not listening to his or her views.**	
4. Ask how the client is doing with home management responsibilities. Questions that may be asked include, "To give me an idea of how you manage at home, what bills do you pay each month; how do you organize yourself?" and "When do you regularly buy groceries and supplies?"	Provides a good comparison of client and family perceptions. Interaction will help to measure short-term memory, judgment, and problem solving.
5. Assess the medications the client takes. Review the number and type of medications, purpose as prescribed, time of day taken, and dosages. Give special attention to pain medications, anticonvulsants, antihypertensives (especially beta-blockers), Lasix, digoxin, aspirin, and other anticoagulants.	Older adults frequently suffer drug interactions from **polypharmacy,** the concurrent prescribing of multiple medications. Select drugs and/or combinations of drugs can place a client at risk for side effects that may increase the chances of injury as a result of physical or cognitive changes.
6. Determine if client has family member or friend who assists with self-care or home management responsibilities. How do that individual and the client perceive satisfaction in supporting the client?	Role of family care giver can be stressful. Determines availability of resource to client and quality of that support.
7. During discussion, observe client's dress, nonverbal expressions, appearance, and cleanliness.	Conditions such as depression and dementia can result in the client's inability to attend to personal appearance.
CRITICAL DECISION POINT **Do not confuse behavioral changes with lack of available resources to maintain hygiene.**	
8. Observe the immediate home environment; is it well kept and orderly?	Behavioral changes associated with cognitive dysfunction may be first detected in a disorderly home and inappropriate placement of objects (e.g., carton of orange juice placed inside kitchen cabinet instead of refrigerator).
9. If you suspect a cognitive or mental status change, complete a Mini–Mental State Examination (see Chapter 11).	Screening exam will measure orientation, attention and calculation, recall, language, and intelligence.

NURSING DIAGNOSIS

Clustering of defining characteristics from the assessment data may reveal the following nursing diagnoses for clients requiring this skill:

- Acute confusion
- Altered health maintenance
- Altered thought processes
- Caregiver role strain
- Impaired home maintenance management
- Impaired memory
- Self-care deficit

Related factors are individualized based on a client's condition or needs.

PLANNING

1. Expected outcomes following completion of procedure:	
➤ Client is able to complete home management responsibilities within existing limitations.	Modifications are made that help client apply remaining cognitive functions.

STEPS	RATIONALE
➤ Client receives appropriate combination of medications for diagnosed conditions.	
➤ Care giver describes techniques to use in helping the client perform self-care and home management activities.	Care giver is a key participant in learning how to support client.
➤ Care giver uses techniques to help client complete self-care and home management activities.	
2. If client has difficulty with self-care skills, refer family to homemaker services and **respite care** as appropriate.	Provides additional resource to either deliver direct personal care to client or to provide care giver temporary rest away from continuous responsibilities.
3. If client has physical disability affecting fine motor skills, consult with physical and/or occupational therapist.	Can offer assistive devices to make bathing, dressing, writing, and feeding easier (see illustration).
4. Consider client's level of cognitive impairment before implementing strategies that will require changes in the living environment. Some clients may only require minor adaptations, and others will depend more on assistance of care givers.	Retention of client's independence and autonomy is ultimate goal.
5. Determine best time of day for approaches that result in desired response.	Client may be more alert and responsive in morning versus afternoon or vice versa.

IMPLEMENTATION

STEPS	RATIONALE
1. If client has difficulty remembering when to perform tasks (e.g., paying bills or taking medicines) help to create a list or post reminder notes in a conspicuous location (e.g., bulletin board, front of refrigerator).	Memory function in older adults tends to be preserved for relevant, well-learned material (Lueckenotte, 1996). Lists will help client overcome memory loss.
2. When client has difficulty completing tasks such as writing checks for bills or bringing groceries into the home to store, reduce the steps it takes to complete the task. Find ways to consolidate steps or simplify the task.	Prevents frustration in completing task and/or forgetting a step that leads to the task being unfinished.
3. Help client and care giver determine a routine schedule for daily activities such as eating, bathing, daily exercise, home management activities, and napping. Have a large calendar posted to write in appointments or special planned events.	Consistency creates a sense of security and keeps the client more easily oriented to daily activities. Routines are important in providing security but client must also have the option of making changes as necessary.

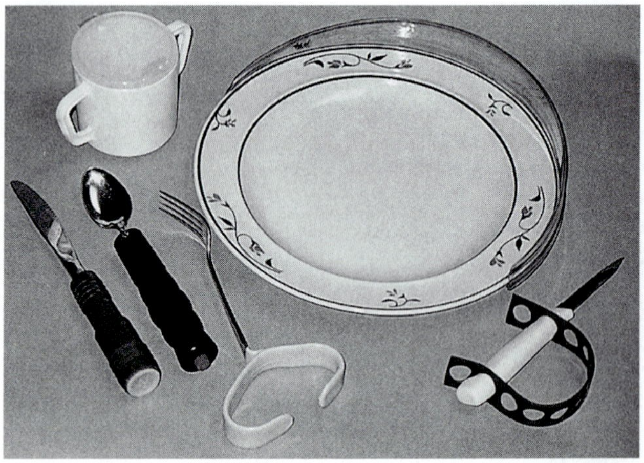

Step 3 Assistive feeding devices.

STEPS	RATIONALE
4. Instruct care giver to focus on client's abilities rather than disabilities.	Helps to retain dominant skills (Burgener, Shimer, and Murrell, 1993).
5. Have care giver assist with setting-up activities so that client can complete task (e.g., chopping up vegetables before actual cooking, placing a wash basin on table in bedroom for a sponge bath, placing clothes to wear for the day on the bed, unpacking groceries on countertop for eventual storage).	Helps client master task even though unable either physically or cognitively to perform all steps.
6. Discuss with client, care giver, and physician or primary care provider options for scheduling multiple medications: a. Administer drugs likely to cause confusion at nighttime.	Drugs may cause physiological changes that create risk for injury.
CRITICAL DECISION POINT Do not recommend this if client has nocturia.	
b. Space antihypertensives and antiarrhythmics at different times to minimize side effects. c. Reduce number of different pain medications used. d. Give Lasix (diuretic) early in day and not at night.	
7. Instruct care giver on how to use simple and direct communication: a. Use a calm and relaxed approach. b. Use eye contact and touch. c. Speak in simple words and short sentences. d. Use nonverbal gestures that compliment verbal messages.	Relays care and support through therapeutic communication techniques.
CRITICAL DECISION POINT Be sure client can contribute to discussion. Care giver should not dominate discussion.	
8. Keep clocks, calendars, and personal mementos (e.g., pictures, scrapbooks, and special personal gifts from loved ones) situated throughout rooms within the home.	Reinforces reality orientation when client's memory is failing.
9. Have the care giver routinely orient the client to who the care giver is and what activities they are going to complete.	This strategy is useful in clients with progressive dementia. This improves their productivity and responses (Lueckenotte, 1996).
10. Be sure client has regular naps or rest periods during the day.	Fatigue can add to any mental status changes. Gives client energy to perform planned activities.
11. Have care giver encourage and support frequent visits by family and friends. Instruct care giver on how to use humor and **reminiscing** of favorite stories to promote social interaction.	Participation in social activities prevents boredom and restlessness.

EVALUATION

STEPS	RATIONALE
1. During a follow-up visit, ask client to review the home management activities completed the morning of that day, as well as the previous day.	Determines client's ability to recall events and evaluates if planned activities were completed.
2. Review with client and care giver revised schedule for medication administration.	
3. Ask care giver to describe ways that will increase client's success in completing home management and self-care activities.	Measures learning.

STEPS	RATIONALE
4. Have care giver show schedules of daily routines and review specific approaches used. Observe environment for presence of reality orientation cues.	Determines care giver's success in applying information and making environmental changes.
5. **Unexpected outcomes** that may occur include:	
➤ Client fails to complete activities as planned.	Further modifications may be needed to help client be successful. Reassess what occurred when a task was not completed. Care giver and client conflict could have played a role rather than client being unable cognitively to complete task.
➤ Client experiences drug interaction from multiple medications.	
➤ Care giver is unable to describe techniques that will improve client's orientation and ability to complete activities.	Reinstruction and discussion will be necessary. Focus on degree of stress care giver is feeling. Support for care giver may be necessary before care giver can learn how to support someone else.

Recording and Reporting

1. Record assessment of client's cognitive and mental status, recommended interventions, and client's and care giver's response in progress notes.	Ensures continuity of care for next home visit.
2. Report to physician any change in client's behavior that might reflect a decline in cognitive or mental status.	Change might warrant further medical evaluation.

Follow-up Activities

1. In the event multiple medications are being taken by a client, consult closely with a physician. Desai, Rajput, and Desai (1990) found in a sample of 100 older adult adults that 39% of the clients had at least one unnecessary drug prescribed. Often clients continue to take medications from physicians who no longer are supervising their medical care.

• • • • •

Special Considerations

➤ Behavior problems and emotions can increase the stress associated with care of clients with cognitive and mental status deficits.

➤ Many clients experience progressive loss of function, requiring constant adaptations and adjustments.

Teaching Considerations

➤ Instruct care giver on signs and symptoms to expect for clients suffering from dementia and Alzheimer's disease. If client's functionality continues to decline, care giver may choose to learn more ADL support skills (e.g., how to assist with hygiene, dressing, transfer and turning, toileting).

Pediatric Considerations

➤ Children with cognitive impairment are often not aware of inherent dangers during play and other activities. Parental supervision is critical.

SKILL 41-3 Medication and Medical Device Safety

Clients frequently must manage the administration of medications, as well as the use of medical devices such as syringes, blood glucose monitoring equipment, dressing supplies, and even intravenous devices. This includes administration, storage, and disposal. Safety is critical in ensuring that medications are administered correctly, devices are used properly, and equipment is cleaned and/or removed as waste. Infection control is just one principle the client and/or care giver must learn to ensure a safe environment within the home.

One of the nurse's responsibilities within the home environment is to assist the client with sensory, mobility, or cognitive deficits. Older adults are again at risk, because they frequently suffer from chronic diseases that leave deficits that make manipulation of medical devices and dispensing of medications difficult. For example, clients with arthritic hands are sometimes unable to open medication containers because of the lack of strength in the hands and the pain created by pressure on the joints. This skill reviews steps to take to ensure safe use of medications and medical devices. Chapter 42 addresses how to instruct clients on medication use.

EQUIPMENT

- **Colored marking pens**
- **Labels**
- **Puncture-resistant sharps container or 2-liter soda bottle with cap**
- **Duct or adhesive tape**

DELEGATION CONSIDERATIONS

Assessment of the client's risks in using medical devices and in administering medications requires problem solving and knowledge application unique to a professional nurse. The RN is best equipped to identify the adaptations needed within the home based on the client's limitations. However, unlicensed assistive personnel, such as home health aides, will frequently be in a situation to be able to see how clients use these adaptations. Unlicensed assistive personnel can learn how to make suggestions that further ensure client safety:

- Use of basic infection control practices
- How to dispose of sharps and needles
- How to dispose of contaminated supplies

STEPS	RATIONALE
ASSESSMENT	
1. Assess client's sensory, musculoskeletal, and neurological function (see Chapter 11).	Helps to reveal any deficits in preparation and use of medications or medical devices.
CRITICAL DECISION POINT If care giver provides most of care, assess care giver's functions.	
2. Assess the client's medication regimen and the length of time client has been receiving each drug.	Determines most current medication regimen.
3. Ask client to show you where medications are stored in the home. Look at each container.	Allows nurse to assess storage conditions and labeling of containers.
CRITICAL DECISION POINT Note temperature of storage area. Medications should not be stored in extreme heat. Insulin should be kept in a cool place.	
4. Have client describe daily schedule for drug administration and whether there are any problems in following that schedule.	Helps to reveal client's compliance or misunderstanding of instructions (see Skill 42-5).
5. If client self-administers injections, ask to see where those supplies are stored and what is used to dispose of used syringes and needles.	Determines sterility of equipment and whether method of disposal creates risk to client or family for needlestick injuries.
6. If client uses a glucose monitoring device, ask to see where the monitor, lancets, and glucose strips are stored. Also ask about how the client disposes of lancets.	Allows nurse to examine cleanliness of equipment, sterility of lancets, and condition of glucose strips. Sharps should be disposed of in puncture-proof container.
7. If client applies dressings to a wound, ask to see where dressings are stored and determine how the client disposes of soiled dressings.	Dressings must be kept in dry storage area to avoid contamination. Soiled dressings should be double bagged and removed to prevent contamination with other items in the home.

NURSING DIAGNOSIS

Clustering of defining characteristics from the assessment data may reveal the following nursing diagnoses for clients requiring this skill:

- Altered health maintenance
- Health-seeking behaviors regarding medication safety
- Risk for infection
- Risk for injury

STEPS	RATIONALE
➤ Knowledge deficit regarding medication and medical device safety	
Related factors are individualized based on a client's condition or needs.	
PLANNING	
1. **Expected outcomes** following completion of procedure:	
➤ Client and care giver will discuss principles of medication safety.	Ensures client is taking correct medications as prescribed.
➤ Client and care giver will be able to prepare medications independently.	Adaptations are made to accommodate client's deficits in handling and manipulating equipment.
➤ Client and care giver will identify the correct conditions for storing medications, medical devices, and supplies.	Instruction focuses on infection control measures.
➤ Client and care giver will dispose of used medical equipment and supplies correctly.	Appropriate receptacles and methods for disposal are made available.
IMPLEMENTATION	
1. Instruct client and care giver on principles to ensure medications are safe to use:	Medications must be of full strength and used for the appropriate pharmacological reason to have therapeutic benefit.
a. Never take a medicine prescribed for another member of household.	
b. Do not take any medicine more than a year old or past the expiration date on the container.	
c. Do not place different medicines in the same container.	
d. Always finish a prescribed medication; do not save for a future illness.	
2. Recommend approaches to facilitate preparation of medications:	
a. For clients with weakened grasp or pain of the hands and fingers, have the local pharmacist place medications in a screw-top or flip-top container.	Child-proof containers are difficult to remove, especially if hand and finger grasp are weakened.
➤ ***CRITICAL DECISION POINT*** **If client has children or grandchildren who have easy access to medication storage area or client's purse, be sure medications are stored in secure place.**	
b. For clients with visual alterations, have pharmacy type larger labels on all medication containers.	Ensures client is able to read drug name and dosage schedule clearly.
c. For clients who are legally blind, have braille labels placed on medication containers.	Label embossed with drug name, strength, and prescription numbers can be easily read by client trained in use of braille.
d. For clients taking multiple medications, a color-coding system may be useful. For example, colors could be used for drugs that are to be taken at the same time. Tops of bottle caps can be marked with a colored marking pen.	May help to ensure drugs and dosages are taken at correct times of day.
e. Provide specially designed syringes with large numerals or syringe magnifier for clients with visual alterations.	Ensures accurate dosage of drug is prepared in syringe.
f. For clients who have difficulty manipulating syringes, offer a spring-loaded needle insertion aid.	Delivers subcutaneous injection safely without manual manipulation of plunger.
g. Have care givers learn how to properly draw up prescribed volume of medication into syringe.	

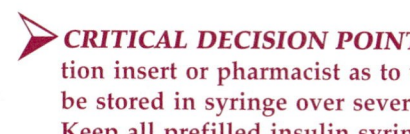

STEPS	RATIONALE
When necessary have care giver prepare extra prefilled syringes for client's use when care giver is absent.	
CRITICAL DECISION POINT **Refer to medication insert or pharmacist as to whether dosages can be stored in syringe over several hours or days. Keep all prefilled insulin syringes refrigerated and use within 21 days (Rice, 1996).**	
3. Recommend approaches to ensure medications and supplies are properly stored:	
a. Store medications in a safe place, preferably in the kitchen.	Moisture in bathroom may cause medications to decompose.
b. Keep liquid medications and parenteral drugs, especially insulin, in a cool place.	
CRITICAL DECISION POINT **Insulin may be stored in a refrigerator, but it is not necessary. The vial in use can be stored at room temperature for up to 30 days without losing potency (Rice, 1996). If stored in refrigerator, be sure drug is kept in a bin or container, away from food. An unused supply of insulin vials should be stored in the refrigerator to maintain potency.**	
c. Keep medical supplies such as syringes, dressing supplies, and glucose meter in an air-tight container (e.g., plastic storage bin) and stored in a cool place, such as a bedroom closet.	Ensures supplies are not exposed to moisture or other contaminants.
4. Review for client and care giver the proper techniques for disposal of medications, "sharps" and disposable medical supplies:	
a. Discard unused portions of drugs or outdated drugs in sink or toilet.	
b. Obtain sharps container from medical supply store or IV equipment supplier. (If finances are limited, have client use a small-neck plastic bottle, such as a soda bottle.) Dispose of all needles and lancets in container.	Puncture-proof container prevents exposure to contaminated needle-stick. Small-neck container makes it difficult for anyone to easily retrieve a used needle or sharp.
c. Caution against filling container to a point where needles protrude out the opening. Discard when three-fourths full, securing top with duct tape or adhesive tape.	Prevents needle-sticks.
d. Store sharps container in an area inaccessible to children.	
e. Dispose of soiled dressings, used glucose testing reagent strips, and IV tubing in a separate, sealed, plastic garbage bag. Then place in second plastic bag and discard appropriately as trash.	
f. Consult local public health department or community authorities regarding proper way to dispose of waste.	
EVALUATION	
1. Have client and/or care giver describe steps to take to ensure medications are safe to use.	Demonstrates learning.

STEPS	RATIONALE
2. Observe client prepare and administer a medication dose.	Evaluates ability to physically manipulate medications and necessary equipment.
3. Observe home setting for location of medications and supplies.	Evaluates client's or care giver's compliance with recommendations.
4. Have client describe how sharps or medical equipment is discarded.	Demonstrates learning.
5. **Unexpected outcomes** that may occur include:	
➤ Client or care giver is unable to recall principles for safe use of drugs.	Reinstruction may be necessary, or client and care giver may need chance to ask more questions regarding the benefit of precautions. Offer written, simple, and clear instructions.
➤ Client has difficulty or is unable to prepare and self-administer a medication.	Further assistance may be necessary in setting up equipment, offering assistive aids, or explaining steps to prepare medication. See Chapter 42 for self-injections.
➤ Medications and medical devices are not stored in a secure or appropriate location.	Resources may be limited in home. Client may choose to store items conveniently rather than safely. Reinstruction and discussion are necessary.
➤ Sharps and disposable medical equipment are not disposed of properly.	Reinstruction is required. Arrange to provide appropriate containers.
RECORDING AND REPORTING	
1. Record recommendations to client and care giver and their response in progress notes.	Ensures continuity in instruction that is reinforced during subsequent home visits.

• • • • •

Special Considerations

- ➤ Use of lancets or application of dressings may cause soiling of client's linen supply. Infected or soiled linen should be kept in a separate, leakproof plastic bag. Contaminated items should be washed separately from household laundry in hot water with one cup of bleach and detergent for **two** regular wash cycles.
- ➤ If client, care giver, or visitor suffers a needle-stick injury, wash the affected area thoroughly with soap and water, then dry. Report incident to physician.

CRITICAL THINKING EXERCISES

1. Miss Rosario has had a repair of her left hip after a fracture. She will return home with crutches. What safety measures might you recommend for Miss Rosario's family to implement in her home?
2. Mr. O'Connor has a progressive memory loss and lives alone. How might you better ensure his ability to self-administer his antihypertensive and diuretic medications safely?
3. If a client tells you that he disposes of insulin syringes and needles in a used milk carton, what advice would you give, and why?

REFERENCES

Burgener SC, Shimer R, Murrell L: Nursing care of cognitively impaired, institutionalized elderly, *J Gerontol Nurs* 17:37, 1993.

Corbett C, Pennypacker B: Using a quality improvement team to reduce patient falls, *JHO* 15(5):38, 1992.

Desai T, Rajput A, Desai H: Use and abuse of drugs in the elderly, *Prog Neuropsychopharmacol Biol Psychiatry* 14(5):779, 1990.

Ebersole P, Hess P: *Toward healthy aging,* ed 4, St Louis, 1994, Mosby.

Lueckenotte A: *Gerontologic nursing,* St Louis, 1996, Mosby.

Maslow A: *Motivation and personality,* ed 2, New York, 1954, Harper and Row.

McDougall GJ: A review of screening instruments for assessing cognition and mental status in older adults, *Nurs Pract* 15:11, 1990.

Palmateer LM, McCartney JR: Do nurses know when patients have cognitive deficits? *J Gerontol Nurs* 11(2):6, 1985.

Rice R: *Home health nursing practice,* ed. 2, St Louis, 1996, Mosby.

Shamberg S, Shamberg A: Reentry begins at home, *TBI Challenge* Winter:4 1994.

Solomon D: National Institutes of Health consensus development conference statement: geriatric assessment methods for clinical decision-making, *J Am Geriatr Soc* 36(4):342, 1988.

CHAPTER 42

Home Care Teaching

OBJECTIVES

Mastery of content in this chapter will enable the nurse to:

- Define key terms.
- Identify factors that alter clients' learning abilities.
- Discuss the collaborative nature of home health care teaching.
- Assess safety factors that may impair or prohibit the client's skill performance in the home setting.
- Discuss situations and conditions that require client/family skills performance to support and achieve health maintenance.
- Understand variances in teaching strategies in the home setting.
- Identify factors influencing attainment of individualized goals for home care clients' learning and skill performance.
- Assess, implement, and evaluate appropriate learning strategies that support positive client outcomes.

KEY TERMS

Antipyretic
Dementia
Enteral nutrition
Febrile
Gastrostomy feeding tube
Hypothermia
Hypoxia
I&O record
Medical asepsis
Nasal cannula
Nasogastric feeding tube
Oxygen therapy
Over-the-counter drug
prn
Transtracheal oxygen therapy

SKILLS

42-1 Teaching Clients to Measure Body Temperature, Blood Pressure, and Pulse

42-2 Using Home Oxygen Equipment

42-3 Teaching Home Tracheostomy Care and Suctioning

42-4 Helping Clients with Self-Medication

42-5 Enteral Nutrition in the Home

Changes in the health care delivery system in recent times have promoted a shift of the site of care delivery from the acute in-patient setting to the home health care arena. Although acute and long-term care settings continue to provide services along the spectrum of the health care continuum, more frequently than in past decades, clients recover from or are treated for illnesses in the home environment. The psychosocial, emotional, and financial issues surrounding the care needs of individuals and families dealing with chronic or episodic illnesses are often seen as being dealt with best in the home setting as well.

The home care nurse is faced with a diverse client population with varying levels of acuity of illness. Techniques and treatments that a few years ago were strictly provided in a general hospital are now commonplace occurrences in home health care.

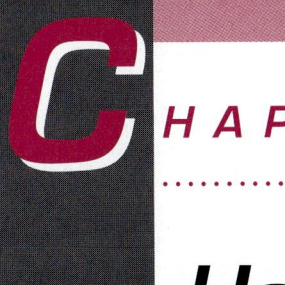

The development and maintenance of successful treatment plans for home care teaching of self-care skills must be done in collaboration with the prescribing physician, the client, family, or designated care givers, pharmacists, organizations that provide and maintain equipment; and very often a variety of other social services and/or health-related organizations that are involved in making the client's home care plan successful. The home nurse not only teaches and assesses the client's health status but also identifies, coordinates, and intervenes with the various services and resources that are required to support the client's successful health maintenance. Teaching techniques will not achieve positive outcomes if the client has an unidentified barrier to following through, such as lack of transportation or inadequate funds for medication and equipment. In addition to the understanding and ability of the nurse to perform the skill and the ability to teach it, the home care nurse must perform global assessments of all intrinsic and extrinsic factors that could affect the client's ability to comply with self-care.

Knowledge of agency policies, regulatory requirements, the nurse practice acts, and laws governing health care providers are important to the home care nurse's knowledge base when delivering or teaching care. Professional organizations, accrediting bodies, and governmental regulations also offer a variety of standards of practice that must be known and incorporated into the performance of home health care services. Client education is a basic component of home health care. By providing services in this setting and successfully teaching aspects of self-care maintenance, clients and families achieve "a better quality of life, fewer hospitalizations, decreased overall costs of therapy, and a greater sense of participation and control over illness" (LaRocca, 1994).

GUIDELINES

1. Consider the client's physical, cognitive, emotional, environmental, social, and resource networks in regard to successful learning and skill performance.
2. Information must be presented in an understandable and orderly manner directed toward the client's learning style and abilities.
3. The teaching care plan must be individualized based on the physical, psychosocial, and comprehension abilities of the client.
4. The safety of the skill performance being done in the home setting must be assessed. A care partner may be required for some skills to be considered as safe in the home setting.
5. Assess the environment for appropriate level of hygiene to support successful self-care management of certain treatment modalities.
6. Consider other persons in the household who influence positively or negatively on the client's self-care modalities.

DELEGATION CONSIDERATIONS

All skills in this chapter have the goal to be delegated to the client, family member, or designated care giver. Delegation of these skills should never be finalized until a complete understanding by the client or care partner regarding actions to take in the event of an unexpected outcome or emergency situation is demonstrated.

- The nurse must assume accountability for appropriate assessment and implementation of the delegation responsibilities.
- Not all home situations will be appropriate for delegation; issues of safety, environment, support networks, and learning abilities will determine appropriateness.
- Client choice of teaching partner is to be considered.
- Depending on the learner, the client, or a care partner, the methodology of a technique may sometimes be altered.
- Some skills are only partially delegated.

SKILL 42-1 Teaching Clients to Measure Body Temperature, Blood Pressure, and Pulse

TEACHING CLIENTS TO MEASURE BODY TEMPERATURE

To practice health maintenance for themselves and their family members, clients need to know how to measure body temperature. An elevation in body temperature can be an early warning sign of serious health problems. Clients susceptible to temperature alterations should know how to measure their temperatures correctly so that they can seek medical attention early when alterations occur. Parents must know how to measure their children's temperature, since children can develop seriously high fevers very quickly. Because older adults have impaired temperature-control mechanisms, the care giver should know the techniques for temperature measurement. Nurses can teach clients the skills of measuring body temperature and lowering temperature when a **febrile** episode occurs at home and medical care is not immediately accessible.

Although there are a variety of body temperature measurement tools now available for use, the most common in the home care setting remains the glass thermometer. The disposable, single-use thermometer and the tympanic membrane thermometer are newer devices with various prevalence in this setting. The small electronic digital thermometers are less expensive and more readily available than some of the newer types mentioned and perhaps allow for safer use than the glass thermometer. This section will deal with the instruction to the client/family on the use of glass thermometers, which most families have or are able to have available in the home. The need for the use of an oral, rectal, or stubby (axillary) thermometer will be determined before use depending on the client's age and status. Having all three types of these inexpensive items at home allows for a variety of client possibilities and needs. (See Chapter 10 for a review of vital signs assessment).

EQUIPMENT

Instruct client on purchase and selection of glass thermometer. Determine need for oral, rectal, or stubby thermometer before purchase if finances are limited.

- **Soft tissue**
- **Lubricant (for rectal measurement)**
- **Paper and pencil if frequent measurements are to be taken**
- **Disposable gloves (for rectal temperature taken by a care giver)**

STEPS	RATIONALE
ASSESSMENT	
1. Assess client's ability to manipulate and read thermometer by having client read temperature values and shake thermometer down. Client who wears eyeglasses should wear them while reading thermometer.	Physical restrictions in handling or reading thermometer may require nurse to instruct family member or significant other instead of client. Visual acuity impairment may prevent client from being able to read thermometer.
2. Assess client's knowledge of normal temperature range and symptoms and common causes of fever and **hypothermia.**	Identifies client's ability to initiate preventive health measures and recognize alterations in body temperature.
3. Assess client's knowledge of criteria to determine appropriate type of thermometer to be used in varying situations (See Chapter 10).	Determines knowledge of age-related or medical conditions that would make oral or rectal temperature measurement detrimental to the client.
4. If client has had experience in measuring temperature, ask for demonstration of technique.	Allows nurse to assess client's knowledge and use of safety precautions, aseptic technique, and time period for insertion.

NURSING DIAGNOSIS

Clustering of defining characteristics from the assessment data may reveal the following nursing diagnoses for clients requiring this skill:

- Impaired home maintenance management
- Health-seeking behaviors
- Hyperthermia
- Hypothermia
- Knowledge deficit regarding specific temperature measurement
- Risk for altered body temperature
- Risk for infection

Related factors are individualized based on a client's condition or needs.

STEPS	RATIONALE
PLANNING	
1. Expected outcomes following completion of procedure:	
➤ Client is able to correctly measure own or family member's temperature.	
➤ Client demonstrates proper cleaning and storage of equipment.	Indicates skills are effectively learned.
➤ Client knows factors affecting temperature, signs and symptoms of fever and hypothermia, and measures to take.	Cognitive learning is achieved.
2. Select setting in home that client is most likely to use when measuring temperature.	Practicing in same environment where skill is routinely performed facilitates comprehension and learning.
3. Discuss and demonstrate with client or family member proper way to position client before thermometer insertions; instruct family member to remain with client if age or physical status requires.	Promotes client's understanding of comfort and safety principles, as well as technique to ensure accurate measurement.

STEPS	RATIONALE
IMPLEMENTATION	
1. Demonstrate steps and provide rationale for the steps to client/care giver.	Demonstration is best technique for teaching psychomotor skill.
2. Have client perform each step with guidance from nurse. Do not rush client.	Nurse is able to correct errors in technique as they occur and discuss implications.
➤ ***CRITICAL DECISION POINT*** **Discuss normal temperature for adult or child.**	Client must be able to identify temperature alterations.
3. Discuss effects of smoking and hot and cold liquids or foods on oral temperature readings.	Client must understand factors that can alter temperature readings.
4. Discuss common symptoms of fever: warm, dry, flushed skin; feeling warm; chills; piloerection; malaise; restlessness.	Client must be able to recognize onset of fever in self or family member.
5. Discuss common signs and symptoms of hypothermia: cool skin, uncontrolled shivering, loss of memory, signs of poor judgment.	Persons with inadequate home heating, older adults, or those unaware of potential dangers of cold conditions are at risk.
6. Discuss importance of notifying physician when temperature elevations occur, and review common therapies for temperature reduction that are safe to perform at home.	Clients must understand danger of high temperature elevations. Use of antipyretics, sponging with tepid water, and drinking fluids are unlikely to cause complications.
7. Create written guidelines for reference to promote client confidence in ability to implement the skill independently, and offer guidance regarding when additional action (such as notifying physician) should be taken.	Some clients need instructions written out in clear, concise statements or pictures to minimize anxiety and support appropriate actions for health maintenance.
EVALUATION	
1. Have client independently demonstrate technique for temperature measurement, including ability to read the thermometer three separate times.	Feedback through independent demonstration of psychomotor skill is best means of evaluating mastery of skill.
2. Ask client to identify normal temperature range and influence of smoking and hot and cold liquids or foods on oral readings; discuss safety implications for temperature measurement.	Measures cognitive learning.
3. Have client describe common signs and symptoms of fever and hypothermia and methods for control.	Measures cognitive learning.
4. **Unexpected outcomes** that may occur include:	
➤ Client is unable to measure temperature or clean thermometer correctly.	May be result of physical weakness, visual alterations, poor motor coordination, poor memory or concentration, anxiety, or lack of interest.
➤ Client is not able to explain factors affecting temperature, common signs and symptoms of fever and hypothermia, or measures to lower fever.	Anxiety, lack of interest, language barrier, or method of instruction may interfere with learning.
RECORDING AND REPORTING	
1. Record information taught and client's response in the home care record.	Documentation of client education is required and will provide continuity of care as the teaching plan progresses.
2. Instruct client to maintain a written record of temperature readings along with time of day measured if routine temperature taking is part of the plan of care.	Variations in temperatures affect the medical and nursing plan of care and can be significant to the treatment ordered.

FOLLOW-UP ACTIVITIES

1. Plan for client to demonstrate next temperature measurement under observation.
2. If home health nurse is visiting client, plan for a repeat demonstration during a scheduled visit.

STEPS | **RATIONALE**

3. Ask client to describe any difficulties experienced while performing temperature measurement and review and/or redesign the learning component with demonstration of that part of the skill.

• • • • •

Special Considerations

- Arthritis or other joint conditions, weakness in finger grasping, or conditions causing pain in upper extremities may prohibit client from being able to shake down thermometer properly.
- Decreased visual acuity or poor lighting in the environment may impair client's ability to properly read the thermometer.
- The client may be unable to safely have temperature measurement taken with a glass thermometer due to physical condition such as **dementia** (does not allow rectal or axillary method, and is at risk for harm if oral route is attempted).
- Clients who are unable to use the glass thermometer may have to use the chemical single-use thermometer strips or the tympanic membrane measurement device.

Teaching Considerations

- Nurse may demonstrate on self or family member. Using client for demonstration prevents client from being able to observe entire procedure.
- Instruct client/family never to use rectal thermometer if post–rectal surgery, with a client who has a rectal disorder such as tumor or severe hemorrhoids, or with clients who cannot be positioned for proper thermometer placement.
- Instruct client/family never to force thermometer into rectum and if client complains of rectal pain after insertion to notify physician and observe for rectal bleeding.
- Use caution in recommending aspirin or any other **over-the-counter drug** or **antipyretic** medicine in clients whose conditions contraindicate their use (e.g., gastric ulcer, bleeding tendencies, risk of Reye's syndrome, allergic reactions, drug interactions, liver or kidney dysfunction). Physician contact before use of antipyretics, even over-the-counter types, is recommended.
- Instruct care giver in safety measures for children and very debilitated clients to include remaining with the client and assisting with maintaining safe and proper placement of thermometer.

Pediatric Considerations

- The stage of growth and development of the child will determine the site of measurement and the type of equipment used (see Chapter 10).
- When using glass thermometers in particular, but as a general rule for any equipment type, the younger child should never be left unattended during the procedure.

Gerontologic Considerations

- The median oral temperature of older adults is 36° C (96.8° F). (Ebersole and Hess, 1994).
- Older adults are more sensitive to temperature changes and have a tendency to demonstrate symptoms of delirium or dementia with variations of body temperature on a more frequent basis than a younger adult.
- Altered internal temperature regulation or dehydration may be seen in frail, debilitated clients. Temperature measurement becomes very important to prevent severe states of hypothermia or hyperthermia.
- Teaching sessions should involve client actively with discussion of activity. Learning will be best accomplished when client is rested and alert. Sessions may be shorter in duration depending on factors such as fatigue.
- Consider common age-related sensory changes in the older adult and direct teaching strategies to compensate for any alterations.

TEACHING CLIENTS TO MEASURE BLOOD PRESSURE

Clients learn to measure blood pressure to assist in the monitoring of health, assessing medication regime effectiveness, or as part of a rehabilitation or exercise program. Clients with underlying physical ailments such as cardiac, kidney, or vascular disease may be susceptible to wide variations in their blood pressure. They should know how to correctly measure this indicator of their health status so they can seek medical attention early when alterations outside their acceptable ranges occur. Nurses can teach clients the skills of measuring arterial blood pressure and the important issues surrounding unusual readings of this measurement. Specific actions to be taken to reduce the chance of negative outcomes that are possible with poorly controlled blood pressure are equally important to the teaching plan. (See Chapter 10.)

EQUIPMENT

- Mercury or aneroid sphygmomanometer
- Bladder and cuff: bladder should completely encircle arm without overlapping; cuff should be secure and fit snugly

Average measurements:

a. Width of bladder
   - Adult: 12 to 13 cm (4.8 to 5.2 in)
   - Obese arm: 15 to 16 cm (6 to 6.4 in)
   - Infant: 6 to 8 cm (2.4 to 3.2 in)

b. Length of bladder:
   - Adult: 22 to 23 cm (8.8 to 9.2 in)
   - Obese arm: 30 cm (12 in)
   - Infant: 12 to 13 cm (4.8 to 5.2 in)

- Stethoscope (two-headed stethoscope ideal for teaching)
- Pen and paper for recording

Various types of electronic blood pressure reading devices are commercially available for home care use. These devices produce a blood pressure measurement without needing to use a stethoscope. A cuff around the arm or even a fingertip device is used and a reading is displayed electronically for the client. When teaching this skill is not possible using the conventional equipment, these types of equipment may be used. Issues surrounding calibration and accuracy of this equipment needs to be investigated before a purchase by the client is made.

STEPS	RATIONALE
ASSESSMENT	
1. Assess client's abilities to manipulate and properly place the cuff, to handle and read the measurement gauge, and to properly place and hear through the stethoscope.	Physical restrictions in handling, seeing, or hearing through the equipment may require the nurse to instruct family member instead of client.
2. Assess client's knowledge of normal blood pressure range and symptoms and common causes of hypotension and hypertension.	Identifies client's ability to know when to initiate preventive health measures and recognize alterations in BP.
3. Assess client's knowledge of what BP measures and any specific medical issues that impact on why an awareness of variations are important to the client's well-being.	Identifies client's understanding of potential cause-and-effect relationships of poorly controlled BP variations for health status.
4. If client has had experience in measuring BP, ask for demonstration of technique.	Allows nurse to assess client's knowledge and skill performance.
5. Determine best site for BP assessment. Avoid applying cuff to arm with IV fluids infusing or with an infusion catheter in place, in the presence of arteriovenous shunt, when breast or axillary surgery has been performed on that side, if arm or hand has been traumatized or diseased, or in presence of lower arm cast or bulky bandage.	Inappropriate site selection may result in poor amplification of sounds, causing inaccurate readings. Application of pressure from inflated bladder can temporarily impair blood flow and compromise circulation in extremity that already has impaired circulation.
6. Assess the home environment for a quiet place for accurate BP measurement.	

NURSING DIAGNOSIS

Clustering of defining characteristics from the assessment data may reveal the following nursing diagnoses for clients requiring this skill:

- Decreased cardiac output
- Fluid volume deficit
- Fluid volume excess
- Health maintenance management
- Health-seeking behaviors
- Knowledge deficit regarding blood pressure monitoring

Related factors are individualized based on a client's condition or needs.

PLANNING

STEPS	RATIONALE
1. **Expected outcomes** following completion of procedure:	
➤ BP is accurately monitored by client.	Learning has occurred.
➤ BP is within range expected for client for client's age and condition.	Cardiovascular status is maintained at a level that is acceptable for the client.

STEPS	RATIONALE
➤ Client explains purpose and implications of therapies and describes which alterations in BP require communication with physician to evaluate changes in treatment regime.	Measures cognitive learning.
2. Encourage client to perform measurements on routine schedule for a long-term monitoring plan.	Daily activities and many extrinsic and intrinsic factors affect BP fluctuations.
3. Encourage client to avoid exercise and smoking for 30 minutes before assessment.	These factors can cause false elevations in BP.
4. Have client perform measurement in a comfortable position and warm and quiet environment.	Maintains client's comfort during measurement.
5. In teaching phase, explain procedure to client and have client rest at least 5 minutes before measurement.	Reduces anxiety that can falsely elevate readings. BP readings taken at different times can be objectively compared when all are assessed with the client at rest.
6. Have client describe symptoms that would benefit from performing a BP measurement to evaluate possible causes of symptoms.	Measures learning of health status alterations that may need medical intervention.

IMPLEMENTATION

STEPS	RATIONALE
1. Discuss with client the best sites for assessing BP: brachial and popliteal artery. For self-measurement, brachial artery is almost always used.	Most accessible sites are easiest to measure for accuracy of assessment.
➤ **CRITICAL DECISION POINT** **Caution client about inappropriate site selection that would result in poor amplification of sounds or compromise circulation in a traumatized limb.**	Appropriate site selection will promote accuracy in reading and minimize potential for trauma.
2. Demonstrate steps for skill performance (see Chapter 10): palpation of artery, positioning of cuff, wrapping of cuff, placement of stethoscope, inflation and release of cuff, listening.	Demonstration is best technique for teaching psychomotor skill.
3. Describe the sounds of measurement and relationship to observation of gauge as BP reading.	Learning is supported with appropriate information being received.
➤ **CRITICAL DECISION POINT** **Caution client about circulation to the limb being used for measurement and the level and length of time appropriate for cuff inflation.**	Prolonged inflation of cuff may damage circulation of limb.
4. Have client manipulate all the equipment away from a limb.	Proper equipment utilization is required for accurate skill performance.
5. Have client attempt each step of the skill on the nurse or a family member.	Nurse can correct any errors in technique as they occur.
6. Have client demonstrate techniques on self. Do not allow multiple repetitive attempts on any one limb.	Repeated attempts may affect measurement due to anxiety and repeated circulatory restriction.
7. Identify that skill performance teaching may need to be accomplished slowly, attempting each step of the skill at different times until comfort is gained.	Psychomotor, cognitive, and affective learning may be impaired if teaching too quickly is attempted rather than in incremental steps.
8. Have client perform skill under observation and record readings. Use a double-headed stethoscope to verify accuracy of reading, or the nurse should perform BP reading after the client's attempt.	Verification of accuracy promotes confidence in client's abilities to successfully measure BP.
9. Utilize instructions with a written or pictorial guide.	References for the client will promote confidence for independent performance.

EVALUATION

STEPS	RATIONALE
1. Observe client demonstrate technique for BP measurement on at least three different occasions.	Feedback through independent demonstration of psychomotor learning is best means to evaluate.

STEPS	RATIONALE
2. If BP is inaudible or difficult to obtain, wait 1 or 2 minutes and repeat attempt.	Prevents venous congestion and false high reading.
3. If pressure is still inaudible or difficult to obtain, try alternative methods: use other arm, attempt palpation, consider other equipment for measurement, or attempt measurement in leg.	Alternative methods can provide accurate measurement of BP.
4. **Unexpected outcomes** that may occur include:	
➤ Client or family member is unable to utilize this measurement method due to inability to manipulate equipment or accurately hear or palpate BP.	Indicates need for alteration in teaching plan.
➤ Client has difficulty in explaining purposes or implications of therapy.	Reinstruction is required.
➤ BP is above or below normal range for client.	Indicates potential for alterations in peripheral vascular resistance, blood volume, or cardiac function.

Recording and Reporting

1. Record teaching and client responses in home care record.	Allows for continuity and progression in teaching plan.
2. Record BP in home care record and home documentation system developed.	Vital signs should be recorded immediately to ensure accuracy.
3. Report abnormal readings to physician.	Abnormalities may necessitate alteration in treatment regime or immediate medical therapy.

Follow-Up Activities

1. Review skill performance and recording of BP measurements client has performed in between home care nursing visits. Demonstrates ability to comply and learned responses to take in event of abnormal reading.

• • • • •

Special Considerations

- ➤ If palpation method is used, palpation of artery should not be done with thumb, because pulse in thumb will confuse palpation.
- ➤ As long as cuff is inflated client will feel numbness or tingling in arm because of reduced blood flow.
- ➤ Auscultation in lower extremity is used when brachial artery is inaccessible or unavailable or in certain clients with BP abnormality that requires a comparison of arm and leg BP.
- ➤ The appropriate cuff size must be used (adult, large adult, thigh, or pediatric) to provide accuracy.
- ➤ If a digital or aneroid sphygmomanometer is used, it should be calibrated to a mercury sphygmomanometer on an annual basis.
- ➤ Improper care and storage of equipment can affect accuracy of measurement.

Teaching Considerations

- ➤ Nurse should demonstrate on self or family member. Using client for total demonstration prevents client from being able to observe entire procedure. Nurse explains rationale for each step during demonstration.
- ➤ Client needs to be educated about risks for hypertension (see Chapter 10).
- ➤ The client needs to understand the specifics of the treatment regime, including potential side effects and interactions of any drug therapies.
- ➤ Instruct that if it is difficult to hear the pressure, the cuff may be too loose or not the correct size; the stethoscope may not be over the arterial pulse, or the tubing may be too long; the cuff may have been deflated too quickly or too slowly; or cuff may not have been pumped high enough for systolic readings.
- ➤ Issues of mobility, movement, and manual dexterity will impact on ability to perform BP measurement.

Pediatric Considerations

- ➤ A newborn's BP range is normally 50 to 52/25 to 30.
- ➤ A 3 year old's BP range is normally 78 to 114/46 to 78.
- ➤ A 10 year old's BP range is normally 90 to 132/56 to 86.
- ➤ An adolescent's BP range is normally 124 to 136/77 to 84 for boys (124 to 127/63 to 74 for girls).

- Understand that accurate BP readings may be difficult if the infant or young child is not cooperative in the procedure. Assistance from others in the form of cajoling or providing diversionary tactics may be needed.
- Young children will be more apt to cooperate if allowed to manipulate and/or play with the equipment before the procedure. Another suggested technique is to perform the procedure first on the parent or other significant person to the child to allow observation of role modeling that the procedure is safe for the child to undergo.

Gerontologic Considerations

- An older adult's BP range is normally 140 to 160/80 to 90.
- Musculoskeletal changes such as arthritis or other joint conditions may impair abilities to position limb comfortably and/or perform the fine motor skills required.
- Possible alterations in hearing or visual acuity associated with changes of aging or disease processes may impact negatively on this skill performance by the client.

TEACHING CLIENTS TO ASSESS THEIR OWN PULSE

Certain clients can benefit from knowing how to assess their own pulse. Persons taking medications that specifically affect heart function are already symptomatic of heart disease and are susceptible to side effects of the medications. By being able to assess their own pulse rate and rhythm correctly, these clients can detect complications of their disease, as well as any undesirable effects of their medications. Clients can thus seek prompt medical attention before serious problems occur.

Another group of clients who should learn how to assess their own pulse are those undergoing cardiovascular rehabilitation. For example, clients who have had myocardial infarction undergo exercise training to improve the strength of their heart muscle. Pulse rate and rhythm are the criteria used to determine how well these clients tolerate exercise.

There are also many healthy persons who actively exercise and who can learn about their health from measuring their own pulse. Exercise tolerance can vary depending on environmental conditions, intake of certain foods, and the overall physical condition of a person. By measuring pulse rate and rhythm, a person can learn how the body responds to strenuous exercise and when to cease further physical activity.

EQUIPMENT

- Wristwatch or clock with second hand
- Paper and pencil

STEPS	RATIONALE
ASSESSMENT	
1. Identify client's knowledge of purpose for assessing pulse and level of interest in performing skill.	Aids in identifying client's motivation to regularly assess pulse after learning skill. Also allows nurse to assess client's understanding of physical conditions and knowledge of medications prescribed.
2. Assess client's ability to feel arterial pulse by having client palpate own or nurse's artery. (Nurse palpates pulse of client or self simultaneously to see if client can successfully feel pulse wave.)	Physical impairment in sensation may necessitate nurse instructing family member or significant other instead of client.
3. If client reports having measured own pulse before, ask client to demonstrate technique for assessing pulse.	Reveals client's level of skill in assessing pulse.

NURSING DIAGNOSIS

Clustering of defining characteristics from the assessment data may reveal the following nursing diagnoses for clients requiring this skill:

- Anxiety
- Decreased cardiac output
- Fluid volume deficit
- Fluid volume excess
- Impaired home maintenance management
- Health-seeking behaviors
- Knowledge deficit regarding obtaining pulse

Related factors are individualized based on a client's condition or needs.

STEPS	RATIONALE
PLANNING	
1. **Expected outcomes** following completion of procedure:	
➤ Client is able to measure own pulse rate and rhythm correctly.	Indicates skill was effectively learned.
➤ Client identifies normal range of pulse rate.	Cognitive learning was achieved.
➤ Client discusses importance of assessing pulse and best time for measurement.	
➤ Client discusses abnormalities and steps to take.	
2. Select setting in home that client is most likely to use when assessing pulse.	Practicing in same environment in which skill is routinely performed facilitates comprehension and learning.
IMPLEMENTATION	
1. Discuss with client the best sites for assessing pulse: radial and carotid.	Most accessible sites are easiest to palpate for accuracy of assessment.
CRITICAL DECISION POINT If carotid is chosen, caution client against vigorously massaging the neck while attempting to locate pulse or attempting to locate both arteries at the same time.	Stimulation of carotid sinus could lead to reflex slowing of heart rate. Simultaneous occlusion of both carotid arteries decreases blood to brain, resulting in fainting.
2. Demonstrate steps for palpating pulse (see Chapter 10): position wrist or neck, locate artery, use fingertips for palpation, compress artery, palpate pulse before counting, count pulse, calculate pulse.	Demonstration is best technique for teaching psychomotor skill.
➤ Instruct use of gentle pressure; reinforce not to press hard over pulses.	
➤ Instruct in use of watch or clock with a second hand to assess pulses.	
➤ Instruct to count for a full 60 seconds, starting with the second hand at the 12:00 position to reduce confusion, forgetfulness about the time period, or starting point used for pulse measurement.	

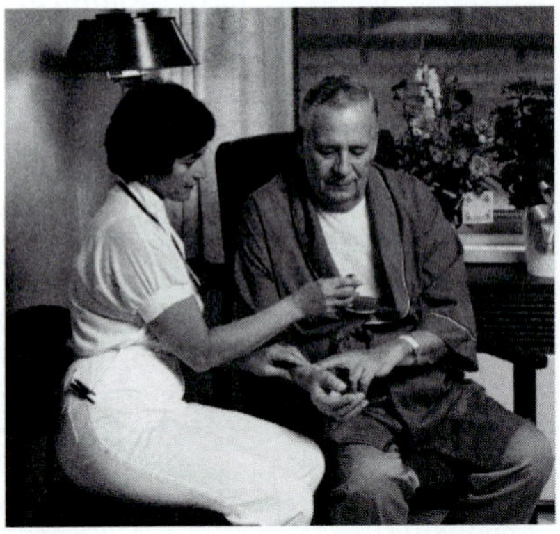

Step 3 Nurse observing client checking pulse.

STEPS	RATIONALE
3. Have client perform each step with nurse's guidance (see illustration).	Nurse can correct any errors in technique as they occur.
4. Discuss normal desired pulse range, purpose for monitoring pulse, and best time to assess pulse.	Client must be able to identify pulse alterations.
CRITICAL DECISION POINT Discuss importance of notifying physician and withholding medication dose when pulse alterations occur.	Client must understand preventive measures to take and physician's directions to be followed if alterations in pulse develop.
EVALUATION	
1. Observe client independently demonstrate technique for pulse assessment and calculate pulse rate and rhythm three times.	Feedback through independent demonstration of psychomotor skill is best means of evaluating learning of skill.
2. Have learner take radial pulse rate of nurse or other person at same time nurse is taking pulse of the individual.	Concomitant pulse taking will verify the learner is able to accurately accomplish this skill.

STEPS	RATIONALE
3. Ask client to identify reasons for assessing pulse, normal pulse rate range, and steps to take when abnormalities are found.	Measures client's cognitive learning.
4. Ask client to reiterate instructions regarding the withholding of medication in response to critical changes in pulse rate.	Confirms understanding of specific medical instructions received regarding the withholding of certain prescribed medications with specific pulse rates.
5. Ask client to state time of day and activity level before pulse taking if purpose of measuring is for possible medication dosage adjustment.	Demonstrates understanding of relationships of time of day and activity levels with pulse rate variation.
6. **Unexpected outcomes** that may occur include:	
➤ Client is unable to palpate pulse or count rate correctly.	May result from sensory alteration or inability to locate artery or palpate it correctly. Clients with preexisting dysrhythmias often have difficulty learning to count pulse correctly.
➤ Client is unable to discuss information related to pulse assessment.	Anxiety, lack of interest, language barriers, or method of instruction may interfere with learning.

Recording and Reporting

1. Record information taught and client's response in home care record.	Health agencies are required to document client education; provides continuity between teaching sessions.
2. Have client develop and use a written record of pulse rate, rhythm, time of taking, and whether medications are to be withheld with certain variations.	A written record of pulse rate will help in assessment of cardiovascular status and understanding of medication compliance.

Follow-up Activities

1. Plan a repeat demonstration during subsequent scheduled home care nursing visits to evaluate client's ability to retain information and skill.
2. Review the client's pulse assessment recording sheet to assess for significant issues or medication noncompliance.

• • • • •

Special Considerations

- A very difficult learning step is that of palpating the artery. Clients tend to obliterate pulse at first. Gripping wrist with use of thumb to palpate pulse is a common action used initially by the learner. The thumb is not the appropriate digit to palpate a pulse. Taking the client's pulse can be an effective way of showing how light palpation with fingers works best.
- Pulse rate is usually assessed before medications are taken and before and during exercise.
- Physicians will recommend whether drug dose should be withheld in the event of pulse alteration. Clients taking thyroid medications are often instructed to withhold medications when pulse is above 100; Inderal or digitalis often is withheld if pulse is below 60. Specific drug dosage instructions are to be confirmed with physician and documented in the home care record, as well as written for the client.

Teaching Considerations

- Nurse may demonstrate on self or family member. Using client for entire demonstration prevents client from being able to observe entire procedure. Nurse explains rationale for each step during demonstration.

Pediatric Considerations

- The femoral pulse is the best site for palpation of pulse for an infant or toddler. Although the carotid pulse is a more easily obtained reading than the radial, which is usually used for adults, when teaching nonmedical care givers, the potential for occluding the carotid artery and creating hypoxia should be avoided.
- In infants, a pulse can be observed (do not palpate) and counted on the anterior fontanelle.
- At birth, the pulse rate averages 120 beats/minute. This rate decreases steadily over the next 4 years until reaching an average pulse rate of 100 beats/minute.
- The normal pulse range by adolescence is within the adult range of 60 to 100 beats/minute.

Gerontologic Considerations

- Musculoskeletal changes such as arthritis or other joint conditions may impair abilities to palpate pulse for 60 seconds due to discomfort caused by positioning. Provide the client with options for comfortable resting position of limbs when measuring pulse.
- Be aware of possible changes in visual acuity and ensure the environment and equipment used (clock or watch) support clear visualization.

SKILL 42-2 Using Home Oxygen Equipment

Home oxygen therapy is usually administered via a **nasal cannula;** and, more recently, is administered through a reservoir nasal cannula, which stores oxygen in a chamber during the expiratory phase of respirations (Rice, 1996), and a Venturi mask. When a client has a permanent tracheostomy however, a T-tube, tracheostomy collar, or **transtracheal oxygen therapy** (TTOT) is used. TTOT is a newer method of oxygen administration that delivers oxygen directly into the trachea using a scoop catheter. In the home, the main consideration is the oxygen delivery source; the three types used are (1) compressed oxygen, (2) oxygen concentrators (Fig. 42-1; Table 42-1), and (3) liquid oxygen (see Fig. 42-2 A-B).

Compressed oxygen requires the delivery of several large oxygen tanks to the home. Each tank lasts approximately 50 hours at 2 liters/minute. Liquid systems use a small portable tank that is filled from a reservoir in the home. The oxygen concentrator method extracts oxygen from the room air and supplies oxygen to the client at prescribed flow rates. Table 42-2 shows how long a liquid oxygen system will last depending on the prescribed flow rate. Home oxygen therapy is often paid for by governmental or private insurances if there are written orders prescribed by the physician. Specific guidelines must be met before Medicare coverage can begin (see the box on p. 1187).

Clients requiring home oxygen need extensive teaching so that they can continue their oxygen therapy efficiently and safely. In preparation the home care nurse must coordinate efforts with the client, physician, care givers, oxygen supply vendor, and payor. The nurse must set aside sufficient time for client and family teaching so proper oxygen therapy can be performed safely and accurately in the home. Ultimately, the home care nurse is responsible and accountable for determining the validity of safe and effective home oxygen administration.

EQUIPMENT

- **Nasal cannula (see Skill 12-1) or other prescribed delivery device**
- **Oxygen tubing**
- **Liquid oxygen**
- **In home: Liberator**
- **Portable system: Stroller**
- **Cylinders**
- **In home: H tanks**
- **Portable system: E cylinder**
- **Concentrator for home system**

Table 42-1 Home Oxygen Systems

Primary Use	Advantages	Disadvantages
Compressed gas cylinders		
Intermittent therapy, such as for exercise or sleep only	100% oxygen, relatively inexpensive, no loss of gas during storage, relatively portable, delivery of up to 15 L/min	Bulky, possibly unsightly, frequent refilling necessary with continuous use
Liquid oxygen systems		
High-liter flows and active clients	100% oxygen, conveniently portable, portable units refilled at home, delivery of up to 6 L/min	Usually weekly delivery necessary for refill, evaporates if not used, potential for frostbite at connections and if liquid is spilled
Concentrators		
Moderate-liter flows and clients with limited mobility inside or outside home	Fixed monthly cost, minimal interruption of household by supplier, no refills of "main tank," most units with delivery of up to 4 or 5 L/min	Oxygen concentration decreases as liter flow increases (usually 85% to 90%), power supply necessary, electric bill increase of $15 to $20 a month, second system for portability necessary (usually gas cylinders)

From Dettenmeier PA: *Pulmonary nursing care,* St Louis, 1992, Mosby.

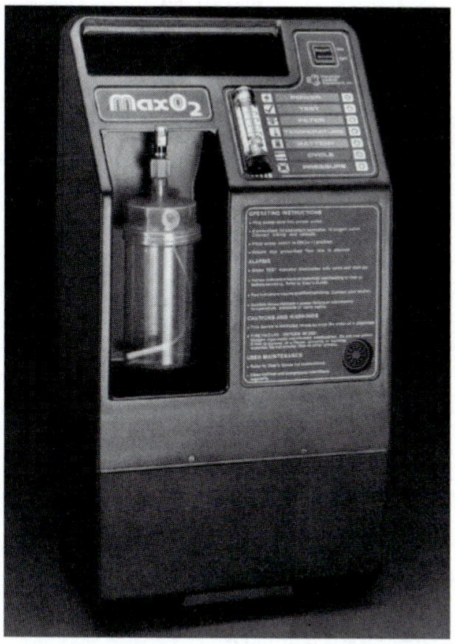

Fig. 42-1 Oxygen concentrator. (Courtesy Mountain Medical Equipment Inc, Littleton, Colo.)

MEDICARE QUALIFICATIONS FOR HOME OXYGEN THERAPY

PaO_2 ≤55 mm Hg or SaO_2 ≤85% or PaO_2 = 56 to 59 mm Hg *and*
Dependent edema suggesting congestive heart failure *or*
Cor pulmonale as evidenced on ECG *or*
Erythrocytosis as evidenced by hematocrit >56%

Nocturnal Oxygen Therapy

PaO_2 ≤55 mm Hg during sleep *or*
PaO_2 falls more than 10 mm Hg during sleep *or*
SaO_2 ≤85% during sleep or falls more than 5% during sleep

Exercise Oxygen Therapy

PaO_2 ≤55 mm Hg during exercise *or*
SaO_2 ≤85% during exercise

PaO_2, Arterial oxygen tension (partial pressure); SaO_2, oxygen saturation in blood; ECG, electrocardiogram.

Table 42-2 Liquid Oxygen Timetable

	Stationary Reservoirs		Portable Units	
L/Min	17,000 L	25,000 L	500 L	1000 L
1	248 hr	396 hr	7 hr	14 hr
2	124 hr	198 hr	3 hr	7 hr
3	83 hr	134 hr	2 hr	4½ hr
4	61 hr	99 hr	1½ hr	3½ hr
5	40 hr	80 hr	—	—
6	—	—	1 hr	2 hr

When oxygen cylinders are used, the following formulas are used to determine the length of time a tank will last.

For E Cylinders
Pressure on cylinder gauge (PSI)—500 psi (safety factor) × 0.3 (E cylinder factor) ÷ L/min = minutes

For H Cylinders
Pressure on cylinder gauge (PSI)—500 psi (safety factor) × 3.1 (H cylinder factor) ÷ L/min = minutes

EXAMPLE: E cylinder reads 1500 psi
Liter flow rate is 4 L/min
1500 − 500 × 0.3 ÷ 4 = ?
1000 × 0.3 ÷ 4 = ?
300 ÷ 4 = ?
75 minutes, or 1 hour 15 minutes

NOTE: Do not allow oxygen cylinder pressure to fall below 500 psi, or the client may run out of oxygen.

STEPS	RATIONALE
ASSESSMENT	
1. Determine client's or family's ability to use oxygen equipment correctly while in hospital (if appropriate and possible), and assess for appropriate use of equipment in the home.	Physical or cognitive impairments may necessitate instructing family member or significant other how to operate home oxygen equipment.
2. Assess the home environment for electrical power if compressor is used.	
3. Assess client's and/or family's ability to observe for signs and symptoms of **hypoxia:** apprehension, anxiety, decreased ability to concentrate, decreased levels of consciousness, increased fatigue, dizziness, behavioral changes, increased pulse, increased respiratory rate, pallor, cyanosis.	Hypoxia can occur at home when client uses oxygen. It can be caused by worsening of the client's physical problem or another underlying condition such as change in respiratory status.
4. Observe client's or family's ability to use prescribed oxygen therapy.	Enables nurse to determine specific components of skill that client or family can easily complete.
5. Determine appropriate resource in the community for equipment and assistance.	Ensures repair service availability, readily available assistance, and additional equipment for clients with home oxygen systems.
6. Determine appropriate back-up system, if compressor is used, in event of power failure.	

NURSING DIAGNOSIS

Clustering of defining characteristics from the assessment data may reveal the following nursing diagnoses for clients requiring this skill:

- Altered peripheral tissue perfusion
- Anxiety
- Impaired home maintenance management
- Ineffective breathing pattern
- Knowledge deficit regarding home oxygen therapy

Related factors are individualized based on a client's condition or needs.

A

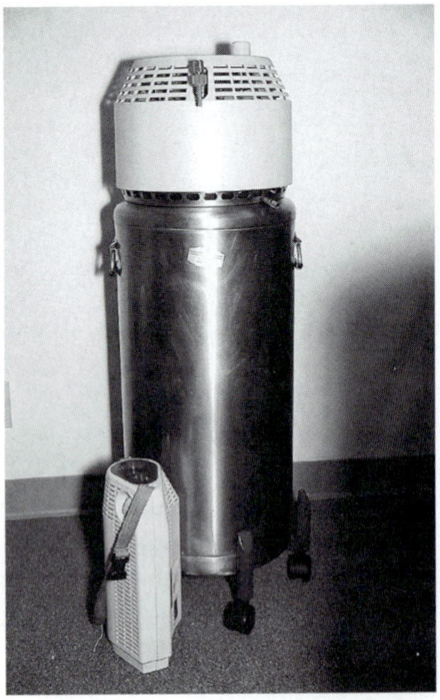

Fig. 42-2A Liquid oxygen container.

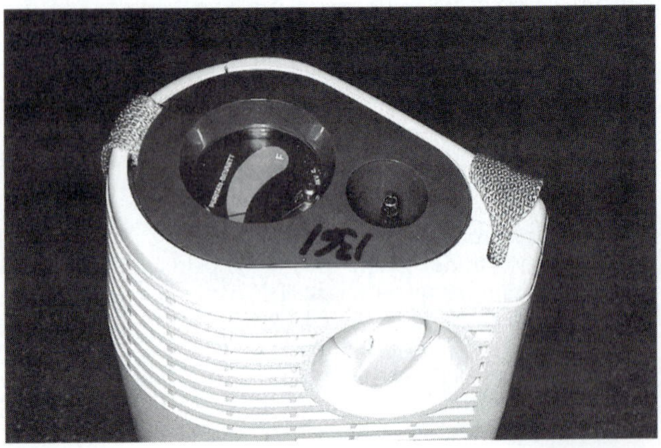

B

Fig. 42-2B Control panel.

STEPS	RATIONALE
PLANNING	
1. Expected outcomes following completion of procedure:	
➤ Client and family will verbalize the purpose and correct use of home oxygen.	Provides measurable criteria to determine the client's and family's level of understanding.
➤ Client and family will demonstrate how to set up the oxygen system.	Provides return demonstration of skills needed to use home oxygen system.
➤ Client and family will be able to verbalize safety guidelines for oxygen use.	Provides measure of client's and family's understanding of oxygen use.
➤ Client and family will be able to verbalize emergency plan of care.	
2. Explain the procedure to the client and family.	Reinforces teaching received. Enables client and family to ask questions.
IMPLEMENTATION	
1. Wash hands.	Reduces transmission of microorganisms.
2. Demonstrate steps for preparation and completion of oxygen therapy.	Demonstration is reliable technique for teaching psychomotor skill and enables client to ask questions.
3. Prepare the Liberator and Stroller for use:	
a. Place Liberator in a clutter-free environment (Fig. 42-2A).	30-L Liberator replaces three-and-one-half compressed oxygen cylinders.
➤ ***CRITICAL DECISION POINT*** **Check oxygen levels of both Liberator and Stroller by depressing button at lower right corner and reading dial (Fig. 42-2B).**	Ensures timely and effective use of remaining oxygen supply and allows time for refill.
b. When necessary, refill Stroller: turn bayonet coupling lock on Stroller 45 degrees. Insert female adapter (Liberator) to male adapter (Liberator) (Fig. 42-3).	Allows secure connection between Liberator and Stroller to prevent leakage of oxygen into room air.
c. Select prescribed rate (Fig. 42-4) and lock flow meter.	Ensures delivery of prescribed amount of oxygen and prevents client from changing oxygen flow rate.

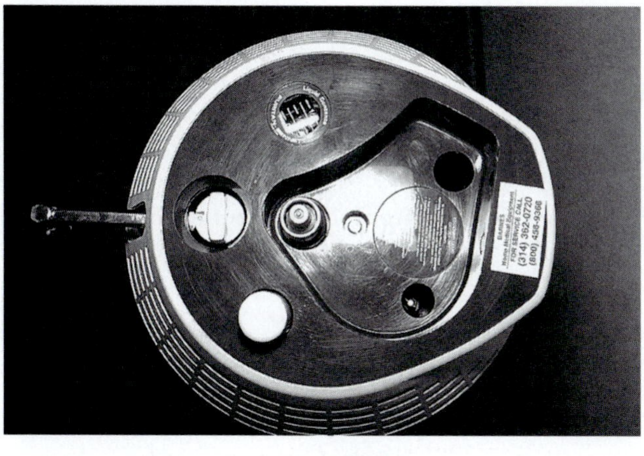

Fig. 42-3

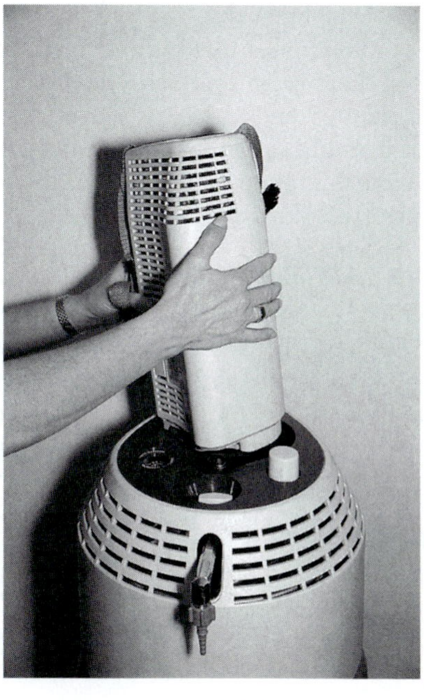

Fig. 42-4

STEPS	RATIONALE
d. Connect appropriate oxygen delivery device and oxygen tubing to Stroller (see Chapter 12)	Connects oxygen source to delivery method.
e. Place Stroller on cart.	Allows client to ambulate freely without expending energy to carry Stroller.
4. Have client or family member perform each step with guidance from nurse. Provide written material for reinforcement and review.	Allows nurse to correct any errors in technique and discuss their implications.
CRITICAL DECISION POINT **Discuss signs and symptoms of respiratory tract infection: fever, increased sputum, change in color of sputum, foul sputum odor.**	
5. Instruct client or family to notify physician if signs or symptoms of hypoxia or respiratory tract infections occur.	Respiratory tract infections increase oxygen demand and may affect oxygen transfer from lungs to blood. Can create severe exacerbation of client's pulmonary disease.
CRITICAL DECISION POINT **Discuss signs and symptoms of mucous plug at tip of scoop catheter: unexplained dyspnea.**	
6. Instruct client or family to irrigate catheter or have client attempt to cough the mucus out. If unsuccessful, put on nasal oxygen cannula and notify the physician.	Mucus plugs decrease oxygen transfer to lungs. Prevents hypoxia.
7. Discuss emergency plan: power loss, natural disaster, acute respiratory distress; call 911, notify physician and agency.	Ensures appropriate response and can prevent worsening of client's condition.
8. Wash hands.	Reduces transmission of microorganisms.
9. Record teaching plan, information given to client, and validation of learning.	Provides written documentation of teaching plan for client and family. Documents client learning.
EVALUATION	
1. Evaluate client's or family's understanding and ability to use oxygen at home.	Determines ability of client or family to deal with stressors associated with home oxygen use. Also indicates client's risk for inappropriate oxygen use.
2. **Unexpected outcomes** that may occur include:	
➤ Signs and symptoms associated with hypoxia (see Assessment, Step 3).	Indicates inadequate oxygen delivery and can result from or lead to worsening of client's condition.
➤ Client uses unsafe practices with oxygen therapy, uses oxygen around fire or cigarette smoking, or sets incorrect flow rate.	Indicates knowledge deficit regarding use of home oxygen.

Recording and Reporting

1. Record in home care record teaching plan preparations for teaching client to use home oxygen.	Provides written documentation for nurses to complete the teaching plan for client or family.
2. Record in home care record information given to client or family and any validation of learning.	Documents client teaching in record.
3. Communicate client's or family's learning progress to other health care providers involved.	Provides continuing feedback to client regarding ability to independently use portable oxygen system.

Follow-up Activities

1. Instruct client and family when to notify physician of signs of hypoxia.
2. Reinforce education and perform follow-up assessment.

Special Considerations

- Sprint has flow rate setting of 0.25, 0.5, 0.75, 1, 2, or 3 L/minute. Standard Stroller has flow rate of 1, 1.5, 2, 2.5, 3, 4, or 6 L/minute.
- Potential for oxygen desaturation and decreased oxygen delivery to brain impairs client's ability to remember previous learning. Thus nurse should provide more opportunity and written or pictorial instructions to reinforce previous learning of teaching plan.
- Some clients are able to manage portable oxygen system but are unable to fill portable system and require assistance.

Teaching Considerations

- Equipment vendor and nurse should instruct client how frequently Liberator and Stroller must be filled. Small Liberator (Sprint) has 4-hour capacity, whereas 9.5 lb Stroller has 8-hour capacity. Refilling occurs automatically and takes a few seconds to a minute, depending on amounts of oxygen required to fill Stroller.
- Identify learning objectives for teaching plan. Client or family will be able to state signs and symptoms of hypoxia and respiratory tract infections, state factors that affect oxygenation, and correctly use prescribed oxygen delivery system (i.e., nasal cannula [see Skill 12-1] or portable oxygen delivery system).
- Instruct client to observe level of oxygen in canister tank and to use portable tank when client goes out.
- Instruct client to fill plastic humidity bottle with distilled water every 24 hours. Tap water should not be used.
- Check mask and tubing by placing hands or face over mask or cannula to feel air flow.
- Check to be sure mask is not too tight; it can leave marks on skin. Apply cotton or gauze sponge at pressure points.
- Instruct client to keep a bell handy for notifying primary care giver when help is needed.

Pediatric Considerations

- Equipment must be kept out of reach of the child and/or other children in the home. Manipulation of dials or flow meters could have disasterous effects on the oxygen delivery process.

Gerontologic Considerations

- Older adults have less efficient respiratory systems and less surface area for gas exchange, so their response to decreased oxygen and infection may cause cerebral anoxia and they may experience confusion. They may be unable to recognize respiratory problems or problems with the delivery system; therefore they must have frequent contact with a designated care giver.
- Provide two complete sets of tubing so that there is equipment available for use while the other is being cleansed or repaired.
- Assess the home for availability of a three-pronged outlet for the compressor to prevent electric shock.
- Keep skin dry under mask; wash with soap and water. Nasal prongs can be cleaned using moistened cotton applicator.
- Maintain constant flow rate: change flow rate only with order of physician.
- Client, family, and visitors must understand danger of and refrain from smoking cigarettes or having any source of fire near oxygen system.

SKILL 42-3 Teaching Home Tracheostomy Care and Suctioning

The indications for performing tracheostomy care and suctioning in the home are similar to tracheostomy care and suctioning in the hospital except for one key variable: the use of principles of medical asepsis or "clean technique." In the hospital, principles of surgical asepsis are used because the client is more susceptible to infection and because more virulent or pathogenic microorganisms are usually present than in the home setting. In the home setting the majority of clients use clean technique.

However, not all home care clients should use the clean technique. The nurse must use good nursing judgment in choosing clients who are candidates for using clean or aseptic technique. The immunocompromised client, who is at risk for severe infections, may need to continue to receive suctioning using principles of surgical asepsis. A client receiving care from visiting nurses or other care givers who have contact with other clients (or institutions) should be suctioned by the nurse using sterile technique. Infected (not colonized) clients should be suctioned using sterile technique until the infection is resolved. Care givers who are infected with viral, bacterial, or fungal microorganisms should suction using principles of surgical asepsis. All care givers should use Standard Precautions when suctioning. Clients living in nonhygienic (nonclean) conditions should be suctioned using sterile technique whenever possible, in hopes of preventing infection.

Caring for a tracheostomy at home begins in the hospital with teaching and return demonstration. The client usually learns better when less invasive techniques such as stoma care precede more invasive techniques such as inner cannula care and suctioning. The nurse continually develops, implements, and evaluates the teaching plan based on client performance. Some clients and their families learn quickly, whereas others do not. Therefore teaching should begin as soon as it is feasible. It is imperative that clients and their families have the ability to suction before discharge; otherwise arrangements to provide 24-hour care are necessary before discharge.

EQUIPMENT

- Suction machine with connecting tube (Fig. 42-5)
- Nonsterile gloves
- 3 Small basins
- Hydrogen peroxide, water (boiled preferred over tap)
- Normal saline
- Clean 4 × 4 gauze pads (nonshredding)
- Appropriate size of sterile or clean and disinfected catheter (diameter should be no greater than half the diameter of the trach tube)
- Tracheostomy care kit *or*
  - Clean 4 × 4 gauze pads (nonshredding)
  - Water-soluble lubricant
  - Small nylon bottle brush or pipe cleaners
  - Cotton-tipped applicators
  - Trach ties (twill 3/8-in preferably)

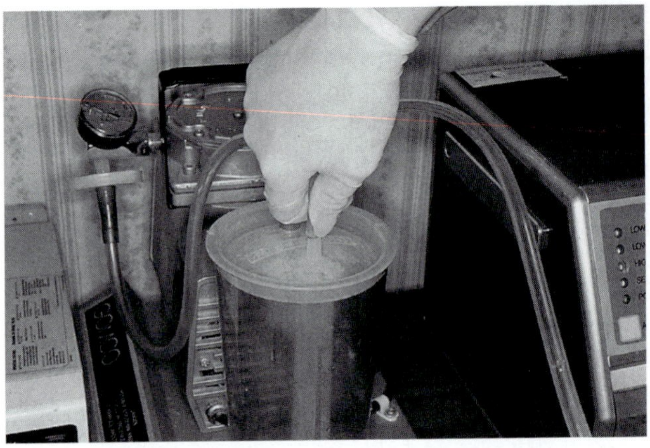

Fig. 42-5

- Mirror
- Wet washcloth or paper towel
- Dry cloth, towel, or paper towel
- Protective eye wear (optional)
- Trash bag (plastic, nonleaking preferred)
- Disposable apron (optional)

STEPS	RATIONALE
ASSESSMENT	
1. Assess client's ability to properly perform tracheostomy care and suctioning.	Physical and cognitive impairment may necessitate instructing family member or significant other to perform tracheostomy care and suctioning. An emergency situation may also necessitate family member or significant other to suction.
2. Assess client and family member's knowledge and ability to observe for signs and symptoms of need to perform:	
a. Tracheostomy care, including excess peristomal secretions, excess intratracheal secretions, soiled or damp tracheostomy dressing/ties, and diminished airway through trach tube.	Signs and symptoms are related to presence of secretions at stoma site or within tracheostomy tube.
b. Suctioning, including gurgling, tactile fremitus, wheezes or crackles on inspiration or expiration, restlessness, ineffective coughing, absent or diminished breath sounds, tachypnea, cyanosis, acutely decreased level of consciousness, hypertension or hypotension, tachycardia or bradycardia, acutely shallow respirations, or acute dyspnea.	Physical signs and symptoms result from lower airway obstruction and tissue hypoxia.
3. Assess client's and family's ability to observe for factors that normally influence tracheostomy airway functioning.	Allows client to accurately evaluate need to perform trach tube suctioning.
4. Assess client understanding of and ability to perform own tracheostomy care and suctioning.	Allows nurse to identify potential need for instruction.
5. Observe client or family member performing complete trach tube care and suctioning.	Allows the nurse to determine which specific components of skill client or family member can easily complete and which are more difficult.

STEPS	RATIONALE

NURSING DIAGNOSIS

Clustering of defining characteristics from the assessment data may reveal the following nursing diagnoses for clients requiring this skill:

- Body-image disturbance
- Caregiver role strain
- Impaired verbal communication
- Ineffective airway clearance
- Ineffective breathing pattern
- Knowledge deficit regarding tracheostomy care
- Risk for infection

Related factors are individualized based on a client's condition or needs.

PLANNING

STEPS	RATIONALE
1. **Expected outcomes** following completion of procedure:	
➤ Client is able to identify signs and symptoms indicating need for trach care and suctioning.	Allows nurse to objectively measure client's learning and to modify teaching plan as necessary.
➤ Client can state factors that normally influence tracheostomy airway functioning.	Tracheostomy can impair normal airway clearance, humidification, and gas exchange.
➤ Client can correctly demonstrate complete trach tube care and suctioning in controlled setting.	Provides documentation of client's ability to perform procedure.
➤ Client is able to identify signs and symptoms indicating need for trach tube care and suctioning, signs and symptoms of stoma inflammation or respiratory tract infection, and when to notify physician.	Measures cognitive learning.
➤ Lower and upper airways are cleared of secretions. Suctioning is successful as evidenced by absent or diminished crackles, wheezes, tactile fremitus, and gurgles in large airways; return of absent or diminished breath sounds; normalization of vital signs; increased depth of respirations; absence of cyanosis; and decreased dyspnea.	Suctioning is successful.
➤ Stoma site is clean and free of infection; inner cannula is free of secretions.	Tracheostomy care is successful.
2. Select setting in home that client is most likely to use when completing trach tube care.	Practicing skill in same setting where skill will be routinely performed facilitates comprehension and learning.
3. Discuss and demonstrate with client proper position for procedure (high Fowler's position in front of a mirror).	Promotes client's understanding of comfort and safety principles, as well as facilitating visibility.

IMPLEMENTATION

STEPS	RATIONALE
1. Demonstrate step by step preparation and completion of tracheostomy tube suctioning.	Demonstration is reliable technique for teaching psychomotor skill and enables client to ask questions throughout procedure.
2. Verify physician orders for suctioning.	
3. Wash hands.	Reduces transmission of microorganisms.
4. Prepare suction equipment according to manufacturer's directions. a. Place machine on level surface. b. Plug into grounded outlet. c. Set suction pressure between 100 and 120 mm Hg.	
5. Place client in semi-Fowler's position.	Promotes lung expansion.
6. Fill basin with ½ cup water or normal saline.	
7. Put on gloves.	

STEPS	RATIONALE
8. Connect suction catheter to suction apparatus and check that equipment is functioning by suctioning small amount of fluid from basin.	Prepares suction. Ensures proper equipment function before catheter insertion and lubricates internal catheter.
CRITICAL DECISION POINT **Encourage client to cough.**	Loosens secretions and facilitates suctioning.
CRITICAL DECISION POINT **If applicable, remove oxygen or humidity source.**	
9. In an adult insert catheter without applying suction. If resistance (carina) is met, pull catheter back 1 cm.	Places catheter to end of trach tube into tracheobronchial tree.
10. Apply intermittent suction, 5 to 10 seconds, by placing and releasing thumb over catheter vent, and slowly withdraw catheter while rotating it between thumb and forefinger (see illustration). Reapply oxygen or humidifying device.	Intermittent suction and rotation of catheter prevent injury to tracheal mucosal lining and hypoxia.
CRITICAL DECISION POINT **Before continuing suction allow client to rest and encourage to take two to three deep breaths.**	Reduces impact of oxygen loss during suctioning and prevents hypoxia.
11. Using continuous suction, rinse catheter with basin fluid until clean. Repeat steps as needed to remove secretions.	Removes secretions from catheter. Promotes patent airway.
12. Suction nasal and oral pharynx if needed (see Chapter 14).	Removes secretions from upper airway.
13. Rinse catheter as described.	Removes secretions from catheter. Reduces transmission of microorganisms.
14. At conclusion of procedure have client take two to three deep breaths.	Reduces oxygen loss and prevents hypoxia.
15. Disconnect suction catheter, coil, and discard. If catheter is to be cleaned and disinfected, set aside.	
Trach Care	
1. To clean inner cannula, place impervious trash bag near work site and create a clean field for equipment; place the three basins on the field.	Ensures maintenance of Standard Precautions.

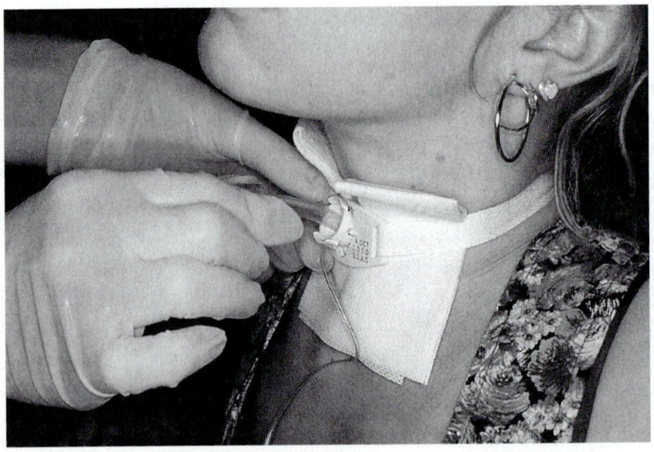

Step 10

STEPS	RATIONALE
2. Pour hydrogen peroxide in one container and water or normal saline in second container. Pour hydrogen peroxide or normal saline in third container with 4 × 4 gauze pads.	
3. Remove old tracheostomy bib or dressing and discard using Standard Precautions.	Reduces transmission of microorganisms.
4. Remove and discard contaminated gloves.	
5. Put on clean gloves.	Reduces transmission of microorganisms.
6. Using presoaked 4 × 4 gauze sponges and damp applicators, gently wash skin around stoma, under trach ties and flanges (see illustration).	Removes secretions that predispose client to localized infection.
7. Dry exposed outer cannula and skin with dry trach gauze/towel.	Prevents moist environment for organism growth.
CRITICAL DECISION POINT **Unlock and remove inner cannula; place in hydrogen peroxide and allow to soak.**	Removes secretions and encrustations adhered to inner cannula.
8. Using nylon brush or pipe cleaners, gently scrub inner cannula.	
CRITICAL DECISION POINT **Rinse inner cannula thoroughly with normal saline or water for at least 15 seconds; shake off excess solution.**	
9. Examine patency of cannula; if not clean, repeat cleansing process. Replace inner cannula in position and lock.	Removes hydrogen peroxide from inner cannula. Remaining solutions could cause airway or stoma irritation.
10. Change ties (see Chapter 14).	
11. Apply fresh trach dressing (see illustration).	Protects skin around stoma from pressure breakdown and collects secretions.
12. Clean reusable supplies in warm soapy water. Rinse thoroughly and dry between two layers of clean paper towels. Store supplies in loosely closed clear plastic bag.	Prevents transmission of microorganisms. Air must circulate or humidity in bag can promote microorganism growth.
13. Remove and discard gloves. Wash hands.	Reduces transmission of microorganisms.
14. **Reusable supplies should be disinfected at least weekly.** To disinfect supplies use one of the methods described here: a. Method 1: Boil reusable (boilable) supplies for 15 minutes. Allow to cool and dry.	

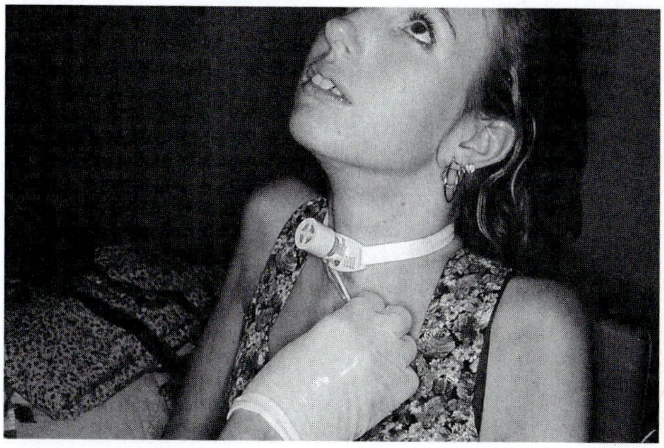

Step 6

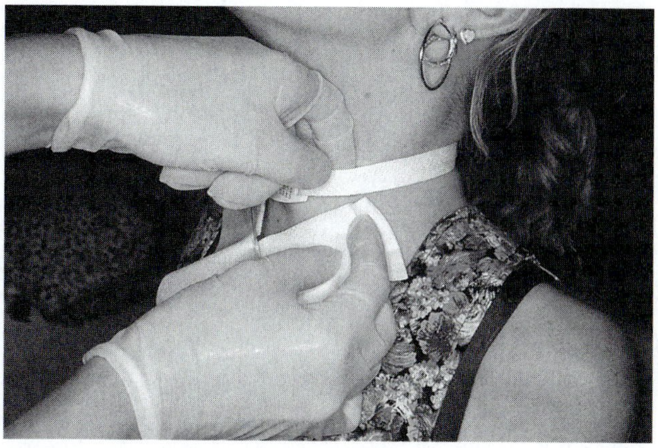

Step 11

STEPS	RATIONALE
b. Method 2: Soak reusable supplies in equal parts of vinegar and water for 30 minutes. Remove, rinse thoroughly, and dry.	Reduces transmission of microorganisms.
c. Method 3: Soak reusable supplies in prepared solutions of quaternary ammonium chloride compounds according to manufacturer's instructions. Rinse and dry.	
15. Have client or family member perform each step with guidance from nurse.	Nurse can correct any errors in technique as they occur and discuss their implications.
16. Discuss signs and symptoms of: a. Stomal infection (redness, tenderness, drainage) b. Respiratory tract infection (fever, increased sputum, change in color of sputum, foul sputum odor, increased cough, chills, nightsweats).	Client must be able to recognize onset of inflammation or infections.
CRITICAL DECISION POINT **Discuss importance of notifying physician when prolonged stoma inflammation or respiratory infection occurs.**	Physician can prescribe medications to alleviate respiratory tract infection and inflammation. Client must understand implications of upper respiratory tract infection.

EVALUATION

1. Ask client to state signs of stomal or respiratory tract infection.	Prompt identification of symptoms results in early treatment and decreases risk of complications that may lead to hospital readmission.
2. Have client demonstrate technique for trach tube care and suctioning.	Feedback through independent demonstration of psychomotor skill is reliable method to evaluate learning.
3. **Unexpected outcomes** that may occur include:	
➤ Stoma site is reddened or hard, with or without drainage.	Tracheostomy site is contaminated.
➤ Copious colored secretions are present around stoma or when client is suctioned.	Infection is present.
➤ Bloody secretions are suctioned.	Sign of denuded cilia and mucosal lining or infection.
➤ No secretions are suctioned.	No secretions are present or secretions are too thick to suction.
➤ Trach tube comes out.	Trach tube is improperly secured.
➤ Skin breakdown is present at stoma site.	Pressure areas have developed from faceplate of trach tube or area has not been kept clean and dry.

RECORDING AND REPORTING

1. Record in client record the teaching done and accuracy of care delivered by client or family member.	Documents type and quality of self-care delivered by client and family.
2. Develop a system of recording to be used by the client/care giver to provide information that compliance is achieved or maintained.	To be effective on a long-term basis, accuracy in technique must be maintained and can partially be monitored by some reporting/recording mechanism.

FOLLOW-UP ACTIVITIES

1. For bloody secretions, evaluate suctioning technique, suctioning frequency, and size of catheter used; identify other signs of infection.
2. For absence of secretions, evaluate fluid status, need for increased humidity, size of suction catheter used, and need for suctioning.
3. For infected stoma site, evaluate cleaning regimen for continued use of "clean technique." Evaluate other possible contaminants, including use of finger to occlude fenestrated trach tube for speech (encourage client to place clean facial tissue between finger and tube) or scratching of dry skin (moisturize skin with lotion). Increase tracheostomy care frequency.
4. For copious yellow secretions, use sterile technique for suctioning and tracheostomy inner can-

STEPS **RATIONALE**

nula care. Evaluate for adequate humidity (use room humidifier or tracheostomy collar humidity, if needed) (see Chapter 12). Notify physician.

5. For displaced trach tube, initiate agency protocol for replacement or resuscitation as needed.

• • • • •

Special Considerations

- Physical limitations or weakness impairs client's motor coordination and prohibits client from being able to remove, clean, and reinsert inner cannula or change tracheostomy ties or suction. Cognitive impairments can result from primary disease or oxygen desaturation.
- Procedure must be performed at least daily in home setting. When tracheal secretions are copious, client or family member must perform procedure more frequently (such as every 4 hours).
- Hydration: inadequate hydration can cause thicker secretions. Humidity: inadequate inspired humidity predisposes client to dry crusted secretions and dry, cracked, possibly infected mucous membranes. Most clients benefit from a room humidifier. Infection: secretions increase in thickness and quantity in infected areas. Nutrition: inadequate nutrition predisposes client to poor wound healing and greater risk of infection. Ability to cough: strong cough effectively removes secretions. Weak cough promotes retained secretions. Coughing is altered in tracheostomy clients.
- Clients usually wear a special bib or handkerchief to warm air and moisture and protect airway from inhalation of dust and germs.
- Clients with the following are at greater risk: impaired or absent cough or gag reflex, decreased level of consciousness, neuromuscular diseases, pneumonia, chronic obstructive pulmonary disease, congestive heart failure, and pulmonary edema. Families of tracheostomy clients must know how to obtain emergency assistance within their community.

Teaching Considerations

- Client may need mirror to visualize stomal area.
- If at all possible, a family member or other care giver in the home should learn the procedure in the event emergency assistance is required, or the client's level of debilitation makes self-care improbable.
- Loss of upper airway functions with tracheostomy can predispose client to greater secretions. Infants and young children have smaller diameter airway. Older adults have lost some properties of elastic recoil and gas exchange.

Pediatric Considerations

- Ideally, the home care nurse should participate in discharge teaching in the hospital at the same time the parents are learning.
- Many physicians order the child to receive 10% to 15% higher oxygen before tracheostomy tube changes.
- Awareness of the level of parent's anxiety surrounding the performance of this skill will require frequent support and assistance by the home care nurse until independence and a comfort level are achieved.
- The emotional, cognitive, and physical abilities of the child must be considered before planning to teach self-care of this procedure.

Gerontologic Considerations

- Manual dexterity may be limited due to arthritic changes of the upper extremities.
- Skin integrity may be compromised and at risk for breakdown from secretions and/or tape.

SKILL 42-4 Helping Clients with Self-Medication

Clients who are prescribed drug regimens at home often fail to take medications correctly. Difficulty in taking prescribed medications regularly exists for several reasons: clients stop taking medications once symptoms subside; regimens involving multiple drugs are confusing; the consequences of not taking medication are poorly understood; prescriptions are costly; and many clients fear addiction. A large portion of clients who do not comply are older adults, who frequently suffer sensory and mobility problems that interfere with the ability to prepare and take medications correctly.

The following skill is actually an outline to help prepare clients for following drug regimens in the home.

EQUIPMENT

- Medication
- Liquid to take with medication
- Medication administration record or computer printout
- Container for daily or weekly preparation
- Measuring devices as needed (e.g., medicine cup, teaspoon)
- Teaching tools (e.g., charts, written instructions, color codes)

STEPS	RATIONALE
ASSESSMENT	
1. Assess if client is able to read, understand, and follow written instructions by asking client to read a teaching pamphlet and explain what was read.	Learning is inhibited if client is illiterate, has difficulty with written instructions, has a language barrier, or has diminished visual acuity; the teaching plan being used relies heavily on the client's ability to follow written instructions.
2. Assess the resources the client has to obtain medications when needed.	Lack of financial resources or transportation are two major factors that will negatively affect compliance with a self-medication regime.
3. Assess client's learning readiness and abilities.	Presence of significant illness, frailty, or the suggestion of or presence of confusion will impact teaching plan. Reliance on care giver for learning and implementation (if available) may be necessary on a short- or long-term basis.
4. Assess client's knowledge regarding drug therapy: names of drugs, how to administer, purpose or action, daily doses and times taken, side effects to expect, and what to do if problems occur	Reveals client's level of understanding and need for instruction.
5. Assess family member's knowledge of drug therapy: why client takes drug, daily doses, side effects, and what to do if problems arise.	Family member or support person is important resource to help client comply with therapy.
6. Assess client's sensory function including sight, hearing, touch, and physical coordination, including ability to self administer injections (when ordered) (see illustration).	Client's sensory impairments create need for specific types of teaching strategies so that nurse can be sure client has capacity to see medication, open prescription bottles, and read labels.
7. Assess client's ability to ambulate and tolerate exercise.	Older adults may have mobility problems that interfere with ability in getting to pharmacy, opening containers, or reaching and manipulating medications and equipment.
8. Assess client's belief in need for drug therapy. Consider cultural values, religious beliefs, personal experiences with medications, and significant others' values about drugs.	Many factors influence client's willingness to follow drug regimen.
9. Check client's prescribed drugs: Has more than one physician prescribed medications? Are medications obviously inappropriate? Are labels clearly marked? Are time schedules confusing? Do different drugs look alike? Does client store medications together or out of original containers?	Assists nurse in determining sources of confusion affecting client's compliance.

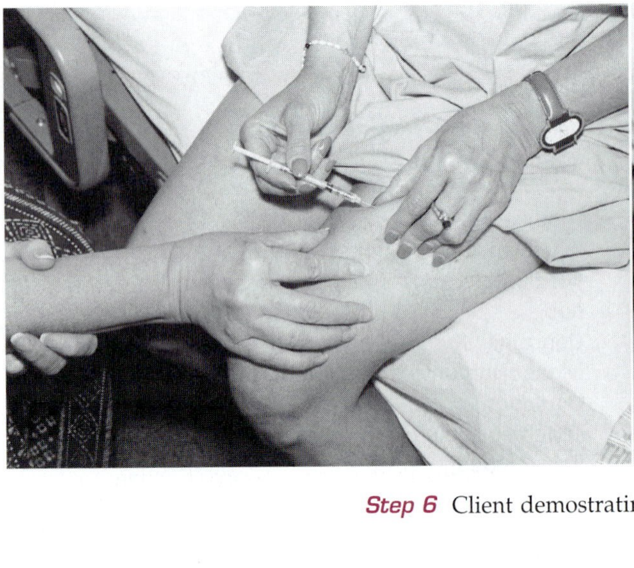

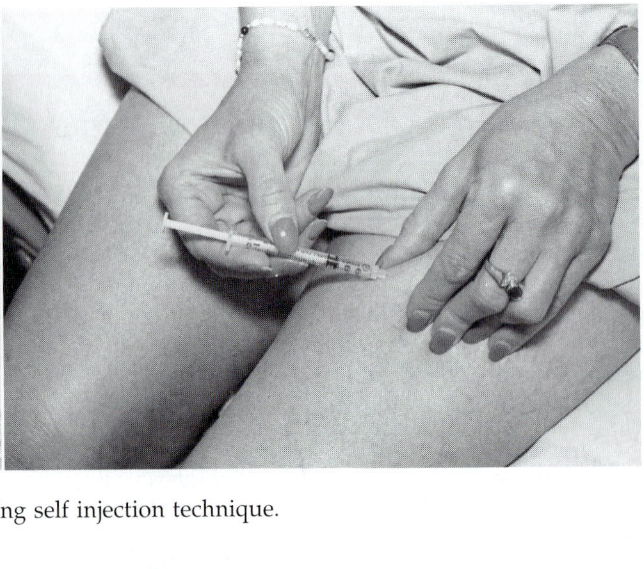

Step 6 Client demostrating self injection technique.

STEPS	RATIONALE
10. Assess client's understanding of effects and interactions between prescribed medications and the ingestion of certain foods, as well as with over-the-counter drugs.	Medication interactions, including with over-the-counter drugs and certain foods, can be serious to the effectiveness and/or create negative side effects.

NURSING DIAGNOSIS

Clustering of defining characteristics from the assessment data may reveal the following nursing diagnoses for clients requiring this skill:

- Anxiety
- Ineffective denial
- Altered health maintenance
- Health-seeking behaviors
- Ineffective management of therapeutic regimen (individual)
- Knowledge deficit regarding drug administration

Related factors are individualized based on a client's condition or needs.

PLANNING

1. **Expected outcomes** following completion of procedure:
   - Client is able to state the purpose of each medication and why it is beneficial.
   - Client identifies common side effects and relief measures.
   - Client is able to state when to notify physician about drug problems.
   - Client reads each label and explains when each drug should be taken.
   - Client demonstrates preparing prescribed drug dose from prescription bottle.

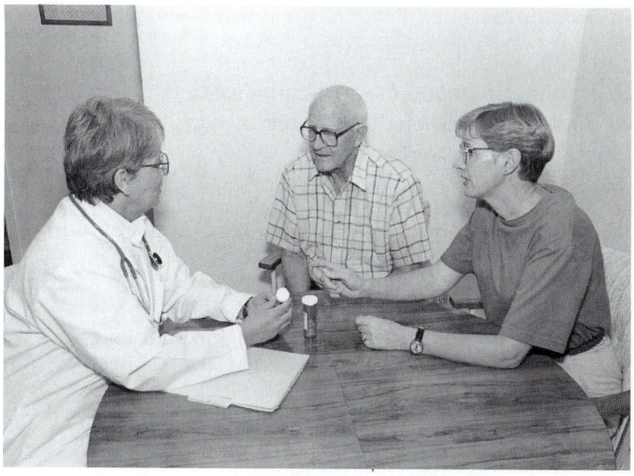

Step 6

STEPS	RATIONALE
2. Prepare the environment for a teaching session: a. Select room that is well lit. b. Provide comfortable seating. c. Be sure client is close and can see nurse clearly. d. Control sources of noise and distractions.	Room environment should be designed to minimize existing sensory alterations. Comfortable environment free of distractions promotes client's attention.
3. Prepare teaching materials: a. Materials should be printed in large bold letters. b. Illustrations of safety guidelines should be provided. c. Written schedules or individualized instruction sheets are helpful.	Teaching materials should be designed to meet client's learning needs, as well as client's capacity to learn.
4. Be sure clients who wear glasses or hearing aids do so during the teaching session.	Use of glasses or hearing aids increases client's sensory perception and increases likelihood of attending to teaching session and understanding content.
5. Consult with the physician to review medications client is receiving and to simplify regimen if possible.	Review of medications can help minimize risk of drug interactions from multiple medications and ensures accuracy of medication regimen. Simplification of regimen can improve compliance, particularly related to the daily frequency of prescribed doses
6. Arrange teaching time so that family members may participate (see illustration).	Family can serve as positive resource to client.

STEPS	RATIONALE
IMPLEMENTATION	
1. Present information clearly and concisely:	
a. Face learner; be sure nurse's face is illuminated. b. Use short sentences and speak in slow, low-pitched voice.	Client with hearing loss or visual problem will be able to see nurse's expressions and hear voice more clearly.
c. Provide descriptions in understandable terms.	Prevents confusion of terminology.
2. Provide frequent pauses so that client can ask questions and express understanding of content.	Increases client's participation in learning process. Ongoing feedback assures nurse that client is acquiring information.
CRITICAL DECISION POINT **Discuss the following content: purpose of drugs and their positive effects, how drug works and why it helps, dosage schedules and rationale, common side effects, what to do to relieve side effects, what to do if dose is missed, when to call with problems, who to call with problems, drug safety guidelines, and implications when medications are not taken.**	Content presented, if learned, improves client's ability to self-medicate correctly. Individualizing dosage schedules makes it easier for client to comply.
3. Provide frequent short teaching sessions. Learning about multiple medication regimen will require several teaching sessions.	Improves client's attention and retention of information discussed.
CRITICAL DECISION POINT **Review previous information and ask client to recall and relay previously taught information before proceeding to new teaching area.**	Client needs to learn extensive amount of information. Reference to charts, written information, and other teaching tools as a resource will assist client in learning.
4. Be sure to include teaching about prescribed and over-the-counter medications that are used on a **prn** basis.	Consideration of knowledge and accessibility of these medications must be given, because prn drugs are not included in routine, prepoured medication delivery systems (i.e., daily or weekly pill box systems).
CRITICAL DECISION POINT **Provide client with special charts, diagrams, or learning aids (Fig. 42-6).**	Simplest mechanism for reminding clients of when to take medications improves compliance.

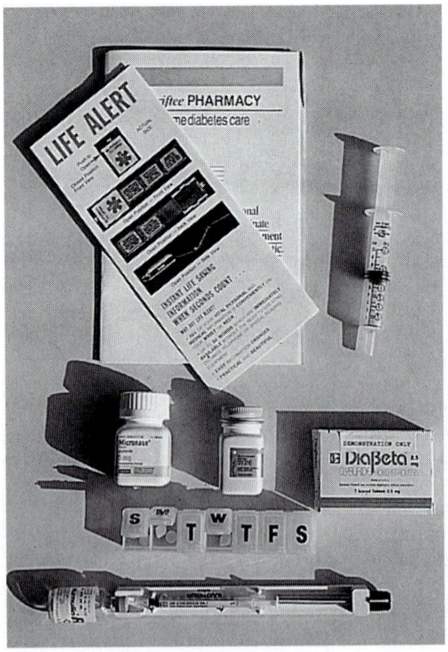

Fig. 42-6

STEPS	RATIONALE
5. Offer assistance as client practices preparing medication (e.g., "Let's prepare the medications you will take with your meals. Prepare the medicines you take first in the morning.").	Nurse can observe client's ability to read labels correctly and prepare all medications for prescribed times.
6. Have pharmacy provide clear, large-print labels for medication bottles if appropriate.	Improves client's ability to read and follow directions.
7. Have pharmacy provide containers that client can open independently if manual dexterity is limited.	Most pharmacies dispense pills in "child proof" containers, which the client with limited mobility of fingers/hands may find difficult to manipulate or open.
8. Facilitate arrangements for pharmacy to receive written prescriptions in a timely fashion if required for dispensing and to deliver medications at home if client is unable to reach facility.	Availability of drugs influences compliance.
EVALUATION	
1. Ask client and family member to explain information about each drug: purpose, actions, reason/maximum frequency of use of either the prescribed or over-the-counter drug, side effects and interactions, and foods or over-the-counter drugs to avoid.	Feedback measures client's cognitive learning.
2. Identify client's problem-solving initiatives if unsure of action to be taken (e.g., call health care provider, refer to printed information for resources).	Developing techniques to gain information and solve problems will assist in client compliance, as well as reduce potential problems from medication regimen.
3. Have client or family member prepare doses for all prescribed medications.	Indicates client's understanding of dosages and schedules.
4. Ask client about any questions.	Offers opportunity for clarification and minimizes any remaining confusion or misunderstanding.
5. **Unexpected outcomes** that may occur include:	
➤ Client makes errors in preparing medications.	May be result of misunderstanding or sensory deficits.
➤ Client is unable to recall and/or explain information discussed in teaching sessions.	Requires additional instruction and/or teaching materials that client could self-reference accurately when information is forgotten or unclear.
➤ Self-medication plan is not possible due to client's self-care deficits—very commonly in relation to changes in mentation.	Alternate plan, which may rely on others, is developed to provide administration of a home medication regimen.
RECORDING AND REPORTING	
1. Document instruction provided and learning outcomes achieved by client in home care record.	Provides continuity of care when other nurses attempt to resume teaching or reinforce client's learning.
2. Develop a system of recording to be used by the client/family member to provide information that compliance is achieved or maintained.	For long-term compliance, accuracy must be maintained and the ability to assess accuracy of the regimen needs to be accessed in some reporting/recording mechanism.
3. Develop a client recording mechanism of dosage schedules and self-monitoring of regimen.	Client self-recording will support accuracy of self-administered drug regimen.

FOLLOW-UP ACTIVITIES

1. Ensure that physician's orders for the client's medication regimen are kept current and reflect all components and changes of the medication care plan. Including over-the-counter medications will reflect the entire plan.
2. Periodically evaluate client's level of understanding and learning retention and detemine if changes between nursing visits have been made. Learning needs to be reinforced. Often home medication plans change via a phone call between the client and physician or a covering physician. By reviewing the plan at each visit, the nurse assesses if additional medications ordered could be problematic.

• • • • •

STEPS	RATIONALE
return gastric contents; and to elevate the client for 1 hour after feedings or maintain at least a 30-degree elevation for continuous feedings.	
5. Observe client and care giver aspirating gastric contents.	Identifies competence and need for further teaching. Allows client/care giver to perform skill with nurse in attendance for guidance.
6. Discuss use of medical asepsis techniques in setting up administration and changing administration sets, mixing formulas (not adding formula to hanging bag), refrigeration of unused formula, limiting amount of formula "hung" at one time to amount that can be infused in a 4- to 6-hour period (less time in warmer weather), and maintenance and care of bag.	Medical aseptic technique minimizes risk of microorganism contamination. Refrigeration and limiting "hang" time reduces microorganism proliferation. Changing administration sets every 24 hours reduces microorganism growth (Doughty and Jackson, 1993).
7. Observe client and care giver mixing, administering, and storing formulas, changing administration sets, and cleaning bags.	Identifies competence and need for further teaching.
CRITICAL DECISION POINT **Discuss mixing and administration of medications via tube and flushing tube after administration.**	Ensures administration of medication dose and prevents clogging of tube.
8. Observe client/care giver administering medications and flushing tube.	Identifies competence and need for further teaching.
9. Discuss and observe use of infusion pump if client is receiving continuous feeding (see Chapter 23).	Infusion pumps provide positive pressure to ensure constant flow and prevent occlusion and gastric distention.
10. Discuss measures to stabilize the feeding tube in clients with abdominal tubes and to protect skin integrity.	Prevents tube from dislodging and prevents skin breakdown.
11. Discuss measures to prevent tube occlusion and aspiration.	Ensures safe home management.
12. Discuss whom to contact for equipment, supplies, or in case of equipment failure.	
13. Discuss emergency plan and actions to take for signs and symptoms of aspiration.	
14. Discuss whom to contact and when for signs of diarrhea, constipation, or weight loss.	Ensures client/care giver's understanding of management of equipment, supplies, emergency plan, and collaboration.
15. Wash hands.	Reduces transmission of microorganisms.

EVALUATION

1. Ask client to state the purpose of home enteral nutrition therapy.	
2. Observe client/care giver performing medical asepsis techniques, checking tube placement, administering medications and solutions, and using equipment.	
3. Assess client/care giver's understanding of measures needed to be used to prevent complications (e.g., verification of tube position before each feeding, elevation of client during feeding, stabilization and flushing of tubing).	Ensures safe home management and identification of areas for teaching.
4. Assess client/care giver's understanding of tube occlusion and handling of formulas.	Ensures safe home management and identification of areas of teaching.

STEPS	RATIONALE
5. Assess client/care giver's understanding of management of complications (e.g., signs of intolerance: nausea, abdominal distention, diarrhea, skin problems, and fluid deficit).	Ensures safe home management and identification of areas of teaching.
6. Ask client about community contacts for supplies, equipment, collaboration, and emergency care.	Ensures safe home management.
7. **Unexpected outcomes** that may occur include:	
➤ Displacement of feeding tube.	May occur when client coughs, vomits, or in the course of certain movements.
➤ Signs and symptoms of aspiration.	May occur when gastric contents or feeding solutions reflux into or are inappropriately placed into respiratory system.
➤ Client develops diarrhea.	Indicates intolerance to formula.
➤ Skin surrounding stoma or tube insertion site (nares) breaks down.	Pressure from tube or presence of gastric contents.

RECORDING AND REPORTING

1. Record in home care record instructions given to client and care givers and their response to them.	Provides continuous documentation of information given to client.
2. Record specifics of enteral feeding plan, including type and size of tube in home, formula, and amounts to be administered in specific time frames.	Documents timely administration of prescribed enteral feedings.
3. Client and care givers need to document I&O, daily weights, amount of gastric fluid aspirated before each feeding (or every 4 hours if receiving continuous feeding), date and time of feedings, amount and type of formula, any additives, and date and time administration sets are changed.	

FOLLOW-UP ACTIVITIES

1. For gastrostomy tubes, have extra Foley catheter and insertion tray available in the home at all times. For displaced or occluded nasogastric or gastrostomy tubes, remove old tube and insert new.
2. Give client and care givers the names, addresses, and phone numbers of equipment and supply companies, agency number, and pharmacist and physician number.

• • • • •

Special Considerations

- Frequent oral and nasal hygiene is required.
- Enteric-coated medications cannot be administered through a feeding tube.
- Medications that cannot be crushed and administered through a feeding tube should be validated by a pharmacist.

Teaching Considerations

- Teaching of enteral therapy skills begins in the hospital.
- Teaching approach must be individualized, and appropriate teaching strategies must be identified that will facilitate client and care giver's learning.
- Carrying out performance of skills without the nurse in attendance is anxiety provoking. Always leave a phone number and instructions about how to reach the nurse if needed.

Pediatric Considerations

- A child's potential risk factor for aspiration and fluid and electrolyte imbalance are great and must be carefully monitored, with precautions incorporated into the care plan.

Gerontologic Considerations

- Changes and limitations in sensory functioning or issues with mobility, dexterity, and fluid and caloric needs must be factored into the plan of care and monitored for needs to alter prescriptions or teaching methods.

CRITICAL THINKING EXERCISES

1. Mrs. Grey is able to demonstrate effective and accurate measurement of her radial pulse when the home care nurse is observing her. When attempting this skill alone she does not accurately perform. What nursing actions would you implement to promote successful, independent skill performance?

2. During your third home care nursing visit for the purpose of teaching the client a self-medication regimen, you note that several types of pills are grouped together in one container. What actions would you take?

REFERENCES

Dettenmeier PA: *Pulmonary nursing care,* St Louis, 1992, Mosby.

Doughty D, Jackson D: *Gastrointestinal disorders,* St Louis, 1993, Mosby.

Ebersole P, Hess P: *Toward healthy aging: human needs and nursing response,* ed 4, St Louis, 1994, Mosby.

LaRocca J: *Handbook of home care IV therapy,* St Louis, 1994, Mosby.

Morse NA: Nurses speak out on patient and drug regimens, *Am J Nurs* 85:51, 1985.

Potter P, Perry A: *Fundamentals of nursing: concepts, process, and practice,* ed 4, St Louis, 1997, Mosby.

Rice R: *Home health nursing practice—concepts and application,* ed 2, St Louis, 1996, Mosby.

Young C, White S: Tube feeding at home, *Am J Nurs* 92(4):46, 1992.

ADDITIONAL READING

Bockus S: Troubleshooting your tube feedings, *Am J Nurs* 91(5):24, 1991.

Eisenberg P: Causes of diarrhea in tube fed patients: a comprehensive approach to diagnosis and management, *NCP* 8(3):119, 1993.

Mattox T: Drug use evaluation approach to monitoring use of total parenteral nutrition. A review of criteria for use in cancer patients, *NCP* 8(5):235, 1993.

McCoy PA, Votroubek WL: *Pediatric home care,* Frederick Maryland, 1990, Aspen Publications.

Metheny N: Minimizing respiratory complications of nasogastric tube feedings: state of the science, *Heart Lung* 22(3):213, 1993.

Pfister S: Home oxygen therapy: indications, administration, recertification, and patient education, *Nurse Pract* 20(7):44, 1995.

Varricchio C: Human and indirect costs of home care, *Nurs Outlook* 42(4):151, 1994.

Visiting Nurse Association of America procedure book, ed 2, Denver, 1994, VNAA.

UNIT XV

Special Procedures

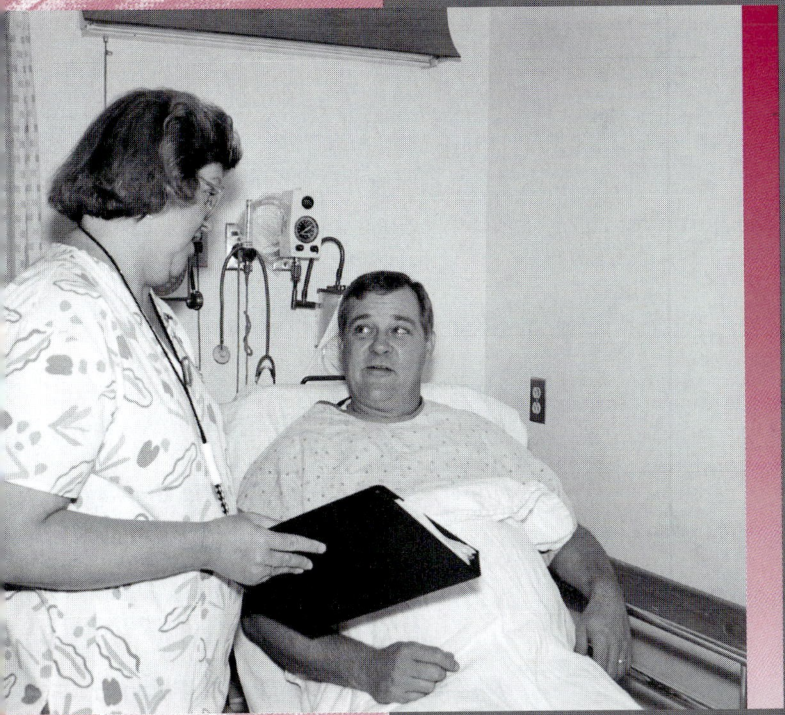

CHAPTER 43

Specimen Collection

OBJECTIVES

Mastery of content in this chapter will enable the nurse to:

- Define key terms.
- Explain the rationale for the collection of each specimen.
- Identify special conditions necessary for satisfactory collection of each specimen.
- Describe instructions to encourage client cooperation for successful collection of the specimen.
- Identify measures to minimize anxiety and promote safety for selected techniques.
- Discuss nursing responsibilities for processing the specimen after collection.
- Chart appropriate information in the client's record after collection of the specimen.
- Discuss precautions to prevent injury to the client during specimen collection.
- Properly collect clean-voided, timed, and catheterized urine specimens.
- Correctly measure specific gravity and pH of urine.
- Correctly measure glucose, ketones, protein, and blood in urine.
- Correctly measure for the presence of occult blood in a stool specimen.
- Properly collect specimens for culture from the nose and throat, urethra and vagina, sputum, and wound.
- Correctly measure for pH and presence of occult blood in gastric drainage.
- Properly perform venipuncture.
- Correctly measure for blood glucose from a blood specimen collected by skin puncture.
- Properly collect an arterial blood sample.
- Utilize measures recommended for preventing transmission of pathogens.

SKILLS

KEY TERMS

Acetest
Aerobic
Allen's test
Anaerobic
Aseptic technique
Aspirate
Autolet
Clean-voided specimen
Clinitest
Culture
Double-voided specimen
Ecchymosis
Expectorate
Feces
Frequency
Glucose monitoring
Guaiac test
Hematemesis
Hematoma
Hematuria
Hemoconcentration
Hemolysis
Hemostasis
Ketones
Meatus
Melena
Midstream
Occult blood
pH
Platelet
Reagent
Refractometer
Renal
Saliva
Sensitivity
Specific gravity
Timed urine collection
Tourniquet
Urgency
Urinometer
Vacutainer tube
Venipuncture
Void

Nurses often assume the responsibility for collection of specimens of body secretions and excretions. Laboratory examination of specimens of urine, stool, sputum, blood, and wound drainage provides important information about body functioning and contributes to the assessment of health status. Laboratory test results can aid the diagnosis of health care problems, provide information about the stage and activity of a disease process, and measure the response to therapy.

Clients often experience embarrassment or discomfort when giving a sample of body excretions or secretions. Most persons believe that excretions should be handled discreetly; therefore it is important to provide the client with as much comfort and privacy as possible. Anxiety is also provoked by the invasive nature of some collection procedures or by fear of unknown test results. Clients who are given a clear explanation about the purpose of the specimen and how it is to be obtained will be more cooperative in its collection. With proper instruction many clients are able to obtain their own specimens of urine, stool, and sputum, thus avoiding embarrassment. Often the success of specimen collection depends on cooperation.

Laboratory tests are often expensive. The nurse can prevent unnecessary costs by using the correct procedure for obtaining and processing specimens. When there are questions about laboratory tests, the nurse should consult the institution's procedure manual or call the laboratory.

Normal values for laboratory tests can be found in reference books, but the nurse should know that each laboratory establishes its own values for each test. These values are usually readily available on the laboratory slips of the agency. Any major deviations should be discussed with the physician immediately.

GUIDELINES

1. Consider the client's need and ability to participate in specimen collection procedures.
2. Recognize that collection of a specimen may provoke anxiety, embarrassment, or discomfort.
3. Provide support for clients who are fearful about the results of a specimen examination.
4. Recognize that children require a clear explanation of procedures and may benefit from support of parents or family members.
5. Obtain specimens in accordance with specific prerequisite conditions (e.g., fasting, NPO [nothing by mouth]) as required.
6. Follow the standard precautions (see Chapter 33) when collecting specimens of blood or other body fluids.
7. Wash hands and other skin surfaces immediately and thoroughly if they are contaminated with blood or body fluids; wash hands immediately after removing gloves.
8. Collect specimens in appropriate containers, at the correct time, in the appropriate amount.
9. Properly label all specimens with the client's identification; complete laboratory requisition as necessary.
10. Deliver specimens to the laboratory within the recommended time, or ensure that they are stored properly for later transport.
11. Use **aseptic technique** in all collections to prevent contamination, which can cause inaccurate test results.
12. Transport specimens under special conditions (e.g., iced specimens or special containers with preservatives) as required.
13. Know institutional policy regarding infection control practices for transportation of all specimen containers of body substances.
14. Be aware that some deviations from normal values occur as a result of medications or dietary intake.
15. Follow precautions for collecting specimen from clients who are in protective isolation.
16. Employ the principles of medical and surgical asepsis whenever necessary in specimen collection.

SKILL 43-1 Collecting a Midstream (Clean-Voided) Urine Specimen

A common test performed on urine is a **culture** and **sensitivity** measurement. A few drops of urine are placed on a special medium to determine if bacteria are present. Readings are made at 24- and 48-hour intervals, and the final reading is made after 72 hours. If bacteria are present, sensitivity testing reveals which antibiotics that will be effective against the microorganisms.

With clients who are able to void voluntarily, the nurse collects a **midstream** urine specimen for culture and sensitivity testing. A client begins the urinary stream and then during the middle portion of voiding collects a specimen. The initial stream flushes the urethral orifice and meatus of any resident bacteria. It is easiest for a client to obtain a **clean-voided specimen** while using toilet facilities rather than a bedpan or urinal.

EQUIPMENT

Commercial Kit for Clean-Voided Urine Containing:*

- Sterile cotton balls and/or 2 × 2-inch gauze pads, cleansing towelette, or 2 gauze pads
- Antiseptic solution (usually povidone-iodine solution)
- Sterile water or saline
- Sterile specimen container
- Sterile gloves
- Soap, water, washcloth, and towel
- Bedpan (for nonambulatory client), specimen hat (if all urine needs to be measured), potty chair (for young child)
- Completed specimen identification label
- Completed laboratory requisition form

*See Fig. 43-1.

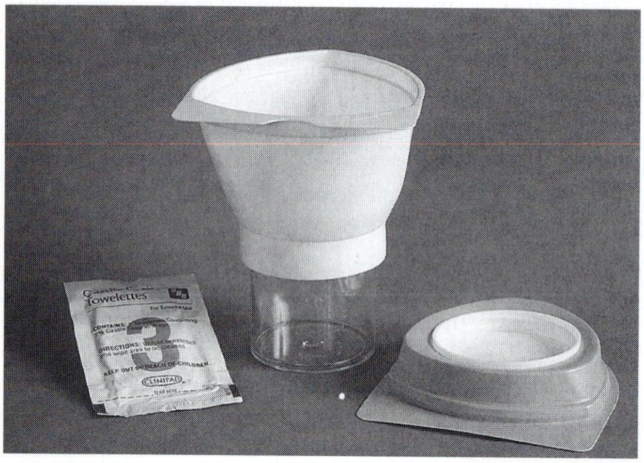

Fig. 43-1 Clean-voided specimen collection kit.

DELEGATION CONSIDERATIONS

The collection of a clean midstream urine specimen may be performed by unlicensed personnel.

- Inform care provider how to instruct client to obtain specimen.
- Inform care provider how to cleanse urethra before obtaining specimen.

STEPS	RATIONALE
ASSESSMENT	
1. Assess client's level of understanding of purpose of test and method of collection.	Information allows nurse to clarify misunderstanding; promotes client cooperation.
2. Assess client's mobility and balance in being able to use toilet facilities independently.	Determines level of assistance required by client.
3. Refer to medical record for indications of urinary infection.	Helps nurse explain purpose of specimen procedure for client.
4. Assess risks for urinary tract infection: e.g., poor perineal hygiene, improperly handled diagnostic instruments, and previous urinary catheterization.	Allows nurse to anticipate need to test client's urine for bacteria.
5. Assess for signs and symptoms of urinary tract infections: frequency, urgency, dysuria, hematuria, flank pain, fever.	Can suggest bacteria in urine.
6. Refer to agency procedures for specimen collection methods.	Agency policies may vary as to proper way to collect or handle specimens.

STEPS	RATIONALE

NURSING DIAGNOSIS

Clustering of defining characteristics from the assessment data may reveal the following nursing diagnoses for clients requiring this skill:

- ➤ Anxiety
- ➤ Knowledge deficit regarding specimen collection
- ➤ Pain
- ➤ Risk for infection

Related factors are individualized based on a client's condition or needs.

PLANNING

STEPS	RATIONALE
1. Expected outcomes following completion of procedure:	
➤ Client produces midstream urine specimen that is not contaminated with feces or toilet paper.	These substances change normal characteristics of urine.
➤ Urine has normal characteristics and does not reveal bacterial growth.	Provides evidence of absence of infection.
➤ Client will discuss purpose and benefits of midstream urine collection.	Identifies that learning has occurred.
2. Offer client fluids to drink (if permitted) before attempting to collect specimen.	Enhances client's ability to void.
3. Explain procedure to client and/or family member: a. Reason midstream specimen is needed. b. How client/family member can assist. c. How to obtain specimen free of feces and tissue.	Promotes cooperation and participation and client may be able to independently obtain specimen. It also prevents accidental disposal of it. Feces and tissue alter chemical composition of specimen.
4. Use visual aids (if available) to explain procedure to client.	Because this method of urine collection is somewhat complicated, clients benefit from illustrations emphasizing midstream collection technique.

IMPLEMENTATION

STEPS	RATIONALE
1. Identify client. Wash hands.	Handwashing reduces transfer of microorganisms.
2. Provide privacy for client who will give specimen in bed by closing curtain around bed or closing room door.	Privacy allows client to relax and produce a specimen more quickly.
3. Give client or family member cleansing towelette or towel, washcloth, and soap to cleanse perineum or assist client to cleanse perineum.	Clients prefer to wash their own perineal areas when possible. Cleansing prevents contamination of specimen after urine passes from urethra.
4. Assist bedridden client onto bedpan (see illustration).	Provides easy access to perineal areas to collect specimen.
5. Using surgical asepsis, open sterile kit or prepare sterile tray.	Maintains sterility of equipment.

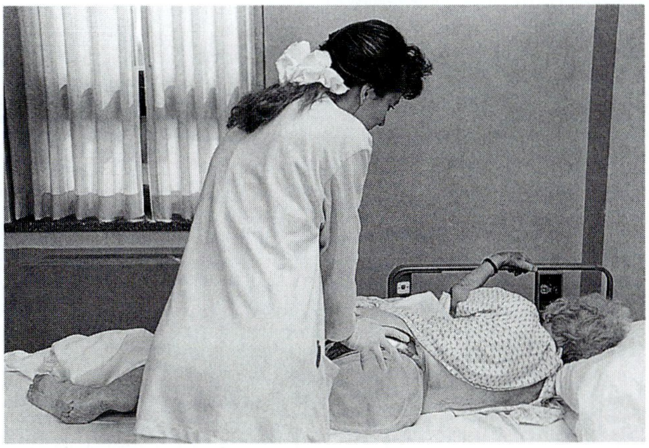

Step 4

STEPS	RATIONALE
6. Don sterile gloves.	Prevents introduction of microorganisms on nurse's hands into specimen.
7. Pour antiseptic solution over cotton balls (unless kit contains prepared gauze pads in antiseptic solution).	Cotton ball or gauze is used to cleanse perineum.
8. Open specimen container and place cap with sterile inside surface up and do not touch inside of container.	Contaminated specimen is most frequent reason for inaccurate reporting on urine cultures and sensitivities.
9. Assist or allow client to independently cleanse perineum and collect specimen.	

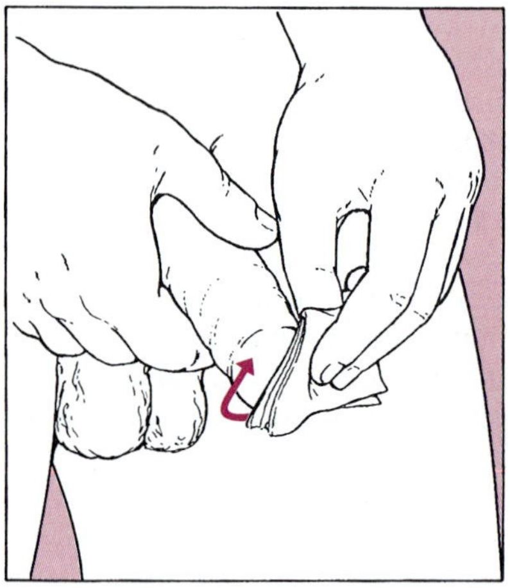

Step 9a(1) (Modified from Grimes D: *Infectious diseases,* Mosby's Clinical Nursing Series, St Louis, 1991, Mosby.)

a. Male.

STEPS	RATIONALE
(1) Hold client's penis with one hand. Using circular motion and antiseptic swab, cleanse meatus, moving from center to outside (see illustration).	Cleanse from area of least contamination to area of greatest contamination to decrease bacterial levels.
(2) If agency procedure indicates, rinse area with sterile water and dry with cotton balls or gauze pad.	Prevents contamination of specimen with antiseptic solution.
(3) After client has initiated urine stream, pass urine specimen container into stream and collect 30 to 60 ml of urine (see illustration).	Initial urine flushes out microorganisms that normally accumulate at urinary meatus and prevents collection in specimen.

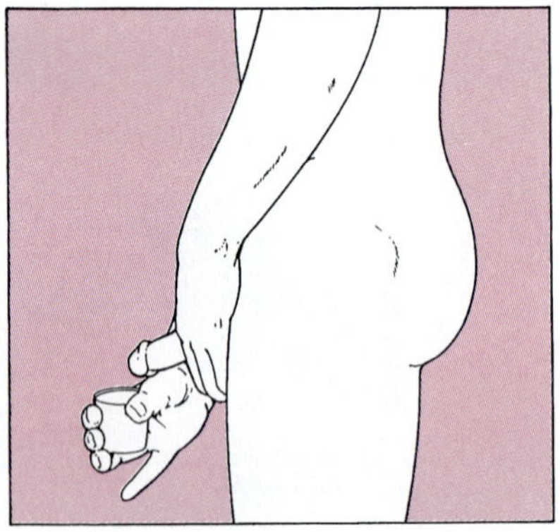

Step 9a(3)

STEPS	RATIONALE
b. Female.	
CRITICAL DECISION POINT Indicate on the laboratory slip if client is menstruating.	
(1) Spread client's labia minora with thumb and forefinger of nondominant hand.	Provides access to urethral meatus.
(2) Use dominant hand to cleanse area with swab (cotton ball or gauze), moving from front (above urethral orifice) to back (toward anus). Using a fresh swab each time, repeat front-to-back motion three times (begin with left side, then do right side, then center (see illustration).	Prevents contamination of urinary meatus with fecal material (see illustration).
(3) If agency procedure indicates, rinse area with sterile water and dry with cotton ball.	Prevents contamination of specimen with antiseptic solution.
(4) While continuing to hold labia apart, client should initiate urine stream; after stream is achieved, pass specimen container into stream and collect 30 to 60 ml (see illustration).	Initial stream flushes out microorganisms that accumulate at urethral meatus.
10. Remove specimen container before flow of urine stops and before releasing labia or penis. Client finishes voiding into bedpan or toilet.	Prevents contamination of specimen with skin flora.
11. Replace cap securely on specimen container (touch only outside).	Retains sterility of inside of container and prevents spillage of urine.
12. Cleanse urine from exterior surface of container.	Prevents transfer of microorganisms to others.
13. Dispose of bedpan (if applicable), remove and discard gloves, and wash hands.	Reduces transmission of microorganisms.
14. Label specimen and attach laboratory requisition.	Prevents inaccurate identification that could lead to errors in diagnosis or therapy.
15. Take specimen to laboratory within 15 minutes or immediately refrigerate.	Since bacteria grow quickly in urine, urine should be analyzed immediately (or refrigerated).

EVALUATION

STEPS	RATIONALE
1. Observe specimen for contaminants such as toilet paper or feces.	
2. Assess client's urine culture and sensitivity report for bacterial growth.	Numbers and type of bacteria present dictate treatment and need for further testing.
3. Ask client to describe midstream urine collection procedure.	Documents learning.

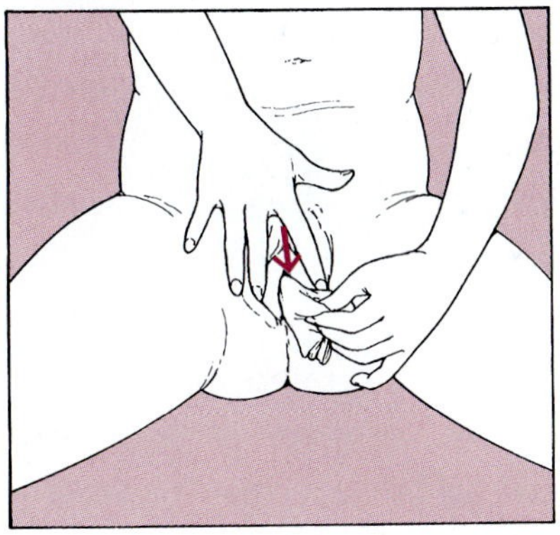

Step 9b(2) (Modified from Grimes D: *Infectious diseases*, Mosby's Clinical Nursing Series, St Louis, 1991, Mosby.)

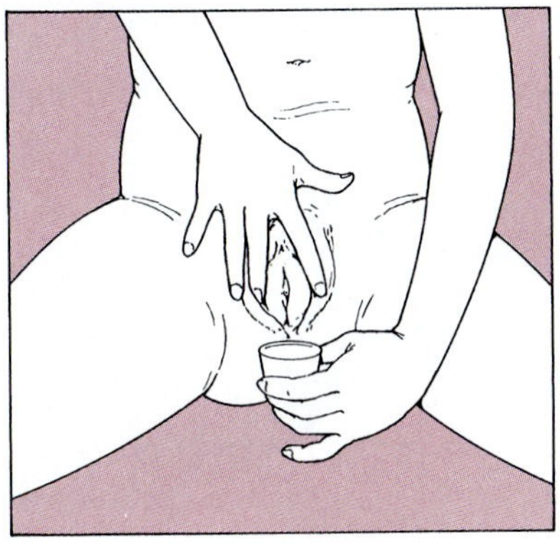

Step 9b(4) (Modified from Grimes D: *Infectious diseases*, Mosby's Clinical Nursing Series, St Louis, 1991, Mosby.)

STEPS	RATIONALE
4. **Unexpected outcomes** that may occur include:	
➤ Urine specimen is accidentally discarded.	Communication regarding urine collection was ineffective.
➤ Urine specimen is contaminated with feces or toilet paper.	Requires repeat of specimen collection procedure.
➤ Client is unable to urinate on demand.	May require more time for urine to accumulate in bladder.
➤ Urine culture reveals bacterial growth (designated by colony count of more than 10,000 organisms/ml).	Evidence of urinary tract infection.

Recording and Reporting

1. Record date and time urine specimen was obtained in nurses' notes.	Documents implementation of physician's order.
2. Record appearance and odor of urine and evidence of dysuria in nurses' notes.	Data can support other evidence of urinary tract infection.
3. Notify physician of any significant abnormalities.	

Follow-up Activities

1. Discuss findings of laboratory test with client and physician.

• • • • •

Special Considerations

- Varying degrees of assistance are required by clients who are seriously ill, have difficulty standing, or are confused. Some clients may need assistance in bathroom, whereas others may require bedpan or urinal in bed.
- In uncircumcised males foreskin must be retracted for effective cleansing of **meatus** and during voiding.
- If specimen is taken from protective isolation room, it should be placed in paper bag according to hospital policy.

A

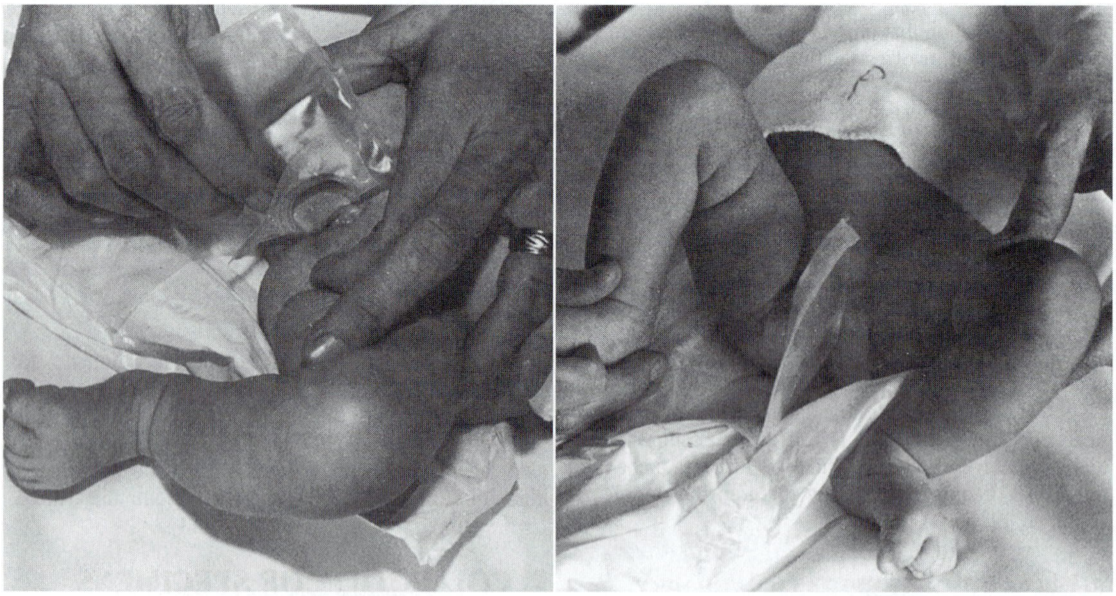

B

Fig. 43-2 Application of urine collection bag. (From Wong DL: *Whaley & Wong's nursing care of infants and children,* ed 5, St Louis, 1995, Mosby.)

- Always cover specimens to prevent carbon dioxide from diffusing into the air, which will result in urine becoming alkaline and fostering bacterial growth.

Teaching Considerations

- Discuss signs and symptoms of urinary tract infection.
- Explain significance of cleansing genital area before collecting specimen.
- Explain to female client importance of cleansing labia from front to back.
- Discuss client's role in collecting specimen.
- Nurses should request feedback to assess client's understanding of purpose of test and directions for collecting specimen (Redman, 1997).
- Use visual aides to describe collection of specimen.

Pediatric Considerations

- It is not possible to obtain a midstream urine collection on a non–toilet-trained child; consequently, urine for culture should be obtained via suprapubic needle aspiration by the physician or use of a sterile plastic urine-collecting bag that adheres to the perineum (Fig. 43-2). The same cleansing procedure should be followed as indicated in Step 9 of Implementation.

Gerontologic Considerations

- Special assistance should be given to older adults. A clear and concise explanation should be given about the procedure and the reason for the sample to be obtained. All equipment should be available at bedside to allow proceeding with obtaining a specimen when the client needs assistance.

Home Care Considerations

- Ideally, a specimen for culture should not be collected at home because the time delay before applying it to a culture medium in a laboratory setting would greatly enhance bacterial growth. If a urine specimen is collected, it should be kept on ice until it reaches the laboratory and is placed on the medium.

SKILL 43-2 Collecting a Timed Urine Specimen

Some tests of **renal** function and urine composition require urine to be collected over 2 to 72 hours. The 24-hour timed collection is most common. The tests allow for the measurement of elements such as amino acids, creatinine, hormones, glucose, and adrenocorticosteroids, whose levels change over time. A **timed collection** can also provide a means to measure the concentration or dilution of urine.

Timed urine collections begin after a client urinates. The nurse discards the first specimen and then collects every successive specimen until the time period has ended. Each specimen is transferred immediately to a large collection bottle kept in the client's bathroom. Any missed specimens make test results inaccurate. The client should always provide the last specimen as close as possible to the end of the collection period.

EQUIPMENT

- Large collection bottle with cap that may contain a chemical for urine preservation (consultation with laboratory is usually necessary to obtain bottle and determine appropriate chemical additive [e.g., toluene or acetic acid])
- Bedpan, urinal, specimen hat, or potty chair if client does not have indwelling catheter
- Graduated measuring cup if intake and output are to be measured
- Basin large enough to hold collection bottle surrounded by ice if immediate refrigeration is required
- Completed specimen identification label
- Completed laboratory requisition with client's name, date, and time of collection
- Signs that remind client and staff of timed urine collection
- Clean disposable gloves

DELEGATION CONSIDERATIONS

A timed urine specimen may be completed by unlicensed personnel:

- Instruct care provider when to begin collection.
- Inform care provider how specimen container is to be stored during collection period.

STEPS	RATIONALE
ASSESSMENT	
1. Determine purpose of timed urine specimen collection for client and period collection is to include.	Most common collections are for 24 hours because this provides average excretion rate for substances such as hormones or proteins excreted in small variable amounts in urine. If these substances are to be accurately measured and yield quantities of diagnostic value, urine must be collected over extended period. Challenge dose of chemical such as insulin may be given, and then timed urine specimen collection may be begun to detect renal disorders.
2. Determine if fluid or dietary requirements or medications need to be administered in conjunction with test.	Certain substances affect excretion and levels of urinary constituents. Glucose solution may be given for glucose tolerance test. Specific amounts of fluid may be required for concentration/dilution tests.
3. Determine that correct diet is being taken by client.	
4. Assess client's ability to collect specimens independently.	Promotes cooperation and determines level of assistance required.
5. Assess client's or family members' understanding of purpose of test and need to collect urine over extended period.	Cooperation is facilitated by degree of understanding.
6. Refer to agency policy for specimen collection procedure.	Agency policies may vary as to proper way to collect or handle specimens.

NURSING DIAGNOSIS

Clustering of defining characteristics from the assessment data may reveal the following nursing diagnosis for clients requiring this skill:

- Knowledge deficit regarding urine collection procedure

Related factors are individualized based on a client's condition or needs.

PLANNING

STEPS	RATIONALE
1. **Expected outcomes** following completion of procedure:	
➤ All of client's urine voided during time period is saved.	Necessary for satisfactory completion of test.
➤ Urine specimen is not contaminated with feces or toilet tissue.	Prevents results of urine test from being adversely affected by these substances.
➤ Urine has normal constituency.	Client is free of urinary alterations.
➤ Client explains purpose of and procedure for urine collection.	Demonstrates learning.
2. Have client drink 2 to 4 glasses of water about 30 minutes before timed collection is to begin.	Enables client to void old urine (collected in bladder) at time test begins.
3. Explain procedure to client and/or family member. Discuss reason for specimen collection and how client can assist. Explain that urine must be free of feces and tissue.	Client who understands procedure is more likely to cooperate and may be able to obtain the specimen independently. It also prevents accidental disposal and chemical changes resulting from feces and tissue.

IMPLEMENTATION

STEPS	RATIONALE
1. Provide privacy for and assist client in collecting specimen.	Clients prefer collecting specimens themselves. Timed specimens are not sterile.
2. Wear gloves when handling urine.	
3. Discard this first specimen as test begins. Print time that test began on laboratory requisition.	Collection period begins with empty bladder.
4. When applicable, have client drink required amount of liquid or take ordered medication.	Required for specific types of tests to measure elimination of urine constituents.
5. Place signs indicating that timed urine specimen collection on client's door, and toileting area.	Prevents uninformed staff and relatives from accidentally discarding urine specimens.

STEPS	RATIONALE
6. Measure volume of each voiding if output is recorded.	Measures client's fluid balance.
7. Place all voided urine in labeled specimen bottle with appropriate additive.	Preserves urine specimen and prevents deterioration.
8. Unless instructed otherwise, keep specimen bottle in specimen refrigerator or in container of ice in bathroom.	Coldness prevents decomposition of urine.
9. Wash hands and discard gloves after collection of each voiding.	Reduces transmission of microorganisms.
10. Encourage client to drink two glasses of water 1 hour before timed urine collection ends.	Facilitates client's ability to void at end of period.
11. Encourage client to empty bladder during last 15 minutes of urine collection period.	Ensures urine collected for precise amount of time.
12. At end of period, send labeled specimen to laboratory with appropriate requisition.	Ensures laboratory results credited to correct client.
13. Remove signs and remind client that specimen collection period is completed.	Allows client to resume usual voiding habits.

EVALUATION

1. Intermittently during collection period, observe client's compliance with saving of all urine.	Clients often benefit from being reminded to save urine.
2. Inspect urine for contamination from feces or toilet tissue.	
3. Compare results of client's urinalysis with normal laboratory values.	Reveals deviations from normal and may indicate need for further testing.
4. **Unexpected outcomes** that may occur include:	
➤ A portion of urine specimen is accidentally discarded.	Test collection period must be restarted.
➤ Urine specimen is contaminated by feces or toilet tissue.	May cause inaccurate test results.
➤ Laboratory results reveal abnormal values for urine constituents.	Alteration in urinary function or metabolism.

RECORDING AND REPORTING

1. Record starting time of urine collection in client's chart.	Documents collection has begun.
2. At completion of test, record time urine collection is finished; appearance, amount, and odor of urine; and disposition of specimen to laboratory.	Documents completion of timed collection of urine.
3. Discuss abnormal test results with physician.	Facilitates appropriate intervention.

• • • • •

Special Considerations

- See Skill 43-1.
- If client leaves unit for test or procedure, be sure that personnel in that area collect urine.
- If client has indwelling catheter, place collection bag in ice-filled container.
- If client's physical condition warrants fluid restriction, be cautious in encouraging fluids.
- If urine is accidentally discarded or contaminated, restart timed period.
- Some references call time collections "composite specimens."

Teaching Considerations

- Explain fluid or dietary requirements or medications related to test.
- Explain significance of collecting all urine for specific period.
- Explain why urine must be kept in special container, with preservative (if used), and cold.

Pediatric Considerations

- For infants and young children who are not yet potty trained, special plastic urine-collecting bags with self-adhesive are designed to attach to the perineal area and have tubing attached that drains urine into a collecting receptacle. (A thin coating of sealant, such as skin-prep, applied to the skin helps to protect it and aids adhesion.)

Gerontologic Considerations

- The older adult may not be given a clear, concise explanation regarding the sample collection. A reminder should be placed in the bathroom on the mirror for the ambulatory client. The verbal reminders will further enhance continuing the sample collection.

Home Care Considerations

- For home care considerations, see Skill 43-1.

SKILL 43-3 Collecting a Sterile Urine Specimen from an Indwelling Catheter

It is often necessary to collect urine specimens from a client who has an indwelling catheter. Strict aseptic technique should be used to ensure sterility and to avoid introducing infection into the urinary tract.

A urine specimen should not be collected for culture tests from a urine drainage bag unless it is the first urine to drain into a new sterile bag. Bacteria grow rapidly in drainage bags and can give a false measurement of bacteria in the urine.

EQUIPMENT

- **3 ml syringe with 1-inch needle (21 gauge) (for culture) or 20 ml syringe with 1-inch needle (21 gauge) (for routine urinalysis)**
- **Metal clamp or rubber band**
- **Alcohol, povidone-iodine, or other disinfectant swab**
- **Specimen container (nonsterile for routine urinalysis, sterile for culture)**
- **Completed specimen identification label**
- **Completed laboratory requisition with client's name, date, and time of collection**
- **Clean disposable gloves**

DELEGATION CONSIDERATIONS

This procedure may be performed by unlicensed personnel:

- Determine that care provider understands sterile technique.
- Inform care provider when to obtain specimen.

STEPS	RATIONALE
ASSESSMENT	
1. Assess client's or family members' understanding of need to collect urine from indwelling catheter.	Reveals knowledge of procedure and willingness to cooperate.
2. Assess for signs and symptoms of urinary tract infection: temperature slightly elevated, hematuria, flank pain, **frequency,** fever, **urgency,** cloudy urine with sediment.	Suggest bacteria in urine.
3. Assess indwelling catheter for built-in sampling port and type of material from which it is made.	Provides appropriate place for removal of urine from catheter. Port prevents leakage of urine from catheter. It is safe to insert needle directly into self-sealing rubber catheter. Silastic, silicone, or plastic catheters are not self-sealing and thus should not be punctured with needle for aspiration of urine.

NURSING DIAGNOSIS

Clustering of defining characteristics from the assessment data may reveal the following nursing diagnoses for clients requiring this skill:

- Pain
- Risk for infection
- Toileting self-care deficit

Related factors are individualized based on a client's condition or needs.

STEPS	RATIONALE
PLANNING	
1. **Expected outcomes** following completion of procedure:	
➤ Urine specimen is obtained from catheter without contamination.	
➤ Urinary catheter and drainage system remain intact.	There is no indication (e.g., leaking of urine) that the catheter or drainage system was punctured by the needle during specimen collection.
➤ Urine has normal characteristics and no bacterial growth.	Client is free of urinary abnormality. No signs of nosocomial infection.
2. Explain why the catheter will need to be clamped for 30 minutes before obtaining a urine specimen and why it is not obtained from drainage bag.	Prevents development of anxiety over catheter clamping and promotes understanding of need for urine to collect within bladder.
3. Explain procedure to client and/or family member. Emphasize that although a syringe with a needle is used to remove the urine from the catheter, the client will not experience any discomfort.	Prevents anxiety when the nurse manipulates the catheter and aspirates the urine with the syringe and needle. Promotes client cooperation.
IMPLEMENTATION	
1. Wash hands.	Reduces transfer of microorganisms.
2. Clamp drainage tubing with clamp or rubberband for 30 minutes (see illustration).	Permits collection of fresh sterile urine in catheter tubing rather than draining into bag.
3. Return to room and inform client that procedure to collect specimen from catheter will begin.	Allows client to anticipate manipulation of urinary catheter and cope more effectively with discomfort that may occur when catheter is moved.
4. Wash hands and put on gloves.	Reduces transfer of microorganisms.
5. Position client so that catheter is easily accessible.	Allows for easy collection of specimen.
6. Cleanse entry port for needle with disinfectant swab.	Prevents entry of microorganisms into catheter.
7. Insert needle at 30-degree angle just above where catheter is attached to drainage tube or at built-in sampling port (see illustration).	Ensures entrance of needle into catheter lumen and prevents accidental puncture of lumen leading to balloon that holds catheter in place in bladder. Aspiration of water from lumen can result in catheter falling out of bladder.
8. Draw urine into 3 ml syringe (for culture) or draw urine into 20 ml syringe (for routine urinalysis).	Allows collection of urine without contamination. Proper volume is needed to perform test.

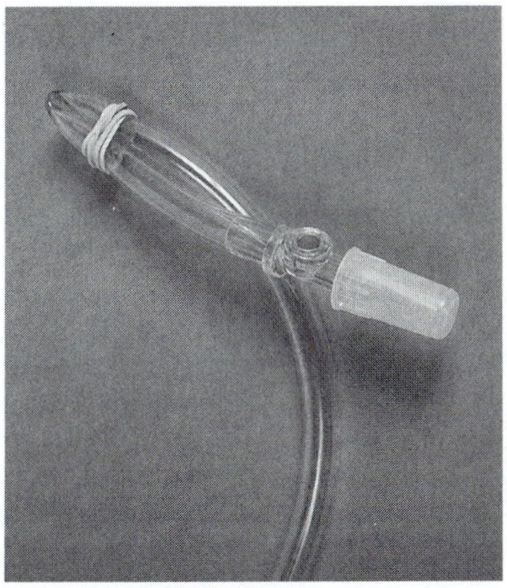

Step 2

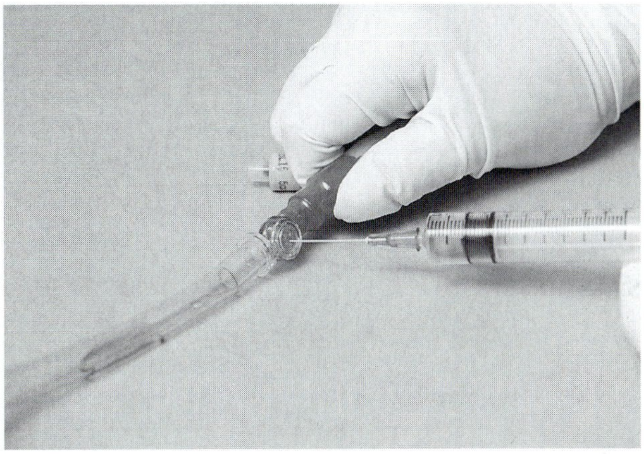

Step 7

STEPS	RATIONALE
9. Transfer urine from syringe into nonsterile urine container for routine urinalysis or transfer urine from syringe into sterile urine container for culture.	Prevents contamination of urine during transfer procedure.
10. Place lid tightly on container.	Prevents contamination of specimen by air and loss by spillage.
11. Unclamp catheter and allow urine to flow into drainage bag.	Allows urine to drain by gravity and prevents stasis of urine in bladder, which can cause much discomfort and potential damage to kidneys.
12. Dispose of soiled supplies, remove and discard gloves, and wash hands.	Reduces transmission of microorganisms.
13. Securely attach properly completed identification label and laboratory requisition to specimen.	Incorrect identification of specimen could result in diagnostic or therapeutic errors.
14. Send specimen to laboratory immediately or place in specimen refrigerator.	Bacteria grow quickly in urine; therefore urine should be analyzed immediately or refrigerated.

EVALUATION

1. Observe characteristics of urine and any signs of client discomfort.	Early clues to urinary tract infection.
2. Observe urinary drainage system to ensure that it is intact and patent.	
3. Compare results of client's laboratory report with normal laboratory values and report any abnormalities to the physician.	Reveals deviations from normal and indicates need for further testing and intervention.
4. **Unexpected outcomes** that may occur include:	
➤ Urine specimen is contaminated during procedure.	Cannot be evaluated unless nurse obviously contaminates equipment.
➤ Lumen that leads to balloon that holds catheter in bladder is punctured.	Will require reinsertion of catheter.
➤ Urine has abnormal constituents.	Indicates infection or other alteration.
➤ Client has pain during procedure.	

RECORDING AND REPORTING

1. Record collection of specimen in nurses' notes or per agency policy; note time and date, appearance, odor and color of urine and disposition to laboratory.	Verifies collection of specimen if report is slow to return to laboratory.
2. Notify physician of any significant differences in urine.	Allows physician to begin therapeutic action if needed.
3. Document any unexpected outcomes.	

FOLLOW-UP ACTIVITIES

1. Check needle insertion site on catheter to be sure it is not leaking.

SKILL 43-4 Measuring Specific Gravity of Urine

Specific gravity, the concentration of dissolved substances in water, can be measured easily by the nurse in any clinical setting. At least three modes currently exist to accomplish this measurement. The most common mode is to place a **urinometer** with a mercury bulb in a cylinder containing urine. The density or concentration of urine determines the level at which the urinometer floats within the cylinder. If the urine is dilute, the urinometer tends to sink. Concentrated solutes in urine raise the level at which the urinometer floats. This test requires only a few seconds to complete and can often provide useful information about the client's state of hydration and or kidney function and provide a parameter for the adjustment of fluid intake. Two other modes for measuring specific gravity are mentioned in the Special Considerations section.

EQUIPMENT

- **Accurately calibrated urinometer (validate by measuring specific gravity of distilled water, which is 1.000)**
- **Clean, dry glass cylinder**
- **20 ml urine or enough volume to fill glass cylinder two thirds full**
- **Clean disposable gloves**

DELEGATION CONSIDERATIONS

The measurement of specific gravity may be performed by unlicensed personnel:

- Instruct care provider how to use calibrated urinometer.

STEPS	RATIONALE
ASSESSMENT	
1. Assess client's or family members' understanding of need to test specific gravity and how test is performed.	Provides nurse with information on which to base teaching.
2. Determine client's ability to collect specimen.	Determines level of assistance required from nurse.
3. Assess client's hydration status: skin turgor, condition of mucous membranes, intake and output, (I&O), integrity of fontanels (infants).	Specific gravity measures concentration of urine solutes and is affected by state of hydration.
4. Assess client's medical history for evidence of renal disease.	Renal tubular disease results in loss of capacity of kidneys to concentrate urine.

NURSING DIAGNOSIS

Clustering of defining characteristics from the assessment data may reveal the following nursing diagnoses for clients requiring this skill:

➤ Fluid volume deficit
➤ Fluid volume excess

Related factors are individualized based on a client's condition or needs.

STEPS	RATIONALE
PLANNING	
1. **Expected outcomes** following completion of procedure:	
➤ Specific gravity is between 1.010 and 1.025.	Normal range of values.
➤ There are no feces, blood, or tissue in urine specimen.	Feces, tissue, and menstrual blood falsely elevate specific gravity reading.
2. Explain procedure to client and/or family member. Explain that urine must be free of feces and tissue.	Understanding promotes cooperation and relieves anxiety.
IMPLEMENTATION	
1. Wash hands and put on clean, disposable gloves.	Reduces transmission of microorganisms.
2. Carefully pour fresh urine specimen into glass cylinder until it is two thirds to three quarters full.	Cylinder must be at least two thirds full to cause urinometer to float.
3. Place urinometer in cylinder of urine and gently twirl top of stem.	Prevents urinometer from adhering to sides of cylinder.

STEPS	RATIONALE
4. Wait until urinometer stops bobbing; then with urinometer scale at eye level, read point where urine level touches calibrated scale. Read scale at lowest point of meniscus for best accuracy (see illustration). Report abnormal reading to physician.	Concentration of dissolved solutes in urine influences depth at which urinometer floats. Point at which urine reaches scale is specific gravity.
5. Discard urine and wash cylinder and urinometer in cool water.	Warm water coagulates proteins in urine and causes them to stick to glass surfaces.
6. Remove and discard gloves and wash hands.	Reduces transfer of microorganisms.

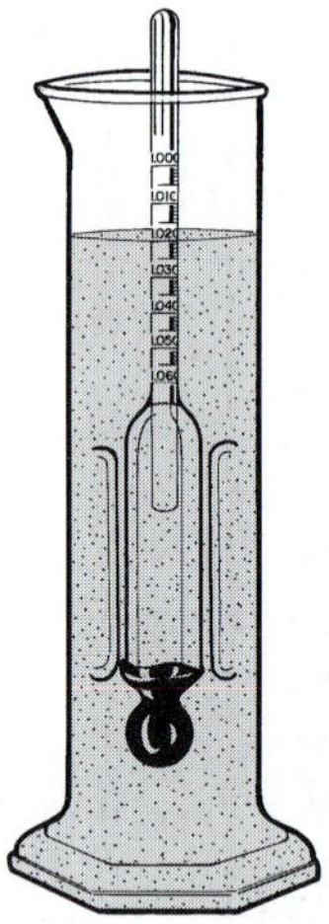

Step 4

EVALUATION

1. Observe specimen for contaminants, feces, or toilet tissue.	
2. Compare results of client's urinalysis with normal laboratory values.	Reveals deviations from normal and indicates need for intervention.
3. **Unexpected outcomes** that may occur include:	
➤ Specific gravity is less than 1.010 or greater than 1.025.	Dilute urine is less than 1.010; concentrated urine is greater than 1.025.
➤ Urine contains feces or blood.	Causes elevated specific gravity reading; repeat with next voiding.

RECORDING AND REPORTING

1. Record specific gravity reading and note character of urine in nurses' notes.	Allows for early treatment intervention.
2. If client's I&O is being monitored, record urine volume on flow sheet.	All urine must be measured to obtain accurate 24-hour output.
3. Report abnormal values to physician.	Results may indicate need for further therapy.

FOLLOW-UP ACTIVITIES

1. Check physician's orders to determine if specific nursing care is required for given reading (e.g., regulate IV rate, administer pitressin, regulate oral intake of diuretics).

• • • • •

Special Considerations

- Urine should be at room temperature for testing because urinometer is calibrated at room temperature.
- Special flow sheets are available for recording frequent measurements of specific gravity.
- Multistix reagent test strip can now be used to measure specific gravity. The end of the test strip is impregnated with a chemical reagent, which is dipped into the urine sample. After a specified time, the color of the strip is compared with the color chart on the bottle.
- Diluted, watery urine results in low specific gravity readings and dark-yellow concentrated urine results in high specific gravity readings.
- For infants and children who are not toilet trained, the urine specific gravity may be obtained if a cotton ball is left in the diaper area. The cotton ball can be removed when it is well saturated to obtain specimen.
- Use of a **refractometer,** a small telescope-like instrument, is a newer technique for measuring specific gravity. One drop of urine is placed on a slide and viewed through refractometer, which allows visualization of density of urine on calibrated scale.

Teaching Considerations

- Instruct client about proper method for collecting random urine specimen.
- Explain reason for measuring specific gravity.
- Discuss significance of test if client shows interest.

Gerontologic Considerations

- When obtaining specific gravity for older adult, note any medications that may influence results of sample. Some medications may cause alteration in true values.
- When older adult is undergoing fluid restrictions, this may also have an impact on true specific gravity of urine.

SKILL 43-5 Measuring Chemical Properties of Urine: Glucose, Ketones, Protein, Blood, and pH

Tests for chemical properties of urine, which are a part of the routine urinalysis done by the laboratory, can be performed quickly. Normally, glucose and ketones are not present in the urine, and the appearance of either element generally indicates that glucose is not effectively reaching the body's cells. When this screening test for the presence of glucose in the urine is positive, other tests are used to determine the diagnosis of diabetes mellitus.

In the past, persons with diabetes mellitus routinely used urine testing of glucose to monitor the effectiveness of their medication, diet, and exercise on their blood glucose levels. Today, this practice has been largely supplanted by determination of blood glucose levels by finger sticks. Nevertheless, this traditional method of testing the urine for glucose is described here.

Urine testing for glucose and acetone has been used for many years to monitor glucose control by diet and insulin. The test is acceptable to clients because it is easily performed and causes no pain; however, it is being replaced by testing capillary blood, which is obtained by skin puncture of the fingertip (see Skill 43-13). This change is being made because capillary blood monitoring directly reflects current serum glucose levels and is not affected by the renal threshold for glucose or fluid volume. Hypoglycemia, which cannot be detected by urine testing, may be identified by sampling of serum glucose.

Assessing the chemical properties of urine can be done by immersing a special chemically prepared strip of paper into a clean urine specimen or by combining drops of urine with chemically prepared tablets. The change in color of the strip or tablet indicates the presence of any of these substances.

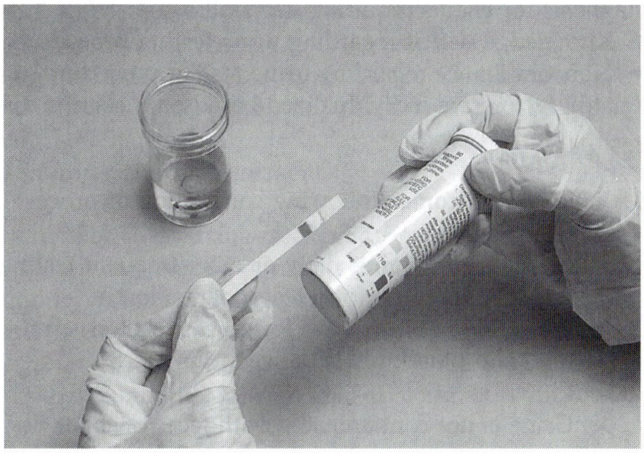

Fig. 43-3 Testing urine using a reagent strip.

STEPS | **RATIONALE**

CRITICAL DECISION POINT Unnecessary if Ketostix, Multistix, or Diastix reagent test strips are used.

a. Place Acetest tablet on white tissue. — Color of tablet changes to shades of tan or gray, which can be seen more easily on white background.

b. Add 1 drop of urine to tablet. — Begins chemical reaction.

c. Time for 30 seconds and compare color of tablet with Acetest color chart. — Time required for reagent to indicate ketone bodies.

d. Discard tablet and tissue in trash. — Reduces transmission of microorganisms.

6. Use Multistix reagent test strip to assess for chemical properties of pH, protein, glucose, ketones, and/or blood simultaneously: — Eliminates need for all previous testing discussed. Presence of these elements may indicate renal or other systemic diseases.

a. Immerse end of chemically impregnated test strip into urine. — Exposes reagent to urine.

b. Remove strip from container immediately and tap it gently against side of container. — Excess urine can dilute reagents.

c. Hold strip in horizontal position. — Prevents possible mixing of chemical reagents.

d. Time for number of seconds specified on container, and compare color of strip with color chart (Table 43-1). — Accurate interpretation of results depends on precise timing.

7. Remove and discard gloves, wash hands. — Reduces transmission of microorganisms.

8. Discuss test results with client. — Client should participate in care to improve understanding and compliance.

Table 43-1 Multistix

Test	When to Read	Range of Results
pH	Anytime	5-9
Protein	Anytime	(1) to +4 (72,000 mg/dl)
Glucose	10 seconds (qualitative)	(−) to +4
	30 seconds (quantitative)	(−) to +4 (270)
Ketones	15 seconds	(−) to +3 (large)
Blood	25 seconds	(−) to +3 (large)

EVALUATION

1. If client is to be responsible for self-testing, have client demonstrate proficiency. — Return demonstration is best evidence of proficiency.

2. Note presence of blood, protein, glucose, or ketones in the urine. — None of these substances should be in the urine; pH should be slightly acidic (average = 6; normal = 4.5-8).

3. Observe that sample is not contaminated with feces or toilet tissue.

4. **Unexpected outcomes** that may occur include:
   - Client or family member is unable to perform urine test correctly. — Indicates need for further teaching.
   - Test results are positive for:
     - Glucose — When blood glucose level exceeds 180 mg/dl (renal threshold), glucose spills into urine. This most commonly occurs in poorly controlled diabetes mellitus, but it also occurs with IV administration of fluids containing dextrose and with hyperalimentation.

STEPS	RATIONALE
• Ketones	Ketones are the end product of fatty acid breakdown; they are excreted in the urine when fat is burned for energy, as occurs in low-carbohydrate diets, starvation, diabetes mellitus, and alcoholism (Pagana and Pagana, 1995).
• Protein	Protein in the urine is indicative of renal dysfunction and occurs only when the glomerular membrane fails to prevent its escape. A transient proteinuria may occur with excess exercise, cold baths, severe stress, and pregnancy.
• Blood	Blood in the urine may be indicative of renal damage, tumors, stones, infection, or trauma in the urinary tract (Pagana and Pagana, 1995).
• Alterations in pH	Urine becomes excessively alkaline with alkalemia, infection of urinary tract, and a diet high in vegetables or citrus fruits. Acidic urine is associated with acidemia, diarrhea, starvation, and a diet high in meat products or cranberries (Pagana and Pagana, 1995).

Recording and Reporting

1. Record results immediately in nurses' notes or glucose testing flow sheet.	Timely documentation ensures accurate therapeutic intervention.
2. Have client in home setting record results of test on flow sheet. Encourage client to take samples at the same time each day.	Allows client to see variations in testing over several days. Provides record of testing between visits to physician.

Follow-Up Activities

1. Consult with physician when results are unexpected.
2. If client is diabetic, nurse should determine if insulin should be given.

• • • • •

Special Considerations

- Clarify with other health team member if Clinitest is to be done with 1 drop, 2 drops, or 5 drops of urine.
- If client has difficulty complying with double-void specimen, check first voided specimen for sugar and acetone; however, this is not an accurate assessment of current blood glucose level.
- Clients receiving high concentrations of glucose (see Chapter 28) often undergo glucose testing.
- Diabetic flow sheets often require charting of medications and amount of urine as well as results of glucose and ketone tests.

Teaching Considerations

- Instruct client about proper method for collecting random urine sample.
- Teach client to check expiration date on bottle.
- Teach client to store tablets in clean, dry area. Moisture can alter chemical makeup of tablets.
- Clients should be taught to close bottles tightly after removing reagent strips to prevent them from absorbing moisture and altering future results.
- Explain rationale for double-voided specimen, and seek appropriate client feedback.
- Explain relationship of urinary findings of glucose with blood glucose when indicated.
- Discuss possible reasons for finding acetone, blood, and protein in urine.
- Discuss relationship of urinary pH to urinary tract infection and formation of renal calculi when appropriate.
- Have client return demonstrations on urine testing until client uses correct technique.
- Discuss client's plans for testing urine at home, if indicated.

Pediatric Considerations

- School-age children can learn to test urine accurately, but parents should continue to provide backup.
- If reagent tablets are used, keep them away from small children. Tablets contain caustic soda, which can burn mouth and oral mucosa.
- Parents are usually very helpful in guiding young children through procedure.

Gerontologic Considerations

- Older adults may have difficulty seeing color chart.
- Older adults with musculoskeletal alterations may not have fine motor coordination necessary to obtain samples on conduct test.

Home Care Considerations

- Most kits sold in drug stores contain all equipment necessary for testing urine except specimen container.
- Clients at home may prefer to use large clock with second hand for timing urine tests.

SKILL 43-6 Measuring Occult Blood in Stool

A common fecal laboratory test is the guaiac test for occult blood. The test measures microscopic amounts of blood in the feces. Normally a person loses small amounts of blood daily in the feces as a result of minor abrasions of the nasopharyngeal or oral mucosa. If greater than 50 ml of blood enters the feces from the upper gastrointestinal tract, the blood can be visualized as **melena** (darkening of feces). The **guaiac test** helps to reveal blood that is visually undetectable. The test is a useful diagnostic tool for conditions such as colon cancer, upper gastrointestinal ulcers, and localized gastric parasitic infections or intestinal irritation.

The test is easy to perform. Clients are often instructed on how to collect fecal specimens for the test in the home. Only a small amount of stool is needed to perform the test successfully. The most common guaiac tests are the Hemoccult slides and the Hematest tablets.

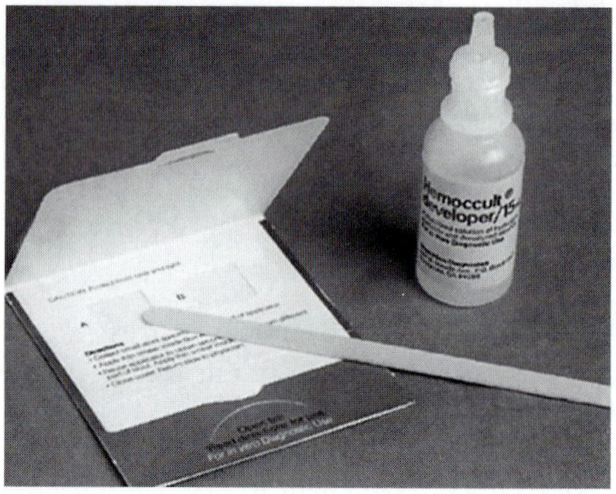

Fig. 43-4 Hemoccult testing kit for measuring occult blood in stool.

EQUIPMENT

- Paper towel
- Disposable gloves
- Wooden applicator

Hemoccult Test (Fig. 43-4)

- Cardboard Hemoccult slide
- Hemoccult developing solution

OR

Hematest

- Hematest tablets (tablets must be protected from moisture, heat, and light)
- Guaiac paper (reagent tablet produces blue reaction on guaiac paper if fecal smear contains blood)
- Sink with running water

DELEGATION CONSIDERATIONS

The obtaining and testing of stool for occult blood may be performed by unlicensed personnel:

- Inform care provider to inform nurse immediately if blood is detected.
- Inform care provider not to discard stool from a positive test, so that the nurse may repeat the testing.

STEPS | **RATIONALE**

ASSESSMENT

1. Assess client's or family members' understanding of need for stool test.
   Provides nurse with data base on which to provide necessary health teaching.
2. Assess client's ability to cooperate with procedure and collect specimen.
   To avoid embarrassment, clients often prefer to collect own stool specimen. Some clients require assistance.
3. Assess client's medical history for bleeding or gastrointestinal disorder.
   Routine screening can be instituted by nurse.
4. Obtain client's medication history. Note drugs that can cause gastrointestinal mucosal bleeding.
   Anticoagulants increase risk of bleeding in gastrointestinal tract, even from minor trauma to mucosa. Long-term use of steroids and acetylsalicylic acid can irritate mucosa.
5. Refer to physician's orders for medication or dietary modifications or restrictions before test.
   Certain medications such as iron supplement and bismuth compounds can cause stools to resemble melena. Rare meats can cause same results.

NURSING DIAGNOSIS

Clustering of defining characteristics from the assessment data may reveal the following nursing diagnoses for clients requiring this skill:

- Bowel incontinence
- Constipation
- Diarrhea
- Knowledge deficit regarding collection and testing of stool specimen

Related factors are individualized based on a client's condition or needs.

PLANNING

1. **Expected outcomes** following completion of procedure:
   - Test for **occult blood** is negative.
     Client has only small amount of blood in feces because of normal nasopharyngeal and oral mucosa abrasions.
   - Client will discuss purpose and benefits of testing stool for blood.
     Documents learning.
2. Explain procedure to client and/or family member. Discuss reason for specimen collection and how client can assist. Explain that feces must be free of urine and tissue.
   Client who understands procedure is more likely to cooperate and may be able to obtain specimen independently. Also prevents accidental disposal of specimen.
3. Arrange for any needed dietary or medication restrictions.
   Ensures accuracy of test results.

IMPLEMENTATION

1. Wash hands and apply clean disposable gloves.
   Reduces transmission of microorganisms.
2. Obtain uncontaminated stool specimen.
   Specimen is obtained in clean, dry container and not contaminated with urine, water, or toilet tissue.

CRITICAL DECISION POINT **Observe fecal specimen. If frank red blood is observed within stool itself, report these findings.**

3. Use tip of wooden applicator to obtain small portion of feces.
   Small specimen is sufficient for measuring blood content.
4. Perform Hemoccult slide test:
   a. Open flap of slide and apply thin smear of stool on paper in first box.
      Guaiac paper inside box is sensitive to fecal blood content. Occult blood from upper gastrointestinal tract is not always equally dispersed throughout stool.
   b. Obtain second fecal specimen from different portion of stool, and apply thinly to slide's second box (see illustration on p. 1230).
      Findings of occult blood are more conclusive for gastrointestinal bleeding when entire specimen is found to contain blood.

STEPS	RATIONALE
ASSESSMENT	
1. Assess understanding of purpose of procedure and ability to cooperate.	Provides basis to determine need for health teaching and need for assistance.
2. Assess condition of and drainage from nasal mucosa and sinuses.	Reveals physical signs that may indicate infection or allergic irritation.
➤ ***CRITICAL DECISION POINT*** **Clear drainage usually indicates allergy. Yellow, green, brown drainage usually indicates infection.**	
3. Determine if client has experienced postnasal drip, sinus headache or tenderness, nasal congestion or sore throat.	Symptoms help reveal nature of problem.
4. Assess condition of posterior pharynx.	
➤ ***CRITICAL DECISION POINT*** **Pay particular attention to areas of inflammation or purulent drainage. Identification of inflamed or purulent areas allows nurse to swab those sites quickly.**	
5. Assess client for systemic signs of infection: fever, chills, fatigue.	Infection originating within nasopharynx can become systemic, requiring antibiotic therapy.
6. Review physician's orders to determine if nose, throat, or both cultures are needed.	Prevents exposing client to unnecessary discomfort of repeated cultures.

NURSING DIAGNOSIS

Clustering of defining characteristics from the assessment data may reveal the following nursing diagnoses for clients requiring this skill:

- Knowledge deficit regarding specimen collection
- Pain
- Risk for infection

Related factors are individualized based on a client's condition or needs.

STEPS	RATIONALE
PLANNING	
1. **Expected outcomes** following completion of procedure:	
➤ There is no bacterial growth in specimens.	Proves absence of infection.
➤ Client does not experience bleeding of nasal mucosa.	Procedure is atraumatic.
➤ Specimen is not contaminated.	Evidenced by results of laboratory analysis.
➤ Client will discuss purpose and benefits of nose and throat cultures.	Documents learning.
2. Plan to do culture before mealtime or at least 1 hour after eating.	Decreases incidence of vomiting.
3. Explain procedure to client and/or family member. Discuss reason for specimen collection and how client can assist.	Understanding of procedure usually decreases anxiety and promotes cooperation.
4. Explain that client may have tickling sensation or gag during swabbing of throat. Nasal swab may create urge to sneeze. Both procedures require only a few seconds.	Nursing research has demonstrated that clients who have been made aware of sensations they will experience are more able to cooperate with experiences that are uncomfortable (Johnson, 1984).
IMPLEMENTATION	
1. Ask client to sit erect in bed or chair facing nurse. Acutely ill client or young child may lie back against bed with head of bed raised to 45-degree angle.	Reduces transmission of microorganisms. Provides easy access to nasal or oral structures.

STEPS	RATIONALE
2. Have swab in tube ready for use. Nurse may wish to loosen top so that swab can be removed easily.	Nurse should be able to grasp swab easily without danger of contaminating it. Most commercially prepared tubes have top that fits securely over end of swab, which allows nurse to touch outer top without contaminating swab stick.
3. COLLECT THROAT CULTURE:	
a. Wash hands and put on gloves.	
b. Instruct client to tilt head backward. For clients in bed, place pillow behind shoulders.	Facilitates visualization of pharynx.
c. Ask client to open mouth and say "ah."	Permits exposure of pharynx, relaxes throat muscles, and minimizes gag reflex.

CRITICAL DECISION POINT **If pharynx is not visualized, depress tongue with tongue blade and note inflamed areas of pharynx or tonsils. Depress anterior third of tongue only. (Illuminate with penlight as needed.) Area to be swabbed should be clearly visualized. Placement of tongue blade along back of tongue more likely initiates gag reflex.**

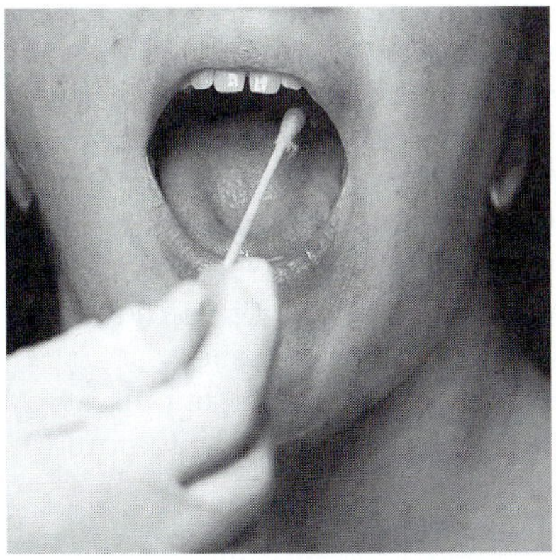

Step 3e

STEPS	RATIONALE
d. Insert swab without touching lips, teeth, tongue, or cheeks.	Touching lips or oral mucosal structures can contaminate swab with resident bacteria.
e. Gently but quickly swab tonsillar area side to side, making contact with inflamed or purulent sites (see illustration).	These areas contain most microorganisms.
f. Carefully withdraw swab without striking oral structures. Immediately place swab in culture tube and crush ampule at bottom of tube. Push tip of swab into liquid medium (see illustration).	Retains microorganisms within culture tube. Mixing swab tip with culture medium ensures life of bacteria for testing.
g. Place top on culture tube securely.	Prevents contamination from microorganisms.
h. Discard tongue depressor into trash.	Reduces transmission of microorganisms.
i. Remove gloves and discard.	

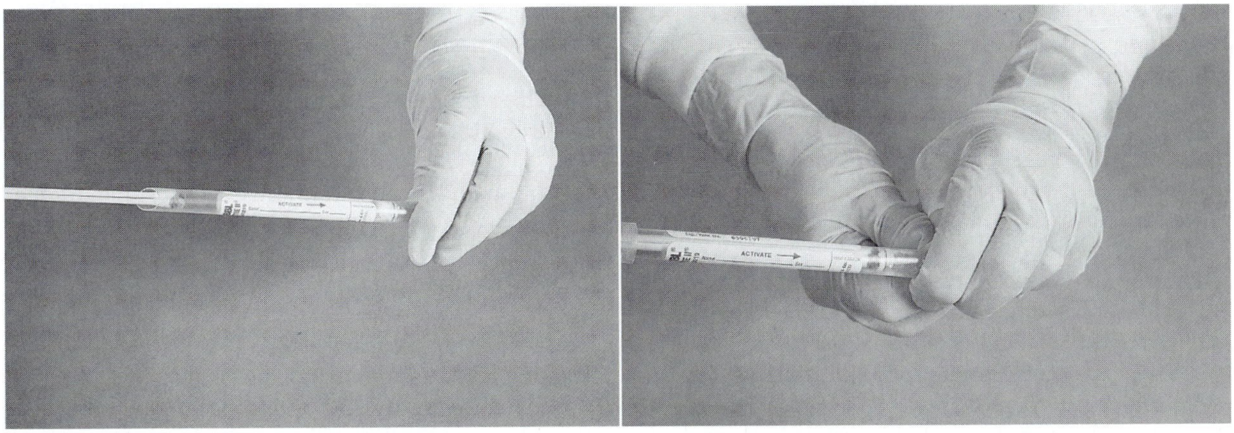

Step 3f

STEPS	RATIONALE
4. COLLECT NOSE CULTURE:	
a. Wash hands and put on gloves.	
b. Encourage client to blow nose and check nostrils for patency with penlight.	Clears nasal passages of mucus containing resident bacteria.
➤ ***CRITICAL DECISION POINT*** **Ask client to alternatively occlude each nostril and exhale. Determines nostril with greater patency, from which specimen will be collected.**	
c. Ask client to tilt head back. Clients in bed should have pillow behind shoulders.	Facilitates visualization of nasal septum and sinuses.
d. Gently insert nasal speculum in one nostril (optional).	Allows retraction of mucosa for easier swab insertion.
e. Carefully pass swab through center of speculum (if used) into nostril until it reaches that portion of mucosa that is inflamed or containing exudate. Rotate swab quickly.	Swab should remain sterile until it reaches area to be cultured. Rotating swab covers all surfaces with exudate.
f. Remove swab without touching sides of speculum.	Prevents contamination of swab by resident bacteria.
g. Carefully remove nasal speculum (if used) and place in basin. Offer client facial tissue.	Minimizes period of time client will experience discomfort.
h. Insert swab into culture tube. Crush ampule at bottom of tube and push tip of swab into liquid medium.	Retains microorganisms within culture tube. Mixing swab tip with culture medium ensures life of bacteria for testing.
i. Place top on tube securely.	Prevents contamination from microorganisms.
j. Remove gloves, discard, and wash hands.	
5. COLLECTION OF NASOPHARYNGEAL CULTURE:	
a. Follow Step 5, a through j, except use a special swab on a flexible wire that can be flexed downward to reach nasopharynx via nose.	Only this specially designed swab allows access to difficult-to-reach nasopharyngeal area.
➤ ***CRITICAL DECISION POINT*** **This swab must advance into the nasopharynx to ensure that the culture has been obtained correctly.**	
6. Remove gloves, discard, and wash hands.	Reduces transmission of microorganisms.
7. Securely attach properly completed identification label and laboratory requisition to culture tube.	Incorrect identification of specimen could result in diagnostic or therapeutic errors.
8. Send specimen to laboratory immediately or refrigerate.	Fresh specimen provides most accurate test results.

EVALUATION

1. Check laboratory record for results of culture test.	Results reveal type of organisms in nose or pharynx and antibiotics most likely to be effective.
2. Inspect client's nose for evidence of bleeding.	Speculum and swab can traumatize sensitive, fragile mucosa.
3. Observe that specimen was not contaminated during procedure by coming in contact with client's teeth, tongue, or cheek.	
4. Ask client about need for obtaining these cultures.	
5. **Unexpected outcomes** that may occur include:	
➤ Nose and throat cultures reveal bacterial growth.	Evidence of upper respiratory or sinus infection.
➤ Client experiences minor nasal bleeding.	Trauma to sensitive mucosa causes bleeding, which should disappear with mild pressure over bridge of nose or application of ice.
➤ Specimen is contaminated.	Result of abundant number of resident bacteria on swab from contact with tongue, cheek, or teeth.

STEPS	RATIONALE
RECORDING AND REPORTING	
1. Record specimen collection, date, time, and disposition in nurses' notes.	All specimens should be documented to verify procedure performed.
2. Describe appearance of nasal and oral mucosal structures in nurses' notes.	Physical signs may add to diagnostic data base.
3. Report unusual test results to physician.	Findings may indicate need for therapy (e.g., antibiotic administration).

• • • • •

Special Considerations

- Nurse often needs assistance to obtain throat cultures from confused, combative, or unconscious clients.
- If client gags, remove tongue blade and allow to relax before reinserting. Place pressure only on anterior third of tongue.
- Most agencies use commercially available culture tubes containing special transport medium.
- Agency policy may dictate type of information to place on label. Note on laboratory requisition if client is taking antibiotic or if specific organism is suspected (e.g., *Bordetella pertussis*).

Teaching Considerations

- Allowing young children to visualize and examine speculum decreases their fear of it.
- Clients should be instructed that procedure is painless but gagging is common.
- Discuss client's role in collecting specimen.
- Explain how and why specimen is being obtained.
- Discuss relationship between culture results and medication.
- Discuss reason for time delay in receiving culture results.

Pediatric Considerations

- Immobilization of child's head and arms is important when obtaining nose or throat culture and should be done in firm, gentle, kind manner. Ask another nurse to assist, if necessary. Ask parents to act as coach with their child.
- Showing tongue blade and penlight to child and demonstrating how to say "ah" helps to decrease anxiety (Fig. 43-5).
- School-age child will be more cooperative if given opportunity to ask questions about procedure and results.

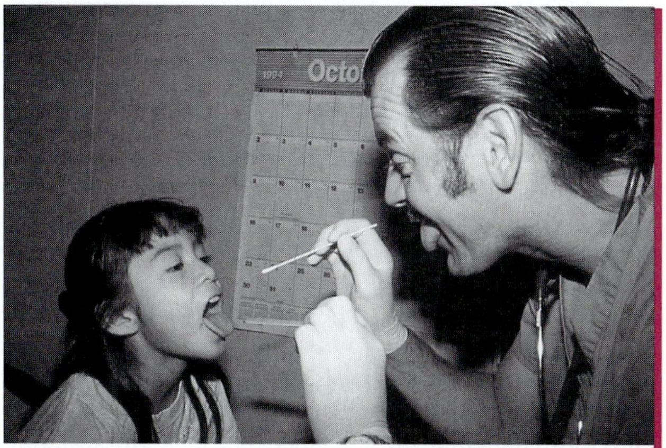

Fig. 43-5 Preparing a child for a throat culture increases cooperation.

- Respiratory syncytial virus is detected directly in respiratory secretions, usually obtained by nasopharyngeal aspiration (American Academy of Pediatrics Committee on Infectious Diseases, 1993). After positioning child in supine position, syringe is used to instill about 2 ml of sterile normal saline into one nostril; then sterile bulb syringe is used to aspirate it. Procedure is repeated in other nostril.
- Throat cultures should not be attempted if acute epiglottitis is suspected because trauma from swab might cause increase in edema and resulting occlusion of airway (Wong, 1995).

Gerontologic Considerations

- Older adults may need assistance in keeping mouth open in order to obtain specimen. In confused clients auxiliary personnel may be necessary to hold client's hands while sample is being obtained.

SKILL 43-8 Obtaining Vaginal or Urethral Discharge Specimens

Normally there is minimal discharge from the vagina or urethra. Poor hygiene practices may cause an accumulation of discharge. However, if a client develops an increased amount of discharge or if there is a change in the character of discharge from the vagina or urethra, medical follow-up is necessary.

Drainage from the vagina or urethra is normally thin, nonpurulent, whitish or clear, and small in amount. A woman will have bloody discharge during menstruation. A newborn infant may have bloody discharge from the vagina for 2 to 4 weeks after birth because of the abrupt decrease in maternal hormones at birth.

The clients most commonly requiring cultures of vaginal or urethral discharge have signs and symptoms of sexually transmitted disease or urinary tract infection. Clients suspected of having a sexually transmitted disease may be embarrassed by their condition. The nurse must show respect and understanding toward the client. If the client undergoes a complete diagnostic workup, the many questions can be exhausting and may cause anxiety. When collecting vaginal or urethral specimens, the nurse should work quickly and calmly, maintaining the client's privacy at all times.

EQUIPMENT

- **Sterile swab in sterile culture tube (commercially available culture tubes have swab and tube with ampule containing special transport medium)**
- **Sheet, blanket, paper drape**
- **Clean disposable gloves**
- **Penlight or gooseneck lamp**
- **Completed identification labels**
- **Completed laboratory requisition (date, time, name of test, type of culture)**

DELEGATION CONSIDERATIONS

The skill of obtaining the vaginal and urethral discharge culture samples requires problem solving and knowledge application unique to a professional nurse. Delegation of this skill is inappropriate.

STEPS	RATIONALE
ASSESSMENT	
1. Assess understanding of need for culture and ability to cooperate with procedure.	Provides data on which nurse develops teaching plan.
2. Assess condition of external genitalia. Observe urethra, meatus, and vaginal orifice for redness, swelling, tenderness, and discharge that is whitish, mucoid, and purulent.	Assessment findings and specimen test results reveal nature of problem.
3. Ask client if dysuria, localized pruritus of genitalia, or lower abdominal pain have been experienced.	Symptoms of urinary tract or vaginal infection.
4. If symptoms suggest sexually transmitted disease, record sexual history of client.	It is important to know nature of client's disease and to what extent sexual partners have been exposed to infection.
5. Refer to physician's order for type of culture.	Client may require one or both types of cultures.

NURSING DIAGNOSIS

Clustering of defining characteristics from the assessment data may reveal the following nursing diagnoses for clients requiring this skill:

- Anxiety
- Pain
- Risk for infection

Related factors are individualized based on a client's condition or needs.

PLANNING

STEPS	RATIONALE
1. **Expected outcomes** following completion of procedure.	
➤ Specimen is not contaminated.	Results on laboratory test can reveal whether skin cells or mucosal cells have contaminated specimen.

STEPS	RATIONALE
➤ Vaginal or urethral cultures do not reveal growth of microorganisms.	Evidence of absence of infection.
2. Explain procedure to client and/or family member. Discuss reason for specimen collection and how client can assist. Instruct female client not to douche before culture is obtained.	Client who understands procedure is less anxious and more likely to cooperate. Douching of vaginal canal would remove discharge containing pathogens.
3. Select area where privacy can be ensured.	Demonstrates respect for client.

IMPLEMENTATION

STEPS	RATIONALE
1. Wash hands.	Reduces transmission of microorganisms.
2. Draw bedside curtains or close room door. Place "Do Not Enter" sign on door (if available).	Provides privacy for client and demonstrates nurse's respect for client's well-being.
3. Assist client to proper position, raise gown, and drape body parts to be exposed: a. **Female:** Dorsal recumbent position with sheet draped over each leg and genitalia. b. **Male:** Sit on chair or bed or lie supine with sheet draped across lower trunk and genitalia.	Provides easy access to perineal area. Draping minimizes exposure of body parts, minimizing anxiety.
4. Apply clean disposable gloves.	Prevents contamination of nurse's hands from discharge.
5. Direct light source onto perineum (may not be needed for male client).	Allows better visualization of urethral or vaginal structures.
6. Open culture tube and hold swab in dominant hand.	Provides for easier manipulation of swab during culture collection.
7. Instruct client to slowly deep breathe.	Helps client to relax. Tensing of muscles around pelvic floor may cause discomfort during swabbing.
8. Obtain necessary specimens:	
a. *Female.*	
(1) With nondominant hand, fully separate labia to expose vaginal orifice.	Exposes perineum and ensures specimen is of vaginal discharge.
(2) Touch tip of swab into discharge pool, being careful not to touch skin or mucosa along perineum or vaginal canal. If no discharge is visible, gently insert swabs 1 to 2.5 cm (½-1 inch) into vaginal orifice and rotate before removal.	Discharge contains the greatest concentration of microorganisms.
(3) To expose urethral meatus, use nondominant hand to pull gently on labia minora upward and back.	Labia are often retracted over urethral orifice.
(4) Use clean swab and gently apply to tip of meatus where discharge is visible. Avoid touching labia.	Discharge contains greatest concentration of microorganisms.

➤ *CRITICAL DECISION POINT* If discharge near vagina appears different from discharge along perineum, collect separate specimens from each area. If there are two organisms present, they are not cross contaminated on a single swab.

STEPS	RATIONALE
b. *Male.*	
(1) Hold client's penis near tip with nondominant hand; if male is uncircumcised, gently retract foreskin.	Provides clear exposure of urethral meatus.
(2) Use dominant hand to hold swab. Apply gently to area of discharge at urinary meatus. If no discharge is apparent, physician may order swab to be introduced into urinary meatus.	Discharge contains greatest number of microorganisms.

STEPS	RATIONALE
(3) Return foreskin to natural position.	Tightening of foreskin around shaft of penis can cause localized discomfort and edema.
9. Return each swab to culture tube and secure top.	Retains microorganisms within tube.
10. Remove and discard gloves.	Reduces spread of microorganisms.
11. If using commercial culture tube, immediately squeeze end of tube to crush ampule (see Skill 43-7, Step 3, p. 1233). Push tip of swab into fluid medium.	Medium supports life of microorganisms until culture is obtained.
12. Label each culture tube with identification label and affix completed requisition.	Incorrect specimen identification could lead to diagnostic or therapeutic error.
13. Send specimen immediately to laboratory or refrigerate.	Bacteria multiply quickly; specimen should be analyzed quickly for accurate results.
14. Assist client to comfortable position, replace gown, and remove drape.	Reinforces client's sense of self-esteem.
15. Wash hands.	Reduces transmission of microorganisms.

EVALUATION

1. Review laboratory results for evidence of pathogens.	Results will reveal type of organisms present. Certain organisms are common to vaginal tract. Urethra should be free of microorganisms.
2. If discharge is present, observe color and amount.	Characteristics of discharge can indicate specific type of infection.
3. Observe specimen for presence of feces.	
4. **Unexpected outcomes** that may occur include:	
➤ Vaginal or urethral cultures reveal growth of pathogenic microorganisms.	Indication of infection.
➤ Specimen is contaminated with epidermal cells.	Poor technique results in inconclusive findings.

RECORDING AND REPORTING

1. In nurses' notes record types of cultures obtained and date and time sent to laboratory.	Documents cultures were obtained.
2. Describe character of discharge and appearance of vaginal orifice or urethral meatus.	Data document infection.
3. Report laboratory results to nurse in charge or physician.	Results may indicate specific therapies such as antibiotic administration.

FOLLOW-UP ACTIVITIES

1. If culture results indicate presence of sexually transmitted disease, develop a plan of care for the client.

• • • • •

Special Considerations

- Most clients wish to discuss reason for vaginal or urethral culture privately, and many fear possible results of test.
- Collection of sexual history must be performed nonjudgmentally.
- Hold male genitalia gently. Excess manipulation can cause erection.
- Some institutions have special bags for specimens. If client is in isolation, specimen container must be placed in bag.

Teaching Considerations

- Discuss symptoms of vaginal or urethral infection with client as appropriate.
- Explain relationship between genital discomfort and infection of vaginal or urinary tract.
- Explain time required to obtain results of culture.
- Discuss sexuality and safe sexual practices with client if appropriate.
- Clients with urethral or vaginal discharge may require instruction about perineal hygiene measures.
- If topical treatments (e.g., suppositories) are ordered, instruct client in proper administration of medication (see Chapter 19).

Pediatric Considerations

- ➤ Young child will probably desire parents' presence, whereas adolescent usually will not.
- ➤ In collection from infant or young child, another nurse can assist with specimen by gently holding child's legs apart in froglike position. Have parent present to encourage cooperation.
- ➤ Parents should understand that obtaining specimen will not affect virginity of child.

Gerontologic Considerations

- ➤ When obtaining a sample from older adults, assist client to comfortable position.
- ➤ Clear explanation regarding importance of obtaining sample is extremely helpful to gain cooperation.
- ➤ Auxiliary personnel may be needed to assist in obtaining the sample.

SKILL 43-9 Collecting Sputum Specimens

Sputum is produced by cells lining the respiratory tract. Although production is minimal in the healthy state, disease states can increase the amount or change the character of sputum. Examination of sputum may aid in the diagnosis and treatment of several conditions ranging from simple bronchitis to lung cancer.

Three major types of sputum specimens are sputum for cytology, culture and sensitivity, and acid-fast bacilli (AFB). Sputum collected for culture and sensitivity testing can be used to identify specific microorganisms and to determine antibiotics to which they are most sensitive. AFB in sputum indicates tuberculosis. Cytological or cellular examination of sputum may identify aberrant cells or cancer.

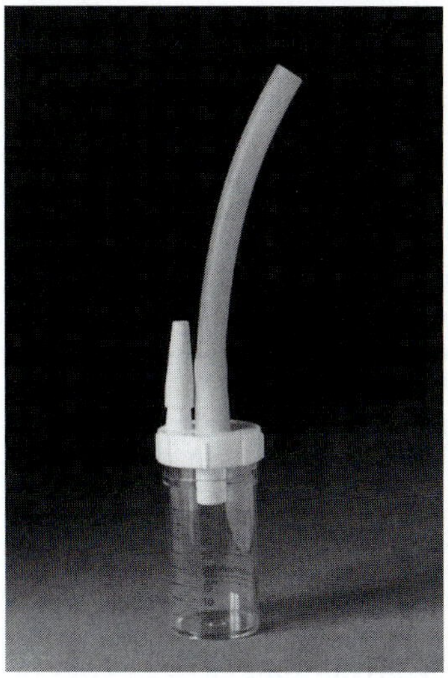

Fig. 43-6 Sputum collection device, also called "Sputum trap", used for collecting specimens.

EQUIPMENT

Expectorated Specimen

- Sterile specimen container with cover
- Clean disposable gloves
- Facial tissues
- Emesis basin (optional)
- Toothbrush (optional)
- Completed identification labels
- Completed laboratory requisition (date, time, name of test, source of culture)
- Small plastic bag for delivery of specimen to lab (or a container as specified by agency)

Suctioned Specimen

- Suction device (wall or portable)
- Sterile suction catheter (size 14, 16, or 18 Fr [not large enough to cause trauma to nasal mucosa])
- Sterile gloves
- Sterile saline in container
- In-line specimen container (sputum trap) (Fig. 43-6).
- Small plastic bag for delivery of specimen to laboratory (or a container as specified by agency)
- Oxygen therapy equipment if indicated
- Protective eye wear (if required)

DELEGATION CONSIDERATIONS

Collection of sputum specimens may be done by unlicensed personnel:

- Inform care giver when sputum should be obtained.
- Instruct care giver to obtain specimen before a meal.
- Instruct care giver about how to position client with impaired mobility.

➤ **CRITICAL DECISION POINT** **If a sterile suction method is needed, this skill then requires problem solving and knowledge application of a professional nurse. Delegation of this skill is inappropriate.**

STEPS	RATIONALE
ASSESSMENT	
1. Check physician's orders for type of sputum analysis and specifications (e.g., amount of sputum, number of specimens, time of collection, method to obtain).	Specific test to be performed may dictate when or how frequently specimens are collected. Ideal time to collect sputum is early morning because bronchial secretions tend to accumulate during night. Bacteria also accumulate as secretions pool.
2. Assess level of understanding of procedure and its purpose.	Provides baseline for nurse to establish teaching plan.
3. Assess client's ability to cough and expectorate specimens.	Adequate cough is essential in production of mucus from tracheobronchial tree. Client may have nonproductive cough associated with abdominal or chest pain. Simple clearing of throat is unacceptable.
4. Determine type of assistance needed by client to obtain specimen.	Positioning, postural drainage, deep breathing and coughing exercises may improve ability to cough productively. Suctioning may be indicated if client is unable to cough and expectorate.
5. Assess client's respiratory status, including respiratory rate, depth, pattern, skin color.	Active coughing may alter respiratory status. Respiratory status can depend on amount of sputum in tracheobronchial tree.

NURSING DIAGNOSIS

Clustering of defining characteristics from the assessment data may reveal the following nursing diagnoses for clients requiring this skill:

- Ineffective airway clearance
- Ineffective breathing pattern
- Knowledge deficit regarding specimen collection procedures
- Risk for infection

Related factors are individualized based on a client's condition or needs.

PLANNING

STEPS	RATIONALE
1. **Expected outcomes** following completion of procedure:	
➤ Client's respirations are same rate and character as before procedure.	Specimen collection did not alter respiratory status.
➤ Client is relaxed, able to answer questions (if no artificial airway present).	Suctioning tends to cause anxiety.
➤ Sputum is not contaminated by saliva or oropharyngeal flora.	Sputum must originate from tracheobronchial tree for accurate results.
➤ Laboratory tests fail to reveal abnormal cells or microorganisms.	Absence of infection or abnormal cells.
➤ Client will discuss purpose and benefit of sputum collection.	Documents learning.
2. Explain steps of procedure and purpose. Specimen should not contain saliva. Secretions from oropharynx contain numerous bacteria that will contaminate sputum. Client who is to be suctioned should breathe normally to prevent hyperventilation.	Promotes understanding and cooperation.

CRITICAL DECISION POINT When client is expectorating sputum, stress importance of deep coughing and need to avoid clearing of throat. If client is to be suctioned, stress importance of relaxing and breathing at normal rate.

STEPS	RATIONALE
3. For expectorated specimen, have client rinse mouth or brush teeth with water.	Reduces number of oral contaminants that can alter test results.

STEPS	RATIONALE
CRITICAL DECISION POINT Mouthwash or toothpaste may decrease viability of microorganisms.	
IMPLEMENTATION	
1. Wash hands.	Reduces transmission of microorganisms.
2. Close curtains or room door.	Provides privacy.
3. Position client: semi-Fowler's position, sitting on side of bed or chair, standing for coughing and expectorating specimen; high or semi-Fowler's position for suctioning.	Promotes full lung expansion and facilitates ability to cough.
CRITICAL DECISION POINT If client has incision or localized area of discomfort, have client place hands firmly over affected area or place pillow over area. Splinting of painful area minimizes muscular stretching and discomfort during coughing and thus makes cough productive.	
4. Collect specimen:	
a. **Coughing and Expectoration:**	
(1) Apply disposable gloves.	Reduces risk of exposure to pathogens.
(2) Provide client with specimen container and instruct client not to touch inside.	Prevents risk of contamination.
(3) Instruct client to take three to four slow deep breaths.	Helps to open airways, loosen secretions, and stimulate cough reflex.
(4) Instruct client to emphasize slow, full exhalation.	Moves secretions into large airways.
(5) After series of deep breaths, ask client to cough after full inhalation.	Full inhalation provides force to move secretions out of airways up to pharynx.
(6) Instruct client to **expectorate** sputum directly into specimen container.	Retains microorganisms in sterile container.
(7) Have client repeat coughing until adequate amount of sputum has been collected.	Usually 2 to 10 ml (½-2 teaspoons) is required to ensure accurate analysis of specimen.
b. **Suctioning:**	
(1) Prepare suction machine or device and determine if it functions properly.	Adequate amount of suction is necessary to **aspirate** sputum.
(2) Connect suction tube to adapter on sputum trap.	Establishes suction that passes through sputum trap to aspirate specimen.
(3) Apply sterile gloves (required only for dominant hand).	Tracheobronchial tree is sterile body cavity. Allows nurse to manipulate suction catheter without contamination.
(4) With gloved hand, connect sterile suction catheter to rubber tubing on sputum trap.	Aspirated sputum will go directly to trap instead of to suction tubing.
(5) Other hand should have glove on for application of suction. Thumb should be on trap to provide suction and trap should be covered.	
(6) Gently insert tip of suction catheter through nasopharynx, endotracheal tube, and tracheostomy without applying suction (see Chapter 14).	Minimizes trauma to airway as catheter is inserted.
(7) Advance catheter into trachea.	Entrance of catheter into larynx and trachea triggers cough reflex.

STEPS	RATIONALE
(8) As client coughs, apply suction for 5 to 10 seconds, collecting 2 to 10 ml sputum.	Ensures collection of sputum from deep within tracheobronchial tree. Suctioning longer than 15 seconds can cause hypoxia.
(9) Remove catheter without applying suction, then turn off suction.	Suction can damage mucosa if applied during withdrawal.
(10) Detach catheter from specimen trap, and dispose of catheter into appropriate receptacle.	Decreases risk of spreading microorganisms.

Step 5

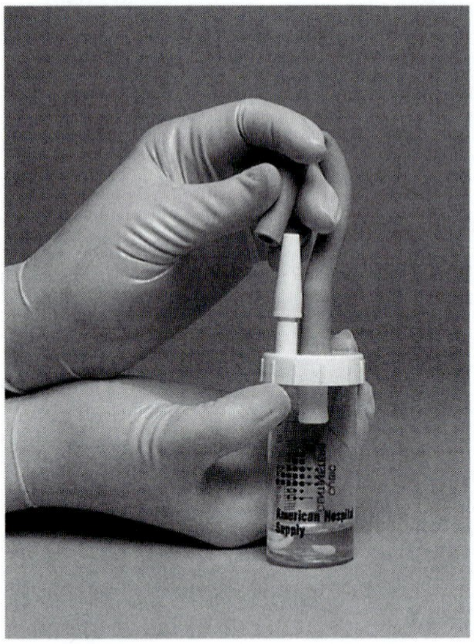

STEPS	RATIONALE
5. Secure top on specimen container tightly. For sputum trap, detach suction tubing and connect rubber tubing on sputum trap to plastic adapter (see illustration).	Contains microorganisms within container, preventing exposure to personnel handling specimen.
6. If any sputum is present on outside of container, wash it off with disinfectant.	Prevents spread of infection to persons handling specimen.
7. Offer client tissues after expectorating. Dispose of tissues in emesis basin or trash container.	Maintains cleanliness and comfort.
8. Remove and dispose of glove(s).	
9. Offer client mouth care, if desired.	Promotes comfort.
10. Wash hands.	Reduces spread of microorganisms.
11. Label specimen with identification label.	Incorrect identification could lead to diagnostic or therapeutic error.
12. Place specimen in small plastic bag (or container specified by agency) and attach requisition.	Plastic bag or container reduces risk of health care worker's exposure to sputum.
13. Send specimen immediately to laboratory or refrigerate.	Bacteria multiply quickly. Specimen should be analyzed promptly for accurate results.

EVALUATION

1. Observe client's respiratory status throughout procedure, especially during suctioning.	Excessive coughing or prolonged suctioning can alter respiratory pattern and cause hypoxia.
2. Note anxiety or discomfort in client.	Procedure can be uncomfortable. If client becomes short of breath, anxiety will develop.
3. Observe character of sputum: color, consistency, odor.	Characteristics may indicate disease entities.
4. Refer to laboratory reports for test results.	Report abnormal cells or microorganisms in sputum.
5. Evaluate client's ability to describe/demonstrate sputum collection process.	

STEPS	RATIONALE
6. **Unexpected outcomes** that may occur include:	
➤ Client becomes hypoxic; increased respiratory rate and effort are necessary; client feels short of breath.	Most common after suctioning. Clients known to have respiratory alterations may be short of breath or dyspneic and may be anxious.
➤ Client remains anxious or complains of discomfort from suction catheter.	Anxiety or discomfort may remain for several minutes until client is able to breathe normally.
➤ Specimen contains **saliva.**	Saliva is watery and clear. Requires specimen collection be repeated.
➤ Inadequate amount of sputum is collected.	Client may be unable to expectorate, or sputum may be very thick or reduced in amount.
➤ Specimen contains blood, pathogenic organisms, or abnormal cells.	Diagnostic of infection or disorders such as malignancy.
➤ Client complains of pain when coughing to produce sputum.	Coughing can cause discomfort from incision or illness may prevent effective coughing.
RECORDING AND REPORTING	
1. Record method used to obtain specimen, date and time collected, type of test ordered, and laboratory receiving specimen in nurses' notes.	Documents that specimens were obtained.
2. Describe characteristics of sputum specimen.	Data can help in diagnosis of alterations and serve as baseline to detect changes.
3. Describe client's tolerance of procedure.	Provides data to measure respiratory status.
4. Report unusual sputum characteristics and client response to nurse in charge or physician.	Findings may require specific intervention.
5. When laboratory reports are available, report abnormal findings.	May require new or revised therapies.

FOLLOW-UP ACTIVITIES

1. If sputum is positive for AFB, initiate appropriate isolation (see Chapter 33).

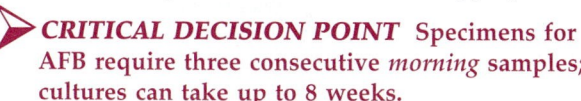

CRITICAL DECISION POINT **Specimens for AFB require three consecutive *morning* samples; cultures can take up to 8 weeks.**

2. If specimen could not be obtained under normal procedures, obtain order to induce specimen (e.g., with use of humidification, aerosol therapy, postural drainage, suction).

• • • • •

Special Considerations

- Postoperative client benefits from splinting surgical wound to cough deeply (see Chapter 35).
- Client who is able to cough effectively may prefer to take specimen container to bathroom.
- Refer to institution's policy and procedure for type of specimen container. Some tests require glass (instead of plastic) containers. Some specimens require additives. Sputum collections taken over 24 hours require special containers.
- Agencies have special bags in which to transport specimens.
- Many agencies require nurse to note on specimen requisition if client is receiving antibiotics.
- If client is undergoing oxygen therapy through tracheostomy or endotracheal tube, nurse can insert catheter without removing oxygen tubing.
- If client appears hypoxic or in distress during suctioning, discontinue procedure and provide oxygen therapy as needed.

Teaching Considerations

- Nurse may demonstrate effective coughing techniques versus clearing of throat.
- Nurse can demonstrate proper splinting technique for postoperative clients.
- Explain purpose of avoiding use of mouthwashes and toothpaste before sputum expectoration (to prevent decreasing viability of microorganisms).
- Explain purpose of obtaining specimen before breakfast (specimen will be most concentrated and free of food particles).

- If aerosol treatment is indicated, teach client purpose of procedure, explaining that it will stimulate coughing and sputum expectoration.
- Nurse can teach client to avoid contaminating outside of specimen cup to reduce risk of spread of infection.

Pediatric Considerations

- Children need very clear instructions or demonstration for deep breathing. Infants and young children will be unable to cooperate; aerosol treatment or suctioning may be indicated.
- Another nurse can assist nurse in restraining young child's head and arms during suctioning, parent may assist to give support.
- Young children often swallow secretions instead of expectorating. Use smaller catheter size for young children.

Home Care Considerations

- If client is to produce sputum specimen at home, instruct client and/or family member regarding proper technique and importance of having specimen sent to laboratory in timely manner.

SKILL 43-10 Obtaining Gastric Specimens

Analysis of gastric contents can aid physicians in diagnosing and treating a number of conditions such as gastric acid irregularities, **hematemesis,** and gastrointestinal bleeding from ulcers or tumors. Gastric pH level determines the acidity of gastrointestinal secretions. Measuring gastric occult blood, which reveals bleeding in the esophagus, stomach, or duodenum, is similar to measuring stool for occult blood.

The testing of gastric specimens for occult blood and pH is relatively easy. The nurse can perform the tests on emesis or on drainage collected from an existing nasogastric tube. Inserting a nasogastric tube solely to collect gastric secretions is very unusual.

EQUIPMENT

- Clean disposable gloves
- Facial tissues
- Emesis basin
- Wooden applicator or 1 ml syringe
- Commercial kit with test paper for pH level and occult blood appropriate for gastric secretions
- Developing solution
- 60 ml bulb or catheter tip syringe
- Nasogastric tube and supplies for insertion (if indicated)

DELEGATION CONSIDERATIONS

Obtaining gastric secretion specimens requires problem solving and knowledge application unique to a professional nurse. Delegation of this skill is inappropriate.

STEPS	RATIONALE
ASSESSMENT	
1. Review physician's order to determine test and source of specimen.	Provides order when regularly testing specimen.
2. Determine presence of nasogastric tube.	Test requires aspiration of gastric secretions from nasogastric tube.
3. Assess level of understanding of procedure and purpose.	Provides baseline for nurse to establish teaching plan.
4. Review medications that client is receiving and foods eaten by client recently.	Some medications and foods can cause false-positive readings for occult blood.
5. Check with laboratory and physician to determine if dietary restrictions or temporary discontinuation of medications is necessary before test.	Gastric analysis for occult blood requires fasting because results depend on peroxidase activity of hemoglobin in red blood cells. Some foods contain peroxidases and cause false results.
6. Assess client for symptoms of abdominal cramping, pain, nausea, vomiting.	Symptoms are characteristic of gastrointestinal alteration.

STEPS	RATIONALE
CRITICAL DECISION POINT Foods that cause false-positive results for occult blood include turnips, horseradish, and red meats. Medications that can cause false-positive results include vitamin C in large doses, aspirin, cimetidine (Tagamet), and iron pills.	

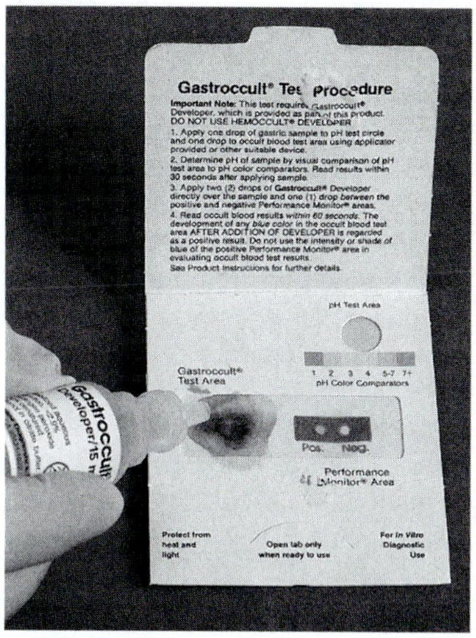

Step 10

NURSING DIAGNOSIS

Clustering of defining characteristics from the assessment data may reveal the following nursing diagnoses for clients requiring this skill:

- Anxiety
- Knowledge deficit regarding gastric specimen collection procedure

Related factors are individualized based on a client's condition or needs.

PLANNING

STEPS	RATIONALE
1. **Expected outcomes** following completion of procedure:	
➤ Gastric secretions are greenish to clear, with no evidence of bleeding or clots.	Greenish color results from bile secreted in duodenum.
➤ **pH** level is 1.5 to 3.0	Gastric secretions are highly acidic. Lower gastrointestinal tract secretions are more basic.
➤ Test is negative for occult blood.	Indicates absence of bleeding in gastrointestinal tract. Positive result indicates bleeding in gastrointestinal tract.
➤ Client will discuss purpose and benefits of gastric analysis.	Documents learning.
2. Institute dietary or medication restrictions as needed.	Ensures accurate test results.
3. Explain steps of procedure to client. Emphasize that test is painless.	Reduces anxiety and promotes cooperation.

IMPLEMENTATION

STEPS	RATIONALE
1. Wash hands before procedure.	Reduces transfer of microorganisms.
2. Apply disposable gloves.	Prevents risk of exposure to pathogens in bodily secretions.
3. Position client in high Fowler's position in bed or chair.	Minimizes aspiration of gastric contents. Position relieves pressure on abdominal organs. If client is nauseated, flat position in bed or one in which client cannot sit straight may cause abdominal discomfort.
4. Close bedside curtains or door to room.	Maintains privacy.
5. Verify nasogastric tube placement (see Chapter 35).	Allows aspiration of gastric contents.
6. Obtain specimen of gastric contents by attaching bulb syringe to nasogastric tube and aspirating 5 to 10 ml; obtain sample of emesis with 1 ml syringe or wooden applicator.	Only small amount of specimen is needed for pH and occult blood testing.
7. Using applicator or syringe, apply 1 drop of gastric sample to pH test paper. Be sure that drop covers paper completely.	Paper should be completely exposed to secretions to ensure full color change.
8. Read color of pH test paper within 30 seconds and compare with pH color guide.	Results range from 1 to 7. Acidic solutions are 4 or less. Basic solutions are 5 or more.
9. Apply 1 drop of gastric sample to Gastroccult blood test paper.	Sample must cover guaiac paper for test reaction to occur.
10. Apply 2 drops of commercial developer solution over sample and 1 drop between positive and negative performance monitors (see illustration).	Developer initiates chemical reaction of solution with guaiac paper.

STEPS	RATIONALE
11. After 60 seconds, compare color of gastric sample to that of performance monitors.	Positive performance monitor turns blue in 30 seconds and negative monitor remains white or beige. If sample turns blue, test is positive for occult blood. If sample turns green, test is negative.
12. Explain results to client.	Immediate results are obtained. Allows client to participate in care.
13. Dispose of test slide paper, wooden applicator, and 1 ml syringe in proper receptacle.	Reduces spread of infection and keeps environment clean.
14. Reconnect nasogastric tube to drainage system or clamp as ordered.	Nasogastric tube serves to decompress abdomen by promoting drainage. Clamping may be ordered to determine tolerance to stomach filling.
15. Remove and dispose of disposable gloves.	
16. Assist client to comfortable position and offer oral hygiene.	After vomiting or removal of tube, oral hygiene promotes comfort and helps to reduce nausea.
17. Wash hands.	Reduces transmission of microorganisms.

EVALUATION

1. Observe quantity, character, and color of emesis or gastric secretions.	Characteristics can reveal abnormal status.
2. Measure emesis for pH and blood.	
3. Compare test findings with normal expected results.	Determines if gastric contents are abnormally acidic or basic.
4. Ask client about purpose of test.	
5. **Unexpected outcomes** that may occur include:	
➤ Gastric secretions may contain clots or blood. Emesis may have "coffee grounds" appearance.	Indicate gastrointestinal bleeding. Bright-red blood indicates active bleeding. "Coffee grounds" emesis indicates slow, less active bleeding.
➤ pH level is above or below desired range.	Each physician may set guidelines on level at which pH should be maintained.
➤ Test is positive for occult blood.	Indicates gastrointestinal bleeding.

RECORDING AND REPORTING

1. Record test performed, source of specimen, results, and disposition of specimen in nurses' notes.	Documents specimen obtained and tested.
2. Describe characteristics of gastric contents.	Provides baseline to determine change in client's condition.
3. Report abnormal results to nurse in charge or physician.	May indicate need for additional therapy.

FOLLOW-UP ACTIVITIES

1. If results are positive for blood, continue to monitor client for gastrointestinal bleeding. Perform guaiac test on all stools.

• • • • •

Special Considerations

- Nurses caring for clients at risk for gastrointestinal bleeding, such as critically ill clients prone to stress ulcers, may screen specimen periodically for occult blood or pH level.
- Dietary restrictions may be necessary 2 or 3 days before testing.
- Gastric secretions vary in color if collected from emesis.
- Test may be repeated to confirm results, especially if client did not fast or if indications causing false results were not withheld.

Teaching Considerations

- Instruct client on foods and medications that may give false test results for occult blood.
- If antacids are ordered, instruct client on proper use.

SKILL 43-11 Obtaining Wound Drainage Specimens

When caring for a client with a wound, the nurse assesses the wound's condition and observes for the development of infection. Localized inflammation, tenderness, and warmth at the wound site, in addition to purulent drainage, usually signify wound infection. Infection cannot be confirmed accurately unless the causative organism is identified. A specimen of wound drainage is analyzed to determine the type and number of pathogenic microorganisms.

The nurse should never collect a wound culture sample from old drainage. Resident colonies of bacteria on the skin grow in wound exudate and may not be the true causative organisms of infection. Separate techniques are used to collect specimens for measuring aerobic versus anaerobic microorganisms. Aerobic organisms grow in superficial wounds exposed to the air. Anaerobic organisms grow deep within body cavities, where oxygen is not normally present.

EQUIPMENT

- Culture tube with swab and transport medium for aerobic culture
- Anaerobic culture tube with swab (tubes contain carbon dioxide or nitrogen gas)
- 5 to 10 ml syringe and 21-gauge needle
- Disposable gloves
- Sterile gloves
- Protective eyewear
- Antiseptic swab
- Sterile dressing materials (determined by type of dressing)
- Paper or plastic disposable bag
- Completed specimen identification label (according to institutional policy)
- Completed laboratory requisition (date, time, name of test)
- Small plastic bag for delivery of specimen to laboratory (or container specified by agency)

DELEGATION CONSIDERATIONS

Obtaining wound drainage specimens requires problem-solving and knowledge application unique to a professional nurse. Delegation of this skill is inappropriate.

STEPS	RATIONALE
ASSESSMENT	
1. Assess client's understanding of need for wound culture and ability to cooperate with procedure.	Nurse uses data to develop teaching plan. Wound is painful site. Collection of specimen may arouse anxiety or fear.
2. Assess client for signs of fever, chills, or thirst. Note in laboratory results if white blood cell count is elevated.	Signs and symptoms indicate systemic infection.
3. Ask client about extent and type of pain at wound site.	Pain at wound site often increases with infection.
4. Review physician's orders for **aerobic** or **anaerobic** culture.	Specimens are taken from different sites and placed in different containers, depending on type of culture.
5. Wear disposable gloves to remove any soiled dressings covering wound. Apply sterile gloves and assess condition of wound carefully. Observe for swelling, opening of wound edges, inflammation, and drainage. Palpate gently along wound edges and note tenderness or drainage.	Surface of open wound is considered sterile. Sterile gloves allow nurse to palpate area without wound contamination. Signs indicate wound infection. Gloves minimize exposure to microorganisms.

NURSING DIAGNOSIS

Clustering of defining characteristics from the assessment data may reveal the following nursing diagnoses for clients requiring this skill:

- Anxiety
- Knowledge deficit regarding wound drainage culture procedure
- Pain
- Risk for infection
- Risk for injury

Related factors are individualized based on a client's condition or needs.

STEPS	RATIONALE
PLANNING	
1. **Expected outcomes** following completion of procedure:	
➤ Wound culture does not reveal bacterial growth.	Wound remains free of pathogenic microorganisms.
➤ Culture swab is not contaminated by bacteria from skin.	Test results indicate type of cells present. Specific cells usually originate from skin.
➤ Client will discuss purpose and procedure for specimen collection.	Documents learning.
2. Determine if client may receive analgesic before dressing change or specimen collection. Administer as ordered.	Minimizes discomfort during procedure.
3. Explain reason for wound culture and how it will be collected.	Promotes understanding and cooperation and eases anxiety.
4. Explain that client may feel tickling sensation when wound is swabbed.	Anticipation of expected sensations minimizes anxiety.
IMPLEMENTATION	
1. Wash hands.	Reduces transfer of microorganisms.
2. Close bedside curtains or door to room.	Avoids embarrassment.
3. Apply disposable gloves and remove old dressing. Observe drainage. Fold soiled sides of dressing together and then dispose of dressing in bag.	Protects hands from contact with drainage.
4. Cleanse area around wound edges with antiseptic swab. Remove old exudate.	Removes skin flora, preventing possible contamination of specimen.
5. Discard swab and dispose of soiled gloves in bag.	Reduces spread of infection.
6. Open packages containing sterile culture tube and dressing supplies.	Provides sterile field from which nurse can pick up and handle sterile supplies.
7. Apply sterile gloves.	Allows nurse to maintain sterility of items while collecting specimen.
8. Collect cultures:	
a. **Aerobic Culture:**	
(1) Take swab from culture tube, insert tip into wound in area of drainage, and rotate swab gently. Remove swab and return to culture tube. Crush ampule of medium and push swab into fluid.	Swab should be coated with fresh secretions from within wound. Medium keeps bacteria alive until analysis is complete.
b. **Anaerobic Culture:**	
(1) Take swab from special anaerobic culture tube, swab deeply into draining body cavity, and rotate gently. Remove swab and return to culture tube. OR: Insert tip of syringe (without needle) into wound and aspirate 5 to 10 ml of exudate. Attach 21 gauge needle, expel all air, and inject drainage into special culture tube.	Specimen is taken from deep cavity where oxygen is not present. Carbon dioxide or nitrogen gas keeps organisms alive until analysis is complete. Air injected into tube would cause organisms to die.
➤ ***CRITICAL DECISION POINT*** **Never collect exudate from skin unless it is separate culture and labeled as such.**	
9. Place each culture tube on correct specimen label.	Maintains sterility of gloves worn. Prevents confusion over aerobic and anaerobic cultures.
10. Ask another nurse to attach labels and proper requisitions to each tube and to send specimens to laboratory immediately.	Bacteria grow rapidly. Cultures should be prepared quickly for accurate results.

STEPS	RATIONALE
11. Clean wound as ordered and apply new sterile dressing.	Protects wound from further contamination and aids in absorbing drainage and debriding wound.
12. Remove gloves by pulling inside out and dispose of gloves in trash. Dispose of soiled supplies according to agency policy.	Reduces spread of infection.
13. Secure dressings with tape or ties.	Keeps dressing securely in place over wound.
14. Assist client to comfortable position.	Promotes client's ability to relax.
15. Wash hands after procedure.	Reduces transmission of microorganisms.

EVALUATION

1. Obtain laboratory report for results of cultures.	Report indicates if pathogenic organisms are identified.
2. Observe character of wound drainage.	Characteristics can reveal abnormal status.
3. Observe edges of wound for redness and bleeding.	Indicates trauma to healing tissue.
4. Ask client about purpose of wound culture.	
5. **Unexpected outcomes** that may occur include:	
➤ Wound cultures reveal heavy bacterial growth.	Wound is contaminated by pathogenic microorganisms.
➤ Wound culture is contaminated from superficial skin cells.	Inaccurate results require repeat specimen.

RECORDING AND REPORTING

1. Record types of specimens obtained, source, and time and date sent to laboratory in nurses' notes.	Documents that cultures were obtained.
2. Describe appearance of wound and characteristics of drainage in nurses' notes.	Data support evidence of infection and provide baseline to determine change in condition of wound.
3. Report any evidence of infection to nurse in charge and physician.	Findings may indicate need for further therapy (e.g., antibiotics or wound irrigation).

• • • • •

Special Considerations

- Wound cultures are often obtained during dressing change (see Chapter 37); thus this step may be performed as part of procedure.
- If client requires analgesic before dressing changes, ideally medication is given 30 minutes before to reach peak effect.
- While dressing is being changed, client may prefer not to see soiled portion of dressing.
- Some agencies require culture tubes to be transported in bags.
- To note on specimen requisition if client is receiving antibiotics.

Teaching Considerations

- Notify client before possible discomfort during procedure.
- Instruct client to inform nurse if procedure causes pain.
- Teach client to assess status of wound for changes.
- Discuss signs and symptoms of infection.

Pediatric Considerations

- If procedure is to be performed on a child and is anticipated to be painful, some agencies prefer performing procedure in area other than child's room, thus maintaining feeling that child's room is safe place.
- Ask parents if they wish to help hold child or if they prefer nurse to do so.

Home Care Considerations

- When applicable, discuss ways to prevent infection.
- Teach client aseptic technique for self-dressing change.

SKILL 43-12 Collecting Blood Specimens by Venipuncture

Blood tests are one of the most commonly used diagnostic aids in the care and evaluation of clients. In any health care setting blood tests can yield valuable information about nutritional, hematological, metabolic, immune, and biochemical status. Tests allow physicians to screen clients carefully for early signs of physical alterations, plot the course of existing disease, and monitor responses to therapies.

The nurse is often responsible for collecting blood specimens; however, many institutions have specially trained technicians whose sole responsibility is to draw blood. Nurses must be familiar with their institution's policies and procedures as well as their state's nurse practice act regarding guidelines for drawing blood samples.

The three primary methods of obtaining blood specimens are venipuncture, skin puncture, and arterial stick. **Venipuncture,** the most common method, involves inserting a hollow-bore needle into the lumen of a large vein to obtain a specimen. The nurse may use a needle and syringe or a special **Vacutainer tube** that allows the drawing of multiple blood samples. Because veins are major sources of blood for laboratory testing and routes for IV fluid or blood replacement, maintaining their integrity is essential. The nurse should be skilled in venipuncture to avoid unnecessary injury to veins.

Skin puncture is the least traumatic method of obtaining a blood specimen. A sterile lancet or needle is used to puncture a vascular area on a finger, toe, or heel. A drop of blood is placed on a test slide or collected within a thin glass capillary tube for laboratory analysis.

Regardless of the method used to obtain a blood specimen, the nurse must anticipate the client's anxiety. The procedures can be painful, and often just the appearance of a needle is frightening, especially to children. The nurse's calm approach and skilled technique helps to limit anxiety.

EQUIPMENT

- Alcohol or antiseptic swab
- Disposable gloves
- Small pillow or folded towel
- Sterile gauze pads (2 × 2 inch)
- Rubber tourniquet
- Band-Aid or adhesive tape
- Appropriate blood tubes
- Completed identification labels according to agency policy
- Completed laboratory requisition (date, time, type of test)
- Plastic bag for delivery of specimen to laboratory (or container as specified by agency)

Syringe Method

- Sterile needles (20- to 21-gauge for adults, 23- to 25-gauge for children, 23- to 25-gauge butterfly for older adults)
- Sterile syringe of appropriate size

Vacutainer Method

- Vacutainer tube with needle holder
- Sterile double-ended needles (20- to 21-gauge for adults, 23- to 25-gauge for children)

DELEGATION CONSIDERATIONS

The phlebotomy trained staff are the personnel used to obtain venipuncture samples. They may be unlicensed or licensed staff. Usually they are intravenous certified by the agency that employs them.

STEPS	RATIONALE
ASSESSMENT	
1. Determine understanding of purpose of procedure and method to be used.	Provides data for nurse to establish teaching plan and provide emotional support. Many clients may have past experiences that increase anxiety.
2. Determine if special conditions need to be met before specimen collection (i.e., client to be NPO [nothing by mouth], specific time for collection after medication or meal).	Some tests require meeting specific conditions to obtain accurate measurement of blood elements (e.g., fasting blood sugar, drug peak and trough level, and timed endocrine hormone levels).

CRITICAL DECISION POINT Some specimens require special collection requirements before or following specimen collection:

- Cryoglobulins: need prewarmed test tubes
- Ammonia levels require tube to be placed in ice for delivery to laboratory
- Lactic acid levels: do not use tourniquet
- Vitamin levels: avoid exposure of test tube to light

STEPS	RATIONALE
3. Assess client for possible risks for venipuncture: anticoagulant therapy, low platelet count, bleeding disorders (history of hemophilia or **ecchymosis**). Review medication history.	History may include abnormal clotting abilities caused by low platelet count, hemophilia, medications that increase risk for bleeding and hematoma formation.
4. Determine client's ability to cooperate with procedure.	Some clients may need assistance of another nurse. Procedure can appear threatening to client.
5. Assess client for contraindicated sites for venipuncture: presence of IV fluids, hematoma at potential site, arm on side of mastectomy, hemodialysis recipient.	Drawing specimens from such sites can result in false test results or may injure client.
6. Review physician's orders for type of tests.	Multiple samples may be needed; physician's order is required.

NURSING DIAGNOSIS

Clustering of defining characteristics from the assessment data may reveal the following nursing diagnoses for clients requiring this skill:

- Anxiety
- Knowledge deficit regarding blood specimen collection process
- Risk for infection
- Risk for injury

Related factors are individualized based on a client's condition or needs.

PLANNING

1. **Expected outcomes** following completion of procedure:	
➤ Venipuncture site shows no evidence of continued bleeding or hematoma.	Indicates hemostasis achieved.
➤ Client denies anxiety or discomfort.	Removal of painful stimulus lessens anxiety. Some clients are not anxious about procedure.
➤ Laboratory tests show normal findings.	No abnormalities are found in blood elements.
➤ Client will discuss purpose, procedure, and benefits of venipuncture.	Documents learning.
2. Explain procedure to client: describe purpose of tests; explain how sensation of **tourniquet,** alcohol swab, and needle stick will feel.	Anticipatory guidance helps to reduce anxiety.

IMPLEMENTATION

1. Wash hands.	Reduces transfer of microorganisms.
2. Bring equipment to bedside.	Ensures organized procedure.
3. Close bedside curtain or room door.	Provides for privacy.
4. Raise or lower bed to comfortable working height.	Reduces strain on nurse's back muscles and improves access to body part.
5. Assist client to supine or semi-Fowler's position with arms extended to form straight line from shoulders to wrists. Place small pillow or towel under upper arm.	Helps to stabilize extremity because arms are most common sites of venipuncture. Supported position in bed reduces chance of injury to client if fainting occurs.
6. Apply disposable gloves.	Reduces risk of exposure to blood-borne bacteria.
7. Apply tourniquet 5 to 10 cm (3-4 inches) above venipuncture site selected (antecubital fossa site is most often used). Encircle extremity and pull one end of tourniquet tightly over other, looping one end under other. Apply tourniquet so it can be removed by pulling end with single motion.	Tourniquet blocks venous return to heart from extremity, causing veins to dilate for easier visibility.

➤ **CRITICAL DECISION POINT** **Palpate distal pulse (e.g., radial) below tourniquet. If pulse is not palpable, reapply tourniquet more loosely. If tourniquet is too tight, pressure will impede arterial blood flow.**

STEPS	RATIONALE
8. Keep tourniquet on client no longer than 1 to 2 minutes.	Prolonged time may alter test results and cause pain and venous stasis (e.g., falsely elevated serum potassium level). Minimizes effects of hemoconcentration.
9. Ask client to open and close fist several times, finally leaving fist clenched.	Facilitates distention of veins by forcing blood up from distal veins.
CRITICAL DECISION POINT **Avoid vigorous opening and closing of fist, which may cause erroneous laboratory results of hemoconcentration.**	
10. Quickly inspect extremity for best venipuncture site, looking for straight, prominent vein without swelling or hematoma.	Straight and intact veins are easiest to puncture.
11. Palpate selected vein with fingers. Note if vein is firm and rebounds when palpated or if vein feels rigid and cordlike and rolls when palpated (see illustration).	Patent, healthy vein is elastic and rebounds on palpation. Thrombosed vein is rigid, rolls easily, is difficult to puncture.
12. Select venipuncture site. If tourniquet on arm is too long, remove and assess other extremity, or wait 60 seconds before reapplying.	Prevents discomfort to client and inaccurate test results.
13. Obtain blood sample:	
a. Syringe Method:	
(1) Have syringe with appropriate needle securely attached.	Needle should not dislodge from syringe during venipuncture.
(2) Cleanse venipuncture site with alcohol swab (70% isopropyl alcohol is recommended), moving in circular motion from site for approximately 5 cm (2 inches) (see illustration). Allow to dry.	Antimicrobial agent cleans skin surface of resident bacteria so organisms do not enter puncture site. Allowing alcohol to dry reduces "sting" of venipuncture. Alcohol left on skin can cause **hemolysis** of sample.
(3) Remove needle cover and inform client that "stick" lasting only few seconds will be felt.	Client has better control over anxiety when prepared about what to expect.
CRITICAL DECISION POINT **Observe needle for defects; such as burrs, which can cause increased discomfort and damage to the client's vein.**	
(4) Place thumb or forefinger of nondominant hand 2.5 cm (1 inch) below site and pull skin taut.	Stabilizes vein and prevents rolling during needle insertion.

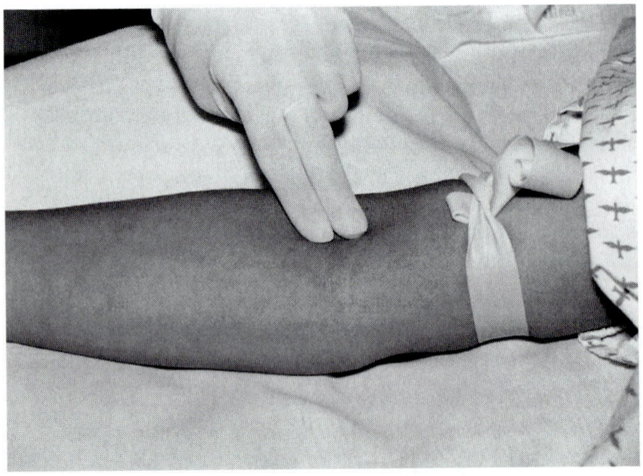

Step 11

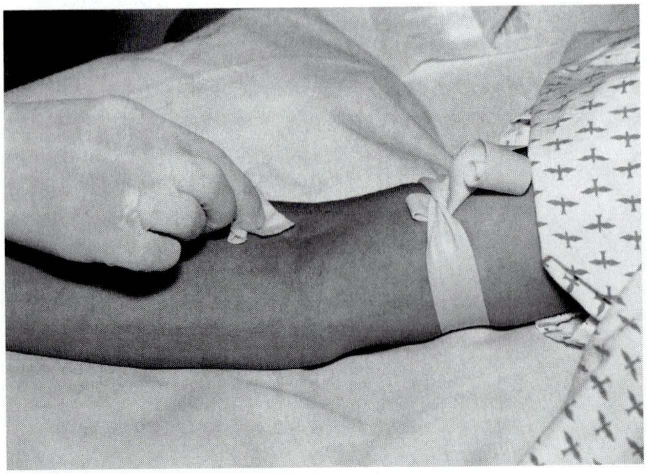

Step 13a(2)

STEPS	RATIONALE
(5) Hold syringe and needle at 15- to 30-degree angle from client's arm with bevel up.	Reduces chance of penetrating both sides of vein during insertion. Keeping bevel up reduces vein trauma.
(6) Slowly insert needle into vein (see illustration).	Prevents puncture on opposite side.
(7) Hold syringe securely and pull back gently on plunger (see illustration).	Syringe held securely prevents needle from advancing. Pulling on plunger creates vacuum needed to draw blood into syringe.
(8) Look for blood return.	If blood flow fails to appear, needle is not in vein.
(9) Obtain desired amount of blood, keeping needle stabilized.	Test results are more accurate when required amount of blood is obtained. Some tests cannot be performed without minimal blood requirement. Movement of needle increases discomfort.
(10) After specimen is obtained, release tourniquet.	Reduces bleeding at site when needle is withdrawn.
(11) Apply 2 × 2–inch gauze pad or alcohol swab over puncture site without applying pressure and quickly, but carefully withdraw needle from vein and apply pressure following removal of needle (see illustration).	Pressure over needle can cause discomfort. Careful removal of needle minimizes discomfort and vein trauma.
(12) Discard needle without recapping in proper receptacle.	Reduces risk of needle stick injury.

Step 13a(6)

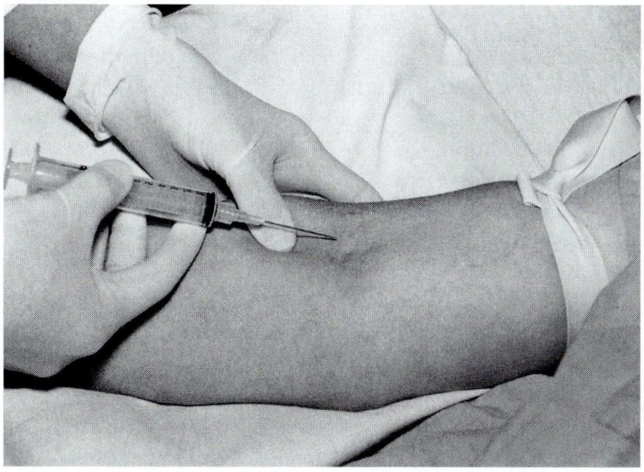

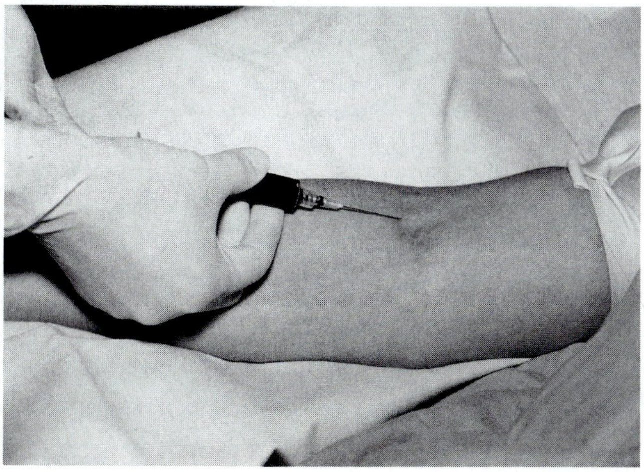

Step 13a(7)

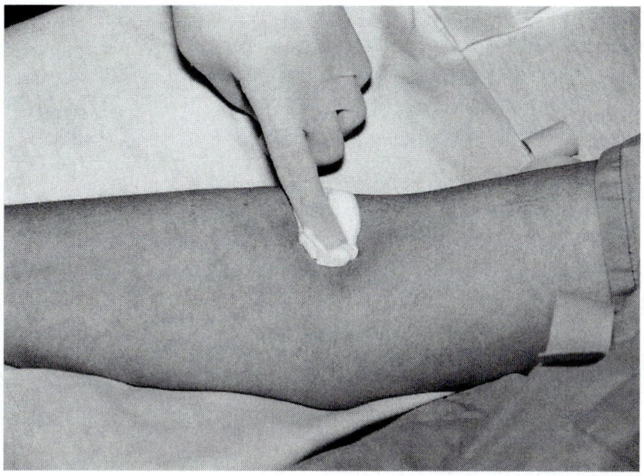

Step 13a(11)

STEPS	RATIONALE
b. Vacutainer Method:	
(1) Attach double-ended needle to Vacutainer tube (see illustration).	Long end of needle is used to puncture vein. Short end fits into blood tubes.
(2) Have proper blood specimen tube resting inside Vacutainer, but do not puncture rubber stopper.	Causes loss of tube's vacuum.
(3) Cleanse venipuncture site with alcohol swab, moving in circular motion out from site for approximately 5 cm (2 inches).	Cleans skin surface of resident bacteria so that organisms do not enter puncture site.
(4) Remove needle cover and inform client that "stick" lasting only few seconds will be felt.	Client has better control over anxiety when prepared about what to expect.
(5) Place thumb or forefinger of nondominant hand 2.5 cm (1 inch) above or below site and pull skin taut. Stretch skin down until vein is stabilized.	Helps to stabilize vein and prevent rolling during needle insertion.
(6) Hold Vacutainer at 15- to 30-degree angle from arm with bevel up.	Reduces chance of penetrating both sides of vein during insertion. Keeping bevel up causes less trauma to vein.
CRITICAL DECISION POINT **Do not push tube past Vacutainer holder before venipuncture because this will cause collection tube to lose its vacuum.**	
(7) Slowly insert needle into vein (see illustration).	Prevents puncture on opposite side.
(8) Grasp Vacutainer securely and advance specimen tube into needle of holder (do not advance needle in vein).	Pushing needle through stopper breaks vacuum and causes flow of blood into tube. If needle in vein advances, vein may become punctured on other side.
(9) Note flow of blood into tube (should be fairly rapid) (see illustration on p. 1255).	Failure of blood to appear indicates that vacuum in tube is lost or needle is not in vein.
(10) After specimen tube is filled, grasp Vacutainer firmly and remove tube. Insert additional specimen tubes as needed.	Prevents needle from advancing or dislodging. Tube should fill completely because additives in certain tubes are measured in proportion to filled tube. Tubes with additives should be inverted as soon as possible.
CRITICAL DECISION POINT **When filling tubes with an anticoagulant additive, let tube fill until the vacuum is exhausted. Ratio of blood to additive is important.**	

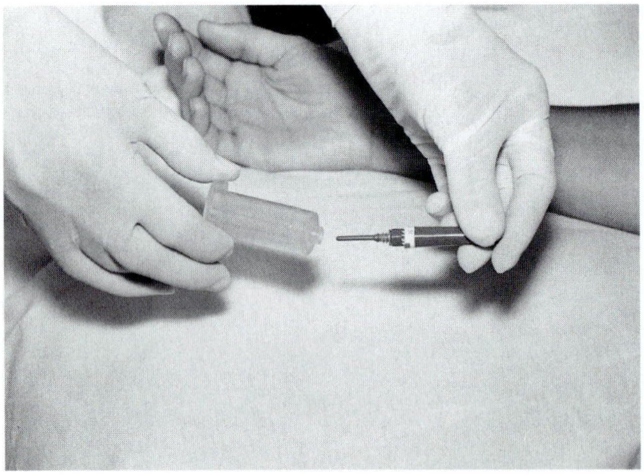

Step 13b(1)

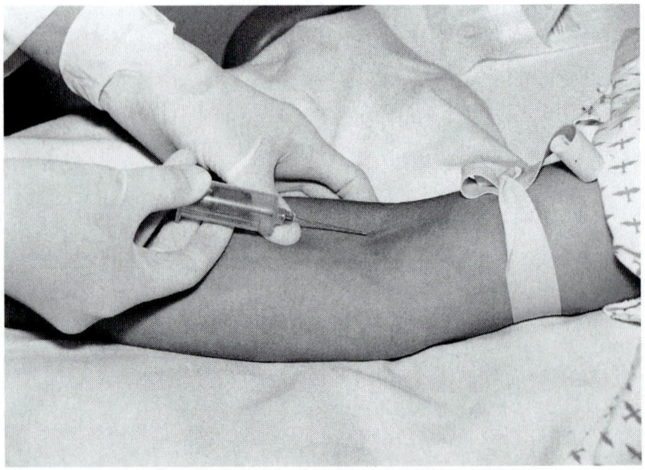

Step 13b(7)

STEPS	RATIONALE
(11) After last tube is filled, release tourniquet.	Reduces bleeding at site when needle is withdrawn.
(12) Apply 2 × 2–inch gauze pad over puncture site without applying pressure and quickly but carefully withdraw needle from vein.	Pressure over needle can cause discomfort. Careful removal of needle minimizes discomfort and vein trauma.
14. Immediately apply pressure over venipuncture site with gauze or antiseptic pad for 2 to 3 minutes or until bleeding stops (see Step 13a(11), p. 1253). Apply pressure over site and tape gauze dressing securely.	Direct pressure minimizes bleeding and prevents hematoma formation. Pressure dressing controls bleeding.
15. For blood obtained by syringe, transfer specimen to tubes.	
a. Using one-handed technique, insert needle through stopper of blood tube and allow vacuum to fill tube. Do not force blood into tube.	Blood should not be forced into tube; this prevents hemolysis of red blood cells. OSHA (1996) recommends one-handed technique to avoid needle-stick injury.
b. Alternative method is to remove needle from syringe and stopper to each test tube. Gently inject required amount of blood into each tube. Reapply stopper.	Blood injected too quickly may cause frothing or hemolysis of red blood cells. Stopper maintains sterility of specimen.
16. Take blood tubes containing additives; gently rotate back and forth 8 to 10 times.	Additives should be mixed with blood to prevent clotting. Shaking can cause hemolysis of red blood cells, producing inaccurate test results.
17. Inspect puncture site for bleeding and apply adhesive tape with gauze.	Keeps puncture site clean and controls any final oozing.
18. Check tubes for any sign of external contamination with blood. Decontaminate with 70% alcohol if necessary.	Prevents cross-contamination. Reduces risk of exposure to pathogens present in blood.
19. Assist client to comfortable position.	
20. Securely attach properly completed identification label to each tube and affix proper requisition.	Incorrect identification of specimen could result in diagnostic or therapeutic errors.
21. Dispose of needles, syringe, and soiled equipment in proper container. Do not cap needles.	Prevents cross-contamination through needle sticks and contact with blood.
22. Place specimens in bag to be sent to laboratory.	
23. Remove disposable gloves after specimen is obtained and any spillage is cleaned.	Reduces risk of exposure to HIV, hepatitis, and other blood-borne pathogens.
24. Wash hands after procedure.	Reduces transfer of microorganisms.
25. Send specimens immediately to laboratory.	Fresh specimen ensures accurate results.

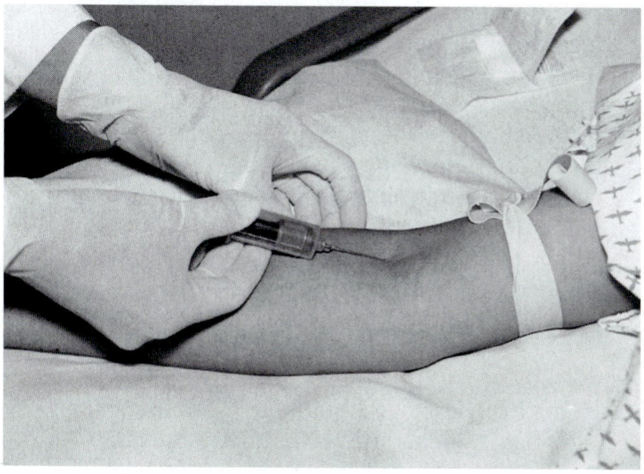

Step 13b(9)

STEPS	RATIONALE
EVALUATION	
1. Reinspect venipuncture site.	Determines if bleeding has stopped or hematoma has formed.
2. Determine if client remains anxious or fearful.	Client may require more blood tests in future. Anxiety or concerns should be expressed.
3. Check laboratory report for test results.	Reveals constituents of blood specimen.
4. Ask client to explain purposes of tests.	
5. **Unexpected outcomes** that may occur include:	
➤ Hematoma forms at venipuncture site.	Blood has escaped from vein and entered surrounding tissues.
➤ Bleeding at site continues.	Clotting mechanisms may be altered.
➤ Client continues to be anxious or fearful.	Level of discomfort experienced can heighten anxiety.
➤ Laboratory tests reveal abnormal blood constituents.	Tests reveal alterations in physiological mechanisms.
RECORDING AND REPORTING	
1. Record date and time of venipuncture, test samples obtained, and disposition of specimen to laboratory in nurses' notes.	Documents samples obtained.
2. Describe venipuncture site after specimen collection and response in nurses' notes.	Documents response to diagnostic therapy. Description of site provides baseline to monitor change.
3. Report any "stat" test results to physician.	Certain tests are ordered stat (immediately) to determine condition immediately so that proper therapies can be selected.
4. Report abnormal test results to physician.	

FOLLOW-UP ACTIVITIES

1. If hematoma develops, obtain order from physician to apply cold compress. After bleeding subsides, order for hot compress can be obtained.
2. Inform clients who are to receive further venipunctures about reasons for tests.

• • • • •

Special Considerations

- ➤ Check with institutional policy regarding designated container for disposal of contaminated needles and syringes.
- ➤ If gloves become contaminated with blood, replace with clean pair after proper disposal of contaminated ones. Touch nothing and do not handle supplies with contaminated gloves.
- ➤ In clinic or physician's office, chair with special arm extension may be used when obtaining blood specimens.
- ➤ If client has large distended veins, tourniquet may not be needed.
- ➤ Clients undergoing frequent venipunctures may have preferred or undesirable site. Most commonly used vein is median cubital in antecubital fossa. In children, use veins on dorsal aspect of foot or scalp veins. Avoid vessels that pulsate; this indicates artery.
- ➤ If vein cannot be palpated or viewed easily, remove tourniquet and apply warm, wet compress over extremity for 10 to 20 minutes. Heat causes local vasodilation.
- ➤ With experience nurse will feel "pop" as needle enters vein. If plunger is pulled back too quickly, pressure may cause vein to collapse.
- ➤ Samples taken from vein near IV infusion may be diluted or may contain concentrations of IV fluids. Postmastectomy client may have reduced lymphatic drainage in arm on operative side, increasing risk of infection from needle sticks. Arteriovenous shunt should never be used to obtain specimens because of risks of clotting and bleeding. Hematoma indicates existing injury to vessel's wall.
- ➤ If drawing sample for blood alcohol level or blood cultures, use only antiseptic swab rather than alcohol swab to ensure accurate test results.
- ➤ Although comparative studies are limited, data suggest that iodine pads may have advantage over alcohol in preparing skin for venipuncture.

Teaching Considerations

- ➤ Instruct client to apply pressure to venipuncture site briefly. Clients with bleeding disorders or those undergoing anticoagulant therapy should apply pressure for at least 5 minutes.

- Instruct client to notify nurse or physician if persistent or recurrent bleeding or expanding hematoma occurs at venipuncture site.

Pediatric Considerations

- At times it is advantageous to draw children's blood specimens in treatment room instead of in bed or room to maintain feeling that room is safe place.
- Ask staff member to restrain child so venipuncture site is immobilized. Prevents sudden movement, which can cause serious injury to vessel wall or soft tissues.
- When performing venipuncture on children, the nurse needs to explore a variety of sources for vein access: scalp, antecubital fossa, saphenous, hand veins.
- Application of Emla Cream may be ordered to reduce pain in infants and young children.

Gerontologic Considerations

- Older adults have fragile veins that are easily traumatized during venipuncture. Sometimes application of warm compresses may help in obtaining samples. Using a small-bore catheter also may be beneficial.

Home Care Considerations

- In the home care setting a blood pressure cuff, rather than a tourniquet, can be used for venipuncture.

SKILL 43-13 Measuring Blood Glucose Level after Skin Puncture

Obtaining capillary blood by skin puncture is an alternative when venipuncture cannot be performed or when reducing the frequency of needle sticks is desirable. The procedure is also less painful than venipuncture, and the ease of the skin puncture method to obtain blood samples makes it possible for clients to perform this procedure. Along with the development of reagent strips and home glucose monitors, the skin puncture method has revolutionized home management care of clients with diabetes. Although not all blood tests can be performed on capillary samples, it is a viable alternative to venipuncture in many situations.

Self-testing of blood glucose can be performed by two methods. Both methods require obtaining a large drop of blood by skin puncture. A hand-held single-use lancet or one of many automatic lancet-holding devices available on the market today may be used. The blood is applied to a specially prepared chemical reagent strip.

The first method involves visually reading the reagent strip by comparing it to the color chart on the container. Examples of such strips include Chemstrip BG, Glucostix, and Trendstrips. If the color on the strip falls between two reference blocks on the chart, the results may need to be estimated. Thus accurate results of blood glucose may not always be obtained.

The second type of blood glucose monitoring is done by the use of reflectance meters. A variety of meters are on the market, including the Glucometer II (Ames), Accucheck III (Boehringer Mannheim), Glucoscan 3000 (LifeScan), and One Touch (LifeScan). After a drop of blood from the skin puncture is dropped onto the reagent strip, the meter provides an accurate measurement of blood glucose in less than 5 minutes.

The meters use a wet-wash or dry-wipe method of testing. To perform a wet wash, the user flushes the blood-coated reagent strip with water before inserting the strip into the glucose meter. The dry-wipe method is somewhat simpler, requiring the user to wipe off the blood-coated reagent strip with a dry cotton ball before making a reading. Some products do not require blood to be wiped before a reading is given. The various methods allow measurement of blood glucose between 20 and 800 mg/100 ml, thus providing a sensitive measure of blood glucose.

The glucose meters are rapidly replacing urine glucose testing in managing clients with diabetes. The skill describes the techniques used to measure blood glucose with a meter using the dry-wipe method. Figure 43-7 depicts

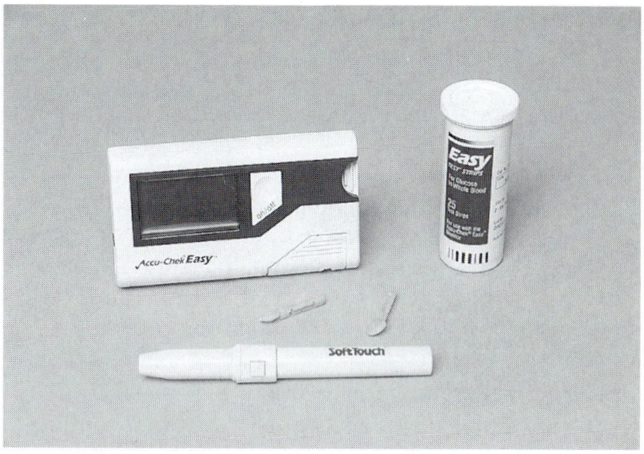

Fig. 43-7 Accu-chek Easy glucose monitoring equipment.

an Accu-Chek Easy glucose monitor. When the nurse measures blood glucose, gloves are worn according to the CDC's standard precautions and OSHA's recommendations (OSHA, 1996).

EQUIPMENT

- Antiseptic swab
- Cotton ball
- Sterile lancet or blood-letting device
- Heel-warming device (optional)
- Paper towel
- Glucose testing meter
- Blood glucose reagent strips (brand determined by meter used)
- Disposable gloves

DELEGATION CONSIDERATIONS

This skill requires problem solving and knowledge application unique to a professional nurse. Delegation of this skill is inappropriate.

STEPS	RATIONALE
ASSESSMENT	
1. Assess understanding of procedure and purpose. Determine if clients with diabetes understand how to perform test and realize importance of **glucose monitoring.**	Data set guidelines for nurse to develop teaching plan.
2. Determine if specific conditions need to be met before sample collection (e.g., with fasting, after meals, or after certain medications).	Dietary intake of carbohydrates and ingestion of concentrated glucose preparations alter blood glucose levels.
3. Determine if risks exist for performing skin puncture (e.g., low platelet count, anticoagulant therapy, bleeding disorders).	Abnormal clotting mechanisms increase risk for local ecchymosis and bleeding.
4. Assess area of skin to be used as puncture site. Inspect fingers, toes, and heel. Avoid areas of bruising and open lesions.	Sides of fingers, toes, and heels are commonly selected because they have fewer nerve endings and are highly vascular. Area should be free of lesions or abnormalities.
5. Review physician's order for time of frequency of measurement.	Physician determines test schedule on basis of client's physiological status and risk for glucose imbalance.
6. For diabetic client who performs test at home, assess ability to handle skin puncturing device.	Client's physical health may change (e.g., vision or from fatigue, pain, disease state), preventing client from performing test.

NURSING DIAGNOSIS

Clustering of defining characteristics from the assessment data may reveal the following nursing diagnoses for clients requiring this skill:

- Altered health maintenance
- Anxiety
- Knowledge deficit regarding blood glucose monitoring
- Impaired sensory perception

Related factors are individualized based on a client's condition or needs.

PLANNING

STEPS	RATIONALE
1. **Expected outcomes** following completion of procedure:	
➤ Puncture site shows no evidence of bleeding or tissue damage.	Hemostasis achieved. Lancet or needle did not puncture skin too deeply.
➤ Blood glucose level is normal.	Normal fasting glucose is 70 to 120 mg/100 ml, indicating good metabolic control.
➤ Client demonstrates procedure.	
➤ Client explains test results.	Shows success of nurse's instructions and demonstration.
2. Explain procedure and purpose to client and/or family.	Promotes understanding and cooperation.

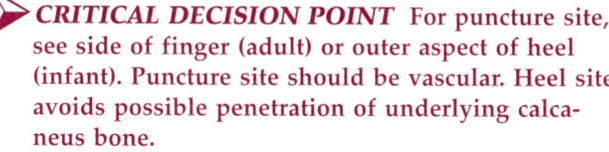

STEPS	RATIONALE
IMPLEMENTATION	
1. Wash hands before procedure.	Reduces transfer of microorganisms.
2. Instruct adult to wash hands with soap and warm water, if able.	Promotes skin cleansing and vasodilation at selected puncture site. Hand washing establishes practice for client when test is performed at home.
3. Position client comfortably in chair or in semi-Fowler's position in bed.	Ensures easy accessibility to puncture site. Client will assume position when self-testing.
4. Remove reagent strip from container and tightly seal caps.	Protects strips from accidental discoloration.
5. Turn on glucose meter.	Activates meter.
6. Insert strip into glucose meter (see manufacturer's directions) and make necessary adjustments.	Some machines must be calibrated; others require zeroing of timer. Each meter is adjusted differently.
7. Remove unused reagent strip from meter and place on paper towel or clean, dry surface with test pad facing up.	Moisture on strip can change its color, altering reading of final test results.
8. Apply disposable gloves.	Reduces risk of contamination by blood.
9. Choose puncture site.	
CRITICAL DECISION POINT For puncture site, see side of finger (adult) or outer aspect of heel (infant). Puncture site should be vascular. Heel site avoids possible penetration of underlying calcaneus bone.	
10. Hold finger to be punctured in dependent position while gently massaging finger toward puncture site.	Increases blood flow to area before puncture.
11. Clean site with antiseptic swab and *allow to dry completely.*	Alcohol can cause blood to hemolyze.
12. Remove cover of lancet or blood-letting device.	Cover keeps tip of lancet/needle sterile.
13. Place blood-letting device firmly against side of finger and push release button, causing needle to pierce skin (see illustration). Hold lancet perpendicular to puncture site, and pierce finger or heel quickly in one continuous motion (do not force lancet).	Blood-letting devices are designed to pierce skin for specific depth, ensuring adequate blood flow. Perpendicular position ensures proper skin penetration.
14. Wipe away first droplet of blood with cotton ball. (See manufacturer's directions for meter used.)	First drop of blood generally contains large portion of serous fluid, which can dilute specimen and cause false results.
15. Lightly squeeze puncture site (without touching) until large droplet of blood has formed.	Ensures proper coverage of test pad on reagent strip.

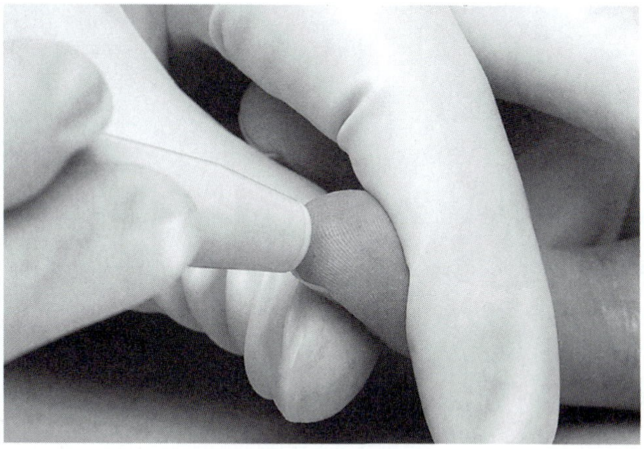

Step 13

STEPS	RATIONALE
16. Hold reagent strip test pad close to drop of blood, and lightly transfer droplet to test pad (see illustration). Do not smear blood.	Droplet must be absorbed by test pad to ensure proper chemical reaction. Smearing causes inaccurate test results.
17. Immediately press timer on glucose meter, and place reagent strip on paper towel or on side of timer. (see manufacturer's directions for meter used.)	Blood must be exposed to test strip for prescribed time to ensure proper results. Strip should lie flat so that blood does not pool on only one part of pad.

➤ CRITICAL DECISION POINT Some meters, (such as One Touch [LifeScan]), require blood sample to be applied to test strip already in meter.

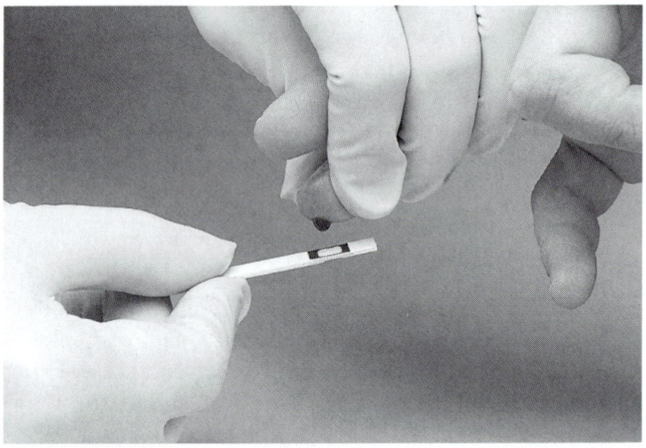

Step 16

STEPS	RATIONALE
18. Apply pressure to skin puncture site.	Promotes hemostasis.
19. When timer displays 60 seconds (for Accu-Check III model), use moderate pressure to wipe blood from test pad with cotton ball. No blood should remain on test pad for some meters. (See manufacturer's directions for meter used.)	For meter to read glucose levels, some strips must be dry. Refer to product directions for timing used with each type of meter.
20. While timer continues to count, place reagent strip into meter (see illustration).	Strip must be inserted correctly to obtain accurate reading.
21. Read meter, noting reading on display (see illustration).	Each meter has specified time for reading glucose level.
22. Turn meter off. Dispose of test strip, cotton balls, uncapped lancet or **autolet,** and platform from lancet device (if indicated) in proper receptacle.	Meter is battery-powered. Propel disposal reduces spread of microorganisms. Lancets and platforms need to be disposed of after each client use (Food and Drug Administration, 1990).

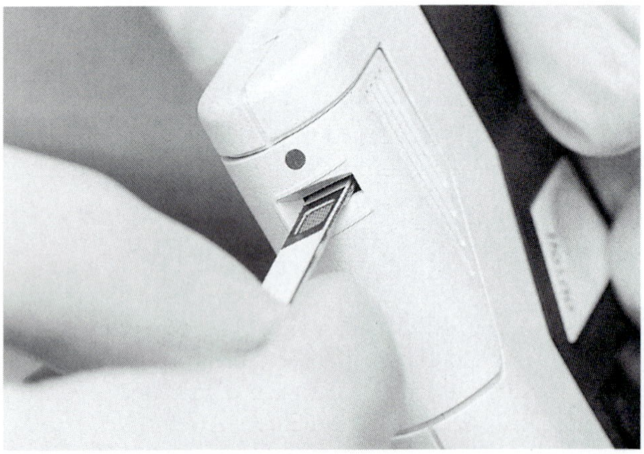

Step 20

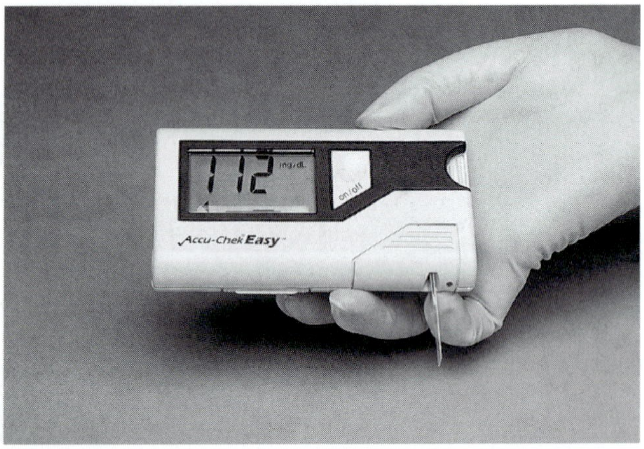

Step 21

STEPS	RATIONALE
23. Remove disposable gloves and dispose of them properly.	
24. Wash hands.	Reduces transmission of infection.
25. Share test results with client.	Promotes participation and compliance with therapy.

EVALUATION

1. Reinspect puncture site for bleeding or tissue injury.	Can be source of discomfort.
2. Compare glucose meter reading with normal blood glucose levels.	Determines if glucose level is normal.
3. Ask client to demonstrate procedure.	Demonstration documents level of learning.
4. Ask client to explain test and results.	Results of test may cause anxiety. Client may misunderstand specific step of procedure.
5. **Unexpected outcomes** that may occur include:	
➤ Puncture site is bruised or continues to bleed.	Adequate pressure may not have been applied to site, or clotting mechanisms may be altered.
➤ Blood glucose level above or below normal range.	Client is hypoglycemic or hyperglycemic.
➤ Glucose meter malfunctions.	Technique has not been followed as directed; battery may be low; instrument may not be clean.
➤ Client expresses misunderstanding of procedure and results.	Lack of motivation or attention span may be lessened. Nurse may not have explained steps clearly.

RECORDING AND REPORTING

1. Record procedure and glucose level in nurses' notes or special flow sheet as well as action taken for abnormal range.	Documents testing.
2. Administer insulin or carbohydrate source as ordered, depending on glucose level.	
3. Describe response, including appearance of puncture site, in nurses' notes.	Documents response to therapy.
4. Describe explanations or teaching provided in nurses' notes.	Ensures continuity of health education.
5. Report abnormal blood glucose levels to physician.	Findings may indicate need for new therapy.

FOLLOW-UP ACTIVITIES

1. Offer client and family opportunity to practice testing procedures.
2. Provide information on where client with diabetes can obtain testing supplies.
3. Provide client with information on where to obtain assistance if glucose meter has malfunctioned.
4. Provide resources and teaching aids for client to assist.

• • • • •

Special Considerations

- Some clients with diabetes may already routinely monitor blood glucose at home and may wish to continue doing so in hospital.
- Blood glucose levels are frequently assessed before meals to help to determine required insulin dosages.
- Clients who undergo frequent skin punctures may develop callous at finger sites they prefer to be used. Nurse performing test should use sites client infrequently uses.
- Repuncturing skin may be necessary if large enough droplet of blood does not form to ensure accurate test results.
- Diabetic clients frequently have peripheral vascular disease, making it difficult to produce a large droplet of blood after a finger stick. Be sure that finger is held in dependent position before stick is done to improve blood flow to area.
- Some agencies use lancet devices with an automatic blade retraction system (Microtainer Brand Safety Flow Lancet, Becton Dickinson). This reduces the possibility of self-sticks, preventing exposure to blood-borne pathogens. The Department of Health and Human Services distributed a Federal Drug Administration Safety Alert (FDA, August 28, 1990) warning of potential risk for transmission of hepatitis B that exists with spring-

loaded lancet devices that are used on multiple clients if the lancet and platform are not removed and discarded after each stick.

- Some agencies use capillary tubes or pipettes to collect the blood sample, reducing risk of direct contact with blood.
- Young children should be allowed to choose puncture site.
- Allow young child with parent to demonstrate technique, incorporate a play activity for further understanding.

Teaching Considerations

- Recommendations have been listed in a position statement developed by the American Association of Diabetes Educators (1988) to address concerns and precautions to be used during blood glucose monitoring.
- Many diabetic aids and products are available for people with visual or physical impairment (Petzinger, 1992). Some products have audio component; some have special features for visually impaired.
- Instruct client about what to do and who to contact if glucose meter malfunctions.

Pediatric Considerations

- Heel and great toe are frequently used as puncture sites in infants.
- Heel warming can be used to facilitate obtaining specimen from neonate.

Gerontologic Consideration

- Warming fingertips may facilitate obtaining specimen.

Home Care Considerations

- Glucose meters may be used routinely by clients in their homes.

SKILL 43-14 Measuring Arterial Blood Gases

Oxygenation and ventilation can be assessed by measuring arterial blood gases (ABGs). Measurement of ABGs provides valuable information in assessing and managing a patient's respiratory and metabolic disturbances (Pagana and Pagana, 1995). The parameters measured include arterial blood pH, partial pressure of oxygen, partial pressure of carbon dioxide, and arterial oxygen saturation. The ABG sample is easily obtained and can be quickly analyzed to provide the nurse with a clear picture of acid-base balance, oxygenation, and ventilation. Alterations from normal show the nurse how the client is adapting to the disease process.

Measuring ABGs aids the nurse in assessment. A decision to draw ABGs frequently may be a direct result of the nurse's physical assessment (see Chapter 11). Nursing diagnosis and interventions can be determined based on the clinical picture and laboratory data.

EQUIPMENT*

- 3 ml heparinized syringe
- 23- or 25-gauge needle
- Syringe cap
- Alcohol swabs (2)
- 2 × 2-inch gauze pad
- Heparin (1 : 1000 solution)
- Cup or plastic bag with crushed ice
- Label with client identification
- Laboratory requisition
- Disposable gloves
- Protective eyewear

*Commercial blood gas kits are available.

DELEGATION CONSIDERATIONS

Obtaining an arterial blood sample requires problem solving and knowledge application unique to a professional nurse. Delegation of this skill is inappropriate.

STEPS	RATIONALE
ASSESSMENT	
1. Determine need to obtain ABG sample and presence of physician's order. Signs and symptoms of alteration in respiratory status requiring sampling may include dyspnea, sudden change in respiratory rate or pattern, unequal breath sounds, unequal chest expansion, cyanosis, change in level of consciousness, self-extubation without need for immediate reintubation, and increased work of breathing.	Some situations and medical conditions place clients at risk for alteration in acid-base balance and ventilation status. Physician's order is required for ABGs.
2. Assess for factors that influence ABG measurements: a. Client has just awakened. b. Immediately after suctioning. c. Less than 20 to 30 minutes after oxygen therapy or ventilator setting change. d. Client whose oxygen has not been in place continually for at least 20 to 30 minutes.	Allows nurse to eliminate factors that cause inaccurate results.
3. Perform physical assessment of thorax and lungs.	Physical signs and symptoms may indicate need for ABG sample.
4. Review criteria for choosing site for ABG sample. a. Assess collateral blood flow. Perform **Allen's** test:	Arterial puncture may result in spasm of artery, clotting, **hematoma;** any of these factors may result in reduced or obstructed blood flow to tissues supplied by vessel. Collateral blood flow availability is essential if complications occur. Determines adequate collateral flow for radial artery.
(1) Have client make tight fist.	Removes as much blood from hand as possible.
(2) Apply direct pressure to both radial and ulnar arteries (see illustration).	Obstructs arterial blood flow to hand.
(3) Have client open hand (see illustration).	Fingers and hand should be pale and blanched, indicating lack of arterial blood flow.
(4) Release pressure over ulnar artery; observe color of fingers, thumbs, and hand. (see illustration).	

CRITICAL DECISION POINT **Fingers and hand should flush within 15 seconds. Flushing is positive Allen's test. If test is negative (no flushing), radial artery should be avoided. Check other hand.**

If collateral circulation is present through ulnar artery, hand and fingers flush. Ulnar artery is capable of supplying blood flow to hand if radial artery is damaged or becomes occluded during procedure.

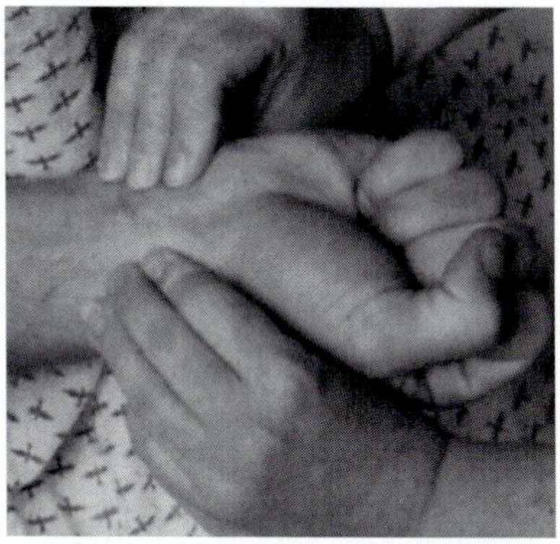

Step 4a(2)

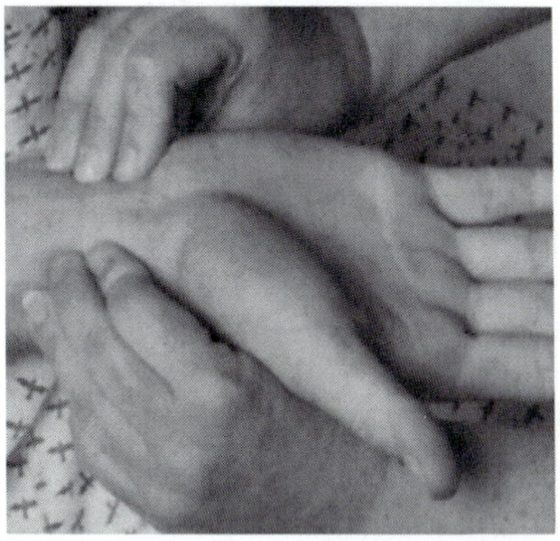

Step 4a(3)

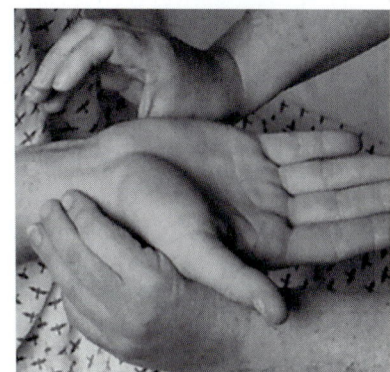

Step 4a(4)

STEPS	RATIONALE
b. Accessibility of vessel.	Palpating, stabilizing, and performing venipuncture of superficial artery is easier. Superficial arteries are located at distal ends of extremities.
c. Tissue surrounding artery.	Muscle, tendon, and fat have decreased sensation to pain. Bony periosteum and nerves are highly sensitive to pain.
d. Arteries surrounded by relatively insensitive tissues.	These are preferred sites; reduces discomfort to client.
e. Arteries not directly adjacent to veins.	Help reduce chance of venous puncture and possibility of inaccurate samples.
5. Assess best arterial sites for use in obtaining specimen.	
CRITICAL DECISION POINT **Previous punctures or preexisting conditions may eliminate potential sites. Artery should be easily accessible.**	
a. Radial artery	Safest, most accessible site for puncture; is superficial, is not adjacent to large veins, usually has adequate collateral circulation by ulnar artery, is relatively painless if periosteum is avoided, is used when Allen's test is positive.
b. Brachial artery	Has reasonable collateral blood flow, is less superficial, is more difficult to palpate and stabilize, carries increased risk of venous puncture, results in increased discomfort for client if brachial nerve is punctured, is used when radial artery is inaccessible or Allen's test is negative.
c. Femoral artery	Should not be used by nurses without specialized training. Has no adequate collateral flow if obstructed below inguinal ligament, is difficult to stabilize, is deep, and directly adjacent to femoral vein. Is best artery to use in emergency (e.g., cardiac arrest or hypovolemic shock when pulses are difficult to palpate).
6. Determine baseline ABGs for client.	Provides basis for comparison and evaluation of therapies.
7. Determine client's knowledge about ABG procedure.	Obtaining blood specimen is painful. Client who is knowledgeable will be more cooperative.

NURSING DIAGNOSIS

Clustering of defining characteristics from the assessment data may reveal the following nursing diagnoses for clients requiring this skill:

- Altered peripheral tissue perfusion
- Impaired gas exchange
- Ineffective breathing pattern
- Knowledge deficit regarding arterial blood gases
- Risk for injury

Related factors are individualized based on a client's condition or needs.

PLANNING

STEPS	RATIONALE
1. Expected outcomes following completion of procedure:	
➤ Client's ABG values are within normal ranges.	Determining normal values is essential for accurate interpretation.
➤ Client's extremity distal to puncture remains warm, pink, and free of pain and has adequate capillary refill.	Documents adequate arterial circulation to extremity.
➤ Client denies anxiety and respiratory rate remains within baseline.	Anxiety can increase respiratory rate, which can alter ABG results.
➤ Client discusses ABG procedure.	Documents learning.

STEPS	RATIONALE
2. Prepare heparinized syringe (if heparinized syringes are unavailable).	
a. Aspirate 0.5 ml sodium heparin (1000 units/ml) into syringe from vial or ampule.	Prevents blood sample from clotting before reaching laboratory. Excessive heparin can affect pH of arterial sample.
b. Withdraw plunger entire length of syringe and maintain asepsis.	Coats barrel of syringe with heparin.
c. Eject all heparin in barrel out of syringe.	0.15 to 0.25 ml of sodium heparin remains in hub of syringe; 0.05 ml of sodium heparin adequately anticoagulates 1 ml of blood; 0.15 ml adequately anticoagulates 3 ml without affecting pH level.
3. Explain steps and purpose of procedure to client.	Reduces anxiety and promotes understanding and cooperation.

IMPLEMENTATION

STEPS	RATIONALE
1. Wash hands and apply gloves.	Reduces transmission of infection.
2. Palpate selected radial site with fingertips.	Determines area of maximal impulse for puncture site.
3. Stabilize artery by hyperextending wrist slightly.	Reduces mobility of artery and makes insertion of needle easier.
4. Clean area of maximal impulse with alcohol swab, wiping in circular motion.	Reduces number of resident bacteria on skin's surface.
5. Hold alcohol swab with same fingers used to palpate artery.	Keeps swab accessible when covering of puncture site becomes necessary.
6. Keep fingertip on artery, just above chosen puncture site.	Maintaining location of artery improves likelihood of successful puncture because multiple sticks are painful.
7. Hold needle bevel up and insert at 45-degree angle into artery, with bevel directed proximally.	Angle allows for better arterial flow into needle. Oblique hole in artery seals more easily.
8. Stop advancing needle when blood is noted returning into hub of needle or syringe.	Quick return of blood indicates that arterial flow is obtained. Prevents completely transversing needle through artery.
9. If using open needle, attach syringe securely.	Prevents air bubbles from entering sample.
10. Use 2 × 2–inch gauze or antiseptic swab to catch blood that may spill when syringe is attached.	Maintains cleanliness.
11. Allow arterial pulsations to pump 2 to 3 ml of blood into heparinized syringe slowly (see illustration).	Allowing pulsations to assist in filling syringe reduces presence of air bubbles in sample. Bubbles can alter ABG results.
12. When sampling is complete, hold alcohol swab over puncture site and withdraw needle.	Swab minimizes pulling of skin as needle is withdrawn.

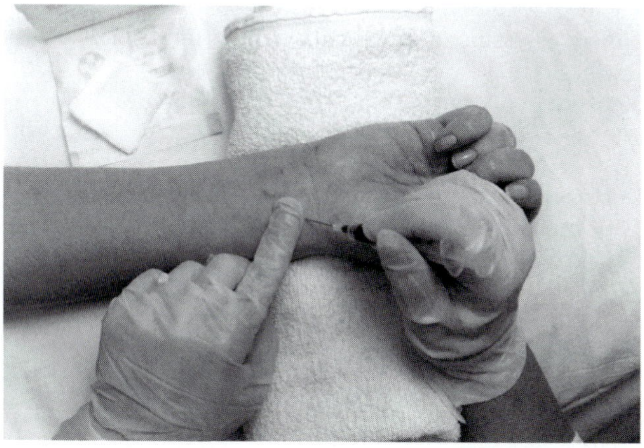

Step 11

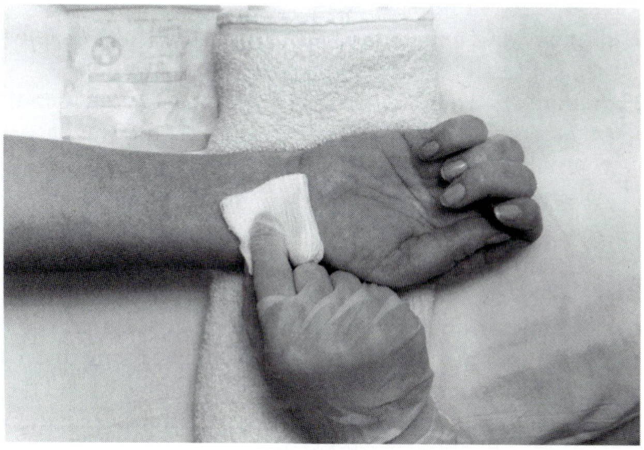

Step 13

STEPS	RATIONALE
13. Apply pressure over and just proximal to puncture site with swab (see illustration).	Insertion of needle into artery is just proximal to insertion site through skin. Gauze absorbs any blood that might ooze from site.
14. Maintain continuous pressure over and proximal to site for 5 minutes (10 minutes if client is undergoing anticoagulant therapy or has bleeding disorder).	Ensures adequate coagulation of arterial puncture site.
15. Visually inspect site for signs of bleeding.	Determines if continued need exists to exert pressure.
16. Palpate artery below or distal to puncture site.	Determines if pulse quality has changed, indicating alteration in arterial flow.
17. Remove gloves and wash hands.	Reduces transmission of microorganisms.
18. Expel air bubbles from syringe.	Air bubbles can falsely elevate arterial oxygen pressure (PaO_2) and lower arterial carbon dioxide pressure ($PaCO_2$).
19. Prepare syringe for laboratory analysis according to agency policy. Common principles include:	
a. Place client identification label on syringe.	Permits proper identification of sample for laboratory.
b. Place syringe in cup of crushed ice.	Reduces blood cell metabolism (e.g., oxygen consumption and carbon dioxide production) within sample.
c. Attach properly labeled requisition to blood gas sample.	Prevents mislabeled specimens in laboratory. Ensures correct results received for correct client.
d. Indicate amount of any supplemental oxygen (e.g., 2 liters O_2, 70% by mask, room air) on requisition.	Essential for proper identification of sample.
e. Indicate client's temperature.	
f. Send sample to laboratory immediately.	Prevents changes in sample resulting from delay in procedure. Provides timely return of results to nurse.

EVALUATION

1. Inspect area distal to puncture site for complications.	Obstruction of artery can develop from hematoma or damage to vessel wall, reducing arterial flow.
2. Review results of sample as soon as possible.	Identifies any abnormality.
3. Obtain client's respiratory rate.	
4. **Unexpected outcomes** that may occur include:	
➤ Client has elevated pH and lowered $PaCO_2$.	Indicates respiratory alkalosis.
➤ Client has lowered pH and elevated $PaCO_2$.	Indicates respiratory acidosis.
➤ Client has elevated PaO_2.	Indicates possible contamination of sample.
➤ Client has lowered PaO_2.	Indicates inadequate FiO_2; client unable to oxygenate efficiently.

RECORDING AND REPORTING

1. Record puncture site and disposition of specimen to laboratory in nurses' notes.	
2. Report ABG results to physician as soon as available.	Timely assessment of results and reporting enable physician to make decisions regarding care.
3. Be sure to include client's FiO_2 and any ventilator settings (e.g., V_T, respiratory frequency [R_F] mode of ventilation).	Necessary to interpret PaO_2 and $PaCO_2$ accurately.
4. Record results of test and condition of puncture site in nurses' notes.	Documents test results and indicates proper evaluation of puncture site.

FOLLOW-UP ACTIVITIES

1. Continue to observe puncture site and assess pulse.
2. If client's oxygenation status is poor, indicated by low PaO_2, lower pH, elevated PaO_2 (respiratory acidosis):
   a. Administer oxygen therapy.
   b. Encourage coughing and deep breathing.
   c. Perform tracheal suctioning.
   d. Elevate head of bed.
   e. Hold pain medication administration if possible.

STEPS | **RATIONALE**

3. If oxygenation status is poor, indicated by elevated pH and low $PaCO_2$ (respiratory alkalosis):
   a. Encourage slow, deep breaths or have client breathe into paper bag.
   b. Administer pain medication.
   c. Talk with client about fears or concerns.

• • • • •

Special Considerations

- Venous sample has low PO_2 and slightly higher PCO_2 compared to arterial sample.
- Factors that contraindicate use of arterial site include amputation, contractures, dressing or cast, arteriovenous shunts.
- Check with laboratory to verify quantity of sample required. Blood should return easily into syringe because of arterial pressure.
- If hyperventilated, client may feel dizzy and confused and may require coaching to begin slow breathing.

Teaching Considerations

- Prepare client for needle stick because radial sticks are painful. Prepared client will not reflexively withdraw arm.
- Instruct client to breathe normally.
- Client is taught to report numbness, burning, and/or tingling in hand that had radial artery puncture.

Pediatric Considerations

- In neonatal and pediatric clients, capillary blood gas may also be used. Procedures are similar to those for obtaining heel sticks.
- When dealing with neonatal clients, especially premature infants, normal values for ABGs may differ from those of adults.

Gerontologic Consideration

- Special attention in interpretation of ABGs must be devoted to clients with chronic pulmonary conditions. In these clients compensatory mechanisms may allow normal pH in face of markedly elevated PCO_2.

CRITICAL THINKING EXERCISES

1. A 37-year-old woman with new-onset insulin-dependent diabetes says that she is "afraid to poke myself" for blood sugars and would like to know more about urine testing. What positive and negative aspects of each method would you review with her? If she opts for glucose testing by the finger-stick method, what points would you review with her to make her testing less traumatic?
2. A 62-year-old man comes in to pick up some guaiac cards for occult blood testing. As part of your assessment, you inquire about medications. He takes "something" but cannot remember the name of it. Which medication(s) and food(s) would have an impact on the occult blood test?
3. An 18-year-old woman is very anxious before an arterial blood gas test. What effect might this have on the results? How could you alleviate her anxiety?
4. What nursing strategies would you need to implement to obtain a clean-voided specimen from a very obese woman confined to bed rest?

REFERENCES

American Academy of Pediatrics Committee on Infectious Diseases: Use of Ribavarin in treatment of respiratory syncytial virus infection, *Pediatrics* (92)(3):501, 1993.

American Association of Diabetes Educators: Prevention of transmission of blood-borne infectious agents during blood glucose monitoring (position statement), *Diabetes Educator* 14(5):425, 1988.

Centers for Disease Control and Prevention: Standard Precautions, *Am J Infect Control,* February:24, 1996.

Dettenmeier PA: *Pulmonary nursing care,* St Louis, 1992, Mosby.

Food and Drug Administration: *FDA safety alert: hepatitis B transmission via spring-loaded devices,* Rockville, Md, August 28, 1990, Department of Health and Human Services.

Johnson JE: Coping with elective surgery. In Werley HH, Fitzpatrick JJ, editors: *Annual review of nursing research—2,* New York, Springer, 1984.

Occupational Safety and Health Administration: Occupational exposure to bloodborne pathogens: final rule, 29 CFR 1919:1030, *Fed Regis* 56:64003, 1991.

Pagana KD, Pagana TJ: *Mosby's diagnostic and laboratory test reference,* ed 2, St Louis, 1995, Mosby.

Petzinger RA: Diabetes aids and products for people with visual or physical impairment, *Diabetes Educator* 18(2):121, 1992.

Redman BK: *The practice of patient education,* ed 8, St Louis, 1997, Mosby.

Wong DL: Diapering choices: a critical review of the issues, *Pediatr Nurs* 18(1):41, 1992.

Wong DL: *Whaley and Wong's nursing care of infants and children,* ed 5, St Louis, 1995, Mosby.

CHAPTER 44

Diagnostic Procedures

OBJECTIVES

Mastery of content in this chapter will enable the nurse to:

- Define key terms.
- Identify physiological factors related to diagnostic procedures.
- Perform physical and psychological assessment related to procedures.
- Demonstrate organizational skills in planning procedures.
- Effectively assist the physician or other health professional with abdominal paracentesis, arteriography, bone marrow aspiration, bronchoscopy, electrocardiogram, endoscopy, lumbar puncture, magnetic resonance imaging, and thoracentesis.
- Demonstrate understanding of follow-up activities of procedures.
- Describe the responsibilities related to the procedure of the nurse, physician, and unlicensed assistive personnel.

SKILLS

44-1 Assisting with Abdominal Paracentesis
44-2 Assisting with Angiography (Arteriography)
44-3 Assisting with Bone Marrow Aspiration/Biopsy
44-4 Assisting with Bronchoscopy
44-5 Assisting with Electrocardiogram
44-6 Assisting with Endoscopy
44-7 Assisting with Lumbar Puncture
44-8 Assisting with Magnetic Resonance Imaging
44-9 Assisting with Thoracentesis

KEY TERMS

Abdominal girth
Ascites
Aspiration
Biopsy
Bone marrow
Cannula
Cerebrospinal fluid
Coagulopathy
Cytologic
Fiberoptic
Foramen magnum
Herniation
Immunocompromised
Intercostal space
Intestinal obstruction
Intraabdominal pressure
Intracranial pressure
Intravenous conscious sedation (IVCS)
Lavage
Lumens
Manometer
Medullary
Megakaryocyte
Occult
Peritoneal fluid
Pleural cavity
Pleural fluid
Portal hypertension
Precordial
Radiopaque
Sigmoid colon
Stopcock
Subarachnoid space
Thrombocytopenia
Tracheobronchial tree
Trochar
Varices
Viscera

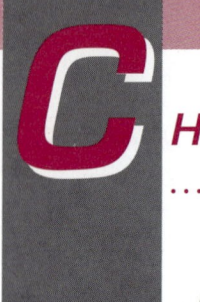

Diagnostic tests may be performed by a physician at the client's bedside or in a room equipped specifically for therapeutic or diagnostic purposes. The nurse is responsible for assessing the client's knowledge of the procedure, preparing the client, providing a safe environment during the procedure, caring for the client after tests are completed, and supervising care provided to the client by unlicensed assistive personnel. The nurse's knowledge of each test and the application of the nursing process ensure safe performance of the procedure.

In the implementation phase of those tests performed by a physician, the physician's responsibility is outlined separately from the nurse's responsibility. There are two main reasons for this separation of duties. First, the nurse anticipates the needs of the physician to have supplies ready. Second and most important, the nurse keeps the client adequately informed of procedural details that could cause discomfort.

The nurse must know legal implications for diagnostic testing. Most invasive diagnostic tests require a signed informed consent. The physician is ultimately responsible for disclosure, but the nurse must be aware of institutional policies regarding consent forms and ensure that informed consent is obtained before the procedure (Cushing, 1991). The nurse must also record and report the client's status before, during, and after the procedure. The nurse assists the client throughout a procedure. Most of these procedures cause moderate discomfort, and the client may tolerate the procedure better if a well-informed nurse stays at the bedside and explains each step.

Certain diagnostic procedures require the client to receive **IV conscious sedation (IVCS).** IVCS is the administration of pharmacological agents to provide a minimally depressed level of consciousness. During IVCS the client independently and continuously maintains an airway and is responsive to physical stimulation and verbal commands. The use of IVCS provides client comfort along with safe and effective performance during the procedure. Although IVCS may be administered by a registered nurse with a physician in attendance, it is the responsibility of the physician to order the appropriate drugs and their dosages. Check agency policy for recommended and maximum doses of medications. After IVCS clients need continuous monitoring of vital signs (pulse, blood pressure, and respiration) and oxygen saturation by pulse oximetry.

Client risks during IVCS include airway compromise, hemodynamic instability, and/or altered level of consciousness. Emergency equipment (see Chapter 16) must be immediately accessible where IVCS is administered. After the administration of IVCS, the client's level of sedation and level of consciousness must be assessed and documented according to agency policy by the RN or delegated to an LPN or respiratory therapist.

GUIDELINES

1. Assess client's baseline vital signs. Invasive diagnostic procedures can cause complications. Deviations from the baseline vital signs can provide early physiological data about potential complications.
2. Determine client's level of anxiety, educational level, previous experience, language barriers, and sensory deficits that may have an impact on the learning process.
3. Determine the client's knowledge and perception of both actual and potential medical diagnoses.
4. Be aware of any abnormal findings that indicate or contraindicate a particular diagnostic test (e.g., prolonged clotting time or prothrombin time).
5. Be aware of a past history of adverse reaction to IVCS (e.g., hemodynamic instability, airway compromise, and/or altered level of consciousness).
6. Clients who have previously experienced diagnostic testing may have preconceived (positive or negative) ideas concerning the test, which may influence the amount of preprocedure teaching and support required.
7. Be aware of clients' disabilities that might affect their ability to be positioned for certain procedures.
8. Be sensitive to cultural patterns that might influence a client's response to various procedures. For instance, clients from the Middle East will not allow male physicians to examine females (Galanti, 1994).
9. Certain diagnostic procedures require that the client remain NPO before testing. When performing the medication history, the nurse assesses whether the client is taking medications that require an uninterrupted dosage schedule (e.g., anticonvulsants, antibiotics, or cardiac medications) and contact the physician.
10. If insulin or oral hypoglycemic medications have been administered to clients before diagnostic testing, arrange to have either the client's meal or other nutritional support available upon completion of the test.
11. Because of age-related cardiovascular changes in the older adult, plan diagnostic testing schedules to provide rest periods.

DELEGATION CONSIDERATIONS

The skills of assisting the physician with diagnostic procedures in this chapter may be delegated to unlicensed assistive personnel if the client is stable. Procedures that require IVCS (i.e., arteriography, bone marrow aspiration, bronchoscopy, endoscopy, and proctosigmoidoscopy) will require the skill and judgment of a registered nurse to ensure client safety.

- Inform and assist care provider in proper way to position client before diagnostic procedure.
- Instruct care provider to take baseline, as well as postprocedure, vital signs and to report these vital signs to the registered nurse.
- Caution care provider to be alert for and report signs and symptoms experienced by the client indicating possible complications of the diagnostic procedure.
- Inform care provider to obtain specimen requisitions and to transport specimens to the laboratory if necessary.
- Unstable clients (e.g., those on ventilatory support or receiving blood products) and those receiving IVCS will need the supervision of a registered nurse during and after the procedure.

SKILL 44-1 Assisting with Abdominal Paracentesis

Abdominal paracentesis is a sterile, invasive procedure performed by the physician to obtain **peritoneal fluid** for diagnostic analyses or for palliative reasons such as to reduce **intraabdominal pressure.** Two types of abdominal paracentesis include peritoneal **lavage** and abdominal **aspiration.** Common medical diagnoses requiring abdominal paracentesis include blunt trauma with possible intraabdominal bleeding and **ascites.**

Peritoneal fluid is obtained by inserting a large-bore needle or trochar and **cannula** into the peritoneal cavity. The fluid aspirated is analyzed to determine the presence of bacteria, blood, fungi, glucose, and protein. Additionally, **cytologic** analyses may be done to detect tumors.

As a palliative measure, paracentesis may be performed to provide temporary relief of respiratory and abdominal discomfort caused by severe ascites. Abdominal paracentesis may be performed in the hospital at the client's bedside, the treatment room, or the physician's office in less than 30 minutes.

EQUIPMENT

- Antiseptic solution for hand washing (e.g., povidone-iodine scrub)
- Paracentesis tray, if available from central supply, which may include:
  - Antiseptic solution (e.g., povidone-iodine solution)
  - Sterile gauze sponges (4 × 4)
  - Local anesthetic solution for injection (e.g., lidocaine 1%)
  - Sterile syringes: two 3-ml, 23- to 25-gauge needles for anesthetic; four 10- to 60-ml, 19- to 21-gauge needles
  - Small, sterile knife blade
  - Two sterile cannula needles; sizes 10 or 12, with inner trochar, or catheter
- 2 to 3 L IV fluids as ordered
- IV tubing, usually macrodrip size
- Sterile specimen containers and bag for containment
- Vacuum bottles as ordered
- Two packages of sterile gloves (check physician's preferred size)
- Masks and goggles for nurse, physician, and unlicensed assistive personnel (check institution's policy)
- Sterile gauze sponges (2 × 2), tape, adhesive bandages, and antiseptic ointment
- Pain medication if ordered (given 30 minutes before procedure)
- Laboratory requisitions and labels
- Measuring tape and marker

STEPS	RATIONALE
ASSESSMENT	
1. Assess whether client has history of being uncooperative or has severe coagulopathy, thrombocytopenia, **intestinal obstruction,** abdominal wall infection, previous multiple abdominal surgeries, or **portal hypertension** with abdominal collateral circulation (SGNA, 1993).	Conditions contraindicate procedure.
2. Wash hands.	Reduces transmission of microorganisms.

STEPS	RATIONALE
3. Assess vital signs, especially blood pressure.	Baseline vital signs detect changes caused by complications from drainage of large fluid volumes.
4. Assess client for bladder distention or time of last voiding.	Chance of bladder trauma is decreased if bladder is not distended.
5. Assess client's medication history. Determine if there are allergies to local anesthetic or antiseptic solutions that may be used or if client is receiving anticoagulants.	Common allergic reactions to anesthetic agents are central nervous system depression, respiratory difficulties, and hypotension. Allergic reactions to antiseptic solutions are usually skin irritations. Client who is receiving anticoagulants may experience hemorrhage.
6. Weigh client, assess abdomen (see Chapter 11), and measure **abdominal girth** in centimeters at largest point of abdomen. Use ink pen to mark where measuring tape lies.	Abdominal girth is measured in same place to accurately note abdominal size before and after paracentesis.
7. Assess client's respiratory rate, diaphragmatic excursion, and chest wall motion.	Excess peritoneal fluid increases intraabdominal pressure, which in turn compromises respiration.
8. Assess client's knowledge regarding procedure.	Client must be informed of impending procedure, its purpose, and its outcomes.
9. Check whether written informed consent has been signed by client.	Most institutions require written permission for procedure.
CRITICAL DECISION POINT **Do not administer an analgesic before the client receives informed consent.**	
10. Administer preprocedure medication if indicated.	Clients who are anxious may benefit from preprocedure medications.

NURSING DIAGNOSIS

Clustering of defining characteristics from the assessment data may reveal the following nursing diagnoses for clients requiring this skill:

- Anxiety
- Fear
- Ineffective breathing pattern
- Knowledge deficit regarding purpose and steps of procedure
- Pain
- Risk for fluid volume deficit
- Risk for infection
- Risk for injury

Related factors are individualized based on a client's condition or needs

PLANNING

STEPS	RATIONALE
1. **Expected outcomes** following completion of procedure:	
➤ Client assumes positions without problems, has few changes in vital signs, and has no complications.	Client tolerates procedure well.
➤ For peritoneal lavage and abdominal aspiration, aspirate is clear or slightly blood tinged.	Slight amount of blood-tinged drainage may be caused by irritation to tissue by needle.
➤ For therapeutic treatment of ascites by paracentesis, amount of fluid drained results in decreased abdominal girth, skin tightness, and weight.	Related to ascitic fluid loss and relief of pressure on diaphragm and abdominal contents.
➤ Client experiences increased comfort.	Distention from buildup of fluid in peritoneal space is relieved.
➤ Client has improved respiratory status.	Abdominal distention can reduce diaphragmatic excursion.
2. Organize equipment on bedside table.	Ensures ease and success of procedure.
3. Prepare client for procedure:	
a. Explain purpose of and steps in the procedure.	Assists in minimizing anxiety and promoting relaxation and cooperation.

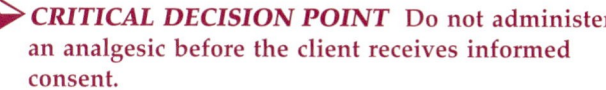

STEPS	RATIONALE
b. Have client void before procedure.	Full or distended bladder increases possibility of puncturing bladder.

CRITICAL DECISION POINT If unable to void and bladder is distended, obtain order to catheterize client.

c. Client assumes position desired by physician, either semi-Fowler's in bed or sitting upright on side of bed or in chair with feet supported. Due to underlying physical condition (i.e., respiratory distress from increased fluid), client may be unable to assume required position for procedure and may require assistance of pillows or other positional devices.	Semi-Fowler's or sitting position is used to drain ascites because of effect of gravity on fluid in peritoneal cavity. Fluid accumulates in lower abdomen and may be drained more easily in these positions (see illustration).

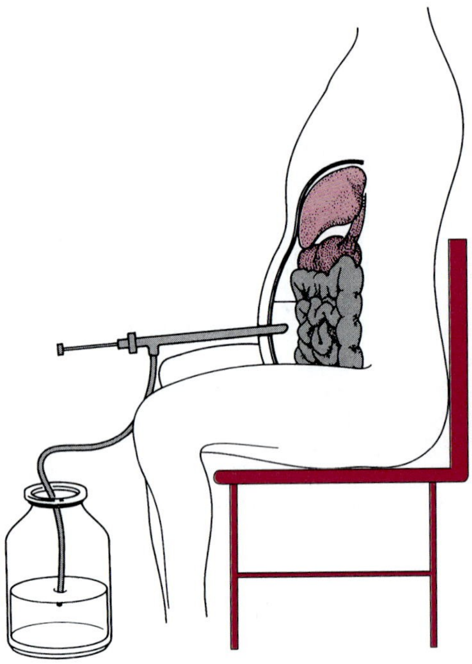

Step 3c Paracentesis. (Modified from Beare PG, Myers JL: *Principles and practice of adult health nursing,* ed 2, St Louis, 1994, Mosby.)

IMPLEMENTATION
Nurse's Responsibility

STEPS	RATIONALE
1. Wash hands.	Reduces transmission of microorganisms.
2. Set up sterile tray or open sterile supplies and make accessible for physician.	Ensures maintenance of sterility throughout procedure.
3. Prepare solution to be used for lavage; attach to IV tubing.	If fluid instillation is to be performed, as with blunt abdominal trauma, fluid is ready to attach to plastic tubing after cannula is in place in abdomen.
4. Assist client through procedure:	
a. Describe steps of procedure as they are implemented by physician.	Allows client opportunity to ask questions and helps to decrease anxiety.
b. Ensure client's comfort and assess for complications.	Assists client in tolerating procedure and identifies need to modify or discontinue procedure.
5. Assess vital signs before, every 15 minutes during, and, every 15 minutes for an hour after the procedure.	Identifies possible complications of procedure, such as shock.
6. Implement fluid instillation for lavage:	
a. Apply clean gloves (and mask and goggles, if required).	Reduces transmission of microorganisms.
b. After IV tubing is attached to cannula; administer physician-ordered amount of fluid at prescribed rate.	Promotes infusion of prescribed fluid into peritoneum.

STEPS	RATIONALE
c. Clamp IV tubing after fluid is instilled and place drainage tubing below client's abdominal level.	Promotes gravitational drainage of fluid from peritoneal cavity.
7. Ascitic fluid is withdrawn by either gravity or vacuum drainage. Maximum amount of ascitic fluid usually allowed to drain is 1500 ml.	Permits flow of fluid or solution from abdomen. Maximum of 1500 ml drainage prevents hypovolemic shock.
8. Collect any necessary laboratory specimens in sterile containers.	
9. Assess client's tolerance of procedure including pain, and mental status.	Enables nurse to evaluate client's tolerance of procedure and detects changes from preprocedure condition.
10. Carefully dispose of equipment, remove gloves, and wash hands. Needles and other sharp objects should be placed in special containers. Dispose of peritoneal fluid not sent to laboratory according to hospital procedure.	Controls transmission of infection. Proper disposal of sharps prevents accidental injury to personnel.
Physician's Responsibility	
1. Wash hands. Prep abdomen with antiseptic solution and 4 × 4 sponges.	Reduces transmission of microorganisms.
2. Wear mask (if required), apply sterile gloves and goggles, and drape client with sterile towels.	Maintains surgical asepsis.
3. Inject local anesthetic and allow to take effect.	Provides local anesthetic to area of puncture or incision.
4. If the purpose of the paracentesis is to drain ascitic fluid or to lavage, insert the large-bore needle or trochar through a small incision between the umbilicus and the symphysis pubis.	Facilitates placement of large-bore needle or trochar into abdominal cavity for instillation and drainage of fluid. Permits the removal of blood and/or fluid specimens.
5. Attach IV tubing to the cannula and allow fluid to drain into a receptacle to a maximum of 1500 ml. (The fluid may also be aspirated, using a 60-ml syringe.) For lavage, instill prescribed amount of sterile fluid and allow it to drain.	Fluid is drained slowly, to a maximum of 1500 ml to prevent hypovolemic shock.
6. If only specimens are needed, and incision is not made, insert 10-gauge needle attached to syringe, aspirate fluid, and place in specimen containers. Remove cannula, needle, or trochar.	Obtains sterile specimens for laboratory analysis.
7. Place manual pressure over insertion site until drainage ceases, or apply pressure dressing.	Prevents excessive drainage from puncture site.
8. Place antiseptic ointment with 2 × 2 gauze sponge over insertion site.	Prevents growth of bacteria at puncture site.

EVALUATION

1. Take vital signs every 15 minutes for 1 hour and then every 30 minutes for 2 hours; check for stability by comparing with preprocedure values.	
2. Monitor urinary output for 24 hours.	Verifies client's physiological status. Hematuria may indicate bladder trauma.
3. Check dressing over insertion site for bleeding or drainage.	Provides for continued observation of puncture site. May indicate accumulation of blood or fluid in abdominal cavity.
4. Measure abdominal girth and weight.	Determines change after fluid drainage.
5. Inspect character of lavage or aspirate.	For peritoneal lavage and abdominal aspiration, aspirate is clear or slightly blood tinged.
6. Observe and question if client is having discomfort.	May indicate puncture of underlying organs.
7. **Unexpected outcomes** that may occur include:	
➤ Changes in vital signs are not within normal limits.	Hypotension may indicate impending hypovolemic shock. Slight hypertension and tachycardia may be caused by anxiety.

STEPS	RATIONALE
➤ In clients with blunt abdominal trauma, injured or perforated contents may bleed into peritoneal cavity, which may be observed through this procedure.	
➤ Aspirate or drained fluid is bloody—bright or dark red.	Indicates blood in peritoneal cavity. Results from irritation and/or trauma of blood vessels during procedure.
➤ Infection	Contaminated techniques or accidental perforation of organs may cause peritonitis.
➤ Laboratory test results, including cell counts, protein levels, and specific gravity, are not within normal limits.	Indicates abnormal process such as infection, cancer, or portal hypertension.

Recording and Reporting

STEPS	RATIONALE
1. Record in client's chart the type of procedure (aspiration or lavage), client's tolerance of procedure (pain level, vital signs), type of dressing over insertion, whether drainage is present, and if specimen sent to lab.	Documents client's response to invasive procedure.
2. Record changes in abdominal girth and weight and amount, color, and clarity of fluid.	Documents outcomes of removal of fluid from peritoneal cavity.
3. Report to physician immediately:	
a. Deviations from client's baseline vital signs.	May indicate hypovolemic shock or peritonitis.
b. Severe abdominal pain.	May indicate perforation of **viscera.**
c. Excessive bloody drainage from insertion site.	May indicate irritation and clotting problem of skin artery. Place manual pressure over insertion site.

Follow-up Activities

1. Assist client in assuming comfortable position in bed.
2. Send appropriately labeled specimens to laboratory.
3. Monitor abdominal dressing for drainage, and document findings.
4. Obtain laboratory data for interpretation by nurse and physician.

• • • • •

Special Considerations

- ➤ If in doubt as to whether laboratory specimen will be needed, collect sterile specimen. Specimen can easily be discarded, at no cost to the client, if it is not needed.
- ➤ IV fluids or albumin may be given to prevent hypotension.
- ➤ In addition to signing consent for procedure, clients who have experienced blunt abdominal trauma should also sign consent for emergency abdominal surgery. Operating room personnel need to be notified of pending emergency surgery before procedure takes place.

Teaching Considerations

- ➤ Explain to client that procedure will be more safely performed if bladder is empty.
- ➤ Explain that although the local anesthetic will eliminate pain at the insertion site, a pressure-type discomfort may be experienced as the needle is inserted.
- ➤ Tell client with ascites that comfort will probably increase and respiration will be easier after paracentesis.
- ➤ Inform client with ascites that the procedure provides temporary decrease in abdominal distention and may need to be repeated.
- ➤ Encourage client to check with physician regarding test results.

Gerontologic Considerations

- ➤ In older adults, skin is normally inelastic and thin; therefore special care should be used when removing adhesive bandages or tape at puncture site.

Home Care Considerations

- ➤ If paracentesis is done on an outpatient basis, inform client to notify physician of fever or any swelling, pain, or drainage at puncture site. In males, scrotal edema should be reported to the physician (SGNA, 1993).

SKILL 44-2 Assisting with Angiography (Arteriography)

Angiography (arteriography) permits radiographic visualization of the vasculature of the heart and arterial system after the intravascular injection of a **radiopaque** contrast medium. Arteriography is most frequently performed to aid in the diagnosis of occlusions, stenosis, emboli or thrombosis, aneurysms, tumors, congenital malformations, or trauma of the arteries of the brain, heart, lung, kidneys, or lower extremities.

A small incision or needle puncture is made in a peripheral artery (femoral, brachial, or carotid), and under x-ray visualization a small radiopaque catheter is threaded through the artery to the site. The iodinated contrast material is injected, and timed x-ray films are taken. The test is usually performed by a radiologist in the x-ray department.

Potential complications of angiography include hemorrhage or thrombosis at the catheter insertion site, infection, allergic reactions to the dye, embolism, and renal failure. Additionally, the nurse must be alert for complications related to IVCS.

Cardiac catheterization is a specialized form of angiography in which a catheter is inserted into either the left or right side of the heart to study pressures within the heart, cardiac volumes, valvular function, and patency of coronary arteries. A contrast medium is injected and the structures and functions of the heart assessed. In right-side heart catheterizations, usually the subclavian or femoral vein is used for vascular access.

Cardiac catheterizations may be contraindicated in clients who would refuse surgery if needed, who are allergic to iodine contrast media, who are uncooperative or who cannot lie still during the entire procedure, or who are susceptible to dye-induced renal failure (Beare and Myers, 1994; Pagana and Pagana, 1995).

For both procedures, the cardiologist or radiologist is usually assisted by a technologist rather than the nurse, and the procedures are done in the radiology department. An exception would be when IVCS is administered by an RN with a physician in attendance. Agency policies may vary.

EQUIPMENT

For either an arteriogram or a cardiac catheterization, special packs are usually available from central sterile supply. The packs contain various sizes and types of catheters for performing the procedures, as well as the necessary specialized equipment.

- Sterile gown
- Sterile gloves
- Mask
- Goggles
- Intravenous equipment for IV start
- Diazepam, midazolam, or other sedative for IV sedation
- Oxygen, resuscitative equipment, pulse oximeter, cardiac monitor for IVCS

STEPS	RATIONALE
ASSESSMENT	
1. Assess client's knowledge of procedure.	Procedure creates physical sensations and involves visual analyses of x-ray/fluoroscope that need to be explained in detail.
2. Assess vital signs and peripheral pulses. Mark client's peripheral pulses before procedure. For cardiac catheterization, also auscultate heart and lungs and obtain weight.	Provides baseline data for comparison with findings during and after procedure. Marking pulses permits quicker postprocedure assessment.
3. Determine type of arteriogram to be performed—carotid, femoral, or brachial. If cardiac catheterization, determine whether right or left heart is being studied.	Enables nurse to anticipate client teaching needs and postprocedure interventions.
CRITICAL DECISION POINT Area of catheter insertion may need to be shaved and prepped with antiseptic just before the procedure.	
4. Assess whether client has signed consent form.	Procedures usually require signed consent form to reduce legal risk to institution.
CRITICAL DECISION POINT Consent form must be completed before administration of preprocedural sedation or IVCS.	

STEPS	RATIONALE
5. Assess that client has been NPO for 6 to 8 hours before the procedure.	Prevents possible aspiration since client is sedated. Excessive hydration causes dilution of the contrast medium, making structures more difficult to visualize.
6. Assess whether client is allergic to iodine dye. If so, notify cardiologist or radiologist. Benadryl IV may be routinely given before the procedure.	An iodine-based radiopaque contrast medium may be used during the procedure; however, a nonionic, hypoallergenic contrast medium is more frequently used (Pagana and Pagana, 1995).
CRITICAL DECISION POINT Clients with allergies to iodine, shellfish, or other contrast media may experience anaphylactic reactions.	
7. Assess CBC, platelets, and prothrombin time, electrolytes, BUN and creatinine levels before the procedure.	Abnormal findings might contraindicate the procedure at that time, since hemorrhage and/or renal failure may be complications.
8. Review physician's orders for preprocedure medications (may be given on nursing unit or in radiology department) and sedative for IVCS:	
CRITICAL DECISION POINT In anxious or confused clients increased sedation may be necessary.	
a. Atropine	Decreases or prevents vagally induced bradycardia; decreases oral secretions.
b. Benadryl	Prophylaxis against allergic reaction to dye.
c. Preprocedural sedative	Decreases anxiety and promotes relaxation.
d. IVCS during procedure	Provides a minimally depressed level of consciousness yet allows client to independently and continuously maintain an airway and respond to physical stimuli and verbal commands.

NURSING DIAGNOSIS

Clustering of defining characteristics from the assessment data may reveal the following nursing diagnoses for clients requiring this skill:

- Altered thought processes
- Anxiety
- Decreased cardiac output
- Fear
- Impaired gas exchange
- Ineffective breathing pattern
- Knowledge deficit regarding purpose and steps of procedure
- Pain
- Risk for aspiration
- Risk for fluid volume deficit
- Risk for infection
- Risk for injury
- Risk for peripheral neurovascular dysfunction

Related factors are individualized based on a client's condition or needs.

PLANNING

1. **Expected outcomes** following completion of procedure:	
➤ Client has no significant changes in vital signs or peripheral pulses, and no allergic response.	Procedure performed without complication.
➤ Client has minimal discomfort.	Client tolerates procedure.
➤ Client experiences soreness at catheter insertion site and possible backache.	These are considered normal and expected.
➤ Client recovers from IVCS without respiratory complications or change in level of consciousness.	Level of sedation is appropriate.
➤ Client has no lab value changes.	
2. Explain to client purpose of the procedure and what will happen during the procedure.	Helps to minimize client's anxiety.

IMPLEMENTATION

Nurse's Responsibility

STEPS	RATIONALE
1. Wash hands and apply clean gloves.	Reduces transmission of microorganisms.
2. For cardiac catheterization, provide IV access using large-bore cannula.	Provides access for delivery of intravenous fluids and/or drugs.
3. Assess vital signs, obtain weight, and palpate peripheral pulses.	Provides baseline data for comparison during and after procedure.
4. Assist client in assuming comfortable position on x-ray table.	Position may need to be maintained for 1 to 3 hours.
5. Provide support to client throughout the procedure and as x-rays are taken, because the client may be frightened by the loud noises (Pagana and Pagana, 1995).	
6. Tell client that during the injection of the dye, there may be a severe hot flash that is quite uncomfortable but lasts only a few seconds (Pagana and Pagana, 1995).	Dye causes vasoactive response.
7. Nurse administering IVCS monitors level of sedation and level of consciousness.	IVCS should not cause loss of consciousness.
8. Note that some clients have a tendency to cough as the catheter is placed into the pulmonary artery (Pagana and Pagana, 1995).	

Physician's Responsibility

STEPS	RATIONALE
1. Wash hands and prep area of catheter insertion (femoral, carotid, or brachial) with antiseptic.	Reduces transmission of microorganisms.
2. Apply mask and goggles, sterile gown, cap, and gloves. (All technologists and assistants do the same.) Drape client with sterile drapes.	Maintains surgical asepsis.
3. Anesthetize the skin overlying the arterial puncture site.	Provides local anesthetic to area of incision or puncture.
4. Perform needle puncture of artery; insert guidewire through needle and angiographic (or cardiographic) catheter threaded over wire.	Permits access to artery and prevents coiling of catheter in artery.
5. Advance catheter to desired artery or cardiac chamber and inject contrast medium.	Permits radiographic visualization of structures, aneurysms, occlusions, or anomalies.
6. During dye injection, specialized machinery takes rapid sequence of x-rays.	Permits radiographic records of visualization of dye through artery, as well as any abnormalities present.
7. For cardiac catheterization, also measure cardiac volumes and pressures, then withdraw catheter and apply pressure to puncture site for at least 5 minutes.	Provides data related to cardiac output, central venous pressure (CVP), ventricular pressures, and pulmonary artery pressure. Pressure on puncture site promotes clotting and prevents bleeding.

EVALUATION

STEPS	RATIONALE
1. Monitor vital signs and assess peripheral pulses (compare right and left), auscultate heart and lungs if cardiac catheterization done, and compare findings with preprocedure values.	Verifies client's physiological status and evaluates effect of procedure.
2. Assess client for possible delayed reaction to iodine dye (if used)—dyspnea, hives, tachycardia, and rash (Pagana and Pagana, 1995).	Reaction may occur up to 6 hours after injection of dye.
3. Assess for level of sedation, level of consciousness, and O_2 saturation.	Determines client's response to IVCS.
4. Assess postprocedure laboratory values—CBC, prothrombin time, electrolytes, BUN, and creatinine.	Changes in laboratory values may indicate the onset of complications.

STEPS	RATIONALE
5. Observe client for signs of discomfort.	May be early sign of complication.
CRITICAL DECISION POINT **Stress the importance of reporting any feelings of pain, dyspnea, numbness or tingling, or other untoward symptoms.**	
6. **Unexpected outcomes** that may occur include:	
➤ Client has marked changes in vital signs or peripheral pulses.	Hypotension and tachycardia may signify hemorrhage or allergic reaction to dye. Diminished or absent peripheral pulses may signify thrombosis or embolism.
➤ Client remains sedated with decreased respiration or blood pressure, decreased oxygen saturation, or decreased level of consciousness.	Continued monitoring is necessary. Reversal agent may be administered if physiological signs continue to decline.
➤ Hematoma or hemorrhage is present at catheter insertion site.	May indicate presence of abnormal coagulation, local trauma, or inadequate pressure being maintained over puncture site.
➤ Client experiences flushing, itching, and urticaria.	Signifies possible allergic reaction to dye.
➤ Test results are not within normal limits.	Indicates abnormal processes, such as obstruction, stricture, aneurysm, tumor, occlusion, or congenital malformation of heart or arteries.
➤ Client experiences the following complications:	
• Cardiac dysrhythmias	Related to conduction disorders induced by catheter or dye.
• Infection/sepsis	Lack of surgical asepsis during procedure may result in local infection or widespread sepsis.

Recording and Reporting

1. Record client's status on return to nursing unit: vital signs, status of pulses, condition of puncture site, presence of dressing, condition of IV site, and client's level of responsiveness.	Documents client's response to invasive sedation.
2. Nurses who monitored IVCS record vital signs, O_2 saturation, airway status, and level of consciousness.	Documents physiological responses to sedation.
3. Record type of dressing and amount and type of drainage; record presence of pain or discomfort.	Provides baseline data for determining client's progress.
4. Report to physician immediately:	
a. Changes in vital signs beyond normal limits for client.	May indicate hypovolemic shock or allergic reaction to dye.
b. Excessive bleeding or increasing hematoma at catheter insertion site.	May indicate trauma to blood vessels or coagulation abnormality.
c. Decreased or absent peripheral pulses.	May indicate thrombus or embolus formation.
d. Altered neurological status; dysrhythmias.	May indicate embolus to brain; conduction disorder.
e. Decreased oxygen saturation or decreased responsiveness after sedation.	May require sedative reversal.
5. Report to nurses on next shift all relevant physiologic data, status of puncture site and dressing.	Ensures continuity of care.

Follow-up Activities

1. Maintain bed rest for 6 to 8 hours or as ordered.
2. Monitor vital signs and peripheral pulses every 15 to 30 minutes for 2 to 3 hours, then every hour for 4 hours, or as ordered. A Doppler may be needed on those clients who do not have strong peripheral pulses. When delegating assessment of vital signs to unlicensed personnel, stress the importance of reporting any changes immediately.
3. Administer analgesics as ordered.
4. Check for bleeding, swelling, or discoloration at catheter site every 30 minutes for 2 to 3 hours, then as ordered. Monitor client for complications.

BARNES

POST-CARDIAC CATHETERIZATION ORDERS
FORM #234A

A-17

1. Notify intern/resident or house physician that patient has returned from the cardiac cath lab.

2. Cardiac catheterization performed by *(please check)*:
   ☐ RFA ☐ RFV
   ☐ LFA ☐ LFV

3. Record blood pressure and heart rate every 15 minutes x 4, every 30 minutes x 2, every 1 hour x 2, then every 4 hours x 24 hours if patient stable, then evey shift.

4. Call house physician stat for: HR > 100 ________ or < 50 ________ bpm.
   sBP > 160 ________ or < 100 ________ mmHg.

5. Mark pedal pulses distal to cardiac cath site. Monitor ☐ Rt. ☐ Lt. groin puncture site and distal pedal pulses every 15 minutes x 4, every 30 minutes x 2, every 1 hour x 2, then every 4 hours x 24 hours if patient stable.

6. Report bleeding, swelling or pain at groin puncture site or reduction or loss of distal pedal pulses to house physician and on-call cardiac cath fellow.

7. Record I & O every 8 hours for 24 hours. Notify house physician if urine output is less than 400cc in 8 hours.

8. Patients with femoral sheaths sutured in place should remain at strict bedrest with HOB < 30° and cath leg straight until sheaths removed by the cardiac cath fellow.

9. For patients with femoral sheaths removed:
   a. Patient to remain at strict bedrest for 6 hours or ________ hours after return from cath lab.
   b. The HOB may be raised to 30° one hour after return from cath lab, if there is no bleeding at puncture site and vital signs are stable.
   c. RN to remove sandbag 4 hours after return from cath lab.
   d. When period of strict bedrest is over, RN to remove groin dressing and observe puncture site for bleeding or swelling.
   e. When groin dressing removed assess puncture site and distal pedal pulse every 2 hours x 2, every 4 hours x 2, every shift for 24 hours, then daily.
   f. If bleeding or oozing noted at puncture site apply firm pressure and call the on-call cardiac cath fellow.
   g. If groin puncture site intact patient may sit at side of bed and ambulate to bathroom with assistance. Apply bandaid to site and change daily for two days.
   h. In AM patient may resume pre-cath activity level if vital signs stable and there is no bleeding or swelling at groin puncture site.

10. Orthopedic bedpan for female patients as needed while at bedrest.

11. Straight cath PRN if patient unable to urinate within 4-8 hours following cardiac cath.

12. Diet post-cardiac cath:
    a. Clear liquids for first hour if patient alert and free from nausea.
    b. Resume previous diet after one hour if patient fully awake and free from nausea, vital signs stable, and groin puncture site intact.

13. Medications post-cardiac cath:
    a. Acetaminophen 300mg and codeine 30mg (acet/codeine #3 tabs) 1 or 2 tablets po every 4 hours PRN for pain at puncture site, back pain, or headache.
    b. If allergic to codeine substitute Darvocet N-100 1 tablet po every 4 hours PRN.
    c. Tigan suppository 200mg for nausea and/or vomiting (stat dose only).
    d. Resume previous oral medications when vital signs stable and patient free from nausea.

14. IV medications post-cardiac cath *(check and fill in blanks)*:
    a. ☐ Heparin 25,000u/250ml 1/2 NS to be resumed at (time) ______ on (date) ______ at ______ U/hr. Avoid heparin boluses for at least 12 hours following cardiac cath.
    b. ☐ Nitroglycerin 50mg/250ml D5W at ______ mcg/min, titrate for sBP > ______ or < ______ mmHg. Wean nitroglycerin off after ______ hours.

15. Post-cardiac cath IV fluids:
    Start 1L NS or ____________ at ____________ ml/hr,
    then 1L NS or ____________ at ____________ ml/hr,
    then 1L NS or ____________ at KVO.

16. In AM: *(check one)* ☐ discontinue post-cath IVFs and resume pre-cath IVFs or
    ☐ replace with saline lock (flush each shift).

17. AM labs:____

18. For chest discomfort/anginal equivalent, shortness of breath, nausea/vomiting, or hypotension obtain a stat ECG and contact the house physician and on-call cardiac cath fellow STAT.

19. For acute cardiac problems or puncture site bleeding contact the cardiology fellow (Dr.______________ Pager:________) or the cardiac cath lab (2-9300). At night contact the on-call cardiology fellow in the CCU (2-5096) or the on-call cardiac cath fellow (2-2284).

20. No patient should be discharged until a note in the chart indicates that the patient's groin puncture site has been examined by the cardiac cath fellow.

21. If patient is to be discharged the morning after cardiac cath, give patient a copy of "Barnes Hospital Nursing Service Cardiac Catheterization Discharge Instructions".

22. Other orders:____

MD: ____________________

Fig. 44-1 Postcardiac catheterization (coronary angiography) patient discharge orders. (Courtesy Barnes-Jewish Hospital, St Louis.)

Continued

BARNES HOSPITAL CARDIAC CATHETERIZATION
DISCHARGE INSTRUCTIONS

C-51

The following information is intended to serve as a guide to assist with your care after discharge following cardiac catheterization.

1. Resume your normal diet immediately, unless directed otherwise by your physician.
2. It is important to limit activity of the limb site used for the catheterization for **3 days.*** This includes, but is not limited to activities such as aerobics, swimming, jogging or running, bicycling, bowling, dancing, rowing, stair-stepping. If you are involved in activities not listed above, please ask your nurse or physician for specific instructions.
3. Avoid lifting for **2 days.***
4. Gentle walking is permissible but only on level ground.
5. No driving for **2 days.***
6. Restrict stair-climbing for **2 days,** if possible. If stair-climbing is essential, climb with your non-catheterized leg, then bring the catheterized leg up to the same step.*
7. Customary sexual activity may be resumed after **2 days.** Use postures that do not place a strain on the catheterized leg.*
8. Avoid straining for bowel movements for **7 days.** If you tend to be constipated and/or regularly strain to pass stool, please inform your nurse of this so that a stool softening medication can be ordered.
9. It is common to have some bruising or purple discoloration of the skin near the puncture site.

***(If you have received an angioplasty, atherectomy, laser, rotoblator or stent procedure extend activity restrictions to 7 days.)**

However, if any of the following occur, immediately contact your own physician, or the Barnes Hospital Emergency Department at **(314) 362-9123.**

a. Bleeding from the catheterization puncture site: apply gentle pressure with a clean gauze or cloth and call your physician or the Barnes Hospital Emergency Room immediately.
b. If a knot or lump under the skin increases in size or,
c. If bruising appears to be worsening or tracking/moving down the leg rather than disappearing.
d. If you have pain at the puncture site or in the leg used for the catheterization.
e. If the leg used for the catheterization appears pale in color and/or feels cooler to touch compared to the opposite leg.
f. If the leg used for the catheterization appears reddened, swollen and/or feels warmer to touch compared to the opposite leg.

10. You may bathe or shower the day following the catheterization. Be careful to avoid slipping as your leg may feel stiff.
11. Resume the same medications you were taking before the catheterization unless otherwise ordered by your physician.
12. If you have any questions or concerns, contact your private physician or call the Barnes Hospital Emergency Department.

My discharge instructions have been explained and a copy has been given to me.

____
Physician's Signature/Date and Time

____
Patient/Significant Other/Signature Date and Time

____
Nurse's Signature/Date and Time

White copy (place in chart)

Yellow copy (patient's copy)

1290-21 Revised 12/94

Fig. 44-1, cont'd Postcardiac catheterization (coronary angiography) patient discharge orders. (Courtesy Barnes-Jewish Hospital, St. Louis.)

STEPS **RATIONALE**

5. Keep the affected extremity extended and immobilized. (Sandbags may be used to apply pressure over puncture site.)
6. Elevate head of bed no more than 30 degrees if femoral artery is punctured.
7. Encourage fluids (unless contraindicated) to maintain hydration and assess output. Dehydration may be caused by the diuretic action of the dye (Pagana and Pagana, 1995).
8. Use orthopedic bedpan for female client as needed while on bed rest.
9. Obtain laboratory data for interpretation by nurse and physician.

• • • • •

Special Considerations

- The procedures are usually elective but may be done on an emergency basis in the event of sudden occlusion of an artery or in the case of myocardial infarction.

Teaching Considerations

- Explain to client that during the procedure, lying in one position for 1 to 3 hours is expected.
- If IVCS is to be used, explain to client purpose and expected effects of sedation and postprocedure instructions regarding client's care and necessary precautions.
- Explain that the client might experience a feeling of falling when the table is rotated from side to side.
- Explain the necessity of bed rest and immobility following the procedure.
- Explain that after the procedure the client's vital signs will be taken and the puncture site will be inspected at frequent intervals.
- Some clients may experience difficulty urinating in a supine position and may require measures that stimulate voiding.
- Encourage client to check with physician regarding test results.
- Some institutions provide written discharge instructions (Fig. 44-1).

Pediatric Considerations

- Increased sedation in children may be necessary.

Gerontologic Considerations

- Since frail older adults may be more susceptible to skin breakdown from lying in one position during this procedure, inspect bony prominences frequently.
- In the older adult, slight alterations in vital signs or behavior may be precursors to impending problems; therefore skilled observations are critical (Phipps et al., 1995).
- Older adult clients may have reduced drug clearance from decreased glomerular filtration rate (GFR) and nephron activity or decreased hepatic function. Therefore the nurse must monitor the effects of narcotics and hypnotics that may interfere with breathing (Phipps et al., 1995).
- Because of the normal aging process, an older adult is at risk for skin breakdown and joint stiffness. The client may require assistance with frequent position changes.
- Offer bedpan/urinal every 2 to 3 hours in the older adult client because of age-related changes in the urinary tract.
- Be aware that NPO status in the older adult client may result in dehydration.
- Because of multiple medications the older adult client may be taking, be aware of alterations in administration schedules necessary due to NPO status for diagnostic test.

Home Care Considerations

- Upon discharge, client will be instructed to contact the physician (or affiliated emergency department) if the following occurs after cardiac catheterization:
  - Bleeding from the catheterization puncture site; apply gentle pressure with a clean gauze or cloth.
  - Formation of a knot or lump under the skin that increases in size.
  - Worsening of a bruise or its movement down the extremity rather than disappearing.
  - Pain at puncture site or in the extremity used for the catheterization.
  - Extremity where arterial puncture is made becomes pale and cool to touch.
  - Appearance of reddness, swelling, or warmth of the affected extremity.
- Although bathing or showering may be allowed the day after the catheterization, the client should be cautioned to avoid slipping, as the leg (if this extremity was used) may feel stiff.

SKILL 44-3 Assisting with Bone Marrow Aspiration/Biopsy

Bone marrow aspiration is the removal of a small amount of the liquid organic material in the **medullary** canals of selected bones, in particular the sternum and the posterior superior iliac crests (Fig. 44-2). In children, the proximal tibia may be used (Pagana and Pagana, 1995). A **biopsy** is the removal of a core of marrow cells for laboratory analysis. Both aspiration and biopsy are used to diagnose leukemias and other malignancies, anemias, and **thrombocytopenia.** The marrow is examined in a laboratory to reveal the number, size, shape, and development of red blood cells (RBCs) and **megakaryocytes** (platelet precursors).

The sterile procedure is usually performed by a physician assisted by a nurse or unlicensed assistive personnel at the client's bedside and takes approximately 20 minutes.

Potential complications of bone marrow aspiration or biopsy are bleeding, especially if a **coagulopathy** is present, infection, and less commonly, organ puncture. The nurse should know normal hematological laboratory values before assisting with the procedure.

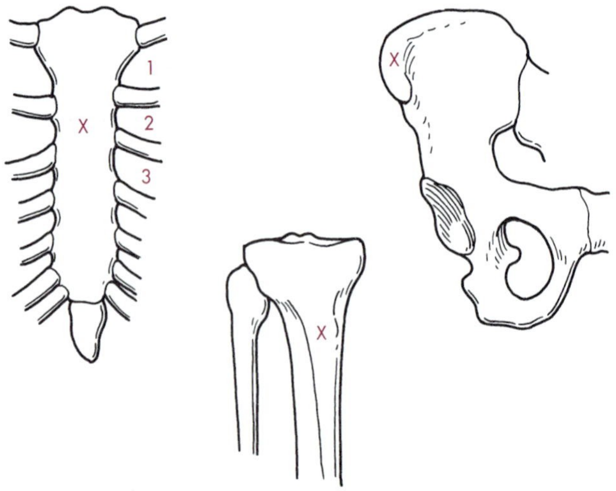

Fig. 44-2 Sites for bone marrow aspiration: sternum, iliac crest (most common), and tibia. (From Phipps WJ et al, editors: *Medical-surgical nursing: concepts and clinical practice,* ed 5, St Louis, 1995, Mosby.)

EQUIPMENT

- Antiseptic solution
- Bone marrow aspiration tray, if available from central supply, which may include:
  - Antiseptic solution (e.g., povidone-iodine)
  - Gauze sponges (4 × 4)
  - Sterile towels for draping
  - Local anesthetic solution (e.g., lidocaine 1%)
  - Sterile syringes: two 3-ml, 23- to 25-gauge needles for anesthetic; two 10- and 50-ml for marrow aspiration
  - Two bone marrow needles with inner stylus
- Test tubes and/or glass slides
- Sterile gloves of proper size for physician
- Masks, goggles, and gowns for physician and nurse (check institution's policy)
- Gauze 2 × 2, tape, and antiseptic ointment
- Pain medication if ordered (given 30 minutes before procedure)

STEPS	RATIONALE
ASSESSMENT	
1. Assess client's knowledge of procedure; observe verbal and nonverbal behaviors.	Determines level of understanding and client's anxiety.
CRITICAL DECISION POINT Obtain a premedication order (i.e., sedative) if client is extremely anxious.	
2. Assess client's ability to assume position required for procedure and ability to remain still.	Required position depends on site used for bone marrow aspiration (e.g., sternum, tibia, or anterior iliac spine—use supine position; posterior iliac spine or iliac crest—use prone or lateral position). Client must maintain position without moving to avoid complications.
CRITICAL DECISION POINT This procedure may be contraindicated in clients who cannot cooperate or remain still during the procedure (Pagana and Pagana, 1995).	
3. Assess vital signs.	Provides baseline for comparison with postprocedure vital signs.

STEPS	RATIONALE
4. Assess client's coagulation status: use of anticoagulants, platelet count, prothrombin time.	Factors that can increase risk of bleeding put client at risk. However, test is performed to diagnose coagulation alterations.
5. Determine purpose of procedure.	Allows nurse to determine whether aspiration or biopsy will be performed to anticipate laboratory requisitions.
6. Check whether client has signed a consent form.	Documents that client has consented to procedure; this reduces institution's legal risk.
7. Determine whether client is allergic to antiseptic or anesthetic solutions.	Decreases chance of allergic reactions.

NURSING DIAGNOSIS

Clustering of defining characteristics from the assessment data may reveal the following nursing diagnoses for clients requiring this skill:

- Anxiety
- Fear
- Knowledge deficit regarding purpose and steps of procedure
- Pain
- Risk for infection
- Risk for injury

Related factors are individualized based on a client's condition or needs.

PLANNING

STEPS	RATIONALE
1. **Expected outcomes** following completion of procedure:	
➤ Client can assume position and has little pain.	Client tolerates procedure well.
➤ Client has no bleeding at needle insertion site.	Precautions during procedure prevent bleeding.
➤ Amount of aspirate is sufficient to perform laboratory testing.	
➤ Client explains steps of procedure and position to be assumed.	Documents learning.
2. Explain steps of skin preparation, anesthetic injection, needle insertion, and position required.	Anticipation of expected sensations and procedural activities reduces anxiety.

IMPLEMENTATION

Nurse's Responsibility

STEPS	RATIONALE
1. Wash hands.	Reduces transmission of microorganisms.
2. Set up sterile tray or open supplies to make accessible for physician.	Maintains integrity of sterile field and promotes prompt completion of procedure.
3. Assist client in maintaining correct position (see Assessment, step 2). Reassure client while explaining procedure.	Decreases chance of complications occurring during procedure. Explanations increase client comfort and relaxation.

CRITICAL DECISION POINT **Emphasize to client to remain very still and avoid sudden movement throughout the procedure.**

STEPS	RATIONALE
4. Assess client's condition during procedure, including respiratory status and vital signs if indicated.	Identifies any changes that may indicate complication.
5. Note characteristics of bone marrow aspirate (e.g., amount, color).	Characteristics are used for observation, reporting, and recording.

Physician's Responsibility

STEPS	RATIONALE
1. Wash hands.	Reduces transmission of microorganisms.
2. Select site to be used for bone marrow aspiration.	Sites are chosen for direct access to area of spongy bone. These sites include anterior and posterior iliac spines, iliac crest, body of sternum, and tibia.
3. Apply sterile gloves. Disinfect skin with antiseptic solution and 4 × 4 gauze sponges. Remove gloves and discard.	Removes surface bacteria from skin at area of puncture site.

STEPS	RATIONALE
4. Apply sterile mask and goggles, then new pair of sterile gloves, and drape client with sterile towels.	Maintains surgical asepsis.
5. Inject local anesthetic and allow it to take effect.	Provides optimal effect of anesthesia at time of bone marrow aspiration.
6. Insert bone marrow needle (see illustration) with inner stylus into bone, then advance needle until it reaches area of spongy bone and remove stylus.	Stylus is stiff and has longer bevel to enter bone with more ease. Spongy bone is location of bone marrow.
7. Attach 10-ml syringe to needle and aspirate bone marrow. For biopsy, screw the core biopsy instrument into the bone and remove plug of tissue.	Amount aspirated is determined by purpose of procedure: small amount (approximately 0.5 to 2.0 ml) is obtained for laboratory test; larger amount, including cells, is obtained by biopsy.
8. Remove needle or biopsy instrument and apply pressure to puncture site. Apply antiseptic ointment and dressing.	Prevents bleeding from puncture site. Antiseptic ointment reduces bacterial growth at puncture site.
9. Place the specimen on glass slides or in test tubes.	Allows specimen to be sent for laboratory analysis.

EVALUATION

STEPS	RATIONALE
1. Monitor vital signs. Check hospital policy; may be as often as every 15 minutes for 2 hours.	Verifies client's physiological status in response to potential blood loss.
2. Inspect dressing over puncture site.	Determines further blood loss from puncture site.
CRITICAL DECISION POINT A pressure dressing may be in place. If so, do not remove.	
3. Observe client's level of comfort.	Client may require postprocedure analgesia.
4. Unexpected outcomes that may occur include:	
➤ Client is unable to assume correct position; moves during procedure.	May contraindicate continuing procedure; untoward reaction or complication may occur.
➤ Tenderness, erythema, decreased blood pressure, and increased pulse indicate complications of procedure.	May indicate infection at site or shock (Pagana and Pagana, 1995).
➤ Client is unable to discuss procedure.	Documents need for more education or explanation during procedure.

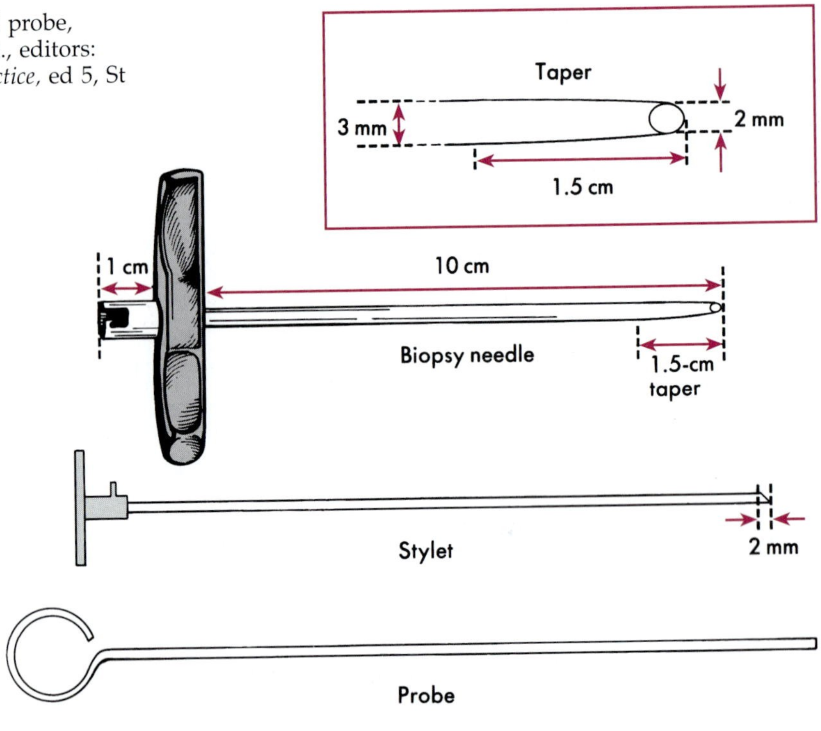

Step 6 Bone marrow biopsy needle stylet, and probe, showing shape and size. (From Phipps WJ et al., editors: *Medical-surgical nursing: concepts and clinical practice,* ed 5, St Louis, 1995, Mosby.)

STEPS	RATIONALE
RECORDING AND REPORTING	
1. Record in client's chart:	
a. Name of procedure, location of puncture site, amount and color of marrow aspirated, duration of procedure, and client's tolerance to the procedure.	Accurate recording of procedure is legal necessity.
b. Vital signs, pain, and complications.	Provides ongoing assessment of client's tolerance to procedure.
c. Laboratory tests ordered and specimen sent.	Documents that specimen was obtained and to which laboratory it was delivered.
d. Type of dressing over puncture site and whether drainage is present.	Provides baseline data for monitoring amount of blood loss and drainage from puncture site.
2. Report to physician immediately:	
a. Change in vital signs beyond client's normal limits.	Could indicate possible complications such as organ puncture or bleeding.
b. Excessive drainage from dressing over puncture site.	Could indicate postprocedure bleeding or localized infection at puncture site.
3. Report results of procedure to nurses on the next shift.	Ensures continuity of care.

FOLLOW-UP ACTIVITIES

1. Assess puncture site for swelling, tenderness, and/or erythema.
2. Assist client in assuming comfortable position in bed.
3. Apply gloves. Clean up area, and discard or send supplies to proper sterilization department. Label and send specimens to laboratory.
4. Obtain laboratory data for interpretation.

• • • • •

Special Considerations

- If client experiences respiratory distress when supine or prone, physician may elect to perform aspiration in semi-Fowler's position.
- When client is uncooperative, procedure may need to be performed in OR or with IVCS.
- Masks are used with **immunocompromised** clients, including those receiving cancer chemotherapy or high-dose steroid therapy.
- Complications are rare but include sternal puncture, heart and lung puncture, iliac crest or spine puncture, and bowel puncture.

Teaching Considerations

- After explaining this procedure, encourage client to verbalize concerns. Many clients are anxious about procedure.
- Emphasize importance of remaining still during procedure.
- Encourage client to contact physician regarding test results.

Pediatric Considerations

- Very young children may receive a general anesthetic for this procedure.
- Allow child to practice procedure beforehand, using doll as a model (Broome et al., 1992).

Gerontologic Considerations

- Older adults with arthritis may have difficulty sustaining the position required for the procedure.

Home Care Considerations

- Instruct client that some clients experience tenderness at the puncture site for several days after this study and that mild analgesia may be ordered by the physician.

SKILL 44-4 Assisting with Bronchoscopy

Bronchoscopy is the examination of the **tracheobronchial tree** through a lighted tube containing mirrors. The tube, or bronchoscope, most commonly used is a flexible **fiberoptic** bronchoscope. The fiberoptic bronchoscope has **lumens** for visualization and for obtaining sputum, foreign bodies, and biopsy specimens. Laser ablation of endotracheal lesions may be performed through the bronchoscope.

Bronchoscopy may be an emergency or elective procedure and is performed for diagnostic or therapeutic reasons. The main purposes of this procedure are to aspirate excessive sputum or mucous plugs that cannot be sufficiently suctioned nasotracheally and to visualize the tracheobronchial tree for assessment of abnormalities of the mucosa. Routine bronchoscopy should be avoided in poorly cooperative clients (Silver and Balk, 1995). This procedure would be contraindicated in clients who could not be adequately oxygenated or ventilated, as well as those experiencing angina, status asthmaticus, severe pulmonary hypertension, coagulopathy, or thrombocytopenia (Pagana and Pagana, 1995; Silver and Balk, 1995). Complications of bronchoscopy may include fever, hypoxemia, laryngospasm, pneumothorax, aspiration, and hemorrhage (after biopsy). The nurse should be able to perform nasotracheal and orotracheal suctioning before assisting with the procedure.

This procedure is usually performed by a specially trained physician and assisted by specially trained health professionals in a designated bronchoscopy room for inpatients or outpatients who are not critically ill (Shrake, 1993). The procedure may also be performed in the intensive care unit, operating room, outpatient facility, or other appropriate clinical area (Shrake, 1993).

EQUIPMENT

- Antiseptic solution for hand washing
- Bronchoscopy tray, if available from central supply, which may include:
  - Flexible fiberoptic bronchoscope (Fig. 44-3)
  - Gauze sponges (4 × 4)
  - Local anesthetic spray (lidocaine)
  - Sterile tracheal suction catheters (see Chapter 14)
  - Diazepam, midazolam, or other sedative for IV sedation
  - Oxygen, resuscitative equipment, pulse oximeter, cardiac monitor for IV sedation
  - Sterile gloves
  - Sterile water-soluble lubricating jelly

CRITICAL DECISION POINT Petroleum-based lubricants should not be used because of hazard of aspiration and subsequent pneumonia.

- Mask and goggles for physician and nurse (check institutional policy)
- Emesis basin
- Oxygen equipment

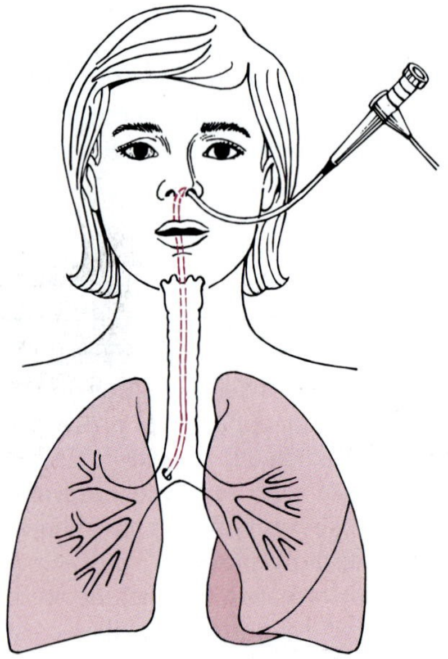

Fig. 44-3 Bronchoscope inserted through nose into trachea and to bronchus.

STEPS	RATIONALE
ASSESSMENT	
1. Assess client's knowledge of procedure; observe verbal and nonverbal behaviors.	Determines client's level of understanding and anxiety.
CRITICAL DECISION POINT Since client may fear the diagnosis that may follow, allow client to verbalize feelings and concerns regarding this procedure.	
2. Assess vital signs.	Baseline data provides for comparison with findings during and after procedure.

STEPS	RATIONALE
3. Assess respiratory status: type of cough, sputum produced, and lung sounds.	Provides for comparison with respiratory status during and after procedure.
4. Determine purpose of procedure: for sputum aspiration, for assessment, for tissue biopsy, or for removal of foreign body.	Enables nurse to anticipate needs of client and physician.
5. Check whether client signed a consent form (check institution's policy). This must be done before administration of preprocedural sedative or IVCS.	Allows client to make an informed decision regarding the procedure.
6. Determine whether client is allergic to local anesthetic used for spraying throat (lidocaine usually used).	Allergy could cause laryngeal edema or laryngospasm.
7. Assess need for preprocedure medication (usually atropine and narcotic or sedative).	Atropine decreases secretions and inhibits vagal stimulation (which induces bradycardia); narcotics or sedatives relieve anxiety and decrease discomfort.
8. If using IVCS, assess pulse and respiratory rate, blood pressure, and oxygen saturation before administration of IVCS.	Provides baseline data.
9. Assess time client last ingested food. Client should have been NPO for 8 hours before procedure.	Reduces risk of aspiration.

NURSING DIAGNOSIS

Clustering of defining characteristics from the assessment data may reveal the following nursing diagnoses for clients requiring this skill:

- Anxiety
- Fear
- Impaired gas exchange
- Ineffective breathing pattern
- Knowledge deficit regarding purpose and steps of procedure
- Risk for aspiration
- Risk for infection
- Risk for injury

Related factors are individualized based on a client's condition or needs.

PLANNING

1. **Expected outcomes** following completion of procedure:	
➤ Client has no respiratory complications.	Client tolerates procedure well.
➤ Client has minimal pain.	Minimal trauma caused by bronchoscope.
➤ Physician is able to observe, suction, and obtain specimens from tracheobronchial tree.	Indicates that purpose of procedure was achieved.
➤ Client recovers from sedation without respiratory complications or change in level of consciousness.	Sedation adequate.
➤ Client is able to describe procedure.	Demonstrates learning.
2. Explain procedure to client.	Reduces anxiety and increases cooperation.
3. Assist client in maintaining position desired by physician: semi-Fowler's or supine.	Provides maximal visualization of lower airways and adequate lung expansion.
4. Remove and safely store client's dentures.	Minimizes chance of airway obstruction.
5. Make sure client is NPO at least 8 hours before procedure.	Decreases risk of aspiration of gastric contents.

IMPLEMENTATION

Nurse's Responsibility

1. Instruct client not to swallow local anesthetic; provide emesis basin for expectoration of local anesthetic.	Anesthetic may be absorbed systemically and cause severe CNS and cardiovascular (CV) reactions.
2. Assist client through procedure with explanations.	Although premedicated and drowsy, clients need to be reminded not to change position and to cooperate.

STEPS	RATIONALE
3. Assess client's respiratory status during procedure: observe degree of restlessness and respiratory rate; observe capillary refill and color of nail beds.	Bronchoscope may cause feelings of suffocation; in addition, because airway is partially occluded, client may become hypoxic during observations.
➤ ***CRITICAL DECISION POINT*** **If needed, oxygen may be administered through bronchoscope.**	
4. Note characteristics of suctioned material.	Information used to record and report and to make further client observations.
➤ ***CRITICAL DECISION POINT*** **Small amount of bleeding in suctioned material is expected because of tissue trauma.**	
5. Using gloved hand, wipe client's mouth and nose to remove lubricant after bronchoscope is removed.	Promotes hygiene and comfort.
6. Do not allow client to eat or drink until the tracheobronchial anesthesia has worn off and gag reflex has returned, usually 2 hours. Use tongue depressor to touch pharynx to test for presence of gag reflex.	Prevents aspiration.
Physician's Responsibility	
1. Wash hands.	Reduces transmission of microorganisms.
2. Spray nasopharynx and oropharynx with topical anesthetic. Lidocaine is commonly used for throat spraying. Anesthetic spray is not needed with intubated spray.	Throat is sprayed early for anesthesia to take effect.
3. Attach bronchoscope to machine for light source.	Another physician, OR personnel, or nurse attaches machine cable to bronchoscope.
4. Apply goggles, mask, and sterile gloves; then introduce bronchoscope into mouth to pharynx, and pass through glottis. May use more anesthetic spray at glottis to prevent cough reflex. Pass tube into trachea and bronchi.	Bronchoscope must be passed through upper airway structures to promote visualization of lower airways. Trachea and bronchi are observed for lesions and obstructions. For intubated client, bronchoscope is passed through endotracheal tube. Adaptor accompanies bronchoscope and may be used for Ambu bag or ventilator use.
5. Obtain cytological specimens with wire brush or curette.	Cytological specimens are obtained to diagnose carcinoma.
EVALUATION	
1. Monitor vital signs.	Verifies physiological response.
2. Observe character and amount of sputum.	Sputum may be blood tinged, which indicates superficial tissue damage. Severe hemoptysis is emergency.
3. Observe respiratory status closely.	May provide evidence of laryngeal bronchospasm.
4. Assess for level of sedation and level of consciousness.	Determines client's response to IVCS.
5. Assess for return of gag reflex.	Reflex return allows client to resume eating and drinking.
6. Ask client to describe postprocedure normal and abnormal symptoms.	Evaluates learning.
7. **Unexpected outcomes** that may occur include:	
➤ Laryngospasm and bronchospasm indicated by sudden, severe shortness of breath.	Constriction of large airways is response to laryngeal or bronchial irritation from bronchoscope or topical anesthetic.
➤ Hypoxemia indicated by gradual shortness of breath and decreasing level of consciousness.	Hypoxemia is caused by occlusion of airways resulting from mucous plug or bronchoscope.
➤ Hemorrhage occurs.	Result of trauma to pulmonary vasculature or trachea.

STEPS	RATIONALE
➤ Client remains sedated with decreased respiration or blood pressure, decreased oxygen saturation, or decreased level of consciousness.	Continued monitoring is necessary. May require administration of narcotic reversal agent.

Recording and Reporting

1. Record in nurse's notes name of procedure (include biopsy if performed), duration of procedure, client's tolerance of procedure and complications, and collection and disposition of specimen.	Accurate recording of procedure is legal necessity. Ensures continuity of care.
2. Report to physician immediately:	
a. Excessive bleeding or respiratory difficulty after procedure.	May indicate tracheal perforation.
b. Changes in vital signs beyond client's normal limits.	May indicate signs of hypoxia.
3. Report results of procedure to nurses on the next shift.	Ensures continuity of care.

Follow-up Activities

1. Apply gloves. Label and send biopsy or other specimens to laboratory.
2. Clean up area and send supplies to proper sterilization area.
3. Assist client in assuming comfortable position in bed.
4. Obtain laboratory data for interpretation.
5. If bronchoscopy is performed on an outpatient basis, client is kept in the department until gag reflex returns and client is able to swallow water easily (Phipps et al., 1995).

• • • • •

Special Considerations

- After bronchoscopy, physician may order serial sputum collections for 24 hours for cytological examination.
- Make sure client knows not to eat or drink until gag reflex returns. Before return of reflex, client could aspirate food or fluids, resulting in chemical pneumonitis.

Teaching Considerations

- After thoroughly explaining procedure, assure that client will be able to breathe during procedure.
- If IVCS is to be used, explain to client purpose and expected effects of sedation and postprocedure instructions regarding client's care and necessary precautions.
- Inform client that a sore throat may be relieved by using warm saline gargles and throat lozenges.
- Instruct client how to perform controlled coughing techniques for obtaining sputum samples, if ordered (see Chapter 43).
- Encourage client to be involved in self-care by contacting physician regarding test results.

Pediatric Considerations

- In children, the procedure is most frequently performed to remove foreign bodies from larynx or trachea and is often done under general anesthesia. Client is placed in the lateral position after the procedure to prevent aspiration.

Gerontologic Considerations

- Be aware that NPO status in the older adult client may result in dehydration.
- Because of multiple medications the older adult client may be taking, be aware of alterations in administration schedules necessary due to NPO status for diagnostic test.

Home Care Considerations

- Outpatients should be instructed to notify the physician if the following symptoms develop: fever, chest pain or discomfort, dyspnea, wheezing, or hemoptysis (Shrake, 1993).
- Written instructions regarding names and phone numbers of persons to contact should reinforce oral instructions (Shrake, 1993).

SKILL 44-5 Assisting with Electrocardiogram

An electrocardiogram (ECG or EKG) is a graphic representation of the electrical impulses generated by the heart during the cardiac cycle. The electrical impulses are conducted to the body's surface, where they are detected by electrodes placed on the limbs and chest. The electrodes carry the electrical impulses to a continuously running graph that plots the ECG wave pattern. The appearance of the ECG pattern helps diagnose whether there are any abnormalities interfering with electrical conduction through the heart. The 12-lead ECG is composed of five electrodes. One electrode is placed on each of the four extremities, and one is successively placed at varying sites on the chest.

If continuous ECG recording is needed over an extended period of time, a Holter monitor is used. A Holter monitor is a small, portable device that records electrical activity of the heart for up to 24 hours. The ECG is recorded on magnetic tape and monitors cardiac rhythm during activity, rest, and sleep.

EQUIPMENT

- **ECG machine**
- **ECG leads or electrodes (self-stick adhesive)**
- **Electrode gel (optional)**
- **Alcohol wipes**
- **Razor**

STEPS	RATIONALE
ASSESSMENT	
1. Determine rationale for obtaining ECG.	ECG represents the electrical impulses during the cardiac cycle and may be done to determine baseline cardiac function (e.g., preoperative, prediagnostic testing) or when client experiences chest discomfort.
2. If client reports chest pain assess character of pain thoroughly.	Pain may be related to any number of factors (e.g., positioning, trauma, GI disturbance). Characteristics will help in determining therapy.
CRITICAL DECISION POINT Crushing substernal chest pain that radiates to jaw or arm may indicate angina or myocardial infarction. Chest pain should be brought to immediate attention of physician.	
3. Assess client's knowledge of procedure; observe verbal and nonverbal behaviors.	Identifies needed education and client's anxiety level.
CRITICAL DECISION POINT Assure the client that the flow of electric current is from the client and that nothing will be felt during the procedure (Pagana and Pagana, 1995).	
4. Obtain baseline vital signs.	Provides for comparison with vital sign data at later date.

NURSING DIAGNOSIS

Clustering of defining characteristics from the assessment data may reveal the following nursing diagnoses for clients requiring this skill:

- Anxiety
- Fear
- Knowledge deficit regarding purpose and steps of procedure

Related factors are individualized based on a client's condition or needs.

PLANNING

STEPS	RATIONALE
1. **Expected outcomes** following completion of procedure:	
➤ Client tolerates procedure without anxiety or discomfort.	Appropriate preparation decreases anxiety.
➤ Client discusses purpose and steps of procedure.	Demonstrates learning.

STEPS	RATIONALE
2. Close room door or bedside curtains.	Provides privacy.
3. Prepare client for procedure:	
a. Remove client's clothing or raise gown from waist up to expose only the client's chest and arms. Keep the abdomen and thighs covered.	Facilitates correct placement of cardiac leads and minimizes client's embarrassment.
b. Place client in supine position.	Exposes client for lead placement.
c. Instruct client to lie still without talking (12-lead ECG only) and to not cross legs.	Prevents recording of electrical artifacts caused by motion of chest wall.

IMPLEMENTATION

STEPS	RATIONALE
1. Wash hands.	Reduces transmission of microorganisms.
2. Cleanse and prepare skin; wipe sites with alcohol. It may be necessary to shave the chest if large amounts of hair are present.	Alcohol defats the skin and promotes adherence of leads (electrodes) to chest or extremity.
3. Apply self-sticking electrode and attach leads. (If self-sticking leads are not available, apply electrode paste to skin before attaching leads.) For 12-lead ECG:	Position of leads promotes proper display of ECG on paper.
a. Chest (**precordial** leads) (see illustration):	
(1) V_1—Fourth **intercostal space** (ICS) at right sternal border.	
(2) V_2—Fourth ICS at left sternal border.	
(3) V_3—Midway between V_2 and V_4.	
(4) V_4—Fifth ICS at midclavicular line.	
(5) V_5—Left anterior axillary line at level of V_4 horizontally.	
(6) V_6—Left midaxillary line at level of V_4 horizontally.	
b. Extremities: one on each extremity.	

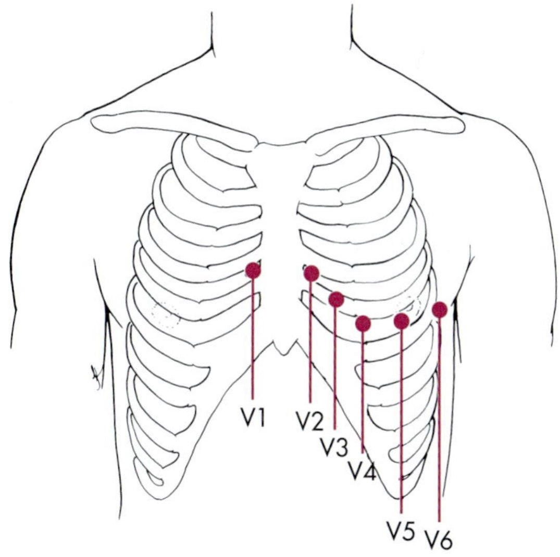

Step 3(a) Placement of chest leads for a 12-lead ECG. (From Phipps WJ et al, editors: *Medical-surgical nursing: concepts and clinical practice,* ed 5, St Louis, 1995, Mosby.)

STEPS	RATIONALE
4. Obtain tracing; 12-lead ECG may be obtained without removing precordial leads.	Transfers electrocardiac conduction on ECG tracing paper for subsequent analysis by cardiologist.
5. Disconnect leads, wipe excess electrode paste from chest, and wash hands.	Promotes comfort and hygiene. Reduces transmission of microorganisms.
6. Deliver ECG tracing to appropriate laboratory or heart station.	Provides for review of ECG by cardiologist.

EVALUATION

STEPS	RATIONALE
1. Although the procedure is painless, it is important to note and document if the client is experiencing any chest discomfort during the procedure.	Determines worsening of condition.
2. Measure vital signs.	Electrocardiac changes may result in vital sign alterations.
3. **Unexpected outcomes** that may occur include:	
➤ Client experiences chest pain (not result of test, but client's condition).	May be related to myocardial ischemia or anxiety.
➤ Client experiences anxiety.	Anxiety may be result of fears regarding test results.

STEPS | **RATIONALE**

RECORDING AND REPORTING

1. Record in nurse's notes when ECG was obtained (date and time) and where tracing was sent; rationale for obtaining ECG (e.g., pain, discomfort, preop, postop); and baseline vital signs. — Documents completion of test and complications.
2. Report any unexpected outcomes immediately. — Indicates whether there is need for prompt medical follow-up.

FOLLOW-UP ACTIVITIES

1. If client experiences severe chest pain, notify physician, continue to monitor cardiac activity with ECG, obtain vital signs, and remain with client.

• • • • •

Special Considerations

- If Holter monitoring is selected, client may require further explanation of how cardiac cycle is monitored.
- In clients who are very thin and emaciated, it may be difficult to secure electrodes because of the bony structure and decreased amount of subcutaneous tissue.

Teaching Considerations

- After explaining procedure, assure client that flow of electric current is from client to machine. Client will not feel anything during procedure.
- Encourage client to contact physician regarding test results.

Home Care Considerations

- If Holter monitoring is selected, instruct the client to maintain an accurate diary of activities (detailed documentation of activities and occurrence of chest pain assists in diagnoses of condition).

SKILL 44-6 Assisting with Endoscopy

Endoscopy is any study that allows direct visualization of an internal organ or structure by means of a long, flexible fiberoptic scope with a light source attached. For visualization of the upper GI tract, esophagoscopy, gastroscopy, or duodenoscopy is performed, or more frequently, esophagogastroduodenoscopy, which permits visualization of esophagus, stomach, and duodenum in one examination. For visual examination of the lower GI tract, a proctoscopy, sigmoidoscopy, or colonoscopy may be performed. Typically, these clients receive IVCS.

Endoscopy of the upper GI tract is indicated to diagnose lesions such as gastric or duodenal ulcers and neoplasms, to locate sources of upper GI bleeding, to study upper GI bleeding, to study upper GI motility and identify strictures and obstructions, and to diagnose hiatal hernias and esophageal and gastric **varices.** Both upper and lower GI endoscopic examinations are performed in a specially equipped endoscopic unit.

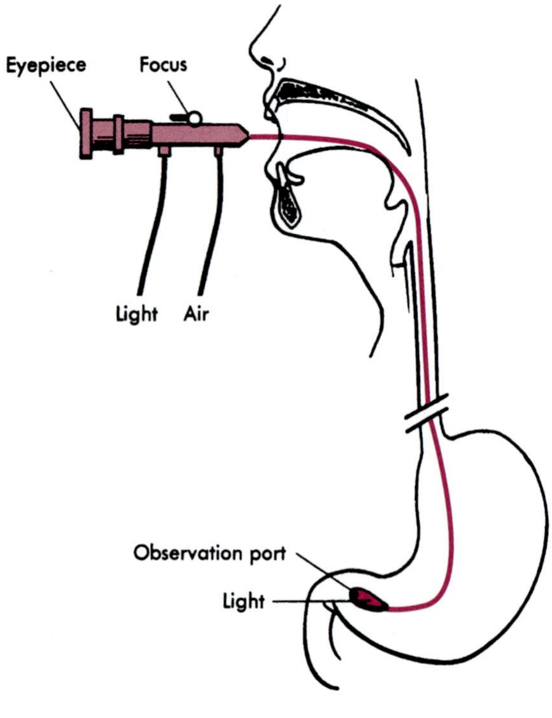

Fig. 44-4 Stomach may be visualized by means of a fiberscope. (From Phipps WJ et al, editors: *Medical-surgical nursing: concepts and clinical practice,* ed 5, St Louis, 1995, Mosby.)

EQUIPMENT

- Antiseptic solution for hand washing
- Endoscopy tray
- Fiberoptic endoscope (Fig. 44-4)
- Camera
- Solutions for biopsied specimens
- Local anesthetic spray
- Tracheal suction equipment (see Chapter 14)
- Blood pressure equipment
- Sterile water-soluble jelly
- Sterile gloves for physician
- Emesis basin
- Intravenous fluid and equipment for IV start (optional)
- Diazepam, midazolam, or other sedative for IV sedation (optional)
- Oxygen, resuscitative equipment, pulse oximeter, cardiac monitor if IVCS is used
- Mask
- Gown
- Gloves
- Goggles

STEPS	RATIONALE
ASSESSMENT	
1. Assess client's knowledge of procedure; observe verbal and nonverbal behaviors.	Determines client's understanding and level of anxiety.
2. Determine if GI bleeding is present. Observe character of emesis, stool, and nasogastric tube drainage.	Test is contraindicated in clients with severe upper GI bleeding, because viewing lens may get covered with blood clots, preventing visualization.
➤ **CRITICAL DECISION POINT** If client is actively bleeding, physician may order stomach be lavaged and aspirated clear of clots before procedure is attempted.	
3. Determine purpose of procedure: biopsy, examination, or coagulation of bleeding sites.	Enables nurse to anticipate equipment needs.
4. Check for completion of signed consent form (check institutional policy).	Invasive procedures require consent form.
5. Verify that client has been NPO for at least 8 hours for endoscopy of upper GI tract.	Introduction of endoscope can induce vomiting. Empty stomach reduces risk of aspiration of stomach contents.
➤ **CRITICAL DECISION POINT** If endoscopy of the upper GI tract is an emergency procedure and client has had something to eat or drink, be sure physician is informed first.	
6. Assess pulse and respiratory rate, blood pressure, and oxygen saturation before administration of IVCS.	Provides baseline data.
7. Verify that client does not have esophageal diverticulum.	Esophageal diverticulum is contraindication to endoscopy because scope can easily fall into diverticulum and perforate its wall.
8. Review physician's orders for preprocedure medication and IVCS.	
a. Diazepam	Decreases anxiety and promotes muscle relaxation.
b. Morphine	Decreases pain and induces sedation.
c. Midazolam (given in endoscopy unit just before examination)	Produces amnesic effect; diminishes recall of events during procedure.

NURSING DIAGNOSIS

Clustering of defining characteristics from the assessment data may reveal the following nursing diagnoses for clients requiring this skill:

- ➤ Anxiety
- ➤ Fear
- ➤ Impaired gas exchange
- ➤ Ineffective breathing pattern
- ➤ Knowledge deficit regarding purpose and steps of procedure
- ➤ Pain
- ➤ Risk for aspiration
- ➤ Risk for infection
- ➤ Risk for injury

Related factors are individualized based on a client's condition or needs.

STEPS	RATIONALE
PLANNING	
1. **Expected outcomes** following completion of procedure:	
➤ Client has little pain or discomfort, does not aspirate, and has no postprocedure bleeding.	Indicates absence of complications and tolerance of procedure.
➤ Client is without respiratory complications or change in level of consciousness.	Recovers from sedation.
➤ Client describes purposes and steps of procedure.	Documents learning.
2. Prepare client:	
a. Explain steps of procedure, including sensations to expect.	Nurse can relieve anxiety and answer client's questions.
b. Explain purpose and effects of IVCS.	
c. Administer pain medication or preprocedure medication.	Promotes relaxation and reduces anxiety.
➤ ***CRITICAL DECISION POINT*** **Be sure informed consent signed before sedative administered.**	
IMPLEMENTATION	
Nurse's Responsibility	
1. Wash hands and apply gloves, goggles, and mask.	Reduces transmission of organisms.
2. Remove client's dentures or other dental appliances.	Prevents dislodgment of dental structures during intubation phase.
3. Assist client in maintaining left lateral position.	Unexpected change of position can cause accidental perforation of esophagus, stomach, or duodenum.
4. Ensure IV line is patent. RN will administer sedation for IVCS (according to institution policy).	Provides route for emergency medications.
5. Assist client through procedure:	
a. Anticipate needs and promote comfort.	Client is unable to speak after tube is passed into throat.
b. Tell client what is happening.	Reassures client about procedure and how long it will last.
6. Place tissue specimens in proper laboratory containers.	Ensures proper labeling and preparation of specimens for microscopic examination.
7. Suction if client begins to vomit or accumulate saliva.	Prevents aspiration of gastric contents or oral secretions. Ensures client safety.
8. Assist client to comfortable position, then wash hands.	Promotes rest and relaxation.
Physician's Responsibility	
1. Wash hands.	Reduces transmission of microorganisms.
2. Spray nasopharynx and oropharynx with local anesthetic (usually xylocaine).	Early application of anesthetic allows for optimal effect. Lidocaine inactivates gag reflex.
3. Apply gown, mask, goggles, and gloves.	Adheres to standard precautions.
4. Attach distal end of endoscope to light source (see Fig. 44-4).	Provides for direct visualization of upper GI tract.
5. With nursing or unlicensed assistive personnel's assistance, position client in left lateral (Sims') position.	Provides for airway clearance if client gags and vomits gastric contents.
6. Slowly pass endoscope into mouth, esophagus, stomach, or duodenum.	Provides visualization of structures.
7. Insufflate air through endoscope into upper GI tract.	Distends GI structures for better visualization.
8. Examine or perform biopsy of structures.	Provides data from which physician makes diagnosis.
EVALUATION	
1. Monitor vital signs and O_2 saturation according to hospital policy. May be as often as every 15 minutes for 2 hours.	Change in vital signs can indicate new bleeding in GI tract or oversedation.

STEPS	RATIONALE
CRITICAL DECISION POINT Initially, after procedure, client may experience internal bleeding without visible signs of blood loss.	
2. Assess for level of sedation and level of consciousness.	Determines client's response to IVCS.
3. Observe for pain.	Sudden abdominal pain can indicate rupture of abdominal organs.
4. Evaluate emesis or aspirate for frank or **occult** blood (see Chapter 43).	Indicates gastrointestinal bleeding.
5. Assess for return of gag reflex.	Determines when effects of anesthetic have disappeared. Gag reflex prevents aspiration.
6. Ask client to state postprocedure dietary and activity limitations.	Evaluates learning.
7. **Unexpected outcomes** that may occur include:	
➤ Client has abdominal pain, fever, or bleeding.	Occurs with perforation of abdominal structures; pain is accompanied by abdominal distention or bleeding.
➤ Client develops dyspnea or aspiration pneumonia.	Caused by aspiration of gastric contents into lungs; may be accompanied by fever, chest pain, and productive cough.
➤ Client remains sedated with decreased respiration or blood pressure, decreased oxygen saturation, and decreased level of consciousness.	Continued monitoring necessary. May require administration of narcotic reversal agent.
➤ Vital signs indicate deterioration of condition.	Results from loss of blood volume related to bleeding or perforation of abdominal structures.

Recording and Reporting

1. Record in nurse's notes the procedure, duration, client's tolerance, and collection and disposition of specimen.	Provides documentation of procedure in client's record.
2. Report onset of bleeding, abdominal pain, dyspnea, and vital sign changes to physician.	May require emergency treatment.
3. Report to nurse in charge the duration of procedure, client's tolerance, and changes in vital signs or condition.	Enables prompt medical follow-up for unexpected outcomes.

Follow-up Activities

1. Do not allow the client to eat or drink anything until the anesthesia has worn off and gag reflex returns (2 to 4 hours).
2. Provide oral hygiene when gag reflex returns.

• • • • •

Special Considerations

- ➤ Procedure may be contraindicated in clients unable to fully cooperate.
- ➤ Know in advance if specimens are to be immediately delivered to laboratory, and have person available to transport specimen.

Teaching Considerations

- ➤ Inform client of preprocedure medication and anticipated effects.
- ➤ Explain method for endoscope insertion.
- ➤ Explain that client will be unable to speak when the endoscope is positioned in the esophagus.
- ➤ Make sure client knows not to eat or drink until gag reflex returns. Before return of gag reflex, client could aspirate and develop pneumonia.
- ➤ Inform client that insertion of endoscope into mouth may cause feeling of inability to breathe. Assure client that suffocation will not occur.
- ➤ Encourage client to contact physician regarding test results.
- ➤ Some institutions may provide written discharge instructions (Fig. 44-5).

DIGESTIVE DISEASE CLINICAL CENTER
ENDOSCOPY UNIT
BARNES HOSPITAL
PATIENT DISCHARGE INSTRUCTIONS

Patient Name: ____________________

OP # ____________________

You have just had a diagnostic and/or therapeutic procedure performed in the Barnes Hospital Digestive Diseaes Clinical Center. Please contact your physician promptly or go to the emergency room if you develop persistent or large amounts of bleeding or persistent or increasing pain.

Private doctor's office # ____________________

Digestive Disease Clinical Center # (314) 362-5673. (8:00 a.m. - 4:30 p.m.)

After 4:30 p.m. call Barnes Hospital Operator #(314)362-5000 and ask for the G.I. Fellow "ON CALL".

Patient Instructions: Follow instructions checked

1) _______ The procedure on your GI tract required medication to assist you in relaxing. Rest at home for the remainder of the day and night. Do not drive or perform any activity that requires you to be completely alert during this recovery period. Alcohol should not be used during this period.

2) _______ Do not eat or drink until you are able to swallow without difficulty.

3) _______ Avoid roughage for 14 days (this includes nuts, popcorn, seeds, fresh fruits and raw vegetables).

4) _______ Do not take aspirin or aspirin-like products (such as Alka Seltzer, Bufferin or Advil) for 14 days.

5) _______ Resume normal activities and diet.

6) _______ Additional instructions: ____________________

____

____

____

____

Follow-up Care:

You should call Dr. ____________________ on ____________________

Ordered by: ____________________

Issued by: ____________________

Signature indicates that you acknowledge receipt of these discharge instructions.

Patient ____________________

Responsible Party ____________________

Relationship to Patient ____________________

Date: ____________________

3160-15 New 5/88

Fig. 44-5 Barnes-Jewish Hospital discharge orders for endoscopy. (Courtesy Barnes-Jewish Hospital, St Louis.)

Gerontologic Considerations

- Removal of dentures may cause embarrassment to client.
- Older adult clients may have reduced drug clearance from decreased glomerular filtration rate (GFR) and nephron activity or decreased hepatic function. Therefore the nurse must monitor the effects of medications given to the older adult client (Phipps et al., 1995).
- Because of age-related changes in the older adult, the gastric mucosa is thinner, which increases the incidence of irritation and ulceration (Phipps et al, 1995).
- Assess skin integrity of client after lying still on examining table. Older adult clients are at greater risk for skin breakdown.
- When older adult client recovers from IVCS, offer bedpan/urinal every 2 to 3 hours because of age-related changes in the urinary tract.
- Be aware that NPO status in the older adult client may result in dehydration.
- Because of multiple medications the older adult client may be taking, be aware of alterations in administration schedules necessary due to NPO status for diagnostic test.

Home Care Considerations

- Explain that client may be hoarse or have sore throat after procedure. Ice chips or anesthetic lozenges can be given after gag reflex returns.
- Instruct client to drink fluids to promote dye excretion.

SKILL 44-7 Assisting with Lumbar Puncture

A lumbar puncture, also called a spinal puncture or spinal tap, involves the introduction of a spinal needle into the **subarachnoid space** of the spinal column. The actual procedure is performed by a physician who may be assisted by a nurse or by unlicensed assistive personnel.

The purposes of a lumbar puncture are to measure **cerebrospinal fluid** (CSF) pressure in the subarachnoid space; to obtain CSF for visual and laboratory examination; and to inject anesthetic, diagnostic, or therapeutic agents.

This procedure is contraindicated if there is evidence of greatly increased **intracranial pressure,** because the sudden release of pressure may cause **herniation** of the brain structures through the **foramen magnum.** This herniation compresses the brainstem, which contains the vital cardiac, respiratory, and vasomotor centers, and sudden death may result.

Lumbar puncture is useful in the diagnosis of meningitis, encephalitis, brain or spinal cord tumors, and cerebral hemorrhage.

EQUIPMENT

- Lumbar puncture tray, including:
  - Antiseptic solution (e.g., povidone-iodine)
  - Ten gauze sponges (4 × 4)
  - Sterile towels
  - Three spinal needles (various sizes) with inner obturators (5 to 12.5 cm long; infants need 5-cm needle)
  - Alcohol swabs
  - Anesthetic agent (e.g., lidocaine 1%)
  - Syringes (3 to 5 ml)
  - Two rolled bath towels
  - Needles (5/8 inch, 25 gauge to 1/2 inch, 21 gauge)
- Sterile gloves (check physician's size)
- Masks (optional)
- Goggles (optional)
- Glass or plastic manometer with three-way stopcock
- Four test tubes
- Antiseptic ointment
- Band-Aids or 2 × 2 gauze dressing
- Straight chair for physician

STEPS	RATIONALE
ASSESSMENT	
1. Assess client's ability to understand and follow directions.	Procedure requires client to follow directions closely and assume proper position. Clients with neurological problems may have reduced level of consciousness.
2. Assess musculoskeletal flexibility of client to assume lateral decubitus (fetal) position.	Lateral decubitus position is important to place spinal needle in proper position.
CRITICAL DECISION POINT Clients who have severe arthritic conditions or who are orthopneic may be unable to assume this position.	

STEPS	RATIONALE
3. Assess degree of cooperation of client to remain in position without excessive movement.	Movement can cause injury from spinal needle.
4. Examine medical record for contraindications of increased intracranial pressure or degenerative joint disease.	Increased intracranial pressure may cause brain herniation. Degenerative joint disease may prevent client from attaining proper position or physician from easily entering subarachnoid space for procedure.
5. Determine whether client is allergic to medication to be used as local anesthetic agent (e.g., lidocaine).	Previous allergies to anesthetic agents should be noted so these agents may be avoided by physician.
6. Assess client's knowledge regarding procedure.	Procedure can create anxiety because of needle placement.
7. Check signed consent form (refer to institution's policy).	Consent forms are required for invasive diagnostic testing procedures.
8. Assess vital signs and neurological status of lower extremities: movement, sensation, and muscle strength (see Chapter 11).	Provides baseline data for comparison with postprocedural measurements.

NURSING DIAGNOSIS

Clustering of defining characteristics from the assessment data may reveal the following nursing diagnoses for clients requiring this skill:

- Anxiety
- Fear
- Knowledge deficit regarding purpose and steps of procedure
- Pain
- Risk for infection
- Risk for injury

Related factors are individualized based on a client's condition or needs.

PLANNING

STEPS	RATIONALE
1. **Expected outcomes** following completion of procedure:	
➤ Small amount (1- to 2-cm circle) (½ to 1 inch) of clear or red drainage is present at puncture site.	Small amount of CSF or bloody drainage is considered normal and expected.
➤ Client does not experience postpuncture headache or herniation.	Without CSF leakage through subcutaneous track, postpuncture headache and herniation do not occur.
➤ Test results of CSF are normal.	Comparison of client's laboratory data with normal laboratory values shows no abnormal pressures, cells, organisms, or other constituents.
➤ Client understands procedure.	
2. Explain procedure to client.	Nurse tells client in understandable terms about potential discomfort associated with procedure and length of procedure.
3. Have client empty bladder and bowels before procedure begins.	Avoids interruption of test and prevents discomfort.
4. Position client in lateral decubitus (fetal) position with head and neck flexed (see illustration, p. 1299).	Flexion of lumbar spine allows easy access to CSF in spinal canal.
a. Bring both arms and knees toward center of body; client may grasp knees with hands.	Gives spinal column full curvature. Spinal column should be flexed as much as possible to allow maximal space between vertebrae.
b. May place pillow between knees.	Prevents discomfort and possibility of upper leg rolling forward.
c. Be sure back is exposed.	Allows easy access to spinal column.

IMPLEMENTATION

Nurse's Responsibility

STEPS	RATIONALE
1. Reexplain that client must lie in flexed position and remain still for entire procedure.	Client must remain still throughout procedure to ensure no movement of spinal needle within spinal column and canal.

STEPS	RATIONALE
2. Position client so spine (dorsal side) is against side of bed. Hold arms and legs in flexed position.	Position allows full flexion of the spine and wider spaces between the vertebrae. Prevents sudden movement by client.
3. Caution client not to cough and to breathe slowly and deeply.	Coughing or changes in breathing increase CSF pressure and give false reading.
4. Explain each step that may give discomfort.	Client should know exactly what is occurring so that discomfort can be anticipated and surprises eliminated.
5. Apply gloves in preparation for assisting with filling test tubes with CSF.	Prevents transmission of microorganisms.
6. Properly label tubes with client information and name of test desired.	Test tubes are numbered in sequence of collection (e.g., 1 through 4).
7. Assist with placement of direct pressure and gauze dressing once needle is withdrawn from puncture site.	Pressure helps minimize CSF loss and bleeding.
8. Remove gloves; wash hands thoroughly after procedure, especially if tubes with CSF have been handled.	Tubes might contain virulent organisms. Proper disposal of gloves reduces transmission of organisms.
9. Assist client in assuming comfortable position.	
10. Ask client to maintain supine or dorsal recumbent position usually 8 to 12 hours. Client may turn from side to side.	Supine or dorsal recumbent position reduces risk of spinal headache, which may result if client sits upright.
CRITICAL DECISION POINT **Explain how to log roll with minimal lifting of head.**	
11. Provide for client's comfort with medication if ordered, desirable, and not contraindicated.	Procedure is usually described as painful by client. Postprocedure headache may require that client be medicated.
CRITICAL DECISION POINT **If client has a CNS disorder a sedative or analgesic may be contraindicated so as not to further cloud client's consciousness.**	
12. During and after procedure, observe client for:	
a. Changes in level of consciousness, pupil size and reaction, respiratory status, and vital signs.	Changes in level of consciousness, pupil size and reaction, respiratory status, and vital signs indicate increasing intracranial pressure.

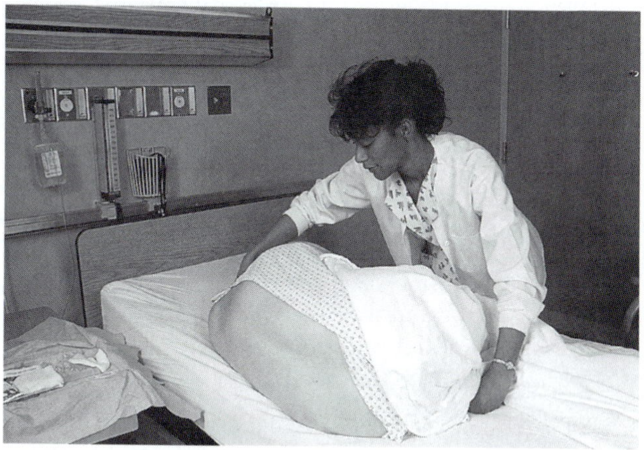

Step 4 Position for lumbar puncture.

STEPS	RATIONALE
b. Respiratory status.	May indicate increasing intracranial pressure.
c. Numbness, tingling, or pain radiating down legs.	May result from spinal nerve irritation.
13. Encourage client to force fluids by mouth using a straw if not contraindicated.	Needed to replace CSF lost and resume hemodynamics. Use of straw allows client to drink while supine.

Physician's Responsibility

STEPS	RATIONALE
1. Wash hands.	Reduces transmission of microorganisms.
2. Set up sterile field of equipment.	Provides sterile work area.
3. Apply sterile gloves (mask and goggles optional).	
4. Prepare lumbosacral area with antiseptic solution and gauze sponges.	Prevents entry of microorganisms from skin to CSF in spinal canal.
5. Inject topical anesthetic agent.	Provides local anesthetic to skin surrounding puncture site.
6. Insert spinal needle containing an inner obturator into subarachnoid space (see illustration).	Care is taken to avoid trauma to spinal nerves.
7. After entering subarachnoid space, obturator is removed.	Allows flow of CSF from subarachnoid space.
8. Attach manometer with stopcock and read manometer for "opening pressure."	Manometer is calibrated in centimeters of water.
9. Turn stopcock to allow CSF to drip into test tubes to send for appropriate testing.	
10. Remove spinal needle and place direct pressure on insertion site.	Decreases or stops CSF leakage from spinal canal and blood from subcutaneous tissue track of needle.
11. Place adhesive gauze or Band-Aid over insertion site.	Ensures sterility of insertion site.

EVALUATION

STEPS	RATIONALE
1. Assess needle insertion site for drainage.	Small amount of CSF (clear) or bloody (red) drainage is considered normal.

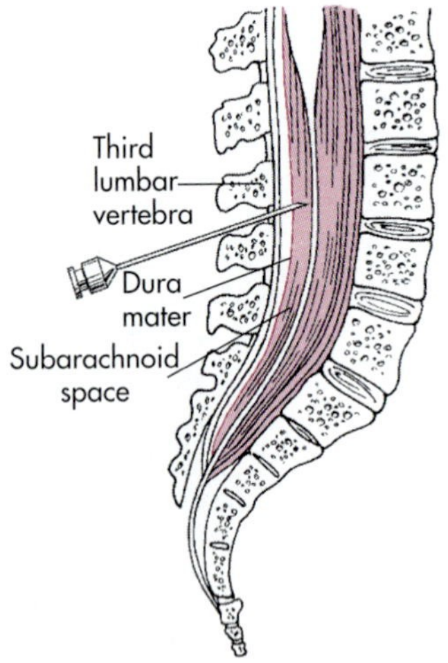

Step 6 Placement of needle for lumbar puncture.

CRITICAL DECISION POINT **Report any excessive drainage (e.g., saturation of gauze dressing) from the insertion site, which may predispose client to postpuncture headache and infection (moisture may function as growth medium for bacteria). If excessive drainage occurs, place pressure dressing on site.**

STEPS	RATIONALE
2. Assess level of consciousness, vital signs, pupils, and respiratory status; assess numbness, tingling, and ability to move the lower extremities.	Changes may indicate complications of brain herniation or irritation of spinal nerves.

STEPS	RATIONALE
3. Ask client to describe postprocedure positioning and activity restriction.	Evaluates learning.
4. **Unexpected outcomes** that may occur include:	
➤ Client has excessive drainage from insertion site.	Indicates CSF or blood leakage through subcutaneous track.
➤ Client has postpuncture headache.	Precise cause of postpuncture headache is unknown, although CSF leak is a theorized cause. Also called spinal headache, it is typically a throbbing, bifrontal, or occipital headache that worsens when the client sits or stands. It appears a few hours to several days after procedure and can be alleviated by bed rest in a dark quiet room and with analgesics (Beare and Myers, 1994).
➤ Client has pain or tingling sensation in lower extremities.	Could be caused by nerve root irritation related to needle trauma to spinal nerves.
➤ Client develops reduced level of consciousness, dilated pupils, and increased blood pressure.	Signs of brain herniation.

Recording and Reporting

1. Record in nurse's notes the procedure performed, including time, physician's name, client's tolerance (e.g., opening pressure, color of CSF, amount of drainage on dressing, and whether headache and leg tingling are present), and specimen sent to lab.	Accurate documentation of procedure is important for legal reasons.
2. Record and report pertinent findings to nurse in charge and to physician: changes in vital signs, nausea, vomiting, and changes in level of consciousness.	May indicate medical emergency.

Follow-up Activities

1. Provide for client's comfort through positioning, relaxation techniques, and analgesics if indicated.
2. Initiate client teaching for usual postlumbar puncture care, including activity and forcing fluids.

• • • • •

Special Considerations

➤ Client's feelings of discomfort may vary depending on tolerance of pain, degree of difficulty in obtaining CSF, and extent of CSF leakage after end of procedure.

➤ Most physicians order bed rest after lumbar puncture. Treatment for headache is bed rest, ice pack applied to head, and analgesia. Analgesia may be restricted in some clients. Forcing fluids helps reestablish CSF level.

➤ Duration of lumbar puncture is 15 to 60 minutes.

Teaching Considerations

➤ Thoroughly explain procedure and postprocedure routine to client. Many clients have misconceptions regarding procedure. Emphasize importance of remaining flat after procedure.

➤ Assure client that insertion of needle into spine will not cause paralysis because needle is inserted into area below spinal cord.

➤ Teach client the importance of forcing fluids after the procedure.

➤ Encourage client to contact the physician regarding test results.

Pediatric Considerations

➤ Lumbar punctures are frequently done on children with cancer. The use of active coping skills, such as relaxation and imagery, have been shown to decrease children's pain perceptions during the procedure (Heiney, 1991; Broome et al., 1990).

Gerontologic Considerations

➤ Older adults may have difficulty assuming the side-lying knee-to-chest position.

Home Care Considerations

➤ If lumbar puncture is done on an outpatient basis, the client lies flat before being discharged and needs to be taught about signs and symptoms of complications to watch for (Phipps et al., 1995).

➤ Provide written instructions to reinforce oral instructions.

SKILL 44-8 Assisting with Magnetic Resonance Imaging

Magnetic resonance imaging (MRI) is a noninvasive scanning technique that provides visualization of the body's organs and structures by means of magnetic forces rather than by ionizing radiation. Magnetic resonance images are picked up by computers once the client is placed inside a large electromagnet (Fig. 44-6). This diagnostic study is based on the alignment of hydrogen atoms in the body and the change in alignment of those atoms by radiofrequency signals. Billions of mathematical calculations are produced and displayed as clear images on a television screen (Phipps et al., 1995).

MRI may be used in the diagnosis of pathological lesions in almost every organ or tissue (Pagana and Pagana, 1995). MRI provides excellent visualization of soft tissue and is useful in detecting circulatory abnormalities and tumors of the eye (Beare and Myers, 1994). The procedure is usually performed by a trained technologist in the MRI department.

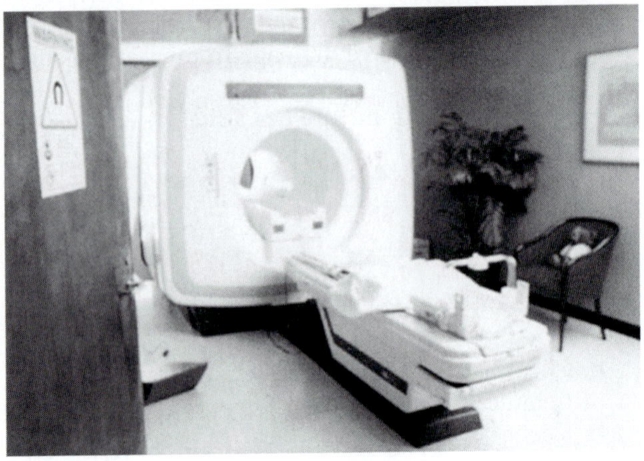

Fig. 44-6 Magnetic resonance imaging is the most precise diagnostic tool available. (From Brundage DJ: *Renal disorders.* St Louis, 1992, Mosby.)

EQUIPMENT

- **Contrast medium gadolinium (Magnevist) (optional); must be ordered by physician**

STEPS	RATIONALE
ASSESSMENT	
1. Assess client's knowledge of purposes of and steps in the procedure.	Helps to reduce anxiety and gain cooperation.
CRITICAL DECISION POINT **MRI is contraindicated in clients who are confused or agitated.**	
2. Assess stability of client's medical condition.	Monitoring equipment and other equipment (that contains metal) cannot be used inside the scanner room.
CRITICAL DECISION POINT **Clients who are medically unstable and require continuous life-support equipment (that contains metal) are not candidates for this procedure unless specially designed monitoring equipment is available.**	
3. Assess client's weight.	Procedure contraindicated in clients over 300 pounds.
4. Assess client for implantable metal objects such as cardiac pacemaker, aneurysm clips, inner ear implants, or history of valve replacement, as well as those clients with medical equipment that contains metal (e.g., infusion pumps, neurostimulator—TENS unit, or implanted insulin/drug pumps). Equipment is available that does not contain metal parts. Additional items that may interfere with magnetic resonance imaging are found on the informational diagram (see illustration).	Procedure is contraindicated if any of these are present, because the magnet may cause movement of metal or electronic objects (Pagana and Pagana, 1995).
5. Assess client for claustrophobia.	Client may become fearful or overly anxious of becoming trapped in an enclosed or narrow place.

ALL INFORMATION IN SHADED BOXED AREA MUST BE FILLED OUT PRIOR TO MRI

THE FOLLOWING ITEMS MAY INTERFERE WITH MAGNETIC RESONANCE IMAGING AND SOME CAN BE POTENTAILLY HAZARDOUS. PLEASE INDICATE IF YOU HAVE THE FOLLOWING:

- Cardiac Pacemaker — YES NO
- Aneurysm Clip(s) — YES NO
- Implanted Insulin/Drug Pump — YES NO
- Neurostimulator (TENS Unit) — YES NO
- Biostimulator/Bone Growth Stimulator — YES NO
- Hearing aid/Cochlear Implant — YES NO
- Gianturco Coil (embolus coil) — YES NO
- Vascular Clip(s) — YES NO
- Heart Valve Prosthesis — YES NO
- Greenfield Vena Cava Filter — YES NO
- Middle Ear Implant — YES NO
- Penile Prosthesis — YES NO
- Orbital/Eye Prosthesis — YES NO
- Shrapnel or Bullet — YES NO
- Wire Sutures — YES NO
- Tattooed Eyeliner — YES NO
- Any type of Dental Item held in place by a Magnet — YES NO
- ANY OTHER IMPLANTED ITEM — YES NO
  TYPE ______________________________
- Diaphram/IUD — YES NO
- Intraventricular Shunt — YES NO
- Wire Mesh — YES NO
- Artificial Limb or Joint — YES NO
- Any Orthopedic Item (i.e. pins, rods, screws, nails, clips, plates, wire, etc.) — YES NO
- Dentures — YES NO
- Dental Braces or any other type of Removable Dental Item — YES NO

Please mark on this drawing the location of any metal inside your body.

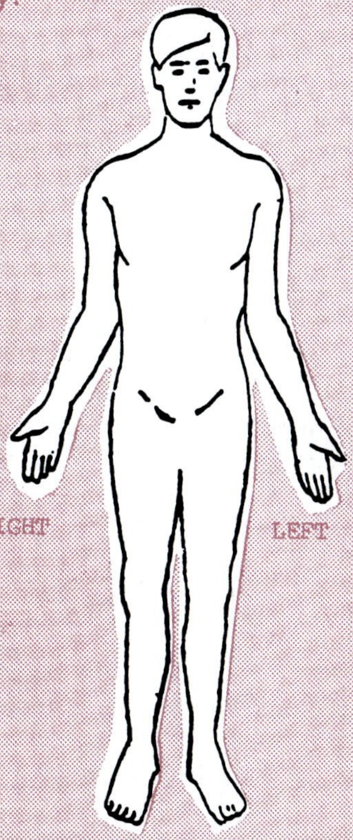

- Have you ever had a surgical procedure or operation of any kind? YES NO
  If YES please list type of operation and the date:
  ____
  ____
- Are you claustrophobic — YES NO
- Have you ever had an injury to your eye involving metal? YES NO
- Is there any possibility you may be pregnant? YES NO

I attest that the above information is correct to the best of my knowledge, understand any risks associated with the above conditions, and consent to undergoing this Magnetic Resonance Imaging examination.

____
(Patient's or Legal Guardian's Signature)

____
(Witness Signature) DATE:

Step 4 Sample check-off sheet for clients having an MRI.

STEPS	RATIONALE
CRITICAL DECISION POINT Procedure may be contraindicated if claustrophobia is severe and/or not relieved by sedation.	
6. Assess client for pregnancy.	The long-term effects of MRI on fetus are currently unknown (Pagana and Pagana, 1995). MRI is contraindicated during pregnancy.
7. Assess client's ability to remain still throughout the procedure. Determine client's understanding of the importance of remaining in one position for the duration of the procedure. Factors that might influence client's inability to remain still include pain, alteration in mental status, claustrophobia, difficulty breathing, polyuria, and restlessness.	Any movement may produce artifacts. Client must remain still for 30 to 90 minutes.
8. Assess for allergies to dye and contrast medium.	Prevents injury to client. If allergy is noted, ensure that client is wearing an allergy wristband and document appropriately.
CRITICAL DECISION POINT Intravenous injection of allergic substance is a life-threatening condition and can result in anaphylactic shock and death.	
9. Assess whether client signed a consent document (check institution's policy).	Minimizes institution's legal risk.

NURSING DIAGNOSIS

Clustering of defining characteristics from the assessment data may reveal the following nursing diagnoses for clients requiring this skill:

- Anxiety
- Fear
- Knowledge deficit regarding purpose and steps of procedure
- Pain
- Risk for injury

Related factors are individualized based on a client's condition or needs.

PLANNING

1. **Expected outcomes** following completion of procedure:	
➤ Client tolerates procedure with minimal discomfort.	
➤ Client can maintain position without moving.	Anxiety or sense of claustrophobia minimized.
➤ If contrast medium is used, client has no reaction to dye.	Indicates absence of complications.
➤ Satisfactory images are obtained.	Indicates that purpose of procedure was achieved.
➤ Client describes purpose and steps of procedure.	Documents learning.

IMPLEMENTATION

Nurse's Responsibility

1. If possible, show client picture of MRI machine and encourage questions (see Fig. 44-6).	
2. Remove all metallic objects from client, such as watch, jewelry, coins, keys, hair pins, credit cards, prostheses, and dentures. Lock away for safe keeping (Pagana and Pagana, 1995).	Metallic objects will create artifacts on the scan, and some metal objects may be moved or damaged by the magnetic field.
3. Have client put on hospital gown without snaps and void before the procedure.	Voiding promotes comfort during procedure.

STEPS	RATIONALE
Technologist's Responsibility	
1. If not previously performed, remove all metallic objects from client (see Step 2 above).	Metallic objects will create artifacts on the scan, and some metal objects may move or be damaged by the magnetic field.
2. Assist client onto padded table and position comfortably.	Provides for correct positioning and for client's comfort.
3. Place special helmet around head if it is to be scanned and secure client on table with Velcro straps.	Allows for accurate imaging and helps to keep client from moving during procedure.
4. Provide client with earplugs and/or intercom or earphones.	Decreases sounds of images and allows for communication between client and technologist.
5. After examination, allow client to sit for a few moments before standing.	Decreases possibility of orthostatic hypotension.
EVALUATION	
1. Evaluate client's level of comfort after procedure.	Determines if complications related to positioning have occurred.
2. **Unexpected outcomes** that may occur include:	
➤ Allergic reaction to contrast medium. Reaction is immediate.	Can result in anaphylactic shock.
➤ Client is unable to maintain position during procedure.	Can result in inaccurate findings on MRI.
RECORDING AND REPORTING	
1. Record in client's chart the date, time, and place MRI was performed; whether contrast medium was used; and client's tolerance of procedure.	Provides documentation of procedure in record.

FOLLOW-UP ACTIVITIES

1. Assist client in assuming comfortable position after procedure.
2. Inform client that no special postprocedural care is needed (Pagana and Pagana, 1995).
3. Encourage client to check with physician regarding test results.
4. If personal items were removed before diagnostic procedure, return them to client.

• • • • •

Special Considerations

- Clients who are severely claustrophobic and in whom diagnostic testing by the scanner is essential may receive antianxiety medications as ordered by the physician (i.e., midazolam or diazepam) before the procedure.

Teaching Considerations

- Inform the client that no food or fluid restrictions are necessary before or after the test.
- Instruct the client to void just before the procedure (Pagana and Pagana, 1995).
- Explain that during the examination the client will hear the hum of the machine and a loud thumping sound when the radiowaves are turned on. Earplugs are usually available.
- Reassure client that a microphone and earphone are present in the scanner to enable communication with the staff during the scan.
- Inform client that make-up should not be worn, because some may contain metallic particles.
- Explain that client must remain motionless throughout this painless study. A slight discomfort may be experienced if contrast medium is injected.
- Inform client that a tingling sensation may be felt in teeth containing metal fillings (Pagana and Pagana, 1995).

Pediatric Considerations

- Parents may remain with children during the scan, because no danger of radiation exists.

Gerontologic Considerations

- The older adult client may experience increased discomfort during the procedure because of lying motionless for an extended period of time.
- Assess skin integrity of client after lying still on hard narrow examining table. Older adult clients are at greater risk for skin breakdown.
- After the procedure, be aware of need to change positions in older adult clients slowly to minimize safety risks and possible postural changes.

- Because of age-related cardiovascular changes in older adults, plan diagnostic testing schedule to provide rest periods.
- If the older adult client was required to remove sensory assistive devices (e.g., glasses, hearing aids) for diagnostic testing, provide measures to compensate for these sensory deficits.

Home Care Considerations

- Inform the client that no food or fluid restrictions are necessary before or after the test.

SKILL 44-9 Assisting with Thoracentesis

Thoracentesis is performed to analyze or remove **pleural fluid** or to instill medications intrapleurally. Specimens are examined for gross appearance and consistency and for protein, glucose, amylase, lactic dehydrogenase (LDH), and cellular composition. Cytologically specimens are examined for malignancy and cultured for pathogens. The procedure is performed by a physician and assisted by a nurse or unlicensed assistive personnel using strict sterile technique. A large-bore needle is passed through the chest wall into the **pleural cavity.** Excess pleural fluid resulting from injury, infection, or disease may be removed. The primary therapeutic purpose of thoracentesis is to relive pain, dyspnea, and other signs of pleural pressure. Diagnostically, the procedure is performed when there is evidence of pleural effusion with unknown etiology. Before the procedure, a decubitus chest x-ray is done to ensure the mobility of pleural fluid and therefore the accessibility of pleural fluid to a needle inserted into the pleural space.

The procedure is usually performed while the client is in a sitting position with one arm held upward from the chest, or more commonly, leaning over a bedside table padded with pillows. A thoracentesis is generally performed in less than 30 minutes at the client's bedside, in a procedure room, or in the physician's office.

EQUIPMENT

- Antiseptic solution for hand washing
- Thoracentesis tray, if available from central supply, which may include:
  - Antiseptic solution (e.g., povidone-iodine)
  - Gauze sponges (4 × 4)
  - Sterile towels
  - Local anesthetic solution for injection (e.g., lidocaine 1%)
  - Sterile syringes: two 3-ml, 23- to 25-gauge needles for anesthetic; two 50-ml, 14- to 17-gauge needles, 5 to 7 cm long (or 2 to 3 inches), for drainage of pleural fluid
  - Receptacle for fluid
  - Three-way stopcock
  - Two-way stopcock with extension tubing
  - Test tubes
- Sterile gloves of proper size for physician
- Masks and goggles for physician, nurse, and/or unlicensed assistive personnel (check institution's policy)
- Gauze (2 × 2), tape, and antiseptic ointment
- Cough suppressant (Pagana and Pagana, 1995) or pain medication if ordered

STEPS	RATIONALE
ASSESSMENT	
1. Assess client's knowledge of procedure.	Determines level of health teaching required.
2. Assess client's ability to assume position required for procedure (see illustration on p. 1307).	Clients with musculoskeletal or respiratory alterations may be unable to sit on side of bed with arms draped over high bedside table.
CRITICAL DECISION POINT Client must remain immobile during the procedure to prevent trauma to visceral pleura.	
3. Assess vital signs.	Provides baseline data for comparison with vital signs.
4. Be aware of client's underlying medical condition that may indicate presence of thrombocytopenia.	May contraindicate procedure due to risk of bleeding.
5. Assess respiratory function: symmetry of chest on inspiration and expiration, respiratory difficulty, and type of cough and sputum produced.	Provides for comparison with respiratory status during and after procedure.

STEPS	RATIONALE
6. Determine purpose of procedure.	Enables nurse to anticipate needed supplies and laboratory requisitions.
7. Assess if client signed a consent form (check institution's policy).	Signed consent is needed to reduce institution's legal risk.
8. Determine whether client is allergic to antiseptic or anesthetic solutions.	Decreases chances of complications.
9. Assess need for preprocedure pain medication.	Procedure can be painful, and client must remain still throughout it because of potential complications.

NURSING DIAGNOSIS

Clustering of defining characteristics from the assessment data may reveal the following nursing diagnoses for clients requiring this skill:

- Anxiety
- Fear
- Impaired gas exchange
- Ineffective breathing pattern
- Risk for infection
- Risk for injury
- Knowledge deficit regarding purpose and steps of procedure
- Pain

Related factors are individualized based on a client's condition or needs.

PLANNING

STEPS	RATIONALE
1. **Expected outcomes** following completion of procedure:	
➤ Client tolerates procedure well.	Client can assume position without problems; has little discomfort.
➤ Respiratory status is improved as evidenced by nonlabored respirations, improvement in arterial blood gases, and improved comfort.	Optimal expansion of lungs improves gas exchange.
➤ Client describes purpose and steps of procedure, as well as proper positioning.	Documents learning.
2. Prepare client:	
a. Explain procedure.	Ensures knowledge of procedure, thus promoting cooperation and relaxation.

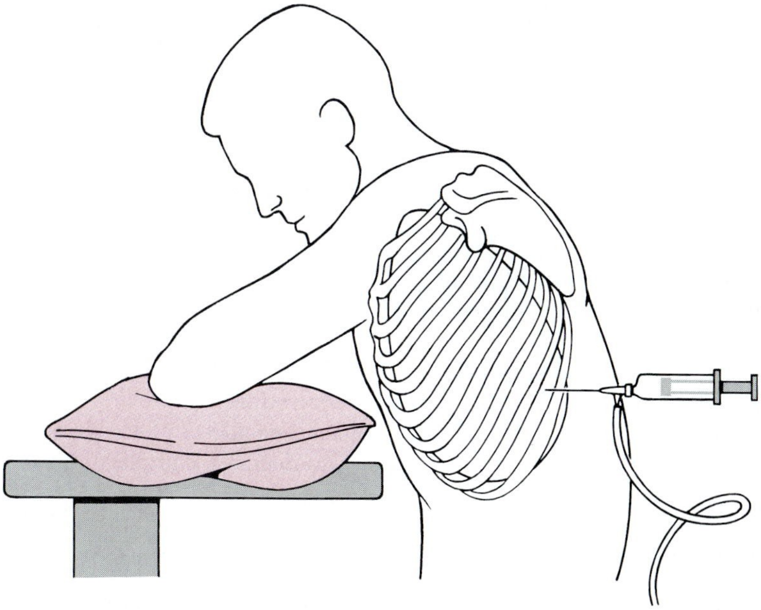

Step 2 Position for thoracentesis. (From Beare PG, Myers JL: *Principles and practice of adult health nursing,* ed 2, St Louis, 1994, Mosby.)

STEPS	RATIONALE
b. Explain that although a local anesthetic will be given at the insertion site, the client may feel a pressure-like pain upon entering the pleura for fluid removal.	
c. Have client void just before procedure.	Prevents interruption of procedure and promotes client's comfort.
d. Assist client in assuming high Fowler's position: sitting on side of bed, leaning over bedside table. Arms are draped over one or two pillows on table to slightly spread intercostal spaces (Pagana and Pagana, 1995).	Provides access to intercostal space to ribs.

IMPLEMENTATION

Nurse's Responsibility

STEPS	RATIONALE
1. Wash hands.	Reduces transmission of microorganisms.
2. Set up sterile tray or open supplies to make them accessible for physician.	Prevents introduction of pathogens into the pleural space.
3. Assist client in maintaining correct position. If necessary, hold client's shoulders or sides and provide reassurance.	Prevents sudden movement on part of client.

CRITICAL DECISION POINT Emphasize the importance of remaining immobile during the procedure to prevent trauma to the visceral pleura. Client must not cough, sneeze, or breathe deeply during procedure because it could cause trauma to visceral pleura (Thompson et al., 1993).

STEPS	RATIONALE
4. Assess client's pulse for reflex bradycardia, diaphoresis, and feeling of faintness (Pagana and Pagana, 1995).	Evaluates tolerance to procedure.
5. Assess client's respiratory status during procedure: rate, effort to breathe, and color of mucous membranes and nail beds.	Enables nurse to detect tolerance to procedure and possible complications.
6. After thoracentesis assist client in assuming comfortable position in bed.	If leakage into pleural space is suspected, client is positioned recumbent with punctured chest side up.

Physician's Responsibility

STEPS	RATIONALE
1. Wash hands.	Reduces transmission of microorganisms.
2. Disinfect skin with antiseptic solution and 4 × 4s.	Removes surface bacteria on skin.
3. Apply mask, goggles, and sterile gloves, and drape client with sterile towels.	Maintains surgical asepsis.
4. Inject anesthetic and allow time for it to take effect.	Provides local anesthesia at needle insertion site.
5. Palpate exact site needed for thoracentesis (most often just below angle of scapula at seventh intercostal space).	If needle is inserted too low, liver or spleen may be punctured, causing serious complications.
6. Attach thoracentesis needle to three-way stopcock, which is turned off to needle lumen.	Ensures that no air enters pleural space when needle is introduced.
7. Insert needle into determined site slowly until pleural space is reached, and slowly aspirate fluid.	Places needle in pleural space. Fluid is aspirated slowly to decrease complications of drawing lung tissue into needle.

CRITICAL DECISION POINT No more than 1500 ml of pleural fluid should be removed in a 30-minute time period because of risk of intravascular fluid shift with resultant pulmonary edema (Phipps et al., 1995).

STEPS	RATIONALE
8. Remove needle and apply pressure and sterile dressing to puncture site.	Pressure assists in sealing puncture site. Dressing ensures sterility of site.
9. Order chest x-ray film and blood work (e.g., hematocrit and hemoglobin, serum electrolytes).	Chest x-ray may show decreased fluid level in pleural space. Blood work is performed to check cell count and electrolytes in case replacement is needed.

EVALUATION

1. Note amount and color of pleural fluid.	Characteristics are used for observation, reporting, and recording.
2. Monitor vital signs and auscultate lung sounds. Compare with prethoracentesis vital signs.	Monitors physiological status.
3. Monitor client for complications from the thoracentesis, which may include pneumothorax (e.g., acute SOB, anxiety, tachypnea), shock (e.g., hypotension, tachycardia, cool clammy skin, altered LOC), subcutaneous emphysema (e.g., swelling of soft tissues and palpation of crepitations over the affected area), and pyogenic infection (e.g., fever, tachycardia, chills).	

➤ *CRITICAL DECISION POINT* The complications of liver and spleen perforation are less common than lung perforation. Symptoms are subtle and may not be noted for several days. Symptoms include decreasing hemoglobin and hematocrit values and possibly abdominal pain.

4. Follow up on postthoracentesis chest x-ray as indicated.	Determines presence of pneumothorax.
5. Note drainage on chest dressing.	Documents leakage of fluid from puncture site.
6. Ask client to describe postprocedure limitations and positioning.	Evaluates learning.
7. **Unexpected outcomes** that may occur include:	
➤ Client does not assume position well.	May be result of anxiety, pain, musculoskeletal alteration, or respiratory distress.
➤ Client moves abruptly or coughs during procedure.	May be result of underlying pathological condition of lungs.
➤ Other complications (e.g., liver or spleen perforation) occur.	Result of improper needle placement or abrupt movement.

RECORDING AND REPORTING

1. Record in nurse's notes the name of procedure, location of puncture site, amount and color of fluid drained, duration, tolerance (e.g., vital signs, pain, respiratory status, complications), laboratory tests ordered and sent, type of dressing over puncture site, and drainage.	Accurate recording of any procedure is legal necessity in nursing.
2. Report to physician immediately:	
a. Decreased respiratory function.	
b. Changes in vital signs beyond normal limits.	
c. Changes in postprocedure hemoglobin, hematocrit, or serum electrolyte values.	
d. Document completion of chest x-ray if ordered after procedure; notify physician if any complications were detected.	Could indicate lung perforation with resultant pneumothorax, hemothorax, or atelectasis.
3. Report to nurses on next shift all data that have been recorded in nurse's notes and reported to physician.	Allows for continuity of care.

STEPS **RATIONALE**

FOLLOW-UP ACTIVITIES

1. Place client on unaffected side for 1 hour to allow puncture site to close (Beare and Myers, 1994).
2. Observe for hemoptysis, anxiety, and restlessness.
3. Send specimens to appropriate laboratory.
4. Clean up area and send supplies to proper sterilization department.
5. Obtain laboratory data for interpretation by nurse and physician.

• • • • •

Special Considerations

- Nurse may need to obtain sterile specimen container for collection of large amount of fluid.
- If client cannot assume high Fowler's position sitting on side of bed, lateral high Fowler's position is used. Affected lung is on top with arm from that side placed up over head.
- Determining exact site for needle insertion is performed by examining chest x-ray film and noting level of fluid in pleural space.
- If lung becomes punctured and air escapes into pleural space, chest tube will need to be inserted as soon as possible.

Teaching Considerations

- After explaining procedure, make certain client knows that movement or coughing could damage lung or pleura. Cough suppressant may be administered before test if client has cough.
- Explain to client that chest x-ray is often ordered after procedure to check for adequate lung expansion.
- Encourage client to report any dyspnea, chest pain, or cough after procedure.
- Inform the client that no food or fluid restrictions are necessary before or after the test.
- Encourage client to check with physician regarding test results.

Gerontologic Considerations

- During all aspects of this procedure, be aware of ineffective breathing patterns in the older adult because of age-related changes such as reduced elastic lung recoil, declining chest expansion, reduced cough efficiency, and weaker thoracic and diaphragmatic muscles (Stanley and Beare, 1995).
- Age-related changes of the musculoskeletal system may restrict movement during positioning and during procedure.
- After the procedure, be aware of need to change positions in older adult clients slowly to minimize safety risks and possible postural changes.

Home Care Considerations

- Teach client symptoms of complications related to liver and spleen perforation that may not present for several days after procedure.
- Encourage client to report any dyspnea, chest pain, or cough after procedure.
- Inform the client that no food or fluid restrictions are necessary before or after the test.

CRITICAL THINKING EXERCISES

1. Your older adult client, Mr. Sanchez, has just had an abdominal paracentesis performed. After assisting the client to a comfortable position, you hear him state he suddenly feels faint and dizzy. You note the client's color to be pale and he appears anxious. What nursing interventions would be appropriate?
2. You are assisting in maintaining the position of the client who is being prepped for a thoracentesis. The physician is preparing to insert the large-bore needle when the client whispers to you, "I'm going to sneeze." What do you do?
3. Ms. Ramirez, who is to have an arteriogram, tells you that although she told the physician that she is not allergic to contrast media that she has in the past had an allergic reaction to it. She indicates that she denied this allergy because she knows that this test is very important in the diagnosis of her condition. What nursing interventions would be appropriate?
4. You have delegated to the unlicensed assistive personnel the task of taking vital signs on the client who has just received a lumbar puncture. This employee questions why it is necessary for the client to lie flat following this procedure. What would be the appropriate nursing response?

REFERENCES

Beare PG, Myers JL: *Principles and practice of adult health nursing,* ed 2, St Louis, 1994, Mosby.

Broome ME et al: Children's medical fears, coping behaviors, and pain perceptions during a lumbar puncture, *Oncol Nurs Forum* 17(3):361, 1990.

Broome ME et al: The use of distraction and imagery with children during painful procedures, *Oncol Nurs Forum* 19(3):499, 1992.

Brundage DJ: *Renal disorders,* St Louis, 1992, Mosby.

Cushing M: Demystifying informed consent, *Am J Nurs* 91(11):1991.

Galanti GA: *Caring for patients from different cultures: case studies from American hospitals,* Philadelphia, 1994, University of Pennsylvania Press.

Heiney S: Helping children throughout painful procedures, *Am J Nurs* 91(11):20, 1991.

Pagana KD, Pagana TJ: *Mosby's diagnostic and laboratory test reference,* St Louis, 1995, Mosby.

Phipps WJ et al, editors: *Medical-surgical nursing: concepts and clinical practice,* ed 5, St Louis, 1995, Mosby.

Shrake K: AARC clinical practice guidelines: fiberoptic bronchoscopy assisting, *Resp Care* 38(11):1173, 1993.

Silver MR, Balk RA: Bronchoscopic procedures in the intensive care unit, *Crit Care Clin* 11(1):97, 1995.

Society of Gastroenterology Nurses and Associates (SGNA): *Gastroenterology nursing: a core curriculum,* St Louis, 1993, Mosby.

Stanley M, Beare PG: *Gerontological nursing,* Philadelphia, 1995, FA Davis.

Thompson JM et al: *Mosby's clinical nursing,* ed 3, St Louis, 1993, Mosby.

ADDITIONAL READING

Aragon D: Cardiac monitoring: follow these leads, *Am J Nurs* 94(12):5A, 1994.

Boraski J, McSwain NE: Vascular injuries and the criteria for arteriography, *Emerg Med* 25(11):91, 1993.

Caffery L, Claussen DS: Inpatient education for fiberoptic/videoptic diagnostic and therapeutic procedures for gastroenterology, *Gastroenterol Nurs* 14(2):106, 1991.

Fullhart JW: Preparatory information and anxiety before sigmoidoscopy: a comparative study, *Soc Gastroenterol Nurs Assoc* 14(6):286, 1995.

Quigly RL: Thoracentesis and chest tube drainage, *Crit Care Clin* 11(1):111, 1995.

Qureshi N, Brandsetter RD: Thoracentesis in clinical practice, *Heart Lung* 23(5):377, 1994.

Schultz SJ, Foley CR, Gordon DG: Preparing your patient for a cardiac PET scan, *Nurs* 21(9):63, 1991.

Weikart CJ: New eye into the heart, *RN* 56(10):36, 1993.

Chapter 45

Care After Death

OBJECTIVES

Mastery of content in this chapter will enable the nurse to:

- Discuss important considerations when working with families and significant others in regard to organ and/or tissue donation.
- Describe the physiological changes after death.
- Describe postmortem care techniques.
- Correctly prepare a client's body after death.

KEY TERMS

Advanced directives
Anorexia
Antiemetics
Autopsy
Epidemiology
Loss
Morgue
Organ/tissue donation
Rigor mortis

SKILLS

45-1 Care of the Body After Death

Dying is a profound process affecting everyone involved: the dying person, significant others, friends, and care givers. Each person's self-concept, past experiences, values, beliefs, and emotions will affect how the person handles the process of dying and death. To be effective in providing care during this time, the nurse needs both a knowledge of the dying process and a degree of personal comfort in addressing death.

As death approaches, the family and significant others need support. Often times family members want to be involved in the client's care (see box). Factual information about what to expect as death draws near can provide some understanding of the unknown. Nurses can give families and significant others information about the signs and symptoms of approaching death (see the box on p. 1313).

The nurse and other members of the health care team need to consider life support and the degree of intervention the person desires at the time of death. The Patient Self-Determination Act of 1991 requires all health care agencies serving Medicaid and Medicare clients to provide clients with information regarding the various advanced directives options. **Advanced directives** are legal documents that allow a person to have a say in the medical treatments the person will receive if unable to make decisions. The person can specify what types of treatments are acceptable or unacceptable, and the person can also designate another person to make treatment decisions if he/she is unable to make decisions. It is the nurse's responsibility to determine if the client's wishes have been assessed and if advanced directives are appropriately documented in the client record. Even though it is legally mandated that health care agencies provide information related to advanced directives, studies suggest that clients often have a limited understanding of advanced directives and their implications. Many clients have not executed advanced directives (Rein et al., 1996). The nurse may well find it beneficial to discuss advanced directives with a dying person and family if the person's wishes are not clearly reflected in the record (Johns, 1996). Because agency policies and state laws differ, nurses need to be familiar with agency policies and the state laws where they are practicing (Badzek, 1992).

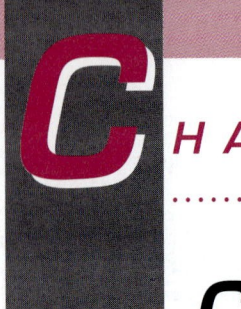

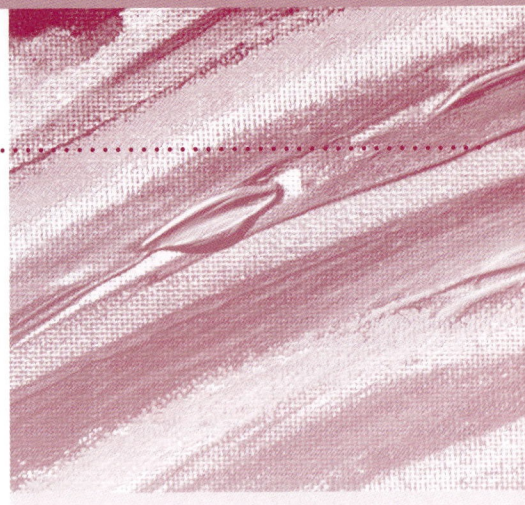

Another consideration as death approaches is one of **organ/tissue donation.** The 1986 Omnibus Budget Reconciliation Act (OBRA) mandates that significant others be offered the option of organ and tissue donation (Chabalewski and Norris, 1994). Gallup polls have consistently reported that the majority of Americans favor organ/tis-

SUGGESTIONS FOR INVOLVING THE FAMILY IN THE CARE OF A DYING CLIENT

- Assist in planning a visitation schedule for family members to prevent client and family from becoming fatigued.
- Allow young children to visit a dying parent or grandparent.
- Be willing to listen to family complaints about the client's care and feelings about the client.
- Help family members learn to interact with the dying person (e.g., using attentive listening, avoiding false reassurances, conducting conversations about normal family activities or problems).
- Allow family members to help with simple care measures such as feeding, bathing, and straightening bed linen. Recognize that family members are often more successful than nursing staff in persuading the client to eat.
- When the family becomes fatigued with care activities, relieve them from their duties so that they can acquire needed rest and support. Refer them to resources for meals and lodging.
- Support the act of grieving between client and family. Provide privacy when preferred. Do not discourage open expression of grief between family and client.
- Provide information daily with regard to the client's condition. Prepare the family for sudden changes in the client's appearance and behavior.
- Communicate news of impending death when the family is together, if possible. Remember that members can provide support for one another. Convey the news in a private area and be willing to stay with the family.
- As death nears, help the family stay in communication with the dying person through short visits, caring silence, touch, and telling the client of their love.
- After death, assist the family with decision making, such as selection of a mortician, transportation of family members, and collection of the client's belongings.

SIGNS AND SYMPTOMS OF APPROACHING DEATH

The arms and legs may become cool to the touch and the underside of the body may become darker in color. These symptoms are the result of the blood circulation slowing down.

The patient will spend more and more time sleeping during the day and at times will be difficult to arouse. This results from slowing of the body's metabolism.

The patient may lose bladder or bowel control, resulting in incontinence.

Oral secretions may become more profuse and collect in the back of the throat, producing what is commonly referred to as the "death rattle." This is a result of decreased fluid intake and the patient's inability to cough up normal saliva.

The patient's vision and hearing decrease slightly, with hearing generally being the last sense to be lost.

The patient may become restless, pulling at bed linen and having visions of people or things. This is the result of decreased oxygen to the brain, as well as the decreased metabolism.

The patient will have a decreased need for food and drink.

The patient's breathing pattern will change during sleep to an irregular pace with 10- to 30-second periods of no breathing.

Signs of death include no breathing, no heartbeat, no response to shaking or shouting, loss of bladder and bowel control, eyelids slightly open with eyes fixed on one spot, and jaws relaxed and mouth slightly open.

NOTE: Not all these symptoms will appear at the same time and some may never appear.

From Long B, Phipps W, Cassmeyer V: *Medical-surgical nursing: a nursing process approach*, ed 3, 1993, St Louis, Mosby.

sue donation and express that they are likely to donate their own organs/tissues when they die. Following donation, most donor families report feeling positive about the donation and report that donation has helped them in working through the grieving process. Families and significant others have indicated a desire for health care providers to approach them regarding organ and tissue donation, to let them know if their dying significant other is a potential donor, and to describe what types of organs/tissues could be donated. Even though organ/tissue donation is favored, there is a shortage of donor organs and tissues. This shortage is partly the result of health care professionals' hesitancy to identify and approach potential significant others and the dying regarding organ/tissue donation (Lindsay, 1995). To help the nurse in approaching families regarding organ/tissue donation, the nurse can contact the Organ Procurement and Transplantation Network, which coordinates donors and transplants. This nationwide organization has within each region of the country local organ procurement organizations (OPAs) that have trained personnel who can offer assistance 24 hours a day to answer questions and coordinate necessary details of the process. Health care agencies have policies and procedures that facilitate interface with this organization (Chabalewski and Norris, 1994).

Table 45-1 Physiological Changes After Death

Change	Related Interventions
Stiffening of body **(rigor mortis)** developing 2 to 4 hours after death; involves contraction of skeletal and smooth muscle owing to lack of adenosine 5′-triphosphate (ATP)	Before rigor mortis develops, position body in normal anatomical alignment, close eyelids and mouth, insert dentures in mouth.
Reduction in body temperature with loss of skin elasticity (algor mortis)	Gently remove tape and dressings to avoid tissue breakdown. Avoid pulling on skin or body parts.
Purple discoloration of skin (livor mortis) in dependent areas caused by breakdown of red blood cells	Elevate head to prevent facial discoloration.
Body tissues soften and liquefy by bacterial fermentation	Store body in cool place in hospital morgue or other designated area.

SIGNS OF DEATH

When death occurs, the traditional clinical signs are cessation of the apical pulse, respirations, and blood pressure. Many clients, however, are maintained on mechanical ventilators, artificial pacemakers, and supportive intravenous medications that maintain respiration and circulation, making the determination of death more difficult. The Uniform Determination of Death Act (UDDA) definition or a similar definition of death is now accepted in all 50 of the United States as valid and legal criteria of death. The UDDA defines death as "irreversible cessation of circulatory and respiratory functions or irreversible cessation of all function of the brain, including the brainstem" (Chabalewski and Norris, 1994).

PHYSIOLOGICAL CHANGES AFTER DEATH

When death occurs, cellular and circulatory changes create alterations in the body's tissues (Table 45-1). These changes influence the manner in which the nurse cares for the body after death. It is important for the nurse to prepare the body for viewing as quickly as possible. The longer a nurse waits to care for the body, the more difficult it is to make the body appear natural.

GUIDELINES

1. As it becomes obvious that a person is facing a life-threatening illness or likely to die following an accident, the nurse needs to establish the status of the person's advanced directives.
2. As a client's death approaches, the nurse needs to consider if the dying person is a candidate for organ/tissue donation.
3. Following a client's death, consult agency policy regarding who is to be notified at the time of death and notify as directed.
4. Following a client's death, the nurse should make contact with significant others to determine their status and to address priority needs.
5. Care for the body needs to be performed in a timely manner. If organ or tissue donation has been made, the OPA should be notified as soon as death is imminent.
6. The needs and desires of the family and significant others should be considered as the body is prepared for transfer to the funeral home or **morgue.** The nurse should consult with significant others about when they want to see the deceased, if or how they want to be involved in caring for the body, and if cultural practices or spiritual beliefs of the deceased impact on care of the body.
7. Consider the well-being of the roommates and others in the unit. Let the roommate know of the death and offer the opportunity to move the roommate to another location while the deceased is prepared to be removed from the room. Close door of other client rooms during body preparation and transfer.
8. Implement Standard Precautions: use protective equipment for the level of anticipated body substance exposure.
9. Ensure that the deceased's belongings are given to significant others. Follow agency policy in documenting the transfer. If there are valuables involved, having a second witness present is always a sound practice.

SKILL 45-1 Care of the Body After Death

When a client's death is pronounced, the physician certifies the death in the medical record and records the time of death and a description of therapies or actions taken. The physician may request permission from the family for an autopsy. An **autopsy** or postmortem examination is performed to confirm or determine the cause of death, gather data regarding the nature and progress of a disease, study the effects of therapies on body tissues, and provide statistical data for **epidemiology** and research purposes. A consent form must be signed by the most immediate family member and the physician or designated requester. Autopsies are required in circumstances of unusual death (e.g., violent trauma, unexpected death in the home) as well as death occurring within a set time frame following hospitalization. Each state has guidelines for when autopsies are required. Autopsies normally do not delay burial.

EQUIPMENT

- Disposable gloves, gown, and other protective clothing
- Plastic bag for hazardous waste disposal
- Washbasin, washcloth, warm water, and bath towel
- Clean gown or disposable gown for body as indicated by agency policy
- Absorbent pads
- Body bag or plastic shroud (consult agency procedure)
- Gauze for ties
- Identification tag(s) as specified by hospital policy
- Small pillow or towel
- Paper tape, gauze dressings
- Paper bag, plastic bag, or other suitable receptacle for client's clothing, belongings, and other items to be returned to significant others
- Valuables envelope

DELEGATION CONSIDERATIONS

Most hospitals and long-term care facilities allow unlicensed assistive personnel to prepare the body for viewing and transport the body to the morgue. When delegating to personnel, the nurse should:

- Review any instruction and reinforce the importance of handling the body with respect.
- Reinforce to staff the importance of following infection control guidelines.
- Inform staff of any special needs the family might have regarding the preparation of the body.

STEPS	RATIONALE
ASSESSMENT	
1. Assess for presence of family members or significant others and whether they have been informed of the client's death. Determine who is legally defined as next of kin.	It is the physician's responsibility to notify significant others of the client's death. Nurse provides emotional support and prepares the body for viewing. Next of kin is approached for tissue donation.
CRITICAL DECISION POINT Observe response of significant others. There is no "right" way to respond. Expression of grief may be very obvious, such as loud screaming or falling on the body, or very subtle and perhaps nondetectable.	
2. Allow time for significant others to ask questions.	Conveys caring and concern for significant others. May provide valuable information about the response of significant others and their needs.
3. Approach next of kin or accompany person who makes requests for tissue donation, and discuss options with family.	Family needs full understanding of tissue donation options and implications.
4. Once family has made decision, complete necessary organ/tissue donation request form.	Federal guidelines require documentation that request has been made.
5. Assess the deceased for general condition of the body and any bandages, tubes, or equipment.	Because of the fragility of tissues following death, tissue damage can occur easily. Most agencies have specific policies about removal of tubes, wires, and equipment.
6. Determine if an autopsy is planned.	If an autopsy is planned, some procedures such as removal of tubes and lines may be altered.

STEPS / **RATIONALE**

NURSING DIAGNOSIS

Clustering of defining characteristics from the assessment data may reveal the following nursing diagnoses for clients requiring this skill:

➤ Risk for impaired skin integrity

For family members or significant others:

➤ Dysfunctional grieving

Related factors are individualized based on the family's and significant others' needs.

PLANNING

1. **Expected outcomes** following completion of procedure:
   - ➤ Deceased's body will be free of skin damage.
     Deceased's skin will be free of additional bruises, lacerations, or abrasions.
   - ➤ Significant others will express grief.
     Significant others acknowledge loss of loved one.
2. Gather or direct assistive personnel to gather needed equipment.
   Because this is often a time of emotional intensity for significant others, organization is particularly important.

IMPLEMENTATION

1. Check with significant others about notifying other significant people.
   Following a death, significant others may have trouble dealing with the concrete details surrounding the death and may need assistance.
2. Discuss procedure of preparing the body with significant others. Inquire if there are particular cultural or spiritual practices that are significant for the deceased or significant others.
   Having some ability to direct what is happening can increase the significant others' sense of control. Consulting with significant others can provide valuable information in regard to specific practices related to culture and spirituality. Discussing these aspects of care with the significant others can convey your caring and concern.

➤ CRITICAL DECISION POINT Significant others may want to be involved with the final preparation of the body. Being able to participate in this final aspect of care can facilitate grieving and acknowledgment of the death.

3. If tissue donation has been made, consult policy for specific guidelines in care of the body.
   Retrieval of tissues (e.g., eyes, bone, skin) may require certain preparation measures.
4. Wash hands.
   Reduces transmission of microorganisms.
5. Close room door or draw bedside curtain.
   Provides privacy for the deceased and significant others. Limits exposure of other clients to the person's death.
6. Apply disposable gloves and gown or protective barriers as applicable.
   Body excretions may harbor infectious microorganisms. Withdrawal of intravenous tubing or other tubing may cause temporary bleeding.

➤ CRITICAL DECISION POINT If significant others are assisting in the preparation of the body, be sure they too are protected from body excretions.

7. Identify the body according to agency policy. Leave identification in place as directed in agency policy.
   Ensures proper identification of the body.
8. If in keeping with agency procedures, remove all indwelling catheters, intravenous, oxygen, and other tubes. **(If an autopsy is to be performed, policy may direct to leave these devices in place.)** Dress puncture wounds with a small dressing and paper tape.
   Creates a normal appearance. Paper tape minimizes skin trauma.

STEPS	RATIONALE
9. If the person wore dentures, insert them. If mouth fails to close, place a rolled up towel under the chin.	It is difficult to insert dentures after rigor mortis occurs. Dentures maintain natural facial expression.
10. Position client as outlined in agency procedures. In general, do not place one hand on top of the other. Placing one hand on top of another can lead to skin discoloration.	Client appears natural and comfortable.
11. Place small pillow or folded towel under the head or elevate head of bed 10 to 15 degrees.	Prevents pooling of blood in the face and subsequent discoloration.
12. Close eyes gently by grasping the eyelashes.	Closed eyes present a more natural appearance. Pressure on the lids can lead to discoloration.
13. Wash body parts soiled by blood, urine, feces, or other drainage. (A mortician will provide a complete bath.)	Prepares body for viewing and reduces odors.
14. Place an absorbent pad under the client's buttocks.	Relaxation of sphincter muscles after death may cause release of urine or feces.
15. Remove soiled dressings and replace with clean gauze dressings. Use paper tape.	Paper tape minimizes skin trauma. Changing dressings helps to control odors caused by microorganisms and to create a more acceptable appearance.
16. Place a clean gown on the client (agency policy may require removal before body is wrapped).	Prepares body for viewing.
17. Brush and comb client's hair. Remove any clips, hairpins, or rubber bands.	During viewing, the client should appear well-groomed. Hard objects such as pins can damage or discolor the face and scalp.
18. If significant others request viewing, place a sheet or light blanket over the body with only the head and upper shoulders exposed. Remove unneeded equipment from the room. Provide soft lighting and offer chairs.	Maintains dignity and respect for the client and significant others. Prevents exposure of body parts.

CRITICAL DECISION POINT **Determine if significant others need time alone with the deceased or would be more comfortable if a staff member remained in the room.**

STEPS	RATIONALE
19. After the significant others have left the room, remove all linen and the client's gown (refer to agency policy). Place body in body bag or apply the shroud as required by the agency (see illustration).	Prevents injury to skin and extremities. Avoids unnecessary exposure of body parts.
20. Label the body as directed by agency policy.	Ensures proper identification of the body.

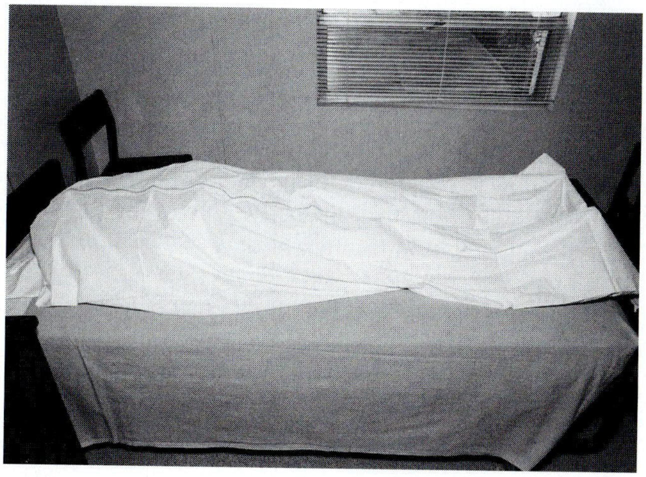

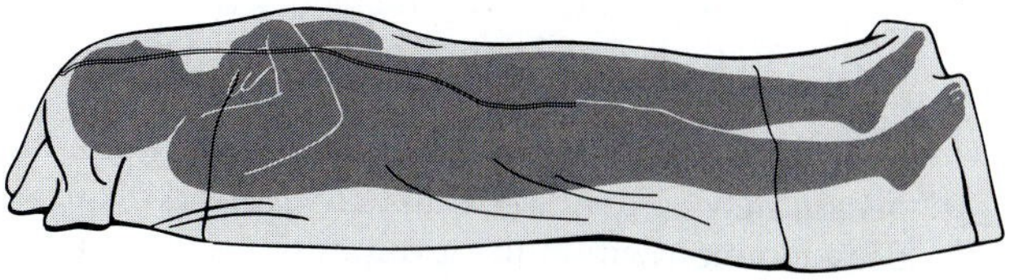

Step 19 Body bag.

STEPS	RATIONALE
21. Arrange transportation of the body to the morgue or mortuary.	If delay is anticipated before the mortician arrives, the body should be cooled in the morgue to prevent further tissue damage.

E VALUATION

1. Observe significant others' response to the loss.	Each person's response to loss is unique, and assessment is necessary to determine the need for referral for assistance.
2. Provide significant others with the opportunity to express feelings.	Significant others often seek the opportunity to express feelings with someone other than an immediate family member.

CRITICAL DECISION POINT **The nurse may need to find a private place for significant others so they can feel free to express their emotions.**

3. Note appearance and condition of client's skin during preparation of the body.	Determines if damage to tissues occurs after preparation.
4. **Unexpected outcomes** that may occur include:	
➤ Significant others become immobilized by their grief and have difficulty functioning.	
➤ Lacerations, bruises, or abrasions are noted on skin surfaces of deceased.	Positioning or preparation of the body results in skin injury.

RECORDING AND REPORTING

1. Record date and time of death, time physician notified, name of physician pronouncing death, delivery of postmortem care, identification of body, consent form signed by significant other, disposition of the body, and information provided to significant others.	Ensures that client's death is accurately and legally recorded.
2. Document any marks, bruises, wounds on body before death or those observed during care of the body.	Reduces risk of liability for creating such marks in the care of the body after death or in transport to the morgue. Certain markings can identify the body if identification tags are lost or destroyed.
3. Document how valuables and personal belongings were handled and who received them. Secure signatures as required by agency policy.	Makes clear how things were distributed if a question arises.

• • • • •

Special Considerations

- Some cultures and religions have specific practices that are performed before or after death. Religions that have practices surrounding death include the Eastern Orthodox Church, Judaism, Christianity, Roman Catholicism, Islamism, and Buddhism.
- Spiritual beliefs are individual. Even though a person may belong to a particular religious group, the person may or may not adhere to particular practices common within the group.

Home Care Considerations

- As death approaches, significant others often need information about what to expect. The information in the box on p. 1313 can be useful.
- As death approaches, the nurse needs to consider the type of support the significant others are likely to need at the time of death and make plans to put this support in place.
- Following death in the home, the nurse will need to follow agency guidelines related to body preparation and transfer of the body.
- For disposable dressings or linens soaked in body substances, the nurse must follow the policies of the agency. The nurse may need to instruct significant others in the handling of body substances in the home.

CRITICAL THINKING EXERCISES

1. You are to prepare a body for viewing. You do not know whether there were any infectious processes involved in the illness. Where would you find that information? How would you protect yourself? What must you do to prepare the body before the significant others are allowed in to see the deceased?

2. Your client died about 2 hours ago. Someone is on the telephone inquiring about your client's condition. How would you handle this situation? Who would be the most helpful individual in your agency to deal with this call?

REFERENCES

Badzek L: What you need to know about advance directives, *Nurs 92* 22(6):58, 1992.

Callanan M, Kelley P: *Final gifts: understanding the special awareness, needs and communications of the dying,* New York, 1992, Simon & Schuster.

Chabalewski F, Norris M: The gift of life: talking to families about organ and tissue donation, *Am J Nurs* 94(6):28, 1994.

Johns J: Advanced directives and opportunities for nurses, *Image* 28(2):149, 1996.

Long B, Phipps W, Cassmeyer V: *Medical-surgical nursing: a nursing process approach.* ed 3, St Louis, 1993, Mosby.

Lindsay K: Assisting professionals in approaching families for donation, *Crit Care Nurs Q* 17(4):55, 1995.

Rein A, et al: Advance directive decision making among medical inpatients, *J Prof Nurs* 12(1):39, 1996.

ADDITIONAL READING

Meyer C: Coming to new terms with death, *Am J Nurs* 92(8):19, 1992.

Ufema J: Insights on death and dying, *Nurs 88* 18(10):97, 1988.

Ufema J: Helping loved ones say good-bye, *Nurs 91* 21(10):42, 1991.

Zerwekh J: The truth-tellers: how hospice nurses help patients confront death, *Am J Nurs* 94(2):31, 1994.

Glossary

abdominal girth The measurement of the abdomen's circumference, taken at the same place with each measurement.

abduction Movement of an extremity away from the midline of the body.

accommodation reflex Adjustment of the eyes for near vision, composed of pupillary constriction, convergence of the visual axes, and increased convexity of the lens.

accurate empathy Communication technique used by nurse to show understanding of client's feelings and experiences.

Acetest A test that measures the presence of ketone (acetone) bodies in the urine. A large quantity of acetone causes rapid change in the color of the Acetest tablet.

active listening An interpersonal process whereby a person hears a message, decodes the meaning, and conveys an understanding about the meaning to the sender.

active-assisted range of motion Exercises of the joints performed by an individual with some assistance.

active range of motion Exercise of the joints performed by an individual without assistance.

activity tolerance Kind and amount of exercise or work that a person is able to perform.

acuity charting Documentation that quantifies the level of care required by a client in a health care setting.

acute pain Severe pain with a rapid onset and of short duration.

adduction Movement of an extremity toward midline of the body.

adjuvant therapy The treatment of a disease with substances that enhance the action of drugs, especially drugs that promote the production of antibodies.

adrenergic drug A medication that mimics the effects of sympathetic nerve stimulation of the autonomic nervous system.

advance directives A written agreement established between a client and physician to withhold heroic measures or life-sustaining treatment if the client's condition becomes irreversible. Advance directives are usually written at a time when clients are healthy or able to make conscious decisions regarding their welfare.

aerobe A microorganism that lives and grows in the presence of free oxygen.

agglutinate A process by which cells that display antigens (red blood cells, bacteria) adhere to each other, or clump together.

air embolus A quantity of air that circulates in the bloodstream to eventually lodge in a blood vessel.

air fluidization The process of blowing warm air through a collection of microspheres to create a fluidlike environment; used in special mattresses designed to reduce pressure against a person's skin.

air suspension bed A device that supports a client's weight on air-filled cushions, minimizing tissue damage from pressure and shear.

airway obstruction An abnormal condition of the respiratory system characterized by a mechanical impediment to the delivery or the absorption of oxygen in the lungs.

aldosterone A steroid hormone produced by the adrenal cortex that causes the kidney tubules to excrete potassium and reabsorb sodium and water.

Allen test This test is performed to determine the collateral circulation supply in the radial and ulnar artery.

allergen A substance that can produce a hypersensitive reaction in the body but that is not necessarily intrinsically harmful.

alopecia Partial or complete lack of hair.

Alzheimer's Disease Presenile dementia, characterized by confusion, memory failure, disorientation, restlessness, and speech disturbances. The disease usually begins in later middle life with slight defects in memory and behavior and occurs with equal frequency in men and women.

Ambu-bag Portable resuscitation device that provides manual inflation of the lungs. An Ambu-bag is usually used with supplemental oxygen.

Ambularm™ Battery operated, position sensitive alarm attached to a client's leg, which alerts the staff when a client attempts to get out of bed.

American Hospital Association (AHA) A not-for-profit association of health care provider organizations that are committed to health improvement of their communities. The AHA is the national advocate for its members, which includes 5,000 hospitals, health care systems, networks, and other providers of care. Founded in 1898, AHA provides education for health care leaders and is a source of information on health care issues and trends (American Hospital Association, 1996).

The American Society of Parenteral and Enteral Nutrition (ASPEN) An organization that provides education, support, and accreditation to individuals in the nutritional support field.

amino acid An organic compound composed of one or more basic amino groups and one or more carboxyl groups. Amino acids are the building blocks that construct proteins and the end products of protein digestion.

amnesic syndrome Memory impairment in the absence of other cognitive impairments.

ampule Small sterile glass or plastic container that usually contains a single dose of solution to be administered parenterally.

anaerobic Pertaining to absence of air or oxygen.

anaphylactic reaction Exaggerated hypersensitivity reaction to a previously encountered antigen. It is a severe and sometimes fatal systemic reaction characterized by itching, hyperemia, angioedema, and in severe cases vascular collapse, bronchospasm, and shock.

anaphylaxis An exaggerated hypersensitivity reaction to a previously encountered antigen. The reaction may be localized or generalized.

anastomosis A surgical joining of two ducts or blood vessels to allow flow from one to the other.

anemia A disorder characterized by a decrease in hemoglobin in the blood to levels below the normal range, decreased red cell production, or increased red cell destruction or blood loss.

anesthesia The absence of normal sensation, especially sensitivity to pain.

anions Negatively charged ions.

anthropometry The science of measuring the human body as to height, weight, and size of component parts, including measurement of skin folds.

antianginal drug A medication that dilates coronary arteries, improving blood flow to the myocardium to prevent angina.

antidysrhythmic A class of medications that possesses properties for controlling abnormal cardiac rhythms, e.g., quinidine and propranolol (Inderal).

antiemetic Of or pertaining to a substance or procedure that prevents or alleviates nausea and vomiting.

antipyretic Pertaining to a substance, such as a medication, that reduces fever.

apical pulse Measurement of the heartbeat as taken with the stethoscope placed over the apex of the heart.

apnea An absence of spontaneous respirations.

approximate To come together, as in the edges of a wound.

aqueous Watery or waterlike; referring to a medication prepared with water.

areola Referring to the areola mammae, the pigmented, circular area surrounding the nipple of each breast.

artificial airway Plastic or rubber device inserted into the upper or lower respiratory tract to facilitate ventilation or secretion removal.

ascites Effusion and accumulation of serous fluid in the abdominal cavity.

asepsis The absence of disease-producing (pathogenic) organisms.

aseptic technique The methods used during client care to prevent microbial contamination. They can be either clean (medical asepsis) techniques or sterile (surgical asepsis) techniques.

aspirant Fluid or particulate that is aspirated.

aspirate Withdrawal of fluid or air into the barrel of a syringe or suction device.

aspiration The inhalation of a foreign substance into the lungs.

astigmatism Abnormal condition of the eye in which the light rays cannot be focused clearly in a point on the retina because the spherical curve of the cornea is not equal in all meridians. Vision is blurred and use of the eyes causes discomfort.

astringent A topical substance that causes constriction of tissues upon application; commonly used for cleansing the skin.

atelectasis An abnormal condition characterized by the collapse of lung tissue, preventing the respiratory exchange of carbon dioxide and oxygen.

atrophy Wasting or diminution of size or physiologic activity of a part of the body caused by disease or other influences.

atmospheric pressure Pressure exerted by the atmosphere. (Atmospheric pressure at sea level is 760 mm Hg.)

auscultation The act of listening for sounds within the body to evaluate the condition of the heart, lungs, pleura, intestines, or other organs or to detect fetal heart sounds. Performed directly or most commonly through use of a stethoscope.

autoclave An appliance used to sterilize medical instruments or other objects with steam under pressure.

autolet A small instrument with a lancet used to obtain a capillary blood specimen.

autologous blood transfusion Transfusion of a client's own blood either through predeposit, blood salvaged intraoperatively by a cell saver, or shed blood postoperatively.

autopsy Examination performed after a person's death to confirm or determine the cause of death.

autotransfusion The collection, anticoagulation, filtration, and reinfusion of blood from an active bleeding site.

axillary Pertaining to the pyramid-shaped space that forms the underside of the shoulder between the upper part of the arm and the side of the chest.

backrub The application of gentle methodical pressure to the back.

bacteremia Presence of bacteria in the blood.

bacteriostatic Inhibits development of bacteria.

bariatric bed A specialized surface, equipped with hand controls to allow for self-positioning, providing a stable, adaptable surface for managing the morbidly obese client.

basal energy expenditure The amount of energy required at rest for basic life processes, such as breathing, maintaining body temperature, and cardiac function. Basal energy expenditure can be estimated or measured.

basal metabolism Energy needed to maintain the body's basic processes such as respiration, circulation, and temperature.

base of support Surface area on which an object rests.

bed rest Placement of the client in bed for a prescribed period for therapeutic reasons.

BEE Abbreviation for Basal Energy Expenditure.

belt restraint Type of restraint used to secure a client on a stretcher.

bile A digestive juice secreted by the liver, stored in the gallbladder, and secreted in the small intestine to digest fat. Bile causes brown color of feces.

binder Bandage made of a large piece of material to fit and support a specific body part.

biopsy The removal and microscopic examination of tissue, performed to establish precise diagnosis.

blood group Classification of blood based on the presence or absence of genetically determined antigens on the surface of the red cell.

blood plasma The liquid portion of the blood, free of its formed elements and particles.

blood transfusion Administration of whole blood or a blood component as cells to replace blood lost through trauma, surgery, or disease.

blood typing Identification of genetically determined antigens on the surface of the red blood cell, used to determine a person's blood group.

blood warming coil Device constructed of coiled plastic tubing used to warm reserve blood before massive transfusion.

body alignment Refers to the condition of joints, tendons, ligaments, and muscles in various body positions.

bolus 1. A round mass, specifically a masticated lump of food ready to be swallowed. 2. A large, round preparation of medicinal material for oral ingestion. 3. A dose of a medication or a contrast material injected all at once intravenously.

bone marrow Specialized, soft tissue filling the spaces in cancellous bone of the epiphyses; responsible for red blood cell production.

borborygmus Audible abdominal sound produced by hyperactive intestinal peristalsis.

bradycardia An abnormality in heart rate in which the heart contracts steadily at a rate less than 60 contractions per minute.

broad-spectrum antibiotic An antibiotic that is effective against a wide range of infectious microorganisms.

bronchophony An increase in intensity and clarity of vocal resonance that may result from an increase in lung tissue density, such as in the consolidation of pneumonia.

bronchospasm Abnormal contraction of the smooth muscles of the bronchi.

bronchus One of several large air passages in the lungs through which pass inspired air and exhaled gases.

bruit Abnormal sound or murmur created by turbulent blood flow heard while auscultating an organ, gland, or artery.

buccal Of or pertaining to the inside of the cheek; surface of a tooth or gum next to the cheek.

cadence Pace or rate of verbal communication.

calorie (Kcal) A calorie is the amount of heat required to raise the temperature of 1 g of water 1° C at atmospheric pressure.

cannula A flexible tube containing a stiff, pointed trocar; the tube may be inserted into the body, guided by the trocar. As the trocar is removed a body fluid may pass through the cannula.

capillary closing pressure The amount of external pressure required to close off the blood flow to the capillaries.

carcinoma Malignant epithelial neoplasm that tends to invade surrounding tissue and spread to distant regions of the body.

cardiac 1. Of or pertaining to the heart. 2. Pertaining to a person with heart disease.

cardiac output Volume of blood ejected by the ventricles of the heart in one minute; equal to stroke volume times heart rate.

cardiopulmonary arrest Sudden cessation of respirations, pulse, and circulation.

cardiopulmonary resuscitation (CPR) Basic emergency procedure for life support, consisting of artificial respiration and manual external cardiac massage.

caries Decay of a tooth; progressive decalcification of enamel and dentin of a tooth.

carminative A solution to provide relief from gaseous distention.

case management The assignment of a health care provider to assist the patient in assessing health and social service systems and to assure that required services are obtained.

cast Rigid plaster or fiberglass application molded over skin tissues to hold musculoskeletal tissues to permit healing of injuries.

cast brace Combination of a brace within a cast at a joint.

cast saw Saw used to cut through plaster to remove cast.

cast shoe Shoe worn over the foot encased in plaster.

cast stabilization Use of rods, pins, broom handles, or sticks to lend stability to a particular cast.
cast syndrome A series of client signs indicative of an untoward (claustrophobic) reaction to being in a cast.
casting tape Rolls of adhesive or resin-impregnated tape for use as lightweight casts.
cathartic Drug that acts to promote bowel evacuation.
catheter hub Plastic threaded connection at end of an intravenous catheter.
catheterization Introduction of a rubber or plastic tube through the urethra and into the bladder.
cations Positively charged ions.
cell cycle The sequence of events that occurs during the growth and division of tissue cells.
center of gravity Midpoint or center of body weight. In the adult it is the midpelvic cavity between the symphysis pubis and the umbilicus.
centigrade Temperature scale in which 0 degrees is the freezing point of water and 100 degrees is the boiling point of water at sea level; also called Celsius.
central venous catheter A catheter that is threaded through the internal jugular, antecubital, or subclavian vein, usually with tip resting in the superior vena cava or right atrium.
central venous pressure (CVP) Pressure in the great veins (superior and inferior vena cava) as blood returns to the heart.
cephalic vein One of the four superficial veins of the upper limb.
cerebrospinal fluid Substance contained within the four ventricles of the brain, the subarachnoid space, and the central canal of the spinal cord.
cerumen Earwax; a waxy secretion produced by apocrine sweat glands in the external ear canal.
cervical halter Support for the head, made of cotton material, used for traction.
chart A client's record; or to note data in a client's record, usually at prescribed intervals.
charting by exception A charting methodology in which data is entered only when there is an exception from what is normal or expected. Reduces time spent documenting.
cheilosis Disorder of the lips and mouth characterized by scales and fissures.
chemotherapeutic agent A medication used to treat cancer, which alters the growth of a cancer cell.
chemotherapy Use of drugs to prevent cancer cells from multiplying, invading adjacent tissue, and metastasizing.
chest physiotherapy Physical maneuvers, including postural drainage, chest percussion, vibration, rib shaking, and cough, to improve airway mucus clearance in clients with retained tracheobronchial secretions.
chest tube Catheter inserted through the chest wall into the intrapleural space by the physician.
chronic pain Continuous or recurrent pain lasting longer than 3 months.
circumduction The circular movement of a limb; the motion of the head of a bone within an articulating cavity, such as the hip joint.
clarification An attempt to put into words vague ideas or unclear thoughts of the client to enhance the nurse's understanding or asking the client to explain what he or she means.
class II biologic safety cabinet A vertical containment or biologic safety cabinet that recirculates air through a high-efficiency particulate air (HEPA) filter.
clean technique (medical asepsis) The purposeful prevention of the transmission of microorganisms by using procedures such as handwashing and disinfection of equipment to reduce the number of microorganismms.
clean-voided specimen A technique used to collect a urine specimen as free from bacterial contamination as possible without catheterizing the client.
cleansing enema An enema, usually soap suds, administered repeatedly until the colon is free of all formed fecal material.
client-centered air leak The entry of air, which originates from the client, into a closed chest drainage system, as opposed to the entry of air originating from the chest drainage system itself.
Clinitest A test that measures the amount of glucose and acetone in a urine specimen.
Clinitron bed A special bed containing an air-fluidization mattress that conforms to the shape of a person's body to reduce pressure exerted against skin and soft tissues.
closed system catheter A suction catheter that is attached to the mechanical ventilator circuit encased within a sterile sheath. The catheter system permits sterile airway suctioning without interrupting mechanical ventilation or requiring the nurse to apply sterile gloves.
coagulopathy A pathologic condition affecting the ability of the blood to coagulate.
colon Portion of large intestine from the cecum to the rectum.
colon conduit A surgical noncontinent (sometimes called incontinent) urinary diversion where the ureters are inplanted into a 4-6 cm piece of large intestine that has been removed from the rest of the bowel and will now serve as a passageway for the urine. The distal end of this piece of colon is sutured closed while the other end of the colon is brought out onto the client's abdomen as a stoma.
colonization The reproduction of microorganisms at a specific site without the signs/symptoms of a disease or tissue invasion.
colonized The presence of bacteria on the surface or in the tissue of a wound without indications of infection such as purulent exudate, foul odor, or surrounding inflammation. All stage II, III, and IV pressure ulcers are colonized (AHCPR, 1994, p. 107).
colostomy Surgical formation of an opening of the colon onto the surface of the abdomen through which fecal matter is emptied.
compartment syndrome Insufficient arterial perfusion to an extremity caused by trauma or stasis; leads to ischemia and tissue necrosis if not reversed.
compatibility The quality or state of existing together in harmony. The formation of a stable chemical or biochemical system, specifically in medication, so that two or more drugs can be administered at same time without producing side effects.
compliance Fulfillment by the client of the caregiver's prescribed course of treatment.
compound A substance composed of two or more different elements, chemically combined, that cannot be separated by physical means.
compress Soft pad of gauze or cloth used to apply heat, cold, or medications to the surface of a body part.
concreteness Communication that includes specific feelings, behaviors, and experiences or situations; communication that is not vague.
conduction Mechanism of heat transfer involving flow of heat from one object to another with which it is in contact.
conduit An artificially created channel for drainage of urine, e.g., ileoloop.
congruent Harmonious and consistent; the verbal and nonverbal message is congruent when the nonverbal message is the same or consistent with the verbal message.
conjunctiva Mucous membrane lining the inner surfaces of the eyelids and anterior part of the sclera.
conjunctivitis A highly contagious eye infection. The crusty drainage that collects on eyelid margins can easily spread from one eye to the other.
consensual light reflex Constriction of the pupil of one eye when the other eye is illuminated.
constipation Condition characterized by difficulty in passing stool, or an infrequent passage of hard stool.
consultation A process in which the help of a specialist is sought to identify ways to handle problems in patient management or in the planning and implementation of health care programs.
contact lens A small, transparent, curved glass or plastic lens shaped to fit over a person's cornea; the lens floats on a precorneal tear film.
contaminated Being soiled, stained, touched, or otherwise exposed to harmful agents, such as by entry of potentially infectious microorganisms into or upon a previously clean or sterile environment.
contamination The introduction of infectious material on normally clean or sterile sites.
continent ostomy or diversion Results from a surgical procedure that leaves the client with an internal pouch where either stool or urine is temporarily stored and the effluent is removed by intubation through the external stoma. It is continent because the effluent does not drain spontaneously from the stoma; instead a catheter must

be inserted through the stoma to drain the effluent from the internal pouch.
contracture Abnormal condition of a joint, characterized by flexion and fixation and caused by atrophy and shortening of muscle fibers or by loss of normal elasticity of the skin.
coping An individual's ability to manage stressful situations.
core temperature Temperature of deep body tissues and organs.
cough Forced exhalation following in order after this normal series of events: (a) partial or full inhalation; (b) closure of the glottis; (c) active contraction of expiratory muscles; and (d) rapid glottic opening.
countertraction Use of client's body weight or other weights, ropes, and pulleys to counter the pull of the traction weight.
crackle Fine bubbling sound heard on auscultation of the lung.
crepitation The sound and/or feeling produced when bone ends rub against each other. The client describes the sound and feeling.
critical pathway A schedule of critical care medical and nursing procedures, including diagnostic tests, medications, and consultations designed to effect an efficient coordinated program of treatment.
crutch gait Gait assumed by a person on crutches by alternately bearing weight on one or both legs and on the crutches.
crutch palsy Temporary or permanent loss of sensation or movement resulting from pressure on axilla from crutch.
culture Laboratory test involving the cultivation of microorganisms or cells in a special growth medium.
cuff A plastic, air or foam and air filled, balloon-like attachment on the distal end of the endotracheal tube or tracheostomy tube that prevents loss of air from the lung and inhalation of foreign bodies around the tube.
cuticle A thin edge of cornified epithelium at the base of a nail.
CVA tenderness Diagnostic sign of kidney inflammation. Tenderness is elicited during light percussion of the costal vertebral angle (CVA).
cyanosis Bluish discoloration of the skin and mucous membranes caused by an excess of deoxygenated hemoglobin in the blood or a structural defect in the hemoglobin molecule.
cycloplegic Pertaining to a drug that paralyzes ciliary muscles of the eye, causing pupillary dilation for ophthalmologic examination or surgery.
cystectomy The surgical removal of the bladder.
cytology The study of cells, including their formation, origin, structure, function, biochemical activities, and pathology.
Dacron cuff A sheath of Dacron surrounding an atrial or venous catheter to prevent ascending infections and accidental displacement of the catheter.
dandruff Scaly material composed of dead, keratinized epithelium shed from the scalp. May also be a mild form of seborrheic dermatitits.
dangling To sit on the side of a bed with legs dependent or feet on the floor.
dead space A cavity remaining in a wound (AHCPR, 1994, p. 108).
debride To remove dead or damaged tissue from a wound; to remove dirt, foreign objects, damaged tissue, and cellular debris from a wound or burn in order to prevent infection and promote healing.
debridement Removal of dead tissue in a wound.
decompression Removal of pressure as from gas and fluid in the stomach and intestinal tract.
de-escalation A communication strategy involving the reduction of anxious and/or agitated behaviors exhibited verbally or nonverbally by the client; using a calm yet firm approach diffuses the client's increasing anxiety and/or agitated state, thereby minimizing potentially violent outbursts.
defecation Passage of feces from the digestive tract through the rectum.
dehiscence The separation or opening of wound layers.
dementia A term used to describe a group of symptoms related to a loss or impairment of mental powers. These symptoms appear in a person who is awake, and are demonstrated by symptoms of mental confusion, memory loss, disorientation, intellectual impairment or similar problems. The origin of the term is from two Latin words meaning "away" and "mind."
dentifrice A pharmaceutic compound used with a toothbrush for cleaning and polishing teeth.
dependent position The lowest position of an extremity or body.
dermatitis An inflammatory condition of the skin, characterized by erythema and pain or pruritis.
devitalized Tissues with reduced oxygen supply and blood flow.
dextrose The hydrated form of glucose.
diagnosis-related group (DRG) Groups of diseases or conditions classified on the basis of primary and secondary diagnosis, primary and secondary procedure, and client age. The assigned length of stay for each DRG is part of the formula used in determining a medical facility's reimbursement for each DRG.
dialysis A procedure that removes fluid and solid wastes from the blood or lymph.
diaphoresis Secretion of sweat typically associated with hyperthermia, physical exertion and emotional stress.
diastolic pressure The lower blood pressure measurement that reflects pressure within the arterial system during the period of ventricular relaxation—diastole.
diluent Agent that makes a solution or mixture thinner or more liquid by admixture.
discharge planning The process by which the nurse plans for a client's eventual release from a health care agency; the process begins on a client's admission to the agency.
don To put on.
dorsal Pertaining to the back or posterior.
dorsiflexion Flexion of the foot at the ankle (or flexion of other joints).
double-void A procedure of discarding the first urine specimen and testing the second urine specimen that was obtained 30 to 45 minutes later; this procedure gives a more accurate amount of glucose being spilled into the urine at that particular time.
drawsheet A special sheet placed over the regular sheet on a bed and used to move a person in bed.
drop factor Refers to the calibration of IV tubing (IV infusion set) in drops per milliliter. For example, the drop factor of microdrip IV tubing is 60 gtt/ml.
drug abuse Use of a drug to obtain effects for which it is not prescribed. May lead to physical, social, and psychologic harm.
drug addiction Inability to control a drive or craving for a chemical substance.
drug dependence Psychologic or physiologic reliance on a chemical substance.
drug interaction The pharmacological interaction of drugs taken concurrently which may result in an antagonistic, synergistic or lethal response.
drug plateau Blood serum concentration reached and maintained after repeated, fixed doses of a medication.
duration A characteristic used in assessing a symptom; the length of time a symptom lasts.
dyspnea Difficulty in breathing.
dysrhythmia An irregularity or deviation from the normal pattern of a heartbeat.
ecchymosis Discoloration of an area of the skin or mucous membrane resulting from extravasation of blood into the subcutaneous tissues as a result of trauma to the underlying blood vessels or to fragility of the vessel walls.
eczema Superficial dermatitis of unknown cause.
edema Abnormal accumulation of fluid in interstitial spaces of tissues.
effective osmolality Osmolality that causes water to move from one cell compartment to another. Effective osmolality is dependent on the number of solutes and on the permeability of the cell membrane to these solutes. Also referred to as tonicity.
effluent The drainage that is normally expected from an ostomy.
egophony A change in the voice sound as heard on auscultation of a client with pleural effusion. When client is asked to make e-e-e sounds, the sound is heard over the peripheral chest wall as a-a-a.
elastic bandage Bandage of elasticized fabric that provides support and allows movement.
electrolyte An element or compound that, when melted or dissolved in water or another solvent, dissociates into ions and is able to carry an electric current.
electronic infusion device (EID) Used to infuse IV fluid at a prescribed rate. There are two types; an infusion pump which is designed to deliver a measured amount of fluid over a period of time, and an IV controller which delivers fluid with the aid of gravity.
embolus A foreign object, a quantity of air or gas, a bit of tissue or

tumor, or a piece of thrombus that circulates in the bloodstream until it becomes lodged in a vessel.

empathy Ability to recognize and to some extent share the emotions and state of mind of another and to understand the meaning and significance of that person's behavior.

endotracheal tube Artificial airway inserted through the mouth into the trachea.

enema Procedure involving introduction of a solution into the rectum for cleansing or therapeutic pur- poses.

enteral nutrition The administration of nutrition via the gastrointestinal tract (i.e., by mouth, tube feeding, or oral supplement).

enteric-coated Tablets coated with a substance that does not dissolve until reaching the intestine. Used when drug constituents are irritating to oral and gastric mucosa.

enterostomy Surgical procedure that produces an artificial anus or fistula in the intestine by incision through the abdominal wall.

enucleation Removal of the eyeball, performed in cases of malignancy, severe infection, extensive trauma, or to control pain in glaucoma.

epidemiology Study of the occurrence, distribution, and causes of disease.

epidural analgesia Administration of local anesthetic by way of a catheter into the epidural space of the spinal column. Designed to produce anesthesia of the pelvic, abdominal, or genital areas.

episiotomy A surgical procedure in which an incision is made in a woman's perineum to enlarge her vaginal opening for delivery of an infant; procedure prevents tearing of perineum.

epithelialization The process by which epidermal cells migrate (move) over the wound's surface to close the top or "resurface" the wound.

erythema Redness or inflammation of the skin or mucous membranes, result of dilatation and congestion of superficial capillaries.

eschar Scab or dry crust that results from excoriation of the skin.

evaporation Mechanism of heat loss whereby moisture from the body's surface changes to vapor and transfers heat to the surrounding air.

eversion Turning outward or inside-out, such as turning the foot outward at the ankle.

evisceration The separation of wound layers with the protrusion of abdominal organs through the wound layers.

excoriation An injury to the surface of the skin or other part of the body caused by scratching or abrasion.

excretion The process of eliminating, shedding, or getting rid of substances by body organs or tissues.

exercise Performance of any physical activity for the purpose of conditioning the body, improving health, maintaining fitness, or as a therapeutic measure.

exit site Point at which a catheter leaves a body site.

exophthalmos Abnormal protrusion of one or both eyeballs caused by trauma, intracranial lesions, intraorbital disorders, or systemic disease, most commonly hyperthyroidism.

expectorant An agent that facilitates removal of bronchopulmonary secretions.

expectoration Expulsion of mucus or sputum from the mouth or lungs.

exploratory laparotomy The surgical exploration or examination of an abdominal organ or part.

extended care facility An institution that provides medical, nursing, and/or custodial care for an individual over a prolonged period, as during the course of a chronic disease or during the rehabilitation phase after an acute illness.

extension Movement increasing the angle between two adjoining bones.

external air leak The presence of air originating from outside of the closed chest drainage system.

external fixation Skeletal traction applied through the use of pins attached to a frame rather than weights.

external jugular vein One of a pair of large vessels in the neck that receive most of the blood from the exterior of the cranium and the deep tissues of the face.

external rotation Rotation of a joint outward.

extravasation The inadvertent infiltration of intravenous fluids or medications into the subcutaneous tissues surrounding the infusion site.

extremity restraints Restraints used to immobilize one or all extremities.

exudate Any fluid that has been extruded from a tissue or its capillaries, more specifically because of injury or inflammation. It is characteristically high in protein and white blood cells (AHCPR, 1994, p. 110).

Fahrenheit Temperature scale in which 32 degrees is the freezing point of water and 212 degrees is the boiling point of water at sea level.

fascia Fibrous connective tissue.

febrile Pertaining to or characterized by fever or an elevation in body temperature.

feces The waste material excreted by the rectum after digestion; stool.

fenestrated drape A drape with a round or slitlike opening in the center.

fenestrated tracheostomy tube A tracheostomy tube containing a hole (fenestration) on the posterior aspect of the outer cannula that allows air flow over the vocal cords and speech in spontaneously breathing clients.

fever An abnormal elevation of body temperature.

fiberoptic Pertaining to fiberoptics; referring to the transmission of an image along flexible bundles of coated glass or plastic fibers having special optical properties.

flatulence Condition characterized by the accumulation of gas within the lumen of the intestines.

flexion Movement decreasing the angle between two adjoining bones; bending of a limb.

floorstock A term applied to medications that are distributed, by the pharmacy, to the nursing unit in bulk. Generally, floorstock medications are ones that are commonly used, and are often obtainable as over the counter preparations. Examples include: Tylenol, Milk of Magnesia, antacids and stool softeners.

flotation device A foam mattress with a gel-like pad located in its center, designed to protect bony prominences and distribute pressure more evenly against the skin's surface.

flora Microorganisms that reside on and within the body to compete with disease-producing microorganisms to provide a natural immunity against certain infections.

flossing Mechanical cleansing of tooth surfaces with the use of stringlike waxed or unwaxed dental floss.

flowsheet A form used to record the same type of repeated measurements, procedures, or observations over time. Data on flowsheets allow the user to see trends over time.

fluid volume deficit An alteration characterized by the loss of fluids and electrolytes in an isotonic fashion.

fluid volume excess An alteration characterized by the abnormal retention of fluids and electrolytes in an isotonic fashion.

focus charting A charting methodology for structuring progress notes according to the focus of the note, for example, symptoms and nursing diagnosis. Each note includes data, action, and client response.

fontanel A space covered by tough membranes between the bones of an infant's cranium.

foramen magnum The large opening in the anterior and inferior part of the occipital bone, interconnecting the vertebral canal and cranial cavity.

foreign body airway maneuver One of three methods used to remove a foreign object that is obstructing the airway.

footboard Board placed perpendicular to the mattress, parallel to and touching the plantar surface of the client's feet and used to maintain dorsiflexion of the feet.

footdrop A falling or dragging of the foot from paralysis of the flexors of the ankle.

four-poster cast Cast placed over the shoulders; contains four vertical posts or poles on the anterior and posterior lateral sides of the head to immobilize the cervical vertebrae.

Fowler's position Posture assumed by a client when the head of the bed is raised approximately 45 to 90 degrees, as though the client is sitting upright.

frail elderly An older adult usually over the age of 75 who may have physical or mental disabilities that interfere with independent performance of ADL's.

frequency Symptom of urinary disorder involving repetitive voidings over a fixed time period.

friction Effect of rubbing, or the resistance that a moving body meets from the surface on which it moves; a force that occurs in a direction to oppose movement; in massage, technique in which deeper tissues are stroked or rubbed, usually through strong circular movements of the hand.

friction rub Dry grating sound heard during auscultation, caused by rubbing of tissue surfaces.

full liquid diet A diet consisting of only liquids and foods that liquefy at body temperature.

gag reflex A normal neural reflex elicited by touching the soft palate or posterior pharynx, the response being the elevation of the palate, retraction of the tongue, and contraction of the pharyngeal muscles. Tests for function of the vagus and glossopharyngeal nerves.

gait Manner or style of walking, including rhythm, cadence, and speed.

gastrostomy feeding tube Long, hollow, flexible tube inserted into the stomach through a stab wound in the upper left abdominal quadrant.

genuineness Communication of authenticity or sincerity.

gingiva The gum of the mouth.

gingivitis Inflammatory condition in which the gums are red, swollen, and bleeding.

glaucoma An abnormal condition of elevated pressure within the anterior chamber of an eye due to obstruction of outflow of aqueous humor.

glucose monitoring A diagnostic test to determine the blood glucose level.

granulation The presence of red, granular, moist tissue that appears during the healing of open wounds; type of tissue containing new blood vessels that bleed readily.

granulation tissue Soft, pink, fleshy projection of tissue that forms during the healing process in a wound not healing by primary intention.

grief Form of sorrow involving the person's thoughts, feelings, and behaviors, occurring as a response to an actual or perceived loss.

guided imagery Technique in which client focuses on an image, becoming less aware of pain.

gurgle Abnormal coarse sound heard during auscultation of the lung; produced by air entering large mucus-containing airways.

gypsum Plaster of Paris; material used for casts as it becomes hard and rigid.

halitosis Offensive breath resulting from poor oral hygiene, dental or oral infections, ingestion of certain foods, or systemic diseases.

hand roll Cylindric roll of cloth or gauze placed against the palmar surface of a client's hand to maintain hand, thumb, and fingers in a functional position.

Harris splint Expandable splint that supports the thigh in skeletal traction.

hazards of immobility Health problems resulting from a decrease in physical mobility or activity.

head tilt–chin lift A method for opening the airway in which the rescuer places one hand on the victim's forehead and applies firm backward pressure with the palm to tilt the head back. At the same time, with the other hand the rescuer places the fingers of the hand under the bony part of the lower jaw near the chin and lifts.

heat stroke Condition characterized by core body temperature of 47 C (113 F).

heave A lift or thrust felt during palpation of the heart.

Heimlich maneuver A method by which a foreign body can be dislodged from the larynx or trachea.

hematemesis Vomiting of blood.

hematology The study of blood cells.

hematoma Collection of extravasated blood trapped in the tissues of the skin or in an organ; results from trauma or incomplete coagulation.

hematopoiesis The formation and development of blood cells in bone marrow.

hematuria Abnormal presence of blood in the urine.

hemiparesis Muscular weakness of one half of the body.

hemiplegia Paralysis of one side of the body.

hemoconcentration The concentration of red blood cells in one area.

hemodialysis A procedure in which impurities or wastes are removed from the blood; used in treating renal insufficiency and various toxic conditions.

hemodynamics The study of movements of the blood and of the forces concerned therein.

hemolysis The destruction of red blood cells.

hemoptysis Coughing up of blood from the respiratory tract.

hemorrhoids A varicosity in the lower rectum or anus caused by congestion in the hemorrhoidal veins.

hemostasis Termination of bleeding by mechanical or chemical means or by the coagulation process of the body.

hemothorax An accumulation of blood in the intrapleural space caused by a pulmonary infarction, tissue damage due to lung cancer or other chest trauma, or a complication of anticoagulant therapy after chest surgery. This condition is characterized by tachycardia, hypotension, diaphoresis, chest pain, dyspnea, asymmetric chest movements, decreased breath sounds on the affected side, and dullness on percussion on the affected side.

hemopneumothorax An accumulation of both air and blood in the intrapleural space. This condition is characterized by the signs and symptoms listed with pneumothorax and hemothorax.

heparin lock An intravenous needle connected to a small "well" that allows for the intermittent injection of medication without the need for repeated venipuncture.

herniation The abnormal protrusion of an organ or other body structure through a defect or natural opening in a covering, membrane, muscle, or bone.

hirsutism Excessive body hair in a masculine distribution, caused by heredity, hormonal dysfunction, or medication.

homeostasis The state of equilibrium (balance between opposing pressures) in the internal environment of the body, naturally maintained by adaptive responses that promote healthy survival.

Hoyer lift Mechanical device that uses a canvas sling to easily lift dependent clients for transferring.

Huber needle Special needle with a deflected point designed to prevent damage to the silicone septum of implanted infusion ports.

hydrocolloid An adhesive, moldable wafer made of a carbohydrate-based material, usually with a waterproof backing. This dressing usually is impermeable to oxygen, water, and water vapor and has some absorptive properties (AHCPR, 1994, p. 109).

hydrogel A water-based, nonadherent, polymer-based dressing that has some absorptive properties (AHCPR, 1994, p. 109).

hygiene The science of health. Self-care measures people use to maintain their health are called personal hygiene.

hypercalcemia Greater than normal amounts of calcium in the blood.

hypercapnia Elevated arterial PCO_2 greater than 45 mm Hg, also called hypercarbia.

hyperemia Increased blood in part of the body, caused by increased blood flow, as in the inflammatory response, local relaxation of arterioles, or obstruction of the outflow of blood from an area.

hyperextension Movement of a body part beyond its normal resting extended position.

hyperkalemia Refers to solutions with potassium concentrations greater than 5.0 mEq/L.

hypermagnesemia Refers to solutions with magnesium concentrations greater than 2.5 mEq/L.

hypernatremia Refers to solutions with sodium concentrations greater than 147 mEq/L.

hyperphosphatemia Refers to a higher than normal range of serum phosphorus. Normal range for serum phosphorus is 2.5 − 4.5 mg/100 ml (1.7 − 2.6 mEq/L).

hypertonic Having a greater concentration of solute than another solution, hence exerting more osmotic pressure.

hyperopia A refractive error of the eye in which parallel rays of light focus behind the retina; causes difficulty seeing near objects.

hyperpigmentation Unusual darkening of the skin.

hypertension Condition characterized by an elevated blood pressure persistently exceeding 150/90 mm Hg.

hyperthermia Condition characterized by body temperature over 38 C (100.4 F).

hypokalemia Refers to solutions with potassium concentrations less than 3.5 mEq/L.

hypomagnesemia Refers to solutions with magnesium concentrations less than 1.5 mEq/L.

hyponatremia Refers to solutions with sodium concentrations less than 137 mEq/L.

hypoosmolar State in which there is an abnormal gain in water or loss of sodium-rich fluids with replacement by water only. As a result, there is a low concentration of solutes in the body fluids.

hypophosphatemia Refers to a lower than noral range of serum phosphorus. Normal range of serum phosphorus is 2.5 - 4.5 mg/100 ml (1.7 - 2.6 mEq/L).

hypotension Condition characterized by a low blood pressure which is inadequate to perfuse and oxygenate body tissue.

hypothermia Condition characterized by body temperature below 36 C (96.8 F).

hypothermia therapy Techniques used to reduce elevated body temperature.

hypotonic Having a smaller concentration of solute than another solution, hence exerting less osmotic pressure.

hypovolemic shock State of physical collapse caused by massive blood loss, circulatory dysfunction, and inadequate tissue perfusion.

hypoxemia Abnormal deficiency of oxygen in arterial blood.

hypoxia Insufficient oxygen available to meet the metabolic needs of tissues and cells.

idiosyncratic reaction A response to a medication or therapy that is unique to an individual.

ileal conduit A method of urinary diversion through intestinal tissue. Ureters are implanted in a section of dissected ileum that is then sewed to an ostomy in the abdominal wall.

ileostomy Surgical formation of an opening of the ileum onto the surface of the abdomen, through which fecal matter is emptied.

immobility Pertaining to the inability of a body part or limb to be moved.

immunocompromised A state of defective or failed immune response that makes a person more likely to acquire an infection.

impaction Presence of large or hard fecal mass in the rectum or colon.

implanted infusion port A self-sealing silicone septum encased in a metal or plastic case with an attached silicone catheter threaded into a large vein. Used to administer chemotherapy and other irritating intravenous medications.

incentive spirometry Method of deep breathing providing visual feedback to clients concerning their inspiratory volume.

incident report Confidential document that describes any client accident while the person is on the premises of a health care agency.

incompatibility Describes two medications of different chemical makeups that cannot be mixed together.

incontinence Inability to control urination or defecation.

induration Hardening of a tissue, particularly the skin.

infection The invasion and reproduction of microorganisms in a body tissue that can result in a local or systemic clinical response such as cellulitis, fever, etc.

infiltration Presence of intravenous fluids within the subcutaneous space surrounding a venipuncture site.

infusate Volume of parenteral fluid infused into a client over an established period of time.

infusion Introduction of a substance such as a fluid, drug, electrolyte, or nutrient, directly into a vein by means of gravity flow.

infusion pump Device designed to deliver a measured amount of fluid over a period of time.

injection Act of forcing a liquid into the body by means of a syringe.

injection cap A rubber diaphragm covering a plastic cap. Permits needle insertion into a catheter or vial.

in-line suction catheter See closed system suction catheter.

insertion site Site of large vein into which a catheter is threaded.

inspection A physical examination skill involving the examiner's looking at external and internal body parts for physical characteristics.

insulation 1. The act of insulating. 2. A nonconducting substance that offers a barrier to the passage of heat or electricity.

intake Measurement of the ingestion or infusion of liquids into the body, including all liquids and semi- liquids, liquid medications, enteral tube feedings, intravenous therapy, blood components, and parenteral nutrition.

intake/output record Measuring and recording of all liquid intake and output over a 24 hour period of time.

integument Skin and its appendages: hair, nails, and sweat and sebaceous glands.

intercostal space Space found between adjoining ribs.

internal rotation Rotation of a joint inward.

intestinal obstruction Any obstruction that results in failure of the contents of the intestine to pass through the lumen of the bowel.

intraabdominal pressure Amount of tension within the abdominal cavity.

intracavitary Within a body cavity

intracellular fluid Liquid within the cell membrane.

intraclavicular fossa Small pocket area or indentation just below the clavicle on both sides of the neck.

intracranial pressure Pressure exerted by cerebrospinal fluid within the subarachnoid space surrounding the brain and spinal cord.

intradermal injection Form of injection in which a solution is introduced into the dermal skin layer.

intramuscular (IM) injection Form of injection in which a solution is introduced into the body of a muscle.

intrapleural Pertaining to, or affecting, the potential space between the parietal and visceral pleurae.

intrapulmonic Pertaining to, or affecting, the spaces within the lungs.

intrathecal Of or pertaining to a structure, process, or substance within a sheath, as within the spinal canal.

intravenous (IV) injection Form of injection in which a solution is introduced into a vein.

introitus An entrance or orifice into a cavity.

intubation Passage of a tube into a body aperture.

invasive Referring to procedures that involve puncture, incision, or insertion of a foreign object into the body.

invasive procedure A procedure where the normal protective barrier of the skin or mucus membrane is broken or compromised, e.g. an intravenous puncture, a bladder catheterization, etc.

irrigate To flush with a fluid, usually with a slow steady pressure on a syringe plunger. Done to cleanse a wound or clear tubing.

irrigation Gentle washing of an area with a stream of solution.

isolation Infection control and prevention methods such as barrier technique that are used to decrease the transmission of microorganisms.

isometric contraction Increased muscle tension without muscle shortening.

isometric exercise The tightening or tensing of muscles without moving body parts.

isoosmotic solution A solution with electrolytes that will exert the same osmotic pressure as the solution it is being compared with, e.g., peripheral vein solution and RBCs.

isotonic contraction Increased muscle tension resulting in muscle contraction and muscle shortening.

isotonic solution Having the same concentration of solute as another solution, hence exerting the same amount of osmotic pressure as the solution.

IVCS The administration of pharmacologic agents to provide a minimally depressed level of consciousness.

IV plug A small rubber or plastic cap that connects to the open end of a patient's IV access catheter. Also referred to as injection cap because a needle can be inserted into the rubber cap for the administration or aspiration of fluids.

jacket restraint Vestlike restraint that usually crosses in the back of the client but may also cross in the front.

jejunal feeding tube A hollow tube inserted into the jejunum through the abdominal wall for administration of liquefied foods.

Joint Commission on Accreditation of Healthcare Organizations (JCAHO) A private, non-governmental agency that establishes guidelines for the operation of health care facilities. The guidelines are the basis of accreditation, generally required for medicare reimbursement. The commission encourages attainment of high standards of institutional care.

Kardex Trade name for card filing system that allows quick reference to the particular need of the client for certain aspects of nursing care.

ketones An organic chemical compound with two compounds attached to it.

kilogram The metric conversion for a pound; weight (lbs.) × 2.2 = kilograms.

kinesthetic Related to the ability to perceive the existence or direction of weight or movement.

knee exercise Mechanical apparatus for passive exercises of the knee joint.

knee sling Support in sling form used under the knee for Russel's traction.
laryngospasm Spasm of the muscles surrounding the larynx causing airway narrowing and stridorous breathing.
lavage The irrigation or washing out of an organ or cavity.
leukopenia A decrease in circulating white blood cells.
let-down reflex A normal reflex in a lactating woman often elicited by tactile stimulation of the nipple, resulting in release of milk from the glands of the breast.
line of gravity An imaginary line that goes from the center of gravity to the base of support.
lipid emulsion A soybean oil– or safflower oil–based solution that is isotonic and may be infused with amino acid and dextrose solution through a central or peripheral line.
lipodystrophy Any abnormality in metabolism and deposition of fat.
loss Absence of a significant other, object, or state of health to which the person must adapt through the grieving process.
lotion Liquid preparation applied externally to protect the skin or treat a dermatologic disorder.
lower airway respiratory system All respiratory structures below the epiglottis, including trachea, bronchi, and alveoli.
lumen The hollow channel within a tube.
lunula A semilunar structure, such as the crescent-shaped pale area at the base of the nail of a finger or toe.
MAC Mid-upper arm circumference. Measurement midpoint between tip of acromion process of scapula and olecranon process of ulna. Measurement value denotes muscle wasting.
macerate To soften, usually by soaking in water.
maceration Skin that becomes abnormally soft and breaks down because of prolonged exposure to moisture.
maculopapular Discolored elevated lesions on the skin.
malabsorption Impaired absorption of nutrients from the GI tract.
MAMC Mid-arm muscle circumference. Calculation obtained by subtracting the triceps skin fold (TSF) from the mid-upper arm circumference (MAC) measurement. Value assists in denoting muscle wasting.
manometer An instrument for measuring pressure or tension of liquids or gases.
mastication Chewing, tearing, or grinding food with the teeth while it mixes with saliva.
meatus Any opening or tunnel through any part of the body, e.g., the point at which the urethra opens to the skin.
medical asepsis The techniques used to reduce and prevent the spread of microorganisms (clean technique).
mediastinal shift A condition in which the mediastinal contents move toward the unaffected side in the presence of a pneumothorax, hemothorax, or hemopneumothorax. The mediastinal shift causes compression of the organs and is a life-threatening situation. This condition is characterized by deviation of the trachea from the midline toward the unaffected side, cardiac dysrhythmias, hypotension, and distended neck veins.
medicated enema Administration of a medication via an enema. Usually used preoperatively with clients scheduled for bowel surgery.
medullary Of or pertaining to the medulla of the brain.
melanin Black or dark brown pigment that occurs naturally in the skin, hair, and iris.
melanocyte A body cell capable of producing melanin, the pigment of the skin.
melena Darkening of the feces by blood pigments.
metastasis Process by which tumor cells are spread to distant parts of the body.
microorganism Any microscopic entity capable of sustaining living processes, such as bacteria, virus, fungi, etc. only some of which typically cause human disease.
microvasculature The portion of the circulatory system composed of the capillary network.
micturition Urination; act of passing or expelling urine voluntarily through the urethra.
mid-arm circumference A measurement of the circumference of the upper arm used to estimate muscle mass.
midstream collection Procedure in which the client initiates a stream of urine, inserts a sterile collection cup into the stream, and then withdraws the cup before the stream of urine stops.
milliequivalent per liter (mEq/L) Number of grams of a specific electrolyte dissolved in 1 liter of plasma.
minerva jacket Cast encasing the head (with face and ears exposed), continuing over the thorax and back to the iliac crests.
minute ventilation The volume of air expired per minute.
mitered corner A triangular folded corner of a bed sheet, used to prevent the sheet from pulling out from the mattress.
mitten restraints Thumbless mitten devices used to restrain a client's hands.
mobility The amount and quality of physical activity.
moleskin Adhesive-backed tape used for some forms of skin traction.
morbid obesity Pathologic state in which an individual weighs greater than 100 pounds (44.5 kg) over ideal weight.
morgue A unit of a hospital with facilities for the storage and autopsy of the dead.
mucociliary transport Process in which cilia lining the tracheobronchial tree sweep mucus upward toward the esophagus to keep airways clear of inhaled particulate.
mucopurulent Characteristic of a combination of mucus and pus.
mummy restraint Blanket or sheet folded in such a manner as to restrain a small child or infant.
mydriasis Dilation of the pupil of the eye caused by contraction of dilator muscles of the iris.
myelosuppression A decrease in the cellular components of the bone marrow.
myopia A refractive error of the eye in which parallel rays of light focus in front of the retina; causes difficulty seeing far objects clearly.
nares The pairs of anterior and posterior openings in the nose that allow for passage of air to the pharynx and lungs.
nasal Of or pertaining to the nose and nasal cavity.
nasal airway Flexible, curved piece of rubber or plastic, with one wide or trumpet-like end and one nar- row end that is inserted through the nose into the pharynx.
nasal cannula A device for delivering oxygen by way of two small, short tubes that are inserted into the nares.
nasal catheter A flexible, small-bore tube inserted into the oropharynx by way of the nose.
nasogastric feeding tube A small tube that is passed via the nares into the stomach.
nasointestinal feeding tube Tungsten-weighted tube inserted through the naris to allow natural peristaltic movement of the tube through the pyloric sphincter into the duodenum or jejunum.
nebulization Vaporization or dispersion of a liquid in a fine spray.
necrotic Related to death of a portion of tissue.
negative pressure Pressure, measured in mm Hg, that is less than atmospheric pressure.
neovascularization The process by which the vascular network in a wound is generated. This can also be called angiogenesis.
neurologic Pertaining to the study and treatment of the nervous system.
neuropathy An abnormal condition characterized by inflammation and degeneration of the peripheral nerves.
neurovascular assessment Series of eight observations (assessments) required to measure neurologic and circulatory status of a client's peripheral tissues.
neutropenia An abnormal decrease in the number of neutrophils in the blood.
nitroglycerin Medication that causes dilation of coronary arteries.
noncontinent (incontinent) ostomy/diverison Results from a surgical procedure that leaves the client with an external stoma through which either stool or urine drains. It is noncontinent/incontinent because the effluent drains spontaneously from the stoma and the client must continuously wear an external ostomy pouch over the stoma.
noncoring needle needle used to access implanted venous access device; it does not result in coring of the rubber diaphragm.
nonpharmacologic aids Interventions used to prevent illness and promote health without the use of or in addition to the use of medications.
nosocomial infection An infection that developed during a stay or work in a health care facility and was not present or incubating at the time of admission.
noxious Harmful, injurious, or detrimental to health.

NPO Nothing to be taken or given by mouth.
nursing home Type of extended-care facility that is licensed to provide nursing and custodial care for persons over a prolonged period of time. Some nursing homes have living quarters that allow residents to continue normal living routines under staff supervision.
objective data Data obtained by an observer (nurse) through direct physical examination, including observation, palpation, and auscultation, and by laboratory analyses and radiologic and other studies.
obturator Small dull-pointed introducer inserted in outer cannula that facilitates insertion of tracheostomy tube by gradually widening or dilating stoma to width of tracheostomy tube.
ocular Of or pertaining to the eye.
occult blood Blood that appears from a nonspecific source, with obscure signs and symptoms. May be detected by means of a chemical test or microscopic examination.
OD Abbreviation for *oculus dexter,* a Latin phrase meaning "right eye."
oil-retention enema An enema containing a small volume (200 to 250 ml) of an oil-based solution; used to soften fecal mass.
ointment A semisolid externally applied preparation, usually containing a drug.
Omnibus Budget Reconciliation Act (OBRA) Act passed by the United States Legislature that set reductions in medicare payments for physician services.
oncology A branch of medicine regarding the study of tumors.
onset of action Period of time after a drug is administered for it to produce a response.
opening pressure The amount of tension measured in a manometer following insertion of a spinal needle into the subarachnoid space.
ophthalmic Of or pertaining to the eye.
ophthalmologist A medical doctor whose practice is limited to diseases, conditions, and trauma to the eyes. An ophthalmologist also prescribes corrective lenses for clients whose visual acuity is impaired.
optometrist A person who practices optometry, tests the eyes for visual acuity, prescribes corrective lenses, and recommends eye exercises.
oral airway Minimally flexible curved piece of plastic extending from the exterior of the lips over the tongue to the pharynx.
orientation phase Period in the nurse-client relationship when the nurse and client first meet and set the tone for the rest of their relationship, assessing the client's situation and setting goals.
orthopedics Branch of medicine devoted to the study and treatment of the skeletal system, its joints, muscles, and associated structures.
orthopnea An abnormal condition in which a person must sit or stand in order to breathe deeply or comfortably.
orthostatic hypotension A drop in blood pressure of 15 mm Hg or more when an individual rises from a sitting to a standing position.
OS Abbreviation for *oculus sinister,* a Latin phrase meaning "left eye."
osmolality The characteristics of a solution determined by the ionic concentration of the solvent.
ostomy A surgical procedure where the elimination of stool or urine is re-routed from the usual exiting part of the client. Instead the stool or urine exits the body through a surgically created opening called a stoma.
otic Of or pertaining to the ear.
otitis media Inflammation or infection of the middle ear, a common childhood affliction.
ototoxic Having a harmful effect on the eighth cranial nerve or the organs of hearing and balance.
OU Abbreviation for *oculus uterque,* a Latin phrase meaning "each eye."
outer cannula Main portion of tracheostomy tube through which client breathes that stays in place at all times. The pilot balloon and faceplate are connected to the outer cannula.
output Includes all liquids excreted, such as urine, vomitus, and diarrhea, and drainage from wounds, fistulas, and suction equipment.
overdose Oral or parenteral ingestion of an excessive quantity of a medication or drug.
over-the-counter drug Drug available to a consumer without a prescription.
over-the-needle catheter (ONC) A type of angiocatheter. The needle used for peripheral IV access is encased in a catheter made of Teflon, plastic or another flexible material. After the needle pierces the skin, the catheter is threaded into a vein and the needle is withdrawn. The catheter remains in the vein for the instillation of fluid.
oximetry Procedure used to measure amount of oxygenated hemoglobin.
oxygen mask A flexible mask that fits snugly and securely over the client's nose and mouth for delivery of oxygen.
oxygen saturation Amount of hemoglobin which is fully saturated with oxygen expressed as percent of total available hemoglobin.
oxygen toxicity Administration of oxygen level greater than 50% for greater than 24 hours resulting in increased permeability of the aveolar wall, aveolar-capillary leakage, non-cardiogenic pulmonary edema, decreased lung compliance and respiratory failure.
oxygen therapy Administration of oxygen by any route to a client, to prevent or relieve hypoxia.
pain Subjective, unpleasant sensation caused by noxious stimulation of sensory nerve endings.
pain intensity The degree or extent of pain perceived by an individual.
pain threshold The amount of pain stimulus required to produce a physical or psychological response.
pain tolerance Point at which a person is not willing to accept pain of greater severity or duration.
pallor Unnatural paleness or absence of color in the skin.
palpate To feel with the hand.
palpation A technique used in physical examination in which the examiner feels the texture, size, consistency, and location of certain parts of the body with the hands.
palpebra Portion of the conjunctiva that lines the inner surface of the eyelids; it is thick, opaque, and highly vascular.
paralysis An abnormal condition characterized by loss of muscle function or the loss of sensation.
paralytic ileus A decrease in or absence of intestinal paralysis that may occur after abdominal surgery, illness, or trauma.
paraphrase Transform the client's words into the nurse's words, keeping the meaning intact.
parenteral Not in or through the digestive system.
parenteral nutrition The administration of nutrition into the vascular system.
paresis Slight or partial paralysis related in some cases to local neuritis.
parietal pleura The pleura membrane that lines the thoracic cavity.
passive range of motion Exercises of the joints performed for an individual by someone else.
patency Absence of obstruction, such as clots within an intravenous needle, or kinks within intravenous tubing.
pathogen Microorganism capable of producing disease.
pathogenic microorganisms Those capable of producing an infection or disease.
Patient's Bill of Rights A list of patient's rights promulgated by the American Hospital Association; it offers some guidance and protection to clients by stating the responsibilities that a hospital and its staff have toward clients and families during hospitalization; it is not a legally binding document.
Patient Self-Determination Act Became effective 12/1/91 and is legislation which requires all Medicare and Medicaid recipient hospitals to provide clients with information on advance directives and their right to accept or reject medical treatment.
peak action Time it takes for a drug to reach its highest effective concentration.
Peak airway pressure The highest amount of positive pressure needed to inflate the lung.
peak expiratory flow rate (PEFR) The maximal flow rate, measured in liters, that can be generated during a forced expiratory maneuver.
Pearson's attachment The support used under the leg in balanced suspension skeletal traction.
pediculosis Infestation of the integument with blood-sucking lice.
pelvic belt Girdle-shaped cotton belt or support that fits around the hips, lumbosacral area, and abdomen for attaching ropes and weights in pelvic belt traction.
pelvic sling A hammock-like sling that fits under the client's lumbosacral area and hips and is then connected to ropes and weights; it

suspends the pelvis off the bed as treatment for fractures of pelvic bones.

perception The conscious recognition and interpretation of sensory stimuli through unconscious associations, especially memory, that serve as a basis for understanding, learning, and knowing, or for the motivation of a particular action or reaction.

percussion A technique in physical examination used to evaluate the size, borders, and consistency of some of the internal organs and to discover the presence and to evaluate the amount of fluid in a cavity of the body.

percutaneous Performed through the skin, such as a biopsy or the aspiration of fluid from a space below the skin using a needle, catheter, and syringe.

perfusion Effect of pulmonary circulation in moving blood to and from the blood-gas barrier so gas exchange can occur.

periodontal Referring to tissues surrounding the teeth, such as the gums and buccal mucosa.

peripherally inserted central catheter (PICC) A peripherally inserted catheter that extends to the superior vena cava or right atrium.

peristalsis The coordinated, rhythmic, serial contraction of smooth muscle that forces food through the digestive tract.

peristomal Referring to the area of skin surrounding a surgically created stoma.

peritoneal fluid Substance in the abdominal cavity for lubrication of peritoneal membrane and internal organs.

peritonitis Inflammation of peritoneum produced by bacteria or irritating substances introduced into the abdominal cavity by a penetrating wound or perforation of an organ in the gastrointestinal or reproductive tract.

PERRLA Acronym for "pupils equal, round, reactive to light, accommodative"; the acronym is recorded in the physical examination if pupil assessment is normal.

PEH Acronym for "pseudoepitheliomatous hyperplasia"; maceration of skin surrounding the stoma.

petaling Finishing the raw or ragged edges of a plaster cast to prevent skin irritation or pressure.

pétrissage A massage technique in which the skin is gently lifted and squeezed.

pH Reflection of the hydrogen ion concentration of a liquid.

pharmacologic agents Oral, parenteral, or topical substances used to alleviate symptoms and treat or control illness.

phlebitis Inflammation of a vein.

phlebitis solution A hypertonic solution capable of causing inflammation of a vein.

phlebotomy The incision of a vein for the letting of blood, as in collecting blood from a donor.

Physician's Desk Reference (PDR) A compendium, compiled annually, containing information about drugs supplied by manufacturers.

PIE An acronym for "Problem, Intervention, and Evaluation," used as an organizing framework for narrative nurses' notes.

piggyback infusion Method for administering intravenous medications intermittently; a piggyback IV set is a supplementary set that connects with the primary IV tubing.

pillating device Commercial devices that contain a sharp blade used to cut tablets in half.

piloerection Erection of the hairs of the skin in response to a chilly environment, emotional stimulus, or irritation of the skin.

plantar flexion Flexion of the foot and toes toward the sole.

plasmaphoresis Laboratory procedure in which the plasma proteins are separated by electrophoresis for identification and evaluation of the proportions of the various proteins.

plaque (dental) A thin film on teeth made up of mucin and colloidal material found in saliva and often secondarily invaded by bacteria.

platelet Formed particle found in blood that relates directly to the ability of the blood to clot.

pleura Delicate serous membrane enclosing the lung.

pleural cavity Space between visceral and parietal pleura; pressure within the cavity is negative when compared with atmospheric pressure.

pleural fluid Substance contained between visceral and parietal pleurae for lubrication of the membranes.

pneumonitis Inflammation of the lung; may be caused by a virus, or may be a hypersensitivity reaction due to allergy to chemical or organic dusts.

pneumothorax An accumulation of air in the intrapleural space caused by a severe blow to the chest, extremely forceful cough, chest trauma, or open chest surgery. This condition is characterized by sudden sharp pain in the chest or referred pain across the chest to the shoulder or abdomen, dyspnea, dry cough, asymmetric hyperresonance on percussion on the affected side, decreased breath sounds on the affected side, and possible subcutaneous emphysema around the neck. A pneumothorax causes air to enter the intrapleural space with each inspiration.

podiatrist A health professional trained to diagnose and treat diseases and disorders of the feet.

point of maximal impulse (PMI) Point at which the heartbeat can most easily be palpated through the chest wall, usually along the left-midclavicular line at the fourth or fifth intercostal space.

polypharmacy Concurrent prescription, administration or use of multiple medications, some of which may not be indicated clinically.

POMR An acronym for "Problem-Oriented Medical Record," used as an organizing framework for a client's complete medical record.

portal hypertension An increased venous pressure in the portal circulation caused by compression or by occulsion at the portal or hepatic vascular system.

positive pressure Pressure, measured in mm Hg, that is greater than atmospheric pressure.

positive pressure ventilation Mechanical ventilation that delivers compressed gas to the airways at greater than ambient pressure.

postcast care Nursing interventions performed for and with clients in casts or after cast removal.

postoperative Period of time after completion of a surgical procedure wherein the nurse monitors the client's recovery.

postural Position of body, usually refers to change of position from supine to sitting, sitting to standing.

postural drainage Gravitational clearance of airway secretions by assumption of one or more of 10 different body positions for 5 to 15 minutes each; each posture corresponds to specific segments of bronchi in the lung.

prealbumin A plasma protein with a half-life of only 2 days used as a marker of nutritional status.

precordial Of or pertaining to the precordium, which forms the region over the heart and the lower part of the thorax.

premature ventricular contraction (PVC) A cardiac dysrhythmia characterized by a ventricular contraction preceding the expected contraction; it appears on an electrocardiogram as an early, wide QRS complex without a preceding P wave.

preoperative The period of time preceding induction of anesthesia and the beginning of a surgical procedure.

presbycusis Loss of hearing sensitivity and speech intelligibility, associated with aging.

presbyopia Farsightedness resulting from a loss of elasticity of the lens of the eye. The condition commonly develops with advancing age.

pressure cycled ventilation Mechanical ventilation in which gas delivery is limited by a preset pressure to achieve a tidal volume.

pressure ulcer A lesion that develops in the skin as a result of prolonged, unreleived pressure.

primary dressing A dressing that comes in direct contact with the wound bed.

primary intention Primary union of the edges of a wound, progressing to complete scar formation with granulation.

PRN Abbreviation for "pro re nata," a Latin phrase meaning "as needed." The times of administration are determined by the needs of the client.

problem-oriented record (POR) Method of recording data about the health status of a client that fosters a collaborative problem-solving approach by all members of the health care team.

pronation Movement of a body part so the front or ventral surface faces downward.

proprioception Sensation achieved through stimuli originating from within the body regarding spatial position and muscular activity.

prospective reimbursement A method of payment to an agency for health care services to be delivered based on predictions of what the agency's costs will be for the coming year.

prosthesis An artificial replacement for a missing part of the body.

pruritus The symptom of itching.

pseudomonas A genus of gram-negative bacteria that includes several free-living species of soil and water and some opportunistic pathogens, isolated from wounds and sputum; may produce blue and yellow pigments.

pulley Mechanical round, grooved disks over which ropes can move freely for traction pull.

pulse deficit Condition characterized by difference between apical pulse rate and peripheral pulse rate which results in a lack of peripheral perfusion.

quality assurance In health care, any evaluation of services provided and of the results achieved as compared with accepted standards.

radiopaque Not permitting the passage of x-rays or other radiant energy. Bones are relatively radiopaque and therefore show as white areas on an exposed x-ray film. Lead is markedly radiopaque and therefore is widely used to shield x-ray equipment and atomic power sources.

random voided specimen A urine specimen obtained at any point of a 24-hour period.

reagent Chemical used to indicate the presence of a particular substance.

rectal tube Flexible tube inserted into the rectum to assist in relief of flatus.

rectum Portion of the large intestine, about 12 cm long, continuous with the descending sigmoid colon, just proximal to the anal canal.

reduction The alignment of fracture fragments through manipulation. Closed reduction is accomplished through manual manipulation and casting or traction.

reflection A communication strategy linking the client's apparent emotion with the content of the client's message; it is used to clarify what the client is feeling and to affirm that the client's feelings are acceptable.

refractive error Condition in which parallel rays of light are not brought to focus on the retina.

re-infusion device An apparatus which is placed, usually intraoperatively during orthopedic or vascular procedures, into a space where significant blood loss is anticipated (e.g., knee cavity or pleural space). This device collects the blood, filters it, and is then used to re-infuse that blood intra-vascularly. An anti-coagulant may need to be added to the blood before re-infusion. (See manufacturer's guidelines.)

relaxation exercise Pain relief treatment in which clients perform controlled breathing and relaxation exercises and concentrate on a pleasant situation when a noxious stimulus is applied.

reminiscence A form of therapy for older adults that provides a life review. Individual talks about remote memories, expression of related feelings, and recognition of positive experiences as well as conflicts. Helps to enhance memory, adaptation and life satisfaction.

remission The partial or complete disappearance of the clinical and subjective characteristics of a chronic or malignant disease.

renal Pertaining to the kidney.

resident A client in a long term or extended care facility.

residual urine Volume of urine remaining in the bladder after a normal voiding; the bladder normally is almost completely empty after micturition.

resistive isometric exercise Contracting of muscles while pushing against a stationary object or resisting the movement of an object.

respect Communication of esteem, honor, or consideration of another.

respiratory arrest Cessation of respirations.

respiratory distress Difficulty breathing that may be associated with abnormal blood oxygen or carbon dioxide levels and may require supportive measures to preserve life.

respite care Provision of short-term relief or time off for people providing home care to an ill, disabled, or frail older adult.

restatement A communication strategy involving the reiteration of the client's verbal statements and/or questions using similar words; this affirms that the message was acknowledged by the nurse.

restraint Device used to immobilize a client or an extremity.

reverse Trendelenburg's position Position in which the lower extremities are low and the body and head are elevated on an inclined plane.

rib shaking Step in chest physiotherapy involving constant downward pressure with an intermittent shaking motion of the hands on the rib cage over the area being drained; it is done with the flat part of the palm of the hand during 4 to 12 prolonged exhalations through pursed lips.

rib vibration Step in chest physiotherapy involving a downward vibrating pressure done only during exhalation by the flat part of the palm of the hand over the lung segment being drained; usually done during 4 to 12 prolonged exhalations through pursed lips over each segment drained.

right atrial catheter An indwelling intravenous catheter inserted centrally or peripherally and threaded into the superior vena cava or right atrium.

rigidity Condition of hardness, stiffness, or inflexibility.

rigor mortis The rigid stiffening of skeletal and cardiac muscle shortly after death.

rooting reflex A normal response in newborns when the cheek is touched or stroked along the side of the mouth to turn the head toward the stimulated side and to begin suck.

Rotokinetic treatment table A special bed equipped with an automatic turning device that completely immobilizes clients while rotating them from 90 to 270 degrees along a horizontal axis.

S_1 Symbol for the first heart sound in the cardiac cycle occurring with ventricular systole; it is associated with the closure of the mitral and tricuspid valves.

S_2 Symbol for the second heart sound in the cardiac cycle; it is associated with closure of the aortic and pulmonary valves just before ventricular diastole.

saline lock See Heparin lock.

saliva A digestive secretion emitted from the salivary glands in the mouth.

sclerosis Condition characterized by hardening of tissue resulting from any of several causes, including inflammation, the deposit of mineral salts, and infiltration of connective tissue cells.

scrubbed team members Includes the surgeon and scrub nurse or technician and assisting physicians who are scrubbed.

sebaceous gland One of the small glands in the dermis that secretes an oily substance (sebum) on the skin's surface and in the hair.

seborrheic dermatitis A common chronic, inflammatory skin disease characterized by dry or moist greasy scales and yellow crusts.

sebum Oily secretion of the sebaceous glands of the skin. When combined with sweat sebum forms a moist, oily, acidic film that is antibacterial and antifungal and protects the skin against drying.

secondary intention Wound closure in which the edges are separated, granulation tissue develops to fill the gap, and, finally, epithelium grows in over the granulation, producing a larger scar than results with primary intention.

secretion A product produced by a gland of the body.

seizure A hyperexcitation of neurons in the brain leading to a sudden, violent, involuntary series of muscle contractions that may be paroxysmal and episodic, as in a seizure disorder, or transient and acute, as in after a head injury. A generalized tonic-clonic seizure is characterized by a loss of consciousness, tonicity (rigidity) and clonicity (jerking).

seizure precautions Measures that protect the client from injury during a seizure.

self-catheterization The ability of an individual to insert a urinary catheter into their urinary meatus.

semi-Fowler's position Placement of client in an inclined position, with the upper half of the body raised by elevating the head of the bed approximately 30 to 45 degrees.

sensitivity Laboratory test used in conjunction with culture; it measures the response of microorganisms to antibiotics that have been placed on a culture plate.

sepsis Infection, contamination.

serology Branch of medicine dealing with serum and blood products.

sharps container A puncture-proof container that is used for the disposal of any used sharp items such as needles, disposable scissors, scalpels, etc.

shearing Pressure exerted against the surface and layers of the skin as tissues slide underneath the body as it moves against a surface.

sheet wadding Stretchable sheets of cotton padding used to cover skin before a cast is applied; the stretching allows for some extremity edema without the cast's becoming too tight.

side effect An effect caused by a drug that is different from the therapeutic (desired) action; the effect may be harmless or injurious.

sigmoid colon The part of the large intestine that extends from the descending colon to the rectum.
sign Objective finding perceived by an examiner, such as a fever, rash, abnormal reflex, or abnormal breath sound.
silicone septum Silicone partition that covers the port chamber housed in the metal or plastic body of the implanted infusion port.
sitz bath Special bath in which only the hips and buttocks are immersed in fluid.
skin barrier An artificial layer of skin, made of plastic or vinyl-like material, applied to skin before application of tape or ostomy drainage bags. Protects skin from chronic irritation.
sling Used to support, limit movement, enhance circulation, and prevent edema of the arm, hand, or wrist.
slough Necrotic (dead) tissue in the process of separating from viable portions of the body (AHCPR, 1994, p. 118).
SOAP Acronym for "subjective, objective, assessment, and plan," the four parts of the written account of a client's health problem in a problem-oriented record.
solute A substance dissolved in a solution.
solute solution Solutes are dissolved particles and are either electrolytes or nonelectrolytes. Solute solution refers to these particles when they are found in body fluids or plasma (i.e., solution).
solution A mixture of one or more substances dissolved in another substance.
spasm Involuntary muscle contraction.
specific gravity The ratio between the density of a solution and that of water.
speculum A retractor used to separate the walls of a cavity, e.g., the vaginal cavity.
sphygmomanometer Device used for noninvasive measurement of arterial blood pressure consisting of cuff, air bladder, inflation bulb and gauge to indicate amount of air pressure being exerted.
spica cast An orthopedic cast applied to immobilize part or all of the trunk of the body and part or all of one or more extremities.
sponge Gauze dressing used to absorb blood in a surgical wound.
spore An inactive but viable state of microorganisms; certain bacteria and fungi will sustain themselves in this form until the environment is favorable for vegetative growth; while in this stage, the microorganism is highly resistant to heat, toxic chemicals, and other methods of destruction.
spreader bar A metal bar with curved hoop areas for attaching hooks or pins for traction.
sputum Lung mucus; normally thin, watery, and white or clear and watery.
standardized care plan Documentation which uses the nursing process format in specifying the plan of care for client problems.
standard precautions Techniques used to reduce the risk of the transmission of blood borne pathogens or microorganisms present in moist body substances regardless of the client's diagnosis or infection status.
staples Stainless steel wire used to close a surgical wound.
stent A straw or tube like device that is placed through the stoma into bowel to keep open the flow of effluent.
sterile Free from all life forms, including spores.
sterile conscience One's personal principles and morals that guide them to maintain strict asepsis and sterile techniques at all times.
sterile field A specified area, such as within a tray or a sterile drape, that is considered free from microorganisms.
sterilization Process by which microorganisms, including spores, are killed.
stockinette Stretchable cotton materials of various sizes and widths used immediately over the skin to protect tissues from the irritation of felt or plaster.
stoma Surgically created opening between a body cavity and the body's surface, such as a colostomy.
stomatitis Any inflammatory condition of the mouth.
stopcock A valve that controls the flow of fluid or air through a tube.
stroke volume The volume of blood ejected from the left ventricle with each ventricular contraction.
strike through Source of contamination by which moisture permeates a sterile field or barrier.
subarachnoid space Situated or occurring between the arachnoid and the pia mater membranes, which cover the brain and spinal cord.
subcutaneous emphysema The presence of free air or gas in the subcutaneous tissues.
subcutaneous (SQ or SC) injection Form of injection in which a solution is introduced into subcutaneous tissues.
subcutaneous tunnel A tunnel under the skin between the exit site of a catheter and the entrance into a body cavity (such as the epidural space) or vein.
subjective data Data collected from a client.
sublingual Route for administering a drug beneath the tongue.
suction The act of sucking up a substance by reducing air pressure over its surface.
suction catheter Thin plastic or rubber tubing used to remove secretions.
summarization Reworking a lengthy interaction or discussion into a few brief sentences.
supination Movement of a body part so the front or ventral surface faces upward.
suppository A solid form of medication inserted into a body cavity, e.g., the rectum or vagina. The drug is absorbed after it dissolves in the cavity.
surgical asepsis Practices or techniques designed to render and maintain objects and areas free from pathogenic microorganisms. Also referred to as sterile techniques.
surgical scrub Process of removing as many microorganisms as possible from the hands and arms by mechanical washing and chemical antisepsis.
suspension A liquid in which small particles of a solid are dispersed, but not dissolved, and in which the dispersal is maintained by stirring or shaking the mixture.
sympathomimetic A pharmacologic agent that mimics the effects of stimulation of organs and structures by the sympathetic nervous system.
synergistic reaction An undesired reaction that occurs when one drug potentiates the effect of another.
systemic Of or pertaining to the whole body rather than to a localized area.
systolic pressure The higher blood pressure measurement; reflects pressure within the arterial system during the period of ventricular contraction (systole).
T binder Bandage in the shape of a letter T; used to support perineal dressing.
T tube A T-shaped device that is attached to an endotracheal or tracheostomy tube for delivery of humidified air.
tachycardia An abnormality in heart rate in which the myocardium contracts regularly, but at a rate over 100 beats per minute.
tachypnea Condition characterized by respiratory rate greater than 20 breaths per minute.
tartar A hard, gritty deposit—composed of organic matter, phosphates, and carbonates—that collects on teeth and gums.
telephone order A physician or nurse practitioner's order for a medication or other therapeutic that is received by telephone to a nurse to be entered into the client's medical records.
TENS Transcutaneous electrical nerve stimulation. A mild electrical stimulation that interferes with the transmission of painful stimuli.
tepid Moderately warm to the touch.
termination phase The period in the nurse-client relationship when the nurse and client examine and evaluate their relationship and its goals and results; the time when they deal with the emotional content involved in saying good-bye.
therapeutic Treatments or interventions implemented to prevent illness and/or promote health.
therapeutic silence The use of silence that encourages verbal description and reflection; avoidance of premature verbal communication that may be due to the nurse's anxiety.
thermoregulation Ability to control temperature within acceptable range.
third party payor An insurance plan, HMO, or PPO that reimburses for health care services.
Thomas splint A long splint with a half or full ring at one end; covered with towels and lined with felt or other soft material, it is used to suspend the thigh in skeletal traction.
thrill A fine vibration, felt by an examiner's hand on the body of a patient over the site of an aneurysm or on the precordium.
thrombocytopenia A decrease in circulating platelets.

thrombophlebitis Inflammation of a vein, often accompanied by formation of a clot.
thrombus Accumulation of platelets, fibrin, clotting factors, and the cellular elements of the blood attached to the interior wall of a vein or artery, sometimes occluding the lumen of the vessel.
tidaling A normal gentle rocking of fluid in a chest tube water-seal system or in the diagnostic indicator of waterless units. Indicates that the system is functioning properly.
tidal volume Amount, in ml, of air inhaled with each breath. Spontaneous tidal volume is 5-10 ml/kg body weight.
timed collection The collection of a substance such as urine or stool for a specific period of time.
tinnitus Ringing heard in one or both ears.
tissue ischemia Decreased blood supply to body tissues.
TLC 1. Abbreviation for total lung capacity. 2. Informal abbreviation for tender loving care.
tongue-thrust reflex An immature form of swallowing in which the tongue is projected forward instead of retracted during swallowing.
topical Of or pertaining to a drug or treatment applied to the surface of a body part.
tourniquet An item used for the compression of blood vessels.
tracheal-esophageal fistula A hole in the posterior wall of the trachea that extends into the anterior wall of the esophagus and permits aspiration of gastric contents into the lung.
tracheal stenosis Narrowing of the trachea due to scarring.
tracheobronchial tree Anatomic divisions of the respiratory tract, including the combination of trachea, bifurcations into the right and left mainstem bronchi, and subsequent bifurcations into smaller bronchi and bronchioles.
tracheomalacia An abnormal softening or sponginess of the tracheal tissue.
tracheostomy Opening through the neck into the trachea with an indwelling tube inserted; created surgically to produce an airway.
tracheostomy collar Curved oxygen delivery device with an adjustable neck strap that fits around the tracheostomy.
traction Force or pull applied to limbs, bones, or other tissues to pull the tissues apart, often for realignment.
traction boot A foam rubber boot shaped to fit a forearm or leg, used for a type of skin traction.
transdermal Refers to a form of medication that is applied to the skin's surface and is absorbed across the dermal or outer skin layer.
transfusion reaction Systemic response by the body to the administration of blood incompatible with that of the recipient.
transmission-based precautions Techniques used to prevent the transmission of microorganisms from clients documented or suspected to be infected with highly transmissible pathogens for which additional precautions are needed beyond Standard Precautions. The three types are: Airborne, Droplet, and Contact Precautions.
transtracheal oxygen therapy (TTOT) A method of administering oxygen to a client by establishing a low-flow catheter route directly in the trachea.
Trendelenburg's position Position in which the head is low and the body and legs are elevated.
triceps skinfold A measurement, with calipers, of the skinfold over the triceps muscle. The measurement is used to estimate body fat stores.
trocar A sharp, pointed rod that fits inside a tube. It is used to pierce the skin and the wall of a cavity or canal in the body to aspirate fluids, to instill a medication or solution, or to guide the placement of a soft catheter. The trocar is usually removed, and the catheter, tube, or instrument is left in place.
TSF Triceps skin fold. Useful in denoting muscle wasting.
tuberculosis A chronic granulomatous infection caused by an acid-fast bacillus, *Mycobacterium tuberculosis,* generally transmitted by the inhalation or ingestion of infected droplets and usually affecting the lungs.
turning sheet Bed sheet folded in half, placed under the client between shoulders and below the hips. Used by health care providers to lift, turn and position the client.
unit dose system System of drug distribution in which a portable cart containing a drawer for each client's medications is prepared by the pharmacy with a 24-hour supply of medications.
unscrubbed team members Includes the anesthesiologist or anesthetist and the circulating nurse, who wear surgical attire but are not gowned or gloved.
upper airway respiratory system All respiratory structures above the epiglottis, including nose, sinuses, mouth, and pharynx.
ureterostomy An ostomy site in which one or both ureters are surgically brought to the abdominal surface for the excretion of urine.
urethral meatus The opening to the canal for the discharge of urine.
uretheral sphincter Voluntary muscle at the neck of the bladder that relaxes to allow micturition.
urgency The need to void immediately.
urinal Plastic or metal receptacle for urine.
urinary diversion A surgical procedure where the ureters are removed from the urinary bladder and surgically anastomosed directly to the skin or to either a conduit or internal pouch made of bowel with the other end brought out onto the client's skin as a stoma so that the urine can exit the body. Urinary diversions can be continent or noncontinent (incontinent).
urinary retention Inability to empty the bladder due to a number of possible causes.
urinary tract infection Greater than normal level of pathogens in the urinary tract.
urine Fluid secreted by the kidneys, transported by the ureters, stored in the bladder, and voided through the urethra.
urine specific gravity Measurement of the degree of concentration of the urine.
urinometer Device used for determining specific gravity of urine.
Vacu-tainer tube A glass tube with a rubber stopper; air has been removed to create a vacuum.
valgus An abnormal position in which a part of a limb is bent or twisted outward, away from the midline, such as the heel of the foot.
Valsalva's maneuver Any forced expiratory effort against a closed airway, as when an individual holds the breath and tightens the muscles in a concerted, strenuous, effort to move a heavy object or to change position in a bed.
variance Positive or negative changes in client progress towards expected outcomes. Deviations from the critical path plan most often used in the case management model of delivering health care.
varices Tortuous, dilated veins.
varus An abnormal position in which a part of a limb is turned inward toward the midline, such as the heel and foot.
vascular access device (VAD) An indwelling catheter, cannula, or other instrumentation used to obtain venous or arterial access.
vasoconstriction Narrowing of the lumen of any blood vessel, especially the arterioles and the veins in the blood reservoirs of the skin and abdominal viscera.
vasodilation An increase in the diameter of a blood vessel caused by inhibition of its vasoconstrictor nerves or stimulation of dilator nerves.
vein lumen Central opening through which blood flows in a vein.
vellus Soft, fine hair covering all parts of the body except the palms, soles, and areas where other types of hair are normally found.
venipuncture Technique in which a vein is punctured transcutaneously by a sharp rigid stylet (such as a butterfly needle), a cannula (such as an angiocatheter that contains a flexible plastic catheter), or a needle attached to a syringe.
ventilation Respiratory process by which gases are moved into and out of the lungs.
ventral Of or pertaining to an anterior position, toward the abdomen.
verbal order A physician or nurse practitioner's order for a medication or other therapeutic that is spoken to the registered nurse to be entered into the client's medical records. Verbal orders are often taken because some mitigating circumstances preclude the prescriber from immediately entering the order into the client's medical record.
vertigo A sensation of faintness or an inability to maintain normal balance in a standing or seated position, sometimes associated with giddiness, mental confusion, nausea, and weakness.
vesicant A drug capable of causing tissue necrosis when extravasated.
vial Glass container with a metal-enclosed rubber seal.
viscera The internal organs enclosed within a body cavity, primarily the abdominal organs.

visceral pleura A serous membrane lining both lungs.

visceral protein status The amount of protein that pertains to the internal organs (e.g., abdominal).

vital signs Physiological parameters which reflect key body processes; refers to temperature, blood pressure, heart rate, respiratory rate and oxygen saturation.

void The process of emptying the bladder of urine; urinate; micturate.

volume-cycled ventilation A specific tidal volume is delivered to the client within a preset pressure range.

walking belt Leather device with handles that enables the nurse to help a client walk.

walking heel Plastic or rubber heel placed in the sole of a leg cast to allow weight bearing.

webril Stretchable cotton material applied over the skin to protect from plaster irritation.

weight Force exerted on a body by the gravity of the earth.

weight holder A metal, T-shaped bar that holds weights for traction.

weights Filled bags or metal disks of varying poundage used for traction.

whispered pectoriloquy The transmission of a whisper through the pulmonary structures so that it is heard as normal audible speech on auscultation.

windowing Cutting a small area of a cast to permit inspection of the tissues below.

working phase The period in the nurse-client relationship when the focus is on communication strategies, interventions for problem resolution, and enhancement of self-concept.

Yankauer suction A large filter tipped rigid plastic suction catheter used mainly in the mouth or other large body cavity.

Z-track Method for injecting irritating preparations into muscle without tracking residual medication through sensitive tissues.

INDEX

B

F

G

J

K

L

T

U